GELLIS & KAGAN'S

CURRENT PEDIATRIC THERAPY

14

FREDRIC D. BURG, M.D.
Vice Dean for Education
University of Pennsylvania Medical Center
Professor of Pediatrics
University of Pennsylvania and
Children's Hospital of Philadelphia
Philadelphia, Pennsylvania

JULIE R. INGELFINGER, M.D.
Associate Professor of Pediatrics
Harvard Medical School
Co-Chief, Pediatric Nephrology Unit
Massachusetts General Hospital
Boston, Massachusetts

ELLEN R. WALD, M.D.
Professor of Pediatrics and Otolaryngology
University of Pittsburgh School of Medicine
Chief, Division of Pediatric and
Infectious Disease
Children's Hospital of Pittsburgh
Pittsburgh, Pennsylvania

GELLIS & KAGAN'S

CURRENT PEDIATRIC THERAPY

14

W.B. SAUNDERS COMPANY
A Division of Harcourt Brace & Company
Philadelphia London Toronto Montreal Sydney Tokyo

W.B. SAUNDERS COMPANY
A Division of
Harcourt Brace & Company

The Curtis Center
Independence Square West
Philadelphia, Pennsylvania 19106

Managing Editor:
CARLA B. HULTMAN
Special Assistant to the Vice Dean for Education
University of Pennsylvania Medical Center

GELLIS AND KAGAN'S CURRENT PEDIATRIC THERAPY 14

ISBN 0–7216–3703–5
International Edition ISBN 0–7216–4806–1

Library of Congress Cataloging-in-Publication card number 93–20473.

Printed in the United States of America.

Last digit is the print number: 9 8 7 6 5 4 3 2 1

Contributors

Richard D. Aach, M.D.

Professor and Vice-Chairman, Department of Medicine, Case Western Reserve University. Director, Department of Medicine, Mount Sinai Medical Center, Cleveland, Ohio.

Viral Hepatitis

Jon S. Abramson, M.D.

Professor and Vice-Chairman, Department of Pediatrics, Bowman Gray School of Medicine of Wake Forest University. Brenner Children's Hospital of Wake Forest University, Winston-Salem, North Carolina.

Rickettsial Infections

Israel F. Abroms, M.D.

Professor of Pediatrics and Neurology, University of Massachusetts Medical School, Worcester, Massachusetts. Director, Division of Pediatric Neurology, University of Massachusetts Medical Center. Consulting Physician, Medical Center of Central Massachusetts (Memorial), Boston, Massachusetts.

Breath-Holding Spells

Raymond D. Adelman, M.D.

Professor and Chairman of Pediatrics, Eastern Virginia Medical School. Vice President for Medical Affairs, Physician-in-Chief, Children's Hospital of the King's Daughters, Norfolk, Virginia.

Perinephric and Intranephric Abscess; Urinary Tract Infections in Children

Joel W. Adelson, M.D., Ph.D.

Professor of Pediatrics and Physiology, Brown University School of Medicine. Director, Division of Pediatric Gastroenterology and Nutrition, Rhode Island and Women and Infants Hospitals, Providence, Rhode Island.

Acute and Chronic Diarrhea in Infants and Children

Hassan H. A-Kader, M.D.

Attending Physician, Division of Pediatric Gastroenterology and Nutrition, Children's Hospital Medical Center, Cincinnati, Ohio.

Unconjugated Hyperbilirubinemia

Steven R. Alexander, M.D.

Associate Professor of Pediatrics, The University of Texas Southwestern Medical Center at Dallas. Director of Dialysis and Renal Transplantation, The Children's Medical Center of Dallas, Dallas, Texas.

Peritoneal Dialysis

D. A. Allen, Ed. D.

Associate Professor in Child Psychiatry, Albert Einstein College of Medicine. Director of Infant and Preschool Therapeutic Nurseries, Albert Einstein and Bronx Municipal Hospital Center, Bronx, New York.

Autism

John A. Anderson, M.D.

Clinical Professor of Pediatrics, University of Michigan. Head, Division of Allergy and Clinical Immunology, Department of Medicine, Henry Ford Hospital, Detroit, Michigan.

Physical Allergy

Ann M. Apalsch, M.D.

Fellow, Pediatric Infectious Disease, University of Pittsburgh. Physician, Children's Hospital of Pittsburgh, Pittsburgh, Pennsylvania.

The Atypical Mycobacteria

Leonard Apt, M.D.

Professor of Ophthalmology, Director Emeritus of the Division of Pediatric Ophthalmology, Jules Stein Eye Institute, School of Medicine, University of California, Los Angeles. Special Consultant in Pediatric Ophthalmology for the Los Angeles City Health Department and the Bureau of Maternal and Child Health, Department of Public Health, State of California, Los Angeles.

The Eye

Billy S. Arant, Jr., M.D.

Professor and Chairman, Department of Pediatrics, Chattanooga Unit, University of Tennessee College of Medicine. Medical Director, T. C. Thompson Children's Hospital, Chattanooga, Tennessee.

Vesicoureteral Reflux

Kenneth A. Arndt, M.D.

Professor of Dermatology, Harvard Medical School. Dermatologist-in-Chief, Beth Israel Hospital.

Disorders of Pigmentation

Stephen Aronoff, M.D.

Associate Professor, Department of Pediatrics and Microbiology/Immunology, West Virginia University School of Medicine. Physician, West Virginia University, Children's Hospital, Morgantown, West Virginia.

Mucormycosis (Zygomycosis)

Anthony Atala, M.D.

Instructor in Surgery, Harvard Medical School. Attending Surgeon, Division of Urology, Children's Hospital, Boston, Massachusetts.

Patent Urachus and Urachal Cysts

Balu H. Athreya, M.D.

Professor of Pediatrics, University of Pennsylvania School of Medicine. Director of Rheumatology Department, Children's Seashore House, and Department of Pediatrics, Children's Hospital of Philadelphia, Philadelphia, Pennsylvania.

Systemic Lupus Erythematosus

Ellis D. Avner, M.D.

Professor of Pediatrics, University of Washington School of Medicine. Director, Division of Nephrology, Children's Hospital and Medical Center, Seattle, Washington.

Renal Hypoplasia and Dysplasia

Felicia B. Axelrod, M.D.

Professor, New York University School of Medicine. Director, Dysautonomia Treatment & Evaluation Center, and Attending Staff in Pediatrics, New York University Medical Center, New York, New York.

Familial Dysautonomia

Carol J. Baker, M.D.

Professor of Pediatrics, Microbiology and Immunology, Baylor College of Medicine. Active Staff, Texas Children's Hospital, Harris County Hospital District and Woman's Hospital of Texas, Houston, Texas.

Group B Streptococcal Infections

William F. Balistreri, M.D.

Dorothy M. M. Kersten Professor of Pediatrics, University of Cincinnati School of Medicine. Director, Division of Pediatric Gastroenterology and Nutrition, Children's Hospital Medical Center, Cincinnati, Ohio.

Unconjugated Hyperbilirubinemia; Cirrhosis

Giulio J. Barbero, M.D.

Professor of Child Health, University of Missouri School of Medicine. Attending Physician, University of Missouri Hospital, Columbia, Missouri.

Pylorospasm; Pyloric Stenosis

Barbara A. Barlow, M.D.

Professor of Clinical Surgery, Columbia University College of Physicians and Surgeons. Chief of Pediatric Surgery, Director of Injury Prevention Program, Harlem Hospital Center, New York, New York.

Penetrating Knife and Gunshot Wounds in Children

Mark L. Batshaw, M.D.

W.T. Grant Professor of Pediatrics, Professor of Neurology, Professor of Rehabilitation Medicine, University of Pennsylvania School of Medicine. Physician-in-Chief, Children's Seashore House; Director, Division of Child Development and Rehabilitation Medicine, The Children's Hospital of Philadelphia, Philadelphia, Pennsylvania.

Mental Retardation

David Baum, M.D.

Professor of Pediatrics and Chief, Division of Pediatric Cardiology, Stanford University School of Medicine. Pediatric Cardiologist, Stanford Medical Center and Lucille Salter Packard Children's Hospital, Palo Alto, California; Consultant in Pediatric Cardiology for the U.S. Army, Silas B. Hayes Hospital, Fort Ord, California.

Acute Rheumatic Fever

Arthur L. Beaudet, M.D.

Professor, Institute for Molecular Genetics and Department of Pediatrics, Baylor College of Medicine. Investigator, Howard Hughes Medical Institute. Chief, Genetic Services, Texas Children's Hospital, Houston, Texas.

Lysosomal Storage Diseases

Douglas W. Bell, M.D.

Clinical Instructor (Otolaryngology), Harvard Medical School. Associate in Otolaryngology, Children's Hospital, Boston, Massachusetts.

Salivary Gland Tumors

John W. Belmont, M.D., Ph.D.

Assistant Professor, Institute for Molecular Genetics, Pediatrics, Microbiology, Immunology at Baylor College of Medicine. Assistant Investigator, Howard Hughes Medical Institute. Staff Physician, Texas Children's Hospital, Houston, Texas.

Lysosomal Storage Diseases

Charles V. Bender, M.D.

Associate Professor of Pediatrics, University of Pittsburgh School of Medicine. Clinical Neonatologist, Clinical Director of Normal Newborn Nurseries, Coordinator of the Magee-Women's Hospital Regional Neonatal Program, and Chairman of the Department of Pediatrics, Quality Assessment and Improvement Committee, Pittsburgh, Pennsylvania.

Preparation of the Neonate for Transfer

Ira Bergman, M.D.

Associate Professor, The University of Pittsburgh. Active Staff, Children's Hospital of Pittsburgh and The Rehabilitation Institute. Courtesy Staff, Magee Women's Hospital, Pittsburgh, Pennsylvania.

Acute Ataxia; Guillain-Barré Syndrome

Shelly C. Bernstein, M.D., Ph.D.

Assistant Clinical Professor of Pediatrics, Harvard Medical School. Assistant in Medicine (Hematology–Oncology), Children's Hospital; Assistant Physician, Pediatric Oncology, Dana-Farber Cancer Institute, Boston, Massachusetts.

Polycythemia

Jorge A. Bezerra, M.D.

Fellow, Pediatric Gastrointestinal and Nutrition William C. Procter Research Scholar, University of Cincinnati, Children's Hospital Research Foundation, Cincinnati, Ohio.

Cirrhosis

Leonard Bielory, M.D.

Associate Professor of Medicine and Ophthalmology, UMD–New Jersey Medical School. Director, Division of Allergy and Immunology, Co-Director, Immuno-Ophthalmology Service, Newark, New Jersey.

Serum Sickness

Amy Louise Billett, M.D.

Instructor in Pediatrics, Harvard Medical School. Clinical Associate in Pediatrics, Dana-Farber Cancer Institute. Assistant in Medicine and Associate Director Oncology Inpatient Service, Children's Hospital, Boston, Massachusetts.

Treatment of Acute Leukemia in Children

Ronald S. Bloom, M.D.

Associate Professor of Pediatrics, Charles R. Drew University. Attending Physician, King/Drew Medical Center, Los Angeles, California.

Management of the Infant in the Delivery Room

Thomas F. Boat, M.D.

Professor and Chairman, Department of Pediatrics, University of North Carolina. Staff Physician, University of North Carolina Hospitals, Chapel Hill, North Carolina.

Bronchiectasis

Margaret L. Bogle, Ph.D., R.D.

Assistant Professor, Department of Pediatrics, University of Arkansas for Medical Sciences. Director, Clinical Nutrition and Research, Arkansas Children's Hospital, Little Rock, Arkansas.

Vitamin Deficiencies and Excesses

Robert Bortolussi, M.D., F.R.C.P.C.

Professor of Pediatrics, Dalhoasie University. Chief of Research and Clinical Staff Physician, Izaak Walton Killam Children's Hospital. Consultant, Grace Maternity Hospital, Halifax, Nova Scotia, Canada.

Listeria monocytogenes *Infection*

John T. Boyle, M.D.

Associate Professor of Pediatrics, Case Western Reserve University School of Medicine. Chief, Division of Gastroenterology and Nutrition, Rainbow Babies and Childrens Hospital, Cleveland, Ohio.

Portal Hypertension

Eileen D. Brewer, M.D.

Associate Professor of Pediatrics, Baylor College of Medicine. Medical Director, Pediatric Dialysis and Renal Transplantation, Texas Children's Hospital, Houston, Texas.

Hematuria and Proteinuria

Itzhak Brook, M.D.

Professor of Pediatrics, Georgetown University School of Medicine. Attending Pediatric Physician, Georgetown University School of Medicine, Washington, D.C. Consultant, Pediatric Infectious Diseases, Naval Hospital, Bethesda, Maryland.

Aspiration Pneumonia

James W. Brooks, M.D.

Professor of Surgery, Medical College of Virginia. Full-Time Attending Physician, Division of Cardiothoracic Surgery, Medical College of Virginia, Richmond, Virginia.

Pneumothorax and Mediastinal Emphysema; Intrathoracic Cysts and Masses

David Brown, M.D.

Associate Professor of Pediatrics, University of Medicine and Dentistry of New Jersey. Attending Neonatologist, Newark Beth Israel Medical Center, Newark, New Jersey.

Feeding the Low-Birth-Weight Infant

Elizabeth R. Brown, M.D.

Associate Professor of Pediatrics, Boston University School of Medicine. Director of Neonatology, Boston City Hospital, Boston, Massachusetts.

Necrotizing Enterocolitis

Beverly S. Brozanski, M.D.

Assistant Professor of Pediatrics, Obstetrics, and Gynecology, University of Pittsburgh School of Medicine. Clinical Neonatologist, Magee-Women's Hospital, Pittsburgh, Pennsylvania.

Bronchopulmonary Dysplasia

Philip J. Brunquell, M.D.

Assistant Professor of Pediatrics and Neurology, University of Connecticut School of Medicine, Farmington, Connecticut. Director, Clinical Neurophysiology Laboratories, Newington Children's Hospital, Newington, Connecticut.

Degenerative Diseases of the Central Nervous System

Jesus Bulux, M.D., M.P.H.

Adjunct Professor, Postgraduate Program in Ophthalmology, "Francisco Marroquín" Medical School. Chief, Task-Force on Vitamin A. Center for Studies of Sensory Impairment, Aging and Metabolism (CeSSIAM). Attending Physician, Nutritional Rehabilitation Ward, Pediatric Hospital of the Guatemalan Institute for Social Security (IGSS), Guatemala City, Guatemala.

Undernutrition

Bruce Camitta, M.D.

Professor of Pediatrics and Medicine, Medical College of Wisconsin. Director, Midwest Children's Cancer Center, and Chief, Hematology–Oncology, Children's Hospital of Wisconsin, Milwaukee, Wisconsin.

Aplastic Anemia

Thomas R. Caraccio, Pharm. D., R.P.H., A.B.A.T.

Assistant Professor of Emergency Medicine, State University of New York at Stony Brook. Assistant Professor of Pharmacology and Toxicology, New York College of Osteopathic Medicine, Old Westbury, New York. Adjunct Assistant Professor of Clinical Pharmacy, Jamaica, New York. Clinical Coordinator, Long Island Regional Poison Control Center, East Meadow, New York.

Acute Poisonings; Chronic Lead Poisoning in Children

Thomas O. Carpenter, M.D.

Associate Professor of Pediatrics, Yale University School of Medicine. Attending Physician, Yale–New Haven Hospital, New Haven, Connecticut.

Parathyroid Disease

Norris C. Carroll, M.D., F.R.C.S.(C.)

Martha Washington Professor of Pediatric Orthopaedics; Professor of Clinical Orthopaedics, Northwestern University Medical School. Head, Division of Pediatric Orthopaedics, The Children's Memorial Hospital, Chicago, Illinois.

Treatment of Bone Tumors and Limb Salvage

William L. Carroll, M.D.

Associate Professor, Program in Human Molecular Biology and Genetics, and Department of Pediatrics, University of Utah. Attending Physician, Division of Hematology/Oncology, Primary Children's Medical Center, Salt Lake City, Utah.

Malignant Lymphoma

Christopher L. Case, M.D.

Assistant Professor of Pediatrics and Co-Director, Pediatric Cardiology Fellowship Program, Medical University of South Carolina. Director, Electrocardiography and Ambulatory Monitoring, South Carolina Children's Heart Center, Children's Hospital, Charleston, South Carolina.

Dysrhythmias

James T. Casper, M.D.

Professor of Pediatrics, Medical College of Wisconsin. Vice Chief of Staff, Children's Hospital of Wisconsin, Milwaukee, Wisconsin.

Neuroblastoma

Helen Butler Casteel, M.D.

Associate Professor of Pediatrics, Chief, Pediatric Gastroenterology and Nutrition, University of Arkansas for Medical Sciences. Staff Physician, Arkansas Children's Hospital, Little Rock, Arkansas.

Recurrent Abdominal Pain

James C. M. Chan, M.D., FAAP

Professor of Pediatrics and Pediatric Nephrologist, Health Sciences Division of Virginia Commonwealth University, Medical College of Virginia, Richmond, Virginia.

Nephrotic Syndrome

Russel W. Chesney, M.D.

Le Bonheur Professor and Chairman of Pediatrics, University of Tennessee College of Medicine. Le Bonheur Children's Medical Center, Memphis, Tennessee.

Disorders of Porphyrin, Purine, and Pyrimidine Metabolism

Thomas McC. Chesney, M.D.

Clinical Professor of Medicine (Dermatology and Pathology), University of Tennessee. Director, Pathology Resident Training Program. Pathologist, Baptist Memorial Hospital, Memphis, Tennessee.

Disorders of Porphyrin, Purine, and Pyrimidine Metabolism

Cindy Christian, M.D.

Clinical Assistant Professor, University of Pennsylvania School of Medicine. Pediatric Consultant, SCAN, Inc. Attending Physician, Children's Hospital of Philadelphia, Philadelphia, Pennsylvania.

Child Abuse

Katherine Kaufer Christoffel, M.D., M.P.H.

Professor of Pediatrics and Community Health and Preventive Medicine, Northwestern University Medical School. Attending Pediatrician, Children's Memorial Hospital, Chicago, Illinois.

Prevention of Injuries

John P. Cloherty, M.D.

Associate Clinical Professor of Pediatrics, Harvard Medical School. Senior Associate in Neonatology, Joint Program in Neonatology, Brigham and Women's Hospital, The Children's Hospital, and the Beth Israel Hospital, Boston, Massachusetts.

Infants Born to Diabetic Mothers

Bernard Cohen, M.D.

Director, Pediatric Dermatology, Johns Hopkins Medical Institutions, Baltimore, Maryland.

Discoid Lupus Erythematosus; Arthropod Bites and Stings

Eric Cohen, M.D.

Clinical Associate Professor of Family Medicine and Pediatrics, University of Southern California School of Medicine. Medical Director, High-Risk Youth Program, Children's Hospital of Los Angeles, Los Angeles, California.

Homosexuality in Adolescents

Harvey J. Cohen, M.D., Ph.D.

Professor of Pediatrics (Hematology/Oncology), University of Rochester; Chief, Division of Pediatric Hematology/Oncology, Associate Chair for Research and Development; and Director, Strong Children's Research Center, Rochester, New York.

Disseminated Intravascular Coagulation

Andrew A. Colin, M.D.

Assistant Professor of Pediatrics, Harvard Medical School, Boston, Massachusetts. Assistant in Medicine, Children's Hospital, Boston, Massachusetts

Primary Pulmonary Hemosiderosis

Janna C. Collins, M.D.

Associate Professor of Clinical Pediatrics and Medicine, College of Physicians and Surgeons, Columbia University. Attending Physician, Babies Hospital and Presbyterian Hospital, Columbia–Presbyterian Medical Center, New York, New York.

Wilson's Disease

George D. Comerci, M.D.

Senior Clinical Lecturer, University of Arizona College of Medicine, Department of Pediatrics. Director of Pediatric and Adolescent Medicine, Desert Hills Center for Youth and Families, Tucson, Arizona.

Eating Disorders

Serge A. Coopman, M.D.

Clinical Consultant, Department of Dermatology, University of Leuven, Belgium.

Disorders of Pigmentation

W. Thomas Corder, M.D.

Assistant Professor, Department of Pediatrics, West Virginia University. Physician, West Virginia University Children's Hospital, Morgantown, West Virginia.

Mucormycosis (Zygomycosis)

Kenneth L. Cox, M.D.

Staff, Department of Pediatrics, California Pacific Medical Center, San Francisco, California.

Pancreatic Diseases

Christopher Crawford

Academic Research Specialist, Division of Pediatric Endocrinology, Cornell University Medical College, New York, New York.

Disorders of the Adrenal Gland

Robert K. Crone, M.D.

Senior Vice President of Medical Operations, Project Hope, Health Science Educational Center, Milwood, Virginia.

Septic Shock

M. Douglas Cunningham, M.D.

Professor of Clinical Pediatrics and Neonatology, Department of Pediatrics, University of California, Irvine, Orange, California. Medical Director, Neonatology, Saddleback Women's Hospital, Laguna Hills, California.

Disturbances of Intrauterine Growth

Michael J. Cunningham, M.D.

Assistant Professor of Otology and Laryngology, Harvard Medical School. Assistant Surgeon in Otolaryngology, Massachusetts Eye and Ear Infirmary. Assistant in Pediatrics, Massachusetts General Hospital, Boston, Massachusetts.

Nasal Injuries and Epistaxis; Peritonsillar and Retropharyngeal Abscess

Shermine Dabbagh, M.D.

Associate Professor of Pediatrics, Wayne State University. Director, End Stage Renal Disease Program, Children's Hospital of Michigan, Detroit, Michigan.

Management of Acute and Chronic Glomerulonephritis

Ronald E. Dahl, M.D.

Assistant Professor of Psychiatry and Pediatrics, Department of Psychiatry, University of Pittsburgh School of Medicine. Director, Child and Adolescent Sleep Laboratory, Western Psychiatric Institute and Clinic, Pittsburgh, Pennsylvania.

Common Sleep Disorders in Children

Giulio J. D'Angio, M.D.

Professor of Radiation Oncology, of Radiology, and of Pediatrics, Department of Radiation Oncology, University of Pennsylvania School of Medicine. Attending Physician, Hospital of the University of Pennsylvania and Children's Hospital of Philadelphia, Philadelphia, Pennsylvania.

Management of Childhood Brain Tumors

Barry Dashefsky, M.D.

Associate Professor of Pediatrics, University of Pittsburgh. Medical Staff Member, Department of Pediatrics, Divisions of Ambulatory Care and Pediatric Infectious Diseases, Children's Hospital of Pittsburgh, Pittsburgh, Pennsylvania.

Rat-Bite Fever; Gonococcal Infections

Murray Davidson, M.D.
Professor of Pediatrics, Albert Einstein College of Medicine, Bronx, New York.
Constipation and Encopresis

G. Michael Davis, M.B., Ch.B.
Assistant Professor, Division of Respiratory Medicine, Department of Pediatrics, McGill University. Physician, Division of Respiratory Medicine, Montreal Children's Hospital, Montreal, Quebec, Canada.
The Croup Syndrome; Cystic Fibrosis

David M. Dawson, M.D.
Professor of Neurology, Harvard Medical School. Chief of Neurology Service, West Roxbury Veterans Administration Hospital, West Roxbury, Massachusetts. Attending Physician, Brigham and Women's Hospital, Boston, Massachusetts.
Myasthenia Gravis

Virginia Delaney-Black, M.D.
Associate Professor of Pediatrics, Wayne State University. Associate Neonatologist, Children's Hospital of Michigan and Hutzel Hospital, Detroit, Michigan.
Neonatal Polycythemia and Hyperviscosity

William H. Dietz, M.D., Ph.D.
Associate Professor of Pediatrics, Tufts University School of Medicine. Director of Clinical Nutrition, Boston Floating Hospital, Boston, Massachusetts.
Obesity

Joan DiPalma, M.D.
Assistant Professor of Pediatrics, Georgetown University School of Medicine. Staff Physician, Georgetown University Medical Center, Washington, D.C.
Pylorospasm; Pyloric Stenosis

Gary Donath, M.D.
Fellow, Hand and Microsurgery, Group, Inc., San Francisco, California.
Congenital Hand and Arm Deformities

John W. Duckett, M.D.
Professor of Urology in Surgery, University of Pennsylvania School of Medicine. Director, Division of Pediatric Urology, Children's Hospital of Philadelphia, Philadelphia, Pennsylvania.
Disorders of the Bladder and Urethra

Lisa M. Dunkle, M.D.
Director, Antiviral Clinical Research, Bristol-Myers Squibb Pharmaceutical Research Institute, Wallingford, Connecticut.
Infections Due to Anaerobic Cocci and Gram-Negative Bacilli

Paul G. Dyment, M.D.
Professor of Clinical Pediatrics, Tulane University. Director, Student Health Center, Tulane University, New Orleans, Louisiana.
The Hip

Morven S. Edwards, M.D.
Professor of Pediatrics, Baylor College of Medicine. Active Staff, Texas Children's Hospital and Harris County Hospital District, Houston, Texas.
Group B Streptococcal Infections; Animal and Human Bites and Bite-Related Infections

Lamia F. Elerian, M.D.
Fellow, University of Texas Health Science Center, Division of Neonatal-Perinatal Medicine, Houston, Texas.
Urinary Tract Infections in Children

Elliot F. Ellis, M.D.
Professor of Pediatrics, Emeritus, State University of New York at Buffalo. Staff, Jacksonville Wolfson Children's Hospital, Jacksonville, Florida.
Atopic Dermatitis

Elizabeth C. Engle, M.D.
Instructor, Harvard Medical School. Research Fellow, Children's Hospital, Boston, Massachusetts.
Benign Intracranial Hypertension; Spasmus Nutans

Tahsin M. Ergin, M.D.
Clinical Affiliate Staff, Children's Hospital of Philadelphia and Graduate Hospital, Philadelphia, Pennsylvania.
Orthopedic Trauma

Robert B. Ettenger, M.D.
Professor of Pediatrics; Head, Division Pediatric Nephrology, Vice Chairman for Clinical Affairs, University of California School of Medicine, Los Angeles, California.
Renal Transplantation in Children

Arthur R. Euler, M.D.
Director, Gastroenterology, Clinical Development, Glaxo, Inc., Research Institute, Research Triangle Park, North Carolina.
Disorders of the Esophagus

J. R. Evans, M.D., F.R.C.P.C., F.A.A.P.
Associate Clinical Professor of Pediatrics, University of California San Francisco. Attending Physician, University of California San Francisco Hospitals and San Francisco General Hospital. Active Staff, Marin General Hospital.
Listeria monocytogenes *Infection*

Owen B. Evans, M.D.
Professor and Chairman, Department of Pediatrics, University of Mississippi Medical Center. Attending Physician, University of Mississippi Medical Center Hospital, Jackson, Mississippi.
Inflammatory Myopathies

Leonard G. Feld, M.D., Ph.D.
Associate Professor of Pediatrics and Physiology, State University of New York at Buffalo School of Medicine and Biomedical Sciences. Chief, Division of Pediatric Nephrology, and Director, Children's Kidney Center, Children's Hospital of Buffalo, Buffalo, New York.
Systemic Hypertension

William S. Ferguson, M.D.
Chief, Pediatric Hematology/Oncology Children's Service, Massachusetts General Hospital, Boston, Massachusetts.
Burkitt's Lymphoma

Gregory A. Filice, M.D.
Associate Professor, Department of Internal Medicine, University of Minnesota. Staff Physician, Infectious Disease Section, Veterans Affairs Medical Center, Minneapolis, Minnesota.
Toxoplasmosis

Stanley M. Fineman, M.D.
Clinical Assistant Professor, Department of Pediatrics, Emory University School of Medicine. Staff Physician, Scot-

tish Rite Children's Medical Center, Northside Hospital, Atlanta, and Kennestone Hospital, Marietta, Georgia.

Urticaria

Lewis R. First, M.D.

Assistant Professor of Pediatrics, Harvard Medical School. Director, Pediatric Group Associates Program and Associate in Medicine, Children's Hospital, Boston, Massachusetts.

Nasopharyngitis; Nausea and Vomiting

Coy D. Fitch, M.D.

Professor of Internal Medicine, Saint Louis University School of Medicine. Chief of Internal Medicine Service, Saint Louis University Hospital, St. Louis, Missouri.

Malaria

Richard E. Fitzpatrick, M.D.

Assistant Clinical Professor, University of California, San Diego. Consultant, University Hospital and Mercy Hospital, San Diego, and Scripps Memorial Hospital, La Jolla, California.

Fungal Infections of the Skin

Larry E. Fleischmann, M.D.

Professor of Pediatrics, Wayne State University. Director, Pediatric Nephrology, Children's Hospital of Michigan, Detroit, Michigan.

Management of Acute and Chronic Glomerulonephritis

Martin T. Fosburg, M.D.

Formerly, Assistant Professor of Pediatrics, Harvard Medical School; and Associate Director, Transfusion Service, Children's Hospital, Boston, Massachusetts.

Adverse Reactions to Blood Transfusion

Katherine B. Freeman, M.D.

Assistant Professor of Pediatrics, Brown University School of Medicine. Attending Physician, Pediatric Gastroenterology and Nutrition, Rhode Island Hospital and Women and Infants Hospital, Providence, Rhode Island.

Acute and Chronic Diarrhea in Infants and Children

Gilbert A. Friday, Jr., M.D.

Professor of Pediatrics, University of Pittsburgh School of Medicine. Physician, Children's Hospital of Pittsburgh, Pittsburgh, Pennsylvania.

Insect Stings

Louis Friedlander, M.D.

Clinical Professor of Pediatrics, University of Southern California School of Medicine. Physician, Los Angeles County University of Southern California Medical Center, Los Angeles, California.

Vaginitis and Urethritis

Ellen M. Friedman, M.D., F.A.A.P., F.A.C.S.

Associate Professor, Department of Otolaryngology and Communicative Sciences and Pediatrics, Baylor College of Medicine. Chief of Service, Texas Children's Hospital, Houston, Texas.

Foreign Bodies in the External Ear; Injuries to the Middle Ear

Cristine Froemming, M.D.

Urologist, Federal Faculty of Medical Sciences, Pôrto Alegre, Rio Grande, Brazil.

Neurogenic Bladder in Children

David R. Fulton, M.D.

Associate Professor of Pediatrics, Tufts University School of Medicine. Chief, Division of Pediatric Cardiology, The Floating Hospital for Infants and Children, Boston, Massachusetts.

Congestive Heart Failure

J. Carlton Gartner, Jr., M.D.

Professor of Pediatrics, University of Pittsburgh School of Medicine. Physician, Children's Hospital of Pittsburgh, Pittsburgh, Pennsylvania.

Fever of Unknown Origin

Karen M. Gaudio, M.D.

Associate Professor of Pediatrics, Yale University School of Medicine. Director, End Stage Renal Disease Program. Attending Physician, Yale–New Haven Hospital, New Haven, Connecticut.

Acute Renal Failure

Bernard Gauthier, M.B., B.S., F.R.A.C.P.

Associate Professor of Pediatrics, Albert Einstein College of Medicine, Bronx, New York. Chief, Division of Nephrology, Schneider Children's Hospital of Long Island Jewish Medical Center, New Hyde Park, New York.

Renal Venous Thrombosis

Mitchell E. Geffner, M.D.

Associate Professor of Pediatrics, University of California School of Medicine, Los Angeles. Attending Physician, University of California Medical Center, Los Angeles, California.

Tall Stature

Robert H. Gelber, M.D.

Clinical Professor, Departments of Epidemiology and Dermatology, University of California, San Francisco. Attending Physician, San Francisco Regional Hansen's Disease Center, San Francisco, California.

Leprosy (Hansen's Disease)

Stephen E. Gellis, M.D.

Assistant Professor of Dermatology and Pediatrics, Harvard Medical School. Director, Dermatology Program, and Associate in Medicine, Children's Hospital, Boston, Massachusetts.

Scabies and Pediculosis; Disorders of the Sebaceous Glands and Sweat Glands

Lynn A. Gershan, M.D.

Assistant Professor of Pediatrics, The Medical College of Wisconsin. Associate Medical Director, Neonatal Intensive Care Unit, Children's Hospital of Wisconsin, Milwaukee, Wisconsin.

Total Parenteral Nutrition in Infants

Anne A. Gershon, M.D.

Professor of Pediatrics, Columbia University College of Physicians and Surgeons. Attending Physician, Babies Hospital, New York, New York.

Varicella-Zoster Virus Infection

Gerald S. Gilchrist, M.D.

Helen C. Levitt Professor and Chairman, Department of Pediatrics, Mayo Clinic and Mayo Medical School. Consultant in Pediatric Hematology and Oncology, Mayo Medical Center, and Director, Mayo Comprehensive Hemophilia Center, Rochester, Minnesota.

Congenital and Acquired Bleeding Disorders

Paul C. Gillette, M.D.

Professor of Pediatrics and Surgery and Clinical Co-Director Heart Development Research School, Medical University of

South Carolina. Director, Pediatric Cardiology, South Carolina Children's Heart Center, Children's Hospital, and Co-Director, Palmetto Heart Institute, Charleston, South Carolina.

Dysrhythmias

Herbert E. Gilmore, M.D.

Assistant Professor of Pediatrics, Tufts University School of Medicine. Attending Staff, Baystate Medical Center, Children's Hospital, Springfield, Massachusetts.

Infantile Hypotonia

Janet R. Gilsdorf, M.D.

Associate Professor, University of Michigan Medical School. Chief, Pediatric Infectious Diseases, C. S. Mott Children's Hospital, Ann Arbor, Michigan.

Coccidioidomycosis; Immunization Practice

Laurence B. Givner, M.D.

Associate Professor of Pediatrics, Bowman Gray School of Medicine, Wake Forest University. Attending Physician, Brenner Children's Hospital, Winston-Salem, North Carolina.

Enteroviruses

Richard B. Goldbloom, O.C., M.D., F.R.C.P.C.

Professor of Pediatrics, Dalhousie University. Director of Ambulatory Care Izaak Walton Killam Children's Hospital, Halifax, Nova Scotia, Canada.

Psychosomatic Illness

Gerald S. Golden, M.D.

Shainberg Professor of Pediatrics and Professor of Neurology, University of Tennessee. Active Staff, LeBonheur Children's Medical Center; Director, Boling Center for Developmental Disabilities, Memphis, Tennessee.

Tics and Tourette Syndrome

Johanna Goldfarb, M.D.

Staff Physician, Department of Pediatrics, Cleveland Clinic, Cleveland, Ohio.

Parvovirus Infection in Children

Deborah A. Goldman, M.D.

Instructor of Pediatrics, Mayo Medical School. Senior Associate Consultant, Mayo Clinic Hospitals (Saint Marys and Methodist), Rochester, Minnesota.

Peptic Ulcer

Maria D. Goldstein, M.D.

Clinical Assistant Professor of Pediatrics, University of New Mexico School of Medicine. District Health Officer, Public Health Division, New Mexico Department of Health, Albuquerque, New Mexico.

Plague

Manuel R. Gomez, M.D.

Professor of Pediatric Neurology, Mayo Medical School. Consultant in Pediatric Neurology, Mayo Clinic, Rochester, Minnesota.

Neurocutaneous Syndromes

Ricardo Gonzalez, M.D.

Professor of Urologic Surgery, University of Minnesota. Director of Pediatric Urology, University of Minnesota Hospital and Clinic. Attending Urologist, Minneapolis Children's Medical Center, Minneapolis, Minnesota.

Neurogenic Bladder in Children

Estherann Grace, M.D.

Assistant Clinical Professor of Pediatrics, Harvard Medical School. Associate, Division of Adolescent Medicine, Children's Hospital, Boston, Massachusetts.

Sex Education

John W. Graef, M.D.

Associate Clinical Professor of Pediatrics, Harvard Medical School. Associate in Medicine and Chief, Lead and Toxicology Clinic, Boston, Massachusetts.

Chronic Lead Poisoning in Children

Sharon Gray, M.P.H., R.D.

Clinical Nutrition Specialist, Children's Hospital, Boston, Massachusetts.

The Hyperphenylalaninemias

Carlos Grazioso, M.D.

Adjunct Professor, Postgraduate Program in Ophthalmology, "Francisco Marroquín" Medical School. Chief, Task-Force on Sensory Impairments, Center for Studies of Sensory Impairment, Aging and Metabolism (CeSSIAM), Guatemala City, Guatemala.

Undernutrition

Michael Green, M.D., M.P.H.

Assistant Professor of Pediatrics and Surgery, University of Pittsburgh School of Medicine. Physician, Division of Infectious Diseases, Children's Hospital of Pittsburgh, Pittsburgh, Pennsylvania.

Aspergillosis

Morris Green, M.D.

Perry W. Lesh Professor of Pediatrics, Indiana University School of Medicine. Attending Pediatrician, James Whitcomb Riley Hospital for Children, Indianapolis, Indiana.

The Child and the Death of a Loved One

John R. Gregg, M.D.

Clinical Associate Professor of Orthopedics, University of Pennsylvania. Attending Physician, Children's Hospital of Philadelphia, Philadelphia, Pennsylvania.

Orthopedic Trauma

Jeffrey K. Griffiths, M.D., M.P.H. & T.M.

Assistant Professor of Medicine and Comparative Medicine, Tufts University Schools of Medicine and Veterinary Medicine. Director of Microbiology and Traveler's Clinic, Division of Geographic Medicine and Infectious Diseases, New England Medical Center, and Division of Infectious Diseases, St. Elizabeth's Hospital, Boston, Massachusetts.

Cholera

Robert C. Griggs, M.D.

Professor of Neurology, Edward A. and Alma Vollertsen Rykenboer Professor of Neurophysiology, Chair, Department of Neurology, University of Rochester. Attending Physician, Strong Memorial Hospital, Rochester, New York.

Periodic Paralysis

Jay L. Grosfeld, M.D.

Professor and Chairman, Department of Surgery, Indiana University School of Medicine. Surgeon-in-Chief, James Whitcomb Riley Hospital for Children, Indianapolis, Indiana.

Intussusception

Alan B. Gruskin, M.D.

Professor and Chairman of Pediatrics, Wayne State University. Pediatrician-in-Chief, Children's Hospital of Michigan, Detroit, Michigan.

Management of Acute and Chronic Glomerulonephritis

Warren G. Guntheroth, M.D.

Professor of Pediatrics (Cardiology), University of Washington School of Medicine. Staff Physician, University of Washington Medical Center, Children's Hospital and Medical Center, Harborview Medical Center, Seattle, Washington.

Peripheral Vascular Disease

James P. Gutai, M.D.

Professor of Pediatrics, Wayne State University, Director of Endocrinology, Children's Hospital of Michigan, Detroit, Michigan.

Precocious and Delayed Puberty

Fouad Hajjar, M.D.

Assistant Professor Pediatrics, Yale School of Medicine. Attending Physician, Yale–New Haven Hospital, New Haven, Connecticut.

Post-splenectomy Sepsis; Indications for Splenectomy

Brian L. Hamilton, M.D., Ph.D.

Provisional Courtesy Staff, Children's Hospital, Oakland, California.

The Immunodeficiencies

Margaret R. Hammerschlag, M.D.

Professor of Pediatrics and Medicine, State University of New York, Health Science Center at Brooklyn. Attending Physician, Pediatric Infectious Diseases, University Hospital of Brooklyn, Kings County Hospital Center, Brooklyn, New York.

Chlamydia *Infection*

Steven D. Handler, M.D.

Associate Professor, Department of Otolaryngology, Head and Neck Surgery, University of Pennsylvania School of Medicine. Associate Director, Otolaryngology, The Children's Hospital of Philadelphia, Philadelphia, Pennsylvania.

Developmental Cysts of the Neck

Catharine Jean Harris, M.D.

Clinical Assistant Professor of Pediatrics, University of Illinois. Director, Division of Genetics, Cook County Hospital, Chicago, Illinois.

Maternal Alcohol Ingestion: Effects on the Developing Fetus

Gregory F. Hayden, M.D.

Professor of Pediatrics, University of Virginia School of Medicine. Attending Pediatrician, Children's Medical Center of the University of Virginia, Charlottesville, Virginia.

Mumps

Thomas A. Hazinski, M.D.

Associate Professor of Pediatrics, Vanderbilt University School of Medicine. Staff Physician, Vanderbilt Children's Hospital, Nashville, Tennessee.

Atelectasis

Gerald B. Healy, M.D.

Professor of Otology and Laryngology, Harvard Medical School. Otolaryngologist-in-Chief, The Children's Hospital, Boston, Massachusetts.

Hearing Loss

Frederick W. Henderson, M.D.

Professor of Pediatrics, University of North Carolina School of Medicine. Attending Physician in Pediatrics, University of North Carolina Hospitals, Chapel Hill, North Carolina.

Viral Pneumonias

John J. Herbst, M.D.

Professor of Pediatrics; Head, Pediatric Gastroenterology, Louisiana State University School of Medicine–Shreveport. Pediatric Department, Louisiana State University Medical Center–Shreveport.

Gastroesophageal Reflux

John T. Herrin, M.B.B.S., F.R.A.C.P.

Associate Clinical Professor in Pediatrics, Harvard Medical School. Chief, Pediatric Nephrology, Massachusetts General Hospital. Chief, Pediatrics, Shriner Burns Institute, Boston Massachusetts.

Hypocalcemia and Tetany; Hydronephrosis and Disorders of the Ureter; Burns in Childhood

Laura S. Hillman, M.D.

Professor of Child Health, University of Missouri Medical School, and Professor of Nutrition, University of Missouri Graduate School. Staff Neonatologist, University of Missouri Hospital and Clinics, Columbia, Missouri.

Breast-Feeding

J. F. Hirsch, C.B.H.

Professor of Neurosurgery, University René Descartes. Staff Physician, Hôpital des Enfants Malades, Chef du Service de Neuro-chirurgie Pediatrique, Paris, France.

Hydrocephalus

Deborah G. Hirtz, M.D.

Medical Officer, Developmental Neurology Branch, National Institute of Neurological Disorders and Stroke, National Institutes of Health, Bethesda, Maryland.

Treatment of Seizure Disorders in Children

Joan E. Hodgman, M.D.

Professor of Pediatrics, University of Southern California School of Medicine. Neonatal Attending Physician, Los Angeles County & University of Southern California Medical Center, Los Angeles, California.

Skin Disorders of the Neonate

David Holtzman, M.D., Ph.D.

Associate Professor, Harvard Medical School. Attending Staff, Children's Hospital, and Associate in Neurology, Boston, Massachusetts.

Benign Intracranial Hypertension; Spasmus Nutans

Ian R. Holzman, M.D.

Professor of Pediatrics, Chief, Division of Newborn Medicine, Mt. Sinai School of Medicine. Attending Neonatologist, Mount Sinai Hospital, New York, New York.

Meconium Aspiration Syndrome

Paul J. Honig, M.D.

Professor of Pediatrics and Dermatology, University of Pennsylvania School of Medicine. Director, Pediatric Dermatology, Children's Hospital, Philadelphia, Pennsylvania.

Drug Reactions and the Skin

E. Hoppe-Hirsch, C.B.H.

Staff Physician, Hôpital des Enfants Malades, Service de Neuro-chirurgie Pediatrique, Paris, France.

Hydrocephalus

Walter T. Hughes, M.D.

Professor of Pediatrics, University of Tennessee College of Medicine. Chairman, Department of Infectious Diseases, St. Jude Children's Research Hospital, Memphis, Tennessee.

Tularemia; Pneumocystis carinii

Sidney Hurwitz, M.D.

Clinical Professor of Pediatrics and Dermatology, Yale University School of Medicine. Attending Physician in Pediatrics and Dermatology, Yale–New Haven Medical Center and Hospital of St. Raphael, New Haven, Connecticut.

Papulosquamous Disorders

Robert N. Husson, M.D.

Assistant Professor of Pediatrics, Harvard Medical School. Assistant in Medicine, Children's Hospital, Boston, Massachusetts.

Acquired Immunodeficiency Syndrome

Iekuni Ichikawa, M.D.

Professor of Pediatrics, Vanderbilt University. Head, Division of Pediatric Nephrology, Vanderbilt University Medical Center, Nashville, Tennessee.

Fluid and Electrolyte Therapy

Laura S. Inselman, M.D.

Associate Professor of Pediatrics, Jefferson Medical College, Thomas Jefferson University, Philadelphia, Pennsylvania. Associate Pulmonologist; Medical Director, Respiratory Care Department and Pulmonary Function Laboratory; and Attending Pediatrician, A.I. duPont Institute, Wilmington, Delaware.

Tuberculosis

Shunzaburo Iwatsuki, M.D.

Professor of Surgery, University of Pittsburgh School of Medicine. Attending Physician, Presbyterian-University Hospital and Children's Hospital of Pittsburgh, Pittsburgh, Pennsylvania.

Tumors of the Liver

Phillip A. Jacobson, M.D.

Assistant Professor of Anesthesia and Co-Director, Children's Hospital and Medical Center, Seattle, Washington.

Anaphylaxis

Michael S. Jellinek, M.D.

Associate Professor of Psychiatry (Pediatrics), Harvard Medical School. Chief, Child Psychiatry Service; Director, Outpatient Psychiatry; Associate Chief, Psychiatry Service, Massachusetts General Hospital, Boston, Massachusetts.

Children of Divorcing Parents

Bernett L. Johnson, Jr., M.D.

Professor and Vice Chairman, Department of Dermatology, and Associate Dean for Minority Affairs and Graduate Medical Education, University of Pennsylvania School of Medicine and Hospital of the University of Pennsylvania, Philadelphia, Pennsylvania.

Treatment of Malignant Melanoma in Children

Charlotte E. Johnson, L.C.S.T., Ph.D.

Clinical Instructor, Department of Communications and Communication Disorders, University of Pittsburgh. Speech Language Pathologist, Department of Audiology and Communication Disorders, Children's Hospital of Pittsburgh, Pittsburgh, Pennsylvania.

Voice, Speech, and Language Disorders

Maureen Jonas, M.D.

Assistant Professor, Department of Pediatrics, Harvard University School of Medicine. Associate in Gastroenterology, Children's Hospital, Boston, Massachusetts.

Disorders of the Biliary Tree

Gilbert N. Jones III, M.D.

Instructor, Washington University, St. Louis School of Medicine. Attending Physician, St. Louis Children's Hospital, St. Louis, Missouri.

Galactosemia

Leonard B. Kaban, D.M.D., M.D.

Professor and Chairman, Department of Oral and Maxillofacial Surgery, University of California, San Francisco. Chief, Oral and Maxillofacial Surgery Service, Moffitt-Long Hospital, San Francisco, California.

Craniofacial Malformations

Bernard S. Kaplan, M.B., B.Ch.

Professor of Pediatrics and Medicine, University of Pennsylvania. Director, Division of Nephrology, Children's Hospital of Philadelphia, Philadelphia, Pennsylvania.

Hemolytic-Uremic Syndrome

Lawrence C. Kaplan, M.D., Sc.M.

Assistant Professor of Pediatrics, University of Connecticut. Director, Center for Children with Special Health Care Needs, and Attending Pediatrician, Newington Children's Hospital, Pittsburgh, Pennsylvania.

Myelodysplasia

Sheldon L. Kaplan, M.D.

Professor and Vice-Chairman for Clinical Affairs, Department of Pediatrics, Baylor College of Medicine. Chief, Infectious Disease Service, Texas Children's Hospital, Houston, Texas.

Bacterial Meningitis and Septicemia Beyond the Neonatal Period

Lefke P. Karaviti, M.D., Ph.D.

Assistant Professor, Baylor College of Medicine. Attending Staff, Texas Children's Hospital, Houston, Texas.

Disorders of the Adrenal Gland

Michael Katz, M.D.

Reuben S. Carpentier Professor Emeritus of Pediatrics, Columbia University. Consultant in Pediatrics, Babies Hospital, a Division of Presbyterian Hospital, New York, New York

Ascariasis

Robert Kaye, M.D.

Professor of Pediatrics, Medical College of Pennsylvania. Senior Physician, Medical College of Pennsylvania Hospital, Philadelphia, Pennsylvania.

Insulin-Dependent Diabetes Mellitus

Edwin L. Kendig, Jr., M.D.

Professor of Pediatrics, Medical College of Virginia, Health Sciences Division, Virginia Commonwealth University. Coordinator of Hospital Affiliations, St. Mary's Hospital, Richmond, Virginia.

Sarcoidosis

Margaret A. Kenna, M.D.

Associate Professor of Otolaryngology, University of Pittsburgh School of Medicine. Co-Director, Pediatric Otolaryngology, Children's Hospital of Pittsburgh, Pittsburgh, Pennsylvania.

Labyrinthitis

Gerald T. Keusch, M.D.

Professor of Medicine, Tufts University School of Medicine. Attending Physician, New England Medical Center, Chief

Division of Geographic Medicine and Infectious Diseases, Boston, Massachusetts.
Cholera

Sigmund Kharasch, M.D.
Assistant Professor of Pediatrics, Boston University School of Medicine. Associate Director, Pediatric Emergency Medicine, Boston City Hospital, Boston, Massachusetts.
Sexual Abuse and Assault

Kwang Sik Kim, M.D.
Professor, Department of Pediatrics, University of Southern California School of Medicine. Head, Division of Infectious Diseases, and Attending Physician, Children's Hospital of Los Angeles, Los Angeles, California.
Candidiasis

Mark W. Kline, M.D.
Assistant Professor of Pediatrics, Sections of Infectious Diseases and Allergy/Immunology, Baylor College of Medicine. Attending Physician, Texas Children's Hospital, Houston, Texas.
Schistosomiasis

William J. Klish, M.D.
Professor of Pediatrics, Baylor College of Medicine. Chief, Nutrition and Gastroenterology Service, Texas Children's Hospital, Houston, Texas.
Entamoeba histolytica *Infection*

Matthew E. Knight, M.D., M.S.
Assistant Professor Pediatrics and Pharmacology, College of Medicine, University of Florida. Active Staff, Shands Hospital, University of Florida, and North Florida Regional Hospital, Gainesville, Florida.
Adverse Drug Reactions

Steve Kohl, M.D.
Professor of Pediatrics, University of California, San Francisco. Chief of Pediatric Infectious Diseases, Moffitt-Long Hospital, and San Francisco General Hospital, San Francisco, California.
Herpes Simplex Virus Infections

H. Kopelman, M.D.
Assistant Professor of Pediatrics, McGill University. Director, Division of Gastroenterology and Nutrition, and Gastrointestinal/Nutrition Consultant, Cystic Fibrosis Clinic, Montreal Children's Hospital, Montreal, Quebec, Canada.
Cystic Fibrosis

Mark S. Korson, M.D.
Instructor in Pediatrics, Harvard Medical School. Assistant in Medicine (Genetics), and Director, Metabolism Service, Children's Hospital, Boston, Massachusetts.
The Hyperphenylalaninemias

Karen L. Kotloff, M.D.
Associate Professor of Pediatrics, University of Maryland School of Medicine. Physician, Division of Infectious Disease and Tropical Pediatrics, Baltimore, Maryland.
Shigellosis; Nontyphoidal Salmonellosis

Martin A. Koyle, M.D., F.A.C.S., F.A.A.P.
Associate Professor of Surgery, University of Colorado School of Medicine. Chief, Pediatric Urology, The Children's Hospital, Denver, Colorado.
Undescended Testes

Peter J. Krause, M.D.
Professor of Pediatrics, The University of Connecticut School of Medicine, Farmington, Connecticut. Chief of Pediatric Infectious Diseases, Hartford Hospital, Hartford, Connecticut.
Babesiosis

Elise E. Labbé, Ph.D.
Associate Professor of Psychology, Department of Psychology, and Adjunct Associate Professor, Department of Neurology, University of South Alabama, Mobile, Alabama.
Headache

David Lacomis, M.D.
Instructor in Neurology, University of Massachusetts Medical School, Worcester, Massachusetts.
Myasthenia Gravis

Ronald V. Lacro, M.D.
Instructor in Pediatrics, Harvard Medical School. Assistant in Cardiology, Children's Hospital, Boston, Massachusetts.
Marfan Syndrome

Joseph W. Landau, M.D.
Associate Clinical Professor of Medicine (Dermatology), Division of Dermatology, Department of Medicine, University of California School of Medicine. Los Angeles, California. Attending Physician, Dermatology Service, Santa Monica Hospital and St. John's Hospital, Santa Monica, California.
Warts and Molluscum Contagiosum

Craig B. Langman, M.D.
Associate Chair of Pediatrics, and Associate Professor of Pediatrics, Northwestern University Medical School. Director, Mineral Metabolism, Childrens Memorial Hospital, Chicago, Illinois.
Rickets

Philip Lanzkowsky, M.D., F.R.C.P., D.C.H.
Professor of Pediatrics, Albert Einstein College of Medicine, Bronx, New York. Chief, Pediatric Hematology–Oncology; Chairman, Department of Pediatrics, and Chief of Staff, Schneider Children's Hospital & Long Island Jewish Medical Center, New Hyde Park, New York.
Megaloblastic Anemia

Alan M. Leichtner, M.D.
Assistant Professor of Pediatrics, Harvard Medical School. Clinical Director of Gastroenterology, Children's Hospital, Boston, Massachusetts.
Inflammatory Bowel Disease

Martha L. Lepow, M.D.
Professor of Pediatrics, Albany Medical College, Albany, New York.
Meningococcal Disease

Melvin D. Levine, M.D.
Professor of Pediatrics, University of North Carolina School of Medicine. Director, Clinical Center for the Study of Development and Learning, University of North Carolina, Chapel Hill, North Carolina.
Disorders of Learning; Attention Deficits

Myron M. Levine, M.D., D.T.P.H.
Professor and Director, Center for Vaccine Development, University of Maryland School of Medicine, Baltimore, Maryland.
Shigellosis; Typhoid Fever

Fiona H. Levy, M.D.
Critical Care Fellow, Children's Hospital and Medical Center, Seattle, Washington.
Septic Shock

Moise L. Levy, M.D.

Assistant Professor of Dermatology and Pediatrics, Baylor College of Medicine. Chief, Dermatology Service, Texas Children's Hospital, Houston, Texas.

Photodermatoses

James M. Lewis, M.D.

Associate Professor of Pediatrics, Marshall University School of Medicine. Active Staff, Cabell Huntington Hospital, St. Mary's Hospital, Huntington, West Virginia.

Lymphedema

Craig W. Lillehei, M.D.

Instructor in Surgery, Harvard Medical School. Assistant in Surgery, Children's Hospital, Boston, Massachusetts.

Congenital Diaphragmatic Hernia

Aldo Vincent Londino, Jr., M.D.

Clinical Assistant Professor of Medicine and Pediatrics, University of Pittsburgh School of Medicine. Director, Pediatric Rheumatology, Children's Hospital of Pittsburgh, Pittsburgh, Pennsylvania.

Erythema Nodosum

Sarah S. Long, M.D.

Professor of Pediatrics, Temple University School of Medicine. Chief, Section of Infectious Diseases, St. Christopher's Hospital for Children, Philadelphia, Pennsylvania.

Infant Botulism

Joseph Loscalzo, M.D., Ph.D.

Associate Professor of Medicine, Harvard Medical School. Director, Center for Research in Thrombolysis, Co-Director, Lipid Clinic, Staff Physician, Department of Medicine, Brigham and Women's Hospital. Chief, Cardiology Section, Brockton/West Roxbury Veterans Administration Medical Center. Consultant, Cardiology Department, Children's Hospital, Boston, Massachusetts.

Hyperlipoproteinemia

Frederick H. Lovejoy, Jr., M.D.

William Berkenberg Professor of Pediatrics, Harvard Medical School. Associate Physician-in-Chief, Children's Hospital, Boston, Massachusetts.

Reye Syndrome

Stephen Ludwig, M.D.

Professor of Pediatrics, University of Pennsylvania School of Medicine. Education Coordinator, SCAN, Inc., Division Chief, General Pediatrics, Children's Hospital of Philadelphia, Philadelphia, Pennsylvania.

Child Abuse

Joseph A. Majzoub, M.D.

Associate Professor of Pediatrics and Medicine, Harvard Medical School. Senior Associate in Medicine (Endocrinology), Division of Endocrinology, Children's Hospital, Boston, Massachusetts.

Diabetes Insipidus

J. Jeffrey Malatack, M.D.

Associate Professor of Pediatrics, Temple University School of Medicine. Director, Pediatric Diagnostic Referral Service, St. Christopher's Hospital for Children, Philadelphia, Pennsylvania.

Toxicara canis *Infections*

Eric S. Maller, M.D.

Assistant Professor of Pediatrics, University of Pennsylvania School of Medicine. Attending Physician, Division of Gastroenterology and Nutrition, Children's Hospital of Philadelphia, Philadelphia, Pennsylvania.

Malabsorptive Disorders

Susan Bayliss Mallory, M.D.

Associate Professor of Medicine (Dermatology) and Dermatology in Pediatrics, Washington University School of Medicine. Chief, Pediatric Dermatology, St. Louis Children's Hospital. Attending Physician, Barnes Hospital, St. Louis, Missouri.

Allergic Contact Dermatitis

James Mandell, M.D.

Associate Professor of Surgery, Harvard Medical School. Associate in Surgery, Children's Hospital, Boston, Massachusetts.

Exstrophy of the Bladder; Penis, Spermatic Cord, and Testis

Joan Mansfield, M.D.

Assistant Professor of Pediatrics, Harvard Medical School. Assistant in Medicine, Department of Endocrinology and Department of Adolescent and Young Adult Medicine, Children's Hospital, Boston, Massachusetts.

Adolescent Gynecology

Herbert C. Mansmann, Jr., M.D.

Professor of Pediatrics and Associate Professor of Medicine, Thomas Jefferson University. Former Director, Division of Allergy and Clinical Immunology, Thomas Jefferson University, Philadelphia, Pennsylvania.

Middle Lobe Syndrome

Andrew M. Margileth, M.D.

Clinical Professor Pediatrics, University of Virginia Medical Center. Charlottesville, Virginia. Physician, University of Virginia Medical Center, Charlottesville, and Mary Washington Hospital, Fredericksburg, Virginia.

Cat-Scratch Disease

Melvin I. Marks, M.D.

Professor and Vice-Chairman, Department of Pediatrics, University of California, Irvine. Medical Director, Memorial Miller Children's Hospital, Long Beach, California.

Pertussis

D. Richard Martini, M.D.

Assistant Professor of Psychiatry and Pediatrics, Department of Psychiatry, University of Pittsburgh School of Medicine; and Western Psychiatric Institute and Clinic. Program Director, Consultation/Liaison Service, Behavioral Science Division, Children's Hospital of Pittsburgh, Pittsburgh, Pennsylvania.

Psychiatric Disorders of Infants and Children

Helen S. Maurer, M.D.

Associate Professor Pediatrics, University of Illinois at Chicago College of Medicine. Attending Physician, University of Illinois Hospital, Chicago, Illinois.

Thalassemia

Anthony R. Mawson, Dr.P.H.

Assistant Research Professor, Department of Ophthalmology, Louisiana State University Medical Center, New Orleans, Louisiana.

Magnesium Deficiency; Zinc Deficiency

Kenneth L. McClain, M.D., Ph.D.

Associate Professor of Pediatrics, Baylor College of Medicine. Staff, Hematology/Oncology, Texas Children's Hospital, Houston, Texas.

Hemolytic Anemia

Julia A. McMillan, M.D.

Associate Professor of Pediatrics, The Johns Hopkins University School of Medicine. Staff Physician, Johns Hopkins Hospital, Baltimore, Maryland.

Mycoplasma *Infections*

Dan G. McNamara, M.D.

Professor of Pediatrics, Baylor College of Medicine. Emeritus Chief of Cardiology, Texas Children's Hospital, Houston, Texas.

Management of Innocent Murmurs in the Young

Teresita L. Melocoton, M.D., F.A.A.P.

Clinical Instructor in Pediatrics and Nephrology, University of California School of Medicine, Los Angeles, California.

Renal Transplantation in Children

Marian G. Michaels, M.D., M.P.H.

Assistant Professor Pediatrics and Surgery, University of Pittsburgh School of Medicine. Physician, Children's Hospital of Pittsburgh, Division of Infectious Diseases, Pittsburgh, Pennsylvania.

Campylobacter *Infections*

Lyle J. Micheli, M.D.

Associate Clinical Professor of Orthopaedic Surgery, Harvard Medical School. Director, Division of Sports Medicine, Children's Hospital, Boston, Massachusetts.

Orthopedic Disorders of the Extremities

Richard J. Mier, M.D.

Associate Professor of Pediatrics, University of Kentucky College of Medicine. Director of Pediatric Services, Shriners Hospital for Crippled Children, and Attending Pediatrician, University of Kentucky Hospitals, Lexington, Kentucky.

Torticollis; Congenital Muscular Defects

Michael E. Mitchell, M.D.

Professor of Urology, University of Washington School of Medicine. Chief, Pediatric Urology, Children's Hospital and Medical Center, Seattle, Washington.

Hernias and Hydroceles

Thomas G. Mitchell, Ph.D.

Associate Professor, Department of Microbiology, Duke University Medical Center, Durham, North Carolina.

Blastomycosis

Howard C. Mofenson, M.D., F.A.A.P., F.A.A.C.T.

Professor of Pediatrics and Emergency Medicine, State University of New York at Stony Brook. Senior Attending Physician in Pediatrics, Nassau County Medical Center, Winthrop University Hospital, East Meadow, New York.

Acute Poisonings; Chronic Lead Poisoning in Children

Susana Molina, M.D.

Adjunct Professor, Postgraduate Program in Ophthalmology, "Francisco Marroquín" Medical School. Research Physician, Center for Studies of Sensory Impairment, Aging and Metabolism (CeSSIAM). Attending Physician, Nutrition Rehabilitation Ward, Department of Pediatrics, "San Juan de Dios" General Hospital, Guatemala City, Guatemala.

Undernutrition

Frederick C. Morin III, M.D.

Associate Professor, School of Medicine, State University of New York at Buffalo. Attending Physician, Children's Hospital of Buffalo, Buffalo, New York.

Treatment of Respiratory Distress Syndrome

Edward A. Mortimer, Jr., M.D.

Elisabeth Severance Prentiss Professor Emeritus of Epidemiology, Case Western Reserve University School of Medicine. Associate Pediatrician, University Hospitals of Cleveland, Cleveland, Ohio.

Measles

Michele Moss, M.D.

Associate Professor of Pediatrics, Critical Care and Cardiology University of Arkansas for Medical Sciences. Medical Director, Pediatric Transplant Service, and Attending Physician, Pediatric and Cardiovascular Intensive Care Units, Arkansas Children's Hospital, Little Rock, Arkansas.

Syncope and Hypotension

Richard T. Moxley III, M.D.

Professor of Neurology and Pediatrics, Director Neuromuscular Disease Center, University of Rochester. Director, EMG-Nerve Conduction Laboratory, and Attending Physician, Strong Memorial Hospital, Rochester, New York.

Periodic Paralysis

Louis J. Muglia, M.D.

Instructor in Pediatrics Harvard Medical School. Assistant in Medicine (Endocrinology), Division of Endocrinology, Children's Hospital, Boston, Massachusetts.

Diabetes Insipidus

David Muram, M.D.

Associate Professor and Chief, Pediatric and Adolescent Gynecology University of Tennessee, Department of Obstetrics and Gynecology, Memphis, Tennessee.

Vulva and Vagina

Pamela J. Murray, M.D., M.H.P.

Associate Professor of Pediatrics, University of Pittsburgh. Director of Adolescent Medicine, Children's Hospital, Pittsburgh, Pennsylvania.

Contraception, Pregnancy, and Abortion

Lawrence S. Neinstein, M.D.

Associate Professor of Pediatrics and Medicine, University of Southern California School of Medicine. Associate Director, Children's Hospital of Los Angeles, Division of Adolescent Medicine, Los Angeles, California.

Homosexuality in Adolescents

Karin B. Nelson, M.D.

Medical Officer, Neuroepidemiology Branch, National Institute of Neurological Disorders and Stroke, National Institutes of Health, Bethesda, Maryland.

Febrile Seizures

Thomas E. Nevins, M.D.

Associate Professor of Pediatrics, University of Minnesota. Attending Pediatrician, Variety Club, Children's Hospital, University of Minnesota Hospital, Minneapolis, Minnesota.

Chronic Renal Failure

Maria I. New, M.D.

Professor and Chairman, Department of Pediatrics; Harold and Percy Uris Professor of Pediatric Endocrinology and Metabolism, Cornell University Medical College. Pediatrician-in-Chief, Chief, Division of Pediatric Endocrinology, The New York Hospital–Cornell Medical Center, New York, New York.

Disorders of the Adrenal Gland

Jane W. Newburger, M.D., M.P.H.

Professor of Pediatrics, Harvard Medical School. Senior Associate, Department of Cardiology, Children's Hospital, Boston, Massachusetts.

Kawasaki Syndrome

Donald H. Nguyen, M.D.

Director of Pediatric Urology, East Tennessee Children's Hospital, Knoxville, Tennessee.

Hernias and Hydroceles

Perry D. Nisen, M.D., Ph.D.

Associate Professor of Pediatrics, University of Texas Southwestern Medical Center at Dallas. Attending Physician, Children's Medical Center of Dallas and Parkland Memorial Hospital, Dallas, Texas.

Malignant Tumors of the Kidney

Jacqueline A. Noonan, M.D.

Professor of Pediatrics, Chief of Pediatric Cardiology, Chairman of the Department of Pediatrics, University of Kentucky. Staff Physician, University of Kentucky Medical Center, Lexington, Kentucky.

Congenital Heart Disease; Pericarditis

John Noseworthy, M.D.

Professor of Surgery, Thomas Jefferson University–Jefferson Medical College, Philadelphia, Pennsylvania. Surgeon-in-Chief, Alfred I. duPont Institute, and Active Staff, Medical Center of Delaware, Wilmington, Delaware.

Neonatal Ascites

Antonia C. Novello, M.D., M.P.H.

Clinical Professor of Pediatrics, Georgetown University School of Medicine and Uniformed Services University of the Health Sciences, Washington, D.C. Surgeon General, U.S. Public Health Service.

Hemodialysis

David G. Oelberg, M.D.

Associate Professor of Pediatrics, University of Texas Health Science Center at Houston. Active Staff, Hermann Children's Hospital and Lyndon B. Johnson General Hospital, Houston, Texas.

Lobar Emphysema

Paul A. Offit, M.D.

Associate Professor of Pediatrics, The University of Pennsylvania School of Medicine. Chief, Section of Infectious Diseases, The Children's Hospital of Philadelphia, Philadelphia, Pennsylvania.

Rotavirus

Richard Olsen, M.D.

Assistant Professor of Pediatrics, Mayo Medical School. Consultant in Pediatrics, Mayo Clinic. Staff Physician, Rochester Methodist Hospital and Saint Marys Hospital, Rochester, Minnesota.

Pica

P. Pearl O'Rourke, M.D.

Associate Professor of Anesthesiology and Pediatrics, University of Washington School of Medicine. Director, Pediatric Intensive Care Unit, Special Care Unit; Associate Director, Respiratory Therapy and ECMO Program, Children's Hospital and Medical Center, Seattle, Washington.

Anaphylaxis

Richard A. Orr, M.D.

Associate Professor of Anesthesiology/Critical Care Medicine and Pediatrics, University of Pittsburgh. Physician, Children's Hospital of Pittsburgh, Pittsburgh, Pennsylvania.

Near-Drowning

John S. O'Shea, M.D.

Professor of Pediatrics, Emory University School of Medicine. Director of Pediatrics, Southeastern Health Services. Attending Physician, Egleston Children's Hospital, Grady Memorial Hospital, Shepherd Spinal Center, West Paces Ferry Hospital, and Scottish Rite Children's Medical Center. Atlanta, Georgia.

Otitis Media

A. Lee Osterman, M.D.

Associate Professor Orthopedics and Hand Surgery, Hospital of University of Pennsylvania. Chief, Orthopedic Hand Surgery, Children's Hospital of Philadelphia, Philadelphia, Pennsylvania.

Congenital Hand and Arm Deformities

Enrique M. Ostrea, Jr., M.D.

Professor of Pediatrics, Wayne State University School of Medicine. Chief, Department of Pediatrics, Hutzel Hospital, Detroit, Michigan.

Infants of Drug-Dependent Mothers

Reynaldo D. Pagtakhan, M.D.

Professor of Pediatrics and Child Health, University of Manitoba, Faculty of Medicine. Pediatric Respirologist, Children's Hospital of Winnipeg, Manitoba, Canada.

Pleural Effusion and Chylothorax

Regina Mary Palazzo, M.D.

Instructor in Pediatrics, Harvard Medical School. Assistant in Medicine, Children's Hospital, Boston, Massachusetts.

Pulmonary Thromboembolism

Amy S. Paller, M.D.

Associate Professor of Pediatrics and Dermatology, Northwestern University Medical School. Head, Division of Dermatology, The Children's Memorial Hospital of Chicago, Chicago, Illinois.

The Genodermatoses

Dachling Pang, M.D., F.R.C.S.(C), F.A.C.S.

Associate Professor of Neurosurgery University of Pittsburgh. Attending Staff, Children's Hospital of Pittsburgh, Presbyterian University Hospital, and Montefiore University Hospital, Pittsburgh, Pennsylvania.

Epidural and Subdural Hematoma; Brain Abscess and Spinal Epidural Abscess; Rhinitis and Sinusitis

Jack L. Paradise, M.D.

Professor of Pediatrics, University of Pittsburgh School of Medicine. Attending Staff Physician Children's Hospital of Pittsburgh, Pittsburgh, Pennsylvania.

Tonsillectomy and Adenoidectomy

Jan E. Paradise, M.D.

Assistant Professor of Pediatrics, Boston University School of Medicine. Director, Child Protection Program, Boston City Hospital, Boston, Massachusetts.

Sexual Abuse and Assault

Robert C. Pascucci, M.D.

Instructor in Anesthesia (Pediatrics), Harvard Medical School. Associate Director, Medical Intensive Care Unit. Sr.

Associate in Anesthesia, Children's Hospital, Boston, Massachusetts.

Malignant Hyperthermia; Heat-Related Illnesses

Mark S. Pasternack, M.D.

Assistant Professor of Pediatrics, Harvard Medical School, Boston, Massachusetts. Chief, Pediatric Infectious Disease Unit, Massachusetts General Hospital, Charlestown, Massachusetts.

Rabies

Howard A. Pearson, M.D.

Professor of Pediatrics, Yale University School of Medicine. Attending Physician, Yale–New Haven Hospital, New Haven, Connecticut.

Post-splenectomy Sepsis; Indications for Splenectomy

Giorgio Perilongo, M.D.

Assistant Professor, University of Padova Medical School, Department of Pediatrics, Division of Pediatric Oncology, Padova, Italy. Attending Physician, Children's Hospital of Philadelphia, Philadelphia, Pennsylvania.

Management of Childhood Brain Tumors

Georges Peter, M.D.

Professor of Pediatrics, Brown University School of Medicine. Director, Division of Pediatric Infectious Diseases, Department of Pediatrics, Rhode Island Hospital, Providence, Rhode Island.

Pneumonia

Michael J. Pettei, M.D., Ph.D.

Associate Professor of Pediatrics, Albert Einstein College of Medicine, Bronx, New York. Co-Chief, Division of Gastroenterology and Nutrition, Schneider Children's Hospital, Long Island Jewish Medical Center, New Hyde Park, New York.

Constipation and Encopresis

Ronald R. Pfister, M.D., F.A.C.S., F.A.A.P.

Professor of Surgery, University of Colorado School of Medicine. Pediatric Urologist, The Children's Hospital, Denver, Colorado.

Undescended Testes

Carol F. Phillips, M.D.

Professor and Chairman, Department of Pediatrics, University of Vermont. Chief of Pediatrics, Medical Center Hospital of Vermont, Burlington, Vermont.

Psittacosis

Philip A. Pizzo, M.D.

Professor of Pediatrics, Uniformed Services University of the Health Sciences. Chief, Pediatric Branch, Head, Infectious Disease Section, National Cancer Institute, Bethesda, Maryland.

Leukopenia, Neutropenia, and Agranulocytosis

Daniel C. Plunket, M.D.

Professor and Chair, Department of Pediatrics, University of Oklahoma College of Medicine, Tulsa, Oklahoma.

Management of the Child Cured of Cancer

Barbara Pober, M.D.

Assistant Professor of Genetics and Pediatrics, Department of Genetics, Yale University School of Medicine. Staff, Yale–New Haven Hospital, New Haven, Connecticut.

Idiopathic Hypercalcemia

William J. Pokorny, M.D.

Professor of Surgery, Baylor College of Medicine. Chief, Pediatric Surgery, Ben Taub General Hospital. Active Staff, Texas Children's Hospital, and Women's Hospital, Houston, Texas.

Lymphangioma

Margaret Polaneczky, M.D.

Assistant Professor of Obstetrics and Gynecology, Cornell Medical College. Attending Staff, New York Hospital/Cornell Medical Center, New York, New York.

Uterus, Fallopian Tubes, and Ovaries

Richard A. Polin, M.D.

Professor of Pediatrics, University of Pennsylvania School of Medicine. Senior Neonatologist, Children's Hospital of Philadelphia, Philadelphia, Pennsylvania.

Birth Injuries

William P. Potsic, M.D.

Associate Professor, Department of Otolaryngology and Human Communication, University of Pennsylvania School of Medicine. Director of Pediatric Otolaryngology, Children's Surgical Associates, Ltd., Children's Hospital of Philadelphia, Philadelphia, Pennsylvania.

Choanal Atresia; Tumors and Polyps of the Nose

Roy Proujansky, M.D.

Assistant Professor of Pediatrics, Jefferson Medical College, Philadelphia, Pennsylvania. Chief, Division of Gastroenterology and Nutrition, Alfred I. duPont Institute, Wilmington, Delaware.

Neonatal Ascites

Michael Radetsky, M.D., C.M.

Clinical Professor of Pediatrics University of California School of Medicine, Davis, California. Director, Pediatric Infectious Disease and Critical Care, Kaiser Permanente Health Care System, Sacramento, California.

Group A Streptococcal Infections

Ben G. Raimer, M.D.

Clinical Associate Professor of Pediatrics, University of Texas Medical Branch. Attending Physician, University of Texas Hospital System, St. Mary's Hospital, and Mainland Hospital, Galveston, Texas.

Diaper Dermatitis

Sharon S. Raimer, M.D.

Professor of Dermatology and Pediatrics, University of Texas Medical Branch. Attending Physician, University of Texas Hospital System, Galveston, Texas.

Diaper Dermatitis

I. Rapin, M.D.

Professor of Neurology and Pediatrics (Neurology), Albert Einstein College of Medicine. Attending Neurologist and Child Neurologist, Einstein Affiliated Hospitals, Bronx, New York.

Autism

James E. Rasmussen, M.D.

Professor, Department of Dermatology, University of Michigan Medical School. Chief, Clinic in Dermatology, and of Dermatology Outpatients and Pediatric Inpatients, University of Michigan Medical Center, Ann Arbor, Michigan.

Erythema Multiforme; Disorders of the Hair and Scalp

James S. Reilly, M.D., F.A.C.S.

Professor of Surgery/Otolaryngology University of Alabama at Birmingham. Chief, Pediatric Otolaryngology, Children's Hospital of Alabama, Birmingham, Alabama.

Disorders of the Larynx

Margaret B. Rennels, M.D.

Associate Professor, University of Maryland School of Medicine. Physician, University of Maryland Hospital, Baltimore, Maryland.

Yersinia enterocolitica ***Infections***

Frederick J. Rescorla, M.D.

Assistant Professor of Surgery, Indiana University Medical School. Attending Surgeon, James Whitcomb Riley Hospital for Children, Indianapolis, Indiana.

Intussusception

Jeffrey I. Resnick, M.D.

Assistant Clinical Professor, Division of Plastic Surgery, University of California School of Medicine, Los Angeles, California. Staff Physician, Saint John's Hospital and Health Center, Santa Monica, California. Staff Physician, Cedars-Sinai Medical Center, Los Angeles, California.

Diseases and Injuries of the Oral Region

Alan B. Retik, M.D.

Professor of Surgery, Harvard Medical School. Chief, Division of Urology, Children's Hospital, Boston, Massachusetts.

Patent Urachus and Urachal Cysts

Arthur R. Rhodes, M.D., M.P.H.

Professor of Dermatology, University of Pittsburgh School of Medicine. Attending Physician, Children's Hospital of Pittsburgh, Presbyterian-University Hospital, Montefiore-University Hospital, and Magee Women's Hospital, Pittsburgh, Pennsylvania.

Nevi and Nevoid Tumors

A. Kim Ritchey, M.D.

Professor of Pediatrics, Chief, Pediatric Hematology-Oncology, West Virginia University School of Medicine. Attending Physician, West Virginia University Hospital, Morgantown, West Virginia.

Anemia and Chronic Disease

Albert P. Rocchini, M.D.

Director of Pediatric Cardiology, Ruben/Bentson Professor of Pediatrics, University of Minnesota. Staff Physician, University of Minnesota Hospitals and Clinic, Minneapolis, Minnesota.

The Child at Risk for Coronary Disease As an Adult

Juan Rodriguez-Soriano, M.D.

Professor of Pediatrics, Basque University School of Medicine. Director, Department of Pediatrics, Hospital de Cruces, Bilbao, Spain.

Renal Tubular Disorders

Frances J. Rohr, M.S., R.D.

Clinical Nutrition Specialist, Children's Hospital, Boston, Massachusetts

The Hyperphenylalaninemias

Jose Luis Romero, M.D.

Head, Clinical Parasitology Service, Infectious Diseases Department, Hospital Infantil de Mexico "Federico Gomez." Assistant Professor of Infectious Disease, Universidad Nacional Autonoma de Mexico.

Trichinosis

Robert L. Rosenfield, M.D.

Professor, Pediatrics and Medicine, University of Chicago, Pritzker School of Medicine. Chief, Section of Pediatric Endocrinology, Wyler Children's Hospital, Chicago, Illinois.

Endocrine Disorders of the Testis (Hypoandrogenism)

Judith L. Ross, M.D.

Professor, Department of Pediatrics, The Medical College of Pennsylvania, Philadelphia, Pennsylvania.

Short Stature

Thomas M. Rossi, M.D.

Associate Professor of Pediatrics, State University of New York at Buffalo School of Medicine and Biomedical Sciences. Division Chief, Gastroenterology and Nutrition, Children's Hospital of Buffalo, Buffalo, New York.

Hirschsprung's Disease

Barry H. Rumack, M.D.

Clinical Professor of Pediatrics, University of Colorado Health Sciences Center. Director Emeritus, Rocky Mountain Poison Center, Denver, Colorado.

Botulinal Food Poisoning

Ab Sadeghi-Nejad, M.D.

Professor of Pediatrics, Tufts University School of Medicine. Chief, Division of Pediatric Endocrinology and Metabolism, New England Medical Center (Floating Hospital for Infants and Children), Boston, Massachusetts.

Treatment of Thyroid Disorders in Children

Xavier Sáez-Llorens, M.D.

Professor of Pediatrics and Infectious Diseases, Hospital del Niño and University of Panama, Panama City, Panama.

Neonatal Septicemia, Meningitis, and Pneumonia

Lisa Saiman, M.D.

Assistant Professor of Pediatrics, Columbia University. Assistant Attending Physician in Pediatrics, St. Luke's–Roosevelt Hospital, New York, New York.

Endocarditis

Jose R. Salcedo, M.D., F.A.A.P.

Associate Professor of Pediatrics, University of Medicine and Dentistry of New Jersey, New Jersey Medical School. Director, Division of Pediatric Nephrology, University Hospital, Newark, New Jersey.

Nephrotic Syndrome

Stephen E. Sallan, M.D.

Professor of Pediatrics Harvard Medical School. Chemical Director Pediatric Oncology Dana-Farber Cancer Institute. Senior Associate in Medicine, Children's Hospital, Boston, Massachusetts.

Treatment of Acute Leukemia in Children

Pablo J. Sánchez, M.D.

Assistant Professor of Pediatrics, Divisions of Neonatal-Perinatal Medicine and Pediatric Infectious Diseases, University of Texas Southwestern Medical Center at Dallas. Attending Physician, Parkland Memorial Hospital and Children's Medical Center, Dallas, Texas.

Syphilis

Douglas H. Sandberg, M.D.

Professor of Pediatrics, University of Miami School of Medicine, Director, Division of Gastroenterology and Nutrition and Division Allergic Disease Unit, Jackson Memorial Hospital, Miami, Florida.

Allergic Gastrointestinal Disorders

Jose Ignacio Santos, M.D.

Head, Research Division and Infectious Disease Department, Hospital Infantil de Mexico "Federico Gomez," Mexico.

Trichinosis

Sharada A. Sarnaik, M.D.

Clinical Professor of Pediatrics, Wayne State University School of Medicine. St. John's Hospital and Medical Center and Children's Hospital of Michigan, Detroit, Michigan.

Sickle Cell Diseases

Lawrence A. Schachner, M.D.

Professor of Dermatology and Professor of Pediatrics; and Director, Division of Pediatric Dermatology, University of Miami School of Medicine. Staff Physician, Jackson Memorial Hospital, Mount Sinai Medical Center, and Cedars Medical Center, Miami, Florida.

Sun Protection in the Pediatric Population

I. Herbert Scheinberg, M.D.

Senior Lecturer in Medicine, Columbia University, College of Physicians and Surgeons. Senior Research Associate, Department of Medicine, St. Luke's/Roosevelt Hospital, New York, New York.

Wilson's Disease

Selva S. Schenkman, M.D.

Assistant Professor of Pediatrics, Seton Hall University of Graduate Medical Education, Orange, New Jersey. Chief, Pediatric Endocrine Section, St. Joseph's Hospital and Medical Center, Paterson, New Jersey.

Ambiguous Genitalia

Roy Schneiderman, M.D.

Instructor in Pediatrics, University of Pennsylvania School of Medicine. Staff Neonatologist, Hospital of the University of Pennsylvania, Philadelphia, Pennsylvania.

Birth Injuries

Kenneth E. Schuit, M.D., Ph.D.

Associate Professor of Pediatrics, University of Pittsburgh. Physician, Children's Hospital of Pittsburgh, Pittsburgh, Pennsylvania.

The Atypical Mycobacteria

Richard H. Schwartz, M.D.

Clinical Professor in Pediatrics, Georgetown University School of Medicine, Washington, D.C. Clinical Professor Family Medicine, Medical College of Virginia, Richmond, Virginia. Director of Research, Department of Pediatrics, Fairfax Hospital, Falls Church, Virginia.

Management of a Drug-Using Adolescent

Robert Schwartz, M.D.

Professor of Medical Science and Pediatrics, Brown University School of Medicine. Staff Member, Division of Pediatric Endocrinology and Metabolism, Department of Pediatrics, Rhode Island Hospital, Providence, Rhode Island.

Hypoglycemia in Metabolic Disorders

Gwendolyn B. Scott, M.D.

Professor of Pediatrics and Director, Division of Immunology and Infectious Disease, University of Miami School of Medicine. Attending Physician, Jackson Memorial Hospital, Miami, Florida.

The Immunodeficiencies

Robert W. Seibert, M.D.

Associate Professor, Otolaryngology and Pediatrics, University of Arkansas for Medical Sciences. Chief, Ear-Nose-Throat Section, Arkansas Children's Hospital, Little Rock, Arkansas.

Recurrent Acute Parotitis

Boris Senior, M.D.

Professor of Pediatrics, Tufts University School of Medicine. Senior Pediatric Endocrinologist, New England Medical Center (Floating Hospital for Infants and Children), Boston, Massachusetts.

Treatment of Thyroid Disorders in Children

Robert C. Shamberger, M.D.

Associate Professor of Surgery, Harvard Medical School. Senior Associate in Surgery, Children's Hospital, Boston, Massachusetts.

Congenital Deformities of the Anterior Chest Wall

Barry Shandling, M.B., Ch.B., F.R.C.S.(Eng.), F.R.C.S.(C)., F.A.C.S.

Professor of Surgery, University of Toronto. Senior Staff Surgeon, Hospital for Sick Children. Director, Bowel Clinic, Hugh MacMillan Medical Center, Toronto, Canada.

Disorders of the Anus and Rectum

Seetha Shankaran, M.D.

Professor of Pediatrics, Wayne State University School of Medicine. Director, Neonatal-Perinatal Medicine, Detroit Medical Center Regional Neonatal Program, Children's Hospital of Michigan Hutzel Hospital, and Grace Hospital, Detroit, Michigan.

Cerebrovascular Disease in Infancy and Childhood

Daniel C. Shannon, M.D.

Professor of Pediatrics, Harvard Medical School. Professor of Health Science Harvard/M.I.T. School of Health Science and Technology. Pediatrician and Chief of Pediatric Pulmonary Unit, Massachusetts General Hospital, Boston, Massachusetts.

Sudden Infant Death Syndrome and Apparent Life-Threatening Events

Michael Shannon, M.D., M.P.H.

Assistant Professor of Pediatrics, Harvard Medical School. Adjunct Associate Professor, Massachusetts College of Pharmacy and Allied Health Sciences. Associate in Medicine, Children's Hospital, Boston, Massachusetts.

Acute Poisonings

Bruce K. Shapiro, M.D.

Associate Professor of Pediatrics, The Johns Hopkins University School of Medicine. Director, Center for Learning and Its Disorders, Kennedy-Krieger Institute, Baltimore, Maryland.

Mental Retardation

Eugene D. Shapiro, M.D.

Associate Professor of Pediatrics and of Epidemiology, Yale University School of Medicine. Attending Physician, Yale-New Haven Hospital, New Haven, Connecticut.

Lyme Disease; Infections Caused by* Haemophilus influenzae *Type B

Gail G. Shapiro, M.D.

Clinical Professor of Pediatrics, University of Washington School of Medicine. Attending Physician, Children's Hospital and Medical Center, Seattle, Washington.

Allergic Rhinitis in Children

Stephen R. Shapiro, M.D.

Assistant Clinical Professor, University of California, Davis, School of Medicine. Senior Staff Physician, Mercy General Hospital and Sutter Community Hospitals. Courtesy Staff Physician, Mercy American River Hospital, Methodist Hospital, Roseville Community Hospital, and Sutter Davis Hospital, Sacramento, California.

Perinephric and Intranephric Abscess

Joseph R. Sherbotie, M.D.

Assistant Professor of Pediatrics, University of Pennsylvania School of Medicine. Pediatric Nephrologist, The Children's Hospital of Philadelphia, Philadelphia, Pennsylvania.

Hemolytic-Uremic Syndrome

Dennis W. Shermeta, M.D.

Attending Surgeon, Phoenix Children's Medical Center and St. Joseph's Hospital, Phoenix, Arizona.

Peritonitis

Vivian E. Shih, M.D.

Associate Professor of Neurology, Harvard Medical School. Pediatrician and Associate Neurologist, Massachusetts General Hospital, Boston, Massachusetts.

Amino Acid Disorders

Benjamin L. Shneider, M.D.

Instructor in Pediatrics, Division of Pediatric Gastroenterology/Hepatology Yale University, New Haven, Connecticut.

Chronic Active Hepatitis

Irwin M. Siegel, M.D.

Associate Professor, Departments of Orthopaedic Surgery and Neurological Sciences, Rush-Presbyterian-St. Luke's Medical Center. Attending Orthopedic Surgeon, Louis A. Weiss Memorial Hospital. Assistant Attending Surgeon, Orthopaedics and Department of Neurological Sciences, Presbyterian-St. Luke's Hospital, Chicago, Illinois.

Muscular Dystrophy and Related Myopathies

Jane D. Siegel, M.D.

Associate Professor of Pediatrics, Division of Infectious Disease, University of Texas Southwestern Medical School at Dallas, Texas.

Neonatal Septicemia, Meningitis, and Pneumonia

Garey S. Simmonds, M.D.

Resident, Phoenix Integrated Surgical Residency Program, Phoenix, Arizona.

Peritonitis

Samuel D. Smith, M.D.

Associate Professor of Surgery and Pediatrics, University of Arkansas for Medical Sciences. Chief of Pediatric Surgery, Arkansas Children's Hospital, Little Rock, Arkansas.

Disorders of the Umbilicus

Thomas F. Smith, M.D.

Associate Professor of Pediatrics and Assistant Professor of Medicine and Microbiology and Immunology, Emory University School of Medicine. Chief of Pediatric Allergy and Immunology, Egleston Children's Hospital at Emory and Grady Memorial Hospital. Consulting Staff, Emory University Hospital and Scottish Rite Children's Hospital, Atlanta, Georgia.

Asthma

O. Carter Snead III, M.D.

Professor and Vice Chairman, Neurology; Professor of Pediatrics, University of Southern California School of Medicine. Head, Division of Neurology, Children's Hospital, Los Angeles, California.

Infantile Spasms

Edna H. Sobel, M.D.

Professor of Pediatrics, Emerita, Albert Einstein College of Medicine, Bronx, New York.

Ambiguous Genitalia

Noel W. Solomons, M.D.

Professor, Postgraduate Program in Ophthalmology, "Francisco Marroquín" Medical School. Scientific Director, Center for Studies of Sensory Impairment, Aging and Metabolism (CeSSIAM), Guatemala City, Guatemala.

Undernutrition

William T. Speck, M.D.

Professor of Clinical Pediatrics, College of Physicians and Surgeons, Columbia University. Executive Vice President and Chief Medical Officer, The Presbyterian Hospital in the City of New York at the Columbia–Presbyterian Medical Center, New York, New York.

Leptospirosis

Mary K. Spraker, M.D.

Associate Professor of Dermatology and Pediatrics, Emory University. Attending Physician, The Emory Clinic and Egleston Hospital for Children, Atlanta, Georgia.

Other Skin Tumors

Sergio Stagno, M.D.

Professor and Chairman, Department of Pediatrics, University of Alabama at Birmingham. Physician-in-Chief, The Children's Hospital of Alabama, Birmingham, Alabama.

Cytomegalovirus Infection

Virginia A. Stallings, M.D.

Assistant Professor, University of Pennsylvania School of Medicine. Director, Nutrition Support Service, Division of Gastroenterology and Nutrition, Children's Hospital of Philadelphia, Philadelphia, Pennsylvania.

Nutrition for Normal Infants, Children, and Adolescents

F. Bruder Stapleton, M.D.

A. Conger Goodyear Professor and Chairman, Department of Pediatrics, State University of New York at Buffalo. Pediatrician-in-Chief, Children's Hospital of Buffalo, Buffalo, New York.

Urolithiasis

Thomas E. Starzl, M.D., Ph.D.

Professor of Surgery, Department of Surgery, University of Pittsburgh School of Medicine. Director, Pittsburgh Transplantation Institute, Attending Physician, Presbyterian University Hospital and Children's Hospital of Pittsburgh, Pittsburgh, Pennsylvania.

Tumors of the Liver

Barbara W. Stechenberg, M.D.

Associate Professor of Pediatrics, Tufts University School of Medicine, Boston, Massachusetts. Director, Pediatric Infectious Disease, Baystate Medical Center, Springfield, Massachusetts.

Diphtheria.

James A. Stockman III, M.D.

President, American Board of Pediatrics, Chapel Hill, North Carolina.

Anemia of Iron Deficiency

Dennis C. Stokes, M.D.

Associate Professor of Pediatrics, Vanderbilt University School of Medicine. Clinical Director, Pediatric Pulmonary Medicine, Children's Hospital of Vanderbilt, Nashville, Tennessee.

Emphysema

Sylvan E. Stool, M.D.

Professor Otolaryngology and Pediatrics, University of Pittsburgh School of Medicine. Director Education Department

of Pediatric Otolaryngology, Children's Hospital of Pittsburgh, Pittsburgh, Pennsylvania.
Foreign Bodies in the Nose and Pharynx

D. Eugene Strandness, Jr., M.D.
Professor of Surgery, University of Washington School of Medicine. Chief, Division of Vascular Surgery, University of Washington Medical Center, Seattle, Washington.
Peripheral Vascular Disease

Richard H. Strauss, M.D.
Assistant Clinical Professor of Pediatrics, University of Wisconsin Medical School, Madison. Co-Director, Pediatric Intensive Care Unit, Gundersen Clinic/Lutheran Hospital, La Crosse, Wisconsin.
Head Injury

Douglas R. Strother, M.D.
Assistant Professor of Pediatrics, Medical College of Wisconsin, Milwaukee, Wisconsin.
Neuroblastoma

Terrence L. Stull, M.D.
Acting Chairman, Department of Pediatrics and Professor, Departments of Pediatrics and Microbiology/Immunology, The Medical College of Pennsylvania. Chief, Pediatric Infectious Diseases, Medical College Hospitals, Philadelphia, Pennsylvania.
Influenza

Dennis M. Styne, M.D.
Professor and Chair, Department of Pediatrics, School of Medicine, University of California, Davis. Chair of Pediatrics, University of California, Davis Medical Center, Sacramento, California.
Hypopituitarism and Growth Hormone Therapy

Frederick J. Suchy, M.D.
Professor of Pediatrics, Yale Medical School. Chief, Pediatric Gastroenterology/Hepatology, Yale–New Haven Hospital, New Haven, Connecticut.
Chronic Active Hepatitis

Ciro V. Sumaya, M.D., M.P.H. & T.M.
Professor of Pediatrics and Pathology and Associate Medical Dean, The University of Texas Medical School. Staff Physician, Bexar County Hospital District, and Santa Rosa Children's Hospital, San Antonio, Texas.
Infectious Mononucleosis and Epstein-Barr Virus Related Syndromes

Robert P. Sundel, M.D.
Instructor in Pediatrics, Harvard Medical School. Director of Rheumatology, Children's Hospital, Boston, Massachusetts.
Kawasaki Syndrome

Robert M. Suskind, M.D.
Professor and Chairman, Department of Pediatrics, Louisiana State University. Staff, Children's Hospital of New Orleans and Medical Center of Louisiana, New Orleans, Louisiana.
Magnesium Deficiency; Zinc Deficiency

Michael D. Sussman, M.D.
Professor of Surgery, Oregon Health Science University. Chief of Staff, Shriners Hospital, Portland, Oregon.
Disorders of the Spine and Shoulder Girdle

Ilona S. Szer, M.D.
Associate Professor of Pediatrics, University of Southern California School of Medicine. Associate Head, Pediatric Rheumatology, Children's Hospital of Los Angeles, Los Angeles, California.
Juvenile Rheumatoid Arthritis

H. William Taeusch, M.D.
Professor of Pediatrics, Charles R. Drew University and University of California at Los Angeles. Director, Division of Neonatology, Department of Pediatrics, King/Drew Medical Center, Los Angeles, California.
Management of the Infant in the Delivery Room

Lawrence T. Taft, M.D.
Professor of Pediatrics, University of Medicine and Dentistry of New Jersey–Robert Wood Johnson Medical School. Attending Staff, Robert Wood Johnson University Hospital, and St. Peter's Medical Center, New Brunswick, New Jersey.
Cerebral Palsy

George Thabit III, M.D.
Fellow in Sports Medicine, Children's Hospital, Boston, Massachusetts.
Orthopedic Disorders of the Extremities

James K. Todd, M.D.
Professor of Pediatrics and Microbiology/Immunology, University of Colorado Health Sciences Center. Director, Epidemiology and Clinical Microbiology, The Children's Hospital, Denver, Colorado.
Staphylococcal Infections

Debra A. Tristram, M.D.
Research Assistant Professor of Pediatrics, State University of New York at Buffalo School of Medicine. Assistant Attending Physician, Children's Hospital of Buffalo, Buffalo, New York.
Bronchitis and Bronchiolitis

Walter W. Tunnessen, Jr., M.D.
Professor of Pediatrics, University of Pennsylvania School of Medicine. Associate Chairman for Medical Education, The Children's Hospital of Philadelphia, Philadelphia, Pennsylvania.
Chronic Nonhereditary Vesiculobullous Disorders of Childhood

Mark W. Uhl, M.D.
Assistant Professor of Pediatrics, Division of Pediatric Critical Care, Medical College of Virginia. Physician, Medical College of Virginia Children's Medical Center, Richmond, Virginia.
Near-Drowning

Andrew H. Urbach, M.D.
Associate Professor of Pediatrics, University of Pittsburgh. Physician, University of Pittsburgh Health Science Center and Children's Hospital of Pittsburgh, Pittsburgh, Pennsylvania.
Pinworms

Pablo Vial, M.D.
Assistant Professor of Pediatrics and Head of Infectious Diseases, Centro de Investigaciones Medicas Escuela de Medicina, Pontificia Universidad Catolica de Chile, Santiago, Chile.
Typhoid Fever

Nancy E. Vinton, M.D.
Assistant Professor of Pediatrics, Thomas Jefferson University, Jefferson Medical College, Philadelphia, Pennsylvania. Chief, Nutrition Support Services, Division of Pediatric

Gastroenterology, A.I. duPont Institute, Wilmington, Delaware.

***Malformations of the Intestine;* Clostridium difficile**

Ellen R. Wald, M.D.

Professor of Pediatrics and Otolaryngology, University of Pittsburgh School of Medicine. Chief, Division of Pediatric and Infectious Disease, Children's Hospital of Pittsburgh, Pittsburgh, Pennsylvania.

Rhinitis and Sinusitis

W. Allan Walker, M.D.

Conrad Taff Professor of Pediatrics, Harvard Medical School. Chief, Combined Program in Pediatric Gastroenterology and Nutrition, Children's Hospital, Boston, Massachusetts.

Disorders of the Biliary Tree

Juan N. Walterspiel, M.D., F.A.A.P.

Assistant Director, Therapeutic Research I–Infectious Diseases, Hoffmann-La Roche, Inc., Nutley, New Jersey.

Giardiasis

Robert W. Warren, M.D., Ph.D.

Associate Professor of Pediatrics, Baylor College of Medicine. Chief, Rheumatology Service, Texas Children's Hospital, Houston, Texas.

Hemolytic Anemia

Jon F. Watchko, M.D.

Assistant Professor of Pediatrics, Obstetrics and Gynecology, University of Pittsburgh School of Medicine. Attending Physician, Magee-Womens Hospital, Pittsburgh, Pennsylvania.

Neonatal Pneumothorax and Pneumomediastinum; Neonatal Atelectasis

John B. Watkins, M.D.

Professor of Pediatrics, Washington University. Director of Ambulatory Medicine, St. Louis Children's Hospital, St. Louis, Missouri.

Malabsorptive Disorders

Hugh G. Watts, M.D.

Staff, Shriners Hospital, Los Angeles, California.

Bone and Joint Infections

Leonard B. Weiner, M.D.

Professor of Pediatrics and Pathology State University of New York Health Science Center at Syracuse, Department of Pediatrics. Director, Division of Infectious Disease, SUNY Health Science Center. Attending Pediatrician, University Hospital, Crouse Irving Memorial Hospital, and Community General Hospital. Consultant, St. Joseph's Hospital, Syracuse, New York.

Aseptic Meningitis

Louis M. Weiss, M.D., M.P.H.

Assistant Professor of Medicine, Division of Infectious Diseases, and Assistant Professor of Pathology, Division of Parasitology and Tropical Medicine, Albert Einstein College of Medicine. Attending Physician, Bronx Municipal Hospital and Jack D. Weiler Hospital of The Albert Einstein College of Medicine, Division of Montefiore Medical Center, Bronx, New York.

Cysticercosis

Marc Weissbluth, M.D.

Associate Professor of Pediatrics, Northwestern University Medical School. Active Attending Pediatrician, Children's Memorial Hospital, Chicago.

Colic

Robert C. Welliver, M.D.

Professor of Pediatrics, State University of New York at Buffalo School of Medicine. Attending Physician, Children's Hospital of Buffalo, Buffalo, New York.

Bronchitis and Bronchiolitis

Richard P. Wennberg, M.D.

Professor in Pediatrics, University of California, Davis, Medical School, Davis, California.

Hemolytic Diseases of the Neonate

Steven L. Werlin, M.D.

Professor of Pediatrics, Medical College of Wisconsin. Chief, Gastroenterology, Children's Hospital of Wisconsin, Milwaukee, Wisconsin.

Total Parenteral Nutrition in Infants; Foreign Bodies in the Gastrointestinal Tract

Bernhard L. Wiedermann, M.D.

Associate Professor of Pediatrics, George Washington University School of Medicine and Health Sciences. Attending Physician in Infectious Diseases and Director, Pediatric Residency Training Program, Children's National Medical Center, Washington, D.C.

Histoplasmosis

Eugene S. Wiener, M.D.

Professor of Pediatric Surgery, University of Pittsburgh School of Medicine. President, Medical Staff, Children's Hospital of Pittsburgh, Pittsburgh, Pennsylvania.

Neonatal Intestinal Obstruction

Murray Wittner, M.D., Ph.D.

Professor of Pathology and Parasitology, Department of Pathology, Division of Parasitology and Tropical Medicine, Albert Einstein College of Medicine. Attending Physician, Jack D. Weiler Hospital of the Albert Einstein College of Medicine, Division of Montefiore Medical Center, and Bronx Municipal Hospital Center, Bronx, New York.

Cysticercosis

Mary Ellen B. Wohl, M.D.

Professor of Pediatrics, Harvard Medical School. Chief, Division of Respiratory Diseases, Children's Hospital, Boston, Massachusetts.

Primary Pulmonary Hemosiderosis

Joseph I. Wolfsdorf, M.B., B.Ch.

Assistant Professor of Pediatrics, Harvard Medical School. Associate in Endocrinology, The Children's Hospital; Associate Physician, New England Deaconess Hospital; and Chief of Pediatrics, Joslin Diabetes Center, Boston, Massachusetts.

Gynecomastia

Francis S. Wright, M.D.

Professor of Pediatrics, Ohio State University College of Medicine; Chief, Division of Neurology, Columbus Children's Hospital, Columbus, Ohio.

Spinal Cord Diseases

Aida Yared, M.D.

Assistant Professor of Pediatrics, Vanderbilt University, Nashville, Tennessee.

Fluid and Electrolyte Therapy

Edward J. Young, M.D.

Professor of Medicine, and of Microbiology and Immunology, Baylor College of Medicine. Chief of Staff, Veterans Administration Medical Center, Houston, Texas.

Brucellosis

Harvey A. Zarem, M.D.

Professor Emeritus, University of California School of Medicine, Los Angeles, California. Staff Physician, Saint John's Hospital and Health Center, Santa Monica, California.

Diseases and Injuries of the Oral Region

Joseph T. Zerella, M.D.

Attending Surgeon, Phoenix Children's Medical Center and St. Joseph's Hospital, Phoenix, Arizona.

Peritonitis

Philip R. Ziring, M.D.

Associate Clinical Professor of Pediatrics, University of California, San Francisco. Chairman of Pediatrics, Pacific Campus, California Pacific Medical Center, San Francisco. Children's Hospital, Oakland, California.

Rubella and Congenital Rubella

Basil J. Zitelli, M.D.

Professor of Pediatrics, University of Pittsburgh School of Medicine. Attending Physician, Children's Hospital of Pittsburgh, Pittsburgh, Pennsylvania.

Lymph Node Infections

James R. Zuberbuhler, M.D.

Professor of Pediatrics, and Vice Chairman, Department of Pediatrics, University of Pittsburgh School of Medicine. Director, Pediatric Cardiology, Children's Hospital of Pittsburgh, Pittsburgh, Pennsylvania.

Cardiomyopathy and Heart Transplantation

Preface

The challenge for all of us who are given the privilege of providing health care to infants, children, and adolescents is to be certain that we are offering our patients and their families the most effective therapy available during a period of enormous growth in knowledge about health and disease. *Current Pediatric Therapy* was developed by two of the great practitioners and writers in the history of pediatrics, Sydney S. Gellis, M.D., and Benjamin M. Kagan, M.D. For 30 years, it has served an immeasurable number of health care workers by providing expert advice on high-quality therapeutic care for our world's most precious asset, our children. Their success in working with thousands of pediatric experts to put forth 13 editions of this book is a contribution that, when put into perspective, is probably one of the most important in the history of child care. It is an honor and an enormous responsibility to embrace the challenge of guiding the future direction of this text and to work with pediatricians everywhere to continue to spread the word on how best to help the children of the world. As these children encounter diseases and a multitude of other health problems, proper management will allow more and more of them to thrive, to move into adulthood, and to face the next century with a promising chance to help our civilization move forward.

During the planning of the 14th edition, it was our goal to identify experts from multiple disciplines concerning the problems of infants, children, and adolescents. As a result, the new text not only includes significant contributions from surgeons, psychiatrists, experts on nutrition, and specialists in child development but also reflects new developments in therapy that have grown from recent advances in molecular biology, bioengineering, and our understanding of the social sciences. Such advances are moving the field of child care forward at a remarkable pace, challenging us all to assimilate this new information, to integrate it into our practices, and to utilize it in the development of new approaches to child care. We hope that you will find the organization and content of this book useful in meeting your needs at the front line of child health care and in helping you to understand cutting-edge new developments in therapy.

We have adopted the philosophy of Drs. Gellis and Kagan in assuming that a correct diagnosis has been made, so that the information presented in this text relates primarily to management. At times we have included other background information, especially in articles in which we believed such detail would provide a sound scientific base for understanding the proper management of a particular condition. Contributors have been asked to describe which treatments have worked for them rather than present a review of therapies. As editors, we recognize that the *absolute truth* on how to treat certain conditions is not known, and thus approaches to some problems are described in various ways in different sections or articles. Clinical judgment is the cornerstone of a great practitioner's skill in enhancing outcomes, and the actual decisions made in planning the management of problems encountered lies in every pediatrician's hands. We hope that this book will be of help to you in making the best possible decisions.

There are two new features of this edition. The first is an accompanying pocket drug handbook that should provide on-the-spot guidance in using the multiple agents available for patient care. The second is the inclusion of a few selected references at the end of many articles. These are meant to provide you with an opportunity to explore in greater detail the foundation for the therapies recommended.

Finally, as our two predecessors have done at the end of their preface, we thank the many contributors to this volume who have taken time to write down and share with all of us their best ideas on how to care for our children.

FREDRIC D. BURG
JULIE R. INGELFINGER
ELLEN R. WALD

Contents

4 RESPIRATORY SYSTEM

5 CARDIOVASCULAR SYSTEM

6 DIGESTIVE TRACT

7 BLOOD

8 SPLEEN AND LYMPHATIC SYSTEM

9 ENDOCRINE SYSTEM

13 BONES AND JOINTS

14 MUSCLES

15 SKIN

16 THE EYE

17 THE EAR

18 INFECTIOUS DISEASES

22 SPECIAL PROBLEMS IN THE ADOLESCENT

1

Nutrition

NUTRITION FOR NORMAL INFANTS, CHILDREN, AND ADOLESCENTS

VIRGINIA A. STALLINGS, M.D.

Optimal nutrition and growth, so basic to the care of all children, are goals for both the family and the medical community. Combining science with sociocultural influences, however, results in a constantly evolving and occasionally divergent set of recommendations. It is likely that recommendations will continue to change, based less on the changes in food safety and the identification of essential nutrients and more on the presence or absence of childhood antecedents of adult diseases such as obesity, atherosclerosis, hypertension, and osteoporosis. This article presents current thoughts on the feeding of healthy infants, children, and adolescents.

INFANCY

Breast feeding is best for an infant, and its success depends on the active support of the new mother by her partner, family, physicians, and nurses. Most obstetric services and newborn nurseries are organized to encourage breast-feeding and provide breast-feeding counselors when problems arise. The immunologic, nutritional, and social advantages of breast milk from a well-nourished mother are established. The few contraindications for breast-feeding are related mostly to maternal health and may include maternal infection with tuberculosis, hepatitis B, human immunodeficiency virus (HIV), or other severe medical or psychiatric illness. Decisions to discourage or discontinue breast-feeding are made on an individual basis, depending on the severity of the maternal illness, its stage of treatment, and the risk to the infant. Drugs are secreted in human breast milk, usually in small amounts, and most are thought to present little risk for the infant. The mother's use of antimetabolites, radioactive drugs, iodides, ergot alkaloids, metronidazole, propylthiouracil, diazepam, chlorpromazine, lithium, chloramphenicol, or tetracycline necessitates temporary or complete discontinuation of breast-feeding. Infant conditions such as the metabolic disorders of galactosemia, phenylketonuria, and maple syrup urine disease, or the anatomic malformations of some types of cleft lip and palate are also contraindications.

The vitamin and mineral supplementation needs for breast-fed and formula-fed infants are described in Table 1. The practice of prescribing vitamins A, C, D, and E and iron for breast-fed infants prior to the introduction of solid food at 4 to 6 months is related more to the history of the use of cod liver oil and to the availability of commercial infant vitamin and mineral supplements than to actual need for nutrient supplementation above that provided by breast milk. Breast-fed infants who do not receive adequate sunlight require vitamin D supplementation. There is no need for supplements of vitamins A, C, and E or iron in healthy breast-fed infants. Malnourished lactating women should receive multiple vitamin and mineral supplementation as well as additional calories and protein to ensure the production of an adequate supply of nutritionally complete breast milk.

Commercial formulas or other alternatives are indicated for infants if mothers do not choose to or cannot breast-feed. Formulas are also used to supplement breast-feeding by choice or when milk production is inadequate in the lactating mother. Modern commercial infant formulas are manufactured from modified cow's milk to simulate the basic composition and digestibility characteristics of breast milk. The standard infant formulas are whey-predominant cow's milk protein, lactose carbohydrate, and a mixture of various fats (soy, corn, coconut, safflower oils).

Currently, 80 per cent of the commercial formula sold is cow milk–based and 20 per cent is made from soy protein. Methionine (an essential amino acid) supplemented soy protein–based formula is an alternative for infants with galactosemia, lactose intolerance, or a vegetarian family. Soy-based formulas are also used for potentially allergic infants, although there is a 10 to 20 per cent cross-reactivity with milk and soy protein. Semielemental protein hydrolysate infant formulas are more hypoallergenic and are indicated for infants with cow's milk protein allergy.

The less expensive, evaporated milk–based formula was commonly used until commercial formula became readily available and required additional supplementation with vitamin C (Table 1). Goat milk–based feedings are occasionally preferred by families and also require supplementation of vitamins D and C and folate. Whole cow's milk is not suitable for feeding of young infants (birth to 6 months) and generally is not recommended until after the child is 1 year of age.

Breast-feeding or formula-feeding as the sole source of nutrition is adequate for most infants until they are 4 to 6 months of age. An indicator of adequacy is normal growth and development, and weight gain should be carefully observed by the physician. Healthy infants usually establish an "on demand" system of feeding, and as long as weight gain is adequate, this system is recommended over a regimented number of feedings per day or specified hourly intervals for

TABLE 1. Considerations for Vitamin and Mineral Supplementation for Healthy Children

	Vitamins				Minerals		
	D	*C*	*B_{12}*	*Folate*	*Iron*	*Calcium*	*Fluoride**
Infants (birth to 6 months)							
Breast milk	+	−	−	−	−	−	±
Vegetarian breast milk	+	−	+	−	−	−	±
Commercial formula	−	−	−	−	−	−	±
Evaporated milk†	−	+	−	−	−	−	±
Goat's milk	+	+	−	+	+	−	±
Cow's milk†‡	−	+	−	−	+	−	±
Older Infants (6 to 12 months)	−	−	−	−	+§	−	±
Children							
Healthy	−	−	−	−	−	−	±
Lactose-intolerant	−	−	−	−	−	+‖	±
Vegetarian¶	±	−	±	−	+	±	±
Adolescents#							
Healthy	−	−	−	−	±	±	±
Lactose-intolerant	−	−	−	−	±	+‖	±
Vegetarian¶	±	−	±	−	+	±	±
Pregnant	−	−	−	+	+	+	±

*Depending on fluoride content of local water supply.
†Assuming vitamin D–fortified evaporated milk and whole cow's milk.
‡Inadequate in linolenic acid: may cause gastrointestinal blood loss.
§Usually supplied by infant cereal or iron-fortified commercial formula.
‖Calcium-containing dairy products are often omitted or limited with lactose intolerance.
¶Supplementation requirements depend on type of vegetarian diet (e.g., use of eggs, milk products) consumed.
#Adolescent diets are frequently inadequate in calcium and iron.
Key: +, supplementation needed; ±, supplementation may be needed; −, not needed.

feedings. The Recommended Dietary Allowances (RDA) for caloric intake for infants and children are presented in Table 2. Note that there are large ranges of caloric intake, reflecting the individual variation within the group of healthy children.

The introduction of solid foods should occur when the infant is developmentally prepared. This occurs as the infant develops head and trunk control, can be fed in a sitting position (in a high chair), and can take food from a spoon and transfer it to the back of the mouth to swallow. This requires the extinction of the extrusion or tongue-thrust reflex. These developmental events usually occur between 4 and 6 months. By this age, the infant can indicate an interest in food by opening the mouth and leaning forward and rejection of the food by turning away, thus allowing the child some control of food intake based on hunger and satiety.

TABLE 2. Recommended Dietary Allowances (RDA)* for Caloric Intake of Infants, Children, and Adolescents

			Caloric Allowance		
Category	Age (Years)	REE† (kcal/day)	*kcal/kg/day‡*	*kcal/day*	*Range*
Infants	0.0–0.5	320	108	kg × 108	(520–780)
	0.5–1.0	500	98	kg × 98	(680–1020)
Children	1–3	740	102	1300	(1040–1560)
	4–6	950	90	1800	(1440–2160)
	7–10	1130	70	2000	(1600–2400)
Males	11–14	1440	55	2500	(2000–3000)
	15–18	1760	45	3000	(2400–3600)
Females	11–14	1310	47	2200	(1760–2640)
	15–18	1370	40	2200	(1760–2640)

Adapted with permission from Recommended Dietary Allowances, 10th ed. Copyright 1989 by the National Academy of Sciences. Courtesy of the National Academy Press, Washington, DC.
*The RDAs for protein, vitamins, and minerals appear in the section "Vitamin deficiencies and excesses."
†Resting energy expenditure (REE) is similar to basal metabolic rate.
‡The calculation of kcal/kg/day in children ≥ 3 years of age is based on the average of a wide range of acceptable intakes. Appropriate rates of growth may occur at energy intake levels above and below this estimate.

The general rule for the introduction of solid foods is to offer one new single-ingredient food at a time and to serve the new food daily for 3 to 5 days to identify any adverse food reaction. The first recommended solid food is a single-grain product. Rice is usually chosen because it is the most hypoallergenic of the grains. Other cereals follow, leaving wheat to be added months later because it is a more common food allergen. Cereals, prepared with formula or breast milk, provide a source of dietary iron, now needed by the infant. Vegetables are introduced next, ensuring a new source of vitamins, particularly vitamin A. Fruits are introduced after most single-ingredient vegetables. Fruits or small amounts of fruit juices become the major source of vitamin C. Meats are the last major food group introduced, and mixed dinners of meats and vegetables are used later. Most families offer the 4- to 6-month old infant solids twice during the day. By the time children are about 10 to 14 months old, they are interested in being at the table with the family and move to a three-meal-a-day schedule. Water is rarely needed while the infant is being exclusively breast-fed or formula-fed, but it should be offered in small amounts as the child moves to ingest solid foods with an increased renal solute load. A serving of juice (3 ounces) each day meets the vitamin C requirement, and ingestion of excessive amounts of juice should be avoided. The caloric content of several types of infant foods is shown in Table 3. Foods that are hard to chew and easy to aspirate should be avoided until the child is older (3 to 4 years) and has the needed oromotor skills. These include hot dogs, peanuts, grapes, carrots, and round candies.

Thus, by ages 6 to 12 months of age, the infant partakes of a mixed diet of formula or breast milk, iron-fortified cereals, vegetables, fruits, and meats. The timing of the introduction of whole cow's milk is controversial. Few suggest its use before 6 months, and because of the possibility of associated gastroin-

TABLE 3. Caloric Content of Some Infant Foods

Type	Kilocalories per Serving (~3 Ounces)
Breast milk or formula	60 (20 kcal/ounce)
Infant cereal with formula	110
Infant cereal with water	50
Infant cereal in jars	55–70
Vegetables	25–70
Fruits and juices	40–80
Meats	90–135
Mostly meat dinners	75–105
Whole cow's milk	57 (19 kcal/ounce)
2% cow's milk	45 (15 kcal/ounce)
Skim cow's milk	30 (10 kcal/ounce)

testinal blood loss, many pediatricians suggest withholding cow's milk until after the first birthday.

CHILDHOOD AND ADOLESCENCE

By age 12 to 24 months, the child will be following a three-meal and two-snack-a-day pattern. The introduction of a wide variety of food flavors, textures, colors, and temperatures is important to establish acceptance of a broad range of foods. Families should be guided to avoid the use of food as reward or punishment and to ensure that mealtimes are as free from conflict as possible. Toddlers frequently have capricious appetites and food preferences, yet almost always continue to eat enough food to maintain normal growth even during the most stubborn phases of their newly found independence. During the childhood years, mealtime becomes more social and must incorporate the schedules of the family, school, and play settings.

Teenagers often develop new eating patterns, including fewer meals and more snacks, and some develop diets that are nutritionally inadequate, especially in iron, calcium, vitamin A, and vitamin E. There are increased nutritional requirements related to adolescent growth and pubertal development with increased needs for calories, nitrogen, calcium, and iron. Most teenagers eat more food during the period of growth, which in turn provides the needed nutrients. Iron deficiency anemia commonly develops in both boys and girls and calcium intake is low in those who decrease the intake of dairy products. Calcium and iron supplementation may be required, depending on the usual dietary patterns (see Table 1).

Parents and physicians have concerns over the lifelong health implications of childhood food practices and attitudes. The public health recommendations for children older than 2 years of age and adolescents are as follows:

1. Maintain normal body weight.
2. Limit dietary fat to 30 per cent of daily calories; distribute the fat calories to 10 per cent each from saturated, polyunsaturated, and monounsaturated fatty acids; and limit dietary cholesterol to 100 mg/1000 kcal.
3. Increase consumption of whole grain and cereal products and vegetables (complex carbohydrate and fiber).
4. Reduce intake of sodium by choosing lower-sodium foods and limiting salt in food preparation and at the table.
5. Reduce sugars, particularly for those who are prone to dental caries.
6. Use fluoride as a supplement when the local water supply does not contain optimal levels for the prevention of dental decay.

These recommendations are appropriate for most healthy children.

REFERENCES

Forbes GB, Woodruff CW: Pediatric Nutrition Handbook. Elk Grove, Ill, American Academy of Pediatrics, 1985.

UNDERNUTRITION

JESUS BULUX, M.D.
CARLOS GRAZIOSO, M.D.
SUSANA MOLINA, M.D.
and NOEL W. SOLOMONS, M.D.

DEFINITIONS

The body requires an adequate and balanced intake of foods to obtain the macronutrients (energy, protein, water) and micronutrients (vitamins, minerals) essential for growth, development, and maintenance of normal metabolic functions. In this article, we focus on *undernutrition.* Deficits in linear and ponderal growth and changes in underlying body composition are hallmark features. Sometimes the term "failure to thrive" is used, emphasizing the growth retardation aspects, whereas "protein-energy malnutrition" (PEM) is employed to recognize that clinical syndromes of kwashiorkor (edematous PEM), marasmus (inanition PEM), and a mixed form exist at the extremity of severity. Because the deficits do not have to reach clinical proportions and because deficiencies of vitamins and minerals coexist with protein and energy depletion, the most useful generic term is undernutrition.

Undernutrition is not synonymous with underfeeding. The latter is the etiologic mechanism for *primary* undernutrition caused by consumption of food below requirement levels. It can result from poverty, cultural practices using foods of low-nutrient density, iatrogeny, child abuse, psychogenic eating disorders, or anorexia of psychic or physical origin. Perhaps in both developing and industrialized nations alike, it is *secondary* undernutrition due to psychosocial problems or organic disease states that predominates. Any condition that reduces the absorption, increases the losses, or interferes with the utilization of nutrients will lead to secondary undernutrition. In affluent countries, congenital defects of anatomy or metabolism, prematurity, acquired immunodeficiency syndrome (AIDS), cystic fibrosis, inflammatory bowel diseases, celiac sprue, and malignancies and their chemotherapy are common contributors to undernutrition, as are psychosocial and family pathology. In poor countries and in underprivileged classes of wealthy nations, the aforementioned conditions are present but are overshadowed by contributions to secondary undernutrition, such as recurrent and persistent diarrheal episodes, intestinal parasitosis, respiratory infections, and viral infections (measles, hepatitis).

Whether undernutrition is primary or secondary, the approach to its evaluation is the same. We should endeavor to gauge cause(s), to quantify the degree of deficit, and to plan comprehensive therapy for recovery and prevention of a recurrence. The clinical evaluation begins with a history (including dietary intake pattern) and includes physical examination, formal anthropometry, and, in the presence of a clinical syndrome, basic laboratory tests: complete hematologic workup, serum protein levels, blood glucose levels, serum electrolyte levels, and urinalysis.

CLASSIFICATION

The anthropometric classification of undernutrition takes into account any deficits of height for that expected for chronologic age (height-for-age); an individual with a height below the 5th percentile of the reference standards of the National Center for Health Statistics (NCHS) is classified as "stunted." Lesser deficits are not unimportant, however, especially if the child has parents and siblings of tall stature. Height retardation or stunting is the *sine qua non* of *chronic* nutritional deficiency states. *Acute* undernutrition manifests as a deficit in body weight in relation to that expected for height (weight-for-height). A child with less than 80 per cent of the weight (50th percentile) associated with his or her actual height is classified as "wasted."

The clinical syndromes of undernutrition can occur in tall, medium, and short individuals and have been classified by McLaren as marasmus, kwashiorkor, and a mixed form, marasmic kwashiorkor. The differential descriptions are found in Table 1.

TREATMENT

The phases of treatment of severe *clinical* protein-energy undernutrition can be divided into three sequential phases: (1) emergent resuscitation and rescue, (2) initiation of nutritional recovery, and (3) consolidation of nutritional recovery and prevention of recurrence.

Emergent Resuscitation and Rescue

In this phase, the fundamental objective is to save the life of the child, as the majority of hospital deaths from clinical undernutrition occurs in the first week of treatment. One treats the acute illness(es) that motivated the hospital admission, such as infection, hepatic failure, fluid electrolyte imbalance, and any underlying conditioning pathology, e.g., blastic leukemic crisis, cystic fibrosis pneumonia, or cardiac failure.

Fluid and electrolyte disorders, usually due to acute diarrheal diatheses, are frequent and can be difficult to detect in the presence of edema. In the edematous state, signs of dryness and skin turgor are invalid; still valid, however, are the signs of decreased urinary output, thirst, tachycardia, hypotension, and altered sensorium. Intravenous therapy should be reserved for cases of vascular collapse (impending shock and shock). In milder forms, oral and nasogastric routes are preferred. The World Health Organization (WHO) formulation of oral rehydration salts is safe in marasmus, but with edematous undernutrition, solutions with lower sodium content are preferable. Strict monitoring of volumes administered is vital. Parenteral albumin administration is not recommended. In the edematous state, serum sodium levels from 120 to 135 mEq/L are "normal" and higher concentrations suggest sodium overload or a free water deficit. Acidosis usually corrects with volume expansion and renal regulation. Only in extreme acidosis should exogenous bicarbonate be administered because it carries a risk of sodium overload. Both potassium and magnesium deficiencies can occur as additional electrolyte disturbances. Potassium (6 to 8 mEq/L) should be provided daily once urinary flow is adequate. A single intravenous injection of 50 per cent magnesium sulfate solution is indicated to prevent tetany, depending on weight: 0.5 ml (<7 kg); 1 ml (7 to 10 kg); and 1.5 ml (>10 kg).

Infections are a major concern in a nutritionally compromised host. Often an infection (e.g., urinary tract infection, otitis, sepsis, or bronchopneumonia) was the precipitating event leading to admission. Nosocomial infections of the same classes represent a risk during hospitalization. *The important caveat is that the undernourished state may mask the signs and symptoms of infections, and vigilance regarding infection in the acute stages of admission must be very high.* Thoracic radiographs should be taken routinely, and blood and urinary cultures are in order.

Because of hypothermia, fevers may not manifest. Skin ulcers and exanthems, jaundice and elevated transaminases, hypoglycemia, hypothermia, severe anemia, severe hypoproteinemia, leukopenia or leukocytosis with a shift to the left, and altered states of consciousness are adverse prognostic signs both for the presence of or risk of overwhelming sepsis.

Severe anemia (hemoglobin levels below 5 g/dl) presents a therapeutic dilemma. Oxygen transport capacity is severely compromised, and high-output cardiac failure can occur. However, the security of the blood supply from human immunodeficiency virus (HIV) and hepatitis B contamination, especially in developing countries, cautions increased reluctance for transfusion therapy. When anemia is life-threatening, minimal amounts of packed red blood cells to provide oxygen delivery should be used.

Glycemia should be monitored in severe, clinical undernutrition, and the levels should be kept above 60 mg/dl with oral or tube feedings of formula or with bolus intravenous glucose. To prevent and combat hypothermia, both the provision of energy sources (fats and/or carbohydrates) and maintenance of the children in a 30° to 33°C environment are recommended.

TABLE 1. Clinical Features of the Classic Protein-Energy Undernutrition Syndromes

Marasmus is a chronic deficiency of protein and energy (along with other micronutrients), characterized by severe deficiency in weight-for-height with losses of both muscle and subcutaneous fat, as assessed by arm circumference and skinfold measurements. The chronicity of its onset allows for adaptation mechanisms, and serum and protein and red blood cell volumes are usually well maintained.

Kwashiorkor is a syndrome of acute onset, in which a diet of low-protein density, with scarce, adequate or excessive energy, often precipitated by an acute infection, leads to an edematous undernutrition condition. The metabolic processes are dysadapted; serum proteins are low and red blood cell turnover is slowed. The hallmark features are hypoalbuminemia and generalized edema along with a scaling skin rash, discolored and easily pluckable hair, organomegaly, diarrhea, apathy, and anorexia.

Marasmic kwashiorkor is a mixed undernutrition condition with features of both classic syndromes, i.e., edema and hypoalbuminemia on a background of extreme tissue wasting.

Initiation of Nutritional Recovery

The introduction of food to the severely malnourished child should be gradual and progressive, but because of the deficits that have been accumulated and the amount of catch-up growth to be accomplished, the diet should eventually reach hypercaloric levels with additional protein, above usual requirements. On the first two days or during the time that major complications are controlled, a diet of 70 kcal/kg/day and 0.7 to 1.0 g/kg of high-quality protein is advised. Subsequently, with 3-day increments, the dietary energy should rise to 100, 150, 200, and, in the case of marasmus, 250 kcal/kg/day. Proteins of high biologic quality (see below) should constitute 12 per cent of total energy intake. If the child takes in less than 75 per cent of the calculated amounts, early introduction of nasogastric feeding is indicated, taking all of the nursing precautions to avoid aspiration complications. If nasogastric volumes cannot be maintained, peripheral intravenous nutrition can be used to complement the enteral intake. Only when anatomic or physiologic barriers to enteral feeding are present should *total* parenteral nutrition be used. After 3 days of tube feeding, appetite should drive adequate intakes. Keeping the child in the antireflux position to prevent vomiting may improve tolerance of energy-dense diets.

Diets can be composed of the numerous commercial diet formulas or from whole or skim milk powder. Additional energy comes from vegetable oil, medium-chain triglycerides, and a source of soluble carbohydrates (sucrose, dextrins). Most children can tolerate the low amounts of lactose that accompany milk protein; during the acute phase, however, hydrolysis of lactose with commercial beta-galactosidase liquid drops reduces stool volumes and promotes loss of edema. In children older than 2 years of age, a mixture of liquid formulas and high-density solid foods can be employed.

A single, high dose of vitamin A at the onset is advisable in areas endemic for hypovitaminosis A. It is advisable to accompany the refeeding phase with a selective vitamin mix, containing two to four times the recommended levels of vitamin C, B vitamins, and the fat-soluble vitamins. From the 8th day of recovery, iron can be given as ferrous sulfate, 50 mg daily on a spoon. Zinc (2 mg/kg/day) and copper (2 mg/day) are recommended to enhance the use of macronutrients for growth and for support of immune function. Because skeletal growth accompanies somatic growth in rapid catch-up weight gain, generous amounts of calcium are required, with supplemental forms, if milk is not the basic protein source for the recovery diet.

The response to a nutritional and supportive treatment plan should be monitored continually by a multidisciplinary team. The weight-gain targets should be a minimum of 4 g/kg/day in marasmatic patients. In children with kwashiorkor or marasmic kwashiorkor, there is an initial loss of edema weight through diuresis up to 2 weeks into treatment. Thereafter, a catch-up weight-gain approximating or surpassing that for marasmatic children should be observed. In edematous forms of malnutrition, serum albumin levels should be monitored serially at weekly intervals and should be rising to normal levels progressively. Signs of favorable evolution and recovery include a progressive increase in appetite and spontaneous intake; increased alertness, curiosity, and activity; and smiling. It is not unusual for the child to experience five to ten liquid stools daily in the first week of therapy for edematous undernutrition; this rate of stooling decreases with therapy.

Common generic causes for failure or delay in the emergent and recovery phases of the hospital treatment of clinically malnourished children may be (1) excessively aggressive early diet therapy, (2) low ambient temperature, (3) unnecessary and imprudent use of transfusions of blood products, (4) repeated fasting for tests and lack of adequate supervision of feedings, (5) lactose intolerance, and (6) transmission of nosocomial infections.

When the recovery parameters are not being met as expected, one should rule out the presence of impediments such as hypothermia, oral lesions, cardiac dysfunction, malabsorption, occult infections, neurologic problems, low intakes or losses of potassium and phosphorus, and lack of loving and affective or emotional support on the part of staff or relatives.

Consolidation of Nutritional Recovery and Prevention of Recurrence

Disappearance of edema and an increase in serum albumin levels to >3 g/dl in kwashiorkor, combined with a weight-for-height of at least 80 per cent in the absence of edema are criteria for hospital discharge. Marasmatic children can be discharged when a similar weight adequacy is achieved. Thereafter, the first 2 to 4 months represent the consolidation of nutritional recovery on an outpatient basis. The dietary guidelines are to provide 150 to 200 kcal/kg and 3 to 4 g/kg of protein based on foods available in the home. If the malnutrition was secondary, medical, psychologic, or social worker attention to the precipitating causes should be continued. Persistence of underlying pathology, recurrent infections, and failure to obtain compliance for improved dietary practices are common reasons for recurrences of clinical malnutrition.

OBESITY

WILLIAM H. DIETZ, M.D., Ph.D.

Obesity is one of the most prevalent forms of malnutrition in children and adolescents in the United States. Obesity is usually obvious. The magnitude of weight excess can generally be estimated by a plot of weight and height on growth charts. In general, weight follows the height percentile. *A weight in excess of 120 per cent of the expected weight for height is generally considered overweight.* Nonetheless, a significant proportion of children who are overweight are not overfat. In these children, measurement of the triceps skinfold thickness will clarify whether the excess weight is fat or fat-free mass. The distinction between overweight and overfatness is crucial because weight loss is difficult and potentially hazardous in children who are overweight but not overfat.

The risk of persistent obesity, and therefore the necessity for weight reduction, is affected by severity and age of onset. At any age, severe obesity has a greater likelihood of persistence. Rates of remission are greatest for young children and decline with age.

HISTORY AND GENERAL APPROACH

The medical approach should be directed by the social history. Because obesity often affects other family members or requires that family practices with respect to food purchasing and consumption be modified, a family interview is essential. To establish the degree of involvement, it is often helpful to ask all members of the family how concerned they are about the overweight child's weight. Families with a low level of concern are unlikely to become more active in management if the child's weight is addressed by the practitioner in a perfunctory fashion. Likewise, if a significant discrepancy exists between the level of concern expressed by the parents, it is *not* likely that recommendations for therapy will be successfully implemented. Obesity in young children may reflect inappropriate limit setting. In families in which adolescents are less concerned about their weight than their parents, the choice of when and how to attend to the problem belongs to the adolescent. Adolescents are generally not motivated to lose weight by an emphasis on the health consequences of obesity, but they may be responsive to a focus on the social consequences, such as discrimination or the difficulty in finding clothes that fit.

A dietary history cannot be used to determine caloric intake accurately but will clarify the pattern of eating and identify high-caloric-density foods that can be reduced or eliminated. Some children who report an unremarkable food intake may consume excessive quantities of milk or juice. A history of inactivity may identify children for whom a reduction in television viewing time is essential in order to increase participation in other endeavors.

Most of the syndromes associated with obesity are readily diagnosed by a careful history and physical examination. Signs of congenital syndromes occur in recognizable clusters. Prader-Labhart-Willi syndrome is associated with a characteristic facies, short stature, small hands and feet, central fat deposition, hypogonadism, and mild to moderate mental retardation. Bardet-Biedl syndrome is associated with retinal dyspigmentation and degeneration, syndactyly or polydactyly, and renal disease. Endocrine diseases such as growth hormone deficiency, hypothyroidism, or Cushing's disease are associated with short stature, whereas obese children tend to be taller than their non-obese peers.

As in the evaluation of failure to thrive, laboratory tests and radiologic examinations are rarely helpful unless specifically suggested by the history and physical examination. Recurrent headaches of increasing severity or duration should prompt a careful funduscopic examination to exclude causes of increased intracranial pressure, such as pseudotumor cerebri or hypothalamic tumor. Shortness of breath with exercise indicates a functional limitation consequent to the disease. Daytime somnolence suggests the possibility of sleep apnea. In children or adolescents with sleep apnea, a tonsillectomy may be curative. However, such children present a high postoperative risk because postoperative edema may occlude the airway. Therefore, if a tonsillectomy is performed, obese children should be observed in an intensive care unit postoperatively for at least 24 to 48 hours. Abdominal pain may indicate gastroesophageal reflux. Abdominal pain in association with the use of commercial, fat-free, low-caloric diets raises the possibility of cholelithiasis. Frequent urination or nocturia suggests the rare possibility of non–insulin-dependent diabetes mellitus, particularly in the presence of a strong family history. Hip pain may reflect imminent slipped capital femoral epiphysis. Sprains may heal poorly in the presence of the increased stress of weight bearing associated with obesity.

PHYSICAL EXAMINATION

The physical examination should focus on the identification of signs that represent causes or complications of obesity. The plot of height and weight on a growth chart reveals the severity of obesity. By extrapolation of weight to the same percentile as height, the duration of weight maintenance required to achieve ideal body weight can be established. Short stature should prompt a careful search for other signs of an underlying endocrine abnormality.

As noted earlier, measurement of the triceps skinfold establishes whether excess weight is attributable to fat or fat-free mass. A triceps skinfold that is within the normal range or only slightly elevated suggests that the majority of the excess weight is fat-free mass rather than fat. Blood pressure should be taken with a cuff that covers two thirds of the arm and with a bladder that is large enough to envelop the arm. A thigh cuff may be necessary for an accurate determination of blood pressure in massively obese older children or adolescents.

Increased pigmentation of the skin of the neck or axilla may result from friction to the skin or acanthosis nigricans. Acanthosis nigricans often indicates glucose intolerance. A funduscopic examination is essential to exclude papilledema. An abdominal examination may reveal right upper quadrant tenderness associated with cholelithiasis. Slipped capital femoral epiphysis is associated with a limp and reduced internal and external rotation of the leg at the hip. Bowing may indicate Blount's disease. Radiologic confirmation is required for diagnosis of both Blount's disease and slipped capital femoral epiphysis.

THERAPY

The goals of therapy depend on the age of the child and on the severity of the problem. Because weight loss and the maintenance of weight loss are equally important, permanent behavioral changes should be sought. Therefore, slow, sustained weight changes are preferable to rapid losses followed by weight regain. For young children with mild weight excesses, weight maintenance may be a reasonable goal. For older children, even those with severe problems, sustained weight losses of 1 to 2 pounds per month, combined with the lack of the anticipated 5- to 10-pound annual weight gain, will achieve a weight change of 20 pounds per year.

The most effective therapy involves a reduction in caloric intake, increased activity, family participation, and behavior modification. In most cases, dietary restriction will achieve a caloric deficit more rapidly than increased activity. Because no accurate clinical method exists for establishing caloric intake, alterations in dietary intake should focus on reduction of dietary fat or elimination of high-caloric-density foods that supply large quantities of calories. Until further studies of the safety of restrictive diets in children and adolescents have been performed, very-low-calorie diets should be reserved for patients for whom rapid weight reduction is essential. When these diets are used, their effects on serum electrolyte levels, hepatic function, and cardiac function must be monitored carefully.

Although increased activity plays a limited role in the genesis of a caloric deficit, alterations in activity may be essential to sustain weight losses. Television viewing constitutes the principal source of inactivity among children and adolescents in the United States. Therefore, reductions in television time may be the most effective approach to increase activity. Few data support the hypothesis that increases in activity maintain fat-free mass or metabolic rate during weight reduction.

Parental involvement and successful behavior modification appear to exert independent effects on weight reduction in children. As indicated above, changes in food purchasing, preparation, and storage can be effected only by parental participation. Severely dysfunctional families may require family therapy to address other needs prior to weight reduction. The major components of behavior modification include contracting to reinforce adherence to recommendations regarding behavior change or weight loss, self-monitoring of intake or activity, praise for changes in eating or exercise behavior, and contingency management. These approaches are most effective in the hands of a behaviorally trained psychologist. Weight losses sustained for 10 years have been observed among children and their parents treated in separate groups with these approaches. Whether these techniques can be adapted to office practice or whether success rates in families will match those in patients and their parents treated in groups remains to be determined.

Commercial approaches rarely incorporate all of the elements necessary to achieve and maintain weight loss. Furthermore, the very-low-calorie diets that many commercial programs employ have not been carefully evaluated in children and adolescents and may cause complications that are worse than persistent obesity.

REFERENCES

Dietz WH: Obesity. J Am Coll Nutr 8(Suppl):135–215, 1989.
Dietz WH: You are what you eat—what you eat is what you are. J Adolesc Health Care 11:76–81, 1990.
Gortmaker SL, Dietz WH Jr, Cheung LW: Inactivity, diet and the fattening of America. J Am Diet Assoc 90:1247–1252, 1990.

VITAMIN DEFICIENCIES AND EXCESSES

MARGARET L. BOGLE, Ph.D., R.D.

Determining adequate levels of intake of vitamins for infants, children, and adolescents is difficult because specific requirements are not known and levels producing toxic effects vary considerably with individual physiologic responses. The best measure available is the text *Recommended Dietary Allowances* (see References). The Recommended Daily Allowances (RDAs) are defined as "the levels of intake of essential nutrients that, on the basis of scientific knowledge, are judged by the Food and Nutrition Board to be adequate to meet the nutrient needs of practically all healthy persons." On the basis of the most current scientific data, the RDAs are considered safe levels of nutrients for maintaining good health and for evaluating the adequacy of food intakes of groups of people. They are not intended to present adequacy for specific individuals or for sick individuals. To use the RDAs to evaluate individual children, the average of several (at least three) days of food intake should be reviewed and compared. This allows an estimate of suggested risk of deficiencies to be made.

The RDAs for infants are based on averages of nutrients consumed by healthy, growing infants breast-fed by healthy mothers. Consumption of 750 ml of breast milk per day for the first 6 months and 600 ml per day for the second 6 months is considered minimal for the RDAs. This suggests that infants consuming less than these amounts could be at risk for vitamin deficiencies even if they consume vitamin-fortified commercial formulas.

Deficiencies of vitamins occur when (1) intakes are inadequate, (2) physiologic requirements are high, (3) losses are excessive, or (4) nutrient-nutrient or drug-nutrient imbalances reduce efficacy. Although vitamin deficiency diseases are rarely seen today, pediatric health care professionals must be aware of those individuals at risk and must be able to recognize symptoms of specific vitamin deficiency. Particularly suspect are infants and children with chronic diseases, digestive or absorptive defects, narrow food choices, and acute illnesses necessitating medications.

Excessive intakes or those producing toxic effects must also be recognized, especially since some vitamin compounds are currently used for therapeutic or treatment purposes, not just to maintain good health. In such instances, the compounds are considered to be drugs or medicines rather than vitamins.

The safe level of some vitamins is quite narrow. In other words, there may be very little difference in amounts necessary to prevent deficiencies and to produce toxic effects. The amounts required to produce toxic effects may vary considerably in individual children of differing age groups, body sizes, and body compositions (amount of fat versus lean body mass).

WATER-SOLUBLE VITAMINS

Included in the list or classification of water-soluble vitamins are the B-complex vitamins—thiamine (B_1), riboflavin (B_2), niacin, pyridoxine (B_6), folates (folic acid and folacin), cyanocobalamin (B_{12}), biotin, and pantothenic acid—and ascorbic acid (vitamin C). The vitamins of the B complex generally function as coenzymes in metabolic processes. Vitamin C functions as an antioxidant as well as a cofactor in several enzymatic processes.

Water-soluble vitamins must be consumed daily because there is limited storage in the body and amounts not used in metabolic processes will be excreted in the urine. Only vitamin B_{12} is retained in the body for long periods of time. Careful diet histories that evaluate food consumed over time are useful in pinpointing individuals at risk for deficiency before blood levels drop or deficiency disease symptoms are evident.

Deficiencies of water-soluble vitamins are rarely seen in infants and children consuming adequate calories from a variety of foods.

Vitamin B_{12}

Infants and young children in families practicing total vegetarianism appear to be at risk for vitamin B_{12} deficiency, although no cases of deficiency symptoms have been documented. On the other hand, infants breast-feeding from vegetarian mothers with low levels of vitamin B_{12} have been shown to have low serum levels and some symptoms of deficiency, i.e., macrocytic, megaloblastic anemia. Other symptoms of vitamin B_{12} deficiency are skin hypersensitivity, glossitis, and neurologic signs due to demyelination of the brain and the optic and peripheral nerves. Cases of vitamin B_{12} deficiency are rare, with most being the result of poor absorption.

No toxic effects of excessive amounts of vitamin B_{12} have been reported. In addition, no benefits have been documented in giving nondeficient children large doses.

Vitamin B_1

Prolonged deficiency of thiamine results in beriberi, a disease characterized by mental confusion, muscle weakness, anorexia, peripheral paralysis, muscle wasting, tachycardia, and enlarged heart. The occurrence of beriberi in the United States is extremely rare, since thiamine is widespread in whole grains and cereals and refined cereals are fortified with thiamine.

There are no documented cases of toxicity of thiamine ingested orally. However, there have been reports of sensitivity or toxicity from large amounts given in parenteral solutions.

Pharmacologic doses of thiamine have been used in the treatment of some inborn errors of metabolism (e.g., maple syrup urine disease and thiamine-responsive lactic acidosis).

Vitamin B_2

No specific deficiency disease is attributed to a lack of riboflavin, although symptoms are sometimes referred to as ariboflavinosis. Clinical symptoms of deficiency have been described as angular stomatitis, cheilosis, a normocytic anemia, seborrheic dermatitis, and scrotal skin changes. Because riboflavin is utilized in the metabolism of niacin and pyridoxine, some of the deficiency symptoms may be due to failure of metabolic processes requiring these nutrients.

There has been no documentation of toxic effects of excessive amounts of riboflavin. Increased amounts of riboflavin given to well-nourished children have no positive health benefits.

Niacin

The requirement for niacin (nicotinic acid and nicotinamide) is complicated because much of the individual's need for niacin is fulfilled by the conversion of tryptophan (amino acid) to niacin. Pellagra, the niacin deficiency disease, is characterized by diarrhea, dermatitis, and dementia. Glossitis or inflammation of mucous membranes may also be present.

Large doses of nicotinic acid (>3 g/day) may cause flushing or vascular dilatation, decreased serum lipids, increased utilization of muscle glycogen stores, and decreased mobilization of fatty acids. Pharmacologic doses of niacin have been used in treating hypercholesterolemia, thereby providing opportunity for toxic side effects.

Vitamin B_6

Deficiency of pyridoxine rarely occurs in isolation but, rather, in conjunction with deficiencies of other B-complex vitamins. In addition, the need for vitamin B_6 is closely related to the amount of protein consumed. As protein intake increases, the deficiency of pyridoxine is exacerbated. Symptoms of deficiency in infants and children include convulsions, abdominal distress, anemia, dermatitis, and hyperirritability.

There has been no documentation of toxicity from excessive intakes in infants and children. However, some adults treated with pharmacologic doses showed symptoms of ataxia and sensory neuropathy. Pyridoxine is used in large therapeutic doses to treat a variety of symptoms (depression, muscular fatigue, heart disease) that could be of concern in children. Indiscriminate use of vitamin B_6, therefore, is not indicated. No benefit for supplementing the well-nourished child has been documented.

Folates

The deficiency disease of macrocytic megaloblastic anemia caused by folate deficiency is rare in infants and children because human and cow's milk are excellent sources of folate and are the major source of nutrients for infants. The interaction of folate and vitamin B_{12} in the development of megaloblastic anemia makes it very difficult to pinpoint the specific deficiency.

Excessive intakes of folic acid may inhibit the positive effects of the anticonvulsant drug phenytoin (Dilantin), which calls for caution in supplementing children with seizure disorders. In addition, excessive amounts of folic acid may actually cause seizures in some children controlled on phenytoin. Therefore, supplemental folate should not be given in large amounts because of the toxic potential and because no documented benefits have been seen in well-nourished children.

Biotin

Biotin deficiencies have been described rarely in infants and children and only in those receiving long-term parenteral nutrition. In adults, deficiency states have been produced by ingestion of large amounts of raw egg whites, which contain avidin, a biotin binder. Symptoms of biotin deficiency include dry, scaly dermatitis; anorexia; alopecia; glossitis; and vomiting.

There are no documented instances or reports of toxicity with ingestion of excessive amounts of biotin.

Pantothenic Acid

There has been no recognized deficiency of pantothenic acid in humans, although deficiency states have been described in animals. Pantothenic acid is widespread in foodstuffs, making deficiency states unlikely. In addition, no toxic effects of pantothenic acid have been reported.

Vitamin C

Scurvy, the clinical presentation of ascorbic acid (vitamin C) deficiency, includes swollen or bleeding gums, petechial hemorrhages, and joint pain with tenderness and swelling of the extremities. Loss of appetite and fatigue are common in older children. With supplementation of most fruit juices and the amount of vitamin C occurring naturally in fresh fruits and vegetables, the incidence of scurvy is rare in children eating a normal diet.

Toxic doses of vitamin C have not been reported in children. There is widespread disagreement on the benefits, if any, of large doses of vitamin C greater than that needed to prevent scurvy. Pharmacologic doses have been prescribed to enhance absorption of heme iron and as an antioxidant to prevent oxidative destruction of fat-soluble vitamins A and E.

FAT-SOLUBLE VITAMINS

The fat-soluble vitamins are vitamin A (retinol, retinal, retinoic acid), vitamin D (cholecalciferol, D_3 and ergosterol, D_2), vitamin E (tocopherols), and vitamin K (menaquinones and phylloquinones). Absorption and transport of these vitamins are associated with lipid absorption and transport. The presence of bile salts is required for absorption. The fat-soluble vitamins are not excreted but are stored in body lipids in varying amounts. This storage allows for accumulation of these vitamins and eliminates the need for daily ingestion. It also presents the potential for toxic effects if large amounts are ingested over time.

Vitamin A

Safe and adequate levels of vitamin A are derived from ingested vitamin A and from carotenoids that are converted to active forms of vitamin A in the body. Deficiency symptoms in children are growth failure, poor adaptation to darkness, conjunctival and corneal xerosis and ulceration (xerophthalmia), hyperkeratosis, increased susceptibility to infections, and keratinization of epithelial cells of the respiratory tract and other organs. Vitamin A deficiency is usually due to fat malabsorption and inadequate intake and is most commonly seen in children younger than 5 years of age.

Numerous toxic signs are related to ingestion of high doses of preformed vitamin A over time. Signs usually appear after long-term daily intakes greater than 20,000 IU per day. Included as signs of vitamin A toxicity are headaches, bone abnormalities, alopecia, vomiting, dryness of the mucous membranes, and liver damage.

The carotenoids (precursors of vitamin A) have not been shown to produce toxic effects, even at high doses. If taken in larger doses over time, they are absorbed into the subcutaneous fat and can color the skin. The skin appears yellow, but the color disappears when the high intakes are discontinued.

Vitamin D

The vitamin D deficiency disease in infants and children is rickets, which is manifested by poor bone mineralization resulting in skeletal deformities. Rickets is rare in the United States because of fortification of milk and other foods with vitamin D. However, some low-birth-weight and other infants who are breast-fed may develop rickets only if no supplement is given or the infants receive no exposure to sunlight. Other children at risk for deficiency include those with chronic fat malabsorption or nephrotic syndrome and some black infants with limited exposure to the sun.

Toxicity from ingestion of excessive amounts is more common with vitamin D than with the other fat-soluble vitamins. Even an excess of 1200 IU/day for white children and 2000 IU for black children is known to produce toxic effects. These include vomiting, hypertension, anorexia, renal failure, and failure to thrive. Hypercalcemia and hypercalciuria lead to deposition of calcium in soft tissues (including the brain). Renal and cardiovascular damage is irreversible.

Vitamin E

Vitamin E deficiencies in children have occurred in premature or very-low-birth-weight infants and in those who malabsorb fat (e.g., patients with cystic fibrosis, biliary atresia, other liver diseases, and lipid transport abnormalities). These deficiencies have been characterized by neurologic defects and hemolytic anemias. The anemias were related to the relationship of vitamin E and dietary polyunsaturated fatty acids (PUFAs). As intake of PUFAs increases, the requirement for vitamin E increases even though most of the oils supplying PUFAs are also good sources of vitamin E.

Toxic effects from excessive oral intakes of vitamin E have not been substantiated. Pharmacologic doses given in treatment regimens over long periods of time have not resulted in serious side effects. Because there are no known health benefits associated with vitamin E supplementation, it is not recommended for well-nourished children.

Vitamin K

Vitamin K is sometimes defined as the antihemorrhagic vitamin because it is necessary for the synthesis of factors required for blood coagulation. Infants are at great risk for vitamin K deficiency because food intake is limited to milk, which is a poor source. Therefore, all newborns are considered to need a supplement of vitamin K soon after birth. Exclusively breast-fed and home-delivered, breast-fed infants require special attention. Other infants and children at risk for vitamin K deficiency are those malabsorbing fat and those treated with anticoagulant drugs or broad-spectrum antibiotics.

Excessive amounts of the natural forms of vitamin K have not been shown to cause toxic effects. However, the synthetic form (menadione) has produced toxic effects when ingested in large amounts. These symptoms are manifested as hemolytic anemia, kernicterus, and hyperbilirubinemia.

SUMMARY

Because of the narrow range of safe levels of intake of most vitamins and the lack of documented benefits of supplementation, routine supplementation is not recommended in infants and children. Only those infants and children at risk of vitamin deficiency or showing clinical signs of deficiency disease should receive supplementation. Thus, parents should be cautioned against indiscriminate supplementation with vitamins. If vitamins are to be used in pharmacologic doses as drugs, careful monitoring of blood levels and side effects in individual children is imperative.

REFERENCES

National Research Council: Recommended Dietary Allowances, 10th ed. Washington, DC, National Academy Press, 1989.

TOTAL PARENTERAL NUTRITION IN INFANTS

STEVEN L. WERLIN, M.D.
and LYNN A. GERSHAN, M.D.

After more than 20 years, parenteral nutrition continues to be a source of learning, investigation, and controversy. This seems appropriate for this medical intervention, which, in many ways, has paralleled the growth of neonatology as a subspecialty. Parenteral nutrition involves a diverse group of patients with varying and dynamic nutritional requirements, perhaps best exemplified by the special needs of the very-low-birth-weight infant. For the purposes of this article, a neonate is defined as an infant younger than 6 weeks old.

INDICATIONS

Parenteral nutrition may be provided to any neonate unable to tolerate full enteral feedings. Complete energy and nutritional requirements may be provided by central venous access in the very-low-birth-weight infant and in the postsurgical neonate. Alternatively, peripheral intravenous nutrient/calorie supplementation may be required in the growing premature infant who is progressing in enteral feeding. Diagnoses involving circulatory compromise, such as patent ductus arteriosus and cyanotic congenital heart disease, may present a specific risk to the mesenteric circulation and thereby obviate enteral nutrition. *Other clinical conditions in which parenteral nutrition may be helpful and life-saving include increased catabolism (septicemia), decreased substrate reserves (premature and small-for-gestational-age infants), and inborn errors of metabolism.* General principles are presented, with special attention to the particular needs of the term, preterm, and small-for-gestational-age (SGA) neonate.

METHODS OF ADMINISTRATION

Parenteral nutrition with concentrations of glucose not exceeding 12.5 per cent and amino acids not greater than 1.5 per cent can usually be infused through a peripheral vein without causing discomfort or phlebitis. If greater than 5 to 7 days of administration is anticipated, insertion of a central venous line should be considered. Broviac or Hickman catheters and, more recently, percutaneously placed Silastic catheters provide reliable central access to the venous circulation, enabling infusion of concentrated solutions over a prolonged period.

REQUIREMENTS (Table 1)

Fluid requirements are extremely variable in the newborn period and depend on such factors as gestational age, transepidermal water loss, degree of success in achieving a thermoneutral environment, and disease state. Accurate measurement of input and output, weight, serum electrolyte levels, and urine specific gravity provide rapid feedback of the appropriateness of the amount and content of intravenous fluids. Parenteral nutrition solutions are designed to provide

TABLE 1. Recommended Baseline Fluid Requirements for Infants (ml/kg/day)

Age	Days 1–2	Days 3–5	Days 10–42	Comments
Preterm				
<1000 g	90–110	110–≥180	130–160	May lose 7–10% body weight in first week of life; avoid fluid overload contributing to symptoms of patent ductus arteriosus, bronchopulmonary dysplasia, and hyponatremia
>1000 g	80–100	100–140	120–150	
Term	60–80	80–120	100–150	Baseline insensible losses 20 ml/kg; less transepidermal loss than in premature
Small-for-Gestational-Age	70–90	100–140	120–160	In general, should not lose weight after birth; avoid dehydration, which could worsen the frequently associated polycythemia

TABLE 2. Factors That May Require Adjustment in Fluid Intake

Increased Requirement
Fever, increase in environmental temperature, radiant heat losses
Open abdominal defect (e.g., omphalocele, gastroschisis)
Phototherapy
Physical activity (e.g., tachypnea, hyperthyroidism)
Prematurity
Third-space losses, including postoperative patients
Decreased Requirement
Congestive heart failure
Humidified isolette
Immobilization (e.g., congenital neuromuscular disease, cast placement)
Mechanical ventilation
Pharmacologic neuromuscular blockade
Symptomatic patent ductus arteriosus

optimal non-protein calorie to gram of nitrogen ratios of 150–220:1, and to be infused at rates of 120 to 175 ml/kg/day. If fluid requirements are in excess of these rates, an appropriate supplemental glucose-electrolyte solution replacing the abnormal losses or increased needs should be administered separately. This will avoid hyperglycemia and protein and calorie excess and will allow adjustments based on changes in clinical conditions without interfering with nutrition. Examples of clinical factors that may alter fluid requirements are presented in Table 2.

Energy (Table 3)

The generally accepted range of calories necessary for growth and maintenance of body tissues appears similar in preterm and term infants, masking the importance of the effects of environmental stressors on the caloric needs of the premature neonate. In the past, vigorous attempts to achieve caloric intake equivalent to in utero accretion rates have resulted in an "overload" state, leading to hyperglycemia, severe metabolic acidosis, and hyperlipidemia. Current recommendations account for differences in amount and composition of weight gain in the ex utero versus in utero environment and balance the provision of adequate nutrition while avoiding untoward side effects. A variety of conditions may change both fluid requirements and caloric needs in an individual infant; these include a thermoneutral environment, use of a heat shield or isolette, the postoperative state, and increased baseline physical activity (as in drug withdrawal).

TABLE 3. Daily Intravenous Requirements for Infants

Component	Premature	Term
Energy	***80–90 kcal/kg***	***80–95 kcal/kg***
Glucose: as tolerated for balance of total kcal	6–9 g/kg/day (4–6 mg/kg/minute)	9–12 g/kg/day (6–8 mg/kg/minute)
Maximum carbohydrate	12–14 g/kg/day (8–10 mg/kg/minute)	14–16 g/kg/day (10–12 mg/kg/minute)
Protein: 10–15% of total kcal	Initial intake: 0.5–1.0 g/kg/day Increase 0.5–1.0 g/kg/day as tolerated	
Maximum protein	2.7 g/kg	2.5–3.0 g/kg
Fat: 33–55% of total kcal	Initial: 0.5 g/kg/day, increase 0.5 g/kg/day as tolerated (Minimum requirement to prevent essential fatty acid deficiency is 0.5 g/kg/day)	Initial: 0.5–1.0 g/kg/day
Maximum fat	2.5–3.0 g/kg/day	3.0–3.5 g/kg/day

Carbohydrate

Avoidance of hyperglycemia-associated osmolar shifts is crucial in the newborn period and is particularly important in asphyxiated and premature infants who are at risk for central nervous system (CNS) hemorrhage. Abnormalities in glucose-insulin response, more common with decreasing birth weight and gestational age, are further exacerbated by the increased fluid requirements in these small babies. Decreased hepatic glycogen stores and diminished capacity for gluconeogenesis are also common in premature and SGA infants. In the intraoperative and postoperative neonate, both stress and anesthesia-related decreases in oxygen consumption may require reduction of the glucose infusion rate to prevent hyperglycemia.

Protein

The modern amino acid solutions now commercially available ensure that both the composition and the quantity of the nitrogen component are consistent and able to be metabolized by the maturing neonate. Adjustments in arginine and chloride content; increased proportions of aspartate and glutamate versus glycine; and provision of taurine, cysteine, and *N*-acetyl-L-tyrosine are some of the most important improvements now found in neonatal formulations. These make allowances for immaturity of amino acid utilization pathways and provide an improved balance of essential and nonessential amino acids. Tolerance to protein intake may be assessed indirectly by measurement of blood urea nitrogen (BUN) and serum bicarbonate, with goals of achieving concentrations of urea nitrogen less than 15 mg/dl and bicarbonate greater than 18 mEq/L. Measurement of ammonia and quantitation of urine and plasma amino acids are also useful if specific questions regarding protein utilization arise.

Fat

The use of 10 and 20 per cent intravenous lipid emulsions has allowed for improvement in caloric density and balance and prevention of essential fatty acid deficiency with only small increments in fluid intake. Associated risks include potential displacement of bilirubin from albumin, lipid deposition in the lungs resulting in decreased pulmonary diffusing capacity and PaO_2, and interference with cell defenses against infection. Sepsis, dysmaturity, extreme prematurity, persistent pulmonary hypertension, acute pulmonary disease, and hyperbilirubinemia are conditions in which lipid clearance may be altered. In these situations, the infusion should be decreased or discontinued. Tolerance of lipid infusion is currently best assessed by measurement of the serum triglyceride level (normal value < 120 mg/dl) before the initiation of an intravenous lipid infusion and after any increase in dose. Plasma lipid level correlates best with the hourly infusion

TABLE 4. Daily Intravenous Major Mineral Requirements (per Kilogram)

Sodium	2–4 mEq (range: 2–8)
Potassium	1–3 mEq (range: 0–5)
Chloride	2–3 mEq (range: 1–5)
Calcium	
Premature	60–100 mg (3–5 mEq)
Term	40–80 mg (2–4 mEq)
Phosphorus	20–45 mg (0.7–1.4 mmol)
Magnesium	0.5–0.9 mEq (6–10 mg)

TABLE 5. Recommendations for Daily Administration of Vitamins and Trace Elements in Infants (per Kilogram)

Vitamins	2 ml of MVI-Pediatric,‡ up to a maximum of 5 ml/day
Zinc	400 μg for infant <37 weeks' gestation 250 μg for term infant <3 months of age
Copper*	20–60 μg
Manganese*	1–5 μg
Chromium†	0.2 μg
Selenium†	2.0 μg
Molybdenum†	0.25 μg (recommended only in long-term total parenteral nutrition)

Data from Shils et al: JAMA 241:2050, 1979; and Grune et al: Am J Clin Nutr 48:1324, 1988.
*Omit in biliary obstruction.
†Reduce in significantly impaired renal function.
‡Rorer Pharmaceuticals, Fort Washington, Pa.

rate and should not exceed 0.15 mg/kg/hour. Continuous 24-hour infusion of lipid may prevent the hypertriglyceridemia seen with cyclic infusions.

Major Minerals, Vitamins, and Trace Minerals

The addition of electrolytes to a dextrose-water solution on day 2 or 3 of life is dependent on the individual patient's renal maturity, acid-base status, and ongoing losses. In general, premature, asphyxiated, or stressed newborns and infants of diabetic mothers need earlier calcium supplementation than do term newborns (Table 4). Vitamins and trace minerals must be added not only to prevent multiple deficiency but also to replete body stores so that deficiency does not occur in the face of rapid growth.

Recommendations for administration appear in Table 5. No multivitamin preparation currently available provides the recommended dose of all vitamins for low-birth-weight infants. The referenced recommendation delivers adequate vitamins E, D, and K; low levels of retinol; and an excess of most of the B vitamins. The issues of photodegradation and adherence to plastic tubing, specifically for vitamin A, have not yet been resolved for the premature infant. Some nurseries, therefore, give supplemental vitamin A as retinyl palmitate. When parenteral nutrition is supplemental or is administered for less than 4 weeks, only zinc need be added to the solution. If total parenteral nutrition (TPN) continues for more than 4 weeks, copper, manganese, and chromium must be added. For stable patients on long-term TPN, multielement solutions are commercially available.

TABLE 6. Laboratory Monitoring Schedule for Infants Receiving Total Parenteral Nutrition

	Baseline and with Any Changes*	Weekly†	Every 2 weeks
Glucose	X		
Electrolytes	X		
Calcium	X		
Phosphate	X		
Urea nitrogen (BUN)	X		
Triglycerides	X		
Albumin		X	
Fractionated bilirubin		X	
Hemoglobin		X	
Aspartate aminotransferase (AST)		X	
Alanine aminotransferase (ALT)		X	
Alkaline phosphatase			X
Creatinine			X
Gamma-glutamyl transferase (GGT)			X

*Minimum twice weekly.
†More often if clinically indicated.

MONITORING

The site of infusion must be observed carefully for signs of infiltration and erythema. When peripheral parenteral nutrition is employed, rapid alternative venous access must be available to avoid hypoglycemia associated with interruption of the infusion. When parenteral nutrition is delivered by a central venous line, increasing pressure in the catheter, as measured by the infusion pump, may provide an early warning of catheter occlusion or kinking and enable rapid intervention. Accurate weight, intake, chemstrip, and urine for glucose should be assessed at least daily, more often in the premature or compromised infant. Recommendations for laboratory monitoring are summarized in Table 6.

COMPLICATIONS AND RISK MANAGEMENT

The risk of complications from the catheter used for TPN administration, the disease processes involved, and the parenteral nutrition itself may be difficult to separate from one another. Table 7 summarizes complications associated with parenteral nutrition and highlights those that are specific to the neonate. Complications of sepsis and thrombosis appear to be directly related to frequency of entering a central venous catheter for administration of medications and blood products and to duration of line placement. Guidelines for reducing risks include:

1. Use of a "designated" line, exclusively for administration of parenteral nutrition.
2. Optimal placement of the central line tip: above the umbilicus—right atrium/superior vena cava junction or in the superior vena cava; below the umbilicus—in the inferior vena cava.
3. Use of central venous access for the shortest possible time.
4. Use of heparin (0.5 to 1.0 unit/ml) to decrease the risk of thrombosis may be considered, although its efficacy is not proven.
5. Maintenance of sterility of central line exit sites and a high index of suspicion for infection.

TABLE 7. Complications Associated with Total Parenteral Nutrition (TPN)

Bone*
- Osteopenia

Catheter-Related
- Thrombosis
- Phlebitis
- Embolism
- Slough
- Extravasation and hemorrhage

Infectious
- Bacterial
- Fungal
- Impairment of cell defenses (?lipid-associated bacteremia)*

Metabolic*
- Electrolyte/glucose abnormalities
- Metabolic acidosis
- Cholestatic jaundice
- Vitamin and trace element deficiencies
- Aluminum toxicity
- Hyperammonemia

Pulmonary*
- Capillary diffusion block

*Indicates higher risk in neonates than in older children or adults on TPN.

6. Judicious and carefully monitored use of all the components of parenteral nutrition.
7. Early and rapid recognition of occlusion from fibrin clots, thrombosis, or precipitant. Decisions regarding treatment with fibrinolytic agents (e.g., urokinase) or catheter removal should be made by experienced personnel.
8. Institution of enteral feedings at the earliest reasonable time, even if they are dilute and in small volumes. Initiation of normal gut secretory and peristaltic activities is vital to full patient recovery.

REFERENCES

Greene HL, Hambidge KM, Schanler R, et al: Guidelines in the use of vitamins, trace elements, calcium, magnesium and phosphorus in infants and children receiving total parenteral nutrition: Report of the Subcommittee on Pediatric Parenteral Nutrient Requirements of the Committee on Clinical Issues of the American Society of Clinical Nutrition. Am J Clin Nutr 48:1324–1342, 1988.
Shils ME, Burke AW, Greene HL, et al: Guidelines for essential trace element preparation for parenteral use. JAMA 241:2051–2054, 1979.

PICA

RICHARD OLSEN, M.D.

In the narrow definition, pica refers to the ingestion of nonedible substances. In the broader definition, it can include excessive ingestion of edible, but often unusual, substances. See Table 1.

Pica is most common in children but may occur in other groups, most notably pregnant women and retarded individuals. The incidence of pica is 30 per cent in black children aged 1 to 6 years and 10 to 18 per cent in white children. Approximately 30 per cent of children with pica have lead poisoning (Danford, 1982). Estimated daily soil ingestion in young children with pica in normal living conditions is 90 mg with 190 mg representing the 90th percentile (van Wijnen et al, 1990).

Possible etiologic factors in pica have included nutritional and psychosocial factors. Iron, zinc, and trace mineral deficiencies have been implicated as nutritional factors. Other studies suggest insufficient or inappropriate maternal-child interaction as a cause. Cultural beliefs and practices may also play a role. No one etiologic factor explains childhood pica, and there may not be a single, underlying cause.

Depending on underlying etiology, complications of pica include anemia, lead poisoning, intestinal parasite infestation, visceral larva migrans, delayed development, and poor weight gain and growth.

Evaluation should include careful history and physical examination, complete blood count (CBC) with differential, and determination of serum ferritin levels. Depending on symptoms and endemic problems in a given geographic area, free erythrocyte protoporphyrin, serum lead, stool for ova and parasites, and serologic assessment for *Toxocara* may be indicated. If psychosocial factors are suspected as a possible cause of pica, an in-depth assessment of the child's development and parent-child interaction is indicated. On-site assessment of home and/or day care setting may be helpful.

TABLE 1. Substances Commonly Ingested

Edible	Inedible
Baking soda	Soil
Ice	Clay
Lettuce	Starch
Raw potatoes	Paint chips
Peanuts	Hair
Butter	Feces
Tomato seeds	

Treatment of pica depends on underlying etiology. If iron deficiency is found, treatment consists of oral iron at 4 to 6 mg/kg/day for 2 to 3 months as well as dietary evaluation to determine whether contributing factors, such as excessive milk intake, are present. Prevention of recurrence includes dietary prescription of iron-rich foods, such as meats and poultry, as well as foods that promote iron absorption, including fruits and fruit juices.

If excessive lead levels are found, treatment will depend on the level of intoxication (Class II through IV.) Chelating agents are useful when lead intoxication falls into Class III and IV (lead levels greater than 50 μg/dl). Chelation may be done if the lead mobilization test is positive or if the patient is at Class IV.

Treatment of intestinal and systemic parasite infections depends on the specific parasites.

Treatment of psychosocial factors, if they are contributing to the pica, is more complicated and requires a multidisciplinary approach, including developmental intervention, treatment of any underlying psychiatric disorder, and intensive support and education of parents. Involvement of social services and public health nursing is often helpful.

If pica is related to cultural practices, it is important to convey respect for cultural beliefs while providing education regarding the risk of pica.

Pica behavior often abates with correction of underlying iron deficiency. Improving mother-child interaction frequently reduces or resolves pica behavior if psychosocial factors are involved.

REFERENCES

Danford DE: Pica and nutrition. Ann Rev Nutr 2:308, 1982.
van Wijnen JH, Clausing P, Brunekreef B: Estimated soil ingestion by children. Environ Res 51:159, 1990.

MAGNESIUM DEFICIENCY

ROBERT M. SUSKIND, M.D.
and ANTHONY R. MAWSON, Dr.P.H.

As the second most abundant intracellular cation (the first being potassium), magnesium plays a critical role in cellular metabolism; its importance in health and disease is increasingly being recognized. Intracellular magnesium is bound primarily to protein, where it acts as an essential cofactor in numerous important enzymatic processes, including all reactions involved in energy production in plants and animals. Homeostasis of magnesium is maintained by the kidney. After glomerular filtration of the diffusible fraction, 60 to 75 per cent is reabsorbed in the ascending limb of the loop of Henle. Loss of magnesium homeostasis often occurs with renal disease.

The Recommended Dietary Allowances (RDA) of magnesium are 40 to 60 mg/day for infants, 170 mg/day for children at 10 years, and 280 to 400 mg/day for adults. For adults, these amounts are supplied by an average diet containing meat and vegetables. Grains, nuts, and green vegetables are particularly rich sources of magnesium. Forty to 50 per cent of ingested magnesium is normally absorbed in the small intestine, little in the colon. Like potassium, but unlike sodium, magnesium is predominantly an intracellular ion; 60 per cent is found in bone and muscle, the remainder in the viscera.

Only 1 per cent of magnesium is found in the extracellular fluid compartment. Hence, the stated normal serum values of 1.5 to 1.8 mEq/L are unreliable as a measure of total body magnesium levels. Intracellular measurements are preferred to serum levels. However, the technology for measuring free magnesium in the tissues is still not universally available. Hypomagnesemia, therefore, remains a clinical diagnosis except in cases of severe deficiency. In one fourth to one third of patients with hypokalemia, hypophosphatemia, hyponatremia, or hypocalcemia, depletion of tissue magnesium is present.

Clinical magnesium deficiency in humans was first described in 1934. Since then, increasing numbers of clinical disorders associated with magnesium deficiency have been recognized, including the effects of certain drugs that induce renal losses of the nutrient. *In general hospital surveys, 6 to 26 per cent of patients have been found to be hypomagnesemic. In view of the high frequency of hypomagnesemia in acute and chronic illness, magnesium determinations should be performed routinely in hospitalized patients.* Patients with poor food intake, malabsorption, hypokalemia, or hypocalcemia and those receiving diuretics or nephrotoxic agents are particularly at risk. Hypomagnesemia is also common in alcoholism and insulin-dependent type 1 diabetes: *More than one third of infants born to diabetic mothers are hypomagnesemic during the first three days of life.* Magnesium deficiency occurs in children with inadequate food intake and in association with malabsorption, persistent vomiting, diarrhea, and infection.

Hypomagnesemia presents with any of the following major manifestations:

1. Central nervous system (CNS)—depression, agitation, or psychosis.
2. Neuromuscular—weakness, tremors, muscle fasciculation, positive Chvostek's or Trousseau's signs, and dysphagia.
3. Cardiac—electroencephalographic changes (namely, prolonged P-R interval, widened QRS complex, prolonged Q-T interval, depressed S-T segment) and arrhythmias.

Convulsions with or without coma appear to occur more frequently in acutely deficient infants than in adults.

Conditions associated with hypomagnesemia are grouped below. The most common causes of hypomagnesemia are those that increase renal excretion or reduce intestinal absorption.

1. Medications—diuretics, antibiotics, cancer chemotherapy, immunosuppressive agents.
2. Gastrointestinal disorders—fat malabsorption, diarrheal diseases.
3. Endocrine disorders—hyperaldosteronism, hyperparathyroidism, hyperthyroidism.
4. Renal tubular disorders—inflammatory, metabolic, hormonal.
5. Inadequate intake—alcoholism, total parenteral nutrition, catabolic states (e.g., trauma, burns), severe infections.

Digitalis toxicity associated with diuretic therapy may result not only from potassium deficiency but also from lack of magnesium. There is some evidence that the arrhythmias complicating heart failure can be successfully treated with magnesium supplementation.

Normal serum magnesium levels in infants and children range from 1.5 to 1.8 mEq/L. However, clinical symptoms can appear in the absence of major alterations in serum magnesium levels. In *acute* hypomagnesemic tetany and convulsions, a 10 per cent solution of magnesium sulfate ($MgSO_4$) should be administered intravenously at a dose of 0.8 mEq/kg of body weight (1.0 ml/kg of 10 per cent $MgSO_4$) up to 20 ml, and at a rate not exceeding 1.5 ml of 10 per cent $MgSO_4$ per minute. This may be followed by a continuous drip of magnesium at a dose of 1 mEq/kg/day up to 40 mEq/day (10 ml of 50 per cent $MgSO_4$) diluted in 5 per cent dextrose or normal saline to make up less than 10 per cent of $MgSO_4$ concentration for the first 24 hours. In *severe* convulsions, in addition to the initial intravenous dose, an equal dose of magnesium (0.8 to 1.0 mEq/kg) may be injected intramuscularly as 20 per cent (0.5 ml/kg) or 25 per cent $MgSO_4$ solution (0.5 ml/kg).

Intravenously administered magnesium has an immediate effect lasting about 1/2 hour; with an intramuscular injection, the effect occurs after an hour and lasts 3 to 4 hours. Intramuscular injections of magnesium sulfate at the dose of 1 mEq/kg (0.5 ml/kg of 25 per cent $MgSO_4$) may be repeated every 4 to 6 hours for the first 24 hours. A magnesium solution may be administered parenterally for 3 to 5 more days (in a dose half that of the first 24 hours), followed by oral therapy using any one of several forms of magnesium salts (Table 1). To minimize the risk of diarrhea, smaller doses should be given initially, then increased gradually to 2 to 3 mEq/kg/day in 3 to 4 doses. Patients who waste magnesium in urine or stool require a larger dose, while those with impaired renal glomerular filtration require as low as one-fourth the normal dose. Progress should be checked by repeated serum magnesium determinations.

The return of serum magnesium to the normal range is relatively rapid, with small amounts of intravenous or intramuscular magnesium being rapidly effective for controlling neurologic signs and restoring serum levels. However, repletion of magnesium lost from bone and other tissues requires more prolonged magnesium therapy. Parenteral administration is recommended at 0.3 to 0.5 mEq (3.6 to 6.0 mg)/kg of body weight as 50 per cent magnesium sulfate for the first few hours, followed by an equal amount given either intramuscularly or intravenously over the remainder of the day. Calcium should also be infused with potassium and other electrolytes, as indicated, if the child is symptomatic. In cases of chronic malabsorption, 1.0 to 1.5 mEq/kg orally in multiple divided doses should be given.

ZINC DEFICIENCY

ROBERT M. SUSKIND, M.D.
and ANTHONY R. MAWSON, Dr.P.H.

Zinc was first recognized as an essential element for animals in 1916, when zinc-deficient baby pigs were found to be growth-retarded, sterile, and suffering from dermatitis. Zinc deficiency was first recognized in humans in 1958, when Prasad discovered that young male Egyptian dwarfs had unusually low hair and serum zinc levels. Zinc supplementation led to dramatic improvement; growth-retarded males averaging 17 years of age grew 5.0 inches/year. In addition, supplemented subjects showed an increase in body weight and gonadal development.

Individuals at increased risk for zinc deficiency include infants, adolescents, women of reproductive age, and the aged. Zinc requirements for growth in early infancy are calculated as approximately 300 μg/day. Urine and sweat losses account for at least 100 μg/day. Net daily requirements are about 400 μg. Premature infants who are at risk of becoming zinc-deficient have a significantly decreased body

TABLE 1. Magnesium (Mg) Salt Preparations

	Amount of Salt to Make Up 100-ml Solution	Amount
Parenteral Solution		
$MgSO_4$ 7 H_2O	10%	0.8 mEq/ml
$MgSO_4$ 7 H_2O	20%	1.6 mEq/ml
$MgSO_4$ 7 H_2O	25%	2.0 mEq/ml
$MgSO_4$ 7 H_2O	50%	4.0 mEq/ml
Tablet		
Mg hydroxide		13.8 mEq/400 mg
Mg gluconate		4.8 mEq/500 mg
Oral Solution		
Mg chloride	4 g of $MgCl_2$ 6 H_2O	2.0 mEq/5 ml
Mg citrate	6 g of $MgHC_6H_5O_7$ 5 H_2O	2.0 mEq/5 ml
Mg chloride and Mg citrate	4 g of $MgCl_2$ 6 H_2O and 6 g of $MgHC_6H_5O_7$ 5 H_2O	4.0 mEq/5 ml
Mg gluconate	4.2 g of $MgC_{12}H_2O$	2.0 mEq/5 ml
Milk of magnesia	7 g of $Mg(OH)_2$ (in suspension)	12.0 mEq/5 ml

content of zinc at birth because two thirds of the maternal fetal transfer of zinc occurs during the last 10 to 12 weeks of gestation.

Zinc deficiency has been reported in infants fed zinc-deficient breast milk and in those with or without short-bowel syndrome receiving long-term parenteral nutrition. Premature infants with zinc deficiency may present with failure to thrive, persistent generalized dermatitis, and diarrhea despite a high caloric intake. Decreased serum zinc concentrations followed by rapid weight gain and complete clearing of persistent skin lesions after administering 150 mg/day of zinc sulfate for 4 weeks suggests zinc deficiency as causative.

The bioavailability of zinc may be negatively influenced by iron and calcium. Iron-fortified formulas may inhibit zinc absorption and contribute to suboptimal zinc nutrition. Studies of zinc uptake with human milk, cow's milk–based formula, and soy-based and casein hydrolysate–based formulas have shown that uptake with cow's milk and cow's milk–based formula is less than one third of that with human milk. Zinc absorption from soy-based and hydrolyzed casein formulas is one sixth of that from human milk. *Routine investigation of preterm infants with decreased growth velocity or failure to gain weight despite adequate caloric intake, with or without skin lesions and diarrhea, should include measurement of plasma or serum zinc levels.*

Zinc deficiency is reflected by a decreased concentration of zinc in plasma, red blood cells, and hair; increased plasma zinc turnover; and reduced zinc excretion in stool and urine. Mild zinc deficiency has been difficult to diagnose. Reduced plasma or urine zinc levels cannot be taken as necessarily indicating decreased body stores of zinc. Zinc in hair and erythrocytes, in addition, does not reflect active or recent body zinc status. Plasma levels of zinc may remain normal in cases of mild zinc deficiency because these tissues have slower zinc turnover. Zinc may be assayed in cells with a more rapid turnover, such as lymphocytes, granulocytes, and platelets. In studies of human volunteers subjected to mild dietary zinc deficiency, the concentration of zinc in lymphocytes, neutrophils, and platelets was significantly decreased. Dark adaptation and lean body mass were also reduced. Hypogeusia (abnormal sense of taste) together with reduced serum thymulin, testosterone, and dihydrotestosterone, was also noted. The recommended treatment of infants with mild zinc deficiency is 1 to 2 mg/kg of elemental zinc orally for 2 to 3 months.

Numerous experimental and clinical reports suggest an association between marginal zinc deficiency and impaired immune function, including decreased natural killer (NK) cell activity and decreased interleukin-2 activity of T-helper cells. Studies in animals indicate that zinc deficiency is associated with significant delays in the onset of autoimmune disease and enhanced survival. It is possible that other factors secondary to the zinc deficiency syndrome such as accompanying caloric deprivation may contribute to the salutory effect of zinc deficiency or autoimmune disease.

Moderate zinc deficiency is associated with growth retardation; intercurrent infection; mental lethargy; impaired taste, smell, and hearing; alopecia; poor appetite; infertility; impotence; prostatic hypertrophy; poor wound healing; psoriasis-like skin lesions; recurrent boils; hyperkeratosis; and disagreeable perspiration, all of which can be corrected with zinc supplementation. Zinc deficiency also results in fragile fingernails, tinnitus, hearing nerve loss, and night blindness. For infants with protein-calorie malnutrition or zinc deficiency secondary to malabsorption, oral replacement can be safely started with zinc at 1 to 2 mg/kg/day.

Altered zinc metabolism may be a serious complication of several diverse diseases, including renal disease, alcoholism, diabetes, and sickle cell anemia, all of which are characterized by impaired immunocompetence. Zinc deficiency in patients with sickle cell anemia is associated with impaired delayed hypersensitivity and reduced NK cell activity that is corrected by zinc supplementation. Some patients with adult sickle cell anemia may be zinc-deficient. In such cases growth retardation, hypogonadism in men, hyperammonemia, abnormal dark adaptation, and cell-mediated immune deficiency may be related to zinc deficiency, since zinc supplementation reverses these effects.

Severe zinc deficiency occurs in patients with acrodermatitis enteropathica and after total parenteral nutrition (TPN) without zinc, excessive use of alcohol, and penicillamine therapy. Acrodermatitis enteropathica and its attendant severe zinc deficiency occur as a result of zinc malabsorption. Recent reviews indicate that symptoms other than dermatitis vary with age. In infancy, diarrhea, mood changes, anorexia, and neurologic disturbances are reported most frequently. In toddlers and schoolchildren, the most commonly reported symptoms are growth retardation, alopecia, weight loss, and recurrent infections. Spontaneous remission often occurs at adolescence. Overall mortality is about 20 per cent higher in males than in females. Hypoglobulinemia and depressed cellular immunity may be associated with zinc deficiency in acrodermatitis enteropathica. In older children, autoimmune phenomena have been described.

Laboratory diagnosis of acrodermatitis enteropathica is sometimes difficult. Mean zinc values in serum, urine, and hair in patients are 50 per cent of normal levels. However, there is a 10 per cent overlap with normal controls. Low zinc levels are also found in other diseases. In cases of doubt, in vitro or in vivo zinc absorption tests using radioisotopes (^{65}Zn or ^{69m}Zn) may be performed. In young infants with one or more symptoms of acrodermatitis enteropathica, the recommended treatment is a dose of 2 to 3 mg/kg/day, to be increased as needed to achieve remission of symptoms. In older children, 30 to 40 mg of zinc daily is recommended for the rapid resolution of signs and symptoms.

Low levels of zinc have been measured in the plasma, hair, and urine of patients with the inflammatory bowel diseases (IBD) ulcerative colitis and Crohn's disease. The symptoms of ulcerative colitis, a recurrent inflammatory disease of the colon and rectum involving diffuse tissue reactions of the mucosa and submucosa, include diarrhea, rectal bleeding, abdominal pain, and weight loss. In Crohn's disease, a chronic inflammatory disease of unknown etiology involving all layers of the bowel wall and often the entire digestive tract, symptoms include fever, diarrhea, abdominal pain, weight loss, and, in children, impaired growth. Severe impairment of linear growth, lack of weight gain, retarded skeletal maturation, and delayed onset of sexual development is seen in 10 to 40 per cent of patients younger than 21 years of age with IBD. Zinc deficiency has been proposed as a contributory factor for several findings that complicate IBD, including growth failure, hypogonadism, altered taste, acrodermatitis, hair loss, and impaired wound healing. Decreased levels of circulating zinc in hospitalized ill patients with Crohn's disease are correlated with increased activity of interleukin-1—a small polypeptide released in infection, fever, and inflammation.

Reduced serum zinc levels are correlated with hypoalbuminemia in patients with IBD. Albumin serves as the primary transport protein for zinc. Plasma proteins such as albumin, transferrin, prealbumin, and retinol-binding protein decrease with zinc deficiency and increase with repletion. Thus, decreased serum albumin levels may be associated with reduced zinc levels in the presence of adequate zinc stores.

No specific recommendations are available for zinc supplementation in IBD patients. Case reports of severe zinc deficiency in IBD have shown that patients respond to oral supplements of 210 to 750 mg of zinc per day.

For treatment of zinc deficiency in children without malabsorption, the Committee on Nutrition of the American Academy of Pediatrics recommends supplementation with 0.5 to 1.0 mg/kg/day.

Intravenous zinc requirements during TPN are 400 μg/kg/day for prematures, 200 μg/kg/day for term infants 0 to 3 months of age, 100 μg/kg/day for older infants, and 50 μg/kg/day for children. Plasma zinc concentrations should be observed. Patients with severe zinc deficiency should receive 300 to 500 μg/kg/day until skin lesions resolve and normal zinc concentrates are restored. Oral zinc sulfate and acetate, both of which are soluble, are the most frequently used zinc salts. Because foods may affect absorption of zinc, zinc should be administered 1 to 2 hours before meals. Serum zinc levels as well as clinical response to therapy should be monitored. An increased growth rate is one of the most sensitive indicators of response to therapy.

Copper deficiency can be induced by excessive zinc therapy. This occurs with as little as 50 mg/day of elemental zinc given to adults and 25 mg given to an infant for several weeks. Depression of high-density lipoprotein cholesterol may occur with excessive zinc therapy.

2

Mental and Emotional Disturbances

MENTAL RETARDATION

BRUCE K. SHAPIRO, M.D.
and MARK L. BATSHAW, M.D.

Mental retardation is defined as significant subaverage general intellectual functioning associated with impairment of adaptive behavior and manifested during the developmental period. Treatment is palliative, as the underlying defect cannot be corrected. However, there are many ways pediatricians can help children with mental retardation reach their potential, aid the family in coping, and, in some cases, prevent the occurrence of mental retardation in future children. The first step is correct and early diagnosis to provide genetic counseling. Next, the pediatrician needs to advise the parents about appropriate expectations. Third, therapy must be directed at the child's educational needs, behavioral problems, and other associated deficits. Finally, there needs to be a periodic review of progress.

EARLY DIAGNOSIS

Early diagnosis allows for the easing of parental anxiety, realistic goal setting, and greater acceptance of the child. Children with severe mental retardation demonstrate major developmental delays at an early age, making the diagnosis straightforward. However, many children with mild mental retardation will not have significant developmental delays during the first year of life. Certain groups of children are at increased risk: premature infants, children who are small for gestational age, and infants who have suffered perinatal insults. However, most children with mental retardation do not fall into an identifiable "at risk" group. Thus, taking a complete developmental history is important for all children with developmental delays.

The parents will usually bring the child to a pediatrician because the child is failing to fulfill developmental expectations. In early infancy, these include questions about hearing or vision and problems in feeding or swallowing. After 6 months of age, motor delay is the most common complaint. Language and behavior problems become prominent between 2 and 4 years, and school failure becomes evident in nursery school or in the early primary grades. Once identified, the child should be referred to an interdisciplinary evaluation center, e.g., school, university-affiliated facility (UAF), hospital-based or state diagnostic and evaluation center. Evaluation should include an examination by a developmental pediatrician and formal psychological testing. In addition to medical consultations, evaluations may be required from experts in behavioral psychology, special education, social work, speech, language and audiology, nursing, and physical and occupational therapies.

The diagnosis of mental retardation is confirmed by standardized measures that assess a child's cognitive function. The test that is most commonly used in infancy is the Bayley Scales of Infant Development. Preschool children may receive either the Stanford-Binet (4th edition) or the revised form of the Wechsler Preschool and Primary Scale of Intelligence (WPPSI-R). Although the Stanford-Binet continues through adulthood, the Wechsler Series is composed of two additional tests—the 3rd edition of the Wechsler Intelligence Scale for Children (WISC-III) and the Wechsler Adult Intelligence Scale (WAIS). Most of these tests do not predict normal or above-normal function very well but are quite good at detecting children with mental retardation. The greater the degree of mental retardation (slower rate of development), the younger the age at which an accurate diagnosis can be made.

Cognitive deficiency is a necessary but not sufficient characteristic for the diagnosis of mental retardation. Deficits in adaptive behavior also need to be demonstrated. These are harder to measure in children because (1) the examiner is dependent on the respondent for accurate information and (2) there may be limited opportunities for the child to perform a task. The Vineland Adaptive Behavior Scale is the major assessment tool, although the Woodcock Johnson Scales of Independent Behavior and the American Association on Mental Deficiency Adaptive Behavior Scales are suitable alternatives.

ETIOLOGY

Most cases of mental retardation remain idiopathic, especially in the mild retardation group, which composes over 85 per cent of the total population with mental retardation. However, among individuals with an intelligence quotient (IQ) less than 50, determination of etiology is possible in about two-thirds of cases. A diagnosis allows the parents to know why their child has mental retardation. It helps to reduce the guilt of "what could I have done differently to prevent our child's disability" and allows association with other parents who have children with a similar diagnosis. It also permits prediction of future outcome based on reported experience with other children having similar diagnoses. Finally, it is important for genetic counseling. Among idiopathic cases of severe–profound mental retardation, the empiric recurrence risk is 3 to 5 per cent. However, in chromosomal or single-gene defects, recurrence risks can be as high as 25 to 50 per cent. Because of the diversity of conditions leading to mental retardation, there is no screening evaluation possible. A complete history and physical may give leads that should then be fully investigated, but "fishing expeditions" should be avoided. For example, skull x-rays, metabolic screens, and brain imaging studies have not proved useful as diagnostic screening techniques in children with mental retardation. However, if there are multiple malformations or signs suggesting a genetic disorder, specific studies, such as brain imaging procedures, metabolic tests, chromosomal analysis or DNA studies for fragile X syndrome, may be warranted.

GENETIC COUNSELING

Various techniques of prenatal diagnosis are available for families with children having mental retardation of genetic origin. For prenatal diagnosis to be successful, three conditions must be met. First, a correct diagnosis must be established. Second, the mother must be known to be at an increased risk for having a disabled child: e.g., the increased risk of Down syndrome in a mother over 35 years old, the recurrence risk in a mother who has borne a child with Down syndrome or fragile X syndrome, or a mother who is a translocation carrier. Third, the disorder must be identifiable by prenatal diagnostic techniques.

The most common forms of prenatal diagnosis are amniocentesis and chorionic villus sampling. The amniotic fluid can be used for alpha-fetoprotein determination of neural tube defects. The fetal cells are studied for karyotyping to determine the sex of the fetus or to detect chromosomal anomalies. Enzyme assays for inborn errors of metabolism can also be performed on the cells. Chorionic villus sampling permits the same types of analyses as amniocentesis (except for measuring alpha-fetoprotein) but can be performed at an earlier stage of gestation (9 to 11 weeks gestation). A less commonly used technique of prenatal diagnosis involves fetoscopy, which allows direct visualization of body parts so that syndromes associated with absent or deformed limbs can be identified. Fetal skin and liver biopsy can also be performed during fetoscopy. Fetal ultrasonography, a method of indirect visualization, is now being used for definition of neural tube defects, microcephaly, and congenital heart defects.

The primary purpose of prenatal diagnosis has been to identify an affected fetus and offer therapeutic abortion. However, it may also influence the timing and mode of delivery or the perinatal care of the infant. For instance, a child with a complete urea cycle enzyme deficiency, organic acidemia, or maple syrup urine disease will become comatose during the first week of life. If diagnosed prenatally or at birth, the child can be started on appropriate therapy and coma can usually be averted. We are even able to perform fetal therapy in certain cases. Thyroxine has been injected into a hypothyroid fetus, and vitamin B_{12} has been given to a fetus with methylmalonic acidemia. Fetal surgery has been used successfully to divert a bladder blockade. Shunting of fetal hydrocephalus has been less successful, probably because of underlying brain malformations.

TREATMENT

General Pediatric Care

Besides special services, the child with mental retardation requires the same basic pediatric supervision as the child with normal intelligence. This includes following immunization schedules, growth parameters, and treating intercurrent infections. However, there may be additional concerns under certain circumstances. Children in classes or institutions where hepatitis B antigen has been identified may require the hepatitis B vaccine. Children with multiple disabilities may be at increased risk for recurrent respiratory infections and may benefit from influenza vaccine.

Weight gain may be deficient or excessive and may require nutritional intervention. Non-ambulatory children (e.g., those with spastic quadriplegia or spina bifida) have decreased caloric requirements. Counseling of parents concerning reduced growth potential is also necessary. Recently, growth hormone treatment has been shown to increase growth potential in children with Turner syndrome and Down syndrome. Dental hygiene needs to be addressed, especially for children who are receiving phenytoin or who are incapable of self-brushing. Preventive dental measures include decreasing the intake of sucrose-containing sweets by substituting noncariogenic snacks such as fruits and potato chips for candy and sugar-laden cereals. Toothbrushing and the use of fluoride should also be emphasized.

Consideration of Associated Dysfunctions

Mental retardation is often accompanied by associated deficits that further limit the child's adaptive abilities. In their most obvious forms, associated dysfunctions can be considered additional diagnoses—cerebral palsy, visual deficits, seizure disorders, speech disorders, autism, and other disorders of language, behavior, and perception. *Formes frustes* of these disorders have also been recognized—clumsiness, attentional peculiarities (including attention deficit hyperactivity disorder), articulation disorders, hyperactivity, and school underachievement. The severity and frequency of the associated dysfunctions tend to be proportional to the degree of mental retardation but may be more incapacitating than the mental retardation itself. Failure to appreciate the effects of associated deficits usually results in unsuccessful habilitation and may heighten behavioral problems.

Early Intervention

Early intervention is based on the assumption that children who receive remedial services at an earlier age will have a better outcome. There is some evidence that this is true for treating former premature infants, but the effects on children with developmental disabilities remain to be established. The Early Intervention Amendments to Education of the Handicapped Act of 1986 (Public Law 99–457) have mandated services to children who demonstrate developmental delays or are at risk for such disorders. Under this law, early intervention services must include, for each eligible child, a multidisciplinary assessment and a written Individualized Family Service Plan (IFSP) developed by a multidisciplinary team and the parents. The IFSP must contain: (1) a statement of the child's present level of development; (2) a statement of the family's strengths and needs related to enhancing the child's development; (3) a statement of major outcomes expected to be achieved for the child and family plus the criteria, procedures, and timelines for determining progress; (4) the specific early intervention services required to meet the needs of the child and family, including the projected dates for the initiation of services, frequency, intensity, and expected duration; (5) the name of the case manager responsible for implementing the plan; and (6) the procedures for transition from early intervention to preschool services. The initial assessment and plan must be reviewed at least semiannually. This program targets children between 3 and 5 years old. It also has created a discretionary program to address the special needs of infants with disabilities from birth through age 2.

Educational Placement

If a child with mental retardation is placed in an inappropriate educational setting, progress will be slowed and behavioral problems are likely to increase. In 1975, Public Law 94–142, the Education for All Handicapped Children's Act, came into force to ensure education for children with developmental disabilities. The provisions of this law include identification, location, and evaluation of all children with disabilities; provision of a full appropriate public education for those children; and preparation and implementation of an individualized educational plan (IEP).

The goals for education should be based on the child's developmental level and the future goals for independence. If the child has mild mental retardation, the prognosis for independence is good. Most of these individuals marry and hold jobs, although they are generally the last hired and first fired. Social-adaptive skills are also impaired, and this results in greater risks of socially deviant behavior and the need for assistance from social agencies. In school, these children need to gain basic academic and vocational skills and training in social interactions. Some may attain functional literacy (defined as a fourth grade education). Some children with severe mental retardation can look toward independence in self-care skills and partial social independence. Others will remain basically dependent throughout life, especially if the child has associated deficits such as cerebral palsy or seizures.

The appropriate placement for each of these groups of children should be guided primarily by their developmental level rather than by their chronologic age. Although mainstreaming into homeroom, art, music, and physical education may be appropriate for the child with mild mental retardation, it has little benefit for children with severe disabilities. The pediatrician should examine the individual educational program (IEP) to see if it appears appropriate in relation to the child's developmental level, especially if behavioral problems or poor school performance become evident.

Recreation is important to the child with mental retardation. Athletics should be encouraged. In general, these children do better in individual or small group activities than in the more complicated team sports. Activities requiring gross motor skills rather than fine motor coordination are most appropriate. Examples include track and field, swimming, and hiking. Although some physical limitations may be medically necessary, they should be as few as possible.

Behavior Management

Behavioral problems occur with greater frequency in these children than in the general population. The causes are complex and may result from the interaction of a variety of factors, including (1) inappropriate expectations of the child's developmental level; (2) organic behaviors: hyperactivity, short attention span, lack of perseverance, self-injurious or stereotypic behaviors; and (3) family problems.

These factors are not mutually exclusive, and multiple causes are the rule. Most behavioral problems can be ameliorated by altering the child's environment, e.g., placing the child in a more appropriate classroom setting and helping the parents understand that although the child is 15 years old, he or she may not have the judgment to cross the street unsupervised. However, behaviors arising from organic deficits are less amenable to treatment by simple means. Two additional methods are employed to treat behavioral problems: behavior management techniques and pharmacotherapy.

Behavior management has proved effective in the control of various behavioral problems: hyperactivity and self-stimulatory, self-injurious, aggressive, and noncompliant behaviors. The basic premise in applied behavior analysis is that behavior is controlled by its consequences. Thus, if a behavior is reinforced, it will occur with greater frequency in the future. If it is not reinforced, it will be less likely to recur. This theory leads to three basic methods of controlling behavior: reinforcement, punishment, and extinction.

Reinforcement leads to an increase in the frequency of a desired behavior. In positive reinforcement, food or social reinforcers, such as hugs, candy, or money, are given contingent on compliant behavior. Punishment differs from reinforcement in that it reduces the frequency of a behavior by use of aversive consequences or by the withdrawal of positive reinforcement. Aversive approaches are used infrequently, primarily to control self-injurious behaviors. The other form of punishment, "timing out," involves placing the child in a situation or room that lacks anything of interest. This isolates the child for 1 to 10 minutes from any social activity that would provide positive reinforcement.

Extinction involves the removal of positive reinforcement from a situation that was previously rewarding. In effect, the prior relationship between the behavior and the consequence is disconnected. An example is ignoring self-stimulatory behavior while providing positive reinforcement as soon as the child stops. Usually, the targeted behavior will increase initially and then gradually diminish. Often extinction is paired with a procedure called differential reinforcement of other behaviors (DRO). While the self-stimulatory behavior is being extinguished, an incompatible behavior, such as stringing beads, is being reinforced. As a group, these behavioral approaches appear to be as effective as psychotropic drugs, although they obviously take more time and effort and long-term outcome studies have not been performed.

Mental retardation does not usually mandate the use of *psychotropic agents.* Drugs should not be used as a substitute for programming but, rather, to facilitate learning and social interactions or to suppress behaviors that are harmful to the patient or others. The drugs most commonly used to control behavior fall into the groups of phenothiazines, butyrophenones, and stimulants. Phenothiazines include chlorpromazine (Thorazine), thioridazine (Mellaril), and trifluoperazine (Stelazine). These drugs act as dopamine antagonists. They result in sedation and decreased levels of motor activity, anxiety, combativeness, and hyperactivity. They also impair attention span. The usual dose in childhood for chlorpromazine or thioridazine is 25 to 200 mg day, but this dosage needs to be individually titrated. The peak drug levels following oral intake occur in 2 to 3 hours. The half-life varies from 2 to 5 days. Common side effects include hyperphagia and lethargy. Uncommon toxic effects include blood dyscrasias, cholestatic jaundice, dermatitis, and increased seizure frequency. After long-term therapy, tardive dyskinesia and akathisia may occur. These symptoms do not always disappear following termination of drug therapy. Haloperidol (Haldol), a butyrophenone, has similar therapeutic effects. However, it produces more frequent extrapyramidal side effects. The usual dosage range is 0.5 to 7.5 mg/day.

Stimulants such as methylphenidate (Ritalin) or dextroamphetamine (Dexedrine) have been shown to be effective in the short-term control of hyperactivity and attentional problems in children with normal intellectual functioning. They also seem to be effective in children with mild mental retardation but are much less effective in children with severe mental retardation. Although the incidence of side effects may be higher than for the general population, stimulants produce fewer severe side effects than phenothiazines and are worth a therapeutic trial in the child with mental retardation. Dosage ranges from 0.5 to 2.0 mg/kg/day for methylphenidate* and 0.25 to 1.0 mg/kg/day for dextroamphetamine.† Peak levels occur in 2 hours, and the half-life is 2 to 4 hours. Antidepressants may be used for affective symptoms; lithium, carbamazepine, or propranolol has been used for aggression.

A 1- to 2-week trial should be sufficient to evaluate the effectiveness of a stimulant medication in controlling behavior. Preferably, the study should be done with the teacher remaining unaware of the drug condition and keeping records of attention, behavior, and hyperactivity (Conner Rating Scale). Drug holidays should be attempted at least yearly to evaluate the need for continued medication. Psychotropic approaches using antihistamines, megavitamin therapy, and caffeine have been found to be ineffective.

Thus, the benefits of psychotropic drugs in children with mental retardation are modest and the risks, especially of phenothiazines and butyrophenones, are not inconsiderable. The risk-benefit ratio is not clearly positive in many children. Psychotropic drugs, then, should be used as a last resort, on a short-term basis, and only in combination with an appropriate behavior management and educational program.

Family Counseling

The emotional impact of having a child with mental retardation is enormous. The stages of grief the family passes through are similar to those of parents who have lost a child. The initial response is one of disbelief. The parents will rarely hear what you say after the words mental retardation are mentioned. Thus, the parents may find it difficult to absorb medical information about their child at this time.

After the initial shock and denial, the parents start to feel guilty. The mother, especially, may feel that she could have done something during her pregnancy to prevent the disability or could have given better care to the child or sought medical attention sooner. Accompanying these are feelings of anger, "Why us?" The parents may direct their anger at each other, at God, at the pediatrician, or even at their child. The parents also feel isolated. They may believe that they are the only ones with this problem. They need reassurance from the pediatrician and may also benefit from a parents' support group.

The next step in coping involves bargaining: "If only we try harder, perhaps he will be normal." The pediatrician needs to help the parents maintain realistic expectations during this time. Some parents may intellectualize, accumulating a great deal of medical information about the child instead of confronting their own feelings. Some parents remain in this stage forever. Others move on eventually to a stage of acceptance.

Having a child with mental retardation also may affect the stability of a marriage and the emotional health of the siblings. It is not uncommon for parents to be at different stages of coping. Further, one parent may want to talk about his or her feelings while the other does not; this leads to feelings of frustration and isolation. The siblings may share this anxiety. They are stigmatized as being the brother or sister of the "mental kid," and they may worry that they can "catch" the mental retardation. While feeling relieved that they do not have mental retardation themselves, the siblings may also feel guilty about being "normal." They may also feel resentful that the parents spend more time with the sibling than with them. They may even be worried that they will have to care for their disabled sibling when they grow up. The grandparents also need to be considered, as they may assume some of the care of the child and will certainly influence the attitudes of the parents. Thus, counseling of the entire family is needed.

Re-evaluations

Although mental retardation is considered a static encephalopathy, there is a need for periodic review. As the child and family grow, new information must be imparted, goals readjusted, and habilitation programming altered. A review requires information about health status, family functioning, child functioning at home and at school, and the nature of the school programs. Other information, such as formal psychologic or educational testing, may be needed. Annual reviews are generally necessary. These reviews should also be undertaken any time the child is not meeting previous expectations.

Life Cycle Issues

As the child grows, he or she moves from one service provision system to another. This also marks the time for a review. Re-evaluation is necessary with the move from preschool to primary grades, from primary to intermediate grades, from intermediate to senior programming, and at the conclusion of school. By this time, the child usually has been abandoned by other adolescents. The disparity between cognitive abilities and chronologic age prevents the adolescent with mental retardation from fitting in. This isolation promotes social awkwardness and diminishes the adolescent's self-esteem. Many parents feel incompetent to deal with issues of emerging sexuality in their child.

The teaching of sexuality, dealing with menses, masturbation, and inappropriate closeness are some of the more common issues brought up by parents of adolescents who have mental retardation. In the patients who have severe mental retardation, sexual drive is limited and few problems other than masturbation develop. These youngsters should be taught that masturbation is acceptable behavior in the privacy of their room but not in public. In the adolescent with mild mental retardation, sexual drive may be normal, although often late in developing. As judgment is limited, close parental supervision is essential. Contraception should be afforded to all individuals who are sexually active.

Late adolescence coincides with the transition from intermediate to senior programs. School will be ending, and long-term planning concerning vocation, living situation, and independence should be in progress. Such planning needs to be based more on achievement than on potential. It is not uncommon to see a leveling off of academic abilities, and this should not be confused with a progressive neurologic disorder. Heterosexual activities, marriage, contraception, and social integration are all common concerns to many at this age. With the completion of school, there is no clearly identified service system for the person with mental retardation. Plans for living arrangements and vocational pursuits should be in place and able to be activated when school is completed.

In the past, the answer to placement for the patient with mental retardation was institutionalization. Many of those individuals are now being de-institutionalized and placed into group homes or smaller institutions or returned to their families. In general, the only patient who will be institution-

*Manufacturer's warning: Safety and efficacy in children under 6 years of age have not been established.

†Dextroamphetamine is not recommended for children under 3 years of age with attention deficit hyperactivity disorder.

alized in the foreseeable future is the child with multiple disabilities whose parents cannot cope with the combined medical, behavioral, and intellectual problems. Many individuals with severe mental retardation still remain at home and attend activity centers or sheltered workshops. However, supportive employment programs have begun to extend to young adults with severe mental retardation. Rather than teach "prerequisite" skills, job "coaches" train people to perform specific tasks (e.g., dish washing) in the actual work setting and help to facilitate the acceptance of the new worker. As a result, people with mental retardation are successfully moving into competitive employment. Alternate living situations, such as group homes and supervised apartments, continue to expand, but the numbers are insufficient to meet the demand and issues of community acceptance and supervision remain controversial.

REFERENCES

Batshaw M, Perret Y: Children with Disabilities, 3rd ed. Baltimore, Brookes Publishing Co, 1992.

Capute AJ, Accardo PJ: Developmental Disabilities in Infancy and Childhood. Baltimore, Brookes Publishing Co, 1991.

PSYCHIATRIC DISORDERS OF INFANTS AND CHILDREN

D. RICHARD MARTINI, M.D.

Research and clinical experience have demonstrated the presence of psychiatric disorders in children, including preschoolers. Young patients have been noted to suffer from more "traditional" childhood behavior problems like attention deficit disorders and separation anxiety disorders as well as a range of affective, anxiety, and impulse control disorders that have been well documented in adults. The symptom pictures are similar to those seen in adults, with modifications for children that take into account developmental stages. For example, depressed children are more likely to describe themselves as angry than sad, a feeling that they may be better able to recognize and explain. Some of these descriptions have come through prospective studies of childhood disorders, a growing body of literature concerning a variety of diagnoses. In addition to the delineation of symptoms, methods of assessment are important variables in the diagnostic formulation. School-aged children have responded favorably to semistructured interviews that are symptom-focused. The options for younger patients are less clearly defined.

Environmental influences not only can lead to psychiatric disorders in children but also may exacerbate behavioral problems that have existed previously. Significant family factors include socioeconomic stressors and parental psychiatric history. Children with learning disabilities are at greater risk for behavioral disorders, and youngsters with psychiatric problems are more likely to suffer academically. Appropriate school placement is, therefore, an important consideration in case formulation. Ultimately, the successful treatment of children with behavioral problems begins with a thorough psychiatric evaluation that reviews all of the pertinent factors in the child's presentation and accurately details the patient's current mental status.

The treatment options available for children with psychiatric disorders are varied and growing. Individual therapies, including play, continue to be effective for a wide range of behavioral problems. Treatment plans may be supplemented by family contacts utilizing parent management training and psychodynamic therapies. Children benefit from peer group approaches that may be educational, social, or psychodynamic. Therapists also have at their disposal a variety of behavioral strategies that can be implemented in session, at home, or in school. The treatment of childhood psychiatric disorders has increasingly involved pharmacologic interventions. The use of psychotropic medications in prepubertal children is limited to specific disorders with guidelines that are sensitive to treatment goals and possible side effects. Psychotropic medications are rarely recommended in children younger than age 6 years and are chosen for particularly severe behaviors.

The following summary of the treatment of more common psychiatric disorders in infants and young children is based on *Diagnostic and Statistical Manual of Mental Disorders,* 3rd ed. rev. *(DSM-III-R)* diagnoses. This article includes a brief description of the disorders as well as a review of possible therapeutic interventions. The treatment of children with autism, developmental delay, and mental retardation is not addressed here.

DISORDERS OF INFANCY AND EARLY CHILDHOOD

Reactive Attachment Disorder of Infancy

Infants may develop abnormal attachment behaviors secondary to an emotionally deprived caretaking environment. They may experience frequent illnesses and weight loss, even when given an adequate opportunity to thrive, and are described as distant, anxious, and withdrawn. The etiology of the disorder varies. Children may be reacting to prolonged medical hospitalization, to extended institutionalization that has resulted in global developmental delay, to a broken and dysfunctional home, to physical abuse, or to multiple separations from primary caretakers. The parents often have a personal history of abuse, neglect, and psychiatric distress.

Therapeutic Approaches

Hospitalization is the treatment of choice for infants and very young children who are suffering from reactive attachment disorder. The admission improves the child's health while addressing the problematic parent-child relationship. Outpatient therapy is recommended only when the parent is likely to be compliant with the treatment and has demonstrated the skills and sophistication to master the treatment program quickly. Parents are supported in efforts to build stronger, more caring interactions with their child and are encouraged to practice the child care skills taught in therapy. Educational programming also includes didactic material and staff modeling and may utilize videotaping as a means of dramatically demonstrating to the parent the areas of concern in their relationship with the child.

Progress in these cases may be slow and difficult. The parents have typically lived from one crisis to another and are left with little sense of consistency or family organization. Mothers and fathers who have had an angry and confrontational relationship with their own parents may see the caretaking professional in a parental role and, therefore, as an adversary. When the home situation is considered detrimental to the safety and welfare of the child, direction from the juvenile court system is necessary as a means of protecting the infant.

Elective Mutism

Elective mutism is the refusal to speak in school or in social situations other than those in the home or in the company of selected adults and peers. These patients are often shy and communicate through a variety of nods, shakes, grunts, and brief verbal spurts. Speech and language skills are frequently delayed, although intellectual development is typically unaffected. The onset of the disorder is usually between the ages of 3 and 8 years and is most often diagnosed at the time of school enrollment. Elective mutism should not be confused with the shyness that naturally occurs in preschool children when they are introduced to new environments and individuals. The disorder is more persistent and is often accompanied by symptoms of social isolation, immaturity, school refusal, obsessive-compulsive disorder, anxiety, depression, and oppositional disorder.

Therapeutic Approaches

Therapeutic approaches include psychotherapy, family therapy, and pharmacologic intervention. Insight-oriented psychotherapy, with a focus on traditional play therapy techniques, explores family conflict as a possible source of anxiety. Behavioral therapies have been most effective when the stimulus for the mutism is presented to the child and then gradually withdrawn in conjunction with the introduction of relaxation techniques. This method is called "stimulus fading." The use of positive reinforcement and contingency management is usually too direct and demanding for a child who is typically withdrawn and uncommunicative.

The need for family participation in therapy is suggested by the symptoms as well as the consequences of the behavior. The patients are typically fearful of situations outside the home and are affected by enmeshed relationships and social isolation within the family. Marital relationships may also be in turmoil. Pharmacologic therapies for elective mutism in young children have not been attempted. However, the adult literature on the treatment of phobic disorders, a diagnosis thought to include elective mutism, demonstrates the effectiveness of a tricyclic antidepressant (TCA)–benzodiazepine combination.

The accompanying symptoms of delayed speech and language skills, persistent enuresis and encopresis, and signs of electroencephalographic (EEG) immaturity all suggest a role for neuropsychiatric dysfunction in the development of elective mutism.

ANXIETY DISORDERS

Anxiety disorders in children have ranged from those that are unique to a young population, i.e., separation anxiety, to ailments like obsessive-compulsive disorder, that have initially been described in adults. The treatment for anxiety disorders in children is determined by the diagnosis and the age of the patient. The prevalence of somatic complaints in the clinical picture of anxiety disorders may lead the child to the pediatrician or family physician for an initial evaluation. Subsequent referrals to mental health professionals should continue to involve the primary physician in the psychiatric treatment plan. Therapists often use multimodal therapies that include individual approaches, family involvement, and contact with systems outside the home (i.e., school).

Behavioral Therapies

A discussion of behavioral therapy recommendations for specific anxiety disorders requires a general review of the methods used in behavioral treatment planning. Classic conditioning methods are among the most basic techniques of behavior therapy. The gradual exposure of a child to the anxiety-provoking situation, either experientially or through the child's imagination, is the hallmark of *systematic desensitization.* These methods are coupled with *relaxation techniques* that gradually decrease the level of the child's apprehension. A more rapid or sudden exposure to stressful situations is characteristic of *implosion,* a technique that, by its nature, is less attractive for children because of the high level of agitation that frequently accompanies it.

The operant techniques are the most widely used by child therapists. With these methods, the frequency and severity of anxiety symptoms are decreased by modifying those situations that lead to and support the behavior. Parents are often taught these techniques as part of a behavior management program. A commonly recommended approach is *contingency management.* This technique adds rewards for desired behavior as reinforcers and decreases the emphasis on anxiety symptoms. Examples of management techniques that use positive reinforcement include the use of star charts, contracts, and token economies. This method is typically followed by a gradual withdrawal of the more tangible reinforcers and replacement with naturally occurring routines, a technique called *extinction.* Occasionally, consequences may be applied when an undesired behavior occurs. For example, rewards that have been gained through appropriate behaviors may be lost through the "*response cost*" behavioral method. Generally, the use of *positive reinforcements* yields greater success than those techniques that penalize.

Children can master anxiety-provoking situations through contact with peers or adults who *model* appropriate behaviors. In treatment, these *social learning techniques* may include group therapies, video sessions, or practical experience. *Cognitive therapies* are an attempt to change the child's emotional response to a situation by understanding and modifying his or her pattern of thinking. Misconceptions are confronted, and the child is encouraged to be more constructive when faced with a challenging circumstance. In addition, the child is taught how to reframe events and repeat self-instruction when upset or anxious.

Simple Fears and Phobias. Children often develop intense fears and phobias to objects, animals, situations, and imaginary creations. Most of these problems resolve spontaneously. Occasionally, a fear will become socially disabling and will necessitate treatment. The use of exposure and extinction is the most effective means of treating the presence of isolated fears and phobias. The child's experience should be gradual, with systematic desensitization and successive approximation used, accompanied by much support from the parents. Parents may also teach their children to manage fears and phobias by modeling appropriate reactions and by praising them when they do well.

Separation Anxiety Disorder. Children who suffer from separation anxiety disorder experience intense distress when separated from a caretaking figure for any length of time. The child may be unable to sleep at a friend's or relative's house, may experience somatic complaints in anticipation of separation, or may resist leaving home for school. Early separation anxiety is usually handled by directing the child to either return to school or to separate appropriately, accompanied by much praise. Occasionally, systematic desensitization may be helpful, along with extinction and modeling.

Avoidant Disorder of Childhood. Children with this disorder are exceedingly shy and avoid most social contact. The goals of treatment include preventing social withdrawal and the feelings of anxiety and inadequacy that result from social situations. The treatment also attempts to minimize the physiologic symptoms of anxiety that tend to reinforce avoidant behavior. Desensitization, modeling, and forms of operant conditioning are most often employed.

Obsessive-Compulsive Disorder. Recent research on obsessive-compulsive disorders notes that the behaviors frequently begin during childhood and adolescence and are accompanied by significant levels of distress. Behavioral interventions are among the few treatment methods studied in children with obsessive-compulsive symptoms. Response prevention is the most common treatment and attempts to limit the tendency either to repeat a behavior or to review a thought (thought stopping). Cognitive therapies that challenge repetitive thinking have been successful in adult patients, but have not been adequately tested in a pediatric population.

Overanxious Disorder. Children with overanxious disorder are uncontrollably anxious and tense, with inappropriate concerns about competence, past and future events, and physical well-being. A combination of cognitive and behavioral interventions is recommended and includes relaxation therapy, role playing, systematic desensitization, and problem solving, which enable the child to master situations in a controlled and comfortable environment.

Panic Disorder. Panic attacks are intense episodes of anxiety that occur without a clear precipitant and are accompanied by physiologic symptoms. Panic in young children is most often associated with depression and separation anxiety disorder. Treatment of these concomitant problems usually leads to a resolution of the panic symptoms. The behavioral treatment of panic disorder is similar to that of overanxious disorder, in that the approach utilizes cognitive-behavioral techniques to decrease the panic episodes and reduce the anticipatory anxiety and avoidant behavior that often accompanies them.

Psychopharmacology (Table 1)

Antidepressants. Antidepressant medications have been effective in the treatment of anxiety disorders. Studies in adult populations, for example, have demonstrated the effectiveness of serotonergic antidepressants (fluoxetine [Prozac] and clomipramine [Anafranil]) in the treatment of obsessive-compulsive disorder. The exact mechanism of action is not known but is thought to involve reuptake blockade of brain neurotransmitters, particularly norepinephrine and serotonin.

TABLE 1. Medications Used in Childhood Psychiatric Disorders

Drug	Indication
Antidepressants	
Fluoxetine (Prozac)	Obsessive-compulsive disorder
Clomipramine	Obsessive-compulsive disorder
Amitriptyline	Depression; Attention deficit hyperactivity disorder
Imipramine	Separation anxiety disorder; Depression; Attention deficit hyperactivity disorder
Desipramine	Separation anxiety disorder; Depression; Attention deficit hyperactivity disorder
Benzodiazepines	Overanxious disorder; Avoidant disorder; Panic disorder; Anticipatory anxiety disorder
Antihistamines	
Diphenhydramine	Anxiety disorder
Hydroxyzine	Anxiety disorder
Buspirone (BuSpar)	Overanxious disorder
Beta-blockers	Extreme agitation and aggression
Monoamine oxidase inhibitors	Depression
Lithium carbonate	Bipolar disorder; Depression; Conduct disorder with irritability and mood lability
Stimulants	
Methylphenidate (Ritalin)	Attention deficit hyperactivity disorder
Dextroamphetamine (Dexedrine)	Attention deficit hyperactivity disorder
Pemoline (Cylert)	Attention deficit hyperactivity disorder
Clonidine	Attention deficit hyperactivity disorder

Prozac selectively inhibits serotonin reuptake in the central nervous system.

These medications may be equally effective in children. The use of TCAs for simple fears and phobias as well as for overanxious disorder and separation anxiety disorder has not been adequately tested, and the results thus far have been mixed. TCAs have been tried on a limited basis in the treatment of panic disorder in children. *Imipramine and desipramine are most commonly used for anxiety disorder at doses that range from 2 to 5 mg/kg/day. The dosage range for Prozac is 0.5 to 1 mg/kg/day with a maximum dose of 40 mg/day.* The recommended dosages in adults are less than for those for depression, a tendency that is likely to apply to children as well. For more details on the use of TCAs, see text on Depression.

Benzodiazepines. The use of benzodiazepines in children has been established for such problems as seizures, night terrors, somnambulism, sleep induction, and muscle relaxation. A few studies have demonstrated drug effectiveness for other anxiety problems, including overanxious disorder, anticipatory anxiety, avoidant disorder, panic disorder, and nonpsychotic anxiety.

Benzodiazepines that are commonly chosen for use in children include long-acting clonazepam (0.01 to 0.04 mg/kg/day), short-acting alprazolam (0.02 to 0.06 mg/kg/day), and short-acting lorazepam (0.04 to 0.09 mg/kg/day). Children with separation anxiety who have responded to TCAs but continue to suffer from anticipatory anxiety have been helped by benzodiazepines. The mechanism of action is unknown, although some believe that the medication disinhibits the behavioral responses that may have been suppressed by earlier traumatic experiences. The result is a more "normal" expression of emotion through verbal expression. The long-term use of benzodiazepines should be monitored in children because of the addictive potential of the drugs and the dangers of withdrawal.

Antihistamines. Antihistamines have effectively treated anxiety disorders in children, primarily through their sedating properties, on both a regular and an as-needed basis. However, no controlled studies exist on the treatment of psychiatric disorders using these medications.

Diphenhydramine and hydroxyzine are the most commonly used antihistamines in clinical practice at doses of 25 to 50 mg twice a day (b.i.d.). Buspirone (BuSpar), a non-benzodiazepine anxiolytic, has been recently introduced as a treatment for overanxious disorder and other anxiety problems and has been attractive because it is not as sedating as the benzodiazepines. The drug does not bind to benzodiazepine receptors or affect the GABA system as do the benzodiazepines; rather, it has a more selective affinity for serotonin and dopamine (D_2) receptors. *Dosages in children range from 5 to 10 mg/day.* However, the drug has not been extensively tested in young populations and should not be the first medication of choice.

Beta-Blockers. Beta-blockers relieve the physiologic symptoms of anxiety both peripherally and centrally. However, studies examining the use of beta-blockers in children have been limited to cases of extreme aggression and agitation that have been unresponsive to other medications.

Psychodynamic Therapies

Fears and phobias develop normally in children, and the mastery of these challenges contributes to the evolving personality. However, when children are affected by stress and unforseen challenges, these fears may persist and become problematic. Anxiety is considered an expression of affect that develops in the face of perceived danger, real or imagined. Theories on the development of separation-individuation consider the fear of loss of the parental figure as a pivotal factor in the evolution of anxiety disorder. Individual therapies explore these issues with the child and are helpful in most anxiety disorders, although with simple fears and phobias psychotherapy may be necessary only in cases of more generalized disability.

Family Therapy

Family dynamics may play a part in the development and maintenance of anxiety symptoms in children and are best approached through family therapy. Treatment encourages members to support the child in attempts at age-appropriate assertiveness and independence while exploring possible psychologic underpinnings of the disorder in the family system. In cases of mild or developmentally appropriate anxiety symptoms, the family may independently be able to implement treatment plans that can quickly alleviate the problems.

Occasionally, the individual psychologic issues of the parents affect not only the development of anxiety symptoms but also the course of treatment. For example, the most common reason for unsuccessful interventions in cases of separation anxiety is the poor compliance of the parent. Parents may be socially isolated, experiencing marital distress, dependent on the child, or suffering from a psychiatric disorder and therefore may be unwilling to change situations that maintain separation anxiety disorder.

DEPRESSION

DSM-III-R does not distinguish between children and adults in the diagnostic criteria for depressive disorders. Symptoms include depressed mood, loss of interest or pleasure, significant weight loss or weight gain (or, in children, failure to meet expected weight gains), insomnia or hypersomnia, psychomotor agitation or retardation, fatigue or loss of energy, feelings of worthlessness or excessive guilt, decreased concentration, and recurrent thoughts of death or suicide. The differential diagnosis includes dysthymic disorder, a chronic mood problem that is of lesser severity and persists for at least 12 months; and adjustment disorder with depressed mood, a problem that follows within 3 months of a significant stressor and continues for less than 6 months. Children may experience uncomplicated bereavement with accompanying decrease in appetite, insomnia, and sadness that usually begins within 3 months after the death. The child should not experience feelings of worthlessness, psychomotor retardation, or a prolonged decrease in level of functioning. These symptoms suggest major depression.

Individual Therapies

The development of symptoms of depression may be the by-product of recurrent self-deprecatory thoughts that maintain the child's dysphoric mood. The object of *cognitive-behavioral therapy* is to develop a positive self-image through the correction or elimination of maladaptive beliefs. The patient is encouraged to express his or her innermost thoughts while the therapist leads the child to replace distortions that support the mood disorder with more reality-based thinking. The limitations of therapy are defined by the cognitive skills of the child.

Depressed children may also have deficiencies in appropriate social interactions that contribute to their isolation. *Social skills training* works with the child on the most basic of social abilities, i.e., talking to other children and adults, accepting frustration and disappointment, requesting assistance, and conversing with others. By improving such skills, the child receives the positive reinforcement from others that is likely to improve self-esteem. This treatment modality is often practiced in a group setting that encourages disclosure and mutual support.

Affective disorders develop in an interpersonal context, influenced by relationships with parents, family members, and peers. *Interpersonal psychotherapy* reviews these situations with the child and inquires about the feelings that they generate. The therapeutic relationship between the child and therapist becomes the method for understanding and treating the emotional underpinnings of the child's depression. The patient should be capable of formal operational thinking before insight-oriented psychotherapy is attempted, a level of intellectual development more often achieved by adolescents than by prepubertal children. Younger children use *play therapy* as a means of communicating a variety of emotions and information. The play presents an opportunity for the child to express feelings in a comfortable yet therapeutic manner.

Family Therapy

The family may play a role in the development as well as the treatment of depression in children. Families with poor intergenerational boundaries, marital instability, rigid and inconsistent rules, and either overinvolvement or underinvolvement by parental figures are more common in children with depressive disorders. Family therapy influences change by exploring factors that may be maintaining the mood disorder, by improving the level of communication within the family, and by increasing the frequency of positive interactions among its members. Psychiatric disorders among family members may also be identified during the course of treatment, increasing the potential for therapeutic intervention.

Pharmacotherapy

Tricyclic Antidepressants. TCA medications have become an accepted means of treating major depressive disorder in children. The literature has not yet supported the effectiveness of such treatment over placebo in pediatric patients, but the assumption that the success rate in adults will be repeated in children has encouraged its use. Tricyclic antidepressants are most effective in prepubertal patients when the blood level is adequate. Studies have suggested that there is a therapeutic "window" at 125 to 250 ng/ml for imipramine; others support a plasma imipramine level of 150 ng/ml or greater for clinical effectiveness.

Dosage guidelines have suggested a maximum imipramine dose of 5 mg/kg/day, which can be administered in a single dose in the evening or in divided doses throughout the day. The medication should be started at a dose of 1 mg/kg/day and gradually increased over a 10- to 20-day period. The child should continue the medication for a 3- to 4-week period at therapeutic doses before treatment success is evaluated.

Precautions to oversee possible side effects should be taken before beginning treatment, and the patient should receive a general pediatric examination, including height, weight, pulse, blood pressure measurements, and electrocardiogram (EKG). The most common side effects include cardiac conduction slowing with mild increases in PR and QRS intervals, tachycardia, and anticholinergic symptoms like dry mouth and constipation. Neurotoxicity, characterized by confusion and seizures, occurs infrequently. A typical medication trial should continue for 4 to 6 months before treatment is discontinued. Withdrawal should be gradual in order to avoid the symptoms of nausea, vomiting, abdominal pain, and lethargy.

Other Medications

Monoamine Oxidase Inhibitors (MAOIs). These drugs are not frequently used as the treatment of choice for depressed children. The dietary restrictions controlling the intake of tyramine limit its effective use in this population. Managing the intake of such items as sausage, pepperoni, aged cheese, and chocolate in a young and sometimes impulsive child is a challenging task.

LITHIUM CARBONATE. Lithium has become an effective treatment in children and adolescents who demonstrate signs of mania, excessive irritability, and depression that is unresponsive to tricyclic antidepressants. Dosages range from 10 to 30 mg/kg/day. Prior to initiation of lithium, the following laboratory work-up should be completed in order to monitor possible side effects on the kidney, thyroid, and white blood cell (WBC) count: blood urea nitrogen (BUN), complete blood count (CBC) with differential, creatinine, creatinine clearance, electrolytes, thyroid function tests, and urine osmolality. Drug levels should be monitored periodically, with a therapeutic range from 0.6 to 1.4 mEq/L. Lithium's use has not been well tested in prepubertal children and should be carefully considered in those rare cases that meet the diagnostic criteria noted above.

SUICIDAL BEHAVIOR IN CHILDREN

The rate of suicidal behavior in prepubescent children has consistently been low. No records are available on self-destructive behaviors or ideation in children younger than age 5. The 5- to 9-year old age group has no more than ten suicides per year in the United States. The rate of suicide in 10- to 14-year-olds is approximately 1 per 100,000. The figures dramatically increase as the child approaches late adolescence, a trend that holds across cultures. Perhaps the cognitive and physical limitations in the youngster controls the success rates in younger populations. The figures for children may be an underestimation, however, because of a tendency to misclassify suicide and suicide attempts as accidents. Generally, any suicidal statement made by a child should be taken seriously.

The effective management of the suicidal child includes the identification of individuals at risk and the development of a treatment program. Factors that affect the relative danger of suicide have been examined. Children are at higher risk for suicidal behavior if they have experienced parental loss, family psychopathology, divorce or family breakup, a recent death, or parental unemployment. Successful suicide is more prevalent in white males. Many of these children have been suffering from an affective disorder at the time of the suicide, complaining of feelings of hopelessness, low self-esteem, depression, and anhedonia. Environmental factors, including the availability of firearms, have affected the lethality of suicidal behavior in adolescents. Publicizing suicidal behaviors, either in the news media or through television drama, has been followed by an increase in the suicide rates among adolescents, suggesting that guidelines for the broadcasting of such information be created with input from mental health professionals. Education in the schools that involves staff and students increases the likelihood of early detection by improving the awareness in children of early warning signs. Children at risk are more likely to discuss their feelings when the environment is sympathetic to their needs, indicating that parental sensitivity is necessary in order to gain a child's confidence.

The assessment of suicidal behavior in children requires an investigation of four areas of functioning: social adjustment, life stressors, family functioning, and psychiatric disorder—as well as an evaluation of suicidal risk. The latter is based on a review of the lethality of the attempt and an understanding of the child's intention both at the time of the attempt and during the evaluation. Children who are actively suicidal during an interview will require inpatient psychiatric hospitalization. Hospitalization may also be considered when the patient does not have the available supports in the family or community to guarantee his or her safety. Outpatient psychiatric follow-up may adequately maintain the safety of the child when the suicidal intent is less serious and when sufficient supports are available. Uncovering the motivation behind the suicide attempt is essential to the treatment. Young patients may impulsively attempt to take their lives in fits of anger, jealousy, and frustration. Others are in such emotional turmoil that suicide may suddenly seem to be the best solution.

Blumenthal and Kupfer (1988) have developed a strategy for the identification of children at risk for suicidal behavior and the application of appropriate therapeutic interventions. Children are placed in three categories based on a combination of psychosocial factors.

The first level comprises children who are not suicidal and are not experiencing psychiatric disorder but who are likely to be influenced by environmental factors. These subjects are children of parents with histories of substance abuse, depression, and suicide; witnesses to significant levels of stress and trauma; or victims of sexual or physical abuse. All of these stressors are out of the child's control. The youngster is genetically vulnerable to psychiatric disorder based on the parental history. Education of the child and caretakers about the relative risk of suicide and the need for therapy is the primary intervention in these cases. The health care professional may be the first person outside the home to learn of the child's problematic history and should, therefore, carefully document concerns and recommendations. Psychiatric distress may initially present as somatic complaints and should be included in the differential diagnosis of those in whom symptoms persist or are poorly explained on an organic basis.

The second level includes children who are affected by stressors but are not yet suffering from a psychiatric disorder. The child may present with changes in academic functioning, problematic social relationships, learning disabilities, conduct problems, and decreased self-esteem. Mental health intervention is recommended and focuses on the assessment of suicidal risk as well as individual psychotherapy, behavioral therapies, special education programs, and group therapies.

The presence of psychiatric disorder is the criterion for inclusion in the third category. These children may suffer from affective disorder, anxiety disorder, conduct disorder, or substance abuse. The factors listed in levels 1 and 2 may also exist in these cases and increase the child's vulnerability to suicidal behaviors. More traditional psychiatric interventions are recommended in these cases, including individual, family, and group therapies; psychopharmacology; inpatient hospitalization; and drug and alcohol programs. These young patients are more likely to remain in the mental health system for extended periods with a course that may be unremitting and complicated.

DISRUPTIVE DISORDERS

Attention Deficit Hyperactivity Disorder

Attention deficit hyperactivity disorder (ADHD) is one of the most frequently diagnosed and closely examined psychiatric problems of childhood. The options for treatment are varied and are usually offered in combination. Intervention begins with the education of the patient and family about the etiology of the disorder, its clinical course, and the choices of treatment. Diagnoses that often accompany ADHD, like enuresis, conduct disorder, and sleep continuity disorder, are approached concurrently. Baseline assessments and evaluations of the success of treatment can be followed through the use of behavior rating scales completed by both parents and teachers.

Therapeutic Approaches

Behavioral therapy with children who suffer from ADHD attempts to balance rewards for appropriate actions with consequences for undesirable behaviors. Generally, behavioral interventions with ADHD children improve the quality of social interactions, academic productivity, and social skills according to parent, teacher, and observer reports. The limitations of the intervention can be found in the lack of generalization to different environments, the lack of consistency in the parents and teachers who utilize the method, and the investment of time, energy, and money necessary to derive benefits from the treatment. The benefits of behavioral interventions have been short-lived, however, and have not yet demonstrated long-term effectiveness.

Cognitive interventions for ADHD decrease the frequency of inappropriate behaviors by challenging the child to review the possible consequences before acting on impulse. This method has not generally been effective in relieving the target symptoms of ADHD. The intervention requires a level of sophistication that may not be evident in the young, often developmentally delayed child who suffers from ADHD.

Children with ADHD frequently have poor social skills because of a history of difficult relationships with peers and adults. Social skills training is a form of cognitive therapy that encourages appropriate responses in these children and has been helpful, particularly when used in combination with behavioral interventions and medication.

Pharmacotherapy

Stimulants. The pharmacotherapy for attention deficit hyperactivity syndromes includes the psychostimulants methylphenidate (Ritalin), dextroamphetamine (Dexedrine), and magnesium pemoline (Cylert). The medications have demonstrated clinical improvement in 75 per cent (versus 20 to 40 per cent in controls) of treated subjects and have been used in patients from prepubescence into adulthood. Use of stimulants in preschool children is indicated only after behavioral and environmental manipulations have failed. Very young children show higher rates of adverse reactions to medication, including sadness, irritability, clinging behaviors, insomnia, and anorexia.

The dosages of psychostimulants are adjusted according to weight. The starting dose of methylphenidate is usually 5 mg each morning for children weighing less than 30 kg. For larger children, the starting dose may be 10 mg; for preschoolers, a starting dose of 2.5 mg is appropriate. Doses of *d*-amphetamine are half those of methylphenidate. Methylphenidate is therapeutic at a dose of 0.3 to 0.7 mg/kg/dose, *d*-amphetamine at 0.15 to 0.5 mg/kg/dose. Pemoline doses begin at 18.75 mg/dose (37.5 for children heavier than 30 mg) and are increased to a target of 0.5 to 3 mg/kg/day. Increases in psychostimulant doses are made after 5- to 14-day observation periods, and the frequency of administration is usually twice per day. The behavioral effects of methylphenidate and *d*-amphetamine are seen within 30 to 60 minutes after administration and last for 3 to 6 hours. The sustained-release preparation of methylphenidate does not produce the kind of consistent therapeutic response that an additional dose of Ritalin in the afternoon would provide. Pemoline requires three weeks of administration to generate a therapeutic response, and its treatment effect lasts 5 to 6 hours. When one stimulant is not successful, 20 to 25 per cent of patients will respond with a medication change.

The most common side effects of stimulant medication are short-lived and include the following: anorexia, weight loss or decreased weight gain, headache, irritability, insomnia, social withdrawal, and abdominal pain. Patients occasionally have a paradoxical response to the stimulant medication and exhibit increased excitability, talkativeness, impulsivity, or insomnia 5 to 20 hours after the last dose. These problems are not simply a return to baseline behaviors, but an exacerbation of symptoms. Children who are given high doses of stimulants (greater than 1 mg/kg/dose) may suffer from a decrease in cognitive performance. Pemoline may adversely and irreversibly affect liver functioning in approximately 3 per cent of patients. In addition, pemoline may also induce movement disorders, night terrors, and lip licking and biting.

More serious medication side effects rarely occur, but these are worth noting. The most significant is the development of a tic disorder or the inducement of Tourette's disorder. The medications should be reduced, changed, or discontinued when such symptoms appear. A history of a tic disorder is a contraindication to the use of stimulants. Children may become depressed or dysphoric either during stimulant treatment or following drug withdrawal. Blood pressure and pulse rate may exhibit transient increases that are not typically clinically significant. Incidents of psychotic or disorganized behaviors are very infrequent but are characterized by hallucinations, delusions, and self-injurious behavior. Patients with psychotic symptoms should not be started on stimulants. Finally, concern has been expressed about growth retardation in patients on stimulants, particularly *d*-amphetamine. The cause of these mild changes is not clear, but the effects are usually temporary in prepubescent children, resolving after the medications are discontinued.

Antidepressants. TCAs have been effective in the treatment of ADHD, although not as successfully as psychostimulants. Studies have involved imipramine, amitriptyline, and desipramine, and the dosages are usually less than for the treatment of affective disorders (3 to 5 mg/kg/day). The effects of these medications may be rapid but short-lived, and patients do not exhibit much improvement in cognitive functioning. Antidepressants are reasonable alternatives to stimulants, but the long-term efficacy has not yet been proven.

Clonidine. Clonidine is an alternative to stimulant medication in the treatment of ADHD. The drug produces clinical improvement in the symptoms of motor activity, frustration tolerance, compliance, oppositionality, and aggression. Clonidine does not, however, improve the child's attentional skills or distractibility as well as psychostimulants do. Children with ADHD, accompanied by aggression and hyperarousal, who are not responsive to psychostimulants should be the target population for this medication. The dose is 5 μg/kg/day, divided into four doses. Sedation and hypotension are the most common side effects.

Additional Treatment Options

The recommendations for the most effective treatment of ADHD include a multimodal method that incorporates behavioral therapies and medication. Studies that have attempted to find some synergism in the combination of treatments, however, have not yet succeeded. Frequently in ADHD, a collaborative effort between the professional and the child's primary caretakers is required. Parent support groups not only provide comfort and reassurance but also educate about methods of intervention and the availability of resources. Special education programs allow the child to receive the tutoring, remediation, and individual attention that may be required in the classroom.

Conduct and Oppositional-Defiant Disorder

Conduct disorder, a set of behaviors that violates the rights of others, is a frequently diagnosed psychiatric problem in prepubescent children. The *DSM-III-R* criteria include stealing with or without confrontation, running away, lying, fire-setting, truancy from school, vandalism, disobedience, aggression, poor self-control, sensitivity to criticism, and poor social skills. Additional psychiatric diagnoses, like ADHD, affective disorder, anxiety, substance abuse, and specific developmental disorders, may occur with conduct problems and affect the course of treatment. Treating the accompanying psychiatric disorder may improve the child's conduct problems. Children with conduct disorder may be neurologically impaired, with evidence of seizure disorder or a history of head trauma. The latter may be secondary to physical abuse.

The treatment of conduct disorders effects change in home, school, and social environments. The assessment, therefore, should identify risk factors in those areas that may predispose the child to behavior problems. Psychopathology in the family system is particularly important. A family history of depression, alcoholism, marital discord, physical or sexual abuse, or criminal behavior increases the risk to the child. Problematic homes are those with increased size, poor organization, inconsistent discipline, and ineffective levels of communication.

Conduct disorder is usually treated on an outpatient basis. The decision for inpatient hospitalization for children rests on the risk of death or significant injury to the patient or to someone else and on the failure of an intensive outpatient or partial hospitalization treatment alternative.

Psychotherapy

Behavioral therapy has been particularly effective in the treatment of conduct disorders. The techniques that are most often recommended include contingency-based reinforcement, modeling, shaping, and consequences for inappropriate behaviors. Children who are less defiant and aggressive may respond to problem-solving skills training, a cognitive therapy that teaches children to anticipate the response that their behavior will generate in others.

Parent-management training educates parents on behavioral interventions that will increase socially appropriate and decrease deviant behaviors. Parents are encouraged to be consistent in reinforcing as well as limiting the children, and are expected to use clearly defined expectations that are well communicated to the child. In the process, the strengths and weaknesses of the family are identified and specific psychiatric problems, e.g., substance abuse, are addressed. Traditional family therapy methods that examine the child's role in the family system have had limited success.

Children may also be helped by social skills training, often conducted in group settings. Individual psychotherapy has not been effective in reducing the dysfunctional behavior in children with conduct disorders. Interventions of this sort require a degree of insight and motivation that these children rarely possess.

Psychosocial Interventions

Symptoms of conduct disorder may be the by-products of the child's environment. Treatment plans, therefore, should include a variety of psychosocial interventions. Children should be guided away from inappropriate peer groups who encourage deviant behaviors. Families under stress may require extensive and coordinated involvement by social welfare agencies. Occasionally, out-of-home placement in a crisis center, group home, or residential center is indicated. Classroom situations may not be providing either adequate education or proper communication between parent and teacher, necessitating consultation before the child's behavior can improve. The nature of the disorder often leads the child to the juvenile court system and requires collaboration between the therapist and officers of the court. Communities frequently provide additional aid to disturbed children through agencies like the Big Brother and Big Sister programs.

Medications

Pharmacotherapy in conduct-disordered children has usually focused on concomitant psychiatric disorders, i.e., stimulants for ADHD, antidepressants for mood disorder, and anticonvulsants for partial complex seizure disorder. Antipsychotic medications, particularly low-dose haloperidol (Haldol), have been used in cases of extreme aggression and psychosis but are not recommended in children because of the risk of extrapyramidal side effects. Lithium carbonate is promising as a treatment for the labile behavior that may accompany conduct disorder.

REFERENCES

American Psychiatric Association: Treatment of Psychiatric Disorders, Vols 1–3. Washington DC, American Psychiatric Association, 1989.

Blumenthal SJ, Kupfer DJ: Overview of early detection and treatment strategies for suicidal behavior in young people. J Youth Adolesc 17:1–23, 1988.

Lewis M: Child and Adolescent Psychiatry: A Comprehensive Textbook. Baltimore, Williams & Wilkins, 1991.

TICS AND TOURETTE SYNDROME

GERALD S. GOLDEN, M.D.

Tics are the most commonly occurring involuntary movements in childhood. They are sudden, rapid, meaningless, highly stereotyped movements that most frequently involve the face, neck, arms, and hands. Although most patients state that the tics occur without any warning, others feel a premonitory sensation that is relieved by making the movement. Some children have partial ability to suppress their tics but then will experience an increase in tic frequency when they relax. As with all dyskinesias, the frequency of occurrence of the abnormal movements is usually increased by stress.

Family studies have demonstrated that the tic disorders fall along a spectrum of severity. The most common and mildest form is *transient tic disorder.* One or more motor or vocal tics occur for longer than 2 weeks but resolve in less than 12 months. Onset is during childhood or early adolescence with a peak incidence at age 7 years. If the tics recur or last longer than 1 year and if motor or vocal tics, but not both, are present, a diagnosis of *transient motor* or *vocal tic disorder* is made. The presence of both motor and vocal tics that have persisted for more than 12 months is diagnostic of Tourette syndrome. In Tourette syndrome, there is a tendency for the pattern of tics to change over time and for the severity to wax and wane.

Many individuals with Tourette syndrome have additional symptoms. The most common of these are complex stereotyped movements, such as jumping, squatting down in place, or touching. Fewer than 20 per cent of patients develop *coprolalia,* the involuntary utterance of obscene words, or *copropraxia,* the involuntary making of obscene gestures. A smaller number of children have *echolalia,* repeating back the words of others, or *echopraxia,* imitating the movements of others. *Palilalia,* repeating one's own utterances, is fairly common. Although these associated features may assist with the diagnosis, they need not be present.

It has become clear that a number of other conditions are frequently associated with the tic disorders, particularly with Tourette syndrome. Patients may suffer more disability from the associated disorders than from the tics and vocalizations themselves. Symptoms of attention deficit hyperactivity disorder (ADHD) are present in 30 to 40 per cent of children with Tourette syndrome. The typical features of short attention span, impulsivity, and motor hyperactivity are present. ADHD typically antedates the onset of the tic disorder. Learning disabilities may be present with or without associated symptoms of ADHD. Although learning disabilities are common and some studies indicate a high incidence of difficulties with arithmetic, no specific pattern has been defined.

Obsessive-compulsive symptoms have recently been recognized as one of the most common associated problems. These often start in late childhood or early adolescence and may progress in severity to the point where a diagnosis of *obsessive-compulsive disorder* can be made. Genetic studies have shown that if obsessive-compulsive disorder and Tourette syndrome are assumed to be manifestations of the same genetic abnormality, the gene would transmit as an autosomal dominant with a penetrance of 1.0 in males and 0.7 in females. Females are more likely to have the obsessive-compulsive symptoms, whereas males are more likely to display the tic disorder.

The pathophysiology of the condition has not been fully defined, but clinical and laboratory evidence suggests that there is supersensitivity of D_2 dopamine receptors. Abnormalities in serotonin metabolism may also be involved, but the role of this and other neurotransmitters is not clear.

TREATMENT

Four critical components are involved in the treatment of children with tic disorders:

1. Treatment of the tics.
2. Treatment of the associated symptoms.
3. Educational placement.
4. Counseling.

Treating the Tic

The presence of a tic disorder is not a mandate for pharmacologic therapy. Tourette syndrome is a social disability, and the level and severity of this disability must be defined by the patient and the patient's family. Some individuals are quite comfortable with their symptoms, even if they are severe. Other children may be almost incapacitated because of the presence of one or two mild tics. Most clinicians are not encouraging the use of medication unless the symptoms cause a significant adjustment problem.

Treatment decisions also do not depend on whether the full diagnostic criteria of Tourette syndrome are present. Chronic motor or vocal tics are amenable to the same treatment strategies, and therapy should be attempted if the tics cause a major handicap in the child's ability to function. It is not appropriate to treat single, mild tics, except under unusual circumstance.

The most useful drugs in the treatment of both motor and vocal tics are the neuroleptics, probably because of their dopamine receptor–blocking action. Haloperidol and pimozide are most commonly used. Haloperidol is typically begun at a dose of 0.5 mg daily and increased by 0.5 mg daily every 4 or 5 days until the desired effect is obtained or further increase is limited by side effects. The average effective dose is 2 to 3 mg/day, and a beneficial therapeutic response is rarely seen at doses higher than 6 mg daily. Pimozide is started at a dose of 1 mg and increased to an average of 5 to 6 mg/day. Doses of pimozide greater than 12 mg daily are rarely useful. Fluphenazine may be better tolerated by some patients. Effective doses range from 1 to 5 mg daily. Neuroleptics produce significant reduction in the severity and frequency of tics in 80 to 85 per cent of patients.

Unfortunately, approximately 50 per cent of patients treated with these drugs will experience undesirable side effects; the most common are lethargy, dysphoria, and depression. Depression may become so severe that the child becomes suicidal. School phobia has also been reported to be a side effect of these drugs. Stimulation of appetite accompanied by excessive weight gain may also be a problem. Although all neuroleptic drugs, and particularly pimozide, may produce prolongation of the QT interval on the electrocardiogram, this does not appear to be a significant problem in the doses typically used. Extrapyramidal side effects of neuroleptic drugs can occur but are uncommon, and antiparkinsonian drugs are not given routinely.

Reports in the literature have suggested that clonidine is useful in the management of patients with Tourette syndrome, although some studies have not replicated the initially reported results. A trial of clonidine may be useful in patients who cannot tolerate neuroleptic drugs or in those who have associated ADHD. The starting dose is 0.05 mg/day, and this is gradually increased to a dose of 0.3 to 0.4 mg/day if tolerated. The major side effects are lethargy and postural hypotension.

Treating the Associated Symptoms

The treatment of ADHD associated with Tourette syndrome presents a therapeutic dilemma, as at least one third of patients show an increase in the severity of their tic disorder when given any of the commonly used psychostimulant drugs. The most conservative approach is to attempt first to manage the ADHD with behavioral strategies and appropriate classroom management techniques. If this is unsuccessful and if the symptoms of ADHD seriously interfere with the child's adjustment in school and at home, a trial of a psychostimulant drug is reasonable. If the tics worsen significantly, a second attempt to use behavioral strategies is warranted. If it becomes clear that the use of psychostimulant drugs is absolutely necessary but the level of tics becomes intolerable, the psychostimulant drugs can be continued and a neuroleptic added to control the movement disorder.

It appears that fluoxetine may be effective for the treatment of obsessive-compulsive disorder in Tourette syndrome. Although side effects are not a limiting factor in most patients, there is little experience with this drug in tic disorders and it has not been approved for use in children. Behavioral approaches have also been used in the management of obsessive-compulsive symptoms.

Educational Placement

School often presents a problem for children with Tourette syndrome because of the disruptive nature of the tics and other manifestations and the frequent association of ADHD and learning disabilities. The health care provider may have to take an active role in educating the school system about the nature of Tourette syndrome and helping them accept the fact that the child cannot control the tics and that it may be impossible to achieve a satisfactory therapeutic result with medication. If the patient is doing poorly in school, full evaluation is important to differentiate behavioral issues from learning disabilities.

Counseling

Many children with tic disorders and their families will require some level of counseling. This ranges in individual cases from nothing but the provision of factual information to intensive family therapy. It should be clear that the goal of counseling is not the elimination of the tic disorder but the resolution of the social and familial problems that arise in response to the tic disorder and its associated symptoms.

Genetic counseling must be based on clinical analysis of the family because the gene for the tic disorders has not been identified yet. Direct observation of family members is important, since it is a common occurrence to see that tics are present while the informant denies that he or she has ever had tics. If a family history of tics can be documented, the assumption of the presence of an autosomal dominant gene should be made. It should also be recognized, however, that the gene appears to have a broad range of expressivity.

SUMMARY

Tourette syndrome was initially considered to be a lifelong condition. It is now clear that most patients will show improvement, and many will go into remission, during the second half of adolescence. It is also common for patients to discontinue treatment with neuroleptic drugs as they approach adulthood even if the tic disorder continues. Follow-up studies have demonstrated that the majority of patients with Tourette syndrome make a reasonably good adult adjustment despite their disability.

The Tourette Syndrome Association* is an excellent source of information for patients, their families, schools, and health care providers.

*Tourette Syndrome Association, Inc., 42–40 Bell Blvd., Bayside, NY 11361. Phone: 718–224–2999.

AUTISM*

D. A. ALLEN, Ed.D.
and I. RAPIN, M.D.

Autism is a pervasive developmental disorder that involves serious deficits in socialization and interpersonal communication accompanied by a variety of perseverative and/or stereotypic behaviors and abnormal preoccupations. Autism is not a disease. Rather, it is a behavioral syndrome that reflects the dysfunction of as yet undetermined brain system(s).

Autism is a variable disorder, inasmuch as children with the diagnosis may exhibit a wide range of abnormal behaviors. The severity of the disorder varies as a function of both the number and kinds of autistic features exhibited and the level of cognitive functioning in a given child. Language disturbances may be manifested by total lack of language or by severely limited verbal output and poor comprehension in some children, whereas other children may exhibit hyperverbosity and large vocabularies that are clearly articulated but lack social appropriateness or conventional use. Some autistic children are totally withdrawn and unresponsive to other people. Others may be indiscriminately friendly or relate selectively to familiar people. Affect may be blunted or unmodulated. Cognitive levels in children with autism range from profound mental retardation in some to normal or even overdeveloped, isolated skills in others.

DIAGNOSIS

Pediatricians have an important role in the diagnosis and management of the autistic child because they are almost always the first professionals to see the child. Many autistic features are observable in infancy, and many parents are quite likely to detect and report to the physician that they are concerned about abnormal behaviors or developmental delays within the first year of life. Other parents report developmental arrest, usually between the ages of 12 and 36 months, after apparently normal early development. This arrest is followed by regression in the areas of language, socialization, and play without discernible cause and without loss of motor skills. The first obligation of the physician is to pay careful attention to such parental concerns. A detailed developmental history is a must.

The second obligation is to confirm as early as possible any suspicions of autistic behaviors by referring the family to a diagnostic center for a full multidisciplinary evaluation to determine more precisely the exact nature and extent of the child's deficits. The workup must include a definitive test of hearing, a full speech-language assessment, neuropsychologic testing, and a thorough behavioral observation, including, whenever possible, a psychiatric evaluation. The physician must ensure that specific genetic abnormalities such as fragile-X syndrome, tuberous sclerosis, phenylketonuria, and Rett syndrome have been considered, since they mandate genetic counseling. Conditions that require specific therapies must also be ruled out, notably absence seizures and hearing loss, because such conditions can co-occur with autism and because they also affect language development. Any autistic child who does not speak well must have a hearing test because failure to identify even a partial hearing loss can jeopardize any therapeutic effort directed at the child's inadequate communication skills. It is an error to ascribe autistic symptoms to lack of hearing and its consequent communication disorder: Even severely hearing impaired children in whom the diagnosis is missed do not evince autistic behaviors. Hearing-impaired children with autistic symptomatology are multihandicapped, with dysfunction of both the brain and the ear (as, for example, in rubella embryopathy). The same is true of blind children: Those with autistic behaviors suffer from both blindness and autism.

TREATMENT

Community Services

Once the diagnosis of autism has been confirmed, the pediatrician should be prepared to assume the responsibility for assisting the parents by coordinating the many services that will be needed throughout childhood. To assume the pediatric management of the autistic child, it is important that the physician be informed of the availability of services in the community.

The Education for All Handicapped Children Act of 1975, which resulted in Public Law 94–142 and the more recent Public Law 99–457, mandates that any child identified as handicapped between the ages of 3 and 21 years is entitled to "specially designed instruction, at no cost to parents or guardians, to meet the unique needs of a handicapped child, including classroom instruction, instruction in physical education, home instruction, and instruction in hospitals and institutions." In addition, related services, including transportation for such services, are to be provided free of charge. These services include speech-language therapy, physical, occupational, and recreational therapies, and psychologic and counseling services. Medical services necessary for diagnosis and evaluation are also provided for under this law.

Parents may not be aware that they are entitled to these educational and therapeutic services. Because the accessibility and means for obtaining these services vary by state and community, it is incumbent on the pediatrician to inform the

*Supported in part by Program Project Grant NS 20489 from the National Institute of Neurologic Diseases, Communication Disorders and Stroke, U. S. Public Health Service. The assistance of Carl Feinstein, M.D., who reviewed the manuscript, is gratefully acknowledged.

parents about how to proceed. Also, because the law provides only for those services required by each individual child, the physician in conjunction with the educational professionals and psychologists in the child's school district must document the need for such services.

The kinds of programs needed for an autistic child are determined by such factors as the age of the child, cognitive status, and physical condition. The severity and type of impairment in language as well as the extent of social, emotional, or behavioral abnormalities must also be considered. Optimally, a child's needs should be met by educators and therapists who are specialists in autism. However, such optimal conditions may not exist within the home community. In such cases, the parents may need the assistance of professionals to lobby for or help to establish appropriate programs or to facilitate admission to an available program in a community nearby.

Special Education

No child is too young to enter a remediation program. Taking a "wait and see" position is not useful for the family. Autism is a chronic, lifelong condition that children do not outgrow. On the other hand, with early intervention, many children can be helped to attain their highest possible level of functioning. Many communities provide infant stimulation programs that work with parents and children together, either at home or in a center. For toddlers and preschool children, a therapeutic nursery or preschool special education program that serves the needs of the autistic child and provides intensive parent counseling is the treatment of choice. These programs regularly address, through a combination of individual and group work, the deficits in language, socialization, and play. Behavioral management and/or behavior modification techniques are used to assist the child to establish mutual focus and self-control. The young autistic child, perhaps more than any other type of handicapped child, poses extraordinary demands on his family. A well-informed, supportive pediatrician can be of great help to the parents in the early years.

By the time an autistic child reaches school age, the parents of children who have received treatment and remediation in the early years often become experts in the care and management of their child. This expertise is frequently accompanied by frustration that the school personnel seem to know less about their child than they do. In addition, as the child becomes physically more mature, the kinds of demands made on the family may be quite different. Some autistic children become quite aggressive with parents and siblings. Here again, parent counseling, in some cases together with adjuvant medication of the child (see below), is often critical to the maintenance of the child in the home setting. Some communities offer sibling support groups as well as parent groups. The physician should become familiar with the Autism Society of America (ASA). This national group provides useful information to parents and professionals through its state and local chapters.

The Family

It is important that the pediatrician monitor the family situation. Although some families are able to function well with their autistic children, in far too many cases parents continue to attempt to care for severely afflicted children until the marriage dissolves and siblings are severely affected. In such cases, the pediatrician should be knowledgeable about alternative living arrangements, such as residential schools, and should be prepared to support the parents in placing the child.

By adolescence it will be clear whether or not the child will be able to function independently. Some high-functioning autistic individuals can be gainfully employed and manage their own affairs. More commonly, they will continue to need some adult supervision. Many communities in metropolitan areas are currently establishing group homes for autistic adolescents and adults. Again, parents should be informed about their child's alternatives.

Medications

It is common for autistic children to have symptoms reflecting the malfunction of other brain systems besides those that characterize them as autistic. Pharmacotherapy may be useful in the treatment of associated disorders such as seizures, tics, attention deficits with or without hyperactivity, explosive or aggressive behavior, mood disorders, anxiety, and self-mutilation. Unfortunately, many of the stigmatizing or troublesome symptoms of autism, such as stereotypy, perseveration, sensorimotor peculiarities, and aberrant social behaviors, are not amenable to pharmacologic intervention today.

A major problem when considering pharmacologic intervention in autistic children is that the disorder almost always reflects a static encephalopathy. Before committing a child to medical intervention, one needs to be sure that one is not buying relief of symptoms for the present at the expense of long-term, permanent side effects. Because some symptoms are often situationally determined and are more likely to occur in the less stringently structured milieu of the family than at school, one must always consider behavioral approaches to management as an alternative to pharmacology.

Seizures

Some 10 per cent of autistic children have clinical seizures, and they must be treated as one would treat a non-autistic child with epilepsy. Autistic children without clinical seizures whose language is very impaired or who are mute, especially those whose parents report deterioration of language in the toddler or early preschool years, must undergo electroencephalography (EEG) while sleeping: Some of them may be suffering from the syndrome of acquired aphasia with epileptiform EEG discharges, a syndrome particularly associated with profound lack of comprehension of acoustic language (verbal auditory agnosia or word-deafness). These paroxysmal EEG abnormalities are usually bilateral and are especially likely to be present during sleep, when they may dominate the tracing. (Nonparoxysmal EEG abnormalities do not warrant anticonvulsant therapy.)

A trial of adequate doses of anticonvulsants, such as carbamazepine, valproate, or phenytoin, documented by blood levels in the therapeutic range, may be justified in children without seizures whose EEG tracing is frankly epileptiform. Recent reports suggest that severe regression of language and behavior with an epileptiform EEG may warrant treatment with adrenocorticotropic hormone (ACTH) or high-dose steroids. This approach may be worth considering in view of the guarded prognosis. The physician must explain to the parents that prescribing anticonvulsants is controversial in the absence of clinical seizure and that the treatment may be ineffective. There is no clear means of determining when to stop therapy in children who do not have clinical seizures because there is likely to be a poor correlation between the appearance of the EEG and the child's language. The recommendation to give anticonvulsants a trial is motivated by the report of an occasional child whose language and behavior do improve with medication.

Tics

Occasionally, autistic children have tics, either isolated tics or the full-blown Tourette syndrome. Medications are used only when tics and vocalizations are severe enough to cause social problems in school or at home. Tics may respond to clonidine (Catapres), clonazepam (Klonopin), or haloperidol (Haldol) used together with benztropine (Cogentin). Haloperidol may produce acute dystonic reactions, parkinsonian side effects, and, in the long run, tardive dyskinesia, which may be irreversible. The dose is increased until the desired effect is achieved, then, after several weeks, decreased slowly to the smallest effective dose. Tics tend to wax and wane so that long-term medication is indicated only in severely affected children. There is no indication that medication alters the natural history of Tourette syndrome.

Attention Deficits

Many autistic children suffer from attention deficit disorder with hyperactivity (ADHD), which is often associated with sleep disturbance. The use of stimulant drugs, the most widely used pharmacologic approach to the treatment of ADHD in non-autistic children, is controversial in autistic patients. As in non-autistic children, methylphenidate (Ritalin), dextroamphetamine (Dexedrine), and pemoline (Cylert) have unpredictable effects. Stimulants may render some children even more hyperactive than before, whereas other children may be overly sedated even on small doses. Large doses of these drugs may exacerbate autistic behaviors and stereotypies or even precipitate a paranoid state with hallucinations. Yet, when stimulants are used cautiously, starting with a small dose that is increased slowly, some autistic children benefit just as much as non-autistic ADHD children, so that a trial is clearly justified. Whether tricyclic antidepressants have beneficial effects in autistic children with ADHD is uncertain as yet.

There is a larger experience with methylphenidate and dextroamphetamine than with pemoline, but long-term stimulant medication appears to be safe, with the notable caveat that it must be discontinued slowly (over several weeks) because children may become depressed if they are withdrawn too fast. The rule is that the smallest dose that produces the desired behavioral effect is the one used.

The starting dose of methylphenidate is 5 mg twice a day (b.i.d.) (morning and midday), increasing at the rate of 5 mg/dose no sooner than once a week so as to have a representative sample of behavior to evaluate effectiveness. Doses larger than 20 mg b.i.d. are rarely used.

Dextroamphetamine is used exactly like methylphenidate, but the effective dose is half that of methylphenidate. Both of these drugs are available in a sustained-release form that has the advantage of smoother release in some children. In others the greater timing flexibility of the short-acting form is preferable.

Pemoline is a longer-acting drug than methylphenidate and dextroamphetamine. The starting dose of pemoline is 18.75 mg in the morning; the maximum dose rarely exceeds 75 mg/day. The sleep disturbances of autistic children do not respond well to chronic administration of chloral hydrate or barbiturates, drugs that often increase agitation in hyperkinetic children. Some hyperkinetic children actually sleep better with stimulants.

Behavior Problems

Aggressive, impulsive behavior is often a major problem in autistic children. Aggression is frequently motivated by frustration but may also occur spontaneously with no obvious precipitant. Parents may lack knowledge of how to manage this kind of undesirable behavior. Autistic children who have not learned that aggression and tantrums will not be tolerated while they are small present severe problems once they are too big to be physically restrained. Physicians are then frequently pressed to prescribe neuroleptics or anticonvulsants to those children whose temper outbursts are mistaken for seizures.

There are anecdotal reports of both carbamazepine (Tegretol) and valproate (Depakote) improving behavior outbursts. Physicians should be aware that large doses of phenothiazines or butyrophenones may be required to decrease severe behavior disturbances, doses large enough to have sedative effects and doses that are likely to produce tardive dyskinesia if taken over many years. These large doses may also lower seizure threshold in the sizable minority of autistic children who have a tendency to seizures. Physicians also need to know that these medications must be withdrawn very slowly, over many weeks, if they have been taken chronically in high doses, in order to avoid severe emergent movement disorders and agitation. Small doses of haloperidol, on the order of 1 to 4 mg/day, are effective in some cases and have less sedative effect than does thioridazine. Small doses of thioridazine (Mellaril), such as 10 mg three times a day (t.i.d.), are marginally effective, so that improvement may be due to a placebo effect. (The same is true of very small doses of stimulant drugs.)

Thioridazine in higher doses, e.g., 50 mg t.i.d. or more, is frequently prescribed to autistic children with severe aggressive or self-injurious behaviors and to hyperactive patients who do not respond to stimulants. Thioridazine is less likely than haloperidol to produce acute dystonic side effects, but it has very significant and undesirable sedative effects. Some child psychiatrists recommend haloperidol in relatively high doses (5 to 8 mg/day) for relatively short courses in autistic children whose behavior is so out of control as to jeopardize school attendance, in the hopes of making the child amenable to behavioral intervention. A number of severely affected older autistic children are chronically medicated with thioridazine, chlorpromazine, and/or haloperidol. Most of these adolescents or young adults are in custodial situations at home, in group homes, or in other institutions. This approach must be considered a solution of last resort.

There was a great deal of hope that fenfluramine (Pondimin) would improve the behavior of autistic children because of its antiserotonergic activity. Although a few children respond to the drug, overall its effect has been disappointing. Clomipramine (Anafranil), a serotonin uptake inhibitor that improves obsessive-compulsive behaviors, may be helpful in some autistic children. Because of the small number of effective drugs to modify behavior in autistic children, other drugs such as hydroxyzine (Atarax) and thiothixene (Navane) are being tried. Thiothixene has the advantage of being less sedating than thioridazine, and it does not carry as much risk of dystonic reactions as haloperidol; its disadvantage is that it may decrease seizure threshold. Clinical experience with all of these drugs is still limited.

Unprovoked explosive behavior and major temper tantrums may respond to propranolol (Inderal) and other beta-blockers in children in whom these drugs are not contraindicated by a history of asthma. This is a novel indication for propranolol. One may start at a dose of 20 mg b.i.d. and work up to the maximum dose that does not produce bradycardia or arterial hypotension. A combination of propranolol and desipramine (Norpramin) may be more effective in some aggressive autistic children than propranolol alone. Beta-blockers are indicated in children in whom panic or extreme anxiety plays a role in precipitating behavioral explosions.

Depression

Some autistic children and adolescents may show signs of depression. They may respond favorably to the use of such antidepressants as imipramine (Tofranil), nortriptyline (Pamelor), desipramine, or amitriptyline (Elavil). Some agitated autistic children, especially if there is a family history of manic-depressive illness, may respond favorably to lithium.

Anxiety

Many autistic children are anxious. Anxiety may contribute to explosive and hyperkinetic behaviors. In addition to the beta-blockers, drugs such as lorazepam (Ativan) and aprazolam (Xanax) are sometimes prescribed by child psychiatrists and physicians familiar with psychopharmacology. As is true of psychotropic drugs in general, anxiolytic drugs produce physiologic dependence, and therefore must be tapered slowly after prolonged administration so as not to precipitate significant worsening of the symptoms for which they were prescribed in the first place.

Self-Mutilation

One of the most distressing symptoms in severely affected autistic children is self-mutilation. Self-mutilation may take the form of head banging, self-biting, or hitting the head with the hands or fists; this behavior may increase when the child is frustrated or anxious. Self-mutilation does not respond well to tranquilizers unless they are prescribed in sedative doses. Propranolol, the antidepressants, and antipsychotic drugs may help some children. Because of the hypothesis that self-mutilation might be due to excessive levels of endogenous endorphins, a trial of the oral opiate antagonist naltrexone (Trexan) has been suggested. Such a use must be considered experimental.

Polypharmacy

Clearly, the average pediatrician will not be familiar with many of these psychotropic agents and will need to seek a consultation with a child psychiatrist with experience in psychopharmacology. A major pitfall, and one to be strenuously avoided, is to try one drug, then add another and another in an attempt to address each of the child's symptoms. Polypharmacy results in dull, overdrugged children and, occasionally, in life-threatening toxicity. As is true in the case of anticonvulsants, one needs to try one drug at a time and push it to result in either clear improvement or undesirable side effects, then withdraw it slowly before trying another one unless symptoms are so severe as to mandate transient drug overlap.

Behavioral Management and Psychotherapy

Child psychiatrists, psychologists, and special educators with training in behavioral management techniques are often helpful in assisting the parents with the management of autistic children. Some high-functioning children and adolescents can benefit greatly from adjunctive supportive psychotherapy. These intelligent autistic children, after appropriate early intervention, may be educated later on with normal or learning-disabled children. Because autism comprises a spectrum of disorders, it is important to prescribe for each individual child, not for the diagnosis. On the other hand, as more severely affected autistic children grow older, some of them become violent or overtly psychotic and therefore require psychiatric hospitalization for optimal management with psychotropic medication in a controlled environment. The most severely impaired cannot be managed in the community and require long-term residential placement.

SUMMARY

Autism is the most complex of the developmental disorders of brain function. It mandates behavioral, educational, and medical interventions. Autism is the result of a multidetermined encephalopathy that is not well understood and is not curable with today's knowledge. This is not to say that it is hopeless, however, since many of its symptoms may be ameliorated. Prognosis is a function of both the severity of the disorder in the individual child and of the effectiveness and timeliness of the interventions provided.

PSYCHOSOMATIC ILLNESS

RICHARD B. GOLDBLOOM, O.C., M.D., FRCPC

The term psychosomatic illness has been used traditionally as the obverse of "organic" disease in explaining symptoms. However, emotional and organic disorders are not mutually exclusive and often coexist in the same child. Abdominal pain, headache, or fatigue of emotional origin is often as real to the child as when the same symptoms arise from inflammatory bowel disease, migraine, or infectious mononucleosis. Psychosomatic illness is not a form of malingering; the suffering is real. A cardinal rule of management, therefore, is not to try to talk the child out of the symptom, which usually disappears spontaneously after the underlying problem is identified and remedied.

For some infants, the earliest psychosomatic disorder may be represented by excessive crying or "colic"—often interpreted by parents and physicians (rightly or wrongly) as indicative of an organic problem (e.g., abdominal cramps or food allergy) and managed empirically and often ineffectively by formula juggling.

Another disorder of infancy and early childhood that appears to comprise a mixture of somatic and psychologic components is *breath-holding spells.* Although these may begin very early in infancy and a positive family history of similar spells is often present, the majority of episodes are typically triggered by conditions that cause the child pain, anger, or frustration. Because there is no reliable method of averting the episodes, the essential components of management are (1) identifying the parents' frequently unverbalized fear that the child is going to die during an episode and reassuring them unequivocally that this will not happen, and (2) explaining the common incidence and natural history of breath-holding spells, which disappear spontaneously during the early years of childhood, leaving no untoward aftereffects.

In pre-adolescents and adolescents, *hyperventilation* and *chest pain* are two of the more common psychosomatic symptoms associated with anxiety. It has been suggested that the "risk factors" for such complaints include above-average intelligence, a tendency to internalize (rather than verbalize) anxiety and anger, and a past history of expressing emotional tensions somatically. This is a widespread clinical impression, but I am not certain that it has been confirmed by properly designed studies. For some reason, hyperventilation appears to occur much more frequently in females than in males.

In adolescents who complain of transient episodes of chest pain without associated symptoms, underlying organic disease is rarely identified. When told that many teenagers experience occasional sudden, sharp chest pain and that many worry that it might mean something serious (especially heart trouble or cancer), adolescents will often acknowledge such anxieties. Further inquiry may disclose that a relative or acquaintance has had a recent myocardial infarction or has been found to have a malignancy. Simply uncovering the roots of the anxiety, coupled with reassurance about excellent general health and a prediction of longevity, may be all the treatment that is required.

It has long been recognized that adolescents or young adults recovering from viral illness (e.g., "flu-like" illnesses, infectious mononucleosis) may complain for long periods of fatigue, lack of energy, and other nonspecific symptoms. Various labels have been applied to such individuals, e.g., *post-flu syndrome, post-viral syndrome,* and, most recently, *chronic fatigue syndrome* or *myalgic encephalomyelitis.* The etiologic diagnostic categorization of this group of patients is still poorly defined. Undoubtedly included are some adolescents with persistent viral infection and others in whom the symptoms are associated with underlying depression or other emotional disturbances. Attaching diagnostic labels to such youngsters can be therapeutically counterproductive unless the evidence to support a specific diagnosis is conclusive.

Eating disorders such as *anorexia nervosa* and *bulimia nervosa* may also be regarded as psychosomatic illnesses, but these are dealt with in detail elsewhere in this book (see Section 22).

In the interests of successful management, psychosomatic illness should never be a diagnosis of last resort or physician frustration, entertained only after a lengthy series of investigations have been performed to exclude an organic cause for the child's symptoms and have produced negative results. When a child complains of recurrent abdominal pain and the history and physical examination offer no immediately obvious explanation, the effects of hospital admission, imaging studies, or laboratory tests can be therapeutically counterproductive, giving mixed messages to the child and family (if the doctor is so sure Johnny's symptoms are psychosomatic, why did he/she do all those tests?). Thus, the child or family may understandably doubt a diagnosis of psychosomatic illness by exclusion and wonder whether the physician has simply failed to discover the cause, which, by the way, the family often suspects to be serious. This sequence of events establishes a shaky foundation for psychotherapeutic intervention, whether by a pediatrician, psychologist, or psychiatrist.

When it is thought that a child's symptoms *may* be psychosomatic, that possibility should be discussed openly with the child and the parents at the very outset, *especially* if any "organic" types of investigation are planned. "I don't know about you, but many youngsters get tummy aches when they are worried or upset, so we have to find out whether that is what your problem is or if something in your tummy needs to be fixed. Either way, we will try to make you better." Treatment as well as diagnosis begins at the start of the history-taking interview.

When symptoms such as headache, "feeling sick," or recurrent abdominal pain are clearly manifestations of school anxiety or school refusal, the first principle of management is to get the youngster back to school immediately and *then* deal with the underlying problem. A telephone call to the child's teacher can be an invaluable aid to rapid, successful treatment, and it provides an opportunity to find out how the youngster is performing academically and is behaving at school; it also allows the physician to enlist the teacher (with the parents' concurrence) as a therapeutic ally. Giving the child a feeling of importance by assigning special classroom responsibilities, laced with extra doses of recognition and praise, may go a long way toward relieving school-generated anxiety and any associated somatic symptoms.

Effective management of psychosomatic symptoms involves identifying and improving the underlying problem rather than focusing on the symptom. The first step is a thorough history and a family interview, preferably involving both parents and, when appropriate, siblings as well. Special emphasis should be placed on the context of the symptom complaint—when does it occur and what are the aggravating and relieving factors? Is there a relationship of symptoms to school? Do the symptoms occur chiefly on school days, in the morning before going to school, or during school hours?

Who is the patient? Is it the child, or is he or she the sounding board for an underlying family problem? A detailed family and psychosocial history is the most essential ingredient of good management. As a minimum, this should include the following important elements:

1. *Domiciliary history.* Description of the home and its inhabitants: documentation of any and all domiciliary moves (often a major source of family dysfunction).
2. *Occupational and employment history of parents.* Are there any financial problems?
3. *Substance abuse.* Alcoholism is an extremely common, often unrecognized source of family tension and of psychosomatic symptoms in children.
4. *Psychiatric illness.* Depression or other.
5. *Recreational history.* An important clue to quality of family functioning. What do they do as a family for recreation, and how often?
6. *History and direct observation of family interaction.* How do they look? What do they say? What do they do? The three key elements of good family function are shared labor, warm and effective communication, and leadership (as opposed to domination). These can be evaluated readily in most families through straightforward questioning and through direct observation of their verbal and nonverbal interactions. It is of great help to have at least some interaction with all caretakers of the patient (remember the increasing use of child care helpers in home).

As with most illnesses, a clear description of the onset and surrounding circumstances may help to identify and deal with causative issues. Major life events, such as significant illness, death, divorce, marital stress, parental absence, or birth of a sibling, may trigger psychosomatic symptoms in susceptible youngsters. *Anxiety* is the most contagious of childhood diseases. Therefore, identifying the presence, nature, and severity of current parental anxieties may be critical to accurate diagnosis and effective management. For school-aged children, the educational history may yield important clues. Is the youngster in the appropriate grade for age? Any repeats? Any help from the resource teacher? Best and worst subjects? Relationships with teachers and peers? (Again, a telephone call to the child's teacher can be extremely valuable.)

Many families harbor secret concerns that they rarely express unless questioned directly; for example, the silent fear that the child's symptoms may signify serious illness (cancer, leukemia, brain tumor, heart trouble). Even when such fears go unmentioned at home, children sense their parents' anxiety, which in turn compounds their own worry. A style of questioning that emphasizes the frequency and acceptability of such concerns often exposes the secret: "I don't know about you, but a lot of parents of youngsters with (e.g.) headaches like Johnny's worry that it might be something serious—like a brain tumor." A short pause allows the parents to confirm or deny, nonverbally or verbally, the existence of such anxieties, which can then be dealt with on the spot.

Abdominal pain and *headache* are two of the most common psychosomatic complaints in children. When headache is the problem, the process is often one of psychosomatic synergism, in that, as in migrainous adults, tension or anxiety may serve as a major trigger for headaches in children who are genetically susceptible to migraine. Good, comprehensive management requires identification and remediation of *all* trigger factors that may initiate the headaches, including foods, exposure to sunlight, and distress over family problems or school.

In children with recurrent abdominal pain, investigative protocols of laboratory tests and imaging studies almost never yield diagnostically useful information unless specifically indicated by the history and physical findings.

Hysterical or conversion symptoms in older children and adolescents occasionally take bizarre forms such as weakness or paralysis. In such instances, the history and physical findings are often inconsistent on logical grounds with each other or with the child's level of anxiety or lack thereof (*la belle indifference* or the "smiling complainer"). However, this particular affect is neither diagnostic nor reliably present in conversion disorders.

When straightforward exposition of the underlying emotional problem and reassurance are insufficient to resolve the problem, there is no all-purpose treatment protocol for children with psychosomatic disorders. The approach must be custom-tailored to the child's age, the severity and duration of symptoms, and the complexity of the contributory factors. Based on these and on the skills and comfort of individual physicians in undertaking treatment, a decision must be made on the issue of the need for psychiatric referral. For those who feel comfortable with undertaking management, the basic principles of the therapeutic contract should be observed, including:

1. Agreement between physician and family on the nature of the problem.
2. Agreement on short-term tasks to be undertaken by the child and/or individual family member, the teacher, or other person.
3. Agreement on a short-term reporting-back arrangement (usually within 7 to 14 days) to report the response to treatment and determine further steps required.

Behavioral monitoring in a way that involves the family on a short-term basis may be a diagnostic revelation as well as a potent mechanism for therapeutic change. Symptom monitoring is well established in psychiatry to reduce symptom level.

COMMON SLEEP DISORDERS IN CHILDREN

RONALD E. DAHL, M.D.

Sleep-related problems occur frequently in children and adolescents. Numerous well-controlled studies have documented prevalence rates for significant sleep problems ranging from 20 to 30 per cent in community samples as well as pediatric clinic populations. In many cases, disturbed sleep is simply a mild behavioral problem in an otherwise healthy child. In other cases, however, sleep-related symptoms may represent a serious disorder, such as narcolepsy, or may be one component in a larger set of emotional or psychiatric symptoms. In addition, the relationship between sleep and behavioral/emotional problems appears complex. That is, behavioral and emotional problems can contribute to sleep disturbances and, conversely, inadequate sleep can adversely affect mood and behavior. Given these complexities, treatment decisions should be balanced with consideration of further assessment, especially in the older child or adolescent with persistent sleep problems.

SLEEPLESSNESS IN THE VERY YOUNG CHILD

Difficulties in going to sleep and staying asleep are most often related to sleep-onset associations (learned and conditioned factors associated with going to sleep). Some infants learn self-comforting behaviors (such as thumb-sucking, face stroking, body rocking, hair twirling); others use transition objects (pacifier, teddy bear, blanket), and others cue to a parental behavior (such as being held or rocked). It is important to understand that all infants and children normally wake up multiple times at night but put themselves back to sleep uneventfully using the same self-comforting techniques or cues used to go to sleep initially. Children who fall asleep while being held, rocked, or fed may require the same parental interaction to go back to sleep following normal nighttime arousals. Optimal treatment for sleeplessness in the young child usually consists of behavioral techniques focussed on helping the child develop *self-comforting behaviors* to substitute for parental comforting behaviors at sleep onset. This topic has been well reviewed by others (Ferber, 1987).

PARTIAL AROUSALS (NIGHT TERRORS, SLEEPWALKING, CONFUSIONAL AROUSALS)

Partial arousals from deep non–rapid-eye movement (non-REM) sleep may manifest as night terrors, sleepwalking, sleeptalking, or confusional arousals. (Enuretic events occurring in the first 1 to 3 hours of the night may also be related to partial arousals.) Partial arousals occur commonly from age 3 to 8 years, developmental ages corresponding with the greatest amount of intensity of deep stage 4 sleep. Stage 4 sleep is the deepest sleep in humans, usually occurring in the first 1 to 3 hours after sleep onset. The transition out of stage 4 to light sleep can fragment into a mixed state of arousal (partially awake and partially in a deep sleep). The character of these partial arousals can vary from mild events (a few awkward movements or calm mumbling) to intense events (a full-blown night terror with agitated running and screaming). The episodes typically last from 30 seconds to 10 minutes and usually terminate with an abrupt return to deep sleep with the child having no memory of the event in the morning.

There are four important factors in treating partial arousals:

1. Reassuring the parents as to what these events are. (The events can be extremely frightening to parents because children can appear awake but confused and unresponsive.)
2. Explaining to the family that the events are physiologic, they terminate spontaneously with return to deep sleep, and there is no advantage to trying to awaken or shake the child during the event.
3. Instructing the family to ensure physical safety for children having frequent or intense events. (Although self-injury is rare, a safe physical environment is required, as these children are essentially asleep and can become agitated.)
4. Ensuring optimal nighttime sleep.

The role of adequate nighttime sleep in partial-arousal events is a crucial point. Any factor that can result in "overtiredness" in a child (such as giving up a daytime nap, erratic changes in bedtime and wake-up time, the need to get up early for day care, or disturbed nighttime sleep) can contribute to partial-arousal events. The physiologic adaptation to getting less sleep (or to chronically disturbed sleep) is an increase in the *depth* of stage 4 sleep. Increased depth of sleep makes the transition out of stage 4 more difficult and is more likely to result in a partial-arousal event. *Thus, increasing the total amount of sleep (by 30 to 60 minutes a day) over 1 to 2 weeks can dramatically decrease the frequency of partial-arousal events.* Similarly, removing the cause of a chronic sleep disturbance (such as a tonsillectomy in a child with sleep apnea) can also produce a rapid resolution of partial arousals. Nighttime medications (e.g., theophylline) and medical conditions (e.g., atopic dermatitis or conditions with chronic pain) can also cause chronic sleep disturbances and resulting partial arousals.

One additional factor that can negatively feed into the cycle of partial arousals is the role of children being overly "wound up" during the day. Although the mechanism is unclear, children with a large degree of unexpressed anxieties and worries are more prone to partial arousals. Helping these children express their anxieties and concerns (therapeutically) has been documented to resolve partial arousals in some of these cases.

When optimal nighttime sleep has been achieved and intense partial arousals continue, medications can be an important adjunct to treatment. Benzodiazepines and tricyclic antidepressants are effective in decreasing the depth of stage 4 sleep and suppressing partial arousals. Diazepam (at a dosage between 1 and 5 mg at bedtime) and imipramine (25 to 50 mg at bedtime) have been used successfully in treating these events. At our Center, we have also had success using clonazepam (0.25 mg at bedtime) in some very severe cases (with multiple partial arousals every night). It is important to caution that there are no controlled trials to guide the use of pharmacotherapy for this disorder. Further, tolerance (the need to increase the dose over time) and rebound effects (severe partial arousals when the medication is discontinued) can be significant.

OBSTRUCTIVE SLEEP APNEA SYNDROME

Children with enlarged tonsils or adenoids often have increased breathing difficulties during sleep (especially during REM sleep, which causes a significant loss of muscle tone to airway and accessory muscles). Children with Down syndrome, micrognathia, hypotonia, some cleft palate repairs, and other maxillofacial conditions are at increased risk for obstructive sleep apnea syndrome (OSAS). Snoring, restless sleep, and signs of chronically disturbed sleep (daytime somnolence *or* irritability) are important signs suggesting OSAS.

Three important points are relevant to treatment decisions in OSAS in children:

1. The size of the tonsils and adenoids alone is *not* a good predictor of which children will have breathing difficulties during sleep.
2. The loudness of snoring is *not* a good predictor of respiratory difficulties, as some children with severe apnea are reported by parents as just "noisy" breathers.
3. There are two domains of disturbances in OSAS—the degree of breathing impairment (number and length of apneic events) *and* the degree of chronic sleep disturbance. This last point is often overlooked in treatment decisions. Chronically disturbed sleep in *prepubertal* children often presents as irritability, difficulty with concentration, emotional lability, and impulsivity. These children are often difficult to awaken in the morning; however, once up, they can appear hyperactive and may not look somnolent during the day. We have seen numerous children with OSAS receiving stimulant medication for their "attention deficits." Although stimulants do improve symptoms resulting from inadequate sleep, proper treatment requires removing the cause of sleep disturbance. *Tonsillectomy and/or adenoidectomy is the treatment of choice for most children with OSAS.* In other cases, nasal continuous–positive airway pressure (C-PAP) or oral devices to maintain airway patency may be indicated. More involved surgery, such as uvulopalatopharyngoplasty (as used in adult apnea), does not have a proven role in childhood OSAS.

SLEEP-WAKE SCHEDULE DISORDERS

Adolescents frequently develop very late sleep-wake schedules during summers, vacations, and weekends, often "sleeping in" until mid-day. For many of these adolescents, trying to realign their circadian systems to early school schedules is analogous to "jet lag." Many of these adolescents have great difficulties falling asleep at night and are unable to get up on time for school. Severe problems can result in repeated school tardiness and school failure. In some cases, the problem is straightforward: the adolescent is having trouble consistently complying with an earlier bedtime. In other cases, however, even though the adolescent and family are highly motivated to shift to earlier hours, the adolescent has difficulty falling asleep because the circadian temperature rhythm (and timing of physiologic "tiredness") has not been successfully shifted to an earlier hour. A central concept in treating this problem is understanding the circadian regulatory system, which has difficulty adjusting to an *earlier* phase unless changes are small, gradual, and *consistent.* As with jet lag, different components of the system can readjust at different rates and may require 2 weeks on a new schedule to *stabilize* at the earlier time. The problem for many adolescents is that after working hard toward an earlier schedule for a few nights, they revert back to their late night (sleeping-in) schedule on weekends. *Successful treatment requires a structured behavioral contract specifying bedtimes (with lights, television, and music out), exact wake-up times, and avoidance of all naps for a 2- to 3-week period including weekends.* Encouraging the adolescent to take responsibility for the schedule with appropriate rewards-consequences is also important. Parents' roles should be simply enforcing the contract, not fighting with the adolescent to get up in the morning. Early morning activity and exposure to bright light (such as a walk outside) are also important adjuncts to shifting rhythms to an earlier phase. In severe cases involving very late schedules, it can be easier to use successive *delays* in schedule by 3 hours a night (essentially going all the way around the clock until bedtime lines up with early clock time). This technique (called chronotherapy) has been used to treat many adults with delayed sleep phase syndrome. A detailed description of a program for adolescents has also been described (Dahl, 1992).

REFERENCES

Dahl RE: Child and adolescent sleep disorders. *In* Kaufman, DM (ed): Neurology for Child Psychiatrists. Baltimore, Williams & Wilkins, 1992, pp 169–194.

Ferber R: Sleeplessness, night awakening, and night crying in the infant and toddler. Pediatr Rev 9:69–82, 1987.

VOICE, SPEECH, AND LANGUAGE DISORDERS

CHARLOTTE E. JOHNSON, L.C.S.T., Ph.D.

Evaluation and treatment of communication disorders is the responsibility of certified, and often licensed, speech-language pathologists. However, physicians have important responsibilities, primarily in (1) prevention, (2) recognition of the need for evaluation, (3) support of appropriate intervention, and (4) advocacy for the child within the family and the community. All four responsibilities are woven through the following discussions, but prevention deserves separate discussion at the outset.

PREVENTION

Five to 10 per cent of preschool children have trouble acquiring language and speech; those with communication disorders are at greater risk for future learning and behavioral problems. Children who have had remediation by age 5½ ultimately show fewer disorders. Therefore, communication problems deserve early recognition and management. The best single resource for finding professionals qualified in evaluation and treatment is the American Speech-Language-Hearing Association (ASHA),* which is the credentialing body for speech-language pathologists in the United States.

The pediatrician (or other primary care provider) can offer valuable advice to parents and caretakers. Children do not learn communication automatically, and the model provided by adults from the beginning is crucial. Parents may need help in understanding and reinforcing their child's attempts to communicate from the earliest days. Such responsiveness is more valuable than any other language teaching technique.

As children become more active communicators, the role of parents as models should continue. Parents should, for example, be careful about (1) not speaking too fast, (2) pausing a few seconds before answering; (3) not changing the topic without warning; (4) taking time to explain plans and changes; and (5) showing the child that he or she is being heard. Many parents need advice about good vocal habits, e.g., keeping the general noise level down so that speaking and hearing take place at comfortable volume levels. A child who learns high-volume conversation as the norm is at greater risk for abuse of the laryngeal mechanism. The pediatrician or other caregiver can guide the parents in these habits and thus perhaps prevent unnecessary problems for the child.

VOICE DISORDERS

Infancy and Early Childhood

A significant deviation in either vocal production or resonance in very young children is generally an indication that something is amiss in the structure or innervation of the voice and resonance system. A weak or hoarse cry should raise questions about laryngeal webbing or stenosis and, if accompanied by inspiratory stridor, may indicate laryngomalacia. Such a child should be referred to an ear-nose-throat (ENT) specialist for further evaluation.

Hypernasality (excessive nasal resonance), especially if accompanied by feeding, swallowing, or choking difficulties, may be an indication of velopharyngeal insufficiency (VPI). Such resonance problems reflect disorder in a complex interactive neuromuscular system and should be managed by a cleft palate team. A referral to the best center nearby that can offer comprehensive evaluation and program planning services should be provided.

School Age and Adolescence

The most common problem in school-aged children and adolescents is vocal cord nodules. There is evidence for a hemorrhagic etiology and an inflammatory process at work in the early period of nodule formation; but once nodules become chronic, various tissue changes take place involving a shift from edema to fibrosis. Nodules are more common in boys than girls, although at puberty the incidence declines in boys. Adolescent female cheerleaders and sports enthusiasts are at risk. Many vocal cord nodules, in the early stages, respond to vocal re-education and therapy. After the nodules become chronic, surgical removal is necessary. However, surgery alone is not the final answer. The nodules are likely to reappear unless the child is led to understand his or her role and responsibility in management of vocal function. The practitioner's responsibility in this disorder is to seek ENT consultation, to support a trial of voice therapy before recommending surgery, and to encourage child and family participation in vocal rehabilitation.

Resonance disorders are more often concerned with hyponasality than hypernasality (which has usually been identified earlier). Decrease in nasal resonance may indicate enlarged adenoidal mass or other obstruction. If surgery is indicated, a possible complication is ensuing hypernasality, particularly following removal of an adenoidal mass that has long been part of the velopharyngeal valving mechanism. It may take the child some time to accommodate to the structural and dynamic change.

One voice disorder of adolescents concerns pubertal voice change. For some young people, therapy directed to the voice itself and to appropriate pitch for gender and age is sufficient. For others, the voice problem may indicate more deep-seated problems, which should be addressed by mental health professionals.

SPEECH DISORDERS (ARTICULATION AND FLUENCY)

Articulation Disorders

Articulation refers to the motor activities involved in speaking, a complex neuromuscular sequence. Difficulty in articulation creates a problem with intelligibility: the child's ability to be understood. Articulation develops over time, and a normal child's ability improves with practice. "Normal" covers a fairly wide range; boys are often slower than girls in achieving clear, intelligible speech. Many parents become frustrated by "error" patterns that are developmentally normal. The physician should be alert to the parent who is overfocused on intelligibility to the detriment of growth in overall language and communication.

Preschool children who sound immature, using sound patterns more typical of a younger child, may benefit far more from nursery school or a play group than from parental attempts to correct them; indeed, such tactics often backfire. Parents should be encouraged instead to provide good communication models by talking more slowly, repeating correctly to the child what they have said, and by having age-appropriate expectations.

There are two major categories of neurologically based articulation problems—dysarthria and dyspraxia. *Dysarthria,* usually characterized by slurred speech patterns and often by disorders of voice production and resonance, indicates problems of neuromuscular coordination and motor performance. It may well be part of a more basic disorder, e.g., cerebral palsy. Children with dysarthria also have trouble with the vegetative aspects of oral motor function and have often had feeding problems since early life. Management of such difficulties is best entrusted to a specialized multidisciplinary habilitative team. In severe cases *(anarthria),* or when respiration, phonation, and articulation are impaired, useful oral language may never develop. Direct or switch access to an electronic communication device is available to almost any child, and a speech-language pathologist will teach the child to converse and learn with a system, much as he or she might teach an oral language user.

In *dyspraxia* or *apraxia,* the ability to plan and perform voluntary complex motor sequences is disrupted. Eating is not a problem because its sequences are organized at an automatic level. But the apraxic child has serious difficulties with sound production, especially with words. The 2-year-old with normal comprehension but no enjoyment of sound, who is silent even at home, should be monitored by a speech-

*ASHA, 10801 Rockville Pike, Rockville, MD 20852.

language pathologist. In some cases, augmentative communication systems (total communication, i.e., combined use of sign and talking or a communication board or device) may be recommended to relieve the child's frustration. Early education programming may need to be based in alternative communication modes, and the family will need support in meeting the child's needs. Many such children eventually become oral communicators. However, early intervention and long-term treatment strategies are critical as these children work to establish motor patterns that come easily to others.

A second group of articulation disorders is *phonologic disorder.* The children have difficulty learning and using the rules for sound families and sound sequences. Sound patterns in their speech do not resemble those of younger children, and their intelligibility problems are usually severe. They may omit initial or final consonants, confuse front and back sounds (e.g., t or k), or omit whole classes of sounds (e.g., no fricatives like s, f, or th).

Such children, by 3 or 4 years of age, can benefit from a therapeutic program based on sound rules rather than on wrong versus right. Remediation prior to kindergarten often produces good communicative and academic results. Those still struggling with sound systems after beginning school are clearly at higher risk for problems in learning to read and write because the essential relationships between sound and symbol will be harder to learn.

Fluency Disorders

Although it is not uncommon for children to experience normal or "linguistic" dysfluency during the years of rapid language expansion (between 2 and 5), some verbal 2- and 3-year-olds have a true fluency disorder, i.e., stuttering. The distinction lies not in age, but in the nature, frequency, and intensity of the dysfluent behaviors. Stuttering is much more common among boys (ratios of up to 8:1 have been cited), and does seem to run in families.

Some typical or normal dysfluencies are occasional interjections, phrase revisions, phrase repetitions, one or two word or syllable repetitions, and unfinished words. The child seems unaware of what he or she is doing. It is as though the child is challenging the communicative system to its limits, using repetition to plan the rest of the utterance without "yielding the floor."

Some less typical dysfluencies are cause for concern and probable referral. They include word and syllable repetitions of more than three; sound repetitions; sound prolongations, sometimes with voice changes; blocking; tensions associated with talking; and avoidance of talking. These are clear signals of anxiety about talking. Children who stutter should be referred for professional treatment immediately, regardless of age. The pediatrician should advise parents that early intervention will involve them to a great degree and may seem to be more parent-oriented than child-oriented.

LANGUAGE DISORDERS

Language disorders are complicated and significant problems that may be difficult to diagnose. The use of the Denver Developmental Screening Scale alone is not enough. The Early Language Milestones Scale is a valuable tool. Further, a period of observation may validate the parents' report of home-based skills or may reveal that parents need to give the child a large number of nonverbal cues.

Language disorders in young children raise diagnostic questions. One is the relationship between language abilities and overall development. Sometimes children with developmental difficulties are first identified by the absence of expressive language. For a nontalking 2-year-old, one should explore the ability to understand and the level of skill in early self-help as well as the ability to hear. If the child has a general lag in development, communication ability may simply parallel overall progress. Parents may need help in understanding this fact. Another group of language disorders may involve the *autistic* or *pervasive developmental disorder* (PDD) spectrum.

The practitioner needs to identify children with mental retardation or PDD and refer the family to an early evaluation and intervention team. For both groups of disorders, the speech language pathologist is an important part of both evaluative and habilitative teams. However, children with these extensive involvements need more than speech and language therapy.

Hearing loss as a factor in language impairment requires alert early recognition. Language acquisition is much more difficult for the hard-of-hearing, and particularly for the deaf. For hearing-impaired children, the question of whether the child will be able to manage oral language or should use sign is thorny. Because early linguistic input to the child is so important, professionals usually recommend total communication, i.e., sign and oral combined. Children who have used both sign and oral usually drop the use of sign spontaneously when they no longer need it. However, this early additional linguistic input often results in better language outcome, including reading and writing.

Family problems that reduce parental response to the child interfere with communication development. A language disorder for which no reasonable cause can be found should alert the pediatrician to considerations of the child's psychosocial well-being. Social service intervention may be helpful.

When other etiologic factors have been excluded, the diagnosis may be that the disorder is specifically neurologically based. Some children with limited sound repertories, reduced comprehension, and sparse and dysfunctional communicative gestures may do much better when given nonverbal opportunities to perform. They often require intensive early intervention and may benefit from augmentative communication systems. Some have significant apraxia, whereas others have more generalized problems. Some continue as users of augmentative communication systems; others may make gains in therapy, becoming good speakers, but still have difficulties with higher-level uses of language for learning. Significant language difficulties in children after the age of 5½ portend future learning problems.

For all these children, the pediatrician should be a major participant in and coordinator of a series of assessments and interventions, sometimes several years apart as different levels of the problem become manifest. The doctor's support of the parents is important, perhaps in acting as an advocate for insurance coverage of the child's early therapy or helping the parents negotiate with the school system for services and supports. If an adolescent child is having academic trouble, the doctor may be the one who recalls early language problems and identifies the present problems as residual disorder, not adolescent rebellion.

SUMMARY

In all the communication disorders discussed, the emphasis has been on early identification and referral. If a child is slow in learning to communicate, this should be cause for concern. Pediatricians should be assertive about monitoring progress and seeking referral. Because communicating is central to the human condition, all children deserve the best opportunities to develop skill in whatever mode is optimal.

DISORDERS OF LEARNING

MELVIN D. LEVINE, M.D.

In recent years, there has been increasing recognition of a group of school-aged children who are said to harbor the low-severity, high-prevalence dysfunctions of childhood. That is, there are many students whose performance in school is substantially compromised because they have subtle central nervous system handicaps that render evolving academic expectations exceedingly hard and often unrewarding for them. These children usually experience specific delays in skill and knowledge acquisition. In some cases, they superimpose behavior problems, a loss of motivation, a decline of self-esteem, and affective disturbances.

A wide variety of learning disorders have been described. They can have their onset at any age and exert a seriously negative impact upon a child's education. A child's academic performance may be impaired by attentional dysfunction (see next article on attention deficits). Others struggle academically because of ineffective language skills. This particular subgroup has trouble keeping pace with the very intense and rapidly expanding linguistic demands imposed by the school curriculum. Some youngsters may have most difficulties with receptive language (i.e., their understanding of verbal inputs); others may be more compromised in their verbal expressive or communicative abilities. Such language problems can seriously deter the acquisition of skills in reading, spelling, and writing. Language difficulties can even create problems in learning mathematics.

Many students exhibit weaknesses of specific forms of memory in school. They may have trouble with the act of memorizing or, alternatively, they may experience difficulty with the precise and rapid retrieval of material learned in the past. Other children have problems with active working memory; that is, it is excessively hard for them to maintain several task components simultaneously in memory while manipulating them. Such shortcomings commonly take their toll on mathematics, on writing, on reading recall, and on the ability to follow directions in school. Other common dysfunctions that impede learning and academic productivity include fine motor deficits, organizational problems, visual-spatial confusion, temporal-sequential disorganization, and a variety of higher cognitive gaps, including difficulty with problem-solving strategies, poor concept formation, problems with brainstorming, and a relative inability to devise, understand, and apply rules.

Children with learning disorders most often demonstrate *clusters* of dysfunctions rather than single discrete deficits. When a child is foundering academically, it is likely that there is more than one reason for underachievement. In most cases, several dysfunctions are operating to obstruct learning and academic output.

No child with learning disorders can be adequately managed without a thorough initial evaluation. Most commonly, such assessments are performed within the school. In the United States, Public Law 94–142 guarantees that children with academic problems will have access to a multidisciplinary evaluation. In some cases, however, parents feel strongly that they would like an independent or outside opinion. In such cases, pediatricians frequently become involved in the referral process, in direct assessment, in ruling out medical contributing factors, and in coordinating and integrating evaluation results. Any such evaluation needs to uncover a child's cognitive and emotional strengths as well as any specific deficits.

TREATMENT

The management of a child with learning disorders includes the following components: (1) demystification, (2) bypass strategies, (3) remedial help, (4) counseling, (5) appropriate treatments, (6) special services, (7) exploitation of strengths, and (8) case management.

Demystification

Children with learning disorders most need to understand the nature of their learning disorders. They must come to recognize that they are not pervasively defective or retarded. The demystification process needs to include a careful explanation of a child's strengths and weaknesses. It should always begin by describing strengths and end on a highly optimistic note. Children need to understand that they can improve significantly, although it is likely to take time and considerable effort. A clinician offering demystification needs to use plain, non-abstract language that can be readily understood and, preferably, even visualized by the child. Thus, for example, a physician might explain to children that they are much better at understanding information that comes through their eyes than information that comes in long sentences and difficult words when a teacher talks. Such an explanation of a language problem can begin to help a child acquire insight into the nature of the disorder.

Bypass Strategies

Bypass strategies are techniques that can be used in the regular classroom to circumvent a learning disorder. Many different options can be pursued by classroom teachers. Sometimes bypass strategies are most readily implemented when a letter is written to a teacher or school administrator by a clinician. The letter can justify the need for such techniques.

Examples of bypass strategies might include giving a child fewer problems on a test, allowing a child to print instead of using cursive writing, permitting the use of a calculator during mathematics tests, postponing a foreign language requirement, or allowing a child to make use of someone else's notes in class. Such interventions, when used with tact and sensitivity, can help alleviate the embarrassment and lessen the toll stemming from a learning disorder.

Remedial Help

Many children with learning disorders require direct remediation, often from a tutor or in a very small group (such as in a resource room or learning center in school). Remediation most commonly focuses upon a particular academic skill deficiency. For example, a child may need remedial help in learning to decode individual words for reading. A reading tutor may work with that child using one or more multisensory techniques to reinforce the associations between sounds and symbols in the English language. This is a common form of tutorial assistance offered to children who are said to have "dyslexia." Children may also need direct remedial help in mathematics, in writing, or in developing appropriate cognitive strategies and study skills. Often such remedial help can be offered in school. However, many children with learning disorders fail to qualify for such services within the school setting. In these instances, if at all possible, outside educational therapy should be made available.

Counseling

Most children with learning disorders do not require any form of psychotherapy. However, if difficulties in school are accompanied by serious family problems, a complete loss of motivation, major behavioral manifestations, or signs of an affective disturbance, some form of counseling may be indicated. Psychotherapeutic intervention can be provided by a psychologist, a child psychiatrist, a social worker, or some other professional trained to deal with psychopathology during childhood. It is especially important that any therapist working with a child with learning disorders be familiar with the nature of that child's learning difficulties. Such a therapist also needs to possess expertise in learning disorders. The therapist must be an individual who is comfortable working closely with school personnel. To be effective, a therapist must be in constant communication with the school. Anyone offering psychotherapy who never visits the school or communicates with a child is, in all likelihood, not providing adequate care.

Medical Interventions

A number of medical interventions have been suggested for children with learning disorders. A complete medical examination should be part of the evaluation of any child with academic underachievement, and there needs to be specific treatment for any causative or complicating medical conditions. Although such specific problems are relatively rare, there is certainly a need to manage any associated seizure disorder, endocrinopathy, or chronic somatic symptom (such as headache, encopresis, or abdominal pain).

In general, stimulant medications are not indicated for children with learning disorders unless attentional dysfunction is a significant part of the picture. In such instances, medication for the attentional problems can be an important adjunct to management. It should be stressed, however, that stimulant medication should never replace individualized classroom management, remedial support, or other services needed by a child with learning difficulties.

There flows a relentless stream of new "medical" interventions for children with learning disorders. Anyone managing such children needs to help parents and teachers sort out the scientific validity of such seductive therapies. These therapies always have staunch advocates (many of whom have a discernible conflict of interest). Included among such advocated treatments are *sensory integration therapy, optometric therapy, colored transparencies for reading problems* (as well as Irlen lenses), *special diets,* and *motor patterning exercises. None of these therapies has been sufficiently validated by unbiased investigators.* Further research is definitely required before such treatments can be recommended by pediatricians. Future investigations need to determine whether these treatments are at all effective and, if they are, in which patients they are most likely to work. Any therapy that purports to be effective in all or most children with learning disorders is clearly suspect owing to the heterogeneity of this population.

Special Services

Some children may need special therapeutic services because of the specific nature of their learning disorders. Most commonly, there are underachieving youngsters who can benefit from specific language therapy to improve their receptive and/or expressive skills. Occupational therapy may be helpful to some students with significant writing deficits on the basis of graphomotor dysfunctions.

Exploitation of Strengths

It is absolutely essential that all children with learning disorders experience mastery. Many of them are chronically success-deprived. Therefore, any management plan needs to exploit the strengths and affinities of underachieving children. Any highly developed ability must be identified and a program developed to make use of it as a means of enhancing self-esteem and helping a child feel effective. Moreover, in many instances, a child's strengths can be used to strengthen weaknesses. For example, if a child is excellent at visualizing, these visual processing strengths can be used to overcome the effects of a language disability that is impeding reading and spelling. Strong areas of interest can also be mobilized. It has been shown that the best way to learn how to read is by reading about a subject area that one knows a lot about. When a child has a passion for a particular area of content, that intense interest can thus be used to facilitate skill development.

Case Management

Learning disorders are inevitably chronic. Their clinical course, however, is notoriously unpredictable. Therefore, every child with a learning disorder should be monitored and managed closely throughout the course of the school years. A pediatrician can play an important role as an advocate and case manager. There should be periodic reassessment of the child's current status and needs. In many instances, pediatricians are working closely with psychoeducational specialists or educational diagnosticians. The latter frequently work within a pediatrician's office (possibly part time) and offer periodic reassessments of a child's educational progress. Such individuals can also serve as an important liaison between the pediatric office and the school. Together with the educational diagnostician, the pediatrician can offer ongoing advice to the child and to the parents while constantly clarifying for them the child's present needs. The clinician needs to foster optimism and hopefulness while offering realistic insights into the child's current and evolving plight.

ATTENTION DEFICITS

MELVIN D. LEVINE, M.D.

Disorders of attention are among the most common causes of academic underachievement and behavioral maladaptation among school-aged children. The diverse group of youngsters affected by attention deficits exhibit a wide range of manifestations. However, they share in common difficulties mobilizing and directing their mental effort, problems being selective in their concentration and choice of behaviors, difficulties with planning and organization, trouble regulating their tempo and persistence, and weaknesses of self-monitoring. Some children with attention deficits display significant behavior problems, whereas others manifest their attentional difficulty primarily or exclusively in the domains of cognition and learning.

The most common traits of attentional dysfunction are listed in Table 1. Many different parent and school questionnaires have been developed to document the presence and degree of severity of these various traits. Most commonly, a

TABLE 1. Common Traits of Children with Attention Deficits

1. Difficulty concentrating
2. Distractibility
3. Impulsivity
4. Behavioral and/or academic inconsistency
5. Poor self-monitoring
6. Poorly regulated activity (overactivity or underactivity)
7. Insatiability, restlessness
8. Vivid imagination
9. Memory problems in school

diagnosis of attention deficit is made by gathering such data, although direct observations of attention (during testing or in a classroom setting) are also utilized.

EVALUATION AND TREATMENT

Attention deficits seldom exist in isolation. They very commonly cluster with specific learning disorders (see previous article), social skill deficits, conduct disorders, and/or affective disturbances (such as depression or bipolar illness). Therefore, the evaluation and treatment of a child with attention deficits must include consideration of associated problems and the interactions between problems and strengths. The management of children with attention deficits may need to include interventions in the following categories: (1) demystification, (2) pharmacotherapy, (3) home management advice, (4) school management advice, (5) counseling, and (6) case management.

Demystification

Every child and every parent of a child with attention deficits must have an excellent understanding of this clinical disorder. A clinician needs to explain the phenomena associated with attentional dysfunction so that an affected child and parents acquire lucid insight into the condition. Many children harboring attention deficits think of themselves as hopelessly incompetent or "crazy." By circumscribing the disorder, the pediatrician may help a child recognize that attention deficits do not portend inevitably negative outcomes in life and that difficulties with attention represent only one of many components of function. The clinician should use concrete, clearly understood language, sometimes making use of diagrams or pictures to clarify key points. The parents should be present during a demystification session so that they too can gain a better understanding of a child's attentional difficulties.

Sometimes it is necessary to demystify an entire school faculty regarding attention deficits. *For this reason, increasing numbers of pediatricians are providing in-service programs at schools, so that teachers can gain more insight and develop more appropriate methods of dealing with the many students who harbor attention deficits.*

Pharmacotherapy

Stimulants

Frequently children with attention deficits benefit from the use of medication to enhance overall alertness and self-control. Stimulant medication, in particular, may enable a child to become more focused in a classroom. In certain cases, it may diminish overactivity and impulsivity. Unfortunately, no hard-and-fast criteria have been validated to identify children for whom stimulant medication is specifically indicated. Such therapy is generally prescribed for patients whose problems with attention and/or behavioral control are significantly impeding their day-to-day function. When a stimulant is prescribed, its justifications, limitations, and actions should be discussed thoroughly with the child and the parents. Side effects should, of course, be explained. Children taking medication should have regularly scheduled follow-up visits with appropriate interval history taking and physical and neurologic examinations.

It is important to recognize that stimulant medication is never the whole answer. It should not be viewed as the exclusive, definitive, or permanent treatment of attention deficits. Instead, such therapy must be considered part of a multimodal approach, one that includes the additional forms of intervention covered in this article.

It is helpful to include periodic "drug holidays" in any stimulant medication regimen. That is, in most cases at certain points in the academic year, a child should spend 1 or 2 weeks off medication while trying to gain spontaneous control over attention as well as other maladaptive traits associated with the attention deficits.

There exists some controversy regarding whether or not stimulant medication should be taken on weekends and holidays. In cases of severe behavioral maladjustment, such daily administration may be indicated. In less severe forms of attention deficit as well as when the attentional problems are having their major impact on school performance, it is desirable to limit stimulant medication exclusively to school days.

Methylphenidate, dextroamphetamine, and pemoline are the most commonly prescribed stimulants.

Methylphenidate (Ritalin). A relatively mild central nervous system stimulant, methylphenidate is usually given in an initial dosage of 0.3 mg/kg/day. It can then be increased gradually to 0.6 mg/kg/day. The short-acting preparation can be administered once or twice daily (generally in the morning and at noon). The maximum dose is approximately 0.8 mg/kg/day. Doses greater than 1 mg/kg/day are often associated with deterioration in behavior and learning. Some children appear to respond best to a long-acting preparation of Ritalin SR (20 mg) tablets. Others seem to need the relatively quick onset of short-acting medication that appears to provide them with a "jump start" on their day at school. It should be stressed that there is wide variation with respect to the dosage requirements and tolerances of individual children with attention deficits.

Most of the time methylphenidate is not recommended for children younger than 6 years of age. However, in some very severe cases of attention deficit complicated by poorly controllable behavior, the drug is employed in this preschool age. The side effects are generally not substantial. Occasionally, children experience anorexia, insomnia, constipation, or hypertension. The insomnia and anorexia may be dose-related and may also spontaneously diminish over time. In some children taking methylphenidate, tics develop. This should be an indication for stopping therapy.

Some controversy exists about the use of methylphenidate in children with diagnosed Tourette syndrome. In such cases, stimulants have been found to elicit or worsen the motor manifestations. In some instances, methylphenidate actually aggravates the symptoms of an attention deficit. When this occurs, the dose should be reduced significantly or the drug should be discontinued.

In a few cases, methylphenidate works too well! It causes a "zombie-like" sedation, resulting in reduced scintillation of a child's personality. This too suggests the need for a lower dose.

Dextroamphetamine (Dexedrine). In its short-acting form, this drug has a peak effect within 3 to 4 hours. Like methylphenidate, dextroamphetamine can enhance attention and reduce impulsivity and distractibility. It can be used in short-acting form or in a Spansule preparation. The long-acting spansule comes in several strengths, making it especially amenable to careful titration.

The dosage is about half that of methylphenidate. It has been found that some older adolescents respond very well to surprisingly small dosages. In some cases, a 17-year-old student requires a lower dose of medication than an 11-year-old.

Side effects are essentially similar to those of methylphenidate.

Pemoline. Pemoline is a long-acting stimulant that appears to be effective in some children with attention deficits. Its dosage is approximately 2 to 3 mg/kg/day. It is said that the clinical effect may not become evident for 3 to 4 weeks. There has been some concern that pemoline may result in transient liver damage. Consequently, it has been suggested that children taking pemoline receive liver function tests approximately every 6 months. Lasting or permanent liver damage has not been reported.

Nonstimulants

Some children with attention deficits are relatively unresponsive to stimulants. Although stimulant therapy should generally be tried first, other options exist.

Antidepressants. The tricyclic antidepressants (TCAs) seem to help certain children. *Imipramine* (Tofranil) and *desipramine* (Norpramin) have been used increasingly. Desipramine is generally given in a dosage of 0.5 to 1.0 mg/kg initially, increasing to 1.0–5.0 mg/kg/day in one or two doses. These medications are slower in their onset and longer-acting in their effectiveness than short-acting stimulants. Not surprisingly, the TCAs are most likely to be useful in patients who exhibit significant emotional lability, sleep difficulty, anxiety, or signs of depression. There appears to be a variable effect on attention. In some cases, the antidepressants enhance attentional strength; in other cases, they may alleviate anxiety without strengthening attention.

There have been a few reported cases of cardiac arrythmias in children on TCAs. Consequently, periodic electrocardiographic (EKG) rhythm strips have been suggested. Blood levels of antidepressants can be monitored. The drug does accumulate, and children vary markedly in their rates of absorption and turnover.

Antihypertensive Drugs. Certain antihypertensive medications have been used in children with attention deficits. *Clonidine* (Catapres) has been most commonly prescribed. This medication has been found to be useful in patients with Tourette syndrome *and* attention deficits. Clonidine can substantially lower the severity and frequency of tics, and in some cases improvements in attention and reduced impulsivity have been observed. The drug is used in small dosage increments (0.05 mg at a time) up to 3 to 6 μg/kg in three doses. The drug can be administered using a transdermal route (skin patch). Side effects include dizziness and hypotension. Some clinicians have used combined therapy, particularly Ritalin and clonidine.

Lithium has been prescribed for some children with attention deficits. These are often youngsters who are diagnosed as being depressed or having bipolar illness in addition to their attentional difficulties. Lithium may also control aggression. In general, lithium should not be prescribed by physicians who have little experience with its administration and monitoring. The use of lithium in the management of attention deficits remains controversial.

Other Medical Therapies

Sometimes alternative medical therapies are recommended for children with attention deficits. These include special diets. The elimination of food additives (such as in the Feingold Diet) and sugars has been recommended. Scientific studies of dietary interventions have not been convincing. There has been some evidence accrued suggesting that for certain children the ingestion of a high-carbohydrate breakfast in the absence of any protein may have a detrimental impact upon attention in school.

Biofeedback and hypnosis have been used in the management of attention deficits. Their efficacy has not been established, although such interventions may turn out to be a useful adjunct to other components of multimodal therapy.

Home Management

Parents often need advice on the day-to-day care of a child with attention deficits. In general, the clinician needs to help parents make a list of maladaptative disturbing behaviors and then establish priorities for their management. Parents need to realize that they cannot change everything all at once; they need to be helped to select those traits that are most troublesome or severe and then need to develop consistent techniques to minimize the effects of these traits. Parents should be helped to strive toward the control of difficult or disruptive behaviors without trying to eliminate them entirely. They need to learn to provide consistent feedback and appropriate forms of praise and reward.

Many parents need help dealing with the issue of homework, such as helping the child get started. The child may need to work in multiple sites during the same evening. There may need to be frequent breaks, music playing in the background, and a set time for cognitive effort each evening. Parents may need to communicate closely with the school to define precisely the expectations or assignments required from a child. Often children with attention deficits do not understand what they are supposed to do at home. This is largely because they tend not to listen in school while assignments are being given! There should not be an insistence on productivity or output regardless of quality. Parents should avoid giving children an incentive to be impulsive. That is, a set amount of time should be dedicated to work rather than telling children that they can watch television as soon as homework is done. The latter bargain encourages children to rush through their work.

School Management

A child's teacher must understand the nature of a student's attention deficits. A letter from a clinician, a telephone call, an in-service education program for the whole faculty, or a meeting at the school can do a great deal to clarify confusion and to dispel misunderstandings. The management of a child with attention deficits in school depends largely upon that child's associated cognitive strengths and deficits. One cannot intervene on a child's attention deficits without also taking into consideration any associated learning disorders as well as learning strengths. Any specific information processing or production problems must be managed along with a child's attention deficits.

In general, children with attention deficits need to sit close to their teachers. They also need to take frequent breaks. Many of these children require tutorial help to develop appropriate study habits and organizational skills. Very commonly, children with attention deficits have a great deal of trouble with writing. They may need special practice in this domain. They also need to develop their computer skills, so that ultimately they can be productive with a word processor. It is also important to recognize that it is very common for children with attention deficits to have difficulty with those aspects of memory that are needed for success in school. Despite the fact that many such students have an excellent memory for trivia, their ability to memorize academic material can be very constricted. Often they need to be helped to develop effective mnemonic strategies.

Counseling

In many cases children with attention deficits can benefit from ongoing counseling. It is often ideal to involve other family members in such therapy. The counseling can be performed by a psychologist, psychiatrist, social worker, or another individual with experience dealing with attention deficits. In relatively mild cases, a pediatrician can offer periodic counseling. Regardless of the provider, counseling must include specific advice on day-to-day management as well as ongoing refinement of the insights of parents and children regarding the manifestations of attention deficits.

It should be stressed that not all children with attention deficits require psychotherapy. In fact, most of them can be managed appropriately by a pediatrician with the cooperation of the parents and the school. When there is substantial depression, family turmoil, as well as multiple other stresses, psychotherapy may be warranted.

Some children have been found to benefit from a form of treatment called *cognitive-behavioral therapy*, which involves ongoing education about a child's attentional dysfunction along with specific exercises or activities that can be pursued to enhance attention and control. It is most commonly administered by a psychologist.

In some instances, children with attention deficits can gain from social skills training. Often such intervention is provided in a small group setting. Children compare notes and obtain advice on the development of effective interpersonal skills; this can be tremendously beneficial to those who exhibit social cognitive deficits in association with their attentional dysfunctions.

Case Management

All children with attention deficits require longitudinal case management. A clinician needs to be explicit in offering this service and level of commitment to the child and parents. The clinical course of a child with attention deficits is intrinsically unpredictable. There needs to be close observation and year-to-year decision making as there would be with any other chronic condition encountered in pediatrics. Children with attention deficits need to visit their pediatricians at least twice a year. Those taking medication may need to be evaluated three or four times a year along with easy telephone access provided. During follow-up visits, a pediatrician should offer ongoing advice on home and school management as well as constant surveillance for complications, such as anxiety, depression, or a loss of motivation. The pediatrician should be available to help a child obtain services in school and in the community. Pediatricians should coordinate data collection during diagnostic evaluations. The pediatrician also needs to serve as an advocate for the child, helping that youngster avoid excessive humiliation in school, assisting the parents in obtaining an appropriate education, and in meeting the other developmental needs of the child. Such consistent long-term follow-up is critical for the effective management of children who exhibit attentional problems.

It should be stressed that children with attention deficits exhibit remarkable strengths. Many of them are unusually creative and refreshingly entrepreneurial. Their affinities and abilities are often somewhat unconventional and therefore quite innovative. While offering longitudinal case management, the clinician must help the parents and the child to mobilize latent strengths, to pursue affinities in depth, and to preserve individuality.

CHILDREN OF DIVORCING PARENTS

MICHAEL S. JELLINEK, M.D.

Divorce remains common and a major source of stress and dysfunction in children and adolescents. The combination of out-of-wedlock births and divorce will result in over a third of all children living with a single parent, 90 per cent of the time with the mother, for some time prior to age 16. The divorce rate since the 1950s has tripled, and more than 1 million children each year endure the divorce process. Because the average length of marriage is between 6 and 7 years, many of these children are young and will experience years of potentially complex parenting (i.e., single parenting, "joint custody," and step-parenting). Divorce may be the only solution to a hostile marriage and eventually may have a beneficial outcome. However, the transitional period following divorce is a searing experience for children, lasting at least a year and even indefinitely, especially with ongoing parental discord.

How do pediatricians first learn of the separation or divorce? Unless a parent volunteers the information or asks directly about their child's emotional difficulties, pediatricians may not be aware of a pending divorce. Despite the impact and high prevalence of divorce, a serious psychosocial issue in 25 per cent to more than 50 per cent of families in their practices, pediatricians frequently do not ask about marital status or parental discord. Pediatricians often believe that they have not been adequately trained, do not have time, or are not fairly reimbursed for dealing with divorce-related stress and family dysfunction. Pediatricians thus often learn of a divorce indirectly and late in the process through a change of address, a request to send records to another pediatrician, or problems in collecting bills as family finances are frozen in negotiations or in hostility. Sometimes the pediatrician, unaware of the parent's motives, is asked by one parent to write a letter or make a recommendation that is more embedded in parental hostility than the child's well-being. For example, the pediatrician will be led into restricting a child's activity or altering a visitation schedule not knowing the overall context or the other parent's perspective.

Once aware that a divorce is in process or has taken place, the pediatrician should consider a number of issues in addressing the development and psychosocial needs of the child or children in the family. Inevitably, divorce represents a loss and this loss must be mourned. However, the nature of this loss is not like that of a death, which is involuntary, irreversible, and relatively unambiguous, and elicits a broad-based, supportive response from the community. Divorce is voluntary, one or both parents separating of their own accord; and the consequent explanations, hostile behaviors, and community reaction may make little sense to the child.

The losses are multiple and pervasive. During the divorce, the initial level of contact between the child and parents is less than when the family was intact, and even this level decreases further, especially for the noncustodial parent (the father in 90 per cent of divorces). There is also a change in the quality of the time spent. Both parents are frequently preoccupied by their own form of mourning the loss of the marriage, trying to manage the rage they feel toward their former spouse, and dealing with the many details of the divorce process. "Visits" that are too brief or tense may feel artificial. The child loses the structure of the family, a structure that supported a view of the world as safe, predictable, filled with expectations, and encouraging of hope.

The financial impact of divorce is frequently severe. Setting up two households and paying for the divorce itself can be overwhelming. The financial consequences for mothers are especially difficult. Following divorce, mothers on average have suffered a much more significant drop in disposable income, sometimes driving them below the poverty line, than fathers, who are more likely to maintain their standard of living. Child support may be used as a method to gain control or as a weapon in the hostilities. Children may be left in doubt as money to fund clothes, summer camp, after-school programs, or lessons is late, erratic, or withdrawn. Only recently has state and federal legislation been in effect that encourages court action to enforce financial agreements locally and across state lines.

If parents need to work harder or longer hours, then again the amount and quality of time available to the child is diminished. If the family's home has to be sold, the child loses his or her room, neighborhood friends, local school, and the community supports (e.g., religious groups, sports teams, familiar routines).

Parental discord, whether leading to divorce, following divorce, or as a constant source of tension within a marriage, is probably the single most damaging factor to the child's well-being and functioning. When there is continuing discord, the parents' priorities and capacity for empathy are consumed by their anger toward one another. The child's sadness, anxiety, self-blame, private tension, and loneliness are a lower priority or go unnoticed. Children exposed to chronic discord are more likely to be depressed, angry, and dysfunctional throughout their day-to-day life in school and with their peers. Other risk factors include clinical depression in the mother, other psychiatric disorders in either parent, and poverty.

DEVELOPMENTAL CONSIDERATIONS

The expectable reactions to divorce depend on the child's developmental level and the quality of the child's relationship to parents.

In one of few prospective studies, Wallerstein and Kelly reported on children of various ages who were observed after divorce. Infants' and toddlers' reactions were most sensitive to the mother's ability to function. Many reacted to the divorce stresses by regression in toilet training, increased irritability, and greater dependency. Children whose homes were characterized by maternal depression and ongoing parental discord had more severe symptoms lasting over a year.

The preschool or young school-aged child is vulnerable because the child's frame of reference has gone beyond the mother to include the entire family. At this cognitive level, the child is confused by the events and length of the divorce process and uses an egocentric explanation of causation. Emotionally, the child is developing a conscience and is thus very ready to accept responsibility and blame for family events. Guilt-ridden fantasies are substantiated in part by arguments about "the children" overheard, often unbeknownst to the parents, prior to the separation and divorce. In addition, the child feels helpless as events beyond the child's understanding and control (e.g., lawyers, courts, real estate agents) dictate new realities. All children, but especially those of early school age, benefit from repeated assurance that they are not to blame but, rather, that they are loved and will be cared for.

School-aged children are more sophisticated and less likely to feel solely responsible for the divorce. Their reactions to divorce are more diverse and indirect. Children of this age feel sad, lonely, and powerless. They present with depressed mood, psychosomatic disorders, problems in peer relationships, and a decrease in school performance. In addition, there is a higher incidence of aggressive behavior in boys who live with their mothers. These boys seem to cope with missing their fathers by taking his place, often behaving "just like his father," which quickly provokes the mother's anger and worst fears. School-aged children frequently consider changing homes to see what life would be like with the other parent and, possibly, in an effort to reunite the family. These real or imagined efforts may not end until one of the parents remarries. The child's expression of anger to the noncustodial parent, most often the father, may be inhibited by the fear that misbehaving or being undesirable may result in even less time together in the future.

The adolescent's developmental task is to separate from the family unit and establish an adult identity. However, this process is meant to be gradual, lasting approximately 10 years, and characterized by intermittent periods of progression and regression. Divorce disrupts and distorts this developmental process. Home is no longer a place for daily contact and identification with one, the other, or both parents. A frequent defensive reaction is the 10- to 11-year-old's early entry into adolescent behavior or the adolescent's premature closure of identity formation, i.e., uncritical adoption of the absent parent's characteristics. The pseudomature adolescent appears aloof, overly controlled, and overly controlling. Peer groups may become a major source of nurturance, and experimentation with drugs and alcohol may become a daily attempt to hide feelings of shame, suppress anxiety, dull depression, and test the limits in the newly structured family. Adolescents, like older school-aged children, may wish to change custody arrangements and "try" out living with the other parent. The teenager who can strategically withdraw from the crisis, yet still derive emotional support from both parents, may be best able to balance developmental needs. The evolution of the adolescent's sexual identity may be accelerated in an effort to find temporary companionship.

An anecdotal but noteworthy follow-up study by Wallerstein indicated that despite the adolescent's cognitive ability, the effect of divorce is surprisingly profound. Adolescents' perspective on intimacy, a capacity emerging in middle and late teenage years, may be especially vulnerable to the unpredictable, hostile nature of the divorce process.

CLINICAL ASSESSMENT AND MANAGEMENT

How should the pediatrician approach the child and family facing divorce? What questions should be asked of all families? Which children are at special risk?

Given the high prevalence of divorce and the serious impact of ongoing discord, the pediatrician should ask about the quality of family life as a routine part of health maintenance. Early in the course of marital problems, the pediatrician may be able to take a preventive stance and refer the couple for counseling. If a separation or divorce has already been implemented, then the pediatrician should assess:

1. How the child is functioning in the major areas of daily life (family, friends, school, play, mood).
2. How the child is reacting to the divorce.
3. Whether the child is at special risk (i.e., ongoing discord, parental depression).
4. Whether the parents have the capacity to meet the child's physical and emotional needs.
5. Whether the child is being used by one parent against the other (almost a sufficient criterion to refer for counseling or mediation). A child used by one parent against the other or constantly torn by divided loyalties pays a terrible emotional price. The pediatrician should definitely repeat this assessment regularly over the following years.

Court-ordered joint custody is a growing trend and potentially very supportive to the child's long-term development. However, joint custody also requires frequent contact and cooperation between parents—the same adults who could not communicate or achieve harmony in their marriage. If joint custody is agreed to by the parents only grudgingly or ordered by the court as an expedient to avoid a bitter trial, the risks of damaging, ongoing discord are very high. Children who have to walk through a "demilitarized" zone from the car to one or another of their parents' front door are clearly at special risk and require efforts to ease the hostility.

In general, pediatricians can be of real help by remembering that parents are under great stress during a divorce. Simple, nonjudgmental listening and emotional understanding can be very supportive and can give the pediatrician a preliminary sense of how well the parent is functioning. Options for referral depend upon the circumstances. Some parents may benefit from a referral to a local self-help group, others by recommendations to facilitate the child's adjustment. A seriously depressed mother may require a psychiatric referral, ongoing discord about parenting issues may need to be referred to a psychologically sophisticated mediator, and the individual child's dysfunctional reaction may need to be evaluated by a child psychologist or psychiatrist.

Although divorce issues are often complex and stressful for the pediatrician to manage, being available for 10 to 15 minutes to listen, assess, refer, and counsel may be among the most gratifying and helpful aspects of pediatric practice.

REFERENCES

Wallerstein J, Blakeslee S: Second Chances. New York, Ticknor and Fields, 1989.

Wallerstein J, Kelly J: Surviving the Breakup. New York, Basic Books, 1980.

CHILD ABUSE

STEPHEN LUDWIG, M.D.
and CINDY CHRISTIAN, M.D.

Child abuse and neglect are major causes of childhood morbidity and mortality in the United States as well as in other developed countries around the world. In the United States, a recent national incidence study showed that annually more than 650,000 abused and neglected children are known to child protective service agencies, police, schools, hospitals, and other professional organizations. Incidence rates for abuse and neglect are 10.5 children per 1000 U.S. children under 18 years. These rates are clearly underestimated, as most abuse occurs in the privacy of family homes and goes unreported. The number of reported abuse cases is usually estimated to be one-half the number of actual cases. The number of child mortalities attributable to abuse has increased during the past two decades. Child homicides by parents and individuals acting *in loco parentis* have increased in actual number and have been seen in more bold relief as the number of deaths due to motor vehicle injuries has diminished.

The therapy of child abuse has many facets. In temporal terms, one can divide the therapies into the *acute* versus *chronic*. By using another categorization, we may consider the *physical* versus the *psychosocial-developmental* injury. Finally, one may look at the forms of abuse—physical, emotional, sexual, neglect. This article focuses on physical abuse and explores the acute and chronic treatments aimed at both physical and nonphysical aspects of child health.

PHYSICAL ABUSE INJURIES

Acute Therapy

In any consideration of the treatment of child abuse, the first step to consider is the recognition of abuse. Therapy cannot begin unless abuse is suspected, recognized, and reported.

Recognizing Abuse

Abuse can be suspected only when the physician believes that such injuries can and do occur. There continue to be some physicians who have not yet realized the pervasiveness of abuse in our society or the possibility of its occurring in any family given the cumulative effects of personal, family, community, and societal stressors. Some physicians maintain a "that kind of thing couldn't happen here" attitude. Such physicians are placing a nonpermeable mask around their diagnostic abilities.

Level of Suspicion and Reporting

For those who have opened themselves to the possibility of abuse, what remains is a difficult task of pulling together historical, physical examination, laboratory, radiographic, and social data. In doing so, the physician is attempting to answer the question, "Is there a suspicion of abuse?" If there is adequate suspicion, the next step in the acute therapy, the institution of a child protective services (CPS) report, must take place. Every state in the United States has a child abuse reporting law. The law indicates what constitutes abuse, how and by whom it should be reported, what the protections are for the reporter, and the penalties for those who fail to report. States vary as to a physician's ability to take protective custody of a child. However, if physicians are not empowered to take custodial action, certainly law enforcement officials are. Beyond the legal mandate for physicians to suspect and report abuse and thereby protect children, there is a moral imperative to do so. Many studies have documented that the failure to report abuse places the child in the position for increased, and at times fatal, injury.

Dealing with Uncertainty

In suspecting abuse and making the decision to report, the physician may experience internal conflict. There may be uncertainty or an insufficient level of suspicion. The physician may feel uncomfortable about making value judgments on a patient's lifestyle. When such conflicts arise, it is best to call on a multidisciplinary team for consultation. This may be a formal child abuse team within an institution or an ad hoc collection of individuals, including physician colleagues, nurses, social workers, and psychologists. By the addition of the knowledge, experience, and perspectives of a multidisciplinary team, a broader-based, fairer decision process will ensue. A larger number of decision makers lessen individual and cultural bias, personal value judgments, and other factors that make the recognition of abuse somewhat subjective.

Protecting the Child

If the suspicion of abuse warrants reporting, the next issue to resolve is the child's need for immediate protection. The child's safety depends on the continued access of an alleged perpetrator to the child, the CPS system's ability to monitor the situation, the stresses on the family system, the severity of abuse, and other factors. If the child is not felt to be safe if returned home, the physician must provide an alternative protective environment, such as the hospital. Hospitalization may be indicated independent of the need for hospital care based on the severity of the injury. Thus, a child with minor soft tissue injuries may need to be hospitalized acutely if the extended family and CPS cannot be counted upon to make the child's home safe. It is better to decide about the need for hospitalization before moving on to the next step.

Informing Parents

The most difficult and often dreaded part of making a child abuse report is the notification of the parents. In some cases, physicians attempt to avoid this step. This is an error. Failure to be honest with parents sets up the next helping professional for a disastrous nontherapeutic relationship. It also destroys the trusting relationship the family and physician may have once enjoyed. Parents must be told. The physician must do so in a nonaccusatory, nonjudgmental way. Remember, for example, that those caretakers present in the medical facility may not know about the abuse and may themselves be confused, upset, and angry. Working directly with a parent whom one suspects is the abuser is one of the major tests of professional behavior. Physicians must recognize yet control their potential personal angry feelings. The focus of attention must be on the child's health and the child's needs. Most abusive parents are not happy with their own conduct. They feel defensive and ashamed of their loss of control. Anything that makes them feel more guilty or more fearful will result in anger and hostility toward the physician, health care staff, or institution. It is best to avoid these emotions if possible. Ultimately, the pediatrician's suspicions may be inaccurate. Thus, each situation must be approached with delicacy, concern, and openness. At the same time, one must remain vigilant for details of history, observing interactions, inconsistencies, and telling emotional responses.

Documentation

Careful documentation is the next important step in the therapy of acute abusive injury. It is very important to document not only the nature and extent of the child's injury but also a very detailed history of injury, associated findings, general growth and developmental status, and the observed interactions between the medical staff, parents, extended family members, and patient. The size, color, pattern, and location of injuries should be carefully documented when possible. It is also important to document certain negative findings.

The medical record in a child abuse matter is also a legal record. Legal proceedings may occur weeks or months after the medical evaluation. Reviewing an incomplete record several months later may be painfully instructive. In some jurisdictions, special child abuse reporting forms need to be completed. Photographing injuries is advised if high-quality photography services are available. Simple drawings and charts may suffice for less complex injuries. Documentation through videotape and audiotape is permissible and usable in the courts of law in some states, although their use remains controversial.

Referral and Follow-up

Although physical abuse is a diagnosis used by physicians, it is also a sign of family dysfunction. Therefore, every acute episode of abuse needs to have carefully arranged follow-up lest the systems lose track of the child and family and more severe or recurrent abuse occurs. Follow-up may be provided by either the CPS or an organized hospital-based child abuse team. In some circumstances (for example, with uncooperative families) police and the court system will be involved in ensuring follow-up.

Chronic Therapy

Common Elements

There are many potential elements of treatment used in the long-term care of the physically abused child. Treatment strategies vary on the basis of the needs of the child and the needs of the family. However, there are some common elements that should be included in any long-term treatment plan. These include a close, supportive, helping relationship, a system of case management, and a multidisciplinary approach to treatment.

Included in all the attempted forms of therapy for child abuse is one consistent theme that enhances success—the formation of a close, supportive relationship. Theorists have pointed to abusive families as being more isolated and abusive parents as not having a support system. Any form of long-term treatment that is to be successful must address these problems and provide the family with a doctor, nurse, social worker, psychologist, or good neighbor who can be trusted and called on when help is needed. Where multiple agencies provide multiple services, there must be someone designated as case manager to coordinate the agencies and services that are provided.

We find that therapy is also aided by the multidisciplinary approach. This helps lead to less judgmental responses on the part of the helping services and provides the family with a range of professionals who the family feels will be helpful.

Psychotherapeutic Services

The long-term therapy of abuse may involve traditional or nontraditional, individual and/or group psychotherapeutic services. These are services that are directed to the individual personality of a parent or the child or to the family's "personality." Although the provision of mental health services may seem intuitive, they are not always used because they are labor-intensive and costly and may not be applicable to individuals not ready to accept them.

Developmental Services

Many abuse programs have services aimed at the developmental needs of the child. Particularly when abuse is tied to neglect, but even when it occurs independently, the child victim may sustain developmental injury, which should be treated with special developmental services. Special day care centers, nurseries, and therapeutic preschools have been used most successfully. The better programs have tie-in programs for parents aimed at teaching realistic, developmentally appropriate expectations, and parenting skills while striving to diminish the parent's social isolation. Drop-in centers and crisis nurseries have been particularly helpful for crisis-prone families who are without adequate resources.

Life Skill Services

For some families there may be the need for more basic therapy that helps in the achievement of normal life skills. Parent aids help to teach how to survive the daily rigors of ensuring food, clothing, shelter and a reasonable amount of safety and control for children in a society that sometimes makes achievement of such goals seem virtually impossible. Parent aid or family workers help families by being both advocates and role models. A senior social worker once told us, "You cannot go to church if you have no shoes." For some families, this form of survival therapy must precede any attempt at developmental or psychotherapy, as it meets the more basic needs of the family and decreases their level of stress. With reduction of stress, there is less likelihood that the stress will be reflected on the child in the form of abuse.

Self-Help Services

A number of self-help therapies have proved to be useful to abusive parents. Parents Anonymous and other groups have been the rallying point for some parents to share their frustrations and successes with others. Parenting is a lonely business, and self-help groups have been helpful for many.

Legal "Therapies"

It must be recognized that some families will be resistant to accepting any form of help. Other families may want help, but appropriate services may not be available. For yet another group of abusive parents, help is no longer an option and legal punishment with removal from society is the only appropriate approach.

In all of the above situations, the force of legal intervention may be necessary either to mandate therapy or to remove a child from the family (or a perpetrator from society) in order to ensure safety. Legal services should also be viewed as therapeutic, although at times it is used as a second level of therapy rather than as a "treatment of first choice." Although our primary goal is to rehabilitate families, there are some abusive parents whose abuse is part of a pattern of violent behavior and whose violence cannot be controlled.

Alternative-Living Placement

In some cases of abuse, alternative-living situations may be required for the child. There are three basic alternatives: (1) foster care, (2) institutional care, and (3) extended family care. All alternative-living situations are compromises from children living in their own family environment. Each arrangement type has advantages and disadvantages which must be considered for a specific child. But issues of child safety or family disintegration may require that one of the alternatives be selected for either short-term placement or a long-term living situation.

NONPHYSICAL ABUSE

Acute Therapy

Nonphysical abuse includes neglect and psychologic and emotional abuse. (Sexual abuse is covered on page 47.) It is even more difficult to recognize these forms of nonphysical abuse because of the lack of physical markers or the inability to link parental behaviors to their psychologic outcomes in the child. The insidious nature of neglect allows it to continue unchecked because no specific event causes identification and action.

Need for Reporting

Despite the difficulty in identifying nonphysical forms of abuse, when it is recognized, it must be reported in the same way a broken bone or cigarette burn would be. The reporting criterion is a suspicion of abuse, and all the same legal cautions and safeguards apply. Neglect may result in the same degree of physical injury in the child as more active forms of abuse. Thus, from the child's perspective, there is no true differentiation. Failure to thrive may be caused by neglect and may be reported under the child abuse statistics. The clinician should not be complacent in allowing a neglectful situation to persist just because no prior actions have been taken or no overt physical injuries have been inflicted on the child.

Ensuring Safety

Once nonphysical abuse has been identified, it must be reported and consideration must be given to the child's safety and the need for hospitalization or an alternative temporary living situation. Children who are abandoned, as well as some of those with less pervasive neglect, are in obvious need for such protection. Children who have been psychologically abused need to be screened for behaviors that threaten themselves or others. If threatened injury is apparent, involuntary psychiatric hospitalization is indicated.

Notifying the Parent

The notification process in nonphysical abuse may be more difficult but in some ways more necessary. Because there are no prescribed areas of parenting, psychologically abusive or neglectful parents may not see their own behaviors as harmful. Thus, they may be more resistant to change and more indignant about being identified. With a parent who has abandoned a child, there are such strong feelings of guilt that the parent often presents to the hospital with a high level of anger. Some of the most difficult family management scenarios have occurred in situations of abandonment.

Documentation

With nonphysical forms of abuse, documentation is also more challenging and more important. There may not be radiographs of broken bones or photographs of blisters to point to for documentation. Psychologic tests, objective growth charts, and developmental scales should be employed. Quotations and notation of actions and inactions are needed to "make the case." For example, a parent who is neglecting a child's medical needs may have to be presented with a listing of what needs to be done, sent by registered mail. A specific time frame to accomplish the task should be presented. Signed parent contracts are another way of documenting that the parent knows what should be done. Later the contract can be compared to what was done for the child.

Chronic Therapy

An approach to the long-term therapy for neglect and psychologic abuse is needed on an individual, community-wide and societal basis.

Individual and Family Treatments

A variety of individual and family-based therapies may be applied in nonphysical abuse situations. For example, psychologic therapy may vary from individual traditional psychotherapy to treatments based on in-home parental modeling programs. Nonphysical abuse therapy may require specific treatments aimed at improving the child's developmental, nutritional, behavioral, and/or psychologic well-being. Families may be failing in one area of their functioning or in many areas. A family evaluation of strengths and weaknesses must take place on a case-by-case basis to determine therapeutic needs and possible avenues of therapy.

Community-Based and Societal Therapies

Beyond those things that must be done for an individual child and family, consideration must be given to community-wide and societal aspects of therapy. Issues such as reasonable minimal entitlements for all children, access to health care, quality education, prohibition of corporal punishment, and child care policies in the work place all reflect the societal value of children and the supports given to their parents. For example, some would argue that parents who medically neglect their child should not be reported as a case of child abuse or neglect until we treat the 13 million children in the United States who have no health insurance and no access to health care. The 13 million children at risk need a societal therapy both to protect them as individuals and to set a standard for all parents and all countries that shows we care about children.

SUMMARY

The current therapy for child abuse and neglect is not a single-agent treatment. It is a broad series of actions, programs, kinds of therapies, and multidisciplinary therapeutic agents. Each abuse episode requires the willingness to consider abuse and astute diagnostic techniques. Once the suspicion of abuse is recognized, it must be reported. Once it has been reported, the family unit and its members must be analyzed for their strengths and weaknesses and proper fit of therapeutic services made or legal separation encouraged. Throughout the process, the primary physician must continue to ask the question, "Is the child safe?" Corrective action may be needed on an individual, family, community, or societal level.

REFERENCES

Bross D, Krusman RD, Lenherr MR: The New Child Protection Team Handbook, 2nd ed. New York, Garland Press, 1988.

Ludwig S, Kornberg A: Child Abuse: A Medical Reference, 2nd ed. New York, Churchill Livingstone, 1992.

U.S. Department of Health and Human Services. National Center on Child Abuse and Neglect. Study of Natural Incidence and Prevalence of Child Abuse and Neglect, 1988.

Wissow LS: Child Advocacy for the Clinician. Baltimore, Williams & Wilkins, 1990.

THE CHILD AND THE DEATH OF A LOVED ONE

MORRIS GREEN, M.D.

Five per cent of children under the age of 15 experience the death of one or both parents, whereas others lose a sibling, a grandparent, or a friend. The manifestations of grief in children differ in many respects from those in adults.

Children under the age of 3 years do not understand what death means beyond a very traumatic separation experience. Preschool children view death as similar to sleep. Those between the ages of 5 and 9 years begin to recognize death as irreversible but not as something that will happen to anyone they know. After the age of 9, children begin to understand that death is irreversible and could happen to them or their loved ones.

Since children and adolescents tolerate grief and depression poorly, they have a short "sadness span." To avoid being overwhelmed, young children try to deflect the frightening impact of their loss by resuming play, reading comic books, watching television, and acting as if nothing upsetting had happened. Some give no outward sign of grief. Adolescents, who may show little inclination to talk about their loss, may deny that they are depressed. The child or adolescent's behavior may be misinterpreted as inappropriate or uncaring, especially when a young child repeatedly asks when he will get a new father or mother. It is important, therefore, that the physician explain to the surviving spouse and other caregivers how the manifestations of grief in children differ from those in adults.

MANIFESTATIONS OF GRIEF IN CHILDREN

In the young child, the symptoms of grief include regression, sadness, fearfulness, anorexia, failure to thrive, sleep disturbance, social withdrawal, developmental delay, irritability, excessive crying, and increased dependency. The preschool child may demonstrate hyperactivity, constipation, encopresis, enuresis, temper tantrums, "out-of-control" behavior, anger, nightmares, and crying spells. The school-aged child's academic performance may decline. Other symptoms may include resistance to attending school, crying spells, lying, stealing, nervousness, and somatic complaints. Adolescents may demonstrate depression, somatic complaints, suicide attempts, and school drop-out.

THE PHYSICIAN'S ROLE

When a parent dies, the physician may express his or her personal condolences to the surviving parent and offer to be of help to the children. A personal note to each of the children is also meaningful and appreciated.

The child should be told of his parent's death by the surviving spouse or someone else whom the child knows well in a manner attuned to his or her developmental age. The explanation should be simple and repeated as needed. It is best not to use the phrase "went to sleep" because the child may then become afraid of going to bed. Since children may also fear that they or the surviving parent may die and that they were somehow responsible for their parent's death, they should be told explicitly that neither the surviving parent nor they are going to die and that the death was not their fault.

Because children worry about food, housing, and school, they need to be reassured that these needs will be met. Continuity should be stressed. If possible, familiar surroundings and routines should be maintained. So much has changed: The child's future seems uncertain, the surviving parent is preoccupied, the child's schedule is disrupted, and there are many visitors, some total strangers to the child. If possible, children should be kept in their own homes with one familiar primary caregiver to read, talk to, and play with younger children. School-aged children need someone with whom to share the news of the day, to answer questions repeatedly, and, as they are ready, to talk about their feelings.

Children may be confused and anxious about the dramatic changes in their surviving parent. Sad, anxious, disorganized, impatient, angry, irritable, and erratic, a grieving parent may simply be unable to cope with the heightened needs of the child. Bereaved parents may be insufficiently aware of their need for someone to talk to and for reassurance. Inappropriate "blurring of the generations" may lead, for example, to a mother clinging to the child, expecting her son to be the "man of the house," discussing money and other personal worries, or overburdening the child with chores.

Because bereaved children are very much affected by the mental health of their surviving parent, continuing symptoms in a child are often linked to the parent's unresolved grief. Problems related to bereavement in a parent may be manifested by persistent depression, failure to participate in outside social activities, somatic complaints, increased smoking, and abuse of alcohol or drugs. Referral of the parent to a mental health professional may be an important contribution of the physician.

RISK FACTORS IN CHILDREN

In children, the long-term outcome cannot be predicted on the basis of the bereaved child's initial response. Such sequelae, which may include an increased predisposition to illness, depression, and suicide, may not appear until the adult years. The Institute of Medicine Committee on the Health Consequences of Bereavement identified the following risk factors in bereaved children: parental death under 5 years of age or in early adolescence; maternal death when a girl is under 11 years of age; the death of a boy's father; a history of emotional problems in the child; an ambivalent relationship with the deceased parent or sibling; excessive parental dependency on the child; absence of a support network; inability of the surviving parent to use that support; multiple caregivers; lack of environmental constancy; a poor relationship with a stepparent; and bereavement due to sudden death, homicide, or suicide.

INDICATIONS FOR MENTAL HEALTH HELP

"Red flags" that suggest the need of a bereaved child for mental health help include severe anxiety, fear or hope of dying, persistent depression, suicide gestures or attempts, continued regressive behavior, a verbalized hope for reunion with the deceased, unremitting guilt and self-blame, aggressive and destructive behavior, delinquency, avoidance of talking about the deceased, expression of only positive or negative feelings about the deceased, school underachievement, school avoidance, promiscuity, unwillingness to separate from the surviving parent, failure to demonstrate any manifestation of grief, inability to form new attachments to other children or adults, excessive daydreaming, and persistent somatic complaints.

ATTENDING THE FUNERAL

Generally, children who can understand the cause of a sibling's or parent's death are old enough to attend the funeral if they wish. Children should not be forced to do so if they are afraid, reluctant, or revolted by the idea. Many children under 6 years of age are too young, whereas those over 9 may be helped by attending, especially if the service is conducted with the child's needs in mind. Preparation prior to the funeral should include being told by the family what the setting will look like and what will happen. It is also a good idea for the children to be accompanied by a relative or close family friend so that they may be accompanied out of the room where the funeral is being conducted if they wish to leave.

REFERENCES

Brent DA: A death in the family: The pediatrician's role. Pediatrics 72:645, 1983.
Osterweis M, Solomon F, Green M: Bereavement: Reactions, Consequences and Care. Washington, DC, National Academy Press, 1984.
Schowalter JE: Children and funerals. Pediatr Rev 1:337, 1980.

SEXUAL ABUSE AND ASSAULT

SIGMUND KHARASCH, M.D.
and JAN E. PARADISE, M.D.

Definitions of sexual abuse and assault vary considerably. Terms such as incest, molestation, and child rape are often used interchangeably and are not specific. The definition of sexual abuse provided by the National Center on Child Abuse and Neglect is clinically useful:

> Sexual abuse consists of contact or interactions between a child and an adult, when the child is being used for the sexual stimulation of that adult or another person. Sexual abuse may be committed by a person under the age of 18 years, when that person is either significantly older than the victim, or when the abuser is in a position of power or control over that child.

This definition properly emphasizes the importance of coercion in the process of sexual abuse and encompasses the many types of abusive sexual interactions that can occur, from outright rape to fondling without genital contact to pornographic videotaping that involves no physical contact at all.

Criminal laws about sexual abuse and assault also vary considerably in the 50 states. Because abuse and assault often require different actions on the part of the physician, it may be worthwhile to review the distinction between the two. The difference lies in the relationship between the perpetrator and the child. Contacts between a child and any caretaker (e.g., parent, babysitter, teacher) are termed *abuse.* The same contacts made by a person who is not responsible for the child's well-being, i.e., a non-caretaker, are deemed *assault.* In all 50 states, physicians are legally mandated to report suspected abuse cases to child protection service (CPS) agencies. Failure by the physician to report such abuse to state CPS agencies can incur legal penalties. A report of sexual assault by a non-caretaker will usually be rejected by a CPS agency's intake unit unless the event involved neglectful failure to protect on the part of the child's caretaker. Physicians are under no similar mandate to report sexual assault by a non-caretaker but should comply with the wishes of the patient and his or her family. Either the physician or the victim can report an alleged sexual assault to law enforcement officials. Such a report does not obligate the family to pursue subsequent prosecution of an alleged assailant. Although patients may choose not to inform the police about a sexual assault, prompt reporting may entitle the patient to counseling or financial assistance provided by victim-witness advocacy agencies, may document the cause of a subsequent pregnancy, and supports law enforcement efforts to keep communities safe. In either case, it is not the physician's task to determine whether or not a crime has occurred. This responsibility rests with legal authorities. The health needs of a victim of sexual abuse or assault remain the physician's primary concern.

Physicians have an important role to play in the evaluation of children and adolescents who present with a complaint of sexual abuse. Sexual abuse and assault occur commonly and are likely to have an impact on the subsequent emotional well-being of young victims. Physicians are frequently asked to evaluate the psychologic and physical status of abused children and occasionally asked to communicate their findings to CPS social workers and prosecutors. Familiarity with the clinical management of sexual abuse and assault is a necessary prerequisite to effective child advocacy.

EPIDEMIOLOGY

Sexual abuse is now a commonly recognized problem among children and adolescents. The National Incidence and Prevalence Study of Child Abuse and Neglect concluded that 2.5 children per 1000 are reported to have been victims of sexual abuse each year—a total of 159,000 cases annually in the United States. Because some cases still go unreported, as many as 350,000 cases may occur annually. Although epidemiologists differ on the question of whether the actual number of sexual abuse cases is increasing, the number of reported cases has risen dramatically in the past two decades.

Most children are sexually abused by people they know well, such as parents, other relatives, or friends. Overall, 85 to 90 per cent of victims of sexual abuse are girls but, particularly among groups of younger children, boys account for 25 to 40 per cent of cases. Although female perpetrators are increasingly recognized, 95 per cent of cases involve male assailants.

PRESENTATION

Children are brought to medical attention for assessment of possible sexual abuse by parents or social service workers because of a child's direct disclosure, an adult's suspicion of abuse, or somatic complaints that suggest abuse. Many presenting behavioral and somatic complaints, including nightmares, school adjustment problems, suicidal behavior, enuresis, encopresis, genital discomfort, and abdominal pain, have been noted to lead upon further inquiry to a diagnosis of sexual abuse. However, nonspecific signs and symptoms like these are common and are at least as likely to indicate physical and emotional disorders other than sexual abuse. Although sexual abuse should be considered in the differential diagnosis of nonspecific complaints, none of them constitutes presumptive evidence of sexual abuse.

A confident diagnosis of sexual abuse rests on specific descriptive statements made directly by the child. The following are general guidelines for interviewing a child who presents with a complaint of alleged sexual abuse:

1. The physician should obtain the history at the time of presentation if the child is able to discuss it, since some children may subsequently retract allegations in response to pressure from the family or perpetrator or because of fear of retaliation. Statements made by the child shortly after the abuse has occurred may be admissible in court as fresh complaints.

2. No part of the interview should be forced upon a child. If the child appears unwilling or unable to discuss the situation, the interview can be deferred until a later time, or the child can be referred to a pediatrician, social worker, psychologist, or psychiatrist who specializes in this area for further evaluation.

3. *The person most trained or experienced in interviewing young children should conduct the interview.*

4. Repeated interviews are usually not necessary and are potentially harmful. If a child has already been interviewed formally about the present allegation by another professional, the physician should confer with the child's parent or social worker to discover what further diagnostic or treatment issues require attention.

PHYSICAL EXAMINATION

The goals of the physical examination of the sexually abused child are the following:

1. To identify both genital and nongenital injuries.
2. To collect forensic specimens, including samples of secretions that may contain evidence of seminal fluid.
3. To evaluate the adolescent patient for possible pregnancy.
4. To obtain specimens for the diagnosis of sexually transmitted diseases.
5. To identify any previously unrecognized health problems.

The evaluating physician should be familiar with the anatomy of the prepubertal female genitalia and comfortable performing pelvic examinations of adolescents. Figure 1 illustrates the anatomy of the prepubertal female genitalia.

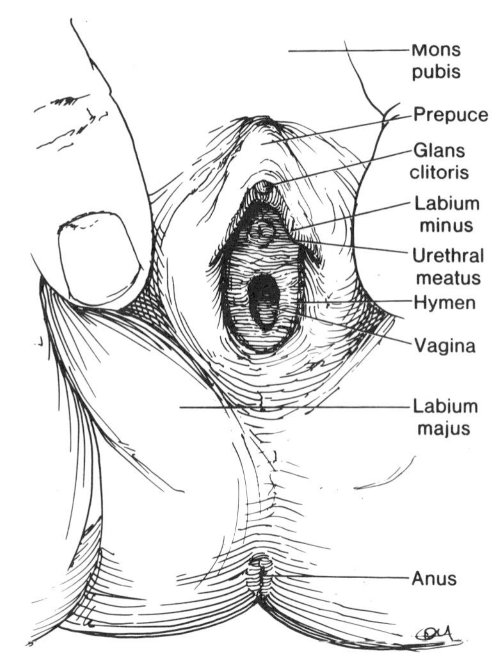

Figure 1. Anatomy of the normal female external genitalia. From Paradise JE: Pediatric and adolescent gynecology. *In* Fleisher G, Ludwig S: Textbook of Pediatric Emergency Medicine, 2nd ed. Baltimore, Williams & Wilkins, 1988, p 710.

EXAMINATION TECHNIQUES

Position

Sexually abused girls should be placed in the frog-leg or knee-chest position for examination of the genitalia (Fig. 2). The latter position allows visualization of the vaginal vault and should be used if intravaginal injury or a foreign body is suspected. In the frog-leg position, gentle superolateral traction should be applied to the labia majora to allow visualization of the introitus. In either position, an otoscope without its speculum or a colposcope (see below) can provide direct illumination and magnification. A careful external examination of the genitalia is usually sufficient to assess the prepubertal girl. In prepubertal boys, the genitalia should be examined with the patient in the supine position. The patient should be placed in the left lateral position with the buttocks gently separated or in the knee-chest position for inspection of the anus.

Colposcopy

Colposcopy can be used to inspect the external genitalia and perineum of sexually abused children under magnified, well-illuminated conditions. Magnified photographs taken by colposcopes with camera attachments can document examination findings and injuries. Because colposcopy is noninvasive and can produce a permanent record of findings, it can also enhance teaching trainees about sexual abuse examinations and can allow examiners to compare their impressions or diagnoses. Drawbacks of colposcopy include the cost of the instrument, the absence of standards for interpreting anatomic variants, and the potential distress experienced by a child if his or her perineal anatomy is scrutinized in the semipublic forum of a courtroom.

INTERPRETATION OF PHYSICAL FINDINGS

Differential Diagnosis

Genital injuries, such as lacerations, abrasions, and contusions, are not difficult to recognize and confirm that physical contact has occurred. Significantly reduced anal tone and anal bruises or hematomas can be seen in both males and females. Minor findings, including vaginal erythema, increased introital vascularity, friability of the vulvar posterior fourchette, anal hyperpigmentation, and perianal tags, are nonspecific and frequently seen in nonabused children. Diagnostic abnormalities—injuries, sexually transmitted infections, and evidence of seminal fluid—have been reported in fewer than 20 per cent of children and adolescents with histories of sexual abuse.

The presence of visible vaginal discharge in a prepubertal girl indicates probable bacterial infection or foreign body. The etiology of vaginitis is discussed elsewhere. Vaginal bleeding in a young girl is always of concern. Besides sexual abuse, other causes of actual or apparent vaginal bleeding include lichen sclerosus, urethral prolapse, foreign body, group A streptococcal or *Shigella* vaginitis, and accidental straddle injuries. Indications for speculum examination are few but include an intravaginal source of bleeding and a history of penetrating vaginal injury. Speculum examination of prepubertal children should be performed using general anesthesia.

Group A beta-hemolytic *Streptococcus* has recently been reported as a cause of balanitis in uncircumcised prepubertal

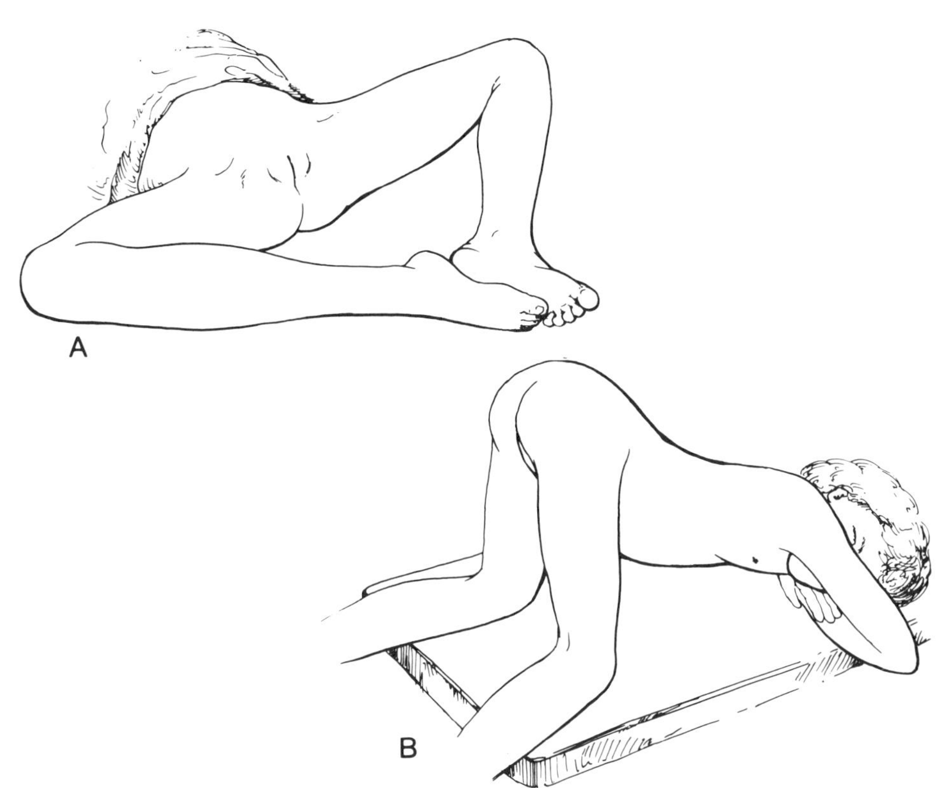

Figure 2. *A*, Girl in the frog-leg position for examination of the external genitalia. *B*, Girl in the knee-chest position with exaggerated lordosis and relaxed abdominal muscles. The examiner can inspect the interior of her vagina by gently separating her buttocks and labia, using an otoscope without an attached speculum for illumination. From Paradise JE: Pediatric and adolescent gynecology. *In* Fleisher G, Ludwig S: Textbook of Pediatric Emergency Medicine, 2nd ed. Baltimore, Williams & Wilkins, 1988, p 711.

boys. This infection is sometimes accompanied by urethral discharge. Venereal causes of urethral discharge in boys are discussed below.

Transverse Hymenal Orifice Diameter

Although the relationship between hymenal orifice diameter and sexual abuse remains somewhat controversial, most experts acknowledge that no single cut-off value differentiates the transverse hymenal orifice diameters of girls with and without histories of genital penetration. The examiner cannot draw any conclusions about sexual contact from the isolated finding of an unexpectedly large hymenal orifice diameter. Several points may be useful in this regard:

1. Changes in observed hymenal orifice diameter in a given child depend on her age and pubertal status, her position during examination, degree of relaxation, the amount of traction applied by the examiner, the method of measurement, and perhaps on whether there has been prior vaginal inflammation or injury.
2. The ranges of transverse hymenal orifice diameters in abused and nonabused children overlap. Small differences are not clinically important.
3. *Many states define penetration as penetration past the labia majora, not of the hymenal ring.* In light of this definition and the many sources of unreliability in measurement, the finding of a hymenal orifice diameter within the range observed in nonabused children is often quite consistent with a history of penetrating sexual abuse or assault.

FORENSIC EVIDENCE

Forensic evidence is collected in cases of sexual assault and abuse in order to corroborate the history of the assault and to identify possible perpetrators. Most hospitals utilize commercially prepared kits with detailed checklists and explanations of proper procedures for evidence collection. Whatever method is used to collect evidence, it is important to minimize the number of personnel handling specimens and to document every transfer of specimens from one person to another, thus maintaining the "chain of evidence." The following items are generally gathered for evidence from patients within 72 hours of the assault if the history indicates that they might provide forensic information:

1. Swabs of secretions from clinically indicated areas (oral cavity, vagina, rectum) to detect evidence of seminal fluid. Sperm can usually be detected microscopically for 12 to 20 hours and occasionally for up to 72 hours after intercourse in the estrogenized vagina. Shorter survival times are found in mouth and rectal specimens as well as in prepubertal girls who lack cervical mucus. Depending on the laboratory, analysis of cervicovaginal secretions may include efforts to detect choline, prostatic acid phosphatase, and P30, a semen glycoprotein of prostatic origin that may be detectable for up to 48 hours after ejaculation. A newer and potentially more sensitive monoclonal antibody test—MHS-5 (mouse anti-human sperm–5)—is an assay for a seminal vesicle peptide. This test is not dependent on the presence of sperm for a positive result and can be positive in cases in which either full ejaculation did not occur or the perpetrator was aspermic. As is true for spermatozoa, evidence of seminal fluid is not usually detectable in vivo for longer than 72 hours after an assault.
2. Clothing worn by the victim. These articles should be stored in sealed bags and labeled. Foreign material or dried semen on clothing may be detectable for many months after an assault.
3. Blood and saliva specimens from the patient. These are used to compare the blood group secretor status of the patient with that of an alleged perpetrator.
4. Specimens for sexually transmitted disease (STD) screening.

PREGNANCY PREVENTION

Although pregnancy resulting from sexual assault is uncommon, it is potentially preventable. Every postpubertal female seen within 72 hours after a sexual assault should be advised about postcoital contraception and offered treatment if she is not currently pregnant. (This should be verified with a pregnancy test.) The combination of ethinyl estradiol and *dl*-norgestrel (Ovral) has proved an effective regimen for pregnancy prophylaxis, reducing the pregnancy rate to less than 2 per cent following unprotected intercourse. To be effective, two Ovral tablets should be given at once and two more tablets given 12 hours later. Treatment must be started within 72 hours after the assault. A second pregnancy test 2 weeks later is recommended to ascertain whether pregnancy has occurred. Patients should be informed in advance of Ovral's possible side effects, principally nausea and vomiting.

ANTIBIOTIC PROPHYLAXIS

Antibiotic prophylaxis is not recommended for most sexually abused children because the abuse has often been chronic, the risk of infection is low, and the customary antibiotic regimen only treats two or, at most, three of the several possible infections. However, if a child or adolescent is a victim of a single, very recent assault or is victimized by multiple assailants, the parents or patient may understandably desire prophylaxis. Antibiotic regimens for prophylaxis are found in Tables 1 and 2. These should not be given until after screening specimens for culture have been obtained. Patients receiving prophylaxis should be retested several weeks later to document therapeutic success or failure.

SEXUALLY TRANSMITTED DISEASES

Screening for STDs is important to guide appropriate therapy and, occasionally, to confirm that sexual contact has occurred. Considerations for proceeding with an evaluation for STDs include the following:

1. Presumptive diagnostic techniques (e.g., Gram stain, rapid antigen detection tests, Tzanck smears) should not be used as the basis for contacting CPS agencies or for confirming a diagnosis of sexual abuse. The risk of both false-positive and false-negative tests, compounded by the potential harm of a premature report of suspected sexual abuse, makes confirmation of any presumptive test by culture mandatory.
2. Although discovery of an STD in a child older than 1 or 2 months is suggestive of sexual abuse, some neonatally acquired infections (e.g., *Chlamydia trachomatis* infection, genital warts, trichomoniasis) can persist for months and produce few or no symptoms.
3. Only a minority (5 to 15 per cent) of sexually abused children acquire STDs. The most common of these infections are often asymptomatic (e.g., gonococcal pharyngitis, chlamydial vaginitis). Thus, all children with histories of sexual abuse should be screened for the most common infections (Table 3).
4. Nonsexual transmission of STDs (fomites, bathing, autoinoculation) is rare.

TABLE 1. Recommended Treatment Regimens for Incubating and Established Gonococcal Infections*

Antibiotic	Regimen by Patient's Weight: ≥45 *kg*	Regimen by Patient's Weight: <45 *kg*	Comments
Amoxicillin† with probenecid	3.0 g p.o. 1.0 g p.o.	50 mg/kg p.o. 25 mg/kg p.o.	Use only when gonococci are known to be penicillin-sensitive; amoxicillin may not treat pharyngeal infection
Ceftriaxone	250 mg IM	125 mg IM	Use when antibiotic sensitivity of organism is unknown
Spectinomycin	2.0 g IM	40 mg/kg IM	Use for patients with penicillin allergy; may not treat incubating syphilis and pharyngeal gonorrhea

Adapted from the Centers for Disease Control: 1989 Sexually Transmitted Diseases Treatment Guidelines. MMWR 38(suppl 8), 1989; and the American Academy of Pediatrics: 1988 Report of the Committee on Infectious Diseases. Reprinted in Paradise JE: The medical evaluation of the sexually abused child. Pediatr Clin North Am 37(4) 839–862, 1990.

**Warning:* Concurrent presumptive treatment for chlamydial infection is recommended. These recommendations are not for patients with suspected or definite pelvic inflammatory disease.

†Other penicillin regimens including benzathine penicillin and penicillin V are not recommended.

Abbreviations: p.o., orally; IM, intramuscularly.

TABLE 2. Recommended Treatment Regimens for Incubating and Established Chlamydial Infection*

Antibiotic	Regimen by Patient's Weight: ≥45 *kg*	Regimen by Patient's Weight: <45 *kg*	Comments
Doxycycline or	100 mg p.o. b.i.d. for 7 days		Tetracyclines are not indicated during pregnancy and for children younger than 8 years of age
Tetracycline	500 mg p.o. q.i.d. for 7 days	40 mg/kg/day in 4 doses for 7 days	
Erythromycin base or	500 mg p.o. q.i.d. for 7 days	40 mg/kg/day in 4 doses for 7 days	Use for pregnant patients and children under 8 years of age
Erythromycin ethylsuccinate	800 mg p.o. q.i.d. for 7 days	40 mg/kg/day in 4 doses for 7 days	

Adapted from the Centers for Disease Control: 1989 Sexually Transmitted Diseases Treatment Guidelines. MMWR 38(suppl 8), 1989; and the American Academy of Pediatrics: 1988 Report of the Committee on Infectious Diseases. Reprinted from Paradise JE: The medical evaluation of the sexually abused child. Pediatr Clin North Am 37(4):839–862, 1990.

**Warning:* These recommendations are not for patients with suspected or definite pelvic inflammatory diseases.

Abbreviations: p.o., orally; b.i.d., twice a day; q.i.d., four times a day.

Gonorrhea

Gonococcal vaginitis produces a copious purulent vaginal discharge. Some, but not all, boys with urethritis have dysuria and urethral discharge. Balanitis and penile venereal edema are uncommon manifestations of gonorrhea in boys. Rectal and pharyngeal infections are almost always asymptomatic.

The treatment regimens for gonococcal infections are outlined in Table 1. Children who are allergic to ceftriaxone or penicillin should be treated with spectinomycin. Because penicillinase-producing *Neisseria gonorrhoeae* strains are increasingly prevalent, an oral treatment regimen should not be used unless the antibiotic sensitivity of the organism has been established in the laboratory. If the organism is penicillinase-negative, an oral regimen can be used to avoid administering an intramuscular injection. Amoxicillin is less likely than ceftriaxone to eradicate pharyngeal and rectal infections. When treatment for gonorrhea is given prophylactically, an

TABLE 3. Common Sexually Transmitted Diseases in Sexually Abused Children

Infection (Incubation Period)	Preferred Method of Diagnosis	Testing Site	Indication for Testing		
			Prepubertal Girls	*Pubertal Girls*	*Boys*
Gonorrhea (2 to 7 days)	Culture	Cervix	No	All	—
		Pharynx	All	All	All
		Rectum	All	All	All
		Vagina or urethra	Sx	No	All
Chlamydial infection (variable)	Culture, or EIA or DFA confirmed by culture	Cervix	No	All	—
		Pharynx	All	Hx	All
		Rectum*	All	Hx	All
		Vagina* or urethra	All	No	All
Trichomoniasis (4 to 20 days)	Microscopy or culture	Vagina or urethra	Sx	Sx	Sx
Genital herpes (2 to 14 days)	Viral culture	Vesicle	Sx	Sx	Sx
Genital warts (1 to 8 months)	Biopsy or inspection	Wart	Sx	All†	Sx

Reprinted with permission from Paradise JE: The medical evaluation of the sexually abused child. Pediatr Clin North Am 37(4):839–862, 1990.
*Fecal flora cross-react with *Chlamydia trachomatis* antisera. Positive vaginal and rectal EIA and DFA test results should be confirmed by culture.
†Screen all with Papanicolaou (Pap) smear. Further investigation as indicated by signs of disease or Pap smear results.
Abbreviations: DFA, direct fluorescent antibody test; EIA, enzyme immunoassay; Hx, if patient describes contact at this site; STD, sexually transmitted disease; Sx, if patient has symptoms or signs of the disease.

antibiotic effective against *C. trachomatis* should be given concomitantly because dual infections are common.

C. trachomatis Infections

The diagnosis of *C. trachomatis* in a child with a history of sexual abuse should depend on tissue culture rather than on the more commonly available and less costly rapid antigen detection tests. The non-culture tests are relatively likely to give false-positive results because the prevalence of infection among abused children is low. Additionally, normal mouth and rectal flora may cross-react with *C. trachomatis* in these tests. If rapid antigen detection tests are employed for initial screening of abused children, positive results should be confirmed by tissue culture.

Treatment regimens for *C. trachomatis* infections are presented in Table 2. Tetracycline and doxycycline should not be given to pregnant patients and children younger than the age of 8 years because of the risk of dental staining. Erythromycin is the preferred alternative antibiotic.

Because erythromycin is less effective than doxycycline, children treated with erythromycin should be retested after 4 to 6 weeks in order to identify treatment failures. (Some delay in assessing cure with enzyme immunoassay tests is desirable because residual chlamydial antigen may produce a positive test for days to weeks after the microorganisms have been killed.) Follow-up tests for adolescent patients treated with tetracycline or doxycyline may also be delayed in order to identify reinfections.

Trichomoniasis

Treatment for trichomoniasis in postpubertal patients can be accomplished with a single dose of 2.0 g of metronidazole orally. Preadolescent children should be treated with 5 mg/kg/day orally of metronidazole in three divided doses for 7 days. Common side effects of metronidazole are nausea, mild abdominal pain, and a metallic taste.

Genital Herpes

Genital herpes simplex virus (HSV) infection is uncommon in children and should be considered a strong indicator of sexual abuse because of its short incubation period. Nonsexual transmission of HSV has not been well studied. Autoinoculation of the virus is a possible explanation for genital lesions that appear simultaneously with or in rapid succession after herpes gingivostomatitis or herpes labialis.

Oral acyclovir shortens the duration of symptoms and viral shedding in adults with initial outbreaks of genital herpes (primary infection), but it does not appreciably alter the clinical course of recurrences. Although experience in treating children is limited, acyclovir may be considered for the treatment of children and adolescents with severe local pain or dysuria, urinary retention, and systemic illness resulting from primary genital infections. The dose of oral acyclovir for adolescents with primary herpes is 200 mg, 5 times daily for 10 days. For children, acyclovir ointment may be applied to lesions topically and may reduce the duration of symptoms and viral shedding.

Genital Warts

The number of treatments available for genital warts underscores how difficult it can be to eradicate this infection. Treatment is complicated by the fact that the virus infects normal-appearing skin adjacent to affected sites. The treatment method currently recommended by the Centers for Disease Control is cryotherapy with liquid nitrogen. Other treatments for genital warts are laser destruction of tissue, trichloroacetic acid, and alpha-interferon in refractory cases.

An alternative regimen is 10 to 25 per cent podophyllin in tincture of benzoin. This can be applied topically to warts on nonmucosal surfaces. The podophyllin should be washed off within 1 to 4 hours after application to avoid damage to normal skin. Recurrences following podophyllin treatment are common. Systemic absorption of podophyllin from mucosal surfaces or treatment of large surface areas can cause bone marrow suppression, peripheral neuropathy, coma, and death. The total volume of podophyllin solution should be limited to less than 0.5 ml per treatment session. Podophyllin treatment is contraindicated during pregnancy.

Syphilis

Syphilis is rarely acquired by sexually abused children. As is the case for other STDs, a child's risk of acquiring syphilis depends on the community prevalence of the disease and on the nature of the physical contacts. If the decision is made to screen abused children for syphilis, serologic tests should not be obtained until 6 weeks or longer after the abuse began. (An incubation period of up to 6 weeks may be required for seroconversion in infected children.)

All of the treatment regimens for gonorrhea outlined in Table 1 except spectinomycin are sufficient to treat incubating syphilis. Spectinomycin, used for children allergic to penicillin or cephalosporins, may be used to treat incubating syphilis, but efficacy is not as certain.

Early syphilis (primary, secondary, and latent syphilis of less than 1 year's duration) must be treated with one intramuscular dose of benzathine penicillin (50,000 units/kg; maximum dose of 2.4 million units). Penicillin-allergic patients younger than 8 years of age should be given erythromycin (30 to 50 mg/kg/day in four divided doses for 2 weeks). Penicillin-allergic older children should be treated with tetracycline (500 mg orally four times a day for 2 weeks) or doxycycline (100 mg orally twice a day for 2 weeks). Because the efficacy of erythromycin and tetracyclines is not assured, consideration should be given to desensitizing infected children to penicillin.

Human Immunodeficiency Virus (HIV)

Acquisition of HIV infection following sexual abuse is rare but has been reported. Many parents are especially anxious about the risk of this infection. The advisability of HIV screening should be reviewed with the parents of all sexually abused children. The very low prevalence of this infection in children makes the occurrence of false-positive antibody tests likely, but if the perpetrator of sexual abuse is judged to be at high risk of being HIV-infected (homosexual, intravenous drug abuse, multiple sexual partners), greater consideration may be given to screening the child. In asymptomatic patients with a positive enzyme-linked immunosorbent assay, Western blot tests for HIV antibody should be used to confirm the presence of the virus.

See Section 18 for a discussion of the treatment of children with HIV infection.

DOCUMENTATION

Medical records are legal documents. A clear and legible medical record can frequently substitute for the physician's testimony in legal proceedings about sexual abuse cases. The identities of involved individuals, quoted statements from the child, and signs found on examination, laboratory tests, treatments, and recommendations should be carefully recorded. When the physician is describing the appearance of the genitalia of girls, phrases such as "hyman intact," "virginal hymen," and "marital introitus" are subjective and vague and should be avoided.

Sexual abuse and assault are legal findings based on accumulated evidence and made only by a judge or jury. Because physicians cannot substitute for a judge or a jury, phrases such as "rape complaint" or "alleged sexual abuse" should be used to indicate the diagnostic impression.

PSYCHOLOGIC TREATMENT

Psychosocial sequelae of sexual abuse and assault in teens and children are unpredictable. Depression, self-blame, fear, and denial are common acute psychologic reactions. In the longer term, some children appear to survive relatively unscathed whereas others develop a syndrome analogous to post-traumatic stress disorder in adults. At the extreme, dissociative and multiple personality disorders have been seen in adults with previously undisclosed childhood sexual abuse. Sexually abused boys in particular appear to be at some risk for incorporating sexual aggression into their behavior and becoming abusers themselves.

It is to be hoped that early recognition and effective, empathetic management of sexual abuse will protect children seen now from long-term distress. Crisis counseling and individual or group psychotherapy should be made available to all victims of sexual abuse and assault. Most parents suffer severely from feelings of anger, guilt, and anxiety after discovering that their children have been sexually abused. Crisis and ongoing counseling for parents may offer an outlet for their intense emotions and may indirectly benefit the abused children themselves.

3

Nervous System

HEAD INJURY

RICHARD H. STRAUSS, M.D.

Five million children suffer head injury in the United States each year, 250,000 of whom are hospitalized; 4000 die and 15,000 have prolonged hospitalization and rehabilitation. Approximately 5 per cent of all hospitalized children are admitted because of head injury. Most of those patients are hospitalized for assessment of neurologic status and for monitoring the development of intracranial complications; less commonly they are hospitalized for immediate treatment of their injuries. Despite these figures, more than 99 per cent of children with head injury have normal outcomes. Most minor head injuries are treated by pediatricians (or parents, babysitters, or school nurses, who may contact a pediatrician) in emergency rooms or in offices. Outcome following major head injury is dependent on the initial level of coma, the severity of intracranial hypertension, the presence of cerebral edema or a mass lesion, and the presence of complications.

EXTRACRANIAL INJURY

Scalp lacerations should be inspected for foreign material, cleaned, and repaired with suture material or sterile tapes to ensure that the apposed wound is free of hair. If lacerations extend to the skull or beyond, further investigation may be warranted to check the integrity of the dura and the brain. Tetanus immunization status should be reviewed and appropriate treatment provided.

Hematomas of the scalp usually resolve within several weeks of the injury (although some go on to calcify). Aspiration of subgaleal hematomas or cephalohematomas is not recommended and may in fact cause further hemorrhage or infection. Some scalp hematomas have sharply edged borders that are so similar to the edges of a depressed skull fracture that a tangential skull x-ray view may be necessary to differentiate the two.

SKULL FRACTURE

Minor Head Injury

Many people who have suffered minor head injury have skull radiographs taken, even though these patients appear normal on physical examination. Those x-rays sometimes demonstrate linear skull fractures. Unless the history of the accident is unusual or unknown or the child has abnormal findings on physical and/or neurologic examinations, hospitalization is not required. Temporal swelling/fracture and swelling/fracture across the sagittal suture are indications for computed tomography (CT) scanning and possible hospitalization in the view of some experts. Guidelines for parents ("head injury sheets"), to be used while observing their child at home, and availability of the pediatrician to answer parents' questions are reasonable alternatives to hospitalization. Observation over a period of several hours in an office or emergency room with repeated neurologic examinations before discharge home with a "head injury sheet" is another acceptable alternative to hospitalization. Skull x-ray examinations are not necessary or diagnostically helpful for patients with minor head injury. Similarly, lumbar puncture is not a useful procedure for diagnosis or treatment of the child with a head injury.

Depressed Skull Fracture

Depressed skull fracture should be considered when a palpable depression or a large swelling is felt on the skull. A tangential skull radiograph is usually adequate for diagnosis unless there are other abnormalities on examination suggesting intracranial injury, which would make emergency unenhanced CT scanning a more desirable examination. Surgical elevation of a depressed skull fracture depends on the depth of the depression (greater than the thickness of the skull), the presence of a dural tear or compound fracture, or the presence of neurologic abnormalities. Whether elevation of a depressed skull fracture stems the occurrence of post–head injury epilepsy is unknown.

Diastatic Skull Fracture

Diastatic fractures occur along the lambdoid and sagittal sutures in young children, and in the absence of other neurologic findings they rarely lead to problems; therefore, no specific treatment other than the guidelines already mentioned is required.

Basilar Skull Fracture

Basilar skull fracture involves the basal sections of the frontal, ethmoid, sphenoid, parietal, or occipital bones. Basilar fractures are more often diagnosed from physical findings (mastoid or periorbital ecchymosis, cerebrospinal fluid (CSF) otorrhea, CSF rhinorrhea, hemotympanum) than from radiographic studies. Basilar skull fracture is associated with dural tear and communication with the paranasal sinuses or the middle ear, and such patients are at risk for the development of meningitis. Studies have not shown that prophylactic antibiotic treatment (against the most common infecting organism, *Pneumococcus*) decreases the incidence of meningitis following basilar skull fracture. Cerebrospinal fluid rhinorrhea and otorrhea usually cease spontaneously by 1 week after the injury. Should a CSF leak persist longer than 2 weeks, radionuclide examination of the CSF can help localize the leak. Patients with hemotympanum should have tympanographic and audiologic evaluation after discharge from the hospital or office. Hospitalization is not necessary when basilar skull fracture is unaccompanied by more serious injuries.

Dural Tear

Children with linear, diastatic, or basilar skull fracture associated with dural tear are at risk for the development of "growing fractures" several months later, and they should undergo periodic clinical and radiographic re-evaluation.

INTRACRANIAL INJURY (Table 1)

Assessing the Severity of Injury

The child who has sustained a mild closed head injury with a period of unconsciousness not longer than 5 minutes can usually be observed at home if the results of physical and neurologic examinations are normal and reliable observation at home can be guaranteed over the next day (with "head injury sheets" that tell parents how to monitor changes in level of consciousness, motor activity, pupillary activity, behavior, sleep habits, and breathing patterns). In addition, parents should be told to observe carefully for neurologic and behavior changes and fever over the next few weeks. If reliable observation in the home cannot be guaranteed, hospitalization is necessary. In either situation, hourly observation over a period of 6 to 24 hours should be instituted, and if the child remains stable, observation may become less frequent. If a deterioration in the level of consciousness or vital signs occurs, neurologic examination must be repeated and CT scanning to check for the presence of intracranial hemorrhage or cerebral edema should be done. The decision to admit a comatose child is not a difficult choice. It is much more difficult to determine the risk for development of an intracranial complication following minor head injury in a healthy-looking child. The child with minor closed head injury who has abnormal findings on neurologic examination even in the absence of obvious head injury should not be sent home. Any child who has altered consciousness, focal central nervous system abnormalities, depressed skull fracture, penetrating head injury, or signs of worsening illness should be hospitalized and should undergo CT scanning. Magnetic resonance imaging (MRI), though not routine in the initial evaluation of head injury, may provide better definition of the posterior fossa than CT scanning and may also have a role in the evaluation of the child during the recovery phase following head injury.

Avoiding Secondary Brain Injury

Severe closed head injury has many anatomic forms, several of which are discussed in other sections of this text. It is frequently (but not always) associated with prolonged (longer than 5 to 10 minutes) loss of consciousness, altered state of consciousness (disorientation, unarousability, delirium), seizures, focal neurologic signs, abnormal vital signs, persistent severe headache, and other physical signs of major trauma. In addition to localizing and describing the intracranial injury by CT scanning and determining whether it is a surgically remediable lesion, intensive care to the injured brain must be provided to optimize oxygen/blood flow to the brain and to minimize secondary injury to the brain: hypoxia, ischemia, edema, increased intracranial pressure (ICP), and herniation. At the same time, support of other body systems must be maintained and neck stabilization must be secured. Endotracheal intubation provides airway protection and a route for pulmonary toilet and mechanical ventilation as well as a means for moderate hyperventilation (P_{CO_2} approximately 25 to 30 mm Hg) to decrease arterial P_{CO_2}, thereby avoiding cerebral vasodilatation and increased ICP (normal is less than 15 mm Hg, or 200 mm H_2O). Intubation itself is a noxious stimulus, and it should be done by the most experienced person present in order to avoid acute severe rises in ICP. Intubation should be preceded by hyperventilation with 100 per cent O_2. If systemic circulation is normal, intubation can be preceded by administration of atropine (0.02 mg/kg IV/IM, minimum dose 0.1 mg), thiopental 2 mg/kg IV), and succinylcholine (2 mg/kg IV/IM for patients under 1 year, and 1 mg/kg IV/IM for patients over 1 year) or (if there are contraindications to

TABLE 1. Drugs Used in Head Injury

Name	Dose	Route	Use	Comments
Oxygen	100%	Mask, ET, cannula	Ensure oxygenation	Pulse oximetry helpful
Atropine	0.02 mg/kg	IV, IM, ET, SC	Dry secretions, prevent bradycardia	Minimum dose 0.1 mg
Thiopental	2 mg/kg	IV	Sedation	May depress circulation
Succinylcholine	2 mg/kg (<1 year) 1 mg/kg (>1 year)	IV, IM	Depolarizing paralyzer	Contraindicated in crush injury, burn, hyperkalemia
Vecuronium	0.1 mg/kg	IV	Nondepolarizing paralyzer	May increase intracranial pressure
Pancuronium	0.1 mg/kg	IV	Nondepolarizing paralyzer	Tachycardia
Midazolam	0.2 mg/kg 0.4–6 μ/kg/minute	IV IV infusion	Sedation	
Diazepam	0.2 mg/kg	IV	Sedation anticonvulsant	Respiratory depression
Mannitol (20%)	0.25–2 g/kg	IV	Decrease ICP	Hyperosmolar state
Furosemide	1 mg/kg	IV		
Ethacrynic acid	1 mg/kg	IV		
Pentobarbital	3–5 mg/kg 1–3 mg/kg/hr	IV IV infusion	Decrease ICP	30–40 μg/ml blood level; CNS and circulatory effects
Phenytoin	15–20 mg/kg	IV	Anticonvulsant	Bradycardia

Abbreviations: IV, intravenous (intraosseous); IM, intramuscular; ET, endotracheal; SC, subcutaneous; ICP, intracranial pressure; CNS, central nervous system.

succinylcholine) vecuronium or pancuronium (0.1 mg/kg IV). Because succinylcholine may increase ICP, it can be given after a defasciculating dose of pancuronium (0.01 mg/kg IV). If systemic circulation is insufficient, midazolam (0.2 mg/kg IV/IM) can be substituted for thiopental. Arterial Po_2 should be maintained at a level greater than 100 mm Hg.

TREATMENT

Fluid and Electrolyte Therapy

Fluid and electrolyte therapy must be titrated to the patient's skin perfusion, heart rate, urine production, insensible water loss, weight change, and degree of cerebral edema/increased ICP, but as a rule, two-thirds fluid maintenance is a reasonable starting point. Hypovolemic shock does not usually result from head injury unless there is excessive scalp bleeding. Shock is treated with volume infusion even in the presence of increased ICP. Serum electrolytes and osmolarity should be monitored frequently in order to avoid (or treat) hyponatremia (caused by inappropriate ADH secretion) or severe hyperosmolarity. There is no evidence that corticosteroids help reduce cerebral edema/increased ICP secondary to severe head injury. Sucralfate (15 mg/kg via nasogastric tube every 6 hours) or antacids (0.5 ml/kg via nasogastric tube to maintain gastric pH at less than 4) may be given to patients with severe head injury.

Treatment of Increased Intracranial Pressure

Increased ICP can be avoided in some patients and treated in other patients by simple maneuvers designed to maintain cerebral perfusion pressure (CPP) over 50 mm Hg. From the equation CPP = mean arterial pressure − ICP, it is apparent that if ICP rises or mean arterial pressure falls, cerebral perfusion pressure and cerebral blood flow may become inadequate. (Invasive monitoring of ICP and arterial blood pressure is necessary if cranial nerve dysfunction, apnea, posturing, and/or Glasgow Coma Score ≤ 8 are present.) Methods to decrease ICP are elevation of the head to 30 degrees; midline positioning of the head so that venous return is not impeded; avoidance of noxious stimuli; a trial of intravenous lidocaine (1.5 mg/kg) before endotracheal suctioning and intubation and chest percussion; endotracheal suctioning that follows hyperventilation; maintenance of normal temperature to avoid shivering; paralysis with vecuronium or pancuronium (0.1 mg/kg IV, given as needed); sedation with midazolam (0.2 mg/kg IV, followed by infusion at 0.4 to 6 μg/kg/min) or morphine (0.05 to 0.1 mg/kg IV every 2 to 4 hours), or diazepam (0.2 mg/kg IV every 1 to 2 hours) unless sedation is believed to interfere with accuracy of the neurologic examination.

Acute ICP elevation over 20 mm Hg can be treated with temporary manual hyperventilation, mannitol (0.25 to 2.0 g/kg IV over 20 minutes every 30 minutes to 4 hours); and drainage of small aliquots (0.5 to 1.0 ml) of CSF. Osmotic agents may be given with furosemide or ethacrynic acid (1 mg/kg IV) to enhance the ICP lowering effect. Craniectomy, hypothermia, and pentobarbital (3 to 5 mg/kg IV over 30 minutes, followed by 1 to 3 mg/kg/hour, to maintain a blood level of 30 to 40 μg/ml) may be considered if other treatments fail. If inadequate mean arterial pressure is the cause of low cerebral perfusion pressure, intravenous fluid administration and inotropic agents may be necessary as well as measurement of central venous or pulmonary artery pressure.

Management of Seizures

Phenytoin (15 to 20 mg/kg IV as a loading dose over 30 minutes, then 5 to 7 mg/kg/day orally or intravenously over 30 minutes, divided in two daily doses) may be useful as an anticonvulsant when seizures occur in children with diffuse cerebral edema, acute subdural hematoma, open depressed skull fracture with parenchymal damage, or severe head injury (Glasgow Coma Score ≤ 8). It is unclear how long anticonvulsant therapy should continue, so patients treated with phenytoin should be evaluated for subsequent seizures even beyond the 6-month seizure-free period of suggested anticonvulsant treatment. Patients with early seizures, those occurring in the first week after head injury, are less likely to develop subsequent epilepsy than those patients with seizures developing after the first week.

Nutritional Support

Nutritional status should be discussed early in the patient's hospitalization, and consideration should be given to nasogastric feeding or total parenteral nutrition when it becomes clear that the patient will not be able to ingest food by mouth.

OUTCOME

Approximately 70 per cent of patients with ICP < 20 mm Hg have good outcomes, whereas only 25 per cent of patients with ICP > 20 mm Hg and ICP reducible with treatment will have good outcomes. If ICP is higher than 20 mm Hg and not reducible with treatment, 90 per cent of those patients will die or be severely disabled. Patients with diffuse cerebral edema generally fare better than patients with mass lesions. Early diagnosis of intracranial injury, cerebral edema, and increased ICP helps lead to definitive care of those problems and avoidance of secondary problems, thereby improving the outcome of patients with severe closed head injury. Some patients with mild or moderate head injury may develop subtle learning disorders and behavioral problems (decreased intelligence, lapses in memory, trouble with verbal fluency, difficulty with cognitive flexibility) despite seemingly excellent recovery; such patients may benefit from psychometric evaluation and appropriate treatment.

REFERENCES

Alberico AM, Ward JD, Choi SC, et al: Outcome after severe head injury: Relationship to mass lesions, diffuse injury, and ICP course in pediatric and adult patients. J Neurosurg 67:648–656, 1987.
Hahn YS, Fuchs S, Flannery AM, et al: Factors influencing posttraumatic seizures in children. Neurosurgery 22:864–867, 1988.
Slater EJ, Bassett SS: Adolescents with closed head injuries: A report of initial cognitive deficits. Am J Dis Child 142:1048–1051, 1988.
Yager JY, Johnston B, Seshia SS: Coma scales in pediatric practice. Am J Dis Child 144:1088–1091, 1990.

EPIDURAL AND SUBDURAL HEMATOMA

DACHLING PANG, M.D.

EPIDURAL HEMATOMA

Large epidural hematomas are uncommon in children with head injury. In adolescents and adults, an underlying skull fracture is present 90 per cent of the time; the bleeding is most often from a lacerated meningeal artery, which gives rise to a rapidly enlarging clot with acute mass effect. Epidural bleeding may also be from the diploic or dural veins, in which case the clot will accumulate slowly and the presentation will be subacute. In young children, more often than not, there is no associated fracture; the bleeding is from capillary oozing after the dura has been stripped off the inner table of the skull, which is malleable enough to inbend with impact but recoils moments later away from the dura. This type of oozing causes slowly accumulating epidural clots, and the child's brain is often able to compensate for the slowly evolving mass effect.

The clinical presentation depends on the severity of the impact injury and the rapidity of clot accumulation. The classic unconsciousness–lucid interval–unconsciousness triad said to be pathognomonic of epidural hematomas is seldom seen, since the initial concussion may or may not occur and has no predictive value for the subsequent development of a clot. Rapidly enlarging arterial clots are poorly tolerated, and patients show signs of impending herniation within hours of the impact injury. These include headache and combativeness, progressing to drowsiness, anisocoria, and decerebration. Slowly accumulating venous clots may not become symptomatic for several days, and the patient may present with nothing more than headache, photophobia, and subtle neurologic deficits. Some moderate-sized venous clots are completely asymptomatic.

The diagnosis of epidural hematoma is best made with computed tomography (CT). Large clots are often associated with significant brain shift, but there are usually remarkably few signs of intrinsic brain injury. The prognosis for large epidural hematomas is therefore excellent, provided that surgical evacuation is done before irreversible brain stem injury occurs. The patient is quickly intubated and hyperventilated. Mannitol (0.5 g/kg) is given intravenously while the operating room is being readied. A large skull flap is created over the site of maximum clot volume, where the bleeding source is usually found and addressed. Venous and capillary bleeders are not usually evident at craniotomy. After evacuation of these subacute clots, the dura is tagged up to the edges of the craniotomy defect to prevent reaccumulation of clot.

Small and moderate-sized subacute or chronic epidural clots in asymptomatic or mildly symptomatic children, without neurologic deficits, can be treated without surgery. Spontaneous resorption of these clots almost always occurs; however, these patients must be observed extremely cautiously in a well-equipped and well-manned neurosurgical unit, where prompt action can be initiated if the patient under observation deteriorates. Overall, the results of conservative treatment in well-selected cases are excellent.

SUBDURAL HEMATOMA

Subdural hematomas are usually caused by closed head injuries. The bleeding is either from the bridging veins between the dura and the brain, torn by sliding motions of the brain relative to the dura, or from cortical lacerations. Both types of injuries result from moderate to severe acceleration-deceleration trauma, which also invariably imparts significant diffuse intrinsic (parenchymal) shearing injuries to brain tissues remote from the subdural clot. The impact predetermines a certain amount of neural damage, which is uninfluenced by the treatment of the subdural clot itself. Consequently, the prognosis of acute subdural hematomas is not so much dependent on the size of the clot or the promptness of its drainage as by the degree of parenchymal brain injury and the response to treatment of the secondary brain edema. In this respect, acute subdural hematomas are very different from epidural clots.

The clinical state of the patient with acute subdural hematoma varies widely, depending on the impact energy. At the very least, the patient has had transient loss of consciousness and presents with progressive combativeness, drowsiness, and focal neurologic deficits, such as hemiparesis or aphasia. Or the patient may remain comatose from the start and present with motor posturing and brain stem findings due to severe brain swelling and severe intracranial hypertension.

Acute subdural bleeding is exceedingly common in nonaccidental shaking injuries in infants. The repetitive acceleration-deceleration forces cause massive shearing injuries to the subdural veins and axons, causing extensive brain disruption, petechial hemorrhages, astroglial and neuronal swelling, and subdural bleeding. Bilateral retinal hemorrhages are likely to be present, and there are frequently coincidental skeletal fractures and cutaneous bruising from contemporaneous battering that must be assiduously looked for and documented. *A very large number of such battered infants will have seizures during the acute phase of the injury, and some will have status epilepticus that is very refractory to treatment.*

CT displays the subdural blood as a radiodense crescentic rim overlying the cerebral hemisphere. The underlying brain shows varying degrees of intrinsic damage, such as punctate hemorrhages, cortical contusions, and heterogeneous regions of lucency indicative of brain necrosis or edema. The total mass effect causing intracranial hypertension is largely due to the brain swelling rather than the volume of the subdural clot.

Treatment for acute subdural hematomas seldom consists of simple evacuation of the blood clot but involves heroic measures to counteract the severe brain edema. These include hypocarbic treatment (P_{CO_2} at 26 to 30 torr), intermittent boluses of mannitol, 0.5 gm/kg per dose, intravenous furosemide, 0.5 mg/kg, every 6 hours, and ventricular drainage via an indwelling ventricular catheter inserted for intracranial pressure monitoring. Occasionally, resection of large areas of hemorrhagic, necrotic brain is necessary to avert fatal brain herniation.

Chronic subdural hematomas are drastically different from acute subdural hematomas, both in pathogenesis and outcome. The chronic clots result from relatively trivial trauma that selectively tears the subdural bridging veins without producing parenchymal brain damage. Such chronic subdurals are more common in infancy and old age (older than 70 years), in both cases because of a wider subdural space for the bridging veins to traverse. The blood accumulates slowly, and the volume expands by a complex cyclic process of local fibrinolytic reactions, repeated microhemorrhages, and further local fibrinolysis. The patient usually complains of worsening headache and displays subtle personality changes. CT shows a low-density, lentiform lesion overlying the brain and causing midline shift.

Treatment is by surgical evacuation via burr holes or small craniotomy. Even in the best of circumstances, the recurrence rate of chronic subdural hematomas is about 5 to 10 per cent.

HYDROCEPHALUS

J. F. HIRSCH, C.B.H.
and E. HOPPE-HIRSCH, C.B.H.

Hydrocephalus is characterized by an excessive accumulation of cerebrospinal fluid (CSF) within the cranial cavity. External hydrocephalus—in which excess fluid is located in the pericerebral subarachnoid spaces—is rare. Hydrocephalus is usually internal and situated in dilated ventricles. Although any brain atrophy, with its attendant reduction in parenchymal volume, can result in a passive CSF accumulation, hydrocephalus, especially in infants and children, usually results from active CSF accumulation under a more or less elevated intracranial pressure (ICP). Therefore, the condition produces a bulging fontanel and an increased head circumference together with a dilatation of the cerebral ventricles in infants. In children, when the disease starts late, the cranial cavity is normal or only slightly increased in volume whereas the ventricles are dilated.

DIAGNOSIS

Ultrasonography, computed tomography (CT), and magnetic resonance imaging (MRI) will allow a recognition of hydrocephalus and, in some cases, its etiology. Brain atrophy is easily distinguished because the head circumference is normal or small, the fontanel does not bulge, and there are no clinical symptoms of increased ICP.

CAUSES OF HYDROCEPHALUS

Theoretically, hydrocephalus can be produced in three different ways:

- CSF hypersecretion
- Impaired CSF resorption at the level of the arachnoid villi
- Impaired CSF circulation due to obstacle in CSF pathways

The first two mechanisms are rare. Choroid plexus papilloma is the only tumor known to secrete CSF. In this case, the logical treatment of such hypersecretion is to remove the tumor. This often is not sufficient, and hydrocephalus has to be shunted as a second-step surgical procedure. An impaired CSF resorption may be the result of an increased venous pressure within the sagittal sinus. This increased pressure is either the consequence of an obstacle in the venous circulation, such as in achondroplasia, or that of an arteriovenous malformation, especially if it is close to the sagittal sinus. However, treatment of the cause may be impossible or insufficient in curing hydrocephalus, so that shunting is again the final solution.

Hydrocephalus is most often related to the third mechanism. When the obstacle is located between the choroid plexus and the foramen of Magendie, hydrocephalus is "noncommunicating"; when this obstacle is located further downstream at the level of the pericerebral subarachnoid pathways, hydrocephalus is "communicating."

Three methods can be used to treat hydrocephalus due to obstructed CSF pathways:

- Remove the obstacle
- Bypass the obstacle
- Establish a new artificial CSF circulation through a prosthesis

Removing the Obstacle. This is the best solution and is possible when a tumor has developed at the level of the foramen of Monro, within the third or fourth ventricle, or, more generally, in the posterior fossa. Even in these cases, a shunt has to be inserted postoperatively in 15 per cent of the cases. Some arachnoid cysts, when located on the midline above the sella turcica or at the level of the tentorial notch, may cause hydrocephalus and can be removed or deflated instead by establishing a free communication between them and the CSF pathways. Hemispheric arachnoid cysts are sometimes associated with hydrocephalus. In these cases, treatment of the cyst does not necessarily cure hydrocephalus that is usually not causally related to the cyst. Finally, it should be pointed out that in aqueductal stenosis some authors advocate the catheterization of the narrow aqueduct. Because this operation needs an opening of the posterior fossa, many neurosurgeons are reluctant to perform it in infants.

Bypassing the Obstacle to CSF Flow. This is feasible in some cases of noncommunicating hydrocephalus, mainly aqueductal stenosis. The modern way to perform this operation is percutaneously under radiologic or endoscopic guidance. This operation works well if the subarachnoid spaces are patent. This is the case in more than 80 per cent of the stenoses that start late and in slightly fewer than 70 per cent of the cases that begin early in life. The postoperative mortality of this technique is less than 1 per cent. The postoperative complications, mainly third nerve palsy, are rare and transitory. The postoperative infection rate is negligible. Recurrence occurs in 15 per cent of the cases, but the patient can undergo reoperation or shunting in a second step. The advantage of this technique is that it re-establishes a physiologic CSF circulation.

Shunting. Unfortunately, in most patients, the techniques just described are not feasible, so that the only solution is to create a new and artificial CSF circulation through a silicone rubber shunt that includes three main parts: a proximal catheter inserted in a ventricle, a one-way valve defined by its opening pressure and its resistance, and a distal catheter that diverts the CSF either toward the peritoneal cavity (in most cases) or toward the atrial cavity (much more rarely). Some surgeons add a reservoir between the ventricular catheter and the valve.

Additional surgery to lengthen shunt tubing during growth is often necessary in ventriculoatrial shunts because the tip of the distal catheter has to remain in or near the atrium. In contrast, this can be avoided in most ventriculoperitoneal shunts because a sufficient tubing length can be inserted in the peritoneal cavity at the time of the first insertion. However, complications, whether infectious or mechanical, are frequent. Therefore children with shunts have to be systematically observed until the end of their growth.

POSTOPERATIVE COMPLICATIONS

Infection

The rate of postoperative infection in most series is close to 5 per cent. These infectious complications are of different types: meningitis, purulent subcutaneous collections along the catheter, septicemia (ventriculoatrial shunts), and peritonitis (ventriculoperitoneal shunts). *Staphylococcus epidermidis* is most often responsible for these complications, most of which usually evolve atypically. In some rare cases, peritonitis is the consequence of a bowel perforation by the distal catheter. All infectious complications should be treated with antibiotics. However, antibiotics alone are always insufficient; the prosthesis should be removed and replaced with a clean shunt. Actually, the best approach to infection is its prevention at the time of surgery.

Mechanical Complications

Mechanical complications are frequent. Eight out of ten children will have undergone reoperation at least once for such a complication during the 10 years following the insertion of the first shunt. Two types of mechanical complications are observed: (1) CSF underdrainage caused by a complete or incomplete obstruction of the shunt, or (2) CSF overdrainage related to the physical properties of the shunt. Obstruction or deconnection of the shunt results in the reappearance of intracranial hypertension and requires emergency operation. CSF overdrainage may be responsible for pericerebral collections that have to be drained through a simple tubing from the subdural space to the peritoneal cavity. Overdrainage may also produce post-shunt craniostenosis, which seldom requires surgery; overdrainage may ultimately result in slit ventricles, which themselves favor the obstruction of the intraventricular catheter or, rarely, are responsible for a "slit ventricle syndrome" characterized by intermittent episodes of increased ICP. The treatment of such slit ventricle syndromes is either to increase the volume of the cranial cavity or to change the shunt, inserting a valve that avoids overdrainage. Such valves are now available and should be inserted at the first operation in order to prevent overdrainage. Their use has halved the rate of these complications.

MEDICAL THERAPY

Medical treatment is only rarely indicated in hydrocephalus. It can be used for a few days when surgery is postponed because of a high risk of infection (meningeal or systemic infection, or infectious disease of the skin). It can also be tried when a prompt stabilization of the disease is likely to occur, as in some cases of post-hemorrhage hydrocephalus in premature infants or some patients with myelomeningoceles. Acetazolamide (Diamox) is known to reduce CSF secretion and is the agent most often used. In some patients, repeated lumbar taps (insertion of an intraventricular reservoir that can be tapped repeatedly) may help. However, these therapeutic means can be used for only a limited period of time before stabilization of the disease or insertion of a shunt.

SUMMARY

The final results of shunting procedures can be summarized as follows. Children requiring shunts have an overall mortality of 10 per cent by 10 years. Roughly 50 per cent of the children needing shunts have an intelligence quotient (IQ) above 80. Although these present results are much better than those observed in the pre-valve era, there is still much room for improvement.

MYELODYSPLASIA

LAWRENCE C. KAPLAN, M.D.

Myelodysplasia represents a heterogeneous group of disorders that results from abnormal development of the neural tube and its derivatives. This relatively common congenital malformation represents a wide spectrum of abnormalities ranging from anencephaly to the caudal regression syndrome and includes defects of the neural tube that are not readily evident by examination alone.

PATHOLOGY

Myelodysplasia may be divided into two general categories: primary neural tube defects and secondary neural tube defects.

Primary Neural Tube Defects. Primary neural tube defects constitute approximately 95 per cent of myelodysplasia cases and result from either primary failure of closure of the neural tube or disruption of an already closed neural tube between 18 and 28 days of gestation. The child's abnormality in this case consists of an exposed mass of neural tissue (the neural placode) along the midline of the back and the Arnold-Chiari type II malformation, which consists of malformation of the pons and medulla and a downward displacement of the cerebellum and stenosis of the fourth ventricle and aqueduct of Sylvius with hydrocephalus. If this rostral abnormality is severe, anencephaly may result, which is always incompatible with life.

Primary neural tube defects include meningomyelocele. This most common neural tube defect causes an outpouching of neural elements through the bone and soft tissues in the thoracic, lumbar, or sacral regions. Hydrocephalus and Arnold-Chiari malformation occur together in more than 85 per cent of cases. The sac typically contains dura mater and arachnoid.

Secondary Neural Tube Defects. Secondary neural tube defects, which make up approximately 5 per cent of all neural tube defects, result from the abnormal development of later cell structures or following primary neural tube closure. Typically, these defects involve the lumbosacral spinal region and are less commonly associated with hydrocephalus or the Arnold-Chiari malformation. The skin is frequently found to be intact over the defect, making the diagnosis more challenging.

Secondary neural tube defects include meningocele, lipomeningocele, sacral agenesis, diastematomyelia, and myelocystocele. The lipomatous tissue usually extends through the defect into the spine and dura and may result in a distortion of the spinal cord or nerve roots. Although secondary neural tube defects are not usually as extensive as the primary types, neurologic manifestations may be present.

EPIDEMIOLOGY AND PREVENTION

The frequency of neural tube defects, which is one in 2000 live births in the United States, appears to be decreasing; but there is an increased incidence among certain ethnic groups as well as a higher incidence among individuals living in parts of Ireland and Wales (4.2 to 12.5 per 1000 live births). The precise mechanism of failed neural tube closure remains unknown. More than 95 per cent of all cases of neural tube defects occur in the children of couples with no family history of such abnormalities. Some reasons for both primary and secondary neural tube defects are maternal alcohol and aminopterin use, thalidomide ingestion by the mother, maternal diabetes, prenatal irradiation, and the amniotic band disruption sequence. Valproic acid, maternal hyperthermia, and other teratogens have also been proposed as causes. Both dominant and recessive mendelian inheritance patterns have been documented in individuals with neural tube defects, and these patterns may also occur in trisomy 18 and other chromosome disorders.

There is mounting evidence that folic acid deficiency is directly related to the occurrence of both primary and secondary neural tube defects, and in well-controlled studies recurrence appears to be reduced with the administration of multivitamins to mothers with affected offspring.

Because of the heterogeneity of the causes that need to be considered, genetic consultation or genetic counseling is critical for parents of a child born with a neural tube defect. In general, primary neural tube defects carry a recurrence risk of 1 in 33 for couples with one affected offspring and a 1 in 10 risk when there are two affected offspring. Before the parents meet with a geneticist, it is important to obtain a detailed prenatal and family history.

A prenatal diagnosis of neural tube defects is facilitated by obtaining maternal serum alpha-fetoprotein (AFP) and a prenatal ultrasonogram. When indicated, AFP determinations in amniotic fluid may also be required. The timing of the AFP sampling is critical to the accuracy of this test, as it is still difficult to base prognosis on the findings of ultrasonography alone.

Initial Evaluation by the Practitioner

With the exception of some secondary neural tube defects, myelodysplasia is generally diagnosable at birth. A thorough physical examination is critical, because other congenital abnormalities can be associated with myelodysplasia. These include congenital heart disease, renal malformations, and malformations of the gastrointestinal tract and bones of the pelvis. In no case should a child be referred for neurosurgical care until the clinician has completed a careful review of systems and diagnostic evaluations to determine the extent of other abnormalities.

The back should be carefully examined, but it is not usually necessary to palpate the lesion. Sterile gloves should be worn if palpation is done, and it is helpful to inform the neurosurgeon if any cerebrospinal fluid (CSF) leaks are seen.

The head circumference should be measured initially as well as serially throughout the hospitalization because macrocephaly—a sign of evolving hydrocephalus—may not be detected until after the immediate newborn period. Close attention should be directed to the anterior fontanelle to look for evidence of increased intracranial pressure. In many cases, the fontanelles appear large in the case of congenital hydrocephalus and the calvarial bones are widely separated.

Deformities of the lower extremities are common in myelodysplasia and often result from limited fetal movement or a lack of movement. As a result, equinovarus (clubfoot deformities) as well as congenital dislocation of the hips may be seen.

It is important to observe the infant's motor function in the immediate newborn period as would be done for any child; but it is misleading to base predictions of ambulation potential entirely on the level of the anatomic defect. Careful monitoring of the child's motor development during growth is needed to assess muscle function realistically.

Very often an anal reflex is present at birth but disappears following the initial back surgery because of postoperative edema.

Although it is currently the practice to consult urologists for the evaluation of bladder and kidney function, the practitioner should look carefully for evidence of abdominal masses, kidney enlargement, or abnormal patterns of urination. If voiding patterns appear irregular, catheterization should be performed to measure the amount of residual urine in the bladder.

EVALUATION AND MANAGEMENT

Specialty Evaluations

Given the complexity of multisystem involvement in the child with myelodysplasia, it is necessary to involve subspecialists early, including a neurosurgeon, an orthopedic surgeon, a urologist, a geneticist, and a social worker as well as nurse specialists and pediatricians who are involved in the care of children with myelodysplasia.

Radiographs of the chest, spine, and hips will assist both the neurosurgeon and the orthopedic surgeon in their evaluations and can also be helpful in determining whether there is a cardiac malformation present or whether the hips are dislocated. Findings from these studies will obviously influence the immediate management of the child.

As early as possible in the newborn period, urodynamic studies should be performed to document bladder and urinary sphincter function as well as to assess the neural function of these structures. Along with this, an intravenous pyelogram (IVP) and/or an ultrasonogram of the urinary tract is usually recommended. A voiding cystourethrogram should be considered if an abnormality is noted on the IVP or in the urodynamic study.

Computed tomography (CT) of the head has been a standard part of the initial assessment of brain anatomy; however, in the hands of a skilled radiologist, ultrasonography of the head can determine the presence and extent of hydrocephalus. In many centers, magnetic resonance imaging (MRI) has supplanted the CT scan because of its ability to define the posterior fossa anatomy and the extent of the Arnold-Chiari type II malformation. Such studies are important, especially in the case of a child who shows evidence of apnea, cyanosis, stridor, or other progressive fontomedullary dysfunctions.

Initial Approach

Of utmost importance in caring for children with myelodysplasia is a respect for the role of the parents. In discussions with them, the practitioner must show respect for the right of every child with neural tube defects to receive planned and consistent care delivered with sensitivity to the child's needs for comfort and dignity. When associated abnormalities are present or a severe disability is evident in the newborn period, it is likely that the practitioner may be challenged with questions related to withholding aggressive surgical management. It is unreasonable and unfair to expect parents to make such decisions on their own; but if the parents can be part of a dialogue based on facts and candor, the pediatrician will be able to help families arrive at a better understanding of prognosis and treatment options.

Most physicians and other health professionals have strong opinions regarding the treatment of infants born with neural tube defects. When the professional staff disagree regarding initial management or if there is a disagreement or communication breakdown with the family, consulting a hospital ethics committee can be critically important and can help establish a forum in which to discuss treatment.

Initial Subspecialty Management

The initial neurosurgical treatment of the open myelomeningocele involves closing the defect to prevent infection and reducing the elevated intracranial pressure. The back is usually repaired on the first day of life or as soon thereafter as possible; skin grafting is often not required, given newer techniques of single-stage closure. If the skin is intact over the back defect, the risk for bacterial contamination is decreased. Repair in this case can be done electively, even after 1 month of age. A continuous ventricular drainage system, usually a ventriculoperitoneal shunt or a ventriculoatrial shunt, reduces intracranial hypertension. Many neurosurgeons may elect either to place this catheter at the time of back closure or to wait and monitor head circumference for evidence of increased intracranial pressure before doing a second procedure to place the shunt. The advantage of this latter approach is that it permits identification of those children who may not require a shunt at all.

Before the child is discharged from the hospital, it is often the practice to obtain brain stem auditory evoked potential studies to assess hearing and to consult a pediatric ophthalmologist. Although blindness and deafness are rare, these evaluations are a necessary part of the developmental follow-up of children with myelodysplasia.

A pediatric orthopedist usually elects to begin treatment of hip dislocation or clubfoot deformity in the newborn period and thus should be involved early on. Serial casting of the feet can begin just prior to discharge, even when the child is recovering from the neurosurgical procedures.

A geneticist should be given the opportunity to meet with the child's family while the child is in the hospital because this is quite often a good time to review the etiology and pathology of myelodysplasia and to begin the process of genetic counseling.

A pediatric urologist may recommend clean intermittent catheterization or Credé's method of expressing urine from the bladder. These techniques require expert teaching by the nursing staff in the neonatal period.

Multidisciplinary Evaluation of Symptomatic Arnold-Chiari Malformation

Although the majority of newborns with primary neural tube defects have the Arnold-Chiari malformation, fortunately few are symptomatic. The presence of symptoms indicates a potential for progressive injury to and dysfunction in the brain stem; if stridor worsens and/or if the child becomes apneic, a repeat MRI scan may be necessary. Treatment options can include posterior fossa decompression and laminectomy, but there remains considerable controversy as to whether this intervention will result in resolution of the symptoms. The prognosis for children with stridor alone remains better than for those with cyanosis and/or apnea.

Further Management and Prognosis

The majority of individuals with myelodysplasia (> 66 per cent) have intelligence within the normal range. This is an important point to make to parents early on and to bear in mind when advocating for children at home and in the school. One can expect a delay in development, but this delay may be modified by bracing, physical therapy, and close monitoring and treatment of scoliosis or kyphosis. The orthopedic prognosis for children with myelodysplasia is not static. Variables such as tethering of the spinal cord, obesity, and decubitus ulcers may delay motor development, and the motivation of a child to remain a "community ambulator" is a very important factor.

Nevertheless, children with myelodysplasia are at risk for mental retardation, and those with mental retardation fall into three subgroups: (1) those with severe hydrocephalus at birth, (2) those in whom infection develops in the central nervous system early in life, and (3) those who have intracranial hypertension not properly controlled. Mental retardation is also encountered more commonly in children with high thoracic level lesions; even here, however, one must be very careful in making a definite prediction or diagnosis of mental retardation without formal developmental testing that carefully assesses visual, perceptual, fine and gross motor, language, and social skills.

Seizures, in particular complex partial seizures, may interfere with intellectual function in some children with myelodysplasia but can be very subtle in their presentation. For example, children in the classroom setting who have progressively diminishing performance in school may be experiencing seizures and will require a careful evaluation by their pediatrician and/or neurologist.

In the 1990s, owing largely to the advances in early neurosurgical care, the effects of progressive hydrocephalus on intellectual function are rarely seen. Shunt malfunction and/or infection, although difficult to define objectively, frequently are of concern to parents of children with myelodysplasia. Parents note changes in sleep patterns, fever, diminishing appetite, lack of attentiveness in school, or irritability and often bring these symptoms to the attention of their pediatrician, who should consider referral to the child's neurosurgeon at that time.

More than 85 per cent of children with spinal lesions in the lumbar region have been reported to complete twelfth grade or beyond. However, young adults and teen-agers with myelodysplasia have multiple and deep needs in such areas as vocational planning, social life, sexuality, body image, and health care planning. The growing population of young men and women with myelodysplasia reports increasing difficulty finding primary care physicians to care for them. Their general adult health care needs are often no different from those of others; however, the need for multidisciplinary care continues throughout their lives and requires considerable coordination by the primary care provider.

Bowel and bladder function continue to be dominant concerns of young adults with myelomeningocele, echoing the concerns frequently expressed by their parents when the child was younger. The dysfunction of bladder and rectum derive from a similar source, namely abnormal innervation or neural function in these structures. Dysmotility of the bowel results in retention of fecal material, subsequent inspissation, and eventual encopresis. Although stool softening and/or lubrication is important, even more important is preventing progressive distention and irreversible stretching of the rectum in the first 5 to 7 years of life. This can generally be managed by the use of stool softeners and hydration, but these interventions are often ineffective if colonic stretching has persisted. Many multidisciplinary myelodysplasia teams have bowel protocols that include educating parents and patients about the physiology of rectal function and rectal dysfunction.

Bladder dysfunction seen in myelodysplasia can lead to two clinical problems. The first of these is recurrent urinary tract infections, and the second is hydronephrosis. Urinary tract infections, which can occur in both hypertonic and hypotonic bladders, represent a distinct entity separate from asymptomatic bacteriuria. The value of urodynamic studies and renal ultrasonography is to identify upper motor versus lower motor neural bladder dysfunction, sphincter dysfunction, or combinations of these patterns that might cause kidney injury through infection or high pressure states. Compared to alpha- or beta-agonist medications, clean intermittent catheterization taught early and maintained as a routine self-help skill has proved to be effective in reducing these complications.

SUMMARY

Remarkable progress has been made over the past two decades in the management and care of children with myelodysplasia. The care of children and adults with this condition is never one-dimensional and requires the coordinated care of multiple specialists both in the tertiary center and in the community. Of pressing importance is the provision of health care services for adults with myelodysplasia because these are the individuals who have benefited from earlier advances in neurosurgical and orthopedic management.

MANAGEMENT OF CHILDHOOD BRAIN TUMORS

GIORGIO PERILONGO, M.D.
and GIULIO J. D'ANGIO, M.D.

The management of primary brain tumors in children has gone through rapid changes in the last few decades. This has occurred through better understanding of the histology and biologic behavior of some of the more common tumors and their therapeutic and prognostic implications. New surgical techniques have made virtually all brain tumors accessible to resection, if not excision. The role of chemotherapy has expanded, and new radiotherapy methods have evolved even as the potentially devastating late effects of conventional treatment methods have been documented. All these advances have made it possible to have a more deliberate approach to children with primary brain tumors than was feasible in the past.

The cell morphology and tissue patterns of childhood brain tumors are heterogeneous. This leads to different opinions among neuropathologists relative to the nature and origin of these neoplasms. Consequently, the development of a uniformly accepted classification system has been difficult. A consortium of neuropathologists was therefore convened by the World Health Organization (WHO) to address this issue and reach a consensus. The classification system that resulted is the one most generally accepted and will be used for this discussion (Rorke et al, 1985). A summary is shown in Table 1.

This classification is based on the appearance of the tumor by light microscopy and on immunohistochemical and electron microscopy findings. A tumor is placed within a specific category according to the predominant cell type, with recognition of the existence of mixed tumors.

The concept of expressing the degree of malignancy in terms of a combination of histologic features (e.g., mitotic activity, presence of necrosis) to grade tumors (e.g. "low-grade" versus "high-grade" glioma or grade I, II, III, and IV tumors) has been abandoned. That is because it is well recognized that brain tumors can be histologically benign but biologically malignant and vice versa. In the WHO classification, categories are subdivided mainly on the basis of the presence or absence of anaplasia. Accordingly, the so-called low-grade and high-grade astrocytomas, for example, will be termed in this discussion simply "astrocytomas" and "anaplastic astrocytomas," respectively. Glioblastomatous tumors represent highly anaplastic glial tumors that are biologically very aggressive.

The WHO experts recognized that there was disagreement regarding the nomenclature of "poorly differentiated or densely cellular neuroepithelial tumors." "Medulloblastoma" is the traditional term used for these tumors in the posterior fossa, and "primitive neuroectodermal tumor" (PNET) refers to those outside the posterior fossa. *It has been proposed that PNET be used to identify all such tumors regardless of their primary location, and the term is used in this way here. The arguments for and against doing so are beyond the scope of this discussion.*

TABLE 1. Classification of Brain Tumors in Children

I. Tumors of Neuroepithelial Tissue
- A. Glial tumors
  1. Astrocytic tumors—astrocytoma, anaplastic astrocytoma, subependymal giant cell tumor, gigantocellular glioma
  2. Oligodendroglial tumors—oligodendroglioma, anaplastic oligodendroglioma
  3. Ependymal tumors—ependymoma, anaplastic ependymoma, myxopapillar ependymoma
  4. Choroid plexus tumors—Choroid plexus papilloma, anaplastic choroid plexus tumor (carcinoma)
  5. Mixed gliomas
  6. Glioblastomatous tumors—glioblastoma multiforme, giant cell glioblastoma, gliosarcoma
  7. Gliomatosis cerebri
- B. Neuronal tumors—gangliocytoma, anaplastic gangliocytoma, ganglioglioma, anaplastic ganglioglioma
- C. Primitive neuroepithelial tumors
  1. "Primitive" neuroectodermal tumors (with or without differentiation)
  2. Medulloepithelioma (with or without differentiation)
- D. Pineal cell tumors
  1. "Primitive" neuroectodermal tumors (see C above; pineoblastoma)
  2. Pineocytoma

II. Tumors of Meningeal and Related Tissues
- A. Meningiomas
  1. Meningioma not otherwise specified (NOS)
  2. "Papillary" meningioma
  3. Anaplastic meningioma
- B. Meningeal sarcomatous tumors
- C. Primary melanocytic tumors

III. Tumors of Nerve Sheath Cells
- A. Neurilemmoma
- B. Anaplastic neurilemmoma
- C. Neurofibroma
- D. Anaplastic neurofibroma

IV. Primary Malignant Lymphomas

V. Tumors of the Blood Vessels
- A. Hemangioblastoma
- B. Hemangiopericytoma

VI. Germ Cell Tumors
- A. Germinoma
- B. Embryonal carcinoma
- C. Choriocarcinoma
- D. Endodermal sinus tumor
- E. Teratomatous tumors
- F. Mixed tumors

VII. Malformative Tumors
- A. Craniopharyngioma
- B. Epidermal cyst
- C. Lipoma
- D. Hamartoma

VIII. Tumors of Neuroendocrine Origin
- A. Tumor of anterior pituitary
- B. Paraganglioma

IX. Local Extension from Regional Tumors

X. Metastatic Tumors

XI. Unclassified Tumors

DIAGNOSIS

Radiology

Once the presence of a neoplasm is strongly suspected or proven, determination of its location and extent (tumor staging) is an essential step in planning workup and appropriate treatment.

Magnetic resonance imaging (MRI) of the brain has revolutionized the diagnosis and management of childhood brain tumors. MRI allows extraordinary and exquisite delineation of the lesions, particularly in areas such as the brain stem and spine, not easily visualized with precision by computed tomography (CT). The introduction into clinical practice of gadolinium (Gd), the intravenous contrast agent for MRI (chelated with diethylenetriaminepentacetic acid [Gd-DTPA]) has further improved the accuracy of this imaging technique. Areas thought to represent tumors that are not suspected on nonenhanced images can now be visualized with accuracy. The sensitivity of Gd-DTPA–enhanced MRI of the spine is replacing myelography in staging tumors such as PNETs, which tend to disseminate along the spine regardless of their primary locations. Finally, radiation therapy planning assumes the MRI to be extremely precise and the margins are tailored to that image because of the sensitivity of the method.

Proton magnetic resonance spectroscopy (H-MRS) provides a noninvasive method to quantify a variety of metabolites in selected regions of the brain using the software available for most clinical MRI units. Such compounds as N-acetylaspartate, choline-containing compounds, lactate, and phosphocreatine and creatinine can be used. The concentration of these compounds can vary from tissue to tissue, and thus they are tissue-specific to some extent. Now under investigation is the possibility of determining the histologic nature of brain lesions. This is being approached by looking for the presence of specific magnetic compounds using resonance spectroscopy (MRS) to differentiate necrosis from tumor and rapidly from slowly replicating tumor cells, for example.

Histology

Determining the histology of a brain lesion is essential for planning the appropriate management. Practically, there are no areas of the brain that cannot be reached surgically. CT-guided stereotactic biopsy has proved to be a safe and relatively reliable technique for the assessment of deeply placed or otherwise poorly accessible lesions. There is a caveat, however; a single tumor can be heterogeneous and can be composed of different histologic patterns so that a small sample can be misleading. Such a biopsy could be from a nonanaplastic area intermixed in an anaplastic one and thus provide inaccurate information on which to base prognosis and therapy. Any histologic specimens should be interpreted cautiously when based on a single sample.

Two exceptions to the rule of obtaining a tissue diagnosis are (1) chiasmatic masses that clearly extend posteriorly along the optic tracts or anteriorly to involve the optic nerves, and (2) diffuse intrinsic brain stem lesions. Chiasmatic tumors are almost always astrocytomas. Tumors of the pons and medulla are often lethal, regardless of their histology, because of their location.

The reasons for obtaining brain tumor tissue go beyond formulating a descriptive histologic diagnosis, important though it be. It is becoming increasingly important not to rely solely on tumor morphology based on light and electron microscopy when the potential aggressiveness of the lesion is being assessed. Other predictors are needed. Preliminary work indicates that ploidy, DNA labeling indices, and oncogene amplification are potentially powerful tools for this purpose. They provide better insights into the molecular genetics and biology of these tumors, and they promise to have an impact on refinements of therapy as well as survival. The well-being of these children will thereby be enhanced by permitting treatments to be modulated in scope and intensity through more precise estimates of risks.

MANAGEMENT

Surgery

The infiltrative growth of many brain tumors and their origin in critical locations limit the curative role of surgery because of the devastating consequences of an aggressive surgical resection.

Nonetheless, the event-free survival time and the cure rate of most brain tumors depend on the extent of surgical resection. Germinomas are notable among the exceptions; they are so sensitive to radiation therapy (and probably to chemotherapy) that the completeness of tumor removal has little, if any, impact on survival.

There have been major advances in surgical techniques to extend those benefits as far as possible. The operating microscope makes it feasible, through better binocular vision, to excise more tumor safely, especially when machines like the Cavitron are used. (The Cavitron employs ultrasonic waves to liquify neoplastic tissue, which is then sucked away, while sparing the normal parenchyma.) Laser beam techniques under study are designed to accomplish the same goals.

Neurosurgeons are also adopting surgical expertise developed by other specialists, such as maxillofacial surgeons, to resect tumors arising in or close to the base of the skull, e.g., chordomas. Suffice it is to say that many other areas, such as the pineal region and the hypothalamus, once considered to be inaccessible, are now being approached with relative impunity. The importance of these surgical advances can be measured by reciting a few facts. No survivors are reported among children with anaplastic astrocytoma or glioblastoma multiforme who undergo only biopsy of the tumor. Some clinicians agree that gross surgical removal is the most important prognostic factor in childhood ependymoma. Incomplete excision is considered a risk factor for tumor recurrence for PNETs, whereas gross resection is accepted as sufficient initial therapy for cerebellar astrocytomas. This probably also holds true for most of the (nonanaplastic) astrocytomas and other histologically benign tumors, such as gangliogliomas, meningiomas, and craniopharyngiomas.

Radiation Therapy

Postoperative radiation therapy (RT) remains the gold standard for the treatment of many childhood brain tumors. Local RT with adequate margins is advocated for most astrocytomas regardless of the extent of surgery. The curative dose is estimated to be in the range of 5400 to 6000 cGy. PNETs have a high tendency to disseminate along the cerebrospinal fluid (CSF) pathways throughout the central nervous system, regardless of their primary location (most commonly the posterior fossa). Thus, prophylactic treatment of the entire craniospinal axis, with a "boost" dose to the primary site, remains the standard for PNETs. Conventional doses are 3600 cGy to the neural axis and 5400 cGy to the posterior fossa. There are, however, severe side effects of those doses on the immature brain. The most important are pronounced learning disabilities and drops in intelligence quotient (IQ) scores. The younger the child, the more profound the problems. Recognition of these deleterious consequences has fostered a series of investigations designed to lessen the complications without compromising therapeutic efficacy. An obvious first step, i.e., lowering the total dose given to the brain of children with PNETs using standard techniques, is under study with contradictory results reported so far. Hyperfractionated RT—typically smaller individual doses of about 100 cGy given twice a day—is another approach. This technique should permit escalation of the dose of RT while reducing the late complications according to radiobiologic theory plus supporting clinical data. Doses of up to 7800 cGy have been safely delivered to children with diffuse pontine gliomas using hyperfractionated regimens. Longer periods of tumor control than usually observed with simple daily doses to totals in the range of 5500 to 6000 cGy are reported. Hyperfractionated RT is also under investigation for the treatment of the neural axis in children with PNETs with the specific aim of minimizing the side effects.

"Radiosurgery" is a relatively recent technical innovation. It uses sharply collimated and angled, converging RT beams delivered through several small ports. A high dose in a well-defined, small volume is thus accumulated while sparing adjacent parenchyma. Treatment is given in a single session. Its use initially was limited to the treatment of vascular malformations, but it is now being extended to the management of brain tumors. Machines specifically for radiosurgery have been constructed or existing machines have been modified, but all have the same aim. The major disadvantage of this technique is that only relatively small lesions in noncritical areas can be treated.

Nonconventional RT methods (e.g., implanting interstitial radioactive sources and using radioactive monoclonal antibodies) are still in an experimental phase in the treatment of childhood brain tumors.

Chemotherapy

Chemotherapy is being given increasing importance in the management of children with brain tumors. A randomized prospective clinical trial by the Children's Cancer Study Group (CCSG) in the early 1980s demonstrated that vincristine (VCR), lomustine (CCNU), and prednisone improved survival of children with anaplastic astrocytoma and glioblastoma multiforme. The 5-year, event-free survival was 46 per cent for patients given RT plus chemotherapy and 18 per cent for the children treated with RT alone. Preliminary data from a later CCSG study seem to confirm this trend.

The role of chemotherapy in children with nonanaplastic astrocytomas is more controversial. The combination of VCR and dactinomycin has been shown to be effective in maintaining tumor control in children with chiasmatic gliomas, thus avoiding or delaying RT in two thirds of the patients. Based on this experience, some centers are exploring the same approach in astrocytomas located outside the optic pathways, especially when young children are affected. The curative role of this treatment modality is far from being demonstrated, but its usefulness in at least delaying RT in some cases of optic nerve gliomas seems convincing.

Studies at the Children's Hospital of Philadelphia indicate a beneficial impact of VCR, CCNU, and cisplatin (CPDD) in children with PNETs. Patients originally considered at high risk, with survivals of 30 to 40 per cent after conventional postoperative RT, are now enjoying 88 per cent 5-year, event-free survival when treated with these three drugs and craniospinal RT. These data overshadow the results of two concurrent prospective, randomized studies conducted in Europe and the United States in the late 1970s to early 1980s. Those failed to demonstrate an improvement in survival when the combination VCR plus CCNU was added to standard RT, except possibly in some subsets of patients.

Chemotherapy is becoming the initial postoperative treatment of choice for brain tumors in infants regardless of histology. The devastating effects of even moderate doses of RT on the developing brain strongly discourage its use in infants. Different multiagent regimens to delay, if not to substitute for, RT are under investigation. The drugs commonly used are VCR, CPDD, cyclophosphamide, etoposide, and CCNU. The combination regimen MOPP (mechlorethamine, Oncovin = VCR, procarbazine, and prednisone) has also been used successfully in infants, initially at the M. D. Anderson Hospital.

Comprehensive Care

Children treated successfully for primary central nervous system tumors may suffer significant unfavorable long-term sequelae. These can be secondary to the tumors themselves, to the means used to control them, or both. The early identification of these sequelae and their timely management, when available, are part of much needed comprehensive care, especially now that better survival rates are being achieved.

Functional handicaps, such as paresis, cerebellar dysfunction, and cranial nerve deficits, can be ameliorated by intensive rehabilitation. Early enrollment in physical, occupational, and speech therapy programs can greatly help to overcome these problems and ensure the best quality of life possible.

Disturbed growth and development can be seen because of direct RT effects on the growing spinal column and because of secondary effects on the hypothalamic-pituitary axis caused by RT, surgery, or the tumor itself. Now that hormone replacement therapy is largely becoming available, an appropriate endocrinologic follow-up is mandatory for all children with brain tumors, especially those who have had cranial radiation.

Profound learning disabilities and overall intellectual developmental disturbances are frequently seen and are irreversible. These and associated neuropsychologic difficulties can be devastating. Special educational and psychologic supportive programs, which can be very beneficial in helping the social adjustment of impaired long-term survivors, are required.

Chemotherapy can cause specific organ damage, sometimes made worse by added RT. For example, CPDD, a drug widely used for many brain tumors, is nephrotoxic and ototoxic, the latter augmented by RT of the inner ear. If not recognized, hearing loss may further compromise the function of children already handicapped by the tumor or iatrogenic effects.

In summary, the management of children with primary central nervous system tumors is an articulated and complex process involving many specialized individuals and services. It is clear that the care of these children is best delivered in centers capable of providing the needed multidisciplinary staff and facilities.

REFERENCES

Packer RJ, Sutton LN, Goldwein JW, et al: Improved survival with the use of adjuvant chemotherapy in the treatment of medulloblastoma. J Neurosurg 74:433–440, 1991.

Rorke LB, Gilles FH, Davids RL, Becker LE: Revision of the World Health Organization classification of brain tumors for childhood brain tumors. Cancer 56:1869–1886, 1985.

Sposto R, Ertel IJ, Jenkin RDT, et al: The effectiveness of chemotherapy for treatment of high grade astrocytoma in children: Results of a randomized trial. A report from the Children's Cancer Study Group. J Neuro Oncol 7:165–177, 1989.

BRAIN ABSCESS AND SPINAL EPIDURAL ABSCESS

DACHLING PANG, M.D.

BRAIN ABSCESS

Four clinical situations predispose to the formation of brain abscesses. In the pediatric population, the majority of brain abscesses arise by direct spread from an adjacent paranasal sinus, middle ear, or mastoid infection, often by way of retrograde thrombophlebitis of the valveless diploic veins. Because the sinus and ear infections are usually chronic and the spread of the organism is slow, enough adhesion forms between the brain surface and the dura-arachnoid that the abscess often forms without signs of meningitis. Such abscesses, from a contiguous infective source, are almost always single, and their locations are predictably close to the source. Thus, frontal and ethmoidal infections cause basal frontal brain abscesses, and otitic infections often percolate through the tegmen tympani to result in temporal lobe abscesses. *The lack of meningitic signs and the common involvement of silent areas of the brain explain why many abscesses reach enormous sizes without focal neurologic deficits. Abscesses from chronic mastoiditis and some cases of otitis are located in the lateral cerebellar hemispheres next to the petrous bone and may present first as acute tonsillar herniation.*

The next most common pathogenetic pathway is hematogenous spread from distant infected sites. Metastatic brain abscesses are particularly common in children with suppurative lung diseases, such as bronchiectasis, lung abscess, and emphysema, and in those with cyanotic congenital heart disease. In the former group, the lung infection dislodges septic emboli directly into the left circulation, which carries them to the brain; in the latter group, the right-to-left shunt allows septic emboli to bypass the filtration system of the lungs and gain brisk access to the cerebral circulation. In both groups, the chronically low oxygen (O_2) tension in the brain substance is especially suitable for seeding of anaerobes and microaerophilic bacteria. Other well-known primary infection sites include skin pustules, dental or tonsillar abscesses, decubitus ulcers, and bacterial endocarditis. Because the regional incidence of hematogenous abscesses depends on the local blood flow, they are most common in the territory of the middle cerebral artery and may also be multiple.

The third and fourth categories of brain abscesses are those following head trauma and brain surgery. Penetrating brain injuries with retained foreign bodies, such as bone fragments, clothing, dirt, and missiles, often provide the nidus for cerebritis, but nonpenetrating basal skull fractures with cerebrospinal fluid (CSF) fistula may also cause silent subfrontal abscesses. Nowadays, brain abscesses are seldom seen in elective, uncontaminated brain operations except in cases of implanted foreign objects, such as CSF shunts and radiation implants; in the latter situation, the local host defense is also compromised as a result of tissue devitalization and the presence of malignant tumor cells.

Last, there is an increased incidence of brain abscess among immunocompromised patients, including those with chronic debilitating diseases such as diabetes and sarcoidosis, those with myeloproliferative conditions such as leukemia and lymphomas, organ transplant recipients receiving immunosuppressive therapy, patients receiving long-term corticosteroids, and those with acquired immunodeficiency syndrome (AIDS).

The pathogenic organism varies somewhat with the primary sites. Organisms isolated from otitis- and sinusitis-related abscesses are anaerobic in more than 50 per cent of cases; these include *Bacteroides* spp., anaerobic streptococci (*Peptostreptococcus*), and *Fusobacterium* spp. Common aerobic organisms include coagulase-positive and -negative staphylococci, aerobic streptococci, and *Haemophilus influenzae*. Metastatic abscesses from pulmonary and cyanotic cardiac sources often grow mixed cultures of the above anaerobes and aerobes plus *Actinomyces* spp., *Pseudomonas aeruginosa,* and the Enterobacteriaceae. *Streptococcus viridans* and beta-hemolytic streptococci continue to be associated with bacterial endocarditis. Posttraumatic and postsurgical abscesses are most likely caused by staphylococci, streptococci, and occasionally *Pseudomonas* spp. In the immunocompromised group, the spectrum of pathogens broadens to include organisms that are usually of low-grade virulence, namely *Nocardia,* fungi such as *Aspergillus* and *Candida,* and parasites such as *Toxoplasma gondii* and *Entamoeba histolytica*.

The most common symptom in brain abscess is progressive headache increasingly refractory to analgesics. This is due to the combined mass effect of the abscess and its surrounding edema. Nausea and vomiting follow the headache, and in 30 to 50 per cent of cases a focal or general seizure heralds the first neurologic crisis. If the mass effect is considerable at this stage, the patient may not regain full consciousness from the seizure and may indeed proceed to show signs of brain herniation. If the abscess involves the dominant temporal lobe, various types of dysphasia may be present or the child may show personality changes secondary to frontal lobe disease. Cerebellar abscesses are the most treacherous, for they may remain silent except for causing a vague feeling of dizziness or disequilibrium until the final catastrophic signs of tonsillar herniation (sudden respiratory arrest, coma, and decerebration).

Diagnosis

The diagnosis of brain abscess is made with computed tomography (CT) or magnetic resonance imaging (MRI). The infusion of intravenous contrast causes enhancement of the abscess capsule, which encloses a lucent, nonenhancing necrotic center and is surrounded by a striking ring of radiolucent edematous brain. The paranasal sinuses and middle ear cavities are also shown to advantage. The MRI is especially suitable for evaluating patency of the large intracranial venous sinuses. A lumbar puncture should never be done regardless of whether or not a specimen is obtainable for culture prior to antibiotic administration.

Treatment

Treatment begins with high doses of antibiotics before identification of pathogen. Because of the frequency of polymicrobial infection, combination therapy is preferable with one of the third-generation cephalosporins with good blood-brain barrier penetration (e.g., ceftazidime, 50 mg/kg, every 8 hours intravenously [IV], or ceftriaxone, 50 mg/kg, every 12 hours IV), and an antistaphylococcal agent such as nafcillin or oxacillin (200 mg/kg/day, given every 6 hours). Vancomycin (10 mg/kg, every 6 hours, IV infusion) is becoming an increasingly useful drug for treating methicillin-resistant strains of coagulase-negative and -positive staphylococci. Metronidazole (15 mg/kg loading dose, 7.5 mg/kg, every 6 hours, all by IV infusion) is also frequently added because of its excellent penetration into brain abscesses and its reliability against anaerobes.

Most large solitary brain abscesses need to be surgically drained. The most effective method and least likely to cause neurologic deficits is catheter puncture using CT stereotactic or intraoperative ultrasound guidance. Continuous catheter drainage is set up for 3 to 5 days or less if drainage is minimal. Postoperative collapse of the abscess cavity is always checked by serial CT scans, as is the effectiveness of medical therapy after removal of the catheter. With successful treatment, the capsule remains collapsed and gradually shrinks, with lessening contrast enhancement and resolution of surrounding brain edema. Antibiotic regimens are adjusted according to culture results and are continued for a total of 4 to 6 weeks.

The mass effect of an abscess is usually adequately treated with simple drainage. In case of continued brain shift due to edema, corticosteroids (dexamethasone, 10 to 12 mg loading dose, followed by 0.5 mg/kg daily in divided doses) can be used to facilitate edema resolution. Anticonvulsants such as dilantin (20 mg/kg loading dose, followed by 5 to 7 mg/kg/day maintenance) or phenobarbital (20 mg/kg loading dose, followed by 3 to 5 mg/kg/day maintenance) should be given prophylactically and continued for 6 months.

Medical therapy without drainage has recently been shown to be successful in treating severely debilitated patients of poor surgical risk and patients with multiple small abscesses. In choosing this modality, one must use serial neuroimaging to monitor the effectiveness of treatment.

SPINAL EPIDURAL ABSCESS

Pyogenic infection of the spinal epidural space is an uncommon infection in childhood but occasionally represents an acute neurosurgical emergency that requires prompt recognition and treatment. More than 50 per cent of the cases of spinal epidural abscess are due to hematogenous spread from remote sites, such as skin pustules, dental caries, suppurative pulmonary conditions, septic thrombophlebitis, and urinary tract infections. Epidural infections may also result from direct extension from decubitus ulcers, psoas abscesses, pelvic abscesses, and mediastinal infections. In addition, epidural abscesses may be an extension of a disc space infection following discectomy.

Acute epidural infections are most commonly caused by *Staphylococcus aureus,* especially those cases following penetrating trauma or disc space surgery. Infections caused by retrograde spread from urosepsis are often due to gram-negative organisms such as *Escherichia coli* and *P. aeruginosa*. Chronic epidural infections, fortunately rare in North America, are almost exclusively due to tuberculous osteomyelitis, which also causes vertebral collapse, relatively rapid kyphotic deformation of the spine, and bony compression of the neural elements. Blastomycosis and other fungal infections are rare and usually occur in diabetics or immunosuppressed patients.

The first symptom of acute infection is usually excruciating pain that is well localized to the affected segments, accompanied by reflex paraspinous muscle spasm and tenderness to percussion. When the nerve roots are involved, radicular pain is common. Myelopathy is usually a late manifestation but may be rapidly progressive; it is thought to be partly due to compression but at least in some cases may be secondary to vasculitis or thrombophlebitis of the cord. Sudden paraplegia has been reported in cases of vertebral collapse and acute angulation secondary to chronic tuberculous abscesses. During the acute infection, systemic signs of sepsis such as fever, leukocytosis, and malaise are usually present in some combination.

The severe local pain, muscle spasm, and percussion tenderness distinguish spinal epidural abscess from transverse myelitis, which is always painless, and from spinal tumors that usually have a chronic or subacute course without spasm or systemic signs of sepsis. Acute epidural hematoma from a vertebral hemangioma or hemorrhage from a spinal cord arteriovenous malformation may present with sudden pain and neurologic deficits, often necessitating imaging studies for differentiation. Acute central intervertebral disc herniation is exceedingly uncommon in childhood but should be thought of in adolescent athletes with a recent history of back trauma.

Plain films are often normal but may show signs of disc space infection or vertebral body end-plate erosion from osteomyelitis. The diagnosis is made with MRI, and the degree of neural compression and spinal cord compromise can be accurately assessed. It is important to evaluate the amount of bony destruction involving the vertebral bodies and neural arches for purposes of predicting stability, and this is best done with CT, with and without intravenous contrast. Contrast myelography is usually not necessary except when MRI is unavailable, and then the contrast should be introduced in the C1-C2 interspinous space, far from the lumbar region, where most of the infections are located. A lumbar puncture is virtually never indicated, for fear of contaminating the CSF and of producing sudden neurologic deterioration from "impaction" at the compressive site.

Treatment

Treatment of epidural abscess is surgical drainage and decompression supplemented by appropriate antibiotics. Liquid pus is sometimes found dorsal to the spinal dura and may be loculated due to adhesions. The laminae may be frankly osteomyelitic, and any sequestra should be removed. Frequently, the mass as shown on MRI may not be a true abscess but a large, friable, vascular mass of granulation tissue densely adherent to the dura. This must be curetted off the dura as much as possible for decompression purposes. An indwelling catheter should be left in for drainage for several days. Postoperatively, the spine should be immobilized by a brace or corset to minimize pain. Late intervertebral fusion is common if disc space infection is also present.

Antibiotic regimens should initially include antistaphylococcal agents such as nafcillin, oxacillin, or vancomycin combined with a broad-spectrum drug, such as the third-generation cephalosporins. Antibiotics should be continued for 2 to 3 weeks.

CEREBROVASCULAR DISEASE IN INFANCY AND CHILDHOOD

SEETHA SHANKARAN, M.D.

ARTERIOVENOUS MALFORMATIONS

The most common cause of brain hemorrhage in infants and children is arteriovenous malformation (AVM). In neonates this lesion occurs at the vein of Galen and presents with congestive cardiac failure and a cranial bruit. In older children, increase in intracranial pressure with headache, vomiting, hydrocephaly, tortuosity of scalp veins, seizures, and nuchal rigidity may be the presenting signs. Cranial bruits are rare. The usual site is the parietal lobe.

Diagnosis can be made with computed tomographic (CT) scanning of the head with contrast as the initial study. A circular homogeneous mass is seen behind the third ventricle. Magnetic resonance imaging (MRI) can demonstrate the malformation with high specificity. Transcranial color flow Doppler imaging and pulsed Doppler are reliable and noninvasive methods for monitoring the hemodynamic effects of the AVM. Digital subtraction angiography (DSA) with magnification is needed to define the feeding vessels and draining veins.

Treatment

Management of the AVM depends on the size and location of the lesion. Accessible lesions can be surgically removed. For larger, deeper lesions, often both interventional radiologic and surgical procedures are required; preoperative and perioperative embolization may be necessary with a staged surgical approach. The embolization may be performed by the transtorcular (a direct neurosurgical approach via the confluence of the venous sinuses) or transarterial approach using balloon embolization or by a percutanous transvenous approach using flexible, flow-guided microcatheters to reach the smaller vessels. The goal of embolization is to occlude the deep feeding vessels, hence reducing dissection of brain tissue during surgery. Embolization is performed with particles (Silastic or silicone spheres, dura), or glues (isobutyl cyanocrylate) that polymerize on contact with blood. Catheter position and deposition of embolic materials need to be monitored closely. Prognosis is poor in children with cerebral tissue damage, gliosis, and atrophy noted at the time of diagnosis of the AVM. Calcification is also a poor prognostic sign, as calcification occurs in areas of tissue anoxia.

Surgical excision may be followed by minor sequelae such as speech disturbance, ataxia, and hypotonia. Large, inoperable lesions are treated by palliative embolization. Encouraging results are now seen when stereotactic radiosurgery is used as an alternative to microsurgery in selected cases of AVM. This approach is closed-skull, single-treatment therapy, using ionizing beams of gamma irradiation from a 10-mV isocentric linear accelerator. More than 50 per cent of reported cases treated in this manner in children were completely obliterated with minimal bleeding during the procedure and no postoperative recurrence. Radiosurgery and interventional radiology are new fields in a process of evolution and may permit more nonoperative approaches for inoperable malformations. It should be noted that the management of the AVM in the pediatric patient should be performed by a multidisciplinary team of critical care, neurosurgery, and interventional radiology specialists. Attention to fluid balance must be maintained during monitoring of side effects of embolization.

Aneurysm

Vascular aneurysms are a rare occurrence in pediatric patients. The most common site is a congenital malformation of the internal carotid artery. The presenting sign is a sudden massive hemorrhage into the subarachnoid space with headache, vomiting, nuchal rigidity, increase in intracranial pressure, retinal hemorrhage, and focal neurologic signs. Diagnosis is made by CT, MRI, and DSA, which gives rapid demonstration of the vascular anatomy free of bony detail.

Treatment

Management involves surgical clipping if the aneurysm is greater than 1 cm in size. Antifibrinolytic therapy (with aminocaproic acid) and calcium channel blockers (nicardipine or nimodipine) have been used with variable results while the patient is awaiting surgery. Complications include neurologic sequelae from brain infarction consequent to delayed vasospasm.

OCCLUSIVE VASCULAR DISEASE

Occlusive vascular disease, or stroke, in infancy and childhood clinically presents as acute hemiplegia and may be due to cerebral arterial or venous thrombosis or emboli. Etiologic factors are often unknown but may include trauma, intracranial infection, hematologic disorders, congenital cardiac disease, metabolic and mitochondrial dysfunction, vasculitis, substance abuse, and migraine.

The hemiplegia following arterial thrombosis is of acute onset with unilateral or generalized seizures, headache, high temperature, obtundation, neuronal dysfunction with disturbances of sensation, dysphagia, and defects in visual fields. Investigations include CT scan of the head indicating initially nonhomogeneous edema of the affected hemisphere and later (within a week) changing to a lucent homogeneous area with well-defined margins. The SPECT (single-proton emission computed tomographic) scan depicting regional cerebral blood flow may demonstrate decrease in vascular distribution in the middle cerebral artery and may be more sensitive than CT. Pulsed Doppler sonography often delineates the site of obstruction in the major vessels. The cerebral arteriogram will locate the site of the occlusion, which may be extracranial in the cervical part of the internal carotid artery or in the vertebral artery. Occlusion of the internal, middle, and anterior cerebral arteries may be seen with extensive telangiectasia: this radiographic picture is termed *moyamoya* ("a puff of smoke") *disease.* Basal arterial occlusion at the origin of the internal carotid artery is less common. Rarely, the arteriogram may be normal.

Treatment

Treatment of acute cerebral thrombosis is aimed at increasing cerebral perfusion and reducing tissue injury. Volume expansion should be administered as needed. Administration of calcium channel blockers can reduce morbidity if they are initiated within 12 hours following diagnosis. Clinical trials are ongoing to assess the role of therapeutic agents such as naloxone (an opiate-antagonist), excitatory amino acid receptors, and salicylates in alleviating tissue injury. Anticoagulants and fibrinolytic agents have not proved to be useful in reducing the severity of the hemiplegia. The role of tissue plasminogen activators is to be explored.

The surgical approach of cerebral vaso-occlusive disease includes either direct or indirect revascularization. Direct vascularization includes anastomosing the superficial temporal artery or occipital artery to the middle cerebral artery. Indirect revascularization includes a temporalis muscle graft EMAS (encephalo-myo-arterio-synangiosus) or EDAS (encephalo-duro-arterio-synangiosus) and placement of the superficial temporal artery directly on the surface of the brain. Direct anastomosis is reserved for patients who have symptoms that persist. Proponents of surgical treatment for moyamoya disease claim significant improvement in symptoms. Alleviation of symptoms is related to development of postoperative collateral circulation. Residual hemiplegia or convulsions are seen in 50 per cent of survivors. No controlled studies have been performed comparing the medical and the surgical approaches to treatment of vaso-occlusive disease.

Neck Trauma

Trauma to the neck result from a blunt injury may cause a contusion or tear of the internal carotid artery leading to aneurysmal dilation or formation of a carotid-cavernous fistula. This may present as pulsating exophthalmos, bruit, and paralysis of the sixth cranial nerve. Thrombosis of the internal carotid artery has been reported in children with a minor injury to the soft palate (with a lollipop stick). The symptoms appear a few hours after injury but may be delayed for months to years.

Treatment

Treatment includes thrombectomy if the site is accessible. Alternatively, anticoagulation can be attempted. The carotid to cavernous fistula can be embolized either through one of the venous effluents or by direct puncture of the cavernous sinus in an effort to preserve the internal carotid artery. Materials used for embolization include Gelfoam, oxidized cellulose, and fiber sealant.

Cyanotic Heart Disease

Congenital cyanotic heart disease (tetralogy of Fallot, transposition of the great vessels) is a frequent cause of cerebrovascular occlusion in the infant younger than 2 years of age. The right to left shunting allows systemic thrombi to embolize to cerebral circulation. Irregular cardiac rhythm and bacterial endocarditis are predisposing factors. Fever, dehydration, and polycythemia also contribute as risk factors. The infant presents with seizures and sudden onset of hemiplegia. Funduscopy is not helpful in assessing intracranial pressure, as dilated vessels and blurred margins are seen in the majority of children as a result of severe hypoxemia and polycythemia.

Treatment

Management includes antibiotic therapy because of the risk of cerebral abscess. Cerebral occlusive disease also can occur in cardiac patients immediately following cardiac-surgical procedures owing to hypoperfusion during cardiopulmonary bypass or to emboli (air, fat, or thrombi). Symptoms may be mild with alteration of consciousness, behavioral changes, decrease in intellectual function, and memory disturbance, with improvement in 3 to 4 weeks. However, a major vascular occlusion may lead to severe brain damage with loss of consciousness and seizures.

Hemoglobinopathy

Hemoglobinopathies are a common cause of stroke in young black children 5 to 7 years of age with sickle cell disease. This is due to occlusive disease of the major vessels at the base of the brain accompanied by an increase of the collateral circulation at the basal ganglia (moyamoya phenomenon). A reduction in capillary flow increases the sickling phenomenon. The onset is sudden and accompanies a sickle cell crisis, which may be precipitated by fever, infection, dehydration, or surgical procedures. Symptoms include seizures, headache, meningeal signs, altered consciousness, hemiparesis, visual defects, and ataxia. Recurrences have been reported to be frequent and occur within 36 months of the initial episode. Diagnostic evaluations include MRI; angiography is contraindicated because contrast medium induces the sickling phenomenon.

Treatment

Treatment includes hydration; correction of acidosis, as acidosis aggravates sickling; and repeated transfusions to maintain the hemoglobin at or above 11 g. Children maintained on a transfusion therapy program in which 2 to 3 units of washed packed red blood cells are transfused every 2 to 4 weeks to maintain hemoglobin at levels where synthesis of sickle cell hemoglobin does not occur have fewer episodes of cerebro-occlusive disease. This therapy also results in normalization of left heart chamber enlargement and decrease in left ventricular mass while stabilizing cardiac output. (See also text on sickle cell, p. 252.)

Hypercoagulable States

In addition to sickle cell disease, other hypercoagulable states that cause occlusive disease and stroke include antithrombin III deficiency, protein C deficiency, nephrotic syndrome, disorders of lipid and lipoprotein metabolism, and acute lymphoblastic leukemia (ALL). The CT scan may be nonspecific, whereas MRI and venous subtraction angiography may be of assistance in the localization of the site of the occlusion.

Treatment

Management, irrespective of etiology, includes supportive care and hydration. The usefulness of heparin therapy has not been proven. Specific therapy includes plasma transfusions in cases of protein C deficiency and antileukemia therapy in ALL.

Hemorrhage

Central nervous system hemorrhage may occur in bleeding disorders such as hemophilia or von Willebrand's disease following head trauma. Therapy includes factor VIII concentrates (cryoprecipitate) and antiplatelet therapy.

Infection

Bacterial and viral central nervous system infections may be complicated by stroke in children. Stroke should also be considered when focal neurologic signs develop in children with human immunodeficiency virus (HIV).

BENIGN INTRACRANIAL HYPERTENSION

ELIZABETH C. ENGLE, M.D.
and DAVID HOLTZMAN, M.D., Ph.D.

The syndrome of benign intracranial hypertension (BIH), or "pseudotumor cerebri," is diagnosed when an alert child has elevated intracranial pressure (ICP > 200 H_2O), normal cerebrospinal fluid (CSF), and normal scans of the brain (no mass or hydrocephalus) by computed tomography (CT) or magnetic resonance imaging (MRI). *BIH is a misnomer, since these children are at significant risk for visual loss and require close neurologic and ophthalmologic care.* Evaluation and rational treatment of BIH require an understanding of etiology, diagnosis, and therapeutic options.

BIH of childhood occurs at all ages and affects males and females equally. Children usually present with a combination of headache, blurred vision, transient visual obscurations, and diplopia. The headache is characteristic of increased ICP and is often associated with vomiting. Signs of BIH include papilledema, unilateral or bilateral sixth nerve palsy (a "false localizing sign"), and deterioration in visual acuity and visual fields. Infants may present only with irritability, lethargy, vomiting, and split sutures and/or a bulging fontanelle without papilledema.

Table 1 lists conditions associated with BIH. In most cases, the etiology remains unknown. Prior to the advent of aggres-

TABLE 1. Conditions Associated with Benign Intracranial Hypertension

Intracranial venous drainage obstruction
- Mastoiditis and lateral (sigmoid) sinus obstruction
- Extracerebral mass lesions
- Congenital atresia or stenosis of venous sinuses
- Head trauma
- Cryofibrinogenemia
- Polycythemia vera
- Paranasal sinus and pharyngeal infections

Cervical or thoracic venous drainage obstruction
- Intrathoracic mass lesions and postoperative obstruction of venous return

Endocrine dysfunction
- Pregnancy
- Menarche
- Marked menstrual irregularities
- Oral contraceptives
- Obesity
- Withdrawal of corticosteroid therapy
- Addison's disease
- Hypoparathyroidism
- "Catch-up" growth after deprivation, treatment of cystic fibrosis, correction of heart anomaly
- Initiation of thyroxine treatment for hypothyroidism
- Adrenal hyperplasia
- Adrenal adenoma

Hematologic disorders
- Acute iron-deficiency anemia
- Pernicious anemia
- Thrombocytopenia
- Wiskott-Aldrich syndrome

Vitamin metabolism
- Chronic hypervitaminosis A
- Acute hypervitaminosis A
- Hypovitaminosis A
- Cystic fibrosis and hypovitaminosis A
- Vitamin D–deficiency rickets

Drug reaction
- Tetracycline
- Perhexiline maleate
- Nalidixic acid
- Sulfamethoxazole
- Indomethacin
- Penicillin

Prophylactic antisera

Miscellaneous
- Galactosemia
- Galactokinase deficiency
- Sydenham's chorea
- Sarcoidosis
- Roseola infantum
- Hypophosphatasia
- Paget's disease
- Maple syrup urine disease
- Turner's syndrome

sive antibiotic therapy, BIH often was associated with otitis media and mastoiditis with secondary venous sinus thrombosis. Today, it is more commonly associated with obesity, chronic steroid use and withdrawal, malnourishment and refeeding, anemia, antibiotics, or megavitamins. One of the first steps in therapy is to eliminate any potential etiologic factors.

In most children, the prognosis of BIH is good. A significant percentage recover after a single diagnostic lumbar puncture (LP), and approximately half are normal by 6 months. Some children experience a progressive or recurrent syndrome and are refractory to medical therapy. Early clinical series found no visual loss in pediatric patients and concluded that children are protected from optic nerve damage. However, subsequent reports have firmly established that children, like adults, are at significant risk for optic neuropathy. The CSF, which is contained within the subarachnoid space between the optic nerve and surrounding dural sheath, transmits the elevated pressure to this compartment. Visual loss occurs when the increased CSF pressure compresses the nerve. The early changes of optic neuropathy are increased size of the physiologic blind spot and constriction of visual fields. Later, decreased visual acuity and blindness develop. Ophthalmologic testing, therefore, must include formal visual field and contrast and color desaturation testing. Visual evoked potentials (VEPs) are abnormal with decreased visual acuity and do not detect the early changes of optic neuropathy. The occurrence and progression of visual loss are unpredictable. Visual loss can progress insidiously or occur suddenly; it may be present at diagnosis, may occur during treatment, or may be found only late in the disease. It does not correlate with the degree of papilledema, the presence of diplopia, or the extent of visual symptoms. Visual loss can improve or can be completely reversed with treatment, even after optic atrophy has developed.

The patient in whom BIH is suspected must undergo neuroimaging for the presence of hydrocephalus, a mass lesion, subarachnoid or intraparenchymal hemorrhage, or demyelination. MRI is recommended over CT because it provides information about the patency of the venous sinuses and abnormalities in the brain.

If the imaging study is normal, a lumbar puncture should be performed. The first LP has both diagnostic and therapeutic benefits. The opening pressure must be recorded with the patient horizontal, breathing comfortably, and relaxed with neck and legs extended. Although premedication and patience may be required, this technique ensures that the pressure is not falsely elevated. Fluid should be determined for cell count and differential, protein, and glucose. Normal CSF is evidence against meningeal infection or inflammation, subarachnoid hemorrhage, or a demyelinating process. Enough fluid must be removed to lower the closing pressure to less than 100 mm of H_2O. This usually ranges from 10 to 30 ml and depends on the size of the patient.

TREATMENT

The two goals of treatment of BIH are relief of symptoms and preservation of visual function. Symptomatic complaints can often be controlled medically by the use of serial LPs, carbonic anhydrase inhibitors, corticosteroids and analgesics, and surgery. *Neuro-ophthalmologists generally agree that a lumboperitoneal shunt or optic nerve sheath fenestration should be performed with any deterioration of vision.* The choice of treatment options is patient-dependent, but general guidelines for each are discussed here.

Lumbar Puncture

The LP provides a nonspecific CSF leak that, if the dura is torn slightly, may continue to drain slowly and lower CSF pressure. Some patients have lasting symptomatic relief. Most clinicians repeat the LP after a day in order to document a persistent elevation in pressure. More than two or three taps, however, becomes painful and frightening to children. Single pressure recordings may not be accurate. If the patient is asymptomatic and frequent ophthalmologic findings remain normal, there is no indication for serial LPs or other treatment. Such a patient still needs monthly neuro-ophthalmologic evaluation.

Medications

When a patient has persistently elevated pressure on two taps and is symptomatic without visual deterioration, it is appropriate to begin acetazolamide (up to a maximum of 60 mg/kg/day), a carbonic acid inhibitor that decreases CSF production. Side effects include acid-base and electrolyte imbalances, renal calculi, gastrointestinal upset, and appetite suppression. Occasionally, furosemide (2 mg/kg three times a day) is used also. Headaches may be controlled by conventional analgesics for tension and/or vascular pain (nonsteroidal anti-inflammatories, amitriptyline, beta-blockers, periactin). It is essential that these be used only if the patient is compliant with frequent ophthalmologic appointments. Freedom from headache does not ensure lack of optic nerve damage.

Steroids

The use of steroids for treatment of BIH in children is very controversial. It is generally agreed that steroids should not be used for more than several weeks. They are associated with severe side effects from chronic use, including weight gain, cushingoid features, acne, and proximal myopathy. If prolonged use appears necessary to control symptoms or if visual deterioration occurs during steroid therapy, the patient should be evaluated for surgery.

Surgery

Surgery is indicated as initial therapy in a patient who presents with visual loss. The first surgical treatment for BIH was a subtemporal decompression. This was abandoned because of failures and complications. *Lumboperitoneal shunts* have been effective for patients with headaches refractory to medical management and no visual loss. The shunt allows CSF to flow down a pressure gradient from the lumbar subarachnoid space into the peritoneum, where it is reabsorbed. When constant drainage is provided, the optic nerve is protected from intermittent pressure spikes. Shunts have the disadvantage of necessitating revisions and serving as a nidus for infection. Low-pressure headaches can occur in shunted patients in whom BIH has resolved.

The most recent advance in treatment of BIH is *optic nerve sheath fenestration.* If the dura and meninges surrounding the optic nerve are opened just behind the globe, CSF can continuously escape and pressure within the subarachnoid space around the nerve is decompressed. In adults, this procedure has yielded stable to improved visual acuity and visual fields in the vast majority of patients, with relief of headache in more than 50 per cent. Unilateral surgery has resulted in improved papilledema bilaterally. Optic atrophy preoperatively does not predict a poor outcome. In children, this procedure is becoming the treatment of choice in any patient who shows deterioration of visual acuity or visual fields.

REFERENCES

Greer M: Benign intracranial hypertension. *In* Gellis SS, Kagan BM: Current Pediatric Therapy, 13th ed. Philadelphia, WB Saunders Co., 1990, pp 61–63.

Lessell S, Rosman NP: Permanent visual impairment in childhood pseudotumor cerebri. Arch Neurol 43:801–804, 1986.

NEUROCUTANEOUS SYNDROMES

MANUEL R. GOMEZ, M.D.

To date more than 50 neurocutaneous syndromes (NCSs) have been described. Some of them are listed under such headings as inherited metabolic diseases, DNA repair disorders, or hereditary neuropathies, among other categories, and are not described in this article.

TUBEROUS SCLEROSIS COMPLEX

Tuberous sclerosis complex (TSC) is a hamartiosis and hamartomatosis of autosomal dominant inheritance, variable expressivity, and high penetrance. The prevalence of TSC is about 1 in 15,000. Approximately half of newly recognized cases are due to new mutation. Through genetic linkage studies, the TSC gene has been mapped to 9q34 (long arm of chromosome 9 near the gene locus for ABO blood types) in certain families, to 11q22-q23 (long arm of chromosome 11 near the NCAM gene) in other families, and to 12q22-q24 in still other families. There are other families informative for markers in these chromosomes, but no linkage has been found.

The symptoms and signs in TSC are caused by the hamartias or the hamartomas located in different organs. The number and size and sometimes the exact location of these lesions determine the presence and severity of the symptoms. The phenotype of patients with cerebral involvement in particular depends on the location of the lesions within the brain. Cortical tubers are associated with seizures and mental retardation, and the subependymal giant cell astrocytomas, truly hamartomas, may cause intracranial hypertension by obstructing the cerebrospinal fluid (CSF) circulation, usually at the foramina of Monro. Cardiac rhabdomyomas may cause arrhythmia or obstruction of blood flow within the heart. By replacing parenchyma, renal angiomyolipomas may lead to chronic renal failure and hypertension, or, by spontaneously rupturing, may cause a potentially serious hemorrhage. Pulmonary lymphangiomyomatosis may lead to pulmonary failure but not before the third decade of life.

Treatment

There is no specific treatment for TSC. Symptomatic treatment listed according to the affected organs is outlined in Table 1.

TABLE 1. Treatment of Tuberous Sclerosis Complex

Clinical Features	Treatment
Seizures	
Infantile spasms	Valproate (VA), adrenocorticotropic hormone (ACTH); see text
Myoclonic	Clonazepam, ACTH, VA
Atonic, tonic	Ethosuximide, acetazolamide, VA
Tonic-clonic	Phenobarbital, phenytoin, VA
Partial seizures	Carbamazepine; surgical treatment may be indicated
Intracranial Hypertension	
Obstructing subependymal giant cell tumors	Surgical removal or shunting; irradiation is contraindicated
Cardiac Rhabdomyoma	
Asymptomatic	No treatment needed
With obstruction	Surgical removal
With arrhythmia	Antiarrhythmic drugs
Renal Angiomyolipomas	
Asymptomatic	No treatment needed
Persistent hematuria	Embolization, partial or total nephrectomy
Retroperitoneal bleed	Nephrectomy
With uremia	Dialysis
Large obstructive renal cysts	Surgical removal
Hypertension	Antihypertensive drugs
Pulmonary Lesions	
Spontaneous pneumothorax	Pleurocentesis
Pulmonary hyperinflation	Respiratory therapy, oxygen
Retinal Hamartoma	None
Skin Lesions	
Facial angiofibromas	Removal with laser beam or abrasion
Shagreen plaques	Cosmetic surgery
Forehead plaques	Cosmetic surgery
Ungual fibromas	Surgical removal

The treatment of infantile spasms and myoclonic seizures should be started as soon as possible after the diagnosis of this symptom is confirmed by electroencephalography. A trial of valproate (up to 60 mg/kg/day), with proper precaution and of no more than 1 week's duration is in order. When it fails, adrenocorticotropic hormone (ACTH) (150 U/m^2/day) should be given intramuscularly (IM) in two divided doses for 7 days, followed by 75 U/m^2/day in a single IM dose for another week, and then 75 U/m^2/every other day for 2 more weeks. After this, the dose should be continued on alternate days, slowly decreasing over a 6- to 8-week period. If there is a seizure relapse as the ACTH is being tapered, the dose should be increased to an amount equal to or greater than the dose that maintained the seizures under good control. After there is again a seizure remission, the dose reduction should continue but by lower or longer steps than before. During the period of ACTH reduction and after its discontinuation, the patient should receive an anticonvulsant medication, preferably with valproate or nitrazepam. Relapses following successful completion of the ACTH course necessitate a second course of ACTH with a longer and more gradual period of withdrawal. Side effects and complications of the ACTH therapy are common but rarely require stopping it; they include hypertension, glycosuria, hypokalemia, irritability with persistent crying, cushingoid features, acne, cataracts, peptic ulcers, osteoporosis, and obesity.

Tonic, atonic, generalized tonic-clonic, partial motor, or complex partial seizure should be treated with anticonvulsant medication: valproate, clonazepam, or carbamazepine. Rarely, acetazolamide has been useful when these drugs have failed. Less often, phenobarbital or phenytoin may be effective, although the former may be accompanied by hyperactivity and the latter with gingival hyperplasia severe enough to require discontinuation. A new anticonvulsant, Vigabatrin, not as yet approved by the Food and Drug Administration (FDA), may be more effective than the above-described medications for the control of infantile spasms.

There is a correlation between early onset, severity of seizures, and mental subnormality with the number of images in magnetic resonance imaging (MRI) head scan believed to represent cortical tubers in patients with TSC. This is frequently demonstrable as, and recognized by, delay in motor and language acquisition. Early-intervention infant stimulation and special education programs should be made available both for the benefit of the patients and the tranquility of the parents, who may find it difficult to cope with retardation and abnormal behavior.

Finally, genetic counseling should be provided to the parents. It is necessary to ascertain whether any parent has TSC by complete examination of the skin and ocular fundi and by imaging the brain with CT or MRI; if findings are negative, the kidneys should be assessed with ultrasound or CT.

NEUROFIBROMATOSIS 1

Neurofibromatosis is the most common of the neurocutaneous syndromes and is reported to have a prevalence of 1 in 3000, or five times greater than that of TSC. It is of autosomal dominant inheritance with high penetrance and variable expressivity. This text refers only to neurofibromatosis 1 (NF1) or so-called von Recklinghausen neurofibromatosis. Neurofibromatosis 2 (bilateral acoustic neurofibromatosis) is a separate entity that rarely causes symptoms during childhood.

A diagnosis of NF1 can be made when a patient has at least two of the following clinical features:

1. Six or more café-au-lait spots larger than 5 mm in greatest diameter in subjects who have not as yet reached puberty and larger than 15 mm in greatest diameter in postpubertal individuals.
2. Multiple axillary or inguinal freckles.
3. At least one plexiform neurofibroma or two neurofibromas of any type.
4. Optic nerve and/or chiasmatic glioma.
5. Two or more iris Lisch nodules demonstrable with slit-lamp examination.
6. Thinning of long bone cortex with or without pseudoarthrosis.
7. Dysplasia of the sphenoid.
8. A first degree relative with NF1 by the above criteria.

These patients also can have significant pruritus.

Treatment

Treatment is always symptomatic and may be medical or surgical. An experimental medical treatment is now under way to control the pruritus with the drug ketotifen. There is no other medical treatment. Anticonvulsant medication may be required in the exceptional patient with NF1 who has seizures.

Surgical treatment may be indicated for cosmetic reasons or to eradicate tumors within the cranium, face, orbits, neck, spinal canal, thorax, or abdomen. Irradiation is contraindicated in the majority of lesions, although it has often been used for treating optic gliomas, astrocytomas, and extracranial lesions. The developing cerebrum of young children is very vulnerable to irradiation, and the resulting postradiation encephalopathy may have worse consequences than an untreated, slow-growing optic glioma. A ventriculoperitoneal shunting procedure or a stereotactic third ventriculostomy may be necessary when there is hydrocephalus secondary to aqueductal stenosis or to ventricular obstruction by a chiasmatic glioma. Tumor removal would be an option if vision has already been lost. When there is pituitary-hypothalamic axis insufficiency, hormonal replacement is necessary.

Malignancy is a complication of NF1. The frequency of malignant transformation of neurofibroma to neurofibrosarcoma has been estimated at about 5 per cent. Other malignant tumors may be angiosarcoma, malignant fibrous histiocytoma, and liposarcoma. Rhabdomyosarcoma, juvenile chronic myelogenous leukemia, and perhaps neuroblastoma have been found with more frequency among NF1 patients than in the general population. The appropriate treatment for the solid lesions is surgical removal. In other cases, radiotherapy or chemotherapy may be necessary.

Patients with NF1 often suffer recurrent headaches in the absence of increased intracranial pressure as demonstrated by head CT or MRI. Some headaches have a vascular characteristic that resembles migraine. Intracranial vascular malformations (IVMs) and vascular occlusions occur with more frequency in NF1 than in the general population. Patients with such findings may present with hemiplegia or other neurologic deficit of sudden onset. Patients with NF1 who have received radiation therapy for intracranial tumors are particularly prone to stroke as a result of added vascular damage.

Special methods of education and behavior modification techniques should be offered to the children with NF1 and learning or behavior disorders. Psychometrics and evaluation by an educational psychologist are often necessary.

Genetic counseling to the patient and family is mandatory. Through linkage studies, the NF1 gene has been mapped to the long arm of chromosome 17, a useful finding that may be applied for prenatal diagnosis in families with informative markers located near the gene locus.

VON HIPPEL–LINDAU DISEASE

Von Hippel–Lindau disease (VHD), also a hamartomatosis, is usually included with the neurocutaneous diseases, although it rarely affects the skin. Like other hamartomatoses, it is of autosomal dominant inheritance.

Characteristically, in patients with VHD, retinal and cerebellar hemangioblastomas, renal, pancreatic, and epididymal cysts, and renal carcinoma develop. The diagnosis can be made when a patient has a hemangioblastoma of the central nervous system (CNS) or retina and one of the other aforementioned visceral lesions or has a direct relative with this disease.

Treatment

Treatment of the intracranial hemangioblastoma and other tumors is surgical. Radiotherapy is of little benefit, but it is recommended for inoperable patients, such as those with a hemangioblastoma in the medulla. Because the disease is autosomal dominant and has a high penetration, individuals at risk should be examined at least once a year to look for the hemangioblastomas; if these are present, they should be surgically eradicated. Head MRI contrasted with gadolinium is the preferred neuroimaging method.

NEVOID BASAL CELL CARCINOMA SYNDROME

This neurocutaneous disease, also of autosomal dominant inheritance, is called by some Gorlin-Goltz syndrome or just Gorlin syndrome. Its characteristic skin lesion—the basocellular nevus on the face, neck, and upper trunk—makes its appearance between puberty and the fourth decade of life, rarely regresses, and may undergo malignant transformation.

The second characteristic lesion, the odontogenic keratocyst, appears in the first decade of life and generally after the age of 7 years. New cysts develop in the second and third decades but remain symptomless unless they become infected. Pathologic fractures of the mandible or the maxilla may occur.

The third characteristic lesion is the palmar or plantar pit. In addition, some patients have one or more of the following tumors: ovarian fibroma or fibrosarcoma, cardiac fibroma, meningioma, cerebellar medulloblastoma, ameloblastoma, leiomyoma, craniopharyngioma, adrenal cortical adenoma, lymphangiomyoma, rhabdomyosarcoma, fetal rhabdomyoma, seminoma, melanoma, neurofibroma, and maxillary fibrosarcoma. These tumors necessitate surgical treatment. In some patients lymphatic cysts of the mesentery, gastric polyps, spindle cell epitheliomas, or hamartomatous cysts of the lung may develop; other patients have congenital blindness due to corneal opacities, congenital cataracts, or glaucoma. Still others may have coloboma of the iris, choroid, or optic nerve; harelip; or cleft palate.

The course of the disease is variable. Only when a medulloblastoma develops is the disease fatal. Its treatment is surgical. The prognosis of medulloblastoma is better than in patients with medulloblastoma but without nevoid basal cell carcinoma syndrome. Even when a fatal neoplasia does not develop, patients may become depressed as a result of the continuous development of malignant tumors of the face, requiring frequent intervention that leaves many facial scars. Psychiatric support may be necessary because the prognosis is relatively good and the patient may live many years. Radiation therapy is contraindicated because it may stimulate the development of new skin lesions.

XERODERMA PIGMENTOSUM

This autosomal recessive inherited disorder is due to a defect in the repair of damaged DNA that causes acceleration in the aging of tissues, particularly after exposure to solar light. There is also premature degeneration of neurons.

Clinical features are hyperpigmented spots on the skin or freckles, hypopigmentation, telangiectasia, xerosis, desquamation, atrophy, and, acutely, erythema bullae following exposure to sunlight. Among the various types of neoplasias and preneoplastic lesions are actinic keratosis, basal and spindle cell carcinoma, malignant melanomas, keratoacanthomas, angiomas, fibromas, and sarcomas. The eyes may be affected by blepharitis; erythema; eyelid pigmentation and keratosis; loss of eyelashes; atrophy of eyelids leading to entropium or ectropium; papillomas or epitheliomas of the lid border; basal or spindle cell carcinomas; conjunctivitis; epiphora; edema; pigmentation; telangiectasias; conjunctival dryness; keratitis; synechiae; and iris atrophy. These lesions appear after exposure of skin and eyes to sunlight, usually in the first months of life. By age 4 years, most of the patients have clinical signs of the disease. A short exposure to sunlight during infancy causes an acute reaction with erythema and vesiculation of the skin. Although this reaction may be transient, subsequently the pigmented lesions appear, increase in number, and become confluent. The skin becomes dry and desquamates, and at the end the neoplasias appear.

Neurologic signs develop in some of the patients. In the most severe form, there is microcephaly, mental deterioration, ataxia, spasticity, choreoathetosis, and hyporeflexia progressing to areflexia as a result of a peripheral neuropathy. There may be also delay in growth and sexual development.

Treatment

Treatment consists of protecting the patients from solar radiation. The diagnosis must be made very early and should be suspected when an infant or small child has suffered an intense erythematous skin reaction after a short exposure to sunlight. Once the diagnosis is confirmed, either because there is a positive family history or diagnostic laboratory testing has shown a deficient DNA repair in cultured fibroblasts, the patient should be well protected from ultraviolet radiation, solar light, and artificial fluorescent light of approximately 313 nm (wavelength). The most damaging radiation energy is a 340-nm wavelength, which penetrates the clouds, although it does not go through ordinary glass. The patient should not be exposed to smoke from cigarettes because it has been demonstrated that cultured fibroblasts of these patients, when exposed to the carcinogen present in tobacco smoke, suffer damage to DNA. Neoplastic skin lesions should be treated with cryotherapy, liquid nitrogen, cryosurgery, electrocoagulation, curetting, or surgical removal. Radiation therapy should not be used to treat the neoplasias.

INCONTINENTIA PIGMENTI

Incontinentia pigmenti affects females almost exclusively and is inherited from the mother. This type of inheritance may be explained by an X-linked dominant gene that is lethal to hemizygotes. Incontinentia pigmenti is manifested by skin lesions that appear in the first days of life as an erythematous macular or papular skin eruption. The lesions are at first vesicular, later bullous, and sometimes pustular. Several crops of lesions appear within the first 2 weeks of life. Between the 3rd and 6th weeks of life, the lesions become keratotic or verrucous. Finally, between the 12th and 36th weeks of life, the skin takes on a dark gray or chocolate color. This pigmentation has the appearance of designs made with a brush on the skin in curious shapes such as streaks, whirls, and flecks. They are seen very often over the lateral surface of the trunk and limbs, more often on the lower than the upper. The pigmentation may persist for several years and disappear by the second decade of life.

In 50 to 80 per cent of patients, there are lesions in the CNS, eyes, teeth, or bony skeleton. The CNS is affected in 30 to 50 per cent of patients. The most common clinical finding is psychomotor retardation of various degrees; generalized or partial seizures may develop early in life. Other findings are spastic diplegia and microcephaly.

Treatment

The treatment of patients with incontinentia pigmenti is symptomatic. For the skin lesions, no treatment other than prophylaxis of infections is needed. For seizures during the acute stage of the disease, anticonvulsant therapy is needed. At a later stage, when the child has developmental retardation, spastic paralysis, or mental subnormality, the appropriate services of education and physical therapy should be offered. Skeletal problems, such as scoliosis, hip dislocation, contractures of tendons, and limb deformities, may necessitate orthopedic treatment. Ophthalmologic service is necessary for refractive errors, strabismus, or cataracts. Finally, genetic counseling should be offered to the parents as well as the children, who may become future parents, before they approach childbearing age.

STURGE-WEBER SYNDROME

Sturge-Weber syndrome (SWS) is a nonhereditary congenital malformation of the cephalic venous microvasculature. The complete syndrome consists of facial, cerebral, and ocular signs resulting from telangiectatic venous angiomas on the face, cranial leptomeninges, and choroid, usually on the same side. In its incomplete form, it may consist of only one or two of these three components.

Skin involvement is recognized at birth. The first cerebral symptoms appear in the first weeks or months of life as partial motor seizures, which may or may not become generalized. As patients become older, seizures may become more frequent and severe. Postictal transient hemiparesis lasting minutes or hours is not unusual and may later become a permanent hemiparesis or hemiplegia.

Buphthalmos or glaucoma associated with choroidal angioma is present in 30 per cent of patients with SWS, and more than 50 per cent of these have buphthalmos. The glaucoma may be bilateral even when the facial nevus is unilateral and vice versa.

Treatment

The prognosis depends on the severity and extension of the cerebral and ocular lesions and not on the cutaneous angiomatous nevus, which may need only cosmetic treatment with laser. Seizures are treated with anticonvulsant medication. If the cerebral lesions are unilateral and associated with intractable seizures, surgical resection of the affected region, lobectomy, or hemispherectomy is an option that should be considered when the patient is still young and before there is neurologic deterioration. Glaucoma is also medically or surgically treated.

REFERENCES

Gomez MR: Tuberous Sclerosis, 2nd ed. New York, Raven Press, 1988.
Horton WA, Wong V, Eldridge R: Von Hippel–Lindau disease: Clinical and pathological manifestations in nine families with 50 affected members. Arch Intern Med 136:769, 1976.
Listernick R, Charnow J: Neurofibromatosis type 1 in childhood. J Pediatr 116:845, 1990.

ACUTE ATAXIA

IRA BERGMAN, M.D.

The most common causes of acute ataxia in childhood are postinfectious acute cerebellar ataxia and drug intoxications. Some causes, such as tumors in the posterior fossa, hydrocephalus, multiple sclerosis, strokes, and hemorrhages, are easily identified by asymmetric clinical findings, associated noncerebellar neurologic signs, and abnormalities on computed tomographic (CT) or magnetic resonance imaging (MRI) scans of the brain. Other causes, such as the paraneoplastic opsoclonus-myoclonus syndrome associated with neuroblastoma, mild inborn errors of metabolism, labyrinthine dysfunction, head trauma, epilepsy, the postictal state, and Guillain-Barré and Miller-Fisher syndromes, are difficult to prove or require special tests for their identification.

POSTINFECTIOUS ACUTE CEREBELLAR ATAXIA

This disorder may follow chickenpox, infectious mononucleosis, or a mild respiratory or gastrointestinal viral illness by about a week. It begins abruptly, causing staggering and frequent falling and can progress to difficulty with standing and sitting. Truncal ataxia may be the only symptom or may be accompanied by dysmetria of the arms, dysarthria, nystagmus, vomiting, irritability, and lethargy. Symptoms usually peak within 2 days, then stabilize and resolve over 1 to 2 weeks. Recovery is usually complete.

Cerebrospinal fluid (CSF) examination sometimes demonstrates a mild lymphocytic pleocytosis or mild elevation of protein content. CT and MRI scans of the brain are usually normal but infrequently demonstrate abnormalities of the cerebellar or brain stem white matter. The pathogenesis of the syndrome is uncertain and may represent either a direct viral infection of the cerebellum or an autoimmune response to the cerebellar white matter precipitated by the preceding viral infection.

No specific therapy is available. In most cases, limitation of activity to prevent injury and reassurance to the parents is all that is required. Symptomatic therapy of ataxia is unsatisfactory. Walkers are tried, but wheelchairs are usually required. Occasionally, nausea and vomiting are severe and intravenous hydration is necessary. If the illness is severe, persistent, and associated with demyelinative changes on CT or MRI scan, a trial of intravenous methylprednisolone (2 mg/kg/day) may be initiated.

DRUG INTOXICATION

Overdosage with any sedative-hypnotic agent can produce ataxia and lethargy, but ataxia without lethargy usually results from intoxication with alcohol, phenytoin, or carbamazepine. When erythromycin is administered to children receiving chronic carbamazepine therapy, the blood levels of carbamazepine often rise into the toxic range, resulting in symptoms of diplopia and ataxia. Treatment is supportive, and the toxic agent is removed.

PARANEOPLASTIC OPSOCLONUS-MYOCLONUS SYNDROME

This syndrome is the initial manifestation of neuroblastoma in 2 per cent of cases. Children 6 months to 2 years of age experience irregular, hyperkinetic, multidirectional spontaneous eye movements; irregular, lightning-like, involuntary movements of the head and limbs; ataxia; dysmetria; and irritability over several days or weeks. *The presence of opsoclonic eye movements demands an intensive search for neuroblastoma, including urinary analysis of catecholamine metabolites; plain x-rays of the chest, abdomen, and skeleton; ultrasound of the abdomen; and contrast-enhanced CT of the abdomen and chest.* This syndrome is usually associated with stage 1 or 2 neuroblastoma, and removal of the tumor results in cure of the cancer in most cases. However, *the neurologic syndrome usually persists despite successful eradication of the tumor and produces disabling symptoms.*

Treatment with oral prednisone (2 mg/kg/day) often relieves the acute neurologic symptoms, but 82 per cent of the children will be left with persistent cerebellar deficits (64 per cent) and/or mental retardation (36 per cent).

INBORN ERRORS OF METABOLISM

Several inborn errors of metabolism can present with intermittent episodes of ataxia as well as somnolence. These include Hartnup disorder, branched chain ketoaciduria (maple syrup urine disease), multiple carboxylase deficiency (biotinidase deficiency), disorders of the urea cycle, and abnormalities of pyruvate metabolism.

Diagnosis is made by analysis of blood gases, ammonia, pyruvate, biotinidase levels, urine amino acids, and organic acids. Treatment involves dietary manipulation and megavitamin therapy.

EPILEPSY AND THE POSTICTAL STATE

Primary generalized epilepsy producing frequent "atypical absence" seizures can manifest with ataxia and confusion that waxes and wanes in severity. The diagnosis is suggested by the clinical findings of brief head drops, eyelid fluttering, nystagmus, and myoclonic jerks of the extremities and is confirmed by electroencephalogram (EEG), which displays generalized spike and wave activity at 2 to 4 hertz (Hz).

The postictal state may be occult when generalized seizures occur at night or when partial complex seizures are subtle and consist of psychic or autonomic phenomena that are not appreciated as seizures. Nighttime seizures are suggested by small amounts of blood on the pillow from tongue or lip biting, incontinence, and unusual difficulty in arousing the child. Partial complex seizures may be indicated by brief lapses of attention; automatisms of chewing, eye blinking, fumbling with clothes, or walking in circles; hallucinations of vision, smell, taste, hearing, or place; or episodic autonomic dysfunction with abdominal pain or dizziness. The EEG may be normal or demonstrate only mild nonspecific background slowing at the time the patient sees the doctor. The diagnosis may be difficult to establish, and repeated re-evaluations, EEG telemetry, or prolonged video recordings may be necessary.

Treatment consists of chronic anticonvulsant therapy with a medication appropriate for either generalized or partial epilepsy.

LABYRINTHINE DYSFUNCTION

Difficulty walking with a severe staggering gait is one manifestation of labyrinthine dysfunction, but the diagnosis is usually clarified by the associated symptoms of a severe sense of spinning dizziness, nausea and vomiting, and the associated signs of pallor, sweating, and nystagmus. Benign paroxysmal vertigo is a disorder of toddlers, 1 to 4 years old, who experience recurrent episodes of vertigo lasting a few minutes each. The children lie still during the attacks, and no other treatment is required. Labyrinthitis is a presumed viral infection of the inner ear that produces hearing loss and intense vertigo on movement of the head. Treatment consists of maintaining the most comfortable resting posture and oral meclizine.

GUILLAIN-BARRÉ AND MILLER-FISHER SYNDROMES

The Miller-Fisher syndrome (ataxia, ophthalmoplegia, and areflexia) is thought to be an acute postinfectious neuropathy, akin to Guillain-Barré syndrome. The symptoms resolve spontaneously over several weeks.

Some children with acute weakness of the legs due to Guillain-Barré syndrome or other causes present with difficulty walking that mimics ataxia. The proper diagnosis is suggested by inability to climb stairs or arise from the ground, inability to elevate the legs from the supine position, and areflexia. Careful monitoring of respiratory function in an intensive care unit is required. The treatment of Guillain-Barré syndrome is discussed on page 96.

DEGENERATIVE DISEASES OF THE CENTRAL NERVOUS SYSTEM

PHILIP J. BRUNQUELL, M.D.

Although degenerative diseases of the central nervous system (CNS) are a heterogeneous group, they share two common features: pathologically there is a progressive, more or less symmetric breakdown of cells in the nervous system, and clinically there is progressive loss of motor and/or intellectual function. Neurons, glia, or myelin sheaths may be primarily affected, but the majority of these conditions represent neuronal degenerations. The ages of onset, rates of progression, and initial clinical manifestations vary. In the later stages of these diseases, however, patients may appear remarkably similar, and therapeutic measures tend to address common clinical problems.

The diseases can be classified into two broad groups: those that are associated with an underlying biochemical defect and those that are not. As research methods become more precise and more biochemical mechanisms are identified, many diseases are being reclassified from the latter category into the former. It is important to distinguish between the two groups because specific therapies are available for some of the disorders in which a biochemical basis is known.

SPECIFIC THERAPY

The goal of specific therapy is to reverse, ameliorate, or circumvent the underlying metabolic defect. Although this approach is currently possible for only some of the diseases, as more biochemical bases are identified, the prospect of having more successful, specific therapies increases correspondingly.

For most of the biochemically based degenerative disorders, an abnormal gene serves as the template for a defective protein, usually an enzyme. The enzyme deficiency may cause accumulation of its substrate, deficiency of the end-product, accumulation of substances via alternate metabolic pathways, or a combination of these factors. Specific therapies have attempted to address each of these biochemical processes.

Gene Manipulation

Currently the most effective way to address biochemically based CNS degenerative disease is to prohibit gene expression through either retrospective or, preferably, prospective genetic counseling. Since many of the biochemical disorders follow mendelian (usually autosomal recessive) modes of inheritance, the risks of recurrence can usually be accurately predicted. Furthermore, for many of these conditions, prenatal detection by transabdominal amniocentesis is possible, and the option of therapeutic abortion can be considered. Prospective counseling depends on screening large populations to detect individuals in the preclinical stages of their diseases (e.g., neonatal metabolic screening programs) or screening segments of the population at risk for transmitting specific disorders (e.g., heterozygous carriers of Tay-Sachs disease).

Beyond genetic counseling, direct gene manipulation holds distinct promise. As gene mapping techniques reveal the chromosomal loci of biochemically based degenerative diseases, and as cloning of "corrected" genes becomes possible, the ultimate goal of gene replacement may not be as unrealistic as once was perceived.

Enzyme Manipulation

Both direct and indirect approaches to this form of therapy have been attempted, with varying measures of success. Indirect approaches include cofactor administration and organ allotransplantation. The direct approach of enzyme replacement remains highly experimental at the current time.

Many enzymes require vitamin or metal cofactors to achieve biologic activity. Cofactor administration may increase a deficient enzyme's catalytic activity and produce clinical improvement, as in the administration of vitamin B_{12} in methylmalonic acidemia and biotin in propionic acidemia. Allotransplantation of an organ that manufactures the deficient enzyme may be limited by the organ's capability for enzyme synthesis: Sufficient enzyme may be produced for its own use but not for other organs of the body, including the brain. Recently, however, encouraging results have been noted in patients undergoing bone marrow transplantation for a number of conditions, including Gaucher's disease and some of the mucopolysaccharidoses. Particular success has been recorded in some patients with the late infantile form of metachromatic leukodystrophy. Bone marrow transplantation has been followed by a rise in leukocyte levels of the deficient enzyme arylsulfatase A, a decline in the accumulation of storage material in biopsied peripheral nerves, improvement in the pattern of central dysmyelination on magnetic resonance imaging (MRI) and an arrest of the expected rapid downhill clinical course. Clinical, radiologic, and biochemical improvement has been documented following bone marrow transplantation for another white matter disease, X-linked adrenoleukodystrophy. Clearly, if such interventions are to succeed, they must be offered early in the course of the disease before extensive destruction of neural tissue has occurred.

Attempts at direct enzyme replacement have been limited by problems with enzyme purification, peripheral inactivation, and tissue targeting. At present, research is aimed at overcoming these obstacles, as in the delivery of enzymes in lipid envelopes (liposomes), the entry of enzymes into the CNS via transient osmotic opening of the blood-brain barrier, and the linkage of enzymes to cell receptor-specific ligands, thus permitting receptor-mediated endocytosis.

Substrate Removal

In many cases, a patient's condition may improve when the accumulating substrate is eliminated or restricted from the diet. Dietary restrictions may be general, such as the reduction of protein in patients who have disorders of the urea cycle, or more specific, such as the elimination of galactose in galactosemia or the reduction of phenylalanine in phenylketonuria. The amount of substrate to eliminate from the diet and the length of time to continue the restriction vary with the underlying metabolic defect; for some disorders there is a lack of consensus on these issues.

Sometimes dietary restriction can be successfully combined with other forms of substrate removal. In Refsum's disease, for example, there is excessive accumulation of phytanic acid, a substance derived exclusively from the diet. Dietary restriction may dramatically reduce phytanic acid levels, but this may take months, presumably because tissue stores are mobilized when intake is reduced. Adding periodic plasmapheresis to the ongoing program of dietary restriction can accelerate phytanic acid removal and help to keep levels low. This arrests the progress of the disease and prevents relapses.

Occasionally, biochemically based degenerative disease may present as an acute, overwhelming encephalopathic illness. This is especially true of conditions presenting in the neonatal period. Emergency removal of excess substrate may in some cases prove life-saving. Peritoneal dialysis, hemodialysis, or exchange transfusion has been useful in a number of disorders of amino acid metabolism, particularly those that are resistant to pharmacologic intervention.

Elimination of Accumulating Substances by Creating Alternate Metabolic Pathways

Administration of certain compounds may permit the disposal of accumulating substances via pathways other than the one catalyzed by the deficient enzyme. In urea cycle disorders, for example, lowering of serum ammonia has been achieved by administering sodium benzoate. Nitrogen-containing compounds that, by virtue of the metabolic defect, cannot be excreted as urea and would ordinarily accumulate as ammonia are conjugated to benzoate to form hippurate, which is then easily excreted in the urine. Another example is the lowering of copper accumulation in Wilson's disease by the administration of the heavy-metal antagonist penicillamine. Penicillamine is a chelating agent that forms a complex with copper, thus competing with body ligands for binding of the cation and permitting enhanced urinary copper excretion.

End-Product Replacement

The clinical symptoms of enzyme deficiency may result not only from substrate accumulation but also from deficiency of the end-product produced by the reaction catalyzed by the deficient enzyme. Replacement of the end-product may, in turn, ameliorate the symptoms or, if administered in the preclinical stage, prohibit the clinical appearance of the disease. Early thyroid hormone replacement in patients with congenital hypothyroidism may, for example, avert clinical catastrophe.

In most cases of biochemically based degenerative disease, the mother's metabolism protects the fetus in utero. Postnatally, when the infant relies on its own metabolism for survival, neural tissue is placed in jeopardy. The effectiveness of the strategies described above depends therefore upon early, accurate diagnosis. Whether the physician is amplifying enzyme activity by cofactor administration, restricting dietary substrate, eliminating accumulating substances by creating alternate metabolic pathways, or supplying missing end-products, intervention must be instituted before irreversible brain damage has occurred.

SYMPTOMATIC THERAPY

The goals of therapy aimed at treating the symptoms of degenerative disease are to maximize remaining function, promote patient comfort, minimize the risk of secondary illnesses, and facilitate nursing care. The implementation of these goals needs to be continually redefined as the patient's disease progresses. The views of the parents or guardians are crucial to this process of redefinition, and therefore it is incumbent upon the physician to discuss with them the clinical manifestations, the therapeutic ramifications, and the natural history of the disease so that they will be equipped to make informed decisions. Plans for emergency management need to be considered prior to any abrupt, life-threatening decline. Some hospitals have guidelines for the selective emergency management of terminally ill children. Such guidelines seek to ally the recommendations of the physician with the desires of the family while providing opportunity for the ongoing reassessment of the management plan as the child's disease progresses.

The remaining text describes issues pertinent to the care of these patients.

Dysphagia

Much of the failure to thrive seen in children with degenerative disease of the nervous system is due to insufficient caloric intake caused by the inability to suck and swallow in a coordinated fashion. Nasogastric feedings are a useful temporary measure, but for chronic use a gastrostomy is usually required. Caloric needs may vary widely. Immobile patients may require substantially less than those who, although bedridden, manifest nearly continual adventitious movements such as chorea or athetosis.

Respiratory Function

With progression of the underlying disease, the child typically becomes prone to episodes of atelectasis and aspiration. Chest physical therapy and postural drainage, amplified by the use of mucolytic agents and expectorants, are frequently required. Tracheostomy may be necessary to promote respiratory toilet. Mechanical ventilatory support is most appropriate during the initial phases of the patient's illness when pneumonia and other pulmonary problems tend to represent transient setbacks.

Seizure Control

Although patients with degenerative disorders of the central nervous system (and gray matter diseases in particular) are prone to seizures on the basis of their underlying condition, seizures secondary to reversible causes, such as hypoglycemia, electrolyte disturbance, or infection, need to be considered because they are unlikely to respond to conventional anticonvulsant therapy unless the precipitating cause is addressed.

For seizures that arise from the primary degenerative process, the choice of a particular anticonvulsant will depend on the clinical and electroencephalographic (EEG) manifestations of the patient's seizures. Because many patients with degenerative disorders exhibit myoclonic seizures, valproic acid may be of particular benefit. However, some children with inborn metabolic errors may be at particular risk for valproate-induced hepatic failure, and therefore alternative anticonvulsants should be considered in this group.

During the evolution of the child's illness, a variety of unusual postures and movements may emerge, not all of which represent seizure activity. Referral of the patient to an EEG-videotelemetry laboratory may be helpful in distinguishing epileptic from nonepileptic behavior. The results of such studies may lead not only to more accurate therapy for seizures but also to the avoidance of unnecessary medication for those events that are not seizure-related.

Behavior

Agitation, irritability, and aggression may become severe enough to require medical management. Before considering whether to administer minor or major tranquilizing agents, the physician needs to rule out the possibility that the patient may be reacting to discomfort from a reversible cause, such as dental abscess, other occult infections, obstipation, or bony dislocation. When tranquilizing agents are indicated, doses need to be carefully titrated to the patient's condition. For example, some patients with degenerative disease may spontaneously and unpredictably alternate between hyperkinetic and hypersomnolent states. The toxic effects of tranquilizing medications may be exacerbated when superimposed on the latter condition.

Neuromuscular Care

Muscle spasticity and contractures are hallmarks of many degenerative diseases of the CNS. Although the maintenance of ambulation may be a viable goal early in the course of the patient's illness, as the disease progresses this expectation becomes increasingly unrealistic. Nonetheless, neuromuscular therapy may still be useful to address separate issues. For example, spasticity with contractures and bony dislocation may cause pain and thus merit treatment, and relief of adductor spasm of the lower extremities may be necessary to permit perineal hygiene.

Overall, management can be viewed in a hierarchical order of invasiveness beginning with physical therapy, advancing to bracing with or without the addition of spasmolytic therapy, and culminating in surgical intervention such as tendon lengthening. Spasmolytic therapy is rarely useful alone and is limited by the occurrence of drug-induced side effects such as sedation from diazepam and baclofen and hepatic dysfunction from dantrolene sodium. Of the surgical procedures, selective spinal dorsal root rhizotomy is currently being evaluated as a promising means of alleviating spasticity. Regardless of which approach is used, care must be taken in those circumstances in which spasticity is necessary to sustain an upright posture or maintain balance in ambulation, as excessive reduction in tone in these instances may further compromise motor function.

Skin Care

Decubitus ulcers should be prevented by proper positioning, frequent turning, protection of bony prominences, treatment of dependent edema, and maintenance of good nutrition. The skin should be kept dry, and a protective ointment, such as petroleum jelly, should be applied to the areas exposed to moisture. If ulcers develop, mechanical and/or lytic enzyme débridement is necessary if necrotic tissue is present. Application of radiant heat and massage around the area of ulcer may improve circulation and facilitate healing. Protective dressings are applied, and use of water- and oxygen-permeable synthetic materials may be helpful (e.g., Op-site).

Bladder Management

Intermittent catheterization is the most common method for managing the neurogenic bladder. Chronic drug therapy is often limited by toxicity. Of the relatively safer medications, imipramine hydrochloride may be useful to reduce detrusor muscle hypertonicity, and oxybutynin chloride* may increase vesical capacity, decrease the frequency of uninhibited detrusor muscle contractions, and delay the initial desire to void in patients with uninhibited neurogenic and reflex neurogenic bladder. Occasionally, a surgical measure such as transurethral resection of the bladder neck is indicated. Because prolonged immobilization may lead to hypercalcinuria, maintenance of a high fluid volume is important to prevent kidney stone formation. Acidification of the urine not only may help to prevent infection but also may keep mineral salts in solution.

Bowel Management

Fecal impaction is very common in patients with CNS degenerative diseases. Adequate hydration, natural dietary laxatives, glycerine or bisacodyl suppositories, and stool softeners such as dioctyl sulfosuccinate are useful measures. Digital removal of stool and enemas may be required.

Infectious Diseases Surveillance

The child's resistance to infection is typically lowered by immobility, poor nutrition, and compromise of protective physiologic functions such as coughing, gagging, and complete bladder emptying. Acute infections, even those outside the nervous system, can produce an abrupt decline from the patient's current level of neurologic functioning, which may often be reversed upon adequate treatment of the infection. The role of occult infections in causing chronic agitation and irritability has already been mentioned.

Psychosocial Support

The presence of CNS degenerative disease in a child places an enormous emotional and financial burden on the family. For the child who is cared for at home, respite care for the parents can be of immense benefit in allowing them to renew their physical and emotional resources. Parent support groups can ameliorate the isolation that families experience in caring for their afflicted child. For some conditions, such as Tay-Sachs disease, national foundations exist that can provide further support services. Financial assistance for such items as adaptive equipment, medications, and nursing care should be explored.

One of the most important therapeutic measures that the physician can employ is to avoid retreating from the patient and the patient's family when the terminal stages of the illness arrive. The presence and concern of the physician are never more fully appreciated than when the technologic methods of treatment are no longer relevant to the destiny of the child.

---

*Manufacturer's precaution: The safety and efficacy of oxybutynin chloride (Ditropan) have been demonstrated for children 5 years of age and older; there are insufficient clinical data for children under age 5, and Ditropan is not recommended for this age group.

CEREBRAL PALSY

LAWRENCE T. TAFT, M.D.

Although cerebral palsy *per se* is a motor disorder, associated nonmotor handicaps, such as mental retardation, often prove more disabling. The specific strategies necessary for cerebral palsied children to develop to their full potential are only partly determined by the type and extent of the cerebral dysfunction. At least as important in the selection of optimal strategies are the child's family and social milieu.

The first goal in pediatric management should be to maximize the coping abilities of the child and family. Several general principles are particularly important in achieving this goal:

1. Past success is a powerful motivator for future effort. Thus, whenever possible, the child should be placed in situations that optimize the chances for success. Failure depresses and tends to lessen motivation; failure must be avoided.
2. The importance of achieving functional motor improvements, such as independent ambulation, should not be unduly stressed.
3. Coordination of the diagnostic and treatment modalities involved is essential.
4. Achievement of the rights of the child and family, *vis-à-vis* governmental and other institutional support, may require active advocacy on the part of the health care provider.

INITIAL DIAGNOSIS

The parents must be told of the problem in a compassionate and empathetic manner as soon as the diagnosis is suspected or confirmed. They should be given as much information about the cause, treatment, and prognosis as is available. When, as frequently occurs, the prognosis for independent ambulation and/or functioning cannot be accurately stated, the parents should be told of the limitations of early prognosis. Upon hearing the words, "Your child has cerebral palsy," the initial reaction of the parents is commonly extreme grief. Listening may continue, but comprehension often suffers. Thus, it is often necessary to repeat the explanations and to answer the same questions over several subsequent sessions to ensure that the parents understand the situation and have no misconceptions.

At the informing interview, physicians should let the parents know that they will be referring the child to a nearby "early intervention center." These centers are available in all 50 states, as mandated by Federal Law PL 99-457. In the majority of states, there is no charge to the parents for these services. Some of these programs are home-based. If the program is center-based, the parent must bring the child to only one session per week. It should be explained that the center will educate the parents further about cerebral palsy, will explore the problems the infant and the family usually have in coping, and will offer intervention strategies to optimize the child's intellectual and motor functioning. The parents will act as therapists, under the tutelage of the intervention center staff. The advantage of immediate referral is that it does not leave the parents with a sense of complete hopelessness after they are informed of the diagnosis. It offers immediate and essential family support.

The Committee on Children with Handicaps of the American Academy of Pediatrics has concluded that early intervention programs mitigate the denial that families experience after learning of the diagnosis and, consequently, allow for an earlier adaptation.

SPECIFIC INTERVENTION STRATEGIES

Motor Performance

Many techniques are used to improve motor function or prevent complications. The purpose may be to modify the dyskinetic movements, to decrease the hypertonus, or to develop specific skills. Treatment includes physical, occupational, and speech therapies, adaptive devices such as braces, medications, chemical neurolysis to decrease tone, and orthopedic intervention to correct the musculoskeletal abnormalities that develop in the growing child with cerebral palsy.

Physical Therapy

Physical therapy for cerebral palsy can be broadly categorized into two major types: The first maintains the range of motion of the joints and increases muscle strength, and the second modifies the abnormal tone and movements favorably.

The first, the most traditional type, includes passive and active stretching of joints to maintain a full range of motion and prevent musculoskeletal deformities, strengthening exercises by active movements against increasingly greater resistance to counteract the weakness of specific muscle groups, and the teaching and encouragement of the voluntary performance of specific tasks, especially those related to daily living. Parents can be taught to be "therapists." As these patients become older, they themselves can assume responsibility for many of these therapies.

Techniques that attempt to influence tone and posture favorably are more controversial. They are best known by the names of the individuals who have described them, e.g., Bobath, Rood, Kabat, Bronstrum, or Fay. Bobath neurodevelopment physical therapy (NDPT) appears to be the most commonly used by physiatrists and physical therapists. This method attempts to inhibit persistent primitive reflexes and to modify tone by the use of applied sensory stimuli—tactile, vestibular, and proprioceptive. An example of the inhibition of a primitive reflex is modification of the dysfunctional posture caused by a persistent obligatory asymmetric tonic neck reflex. When this reflex is present, the trunk extension that often occurs in these children activates extension of the upper extremities. This latter posture does not allow the child to engage in hand-to-mouth activities or to learn eye-hand coordination. With the Bobath technique, the child is placed in a position that encourages trunk flexion. This activates the symmetric tonic neck reflex in a manner to cause flexion of the upper extremities, thereby facilitating the child's use of the hands and, it is hoped, making the child more functional. With active use of the hands, the patient can improve eye-hand coordination and also increase sensory experiences.

A recent clinical trial concluded that short-term motor outcome in infants with spastic diplegia who were given 12 months of NDPT was not improved over a control group who were given 6 months of infant stimulation plus 6 months of NDPT.

Occupational Therapy

Occupational therapy is often prescribed to improve a youngster's ability in self-help activities. Adaptive equipment may be recommended to facilitate functional use of the hands. Adaptive seating is used to maintain trunk stabilization, allowing better use of the upper extremities. With stability of trunk and shoulders, the child is encouraged to attempt developmentally appropriate skills, such as buttoning. Normal children as well as those with neuromotor handicaps may improve their skills with practice but only if the movements are self-directed. For a child with cerebral palsy, "practice may not make perfect" but it definitely increases functional abilities.

Unfortunately, there is no evidence that training to do one task can lead to a more generalized improvement in functioning. For example, a child with poor ability to throw a ball through a hoop will still find this task difficult even though, after practicing on a Nintendo game, eye-hand coordination has improved.

Speech and Language Therapy

Many infants with cerebral palsy have difficulty sucking, chewing, and/or swallowing. This may result in markedly slow feeding, aspiration, and poor weight gain. Speech therapists with training and experience with infants utilize proper positioning and sensory stimulation of the oropharyngeal areas to help ameliorate the problem. Empirically, there appear to be successes that cannot be explained by maturation. Also, coping by infant and mother is made easier when feeding becomes a pleasurable activity.

Early identification of a delay in expressive language is important, and these infants should receive the benefit of a referral to a speech therapists. The mother is taught how to stimulate language development as part of the daily routine care of the infant. A hearing loss must be ruled out.

If articulation is abnormal, a speech therapist should be consulted.

Drug Modification of Tone

Successful use of medication to decrease tone, with the hope of thereby improving voluntary control of movement, has been limited by drug side effects. Diazepam (Valium) usually has a marked sedative effect before it favorably ameliorates hypertonus. However, when anxiety increases involuntary movements, especially noted with athetoid cerebral palsy, diazepam may be beneficial.

Dantrolene, which acts directly on the muscle to limit its contractibility, also may cause sedation. However, the major concern with dantrolene is that the desired decrease in muscle tone is often associated with marked muscle weakness. Dantrolene usually causes transient elevation of liver enzymes, and therefore liver function studies must be monitored while the child is taking this drug. Chronic or fatal liver disease has not occurred in children taking dantrolene.

Baclofen, a gamma-aminobutyric acid derivative, is believed to inhibit neurotransmitter impulses. It has mild sedative effects with no significant toxic effects. Studies on children are limited and have not proved the effectiveness of this drug in improving motor function. A trial of therapy with baclofen may be indicated, especially in children with severe hypertonia.

Use of a muscle relaxant may also benefit the caretaker of the cerebral palsied child. For instance, a child with severe adductor spasticity is difficult to diaper. The spasticity may be minimized by the use of the appropriate drug.

Local therapy to improve tone has included the use of phenol or alcohol. Because of the neurolytic properties of these agents, injection of the drug around the motor nerve results in partial denervation. This effect may last from a few weeks to a few months. It may especially help to alleviate a spastic equinus foot or severe hip adductor spasm. Use of these agents may allow a more accurate prediction of the functional result achievable through surgery.

Orthotic and Adaptive Equipment

Bracing is used for two purposes: to prevent contractures and to maintain joint stability as an aid in achieving an erect posture. Although lightweight braces are now available, bracing is becoming a less popular mode of therapy. Resting or night splints are often used to maintain a range of motion and are often a prerequisite after surgical releases of joint contractures.

There are numerous adaptive devices to aid in independent functioning. Occupational and physical therapists can evaluate the patient to determine the need for these devices and the type that would provide more independent self-care activities.

In the past decade, computers have made it possible to develop electronic aids that may permit the most severely motor handicapped individuals to gain more control of their environment. A movement of the head or an eye blink can permit a severely quadriplegic individual to turn a page or open a door. Rehabilitation engineers are being utilized on rehabilitation teams to assess each individual as to whether a specifically designed environmental control apparatus will aid the individual to function more independently.

Wheelchairs may be self-driven or propelled by caretakers. The latter are called "travel-chairs" and usually are more appropriate for the severely handicapped child. The chair can be aligned to permit maximal stability of the trunk and to minimize reflexive spastic responses such as hyperextension. The traditional, independently propelled wheelchair has segments to support the leg, seat, and back. These can be adjusted to minimize abnormal postures. The specific type of wheelchair and adaptive equipment should be prescribed by an experienced professional.

Biofeedback

Biofeedback involves the patient's active participation in an attempt to control motor activity through a sensory feedback mechanism. There are very few controlled or long-term studies of the duration of the effects achieved. However, there have been some suggestions that biofeedback has helped hemiplegic cerebral palsied children of normal intelligence to attain a more symmetric, more cosmetic gait.

Electromyographic auditory feedback training of the orbicularis oris and an auditory signal to cue swallowing have been shown to be effective in decreasing drooling. Further experience with this technique is necessary before its therapeutic value can be endorsed. However, a trial of therapy is indicated as a first endeavor to correct drooling, since there are no complications. Drugs and surgical interventions have many associated risks.

Inhibitory Casting

Attempts have been made to realign partially deformed ankles by use of a walking cast applied for a period of 4 to 6 weeks. The foot is maintained in a more normal anatomic position which, in spastic cerebral palsy, necessitates sustained stretching.

There is clinical evidence to indicate that inhibitive casting does result in an increase in ankle dorsiflexion and range of motion. However, this gain is usually lost after 4 to 5 months in spite of the use of rigid ankle orthoses worn during waking hours.

Orthopedic Surgery

Orthopedic surgery is often recommended to correct deformities due to the neuromuscular imbalance of cerebral palsy. Heel-cord lengthening, adductor tenotomies, and hip flexor and hamstring releases are done to improve posture and function. There is still controversy regarding the optimal timing of these procedures as well as which procedures are most effective.

Many cerebral palsy centers have a gait analysis laboratory and utilize this type of evaluation to assist in the decision making as to the type of orthopedic surgery that might offer the best result. The gait analysis is also used to monitor the results of the intervention.

Neurosurgery

Selective posterior rhizotomy to reduce hypertonus and therefore to facilitate movement is being done at many neurologic centers. The posterior roots of the lumbar plexus are exposed and stimulated. The observed electromyographic response aids in identifying those fibers that appear to be facilitating muscle responses. These fibers are resected. Spastic diplegic children who are ambulatory and of good intelligence reportedly have benefited most from this type of procedure. Postoperatively, rigorous physical therapy on a daily basis for a period of 6 to 12 months is usually required. Results of the operation are still being assessed in many centers. Decreased spasticity has been evident, with improvement in stride length and speed noted on gait analysis. Complications have been rare but have included loss of ambulatory ability and hip subluxation.

Selective posterior rhizotomy is now being tried on spastic quadriplegics. Preliminary results indicate that these individuals have not improved functionally.

Health Maintenance

Cerebral palsied children should benefit from the health maintenance routines offered to children without handicaps. For example, they should be immunized according to the standard recommended schedule. In addition, a number of screening tests and areas of anticipatory guidance are particularly relevant to the care of disabled children.

Routine screening for auditory abilities is essential. More than 70 per cent of athetoid cerebral palsied youngsters, secondary to bilirubin encephalopathy, have high-frequency hearing loss. Thirty per cent of all other cerebral palsied children have sensorineural hearing impairment. Early recognition of and appropriate intervention for these problems are important for the prevention of additional difficulties.

Vision screening should be stressed during routine examinations. Strabismus is present in more than 75 per cent of cerebral palsied individuals. Early recognition and referral to an ophthalmologist will help to prevent amblyopia ex anopsia. Ophthalmoscopic examination should be done to evaluate for cataracts and to judge whether a refractive error exists. Nearsightedness is commonly found. When the child is cognitively ready, visual acuity should be tested with the use of "E" or Snellen charts.

There should be routine assessments of the range of motion of spastic joints. Tightness or limitation in the full range of joint motion requires a referral to a physical therapist. The parents can be taught to passively stretch the child's joints to prevent irreversible contractures.

The presence of scoliosis must be monitored. A high prevalence is noted, especially in quadriplegic patients.

Leg length discrepancies should be assessed in hemiplegic infants and children. More than 50 per cent of patients with hemiparesis due to congenital insult have a leg length discrepancy. In an ambulatory child, early recognition and correction of an inequality of leg length by the use of a sole lift help to prevent the development of scoliosis.

Advice must be given to parents regarding the importance of preventing obesity in the child. The limitation of physical activity that results from a neuromotor handicap often results in excessive weight gain.

During each health maintenance visit, the parents should be asked whether there are any recurrent episodes in which the child appears to be unaware of his or her surroundings. These may be seizure manifestations. In more than 50 per cent of children with cerebral palsy, epilepsy develops. Some types of psychomotor seizures may not be recognized as such, being attributed to aberrant behavior.

Mental retardation is seen in 50 per cent of children with cerebral palsy. Many of those with normal intelligence have learning disabilities. There is always concern that formal intellectual testing may demonstrate poor cognitive ability, but the results are spurious because of motor limitations and/or expressive language problems of the child.

Assisting Psychosocial Adjustment

Anticipatory guidance of the parents may help to minimize adverse psychosocial adjustment of the child and family members. Parents should be advised not to act solicitously toward the child. Doing so can cause the child to develop a self-concept of dependency and helplessness. Parents should be encouraged to discipline the child as they would a healthy youngster.

Preschool children frequently believe that their handicap is punishment for some wrongdoing. The pediatrician should explore this issue with the child, and if there is evidence that this is the case, the youngster should be informed that the problem is not related to a punishment or previous bad behavior. As children grow older, their inability to compete physically and socially may lead to isolation from their peers. Attempts should be made to find recreational or social activities in which youngsters may successfully interact with peers and, it is hoped, develop more positive social relationships.

Education

Early intervention centers for infants are quite abundant. In almost all states, mandatory education for handicapped youngsters from 3 years of age must be offered. Parents of young cerebral palsied children should be encouraged to enroll their child in these preschool programs. However, if the disability is minimal, as is often found in hemiplegic patients, and if the youngster does not have a significant cognitive deficit, a normal nursery school placement is preferable.

Mainstreaming children who are capable of competing with their normal peers is preferable to special class placement. However, if there is any suggestion that these children are finding it difficult to maintain self-esteem because of an inability to compete academically with peers, they should be placed in a class where they can experience success and better maintain self-esteem. Children in wheelchairs can be successfully mainstreamed if they have the necessary cognitive abilities.

Nonverbal Communication

Many children with cerebral palsy have difficulties with expressive language, owing to severe dysarthria, verbal dyspraxia, or expressive aphasia. The inability to control one's environment through the use of language can be very depressing. With the use of communication devices as substitutes for spoken or written language, significantly language-impaired children can make themselves understood. There are many devices that resemble calculators, which the child can use to make selected inquiries or responses. The use of nonverbal communication has had amazing success. Many children who are thought to be retarded or withdrawn have demonstrated unexpectedly high cognitive abilities. Successful nonverbal communication has also resulted in positive personality changes. The children become more interested in relating to their peers and caretakers. An infant who has evidence of a severe motor dysfunction of the oropharyngeal muscles should be offered nonverbal communication aids. This will not inhibit later development of the ability to communicate verbally.

Drooling

Oromotor dyspraxia, or pseudobulbar palsy, may cause persistent drooling. Drooling should cease by the age of 3 years. If not, it causes significant embarrassment to the child and family. Most persistent droolers cease doing this by 5 to 10 years of age. However, if it persists, a number of procedures can be tried, although there may be varying results and complications. These include removal of the submandibular glands and repositioning of the parotid ducts more posteriorly; resection of the chorda tympani and tympanic plexus nerves; parotid duct ligations; transposition of the submandibular ducts; oral anticholenergic drugs (benztropine or benzhexol); and behavioral management.

Recreation

Recreational and social programs geared to the handicapped are necessary so that the child does not become homebound. Parents should be referred to the regional voluntary health agency, such as the United Cerebral Palsy Association or the state Developmental Disability Council, to learn what programs exist and where they are located.

Day care and sleep-away camps are also available and should be utilized.

Vocational Training

Adolescents should receive vocational training. Parents should be advised to urge their child's educators to find a suitable vocational training program. If the handicap is so great as to preclude functioning in competitive employment, sheltered workshops should be considered.

SPINAL CORD DISEASES

FRANCIS S. WRIGHT, M.D.

The spinal cord may be affected by several pathologic conditions, all resulting in varying degrees of weakness, sensory loss, bowel and bladder dysfunction, and other autonomic symptoms. The major objectives in the treatment of spinal cord diseases are to prevent further neurologic impairment, avoid non-neurologic complications that interfere with recovery, maximize neurologic functional recovery, and provide early rehabilitative procedures.

In patients presenting with signs and symptoms of spinal cord dysfunction, it is essential that spinal cord tumor, epidural abscess, and arteriovenous malformation (AVM) be excluded. These entities are best diagnosed by magnetic resonance imaging (MRI) techniques but also may be detected by myelography and metrizamide computed tomography (CT) scanning.

SPINAL CORD TRAUMA

Any patient who is unconscious or has multiple injuries should be suspected or assumed to have a spinal cord injury until proven otherwise. Consequently, the initial treatment should provide spinal column immobilization with a soft cervical collar and sandbags placed on either side of the neck to prevent possible cervical spine injury, and the patient should be supported on a rigid frame with shoulder and pelvic girdle support for possible thoracic and lumbar injury. The cervical spine must be protected during airway stabilization. If respiratory function is deteriorating as a result of intercostal and/or diaphragmatic dysfunction, intubation should be performed by the nasotracheal route if possible, with the head supported in a neutral position to avoid any manipulation of the head. If the nasotracheal route is inadequate, a tracheostomy may be necessary. Cardiovascular status needs to be monitored continuously. Careful attention should be given to blood pressure, oxygen and carbon dioxide concentration, and possible anemia. Acute spinal cord injury often results in a loss of autonomic nervous system function with an impairment in vasomotor and sympathetic tone. Consequently, bradycardia, functional hypovolemia, and hypotension frequently develop. These effects may be initially treated with intravenous atropine followed by dopamine or dobutamine. The hypovolemia is treated with volume expansion.

Once the patient's condition is stabilized, radiographic examination of the spine should be performed in areas of suspected injury. Cervical spinal radiography should be performed in all patients with multiple trauma or major head injury. The cervical spine should be immobilized and a lateral cervical spinal radiograph obtained. A CT scan may provide additional information. In severely injured patients, neurosurgical, orthopedic, and general surgical management is essential.

The initial neurologic examination should assess the extent of spinal cord injury. Special attention should be given to respiratory movements to detect the typical "see-saw" respirations characteristic of intercostal muscle paralysis. This pattern may be recognized by the failure of the rib cage to expand in conjunction with the abdominal expansion during the inspiration phase so that the chest appears to sink while the abdominal wall is rising, resulting in a see-saw movement. The neurologic examination should include assessment of the level of consciousness. Cranial nerve function should be evaluated. The extent of motor weakness should be documented. Spontaneous movements may indicate the level of dysfunction. If the spinal cord injury is at the thoracic level, the patient moves only the upper extremities and demonstrates a paraplegia. In addition, the patient does not experience pain or discomfort during painful procedures, such as bladder catheterization, or movement of an obviously fractured leg. Response to touch and pin prick should be assessed to establish a sensory level. Position and vibration senses should be evaluated for posterior column function. To test the integrity of the sacral cord, perianal sensation and rectal tone should be evaluated. Generally, in acute spinal shock the tendon reflexes are depressed or absent.

In addition, a sweat level may be detected by stroking the skin upward over the trunk with the dorsum of the hand until an increase in resistance is perceived, which indicates the autonomic sweat level. Hypothermia is common in children with spinal cord injury. This may be managed with a hyperthermia blanket.

The bladder size should be evaluated, since acute urinary retention is very common. A greatly dilated bladder may interfere with respiration in a patient who is dependent solely on diaphragmatic movement. An indwelling catheter should be placed.

Axial skeletal traction is needed if there is any bony vertebral malalignment and for stabilization of the spinal column. Surgery may be necessary for decompression of the spinal cord or to achieve better alignment of the spinal column. General care for the spinal cord–injured patient is similar to that described for the patient with acute myelitis.

Advances in our knowledge of the fundamental biochemical changes associated with acute spinal cord injury have led to clinical trials of pharmacologic treatment. *One study has sug-*

gested that high-dose methylprednisolone given within 8 hours of acute spinal cord injury results in improved neurologic status. Whether practical functional improvement occurs is not firmly established. This study was conducted with adult patients, and more data are needed to assess the treatment of acute spinal cord injury in children.

SPINAL CORD TUMOR

Extramedullary tumors affecting the spinal cord usually can be completely removed surgically. Intramedullary tumors of the spinal cord may benefit from neurosurgical decompression, especially with the improved surgical capability of the operating microscope and with ultrasonic aspirator removal of tumor, leading to subsequent improvement in spinal cord function. Additional chemotherapy or radiation treatment may be indicated. Prior to surgery, spinal cord edema resulting from the mass lesion may be treated with dexamethasone (0.5 to 1.5 mg/kg/day in four divided doses).

TRANSVERSE MYELITIS (MYELOPATHY)

This syndrome is characterized by sudden, progressive weakness and impaired sensation of the legs that evolve over hours to days, and it is associated with bowel and bladder dysfunction. It is essential that spinal cord compression resulting from a tumor, epidural abscess, or AVM be excluded.

The acute management of this condition involves continued assessment of vital signs and evaluation for neurologic progression. In addition, early rehabilitative procedures should be performed that will diminish long-term disability. The vital signs should be monitored every 2 hours or more frequently if they are changing rapidly. Because myelitis often involves the thoracic cord, there may be impairment of respiratory function. Cardiac monitoring should be instituted, and the vital capacity should be measured at frequent intervals. Blood gas determinations may be useful in assessing respiratory function. Neurologic function should be assessed at frequent intervals with regard to progressive weakness and ascending sensory level. Maintenance intravenous fluids should be administered. Because the patient has urinary incontinence, an indwelling catheter should be inserted. Urinary tract infections should be treated with appropriate antibiotics. Because of the sensory loss over the trunk and pelvis, pressure sores may develop. Consequently, the patient should be placed on an air mattress and turned frequently. Heel pads may be used to prevent further skin injury.

Physical therapy should be initiated as soon as the patient's condition is stabilized. The goals of physical therapy are to maintain flexibility in the extremities, increase strength in all extremities with resistive exercises, and develop independent ambulation with minimal assistive devices. The patient's nutritional status should be monitored with regard to caloric intake during the period of inactivity to provide sufficient nutrition while preventing excessive weight gain. If the patient is experiencing pain, analgesics should be prescribed.

Patients often experience a reactive depression, and psychologic intervention is appropriate. Complete or good recovery is expected in more than 50 per cent of the patients.

CONGENITAL DEFECTS

Atlantoaxial instability, syringomyelia, diastematomyelia, narrowed lumbar spinal canal, and tethered cord syndrome all may produce static or progressive spinal cord symptoms and signs. These are diagnosed by MRI techniques. Atlantoaxial instability may be diagnosed by upper cervical spine radiographs demonstrating an increased (5 mm or more) atlantodens interval. Neurosurgical treatment is indicated if there is evidence of spinal cord compression or progressive symptoms.

REFERENCES

Bracken MB, Shepard MJ, Collins WF, et al: A randomized, controlled trial of methylprednisolone or naloxone in the treatment of acute spinal-cord injury: Results of the Second National Acute Spinal Cord Injury Study. N Engl J Med 322:1405–1411, 1990.

TREATMENT OF SEIZURE DISORDERS IN CHILDREN

DEBORAH G. HIRTZ, M.D.

There are a number of different types of seizures, as well as epileptic syndromes, and children with epilepsy may have more than one type of seizure. The clinical manifestations of a seizure range from brief disturbances in consciousness to motor contractions of the whole body with prolonged loss of awareness. Abnormal and excessive electrical discharges in the gray matter give rise to these symptoms, which depend on the location and the extent of the electrical abnormality. Some seizure types in children are age-related and reflect different stages of organization of the developing nervous system.

Epilepsy is defined as the occurrence of at least two nonfebrile seizures. Etiology may often be unknown and may be related to both genetic and acquired factors. Seizures that occur directly in response to a specific immediate cause, such as fever, trauma, central nervous system (CNS) infection, or electrolyte imbalance, are not considered epileptic. All people are capable of having a seizure given the right precipitants, but children are more susceptible than adults.

In older terminology, seizures were classified as "big" *(grand mal)* and "little" *(petit mal)*. The revised classification from the International League Against Epilepsy (1981), which is based on clinical patterns supplemented by electroencephalographic (EEG) findings, divides seizures into two basic types: partial and generalized (Table 1). *Partial seizures* are subdivided into *simple* (there is no disturbance of consciousness) and *complex* (consciousness is lost). Correctly classifying the type of seizure is important for treatment and for prognosis. In children, the most difficult to diagnose may be staring spells, which may indicate absence or atypical absence, complex partial seizures, or simply daydreaming. The primary means of establishing the seizure type is the clinical history. Some seizures that appear generalized actually may be partial at onset, which is determined from simultaneous EEG recording with videotaping of clinical events.

Specific epileptic syndromes, some of which involve more

TABLE 1. Classification of Seizures

Partial seizures
Simple (consciousness preserved)
Complex (consciousness impaired)
Secondarily generalized
Generalized seizures
Absence
Atypical absence
Myoclonic
Clonic
Tonic
Tonic-clonic
Atonic

than one type of seizure, are based on the type of seizure, age, neurologic examination, family history, and EEG findings. Causes may be diverse for the same syndrome. Syndromes such as infantile spasms, Lennox-Gastaut, and most myoclonic epilepsies carry an unfavorable prognosis. Children with other syndromes, such as rolandic epilepsy and benign occipital epilepsy, are usually associated with a good outcome. Children with generalized tonic-clonic seizures alone who are neurologically normal tend to do well, but if additional seizure types are present, the prognosis for intellectual outcome and remission of epilepsy depends on the type of additional seizures.

DIAGNOSIS AND EVALUATION OF A FIRST SEIZURE

Not all disorders characterized by episodic attacks are epilepsy. Three of the most common events confused with seizures are (1) convulsive syncope, (2) breath-holding spells, and (3) hysterical seizures. Others are listed in Table 2.

In *convulsive syncope,* brief generalized tonic-clonic motor activity is seen following syncope or a vasovagal episode. There is usually either a cardiac etiology or a precipitating event causing injury or fright. The child becomes pale, loses consciousness, and has some brief tonic-clonic or clonic movements. These movements result from transient cerebral anoxia. Consciousness is quickly regained.

Breath-holding spells, which occur most commonly between the ages of 8 months and 3 years, may be associated with some seizure-like movements in very young children. Extreme fright or anger usually precipitates the attack. Brief apnea results in cyanosis and sometimes a loss of consciousness with opisthotonus, a few convulsive jerks of the extremities, or tonic-clonic movements. Children are alert but may often be irritable following these episodes.

Hysterical seizures or *pseudoseizures* may be difficult to distinguish from true seizures. They are most frequently seen in teenaged girls and usually consist of generalized movements associated with an apparent loss of consciousness. There may be rhythmic jerking or a combination of unusual movements or posturing. Incontinence, bodily injury, and postictal drowsiness are not characteristic of these attacks. Hysterical seizures may also mimic psychomotor seizures. There is often an underlying emotional disturbance, and a careful psychosocial history should be obtained.

Simultaneous EEG and videotape monitoring may be necessary to differentiate these seizures from true epileptic seizures. The use of a post-seizure prolactin level has been suggested because levels of this hormone have been shown to be elevated 15 to 20 minutes following generalized tonic-clonic seizures but not following pseudoseizures; however, this has limited practical application. In some cases, children may have true epileptic seizures as well as pseudoseizures, and dosage increases leading to medication side effects may result.

TABLE 2. Disorders That Can Be Confused with Epileptic Seizures

Breath-holding spells
Pseudoseizures or hysterical seizures
Migraine
Cardiovascular events (pallid syncope, vasomotor syncope, cardiac arrhythmias)
Sleep disorders (night terrors, sleep walking)
Panic attacks
Hyperventilation
Rage attacks (episodic dyscontrol)
Gastroesophageal reflux
Benign paroxysmal vertigo
Daydreaming (attention deficit disorder)
Movement disorders (paroxysmal choreoathetosis, tics, dystonia)

In initial medical evaluation for possible seizures, it is imperative that a detailed clinical description of the event be obtained from an eyewitness source, including details regarding the sequence of motor and autonomic events, any initial localizing motor signs, the length of the seizure, and the presence of a postictal state. If the child is old enough, questions should be asked regarding the possible presence of an aura.

A detailed history and examination may reveal an etiology. Seizures accompanied by fever in the absence of CNS infection or acute metabolic cause and without a previous history of nonfebrile seizure are considered *febrile seizures,* a common and benign disorder to be discussed separately. Seizures that have an acute precipitating cause, such as toxins or trauma, are considered symptomatic. Nonsymptomatic seizures may or may not have an identifiable etiology, such as tuberous sclerosis, or risk factor, such as positive family history. Details of developmental history and school performance should be obtained. Findings such as spasticity or microcephaly suggest pre-existing neurologic disease. In most metabolic disorders, myoclonic seizures are prominent. Asphyxia during the birth process is a risk factor for later seizures only if the child was clinically affected immediately after birth, with abnormal neurologic signs and seizures in the neonatal period.

On physical examination, café-au-lait spots, shagreen patches, depigmented macules, or adenoma sebaceum may suggest tuberous sclerosis or neurofibromatosis. Head circumference abnormalities may suggest congenital infection (microcephaly), hydrocephalus, or subdural effusions (macrocephaly). The funduscopic examination may indicate congenital viral infection or recent trauma. An infectious illness may cause seizures by direct CNS involvement or by dehydration and fever, leading to electrolyte imbalance or, rarely, cerebral venous thrombosis.

A lumbar puncture should be performed if there are any possible indications of meningitis. Laboratory evaluation, including a complete blood count, electrolytes, calcium, toxic screen, blood glucose, and hepatic and renal function, may be advised in new-onset seizures. If the seizures occur in the setting of progressive neurologic deterioration, appropriate evaluation should be undertaken for metabolic or degenerative disorders, such as organic acidurias, lysosomal enzyme deficiencies, and peroxisomal disorders.

Cranial imaging should not be ordered routinely. If the history or examination suggests focal features, if the seizures are partial, if the EEG is focally abnormal, or if there are significant changes in school work or personality reported, computed tomography (CT) or magnetic resonance imaging (MRI) may be ordered. The MRI is generally more sensitive than CT in detecting cerebral lesions related to epilepsy, but a CT scan is adequate in most cases. Surgically treatable lesions, such as brain tumors or vascular malformations, cause less than 1 per cent of childhood epilepsy. Other new techniques include PET (positron-emission tomography), SPECT (single-photon emission CT), and xenon-enhanced CT. These modalities allow functional views of the brain but are not yet generally available.

Epilepsy is a diagnosis based on clinical findings; however, ictal or interictal epileptic discharges may offer supporting evidence and the EEG pattern may help to classify the seizure disorder. The EEG, therefore, should be ordered after all first afebrile seizures or if there is a marked change in pattern or frequency of seizures. A normal interictal EEG does not rule out a seizure disorder. Conversely, an abnormal EEG does not establish a diagnosis of epilepsy unless it is obtained during an actual seizure.

COMMON SEIZURE SYNDROMES

Infantile Spasms

Infantile spasms are a form of generalized epilepsy usually beginning between ages 4 and 12 months. Massive flexor spasms may occur with doubling over and crying, which may lead to a misdiagnosis of colic. Other seizures may be extensor or mixed. Seizures occur in clusters of a few to hundreds a day, frequently just after arousal. The EEG classically shows hypsarrhythmia, which is a pattern of high-voltage bursts accompanied by transient, generalized slowing. *West syndrome* is defined by infantile spasms, hypsarrhythmic EEG, and mental retardation.

The etiology is diverse and includes intrauterine or perinatal infections, inborn errors of metabolism, neurocutaneous disorders such as tuberous sclerosis, cerebral dysgenesis, and perinatal ischemic-hypoxic injury. *For up to one third, no etiology is known.* Although diphtheria, pertussis, and tetanus (DPT) immunizations are given at the time infantile spasms typically begin, studies have indicated that the association is temporal rather than causal.

The seizures gradually resolve if untreated, usually by age 2 years. About 80 per cent will have epilepsy later in life. The prognosis for normal development is poor; 75 per cent to 90 per cent are abnormal, often markedly so. For those whose seizures are cryptogenic, there is a better chance for normal outcome.

Some controversy exists concerning the preferred treatment. Most clinicians prefer intramuscular (IM) adrenocorticotropic hormone (ACTH) gel, although one well-controlled study indicated equal effectiveness with ACTH, given 20 to 30 units per day IM, and prednisone, given 2 mg/kg/day orally. The response to ACTH is all or none, and once improvement occurs, the drug should be tapered. Neither etiology and/or delay in treatment is a generally useful predictor of response. Treatment failure with ACTH does not imply that response will not occur to prednisone.

One recommended regimen is 150 units/m^2/day of ACTH (80 units/ml) in two divided doses for 1 week, half the dose the following week, followed by gradual taper over the next 2 months. If a low dose is preferred, ACTH should be given IM 20 units/day for 2 weeks, then tapered over 2 weeks. If there is no response, the dose can be increased to 30 units/day for 4 weeks. Spasms should decrease, and the EEG will probably, but not always, also improve. It is not known whether higher doses for a longer time confer any additional benefit. Children treated with ACTH should be hospitalized initially because of the risk of side effects and to teach parents to properly administer medication. Serious problems with hypertension, electrolyte imbalance, hyperglycemia, glycosuria, gastrointestinal bleeding, congestive heart failure, and infections may occur in up to one third of children. If hypertension occurs, salt restriction and diuretics should be attempted before administration of ACTH is stopped.

If recurrences of spasms occur after a course of ACTH, children should be given prednisone (2 mg/kg/day divided in two doses for 4 weeks), followed by tapering regardless of response. In a few children refractory to steroid therapy, nitrazepam and valproate have been used for infantile spasms, with a few successes.

Lennox-Gastaut Syndrome

Children with the Lennox-Gastaut syndrome have severe and intractable seizures beginning between 1 and 8 years; the most common age of onset is 3 to 5 years. There is no presumptive cause in one third, and about 50 per cent of patients have accompanying abnormal neurologic findings or history. The syndrome includes mental retardation and a characteristic EEG pattern of generalized slowing and spike waves. Twenty per cent have a history of infantile spasms. The most common seizure types are tonic, atonic, and atypical absences. Generalized tonic-clonic seizures occur in more than 50 per cent; these are frequently nocturnal and tend to disappear. As children grow older, the developmental lag becomes more evident. More than 80 per cent will have seizures into adulthood.

The treatment of this disorder is frustrating because seizures tend to recur and are very resistant to treatment. Ideally, only one drug should be used, and valproate has the most chance of being successful as monotherapy. But because of frequency of seizures and mixture of seizure types, there is a tendency to prescribe more than one drug. Carbamazepine, phenytoin, or phenobarbital may be used for generalized seizures, but the combination of carbamazepine and valproate may cause an increase in seizures. Benzodiazepines may be effective early in the course but may precipitate tonic status epilepticus. Other possible treatments include ACTH, steroids, and a ketogenic diet.

The ketogenic diet is a high-fat, carbohydrate-restricted diet that is difficult to initiate and maintain but may be highly effective, at least temporarily. Up to 50 per cent may obtain complete seizure control, and half the remainder show some improvement. After a period of fasting in the hospital, a diet that contains three to four parts fat to one part non-fat is initiated. Carbohydrate restriction must be severe, and 1 g of protein/kg/day should be eaten. Supplemental vitamins and minerals are needed. An easier alternative involves medium-chain triglyceride (MCT) oil given with each meal, which allows for less restriction of carbohydrates and protein. Therapeutic anticonvulsant levels should be established before the diet is cautiously discontinued. The diet should not be maintained beyond 1 year because of concerns about decreased growth.

Myoclonic Epilepsies

The myoclonic epilepsies constitute a heterogeneous group of clinical syndromes, overlapping with the Lennox-Gastaut syndrome. The etiology may be multifactorial and may include brain damage and genetic factors. Repetitive myoclonic seizures consisting of brief muscle contractions or loss of tone often result in falls. These seizures are associated with varying degrees of mental retardation. True myoclonic seizures are accompanied by ictal or interictal fast spike wave complexes on EEG. Outcome is least favorable when a mixture of seizure types occurs. Treatment is often unsuccessful, but valproate and benzodiazepines may be useful.

Juvenile Myoclonic Epilepsy of Janz

This syndrome is to be distinguished from the myoclonic epilepsies of early childhood. Brief, bilaterally symmetric myoclonic jerks usually occur after awakening, often followed by generalized tonic-clonic seizures. The family history is frequently positive; the gene has been localized to the short arm of chromosome six. Onset is from 8 to 18 years. The EEG shows bilaterally symmetric, frontocentral polyspike and waves, and photosensitivity is seen in 30 per cent. Seizures may be precipitated by sleep deprivation or disruption and by alcohol; this is important to stress to adolescent patients. Valproate is the drug of choice, but relapse may occur when it is discontinued even if there have been no seizures for many years. Prognosis is generally favorable.

Other seizure syndromes of adolescence include awakening grand mal epilepsy and late-onset absence. All three primary generalized epilepsies of adolescence tend to run in families.

Generalized Tonic-Clonic Seizures

Generalized tonic-clonic seizures are the most common type of childhood seizures and may often occur in combination with other seizure types. Seizures are more likely to occur just before or after one falls asleep or awakens. Most often there is no known cause, although precipitating factors may include excessive fatigue, infectious illness, and withdrawal from anticonvulsant medication. The EEG demonstrates generalized, repetitive spikes during the tonic phase with periodic bursts in the clonic phase. Effective antiepileptic drugs (AEDs) include carbamazepine, phenobarbital, and phenytoin.

Complex Partial Seizures

Less common in children than in adults, complex partial seizures usually begin in adolescence. Most are brief, lasting 1 to 2 minutes, and they are sometimes preceded by an aura. Staring is associated with automatic behaviors and facial grimacing, followed by postictal confusion and lethargy. The more gradual onset and ending help to distinguish this type of seizure from absences.

Etiology is usually not known. *Magnetic resonance imaging has led to diagnosis of focal microdysgenesis or low-grade gliomas in some children with hard-to-control complex partial seizures.* Carbamazepine is the treatment of choice, but phenytoin, primidone, and phenobarbital may also be effective for seizure control.

Absence Seizures

Classic absence seizures usually begin between ages 4 and 10, are unique to children, and consist of unprovoked, brief staring of sudden onset. Many seizures may occur every day. Spells can be provoked by a few minutes of hyperventilation. The EEG demonstrates 3- to 4-second spike and slow-wave activity accompanying the staring spell. Background is normal, and there is no postictal slowing. Eye blinking or mouth twitching may accompany the staring spell.

In atypical absence seizures, there may be more pronounced changes in tone and the EEG may have more irregular spike and slow-wave complexes. Treatment is necessary to prevent school problems and possible accidents. Ethosuximide and valproate are both effective, but ethosuximide is usually the first drug chosen. There is usually no specific etiology. Fifty per cent of children become seizure-free after 2 to 4 years, but tonic-clonic seizures or other seizure types may develop in the remainder. Those with normal intelligence and no other seizure types do well; in others, however, epilepsy may continue to be a long-term problem.

Benign Partial Epilepsy

Benign focal or partial epilepsy of childhood (or benign rolandic epilepsy) usually begins between 5 and 10 years of age. It is a common epileptic syndrome of childhood, *occurring with an annual incidence of 21 per 100,000, and is carried as an autosomal dominant trait with age-dependent penetrance.*

Seizures consist of motor, sensory, and autonomic manifestations with twitching of one side of the face and paresthesias of the face, gum, and tongue that may be followed by hemiclonic movements and do not involve loss of consciousness. Of these seizures, 75 per cent occur at night and most spontaneously remit during adolescence. The EEG shows focal spikes and sharp waves in the central and midtemporal regions.

Some children need not be treated at all, particularly those whose seizures are infrequent and only at night; the minority, with early-onset and repeated attacks, are usually treated with carbamazepine, and seizures are usually controlled with low doses. Generalized tonic-clonic seizures may later develop in a small minority. Children with benign focal epilepsy perform similarly to age-matched controls in school adjustment and on intelligence tests.

Benign Occipital Seizures

The syndrome of benign occipital seizures is less common than benign partial epilepsy. Seizures usually first occur in children ages 2 through 8. The initial symptoms overlap with those of migraine and consist of nausea, headache, and visual disturbances, followed by hemisensory, hemimotor, or generalized motor symptoms. The EEG shows bilateral occipital spike-wave runs that are enhanced by hyperventilation. The seizures generally resolve in adolescence. A family history of epilepsy is present in about 50 per cent of children, and seizures responded to a variety of anticonvulsant agents in one reported series.

Impact Seizures

Impact seizures occur in children *immediately* after a serious fall or blow to the head, especially to the occiput. There are tonic-clonic or tonic motor movements lasting usually only a minute or less that occur as a direct response to the blow. These seizures are not associated with a higher incidence of post-traumatic epilepsy and do not mandate hospitalization or anticonvulsant treatment. Other clinical circumstances, such as loss of consciousness or skull fracture, may dictate specific management.

NEONATAL SEIZURES

The single most common cause of neonatal seizures is thought to be hypoxic-ischemic injury; other etiologic factors include inborn errors of metabolism, sepsis, meningitis, hypoglycemia, hypocalcemia, drug abstinence syndromes, structural brain abnormalities, hemorrhage, and intrauterine infection. The incidence is cited as between 5 to 20 per 1000 live births. More than one third survive with major neurologic disabilities, and the mortality rate is 15 per cent. There is a benign familial form of neonatal convulsions with an autosomal dominant inheritance. These seizures stop by the age of 6 months, and development is normal.

Some clinically recognized neonatal seizures, such as clonic jerking movements, are associated with simultaneous EEG discharges. Other movements commonly called seizures, such as tonic episodes or "subtle" seizures, may arise from nonepileptic brain dysfunction at subcortical or brain stem levels. Video–EEG monitoring is often necessary to distinguish these from epileptic events.

Initial management should be directed at finding potentially treatable etiologic factors such as hypoglycemia or meningitis. Anticonvulsant treatment is usually initiated with a loading dose of phenobarbital (20 mg/kg intravenously [IV]). Plasma levels of phenobarbital as high as 40 μg/ml may be necessary. Phenobarbital may be used in combination with shorter acting intravenous lorazepam as a single bolus at a dose of 0.05 to 0.1 mg/kg. Phenytoin (Dilantin, 20 mg/kg IV given as a loading dose at a rate not to exceed 1 mg/kg/minute), is preferred by some neonatologists. AED absorption, protein binding, clearance, and half-life in neonates may vary widely. Drug levels should be obtained before maintenance doses are initiated.

Because numerous animal and in vitro studies have suggested that anticonvulsants are potentially harmful to the developing brain, it is important to discontinue them as soon as possible. If seizures stop, medication can be discontinued after 1 week of seizure control or at nursery discharge. Normal examination and EEG are favorable prognostic signs. Except in unusual very-high-risk cases (such as cerebral malformations) or when frequent seizures continue, anticonvulsants should be discontinued within a few months.

Pyridoxine dependency is an autosomal recessive disorder in which seizures, usually clonic, begin in the neonatal period. These seizures are diagnosed by giving 100 mg IV pyridoxine during EEG monitoring. The seizures should stop within minutes, EEG abnormalities within hours.

STATUS EPILEPTICUS

Status epilepticus is defined as a continuous convulsion or a series of convulsions without complete recovery between attacks and lasting 30 minutes or more. The seizure is usually major motor but may be any type. Causes include meningitis, encephalitis, cerebral anoxia, and sudden withdrawal of anticonvulsants. The goal of treatment of status epilepticus should be to terminate electrical seizure activity after first ensuring adequate brain oxygenation and cardiorespiratory function. A precipitating cause should be aggressively sought; factors such as metabolic imbalances, hypoglycemia, infection, and fever should be identified and treated.

Once an airway is established, a secure intravenous line should be placed, and appropriate diagnostic studies drawn, for example, complete blood count (CBC), electrolytes, cultures, glucose, toxicology, anticonvulsant blood levels, calcium, magnesium and blood urea nitrogen (BUN). If hypoglycemia is a possibility, 25 per cent glucose should be given by bolus (2 to 4 ml/kg). Blood gas levels should be obtained and adequate ventilation ensured. A lumbar puncture should be considered if there is any possibility of meningitis, but first the risk of increased intracranial pressure must be assessed and a CT scan performed if indicated. The EEG should be continuously monitored, ideally by means of a bedside video monitor.

Initial therapy consists of diazepam (0.2 to 0.4 mg/kg IV at a rate of 1 mg/minute to a maximum of 10 mg) (Table 3). Seizures may recur in 15 to 20 minutes, and the dose can be repeated. If an intravenous line is delayed, liquid diazepam may be given rectally as a 0.5 mg/kg bolus and will reach adequate serum levels in 4 to 10 minutes. Alternatively, lorazepam has more rapid onset and longer duration than diazepam. A bolus of 0.1 mg/kg up to a total of 5 mg can be given. Both these drugs can cause hypoventilation, ataxia, and lethargy, and respiratory depression is a risk, particularly when both drugs are used with barbiturates.

If seizures resume after diazepam is given, a longer-acting drug, such as phenobarbital (20 mg/kg as a bolus) should be given. Potentially troublesome side effects are hypotension and respiratory depression. Maintenance therapy can begin 12 to 24 hours later. A combination of diazepam and phenytoin may also be used. Phenytoin can be used for partial and generalized seizures but not for absence status. In young children, 15 to 20 mg/kg IV as a slow bolus is given at a rate not to exceed 1 mg/kg/minute and the electrocardiograph (EKG) should be monitored for arrhythmias. The advantage over phenobarbital is less depressant effect, and it is useful in trauma when mental status examination may be important. Side effects include hypotension and cardiac conduction defects. Maintenance phenytoin (6 mg/kg/day) can be started at 6 hours later. Drug levels should be followed closely and maintenance phenobarbital or phenytoin adjusted accordingly.

If status epilepticus cannot be controlled, as a last resort an anesthesiologist may induce coma with a pentobarbital drip as a loading dose (20 mg/kg), followed by a continuous drip (1 to 2 mg/kg/hour). This infusion should be stopped in 24 hours to see whether seizures have abated. After several days, mild pulmonary edema can result. Respiratory and cardiac depression are potential side effects.

The outcome of status epilepticus is related to the underlying cause. Although death can result, the prognosis has been improving recently. The mortality rate is lower for children than for adults; recent figures have put the mortality for children at 3 to 6 per cent.

TABLE 3. Treatment of Status Epilepticus

Drug	Dose	May Be Repeated?
First Resort		
Diazepam	0.2–0.4 mg/kg IV at 1 mg/minute, maximum dose 10 mg	Yes, after 15 minutes
Lorazepam	0.5–0.1 mg/kg IV over 1–2 minutes, maximum dose 5 mg	Yes, but loses effectiveness
Phenobarbital	20 mg/kg IV given at 100 mg/minute, maximum dose 300 mg	Yes
Phenytoin	20 mg/kg IV at 50 mg/minute, maximum dose 1000 mg	No
Last Resort		
Pentobarbital	20 mg/kg loading dose, then continuous IV drip of 1–2 mg/kg/hour	

INITIAL ANTICONVULSANT TREATMENT

Certain seizure disorders are brought to medical attention only when multiple attacks have already occurred, as in absence or myoclonic epilepsy. For children who present with a single generalized motor or partial afebrile seizure, the risk of recurrence is fairly low and treatment may be deferred until after a second seizure. Some seizures may not necessitate treatment even if several events have occurred; e.g., benign forms of epilepsy, such as rolandic epilepsy, seizures that occur only at night, and certain seizures that occur in response to stimuli that can be avoided. In addition, the risks of anticonvulsants may outweigh the benefits in the child with infrequent nocturnal, generalized, tonic-clonic seizures whose EEG and neurologic examination are normal. In any case, the physician must make especially sure that the family knows what to do in the event of a recurrence and how to avoid potentially risky situations without overprotecting the child.

A lower likelihood of recurrence is associated with normal EEG and neurologic findings and a generalized seizure type. If the examination and EEG results are abnormal, seizures are likely to recur and more so if seizures are partial. The majority of recurrences occur within 6 to 12 months of the first seizure. Once a second seizure occurs, additional recurrences are likely. Seizures that are precipitated by acute events, such as toxins or metabolic derangements (symptomatic seizures), are associated with less likelihood of recurrence.

Seizures that are initially difficult to control may be associated with a poorer prognosis. However, there is no convincing evidence that relatively brief seizures cause brain damage and we do not know that treatment can prevent future epilepsy; we know only that it can prevent some seizure recurrences at the time of adequate circulating anticonvulsant levels.

The decision to initiate AEDs should be based on consideration of the risks and benefits of medication. Factors to be weighed in the decision include the child's age, timing of seizures, predisposing factors, possible precipitants, and possible physical and emotional consequences of further seizures. Even when AEDs are prescribed, there may still be recurrences. In one prospective study of newly treated children with epilepsy, more than 40 per cent experienced a recurrence within 6 months despite "therapeutic" drug levels and an additional 16 per cent had unacceptable side effects.

The choice of drug is guided by seizure type (Table 4) and potential side effects (Table 5). For absence seizures, ethosuximide is preferred as a first-time drug. Valproate is equally effective; however, it has the disadvantage of producing very rare severe side effects. Valproate is also effective against tonic-clonic seizures. For generalized convulsive seizures, carbamazepine, phenytoin, and phenobarbital are equally effective but carbamazepine is usually preferred as the initial drug because of fewer troublesome side effects.

Therapy should always be initiated with one drug. Multiple drugs increase cost and the risk of toxicity. Because of drug interactions, higher doses may be needed. Although the clearance of drugs is more rapid in children than in adults and dosing intervals therefore are shorter, compliance is better if the drug can be taken no more often than twice daily. Medication should be introduced at low doses that can be increased over intervals of 2 to 7 days until seizures are controlled or until there are significant side effects. A drug should not be considered ineffective unless seizures are still occurring when toxic symptoms develop. Observation for a few weeks may be necessary before one tries a second drug, which should replace but not be added to the first. Exceptions include drug-resistant syndromes, such as Lennox-Gastaut, or situations in which a combination of valproate and ethosuximide is effective for absences but neither drug alone suffices.

Although 3 or 4 years of remission has previously been the standard, recent evidence indicates that prognosis after two seizure-free years in most cases is similar to longer periods of remission. Anticonvulsants should be withdrawn gradually over several months. It is important to avoid sudden withdrawal from anticonvulsant medication because this may cause a prolonged seizure. The risk of relapse is greatest if seizures occurred for several years before they were controlled and if there are other neurologic abnormalities present. If children have remained seizure-free for 2 to 4 years, AEDs can be discontinued without recurrence in 75 per cent of cases. If the EEG shows spikes or focal discharges and if it is worse or unimproved compared with the initial EEG, the prognosis for remission is less favorable. Certain seizure types are likely to be associated with a higher remission rate, such as absence or benign rolandic epilepsy. The discontinuation of anticonvulsants during puberty versus other times has no bearing on the relapse rate.

Plasma Levels

Plasma levels should be determined when seizures are not well controlled, when there are toxic side effects, or when compliance is questioned. In some patients, levels may be controlled above or below the established therapeutic range and the clinical picture is more important than the plasma levels. Levels are routinely indicated in children taking more than one drug. The levels measured are of both bound and free drug, but only the free drug enters the cerebrospinal fluid (CSF). *Drugs that are highly protein-bound, such as phenytoin, carbamazepine, and valproate, may become toxic if a competitive protein-binding substance is given, for example, acetylsalicylic acid (ASA) for fever.* Because acetaminophen has little or no protein binding, it is a better antipyretic for children taking AEDs.

TABLE 4. Choice of Drug and Seizure Type

Drug	Seizure Type	Dose (mg/kg per 24 Hours)	Preparation	Frequency per 24 Hours	Plasma Level (μg/ml)	Half-Life (Hours)
Carbamazepine (Tegretol)	Partial Secondarily generalized	10–25	200 mg tablets 100 mg chewable tablets 100 mg/5 ml suspension	2 or 3	4–12	6–12
Ethosuximide (Zarontin)	Absence	15–40	250 mg capsules 250 mg/ml liquid	2 to 3	40–100	24–36
Phenobarbital	Primary generalized Secondary generalized Partial Status	4–8	Tablets 15 mg, 30 mg, 60 mg; 20 mg/5 ml suspension	1 or 2	15–40	48–100
Phenytoin (Dilantin)	Primary generalized Secondary generalized Partial Status	4–8	100 mg capsules 50 mg chewable tablets 100 mg/5 ml suspension	1 or 2	10–20	6–30
Primidone (Mysoline)	Primary generalized Secondary generalized	10–25	50 mg tablets 250 mg tablets 250 mg/5 ml suspension	3–4	5–12	10–36
Valproate (Depakene)	Primary generalized Absence Myoclonic Partial Atypical absence	20–60	250 mg capsules 125, 250, 500 mg tablets 125 mg sprinkle capsules 250 mg/5 ml liquid	2–3	40–150	6–12
Clonazepam (Klonopin)	Absence Primary generalized Partial Myoclonic	0.05–0.3	0.5, 1 and 2 mg tablets	2–3		24–36

TABLE 5. Side Effects of Commonly Used Anticonvulsants

Drug	Predictable	Idiosyncratic
Carbamazepine	Diplopia Dizziness Drowsiness Nausea Headache Hyponatremia	Agranulocytosis Lupus-like rash Aplastic anemia Pseudolymphoma Hepatotoxicity Photosensitivity Stevens-Johnson syndrome
Ethosuximide	Anorexia Nausea Vomiting Agitation Drowsiness Lethargy	Rash–erythema multiforme Lupus-like syndrome Stevens-Johnson syndrome Agranulocytosis Aplastic anemia Dystonia
Phenobarbital	Sedation Depression Distractibility Poor memory Hypocalcemia Osteomalacia Irritability	Rash Toxic epidermal necrolysis Hepatic toxicity
Phenytoin	Ataxia Gum hypertrophy Nausea Coarse facies Vomiting Hirsuitism Anorexia Megaloblastic anemia Drowsiness Hypocalcemia Nystagmus Osteomalacia Mental slowing	Blood dyscrasias Lupus-like syndrome Rash Peripheral neuropathy Hepatotoxicity Stevens-Johnson syndrome
Primidone	Nausea Vomiting Weakness Dizziness Diplopia Nystagmus Psychosis Hypocalcemia Osteomalacia Anemia	Rash Agranulocytosis Thrombocytopenia Lupus-like syndrome
Valproate	Anorexia Tremor Sedation Nausea Vomiting Hair loss Drowsiness Weight gain	Acute pancreatitis Hyperammonemia Acute liver toxicity Encephalopathy Rash Thrombocytopenia Neutropenia
Clonazepam	Drowsiness Ataxia Behavior disturbance Increased salivation	Rash Leukopenia Thrombocytopenia

Because children may have a relatively high metabolic rate, the dose necessary in children per body weight may be several times higher than for adults. If levels are low, poor compliance may be suspected; however, the capacity to metabolize drug faster due to enzyme induction may occur after a steady state has been reached. Especially with phenytoin, a nonlinear relation may exist and unexpected levels may occur after a change in dose. Most side effects are dose-related, but a few are idiosyncratic, such as a stuporous state secondary to valproate (Table 5).

Laboratory Monitoring

Asymptomatic and stable patients do not necessarily benefit from routine screening of blood and urine. Transient phenomena, such as leukopenia or mildly elevated liver enzymes, can be identified, but very few, if any, severe adverse reactions can be avoided. Baseline laboratory screening before initiation of AEDs should be performed, however, so that pre-existing abnormalities are known and can be compared to later results. These should include liver and renal function tests, and a CBC and platelet count. Parents and families should be informed about possible severe reactions and their early symptoms, including rash, vomiting, anorexia, lethargy, bruising, and symptoms of anemia, and they must understand that prompt reporting of these or any other unusual symptoms is essential.

Specific Anticonvulsants

Phenobarbital

Phenobarbital has been in clinical use since 1912. It is a relatively inexpensive and medically safe drug used chronically primarily for generalized motor and simple partial seizures as well as for neonatal seizures and status epilepticus. It has the disadvantage, particularly for pediatric patients, of possibly producing adverse cognitive and behavioral side effects. In one randomized, controlled study of children treated for febrile seizures, children assigned to phenobarbital scored lower on intelligence tests; in another study, epileptic children had decreased scores on tests of neuropsychologic function associated with phenobarbital. Depression secondary to phenobarbital can be a problem in certain predisposed children and adolescents, particularly in those with a personal or family history of affective disorder.

The oral maintenance dose in children is 2 to 5 mg/kg/day; infants should receive doses in the higher range. Phenobarbital has a long half-life and can be given once a day. A steady-state level is reached in 2 to 3 weeks. Sedation is common at first, but tolerance develops. Allergic reactions and Stevens-Johnson syndrome may occur.

Primidone

Primidone has the same spectrum of action as phenobarbital and is partially metabolized to phenobarbital by the liver. Idiosyncratic effects include sedation and acute psychotic reactions. Side effects are more common than with phenobarbital and include sedation, nausea, vomiting, diplopia, dizziness, and ataxia. A low dose (10 mg/kg/day) should be started initially, which can be gradually increased to a maximum of 25 mg/kg/day.

Phenytoin

Phenytoin is useful in generalized tonic-clonic seizures and partial seizures, both simple and complex. A pediatric oral suspension is available but not recommended because the concentration varies unless the bottle is very well shaken. The half-life is 5 to 18 hours in younger children, longer in adults. Steady-state levels are reached in 7 to 10 days.

The usual pediatric dose is 4 to 5 mg/kg/day. Because as the concentration of phenytoin in the blood increases, the enzymes metabolizing the drug may become saturated, a small increase in dose may cause a large increase in serum level. It can be given parenterally and may be given in a loading dose via the oral or intravenous route. Phenytoin is relatively safe and inexpensive. In adults, it has been associated with some decreases in cognitive performance, especially through impairment of speed at certain tasks. It may cause a mild elevation of liver enzymes, which does not require that the drug be discontinued if there is no other evidence of liver disease. Symptoms of toxicity include mental slowing, unsteadiness, nystagmus, and ataxia. Therapeutic blood levels are approximately 10 to 20 μg/ml but can be higher or lower. Degree of seizure control and symptoms of toxicity, rather than blood level, should govern dosage adjustments.

There is a relatively high incidence of annoying side effects with chronic administration of phenytoin, including acne, coarsening facial features, and gingival hyperplasia, making it a particularly unpopular drug for adolescents. If a rash appears, the drug should be discontinued to avoid the serious reaction of Stevens-Johnson syndrome. Other very rare but serious reactions include thrombocytopenia, leukopenia, and lymphadenopathy.

Carbamazepine

Carbamazepine is effective in partial seizures, both simple and complex, and in generalized tonic-clonic seizures. Efficacy is similar to phenobarbital and phenytoin. It is available as 100- and 200-mg tablets and in a suspension of 100 mg/5 ml that results in less consistent blood levels. The dose is 20 to 40 mg/kg/day, and because of a relatively short half-life it should be administered at least twice and preferably three times a day. Peak serum levels are reached in 4 to 5 hours. The target serum level is 8 to 12 mg/ml. There is no parenteral dose available. If the drug is introduced at a lower dose (10 mg/kg/day) and gradually increased, the risk of side effects is lower. Interactions are complex; clearance of ethosuximde, valproate, and benzodiazepines may be changed. Initially, it may inhibit metabolism of phenytoin. Erythromycin inhibits the metabolism of carbamazepine and may cause toxic levels. Sometimes substitution with a generic preparation may cause undue fluctuation in plasma levels.

Common and troublesome side effects include diplopia and blurred vision. Periodic monitoring has been recommended in the first several months, primarily to screen for bone marrow suppression, but the need for routine monitoring is now coming under question. Aplastic anemia (less than 1:100,000) and serious liver toxicity have been reported but are extremely rare and cannot be prevented by routine monitoring. Baseline CBCs and blood chemistries should always be obtained. At high concentrations, antidiuretic hormone (ADH) secretion may produce fluid retention and mild hyponatremia.

Adverse effects on cognitive function are minimal with carbamazepine, and there is less sedation or effect on intellectual function than with phenytoin or phenobarbital. There may be an antidepressant effect; the compound is chemically related to the tricyclics. Improvement seen in some studies with carbamazepine actually may have been caused by withdrawal of other sedating drugs and/or better seizure control. In one report, seven of 200 children were agitated right after beginning the drug; four of these seven children were mentally retarded.

Ethosuximide

Ethosuximide for absence seizures may be started at 500 mg/day, to which 250 mg/day should be added in weekly intervals to reach a dose of up to 1 g/day. Ethosuximide is equally effective as valproate for absence seizures, but it is less likely to produce serious side effects and is less expensive. It is well absorbed, with a peak level at 1 to 4 hours and a half-life of 24 to 36 hours in children. Although the half-life is long, it should be given two to three times a day because a single large dose may cause gastrointestinal distress.

Interference with other drugs is minimal, since ethosuximide does not induce or inhibit drug metabolism. Therapeutic blood levels are 40 to 80 μg/ml. Dose-related side effects include nausea, fatigue, headache, and dizziness. Rare idiosyncratic reactions occur, including rashes, leukopenia, and pancytopenia.

Valproate

For children who have both absence and generalized tonic-clonic seizures, valproate is the drug of choice. It is also effective for myoclonic seizures and partial seizures with secondary generalization and in most mixed seizure disorders. The recommended dose is 20 to 30 mg/kg/day in two to three divided doses, which can be increased up to a maximum of 60 mg/kg with plasma levels up to 100 to 150 μg/ml if used as monotherapy and if the dosage is gradually increased. Efficacy does not necessarily relate to serum levels, however. Peak levels occur in several hours. It is available as a sprinkle capsule (125 mg), which is useful for young children; an enteric-coated tablet (125, 250, and 500 mg); and a liquid (250 mg/5 ml). Because it is a minor inhibitor of oxidative metabolism, it may increase serum concentration of other drugs. Valproate given with benzodiazepines may increase seizure frequency.

Although behavior problems, including sedation, hyperactivity, and aggression, have been reported, they are infrequent and there is little impact on cognitive function. Mild and usually transient side effects include sedation, nausea, vomiting, and anorexia. A mild liver enzyme elevation is usually dose-dependent and returns to normal if dosage is lowered.

Very rarely, acute liver failure and death result from an idiosyncratic reaction to valproate. The risk is 1 per 45,000 for children older than age 2 on monotherapy, and is higher for children younger than age 2, with no reported cases in children over age 10. The risk is increased to 1:500 in mentally retarded children younger than 2 years old receiving polytherapy. Serious hepatotoxicity may in some children be reversible. Symptoms are malaise, weakness, anorexia, vomiting, loss of seizure control, vertigo, ataxia, and nystagmus. Serum transaminase (SGOT and SGPT) levels should be determined prior to treatment. Routine screening has not proved effective in preventing serious reactions, although it has been recommended that patients be tested monthly for 4 months and at regular intervals every 4 to 6 months thereafter. If liver enzymes are twice the normal levels or there are signs of liver dysfunction, the drug should be stopped. Recently, reports of fatal hepatotoxicity have decreased, probably as a result of an increase in monotherapy. A few patients with fatal reactions to valproate were subsequently found to have underlying metabolic abnormalities, such as urea cycle defects, including ornithine carbamyl transferase deficiency.

Lethargy and coma may occur secondary to hyperammonemia, which occurs independently of hepatotoxicity. This may be mediated through a relative carnitine deficiency that causes organic acids to accumulate, inhibiting the urea cycle enzymes. An ammonia level should be determined, and a decrease in dose may lead to improvement. Pancreatitis has been reported, and serum amylase should be checked if there is severe abdominal pain. Other serious allergic or idiosyncratic reactions include agranulocytosis (usually associated with hepatitis), thrombocytopenia, and aplastic anemia.

Benzodiazepines

Lorazepam and nitrazepam have been used for neonatal seizures and in status epilepticus. Clonazepam is relatively broad spectrum but produces significant behavioral disturbances, and it is rarely used initially. Serum levels of clonazepam are not useful and do not relate directly to seizure control.

Rectal diazepam administered at home by parents has been used successfully to terminate seizures in some children. It may be especially useful if the family is far from medical care or if prolonged seizures are a potential problem. A dose of 0.5 mg/kg up to a maximum of 15 mg per episode is used in a liquid preparation administered into the rectum either directly from a syringe or via tubing. It may be useful to give a test dose under medical supervision to ascertain whether side effects occur and to teach parents how to administer the drug.

SURGERY

Certain neurosurgical procedures, such as partial hemispherectomy, temporal lobectomy, or corpus callosotomy, offer reduction of seizure frequency, which is of significant clinical benefit to selected children with intractable seizures. Referrals may be considered for children with uncontrolled seizures despite adequate drug trials and whose seizures are of a frequency and intensity to significantly interfere with daily living. There are a number of referral centers whose growing experience now reflects a successful outcome from epilepsy surgery in children.

PSYCHOSOCIAL ASPECTS

Children with epilepsy are at higher risk for learning disabilities and behavior problems. An important task of the treating physician is to make sure that assessment of academic achievement and proper school placement are carefully monitored. A recent study showed that underachievement in school was not related to the duration or severity of the seizure disorder or exposure to AEDs but that family environment was an important factor. There is no indication that the seizures actually cause intellectual deterioration. Rather, the underlying brain disorder probably accounts for both.

In addition, children who have epilepsy may have low self-esteem and low expectations for the future. With low self-esteem come higher levels of anxiety. Through counseling and education, some feeling of control can be achieved.

Patients and their parents need to understand this condition. Parents should be encouraged to tell the doctor whether the child is experiencing more seizures or possible side effects from medication. Other family members and teachers should be educated. Teachers should be prepared to deal with a seizure and to assist the other children in the classroom to handle the situation as well. The entire family needs to be guided to avoid excessive anxiety and overprotection and to use rational judgment. In children with epilepsy, excessive fatigue or infectious illness may increase seizure frequency, but generalized stresses, such as strenuous physical activity or emotional upset, rarely cause seizures. Avoiding situations leading to such stress would be destructive emotionally and probably impossible at any rate. Restrictions on normal activity are necessary only during times when seizures are not well controlled. For example, children with epilepsy can swim if well supervised and, ideally, if they are using a "buddy" system. Bathing should be carefully supervised in young children and showers encouraged in the older child. Sports need not ordinarily be restricted. Problems specific to adolescents, such as drugs, driving, alcohol, and the effects of sleep deprivation, should be addressed. Guidelines for emergency care and an explanation of what is happening during a seizure, which can be extremely frightening, should be offered.

The Epilepsy Foundation of America (Phone: 800–EFA–1000) and its local affiliates provide a variety of helpful information to families, such as a school alert program and video series for families.

FEBRILE SEIZURES

KARIN B. NELSON, M.D.

At the onset of acute febrile illness that does not affect the brain directly, young children may experience seizures. Two to 5 per cent of youngsters experience at least one such seizure, commonly between the ages of 6 months and 4 years. The peak age of onset is 18 to 20 months. Seizures accompanying intracranial infection or toxic or metabolic illness, such as lead poisoning or marked hypernatremic dehydration, are excluded by definition. Febrile seizures are to be distinguished from epilepsy, which is characterized by recurrent unprovoked seizures.

Most febrile seizures are brief generalized convulsions occurring in otherwise healthy young children, and the outlook is generally favorable.

TREATMENT

The Acute Attack

A child who is still convulsing when he or she reaches medical attention should be treated as for any other seizure in progress (see text on status epilepticus, p. 84). The chief concerns are maintenance of the airway, prevention of injury, and termination of the seizure as rapidly as is consistent with safety, given the facilities and personnel available. Uncovering, tepid sponging, maintenance of hydration, and antipyretics such as acetaminophen may help to control fever. Diagnostic evaluation is required in order to identify the source of fever, the most urgent consideration being assessment as to whether meningitis is present. Even in a child with a personal or family history of febrile seizures in the past, any new episode of fever and seizure raises the possibility that the current illness is meningitis.

Meningeal or neurologic signs or depression of consciousness or a full fontanelle indicate a need for immediate assessment for meningitis. In the child older than about 18 months, the absence of findings suggestive of meningitis and the return of the child to alert responsiveness on awakening after the seizure will identify youngsters who do not need immediate lumbar puncture. If there is doubt of the child's status or the parents' ability to observe and return quickly for medical care if new signs appear, lumbar puncture may be wise. In a toxic young infant under 6 months of age, blood cultures and further observation are necessary. Laboratory investigation should be directed at recognizing specific disorders causing seizures, including hypoglycemia and toxic encephalopathies (i.e., attempting to make an etiologic diagnosis other than febrile seizures), and also at finding a cause for the fever; both of these searches should be based upon clinical indications derived from the history and physical examination.

In children with a postictal paresis or other fresh neurologic signs following a seizure, a neuroimaging procedure may be performed to look for a structural lesion; in the absence of such new signs, neuroimaging is probably unnecessary. Plain skull films are seldom helpful.

A week or so after the fever has abated, an electroencephalogram (EEG) may be requested for children who had lengthy focal seizures to rule out underlying structural abnormality. Paroxysmal features of the EEG occur with considerable frequency in the years after febrile seizures or in siblings, perhaps permitting recognition of genetic subsyndromes; however, the EEG is probably not helpful in predicting later epilepsy or recurrent febrile seizures.

A history of recurrent infections and the presence of alopecia and ataxia suggest *biotinidase deficiency,* a disorder that can be progressive and lethal if not recognized and treated in time. Febrile seizures beginning in the middle of the first year of life with prolonged or focal and recurring seizures, with seizures associated with lower degrees of fever or none, and development of myoclonic jerks and developmental slowing suggest the possibility of the syndrome of *severe myoclonic epilepsy of infancy.* Children whose course is compatible with either of these syndromes warrant careful evaluation or consultation.

Hospitalization is appropriate for the very toxic young infant with a seizure and fever or for the family living far from medical facilities or unable to cope for other reasons. In general, it is preferable to observe the child until it can be ascertained that he or she is alert, responsive, and free of fresh neurologic signs and then to release the child to the family. That second physical examination, performed after the child awakens from the seizure, is perhaps the most important diagnostic tool in febrile seizures. The interval for observation can also provide the first opportunity to explain febrile seizures to the family, who are likely to be distressed and shaken by the experience.

Management after the Acute Attack

Once the acute episode is over and a diagnosis of febrile seizures made, the task is to evaluate the risk facing the child, decide on a course for long-term management, and counsel the family fully.

Evaluating the Risk Facing the Child

Febrile seizures in general are benign. They are not associated with a substantial risk of death or permanent motor impairment. Children with this syndrome do not later in childhood have more problems in behavior, school achievement, or intelligence than seizure-free siblings or schoolmates. Most children with febrile seizures were neurologically and developmentally normal before the first seizure, but children who were not neurologically or developmentally normal may also experience febrile seizures; such children are at increased risk for later nonfebrile seizures and are more likely to be limited intellectually.

There is a higher rate of later epilepsy (recurrent nonfebrile seizures) in children with febrile seizures, and that increase persists into adult life; the increase in risk is small in magnitude for the majority of children. The risk tends to be concentrated in those who have two or more of the following: neurologic or developmental abnormality before any seizure; family history of nonfebrile seizures; or a first seizure that was focal, multiple in 24 hours, or over 15 minutes in duration. The presence of a single one of the named features is not associated with much increase in risk. For that largely majority of children with febrile seizures who do not have the risk factors mentioned, the risk of epilepsy is 2 to 3 per cent by age 25. The small subgroup with multiple risk factors has a substantially higher rate of later epilepsy; medical treatment has not been shown to alter that risk.

Overall, about a third of children with one febrile seizure have at least one recurrence. Children who experience their first febrile seizure early in the period of vulnerability, especially in the first year of life, those who have seizures with low fevers, and those who are in day care may be especially likely to have recurrences. Three quarters of recurrences take place in the year after the first attack, 90 per cent within 2 years.

Even prolonged febrile seizures are not associated with substantially greater risk of subsequent febrile or nonfebrile seizures except in children who were neurologically abnormal before the first seizure.

Goals of Long-Term Management

Because recurrent seizures may take place whether or not medication is prescribed, a major realistic goal is to prevent any seizure that occurs from becoming prolonged, more than half an hour or so. Counseling of the family (see later) is of great importance in this regard. The other major goal is to normalize life for parents and child.

In general, the more typical the history of and evaluation of the child with febrile seizures—age 6 months to 4 years, previously developmentally and neurologically normal, no Todd's paresis, only a few seizures all of which were brief and nonfocal, no history of epilepsy in the immediate family—the more it is possible to be confident that the reassuring results of the large population studies apply to that child and the less the need to consider daily pharmacotherapy. Children with a first uncomplicated febrile seizure are seldom appropriate candidates for continuous medical treatment.

Medications Available for Long-Term Daily Therapy

Diphenylhydantoin and carbamazepine are apparently ineffective for daily administration in febrile seizures. Valproic acid has been reported to reduce the risk of recurrences, but recent evaluation of pooled information from British trials of treatment have questioned that conclusion. In addition, rare but life-threatening reactions can occur with valproic acid, raising doubts that it is an appropriate agent for the treatment of a benign disorder.

Surveys of pediatricians, neurologists, pediatric neurologists, and family practice physicians indicate that the agent used most commonly for the long-term therapy of febrile seizures is phenobarbital. A number of studies have reported that continuous treatment with phenobarbital decreases the risk of recurrences.

Most of these studies have involved children with a first uncomplicated febrile seizure. *As a group many authors, and a National Institutes of Health consensus development panel, believe such children to be inappropriate candidates for continuous anticonvulsant therapy.* Most trials have been small, and most have excluded data on children who withdrew from the study, experienced side effects, or had blood drug levels not considered to be adequate, procedures that may permit the entry of important bias and thus lead to results that cannot be interpreted. Pooled analysis of British trials of treatment with phenobarbital or valproate, including both published and previously unpublished trials, did not show significant reduction in recurrent seizures with either agent. Two new randomized trials that examined populations of children at special risk of subsequent seizures and analyzed according to intention to treat do not demonstrate efficacy for phenobarbital or valproate in the chronic treatment of febrile seizures.

Phenobarbital is familiar, inexpensive, convenient, and uncommonly associated with major hypersensitivity reactions. It is also a potent pharmaceutical agent with a variety of effects and interactions with other medications and with exogenous and endogenous hormones. Overdosage and accidental poisonings may occur, and abrupt withdrawal of phenobarbital may increase the likelihood of seizures.

Experimental and clinical studies have suggested adverse influences on developing neuronal systems. Reported unwanted effects on behavior and mood are frequent with phenobarbital treatment and include overactivity, excitement, irritability, sleep disturbance, aggression, and tearfulness. Such reactions may decrease with continued treatment. In older children and adults, depression may occur and continue throughout therapy. A recent randomized clinical trial found mean intelligence quotient (IQ) to be 7 points lower in children with early, complex, or repeated febrile seizures who were randomly assigned to treatment for 2 years with phenobarbital as compared with children assigned to placebo. Thus, one study in children with febrile seizures whose characteristics make them candidates for consideration of long-term medical therapy suggests that lengthy administration of phenobarbital may be harmful, and two studies of children who might be candidates for therapy indicate that phenobarbital may not significantly alter the risk of further seizures.

If phenobarbital is prescribed, it may be given as 4 to 5 mg/kg/day in a single bedtime dose. Some authors suggest its use for 2 years or until the child reaches the age of 4 or 5 years, past the period of maximal vulnerability to febrile seizures. Recent evidence that treatment for 2 years was associated with depression of IQ may suggest a need for rethinking the desirability of lengthy treatment for most children with febrile seizures and consideration of a briefer course of therapy even when treatment is felt to be warranted by an atypical clinical history.

Approaches for Intermittent Therapy

Except in loading doses, phenobarbital—administered at the time of febrile illnesses—is ineffective because it requires days for a stable blood level to be achieved. Rapidly absorbed anticonvulsants, especially benzodiazepines, administered orally or rectally provide an attractive therapeutic option and can be used either at the onset of febrile illness in order to prevent seizures or to terminate a seizure that is not rapidly self-limited. For the prevention of seizures, there is the problem that the seizure is fairly often the first indication of illness in the child, so that it is inevitable that intermittent therapy will miss some cases even if otherwise effective. However, that fact is counterbalanced by problems in achieving compliance with chronically administered medications.

In other countries, there is now considerable and generally favorable experience with the use of rectal diazepam at the onset of fevers to prevent seizures or to terminate a seizure once it has begun. This approach requires a competent family with few caregivers. After the seizing child has been tended and properly positioned, the solution regularly used for intravenous or intramuscular injection (5 mg/ml) can be drawn up in a disposable tuberculin syringe and administered per rectum, 0.5 mg/kg up to 15 mg total dose, for administration if the seizure continues more than 5 or 10 minutes. This dose can be repeated in 12 hours. A first test dose should be administered under medical supervision so that the tolerance of the individual child can be established and medical personnel can be assured that the parents have mastered the technique. Complications have been few with this approach, but the child must be watched carefully for respiratory depression or for unsteadiness that might lead to injury from falls after drug administration. The use of liquid diazepam for rectal administration in febrile seizures has not been approved in the United States. Rectal suppositories of diazepam, available in other countries, are associated with slow and irregular release of drug and are not available in the United States.

Diazepam administered orally produces rapid and sustained serum levels. A recent European trial of this potentially attractive approach found that, as actually used, oral administration of diazepam did not lead to a significant reduction in recurrences. A North American clinical trial is under way.

COUNSELING THE FAMILY

Although febrile seizures are in general benign, their occurrence may terrify the family. Realistic reassurance is appropriate and may have to be repeated, both to parents and to other family members. The counseling of the family has several additional objectives; these include preventing status epilepticus; normalizing life; reducing the risk of recurrent febrile seizures; and, with input from the family, deciding whether to employ anticonvulsant therapy either continuously or intermittently.

Whether or not medication is prescribed, recurrences may take place. The siblings of children with febrile seizures face a risk of about 10 per cent for febrile seizures. Therefore, it is important that parents and other caregivers be counseled in the care of children with fever and in first aid for seizures and that they be helped to plan how to get to competent emergency care for any seizure that does not end quickly and spontaneously. Consideration may be given to supplying rectal diazepam to selected families who are responsible and well instructed in its use, especially if they live far from medical care or often travel or camp.

Febrile seizures may be more common in children in day care and in children of mothers who smoke, especially those who smoke heavily, the latter effect perhaps related to the increased frequency of respiratory illnesses in young children exposed to cigarette smoke. For the child with frequent respiratory infections, the feasibility of reducing exposure to ambient smoke warrants consideration. Children subject to febrile seizures should not be too warmly covered, especially early in illness. Oral hydration should be maintained. Although sponging and oral antipyretics at the onset of acute feverish illnesses have not proved effective in preventing recurrent febrile seizures, this generally safe approach seems sensible for the child with previous febrile seizures when fever is first recognized or when fever can be anticipated, as after immunizations. However, parents should be helped to avoid an excessive preoccupation with preventing fevers, which is not always possible.

Febrile seizures are usually benign, and most predictors of the unusual unfavorable outcome are characteristics present or not present in the child by the time he or she is first brought for medical attention for febrile seizures. Prolonged continuous treatment may be harmful and is of questionable efficacy. It is important for medical caregivers to provide information and realistic reassurance, to help to prevent any seizure that occurs from becoming prolonged, and to assist families in comfortable adaptation to the period of vulnerability to this common age-related propensity to experience seizures early in the course of feverish illness.

INFANTILE SPASMS

O. CARTER SNEAD III, M.D.

Infantile spasms represent an infantile myoclonic seizure disorder that is often progressive, associated with a high incidence of neurologic sequelae, and almost always refractory to anticonvulsant drug treatment. These seizures may be classified as *flexor, extensor,* and *mixed* spasms, with the latter being the most common and extensor spasms the least common.

Flexor spasms consist of flexion of the neck, trunk, arms,

and legs. Abdominal flexion may be massive, giving rise to the "jack-knife" or "salaam" seizures that are the hallmark of infantile spasms. During extensor spasms, there is abrupt extension of the neck, trunk, and legs. The mixed flexor-extensor spasms are characterized by flexion of the neck, trunk, and arms, and extension of the legs. The spasms often occur in clusters several times a day, particularly upon awakening, and are often associated with a cry. The doubling over and crying seen with massive abdominal flexor spasms may lead to a misdiagnosis of colic.

Infantile spasms may be classified as either *cryptogenic* or *symptomatic*, depending upon whether an etiology can be identified. Those patients in whom there is a clear-cut etiology (e.g., congenital malformation of brain, perinatal asphyxia, tuberous sclerosis) are termed symptomatic, whereas those in whom no etiology can be found are cryptogenic.

Infantile spasms are associated with a mortality of 10 to 20 per cent and a morbidity which ranges from 75 to 90 per cent. The morbidity consists of mental retardation that is frequently moderate to severe. The incidence of retardation is greater than 90 per cent in the symptomatic cases and 60 to 70 per cent in cryptogenic spasms. Infantile spasms are quite age-specific, usually occurring within the first 6 months of life. The incidence drops off rapidly after 12 months, and the spasms rarely, if ever, occur after the age of 4 years. The electroencephalographic (EEG) abnormality classically associated with infantile spasms is described as hypsarrhythmia. This term refers to high-voltage chaotic slowing, multifocal spikes, and a marked asynchrony. *West syndrome* alludes to those children who have infantile spasms, a hypsarrhythmic EEG, and mental retardation.

TREATMENT

Infantile spasms are intractable to treatment with standard anticonvulsant drugs, but either adrenocorticotropic hormone (ACTH) or oral steroid therapy results in a significant reduction of seizures in 50 to 65 per cent of patients. There seems to be an inverse relation between response to treatment and age, with younger patients having a better therapeutic response. The ultimate prognosis for most of these patients is dismal and depends heavily on the etiology of the spasms, the pre-existing neurologic and developmental status, the presence or absence of other seizures, and the age of the patient at the onset of seizures. The patient with the best prognosis is between 3 and 12 months of age and neurologically normal at the onset, with no other kind of seizure, and without a demonstrable etiology for the spasms.

The literature is conflicting on the question of whether early treatment of spasms makes a difference in the ultimate outcome; however, I favor an aggressive approach in which high-dose ACTH is used in all patients as soon as the diagnosis is established by a clinical description of the seizure, a hard-copy EEG, and EEG-videotelemetry monitoring for 24 hours. The telemetry allows characterization and quantitation of the seizure and also observation of the sleep record. Once the diagnosis is made, the child is admitted to the hospital in order to (1) begin the ACTH therapy; (2) monitor blood pressure, urine, and electrolytes; and (3) teach the parents to give the ACTH intramuscularly (IM), measure urine glucose three times daily with Chemstix, and recognize spasms so that they can keep an accurate seizure calendar. In addition, any diagnostic work-up indicated by clinical circumstances is carried out during this hospitalization. An endocrine profile, complete blood count (CBC), urinalysis, electrolytes, baseline renal function, and calcium, phosphorus, and serum glucose levels are obtained prior to starting ACTH. The drug is not instituted if any of the findings are abnormal.

The initial dose of ACTH is 150 units/m^2/day of ACTH gel [Acthar gel (Armour), 80 units/ml] IM in two divided doses, for 1 week. Synthetic ACTH is not used because of the higher incidence of side effects with this preparation. During the second week, the dose is 75 units/m^2/day in one daily dose for 1 week; the third week, the dose is 75 units/m^2 every other day for 1 week. Over the next 9 weeks, the ACTH is gradually tapered. The lot number of the ACTH gel is carefully recorded. Usually, a treatment response is seen within the first 7 days; if no response is seen in 2 weeks, the lot is changed.

The patient is discharged on day 3 of therapy, and arrangements are made for daily blood pressure measurement the first week, then three times weekly after that. If hypertension occurs, attempts are made to control it with salt restriction and diuretic therapy rather than stopping the ACTH. The patient is observed in the outpatient clinic weekly for the first month and then biweekly. A waking and sleeping EEG is obtained at 1, 2, and 4 weeks after the start of ACTH to determine the treatment response.

We have observed a high relapse rate (50 per cent) during the tapering period, particularly in the symptomatic patients. When this occurs, the dose is increased to the previously effective dose for 2 weeks and then another taper begun. If the seizures continue in the face of such a dosage increase, the dose is increased to 150 units/m^2/day and the regimen is begun again.

It is also possible to treat infantile spasms with oral corticosteroids if it is not feasible for the parents to give injections at home; however, in my experience, corticosteroids are somewhat less effective than ACTH. If the decision is made to use these compounds, the initial dose is 3 mg/kg/day of prednisone in four divided doses for 2 weeks followed by a 12-week tapering period.

Both ACTH and corticosteroids are dangerous drugs at these high doses, with ACTH probably resulting in a higher incidence of side effects. In virtually all these children, cushingoid features develop. Many patients show extreme irritability early in the course, and a few will have hypertension. When using such treatment, one should be constantly alert for sepsis; glucosuria; metabolic abnormalities involving electrolytes, calcium, and phosphorus; and congestive heart failure. An additional reversible side effect of ACTH is cerebral ventriculomegaly. The etiology is unknown, but it points up the importance of doing diagnostic computerized tomographic scans in children with infantile spasms prior to initiation of ACTH.

Finally, some authors advocate the use of valproic acid or the benzodiazepine nitrazepam in the treatment of infantile spasms. Valproic acid is particularly toxic in this age group and should not be a first-line drug for this disorder. Nitrazepam is effective to some degree against infantile spasms but is currently unavailable for use as an anticonvulsant in the United States.

SPASMUS NUTANS

ELIZABETH C. ENGLE, M.D.
and DAVID HOLTZMAN, M.D., Ph.D.

Spasmus nutans (from Greek, nodding spasms) is a transient disorder of infancy classically characterized by the triad of nystagmus, head nodding, and, less frequently, head tilt. It is imperative to determine that the patient has no neurologic or ophthalmologic abnormalities presenting as spasmus nutans. The literature on spasmus nutans is confused by a lack of uniform diagnostic criteria and a frequent lack of long-term patient follow-up. In the last decade, there has been increasing information about this condition as a result of the use of computed tomography (CT), magnetic resonance imaging (MRI), and oculographic studies. However, we know of no series of patients presenting with spasmus nutans in which MRIs have been obtained routinely in order to determine the incidence of structural lesions in this functional disorder.

SYMPTOMS

Nystagmus

The first of these symptoms, head nod or nystagmus, typically begins between 3 and 8 months of age but has been reported as early as 2 weeks and as late as 3 years. The duration of symptoms is typically 4 to 36 months. Full clinical recovery by 3 years is generally the rule. Oculographic studies, however, have shown residual nystagmus in "recovered children." The incidence is estimated to be 3 per 1000 and shows no sex or race predilection. There have been several case reports of concurrence in monozygotic twins, but no clear genetic or familial pattern has been determined.

The nystagmus of spasmus nutans often is notable for its variability both within a single examination and between examinations in a given patient. It is of rapid frequency (7 to 11 cycles per second [Hz]), of small amplitude (usually less than 3 degrees), and pendular. It is usually horizontal but may have a vertical or rotary component. It can be monocular or bilateral, with variable asymmetry of amplitude and periods of dysconjugate nystagmus between the eyes. The nystagmus can be intermittent and may be influenced by direction of gaze, head movement, or close fixation.

Head Nod

Head nod is present at some point in about 80 per cent of cases. It is often the first symptom reported, is more commonly horizontal than vertical, changes with head position, and ceases in sleep. Recent studies have shown that the head nodding reduces nystagmus, presumably allowing better visual fixation by the patient.

Head Tilt

Head tilt is present in one third to one half of cases. It must be differentiated from the head tilt that is due to a posterior fossa mass, cranial nerve dysfunction, or structural abnormalities of the neck or extraocular muscles. In spasmus nutans, there is no consistent direction of head tilt. Movement from primary position to the turned position may transiently dampen the nystagmus. Some children are noted to move their head to the tilted position when fixing on a near object.

ETIOLOGY

The etiology of spasmus nutans is not known. In addition to the classic triad, 25 to 50 per cent of patients with spasmus nutans have strabismus or amblyopia. The symptoms and signs of the disease can be localized to the midbrain and pons and may be associated with an optic glioma or a hypothalamic tumor. A maturation disorder of control of ocular fixation and voluntary movements of the head and eyes has been suggested.

DIFFERENTIAL DIAGNOSIS AND TREATMENT

Spasmus nutans can usually be clinically differentiated from congenital nystagmus. Congenital nystagmus tends to be of earlier onset (<6 months); is characterized by a less marked head nod; tends to be constant, bilateral, symmetric, conjugate, and jerk-like rather than pendular; and is of slower frequency and larger amplitude than the nystagmus of spasmus nutans. Congenital nystagmus does not resolve with time.

Treatment of children with spasmus nutans is directed toward the associated ophthalmologic and neurologic abnormalities. In the last two decades, there have been multiple reports of infants and children diagnosed with spasmus nutans who were subsequently found to have optic gliomas or hypothalamic tumors. There also have been single case reports of spasmus nutans in association with an empty sella, an arachnoid cyst, a porencephalic cyst, cerebrocerebellar degeneration, and also Leigh's disease. These diagnoses may be suspected when the examiner finds decreased visual acuity, optic atrophy or papilledema, an afferent pupillary defect, abnormal visual fields or optokinetic nystagmus, increasing head circumference, or symptoms of the diencephalic syndrome (failure to thrive, hyperactivity, and neuroendocrine dysfunction). Only a very small percentage of cases of spasmus nutans are secondary to an otherwise occult neoplasm. However, the inability to differentiate them clinically makes it imperative that all patients diagnosed with spasmus nutans undergo MRI. Once a normal scan is obtained, the patient should be routinely evaluated by an ophthalmologist for treatment of abnormal visual acuity and/or strabismus.

HEADACHE

ELISE E. LABBÉ, Ph.D.

Headache is a frequent complaint reported by children. The most commonly diagnosed type of headache is migraine. Other types of headache disorders include muscle contraction, mixed (child reports migraine and muscle contraction headache symptoms), postconcussive, and sinus. Migraine headaches can be further subdivided into classic and common.

TYPES OF HEADACHE

Migraine

About 5 per cent of children aged 7 to 15 seen in a pediatric practice may be diagnosed as having migraine. In classic migraine, prior to the onset of head pain, the child will report unusual symptoms such as scotomata, paresthesias of the face and hands, and vertigo. Within minutes the child will report unilateral head pain, describing it as pulsating or throbbing; the child may also experience nausea, vomiting, and photophobia. Headaches last 4 to 12 hours, although this can vary. Rest and sleep can reduce the head pain. Children usually report two to eight headaches per month, although the frequency can vary greatly between children and over the years for a given child. Head pain is usually described as moderate to severe. A family history of migraine has been reported for 66 to 90 per cent of children in several studies. Common migraine is more frequently diagnosed and includes varying combinations of the above-mentioned symptoms, often bilateral pain, without the prodromes. There is some evidence that a subgroup of children may experience recurrent abdominal pain, with vascular changes (pallor or flushing), loss of appetite, and vomiting. These children may also experience migraine symptoms or migraines later in life.

A variety of factors may trigger a migraine, including fatigue, emotional and psychologic stress, certain foods, changes in the menstrual cycle, and allergy. Although it has long been assumed that certain personality traits are associated with migraine, recent research has not been able to demonstrate a consistent personality type or behavioral characteristics associated with childhood migraine. However, psychologic factors can play a role, as home or school stressors may elicit headaches and parental or teacher responses may increase or maintain pain behavior.

To date, no definitive statement can be made on the pathophysiology of migraine. There is evidence for biochemical, neural, and vascular changes in response to environmental, psychologic, or other physical factors. The model most often offered to explain migraine proposes that triggering events cause intracranial and extracranial arteries to the brain to constrict; in response to this vasoconstriction, some extracranial arteries dilate, causing pressure in surrounding tissue, sterile inflammation, and biochemical changes, resulting in pain. More recent studies report that changes in levels of endogenous opiate peptides are associated with reports of head pain; it appears that decreases are related to headache experience.

Long-term prognosis is controversial, with estimates that up to 80 per cent of children will be symptom-free or improved within an 8-year period and others reporting that at least 60 per cent of individuals treated for migraine in childhood continued to have headaches as adults. Many children experience long periods of remission and often report lower headache activity during the summer months.

Muscle Contraction

Most of the medical literature on childhood headache focuses on migraine headache. Controversy appears to exist on the prevalence of muscle contraction headaches. Children are rarely diagnosed with tension headache before puberty, although these headaches may be common. However, adolescents are more likely to seek treatment for muscle contraction headache.

Symptoms include mild to moderate head pain described as pressure, an ache or tight band around the head or base of the skull. Often these headaches last for days. Frequency and duration of muscle contraction headache symptoms vary greatly from individual to individual and within an individual. Physical findings upon medical evaluation are usually minimal and may include tenderness over the cervical muscles and occipital scalp. Most models of pathophysiology of muscle contraction headache include not only muscular but also vascular and biochemical factors. Various emotional or environmental events may trigger or cause scalp and neck muscles to contract for prolonged periods of time, resulting in pain. Vasoconstriction in contracted muscles might also contribute to the pain experience by producing ischemia. Abnormal vascular reactivity in the muscles with accumulation of pain-provoking substances in the muscle or a central deficiency of inhibiting neurotransmitter substances has also been proposed as a possible contributor to the headache. These models, although commonly supported, have not been experimentally validated.

It is often assumed that children with tension headaches experience significant school or family stress or are unable to cope with stress. At present, questions remain as to what role stress does play in the development and maintenance of tension headache. However, factors such as family conflict, school problems, depression, anxiety, and secondary gain may play a significant role in contributing to the headaches and should be evaluated. Care should be taken to not suggest to the parents that the child's headaches are not real, but that for many children these psychologic factors may need to be addressed if symptoms are to be reduced on a long-term basis.

Mixed

Children may experience both tension and migraine headache symptoms simultaneously or at different times.

Other Headache Types

Other types of headache that come to the attention of the pediatrician are post-traumatic headaches; headaches associated with seizure disorders, sinus disease, metabolic disorders, or infections; or those that are drug-related. These types of headaches are usually part of other syndromes and are not discussed here.

GENERAL TREATMENT ISSUES

Several issues should be considered regardless of headache type or therapeutic approach. These include (1) assessment of the child's pain, (2) evaluation of parental concerns, (3) provision of the treatment rationale for parents and child, and (4) fostering the child's participation in the treatment regimen.

Children may not be able to verbalize their experience of pain or to describe the duration and intensity of the pain accurately. A useful procedure is to have the child keep a daily record of headache pain for 2 weeks. Patients can be asked to indicate whether they are having a headache and, if so, to rate it on a 5-point Likert-type scale. A rating of 0 = no head pain, 1 = mild head pain, 2 = moderate head pain, 3 = severe head pain, and 4 = very severe head pain. To facilitate record-keeping, the child can rate the headache four times a day, for example, at breakfast, lunch, dinner, and bedtime. Any prodromes experienced, what things are thought to have triggered the headache, what things made the pain worse, and what decreased the pain can be indicated in the log. The parents can also be asked to keep a log in which they record any times during which the child complains of headaches, pain behavior observed, and anything that they think increased or decreased the pain. Parents can ask the child to describe the head pain during a headache episode because many children forget how it feels when the headache is over. If a child is having difficulty verbally describing the pain, he or she can be asked to draw a picture of it (Fig. 1). The headache log not only allows the gathering of useful and more reliable information about the child's symptoms but can also serve as an estimate of how well the family will comply with behavioral or psychologic treatment approaches, as these require active participation from child and parents.

When a child reports frequent headaches that are severe enough to warrant seeking medical intervention, the parents are usually very concerned. Often they fear that the child may have a tumor or other serious problem. Many parents are relieved when told that the child has migraine or tension headaches after significant pathology has been ruled out. Some parents, however, continue to be concerned and request further medical evaluation, such as magnetic resonance imaging (MRI) scans. The pediatrician can discuss assessment to date, explain to the parent why further diagnostic procedures are not necessary, and discuss the benign nature of migraine or tension headaches. Parents can also be reassured that long-term prognosis is good. Parents can be encouraged to be supportive of the child but to be careful not to reinforce pain behavior. Headaches should be treated in a matter-of-fact manner, prompting the child to employ strategies to prevent or reduce the head pain. Whenever possible, the child should be encouraged to continue school or homework; if this work is missed, parents should make sure that the child makes it up.

To enhance treatment compliance by parent and child, a rationale for choice of treatment should be provided. By

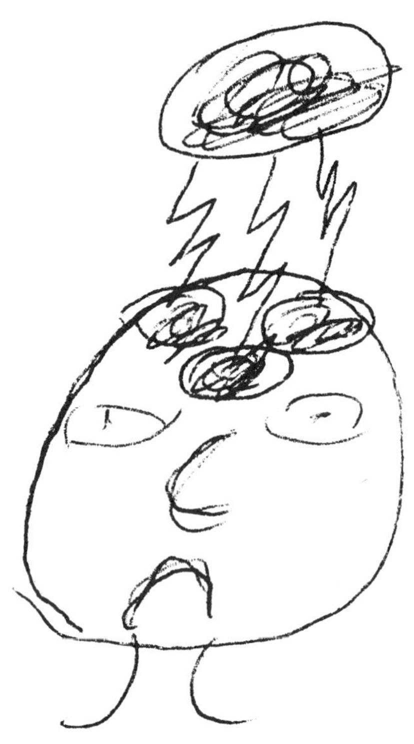

Figure 1. Drawing by an 8-year-old boy diagnosed with migraine headache.

increasing the family's understanding of why either pharmacologic or nonpharmacologic treatment is prescribed, the parent and patient are more likely to comply with treatment consistently over a long period of time. To make sure the child understands, the child should be asked to respond to the pediatrician as to why headaches are occurring and how treatment will be helpful.

Changing the behavior and attitudes of parents and children is an important aspect of treatment effectiveness. Therefore, it is wise to address these issues early in the treatment regimen. When one is dealing with a chronic recurrent problem such as migraine headache, children should be encouraged to adopt an attitude in which they take active responsibility for coping with their headaches. Often triggering events or situations can be identified by the child; when possible, these events should be avoided or modified by the child, sometimes with the help of the parents. An example of this is a child who was a straight A student and a member of the school safety patrol. She took dance and piano lessons several days a week and participated in student government activities, advanced classes, and several other competitive activities. The child believed that she had to be the best at all of these activities. In time she experienced chronic fatigue and severe migraine headaches. Her parents were encouraged to help her manage her time and to reduce her extracurricular activities to a few that were the most important to her. Within a few months, her headaches had decreased significantly in frequency and intensity. Other potential triggers, such as diet and physical exertion, can also be identified by the child and avoided.

Finally, for many treatment regimens, the child can be encouraged to be actively involved, particularly in the nonpharmacologic approaches that require children to integrate new coping behaviors within their daily routine. Parents can remind the child to comply with the treatment programs but should avoid nagging or allowing the child to become overly dependent (thereby creating one more stressful situation). Incentives can be established to motivate children to actively use their new skills or reward them when they cope in an adaptive manner. In some cases (such as very young children or children who have severe symptoms and need someone to help focus attention), parents can be trained to coach the child, for example, by using relaxation phrases.

Treatment of Migraine

Pharmacologic Therapy

Many individual drugs or combinations of drugs have been used in the treatment of migraine headache. These drugs can be generally grouped into two categories: symptomatic or abortive therapy and prophylactic therapy.

Symptomatic Approach. For an abortive or symptomatic approach, an ergot preparation such as Cafergot is often used. Ergot is used to prevent the initial vasodilation; thus, to be effective the ergot must be given early during the prodromal phase. This can be problematic for children because they may not recognize the prodromal phase and many do not experience prodromes. Toxicity can also occur when ergot is overused, as evidenced by drowsiness and diminished pulses. Ergots are not often recommended for younger children. However, Silberstein (1990) reports that pediatric neurologists are now using dihydroergotamine (DHE) alone or with metoclopramide or promethazine. He also reports good success with intravenous (IV) DHE and metoclopramide for children aged 6 to 16. Dosages are as follows:

- Ages 6 to 9: promethazine (0.25 mg/kg or 0.5 mg/kg, maximum dose 25 mg); IV DHE (0.1 to 0.15 mg)
- Ages 9 to 12: promethazine (maximum dose 50 mg); IV DHE (0.2 mg)
- Ages 12 to 16: promethazine (maximum dose 50 mg); IV DHE (0.25 mg to 0.5 mg)

Another approach combines an analgesic plus a sedative or antinausea agent. Acetaminophen may also be helpful for symptomatic relief. An additional frequently prescribed combination is butalbital with aspirin (e.g., Fiorinal) or butalbital with acetaminophen (e.g., Fioricet). For the nauseated or vomiting patient, injectable or suppository formulations of these drugs may be needed. For children whose headaches are infrequent or mild to moderate, a symptomatic approach may be all that is required. However, if a child has weekly or more severe headaches, particularly during the school year, a prophylactic approach may be considered.

Prophylactic Approach. A prophylactic approach includes the use of such medications as beta-blockers (propranolol [Inderal]), anticonvulsants (phenytoin [Dilantin Infatab]), antihistamines (cyproheptadine [Periactin]), antidepressants (amitriptyline), ergot derivatives (methysergide [Sansert]), and calcium channel blockers (Flunarizine). Generally, the chosen drug is prescribed at an average dose based on the child's age or size and increased every 4 to 7 days until some evidence of headache control is established or until side effects or toxicity limits its use. More often than not, these medications do not completely rid the child of headaches but reduce the headache activity to more manageable frequency and intensity levels. Furthermore, because of side effects and unknown long-term effects of prophylactic medications, these drugs can be tapered at the end of the school year and discontinued during the summer vacation or discontinued every 3 to 6 months. Often children experience long periods of remission. There are few controlled studies evaluating the use of medication for children with migraine headaches. The few that have been reported raise questions as to the overall effectiveness of the medications described above, particularly in relation to the negative side effects often experienced and unknown long-term effects on the developing child.

Nonpharmacologic Therapy

Several nonpharmacologic approaches have been reported to be useful with childhood migraine. Relaxation training and skin temperature biofeedback have been well documented as significantly reducing headache activity for the majority of children studied. There have been no reports of detrimental side effects.

Relaxation Training. Relaxation training involves teaching patients to identify when they are physiologically aroused, to become physiologically relaxed, and then to become relaxed when they perceive tension or anxiety. The rationale provided to parents and child is that stress and negative emotional states can trigger or worsen headaches. Relaxation training can reduce or prevent stressful responses and therefore prevent or reduce headache activity. The most common form of relaxation taught is progressive muscle relaxation. The child is shown how to tense and relax 16 muscle groups (Table 1). Once the child is able to do that, the 16 muscle groups are combined into four groups. After the child is able to relax the four muscle groups, the muscles are then divided into two muscle groups. Once the child can completely relax these two groups, the child is taught to relax the entire body.

The goal of the relaxation training is quick relaxation of the entire body within a few moments. This goal can usually be achieved within six to eight treatment sessions, including practice at home for about 20 minutes daily. By tensing different muscles, the child also learns to identify when the muscles are becoming tense during stressful situations. The patients are also encouraged to identify stressors that may initiate a headache episode and to use the relaxation if they feel tense or anxious or when prodromes are experienced. The therapist can help the child develop strategies to relax in situations that are inherently arousing, such as during a sports event or a school test.

For younger children, the parent is encouraged to become familar with the technique and to cue the child to relax if the child appears to be overly aroused or if a headache seems imminent. Audio tapes can also be made to help the child practice the relaxation exercises at home.

Biofeedback. Two types of biofeedback treatments are useful with migraine headaches. These are skin temperature biofeedback and cephalic vasomotor feedback.

SKIN TEMPERATURE BIOFEEDBACK. This modality involves teaching the child to raise the skin temperature, usually on the hand or finger. The rationale behind using skin temperature is that prior to the head pain the child may be experiencing vasoconstriction, particularly in the cranial region. The central nervous system's response to this vasoconstriction is vasodilation, subsequent sterile inflammation, and resulting head pain. By increasing body surface temperature, the child is encouraging general vasodilation, which may prevent or reduce the vasoconstriction and resulting head pain. Most children respond to skin temperature biofeedback after six to eight sessions. Treatment sessions involve teaching the child to warm the hand using a biofeedback device. The device gives audio or visual signals to the child that indicate whether skin temperature is increasing or decreasing. Prior to the feedback, the child is asked to sit quietly for about 5 minutes, during which the skin temperature is allowed to stabilize. This baseline period is followed by 15 to 20 minutes of feedback. Finally, the feedback is turned off and the child is encouraged to continue to try to warm the hands without the feedback. This is called the *self-control phase*, as the goal of biofeedback is for the child to eventually raise the skin temperature without the feedback. The child is instructed to practice warming the hand at least once daily during the treatment phase. As with the relaxation exercise, the child is taught to recognize potential stressors and to warm the hand when feeling stressed or experiencing prodromes. Most children are able to learn to raise their skin temperature in the first few sessions as much as 2° to 4°F.

CEPHALIC VASOMOTOR FEEDBACK. This modality has been used with adults but may also be used with children. The child is taught to directly constrict the temporal artery during a headache episode. A plethysmograph is used to detect blood flow. Audio or visual feedback tells the child whether the blood flow is increasing or decreasing. The goal is to decrease the blood flow when head pain is experienced or increase the blood flow during prodromes. As with skin temperature biofeedback, the child receives several sessions of biofeedback with opportunities to demonstrate self-control of blood flow. The child is also instructed to practice daily and when experiencing head pain.

Cognitive Coping Techniques. These methods are often incorporated into biofeedback or relaxation treatment protocols. Cognitive coping techniques focus on the child's ability to think about the experience of pain and stress and to use thoughts and behaviors that reduce the impact of the pain. For example, through learning skin temperature biofeedback, children are able to learn that they have some control over the body's response. Children are encouraged to use this thought in dealing with stress, so that instead of feeling fear or helplessness, they can relax and do things to prevent or at least reduce the pain. Children are also taught to identify thoughts they may have that in themselves can be stress-inducing. For example, these patients often believe that they have to be perfect. They are extremely achievement-oriented and become overly committed to extracurricular activities. Children may become very upset if they fail or do not do well. These children are then encouraged to modify their expectations to a more realistic but positive level and are taught ways to keep their failures in perspective. They may be taught time management techniques and simple problem solving.

TABLE 1. Muscle Groups Emphasized in Relaxation Training

Group I	*Group III*
1. Hands	9. Upper back
2. Forearms	10. Chest
3. Upper arms	11. Shoulders
4. Feet	12. Neck
Group II	*Group IV*
5. Lower legs (calves)	13. Forehead
6. Upper legs (quadriceps)	14. Eyelids
7. Abdomen	15. Upper cheeks and nose
8. Lower back	16. Lower face and mouth area

Treatment of Muscle Contraction Headache

Pharmacologic Therapy

Symptomatic treatment using pain medication such as aspirin, acetaminophen, or codeine is often utilized. Local anesthetic blocks are occasionally performed in adults but rarely with children. Sedative-hypnotic medications with muscle relaxant properties (e.g., diazepam) may be effective. The dose is 1 to 2 mg three times daily (t.i.d.) in children under 30 kg, and 2 to 5 mg t.i.d. for heavier children.

Antidepressants are also commonly used. Medication should be used as adjunctive therapy because of the potential abuse with some of these drugs. Focusing on the child's symptoms with a daily consistent medication regimen for 4 to 12 weeks can be beneficial. However, emphasizing only pharmacologic management and increasing the use of powerful pain relievers usually are not effective. Massaging the child's muscles and local heat or cold packs can also help reduce the pain. Finally, nonpharmacologic treatments may prove to be effective as either the sole treatment offered or as an adjunct to pharmacologic treatment.

Nonpharmacologic Therapy

Few studies have been reported evaluating pharmacologic and nonpharmacologic treatments for muscle contraction headaches. Relaxation training, electromyographic (EMG) biofeedback, and operant conditioning procedures have been reported to reduce tension headaches in children. However, unlike studies of migraine, only a handful of studies have evaluated these approaches.

Relaxation Training. Progressive muscle relaxation training is the most commonly prescribed treatment for tension headache. The procedure is the same as described for migraine headache.

Biofeedback. The focus of biofeedback therapy for muscle contraction headache is to teach the child to relax the muscles in the region of the head pain and surrounding areas. The most commonly monitored muscles are frontalis, masseter, and trapezius. EMG feedback is used. Most children respond after six to eight sessions of EMG biofeedback. Sessions involve teaching the child to decrease muscle tension using a biofeedback device. The device gives audio or visual signals to the child that indicate whether muscle tension is increasing or decreasing. Prior to the feedback, the child is asked to sit quietly for about 5 minutes, during which a baseline recording is made. This baseline period is followed by 15 to 20 minutes of feedback. Finally, the feedback is turned off and the child is encouraged to continue to try to decrease muscle tension without the feedback. The child is instructed to relax his muscles at least once daily during the treatment phase. As with the relaxation exercises, the child is taught to recognize potential stressors and to decrease muscle tension when feeling stressed or experiencing the muscles begin to tighten.

Operant Conditioning. Children are often subtly rewarded for pain behavior associated with headaches. The child receives special attention from family, teachers, and friends. Often the child is allowed to go home from school or be relieved of household responsibilities. Although operant conditioning is not the sole cause of headaches for most children, it does play a role in maintaining or exacerbating the headache. Treatment can involve having children make up missed school work or do other household chores to replace the ones they were forgiven. Children can be rewarded for positive coping behaviors and utilizing treatment options. One study reported that rewarding the child for headache-free days was successful in reducing headache episodes.

Treatment Expectations and Follow-up

Changes in headache activity usually do not begin to occur until 4 to 6 weeks into treatment when relaxation or biofeedback techniques are used. Thus parents and children are encouraged to be patient and not to expect immediate change. Research indicates that home practice is important for headache reduction to occur. Thus, therapists can emphasize daily practice in the child's natural environment. The therapist can do this each session by discussing how frequently the child practiced during the past week, how it felt and if there were any problems. Strategies can be suggested to help deal with problems that may arise in the upcoming week. The child can be asked to keep a record of practice times.

Children who are competitive or achievement-oriented often have difficulty relaxing because they try too hard to relax or to change the feedback signals. In their efforts to do well, they become overly aroused, making it even more difficult for them to relax. Therapists should encourage the child to try, but not too hard, and not to expect immediate success with the feedback or relaxation. Like most skills, these techniques take time to learn and one often makes mistakes.

Finally, a realistic goal of treatment may be to reduce headache intensity, frequency, and/or duration or medication usage. Complete headache remission may not occur, but the child can learn to cope with the pain in a healthy manner. Employing constructive coping techniques can prevent chronic drug abuse, depression, or anxiety, which often may be associated with recurrent chronic pain conditions in adulthood.

Follow-up visits should be planned, as studies indicate that children need to be periodically reminded to practice coping skills or to re-evaluate whether skills are being effectively used. Booster sessions in which the child receives brief treatment every 3 to 4 months might help maintain treatment gains.

REFERENCES

Silberstein S: Thirty questions about headaches in children and adolescents. Headache 30:716–724, 1990.

GUILLAIN-BARRÉ SYNDROME

IRA BERGMAN, M.D.

The Guillain-Barré syndrome (GBS) is an idiopathic peripheral neuropathy that often follows a respiratory or gastrointestinal infection and presents most characteristically with areflexic, flaccid, relatively symmetric weakness beginning in the legs and ascending to involve arms, trunk, throat, and face. Progression can occur rapidly, in hours or days, or more indolently, over 2 to 4 weeks. Numbness, paresthesias, and crampy muscular pain may be prominent symptoms early in the illness, but objective signs of sensory loss are usually minor compared with the dramatic weakness. Dysfunction of autonomic nerves can lead to hypertension, hypotension, orthostatic hypotension, tachycardia and other arrhythmias, urinary retention or incontinence, stool retention or episodes of abnormal sweating, flushing, or peripheral vasoconstriction. The illness resolves spontaneously, and 75 per cent of patients recover to functional normalcy within 1 to 12 months. Twenty per cent of patients are left with mild to moderate residual weakness in the feet and lower legs. Mortality is 5 per cent and is caused by respiratory failure or complications of mechanical ventilation, cardiovascular collapse, or pulmonary embolism. The pathologic changes of GBS involve inflammation and segmental demyelination in the peripheral nerves.

TREATMENT

Treatment of GBS with plasma exchange (PE) begun within 1 to 2 weeks of the onset of weakness produces mild hastening of the recovery process. In one large, United States multicenter, randomized, controlled but not blinded study of patients older than 12 years old, the time to recover the ability to walk without assistance was 53 days in patients treated with plasmapheresis and 85 days in control patients. However, there is no evidence that long-term outcome is improved in patients receiving PE and the procedure itself may result in morbidity and, rarely, mortality. Complications include fever, chills, skin rash, venous thrombosis and thrombophlebitis, hemorrhage, pneumothorax, and bradycardia. The technical difficulties and risks of exchange will be greater in children than adults because of their smaller blood vessels and blood volume, and the benefits will be fewer because prognosis is better in younger patients. *It is this author's opinion that the small benefits attributable to plasma exchange do not justify its use in children with GBS.*

There are anecdotal reports that intravenous (IV) immunoglobulin therapy (1 g/kg over 2 consecutive days) speeds recovery in children with GBS. Intravenous immune globulin has proved safe and efficacious in several immunoregulatory disorders of childhood, including Kawasaki syndrome and immune thrombocytopenic purpura, but controlled studies of its use for GBS have not been reported.

Required therapy is symptomatic, prophylactic, and rehabilitative and directed to the following areas: ventilation and airway; hypertension, hypotension, and cardiac arrhythmias; venous stasis; nutrition, fluids, and electrolytes; pain; skin, cornea, and joints; bowel and bladder; infection; psychologic support, communication, and rehabilitation. *Patients with moderate or severe weakness or rapidly progressive weakness are best managed in a pediatric intensive care unit.*

Ventilation and Airway. Endotracheal intubation should be performed electively in patients who exhibit either early signs of hypoventilation, accumulation of bronchial secretions, or obtunded pharyngeal or laryngeal reflexes. Ventilation is monitored by frequent spirometric studies, including vital capacity (VC) and maximum inspiratory force (MIF). The indications for intubation include VC less than 12 to 15 ml/kg; MIF less negative than −20 to −40 ml of water; weak cough, voice, or cry; difficulty swallowing; drooling; and aspiration. Prolonged airway intubation lasting 3 weeks to 7 months is often required; the care and comfort of the patient may be facilitated by early tracheostomy.

Hypotension, Hypertension, and Cardiac Arrhythmias. All patients with Guillain-Barré syndrome require continuous cardiac monitoring and frequent blood pressure determinations during the acute phase of their illness. Mild to moderate hypertension is common but usually transient, lasting 2 to 21 days, and does not require treatment. Malignant hypertension should be treated with a drug of rapid onset and short duration, such as sodium nitroprusside. Blood pressure is often labile, and severe hypotension can strike unexpectedly and be difficult or impossible to reverse in the patient taking chronic antihypertensive medication. Maneuvers that decrease venous return to the heart, such as sudden elevation of the patient, straining to pass bowel movements or urine, and use of high positive end-expiratory pressure, should be avoided.

Venous Stasis. Pulmonary embolism can cause sudden death in either the acute or chronic phase of the illness. All patients must be encouraged to exercise their legs and feet to the limits of their ability, receive passive physiotherapy to the legs when voluntary movement is not possible, and wear thigh-length elastic stockings. Treatment with low-dose subcutaneous or IV heparin should be strongly considered in older children and adolescents who have very poor or absent voluntary movement of their legs.

Nutrition, Fluids, and Electrolytes. Patients who require intubation are also likely to experience prolonged pharyngeal weakness. Adequate nutrition should be ensured immediately with nasogastric or gastrostomy feedings. Hyponatremia caused by the syndrome of inappropriate secretion of antidiuretic hormone (IADH) is a complication that can be detected promptly by daily assessment of body weight, fluid intake, urine output, and serum and urine sodium concentration and can be managed by restriction of free water. The patients should be provided with a low-calcium diet because prolonged immobilization can lead to hypercalciuria.

Pain. Crampy muscular pain is treated with mild analgesics such as aspirin or acetaminophen. Painful dysesthesias or lancing pain may require continuous prophylactic therapy with carbamazepine (10 to 20 mg/kg/day), phenytoin (5 mg/kg/day), or amitriptyline.

Skin, Cornea, and Joints. Skin breakdown and pressure palsies in the immobile patient can be avoided by use of a water or air mattress, soft pads at pressure points, frequent turning, and positioning in different postures. Facial palsy may prevent lid closure in some patients with GBS. Patching or treatment with artificial tears during the day and ophthalmic ointment at night is required for protection of the cornea. Physical therapy using exercises and splints to maintain full range of motion and functional positions at all joints is an integral part of therapy.

Bowel and Bladder. Urinary retention or incontinence is usually a transient problem that necessitates either the Credé maneuver or intermittent or constant bladder catheterization. Constipation is frequent, and stool softeners, rectal or oral purgatives, or enemas are required. Adynamic ileus and gastric dilatation are rare complications. Abdominal distention is relieved by continuous nasogastric suctioning.

Infection. Urinary retention and bladder catheterization increase susceptibility to urinary tract infections. Prolonged immobilization, impaired coughing, and low tidal volumes increase the risk of developing pneumonia. Appropriate antibiotic treatment should be promptly instituted when bacterial infection is documented. Chest physical therapy with percussion, postural drainage, and appropriate suctioning must be aggressively pursued, both as a prophylactic and as a therapeutic effort.

Psychologic Support, Communication, and Rehabilitation. Inability to care for one's own basic needs, inability to communicate easily and effectively, and worry about prognosis pose a tremendous psychologic strain on the patient with severe weakness. Frequent reassurance regarding the good long-term prognosis, help in doing as much for oneself as possible, and development of an effective means of communication with a communication board or other system can help relieve some of the distress. Constant attendance by family, visitors, nurses, therapists, or "foster" grandparents may reduce anxiety and the sense of isolation. Occasionally, professional psychologic counseling is necessary.

FAMILIAL DYSAUTONOMIA

FELICIA B. AXELROD, M.D.

Familial dysautonomia (FD) is an inherited disease affecting the development and survival of sensory, sympathetic, and some parasympathetic neurons. Although the primary abnormality in familial dysautonomia is anatomic depletion of unmyelinated sensory and autonomic neurons, the clinical manifestations are the concern of the treating physician. The pervasive nature of the autonomic nervous system results in protean functional abnormalities. Signs of the disorder are present from birth, and neurologic function slowly deteriorates with age so that symptoms and problems vary with time. Frequent manifestations include feeding difficulties, hypotonia, delayed developmental milestones, labile body temperature and blood pressure, absence of overflowing tears and corneal anesthesia, marked diaphoresis with excitement, recurrent aspiration pneumonia, breath-holding episodes, ataxia, spinal curvature, and intractable vomiting.

The disease process cannot be arrested. Treatment is preventative, symptomatic, and supportive. It must be directed toward specific problems that can vary considerably among patients and with different ages.

MANIFESTATIONS

Feeding Problems

Oropharyngeal incoordination is one of the earliest signs. Poor suck or discoordinated swallow is observed in 60 per cent of infants in the neonatal period. Feeding problems are treated with various maneuvers to improve feeding and nutrition and to avoid aspiration. Feeding therapy and experimentation with different nipples and thickened formula should be tried. If weight gain is not adequate, if respiratory problems persist, or if the infant has an elevated blood urea nitrogen (BUN) gastrostomy may be necessary.

Oral incoordination can persist in the older patient and be manifested as a tendency to drool. Cineradiographic swallowing studies using various food consistencies can determine whether particular types of food are more apt to be aspirated. It is not uncommon that liquids will continue to be aspirated but that solids are consumed safely. Even when the patient is able to eat orally, it is not unusual to retain a preference for softer foods.

Vomiting

Dysautonomic patients have abnormal gastrointestinal motility, making them prone to vomiting. Vomiting occurs intermittently in some patients as part of a systemic reaction to infection or stress, either physical or emotional. Gastroesophageal reflux is also a common problem and should be considered in patients with frequent vomiting. About 40 per cent of patients have a pernicious type of vomiting, prolonged episodes occurring in a cyclic pattern. These vomiting crises are often associated with hypertension, tachycardia, diffuse sweating, and even personality changes. The cyclic pattern can be quite striking, weekly or monthly, and is usually characteristic for a particular patient. The crises can last from 3 to 72 hours. Dehydration and aspiration are ever-present risks.

If gastroesophageal reflux is identified, medical management with prokinetic agents, H2 antagonists, thickening of feeds, and positioning should be tried. However, if medical management is not successful, using the criteria of persistence of pneumonia, hematemesis or apnea, then surgical intervention (fundoplication) is performed. After surgery, crises may continue but retching will be substituted for vomiting.

Vomiting or retching in a dysautonomic patient, irrespective of the cause, is managed with diazepam. Diazepam is now considered to be the most effective antiemetic for the dysautonomic crisis. Diazepam can be administered orally, intravenously, or rectally at 0.2 mg/kg/dose. The initial dose of diazepam should be effective in stopping the vomiting, normalizing the blood pressure, and decreasing agitation. If agitation or hypertension is not eliminated, chloral hydrate, 30 mg/kg, can be given as a rectal suppository. Subsequent doses of diazepam are repeated at 3-hour intervals until the crisis resolves. Chloral hydrate can be repeated at 6-hour intervals. Ranitidine (2 mg/kg every 24 hours) is a useful adjunct in reducing emesis volume. Cimetidine should not be used because it slows renal clearance of diazepam. The crisis usually resolves abruptly and is marked by normalization of personality and return of appetite. At this point, the patient may be allowed to resume a normal diet.

A crisis can be usually managed at home, especially if the child has a gastrostomy, which facilitates hydration and giving of medications. Hospitalization is indicated, however, if the expected positive response to medication does not occur by 12 hours, if serious infection is suspected because of high fever or uncharacteristic behavior, if blood or coffee-ground material is vomited, or if dehydration is suspected.

Pneumonia

Recurrent pneumonia is frequent. The major cause of lung infection is aspiration, with most of the damage to the lung occurring during infancy and early childhood, when oral incoordination is extremely poor. If gastroesophageal reflux is present, the risk for aspiration increases.

The signs of pneumonia may be subtle. Cough is not consistently present and is rarely productive. The child is more likely to vomit increased pulmonary secretions. Tachypnea is generally not evident, and auscultation may be unrevealing because of decreased chest excursion. Radiographic examination is helpful in documenting infection. Because of the increased likelihood of aspirating gastric contents, pathogens in cultures from tracheal aspirations can be uncommon agents, such as *Escherichia coli* or *Proteus mirabilis*. Broad-spectrum antibiotics should be used until bacteriologic study guides specific therapy. In the seriously ill child, blood gases must be monitored because respiratory control is abnormal in dysautonomic patients. The ventilatory response to hypercapnia and hypoxia may be inappropriate, resulting in excessive carbon dioxide accumulation; this can be severe enough to cause coma and require assisted ventilation.

Because many of the respiratory problems are avoided when gastrointestinal dysfunction is well managed, patients who have had pneumonia require careful evaluation. For those individuals who misdirect swallows, advice should be provided as to which consistencies are safe or if gastrostomy is indicated. If the aspirations are believed to be secondary to gastroesophageal reflux, appropriate medications should be started or fundoplication performed.

Chest physiotherapy, consisting of postural drainage and inhalation of bronchodilators, is helpful not only in the acute situation but also as a daily routine for children with residual effects from previous aspirations or infections. Suctioning is often required in the individual who has an ineffective cough. Chest therapy should be administered at home by the parents on a regular basis. Chest surgery is rarely indicated, since the disease is usually diffuse. In patients with gastroesophageal reflux, xanthine derivatives are avoided.

Owing to the lack of appropriate response to hypoxia and hypercapnia, all dysautonomic patients must be cautious in settings where the partial pressure of oxygen is decreased, such as at high altitudes or during airplane travel. If the airplane's altitude exceeds 39,000 feet, the cabin pressure will be equivalent to more than 6000 feet and supplemental oxygen probably will be necessary. Diving and underwater swimming are also potential hazards and should be performed with care.

Breath-Holding (Seizures)

The phenomenon of prolonged breath-holding with crying is frequent in the early years. It has occurred at least one time in 63 per cent of patients. It can be severe enough to result in cyanosis, syncope, and seizure activity. This is due to lack of awareness that it is necessary for the next inspiration to be initiated; i.e., the patients are manifesting insensitivity to hypoxia and hypercapnia. This may become a manipulative maneuver with some children. Such an episode is frightening but self-limited and, in our experience, has never been fatal. The cyanosis of breath-holding must be differentiated from that which occurs with mucus plugs. These spells occur suddenly and can be associated with choking. Often the child will be pale and sweating and will require suctioning. Both types of cyanotic spells can produce seizure-like movements and decerebrate posturing. Electroencephalograms (EEGs) usually are normal or nonspecific, and the frequency of either type of spell is unaffected by anticonvulsant therapy.

About 25 per cent of FD patients have abnormal EEGs, but fewer than 10 per cent actually have a true seizure disorder. Within this special population of patients, the incidence of an abnormal EEG rises to 65 per cent. The average age of onset of seizures is 12 years. Anticonvulsant therapy should be used in these cases. The dosage of anticonvulsants is the same as for any other child. Most of the anticonvulsants are tolerated well.

Fever

Labile body temperatures result in brief, episodic fevers in response to dehydration, mucus plugs in the bronchi, excessive external temperature, and even stress. Fever is often preceded or accompanied by shaking chills, cold extremities, and lack of sweating. Antipyretics may not suffice. Cool extremities should be massaged while cooling the trunk by sponging or even with a hypothermic mattress.

A muscle relaxant often is helpful in reducing anxiety and muscular spasms during hyperpyrexia. Diazepam (0.1 mg/kg/dose) has been found effective.

Dysautonomic children are at greater risk for having febrile convulsions; 32 per cent will have at least one febrile seizure. However, the shaking and muscle spasms should not be considered febrile convulsions and should not be treated with anticonvulsant therapy. A persistent fever lasting more than 24 hours necessitates a search for a source of infection.

Spinal Curvature

Spinal curvature (kyphosis and/or scoliosis) develops in 95 per cent of dysautonomic patients by adolescence. Spinal curvature may start as early as 3 years or as late as 14 years. There may be rapid progression at any time. The completion of puberty generally halts the progression of scoliosis, as it does in the idiopathic adolescent form, but puberty is commonly delayed in dysautonomia. Spinal curvature further compromises respiratory function, adding the component of restrictive lung disease to interstitial disease.

Annual examination of the spine will allow early diagnosis of scoliosis and permit appropriate institution of brace and exercise therapy. The latter is helpful in correcting or preventing secondary contractures in shoulders and hips. Extreme care is required in fitting of braces because decubiti may develop on the dysautonomic patient's insensitive skin at pressure points. Braces may also inhibit respiratory excursion and induce gastroesophageal reflux if there is a high epigastric projection. If the brace is not successful in halting progression or if the curve is severe, spinal fusion is recommended.

Corneal Abrasions

Individuals with dysautonomia have diminished baseline eye moisture and do not cry with overflowing tears; this causes the eyes to be drier than normal. Treatment is directed toward keeping the eye as moist as possible because drying results in corneal damage or ulceration.

Corneal complications have been decreasing with the regular use of topical lubrications such as artificial tear solutions. These solutions often contain methylcellulose or are equivalent to hypotonic saline. Preparations without preservatives are also available. During sleep, a thicker preparation or an ointment may be used. The frequency with which tear solutions are instilled depends on the child's own baseline eye moisture and corneal sensitivity, which regulates the blink frequency. In addition, environmental conditions and the child's state of health are influencing factors. Moisture chamber attachments to spectacles and goggles have been used to help retain eye moisture and protect the eye from wind and foreign bodies.

If an abrasion does occur, the frequency of artificial tear use should increase. Often the eye can be helped by patching. Extreme care is necessary in applying a patch. To prevent the child from opening the eye under the patch and allowing the insensitive cornea to be damaged further by the patch, the eye should be taped closed first. Tarsorrhaphy of the medial or lateral part of the palpebral fissure has been reserved for unresponsive or chronic situations. An alternative to the patch is the soft contact lens, which applies gentle pressure and promotes healing. Other methods of increasing baseline moisture include tear duct cautery or narrowing the palpebral angles.

Tarsorrhaphy can be done on a temporary basis by use of glue on the lashes. Permanent tarsorrhaphy has been reserved for unresponsive and chronic situations. Corneal transplants have not been very successful.

Blood Pressure Lability

Orthostatic changes in blood pressure constitute a cardinal sign of autonomic insufficiency and are present in all patients with dysautonomia. Clinical manifestations of postural hypotension include episodes of lightheadedness or dizzy spells. Some patients complain of "weak legs." On occasion, there may be syncope. Symptoms tend to be worse in the morning, in hot or humid weather, when the bladder is full, prior to a large bowel movement, after a long car ride, coming out of a movie theater, or with fatigue. In general, low blood pressure is more troublesome during periods of rapid growth or in the adult years. Postural hypotension is treated by maintaining adequate hydration as monitored by BUN levels. Exercise of the lower extremity is encouraged to increase muscle tone and promote venous return. Elastic stockings and fludrocortisone (Florinef), a mineralocorticoid, have also been of some benefit.

When patients are agitated or in the supine position, blood pressures are often in the hypertensive range, but patients still demonstrate postural hypotension changes without compensatory tachycardia when the erect position is assumed. Hypertension can be quite striking during periods of stress. Because blood pressure is so labile, treatment should be directed to factors precipitating the hypertension rather than the use of blocking agents.

General anesthesia has caused profound hypotension and cardiac arrest. With greater attention to stabilization of the vascular bed by hydrating the patient prior to surgery and titrating the anesthetic, the risk of these problems can be greatly reduced.

Azotemia

It is not uncommon for patients to exhibit azotemia and variable values for creatinine clearance. Although clinical signs of dehydration may not be present, the urea nitrogen often can be reduced by simple hydration. Renal function appears to deteriorate with advancing age, so that about 20 per cent of adult patients have reduced renal function. Pathologic studies reveal excess glomerulosclerosis. Renal biopsy specimens from individuals with uncorrectable azotemia reveal significant ischemic-type glomerulosclerosis and deficient vascular innervation. The high prevalence of the renal lesion has been confirmed by retrospective analysis of autopsy material. Although the cause of the progressive renal disease is not certain, hypoperfusion of the kidney seems a likely explanation. Hypoperfusion may occur because of dehydration, postural hypotension, or vasoconstriction of renal vessels as a result of sympathetic supersensitivity during vomiting crises.

Patients are being encouraged to maintain adequate hydration, especially during warm weather. Treatment of postural hypotension has become more aggressive (see above), and blood pressures are carefully monitored during crises.

Anesthesia

Anesthesia for surgical procedures is associated with an increased risk because of extreme lability of blood pressure and diminished responsiveness to hypoxia and hypercapnia. Although local anesthesia with diazepam as preoperative sedation is preferred whenever possible, procedures requiring general anesthesia can be performed with less risk because homeostatic mechanisms in dysautonomia are now better understood.

Large amounts of epinephrine should not be infiltrated because of the exaggerated response to sympathomimetic drugs. Gas anesthetics have been useful because of the rapid reversibility of their effects. One of the most important factors in reducing risk is maintenance of an adequate circulating volume as vasodilatation during anesthesia may be extreme. The patient is prehydrated the night prior to surgery with intravenous fluids. Arterial blood pressures and blood gases are monitored throughout surgery via an arterial line. Hypotension should be corrected by decreasing the percentage of gas anesthetic and the provision of volume expanders. Rarely has a pressor, such as Neo-Synephrine, been required. Postoperative management can be extremely challenging. Gastric secretions tend to be copious during excitatory anesthetic phases. To avoid postoperative aspirations, ranitidine can be given and the stomach should be kept decompressed. Patients will require vigorous chest physiotherapy, as there is a tendency toward development of mucus plugs and exacerbation of pre-existing lung disease. Intubation may need to be extended until the respiratory status stabilizes or there is less reliance on pain medication. Visceral pain is appreciated so that narcotic pain medication may be required for intra-abdominal or intrathoracic procedures. In orthopedic cases, minimal pain medication is required.

Decreased Sensation (Injuries)

Although internal pain (e.g., stomachache, chest pain) is felt by dysautonomic children, pain and temperature sensations are diminished. Burns, pressure sores, and even broken bones may go unnoticed. Pain insensitivity also results in inadvertent trauma to joints. Charcot joints and aseptic necrosis have been reported. Swelling or mild discomfort with movement may be the only sign of a fracture.

As the children with dysautonomia do not instinctively avoid harmful situations, they must be taught to protect themselves. For example, thermometers can be used to test bathtub water temperature and the child can look for steam from a coffee cup. If there is any reason to believe a fracture has occurred, a radiograph should be taken. Care must be taken in casting, as in bracing, to prevent the development of pressure sores. If possible, complete immobilization should be avoided because children with neurologic problems experience muscle weakness rapidly with disuse. Chest physiotherapy during immobilization and physical therapy after the cast is removed are very important.

SUMMARY

Dysautonomia can no longer be considered only a disease of childhood. With greater understanding of the disorder and development of treatment programs, survival statistics have markedly improved, so that increasing numbers of patients are reaching adulthood. For this type of success to occur, a great deal of effort is necessary. The parents must cope with the care of a chronically handicapped child who may have repeated life-threatening crises. The physician has to become familiar with the varied manifestations of a multisystem disorder. The parents and child will rely on the long-term commitment of the physician for guidance, support, and reassurance.

REFERENCES

Axelrod FB, Donenfeld RF, Danziger F, Turndorf H: Anesthesia in familial dysautonomia. Anesthesiology 68:631–635, 1988.
Axelrod FB, Porges RF, Sein ME: Neonatal recognition of familial dysautonomia. J Pediatr 110:946–948, 1987.

REYE SYNDROME

FREDERICK H. LOVEJOY, JR., M.D.

In 1963 Reye and colleagues decribed a constellation of autopsy findings in children consisting of cerebral edema (without perivascular or meningeal inflammation) and fatty infiltration of the liver (and, to a lesser extent, the pancreas, kidneys, and heart). The disease, Reye syndrome, even today is of unclear etiology. Cases were recognized with increasing frequency throughout the 1970s, reached a peak incidence of 0.88 cases per 100,000 in 1980, followed by a progressive decline to 0.15 cases per 100,000 in 1985. Case fatality rates range from 10 to 40 per cent, with reduced mortality ascribed to early recognition and improved intensive care management.

Predominantly a childhood illness, the median age for cases is 8 years. A viral illness, generally varicella or influenza A or B, precedes. Since 1980, attention has focused on the strong association observed between Reye syndrome and aspirin, with the result that labeling of aspirin noting this association is now required by federal law.

Criteria for the diagnosis of Reye syndrome include:

1. A mild antecedent respiratory or gastrointestinal illness.
2. Hepatic dysfunction defined by a blood ammonia greater than 50 μ/dl or an increase in serum liver enzymes and a prolonged prothrombin time.
3. Objective evidence of central nervous system dysfunction (abnormalities on neurologic examination and electroencephalogram [EEG] with *normal* cerebrospinal fluid findings).
4. Liver biopsy revealing microvesicular fat with no displacement of the central nucleus and diagnostic mitochondrial alterations seen under electron microscopy.
5. Exclusion of other diseases with a similar clinical presentation (chronic salicylate and acute acetaminophen poisoning, viral encephalitis, lead poisoning, viral hepatitis).

A national staging system has been useful in describing the clinical and biochemical course and in following and grading its severity:

Stage I—lethargy, drowsiness, vomiting, elevation in serum liver enzymes, normal blood ammonia level, and grade I EEG (Lombroso grading).

Stage II—disorientation, combativeness, hyperventilation, tachycardia, pupillary dilation, hyperactive reflexes, purposeful response to painful stimuli, bilateral Babinski reflex, elevation in blood ammonia and serum liver enzymes, and grade II or III EEG.

Stage III—coma, upper midbrain involvement (loss of ciliospinal reflex, pupillary dilation, decorticate posturing in response to painful stimuli, bilateral Babinski reflex), persistent elevation in blood ammonia and serum liver enzymes, and grade III or IV EEG.

Stage IV—deepening coma, further rostrocaudal progression of midbrain involvement (loss of doll's head maneuver, sluggish pupillary response to light, decerebrate rigidity and posturing to painful stimuli, bilateral Babinski reflex), decreased blood ammonia and serum liver enzyme activity, and grade III or IV EEG.

Stage V—coma, loss of response to stimuli and to light or doll's head maneuver, cessation of spontaneous respiration, continued improvement in blood ammonia and serum liver enzyme activity, and grade IV or electrocerebral silence on EEG.

The disease occurs in several discrete stages and can be limited in severity to any stage. Recovery is invariable when illness is limited to stage I through III and recovery from stage V does not occur. Other indices associated with poor outcome include rapid passage through clinical stages, a blood ammonia level greater than 300 μ/dl, a prothrombin time two times greater than control, and an increase in liver and skeletal creatine phosphokinase.

Diagnosis is made by clinical and laboratory findings. A lumbar puncture is relatively contraindicated and should be preceded by cranial tomography to rule out cerebral edema. Liver biopsies should be reserved for patients in whom the diagnosis is unclear. Early diagnosis appears to improve clinical outcome. Suspicion should be raised in children who present with altered mental status and severe vomiting after a viral illness (varicella or use of aspirin).

TREATMENT

To date there is no specific treatment for Reye syndrome. Fluid and electrolyte balance and monitoring of increased intracranial pressure must be performed simultaneously. Because of the striking increase in arterial blood ammonia, lactulose and neomycin to decrease its generation by enteric bacteria and administration of citrulline and arginine have been used. There are no data indicating that these maneuvers affect outcome. Exchange transfusion and peritoneal dialysis have also been abandoned because of lack of change in outcome. Children with Reye syndrome are best cared for in a pediatric intensive care unit.

With the basic pathophysiologic derangement and cause of death being cerebral edema, therapy directed toward correcting this abnormal physiology has been pursued. The use of intracranial monitoring devices has made assessment of intracranial pressure more objective. With such devices, mannitol to maintain serum osmolarity between 300 and 320 mOSM/kg and nasotracheal intubation with ventilatory control to maintain P_{CO^2} between 20 and 30 mmHg can maintain the intracranial pressure below 15 torr and the cerebral perfusion pressure at 40 torr or better. These maneuvers are ideally instituted in stage II patients with ominous prognostic signs or in stage III patients. Steroids have not proved useful in managing (cytotoxic) cerebral edema. Barbiturate-induced coma has been used in cases of uncontrolled cerebral edema in an effort to decrease cerebral metabolic demands. A clear benefit from this approach has not been shown.

Other therapies for Reye syndrome include judicious use of fluids with dextrose concentrations of at least 10 per cent, vitamin K to correct prolonged prothrombin time, and phenytoin to control seizures. Children must have careful outpatient follow-up. They may recover fully neurologically but have behavioral and educational sequelae.

REFERENCES

Aoki Y, Lombroso CT: Prognostic value of electroencephalography in Reye's syndrome. Neurology 23:33, 1973.

Consensus Conference. Diagnosis and treatment of Reye's syndrome. JAMA 246:2441–2444, 1981.

NEUROBLASTOMA

DOUGLAS R. STROTHER, M.D.
and JAMES T. CASPER, M.D.

Neuroblastoma is a tumor of variable biologic behavior in that a subgroup of patients experience spontaneous regression of disease whereas another significant proportion fail to respond to intensive therapy. In order to understand better these differences in behavior, the molecular biology of neuroblastoma is being extensively studied. Although patient age and tumor stage have traditionally been the most important factors determining therapy and outcome, other indices, such as the DNA index and N-myc expression of the tumor, have recently been found to be of prognostic value and may be more important than clinical parameters. By incorporating new knowledge of this tumor into treatment planning, patients with lower stages of neuroblastoma may have an excellent chance of being cured with a minimum of therapy and newer strategies may be of benefit to the patients with advanced stages of disease. These issues are discussed in this article.

Neuroblastoma is the second most common solid tumor in childhood, with approximately 500 new cases diagnosed annually in the United States. The median age at the time of diagnosis is 2 years. The primary tumor is usually located in the thorax or abdomen. Metastases to bone marrow, bone, liver, and skin and to local, regional, or distant lymph nodes may occur. Knowledge of potential metastatic sites is crucial in determining the stage, or extent, of disease at diagnosis. The purpose of staging is to predict the likelihood of a lasting response to therapy and to select the treatment regimen that will provide the most favorable response with the minimum of adverse side effects.

Two staging systems presently used are those of Evans and of the Pediatric Oncology Group (POG), itself a revision of the St. Jude Children's Research Hospital staging system[1]; a new international staging system has been developed that combines features from both of these.[2] Briefly, POG designates *stage A* as complete gross excision of all tumor. Intracavitary lymph nodes and the liver must be free of disease. *Stage B* indicates incomplete excision of tumor with lymph nodes and liver free of disease as in stage A. *Stage C* patients have regional lymph node metastases, and *stage D* patients have disease spread beyond intracavitary regional lymph nodes (i.e., distant nodes, bone, bone marrow). Based on POG staging, the likelihood of long-term survival for patients with stages A, B, C, and D disease are 92, 80, 50, and 15 per cent, respectively. The infant with POG stage DS (metastatic disease sparing bone) has an 85 per cent chance of long-term survival.

EVALUATION

A patient suspected of having neuroblastoma should be referred to a pediatric cancer center for confirmation of the diagnosis and therapy planning. Treatment of this disease requires an interdisciplinary team with experience in childhood cancer. Staging must include computed tomography (CT) or magnetic resonance imaging (MRI) of the primary lesion, bone scan, skeletal survey, evaluation of the liver with CT scan, bone marrow aspiration from at least two sites, complete blood count with differential, and a chemistry profile, looking especially at levels of serum lactate dehydrogenase. Urinary catecholamine levels may be elevated and used as a tumor marker, and they should also be determined at diagnosis.

In Japan, screening of young infants for elevated levels of urinary catecholamines has been advocated as a means to detect neuroblastoma at early stages. Surgical removal of neuroblastoma has been curative for affected children identified in this manner. Whether the overall incidence of neuroblastoma can be decreased through such screening or whether it is simply that curable patients are detected at an earlier age remains to be seen.

The diagnosis is usually confirmed by tissue biopsy of the primary tumor. In children with extensive disease, however, bone marrow aspirates unequivocally demonstrating tumor along with elevated urinary catecholamines are adequate for diagnosis; these patients do not need a thoracotomy or laparotomy to obtain additional tissue for diagnosis.

Once the diagnosis is confirmed, the patient will be treated according to a clinical therapeutic protocol, or treatment plan. Referral of a patient to a pediatric cancer center and subsequent placement of the patient on a cooperative group clinical protocol are crucial for continuing to increase our knowledge of the tumor and therapy. Protocols are based on knowledge gathered up to the moment; physicians and parents can feel confident that they are giving and receiving, respectively, state-of-the-art comprehensive cancer care.

TREATMENT

Surgery

The role of surgery in neuroblastoma therapy differs with the patient's stage of disease. For patients in whom it is necessary, surgery will serve to confirm the diagnosis and to procure tissue for biologic studies. For patients with localized, potentially resectable tumor, total gross resection of the tumor should be encouraged because it may render the patient to stage A. In these patients, microscopic residual tumor does not appear to be important for survival because more than 90 per cent of stage A patients are cured of disease with surgery alone. For patients with larger tumors, maximum surgery is recommended, but not that which is disfiguring or potentially life-threatening. Residual gross disease (POG stage B) is usually responsive to multiagent chemotherapy that is well tolerated by patients. Radical surgery for these patients at diagnosis, therefore, is not indicated.

For the patient with clearly unresectable disease on the basis of size or location or in a patient with regional lymph node or other distant metastases, surgery should not be so extensive as to delay or interfere with potentially curative chemotherapy and/or radiotherapy. These patients require intensive, multiagent chemotherapy; in many, a second operation may then be feasible to totally remove or substantially debulk residual tumor. Second-look surgery is also helpful to identify residual masses, because it is possible for therapy to induce maturational changes to ganglioneuroma, a benign tumor for which additional intensive treatment is not indicated.

Chemotherapy

The chemotherapeutic agents most active against neuroblastoma appear to be cyclophosphamide, doxorubicin, *cis*-platinum, and etoposide. Melphalan, vincristine, dacarbazine, and teniposide are also used. Therapy is limited primarily by myelosuppression; more serious late effects on hearing and renal function may occur after *cis*-platinum. Relatively benign chemotherapy may be used to treat the lower-stage patients (stages A and B) with excellent results. For the advanced-stage patient, more intensive chemotherapy is the backbone of treatment. Intensification in recent protocols, however, has primarily lengthened the period of disease-free survival rather than increased the cure rate. Unfortunately, only 10 to 15 per cent of stage D patients are truly cured. A new strategy has been used recently in the POG to test phase II agents in newly diagnosed patients. In an "up-front window," two courses of the test drug are given and the patient is then evaluated for response prior to placement on a standard protocol. This strategy has identified ifosfamide and carboplatinum (a *cis*-platinum analog) as excellent agents against neuroblastoma. Different combinations of well-known drugs or increased intensity of drug dose may provide additional improvement in treatment results. The use of colony-stimulating factors (G-CSF, GM-CSF) may help to alleviate the dose-limiting myelosuppression that occurs with most of these chemotherapy agents.

The infant with stage DS disease, that is, one with metastatic disease sparing bone, may be chosen for observation as initial treatment or to receive chemotherapy immediately. Long-term survival rates are similar for those treated at diagnosis and those treated only at progression of disease. Further insight into intrinsic tumor characteristics may help to better define those children whose tumors are likely to regress spontaneously without chemotherapy. Why the child older than 1 year of age with equivalent disease has a significantly poorer prognosis is not fully understood.

Radiation Therapy

For the infant with stage DS disease, low-dose radiation instead of chemotherapy has been given with equivalent results. The use of radiation in the very young child must be carefully considered in the context of late term effects, particularly somatic. For patients with higher stages of disease, radiation may be used to decrease tumor bulk to render the tumor more amenable to surgical resection. For patients older than the age of 1 year with POG stage C disease, the early use of radiation therapy with chemotherapy provides superior disease control when compared with the same stage with chemotherapy used alone. Occasionally, children may present with tumors impinging on the spinal cord and compromising cord function. Radiation therapy and chemotherapy are equivalent in the immediate management of these patients. Subsequent vertebral body abnormalities may result from irradiation of the very young child and may be avoided by the use of chemotherapy. Finally, radiation may be used for palliation as well, particularly to control pain caused by tumor metastatic to bone.

Bone Marrow Transplantation

The use of autologous or matched allogeneic bone marrow transplantation for advanced-stage disease has been increasing steadily as a form of consolidating therapy. Early results were encouraging and have prompted larger cooperative group trials. Unfortunately, long-term results from European trials have identified relapses in patients 4 to 5 years after their transplants. In transplantation regimens, patients are treated prior to marrow infusion with intensive chemotherapy, debulking surgery, radiation therapy, and myeloablative chemotherapy with agents known to be active against neuroblastoma but whose doses are limited by myelosuppression.

Alkylating agents, such as cyclophosphamide, melphalan, and, more recently, thiotepa, form the bases of such treatment.

Biologic Factors

The amount of genetic material (chromosomes) within the neuroblastoma cell may be equivalent to or exceed that of the patient's normal cells. The DNA Index (DI) is the ratio of the amount of DNA present within the resting tumor cell (cell phase G_0) to that of the normal resting cell. This ratio appears to have prognostic significance in a subgroup of neuroblastoma patients. Specifically, a DI of greater than 1 may portend a better prognosis for long-term survival than a DI equal to 1. The importance of this ratio may exceed that of age and stage and may help to identify those patients, particularly infants under the age of 1 year, who will require more intensive therapy to achieve a disease-free status.

An area on the short arm of chromosome number 2, known as the N-myc oncogene, appears to be involved in the genesis of neuroblastoma. N-myc may be expressed (may be present) in the tumor cell in single or multiple copies. Like the DI, the copy number of N-myc has prognostic value. When present in more than a single copy in the tumor cells, prognosis for patients is very poor. Again, these patients may be selected for more intensive or experimental therapy.

Because a significant proportion of patients with neuroblastoma are not cured, other treatment modalities have been explored. These include the use of biologic response modifiers (BRM) such as monoclonal antibodies and interleukin-2. Monoclonal antibody has been generated to cell surface antigens of human neuroblasts, which are in many cases a ganglioside. Responses have been noted in patients treated with monoclonal antibody alone. Because the monoclonals are developed from mouse hybridomas, one problem in the clinical use of these antibodies has been the development of human anti-mouse antibodies in the patient. The development of chimeric human-mouse monoclonals may alleviate this problem.

Another BRM, interleukin-2, is also being clinically tested as a single agent in combination with tumor-infiltrating lymphocytes (TILs) and in combination with a monoclonal antibody.

Differentiation agents, most notably *cis*-retinoic acid, have been associated with limited anecdotal responses. The recent success of *trans*-retinoic acid in inducing remissions in patients with promyelocytic leukemia may open the way for using this agent against neuroblastoma.

SUMMARY

Therapy for patients with neuroblastoma is evolving with our growing knowledge of the intrinsic biologic characteristics of the tumor. The importance of having every patient with this diagnosis enrolled in prospective, multi-institutional studies cannot be overemphasized. Only through that experience can new prognostic factors and effective therapies be identified. For infants and for children with lower-stage disease, therapy will focus on reducing adverse long-term effects without compromising outcome. For the child with metastatic disease, continuing exploration of new and existing treatment modalities is needed to improve survival.

REFERENCES

1. Hayes FA, Green A, Hustu O, et al: Surgicopathologic staging of neuroblastoma: Prognostic significance of regional lymph node metastases. J Pediatr 102:59–62, 1983.
2. Brodeur GM, Seeger RC, Barrett A, et al: International criteria for diagnosis, staging, and response to treatment in patients with neuroblastoma. J Clin Oncol 6:1874–1881, 1988.

BREATH-HOLDING SPELLS

ISRAEL F. ABROMS, M.D.

Breath-holding spells occur in 4 to 5 per cent of all children. The more common form is the cyanotic or "blue spell." This occurs following an emotional event and vigorous crying. The child holds his or her breath, becomes cyanotic, and loses consciousness. The last is probably due to hypoxic ischemia involving the brain stem. Occasionally, a generalized tonic-clonic seizure may occur, followed by limpness. Breath-holding spells usually occur between the ages of 4 months and 4 years. Occasionally, they persist to 6 years of age. The frequency of cyanotic breath-holding spells can be reduced if a concomitant anemia (usually an iron-deficiency anemia) is treated with oral iron preparations. A misdiagnosis of epilepsy can be made, but the electroencephalogram (EEG) in cyanotic breath-holding spells is normal.

There is no specific treatment for cyanotic breath-holding spells; parents need to be reassured that these episodes will eventually disappear. Some parents are reluctant to discipline their child when necessary for fear of precipitating a cyanotic breath-holding episode. It is most important that the child's consultant address this issue by reassuring the family that they should treat this child as any other.

A less frequent type of breath-holding spell is the *pallid form,* also called a "vagal attack." The child often has a mild injury, and within seconds, even without any true breath-holding, pallor, bradycardia, and unconsciousness will develop. Because of cerebral hypoxic ischemia, a generalized tonic-clonic seizure may ensue followed by limpness. Often there is a family history of syncope. Occasionally, prolonged seizures occur. This usually is associated with a family history of a lowered seizure threshold.

The EEG in these children is normal. With electrocardiographic (EKG) monitoring, ocular compression for 10 seconds performed during the EKG may result in bradycardia or even asystole that will last beyond 4 seconds. This test is not always confirmatory, however, and should be performed with care because prolonged asystole can occur.

A fair number of children exhibit both the cyanotic and pallid forms of breath-holding spells. An EKG or a prolonged period of Holter monitoring may be required to distinguish these from cardiac events.

In the pallid form, the differential diagnosis should include cardiac arrhythmias, such as sinus node dysfunction with either bradyarrhythmia or tachyarrhythmia. Sinus node disease occurs following surgical correction of congenital heart defects or may be associated with neuromuscular disorders, such as myotonic dystrophy, limb girdle muscular dystrophy, or Friedreich's ataxia in the older child. Cardiac inflammatory disorders need to be ruled out, such as acute rheumatic fever, viral myocarditis, and diphtheria. However, in many patients with sinus node disease, no definitive etiology is recognized. Intermittent atrial ventricular block may be present and the syndrome of prolonged Q-T interval may be found on the EKG. The latter can be associated with congenital nerve deafness. It is frequently familial with the disturbing history of recurrent seizures and sudden cardiac deaths.

If any of these cardiac conditions are suspected, the child requires a cardiologic consultation, an EKG, and an echocardiogram. Radiologic studies may be indicated.

If pallid breath-holding spells are occurring frequently, the infant or child may benefit from treatment with oral atropine sulfate (0.01 to 0.02 mg two or three times daily). Occasionally, these spells are so prolonged that the infant requires a cardiac pacemaker.

4

Respiratory System

CHOANAL ATRESIA

WILLIAM P. POTSIC, M.D.

Choanal atresia occurs in approximately 1 in 7000 live births, is more common in females, and is most frequently unilateral. The atresia plate is most often bony but may be membranous. A computed tomographic (CT) scan best defines the configuration of the nasal cavity and atresia plate. Unilateral choanal atresia creates no acute problem, and repair can be performed to eliminate unilateral rhinorrhea before the child enters school. Bilateral choanal atresia causes acute respiratory distress immediately after birth, and an oral airway is required. A neonatal oral airway tied or taped in place relieves the airway obstruction, and orogastric tube feeding maintains hydration.

After the child is stable for a few days, surgical correction is performed using general anesthesia. If there are other conditions that make general anesthesia unwise, the child can be managed with the oral airway and tube feeding until mouth breathing occurs at 4 to 6 weeks of age.

The surgical correction is accomplished using microsurgical or endoscopic techniques to open the atresia plate by the transnasal route. Stents are sutured in place and left for 6 weeks. During the time in which the stents are in place, they are kept patent with saline washes and suction. After the stents are removed, a few choanal dilatations are usually required to keep the choanae open.

If the transnasal correction and dilatations are unsuccessful in keeping the choanae open, a transpalatal correction is performed. The transpalatal approach, although a more extensive operation, provides greater exposure to open the choanae by removing the surrounding bone.

TUMORS AND POLYPS OF THE NOSE

WILLIAM P. POTSIC, M.D.

Tumors of the nose are uncommon in children and adolescents. Benign tumors, such as hemangiomas and lymphangiomas, are the most frequently seen but are rarely confined to the nose itself. They usually are nasal extensions of larger lesions in the region of the nose. Hemangiomas and lymphangiomas may be debulked surgically to relieve nasal obstruction and to improve the appearance of the nose.

Intranasal papillomas are found in the nasal vestibule and are easily removed by local excision. Occasionally, granulomas from trauma (nose picking or nasal foreign body) or granulomatous diseases are found. These are removed by curettage and cauterization.

Fibro-osseous tumors of the facial skeleton may present in the nose or impinge on the nasal cavity, causing airway obstruction. These tumors should be surgically excised. Other extremely rare benign tumors may occur and should be excised or a biopsy specimen obtained for histologic diagnosis.

Malignant tumors are rarely confined to the nasal cavity and frequently remain undiagnosed for months to years. In their early phases, they mimic benign conditions like nasal congestion. Rhabdomyosarcoma and lymphoma are the most common of these malignancies. They usually are extensive in the sinuses and nasal cavity. Computed tomography and biopsy of these tumors direct a multidisciplinary, multimodality therapeutic approach. Surgery for residual or recurrent disease may be required. Neuroblastoma also necessitates surgical excision, and additional treatment modalities may be needed.

Nasal polyps in children and adolescents are caused by chronic inflammation that may indicate the presence of cystic fibrosis, chronic infection, or allergic rhinitis. Nasal polyps may shrink temporarily with the use of nasal steroid sprays, but surgical therapy is usually required to relieve nasal obstruction. Treatment of the underlying medical conditions predisposing to polyposis prevents or delays recurrence.

Intranasal functional endoscopic sinus surgery is utilized to remove nasal polyps and clear the underlying sinus cells of disease. Computed tomography is essential to the surgeon to define the involved sinuses and extent of the disease. Antrochoanal polyps have their origin in the maxillary sinus. A maxillary sinusotomy (Caldwell-Luc) may be needed to release the attachments to the lateral wall of the sinus.

NASAL INJURIES AND EPISTAXIS

MICHAEL J. CUNNINGHAM, M.D.

NASAL INJURIES

Pediatric nasal injuries are best divided into those that occur at birth and those that occur later in childhood.

Minor injuries to the nose, principally dislocation of the septum, can occur during delivery. A grossly disfigured nose warrants consultation. Many neonatal septal deviations can be corrected by manual manipulation or simple closed reduction. Nasal disfigurements not responsive to these conservative treatments should be given a chance for spontaneous improvement. Surgical intervention should be considered only for those infants with severe functional airway compromise as a result of the nasal deformity.

In contrast to an adult's nose, the child's nose has less frontal projection and the framework is proportionately more cartilaginous than bony. Isolated nasal injuries in children principally involve the cartilaginous structures; a bony nasal complex fracture tends to occur more often in the setting of significant maxillofacial trauma.

In children with nasal injuries, it is initially necessary to ensure an adequate airway, arrest any associated epistaxis, and assess for any associated soft tissue trauma. The nose, facial bones, and cranium should be gently palpated. Examination of the nares using either an otoscope or speculum and headlight is necessary to rule out a septal hematoma, which, if present, requires drainage. This evaluation can usually be performed in an ambulatory setting. Severe midfacial swelling, extensive soft tissue injury, or fulminant epistaxis may dictate an assessment using general anesthesia, especially in an uncooperative younger child. Radiographic assessment is useful in generalized maxillofacial trauma but is of little help in isolated nasal injuries.

Traumatic nasal deformities that significantly interfere with respiration should be corrected. Such injuries, if left untreated, can result in abnormal nasal development and anatomic airway obstruction in later years. Conservative surgical management includes repositioning the septal cartilage and nasal bones; resection of cartilage or bone is avoided unless absolutely necessary. Sublabial and external approaches provide better visualization and access to the nasal structures when more extensive septorhinoplasty work is required.

In the absence of functional compromise or gross nasal deformity, observation is the rule. Correction of minor cosmetic deformities is typically delayed until ages 16 to 18 years in boys and 15 to 17 years in girls. Anticipated participation in contact sports as well as social and developmental maturity all play a role in the timing of such an operative decision for each particular child.

EPISTAXIS

Epistaxis in children between the ages of 2 and 10 years is a common problem. It is rarely encountered during infancy and becomes less prevalent after puberty. There are many potential local and systemic causes of epistaxis. The vast majority of childhood cases, however, occur secondary to inflammation and excoriation of the anterior septal nasal mucosa. This region is highly vascular and is within direct reach of a child's finger during nose picking or rubbing. Such local trauma enhances the possibility of bleeding from inflamed mucosa.

The evaluation of a child with epistaxis begins with a careful history. Inflammatory, infectious, and traumatic causes are often bilateral and readily diagnosed with proper questioning. Antecedent unilateral nasal obstruction suggests an anatomic abnormality, mass lesion, or foreign body. Children with systemic diseases, including bleeding disorders, usually report additional signs and symptoms. Epistaxis, however, may be the sole initial manifestation of an underlying bleeding diathesis. A drug exposure history is also important. Many systemic medications may impair hemostasis, and both the excessive overuse of topical vasoconstrictor medications and the use of recreational drugs like cocaine and cannabis can cause local mucosal irritation.

The initial physical examination should include vital signs with blood pressure determination in addition to a careful anterior inspection of the nose. A halogen-illuminated otoscope with a large speculum is sufficient for this purpose. A detailed examination of the posterior nares and nasopharynx by an otolaryngology consultant is warranted in cases of recurrent and persistent bleeding or local and systemic disease concerns. Certain screening laboratory tests—a complete blood count, platelet count, bleeding time, prothrombin time, and partial thromboplastin time—can be useful when the history is suggestive of a bleeding diathesis. More specialized blood work, radiographs, and histopathologic studies should be ordered as needed with the assistance of the appropriate consultant.

Uncomplicated anterior epistaxis most often stops spontaneously or responds to conservative measures, such as head elevation and firm local pressure by pinching of the nose for 5 to 10 minutes. Such pressure may need to be applied successively two or three times. The child should be encouraged to sit with his or her head forward to avoid bleeding into the pharynx with its possible risk of aspiration.

A child who does not respond to these simple measures requires a careful nasal examination to identify the site and cause of bleeding. Again, it needs to be emphasized that the location will be the anterior septal region in the vast majority of children. Good lighting is mandatory. This is best provided by a headlight that also frees up both hands for holding necessary instruments. Pledgets soaked in either 1:10,000 epinephrine, 0.25 per cent phenylephrine, or 0.025 per cent oxymetazoline are firmly applied for mucosal shrinkage and hemostasis; topical 4 per cent lidocaine or 1 per cent tetracaine can be added for local anesthesia; 4 per cent cocaine solution is an alternative agent that achieves both these effects. Topical anesthesia enhances the child's cooperation and is absolutely necessary if topical cauterization proves necessary. *Most cases of uncomplicated anterior septal mucosal bleeding will respond to these measures following the suction removal of old blood and secretions.* If a specific focal point of hemorrhage persists, chemical cautery with a silver nitrate stick may be attempted. Diffuse cauterization of the anterior septal region should *not* be performed. Young children in whom a sufficient nasal examination is not possible or an older child with a very large septal vessel that does not respond to chemical cautery may occasionally require an examination under anesthesia for selective electrocautery and hemorrhage control.

Immediately following epistaxis control by any of the above methods, some form of packing to prevent recurrent hemorrhage and promote mucosal healing is applied. Absorbable packing, such as gelatin sponge (Gelfoam) or oxidized cellulose (Surgicel), is preferred. This obviates the need for packing removal, which in and of itself can be traumatic to local tissues. This is a particularly important issue in hematologically compromised children in whom the slightest amount of nasal mucosal manipulation may promote further bleeding. Coating the Gelfoam or Surgicel with microfibrillar collagen flakes (Avitene) or topical thrombin (Thrombostat) may provide additional hemostasis in these patients.

Children rarely require the placement of a standard anterior or posterior nares pack using petroleum jelly (Vaseline)–impregnated gauze ribbon, an absorbable nasal tampon, or a commercial balloon catheter device. Any child who requires packing of this nature should be hospitalized to allow initiation of antibiotic therapy as sinusitis prophylaxis and to avoid complete sedation, thereby preventing airway obstruction. Thorough pediatric and otolaryngologic work-up is necessary to determine the source of bleeding because the suspicion of a local or systemic neoplastic process is high in such children.

The nasal packing removal in such cases should be performed in the operating room. Arterial ligation of the anterior ethmoid, internal maxillary, and/or external carotid arteries or angiography with selective embolization of the involved vessels is an alternative therapy that may be necessary in refractory cases.

The prevention of recurrent bleeding depends on the underlying etiology. Local mucosal excoriation is treated by behavioral control to avoid finger trauma, daytime applications of saline mist, nighttime bedside humidifier use, and the direct application of antibiotic ointments to the anterior septal mucosa. Allergic rhinitis is treated best with allergen avoidance and desensitization therapy. The abuse of topical vasoconstrictor agents or recreational drugs is treated by discontinuing the offending agent and instituting intranasal steroids. Anatomic abnormalities may require surgical correction, and systemic or hematologic disorders require the expertise of the appropriate pediatric specialist(s). In children with hereditary hemorrhagic telangiectasia or refractory bleeding diatheses who fail to respond to all conservative measures, septal dermoplasty with resurfacing of the anterior nasal cavity with skin or dermal grafts is an alternative surgical option.

REFERENCES

Nasal Injuries

Gussack GS, Luterman A, Powell RW, et al: Pediatric maxillofacial trauma: Unique features in diagnosis and treatment. Laryngoscope 97:925–930, 1987.

Farrior RT, Connolly ME: Septorhinoplasty in children. Otolaryngol Clin North Am 3:345–364, 1970.

Epistaxis

Keen M: The Avitene pack: A new method to control epistaxis in a patient with poor platelet function. Laryngoscope 96:1411, 1986.

Koltai PJ: Nose bleeds in the hematologically and immunologically compromised child. Laryngoscope 94:114–115, 1984.

Letson JA, Binck HG: Septal dermoplasty for von Willebrand's disease in children. Laryngoscope 83:1078–1083, 1973.

FOREIGN BODIES IN THE NOSE AND PHARYNX

SYLVAN E. STOOL, M.D.

The variety of materials that young children can insert or ingest into the air and food passages is endless. Several general principles should be emphasized in this regard. Prevention is preferable to remediation. The physician should suspect foreign body in any diagnostic dilemma or enigma involving the nose and throat and should not make the situation worse with inappropriate manipulation.

The symptoms and signs are influenced by the nature of the material, its composition and size, and the duration in situ. Organic and porous materials usually cause a foul smell, especially when they have been lodged in the nose for prolonged periods. In contrast, plastic and many metals may remain in place for long periods without causing intense inflammation or odor. Eventually, a mass may develop that will cause obstruction and granulation tissue with bleeding. In many instances, the foreign body causes unilateral nasal discharge; however, if the foreign body is in the nasopharynx, the drainage may be bilateral. A major difficulty in the diagnosis is that the incident is infrequently witnessed and the young child does not inform the parents of the event.

Radiographic examination is of value if the object is radiopaque. In some instances, inflammatory reaction surrounding the object may be a clue to the nature of the foreign body.

When the physician is evaluating or attempting to remove a foreign body, it is wise to advise the parents that the examination will be an assessment and not to promise that the object will be removed. The examination may be difficult in young children, as they may be frightened and uncooperative. It is mandatory that the examiner control the situation by restraint, sedation, or general anesthesia. Adequate illumination is necessary. Most physicians are familiar with using the otoscope, and this may be a satisfactory examination instrument with a speculum of adequate size. In many instances, it is desirable to have a head light with coaxial illumination.

Instruments that should be available include a nasal speculum, a small alligator forceps that can grasp the leading edge of a foreign body, and a hook that can be inserted into soft foreign bodies. In all instances in which foreign bodies will be removed, suction should be available to remove secretions or blood so that the object can be adequately visualized. Physicians are familiar with cerumen curets; these may be helpful with small or soft foreign bodies.

Small infants may feel comfortable sitting on the parent's lap. The parent should immobilize the child by putting his or her arm across the child's chest and holding the child's forehead with the other hand. It may be necessary to wrap the child in a sheet, and in recent years the Olympic papoose board has been of value in immobilizing the child. After the child is adequately immobilized, vasoconstrictor can be instilled into the nose so that it is easier to visualize the foreign body. At that time, the foreign body should be inspected and a decision must be made. If the physician is not sure that the foreign body can be removed, it is better to stop at this point and provide general anesthesia or refer the patient so that extraction can be performed.

When the foreign body is visualized in the nose, it may be very mobile. Therefore, it is desirable to get either the hook or curet behind it and pull forward so that the foreign body can be removed from the nares. In some instances when the foreign body has been pulled forward, application of suction will aid in its removal. Foreign bodies that appear to have a leading edge and are soft enough to permit a hook to be inserted or an alligator to be applied are usually relatively easy to remove.

Foreign bodies in the mouth and pharynx may constitute a life-threatening event—especially objects that are round, such as balls and marbles, and foreign bodies that conform, such as balloons. Both of these types of foreign bodies have resulted in suffocation.

Prevention is certainly desirable in dealing with foreign bodies. Parents should be counseled that children younger than 3 years of age should be prevented from playing with these objects. A cylinder test fixture available for small parts can be purchased from many toy stores and is designed so that if the small part fits within the cylinder, it should not be in the hands of children under 3 years of age. The Consumer Product Safety Commission monitors many of the toys; however, some toys are imported and do not come to the Commission's attention.

When a foreign body is lodged in the pharynx of a young child, it is most important that the object not be pushed further down, possibly causing respiratory obstruction. One should first ascertain whether respiration is adequate. If respiration is not adequate and if there is obstruction, blows on the back or turning the child upside down with back blows may dislodge it. In some instances, a subdiaphragmatic thrust, which is a modification of the Heimlich maneuver, can be used to dislodge the foreign body so that the airway is adequate. Obviously, with pharyngeal and hypopharyngeal foreign bodies it is most important to protect the airway.

When a foreign body is observed, it is important to ascertain whether adequate instrumentation and visualization are available. Usually, the physician has only one good opportunity to remove a foreign body in a young child and the first attempt is the one that is most likely to succeed. Therefore, the approach to a foreign body in the pharynx is similar to that in the nose. If a leading edge can be visualized and grasped with forceps, the object usually is easily removed. Hard or round foreign objects should be removed by inserting an instrument behind them and pulling forward. In some instances, the use of Foley catheters to remove foreign bodies in the hypopharynx has been advocated; however, it probably should not be attempted unless enough support personnel are available to establish an airway if the foreign body occludes the upper respiratory passages.

It is not unusual for multiple foreign bodies to occur in a child's air passages, and it is wise if anesthesia is employed for the removal of a foreign body to inspect other areas for concomitant objects. When radiographic examination is performed, the region from the nasopharynx to the pelvis should be included; when general anesthesia is employed, the nose, nasopharynx, and oropharynx should be examined.

NASOPHARYNGITIS

LEWIS R. FIRST, M.D.

Nasopharyngitis, or "the common cold," characterized by inflammation and congestion of the nasal passages and oral pharynx, is perhaps the most frequent illness occurring in childhood. Symptoms consist of nasal discharge, sore throat, malaise, low-grade fever, sneezing, and cough (particularly at night) and are primarily attributed to more than 200 viruses, with rhinovirus, parainfluenza virus, and respiratory syncytial virus (RSV) being the most common instigators of the illness.

Nasopharyngitis occurs anywhere from three to eight times per year in children and approximately two to four times a year in adults. The incidence may increase by 50 per cent if the child is in day care and may also increase in the setting of parental smoking or crowding in a home environment. When nasopharyngitis is due to a viral origin, it usually spreads by respiratory secretions or via contact between nasal secretions and a susceptible person.

An approach to appropriate therapy for nasopharyngitis is based on an understanding of the physiology of the disease process following inoculation by a virus that will in turn invade the epithelia of the nasopharynx, sinuses, and upper respiratory tract. Such invasion results in release of inflammatory mediators in nasal secretions that will increase vascular permeability in the nasal cavity, resulting in mucosal edema, nasal stuffiness, and, subsequently, rhinorrhea. In addition, cholinergic stimulation precipitated by epithelial invasion results in increased mucus production, enhancing the rhinorrhea and facilitating postnasal drip, and subsequent cough. Finally, direct cellular damage to the nasopharyngeal cavity can result in localized inflammation and sore throat. The cough functions on a reflex basis to help clear debris and secretions from the inflamed areas. Cough should not be suppressed in the acute phase of nasopharyngitis. Otherwise, posterior nasal drainage could progress downward to involve the lower respiratory tract, creating mucus plugging and worsening pulmonary disease.

It is important to realize that purulent nasal drainage, which usually occurs in nasopharyngitis, follows at least 2 to 3 days of nasal irritation, scratchy throat, and clear rhinorrhea and does not necessarily signify a bacterial superinfection. It may simply be the result of resolving inflammation of epithelial cells from the inflamed area. A bacterial superinfection can occur, however, particularly if there is a change in the character and severity of the illness late in its stage, i.e., toward the end of 5 to 7 days. Such a bacterial superinfection usually results in a complication in an area of the upper respiratory or lower respiratory tract surrounding the nasopharynx. For example, it is not uncommon to see otitis media, sinusitis, pneumonia, bronchitis, or asthma follow an episode of nasopharyngitis. Although a bacterial source might be a primary etiologic factor in nasopharyngitis, this is extremely rare. In fact, bacterial growth on a nasopharyngeal culture does not necessarily represent a pathogen but, rather, an "innocent bystander" or carrier organism. For example, culture specimens of *Streptococcus pneumoniae* may be obtained from the nasopharynx in an equal number of patients with or without respiratory symptoms.

DIAGNOSIS

Diagnosis of nasopharyngitis is based largely on a fairly classic history consisting initially of nasal irritation, scratchy throat, followed by progressive, clear bilateral nasal discharge, sneezing, and cough (often worse at night) over the initial week of the illness. The color and thickness of nasal discharge cannot help one to differentiate a bacterial from a viral illness. Usually, the posterior pharynx shows extensive erythema or sometimes ulcerative lesions, but it lacks exudate. Therefore, in the presence of significant rhinorrhea without an oral pharynx full of exudate, throat cultures and nasopharyngeal cultures for bacteria are usually not indicated because bacteria are not likely pathogens and antibiotic therapy is not required. Given the usual brief duration of the symptoms, which usually resolve spontaneously, it is not cost-effective to diagnose a particular viral etiology because routine therapy is not directed toward a specific pathogen.

Other diagnostic possibilities, however, do need to be considered. Group A streptococcal illness is usually not associated with nasal symptoms in children over 5 years of age. A nasal foreign body is usually associated with unilateral rhinorrhea. A Wright stain of a nasal swab for eosinophils may help to confirm a diagnosis of allergic rhinitis, an entity often considered in the differential diagnosis of nasopharyngitis. In an unimmunized child who has rhinorrhea and subsequent cough, the diagnosis of pertussis should be considered. If the child has been symptomatic with very copious, thick, discolored discharge and/or fevers, headaches, facial pain, or swelling, one might consider the possibility of sinusitis.

TREATMENT

Nonpharmacologic Therapy

Before pharmacologic therapy is discussed here, it is important to remember that nonpharmacologic therapy can also bring relief of symptoms, particularly in infants and young children. For example, good hydration allows better clearing of nasal secretions. If the infant appears unable to feed because of nasal stuffiness, a bulb syringe can help to remove some of the thicker or drier secretions. Clearing of secretions can be further assisted by the use of saline nose drops, which can be either purchased over the counter under a variety of trade names or made at home using 1 teaspoon of salt in 8 ounces of water. Two drops are applied to one nostril at a time and allowed to sit in the back of the nose for 2 to 3 minutes prior to suctioning, at which point the drops are applied to the other nostril. Saline nose drops can be useful before meals and before the child goes to sleep. In addition, elevating the head of the bed or putting books under the head of the crib can enhance posterior nasal drainage. A child with a sore throat can certainly benefit from warm saline gargles and, if necessary, over-the-counter throat lozenges, which lubricate and soothe the surface of the posterior pharynx. Finally, the addition of a cool mist vaporizer or humidifier can also prevent the drying of nasal secretions and subsequent nasal obstruction.

From a prevention standpoint, it is appropriate to reinforce measures such as avoidance of smoking and good hand washing to prevent the spread of nasopharyngitis. One cannot exclude all children with colds from day care, and there is really no contraindication to their presence, assuming that day care providers continue to practice careful hand washing throughout the course of the day. Although there is some suggestion that breast-feeding may provide some immunologic protection, this practice has not been noted to be particularly effective in decreasing the frequency or duration of nasopharyngitis. The use of alpha$_2$-interferon intranasally may be helpful in decreasing an acquired rhinovirus infection when there is a primary exposure to another household member but has not been found to benefit other respiratory viruses.

Pharmacologic Therapy

If a child appears to be well hydrated with no evidence of respiratory distress due to significant nasal obstruction, no further therapy is needed beyond that mentioned above. However, should the child experience discomfort from fever, congestion, rhinorrhea, or cough, pharmacotherapy might be considered. The nature of pharmacotherapy should be symptom-specific rather than a broad combination of decongestants and antipyretics.

The four classes of pharmacotherapy available as over-the-counter agents are shown in Table 1. Multiagent decongestants usually do not achieve the desired effect in children because of their having lower doses of individual agents when used in combination to minimize side effects such as sedation. Acetaminophen remains the first line for fever if the child appears uncomfortable as a result of high fever. Acetaminophen (10 to 15 mg/kg per dose every 4 to 6 hours) is usually successful in reducing the body's temperature in this setting.

TABLE 1. Classification of Over-the-Counter Cold Medicines

Class	Examples	Side Effects
1. Sympathomimetics	Phenylpropanolamine Pseudoephedrine Phenylephrine	Excess stimulation; irritability; hypertension; insomnia
2. Antihistamines	Ethanolamines (diphenhydramine) Alkylamines (chlorpheniramine, brompheniramine)	Sedation; paradoxical central nervous system stimulation
3. Expectorants	Guaifenesin	Gastric upset
4. Cough suppressants	Codeine	Drowsiness; respiratory depression
	Dextromethorphan	Sedation; gastrointestinal upset

Nasal Congestion

For nasal congestion, there are the sympathomimetic decongestant agents and the antihistamines.

Sympathomimetics (Decongestants). The decongestants vasoconstrict nasal blood vessels and therefore help to open an otherwise congested nose. Most of these agents are available orally or nasally. The oral agents provide less intense vasoconstriction but have a longer duration of action and are associated with more systemic side effects. The nasal agents do provide more significant vasoconstriction in the nasal cavity, but they can result in significant "rebound" in nasal congestion, particularly if they are used more than three to four times a day for 3 days.

Major side effects of the sympathomimetics include hyperstimulation, irritability, sleeplessness, and, occasionally, mild hypertension and hyperglycemia. Rarer side effects include dysrhythmias, seizures, and significant hypertension, less commonly found in children.

The three most common agents are as follows:

1. *Phenylpropanolomine* is available only in combination with antihistamines, the latter of which may be serving via a sedating effect to counteract any hyperstimulation from the sympathomimetic.
2. *Pseudoephedrine* is available as a single agent and provides less stimulation, making it the most benign of these agents to use in terms of side effects.
3. *Phenylephrine* is available orally, again in combination with an antihistamine, but it is most popular as a nasal agent—although it can have unpredictable absorption. The infant dose (0.125 per cent two to three times a day) has been found to be efficacious when used in infants older than 1 year of age.

There is no clear evidence of significant benefit in the use of any of these decongestant agents in children younger than 6 months. In fact, cases of cardiovascular complications have been reported with their usage in children in this age bracket. It is recommended, therefore, that these drugs be used only in children older than 6 months according to appropriate dosage for 3 days (before bed or perhaps before school) and discontinued if no benefits have been noted by the end of that time.

Antihistamines. Theoretically, antihistamines are thought to decrease the extent of rhinorrhea by blocking cholinergic effects, but given the dosages of these agents in over-the-counter preparations, the anticholinergic effect is weak, if at all significant. In addition, histamines are not released as mediators in the setting of a viral nasopharyngitis and therefore antihistamines are not useful with viral illnesses. The antihistamines as a group result in significant sedation, although occasionally one may have a paradoxical reaction of excitation, or hyperactivity. In addition, antihistamines are not recommended in children with seizure disorders.

Most common are the *ethanolamines* (of which diphenhydramine is the most common), which are also the most sedating. The *alkylamines* (chlorpheniramine, bronpheniramine) are less sedating and no more efficacious than diphenhydramine. Although some adult studies suggest there may be a slight benefit in decreasing the volume of nasal secretions with chlorpheniramine the maximal clinical effect is small, and usually no greater than 20 per cent over placebo.

Cough

Expectorants. Should cough occur in the setting of nasopharyngitis, one turns to expectorant cough suppressants. Most cough in this setting is secondary to postnasal drip, which can be worse at night. The expectorants, such as guaifenesin, decrease the surface tension in mucus and increase the production of respiratory secretions. However, no clinical studies have demonstrated the benefit of expectorant in decreasing the viscosity of sputum or easing expectoration when compared with simply using good hydration and cool mist.

Cough Suppressants. Because the cough in nasopharyngitis is usually nonproductive and may be associated with emesis, exhaustion, or poor sleep, it may be useful to use a cough suppressant in the evening rather than an expectorant. In the first few days of the illness, however, the cough may be useful to help clear some of the cellular debris and inflammatory secretions. Perhaps one should therefore withhold cough suppressants, except for nighttime use. If the cough is persistent for more than 7 days—which can be the case with coughs of viral origin as well as with *Mycoplasma* and sinusitis—a cough suppressant might be tried at night.

The three most common cough suppressants include codeine, dextromethorphan, and antihistamines. Antihistamines, however, as a result of their anticholinergic effects, dry secretions and thus hamper their removal. They are not indicated for cough in the setting of nasopharyngitis and are useful only if the rhinitis is due to an allergic precipitant.

Codeine and *dextromethorphan* act essentially by depressing the medullary cough control center and may also have a direct effect on respiratory mucosa by increasing the viscosity of bronchial secretions, making them harder to remove. Codeine as a narcotic carries with it the significant side effects of nausea; drowsiness; lightheadedness; and, with chronic use, constipation. At toxic levels, certainly respiratory depression and apnea are a factor. Therefore, codeine, although efficacious, should be used only in school-aged children or if symptoms are extremely severe. The dose is 1 to 2 mg/kg/day, divided four times daily up to a maximum of 30 mg/day. Codeine has a peak effect within 1 to 2 hours and lasts for 4 hours. Lethal doses in children have been reported at as low as 7 mg/kg/day.

Dextromethorphan is a narcotic analogue that retains only the antitussive properties of the opiates and thus carries with it no significant physical dependence. When used in appropriate dosages, it does not cause central nervous system (CNS) depression and can be as effective as codeine in its results. It may produce some mild CNS depression at high doses. It is rapidly absorbed and has a rapid onset of action within 15 to 30 minutes and will last 3 to 6 hours. Overdoses of 100 times the recommended adult dose have not resulted in respiratory depression or fatalities, and if these occur, there has been improvement with treatment with naloxone. The dose of dextromethorphan is 1 mg/kg/day divided three times a day up to 30 mg per dose. Again, milligram for milligram, dextromethorphan and codeine are equal in their ability to suppress cough and can therefore be given similarly.

SUMMARY

In conclusion, it is much better to consider using a sympathomimetic or cough suppressant for particular symptoms, rather than buying them in a combination when the dosage of each of these agents may be inadequate, thus decreasing their efficiency. In regard to other therapeutic regimens, the use of antibiotics is certainly not recommended in treating nasopharyngitis unless there is clear evidence for a complication due to bacterial superinfection. Antibiotics have not been found to decrease the duration of a cold or to decrease the risk of complications from superinfection should they occur. The use of vitamins, although controversial, has not been found in pediatric studies to be successful in decreasing the duration of cold symptoms. There has been no formal study on the efficacy of chicken soup in toddlers and older children.

In fact, the best treatment for nasopharyngitis is probably no pharmacologic treatment at all but simply supportive therapy, especially if the child does not appear significantly ill. One should remember that the side effects of pharmacotherapy may be worse than the cold symptoms itself. A final warning: Be aware of the alcohol content in over-the-counter cold and cough products.

RHINITIS AND SINUSITIS

DACHLING PANG, M.D.
and ELLEN R. WALD, M.D.

Infections of the upper respiratory tract are the most common reason for seeking medical care. Most of these infections are caused by viruses and require no specific therapy; symptomatic treatment may increase patient comfort. However, other respiratory infections, such as otitis media and sinusitis, may be primarily bacterial or may be complicated by impaired local drainage resulting in bacterial superinfection.

RHINITIS

Rhinitis, when acute, is almost exclusively caused by respiratory viruses and as such requires no antimicrobial treatment. However, in the newborn period rhinitis may be due to congenital syphilis.

Persistent rhinitis in infants or young children (younger than 3 years old) suggests the possibility of group A beta-hemolytic streptococcal infection, or "streptococcosis." Streptococcal infection in this age group often fails to localize in the throat and instead causes a clinical picture of a protracted cold. Occasionally an older child (older than 5 years of age) with streptococcal infection presents with persistent nasal discharge and cough.

If streptococcal infection is documented by culture of the nasopharynx or throat, treatment with penicillin for 10 days is appropriate. Dosages of phenoxymethyl penicillin of 125 mg three or four times daily for those weighing under 60 pounds and 250 mg three or four times daily for those weighing more than 60 pounds are recommended. In penicillin-allergic patients, erythromycin at 40 mg/kg/day in four divided doses is a suitable substitute.

In both infants and older children, paranasal sinusitis should be considered as a cause of persistent nasal discharge (see discussion on sinusitis below). Purulent rhinorrhea may also be indicative of an intranasal foreign body, especially if fetor oris is prominent or if the discharge is unilateral or bloody or both.

Whether bacteria other than group A streptococci may cause purulent rhinitis has not been adequately evaluated. The use of antimicrobial preparations cannot therefore be recommended in the management of the routine upper respiratory infection. However, there are data suggesting that antibiotic prophylaxis (daily or during the course of a cold) may be effective in preventing symptomatic episodes of acute otitis media in otitis-prone children.

Children with persistent rhinitis may be demonstrating symptoms of allergic inflammation or vasomotor rhinitis. Children with the former problem may have a positive family history of allergies or the physical stigmata of allergic problems. Symptomatic treatment with oral antihistamines or decongestants or combination agents may result in prompt improvement. Cromolyn sodium and aerosol steroid preparations may be helpful in older patients with chronic allergic nasal symptoms. Reduction of environmental allergens should always be undertaken. If simple measures of avoidance and symptomatic therapy fail, desensitization may be necessary.

SINUSITIS

The agents causing bacterial sinusitis in childhood are *Streptococcus pneumoniae* (30 per cent), nontypable *Haemophilus influenzae* (20 per cent), and *Moraxella catarrhalis* (20 per cent). The recommended treatment is amoxicillin (40 mg/kg/day in three divided doses) or ampicillin (100 mg/kg/day in four divided doses). Both these drugs are relatively safe, inexpensive, and active against the common bacterial pathogens as well as most anaerobic organisms found in the sinuses.

Alternative antimicrobials, which may be useful if the patient is allergic to penicillin or if there is a high local prevalence of beta-lactamase–producing *H. influenzae* or *M. catarrhalis,* are trimethoprim-sulfamethoxazole* (8 and 40 mg/kg/day, respectively, in two divided doses) or erythromycin-sulfisoxazole* (50 and 150 mg/kg/day in four divided doses) or cefaclor (40 mg/kg/day in three divided doses). Trimethoprim-sulfamethoxazole is not optimal therapy for *Streptococcus pyogenes* and is therefore not the best choice as an amoxicillin alternative in the 5- to 15-year age group, an age group in which *S. pyogenes* is most likely to be encountered. Cefaclor, while a reasonable substitute for amoxicillin in selected patients, has been noted to be ineffective in vitro against the majority of the beta-lactamase–producing *M. catarrhalis.* A drug combination consisting of amoxicillin and potassium clavulanate (Augmentin) is also suitable for use in patients who have sustained a clinical failure with amoxicillin or reside in geographic areas where there is a high prevalence of beta-lactamase–producing bacterial species. Potassium clavulanate is an irreversible beta-lactamase inhibitor. If this drug combination is used in treating an infection with a beta-lactamase–producing bacterial species, the beta-lactamase will be bound by the inhibitor and the amoxicillin restored to its original spectrum of activity.

Cefuroxime axetil is a second-generation cephalosporin with a spectrum of activity that includes all the usual sinus pathogens. Unfortunately, it is available only in tablet formulation and should be reserved for children older than 5 years. Cefixime is a third-generation cephalosporin that is active against beta-lactamase–producing *H. influenzae* and *M. catarrhalis.* It is not very active against *S. pneumoniae* and should be reserved for situations in which *S. pneumoniae* is unlikely.

In pediatric patients who require parenteral therapy for acute sinusitis but who do not have intracranial or intraorbital complications, cefuroxime at 150 mg/kg/day in 3 divided doses given intravenously is ideal. This agent is suitable for *S. pneumoniae* and both beta-lactamase positive and negative *M. catarrhalis* and *H. influenzae.* Cefuroxime is also adequate, although perhaps not ideal for *Staphylococcus aureus* and anaerobes of the upper respiratory tract.

The use of antihistamines and decongestants in the treatment of sinusitis is controversial. There has been no evaluation of the efficacy of these preparations in acute or chronic sinusitis. Although the topical decongestants phenylephrine and oxymetazoline produce potentially undesirable local effects such as ciliostasis, they may provide dramatic symptomatic relief. The effectiveness of these agents with respect to shortening the clinical course of illness in acute sinusitis or preventing suppurative complications is unknown.

*Manufacturer's warning: Contraindicated in children younger than 2 months of age.

Sinus puncture with irrigation and drainage (usually best accomplished by a transnasal approach) often results in dramatic relief from pain and provides material for definitive culture and sensitivity (cultures of the nose and throat correlate poorly with sinus aspirate cultures). In experienced hands and with proper sedation, the procedure is safe and can be accomplished with minimal discomfort. Although a sinus aspiration is not necessary for the management of an uncomplicated case of acute sinusitis, indications for sinus aspiration include clinical unresponsiveness to conventional therapy, sinus disease in an immunosuppressed patient, severe symptoms such as headache or facial pain, and life-threatening disease at the time of clinical presentation.

Orbital Complications

Orbital cellulitis is the most frequent serious complication of acute sinusitis. Despite antimicrobial therapy, it is a potentially life-threatening infection.

Children with stage I disease (Table 1) can be managed as outpatients by the usual regimen for acute sinusitis, provided the parents are cooperative and cognizant of the serious implication if prompt alleviation of symptoms does not occur. If the infection has progressed beyond stage I, hospitalization and intravenous antibiotics are mandatory. The choice of antibiotics is guided by knowledge of the usual bacteriology of acute sinusitis. Blood cultures and sinus aspirate should be obtained aerobically and anaerobically, and appropriate antimicrobials should be added if unsuspected organisms are isolated. Surgical drainage is required if there is a subperiosteal or orbital abscess, but orbital cellulitis may respond to antimicrobials without surgical intervention. The prognosis for stages I and II is usually good if diagnosis and appropriate therapy are carried out promptly, but residual visual loss due to infarction of the optic nerve may complicate frank ab-

TABLE 1. Clinical Staging of Orbital Cellulitis*

Stage I	Inflammatory edema	Inflammatory edema beginning in medial or lateral eyelid; usually nontender with only minimal skin changes. No induration, visual impairment, or limitation of extraocular movements.
Stage II	Orbital cellulitis	Edema of orbital contents with varying degrees of proptosis, chemosis, limitation of extraocular movement and/or visual loss.
Stage III	Subperiosteal abscess	Proptosis down and out with signs of orbital cellulitis (usually severe). Abscess beneath the periosteum of the ethmoid, frontal, or maxillary bone (in that order of frequency).
Stage IV	Orbital abscess	Abscess within the fat or muscle cone in the posterior orbit. Severe chemosis and proptosis; complete ophthalmoplegia and moderate to severe visual loss present (globe displaced forward or down and out).
Stage V	Cavernous sinus thrombophlebitis	Proptosis, globe fixation, severe loss of visual acuity, prostration, signs of meningitis; progresses to proptosis, chemosis, and visual loss in contralateral eye.

*Modified from Chandler JR, Langenbrunner DJ, Stevens EF: The pathogenesis of orbital complications in acute sinusitis. Laryngoscope 80:1414–1428, 1970.

scesses. Severe neurologic sequelae or death may follow cavernous sinus thrombophlebitis.

Intracranial Complications

Intracranial extension of infection is the second most common complication of acute sinusitis. Although the incidence of suppurative intracranial disease in patients with sinusitis is unknown, paranasal sinusitis is the source of 35 to 65 per cent of subdural empyemas. Intracranial infection should be suspected if signs of systemic toxicity and headache do not improve after an adequate course of oral antibiotics and decongestant has been given for the original sinusitis.

Treatment of sinusitis-related intracranial suppuration requires antimicrobials, drainage, and excellent supportive care. There is evidence that preoperative meningitic doses of antibiotics may improve the chances for survival. Since the predominant organisms isolated from sinusitis-related subdural empyema include anaerobic and microaerophilic streptococci, non–group A streptococci, *S. aureus*, and a mixture of *Proteus* and other gram-negative rods, the initial antibiotic regimen prior to culture and sensitivity results should be a combination of penicillin and chloramphenicol. The third-generation cephalosporin cefotaxime (Claforan) may be used in place of chloramphenicol to avoid hemopoietic complications in young infants, although experience with this drug is limited.

Hyperosmolar agents should be given if high intracranial pressure threatens brain herniation. Systemic doses of steroid are prescribed with caution because of the theoretical suppressive effect on granulocytic and immune functions. Anticonvulsants should be given prophylactically to protect against a 79 per cent incidence of associated seizures.

Extradural and subdural empyemas should be drained through a generous craniotomy. The entire collection of pus can be evacuated and the infected bed profusely irrigated with bacitracin solution under direct vision, and with a judiciously fashioned flap the opposite parafalcine space can be explored. Extradural and subdural drains are left in place for 3 to 5 days for continuous drainage and intermittent antibiotic lavage. An underlying brain abscess is best handled by intracapsular evacuation and catheter drainage to avoid unnecessary brain damage associated with radical excision of deep-seated lesions within eloquent areas of the brain. In some cases of subdural empyema, the underlying brain is so swollen that the bone flap must be left out for external decompression. Following radical débridement of all osteomyelitic sequestra, the frontal sinus is opened widely, its content exenterated, and its cavity drained.

Postoperatively, intravenous administration of antibiotics should be maintained for a minimum of 2 to 3 weeks. Intermittent antibiotic irrigation of the infected cavities can be done through the catheters until their removal in 3 to 5 days. The shrinking of the abscess or empyema can be followed accurately by serial computed tomographic scans.

Despite modern diagnostic and surgical capabilities, the mortality associated with subdural empyema and brain abscess remains over 20 per cent. Causes of death and permanent morbidity are related to delayed diagnosis, recurrent suppuration, missed concomitant lesions, extensive cortical and dural sinus thrombophlebitis, and fulminant bacterial meningitis in infants. Early diagnosis remains the most effective way for improving survival.

PERITONSILLAR AND RETROPHARYNGEAL ABSCESS

MICHAEL J. CUNNINGHAM, M.D.

The peritonsillar and retropharyngeal spaces are two potential sites of acute abscess formation and upper airway obstruction in children. Despite their anatomic proximity, the etiology, clinical presentation, and treatment of peritonsillar and retropharyngeal abscesses differ significantly.

PERITONSILLAR ABSCESS

Peritonsillar abscess typically occurs as a complication of acute tonsillitis. Despite the broad age distribution of pharyngotonsillitis, peritonsillar abscess is more common in adolescents than younger children. The severity of the clinical presentation is characteristically out of proportion to that expected of a standard tonsillitis episode. High fever, severe throat pain, dysphagia for solids and liquids, and impaired vocal quality—a garbled, so-called "hot potato" voice—are common. The abscess is almost always unilateral. Physical examination typically reveals bilateral tonsillitis and an erythematous mass effect lateral to only one tonsil. Large abscesses push the involved tonsil medially with displacement of the uvula toward the uninvolved side. Trismus due to inflammation of the adjacent pharyngeal wall musculature may limit the oral examination in some cases.

The optimal management of peritonsillar abscess remains controversial. In the older child without significant trismus, transoral permucosal needle drainage will confirm the diagnosis and often provide immediate symptomatic relief. Intravenous volume repletion and parenteral antibiotic therapy are initiated in an ambulatory setting; if the patient is capable of oral intake following needle drainage, treatment is continued on an outpatient basis. Penicillin or an equally appropriate anti–group A beta-hemolytic streptococcal agent is the antibiotic of choice. In young children or in patients with severe trismus in whom an adequate oropharyngeal evaluation is not possible, an examination using anesthesia with incision and drainage of the peritonsillar region is undertaken. Such patients are usually hospitalized 24 to 48 hours postoperatively. A concurrent tonsillectomy is not typically performed unless there is a significant history of prior tonsillitis, and even in these children tonsillectomy may be deferred to a later date to avoid the increased risk of acute complications. A single episode of peritonsillar abscess in the absence of a prior history of chronic, recurrent tonsillitis does not necessitate a tonsillectomy; estimates of the risk of abscess recurrence in such patients range from 7 to 28 per cent.

RETROPHARYNGEAL ABSCESS

Retropharyngeal abscess, in contrast to peritonsillar abscess, is a disease of young children, 70 per cent of the cases in one large series occurring in children younger than 6 years of age. Abscess formation results from a suppurative adenitis of the retropharyngeal lymph nodes. Many children with retropharyngeal abscesses have an antecedent history of upper respiratory tract infection. They acutely present with toxicity and high fever. Older children complain of painful swallowing; younger children simply refuse oral intake. Drooling is common, and inspiratory stridor is reported in 25 per cent of cases, not dissimilar to the presentation of supraglottitis.

Physical examination typically reveals cervical fullness and resistance to neck movement. Oropharyngeal examination is difficult and may actually be contraindicated in stridulous cases; the pathognomonic bulge or swelling of the posterior pharyngeal wall is rarely visualized. A widened retropharyngeal space on a lateral neck radiograph performed during inspiration with the neck fully extended is strongly suggestive of the diagnosis. Fluoroscopy or ultrasonography can be useful in very young children whose pliable pharyngeal wall soft tissues may make plain film interpretation difficult.

In the absence of impending airway obstruction, intravenous rehydration and antibiotics are the initial line of therapy. Potential etiologic organisms include streptococci and staphylococci alone or in combination with anaerobic bacteria. Coverage with early-generation cephalosporins or clindamycin will be appropriate in the majority of cases. The development of airway compromise or a failure of clinical response necessitates airway support and surgical drainage. Care must be taken during intubation not to cause abscess rupture with aspiration. Drainage is performed by either a transoral or external lateral neck approach, depending on the exact location and extent of the abscess. Surgical cultures can guide the selection and duration of postoperative antibiotic therapy. Complete recovery can be anticipated in most patients.

REFERENCES

Stringer SP, Schaefer SD, Close LG: A randomized trial for outpatient management of peritonsillar abscess. Arch Otolaryngol Head Neck Surg 114:296–298, 1988.

Thompson JW, Cohen SR, Reddix P: Retropharyngeal abscess in children: A retrospective and historical analysis. Laryngoscope 98:589–592, 1988.

TONSILLECTOMY AND ADENOIDECTOMY

JACK L. PARADISE, M.D.

GENERAL CONSIDERATIONS

Tonsillectomy and adenoidectomy have long been the most common major operations performed in children, yet uncertainty and controversy about their indications have yet to be fully resolved. Historically, the often indiscriminate resort to these operations, particularly during the early and middle decades of this century, led many pediatricians to oppose their performance under any and all circumstances. On the other hand, the operations have retained support throughout the professional and lay communities for a variety of reasons. First, many clinicians remained convinced—based on their training or experience or, more recently, on evidence from clinical trials—that the operations were efficacious in relieving certain recurrent or persistent upper respiratory and middle-ear disorders. Second, a number of reports made it clear that obstruction of the upper airway by hypertrophied adenoids or tonsils, or both, could become so extreme as to result in alveolar hypoventilation and cor pulmonale, conditions that responded promptly to surgical removal of the offending tissue. And third, many orthodontists have believed, despite lack of conclusive evidence, that chronic upper airway obstruction results in abnormal craniofacial and dental growth—the "adenoid facies"—and that this too can be modified favorably by adenoidectomy or adenotonsillectomy.

Tonsillectomy and adenoidectomy are often thought of, and most commonly performed in children, as a single, combined procedure (T & A), but each of the two components must be considered separately. At present it is possible to define indications for tonsil and adenoid surgery that are absolute and other indications that are well founded and reasonable but whose application requires individualized judgments and decision making. Still other indications in general use have as yet been neither validated nor discredited.

INDICATIONS FOR SURGERY

Absolute Indications

Absolute indications for adenoidectomy and/or tonsillectomy are likely to be encountered infrequently. They consist of:

1. Obstruction of the nasopharyngeal or oropharyngeal airways—by adenoids, tonsils, or both—severe enough to cause unquestioned discomfort in breathing, or frequent episodes of apnea during sleep or, more extremely, alveolar hypoventilation or cor pulmonale.
2. Obstruction by tonsils of the oropharyngeal deglutitory pathway severe enough to interfere with swallowing.
3. Malignant tumors of the tonsil.
4. Uncontrollable hemorrhage from tonsillar blood vessels.

Because vigorous antimicrobial treatment may sometimes be followed by substantial improvement in even severe obstructive symptoms—presumably by reducing edema due to inapparent, low-grade, chronic infection—a trial of such treatment is usually appropriate before a decision on surgery is reached.

Reasonable Indications

Recurrent Throat Infection As an Indication for Tonsillectomy. It is now clear that tonsillectomy is highly efficacious in children defined as "severely affected" with recurrent throat infection on the basis of meeting four criteria:

1. At least three episodes in each of three successive years, or five episodes in each of two successive years, or seven episodes in one year.
2. Each episode characterized by one or more of the following: oral temperature ≥101°F (38.3°C); enlarged (>2 cm) or tender anterior cervical lymph nodes; tonsillar exudate; or a positive culture for group A beta-hemolytic *Streptococcus*.
3. Apparently adequate antibiotic therapy for proven or suspected streptococcal episodes.
4. Each episode confirmed by examination, with qualifying features documented at the time of occurrence.

On the other hand, some of the children who meet these criteria will improve spontaneously, without intervention. Accordingly, tonsillectomy for such children may be considered a reasonable option but by no means is mandatory.

Importantly, children with histories that meet all of the above-listed criteria except full documentation have been found not to be at substantial risk of developing throat infection subsequently. Decisions about tonsillectomy in such children should therefore usually be deferred until at least two additional episodes have been reliably observed and documented. Because the parents of such children often are desirous of obtaining tonsillectomy, they are more likely to accept a "let's wait and see" response from the physician than an unqualified "no."

Whether or not tonsillectomy is justified in children meeting criteria less stringent than those listed above may be clarified by results from an almost completed clinical trial at the Children's Hospital of Pittsburgh. In the meantime, little is lost and much may be gained by restricting consideration of tonsillectomy for recurrent throat infection to children who meet all of the above-listed "severely affected" criteria.

Other Indications for Tonsillectomy. Based on cumulative clinical experience rather than experimental data, the following conditions also may be considered reasonable indications for tonsillectomy:

1. Peritonsillar abscess.
2. Chronic (as distinct from recurrent acute) tonsillitis—a

condition more likely to be found in adolescents than in younger children.

3. Muffled, "hot potato" voice caused by marked tonsillar hypertrophy.

4. Halitosis due to debris in tonsillar crypts and not responsive to gargling or pharyngeal douche.

5. Chronic cervical lymphadenitis, provided that specific causes such as dental infection, cat-scratch disease, mycobacterial infection, and lymphoproliferative disease have been ruled out.

Recurrent Otitis Media As an Indication for Adenoidectomy. In children previously treated with tympanostomy-tube placement who have recurrent otitis media after extrusion of the tubes, adenoidectomy provides limited effectiveness for at least 2 years in reducing both the number and the duration of subsequent recurrences. Cumulative time with middle-ear effusion appears to be reduced to a greater extent than the number of episodes of acute middle-ear infection. Although adenoidectomy is not a sure-fire corrective in such children, the likelihood of even limited benefit would appear to justify its performance when otitis continues to a troublesome degree.

In children not previously treated with tube placement who have long-standing middle-ear effusion, adenoidectomy combined with myringotomy or with tube placement provides better 2-year otologic outcomes than myringotomy or tube placement alone. However, the marginal advantage offered by adenoidectomy suggests tube placement alone as the preferable initial surgical recourse in such children unless adenoidal obstructive symptoms are also present. In children not previously treated with tube placement who have recurrent acute otitis media, the efficacy of adenoidectomy with or without tonsillectomy remains to be determined.

Nasal Obstruction and Related Conditions As Indications for Adenoidectomy. In children with moderate—as distinct from severe—nasal obstruction due to adenoid hypertrophy, in whom obstructive symptoms (mouth breathing, hyponasal speech) have been present for at least 1 year and have not responded to sustained antimicrobial treatment, adenoidectomy is a reasonable option. Possible detrimental orthodontic effects of long-standing nasal obstruction and possible beneficial orthodontic effects of adenoidectomy have been neither proven nor disproven but seem credible on the basis of limited available evidence. However, adenoidectomy is not justified on orthodontic grounds in the absence of symptoms of nasopharyngeal obstruction. The efficacy of adenoidectomy in children with chronic sinusitis is uncertain; however, in such children with adenoids large enough to produce obstructive symptoms, adenoidectomy would constitute a reasonable adjunct to other treatment measures.

RISKS OF TONSIL AND ADENOID SURGERY

Tonsillectomy and adenoidectomy are major operations that require general anesthesia. They are thus attended by the risk of various complications, some of which are potentially fatal and not all of which are preventable under even ideal circumstances of care. Anesthetic complications include malignant hyperthermia, cardiac arrhythmia, vocal cord trauma, and aspiration with resulting bronchopulmonary obstruction or infection; surgical and postoperative complications include hemorrhage, airway obstruction due to postoperative edema or retropharyngeal hematoma, palatopharyngeal insufficiency, otitis media, and, rarely, nasopharyngeal stenosis, refractory torticollis, and facial edema. To minimize the risk of hemorrhage, surgery should be postponed whenever possible until at least 3 weeks after an episode of pharyngitis and aspirin use should be avoided. No firm evidence exists that tonsillectomy or adenoidectomy results in immunologic risks to children, provided that they have been immunized against poliomyelitis.

FACTORS IN SURGICAL DECISION MAKING

Decisions about surgery in children with "reasonable" (as distinct from "absolute") indications must be individualized. At the outset, parents must be made aware of potential risks of surgery, including the remote possibility of severe or catastrophic complications. Parents also should be reminded that most tonsil-related and adenoid-related problems decline naturally with increasing age—although admittedly not predictably within given periods of time. Factors that should influence individual decisions include the apparent degree of impact of the problem on the child and the family, the child's tolerance of antimicrobial drugs, and the nature of available anesthetic and surgical services.

CONTRAINDICATIONS TO SURGERY

Any condition that causes or predisposes to palatopharyngeal insufficiency constitutes a contraindication to adenoidectomy. In children with such conditions, adenoid tissue may serve to partially or completely bridge the gap that might otherwise exist on phonation between the soft palate and the posterior pharyngeal wall. Conditions likely to cause palatopharyngeal insufficiency include:

1. Overt cleft of the soft palate.
2. Submucous (covert) cleft of the soft palate—to be suspected when a bifid uvula or attenuation of the median raphe of the soft palate is present, and confirmed by finding on palpation that the posterior edge of the hard palate is V-shaped rather than curved.
3. Neurologic or neuromuscular abnormalities causing impaired palatal function.
4. The unusually capacious pharynx.

Each of these conditions is likely to be associated with *hypernasality* of speech, which it is crucial to distinguish from the much more common *hyponasality* found in children with nasal obstruction. Any child suspected of having palatopharyngeal insufficiency should be referred to a speech pathologist or other professional experienced in evaluating the problem.

Hematologic contraindications to tonsil or adenoid surgery consist of anemia and disorders of hemostasis. When surgery is being considered, inquiry should be made about a family or past history of unusual bleeding or bruising, as certain rare hemostatic disorders may not be detectable with routine preoperative tests.

Untreated upper respiratory allergy cannot properly be considered an unequivocal contraindication to tonsil or adenoid surgery; however, in clearly allergic children, a reasonable trial of antiallergic management appears advisable before a decision is made to embark on surgery.

Finally, tonsillectomy or adenoidectomy should not be undertaken in the face of local infection unless urgent obstructive symptoms are present; unless appropriate antimicrobial treatment has been administered for a reasonable period; or, in the view of some, unless a peritonsillar abscess is present. Delaying surgery for at least 3 weeks following an episode of infection permits recuperation and also reduces the risk of postoperative hemorrhage.

PSYCHOLOGIC NEEDS BEFORE AND AFTER SURGERY

Children scheduled for surgery should be fully informed in advance about the expected course of events. A parent or parent-surrogate should room-in with younger and with apprehensive older children and should be present without fail immediately before and after the trip to the operating room.

Thoughtful and kind management throughout the hospital and surgical experience should keep the child from being unduly harmed emotionally.

REFERENCES

Paradise JL. Tonsillectomy and adenoidectomy. *In* Bluestone CD, Stool SE (eds): Pediatric Otolaryngology, 2nd ed. Philadelphia, WB Saunders Co, 1990, pp 915–926.

Paradise JL, Bluestone CD, Bachman RZ, Colborn DK, Bernard BS, Taylor FH, Rogers KD, Schwarzbach RH, Stool SE, Friday GA, Smith IH, Saez CA. Efficacy of tonsillectomy for recurrent throat infection in severely affected children: Results of parallel randomized and nonrandomized trials. N Engl J Med 310:674–683, 1984.

Paradise JL, Bluestone CD, Rogers KD, Taylor FH, Colborn DK, Bachman RZ, Bernard BS, Schwarzbach RH. Efficacy of adenoidectomy for recurrent otitis media in children previously treated with tympanostomy-tube placement: Results of parallel randomized and nonrandomized trials. JAMA 263:2066–2073, 1990.

DISORDERS OF THE LARYNX

JAMES S. REILLY, M.D.

EVALUATION

Evaluation of the infant or child with laryngeal disease should focus first on the history. Specific information about respiration, deglutition, and phonation is obtained. The physician should include questions on noisy respirations, particularly stridor; air hunger; cyanosis; aspiration; difficulty feeding or swallowing; and/or abnormal or weakened voice or cry. Each of these symptoms is quite specific for laryngeal disease.

If there are symptoms or signs of air hunger and/or airway distress, the examiner must avoid agitating the child and perhaps worsening the respiratory distress. Oftentimes, simple observation of respiratory rate, intercostal or clavicular retractions, nasal flaring, fatigue, or lethargy will direct one to decide whether prompt intubation and/or radiographic evaluation is the next immediate step. In the more chronic cases, associated either with mild voice change and/or feeding difficulty, a more thorough history and physical and radiographic examination can be undertaken.

Inspect the child for an increased respiratory rate of greater than 40 breaths/minute. Listen carefully to the quality of the cry and voice. Subtle, but very important abnormalities, e.g., weak, breathy, harsh voice, or more striking examples of biphasic ("to and fro") stridor, should be noted. In small infants, the cry may demonstrate weakness, high pitch, stridor, and/or cyanosis. All extra airway sounds result from a structural abnormality of the airway, and the cause must be located.

A brief word about laryngeal examination. Laryngoscopy is now routinely performed in two ways. Flexible laryngoscopy/bronchoscopy (FL/B) uses a small (3.0 mm) fiberoptic bundle instrument that can provide quick and easy inspection for virtually all interested physicians. Small laryngoscopes or bronchoscopes can be passed through the nasal cavity, and a quick and thorough inspection will reveal any gross lesions or injury.

Rigid laryngoscopy/bronchoscopy (RL/B) uses glass rod lens telescopes to provide better laryngeal examination and visualization. Careful RL/B is now the best method for evaluating the airway in infants and children. Video cameras permit recording and documenting of photos, slides, and videos for review and analysis. Both experience and skilled training are essential to safely perform RL/B. RL/B is the method of choice in children when there is air hunger, cyanosis, or any critical symptoms that should be handled in an operating room setting. Modern-trained pediatric anesthesiologists and pediatric otolaryngologists ensure safe procedures. Early diagnostic intervention permits initiation of therapy to maintain an open airway and avoid tracheotomy in most cases.

CONGENITAL DISORDERS

Most neonatal airway disorders present in the first hours to days of life. Atresia, severe stenosis, or large webs are associated with either severe air hunger or cyanosis in the delivery room. Although neonatal airway abnormalities are rare, they must be carefully evaluated by a specialist familiar with these types of disorders. The small size of the infant airway precludes a casual approach because minimal decreases in diameter from edema alone can completely block the airway.

Laryngomalacia

The most common and generally benign disorder causing stridor is known as laryngomalacia. Symptoms generally commence at 2 to 4 weeks of age and include intermittent stridor that is worse with agitation and generally disappears at rest. Respiratory rate, birth weight, and weight gain are normal. There is no cyanosis. Laryngomalacia is associated with excessively flaccid and edematous arytenoids and with infolding of the epiglottis. The depth of the vocal folds appears to be exaggerated, and the ability to support the supraglottic tissue during inspiration is poorly controlled. This reflects a generalized neurologic immaturity of the infant's aerodigestive tract development. Skilled pediatric airway fluoroscopy can also suggest this diagnosis. The diagnosis must be confirmed by FL/B.

When laryngomalacia is not associated with any severe cyanotic spells, examination with FL/B is appropriate. Children with recurrent hospitalizations for "croup" warrant a more complete examination with RL/B to rule out any synchronous lower airway abnormality that may provoke a hyperdynamic laryngeal state, producing laryngomalacia.

Treatment of the infant with laryngomalacia is generally focused on reassurance to the parents by the specialist and periodic examination at monthly intervals by the primary physician. As long as the child continues to show good weight gain, further intervention is not needed. Rarely, there are small infants with severe laryngomalacia and poor weight gain who would benefit from surgical epiglottoplasty. This avoids the need for tracheotomy and permits the redundant, obstructing supraglottic structures to be surgically trimmed by an endoscopic technique.

Subglottic Stenosis

Subglottic stenosis (SGS) is the most serious laryngeal disorder in infants and children and now appears most often as a sequela of prematurity and prolonged intubation. Evaluation of infants and ex-"preemies" with recurrent croup must include RL/B. This is the procedure of choice to define the size of the SGS. Initial evaluation must involve satisfactory inspection of the size, shape, and degree of obstruction. The circumferential obstruction is divided into four categories according to the staging system of Cotton: lumen blockage of 70 per cent or less (grade I); 70 to 90 per cent (grade II); 90 per cent or greater (grade III); and complete blockage (grade IV).

Most significant degrees of SGS (grades I to III) require prompt intervention by surgically opening the larynx. This is done in two stages to try to reduce the need for a tracheotomy. The first is an anterior cricoid-splitting procedure for grade I. Division of the cricoid cartilage dramatically increases the size of the cricoid ring and permits stenting with a larger endotracheal tube for 7 to 10 days. The child remains paralyzed as the wound heals. The newly reformed and enlarged larynx often permits extubation without further procedures. However, recurrent granulomas at the cricoid incision may necessitate some monitoring and endoscopic removal.

More obstructed cases (grades II and III) require laryngotracheoplasty. This is a more invasive procedure that involves not only splitting the cricoid and thyroid cartilage but also interposing a piece of rib to hold and support the area in an enlarged fashion. A tracheotomy is always inserted in grades III and IV and may be required in grades I and II.

Vocal Cord Paralysis

Children with *bilateral* vocal cord paralysis generally have chronic, intermittent stridor. Often there are neurologic abnormalities, such as Arnold-Chiari malformation, worsening hydrocephalus, and stretching of the vagus nerve as it leaves the skull. Absence of vocal cord movement is confirmed by FL/B examination. A new and safe technique uses ultrasound to image the vocal cords and confirm the diagnosis.

Unilateral vocal cord paralysis presents as coughing with liquids and as recurrent aspiration that may produce pneumonia. Barium swallow demonstrating aspiration and ultrasonography are also used to make the diagnosis. FL/B confirms the diagnosis. Diet is modified by thickening all liquids and by offering semisolid food when appropriate. Trauma from retractors during heart surgery is a very common cause. Cystic fibrosis patients with pulmonary artery dilatation may also have unilateral left vocal cord paralysis. Recovery is anticipated in 9 to 12 months if the nerve has not been severed and if the force that is stretching the nerve is removed or reduced dramatically.

Laryngeal Cleft

Posterior laryngeal clefts are extremely rare and are caused by an absence of part of the posterior cervical cartilage, muscle, or upper esophageal wall. Recurrent aspiration of liquids commonly occurs, and mimics vocal cord paralysis. A gastrostomy is placed if thickened feeds do not prevent aspiration. Open repair with a posteriorly placed rib graft is advocated. A high cervical tracheoesophageal fistula can appear similar to a posterior laryngeal cleft.

Subglottic Hemangioma

Subglottic hemangioma (SGH) may arise during the first 3 to 6 months of life and mimic SGS. Both stridor and air hunger occur, worsening as the child and the SGH grow. Recurrent episodes of croup may prompt emergency room visits or hospital admissions. Temporary shrinkage of SGH from vaporized racemic epinephrine can mislead the physician away from the correct diagnosis. The diagnosis is made by airway films demonstrating a noncircumferential, generally left-sided, small hillock encroaching the airway. RL/B confirms the localized lesion and permits assessment of airway size. I prefer a systemic steroid (prednisone, 2 mg/kg/day) as an initial treatment. If airway symptoms decrease, the steroid is reduced to an every-other-day schedule and tapering is considered; however, this is not always practical. Cushingoid appearances occur less often with alternate-day therapy.

Cysts

Single or multiple *subglottic cysts* (SGCs) have recently been reported in ex-preemie neonates. Small, round areas are seen on radiographs located below the vocal cords and may mimic an SGH or even an SGS. However, SGCs are more often multiple and are easily treatable. RL/B is necessary to confirm the diagnosis and to open (marsupialize) the SGC by forceps, laser, or direct pressure. Respirations are quickly improved following surgery. If airway symptoms recur, follow-up airway films and RL/B are repeated to reopen the recurrent SGC. Parents must be instructed to report any recurrence of symptoms promptly.

Vallecular cysts (VCs) are also common neonatal lesions that occur as fluid-filled cysts arising on the front (anterior) surface of the epiglottis. Lateral radiographs of the neck demonstrate the round cysts in front of the epiglottis. The VC must be opened or ruptured and then evacuated, but there may be recurrence. The infants have feeding difficulty and noisy respirations from secretions, but they do not have true stridor.

TRAUMA

Direct laryngeal trauma to children has increased because of the growing use of all-terrain vehicles and snowmobiles in rural areas and bicycles and automobile accidents in congested urban environments. Blunt or penetrating trauma to the anterior neck from a wire fence, trampoline, handlebar, or dashboard is an emergency and can cause aphonia, hemoptysis, stridor, or air hunger. Examination reveals ecchymosis of the skin of the neck, subcutaneous air, or loss of normal laryngeal cartilage contour. Lateral neck films can confirm the presence of free air and are essential to evaluate the cervical vertebrae for injury. Prompt computed tomographic (CT) examination is also essential to evaluate laryngeal fractures and hematomas.

Complete loss of a patent airway is a very real danger, and prompt RL/B or tracheotomy is indicated if any abnormality is found on physical or radiologic examination. Open repair of soft tissues, vocal cords, or cartilage is essential to promote healing and to avoid a secondary web, stenosis, or paralysis. Intubation may be essential in an emergency but should be judicious to avoid a tear that may separate the upper from the lower trachea.

House fire smoke and steam fumes can cause thermal damage and significant injury with progressive aphonia and stridor. Acid-alkali ingestion (accidental or suicidal) can cause similar symptoms. Radiographs are not helpful; FL/B or RL/B is always necessary. Tracheotomy is indicated in all severe burns.

IATROGENIC DISORDERS

The critical need for airway support during severe illness or injury may cause damage to the larynx from the endotracheal (ET) tube. Unique host factors in the child contribute equally. Down syndrome children and premature children have smaller cricoid rings than other children of the same age. Gastroesophageal reflux (GER) into the larynx, seizures, agitation, or other hypermetabolic states initiate the injury.

Injury can be reduced by:

1. Using smaller-diameter ET tubes.
2. Checking for air leakage at 20 mm H_2O pressure.
3. Avoiding or deflating any cuffed ET tube.
4. Reducing GER by H_2 blockers or antacids.
5. Converting to a tracheotomy if ET extubation in 7 to 14 days seems unlikely.
6. Extubating under "ideal" conditions, including (a) steroids (Decadron, 1 mg/kg up to 10 mg at 6-hour intervals, starting 8 hours before extubation and continuing 36 to 48 hours afterward); (b) aerosolized, racemic epinephrine (a mixture of 2.5 per cent epinephrine diluted 1:8 with saline) immediately at extubation and every hour as needed; and (c) absence of any relaxants, narcotics, or oxygen requirements (<30 per cent).

Special mention must be made of children who are accident victims and who are emergently intubated (e.g., at the roadside or in an emergency vehicle). Critical life-saving placement of an ET tube under difficult or dangerous conditions may result in injury to the vocal cords or to their supporting arytenoids. Persistent hoarseness or weak voice after extubation and recovery should prompt a careful laryngeal examination by a throat or voice specialist. Older children and adolescents should be examined by stroboscopic laryngoscopy—a new technique that demonstrates both vocal cord movement and wave formation not visible to the naked eye.

INFECTION

Croup

The most common infection causing reduced airflow through the larynx is laryngotracheobronchitis (infectious croup). (Management is discussed in the following article.) I would emphasize only that recurrent croup in children younger than 12 months of age suggests laryngeal narrowing (SGS, SGH, SGC). These children, when stable, should undergo RL/B if possible.

Epiglottitis

Epiglottitis is the most precipitous and life-threatening laryngeal infection, caused by *Haemophilus influenzae* type B (HIB). Rapid onset of fever, drooling, and air hunger warrant ET intubation by a pediatric airway specialist. Recent HIB vaccination programs appear to be reducing the frequency and severity of this condition. Accurate diagnosis (swollen epiglottis on a lateral neck film) is more difficult to recognize because of a decrease in clinical experience by physicians and other house officers. Thermal laryngeal injury from food that has been microwaved (e.g., formula) has been shown in recent reports to mimic infectious epiglottitis.

NEOPLASMS

Papilloma

Benign squamous papilloma (recurrent respiratory papilloma or juvenile papilloma) is very rare but, when present, is relentlessly recurrent. Once the diagnosis has been established by biopsy, any recurrent airway symptoms (e.g., stridor, retractions, aphonia) must not be ignored. Laryngeal surgery to keep open the airway may be required as often as weekly, monthly, or yearly. "Cure" is very rare prior to puberty. The papovavirus may be transmitted to the infants from vaginal condylomata in their mothers.

Patency of the laryngeal lumen is re-established either by carbon dioxide laser or by skilled forceps. Both methods are acceptable and sometimes are combined. Complete removal is impossible without injury to laryngeal tissue. Carbon dioxide lasers with microdot and superpulse have refined removal in many cases. Judicious removal and vigilant monitoring by parents and physicians avoid tracheotomy placement. Immunotherapy (interferon) has not gained acceptance because of temporary (less than 1 year) response and painful injections.

Polyps and Other Neoplasms

Pyogenic *granuloma* may result from an ET tube placement. Polyps, another benign neoplasm, are common in young boys (aged 4 to 6 years) or in teenagers who cheerlead or overuse the voice.

Malignant conversion of *squamous papilloma* and oral *carcinoma* caused by tobacco chewing or smoking should also be considered in individual children with a predisposing problem.

ALLERGY

Highly allergic children may have localized edema of the larynx, which can cause air hunger, stridor, or airway collapse. *Angioedema* is a specific abnormality in the complement cascade (C3) that is extremely rare before adolescence. Subcutaneous edema of the lips, tongue, or other body parts should prompt administration of adrenalin subcutaneously (1:1000, 0.1 to 0.2 ml). All patients with serious disease should also be given intravenous hydrocortisone (100 mg) or decadron (10 mg). If airway symptoms worsen and oral edema increases, ET tube placement may be necessary and very difficult. If the oral cavity cannot be seen because of edema, tracheotomy under local or by mask ventilation may be the only alternative.

VOICE DISORDERS

Voice straining by excessive volume (cheerleading, pop singing, projections of the voice at an abnormal pitch) causes trauma to the edge of the vocal cords. This leads to edema, thickening, polyps, and eventually to the formation of "singer nodes" (calluses). Hoarseness is of variable duration but may persist from 2 weeks to several months. GER probably has a role. Arytenoid erythema is pathognomonic but not exclusive of GER, and GER can be present without erythema. Direct inspection of the vocal cords by FL/B is suggested.

Initial therapy has always focused on speech therapy through school specialist or clinic-based speech therapists. Response rate to speech therapy is variable (50 to 80 per cent). Severe, persistent, distressing voice changes that last 6 to 12 months can be improved by surgical removal of the singer's nodes in more than 50 per cent of affected children. This more aggressive approach is advocated only when speech therapy has failed, parents concur, and predisposing factors have been investigated and control initiated.

Hysteria may cause a conversion reaction in preadolescent or adolescent children. Chronic daytime cough or unexplained sudden onset of aphonia can prompt excessive school absence, parental anxiety, and expensive, protracted medical and radiographic evaluations. In the office FL/B will reveal normal vocal cords that move correctly with respiration and oppose during voluntary cough. Psychologic evaluations, frank discussions with parents or caretakers, and eventual confrontation of the child are all necessary elements in the treatment to arrest the process and return the child to normalcy.

REFERENCES

Cotton RT: Management and prevention of subglottic stenosis in infants and children. *In* Bluestone CD, Stool SE (eds): Pediatric Otolaryngology. Philadelphia, WB Saunders Co, 1990.

THE CROUP SYNDROME

(Viral Laryngotracheobronchitis, Spasmodic Croup, Epiglottitis, Bacterial Tracheitis, Laryngeal Injuries)

G. MICHAEL DAVIS

The term *croup syndrome* denotes a group of conditions of viral, bacterial, or traumatic origin that all occur at the point of the narrowest cross-sectional area of the tracheobronchial tree. The characteristic features are a very rapid, acute, upper airway obstruction at this critical orifice (the larynx) that leads to a prominent inspiratory stridor; a harsh, barking cough ("seal's cough"); and, usually, tonal changes in voice or cry. If the partial airway obstruction is of infectious origin, fever and signs of systemic illness usually are present. The airway obstruction in croup may be supraglottic (involving the epiglottis, the arytenoids, and the aryepiglottic folds [false cords]) or subglottic (following intubation) or may involve the true vocal cords. Because this region of the airway is the flow-limiting orifice, minor changes in aperture may result in severe airflow limitation, air hunger, and hypoventilation. Young children are most frequently afflicted with croup because the size of the larynx is small and minor changes in wall thickness from edema radically change the cross-sectional area of the aperture.

ACUTE VIRAL CROUP (Laryngotracheobronchitis)

Croup, the most common cause of acute partial upper airway obstruction, is most frequently caused by parainfluenza viruses types 1, 2, and 3 (approximately 50 per cent) and, less commonly, respiratory syncytial virus (RSV), rhinovirus, and adenovirus. The peak incidence is during the first and second years of life: The disease is most likely to occur either late fall or early winter, although sporadic outbreaks occur throughout the year. Typically, the child has signs of mild upper respiratory tract infection (URTI) 1 to 2 days before there is lower respiratory tract involvement with a harsh, barking cough and hoarseness. The cough is more prominent during the night, and inspiratory stridor develops rapidly from (sub)glottic edema. Fever is variable but usually less than 39°C. Normally, the symptoms last 1 to 2 days but in rare instances cough persists for up to 2 weeks.

This partial upper airway obstruction results in increased work of breathing, with stridor varying according to effort. Rarely, severe obstruction can lead to muscle exhaustion; in the most severely affected infants, however, an elevated Pa_{CO_2} is the direct result of the airflow obstruction causing alveolar hypoventilation. Stridor may decrease in intensity because of either increasing obstruction or relief of the obstruction: The degree and severity of distortion of the chest remain important clinical signs because they reflect the intrathoracic pressure swings generated by the muscles of respiration.

The diagnosis of croup is usually not difficult, although it must be differentiated from bacterial epiglottitis (see later). In the unusual case without preceding coryza, alternative diagnoses, such as spasmodic croup (see below), foreign body in either the larynx or esophagus, or, rarely, diphtheria in this affluent immunized community, must be considered.

The vast majority of children with viral croup who have only mild obstruction can be managed very successfully at home. Usually, relief can be obtained in a closed bathroom filled with steam from hot water. Alternatively, some children benefit from cold, dry air, with the parents remarking upon the dramatic improvement while being transported to the emergency room.

The first step in the treatment of any infant or child with airway obstruction is to assess the adequacy of the airway by examining color, respiration, pulse rate, and severity of retractions. Patients who need an emergency airway must be transported rapidly to a setting where a skilled experienced team (which may include an anesthesiologist, otolaryngologist, pediatric surgeon, or intensivist) is available to place an emergency airway (by endotracheal intubation, tracheostomy, or cricothyroidotomy).

Minimal disturbance to the child is important: Anything that causes hyperventilation is deleterious, so that investigations and nursing procedures should be kept to a minimum with humidification by cool mist from a vaporizer. In addition to humidification, hospitalized patients may require supplemental oxygen because of the frequent hypoxemia (which, presumably, is due to diffuse airway involvement). A quiet environment (but not at the expense of careful observation) and adequate hydration should be provided. Racemic *epinephrine* delivered by oxygen-driven nebulizer (0.25 to 0.5 ml of a 2.5 per cent solution of epinephrine diluted in 3.0 to 4.0 ml normal saline) often provides short-term relief (generally less than 2 hours) of airway obstruction in patients with moderate distress, but a return of the severity of the obstruction may occur when the drug action has ceased. Epinephrine should never be used in ambulatory patients who are to be sent home shortly after receiving the medication.

If the child is exhausted, as assessed clinically by evidence of paradoxical motion of the rib cage and abdomen with decrease in air entry, associated with hypoxemia or hypercapnia, prompt relief of the mechanical obstruction to the upper airway is indicated. The preferred method is placement of a nasotracheal intubation under inhalational general anesthesia by a skilled anesthesiologist. Muscle paralysis is to be avoided, and a smaller than normal endotracheal tube is placed to avoid trauma to the swollen subglottic space. Tracheostomy should be performed in those children whom it is impossible to intubate or if skilled personnel are not available for nasotracheal intubation.

Subsequently, mechanical ventilation is usually not necessary, as the obstruction is relieved, although a brief period of pressure support may be necessary because of the ill-understood phenomenon of post-intubation pulmonary edema. Because croup involves all the tracheobronchial tree, frequent suctioning to remove excessive secretions and supplemental oxygen may be necessary in some children. The endotracheal tube should be removed if the child is afebrile, if the child is coughing around the tube, and if secretions are thin. This is usually 2 to 3 days later, although intubation may occasionally be necessary for 7 to 10 days. Care must be taken to avoid accidental extubation, and the use of arm (elbow) restraints and/or sedation may be necessary.

The role of steroids in the treatment of croup is controversial. Dexamethasone (0.2 to 0.5 mg/kg for two to three doses) is being advocated in the absence of studies that clearly demonstrate either benefits or adverse effects from this treatment. Steroids may also be used at the time of extubation, although no clear advantage has been proven. Antibiotics are not indicated in uncomplicated viral croup, as distinguished from the severe form of obstruction seen in bacterial tracheitis. *Ribavirin* has in vitro activity against parainfluenza, but there is no evidence that it is effective in viral croup.

RECURRENT (SPASMODIC) CROUP

About 5 per cent of children experience recurrent episodes of acute upper airway obstruction that are spasmodic, recurrent, and not associated with URTI. Typically, these patients are older and, having gone to bed perfectly well, awake with harsh, barking cough; dyspnea; hoarse voice; and inspiratory stridor. These signs of partial laryngeal obstruction may last for hours but clear by morning, although they may recur the subsequent few nights. Frequently, these patients respond dramatically to a warm, moist atmosphere.

The nature of the illness is obscure. Direct laryngoscopy during the episode demonstrates a pale, watery edema of the subglottic tissues. There appears to be a relationship with an allergic diathesis epidemiologically, and undoubtedly some of the children progress to hyperreactive airways disease. A histamine challenge test in older children may produce a clinical disease indistinguishable from croup. It is more common in boys, and often there is a familial disposition.

Congenital abnormalities, such as hemangiomas and mucoceles, often present with recurrent and unusually severe episodes of croup. Recurrent stridor, usually with infections, is common among graduates of neonatal nurseries with mild acquired subglottic stenosis. Management of these forms of recurrent croup depends on recognition of these lesions by a careful history, physical examination, and use of diagnostic procedures, such as radiography, followed by referral to an experienced otolaryngologist.

The approach to treatment is the same as for viral croup. There is no evidence that β-agonists or antihistamines are useful, although corticosteroids and α-adrenergics (*pseudoephrine*) may have a therapeutic role. Occasionally, patients with this disease may require intubation.

EPIGLOTTITIS (supraglottitis)

Epiglottitis is an acute infectious disorder of the upper airway, generally caused by *Haemophilus influenzae,* type b, that primarily involves not only the epiglottis but also the adjacent areas (supraglottis). This is the most serious type of acute laryngeal obstruction, accounting for about 5 per cent of admissions for laryngeal obstruction. Typically, the patient with epiglottitis is older (3 to 6 years) and presents with an acute febrile systemic illness, pharyngitis with a rapid onset of dysphagia, inability to control oral secretions, aphonia, and anxiety. Cough is not a prominent sign, and the child prefers to sit up with mouth open to breathe. Signs of airway obstruction may be surprisingly mild initially but rapidly progress to complete airway obstruction. Epiglottitis should never be excluded as a diagnosis on the basis of age; it has been reported both in the newborn and in adults.

Epiglottitis is a true medical emergency because of the suddenness with which complete airway obstruction can occur. A patient suspected of having epiglottitis, seen in a private office, should be transported *accompanied by the physician* to the nearest facility equipped to perform emergency intubation in children. Every emergency room should have a protocol for managing suspected epiglottitis with a team that includes an anesthesiologist, otolaryngologist, and operating room personnel. This team should be assembled as soon as possible after patient arrival.

The child with suspected epiglottitis must be kept in a comfortable environment, such as the parent's arms for all examinations, and painful procedures should be deferred until after the airway is secured. Arterial blood gas determinations are *not* indicated in the severely affected child, although pulse oximetry may offer an atraumatic assessment of oxygenation. Some children may be cooperative and may allow a quick visualization of the epiglottis, but no attempt should be made to force a view of the epiglottis with a tongue depressor because of the risk of precipitating complete airway obstruction. The failure to visualize the classic "cherry-red," swollen epiglottis does not rule out epiglottitis because other structures may be more severely involved with edema and inflammation.

The treatment of acute epiglottitis involves direct visualization of supraglottic structures using inhalational anesthesia and endotracheal intubation if findings are positive. A lateral soft tissue radiograph of the neck has been advocated if the patient's condition is stable and the diagnosis is uncertain, but *a physician competent in intubation must be present at all times.* The child should never be sent to radiologic examinations, but in all cases the technology comes to the child in a setting where intubation is possible if complete obstruction is precipitated by the examination. This is a risky procedure, and direct visualization is generally the more appropriate means of confirming or excluding the diagnosis. Negative or equivocal radiographic studies should never rule out the diagnosis when clinical suspicion of epiglottitis is strong.

In the operating room, every attempt must be made to keep the child comfortable and to reduce anxiety by allowing a parent to stay with the child. Inhalation anesthesia is induced with halothane-oxygen by face mask, with the child sitting in the parent's lap. Intravenous (IV) induction is generally contraindicated because complete airway obstruction may be precipitated during insertion of an IV line, rendering intubation difficult, if not impossible. When swelling of the supraglottic structures is severe, application of pressure on the chest may force bubbles of secretions out of the glottic opening to help guide intubation of the trachea. Preparations for emergency tracheostomy must always be made in case of complete airway obstruction. After examination utilizing anesthesia and confirmatory cultures of the epiglottis and supraglottic structures, the orotracheal tube should be changed to a cuffless nasotracheal tube, smaller than ordinarily used, to minimize the trauma to the swollen edematous tissues.

The management of the patient after intubation requires a pediatric intensive care unit (ICU) team skilled in managing a child with a nasotracheal tube, the prevention of accidental extubation, and the ability to reintubate if necessary. This may require the transfer of the patient to a tertiary care center with this capability. Sedation and restraints may be desirable to prevent accidental extubation, but paralysis and mechanical ventilation generally are not required. Intubation followed by tracheostomy is a much less desirable alternative because of the potential for subglottic damage, although under some circumstances it may be the only available technique to maintain a patent airway.

As soon as the diagnosis of epiglottitis is made and blood specimens obtained for culture, the patient should receive antibiotic therapy against *H. influenzae.* The current recommendation for treatment is cefotaxime (200 mg/kg/day IV in divided doses every 6 hours). The actual choice of antibiotic is predicated upon the sensitivities of *H. influenzae* locally, and alternative effective treatments include ampicillin (200 to 300 mg/kg/day IV) or chloramphenicol (50 to 75 mg/kg/day IV) and should be continued for a minimum of 7 days. These antibiotic choices should provide coverage for the other possible causes of bacterial epiglottitis (*Streptococcus pneumoniae,* group A, β-hemolytic streptococci).

After 1 to 3 days of antibiotic therapy, extubation is generally possible. This determination can usually be made by the presence of a sizable leak around the endotracheal tube and by direct examination of the epiglottis by flexible fiberoptic nasopharyngoscopy.

Epiglottitis secondary to *H. influenzae* type b usually is associated with a bacteremia and may occasionally be accompanied by pneumonia, meningitis, and septic arthritis. Rifampin prophylaxis should be provided to households that include a non-immunized child younger than 5 years. Because most children now receive immunization for *H. influenzae* type b, the development of epiglottitis in an immunized child should prompt further investigation of the child's immune status to assess the possibility of an immunodeficiency.

BACTERIAL TRACHEITIS (Necrotizing Tracheitis, Pseudomembranous Croup)

Bacterial tracheitis (necrotizing tracheitis, pseudomembranous croup) is a severe but localized inflammatory condition of the trachea and main bronchi. It is generally due to bacterial pathogens, principally *Staphylococcus aureus,* as well as group A β-hemolytic streptococci, *S. pneumoniae, H. influenzae,* and some viruses. The acute airway obstruction is caused by necrosis and sloughing of airway mucosa, filling the lumen with inflammatory exudate (the "pseudomembrane"). This may present de novo or as a complication of croup in an older child who becomes toxic and febrile, more reminiscent of epiglottitis. The copious, thick secretions cause severe airway obstruction that constitutes an airway emergency. The diagnosis is generally made by the presence of large amounts of purulent tracheal secretions at intubation and the presence of a "pseudomembrane" over the larynx and trachea. Radiographs may show airway narrowing or abnormal ragged shadows within the tracheal air column.

Treatment includes aggressive airway management to remove secretions and broad-spectrum antibiotic coverage for possible bacterial pathogens. If intubation is required, the endotracheal tube must extend beyond the region of obstruction, which is usually lower than that found with croup or epiglottitis.

ACUTE LARYNGEAL INJURIES

Similar to other diseases in this group, the cardinal signs of acute laryngeal injury include partial airway obstruction and inspiratory stridor, with or without changes in voice or ability to swallow normal pharyngeal secretions.

Foreign Bodies. Acute inspiratory stridor from a foreign body lodged at the larynx, in the trachea, or in the esophagus at the level of the cricopharyngeus occasionally occurs. Like bronchial foreign bodies, the diagnosis is dependent on a high index of suspicion, a history compatible with foreign body aspiration, recognition of an atypical croup history, and careful radiologic examinations. Sometimes the diagnosis can be excluded only by direct examination under anesthesia. The foreign body must be carefully removed by an experienced otolaryngologist to prevent possible distal dislodgment and complete obstruction of the larynx or trachea.

Burns. Any injury to the epiglottis can produce acute upper airway obstruction similar to that seen with bacterial epiglottitis. Hot water scalds, burns, and ingested caustic agents are the most common causes of the injury. A high degree of suspicion is needed because an undamaged oropharynx does not exclude more distal damage. As in the case with epiglottitis, securing the airway by nasotracheal intubation is a major and immediate concern.

Post-intubation Croup. Prolonged endotracheal intubation can result in subglottic edema. Various therapies have been recommended to reduce or prevent this sequela, including corticosteroids, racemic epinephrine, furosemide, and other α-adrenergic vasoconstricting agents. Although none of these agents is associated with major side effects, their effectiveness, in contrast to that of humidification, has not been proven in carefully controlled studies.

CROUP IN THE IMMUNOCOMPROMISED HOST

Croup in the immunocompromised host, such as patients with cancer or acquired immunodeficiency syndrome (AIDS) or those who have undergone bone marrow transplantation, is likely to be due to unusual opportunistic pathogens like *Candida albicans.* An aggressive approach to diagnosis, including the use of flexible fiberoptic endoscopy (with cultures and biopsies), is necessary to guide appropriate therapy.

PNEUMOTHORAX AND MEDIASTINAL EMPHYSEMA

JAMES W. BROOKS, M.D.

The pleurae, both visceral and parietal, are composed of mesothelial cells. The visceral and parietal pleurae are separated by a very thin layer of fluid that lubricates the two surfaces so that they can slide over one another during the phases of respiration without friction.

Air in the pleural space separating the visceral and parietal pleurae is termed a *pneumothorax.* This may anatomically involve the entire hemithorax or only a portion. It may be bilateral or unilateral. It is a simple pneumothorax if the intrapleural pressure remains negative. It is a tension pneumothorax if the intrapleural pressure becomes positive.

The parietal pleura is innervated by the phrenic nerve. The visceral pleura is not innervated by any pain fibers. When air enters the pleural space, it frequently causes discomfort by irritation of the nerve endings in the parietal pleura. If the source of air entry into the pleural space stops, all of the air can be absorbed through the pleural surface in a matter of days (the pleural membranes are permeable to gases)—oxygen and carbon dioxide rapidly, nitrogen more slowly. The inhalation of 100 per cent oxygen after the pneumothorax is discovered facilitates reabsorption.

Depending on the child's condition and the cause of the air escaping into the pleural space, removal of the pneumothorax may be urgent or may proceed at a calmer pace. The object of treatment is total and continuous removal of air allowing maximum function of the lung by preventing collapse of alveoli by the intrapleural air. Treatment also guarantees that lung function will not be sacrificed by adhesions and entrapment of the lung.

Tension pneumothorax must be rapidly removed because it threatens life. In patients with tension pneumothorax, the ipsilateral lung may be totally collapsed and accompanied by a shift of the mediastinum, thus involving the contralateral lung, depression of the diaphragm, greater separation of the ribs, and interference with venous return to the right side of the heart resulting from kinking of the great veins secondary to the mediastinal shift.

Congenital pulmonary disorders (hyaline membrane disease, meconium aspiration), acute pneumonia, chronic pneumonitis with fibrosis, and trauma may alter pulmonary tissue, causing "stiffness" and resistance to total collapse, but the respiratory reserve still suffers the ill effects of simple or tension pneumothorax.

Because of the probability of a continuous air leak, removal of air is best accomplished by chest tube insertion (in the second intercostal space, midclavicular line) rather than needle aspiration, although the initial attempt at removal may be needle thoracentesis and aspiration. Transillumination, whereby a pocket flashlight is held against the chest, helping to visualize lung edge and air space, and/or sonogram may assist in preventing lung injury by providing visual guidance during insertion of the needle in difficult cases.

Air may enter the pleural space from the respiratory system (most common), from the intestinal tract, from the outside following trauma, or, rarely in the child, secondary to empyema from gas-forming bacilli.

A disease process within the lung or trauma may cause rupture of alveoli, allowing the intra-alveolar gas to escape into the perivascular space and dissect to the hilum and into the mediastinum producing *pneumomediastinum.* The rupture may also occur from the alveoli into the pleural space, or from the mediastinum into the pleural space. If the air leak from injury to the alveoli is only within the parenchyma of the lung, *pulmonary interstitial emphysema* is present. This may lead to mediastinal emphysema or rupture into the pleural space with resulting pneumothorax.

Excessive volume distention may cause rupture, usually at the base of a cluster of alveoli, into the periarterial sheath in the center of the pulmonary lobule. Alveolar pressures are more likely to be excessive when neighboring airways are closed by disease because the pores of Kohn are poorly developed. The newborn lung has little collateral ventilation and is, therefore, likely to rupture. When terminal air spaces are collapsed, as in hyaline membrane disease, rupture may occur in the highly distensible distal conducting airways.

Once air has entered the mediastinum (pneumomediastinum), it generally dissects upward to the highest point and presents in the high retrothymic anterior mediastinum or suprasternal notch area, giving rise to subcutaneous emphysema. Air dissection around the thymus produces the classic radiographic "spinnaker sail sign." This subcutaneous emphysema may extend widely through the upper half of the body and may even dissect downward into the area of the lower abdomen and upper thighs. Dissection from the mediastinum into the peritoneal cavity produces *pneumoperitoneum.*

Air tends to dissect into or around the pericardium more frequently than into the neck. Extension of air into the neck occurs less frequently in infants than older children. Occasionally, the aortic arch, azygos vein, main pulmonary artery, and superior vena cava are outlined by mediastinal air.

In the much less common *pneumopericardium,* air is visible in the pericardial sac between the central tendon of the diaphragm and inferior heart border and within the pericardial reflections over the great vessels. In contrast to the position of the thymus in mediastinal emphysema, the thymus remains approximated to the pericardium. Air may go between the parietal pleura and the diaphragm, enter the retroperitoneal space, and at times go around the mesentery and subserosa, giving the appearance of enterocolitis.

Clinical conditions that favor the development of pulmonary interstitial emphysema, pneumomediastinum, or spontaneous pneumothorax are meconium pneumonitis, hyaline membrane disease, asthma, mucoid impaction, or any disease giving rise to pneumonitis or the need for mechanical ventilation or resuscitation. Primary or metastatic tumors may lead to alveolar breakdown, pneumomediastinum, and pneumothorax. Cystic fibrosis may give rise to pneumothorax because of rupture of subpleural blebs or large bullae. Chronic air trapping from any disease increases the likelihood of pneumothorax.

Symptoms of pneumothorax vary with extent of lung collapse, degree of pulmonary disease, age of patient, and rapidity of lung collapse. Pulmonary venous air embolism is rare and is usually a fatal complication.

Pulmonary interstitial emphysema may be lobar or segmental or diffuse or localized. It occurs mainly in small premature infants with abundant interstitial tissue, but it is nearly always associated with underlying lung disease or mechanical ventilation where the use of positive end-expiratory pressure (PEEP) and inflation pressures over 15 to 20 cm of water favor dissection and accumulation of air. Interstitial blood vessels and airways are compressed as dissection continues and the air accumulates. Pulmonary edema and reduced lung compliance develop as a result of pulmonary lymphatic obstruction.

If pulmonary interstitial emphysema is decompressed by the occurrence of pneumomediastinum or pneumothorax, temporary clinical improvement may be observed.

Pulmonary interstitial emphysema may be best managed by jet ventilation, which reduces mean airway pressure and increases ventilator frequency and oxygen concentration in newborns. Breathing 100 per cent oxygen creates a large gradient between tissue and vascular nitrogen and thus promotes a more rapid resolution. This approach cannot be recommended in small premature infants predisposed to retinopathy because high concentrations of oxygen in solution in plasma enhance retinal damage.

Mediastinal air can be best viewed on a lateral chest radiograph as it tends to collect anteriorly between the heart and the sternum. Air in the mediastinum easily ruptures to produce a pneumothorax. Rarely, if ever, does pneumomediastinum compress venous return to the heart.

The lungs of premature newborns have so much interstitium and fluid that they often do not collapse easily and mediastinal shift is deceptively small. The decubitus view is invaluable for distinguishing pneumothorax from pneumomediastinum.

Some pneumothoraces are asymptomatic, but often there is increased respiratory distress. Patients may have distention of the chest, tachycardia, bradycardia, increased respiratory distress, increased irritability, poor perfusion, hypotension, cyanosis, metabolic acidosis, and hypercarbia. Infants with a thick chest wall may need transillumination with a fiberoptic light to confirm a pneumothorax at the bedside. Only in an emergency is needle aspiration without prior diagnosis of a pneumothorax an acceptable diagnostic procedure.

TREATMENT OF PNEUMOTHORAX

Asymptomatic patients may be managed expectantly by using 100 per cent oxygen; those with very mild symptoms may be managed by needle aspiration; care must be taken not to damage the lung with the needle. In obviously symptomatic patients, the pneumothorax should be managed with insertion of chest tube and underwater seal with suction.

Traumatic tension and open pneumothorax are rare in infants and children. Both types of injuries are formidable, and specific maneuvers are necessary to reverse a malignant chain of events.

Other conditions that give rise to tension pneumothorax are rupture of the esophagus, rupture of a pulmonary cyst, rupture of an emphysematous lobe, and postoperative bronchial fistula. These latter entities frequently require thoracotomy for control.

In cases of trauma, clinical findings include external evidence of a wound, tachypnea, dyspnea, cyanosis with hyperresonance, absence of transmission of breath sounds, and dislocation of the trachea and the apical cardiac impulse. The hemithoraces may be asymmetric, with the involved side being larger. X-ray will confirm the diagnosis. Transillumination by fiberoptic light may be helpful by helping to visualize air space. Chest tube insertion is indicated. Any chest wall defect should be surgically repaired.

An open sucking pneumothorax must be closed promptly and the chest cavity drained. No operative therapy is necessary for treatment of pneumomediastinum.

REFERENCES

Chernick V: Kendig's Disorders of the Respiratory Tract in Children, 5th ed. Philadelphia, WB Saunders Co, 1990.
Sabiston DC, Spencer FC: Surgery of the Chest, 5th ed. Philadelphia, WB Saunders Co, 1990.

PLEURAL EFFUSION AND CHYLOTHORAX

REYNALDO D. PAGTAKHAN, M.D.

A rational approach to therapy of pleural effusion requires a clear understanding not only of normal pleural liquid transport and how various clinical disorders alter it (Table 1) but also of the physical and chemical characteristics of the excess liquid. In addition, a knowledge of the spectrum and degree of the ensuing functional disturbances and the contributory role played by other factors helps to determine the type and tempo of therapeutic intervention initially and subsequently required.

TABLE 1. Pathophysiology of Pleural Liquid Accumulation

Primary Mechanism	Clinical Disorders	Pleural Effusion
Altered Starling Forces		
Increased capillary permeability	Pleuropulmonary infection; circulating toxins; systemic lupus erythematosus; rheumatoid arthritis; sarcoidosis; tumor; pulmonary infarction; viral hepatitis	Exudate
Increased capillary hydrostatic pressure	Overhydration; congestive heart failure; venous hypertension; pericarditis	Transudate
Decreased hydrostatic pressure of the interstitial space	Trapped lung with chronic pleural space; post-thoracentesis	Transudate
Decreased plasma oncotic pressure	Hypoalbuminemia; nephrosis; hepatic cirrhosis	Transudate
Increased oncotic pressure of interstitial space	Pulmonary infarction	Exudate
Inappropriate Lymphatic Flow		
Inadequate outflow	Hypoalbuminemia; nephrosis	Transudate
Excessive inflow	Hepatic cirrhosis with ascites; peritoneal dialysis	Transudate
Impaired flow (mediastinal lymphadenopathy and fibrosis; thickening of parietal pleura; obstruction of thoracic duct; developmental hypoplasia or defect)	Mediastinal radiation; superior vena caval syndrome; pericarditis; tuberculosis; lymphoma, mediastinal hygroma; hereditary lymphedema; congenital chylothorax	Exudate or transudate or chyle
Disruption of diaphragmatic lymphatics	Pancreatitis; subphrenic abscess	Exudate
Vascular Leak	Trauma; spontaneous rupture, vascular erosion by neoplasm; hemorrhagic disease	Blood

From Pagtakhan RD, Chernick V: Liquid and air in the pleural space. *In* Chernick V (ed): Kendig's Disorders of the Respiratory Tract in Children, 5th ed. Philadelphia, WB Saunders Co, 1990, p 547.

Fundamentally, pleural effusion results whenever liquid formation (filtration) exceeds removal mechanisms (absorption) and occurs as a consequence of either (1) increased filtration associated with normal or impaired absorption or (2) normal filtration associated with inadequate capacity for removal. The excess liquid may be an exudate, a transudate, chyle, or blood, depending on the underlying etiology and pathogenesis. They are differentiated from each other by their physical and chemical characteristics (Tables 2 and 3).

Pleural exudation results either from inflammatory diseases that increase capillary permeability due to alterations of the pleural surfaces or from disorders that impede lymphatic drainage (see Table 1). In contrast, transudation occurs as a result of (1) increased pulmonary capillary hydrostatic pressure, (2) decreased plasma oncotic pressure, (3) markedly subatmospheric pleural pressure, (4) excessive lymphatic inflow, or (5) inadequate lymphatic drainage (see Table 1). Because the pleural membranes remain basically healthy in pleural transudation, pulmonary capillary permeability remains normal.

TABLE 2. Chemical Separation of Transudates and Exudates

	Pleural Concentration		Pleural/Serum Concentration Ratio	
Type of Effusion	*Protein*	*LDH*	*Protein*	*LDH*
Transudate	< 3 g/100 ml	< 200 IU	< 0.5	< 0.6
Exudate	≥ 3 g/100 ml	≥ 200 IU	≥ 0.5	≥ 0.6

From Pagtakhan RD, Chernick V: Liquid and air in the pleural space. *In* Chernick V (ed): Kendig's Disorders of the Respiratory Tract in Children, 5th ed. Philadelphia, WB Saunders Co, 1990, p 548.
Abbreviation: LDH, lactate dehydrogenase.

TREATMENT

Therapy is directed at (1) relief of the functional disturbances due to the liquid accumulation irrespective of type, and (2) specific management of the underlying disorder. The spectrum of functional disturbances encompasses chest pain, dyspnea, impaired alveolar gas exchange, increased work of breathing, and other general systemic manifestations, such as fever, irritability, and fluid loss. The degree of functional disturbance is determined by the rapidity of liquid accumulation, duration and stage of its development, extent of pleural involvement, attendant complications, status of cardiopulmonary reserve, and nature of the inciting process.

Clinical Disturbances

Irrespective of the underlying disorder and the nature of effusion, certain clinical disturbances merit specific treatment interventions, as shown in Table 4. When repeated thoracenteses become necessary to relieve dyspnea, continuous chest tube drainage is indicated in order not to upset the patient with repeated needle drainage. *It is also imperative to recognize that irritability and restlessness may be due to high fever, increased work of breathing, hypoxemia, or distressing cough so as not to rely wholly on chloral hydrate.* Although the administration of oxygen may be required in hypoxemia, it may also be indicated to decrease the work of breathing. Oxygen should also be administered during the transition period from the clinical diagnosis through the thoracentesis to minimize extreme respiratory distress. The increased work of breathing and high fever contribute to fluid loss, which must be replaced.

TABLE 3. Certain Physical and Chemical Characteristics of Chyle

Sterile
Ingested lipophilic dyes stain the effusion
Cells predominantly lymphocytes
Sudan stain: fat globules
Total fat content exceeds that of plasma (e.g., up to 660 mg/100 ml)
Protein content = ½ or same as that of plasma (usually ≥ 3.0 g/100 ml)
Electrolytes = same as plasma
Blood urea nitrogen = same as plasma
Glucose = same as plasma

From Pagtakhan RD, Chernick V: Liquid and air in the pleural space. *In* Chernick V (ed): Kendig's Disorders of the Respiratory Tract in Children, 5th ed. Philadelphia, WB Saunders Co, 1990, p 548.

TABLE 4. Therapeutic Interventions for Specific Clinical Situation in Patients with Pleural Effusion

Clinical Situation	Therapeutic Intervention
A. General Manifestations	
Acute ill patient	Bed rest
Dyspnea	Thoracentesis
Restlessness, irritability	Chloral hydrate
Increased work of breathing	Oxygen
Hypoxemia	Oxygen
High fever	Acetominophen
Dehydration	Fluid and electrolytes
Moderately severe chest pain	Acetominophen; lying on affected side
Dry irritating cough	Codeine
Severe chest pain	Codeine; lying on affected side
Excruciating chest pain	Lidocaine intercostal nerve block (morphine only in terminal cases)
B. Transudative Effusion	
Without reaccumulation	Treat underlying causes Induce diuresis
With rapid reaccumulation	Continuous chest tube drainage
C. Hemorrhagic Effusion	
In shock	Immediate expansion of vascular volume and direct surgical repair of bleeders
Small clots	Evacuate clots
D. Chylous Effusion	
Life-threatening	Thoracentesis (repeat as necessary)
Non–life-threatening	Single thoracentesis with complete drainage; replace nutrients and electrolytes vitamin supplement; medium-chain triglyceride diet; avoid fatty meals containing long-chain fatty acid
E. Exudative Effusion	
Grossly purulent, free-moving, and/or positive Gram stain, pH above 7.30, LDH < 1000 units/L	Start antimicrobial treatment Repeat thoracentesis as required
Massive effusion, pH < 7.30, overwhelming sepsis	Closed-tube thoracotomy drainage; antimicrobials continued
Frankly purulent, pH < 7.20, LDH > 1000 units/L	Closed-tube thoracotomy drainage; antimicrobials continued
Thick, loculated empyema	Open thoracotomy drainage; antimicrobials continued

Abbreviation: LDH, lactate dehydrogenase.

In addition to analgesics, lying on the affected side by splinting the involved chest wall may provide temporary relief from chest pain. Morphine for excruciating pain should be reserved only for patients with terminal illness.

The Underlying Disorder

Management of the underlying disorder re-emphasizes the need for careful attention to history taking and physical examination and for certain diagnostic procedures, such as a chest radiograph, after thoracentesis to unmask an underlying parenchymal pathology; examination of the pleural liquid for gross appearance, Gram stain, cytologic test, biomedical determination and microbiologic culture; percutaneous pleural biopsy, tuberculin test, blood culture, and other tests. These examinations help to diagnose the nature and clarify the causative role of the underlying disorder. Viewed with the type of the effusion, the differential diagnoses are narrowed to a few conditions (see Table 1). Some of those associated with a transudate (e.g., fluid overload from intravenous infusion or peritoneal dialysis) may require only diuresis or may resolve spontaneously on removal of the inciting cause. Nevertheless, continuous chest tube drainage may be required for rapid reaccumulation of effusion until the underlying disorder is placed under control. Some specific situations warrant a special approach. *For example, irradiation of the involved mediastinal nodes in lymphoma may be necessary to control the attendant effusion.*

Massive hemothorax associated with shock demands immediate expansion of vascular volume and direct repair of bleeders. Even small clots are best evacuated to prevent adhesions during healing.

Management of chylous effusion in the neonate is almost always nonsurgical because overt trauma and underlying pathologic states are seldom identifiable. Immediate and, when required, repeated thoracenteses are done in the pres-

TABLE 5. A Guide to Antimicrobial Therapy of Bacterial Pleurisy and Empyema

Infecting Agent	Drug and Dosage (per kg per day) Route and Duration*
A. Aerobic bacteria	
1. Staphylococci	1. a. Methicillin, 200–400 mg divided in 3–4 doses IV initially; for 3–4 weeks b. Cloxacillin, 100–200 mg divided in 3–6 doses IV initially; for 3–4 weeks
2. *Haemophilus influenzae*	2. a. Ampicillin, 100–200 mg divided in 2–4 doses IV initially; for 1–2 weeks or b. Chloramphenicol, 50–100 mg divided in 4 doses IV initially; for 1–2 weeks or c. Cefuroxime, 75–225 mg divided in 3 doses IV initially; for 1–2 weeks
3. Pneumococcus and streptococci	3. Penicillin G, 50,000–300,000 units divided in 3–4 doses IV or IM; for 7–10 days
4. *Escherichia coli* and *Klebsiella*	4. Gentamicin, 5–7 mg divided in 2–3 doses IV; for 14 days or longer
5. *Pseudomonas*	5. a. Carbenicillin, 100–600 mg divided in 4 doses IV; for 10 days or longer or b. Ticarcillin, 400 mg, divided in 4 doses IV; for 10 days or longer c. Tobramycin, 5–7 mg divided in 2 doses
B. Anaerobic bacteria	
1. *Bacteroides fragilis*	1. Chloramphenicol, same as A.2.b
2. All except *B. fragilis*	2. a. Penicillin G, same as A.3 b. Ampicillin, same as A.2.a

From Pagtakhan RD, Chernick V: Pleurisy and empyema. *In* Chernick V (ed): Kendig's Disorders of the Respiratory Tract in Children, 5th ed. Philadelphia, WB Saunders Co, 1990, p 443.

*The lower dose in the dosage range and less frequent intervals of administration are recommended for neonates.

Duration of therapy for anaerobic pneumonitis requires an adjustment if the lung lesions go on to cavitate. Often, 6 to 12 weeks are required before the lung lesions clear or only a small stable residual disease is left.

Abbreviations: IV, intravenously; IM, intramuscularly; CNS, central nervous system; kg, kilogram body weight.

ence of life-threatening cardiorespiratory difficulty. In the absence of a life-threatening situation and after nearly complete drainage of chyle, a medium-chain triglyceride diet, and replacement of nutrient and electrolyte losses along with vitamin supplementation are continued for about 2 weeks when chylous effusion largely ceases. A subsequent trial of fasting and parenteral alimentation via a vein other than the left subclavian is started in those who relapse and continued for about 5 weeks to allow for closure of lymphatic channel fistulas.

In the older child, chylothorax due to surgical trauma may also benefit from the foregoing approach. A few cases may require thoracotomy to control the disorder.

Exudative effusion may be infectious or noninfectious in origin. Noninfectious exudates, particularly if not associated with respiratory distress, usually resolve with improvement in the underlying disorder. Hence, only the underlying disease needs to be treated.

In contrast, antimicrobial therapy (Table 5) and certain thoracic surgical procedures (Table 6) are required to treat infectious exudative effusion. In fact, antimicrobial agents are initiated when the liquid is grossly purulent and the Gram stain is positive. The clinical data and the bacterial epidemiology in the community dictate the initial choice of antimicrobials, usually more than one, which are administered initially by intravenous route. Duration of drug therapy must be long enough for the suspected or identified bacteria in order to avoid relapse.

In addition to continuing the antimicrobial umbrella, drainage of the exudate is essential. Repeated thoracenteses suffice when the liquid is free-moving, its pH above 7.30 and lactate dehydrogenate (LDH) under 1000 units/L. Closed-tube thoracotomy drainage is indicated when the liquid is frankly purulent with the pH less than 7.20 and LDH greater than 1000 units/L. It is also indicated even when pH is greater than 7.20 but lower than 7.30 in the presence of massive effusion. For thick, loculated empyema, open thoracotomy drainage with applied suction is required. Instillation of streptokinase (250,000 units diluted in 100 mL of normal saline) into the empyema cavity, where it is kept for approximately 4 hours prior to resuming drainage, helps to lyse adhesions and enhances subsequent evacuation of the empyema.

Timely provision of appropriate pleural drainage and specific antimicrobial therapy decrease fatalities and offer the pediatric patient normal lung growth and function in later life.

TABLE 6. Surgical Management of Bacterial Pleurisy and Empyema

Procedure	Rationale and Comments
Thoracentesis (needle aspiration)	For prompt relief of dyspnea and initial step for diagnostic study of the liquid. May be repeated two or three times and most of effusion removed during tap.
Intercostal tube drainage (closed thoracotomy)	For massive, relatively thin effusion in the presence of overwhelming toxicity (e.g., secondary to lung abscess).
Tube thoracotomy with rib resection (open thoracotomy)	For symptomatic thick, encapsulated empyema not controlled by antibiotics and when early obliteration of empyema cavity is expected (e.g., post-lobectomy empyema).
Open flap drainage	For larger symptomatic empyema (e.g., post-pneumonectomy empyema). Easy to care for technique for septic and debilitated patients.
Pleural decortication	For removal of restrictive fibrous tissue layer on surface of lungs. Indicated for symptomatic chronic empyema with lung entrapment.

From Pagtakhan RD, Chernick V: Pleurisy and empyema. *In* Chernick V (ed): Kendig's Disorders of the Respiratory Tract in Children, 5th ed. Philadelphia, WB Saunders Co, 1990, p 444.

INTRATHORACIC CYSTS AND MASSES

JAMES W. BROOKS, M.D.

Intrathoracic cysts, congenital or acquired, occur both in pulmonary parenchyma and within the mediastinum. Most are asymptomatic. Symptoms may be caused by pressure on surrounding structures, erosion into surrounding structures, hemorrhage, secondary infection, or malignant change.

INTRAPULMONIC CYSTS AND MASSES

Congenital Cystic Disease of the Lungs

Congenital cysts are more rare than acquired cysts of the lung and may be bronchogenic, alveolar, or a combination of both. Congenital cysts may be multiple or single and are usually limited to one lobe. Cysts have been recorded in late embryos and in newborns. They are air-filled and do communicate with the tracheobronchial tree. Chest x-ray before infection shows a cyst occupying a portion of one pulmonary lobe and appearing as oval, thin-walled, and air-filled. Pus may be present because of the ease with which these congenital cysts become infected. The wall of the congenital cysts usually contains bits of smooth muscle and cartilage and is lined by columnar epithelium. (Most acquired cysts have a lining of squamous epithelium.) Because of infection, infected congenital cysts, acquired cysts, and lung abscesses may be indistinguishable pathologically and clinically.

The cyst airway connection may be direct with the bronchial tree or through the pores of Kohn. This air access is free on inspiration, but obstructed during expiration ("ball-valve"). The air trapping causes compression of the ipsilateral lung, depression of the diaphragm, contralateral mediastinal shift, and thus contralateral pulmonary involvement. If the cyst drainage is poor, suppuration develops. Progressive tension within the congenital cyst may lead to respiratory and circulatory problems. By late infancy and childhood, infection is almost invariably present, and cough, fever, and occasionally hemoptysis occur. The cyst may evolve into a lung abscess.

Congenital pulmonary cystic disease is rarely characterized by spontaneous regression. The untreated cyst may result in empyema with tension, infection with abscess, recurrent disabling pneumonia, bronchopleural fistula, hemorrhage, and cystic expansion with possible suffocation. Accordingly, thoracotomy with lobectomy is the preferred form of treatment.

Congenital Cystic Adenomatoid Malformation

Congenital cystic adenomatoid malformation has been called "cystic adenomatoid pulmonary hamartoma." The finding of skeletal muscle in specimens suggests that the lesion is not a hamartoma. Respiratory symptoms may be caused by tension within the cysts and/or secondary infection. Pathologically, an overgrowth of pulmonary tissue in the region of the end bronchioles with suppression of the alveolar growth may be the cause of this congenital cystic malformation. The abnormality is usually unilobar but has been described bilaterally. Prematurity, hydramnios, and anasarca are frequently associated findings. Respiratory distress is manifested soon after birth.

Early surgical excision is the treatment of choice and lobectomy usually is curative. In later life, secondary infection constitutes an indication for thoracotomy.

Pulmonary Sequestration

Pulmonary sequestration represents pulmonary tissue that is embryonic and cystic and does not function. *Males are affected three to four times more frequently than females.* The sequestration is isolated from normal functioning lung, communicating only through the pores of Kohn. Its arterial blood supply is systemic, arising from either the thoracic or the abdominal aorta. There are two types of pulmonary sequestration: (1) the intrapulmonic and (2) the extrapulmonic.

Because of its communication with normal lung, by way of the pores of Kohn, an intrapulmonic sequestration may contain air, may be cystic in nature, and may harbor recurrent infections (the most common denominator in its clinical picture). More sequestrations are located in the posterior basilar segment (left lower lobe), than in any other area of the lungs bilaterally. The appearance on x-ray may result in confusing this congenital anomaly with congenital pulmonary cystic disease. Intralobar sequestrations usually require surgical resection.

Extrapulmonic sequestration is frequently associated with a Bochdalek hernia, and communications have been reported with the trachea, bronchi, esophagus, stomach, and small bowel. The venous drainage is through the azygos system. Simple surgical resection of the sequestered tissue is often possible.

Fistulas

A congenital pulmonary arteriovenous fistula represents a direct communication between pulmonary artery and vein without the intervening capillary bed. Cyanosis, an elevated hematocrit level, and an audible machinery murmur over the lesion are features that should differentiate it from other pulmonary masses. Selective pulmonary angiograms confirm the diagnosis. Embolization, if possible, is the therapy of choice; otherwise, surgical resection is indicated.

Pneumatoceles

Acquired cysts of the lung (pneumatoceles) are lesions that usually follow pulmonary infection. The most common organism is *Staphylococcus aureus.* Invasive therapy is seldom necessary.

Acquired cysts can follow blunt trauma. Occasionally, penetrating injuries of the lung result in a hematoma, which, when absorption occurs, leaves a pneumatocele that will eventually disappear. Rarely, an acquired cyst may rupture into the pleural space, giving rise to a pneumothorax and the necessity for chest tube insertion.

PULMONARY TUMORS

Benign Pulmonary Tumors

Hamartoma. Hamartomas in children, unlike those described in adults, have been very large. They consist mainly of cartilage, epithelium, fat, muscle, and glandular tissue. Surgery is the treatment of choice, and the diagnosis usually is not made prior to excision.

Plasma Cell Granuloma. Plasma cell granuloma of the lung is rare in the pediatric age group, but it has been reported.

Bronchial Adenoma. A low-grade adenocarcinoma, bronchial adenoma is one of the more common pulmonary tumors found in the pediatric age group. Both carcinoid and cylindromatous type adenomas are described; the carcinoid tumor accounts for the greatest number. The child usually has symptoms of recurrent or persistent pneumonitis because the adenoma is intraluminal, causing atelectasis and pneumonitis. The diagnosis can be made by bronchoscopy. The treatment is thoracotomy and resection of that portion of lung involved, usually a lobectomy.

Other Benign Tumors. Primary bronchogenic carcinoma of the lung is rare in the pediatric age group. The youngest patient recorded is a 5-month-old girl with malignancy in her left lung.

Every cell type except alveolar cell carcinoma, giant cell carcinoma, and carcinosarcoma has been seen in the pediatric age group.

Fibrosarcoma of the bronchus, leiomyosarcoma of the bronchus, plasmacytoma, and chorioepithelioma have all been described in isolated cases in the pediatric age group. Resection by lobectomy is required.

Metastatic Pulmonary Tumors

Primary sarcoma of the kidney (Wilms'), primary malignant skeletal tumors (chondrosarcoma and osteogenic sarcoma), Ewing's tumor, reticulum cell sarcoma, and soft tissue sarcomas (fibrosarcoma, rhabdomyosarcoma, liposarcoma, malignant neurilemoma, and synovioma) may metastasize to the lung. In general, the indication for resection of metastatic pulmonary disease should be based on (1) unilateral pulmonary involvement and (2) evidence of local control of the primary malignancy for a period of 1 year. However, recent developments in the chemotherapeutic management of pulmonary sarcomas in children have produced data that strongly support an aggressive approach to this malignancy, whether primary or metastatic. Vigorous attack, using chemotherapy, irradiation, and surgical resection of unilateral or bilateral pulmonary metastases, is now advocated, regardless of the interval between the diagnosis of the primary sarcoma and recognition of the pulmonary metastasis. Conventional chest x-ray and, in particular, computed tomography (CT) of the lung, serve to map bilateral pulmonary lesions in preoperative evaluations and postoperative follow-up. Repeated thoracotomies for removal of recurrent lesions are acceptable.

CYSTS AND TUMORS OF THE MEDIASTINUM

Congenital Mediastinal Cysts

Structures that arise from the foregut are the pharynx, thyroid, parathyroid, thymus, respiratory tract, esophagus, stomach, upper part of the duodenum, liver, and pancreas; thus, abnormal development at this stage may give rise to *bronchogenic cysts, esophageal duplication cysts,* and *gastroenteric cysts.*

Bronchogenic Cysts. The most common congenital mediastinal cysts are bronchogenic cysts. These are benign. Primary mediastinal cysts of bronchogenic origin probably represent abnormalities in embryologic development at the sight of the foregut just where the separation of esophageal and lung buds occurs. Bronchogenic cysts are classified according to location: tracheal, hilar, carinal, esophageal, or miscellaneous. The usual location of bronchogenic cysts is mid-mediastinal. The cyst may be filled with clear fluid or thick, gelatinous material.

Symptoms due to a bronchogenic or foregut cyst are rare but, when present, are related to pressure on surrounding structures, commonly the respiratory system. Hemoptysis is rare; infection can occur but is rare.

Bronchogenic cysts should be removed surgically. Without rapid removal, infection or intracystic hemorrhage may cause rapid, severe symptoms of respiratory distress and continued growth will embarrass surrounding vital structures.

Esophageal Duplication Cysts. Esophageal duplication cysts are always located in the posterior mediastinum. They appear usually on the right side and are intimately associated with the wall of the esophagus. Esophageal cysts may be associated with mild dysphagia and regurgitation, but most frequently they are asymptomatic. Removal by thoracotomy is indicated for the same reasons as noted in the discussion of the therapy of bronchogenic cysts.

Gastroenteric Cysts. These cysts arise from the foregut and are usually located in the posterior mediastinum. The cyst lies against the vertebrae and is posterior or lateral to and usually free from the esophagus. Gastroenteric cysts are usually symptomatic. The symptoms are due to pressure on thoracic structures or rupture into the bronchi with massive hemoptysis.

Penetration of the diaphragm by a cyst arising primarily from the thorax may occur; conversely, penetration of the diaphragm by the free end of an intramesenteric intestinal duplication is also possible.

A survey of the literature on gastroenteric mediastinal cysts combined with vertebral anomalies reveals that hemivertebra, spina bifida, or infantile scoliosis has been reported in a high percentage of cases.

Most of these vertebral lesions involve the upper thoracic and lower cervical vertebrae, and the cysts tend to be caudad to the vertebral lesion. CT and/or magnetic resonance imaging (MRI) may be necessary for the diagnosis.

Gastroenteric cysts may communicate with the intestinal tract below the diaphragm or with remnants of the embryonic neuroenteric canal, which arises in the upper thoracic vertebrae. Even when the enteric cyst does not communicate with the spinal canal, a vertebral malformation is usually evident by x-ray examination.

Because enteric cysts may present as lesions with an air-fluid level, these cysts may be confused with lung abscesses or empyema. *At the time of surgery for removal, extensions to the intestinal tract below the diaphragm and to the spinal canal in the chest must be located and removed appropriately. Surgery is the treatment of choice.*

Pericardial Coelomic Cysts

These mesothelium-lined cysts are developmental in origin, and formal genesis is related to the pericardial coelom. The cysts are usually located anteriorly in the costophrenic angles, more frequently on the right and occasionally on or in the diaphragm. They are usually asymptomatic and are discovered on routine x-ray. Resection is required by open thoracotomy.

Intrathoracic Meningoceles

Intrathoracic meningoceles are not true mediastinal tumors or cysts. They are rare in the pediatric age group. They are diverticula of the spinal meninges that protrude through the neuroforamen adjacent to the intercostal nerve and manifest beneath the pleura in the posterior medial thoracic gutter. There is no indication for removal unless the lesion is symptomatic (not described in pediatric literature).

Miscellaneous Cysts

Other mediastinal cysts seen more commonly in adults, but occasionally in the pediatric age group, are *cystic hygroma, (lymphangioma), thymic cysts,* and *cystic teratoma.* All three of these are located in the anterior mediastinum. Excision is required for specific diagnosis. The teratomas and the thymic cysts have a rare potential for becoming malignant later.

Mediastinal Tumors

Thymic Mediastinal Tumors

The thymus is located in the anterior superior mediastinum; however, abnormalities of the thymus have been reported in all areas of the mediastinum.

Thymic masses are the most common of the mediastinal masses in children; of these, hyperplasia of the thymus is most frequent. The thymus gland varies greatly in size in the pediatric age group. Stimuli that cause it to increase in size are not understood; however, steroids, infections, androgens, and irradiation may make the thymus smaller.

Malignant thymic tumors in children are very rare. Lymphosarcoma is the most frequent of those. Primary Hodgkin's disease of the thymus, teratoid, and carcinoma have been described. None of these cases in the pediatric age group has been associated with myasthenia gravis.

Benign thymic tumors are rare in children. Treatment is by open thoracotomy, usually through median sternotomy approach. If the tumor is malignant, postoperative management may include irradiation and/or chemotherapy.

Teratoid Mediastinal Tumors

Teratoid tumors of the mediastinum may be classified as (1) benign cystic teratomas, (2) benign teratomas, solid, or (3) teratoids (carcinoma). Teratoid mediastinal cysts contain elements of the ectoderm, mesoderm, and endoderm. If only ectodermal tissue is seen, the lesion is classified as a *dermatoid cyst,* which commonly contains hair, sweat glands, sebaceous cysts and teeth.

Cystic teratomas are more common than solid ones, whereas malignant degeneration is the least common. Most, if not all, mediastinal teratomas are present at birth. Cystic teratomas located in the anterior mediastinum may cause symptoms because of pressure or erosion into the adjacent respiratory system. On x-ray the lesion is well outlined with sharp borders. A definitive diagnosis cannot be established unless teeth can be demonstrated in the mass. Calcification, which is not unusual, appears as scattered masses rather than diffuse small densities. Benign cystic teratomas should be removed. If infection, perforation, intracystic hemorrhage, or malignant degeneration has occurred, complete removal may be difficult or impossible owing to extensive surrounding reactions.

Benign and/or malignant *teratoma* is the most common solid tumor occurring in the anterior mediastinum of infants and children. The solid tumors of the teratoid group are much more complex and have a greater propensity for malignant change (20 per cent). The solid teratoid tumors of the anterior mediastinum reveal microscopic evidence of all layers, including ectoderm, endoderm, and mesoderm with their various structures, such as hair, skin, teeth, skin appendages, bone cartilage, intestine, and respiratory and pancreatic tissue. Treatment is surgical resection by thoracotomy or median sternotomy incision.

Neurogenic Mediastinal Tumors

Neurogenic tumors are by far the most common tumors with a posterior mediastinal origin. Frequently, neurogenic tumors are found incidentally when the infant or child with respiratory symptoms is being evaluated by chest films. Except for massive tumors and those dumbbell-type tumors that involve the spinal canal and cause cord compression, mediastinal neurogenic tumors rarely cause symptoms.

In the younger child, *neuroblastoma* is the predominant histologic type. The primary treatment is surgical excision. If the tumor is completely excised, no chemotherapy or irradiation therapy is indicated. For the child with a dumbbell neuroblastoma, the treatment varies, depending on signs and symptoms of cord compression. In the case of cord compression, emergency laminectomy is necessary as the first step; at the time of thoracotomy 7 to 10 days later, the intrathoracic portion of the mass is removed. This order of surgery is reversed when the intrathoracic spinal component of the tumor is small and there are no signs of cord compression.

Radiation therapy and chemotherapy are employed when the entire tumor cannot be excised.

Ganglioneuroma is the benign variant of neuroblastoma and is usually found in the older child. It may represent maturation of a neuroblastoma. Surgical excision is curative.

Neurofibroma, neurilemma, malignant schwannoma, ganglioneuroblastoma, pheochromocytoma, and chemodectoma (usually located anteriorly) are rare in children. Excision, where possible, is the treatment of choice. These tumors are removed because they are an unknown mass.

Mediastinal Lymph Node Abnormalities

Abnormalities of the lymph nodes of the mediastinum may occur. Any lymph node enlargement in the child should be viewed with suspicion. The diagnosis is made by biopsy.

Lymphoma is the most common tumor in the middle and anterior mediastinum of children. Biopsy for diagnosis, not curative excision, is the usual surgical approach.

Leukemia, Hodgkin's disease, sarcoidosis, tuberculosis, fungus infection, and nonspecific enlargement of nodes have been reported and must be considered in any enlargement suspected of being lymph node only. (See article on malignant lymphoma, p. 278.)

Cystic hygromas are relatively rare. These tumors consist of masses of dilated lymphatic channels containing clear, watery fluid; they are lined with flat endothelium and are usually multilocular. They may appear to be isolated in the mediastinum, but more often they have an associated continuation into the neck. They may be rather large and unilateral with lateral masses in the superior mediastinum. Treatment is by surgical incision.

PRIMARY CARDIAC AND PERICARDIAL TUMORS

Rhabdomyoma appears to be the only cardiac tumor showing a definite predilection for the younger age groups. This is particularly true of children with tuberous sclerosis. It is not unusual for rhabdomyoma to regress spontaneously without having caused any appreciable impairment of cardiac function.

Myxoma is by far the most common primary tumor of the heart. It may be encountered at almost any age. Most myxomas are located in the atria, more on the left than on the right. The origin appears to be the septa. Surgical removal is indicated.

Primary sarcoma of the heart is less common than myxoma but may occur at any age. It tends to infiltrate the wall of the myocardium and extends into the pericardial cavity; however, it does not proliferate into the lumina of the heart.

Other primary tumors of the heart are angioma, fibroma, lipoma, and hamartoma. All are rare.

Primary neoplasms of the pericardium are rare. On histologic examination, the predominant tumors are mesotheliomas (endotheliomas) and sarcomas, but leiomyomas, hemangiomas, and lipomas occasionally occur. Treatment is by thoracotomy.

TUMORS OF THE DIAPHRAGM

Benign and malignant tumors of the diaphragm have not been described in children. If present, they again would cause symptoms secondary to pressure on adjacent structures. Treatment is by thoracotomy.

CHEST WALL TUMORS

Benign and malignant chest wall tumors in the pediatric age group are extremely rare, if they occur at all. The most common benign chest wall tumor is a simple lipoma. Treatment is by local excision. If the tumors are malignant, a wide (2- to 3-inch) margin is desirable.

REFERENCES

Arciniegas E, Hakimi M, Farooki ZQ, et al: Primary cardiac tumors in children. J Thorac Cardiovasc Surg 79:582, 1980.

Chernick V: Kendig's Disorders of the Respiratory Tract in Children, 5th ed. Philadelphia, WB Saunders Co, 1990.

Kirks DR, Korobkin M: Computed tomography of the chest in infants and children: Techniques and mediastinal evaluation. Radiol Clin North Am 19:409, 1981.

MIDDLE LOBE SYNDROME

HERBERT C. MANSMANN, JR., M.D.

DIAGNOSIS

Modern medical advances have significantly reduced the incidence, duration, and outcome of the atelectasis associated with middle lobe syndrome (MLS). The typical roentgenographic change is diagnostic in the form of a triangle-like increase in density resulting from the loss of air in the middle lobe (ML) area of the right lung. The apex is at the hilum, and the base is at the convergence of the diaphragm with the anterior thoracic wall in the lateral view of the chest. Rarely, incomplete obstruction results in a blurred cardiac border or increased bronchial marking, which may require a tomogram to outline the ML.

ETIOLOGY

Initially, this lesion was a manifestation of mediastinal lymphadenitis due to tuberculosis. Obviously, this must still be considered in certain high-risk situations, such as a child of recent immigrants to the United States, a child living in a home with a patient with acquired immunodeficiency syndrome (AIDS), or a child who visits a coughing grandparent in a nursing home. At present, invasive procedures and surgery are rarely required.

Asthma

Most patients respond to aggressive medical therapy of the inflammatory component (see asthma, Section 19). Moreover, the inflammation should also be preventable by early outpatient management of the bronchial asthma. Because this reversible component of the asthmatic airflow illness is the last to heal, early interventions with anti-inflammatory agents, in addition to the bronchodilators, are essential. For the next year or so, chest radiography must be performed after each episode because recurrence will ultimately lead to resection. Particular care must be exercised to adequately treat and suppress the inflammatory component of asthma for the first several months, as this lesion may be silent in the absence of signs and symptoms of bronchospasm. Yet MLS probably can occur only when airflow limitations are present; therefore, determination of peak expiratory flow rates three times a day at home is necessary. Optimally, small airway parameters of pulmonary function tests should be repeated monthly until findings are normal on two successive occasions and then repeated after any acute exacerbation of the asthma.

Once this diagnosis has been made, prevention and adequate care of all asthma recurrences are mandatory. Short courses of oral steroids may be necessary to reverse the occlusion. It is important to realize that the chronic use of inhaled β_2-agonists alone is now unacceptable, because an increase in bronchial hyperreactivity has been well documented after prolonged use.

Because the specific etiology of this inflammation must be identified, each patient with this complication of asthma must have a consultation with an experienced and competent pediatric allergist and immunologist. Specific inhalant allergen sensitivities must be determined and avoided when possible. No asthmatic child should ever have to undergo surgery for this lesion without the benefit of optimal allergic management, including elimination of pets or smoking in the house, in addition to immunotherapy for unavoidable inhalant allergens.

In those children who are neglected, in the form of "too little and too late" bronchial airway therapy, MLS is a distinct possibility. Those with three episodes should undergo bronchoscopy. Bronchography should be reserved for those who are scheduled for surgery.

Other Causes of Middle Lobe Syndrome

Appropriate therapy for the other causes of MLS might include antibiotics, especially if there is associated loss of immune competency. Central cough suppressants must be avoided because cough facilitates mucus evacuation, which must be permitted to occur. The anti-inflammatory action of simple antihistamines might be necessary to reduce rhinitis, sinusitis, bronchial mucosal edema, and bronchorrhea. Yet, many mixtures contain dextromethorphan, which also must be avoided because this is a codeine derivative with the inherent problem of the parent compound.

REFERENCES

Altamirano HG, McGeady SJ, Mansmann HC Jr: Right middle lobe syndrome in asthmatic children. Pediatr Asthma, Allergy Immunol 5:33–37, 1991.

Livingston GL, Holinger LD, Luck SR: Right middle syndrome in children. Intern J Pediatr Otorhinolaryngol 13:11–23, 1987.

BRONCHITIS AND BRONCHIOLITIS

DEBRA A. TRISTRAM, M.D.
and ROBERT C. WELLIVER, M.D.

BRONCHITIS

Acute bronchitis is a commonly encountered illness in pediatric practice. It is characterized by upper respiratory symptoms (rhinorrhea, pharyngitis), fever, rhonchi on chest auscultation, and, most important, a prominent cough. Wheezing and crackles suggestive of pneumonia are usually absent. Most cases resolve within a week without sequelae, but the cough may persist for several weeks. Pathologically, bronchitis represents inflammation and edema of the larger airways (trachea and bronchi) in contrast to bronchiolitis, which affects the smaller airways. At all ages, viruses are the most common pathogens responsible for bronchitis: Adenoviruses, influenza and parainfluenza viruses, and, less commonly, respiratory syncytial virus (RSV) are recovered from respiratory secretions. In a school-aged child or a younger child with older siblings, *Mycoplasma pneumoniae* may be a frequent culprit. Although concomitant bacterial infection is unusual, persistent fever beyond 6 or 7 days or continued deterioration in clinical status should suggest the possibility of secondary bacterial infection.

Treatment

Because most episodes of bronchitis are caused by viral agents, no specific therapy is generally warranted. Symptomatic therapy aimed at fever and control of pain due to coughing with oral acetominophen (Tylenol) (10 to 15 mg/kg per dose given every 4 to 6 hours) is sufficient in most cases. The routine use of antibiotics is unwarranted. However, if *M. pneumoniae* is suspected, erythromycin (30 to 50 mg/kg/day divided into four equal doses for 10 to 14 days) may shorten the clinical course. For patients whose cough interferes with sleep, or causes post-tussive emesis, cough suppression with dextromethorphan- or codeine-containing compounds may be considered. However, codeine preparations should not be prescribed in children younger than 3 years of age or in those with productive coughing. Adequate hydration should be maintained, and the use of antihistamines and decongestants is discouraged because they may possibly dry secretions and delay mucus clearance from the airways. A trial of an inhaled bronchodilator may be warranted.

BRONCHIOLITIS

Bronchiolitis is an acute infectious illness occurring most commonly in infants 2 to 12 months of age. The illness is characterized initially by upper respiratory symptoms with copious clear nasal discharge and variable degrees of fever. There is progression over 3 to 7 days to lower respiratory infection manifested by tachypnea, wheezing, and lung hyperinflation. In the majority of infants, involvement of the lower respiratory tract is mild. Illness occasionally can be severe with impaired oxygenation and ventilation, requiring mechanically assisted ventilation. This is particularly true for infants younger than 6 weeks of age and in young infants and children with underlying cardiac, pulmonary, or immune defects. Respiratory syncytial virus is the most common pathogen, causing 50 to 75 per cent of all bronchiolitis. Parainfluenza, influenza, and adenoviruses comprise the rest of the viral agents responsible for this clinical picture.

Treatment

The mainstay of treatment for bronchiolitis remains supportive care. Most infants can be managed at home if the respiratory distress is mild and if oral intake is adequate to maintain hydration. If the infant is unable to take adequate fluids orally or if the tachypnea and respiratory distress are of a degree to make aspiration a clear possibility, hospitalization and intravenous hydration are necessary. Maintenance fluids should be provided with correction for increased fluid requirements due to fever or hyperventilation. Infants should not be overhydrated because pulmonary interstitial edema is generally present.

Supplemental oxygen is necessary for hospitalized infants with respiratory distress or hypoxemia. Initial and subsequent monitoring of oxygenation by pulse oximetry facilitates appropriate management of hypoxia. An Oxy-Hood oxygenator or tent with humidified oxygen at an FIO2 of 30 to 40 per cent is often sufficient to maintain an oxygen saturation of greater than 90 to 92 per cent or an arterial PaO_2 of 70 mm Hg or greater. However, the infant at risk for respiratory failure or with elevated Pco_2 concentration may need serial arterial blood gas sampling. Infants with persistently increasing oxygen requirements or progressively rising Pco_2 levels may require intubation and assisted ventilation.

Ribavirin (Virazole) is an antiviral agent that is active against RSV. In early clinical trials, improvement in clinical illness and viral shedding was noted in infants treated with aerosolized Ribavirin; however, the magnitude of the responses was small. For this reason and because of the high cost of the drug, the routine use of Ribavirin is not encouraged for mild to moderate, uncomplicated cases of RSV bronchiolitis. The most current recommendations (1990) of the American Academy of Pediatrics for the use of Ribavirin were as follows: infants at risk for severe disease (i.e., infants with congenital heart disease, bronchopulmonary disorders, or immunodeficiencies); infants younger than 6 weeks of age; and infants severely ill at presentation with PaO_2 less than 65 mm Hg in room air or an increasing $Paco_2$. Ribavirin can be nebulized into an oxygenator, tent, or mask from a solution of 20 mg of Ribavirin per milliliter of sterile water by a special small-particle aerosol generator supplied with the drug by the manufacturer. The treatment is administered for 12 to 18 hours per day for 3 to 7 days. Ribavirin is currently not licensed for use in intubated patients because of problems with precipitation of the drug in the ventilatory tubing. Several studies have demonstrated that such patients can be treated safely with Ribavirin, and this is done frequently at the authors' institution. However, this should be attempted only by personnel who are skilled in the use of ventilators and in the care of small, severely ill infants.

The use of aerosolized bronchodilators, such as albuterol sulfate (Proventil), may be beneficial in certain patients with RSV-associated bronchospasm. Nebulized albuterol in saline can be administered by face mask or by inhaler every 2 to 4 hours. Initial decreases in PaO_2, followed after approximately 30 minutes by improvement in oxygenation, have been noted following this regimen in some infants. Oral or intravenous bronchodilators (oral theophylline preparations and aminophylline drips) have been less effective at producing improvements in oxygenation and are associated with more undesirable side effects—tachycardia, restlessness, and irritability. The use of corticosteroids in bronchiolitis has never been adequately evaluated. Most patients treated at our institution receive a brief trial of aerosolized β-adrenergic agents, but theophylline and corticosteroids are used infrequently.

Because RSV is contagious, children hospitalized for bronchiolitis should be isolated from other children, particularly those with chronic diseases that may predispose them to severe RSV disease. If possible, patients with acute respiratory illnesses should be cohorted. Visitation by siblings who may have respiratory illnesses should be limited during RSV season, and children admitted for reasons other than respiratory infection should perhaps be screened for RSV if a rapid diagnostic test is available. These measures may be helpful in the prevention of nosocomial spread of RSV disease.

ASPIRATION PNEUMONIA

ITZHAK BROOK, M.D.

Aspiration pneumonia involves an inflammatory reaction in the lung parenchyma following entrance of foreign material. Aspiration can be acute or chronic. Following aspiration of food, vomitus, or secretions, the initial reaction is chemical, with edema and cellular infiltrations accompanied by acute respiratory distress. In instances in which mucus secretions containing oral flora are also aspirated, these microorganisms may initiate an infectious process that ranges from aspiration pneumonitis to lung abscess.

MILK, FOOD, AND VOMITUS

Aspiration of milk, food, and vomitus is common in pediatric patients who tend to aspirate because of debilitation, tracheoesophageal malformations, central nervous system disorders, and altered consciousness. Aspiration of food and vomitus rarely causes asphyxiation and death. More often, there is a short latent period of 1 to 2 hours prior to onset of pneumonia. The pneumonia is characterized by tachypnea and fever; rarely do apnea and hypotensive shock occur.

Prevention of aspiration is of particular importance. Overfeeding should be avoided, and the child should be placed on the abdomen with the head elevated. If a large amount of material or material that includes large particles has been aspirated, laryngoscopy or bronchoscopy and direct suctioning of the airway should be initiated as soon as possible. Oxygen saturation greater than 90 per cent should be achieved. Intubation and mechanical ventilation may be required. A program of chest percussion and postural drainage with or without suctioning should be instituted.

Bronchodilatory therapy with theophylline and β-agonists may be useful in improving airway patency. Inhaled β-adrenergic bronchodilators may be used for bronchospasm in standard doses up to every 4 hours. Intravenous aminophylline or oral theophylline may be useful, although such an agent may induce gastroesophageal reflux. The administration of corticosteroids and prophylactic antibiotics is advocated by some; however, their usefulness is not proven.

Bacterial pneumonia is uncommon in the first 48 hours after aspiration, although acute aspiration may suggest the presence of infection (i.e., fever, leukocytosis, and pulmonary infiltrates). Therefore, antimicrobials are not immediately indicated unless the aspirate is contaminated (i.e., pus). Subsequent close monitoring of the patient may reveal signs of superinfection. Signs of infection are a change in the pulmonary infiltrates, recurrent fever or leukocytosis, and clinical deterioration. If superinfection is suspected, Gram stain and culture of tracheal secretion should be performed and antimicrobial therapy should be initiated.

SALIVA AND OROPHARYNGEAL SECRETIONS

Because human saliva and oropharyngeal secretions contain many aerobic and anaerobic bacteria, their aspiration may contaminate the lower respiratory tract. Children with periodontal disease are at particularly high risk. The mixed aerobic-anaerobic infection that usually occurs after aspiration of oropharyngeal secretion into a dependent segment of the lung commences as pneumonitis with relatively mild symptoms. If infection remains unresolved, liquefaction, abscess formation, and empyema occur within 7 to 14 days. Excavation may lead to solitary lung abscess or multiple small areas of necrosis of the lung (necrotizing pneumonia). The severity of the illness varies considerably. Patients with necrotizing pneumonia are often quite ill, and their illness is relatively prolonged. Patients with only parenchymal disease require antibiotic therapy of 3 to 8 weeks for complete cure. A much longer time—perhaps 3 to 4 months—is required for patients with empyema.

THERAPEUTIC DECISIONS

The selection of antimicrobials is guided by age, history, and physical and radiographic findings and by recovery of an organism from the blood, lungs, or pleural space. Nasopharyngeal or sputum aspirates cannot provide reliable specimens for the identification of pathogens because the samples are contaminated by bacteria present in the oropharynx. Interpretation of findings from bronchoalveolar lavage, repeated tracheal washings, or quantitative culture of the sputum may also be confounded by contamination of the specimen by oropharyngeal organisms. Attempts should be made, if experienced personnel are available, to avoid such contamination by sampling the lower respiratory tract by direct lung puncture or transtracheal aspiration (TTA).

Because of the small risks (occurring in fewer than 1 per cent of patients) of bleeding, pneumothorax, and subcutaneous or mediastinal emphysema involved in TTA or lung puncture, even when performed by experienced persons, the decision to perform an invasive diagnostic procedure should be weighed against the potential benefit. In most instances, selection of antimicrobials can be made without any of these procedures. However, in patients who do not respond to therapy or who are at risk of harboring unusual or resistant pathogens, obtaining culture specimens through these procedures should be considered. Transtracheal aspiration is contraindicated in uncooperative patients and in those with bleeding diatheses, severe coughing, and serious dyspnea and hypoxemia requiring positive-pressure ventilatory aid.

The organisms recovered from the infected lungs consist of mixed flora of aerobic and anaerobic bacteria. The number of organisms that can be isolated from these infections varies between three and ten (average of three anaerobes and two aerobes). The predominant anaerobes include anaerobic or microaerophilic streptococci, pigmented *Prevotella* and *Porphyromonas* species (previously called *Bacteroides melaninogenicus* group), *Fusobacterium, Clostridium* sp., and *Bacteroides fragilis* group. The major aerobic pathogens are *Staphylococcus aureus, Klebsiella pneumoniae,* and *Pseudomonas aeruginosa.*

Antimicrobial therapy may be guided by Gram stain of appropriate material but should not be withheld pending culture results in severely ill patients. Although penicillin G may be effective, increasing numbers of oral pathogens (i.e., *Prevotella, Porphyromonas, Fusobacterium, Haemophilus, S. aureus*) are capable of resisting penicillin mostly through the production of beta-lactamase. These resistant strains are often found in patients who have recently been treated with beta-lactam antibiotics.

Clindamycin and cefoxitin are effective alternatives to penicillin in the treatment of anaerobic pleuropulmonary infections. In addition to their effectiveness against beta-lactamase–producing anaerobes, clindamycin and cefoxitin are also effective against various aerobic organisms, including *S. aureus* and *Streptococcus* whereas cefoxitin is also effective against Enterobacteriaceae. Carbenicillin and ticarcillin are effective against *Bacteroides* as well as many anaerobic and aerobic gram-negative rods and manifest synergy with aminoglycosides against aerobic organisms. This factor should be considered when such organisms, especially *Pseudomonas,* are recovered. Imipenem-cilistatin and the combination of a penicillin (i.e., amoxicillin) and a beta-lactamase inhibitor (i.e., clavulanic acid) are active against most pathogens isolated from this infection, including those that produce beta-lactamase. However, the addition of agents effective against enteric gram-negative rods may be needed when these organisms are also present. These include aminoglycosides (i.e., gentamicin, tobramycin) or the quinolones (in children older than 16 years).

Prevention of further aspiration following appropriate diagnostic studies to identify the specific cause is the most important aspect of management. This may be accomplished by correction of reflux, gastric tube feeding, and improved oral feeding strategies.

HYDROCARBONS

Aspiration of hydrocarbons, such as kerosene, gasoline, and turpentine, can cause a secondary pneumonitis. Following accidental or intentional ingestion, the child gags, coughs, and sometimes vomits. All these can induce direct aspiration of the ingested hydrocarbon. Pulmonary symptoms in extensive aspiration can be observed within hours; however, in cases of minimal aspiration they may be delayed up to 1 day. These symptoms include tachypnea, dyspnea, cough, and fever. Radiographic changes, which are usually in the lung bases, may also be delayed in appearance up to 48 to 96 hours.

No therapy is indicated prior to appearance of symptoms. In those with mild or no respiratory symptoms, close observation for 4 to 6 hours may be sufficient. Induction of vomiting or gastric lavage is generally contraindicated because of the risk of further pulmonary aspiration. Therefore, gastric emptying is indicated only when the material ingested includes other toxic substances or when an unusually large volume of hydrocarbons has been ingested (more than 1 ml/kg). Gastric lavage should be performed, preferably after tracheal intubation, to minimize further aspiration. If dyspnea or cyanosis develops, patients should be hospitalized and supportive therapy is indicated. This includes supplemental oxygen, tracheal intubation, and mechanical ventilation with positive end-expiratory pressure, physiotherapy, and bronchodilation with intravenous theophylline and inhalation of β-adrenergic bronchodilators. Antimicrobial therapy is indicated only when secondary bacterial infection develops. This can be suspected when fever reappears and symptoms and signs worsen. Administration of corticosteroids has not been shown to be helpful. Prevention of ingestion by small children should be emphasized to parents in health maintenance visits.

BRONCHIECTASIS

THOMAS F. BOAT, M.D.

ETIOLOGY

Bronchiectasis is defined pathologically as an abnormal and permanent dilation of cartilaginous airways at the subsegmental level and more peripherally. Bronchiectasis is often accompanied by bronchiolectasis, and in fact the two conditions undoubtedly have a common etiology in individual patients. Although in the past many cases of bronchiectasis were termed idiopathic, a specific etiology can now be assigned with increasing frequency. Etiologic factors included genetic disorders, such as cystic fibrosis; Young's syndrome, one of the immune deficiency states; primary ciliary dyskinesia; and the Campbell Williams syndrome. Causes of acquired bronchiectasis included asthma with allergic bronchopulmonary aspergillosis, severe adenovirus and other viral airways infections, improperly treated acute bacterial infections, endobronchial tuberculosis, foreign body aspiration, other aspiration syndromes (as in gastroesophageal reflux), and bronchopulmonary dysplasia.

DIAGNOSIS

Bronchiectasis is best detected and assessed by imaging techniques. Routine chest x-rays can demonstrate advanced bronchiectasis. High-resolution computed tomographic (CT) imaging is more sensitive and may now be the procedure of choice, even for smaller children. The diagnostic standard in the past, bronchograms are still used occasionally to define the airways anatomy prior to surgical therapy.

TREATMENT

The initial treatment for bronchiectasis should be medical. Failure of medical therapy to control symptoms and stabilize lung function should raise the question of surgical removal of the involved area(s). Two major objectives of medical therapy are to assist in the clearance of secretions and to control infection or noninfectious inflammation. The mainstay of therapy to clear secretions is chest physical therapy (postural drainage and chest percussion). For example, in patients with cystic fibrosis, this procedure is effective in maintaining pulmonary function when performed on a daily basis. Chest physical therapy can be delivered manually or with a number of mechanical devices that should be effective if properly used. Maintenance of adequate hydration and prompt treatment of dehydration are important, as dehydration promotes removal of water from the secretions and interferes with their clearance. In general, expectorants such as guaifenesin or iodides and mucolytic agents are not useful. *For example, current formulations of N-acetyl cysteine aerosolized into the airways are toxic for ciliated cells and cause an impressive inflammatory response when used more than several days at a time.* More harm than benefit may be done. One exception may be recombinant human DNase, which has recently become available for study and which may be useful for liquifying purulent secretions that contain large amounts of DNA. Aerosol therapy, especially if combined with chest physical therapy, may add additional water, at least in small amounts, to airways secretions and assist their removal. In addition, delivery of a bronchodilator by this route may dilate airways and promote expectoration if the patient can be shown to have reactive airways (15 per cent improvement of FEV_1) as well as improved mucociliary clearance. A substantial shortcoming of all aerosol therapy for bronchiectasis is that drug is not delivered to those areas of the lung that are most involved with mucus plugging.

A second major mode of medical treatment is antibiotic therapy of infection. Use of antibiotics should be determined by the severity of lower respiratory tract symptoms, presence of purulent secretions, and identification of specific pathogenic organisms in sputum or other respiratory cultures as well as their sensitivity patterns. Treatment consists of maximal doses of an antibiotic administered for a relatively long period of time, usually 2 to 4 weeks or until symptoms are controlled. Even using large doses, it is difficult to achieve effective levels of antibiotic in the airways lumen. In general, small doses of antibiotics over long periods of time to "suppress infection" are not useful, in that effective levels of antibiotic in airways secretions cannot be achieved. This approach may also promote the emergence of resistant bacterial strains. Adequate immunization to protect against respiratory pathogens, such as the measles virus and *Bordetella pertussis,* is mandatory. Yearly doses of influenza vaccine are recommended. In addition, careful avoidance of cigarette smoke, both active and passive exposure, and other noxious inhalants is an important component of therapy.

Other medical therapy should be tailored to deal with the specific etiology of bronchiectasis. For example, immunoglobulin replacement therapy for immunodeficiency problems, treatment with steroids for proximal bronchiectasis associated with allergic bronchopulmonary aspergillosis, antimicrobial treatment of tuberculosis, and removal of an undetected foreign body are essential to prevent progressive destruction of airways and loss of function.

If bronchiectasis is progressive and symptoms such as severe cough and fever cannot be controlled medically, surgical therapy should be considered. Lobectomy has been a frequent treatment of bronchiectasis in the past and continues to be an important consideration in selected cases. Lobectomy generally should be reserved for patients who have localized bronchiectasis (confined to one or at the most two lobes) and for whom an underlying progressive condition is not responsible for the bronchiectasis. For example, removal of an area of bronchiectasis in a patient with cystic fibrosis is at best a temporizing measure, in that generalized bronchiectasis occurs in nearly all patients with time. Recent advances in lung transplantation offer hope for a number of children with generalized bronchiectasis and end-stage lung disease. An increasing number of older children with cystic fibrosis have received lung transplants. Although most of these procedures can be accomplished successfully, graft-versus-host reactions and other problems have limited long-term normal functioning of many transplanted lungs.

The complications of bronchiectasis also deserve therapeutic consideration. Heavy and disabling cough may lead to emesis and weight loss and is certainly uncomfortable for the patient. Control of severe cough should be approached through aggressive medical therapy and, if necessary, surgical therapy. The use of antitussives is in general contraindicated. Cough is a necessary and important mechanism for removing secretions when the usual clearance mechanisms are compromised. Hemoptysis is a common complication of bronchiectasis and can be treated with more vigorous medical therapy, with bronchial artery embolization, and with lobectomy in very carefully selected cases. Other complications, such as pneumothorax, cor pulmonale, and respiratory failure, are treated as in other lung conditions and are discussed elsewhere in this volume (see pp. 119 and 137).

ATELECTASIS

THOMAS A. HAZINSKI, M.D.

The term "atelectasis" is used to describe the collapse of alveoli that occurs when an airway is completely obstructed and trapped alveolar gas is reabsorbed. Like fever, it is a clinical sign and not a disease itself. In normal individuals, atelectasis may occasionally be detected by auscultation as transient rales or crackles accompanying a deep inspiration over dependent lung regions. In this situation, the sounds arise from re-expansion of a previously atelectatic area. However, atelectatic regions are usually difficult to detect by clinical examination unless an entire lobe is collapsed; in this case, breath sounds will be absent or diminished over the affected area.

Unless a large airway is abruptly obstructed, atelectasis rarely leads to gas exchange impairment because perfusion is symmetrically reduced to the affected area and ventilation-perfusion matching is maintained.

Practically speaking, the diagnosis of atelectasis is most often considered when one or more patchy densities are seen on plain radiographs of the chest. When the atelectatic area is focal and large, adjacent lung regions are overinflated and the mediastinum shifts toward it; these two findings are absent when the lung is consolidated, as seen in lobar pneumonia. Atelectasis may be *diffuse,* such as that seen with hyaline membrane disease, hydrocarbon ingestion, or neuromuscular disorders. It may also be *focal,* such as that seen in bronchial obstruction due to foreign body; extrinsic airway compression due to nodes, tumors, blood vessels, or a dilated heart; or diseases that cause mucus impaction of bronchi (asthma, cystic fibrosis, or bronchopulmonary aspergillosis).

It may be difficult to differentiate atelectasis radiographically from focal edema, inflammation, or nonpulmonary masses. As a result, atelectasis may be erroneously interpreted as persistent or recurrent pneumonia and treated with repeated courses of antimicrobial therapy. In these instances, review of previous chest radiographs as well as a chest radiograph taken when the child is clinically asymptomatic may allow differentiation between recurrent and persistent disease. Persistent atelectasis at one site in all radiographs suggests the presence of congenital or acquired bronchial obstruction, stenosis, or postinflammatory bronchiectasis. In addition, congenital malformations, such as an H-type tracheoesophageal fistula, esophageal duplication, sequestered lung, lung abscess, or infected lung cyst, may present as persistent focal atelectasis. Radiographic shadows caused by thoracic tumors, such as neuroblastoma and teratoma, may also be interpreted as atelectasis. Recurrent or wandering infiltrates suggest the presence of mucus impaction (cystic fibrosis or asthma), chronic aspiration, pulmonary hemorrhage (hemosiderosis), or gastroesophageal reflux. In these patients, an esophagogram, sweat test, technetium lung scan, and a search for hemosiderin-laden macrophages in gastric aspirate or lung lavage may be useful in establishing an etiology.

The availability of high-resolution chest computed tomography (CT) has proved useful in the evaluation of persistent or recurrent atelectasis. Improvements in technology permit high-resolution imaging of the chest even in uncooperative or tachypneic patients. These studies may reveal a generalized parenchymal abnormality when only focal abnormalities have been initially suggested by routine chest radiographs.

CLINICAL CONDITIONS ASSOCIATED WITH ATELECTASIS

Patients Receiving Mechanical Ventilation

Atelectasis often develops in individuals who are receiving intermittent mandatory ventilation. In these patients, mucociliary clearance and lung fluid balance are impaired whereas sedation and immobility promote stasis of secretions in dependent lung regions. Moreover, some mechanically ventilated patients may have reduced immunity as a result of their underlying disease or its therapy. Inadvertent or intermittent intubation of a mainstem bronchus may cause complete atelectasis of an entire lung and profound hypoxemia. Although vigorous deep suctioning may prevent atelectasis in these patients, it may also cause mucosal damage and stimulate mucus secretion, which may in itself lead to further mucus plugging. For this reason, proper airway suctioning should be performed (i.e., passing the side hole of the suction catheter just below the tip of the endotracheal tube and no further) to ensure the effectiveness of this procedure.

In mechanically ventilated patients, it may be especially difficult to differentiate pulmonary infection from focal atelectasis. Studies in adults indicate that the probability of developing a ventilator-associated pneumonia rises by 1 per cent per day after 7 days of mechanical ventilation. Tracheal aspirate cytologic and culture specimens, while easy to obtain, are often misleading and lack specificity. In these patients, bronchoalveolar lavage via flexible fiberoptic bronchoscopy may be a more accurate way to determine the presence or absence of infection. Even with equivocal lavage data, however, the ventilated patient with new pulmonary infiltrates, worsening gas exchange, and constitutional symptoms deserves treatment with broad-spectrum antimicrobial therapy.

Bronchial Asthma and the Right Middle Lobe Syndrome

Bronchoconstriction, airway infection-inflammation, and increased mucus secretion in the asthmatic child may cause distal airway obstruction and patchy atelectasis where the obstruction is complete. The right middle lobe bronchus is especially vulnerable to persistent recurrent obstruction. Although bacterial pneumonias rarely trigger asthma, asthmatic patients with diffuse infiltrates are usually treated with antimicrobial agents. However, when these infiltrates clear rapidly, a retrospective diagnosis of atelectasis can be made.

The combination of diffuse atelectasis and high-dose bronchodilator therapy may present an unusual paradoxical syndrome in some asthmatic patients. Some patients with respiratory distress and wheezing promptly respond to bronchodilator therapy but still require high-dose oxygen therapy to maintain oxygen saturation. This occurs because β_2-agonist bronchodilator agents are also vasodilators, and these patients may therefore overperfuse unventilated atelectatic lung regions. This leads to the development of right-to-left intrapulmonary shunts and is clinically seen as an increased oxygen requirement with little evidence of respiratory distress. In these instances, a reduction of bronchodilator therapy may permit a reduction in oxygen therapy.

Cystic Fibrosis

Atelectasis occurs when small airways become obstructed by thick mucus or by secretions infected by *Staphylococcus* or *Pseudomonas* bacteria. These infiltrates may be clinically asymptomatic. In these patients, chest physiotherapy, antibiotics, and perhaps the inhalation of mucolytic agents are useful.

Cardiac Causes of Atelectasis

A dilated heart or dilated great vessels can cause airway compression and atelectasis. If the left atrium is enlarged (from congestive heart failure, mitral valve disease, aortic stenosis, or coarctation of aorta), the left mainstem or lower lobe bronchus may become completely obstructed. Hypertensive pulmonary arteries may cause obstruction of the left upper lobe or right middle lobe bronchus.

In these cases, treatment should be directed toward the underlying cause with anticongestive therapy and surgery if indicated. Treatment of atelectasis with chest physiotherapy, bronchodilator inhalation, or bronchoscopy may also be used if gas exchange is impaired.

PREVENTION AND TREATMENT OF ATELECTASIS

In a patient receiving mechanical ventilation, positive end-expiratory pressure (PEEP), ventilator-generated sighs, and voluntary deep breathing may be effective in reversing or preventing atelectasis. In the surgical patient, analgesic administration must be sufficient to permit deep breathing and cough yet not suppress ventilatory drive. In young patients, incentive spirometers are useful in encouraging deep breaths and are available in game-like configurations.

Although chest percussion and other forms of chest physiotherapy are thought to be useful for patients with chronic suppurative diseases, such as cystic fibrosis, the value of these methods in treating diffuse or acute atelectasis is unproven. In these patients, frequent changes of position, coughing, and deep breathing may be all that is necessary. Patients with chronic focal atelectasis should receive a therapeutic trial of chest physiotherapy to the affected site. In addition, the patient can be positioned so that ventilation is optimal to the atelectatic area (i.e., the atelectatic lung should be placed superiorly). The inhalation of β_2-agonists may speed the resolution of atelectasis, but no relevant controlled trials are available to address this issue. Bronchoscopic evaluation of the atelectatic lung segment is useful to define a cause and to obtain secretions for culture and staining. However, if the atelectasis is due to conditions other than a simple mucus plug, a single bronchoscopy may not hasten the resolution of a chronically atelectatic area. Bronchoscopy should be reserved for patients with refractory atelectasis or suspected intrabronchial lesions.

If anatomic obstruction and congenital malformations have

been ruled out and gas exchange is unimpaired, patients with atelectasis can be observed as outpatients. Most studies have shown that atelectasis responds to conservative measures. Depending on the severity of the atelectasis, chest physiotherapy alone or in combination with bronchodilator inhalation may be tried for weeks. Persistent atelectasis of greater than 6 weeks' duration unresponsive to outpatient management may require more intensive investigation. Surgical excision of atelectatic lung, usually secondary to segmental bronchiectasis, is rarely required.

EMPHYSEMA

DENNIS C. STOKES, M.D.

DEFINITION

The pathologic process of emphysema refers to the permanent dilation of peripheral airways and alveoli with destruction and loss of connective tissue so that alveolar spaces are enlarged. Typically, emphysema is accompanied by loss of lung elasticity, airflow obstruction, and gas trapping. This classic definition applies to a form of emphysema that is most commonly found in adults with chronic obstructive pulmonary disease (COPD), generally related to cigarette smoking. Although strictly speaking emphysema is a pathologic diagnosis, the diagnosis is most often made on the basis of clinical and radiographic findings. Emphysema is often used to describe any clinical process that results in increased radiolucency of the lung. This may occur as a result of increased air trapping in the lung, air in the interstitial space, actual destruction of lung tissue in true emphysema, or decreased blood flow (which usually accompanies alveolar hypoxia in emphysema).

PATHOLOGIC FEATURES

Alpha$_1$-Antiprotease Deficiency

Alpha$_1$-antiprotease (also known as alpha$_1$-antitrypsin) deficiency is the prototypical form of emphysema in adulthood, but it has only very rarely been associated with emphysematous changes in the lung in the first two decades of life. In alpha$_1$-antiprotease deficiency, there is a congenital absence of A$_1$-AP, a major protease inhibitor synthesized in the liver that circulates and protects the lungs from proteases derived from neutrophils and other inflammatory cells. These unopposed proteases can then produce lung destruction and emphysema due to destruction of elastin and other connective tissue elements. Typically, the emphysema is of the panacinar, basilar type and occurs primarily in individuals who smoke. Alpha$_1$-antiprotease deficiency also predisposes to development of liver disease, particularly in infants and children, because of the build-up of defective alpha$_1$-antiprotease in the hepatocyte.

Alpha$_1$-antiprotease exists as several variants by protein electrophoresis, also known as Pi types, with varying degrees of enzymatic activity. These include M, S, and Z Pi types, with most individuals having MM genotype and normal levels of activity. ZZ individuals have the lowest activity, and generally emphysema develops in the third and fourth decades of life, particularly when lung inflammation is aggravated by smoking. A$_1$-AP is only one of several antiproteases present in the lung-lining fluid. Other types of antiproteases, such as secretory leukocyte protease inhibitor (SLPI), are also important in preventing lung destruction from proteases derived from inflammatory cells. Inactivation of A$_1$-AP and SLPI by bacterial toxins and proteases in chronic inflammatory states like cystic fibrosis (CF) and bronchopulmonary dysplasia may contribute to development of airway damage and localized emphysema in those disorders.

Congenital Lobar Emphysema

Patients with congenital lobar emphysema are among the most common pediatric patients with emphysema, but in fact most of these patients do not fit the true pathologic definition of emphysema. There are several varieties of congenital lobar emphysema, and presentation may be a severe life-threatening overdistention of a lobe or lung. Most patients with congenital lobar emphysema will require surgery soon after diagnosis. In rare instances, this form of emphysema may remain relatively asymptomatic. Pathologic examination of the excised lobe will help classify the pathogenesis of the hyperinflation as extrinsic compression of the bronchus, intraluminal abnormalities (such as incomplete cartilage), or (rarely) intrinsic abnormalities of the pulmonary parenchyma. In up to 50 per cent of reported cases, no clear abnormality is demonstrated.

Cystic Adenomatoid Malformation and Lung Cysts

Cystic adenomatoid malformation generally presents as a unilobar collection of cystic lesions that can cause respiratory distress as air is trapped. Other single cysts can be found in pediatric patients as congenital or acquired lesions with a hyperlucent appearance and can generally be distinguished from emphysematous enlargement of lung by their pathologic appearance and the lack of blood vessels within the cyst.

Pulmonary Interstitial Emphysema

Pulmonary interstitial emphysema (PIE) is typically seen in premature newborns with hyaline membrane disease who require high pressures for ventilation. Air begins to dissect along interstitial tissue planes, producing a typical radiographic appearance. Airways and vessels are compressed as the air accumulates in the interstitium. If therapy is not instituted, this process will progress to worsened respiratory failure, pneumothorax, or pneumomediastinum. Mean airway pressure must generally be reduced to manage PIE effectively, by decreasing peak pressure and positive end-expiratory pressure (PEEP) or by shortening inspiratory times. This may require increased rates of ventilation and/or increased inspired oxygen concentration to maintain adequate gas exchange. If PIE is unilateral, the affected lung can be placed in the dependent position, favoring ventilation to the normal lung; or the unaffected lung can be intubated and ventilation maintained using that lung until PIE resolves in the contralateral lung. Various forms of high-frequency ventilation have also been used successfully in PIE.

Secondary (Compensatory) Emphysema Following Airways Obstruction

Compensatory emphysema is the most common form of emphysema in childhood and is seen in a variety of disorders, including foreign body aspiration, cystic fibrosis, asthma, and endobronchial obstructing lesions (such as a bronchial adenoma or granulation tissue resulting from a long-standing foreign body). With complete obstruction of a major bronchus, the lung beyond the bronchus becomes atelectatic and the unaffected lung usually expands and becomes more radiolucent. If there is partial obstruction and "ball valving," the lung beyond the obstruction develops air trapping and an emphysematous appearance. Fluoroscopy or inspiratory-expiratory radiographs are very useful in these cases in demonstrating air trapping as the mechanism for "emphysema."

Swyer-James Syndrome (Unilateral or Lobar Emphysema)

Swyer-James syndrome (unilateral or lobar emphysema, or unilateral hyperlucent lung) refers to a radiographic appearance of the lung that has been described following a variety of insults, including measles, adenovirus, *Mycoplasma,* and hydrocarbon pneumonias. In this disorder, a lung or portion of lung shows major destruction of small airways with bronchitis, bronchiectasis, and bronchiolitis obliterans, which result in secondary emphysematous changes. Because this lung or portion of lung is also hypoxic, there is blood flow shunting away from the area and this is a major contributor to the characteristic hyperlucent appearance on chest radiographs rather than increased air or loss of lung tissue. The asymmetry is most marked in expiratory films, and typically the lung is normal or reduced in size and is never increased in volume. Early insults that lead to reduced lung growth produce the greatest reduction in lung size. Lung scans show reduced perfusion and ventilation; pulmonary arteriograms, although rarely necessary, show a typical "pruned tree" appearance of reduced peripheral pulmonary blood flow.

Swyer-James syndrome must be distinguished from endobronchial partial obstructing lesions, congenital hypoplastic pulmonary artery, and previous massive pulmonary embolism. Clinical manifestations are highly variable and may include localized wheezing, relative hyperresonance, and diminished chest expansion.

TREATMENT

Therapy of emphysema depends on determination of the cause. Significant lobar emphysema in the newborn period generally warrants surgical removal, although occasionally a patient can be managed with conservative therapy. Management of secondary obstructive emphysema depends on the etiology. If a foreign body or an endobronchial lesion, such as granulation tissue or bronchial adenoma, is suspected, diagnostic bronchoscopy should be performed. Generally, rigid bronchoscopy should be performed if a foreign body or obstructing endobronchial lesion is suspected. Secondary obstruction in asthma or CF usually responds to more conservative therapy with chest physiotherapy and bronchodilators. Although it is rare in childhood, $alpha_1$-antiprotease deficiency is now being treated with replacement therapy using both intravenous and aerosol $alpha_1$-antiprotease; however, efforts should primarily be directed at avoidance of smoking in young adults with $alpha_1$-antiprotease deficiency. Antiprotease therapy with $alpha_1$-antiprotease and SLPI produced by new genetic technologies are under investigation for CF and other diseases associated with lung destruction by chronic inflammation.

PULMONARY THROMBOEMBOLISM

REGINA MARY PALAZZO, M.D.

Pulmonary thromboembolism is a rare, albeit underdiagnosed complication of childhood disease. Primary pulmonary thrombosis may occur in functional protein C deficiency, antithrombin III deficiency, in the presence of lupus anticoagulant, and in sickle cell disease. More often, pulmonary thromboembolism is secondary to extra-pulmonary emboli, reaching the pulmonary arteries via the venous system. Identifying the source of the pulmonary thromboembolic disease and initiating appropriate therapy are integral to managing the disease.

DIAGNOSIS

Risk factors for thromboembolic events include indwelling catheters, ventriculoatrial shunts, congenital heart disease, recent surgery, sepsis, hemangiomas, arteriovenous malformations, occult malignancy, and prolonged immobility. The patient's history and physical examination findings are nonspecific. The sudden onset of shortness of breath, anxiety, and, less frequently, chest pain are reported by most patients. Tachypnea and tachycardia represent the most consistent physical findings. Although hypoxemia is frequent, as evidenced by an increased alveolar-arterial oxygen difference, the oxygen saturations may be within a normal range. The alveolar-arterial oxygen difference is a more sensitive assessment of pulmonary ventilation than is oxygen saturation. The chest radiogram may be normal or may demonstrate an infiltrate (the classic wedge-shaped defect is not always appreciated); effusion, if present, is usually ipsilateral. An awareness of the risk factors, coupled with the physical findings and laboratory assessment, can direct a further diagnostic work-up.

Duplex studies (ultrasound combined with Doppler studies) of the deep venous system in the legs are as helpful as contrast venography with less risk. Although pulmonary arteriography is the gold standard for the diagnosis of pulmonary emboli, a perfusion lung scan supported by the findings on a xenon ventilation scan (accompanied by the results of duplex studies) may obviate the need for pulmonary arteriography. If ventilation-perfusion scans of the lungs in conjunction with venous studies of the legs do not clearly direct therapy, pulmonary arteriography is indicated.

TREATMENT

Identification of risk factors and attempts to prevent the development of extrapulmonary thrombi constitute the best therapy. Supportive therapy in the form of supplemental oxygen, inotropic support of systemic blood pressure, and analgesic control of chest pain along with the immediate institution of anticoagulant therapy with heparin is indicated upon the diagnosis of pulmonary embolism.

In the unstable, critically ill patient, surgical embolectomy carries substantial mortality. Thrombolytic therapy with urokinase, streptokinase, or tissue plasminogen activator along with heparin increases the rate of resolution of the pulmonary embolus but has not had statistically significant effects on survival or recurrence rates compared with heparin alone. Recurrent emboli are the primary cause of death in most patients with massive pulmonary emboli; therefore, the placement of a Greenfield filter in the inferior vena cava in conjunction with heparin therapy has a role with this group of patients.

Heparin is the mainstay of therapy in stable patients. Heparin arrests growth of the thrombus and prevents platelet aggregation. Therapy should be initiated with a dose of 50 to 75 units/kg, and activated partial thromboplastin time (APTT) is maintained at 1.5 to two times control values with 25 units/kg. Anticoagulant therapy with heparin should be continued for 5 to 14 days. Long-term anticoagulant therapy with subcutaneous heparin or warfarin is guided by evidence of resolution on the lung scan as well as the need for continued therapy for the deep vein thrombosis.

Patients in whom there is poor resolution of the thromboembolic event and who have pulmonary hypertension or dyspnea at rest should be suspected of having chronic thromboembolic occlusion. If this condition is diagnosed early, it may be amenable to pulmonary endarterectomy.

OUTCOME

The incidence of chronic thromboembolic occlusion is very low. The rule for patients surviving the acute event is complete resolution. Recurrence rates are highest in those with ongoing risk factors for extrapulmonary thrombus formation. In that group of patients, longer-term prophylaxis with anticoagulant therapy is indicated.

REFERENCES

Moser KM: Venous thromboembolism. Am Rev Respir Dis 141:235–249, 1990.

PRIMARY PULMONARY HEMOSIDEROSIS

ANDREW A. COLIN, M.D.
and MARY ELLEN B. WOHL, M.D.

Primary (idiopathic) pulmonary hemosiderosis (PPH) is one of several conditions associated with bleeding into the lung. The classic presentation of diffuse pulmonary hemorrhage is the triad of hemoptysis, anemia, and diffuse alveolar infiltration. The three elements rarely coexist, however, and thus a fall in hematocrit value with the onset of respiratory disease should suggest pulmonary bleeding.

The initial presentation is variable, ranging from a fulminant onset with acute, occasionally fatal hemoptysis to an insidious presentation characterized by anemia, pallor, weakness, and poor weight gain. Some patients vomit swallowed blood and do not have hemoptysis.

Physical examination is nonspecific, ranging from dyspnea, with crackles and wheezing on lung auscultation to the physical findings associated with pulmonary hypertension or frank respiratory failure. Fever and chest pain are sometimes associated with the bleeding episode. Similarly, radiographic abnormalities are not specific and vary from minimal fleeting infiltrates to massive parenchymal involvement and may change in the individual patient with recurrent bleeding. In patients with small, frequent episodes of bleeding, the radiographs may reflect chronic diffuse interstitial involvement and may change only minimally with an acute episode of bleeding. Computed tomography (CT) appears to offer no better specificity. Magnetic resonance imaging (MRI) of the lung may prove more useful in defining the presence of blood, showing decreased signal on the T2-weighted images.

Bronchoscopy usually establishes the diagnosis of pulmonary bleeding. Careful examination of the airway will exclude sites in the nasopharynx, trachea, and bronchi, whereas bronchoalveolar lavage will show iron-laden macrophages. The demonstration of iron-laden macrophages by gastric lavage is a useful test in infants. Occasionally, endoscopy of the gastrointestinal (GI) tract will be necessary to exclude GI bleeding with aspiration of blood as the cause of apparent pulmonary hemorrhage.

The hematologic work-up typically reveals hypochromic, microcytic anemia with relatively low serum iron, reflecting prolonged blood loss into the lung with the iron being sequestered by pulmonary macrophages. Coagulation studies will rule out pulmonary hemorrhage of potentially treatable cause. Cardiac evaluation, including electrocardiography and echocardiography, seeks to find evidence of pulmonary hypertension and to rule out cardiac conditions occasionally associated with pulmonary bleeding, such as myocarditis, mitral stenosis, and chronic left heart failure.

Once bleeding has been localized to the lung parenchyma, a lung biopsy will be helpful in defining its etiology. Light microscopy will address the possibility of a veno-occlusive malformation, an infectious cause, or a vasculitis (indicating the presence of connective tissue disease). Immunofluorescence studies will further support the latter diagnosis and reveal deposits of immunoglobulin and complement along the basement membrane that will point to the diagnosis of Goodpasture's syndrome. Electron microscopy may reveal breaks along the capillary endothelial lining.

Classifications of conditions associated with diffuse pulmonary hemorrhage (DPH) have been attempted. Although such classifications constitute a helpful methodologic approach to the pursuit of a diagnosis, it is important to point out that only rarely can a pediatric patient be classified into a well-defined nosologic entity. In most cases, PPH represents a variety of conditions that elude definition and have variable and unpredictable prognoses. Patients with PPH, therefore, need to be observed at regular intervals for subsequent involvement of other systems, such as heart, kidney, thymus, and joints, which can become abnormal in immunologically mediated disease. Because chronic or recurrent bleeding into the lung can be associated with the development of pulmonary fibrosis, regular measurements of lung function are indicated when patients are "well." These studies include spirometry, lung volumes, diffusing capacity (DLCO), and oxygen saturation during exercise. The studies are useful for estimating the degree of respiratory impairment prior to further acute episodes of bleeding, for detecting subsequent ongoing low-grade bleeding, and for evaluating therapeutic interventions.

The immunologic evaluation and follow-up throughout the life of the patient should include immunoglobulins and IgG subclasses (since IgA and IgG_4 were found to be sometimes reduced), serum antibodies to cow's milk protein, and serial measurements of anti–basement membrane antibody, anti-neutrophil cytoplasm antibody (ANCA), immune complexes, and complement.

The laboratory follow-up of patients with PPH includes (in addition to hemoglobin and hematocrit determinations) repeated urinalyses and renal function studies. Minimal indication of renal function impairment should lead to the consideration of renal biopsy because a combined pulmonary-renal disease may be late in revealing itself and severe renal changes can evolve with little warning.

The treatment of PPH in the acute stage is largely supportive, consisting of oxygen administration or mechanical ventilation, preferably with positive end-expiratory pressure (PEEP) in severe episodes. Blood transfusion is indicated in severe anemia or shock.

The evaluation of therapeutic modalities of PPH is complicated by the variable prognosis and by spontaneous resolution in many childhood cases. Few of the therapeutic modalities adopted in the treatment of PPH have proved to be effective, and none has been evaluated by strict scientific criteria. Avoidance of milk is suggested in babies, but this measure probably has no role in older children. Other elimination diets have been advocated with anecdotal success as has inhaled sodium cromoglycate. *Deferoxamine,* an iron-chelating agent, has shown little promise when used. In cases of IgA or IgG_4 deficiency, gamma globulin replacement has proved effective.

The most widely accepted and successful therapies adopted in patients with PPH indicate that although immune processes are not well defined, suppression of a putative immunologic mechanism is the goal of therapy. Most commonly used are corticosteroids, which are administered parenterally at a high dose in the acute phase and later replaced by oral therapy for periods tailored to the needs of the individual patient. Immunosuppressant drugs, such as azathioprine (Imuran) or cyclophosphamide (Cytoxan), have been widely used in combination with corticosteroids in more severe cases. A recently advocated method is plasmapheresis, sometimes combined with gamma globulin replacement immediately following the procedure. The absence of an immunologic marker indicating the activity of the disease or its response to therapy is the main obstacle to the assessment of the efficacy of any of these approaches.

CYSTIC FIBROSIS

H. KOPELMAN, M.D.
and G. MICHAEL DAVIS, M.B. Ch.B.

Cystic fibrosis (CF) is the most common lethal genetic disorder in Caucasians, inherited in autosomal recessive fashion, with an estimated incidence of 1 in 2000 to 1 in 2500 live births. It is the most frequent cause of pancreatic insufficiency and of chronic lung disease with progressive pulmonary failure in childhood.

Although pulmonary and pancreatic manifestations are the most prominent, CF is a multisystem disorder, affecting many different exocrine glands and organs lined by epithelial surfaces. Involvement of the sweat glands is almost universal and is the basis for the sweat test, used worldwide in the diagnosis of CF. In the appropriate clinical setting, a sweat chloride concentration of greater than 60 mEq/L on two occasions in a sample of 100 mg of sweat confirms the diagnosis of CF.

During the more than 50 years since the original description of CF, increasing knowledge has altered the approaches to management of this disorder. Improvements in antibiotics and chest physiotherapy, enzyme, vitamin, and nutritional therapy, early recognition of complications, and more aggressive management have been associated with an increasing life expectancy. By the 1980s, almost 80 per cent of affected individuals were living beyond their 20th birthday.

Over the past decade, research has rapidly advanced our understanding of the basic genetic, biochemical, and physiologic defect in this disorder: the demonstration of faulty regulation of epithelial cell chloride transport in CF; its role in decreased epithelial fluid secretion accounting for the clinical manifestations of the disease; identification of the CF gene on chromosome 7; the recognition that its gene product, the protein CFTR, is responsible for the chloride transport defect; and the association of different allelic mutations in the CF gene with variability in clinical expression. This new information is already being used to try to develop newer diagnostic and prenatal testing and newer treatment approaches to CF for the future.

GENETICS

Cystic fibrosis is an autosomal recessive disorder. The CF gene has now been cloned, and the most common mutation has been identified as a 3 base pair deletion, causing a deletion in the amino acid *phenylalanine* at position 508. This mutation accounts for approximately 70 per cent of all CF genes. Unfortunately, many additional uncommon mutations exist and not all have been identified. It is, therefore, difficult to detect all carriers using mutation analysis, and population screening for CF is not yet recommended. However, testing for carriers and prenatal diagnosis in a family in whom the disease has occurred are almost 100 per cent informative, provided that a DNA sample is available from the affected person in the family. It is, therefore, mandatory to offer prenatal diagnosis and carrier screening to couples with a family history of CF. Genetic counseling by qualified professionals in a supportive and nondirective fashion is an integral part of the education and management of this disorder.

GENERAL ORGANIZATION OF CARE

Education of the parents and patients about the disease, its manifestations, treatments, prognosis, and genetics becomes a crucial part of the approach to this disorder. Appropriate medical, emotional, and financial support for families and an ongoing awareness and experience with the development of very specialized, tertiary care approaches have required a multidisciplinary team composed of personnel from medical, nursing, physiotherapy, dietetic, psychologic-psychiatric, and social service fields, with access to the special expertise from pulmonary, gastrointestinal, nutritional, metabolic, genetic, and surgical physicians. Optimum care is thus best provided within an academic center devoted to the development of a multidisciplinary CF clinic.

At the time of diagnosis, parents and patients are introduced to the different members of the multidisciplinary team and provided with a great deal of new information. The initial weeks and months following diagnosis and commencement of treatment are a time of great anxiety for the parents, especially with the first viral respiratory infection or gastroenteritis. Our practice has been to maintain frequent telephone contact during this time to reinforce information and support and to reassure.

Regular clinical visits are organized every 2 months. At each visit, height and weight are measured; inquiries are made about general well-being, activity, school attendance (if applicable), cough and sputum production, and specific respiratory and gastrointestinal symptoms; and current therapy is reviewed. This is followed by a general physical examination with special emphasis on respiratory signs (including examination for nasal polyps and digital clubbing) and the presence of hepatosplenomegaly. In a well child, laboratory examination is limited to chest radiographs and pulmonary function tests (if older than 6 years) twice a year, and hematologic testing once per year, although this may vary during acute exacerbations. Urine is tested for the presence of glucose at each clinic visit. Routine immunizations and the administration of influenza vaccinations each fall are part of the treatment regimen provided.

Pulmonary Management

Although pulmonary involvement is the most common manifestation of CF, present in approximately 95 per cent of patients, for unknown reasons there is a marked heterogeneity in the severity of pulmonary disease even within the same family. Because the spectrum of the disease varies from infants younger than 6 months of age who present with severe ventilatory failure during respiratory syncytial virus (RSV) bronchiolitis, through to the asymptomatic adult recognized through an infertility clinic, the treatment must be individualized. In general, all patients receive regular physiotherapy at least once a day and continuous oral antibiotics if there are pulmonary symptoms. In asymptomatic children, antibiotic therapy is not regularly administered but is commenced early with each pulmonary exacerbation.

For exacerbations of pulmonary symptoms—principally increasing cough, increasing volume of sputum produced, or change in color and/or consistency of sputum—intensification of therapy at home is instituted. Physiotherapy is increased to two to three times per day; oral antibiotic therapy is started or changed and continued for 2 to 3 weeks at home. If the symptoms progress or fail to resolve, admission for intensive intravenous antibiotic therapy and physiotherapy is considered.

Chest Physiotherapy. Along with postural drainage, chest physiotherapy is used to facilitate mobilization of the increased volume of thick, mucopurulent pulmonary secretions. It is our practice to teach and use physiotherapy in all patients, regardless of age, and to precede the treatment by the administration of an inhaled bronchodilator. A treatment, which consists of postural drainage, vibrations, and percussion, usually takes 20 to 30 minutes to perform and from adolescence can be supplemented by "huffing" during the day. From about the age of 12 years, it is possible for patients to perform their own physiotherapy, often with the aid of a mechanical percussor. Compliance with this regimen is often poor, especially in the totally asymptomatic patient. However, it is not adequately replaced by increased physical activity alone and is invaluable during exacerbations or with the progression of the underlying disease.

Aerosol Therapy. Aerosol therapy is aimed at the clearance of obstructive secretions and appears to be beneficial, especially in patients with a cough with or without sputum production. A bronchodilator (Albuterol) is used by aerosol prior to postural drainage in an attempt to augment secretion clearance, although this is modified if the patient has experienced unacceptable side effects from the medication. There is in vitro evidence of increased ciliary beat frequency with β_2-agonists, but the clinical significance of this effect has not been confirmed by in vivo studies. Particle size determines the site of delivery within the lung; therefore, devices that generate small aerosol particles (mostly ultrasonic) appear to be the most effective. Although aerosol is a convenient method of delivering therapeutic agents to the airway, the actual role of the liquid in altering viscosity is controversial. Mucolytic agents such as N-acetyl-L-cysteine are not effective, but they function as hyperosmolar irritants to increase volume and water content in the mucus. This has infrequently resulted in acute bronchospasm or a rapid mobilization of large volumes of secretions and severe impairment of gas exchange. For this reason, mucolytic agents are not recommended.

Oral Antibiotic Therapy. This measure is used to limit the progressive destruction of lung tissue initiated by the recurrent infection in the obstructed areas of the lung. Because a variety of bacteria may be the infective agent, frequent cultures of secretions (sputum in the older patient, nasopharyngeal aspirate during coughing in the younger) are indicated to guide therapy. It is our practice at all clinic visits to routinely obtain culture specimens and determine antibiotic sensitivities from the respiratory tract.

Because the most common isolates in the younger patient are *Staphylococcus aureus* and *Haemophilus influenzae*, amoxicillin-potassium clavulanate (40 mg/kg/day) or trimethoprim-sulfamethoxazole (Septra, 8 to 10 mg/kg/day) is the basis of outpatient antibiotic treatment. Septra is preferred by parents because of taste and the twice-daily dosage schedule. *Pseudomonas aeruginosa* frequently becomes the predominant organism in culture, although many authors consider *P. aeruginosa* to be only part of a micromilieu contributed to by many organisms. The recently released oral antibiotic ciprofloxacin (20 to 30 mg/kg/day) has activity against *Pseudomonas* species; however, it is contraindicated in children younger than 12 years because it can cause abnormalities in the cartilaginous growth plate of bone, and our experience has been that the rapid acquisition of antibiotic resistance limits its usefulness. Fortunately, the empiric use of antibiotic therapy directed against *S. aureus* and *H. influenzae* during a pulmonary exacerbation often proves effective despite the presence of *P. aeruginosa* only in culture. *Pseudomonas cepacia,* a strain resistant to many antibiotics, has appeared in some patients with advanced disease and is associated with a guarded prognosis and, occasionally, overwhelming invasive infection.

Intravenous Antibiotics. With more severe pulmonary disease and continuous symptoms of cough and sputum production, oral antibiotics are administered on a continuous basis. Under these circumstances, intravenous antibiotics are necessary for most exacerbations. Our practice is to administer an aminoglycoside (usually tobramycin) in sufficiently large dosages to achieve adequate blood levels—peak 6 to 10 μg/ml, trough less than 2 μg/ml—in combination with either a fourth-generation cephalosporin or a semisynthetic penicillin (ticarcillin, 300 mg/kg/day; piperacillin, 300 mg/kg/day; or ceftazidime, 200 mg/kg/day) according to antibiotic sensitivities for 10 to 14 days. Single-drug therapy is never used because of acquisition of antibiotic resistance; occasionally, in the very ill patient, three medications are used simultaneously, guided by antibiotic sensitivities.

In general, oral antibiotics are stopped but will be re-started upon patient discharge. For older patients in whom intravenous therapy is frequent or venous access is difficult, permanent central venous access may be established using an implanted device. Home intravenous antibiotic therapy programs have been successfully established and may obviate the need for frequent hospitalizations.

Inhaled Antibiotics. The role of this mode of therapy, which is undergoing a resurgence at this time, remains controversial. Two different groups of patients have been reported to improve with this therapy: the young child with frequent repeated exacerbations that are not responsive to oral antibiotics, and adolescents with more advanced disease who stabilize with long-term (~2 years) continuous treatment at home with inhaled antibiotics. The most frequently used inhaled antibiotics are tobramycin and gentamicin (40 to 80 mg twice a day, depending on patient size). Semisynthetic penicillins and cephalosporins are not used because of the time needed for aerosolization (~40 minutes) and the offensive smell. It is prudent to initiate this treatment under controlled conditions because acute bronchospasm has been reported in response to the first dose of inhaled antibiotic. A multicenter trial currently being conducted may answer outstanding questions about appropriate dosage, frequency, patient selection, and mode of delivery.

Atopic Complex. The incidence of atopy in CF patients is similar to that in the general population. Reversible airway obstruction (asthma) may coexist with CF and can be effectively treated with bronchodilator agents. Patients with established bronchiectasis (see later) may have reversible airway obstruction secondary to chronic inflammation, which may be responsive to bronchodilators. In all cases, the reversibility of the airway obstruction should be confirmed by pulmonary function tests because a decrease in pulmonary function (negative flow recruitment) may also be seen following bronchodilator therapy and represents dynamic airway compression exacerbated by loss of airway muscle tone. Allergic rhinitis may be treated with antihistamines but at a cost of desiccating bronchial secretions. Rhinitis must be differentiated from nasal polyps, a direct complication of CF. Although both conditions may respond to nasal corticosteroids, surgical excision is usually required for nasal polyps.

Bronchial Lavage. The use of this modality to clear mucopurulent secretions is inefficient, and repeated treatments are necessary. In the severely ill patient, significant hypoxia inevitably occurs without change of progression of the underlying disease. This treatment is never used within our clinic practice.

Expectorants and Cough Suppressants. Expectorants are not effective in clearing pulmonary secretions. Cough suppressants are contraindicated because they interfere with the clearance of secretions. As well, these preparations contain antihistamines, which lead to desiccated secretions, increased mucus viscosity, and poor clearance.

Lung Transplantation. This is a relatively new treatment modality for advanced pulmonary disease. As yet, the treatment has been performed in only a small number of highly selected patients; however, survival rates appear to be 60 to 80 per cent and the transplanted lung does not develop CF. Tissue rejection, superinfection during immunosuppression, and the difficulties in sterilizing the sinus cavities are common problems following transplantation. At present, this therapy is not widely available and strict criteria are applied to determine eligibility for the treatment. When lung transplantation is successful, the transformation in patients and their lifestyle is remarkable.

Pulmonary Complications

Atelectasis. Minor and major areas of atelectases are frequently seen at any stage of the progression of the disease process. This usually results from inspissated secretions blocking an airway and may be recognized only by a pulmonary radiograph. Physiotherapy and bronchodilators are the mainstay of treatment, although antibiotics may be helpful in the presence of acute exacerbation of infection. Re-expansion may not occur despite vigorous physiotherapy, and bronchoscopy is usually ineffective, especially if the site of obstruction is peripheral.

Bronchiectasis. Bronchiectasis is not truly a complication of the disease but an indicator of the progression in severity. The recurrent infections are believed to progressively destroy the structural elements in the bronchi, resulting in fusiform dilatation, easily recognizable, especially in peripheral airways by chest radiograph. Most commonly, this occurs in the bases but may be present in any area of the lung field. Early in the course, when this process is presumably mediated by chronic inflammation, it may be reversible but rapidly this becomes a self-sustaining, irreversible chronic process. As a result of the bronchiectatic segments, cysts develop distally and are often filled with inspissated secretions.

Hemoptysis. Hemoptysis (bleeding from the tracheobronchial tree) is rare and represents active bleeding from increased tortuous bronchial vessels. Bleeding may be spontaneous or may occur in the presence of active infection. It is usually restricted to those patients with severe pulmonary disease, and the term is generally reserved for massive pulmonary bleeding (>300 ml at any time, or >100 ml for 3 consecutive days). Following fluid resuscitation, percutaneous angiographic embolization with absorbable gelatinous sponge (Gelfoam) is the treatment of choice and may need to be repeated on several occasions to achieve hemostasis. Blood-streaked sputum is much more common and represents mucosal capillary bleeding often in the presence of acute infection. This does not have the ominous overtones of pulmonary hemorrhage in the presence of normal clotting times. Usually, this is treated by antibiotics for the treatment of infection, administration of vitamin K if necessary, and cessation of chest physiotherapy for 24 hours.

Pneumothorax. Spontaneous pneumothorax is a complication seen in those with extensive pulmonary disease. A small pneumothorax (<10 per cent of lung volume) does not necessarily require active treatment because spontaneous resolution is likely to occur. If a large or tension pneumothorax is present, active treatment with an intercostal tube is necessary. Previously, chemical pleurodesis had been advocated; however, this procedure may jeopardize later lung transplant, and the decision needs to be carefully examined with this fact in mind.

Cor Pulmonale. Cor pulmonale, defined as right ventricular hypertrophy, can be detected by electrocardiography or echocardiography in moderately to severely affected patients. In patients with advanced disease who are symptomatic, the pulmonary vascular resistance is elevated by both destruction of the vascular bed and hypoxic vasoconstriction, exacerbated by increased hypoxemia during sleep or exercise. Treatment of this complication includes continuous "low-flow" nasal oxygen, especially during sleep, diuretics, and salt restriction. The use of digitalis is controversial. Oral vasodilators (hydralazine, nifedipine) may be effective, but supplemental oxygen therapy is essential.

Pulmonary Osteoarthropathy. The most common manifestation—digital clubbing—is frequently seen but is not associated with symptoms. In advanced disease, a periostitis of long bones may occur with pain and limitation of movement. This usually responds to aspirin or nonsteroidal anti-inflammatories, especially when it is associated with acute pulmonary exacerbations.

Aspergillosis. Incidental cultures of *Aspergillus* in sputum samples represent colonization rather than infection and do not need to be treated. In contrast, hypersensitivity pneumonitis (allergic bronchopulmonary aspergillosis) usually is manifested with increased pulmonary symptoms, central airway dilatation, bronchiectasis, and a markedly elevated immunoglobulin E (IgE). Aspergillosis will respond to steroid treatment.

Respiratory Failure. Acute, rapidly progressive respiratory failure (ARF) may occur unexpectedly in the presence of acute severe pulmonary infection. Vigorous measures, including assisted ventilation, should be instituted because ARF is potentially reversible with effective treatment. On the other hand, the slow, relentless progression to ventilatory failure is the result of the basic disease process. This decline is often heralded by increasingly frequent admissions, bronchiectasis, hypoxemia, and carbon dioxide retention, and the development of cor pulmonale. There is no effective therapy for this end-stage lung disease, short of lung transplant. Under these circumstances, we do not think that mechanical ventilatory assistance is warranted. Treatment options should be discussed with the patient and parents when the inevitable decline is obvious, preferably before acute deterioration necessitates major therapeutic decisions.

Gastrointestinal Management

Pancreatic Therapy

Pancreatic Insufficiency. The earliest lesion in the pancreas in CF is stasis of concentrated secretions within ductules, causing obstruction, subsequent tissue damage, fibrosis, and progressive loss of functioning acinar tissue. Variability in the degree of pancreatic tissue destruction, in part genetically determined, accounts for the differences in clinical presentation and severity of pancreatic manifestations. The majority of patients (80 to 85 per cent) demonstrate virtually complete loss of acinar tissue, an inability to secrete sufficient digestive enzymes, and consequent nutrient maldigestion and malabsorption. They present clinically with large, frequent, greasy stools and poor weight gain or frank weight loss; in infants younger than 6 months, hypoalbuminemia, edema, and anemia are noted. This pancreatic insufficiency can usually be suspected by observing a large number of neutral fat droplets on microscopic examination of a stool smear, by measuring a low stool chymotrypsin activity, or by noting a low plasma para-aminobenzoic acid (PABA) level after administration of N-benzoyl-L-tyrosyl-PABA. The diagnosis is confirmed by quantitation of 72-hour fecal fat excretion on a known fat intake or low duodenal enzyme output from the pancreas during stimulation with secretin and cholecystokinin.

Pancreatic insufficiency can usually be successfully managed by supplementation of meals and snacks with commercial preparations of pancreatic enzymes. The enzyme dose required to maximize digestion and absorption is empiric and dependent on a number of variables, including dietary fat intake and gastric acid denaturation of enzyme activity. One capsule of powdered enzyme (Cotazym) per 120 ml of infant formula is prescribed for infants. The enzyme should not be added to the formula; rather, it is mixed with a few teaspoons of strained foods. An enteric-coated enzyme preparation to avoid gastric acid inactivation of enzyme activity is prescribed for older children. An empiric starting dose is approximately 12,000 to 18,000 units of lipase per meal and 4000 to 6000 units per snack; however, patients not infrequently require up to 30,000 to 40,000 units per meal and 10,000 to 18,000 units per snack.

Despite high levels of enzyme supplementation, some patients remain steatorrheic. If this state is associated with clinical problems, such as poor weight gain, patients may benefit from pharmacologic attempts to (1) counteract gastric acid inhibition of enzyme activity, using H_2 antagonists, acid buffering, or prostaglandin analogues or to (2) replace deficient taurine stores with oral taurine supplementation to enhance taurine-conjugated bile salt secretion and thus intraduodenal lipolytic activity. Most CF patients do not require these additional supplements.

The diagnosis of pancreatic insufficiency does not necessitate the use of special infant formulas containing hydrolyzed proteins and medium-chain triglycerides (e.g., Pregestimil, Portagen, Alimentum). These formulas are more expensive, sometimes less palatable, and do not obviate the need for pancreatic enzyme supplementation. Most infants thrive on any infant formula, provided that sufficient energy intake and enzyme supplementation are prescribed appropriately. Similarly, low-fat diets are no longer recommended because they limit total energy intake and contribute significantly to the development of essential fatty acid deficiency in these patients.

Pancreatic Sufficiency. Fifteen to 20 per cent of CF patients retain sufficient residual pancreatic acinar tissue to digest and absorb nutrients without steatorrhea and do not need pancreatic or vitamin supplementation. However, at least some of these individuals continue to show progressive destruction of acinar tissue with time. Because residual pancreatic exocrine function is extremely variable, those patients with function at the lower end of the spectrum may eventually experience malabsorption and may require enzyme supplementation.

Pancreatitis. Patients with pancreatic sufficiency are at risk for pancreatitis. This presentation may be acute or recurrent. Because pancreatic sufficient patients tend to have a milder clinical course, they may lack the other hallmarks of CF and present with pancreatitis prior to the diagnosis of CF. Sweat testing confirms the diagnosis. Management of pancreatitis in CF is no different from the usual approach to pancreatitis.

Diabetes Mellitus. Because of the extensive pancreatic fibrosis and disruption of normal islet tissue, at least 30 per cent of CF patients will show abnormal glucose tolerance when challenged with glucose loads. Reports show development of an adult-onset type diabetes mellitus in 1 to 13 per cent of patients, with insulin and/or dietary manipulation required. The development of diabetes in CF may account for poor weight gain in some individuals. Its recognition and appropriate management frequently correct the situation.

Intestinal Therapy

Meconium Ileus. The earliest clinical manifestation of CF, occurring in 10 to 15 per cent of individuals, is the result of neonatal intestinal obstruction by inspissated meconium. Neonates present within the first 48 hours of birth with a failure to pass meconium and progressive abdominal distention and bilious vomiting. In uncomplicated meconium ileus, nonsurgical relief of obstruction may be achieved with water-soluble hypertonic enemas (Gastrografin, Hypaque) administered by experienced staff under fluoroscopic control. If this measure is unsuccessful, operative intervention to relieve the obstruction may be necessary. If meconium ileus is complicated by intestinal perforation, meconium peritonitis, volvulus, or atresia, operative intervention is mandatory.

Distal Intestinal Obstruction Syndrome (DIOS). Approximately 10 to 20 per cent of patients beyond the neonatal period experience a spectrum of symptoms attributable to partial or complete intestinal obstruction by inspissated intestinal secretions secondary to pancreatic insufficiency and hyperconcentrated intestinal mucoproteinaceous contents. Crampy abdominal pain and palpable stool masses of a chronic nature, or acute intestinal obstruction with pain, distention, and vomiting, may be the presenting complaint. One per cent of patients may have intussusception, usually ileocolic, with a fecal mass acting as lead point. Surgical intervention is rarely required. Management chronically consists of regular or increased pancreatic enzyme replacement, stool softeners such as mineral oil and psyllium hydrophilic mucilloid (Metamucil), and dietary fiber. Nasogastric suction and intravenous hydration are necessary in acute complete obstruction while the physician attempts to relieve the obstruction with enemas. Both oral and rectal N-acetylcysteine (Mucomyst) administration are sufficiently irritating to facilitate dislodgment of fecal material. Hypertonic enemas (Gastrografin, Hypaque) may also be used, but in older individuals the very large quantities of these agents that are necessary may become costly. In the absence of complete intestinal obstruction, the administration of large volumes of a balanced isotonic electrolyte solution for gastrointestinal lavage, either orally or by nasogastric infusion, has given excellent results.

Constipation. This occurs in CF far more frequently than the classic DIOS. *Management by reducing the dose of pancreatic enzyme replacement, as is frequently done, is not recommended.* Although it may alleviate the constipation by inducing fat malabsorption, it causes the loss of energy, fat-soluble vitamins and micronutrients and may sometimes precipitate an episode of DIOS. Constipation should be managed as in the general population, with stool softeners or lubricants, enemas, and dietary fiber.

Rectal Prolapse. Approximately 20 per cent of patients with CF have rectal prolapse, usually in the first few years of life, often prior to diagnosis and management of CF. Rectal prolapse often improves once pancreatic insufficiency is managed and frequently can be reduced and controlled by the child and family at home. Surgical intervention is necessary in only a minority of cases.

Pneumatosis Intestinalis. Intramural intestinal gas can be seen in patients with CF and advanced pulmonary disease. It is not a danger to the patient, nor is any management required.

Gastroesophageal Reflux. This disorder and the associated esophagitis occur not infrequently in CF patients, presumably secondary to their chronic pulmonary disease and medications, and may cause anorexia, weight loss, and anemia. Management should include elevation of the head of the bed; smaller, more frequent meals; antacids; H_2 antagonists, and motility agents.

Hepatobiliary Therapy

Liver Disease. In CF, liver disease represents a spectrum of disorders of varying frequency and clinical significance to overall health. Prolonged cholestatic jaundice in the neonatal period may occur and frequently resolves within the first months of life. Hepatic steatosis may present with an enlarged liver and normal or mildly elevated transaminase levels and may suggest significant malnutrition. Hepatic congestion secondary to cor pulmonale may be seen in those patients with severe pulmonary disease. Twenty-five to 50 per cent of autopsy cases demonstrate a characteristic histologic focal biliary cirrhosis consisting of eosinophilic ductular plugging, dilatation, portal tract inflammation and fibrosis, in the absence of clinical, radiographic, or biochemical evidence of liver disease. Clinically significant multilobular biliary cirrhosis and portal hypertension develop in only 2 to 5 per cent of patients. These patients present with hepatosplenomegaly, mildly elevated transaminase levels, elevated gammaglutamyl transpeptidase levels, and/or variceal bleeding. Severe hepatocellular dysfunction with jaundice, vitamin K–independent coagulopathy, ascites, and hepatic encephalopathy are unusual.

Management should be supportive as for other forms of liver decompensation. Portal hypertension causing variceal bleeding is effectively managed with injection sclerotherapy, and portosystemic shunting is rarely recommended. Liver transplantation has been successfully performed in patients with CF but should be reserved for those with decompensated hepatocellular function and mild pulmonary involvement. No definitive treatment is currently available for liver disease in CF, although uncontrolled trials have reported improvement with the use of ursodeoxycholic acid supplementation.

Biliary Tract. Patients with CF have an increased incidence of biliary stones, probably secondary to excessive intestinal bile salt loss in CF and consequent lithogenic bile production. Excessive fecal bile salt losses may be partially correctable by improving malabsorption with pancreatic enzyme supplementation, and this may decrease the risk of biliary stones. Most stones are detected by ultrasound in asymptomatic individuals, and no treatment is required. However, upper abdominal pain, symptomatic cholelithiasis, and cholecystitis require intervention. Recently, extrahepatic biliary tract obstruction was detected by hepatobiliary scintigraphy and percutaneous cholangiography in a large number of patients with hepatomegaly. Surgical correction of common duct strictures in symptomatic patients with abdominal pain led to complete symptomatic relief. The frequency of these strictures and their role in the etiology of CF liver disease remain to be explored.

Nutritional Therapy

Patients with CF are at increased risk for malnutrition and specific micronutrient deficiencies as a result of three contributing factors: (1) *energy and micronutrient losses,* secondary to malabsorption; (2) *increased energy expenditure,* largely due to chronic pulmonary disease, recurrent infections, and the use of long-term bronchodilator therapy; and (3) *inadequate energy intake,* due to a combination of anorexia, vomiting induced by coughing, and gastrointestinal pathology, including gastroesophageal reflux, esophagitis, and DIOS. Loss of body fat, muscle wasting, poor growth and weight gain, and delayed pubertal development are seen. Micronutrient deficiencies may include fat-soluble vitamins; minerals such as iron, zinc, and selenium; essential fatty acids; and taurine.

Because dietary preferences are established early and may be difficult to change, from the outset parents and patients should all be taught and encouraged to take a high-energy diet, liberal in fat, with larger portions at meals and high-energy snacks between meals and before bed. Pancreatic enzyme and fat-soluble vitamin replacement should be maximized and monitored. Oral liquid energy supplements and supplemental polysaccharides or medium-chain triglycerides can be encouraged in those instances in which diet is not meeting energy requirements. Unfortunately, as the disease progresses, a small proportion of patients become increasingly malnourished as their intake fails to meet their requirements. More aggressive long-term approaches to nutritional therapy, including parenteral nutrition and nasogastric, gastrostomy, and jejunostomy feedings overnight, are being used successfully at home. The use of elemental enteral preparations ensures maximum absorption without the need for pancreatic enzyme supplementation overnight and is usually well tolerated. It is usually possible to administer 1200 to 2400 calories overnight to supplement daytime oral consumption. In addition to improved weight gain, growth, and development, it appears that nutritional rehabilitation improves patient well-being, may slow the deterioration of pulmonary function, and has beneficial effects on exercise capacity and respiratory muscle strength. The long-term effects on pulmonary status and ultimate prognosis remain to be clarified.

SALT DEPLETION

Hyponatremia, hypochloremia, and metabolic alkalosis may occur in CF patients during the summer months in tropical and subtropical climates as a result of excessive losses of electrolytes in sweat. Anorexia, lethargy, vomiting, and dehydration may occur. Prophylactic treatment with supplemental electrolyte solutions has been suggested for all infants at risk of this complication.

REPRODUCTION

Puberty may be delayed in symptomatic patients with CF secondary to nutritional factors. Most, but not all, males with CF have aspermia as a result of obstruction of the vas deferens. Nonetheless, secondary sexual characteristics develop normally and sexual function is unaffected. Females with CF have reduced fertility, although increasing numbers of patients with mild disease have had a successful term pregnancy with minimal change in pulmonary function. In patients with advanced disease, the normal cardiorespiratory adaptations necessary for pregnancy have resulted in a major deterioration in pulmonary function. Individual counseling of each prospective mother with CF, therefore, is warranted.

SARCOIDOSIS

EDWIN L. KENDIG, JR., M.D.

Sarcoidosis is a multisystem granulomatous disease of unknown cause. It is relatively rare in children, with incidence peaking at 13 to 15 years of age. Because the disease process displaces normal tissue by sarcoid tissue, symptoms and signs depend on the organ or tissue involved. Most commonly affected are the lungs, lymph nodes, eyes, skin, liver, and spleen. Bones may also be involved, although this occurs less often; indeed, any organ or tissue may be affected.

Because the causative agent of sarcoidosis is not known, there is no recognized specific therapy. Adrenocorticosteroids are the only agents currently available that can suppress the acute manifestations of the disease. These agents are utilized only during acute and dangerous episodes.

Adrenocorticosteroid therapy is indicated in patients with intrinsic ocular disease, diffuse pulmonary lesions, central nervous system lesions, myocardial involvement, hypersplenism, and persistent hypercalcemia. Relative indications include progressive or symptomatic pulmonary disease, constitutional symptoms, joint involvement, disfiguring skin and lymph node lesions, persistent facial nerve palsy, and lesions of the nasal, laryngeal, and bronchial mucosa.

Fresh lesions appear to be more responsive to adrenocorticosteroid therapy than older ones. Although the suppressive action is often temporary, it is beneficial when the unremitting course of the disease will result in loss of organ function. For example, adrenocorticosteroid therapy can reduce the level of serum calcium and may thus help to prevent nephrocalcinosis, renal insufficiency, and, possibly, band keratitis. The use of adrenocorticosteroids in the treatment of patients with only asymptomatic miliary nodules or bronchopneumonic patches in the lung fields is debatable.

Prednisone or prednisolone (1 mg/kg/day in three or four divided doses) is continued until clinical manifestations of the disease disappear. A maintenance dose (15 mg every other day) is then given until a course of at least 6 months' treatment has been completed.

Temporary relapse may occur following the discontinuation of adrenocorticosteroid treatment, but improvement usually follows without resumption of therapy. In the management of ocular disease, adrenocorticosteroids in the form of either ointment or drops (0.5 to 1 per cent) are utilized in conjunction with systemic treatment. During the course of local therapy, the pupils are continuously dilated by use of an atropine ointment (1 per cent).

Adrenocorticosteroid ointment may also be used in the treatment of cutaneous lesions, but only in conjunction with systemic therapy; better results are obtained with the latter.

Other drugs occasionally used in the treatment of sarcoidosis in adults (oxyphenbutazone, chloroquine, potassium para-aminobenzoate, azathioprine, and chlorambucil), as well as transfer factor, have seldom been used in children.

5

Cardiovascular System

CONGESTIVE HEART FAILURE

DAVID R. FULTON, M.D.

When ventricular dysfunction causes symptoms of exercise intolerance, pulmonary congestion, or growth failure, congestive heart failure is present. The therapeutic approach is dependent on identification of the underlying cause of the myocardial dysfunction. Structural heart disease is the most common etiology for congestive failure and in the case of congenital disease generally presents within the first several months of life. Viral myocarditis, pericarditis, Kawasaki disease, acute rheumatic fever, acute bacterial endocarditis, toxic shock syndrome, sepsis, and anthracycline toxicity are common causes of acquired congestive failure. When possible, treatment of the underlying abnormality may hasten resolution of the cardiac symptoms and should be used in conjunction with other pharmacologic support. Rhythm disturbances may lead to acute congestive heart failure, and their therapy is discussed elsewhere.

ACUTE CONGESTIVE FAILURE

Viewed most simply, congestive failure is either acute or chronic. In acute disease, the cause may be volume overload, pressure overload, or primary myocardial or pericardial disease.

Inotropic Therapy

The rapid onset of congestive heart failure is frequently accompanied by altered myocardial contractility with diminished myocardial performance. Improvement is most rapidly accomplished by intravenous inotropic agents. Dopamine and dobutamine are preferred because of their rapid onset of activity, minimal proarrhythmogenic effect, potential for titration, and often predictable alpha-adrenergic effect on peripheral vasculature. Dopamine at low doses of 3 to 5 μg/kg/minute potentiates renal vasodilatation, which can improve renal blood flow and subsequent diuresis. In mid-range doses (5 to 15 μg/kg/minute), dopamine has positive inotropic effect on the myocardium, with positive chronotropy as well. At doses beyond 15 μg/kg/minute, dopamine may exert alpha-adrenergic activity, raising systemic or pulmonary vascular resistance. To minimize this effect, dobutamine (5 to 10 μg/kg/minute) can be added to the lower doses of dopamine (2 to 7.5 μg/kg/minute). Isoproterenol, a potent beta-agonist, may be utilized for acute failure at 0.1 to 2.0 μg/kg/minute, but its chronotropic and arrhythmogenic effect may exacerbate symptoms, so doses must be titrated carefully. Amrinone, a nonglycosidic, phosphodiesterase inhibitor, exhibits potent inotropic and vasodilatory effects. In postoperative cardiac patients, an intravenous loading dose of 0.75 μg/kg per bolus over 5 minutes, followed by continuous infusion at 5 to 10 μg/kg/minute, is used. Platelet counts should be monitored for thrombocytopenia, which is reversible after discontinuation of the drug. Digoxin is usually not favored for acute congestive heart failure, particularly in the presence of metabolic derangements or acute myocarditis, which increase myocardial sensitivity to the drug.

Diuretics

The use of diuretic therapy in acute congestive heart failure (CHF) should be prudent and based upon the underlying diagnosis. In the case of volume-overload lesions, such as left-to-right shunts at the ventricular or ductal level, furosemide (1 mg/kg per dose) may improve cardiac function and congestive symptoms of pulmonary edema by decreasing preload. The same may be true in acute pressure-overload lesions, such as left ventricular outflow tract disease, i.e., critical aortic stenosis or coarctation of the aorta; however, volume preservation may be advantageous in these settings, and furosemide should be used cautiously. In the case of impaired primary myocardial dysfunction in acute myocarditis with cardiac decompensation, the use of diuretics should not be considered initially because maintenance of ventricular preload may be essential for preservation of adequate cardiac output.

Afterload Reduction

In the presence of impaired myocardial function with low cardiac output and elevated systemic vascular resistance, various arteriolar vasodilators have been of great benefit. In the acute setting, intravenous nitroprusside (0.25 to 5.0 μg/kg/minute) is used while monitoring heart rate, blood pressure, atrial filling pressures (central venous pressure [CVP] or pulmonary capillary wedge tracings), and urine output. The blood pressure and filling pressures may fall after starting therapy owing to arteriolar vasodilatation and venous pooling. Volume challenges should be used to raise filling pressures in order to sustain cardiac preload. Use of a thermodilution pulmonary artery catheter to measure cardiac output during nitroprusside infusion should be mandatory. Measurements of cardiac output and systemic vascular resistance permit judicious titration of inotropic agents, vasodilators, and fluid replacement. When nitroprusside is used beyond 24 hours, serum thiocyanate and cyanide levels must be monitored for proper dose adjustment.

Transfusion

Increasing the hematocrit for patients with congestive heart failure improves the oxygen-carrying capacity to tissues whose perfusion may be inadequate. In addition, raising the hematocrit increases blood viscosity and has been shown to result in an increase in pulmonary vascular resistance, which in turn decreases the magnitude of left-to-right intracardiac shunting.

Prostaglandin E

In the newborn period, left ventricular outflow tract obstruction is a frequent cause of myocardial decompensation. In particular, aortic arch lesions—severe coarctation and interrupted aortic arch—may produce severe left ventricular dysfunction as the ductus arteriosus narrows and cardiac output falls. Ensuing metabolic acidosis from diminished tissue perfusion may aggravate congestive failure. When the diagnosis is established, prostaglandin E_1 (PGE_1) is started immediately at 0.05 to 0.1 μg/kg/minute. Because central apnea may occur during the initial 30 minutes of use, preparation must be made for possible intubation. Prophylactic intubation prior to interhospital transport is well warranted. Peripheral vasodilatation is frequently seen and may result in hypotension. Initial treatment should be fluid bolus rather than discontinuation of the drug. Titration of the dose may be necessary to avoid persistent hypotension. Concomitant administration of sodium bicarbonate (0.5 to 1.0 mEq/kg per dose) is indicated until improved peripheral perfusion reverses lactic acidemia.

Surgical Therapy

When the primary cause of congestive heart failure is identified, surgical intervention is indicated as soon as practical. When cardiothoracic surgery in infants is not available, arrangement for transport to an identified center is crucial. Balloon dilatation valvuloplasty and surgical valvotomy for critical aortic stenosis, as well as surgical repair of coarctation of the aorta and interrupted aortic arch, are life-saving procedures. Stabilization with inotropic agents and PGE_1 and correction of acid-base balance for a short period of time before proceeding to surgery may improve the outcome.

Pericardiocentesis

Acute hemodynamic decompensation may occur in the presence of acute pericardial fluid collection or progressive constrictive pericarditis. The causes are varied, but in younger children most often the etiology is viral or bacterial. Compression of the cardiac chambers leads to impaired diastolic ventricular filling with resulting diminished cardiac output. When hypotension is present, immediate intervention is indicated. Intravenous access is mandatory, and volume infusion should be, as a minimum, 10 ml/kg over 15 to 30 minutes. A pericardiocentesis should be performed by a skilled operator. Utilizing a long spinal needle or angiocatheter, the pericardial space is entered from either the subxiphoid position or the fifth left intercostal space in the mid-clavicular line. Ideally, an exchange J-wire can be advanced through the needle to the pericardial space and a multiperforated side hole catheter advanced over the wire. This maneuver permits stabilization of access through which large amounts of fluid can be removed. During evacuation of the pericardial space, vital signs must be carefully monitored. Fluid bolus is required if the blood pressure falls further during fluid removal. If the effusion is purulent, antibiotic therapy should be started and consideration given to surgical evacuation of the abscess. If the effusion is serous or serosanguineous, the catheter may be left in place in sterile fashion and used for further fluid removal.

CHRONIC CONGESTIVE HEART FAILURE

Following stabilization of the acutely ill child with congestive heart failure, therapy is directed toward chronic management. As in acute decompensation, selection of therapy depends on the underlying etiology.

Inotropic Support

The standard therapy for inotropic support is digoxin. Although its efficacy for volume overload lesions has been challenged, digoxin is still used almost universally. Loading doses of digoxin are based on body weight, but owing to pharmacokinetic differences for age, various regimens are employed (Table 1). In general, digitalization is scheduled over a 16- to 24-hour period with one half of the total digitalizing dose given initially, followed by one fourth of the dose given 8 to 12 hours later and an equivalent amount 8 to 12 hours after the second dose. Maintenance doses can be started 12 hours after digitalization and are divided into two equal daily doses. In situations in which gastrointestinal absorption is uncertain, the intravenous route is preferable, noting that the oral dose is 75 per cent of the parenteral dose. When not needed acutely, oral digitalization can be performed by starting maintenance doses without loading. In cases of renal insufficiency, maintenance doses should be adjusted according to parameters of renal function. Assessment of digoxin effect by electrocardiographic tracings is important, particularly after completion of digitalization. Digoxin effect is often manifested by prolongation of the P-R interval with changes in S-T segments and T waves and should not necessarily be considered a sign of toxicity. Toxicity in children is not common but includes gastrointestinal symptoms—anorexia, nausea, vomiting. Other symptoms include drowsiness and visual changes. Rhythm disturbance may often be the first and only indication of toxicity and may be either supraventricular, ventricular, or conduction abnormalities. When new rhythm abnormalities occur after starting digoxin, toxicity should be suspected and serum potassium, blood urea nitrogen (BUN), and creatinine should be determined and corrected when possible. Discontinuation of digoxin should occur if any rhythm is thought to be toxic in origin.

Diuretic Therapy

Chronic diuretic therapy is a useful adjunct to digoxin in the management of chronic CHF. Use of diuretic enables moderation of fluid restriction, which secondarily permits optimization of caloric intake. Various combinations are possible; however, chronic therapy with either furosemide (1 to 2 mg/kg/day) or chlorthiazide (20 to 30 mg/kg/day) must be

TABLE 1. Digoxin Doses in Pediatric Practice (IV)

	Loading (μg/kg/day)	Maintenance (μg/kg/day)
Prematures	15–20	5
Neonates* (0–1 month)	20–30	5–10
Infants (1–12 months)	40	10
Children (>12 months)	40	10–15

Data from Nyberg L, Wettrell G: Digoxin dosage schedules for neonates and infants based on pharmacokinetic considerations. Clin Pharmacokinet 3:453–461, 1978, with permission.

*Full-term newborns birth to 1 month of age.

accompanied by potassium supplementation (1 to 2 mEq/kg/day); alternatively, a potassium-sparing diuretic (spironolactone, 2 to 3 mg/kg/day) should be used. Serum electrolytes should be monitored after introduction of combined therapy until a stable state is reached. These drugs may need to be discontinued during acute gastrointestinal losses.

Afterload Reduction

Maximization of therapy to reduce preload and enhance inotropy may not improve CHF sufficiently to permit growth or reduce symptoms of exercise intolerance or dyspnea. A rise in afterload results in increased vascular wall stress and in turn myocardial wall stress, further limiting myocardial performance. In the chronic setting of congestive failure from left-to-right intracardiac shunts or dilated congestive cardiomyopathy, hydralazine, a vasodilator that acts to relax smooth muscle and produces selective arteriolar vasodilation, is given orally as 0.25 to 2.0 mg/kg per dose every 6 hours. The most frequently noted side effects include reflex tachycardia, postural hypotension, and gastrointestinal complaints. A lupus-like syndrome may occur in children as in adults and appears to respond to discontinuation of the drug. Captopril, an angiotensin-converting enzyme inhibitor, promotes vasodilation by decreasing angiotensin. The dose for children is 0.1 to 2.0 mg/kg per dose orally given every 8 hours. Side effects include hypotension with dizziness, rash, and neutropenia.

Nutrition

Children with chronic congestive heart failure have increased caloric requirements to achieve adequate growth. Failure to thrive is a common occurrence in infants with large left-to-right intracardiac shunts as well as in those with dilated cardiomyopathy. Often growth is insufficient with caloric intake of less than 150 to 175 kcal/kg. Early supplementation of formula to 28 to 30 kcal/ounce by addition of polycose, medium-chain triglyceride, or rice cereal is beneficial. If volume increases are not possible because of tachypnea, fatigue, or pulmonary edema, then further slow increase in caloric density to 36 kcal/ounce is indicated. Diuretic therapy is a valuable adjunct in maximization of calories when volume restriction is not practical. If oral feeding is not well tolerated, other routes of alimentation are used, including bolus nasogastric or continuous nasojejunal feeding. When possible, oral feeding is continued to prevent loss of this skill. Rarely, gastrostomy tube or central intravenous alimentation is necessary.

Transplantation

In cases of refractory congestive heart failure from severe left ventricular dysfunction, cardiac transplantation is becoming an accepted alternative. Challenges remain in improving transplant immunology and increasing public awareness to provide for donor sources. Success in the adult population will continue to stimulate efforts for similar results in children.

CONGENITAL HEART DISEASE

JACQUELINE A. NOONAN, M.D.

Since Drs. Gross and Hubbard ligated the first patent ductus arteriosus in 1939, the treatment of congenital heart disease has undergone remarkable changes. In the 1940s and 1950s, only resection of coarctation of the aorta, ligation of patent ductus arteriosus, and palliative surgery for blue babies in the form of a systemic to pulmonary artery shunt were available for children born with heart disease. With the development of cardiopulmonary bypass, open heart surgery to correct intracardiac defects became possible, and in the 1960s and 70s, more and more defects were successfully repaired.

By the 1980s, open heart surgery largely replaced palliation as newborns and young infants were successfully "corrected." The 1980s also saw the development of cardiac transplantation as a treatment for previously inoperable forms of congenital heart disease. Remarkable advances were also made in interventional cardiac catheterization techniques. Dr. William Rashkind in 1966 had pioneered this technique with the development of the balloon catheter to perform an atrial septostomy, which dramatically improved the prognosis for infants born with transposition of the great arteries. Balloon dilatation of the pulmonary valve in the 1980s was followed by balloon dilatation of the aortic valve, coarctation of the aorta, and pulmonary artery stenosis as well as obstruction of other vessels. Since the late 1980s, occlusive procedures to close atrial septal defects, patent ductus arteriosus, and some cases of ventricular septal defects have been developed.

What can we expect, then, for current therapy of congenital heart disease in the 1990s? I believe that we will see an increase in the use of interventional cardiac catheterization and that we will continue to see an aggressive approach to the treatment of congenital heart disease in infancy.

OVERVIEW

Approximately eight out of every 1000 live-born infants will be born with some form of congenital heart disease, and three of these will have such a serious defect that symptoms will occur within the first year of life. The highest mortality from congenital heart disease is in the first month of life. Such infants will present with either cyanosis or cardiac failure. Prompt recognition and appropriate management have greatly reduced the mortality of congenital heart disease in the young infant.

Although there is no medical treatment to cure congenital heart disease, the management of the symptomatic newborn since 1975 has been dramatically improved by the use of prostaglandin E (PGE) to dilate or continue patency of the ductus arteriosus. Infants born with marked obstruction of pulmonary blood flow, such as pulmonary valve atresia or tricuspid atresia, are often dependent on a patent ductus arteriosus for *pulmonary* blood flow. After birth, the ductus tends to constrict and this results in severe hypoxia. An infusion of PGE usually increases oxygen saturation so that diagnostic studies, such as cardiac ultrasound, cardiac catheterization, and the needed surgery, can be carried out on a stable rather than moribund infant. Other neonates with severe left-sided obstruction, such as aortic atresia, aortic arch atresia, or coarctation of the aorta, may be dependent on a patent ductus for *systemic* flow. These infants present with evidence of very low cardiac output and metabolic acidosis. Prostaglandin E often dramatically improves systemic blood flow so that renal function is restored and the infant can be stabilized to undergo the appropriate diagnostic studies and surgery. With the remarkable improvement in cardiac ultrasound techniques and now Doppler flow studies, it is possible to diagnose anatomic defects in newborn infants with remarkable accuracy. The need for cardiac catheterization and angiography has significantly decreased because of the diagnostic accuracy of cardiac ultrasound.

The management of an infant born with congenital heart disease depends largely on the specific anatomic defect and the known natural history of the lesion. Symptomatic infants generally require some form of surgical management. If the defect lends itself to complete repair, this is generally the preferred treatment option. Unfortunately, for many infants, a number of staged operative procedures may be necessary to improve symptoms when the nature of the heart defect does not lend itself to "complete" correction. Fortunately, many infants born with congenital heart disease remain asymptomatic. Some of the lesions may be so mild that no treatment is necessary. Knowledge of the known natural history of many of these cardiac defects prompts the recommendation for surgical repair in childhood, even if such children are "asymptomatic." A brief discussion of the more common cardiac lesions follows.

VENTRICULAR SEPTAL DEFECTS

Over the past 40 years, much has been learned of the natural history of ventricular septal defects. We know that many defects become smaller or undergo spontaneous closure so that no specific treatment is needed. Large ventricular septal defects, however, may cause congestive heart failure in infants and, if left untreated, lead to pulmonary vascular disease.

Appropriate treatment today for infants with a large ventricular septal defect is surgical repair. This can be accomplished with a low mortality (under 5 per cent) and a low morbidity. Infants who are symptomatic because of a moderate or small ventricular septal defect can be safely observed in hopes that the ventricular septal defect will become smaller or will undergo spontaneous closure. If the ventricular septal defect remains functionally significant, surgery can be performed electively later in childhood with a very low risk.

Pulmonary artery banding, which had previously been performed as a palliative treatment for heart failure in a young infant with a large ventricular septal defect, has been largely replaced by early surgical repair. Catheter closure of a ventricular septal defect is being aggressively researched, but it is unlikely that catheter closure will replace surgical repair of a large ventricular septal defect in infancy in the near future.

ATRIOVENTRICULARIS COMMUNIS (Complete AV Canal)

Complete atrioventricular (AV) canal is a serious lesion that is frequently noted in infants with Down syndrome. The anatomy is complex, and surgical repair is difficult. However, today's cardiovascular surgeon trained in congenital heart disease is able to repair this lesion with remarkable success. The mortality rate for this serious lesion has decreased dramatically in the past few years, and in most centers early repair of a complete AV canal is possible with the mortality rate between 10 and 15 per cent. Untreated, such patients are at risk for pulmonary vascular disease and soon become inoperable. Although pulmonary artery banding may still be indicated for the rare patient with an AV canal who has a hypoplastic left ventricle, the majority will be candidates for corrective surgery sometime in the first year of life.

Some patients have a milder or partial form of an AV canal. Surgery can be safely postponed in these patients until later in childhood, when the mortality rate is quite low.

ATRIAL SEPTAL DEFECTS

An isolated atrial septal defect seldom necessitates treatment in early infancy. The defect is generally recognized in early childhood. Surgical repair can be performed with a very low risk (in the range of 1 per cent mortality). This is a lesion that may go undiagnosed until adolescence or adulthood. Echocardiography provides excellent visualization of an atrial septal defect, in many cases obviating the need for cardiac catheterization. Catheter closure of atrial septal defects is carried out in a few institutions at present, but this technique may become more widespread in the 1990s.

PATENT DUCTUS ARTERIOSUS

Delayed closure of a normal patent ductus arteriosus is sometimes a serious problem for the small premature infant. Indomethacin, which blocks prostaglandin production, often accelerates closure of a patent ductus and is used widely in many nurseries for prematures. Some premature infants will require surgical ligation if indomethacin is ineffective or is believed to be contraindicated. For those infants or children who have a persistent patent ductus arteriosus unrelated to prematurity, indomethacin is not effective and surgical ligation is recommended. Many children with patent ductus arteriosus are asymptomatic, but surgery should be performed because of the known long-term complications. The mortality for surgery is under 1 per cent. Catheter closure of a patent ductus arteriosus is now possible and may become more widely used.

TOTAL ANOMALOUS PULMONARY VENOUS RETURN

This is a relatively uncommon disorder that may present a difficult diagnostic problem in early infancy. Infants with obstruction to pulmonary venous return may be confused with infants with lung disease or persistent fetal circulation. Two-dimensional echocardiography with Doppler flow, with particular attention being paid to the course of the pulmonary veins, has greatly improved the diagnosis of this condition in the symptomatic newborn. Some patients with unobstructed pulmonary veins do not have symptoms until later on in infancy or childhood. Surgery is necessary to correct this defect, and an overall mortality of less than 10 per cent is expected.

AORTIC STENOSIS

Critical aortic stenosis in the newborn remains a serious problem. There is significant mortality associated with treatment by surgical valvotomy or balloon valvuloplasty. The high mortality can be attributed to the very abnormal aortic valve, the often hypoplastic left ventricle, and the association of endocardial fibroelastosis. Severe aortic stenosis causing symptoms in the newborn does require treatment either by surgery or balloon valvuloplasty. In either case, the treatment of aortic stenosis is considered palliative, not curative. Fortunately, for most children born with aortic stenosis, symptoms do not develop in the newborn period. Previously, cardiac catheterization was necessary to evaluate the severity of the aortic valve obstruction. Echocardiography with Doppler studies now allows a noninvasive periodic follow-up of children with aortic stenosis. Beyond the newborn period, surgical valvuloplasty for congenital aortic stenosis can be accomplished with a very low operative risk. These children, however, require long-term follow-up because aortic stenosis may recur or progressive aortic insufficiency may develop. Reoperation later on in life is common, and some patients eventually require aortic valve replacement.

PULMONARY STENOSIS

Critical pulmonary stenosis can present in the newborn period often associated with cyanosis from a right-to-left shunt at the atrial level. Such infants require prompt relief of the pulmonary stenosis by balloon valvuloplasty or surgical valvotomy. Most children born with pulmonary stenosis, however, are asymptomatic in infancy, and the degree of pulmonary stenosis can now be determined quite accurately by use of echocardiography with Doppler studies. Most children with valvar pulmonary stenosis will be candidates for balloon valvuloplasty if Doppler studies indicate significant obstruction. If the pulmonary valve is very dysplastic, balloon valvuloplasty may not suffice and surgical resection of the valve may be needed. Surgical repair may also be indicated if other lesions are present that require repair. Both balloon valvuloplasty and surgical relief of pulmonary stenosis carry a minimal mortality.

COARCTATION OF THE AORTA

Surgical repair of coarctation of the aorta has undergone a number of changes. Resection of the coarctation with end-to-end anastomosis was initially the widely accepted procedure. As more infants with coarctation of the aorta underwent surgery, it was apparent that re-coarctation at the site of the end-to-end anastomosis was relatively common in those infants operated on in the first few months of life. It was also noted that many infants had hypoplasia of the aortic arch and that a simple resection of the coarctation did not completely relieve the obstruction. A subclavian flap operation using the subclavian artery to patch the arch and the area of coarctation became popular and is still widely used in infants. Patch repair of the coarctation became an alternative to end-to-end anastomosis; on follow-up, however, aneurysms developed in some of these patients at the site of the previous repair.

Although there is still controversy, balloon angioplasty has been shown to be effective both for native coarctation of the aorta and for relief of re-coarctation. It is likely that in the 1990s balloon angioplasty for coarctation of the aorta will continue to be evaluated and will be used frequently as the initial treatment for coarctation. Infants with symptoms resulting from coarctation of the aorta should gain relief of the obstruction either by surgical repair or by balloon angioplasty, depending on the experience of the center. Older children will likely undergo balloon angioplasty; if they undergo surgery, it is likely that the procedure will consist of resection with end-to-end anastomosis.

MITRAL VALVE PROLAPSE

Mitral valve prolapse (MVP) was first recognized in the mid-1960s. Although the true incidence is unknown, a conservative estimate of 5 per cent makes it by far the most common of congenital cardiac abnormalities. Prolapse refers to the abnormal protrusion of the mitral valve leaflets into the cavity of the left atrium during ventricular systole. Distinctive physical findings include a mid-systolic mitral click with or without a late systolic apical murmur. The abnormality can be confirmed by echocardiography. Primary MVP is now considered to be an autosomal dominantly inherited disorder related to some abnormality in connective tissue. Thoracic skeletal deformities, slender build, and lax joints often accompany the abnormal mitral valve, which is redundant and may show a spectrum of myxomatous change.

The vast majority of children with MVP are asymptomatic and, except for prophylaxis to prevent infective subacute bacterial endocarditis (SBE), may be treated as normal. Occasionally, a child and, more commonly, an adult may display symptoms of chest pain, palpitations, dyspnea, exercise intolerance, and presyncope that cannot be attributed to the mitral valve abnormality. Recent studies suggest that some patients with MVP also have a hyperadrenergic state, autonomic dysfunction, or an abnormal metabolic state, which is a more likely explanation for the symptom complex. Patient education and reassurance as well as prevention of volume depletion and avoidance of stimulants should be tried before drug treatment is recommended. If severe symptoms persist, beta-blocker therapy is sometimes helpful. Although severe progressive mitral regurgitation is very rare in childhood, it may develop in later life, necessitating mitral valvuloplasty or mitral valve replacement. Unfortunately, sudden death has been reported in a rare case of MVP and attributed to a ventricular arrhythmia. A prolonged Q-T interval or frequent premature ventricular beats that increase with exercise have usually been recognized in such patients prior to death. Therefore, patients symptomatic from palpitations or syncope should undergo electrocardiographic monitoring and stress testing before engaging in strenuous activity. Appropriate antiarrhythmic medication should be prescribed if any of these abnormalities are found.

TETRALOGY OF FALLOT

Most children born with tetralogy of Fallot are relatively asymptomatic in early infancy. With increasing obstruction to the pulmonary outflow tract, cyanosis may become prominent and "hypoxic spells" may develop. Previously, there had been reluctance to perform corrective surgery in young infants with tetralogy of Fallot. When the "hypoxic spells" developed, some cardiologists advocated the use of propranolol as medical management of the spells in hopes that the child would grow and become a candidate for surgical repair. Others recommended that a systemic-to-pulmonary artery shunt operation be done if symptoms developed. Such palliative surgery often relieved the cyanosis but, unfortunately, had adverse effects on the pulmonary artery.

As the 1990s approached, primary repair of tetralogy of Fallot has become common even in the young infant. With more surgical experience, it is apparent that if an infant has adequate pulmonary arteries, surgical repair can be performed even in the first year of life with an acceptable mortality and a good result. If an infant is doing well, surgery certainly can be delayed until later childhood. It is expected that most children with tetralogy of Fallot will undergo primary repair rather than palliative surgery. For those children born with complete pulmonary valve atresia or marked hypoplasia of the pulmonary arteries, primary repair may be more difficult; such infants or children may undergo a number of staged operations before complete repair can be accomplished.

TRANSPOSITION OF THE GREAT ARTERIES

The Rashkind balloon septostomy procedure in the 1960s for correcting transposition of the great arteries was followed by the Mustard operation a few years later. Thus, transposition of the great arteries, previously a lethal condition, was changed to one associated with a relatively good prognosis. The Mustard, and later the Senning, operation redirected venous return to the appropriate cardiac chamber but left the right ventricle as a systemic ventricle. Both operations carry a surprisingly low early mortality rate; however, they carry a risk of creating rhythm disturbances. There is concern that right ventricular failure will develop in some patients on long-term follow-up. The arterial switch operation, therefore, is now an alternative to the Mustard and Senning operations. Such surgery is performed in the newborn period, when the left ventricular pressure is still at a systemic level.

Although the early mortality with the arterial switch operation is higher than that of the Senning or Mustard procedure, the long-term results are expected to be better but are unknown. It is likely that more centers will switch to the arterial switch operation for transposition of the great arteries and that with more experience the mortality rate will fall to a lower level. The long-term results will need to be evaluated, since in some instances obstruction develops at the site of the pulmonary artery anastomosis and the long-term fate of the transplanted coronary arteries is still uncertain.

TRICUSPID ATRESIA

Patients with tricuspid atresia have a very hypoplastic right ventricle, so that complete surgical repair is not possible. Previously, shunt operations were carried out once symptoms developed; however, left ventricular failure in the second to third decade of life was common, and the long-term prognosis for patients born with tricuspid atresia remained poor. The *Fontan operation* was developed, essentially bypassing the right ventricle, directing systemic venous return directly to the pulmonary arteries, and separating the two circulations. Cyanosis is relieved, but it is difficult to consider this a truly corrective operation. The mortality rate associated with a Fontan operation in early infancy is high, so that most infants with tricuspid atresia undergo a shunt operation prior to a Fontan operation.

Over the past few years, a number of modifications have been made in the operation and a so-called two-staged Fontan procedure has been developed. It is now possible to accomplish the first stage of a Fontan operation in young infants with completion of the second stage by age 2 years. It is likely that in the 1990s there will be fewer shunts performed in infants with tricuspid atresia as more infants undergo an earlier Fontan procedure.

PULMONARY ATRESIA WITH AN INTACT VENTRICULAR SEPTUM

This serious form of congenital heart disease still remains a problem in management. In infants who have a very hypoplastic right ventricle, complete surgical repair may never be possible. Such infants often undergo a palliative shunt procedure in the newborn period followed by a pulmonary valvectomy in hopes that the right ventricle may grow. These infants often require a Fontan procedure later on in life. Some patients with pulmonary atresia and an intact ventricular septum, however, will have an adequate right ventricle, and early relief of the outflow obstruction is indicated. Treatment will be variable with such infants. It is expected that the mortality and morbidity will remain high for this unfortunate group of infants.

HYPOPLASTIC LEFT HEART SYNDROME

Hypoplastic left heart syndrome involves atresia of the aortic valves with a very hypoplastic ascending aorta, hypoplastic mitral valve, and hypoplastic left ventricle. Although the infant appears quite normal at birth, as soon as the ductus begins to close, metabolic acidosis and congestive heart failure with low cardiac output develop. An echocardiogram is very helpful in establishing this diagnosis. Untreated, such infants usually die within days or weeks of birth.

Management of hypoplastic left heart syndrome remains somewhat controversial. An operative approach still considered experimental, the *Norwood operation,** carries a high, early mortality, but with increased experience the mortality from the Norwood operation has decreased. A first-stage Fontan operation† may then be done when the patient is at about six months of age, followed months later by a second operation to complete the Fontan. Although the mortality rate for the combined operative procedures remains high, a number of long-term survivors are doing well.

Another approach for treatment of hypoplastic left heart has been heart transplantation. This technique has been highly successful in a number of centers, but, unfortunately, more babies are born with hypoplastic left hearts than there are donors. Given the high mortality and morbidity of the operative procedure and the scarcity of donor hearts for transplantation, as well as the uncertain long-term prognosis, these babies are made as comfortable as possible and die without any intervention in many centers. This lesion remains a challenge for the 1990s.

*In the Norwood operation, the ascending aorta is anastomosed to the pulmonary artery, the atrial septum is resected, and a shunt is performed between the "new" aorta and pulmonary artery branches.

†In the Fontan operation, systemic venous return is directed to the pulmonary arteries bypassing the right ventricle and pulmonary venous blood is directed to the right ventricle, which is the systemic ventricle in patients with a hypoplastic left heart.

OTHER COMPLEX LESIONS

For those infants born with other forms of complex heart disease, surgical management remains a challenge. For example, an infant recently presented at 7 weeks of age in our center with mild cyanosis and no heart murmur. An echocardiogram showed atresia of the mitral valve with both aorta and pulmonary artery arising from the right ventricle. An atrial opening was relatively small. For survival of this child, an atrial septal defect or widely patent foramen ovale is necessary for blood to exit the left atrium in view of the mitral valve atresia. The pulmonary artery pressure arising from the systemic right ventricle is at a systemic level. Pulmonary vascular disease is destined to develop with time in this case and would preclude any further attempts at a Fontan operation. Although this infant cannot undergo "corrective" surgery, opening the atrial septum to allow good mixing and to prevent pulmonary venous hypertension and banding the pulmonary artery to reduce the pulmonary artery pressure will palliate this infant and permit a Fontan operation to be carried out at a later time.

Truncus arteriosus is another lesion that previously carried a very high mortality in infancy. This lesion can now be repaired even in infancy. A conduit is required between the right ventricle and pulmonary artery. If this is placed in infancy, it is likely that additional surgery to replace the conduit will be required as the child grows.

Today, children born with complex lesions that defy complete surgical correction are often candidates for palliative procedures to improve symptoms and to offer hope for more definitive surgery in the future. For some infants with complex lesions, transplantation of the heart is another option.

THE CHILD AT RISK FOR CORONARY DISEASE AS AN ADULT

ALBERT P. ROCCHINI, M.D.

ETIOLOGY AND RISK FACTORS

Coronary artery disease has its origin in childhood. Coronary atherosclerotic fatty streaks appear in Americans as early as the second decade of life, and fibrous plaques have been found at autopsy in adolescents and young adults who have died accidentally. Epidemiologic and clinical studies in adults with coronary heart disease have made it possible to develop a list of risk factors that can help to identify individuals susceptible to the development of coronary heart disease. The risk factors that have been identified include increased blood levels of cholesterol, elevated blood pressure, cigarette smoking, obesity, and poor physical fitness. This article describes how four of these risk factors (cigarette smoking, elevated lipid levels, reduced physical activity, and obesity) impact on the development of cardiovascular disease and what types of therapy are currently being used to modify them.

Smoking

Cigarette smoking is the major avoidable cardiovascular risk factor. One of the most disturbing features about smoking is that since 1964 more than 30 million Americans have stopped cigarette smoking, yet cigarette smoking has not decreased in its prevalence rate among adolescents. Thus, adolescent subjects represent the largest group of individuals at risk to start cigarette smoking. Smoking is known to increase cardiovascular risk directly by altering blood pressure regulation, increasing total serum cholesterol levels, and decreasing high-density lipoprotein (HDL) cholesterol levels.

The most effective way to treat smoking is through its prevention. Because the incidence of smoking is highest among adolescents, it is, therefore, critical to prevent smoking in this very age group. Most studies have shown that a school-based prevention program, beginning in grade 6 with booster sessions throughout the remaining 6 years of secondary education, can result in a significant reduction in the incidence of adolescent smoking.

Lipids

On the basis of numerous epidemiologic surveys, hyperlipidemia is known to be an important risk factor for the development of adult-onset heart disease. To understand abnormalities of lipid metabolism and their treatment, it is important to understand the process by which the body handles cholesterol. Cholesterol from dietary fat is digested, absorbed, and reprocessed in the liver. The liver then secretes the reprocessed cholesterol either into the intestines as bile or into the blood stream in combination with triglycerides as very-low-density lipoprotein (VLDL) particles. The VLDL particles are converted in the plasma to low-density lipoproteins (LDL), which can then be taken up by the cells and reconverted back into cholesterol. The LDL particles are guided by *apoproteins* (lipoprotein surface proteins) to the LDL receptor sites on the cell. *The number of LDL receptors and their affinity for apoproteins determines the level of cholesterol in the blood.*

Cells prefer to use exogenous cholesterol rather than to manufacture it themselves. This preferential usage depends on a biochemical feedback system whereby raising intracellular cholesterol levels reduces cholesterol production by inhibiting the enzyme 3-hydroxy-3-methylglutaryl coenzyme A (HMG CoA) reductase and by activating the enzyme acyl-coenzyme A transferase (ACAT), which esterifies cholesterol for storage. Increased intracellular cholesterol also reduces cellular LDL cholesterol uptake by blocking formation of LDL receptor proteins and by inhibiting LDL receptor gene expression.

Intracellular cholesterol that is not used or stored by the cell is passed out of the cell and combines with recycled LDL particles to form HDL particles. These HDL particles eventually are removed from the circulation by the liver. The formation of HDL cholesterol is the major means by which excess cholesterol is removed from cells.

Abnormalities in the method by which the cell handles LDL receptor formation is the cause of one of the common genetic forms of hyperlipidemia—*familial hypercholesterolemia.* In this disease, there is an alteration in either the number or the function of LDL receptors, leading to a reduced binding of LDL cholesterol to the receptors; a higher serum LDL cholesterol concentration; a higher plasma cholesterol level; and atherogenesis. Table 1 summarizes the various known genetic forms of hyperlipoproteinemia.

Historical information is of prime importance in determining which children should be screened for hyperlipidemia. The most important feature is a family (parent or grandparent) history of premature atherosclerotic disease, defined as the appearance of clinical manifestations of atherosclerosis prior to 50 years of age for men and 60 years in women. Several other historical features also can suggest the presence of hyperlipidemia. These include (1) a history of recurrent unexplained pancreatitis or abdominal pain (seen with exogenous hyperchylomicronemia, familial hypertriglyceridemia, or familial combined hyperlipidemia); (2) a history of an abnormal glucose tolerance or hyperuricemia (seen with all types of hypertriglyceridemia); (3) a history of xanthoma (seen with familial hypercholesterolemia); and (4) information suggesting a systemic disease that is secondarily associated with hyperlipoproteinemia, such as thyroid disease, liver disease, renal disease, or diabetes. *Lipid screening is currently recommended only if a child has a history compatible with hyperlipidemia.*

TABLE 1. Genetic Forms of Hyperlipidemia

Disorder	Phenotypes*	Mode of Inheritance
Exogenous hypertriglyceridemia	Type I	Autosomal recessive
Familial hypercholesterolemia	Types IIA, IIB	Autosomal dominant
Familial hypertriglyceridemia	Types IV, V	Autosomal dominant
Familial combined hyperlipidemia	Types IIA, IIB, IV, V	Autosomal dominant
Polygenic hypercholesterolemia	Types IIA, IIB	Polygenic
Sporadic hypertriglyceridemia	Types IV, V	Nongenetic
Broad β disease (dysbetalipoproteinemia)	Types III, IV	Autosomal dominant

**Phenotypes:* type I, inc chylomicrons; type IIA, inc low-density lipoprotein (LDL); type IIB, inc LDL and very-low-density lipoprotein (VLDL); type III, abnormal lipoprotein; type IV, inc VLDL; type V, inc chylomicrons and VLDL.

Plasma levels of lipoproteins ultimately are the method for determining the presence or absence of hyperlipidemia. Ideally, a blood sample should be drawn after a 12- to 14-hour fast. Interpretation of the plasma values of these lipoproteins should be made with the consideration of what constitutes normality. As with most clinical laboratory tests, "normals" are based on a statistical distribution of values in the general population. Traditionally, values greater than 90th percentile cutoff have been employed for defining abnormal cholesterol and triglyceride levels (Table 2).

The cornerstone of lipid management, regardless of cause, is diet. Both the saturated fat content and the cholesterol content of the diet must be reduced in order to obtain maximum dietary benefit. Saturated fat appears to increase the synthesis of LDL cholesterol and to decrease LDL cholesterol disposal. Polyunsaturated fat decreases VLDL triglyceride, cholesterol, and apoprotein-B synthesis. Monounsaturated fats, such as canola oil, olive oil and peanut oil, are especially beneficial in that they reduce not only LDL cholesterol but also the LDL cholesterol/HDL cholesterol ratio. Other ways in which changes in diet can lower cholesterol are to increase the intake of high-fiber foods, such as oat bran, beans, and other water-soluble fibers. Marine or omega 3 fatty acids also can result in a reduction in VLDL triglycerides, primarily by decreasing VLDL synthesis. With dietary management alone, one can expect a 5 to 20 per cent decrease in cholesterol. The standard dietary recommendation is an American Heart Association phase I diet, which contains 30 per cent of calories as fat, 55 per cent as carbohydrates, and 15 per cent as protein. The fat should be approximately

TABLE 2. Values in the 90th Percentile for Cholesterol, LDL Cholesterol, and Triglycerides and in the 10th Percentile for HDL Cholesterol by Age and Sex

	White Males				White Females			
Age (Years)	*5–9*	*10–14*	*15–19*	*20–24*	*5–9*	*10–14*	*15–19*	*20–24*
Total cholesterol	191	190	183	204	195	190	191	214
LDL cholesterol	117	122	123	138	125	126	129	141
Triglycerides	85	102	120	165	90	114	114	141
HDL cholesterol*	42	40	34	32	38	40	38	37

Modified from The lipid research clinics' population studies data book, Vol 1. The prevalence study. Lipid Metabolism Branch Division of Heart, Lung and Vascular Disease; National Heart, Lung and Blood Institute; U.S. Department of Health and Human Services; Public Health Services; National Institutes of Health. NIH Publication No. 80-1527. Government Printing Office, 1980.

*10th percentile.

Abbreviations: LDL, low-density lipoprotein; HDL, high-density lipoprotein.

equally divided between polyunsaturated, monounsaturated, and saturated fats. The major source of carbohydrates should be complex carbohydrates, and the cholesterol intake should be below 300 mg/day. If cholesterol elevation persists, the next approach involves a phased reduction in cholesterol intake to 100 mg/day, with 20 per cent of the calories as fat with equal components of saturated, monounsaturated, and polyunsaturated; 65 per cent as carbohydrates; and 15 per cent as protein. Other than diet, the other two nonpharmacologic forms of therapy for hyperlipidemia are weight reduction and exercise.

The goal of therapy should be to reduce total cholesterol below 200 mg/dl and LDL cholesterol below 120 mg/dl, while maintaining HDL cholesterol levels greater than 40 mg/dl. If these goals can not be reached by nonpharmacologic therapy alone, pharmacologic agents need to be considered. However, because pharmacologic agents are not without side effects, especially in the growing child, most pediatric lipid specialists do not recommend adding lipid-lowering drugs unless dietary means are unable to reduce total cholesterol below 250 mg/dl and LDL cholesterol to below 175 mg/dl.

Table 3 lists some of the drugs currently used to treat hyperlipidemia. In the pediatric population, bile acid resins are the most commonly used first-line lipid-lowering drug. The bile acid resins bind bile acids in the intestines and prevent their reabsorption. As a result, there is increased conversion in the liver of cholesterol to bile acid, which ultimately leads to the reduction in hepatic cholesterol content and to an up-regulation of LDL receptor synthesis and an increased disposal of LDL cholesterol from plasma. Unfortunately, as the intracellular content of cholesterol decreases, cellular cholesterol synthesis increases, thus reducing the cholesterol-lowering efficacy of the resins. Therefore, to further lower LDL cholesterol levels, it may be necessary to use a resin in combination with one of the other drugs that blocks cholesterol synthesis, such as niacin or Lovastatin.

It is important to remember that although there is now increasing evidence in the adult that treatment of hyperlipidemia can result in a reduction in coronary mortality and even regression of atherosclerotic lesions, few to no data on the efficacy of long-term treatment of mild to moderately elevated cholesterols to prevent atherosclerosis later in life are available in the pediatric age group.

Physical Exercise

Reduced amount of physical exercise has been documented to be an important cardiovascular risk factor. The amount of exercise an individual regularly performs inversely correlates with cholesterol and triglyceride levels and with obesity. In addition, habitual exercise can normalize triglyceride levels; can increase HDL cholesterol levels; and, in some individuals, also may reduce LDL cholesterol levels. Although it is clear in the adult that physical activity can reduce coronary risk, there is little to no information concerning the long-term effect of childhood exercise programs in reducing the risk for development of cardiovascular disease.

For children, 30 to 60 minutes of exercise four times per week is sufficient to maintain cardiovascular fitness. The exercise must be individualized by considering the type of exercise the child best enjoys and the facilities and equipment available. Not all types of exercise are equally useful for becoming cardiovascularly fit. Activities requiring effort against heavy resistance, such as weight lifting, can cause increased efficiency of certain muscle groups but do little to improve cardiovascular fitness. To achieve the desired degree of cardiovascular adaptation and conditioning, aerobic exercise is necessary. Any activity that can be maintained continuously, is rhythmical, and uses large groups of muscles is aerobic. Vigorous walking, jogging, skating, skiing, aerobic dance, and bicycling are a few of such recommended activities. Despite the reported benefits of regular aerobic exercise training, the drop-out rate among those beginning regular exercise is high. Support from family and friends is critical to maintain continued compliance.

Obesity

Obesity is a complex and difficult clinical problem. It is probably the most prevalent and serious nutritional disease in the United States. Childhood obesity is known to exert a major impact on cardiovascular risk. We have documented that 97 per cent of obese adolescents had four or more of the following risk factors: elevated serum triglyceride levels, decreased HDL cholesterol levels, increased total cholesterol level, elevated systolic and/or diastolic blood pressure, a diminished maximum work capacity, and a strong family history of coronary heart disease.

Before a description on how to treat obesity is presented, it is important to give a brief definition of obesity. In both adults and adolescents, obesity is defined as an accumulation of body fat greater than 22 per cent of total body weight for men and greater than 30 per cent of total body weight for women. Weight for height standards are also useful in defining obesity. A commonly accepted definition for childhood obesity is the combination of triceps and subscapular skinfolds being greater than the 80th percentile and weight for height being greater than the 75th percentile for age and sex. Obesity, as defined by these criteria, is present in 15 to 20 per cent of all school-aged children.

Treatment modalities employed in obese children and adolescents can be categorized into one of a combination of six basic approaches:

- Caloric restriction
- Increased physical activity
- Habit pattern changes based on social learning therapy

TABLE 3. Therapy of Hyperlipidemia

	Mechanism	% Reduction in Cholesterol	Effect of VLDL	Effect on HDL	Side Effects	Dose
			Nonpharmacologic Therapy			
AHA Prudent Diet	Limits exogenous cholesterol	10–15%	Decrease	Decrease	—	
Exercise	Improves insulin resistance	Some decrease	Decrease	Increase	—	
Weight loss	Improves insulin resistance	Some decrease	Decrease	Mild increase	—	
			Pharmacologic Therapy			
Bile acid resins	Accelerates LDL disposal	20–30%	Mild decrease	Mild increase	Epigastric distress, constipation, bloating, interferes with some drug absorption	Up to 24 g/day of cholestyramine in divided doses
Nicotinic acid or niacin	Reduces VLDL and LDL synthesis; increases HDL	25%	50% decrease	30–40% increase	Flushing, headache, tachycardia, GI distress, activation of peptic ulcer disease and inflammatory bowel disease, hepatic dysfunction	Titrate up to 1 g 3 times a day
Probucol	Increases LDL disposal; reduces HDL/LDL ratio	5–15%	—	Decrease	Nausea, diarrhea, flatulence, eosinophilia, hepatic dysfunction, prolong Q-T interval	0.5 g twice a day
Gemfibrozol (Lopid)	Enhances VLDL breakdown and decreased VLDL production	Decrease	40–50% decrease	20–30% increase	Rarely myositis, should not be used in patients with renal disease, cholelithiasis, or liver dysfunction	600 mg twice a day
HMG-CoA reductase inhibitor (Lovastatin)	Inhibits cholesterol synthesis and increases LDL disposal	30–40%	—	—	Elevated liver enzymes, myositis, cataracts in animals	20–40 mg twice a day

Abbreviations: AHA, American Heart Association; HMG-CoA, 3-hydroxy-3-methylglutaryl coenzyme A; LDL, low-density lipoprotein; HDL, high-density lipoprotein; VLDL, very-low-density lipoprotein; GI, gastrointestinal.

- Anorectic drugs
- Therapeutic starvation
- Bypass surgery

Certainly drugs, starvation, and surgery are unacceptable treatment strategies for the majority of children.

A practical weight loss program is outlined in Figure 1. In order to assess the child's ability to comply with a weight loss program, we believe it is advisable to utilize a trial diet for 2 to 3 weeks. If the child is successful with this trial diet, loses at least 1 to 2 pounds in 2 to 3 weeks, he or she is likely to benefit from a weight loss program. If the child is unsuccessful, the family and child should be counseled and asked to return in 3 to 6 months or sooner if there is a change in attitude toward weight loss.

The weight loss program itself consists of three components: diet, behavior change, and exercise. The caloric requirements necessary for a child to lose 1 to 2 pounds per week are determined by reducing the current level of calories by 500 to 1000 calories/day. We believe that adolescent weight reduction diets should not contain below 1200 calories/day because it then becomes difficult to provide adequate vitamins and nutrients to promote normal growth and development. On the other hand, calorie levels should never exceed 2500 calories/day because the child is unlikely to take the diet seriously if allowed too large a caloric intake. An exchange type diet is recommended, since it teaches children the essentials of good nutrition and gets them actively involved in determining their own diet. The behavior change component of the program includes 1 hour weekly class for 20 weeks, then every other week until the child has maintained a goal weight for at least 1 month. The classes should center around (1) nutrition education, (2) record keeping, (3) stimulus control for restricting the external cues that set the occasion for eating, and (4) reinforcement of altered behavior. The purpose of the behavioral change component is to help the obese child learn to eat like a non-obese person, to become aware of current habits, and to normalize and accept responsibility

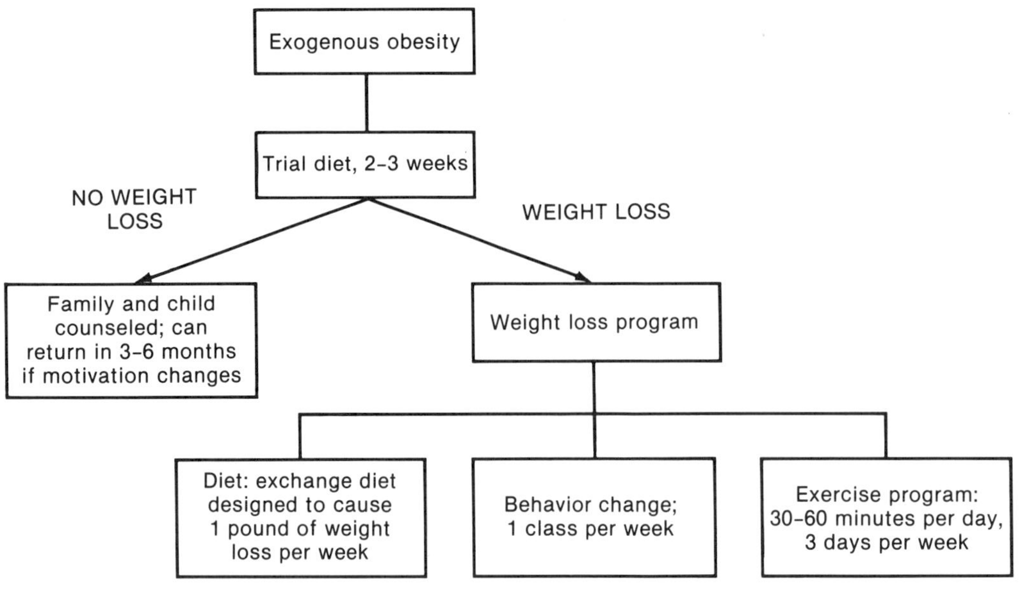

Figure 1. Pediatric weight loss program.

for their eating behavior. All children are also encouraged to exercise for 30 to 60 minutes a day on at least 3 days a week. The weight loss program should have a built-in reinforcement system to help the child establish and maintain new habits. Finally, in addition to the child's structured portion of the program, family support is critical. The family needs to be taught how to give the child positive support without nagging or taking over the child's weight loss program.

Using this type of program, we have been able to achieve adequate weight loss in adolescents who are motivated to lose weight. When dealing with childhood obesity, one must remember that if the child does not want to lose weight, no weight loss program regardless of its approach, organization, or cost will be successful.

SUMMARY

Because coronary artery disease has its origins in childhood, it is critical that the pediatrician become involved in the identification and treatment of the child at risk for the early development of cardiovascular disease.

DYSRHYTHMIAS

PAUL C. GILLETTE, M.D.
and CHRISTOPHER L. CASE, M.D.

FETAL DYSRHYTHMIAS

Cardiac dysrhythmias (abnormal rhythms) are increasingly the concern of pediatric health care practitioners in the care of the fetus as well as the neonate, infant, and child. Many dysrhythmias are first diagnosed in the fetus by ultrasound techniques and confirmed by detailed fetal echocardiography. Patients who survive subsequent cardiac surgical procedures remain at risk for development of important cardiac dysrhythmias for the rest of their lives.

The most frequently diagnosed fetal dysrhythmia is premature atrial contractions (PACs), which do not require treatment unless they lead to supraventricular tachycardia, an infrequent occurrence. Fetal premature ventricular contractions (PVCs) likewise do not require treatment.

Fetal tachycardias, on the other hand, can rapidly lead to fetal congestive heart failure, hydrops fetalis, and death and vigorous treatment and monitoring are therefore mandatory. Most fetal tachycardias, including atrial flutter, are supraventricular. There is usually a 1:1 or 2:1 atrioventricular relationship. A tachycardia with more ventricular contractions than atrial is likely ventricular in origin or due to junctional automaticity. Fetal supraventricular tachycardia is initially treated with maternal digoxin administration. A mid-range serum digoxin concentration (i.e., 1.2 to 1.7) is optimal. Intravenous administration is preferred. This is accomplished during hospitalization using close maternal and fetal monitoring. Digoxin is more effective against supraventricular tachycardias than atrial flutter. If digoxin is ineffective, propranolol may be added if fetal ventricular function is good by echocardiography. The third drug to be tried may be flecainide, again if the fetal ventricular function is adequate. It is given by itself as a single drug.

Amiodarone (a class III antiarrhythmic drug effective against a broad spectrum of arrhythmias by slowing conduction) may also be used, but oral maternal administration has a slow onset of action. European perinatologists have used direct fetal umbilical vein puncture to administer amiodarone. Because hydropic fetuses absorb oral drugs less well, intravenous amiodarone is especially useful.

Chronic fetal bradycardia is most often due to congenital complete atrioventricular (AV) block. This occurs frequently in mothers with connective tissue diseases, although they may not have been diagnosed prior to the fetal bradycardia. Additional fetal cardiovascular malformations are frequent in fetuses of mothers without connective tissue disease and significantly complicate management. Delivery in a center capable of immediate pacemaker placement is indicated. Delivery by cesarean section may be indicated in fetuses with rates below 50 because they may have little or no heart rate response to the stress of labor. Fetal pacing has been attempted, and its use will probably increase in the future. Fetal pacing could be accomplished by direct application of an electrode to the fetal myocardium and implantation of the pulse generator in the abdomen.

NEONATAL AND INFANTILE DYSRHYTHMIAS

Neonatal dysrhythmias are, for the most part, extensions of fetal dysrhythmias. Neonatal PACs may require treatment if (1) they are frequent and not decreasing over several days, (2) they are blocked, particularly with atrial bigeminy resulting in bradycardia, or (3) they occur two or more in a row. The reason for treatment is that PACs may result in atrial flutter. Digoxin, propranolol (Table 1), or both will decrease the number of PACs or prevent or ameliorate the atrial flutter. Neonatal PVCs are less common. If contractions are infrequent, these do not require treatment; if they are frequent or coupled, propranolol (Table 1) treatment is usually successful.

Supraventricular tachycardia is the most frequent dysrhythmia of neonates and infants. Adenosine is the acute treatment of choice. It works by slowing conduction in the AV node, and may be repeated as necessary. It is given intravenously at a dose of 50 to 250 μg/kg as a bolus into a large vein. Adenosine is metabolized in less than 10 seconds by red blood cell esterases. It causes block in the AV node, which breaks the re-entry circuits that cause most supraventricular tachycardias. A few blocked sinus beats after conversion are common. If the tachycardia was atrial flutter or atrial automatic, it continues but AV conduction is temporarily blocked. If the tachycardia was ventricular, it will continue but no harm will result. Thus, adenosine is a safe and effective drug. Verapamil, used in the past, is no longer given routinely.

Because adenosine is so rapidly metabolized, a chronic drug must be chosen and begun promptly. If the post-conversion electrocardiogram (EKG) shows the Wolff-Parkinson-White syndrome, propranolol should be used. If Wolff-Parkinson-White syndrome is not observed, digoxin is the drug of choice (Table 1). Prophylactic treatment for 9 to 12 months is recommended for each neonate or infant with supraventricular tachycardia. Close follow-up and increases in drug dosage with growth are also necessary. Patients with complex cases are best observed in pediatric cardiology centers. Catheter ablation or surgery may be necessary in 5 to 10 per cent of patients.

If adenosine fails to convert the dysrhythmia, referral to a pediatric cardiology center is warranted. If a low cardiac output is present, direct current (DC) cardioversion is indicated if adenosine unmasked atrial flutter. If the P-waves during adenosine induced AV block were normal, low atrial, or left atrial, the likely mechanism is an automatic focus that does not respond to cardioversion.

Neonatal ventricular tachycardia (VT) is unusual and in many cases may be due to hypoxia or electrolyte imbalance. Thus, the first treatment is a search for the cause. Cardiac causes include tumors and the long Q-T interval syndrome.

TABLE 1. Antiarrhythmic Drug Dosages

Adenosine	50–250 μg/kg rapid IV
Esmolol	500 μg/kg IV over 5 minutes, then 200–500 μg/kg/minute infusion IV
Digoxin (Lanoxin)	Oral digitalization 20–50 μg/kg given ½, ¼, ¼ every 8 hours over first 24 hours
Propranolol	2–8 mg/kg/day p.o. in 4 doses; 1 dose per day of long-acting form.
Atenolol	1–2 mg/kg/day p.o. in 1 dose
Phenytoin	3–5 mg/kg/day p.o. in 1 or 2 doses; always use infatabs; maintain serum concentrations >10 <20 μg/ml
Lidocaine	1 mg/kg rapidly IV; maintain 30–50 mg/kg/minute
Procainamide	1 mg/kg IV every 5 minutes × 15 for loading; then maintain 30–50 mg/kg/minute
Flecainide	100–175 mg/M²/day p.o. divided in 2 doses
Amiodarone	10 mg/kg/day p.o. × 10 days, then 5 mg/kg/day in 1 dose

Ventricular tachycardia due to tumors may be insidious, in that it may present with single or multiple PVCs or short runs of nonsustained VT. Under the stress of a mild infection in infancy, it may degenerate into fatal VT or ventricular fibrillation (VF). The prolonged Q-T interval syndrome may present with episodes of multiform VT, "torsade de pointe." Mistreatment of either of these dysrhythmias often leads to sustained VF and death. Digitalis and verapamil are the most frequently *misused* agents. Propranolol (Table 1) given orally is the safest agent and is frequently successful in the prolonged Q-T interval syndrome. Propranolol need no longer be given intravenously, since esmolol is available and is much safer because of its short (10 minutes) half-life. Each of these dysrhythmias is difficult to manage, and the patient should be referred to a pediatric cardiology center. Flecainide and amiodarone (Table 1) are the most frequently successful drugs for infantile VT due to causes other than the prolonged Q-T syndrome. In our referral practice, surgery has been necessary in 50 per cent of cases. In medically controlled cases with normal Q-T intervals, resolution may be expected at a mean of 2 years.

The dysrhythmias just described may be treated in infants in a similar fashion as in neonates. The most important caveat is that any *different* QRS morphology probably indicates ventricular origin of a tachydysrhythmia. In neonates and infants, an abnormal QRS complex may not be wide; rather the size and shape of the Q, R, or S wave may be different. In our experience, only 4 per cent of pediatric supraventricular tachycardias showed aberrant conduction.

Congenital complete AV block is the most common cardiac cause of neonatal or infantile bradycardia. In a neonate with a normal heart, permanent cardiac pacing is indicated if the ventricular rate is less than 55 beats/minute, even if the baby appears clinically stable. In the baby with congenital heart disease or in a stress situation (i.e., hyaline membrane disease) pacing is indicated for a ventricular rate of 65 beats or less. Congestive heart failure, wide QRS (>100 msec), or markedly prolonged QT_C (>490 msec), requires pacing. The epicardial dual chamber approach is favored because the size of the pacemaker is the same. This is accomplished by a subxiphoid incision.

DYSRHYTHMIAS IN CHILDREN

The Child with a Normal Heart

Cardiac dysrhythmias in children are treated in a similar fashion as in infants if cardiac structure and function are normal. Supraventricular tachycardia may be treated with vagal maneuvers acutely, including use of the diving reflex. Consideration should be given to surgical or catheter ablative treatment if two drugs fail to control the tachycardia or result in side effects. The long-term problems of drug therapy must be weighed against the immediate risks of surgical or catheter ablative treatment. The small risk of sudden death in children with the Wolff-Parkinson-White syndrome must be kept in mind, particularly those with syncope or atrial fibrillation.

Single premature atrial or ventricular beats are usually benign in children with normal hearts. *If the beats are suppressed during exercise and the heart structure and function are truly normal, no special follow-up is necessary.* If they do not suppress, a full work-up by a pediatric cardiologist is indicated. Ventricular tachycardia is usually significant in children. Often, signs of cardiac disease are subtle. Angiography and myocardial biopsy are necessary. Sports participation is allowed in children with normal hearts and supraventricular dysrhythmias or exercise-suppressible PVCs.

Congenital complete AV block is often followed into childhood. Pacing is indicated for syncope, near syncope, exercise intolerance, a ventricular rate lower than 40 beats/minute, extreme pauses on ambulatory monitoring, or ventricular ectopy. Dual-chamber transvenous pacing is preferred to achieve the most normal cardiac function possible. This is accomplished by a small incision in the cardiac catheter laboratory followed by puncture of the subclavian vein. Two leads are positioned: one in the right atrium and one in the right ventricle.

The Child with Heart Disease

In this setting, dysrhythmia may indicate myocardial stress. Few children are in this category because most congenital heart disease is "corrected" in infancy. In general, the patient is treated in a manner similar to that in the child with repaired congenital heart disease.

The Child After Heart Surgery

In this setting, dysrhythmias are of great concern. Most cardiac operations leave residua or sequelae that can result in significant dysrhythmias and sudden death. Surveillance and treatment are part of the follow-up after surgery. Treatment is warranted for lesser dysrhythmias than in the child with a normal heart. Asymptomatic dysrhythmias must be treated in many situations.

Pacemaker treatment is indicated for each patient with surgical complete or second-degree AV block that persists for 10 to 14 days. Dual-chamber, rate-responsive pacing is used because the sinus node may also have been damaged. Patients after atrial surgery that results in bradycardia with or without tachycardia are treated with atrial pacing with either rate-responsive or antitachycardia function, depending on the circumstance.

Drug treatment of tachycardias in postoperative patients with known or suspected sinus node dysfunction should be limited to digoxin, phenytoin, or mexilitine unless a pacemaker is inserted. Digoxin is often effective for postoperative supraventricular tachycardia. Phenytoin is extremely effective in suppressing postoperative ventricular dysrhythmias. Atrial antitachycardia pacemakers often prevent the need for drugs.

SUMMARY

Dysrhythmias are treated in a stratified manner in fetuses, infants, and children according to (1) symptoms, (2) normalcy of the heart, and (3) likelihood of sudden death. Definitive treatment, when possible, is becoming the preferred modality.

PERICARDITIS

JACQUELINE A. NOONAN, M.D.

Pericarditis implies inflammation of the parietal and visceral surfaces of the pericardium. Depending on the etiology, the fluid may be serofibrinous, hemorrhagic, or purulent. The hallmark of pericarditis is a friction rub. This is a scratchy, to-and-fro sound heard along the left sternal border, sometimes transmitted over the whole precordium, which is pathognomonic of pericarditis but is not always present. Dull or stabbing chest pain often referred to the shoulder is a characteristic symptom. The child is often pale and anxious and prefers to sit up and lean forward. With rapid accumulation of fluid, the pericardium does not stretch and tamponade may result. This limits cardiac inflow, with resulting pallor, small pulse, narrow pulse pressure, low systolic pressure, and exaggeration of the normal drop in pulse pressure with respiration termed pulsus paradoxus. Regardless of the cause, treatment of tamponade involves the prompt removal of pericardial fluid either by needle aspiration or by a direct surgical approach. Cardiac ultrasound is very helpful in establishing the diagnosis of a pericardial effusion. Fortunately, most patients with pericarditis do not develop tamponade and require no specific therapy. It is important to establish the etiology of pericarditis.

PYOGENIC PERICARDITIS

Pyogenic pericarditis is an uncommon but potential complication of many bacterial infections, especially *Staphylococcus aureus, Streptococcus pneumoniae, Haemophilus influenzae,* and *Neisseria meningitidis.* Pyogenic pericarditis generally occurs in association with meningitis, osteomyelitis, or pneumonia. Muffled heart sounds and a large cardiac silhouette should suggest this diagnosis. A friction rub is present only occasionally in pyogenic pericarditis. Cardiac ultrasound is diagnostic. Cardiac tamponade is a frequent complication of pyogenic pericarditis.

Bacterial pericarditis should be treated with adequate drainage and appropriate antibiotics. Occasionally, a surgical pericardiectomy will be warranted. Tuberculosis may also cause pericarditis but is, fortunately, a rare condition in the United States at this time. Antituberculous therapy and, occasionally, surgical drainage are required.

COLLAGEN VASCULAR DISEASE, RHEUMATOID ARTHRITIS, AND KAWASAKI DISEASE

All of these conditions may feature pericarditis as part of the widespread inflammatory process. Tamponade is rare, and treatment should be directed at the underlying disease.

RHEUMATIC FEVER

Pericarditis is an uncommon, but well-recognized manifestation of rheumatic fever and usually occurs in association with severe valvulitis and myocarditis. Tamponade is rare. If there is severe carditis with cardiac failure, steroids are warranted. Otherwise, the anti-inflammatory effects of aspirin will suffice.

COXSACKIE MYOPERICARDITIS

A number of viruses, especially coxsackievirus, are known to cause myocarditis as well as pericardial inflammation. A cardiac ultrasound helps to define the degree of myocardial dysfunction and also will demonstrate the pericardial effusion. Rest is essential if there is significant myocarditis. Tamponade is rare, and pericarditis is usually self-limited and responsive to anti-inflammatory therapy.

BENIGN OR IDIOPATHIC PERICARDITIS

This is the most common form of pericarditis occurring in children. It is often mild enough to be overlooked. Benign pericarditis is probably viral in origin, but usually no specific diagnosis can be made. It is generally a self-limited disease that can be treated symptomatically by aspirin or other anti-inflammatory drugs. *Although this condition does respond to steroids, relapse is frequent when steroids are discontinued; thus, steroids should be avoided.* An occasional patient will have a chronic course with multiple relapses, and surgical pericardiectomy may be required to effect a cure.

POST-PERICARDIOTOMY SYNDROME

This well-recognized syndrome occurs in some children 1 week or more following surgery in which the pericardium has been opened. This is a febrile illness with pericardial and pleural reaction and effusion. Because this happens in children who have had surgery for heart disease, it may be difficult to distinguish this syndrome from cardiac failure. The echocardiogram is helpful in the differential diagnosis. Should signs of tamponade occur, pericardiocentesis is indicated.

Salicylates in therapeutic doses for several weeks are generally sufficient to relieve the symptoms; however, an occasional patient will have a severe illness and the use of steroids may be justified. Steroids should be avoided, if possible, because there is the tendency for rebound to occur when steroids are discontinued.

OTHER CAUSES OF PERICARDITIS

Uremic pericarditis is best managed by treatment of underlying renal failure with dialysis. I have seen tamponade develop in one patient with uremic pericarditis when hemorrhage occurred into the pericardium; the patient had been heparinized while undergoing dialysis. Both primary and metastatic tumors of the heart can also result in pericardial effusion.

CONSTRICTIVE PERICARDITIS

"Acute" constrictive pericarditis is a rare complication of pyogenic pericarditis. I have seen two children in whom constriction developed within 3 weeks of acute pericarditis secondary to *H. influenzae.* These children showed signs of increased venous pressure, an enlarged liver, and a very low cardiac output. Surgical treatment with pericardial resection restored both to good health.

"Chronic" constrictive pericarditis has a more insidious onset. The cause is usually unknown.

Previously, most cases of constrictive pericarditis were attributed to tuberculosis but this is no longer true. The diagnosis of chronic constrictive pericarditis is often delayed and may be misdiagnosed as liver disease. The hallmark of this condition is ascites with a normal-sized heart and increased venous pressure.

Treatment involves surgical resection of the pericardium. If there is underlying myocardial disease, cardiac failure may occur following surgery. There may be an occasional death from cardiac failure following pericardiectomy.

ENDOCARDITIS

LISA SAIMAN, M.D.

The management of endocarditis presents considerable challenges. Changes in medical and surgical practices during the past two decades have led to new groups of children at risk for development of endocarditis. These new risk groups include children with complex cyanotic heart disease, often with shunts and prosthetic valves; premature infants and older critically ill children in intensive care units with central venous catheters; and adolescents with mitral valve prolapse. Such children are often infected with predictable pathogens, and knowledge of these can be used to guide initial therapy.

Medical management with antimicrobials remains the cornerstone of therapy. However, daily monitoring of hemodynamic status, careful observation of the patient for evidence of embolic complications and, when indicated, timely surgical intervention are critical to ensure the best possible outcome. Thus, optimal therapy depends on collaboration between several subspecialists, including infectious disease physicians, cardiologists, cardiothoracic surgeons, neurologists, and the clinical microbiology laboratory staff.

MEDICAL MANAGEMENT

General Principles

An understanding of the basic principles of antibiotic therapy for endocarditis requires knowledge of the pathology of the thrombus.[1] Bactericidal, not bacteriostatic, antibiotics are imperative because the organisms within the infected thrombus grow slowly; antibiotics do not diffuse well into the thrombus; and complement, antibodies, and inflammatory cells are often excluded from the avascular thrombus. Adequate therapy necessitates long courses of parenteral antibiotics to achieve higher and more predictable blood levels.

Initial antimicrobial management is empirical until a positive blood culture specimen is obtained. The initial choice of antimicrobials is guided by four factors: (1) risk factors of the infected patient, (2) clinical presentation, (3) knowledge of the pathogens that cause endocarditis in specific settings, and (4) antibiotic sensitivities of specific organisms in either community acquired or nosocomial endocarditis. Subsequent modifications in antibiotic therapy are made when the pathogen is identified and in vitro sensitivity profiles are determined by the clinical microbiology laboratory. The treatment durations for pediatric patients with endocarditis are extrapolated from recommendations for adult patients despite the fact that adult patients often have different risk factors, such as calcified or artificial valves, intravenous drug abuse, or rheumatic heart disease.[2]

Most experts recommend obtaining peak serum antibiotic cidal levels when treating a patient with endocarditis. There are no convincing data to indicate that trough serum cidal levels are more predictive of therapeutic efficacy than peak values. To perform serum cidal levels, the patient's serum is obtained immediately following infusion of a dose of antibiotic. A standard inoculum of the patient's organism (5×10^5 colony-forming units/ml) is added to twofold dilutions (1:2, 1:4, 1:8, 1:16, 1:32, 1:64, 1:128, 1:256, 1:512, 1:1028, 1:2056) of this serum and incubated for 24 hours. The tubes are examined for turbidity and the most dilute serum (i.e., that serum containing the least antibiotic) wherein the tube appears clear is considered the serum inhibitory concentration. A loopful of broth from each of the tubes without visible growth is then streaked on an agar plate and incubated for an additional 24 hours to detect viable organisms. The plate containing the lowest dilution of antibiotic without growth is the serum cidal concentration. The serum inhibitory concentration should be no more than fourfold more dilute than the serum cidal concentration. If these two values are more than two tubes apart, the organism is tolerant and thus may be harder to eradicate.

Most experts agree that peak serum cidal levels equal or greater than 1:8 are desirable. However, the use of serum cidal levels has never been subjected to a well-designed clinical trial to demonstrate whether their use is associated with faster microbiologic cure or improved survival. Most patients treated with the antibiotic doses suggested in Table 1 will achieve adequate serum cidal levels. Serum cidal levels will be especially helpful in patients having unusual organisms, those being treated with an unconventional treatment regimen, or those showing slow response to treatment (as evidenced by persistently positive blood cultures, a persistently elevated erythrocyte sedimentation rate [ESR], or high white blood cell count). Serum cidal levels do not replace measuring peak antibiotic levels. Weekly vancomycin and/or gentamicin levels need to be determined if these antibiotics are used.

TABLE 1. Recommended Therapeutic Regimens for Endocarditis

Organism	Sensitivity	Antibiotic (Dosage)	Duration
Streptococci			
On native valve	MIC < 0.1 μg/ml*	Penicillin G (200,000–250,000 units/kg/day IV div q 4 hr) *or*	4 weeks
		Penicillin G (200,000–250,000 units/kg/day IV div q 4 hr) + Gentamicin (1 mg/kg/dose IV q 8 hr)	2 weeks†
	MIC > 0.1 μg/ml	Penicillin G (200,000–250,000 units/kg/day IV) + Gentamicin (1 mg/kg/dose IV q 8 hr)	4 weeks
In penicillin-allergic patient		Vancomycin (40–60 mg/kg/day IV div q 6 hr) + Gentamicin (1 mg/kg/dose IV q 8 hr)	4 weeks
On prosthetic valve		Vancomycin and gentamicin (as in penicillin-allergic patient)	6 weeks
Enterococci		Penicillin G (200,000–250,000 units/kg/day IV div q 4 hr) + Gentamicin (1 mg/kg/dose IV q 8 hr)	6 weeks
Staphylococci	Oxacillin-sensitive	Oxacillin or nafcillin (150–200 mg/kg/day IV div q 6 hr) +	4–6 weeks
		Gentamicin (1 mg/kg/dose IV q 8 hr)	1–2 weeks
		Consider rifampin (20 mg/kg/day p.o. div q 12 hr)‡	2–4 weeks
	Oxacillin-resistant *or* In penicillin-allergic patient	Vancomycin (40–60 mg/kg/day IV div q 6 hr) +	4–6 weeks
		Gentamicin (1 mg/kg/dose IV q 8 hr)	1–2 weeks
		Consider rifampin (20 mg/kg/day p.o. div q 12 hr)	2–4 weeks
Gram-negative organisms		Consult microbiology laboratory sensitivities	6 weeks
Fungi		Amphotericin B 1 mg/kg/dose/day IV + flucytosine 50 mg/kg/day p.o. div q 6 hr Surgery	6 weeks minimum

*Minimum inhibitory concentration to penicillin.
†Consider two additional weeks of treatment with amoxicillin.
‡If slow clinical response or abscess suspected or if coagulase-negative *Staphylococcus* infection of prosthetic valve.
Abbreviations: MIC, minimum inhibitory concentration; IV, intravenous; p.o., by mouth; q, every; hr, hour; div, divided.

Subacute Bacterial Endocarditis

The most common cause of subacute, community-acquired endocarditis in children with congenital heart disease or rheumatic heart disease is *Streptococcus viridans.* In the hemodynamically stable patient with subacute endocarditis, antimicrobial treatment can be delayed until specimens from several sets of blood cultures are obtained over 24 to 48 hours to ensure recovery of an organism. It has been our experience that *Staphylococcus aureus* can also cause a surprisingly indolent course in children with congenital heart disease. Thus, empiric antimicrobial therapy for community-acquired endocarditis in a child with congenital heart disease should include penicillin; a semisynthetic beta-lactam, such as oxacillin or nafcillin; and low-dose gentamicin. Subacute endocarditis in a child with rheumatic heart disease can be treated initially with penicillin and gentamicin. Suggested doses for antimicrobials are listed in Table 1. Streptomycin should not be used because of the increased incidence of ototoxicity. Vancomycin can be used in place of penicillin or oxacillin in penicillin-allergic patients.

Following identification of the pathogen, antibiotic therapy can be modified. *S. viridans,* alpha-hemolytic, and nonhemolytic flora of the oral cavity and gastrointestinal tract, are usually quite sensitive to penicillin with minimum inhibitory concentration (MIC) values obtained by the clinical microbiology laboratory of less than 0.1 μg/ml. Uncomplicated *S. viridans* endocarditis of natural valves can be treated with 2 weeks of penicillin G and low-dose gentamicin or 4 weeks of penicillin G alone when the MIC to penicillins is lower than 0.1 μg/ml. It has been the practice of some clinicians to treat patients who have received only 2 weeks of parenteral antibiotics with an additional 2 weeks of oral amoxicillin and probenecid. Streptococci are considered relatively resistant when the MIC is higher than 0.1 μg/ml. Patients infected with these organisms should be treated with 4 weeks of penicillin G and low-dose gentamicin. Streptococcal infection of prosthetic valves should be treated for 6 weeks. Enterococcal endocarditis may occasionally present subacutely and should be treated with 6 weeks of penicillin, ampicillin or vancomycin and low-dose gentamicin. Courses of intravenous antibiotics may be completed at home in the very stable patient.

Acute Bacterial Endocarditis

S. aureus is the most common cause of acute bacterial endocarditis, and infection can occur on normal heart valves, valves with mitral valve prolapse, or prosthetic valves. Thus far, community-acquired *S. aureus* at Columbia–Presbyterian Medical Center has been sensitive to beta-lactamase–stable, semisynthetic penicillins and can be treated with oxacillin and nafcillin. Methicillin should not be used because of the high incidence of interstitial nephritis.

Treatment of *S. aureus* endocarditis should initially include low-dose gentamicin and/or rifampin. In general, oxacillin and gentamicin are used for 1 to 2 weeks or until blood culture specimens are negative, after which most authors would discontinue gentamicin. Rifampin can then be added, usually after discontinuation of gentamicin, especially when there is suspicion that an abscess has developed in the myocardium or in the periphery secondary to embolization of the infected thrombus. A shorter duration of bacteremia and improved clinical outcome may be achieved by combination therapy. However, there are only limited data in humans to suggest that combination therapy is better than monotherapy with a semisynthetic beta-lactamase–stable penicillin alone. Uncomplicated endocarditis due to *S. aureus* can be treated with oxacillin or nafcillin for 4 weeks if there is a rapid clinical response. Antimicrobial therapy should be continued for 6 weeks or occasionally longer in the patient with a slow clinical response and/or complications such as persistently positive blood culture specimens, intracardiac extension, valve replacement, or embolic phenomena. *S. aureus* endocarditis is often complicated by embolic events, especially to the lungs in patients with right-sided infection or to the central nervous system in left-sided infection. Any patient with left-sided endocarditis should undergo an initial neurologic evaluation and follow-up examinations when there is any evidence of embolization. Throughout treatment, urinalysis and liver function tests need to be monitored weekly because of the risk of interstitial nephritis and hepatitis. For patients taking vancomycin and gentamicin, weekly peak and trough levels must be assessed as well.

Endocarditis caused by methicillin-resistant staphylococci has become an increasingly common problem. Methicillin resistance is defined as growth of the organism on an agar plate containing oxacillin, 6 μg/ml, and resistance to imipenem and augmentin. These organisms are not sensitive to cephalosporins or the macrolides erythromycin and clindamycin. In my experience, hospitalized premature infants and older children with central venous catheters and early postoperative endocarditis following open heart surgery represent the three groups at risk for infection with these nosocomial pathogens. These organisms are treated with vancomycin for 6 weeks and low-dose gentamicin for 1 to 2 weeks. Rifampin may be added if blood cultures are persistently positive or an abscess is suspected as described above. Thus far, methicillin-resistant strains have not been associated with increased morbidity and mortality when compared with methicillin-sensitive strains.

Endocarditis of normal valves can also be caused by enterococcus, *S. pneumoniae,* and, rarely, group A *Streptococcus.* Initially, the diagnosis of endocarditis may not be suspected because these patients appear septic and often present with meningitis and pneumonia. Initial empiric antimicrobial therapy should be vancomycin and gentamicin pending culture results if endocarditis is suspected. As these organisms tend to be associated with large, friable vegetations, there is a high incidence of embolic complications; thus, the patient's clinical course should be closely monitored.

Postoperative Endocarditis

Modern surgical sterilization procedures have dramatically reduced the incidence of early postoperative endocarditis (within 2 months of surgery) in children with congenital heart disease. When early postoperative endocarditis does occur, the most common pathogens causing infection are *S. aureus,* coagulase-negative *Staphylococcus,* and, more rarely, Enterobacteriaceae, diphtheroids, or fungi such as *Aspergillus* or *Candida* species. Empiric antibiotic therapy following at least two sets of blood cultures should usually consist of vancomycin and gentamicin because of the high incidence of methicillin-resistant *Staphylococcus* in many hospitals. Rifampin should be added if a prosthetic valve is infected with coagulase-negative *Staphylococcus.* Nosocomial pathogens vary at individual centers however, and this should be considered when selecting empiric antimicrobial therapy in early postoperative endocarditis. When a bacterial pathogen is identified, the duration of treatment should be 6 weeks. Clinical cure in early postoperative endocarditis may require removal of the prosthetic valve or shunt.

Fungal endocarditis is very difficult to diagnose and treat effectively. Blood cultures are often negative, and a high index of suspicion is required for diagnosis (e.g., when there is a large friable vegetation without a positive blood culture or there has been a recent outbreak of nosocomial fungal infection in postoperative patients). Both amphotericin and flucytosine are used to treat either *Candida* or *Aspergillus* endocarditis. The toxicities of these drugs are considerable, and the patient's renal function and blood counts must be carefully monitored. In some centers, it is possible to obtain serum levels of flucytosine to minimize toxicity. However, the only hope for cure requires surgical excision of the vegetation and removal of the prosthetic valve. Even when managed both surgically and medically, fungal endocarditis carries a mortality rate of 50 to 90 per cent.

Nosocomial Endocarditis

Occasionally, nosocomial endocarditis develops in hospitalized patients and is usually caused by predictable pathogens. Premature infants with normal hearts and central venous catheters are at increased risk for nosocomial endocarditis usually caused by methicillin-resistant *S. aureus* or coagulase-negative *Staphylococcus.* The pathogenesis appears to be formation of a sterile thrombus on the endomyocardium secondary to damage from the central venous catheter. During episodes of bacteremia, the thrombus becomes colonized. Endocarditis may not initially be recognized until persistently positive blood cultures alert the physician to this possibility and echocardiogram reveals a right-sided vegetation. Initial therapy includes vancomycin with gentamicin. Subsequent adjustments in antibiotics are guided by the sensitivity patterns of the organism isolated. The central venous catheter must be removed. It has been our experience that these children experience an excellent outcome.

Unfortunately, it has been noted that nosocomial endocarditis has developed in several critically ill children (8 of 54) with central venous catheters and prolonged hospitalizations. Endocarditis remained undiagnosed in these children until autopsy, when they all demonstrated evidence of systemic embolization. The most frequent organisms isolated at autopsy were nosocomial gram-negative bacilli and *Aspergillus* and *Candida* species. Thus, prolonged bacteremia or clinical sepsis without an organism should alert the physician to the possibility of nosocomial endocarditis.

Culture-Negative Endocarditis

Culture-negative endocarditis occurs in an estimated 5 to 15 per cent of cases of endocarditis and is most often secondary to pretreatment with antibiotics. Blood cultures must be held for 4 weeks to ensure growth of the nutritionally fastidious streptococci and the HACEK (*Haemophilus, Actinobacillus, Cardiobacterium, Eikenella,* and *Kingella*) organisms. These pathogens are very infrequent in pediatric cases of endocarditis. Fungi, chlamydiae, rickettsiae, and viruses may also cause culture-negative endocarditis.

Therapy of community-acquired, culture-negative endocarditis should include ampicillin, oxacillin, and low-dose gentamicin. Gram stain and subculture of the original blood cultures, culture of peripheral emboli or the resected valve, teichoic acid antibodies that measure a cell wall component of *S. aureus,* and bacterial antigen detection of *S. pneumoniae* may occasionally reveal a pathogen, although generally these studies are not helpful. If all these findings remain negative, continual surveillance of the clinical course is imperative to demonstrate response to the initial choice of antimicrobials.

TABLE 2. American Heart Association Recommendations for Prophylaxis of Endocarditis*

Procedure	Antibiotic	Dosage
Dental, oral, upper respiratory tract	Amoxicillin p.o.	50 mg/kg 1 hr before procedure (max 3.0 g) 25 mg/kg 6 hr after procedure (max 1.5 g)
In penicillin-allergic patient	Erythromycin p.o.	20 mg/kg 1 hour before procedure; 10 mg/kg 6 hr after procedure
	or	
	Clindamycin p.o.	10 mg/kg 1 hour before procedure 5 mg/kg 6 hr after procedure
Genitourinary/ gastrointestinal	Ampicillin IV	50 mg/kg 30 minutes before procedure (max 2.0 g)
	+	
	Gentamicin IV	2.0 mg/kg 30 minutes before procedure (max 80 mg) Repeat this regimen 8 hr after procedure
In penicillin-allergic patient	Vancomycin IV	20 mg/kg 1 hr before procedure (max 500 mg)
	+	
	Gentamicin IV	2.0 mg/kg 1 hr before (max 80 mg) Repeat this regimen 8 hr after procedure
If low risk†	Amoxicillin p.o.	50 mg/kg 1 hr before procedure (max 3.0 g) 25 mg/kg 6 hr after procedure (max 1.5 g)

*These are the 1990 recommendations, and revisions are made frequently.

†Procedures and lesions are described in American Heart Association recommendations adapted from JAMA 264:2919–2922, 1990. Copyright 1990, American Medical Association.

SURGICAL MANAGEMENT

Surgical intervention in endocarditis can be considered according to two categories: absolute indications and relative indications.[3] Absolute indications include intractable heart failure secondary to valvular obstruction, prosthetic valve dehiscence, fungal endocarditis, or, most commonly, persistently positive blood cultures for more than 1 week despite appropriate antibiotics. Intracardiac extension causing myocardial abscess, rupture of the papillary muscles, chordae tendineae, and ventricular septum are also clear indications for emergent surgical intervention. Early postoperative prosthetic valve endocarditis is usually an indication for surgery. However, these complications of endocarditis are, fortunately, quite rare.

One of the most difficult management decisions is whether or not to remove the vegetation surgically. The presence of a large vegetation, even when found on the left side of the heart, is not an absolute indication for surgery. Several studies have addressed whether size is predictive of future embolization and have concluded that size alone is not an indication for removal of the vegetation. Likewise, with the exception of fungal endocarditis, the infecting organism does not dictate surgery. The timing of embolization is also somewhat variable, in that vegetations can embolize at presentation or during or following the successful completion of therapy. Pulmonary emboli, even when multiple, rarely cause life-threatening complications necessitating surgical excision of the vegetation. However left-sided embolic events, usually to the central nervous system, do represent relative indications for surgery. However, because of the enormous surgical risks associated with these patients, many authors will wait until a second embolic event occurs before recommending surgery.

PROGNOSIS

The outcome for patients with known endocarditis is usually fairly good. In the late 1970s and 1980s, the mortality rates in published series of endocarditis in pediatrics patients ranged from 14 to 22 per cent.[4–6] Children with endocarditis due to *S. aureus* have the highest risk of morbidity and mortality, as do children with fungal endocarditis and gram-negative endocarditis. It is important to note that approximately 15 to 25 per cent of adult patients who have been cured with medical management alone eventually require cardiac surgery to repair damaged valves. Streptococcal endocarditis is associated with excellent outcomes and minimal morbidity. Relapse is fortunately rare and, not surprisingly, most often occurs in patients with complex, congenital, cyanotic heart disease with prosthetic valves and shunts. Children who have had one episode of endocarditis have about a 5 to 10 per cent chance of a recurrent infection; therefore, blood culture specimens should be obtained during subsequent febrile illnesses.

PROPHYLAXIS

The most recent recommendations for prophylaxis by the American Heart Association attempt to simplify the regimens (Table 2), clarify the lesions, and shorten the list of procedures for which prophylaxis is indicated.[7] These recommendations are continually being updated, and physicians should review the literature periodically. The rationale for antimicrobial prophylaxis for patients at risk for endocarditis is based on many assumptions, and an adequate clinical trial to prove its efficacy will probably never be done. Most of the studies of prophylaxis have been performed in animal models, and most of the episodes of endocarditis are not preceded by an antecedent event that can be pretreated. Furthermore, adequate prophylaxis can fail to prevent endocarditis, and only

Streptococcus and Enterococcus are sensitive to the oral antimicrobials used. Despite these limitations, antimicrobial prophylaxis to prevent endocarditis has been established as routine medical practice.

REFERENCES

1. Saiman L, Prince A: Infections of the heart. *In* Aronoff SC, et al (eds): Advances in Pediatric Infectious Diseases. Chicago, Year Book Medical Publishers, 1989, pp 139–155.
2. Bisno AL, Dismukes WE, Durack DT, et al: Antimicrobial treatment of infective endocarditis due to viridans streptococci, enterococci, and staphylococci. JAMA 261:1471–1477, 1989.
3. Alsip SG, Blackstone EH, Kirklin JW, Cobbs CG: Indications for cardiac surgery in patients with active infective endocarditis. Am J Med 78(Suppl 6B):138–148, 1985.
4. Johnson CM, Rhodes KH: Pediatric endocarditis. Mayo Clin Proc 57:86–94, 1982.
5. Stanton BF, Baltimore RS, Clemens JD: Changing spectrum of infective endocarditis in children: Analysis of 26 cases, 1970–1979. Am J Dis Child 138:720–725, 1984.
6. Van Hare GF, Ben-Shachar G, Liebman J, Boxerbaum B, Riemenschneider TA: Infective endocarditis in infants and children during the past 10 years: A decade of change. Am Heart J 138:1235–1240, 1984.
7. Dajani AS, Bisno AL, Chung KJ, et al: Prevention of bacterial endocarditis. Recommendations by the American Heart Association. JAMA 264:2919–2922, 1990.

CARDIOMYOPATHY AND HEART TRANSPLANTATION

JAMES R. ZUBERBUHLER, M.D.

Cardiomyopathy is strictly defined as cardiac muscle dysfunction of unknown cause. However, specific cardiac muscle diseases of known etiology may have similar clinical presentations and may require similar therapy. They will therefore be included in the following discussion. Cardiomyopathies are classified as dilated, hypertrophic, and restrictive.

FORMS OF CARDIOMYOPATHY

Dilated Cardiomyopathy

In children, dilated cardiomyopathy is most often primary and of unknown etiology but also occurs as a consequence of myocarditis following chemotherapy with doxyrubicin (Adriamycin) and in patients with congenital heart disease, particularly in those who have undergone multiple open heart procedures. Dilated cardiomyopathy is not "curable," but symptoms of congestive heart failure and low cardiac output may be ameliorated, at least for a time, with medical therapy.

The major therapeutic modalities include diuretics, vasodilators, and positive inotropic agents. If congestive heart failure is present, furosemide should be given in a dose of 1 to 2 mg/kg per dose, once or twice daily. If more than 1 mg/kg/day of furosemide is used, supplemental potassium or a potassium sparing diuretic, such as spironolactone, should be added, the latter in a dose of 2 to 3 mg/kg/day in two divided doses. Zaroxylin can be used to potentiate diuresis in diuretic-resistant individuals. The dose is 1.25 to 5.0 mg orally once daily. If there are signs and symptoms of low cardiac output, afterload reduction can be tried with an angiotensin-converting enzyme (ACE) inhibitor, such as captopril. The dose of captopril must be titrated, beginning with 0.5 to 1.0 mg/kg/day in three divided doses and increasing as needed to a maximum of 6 mg/kg/day. The usual dose range in the adolescent is 6.25 to 25 mg three times daily. Afterload reduction is contraindicated if there is pre-therapy hypotension, and the dose must be reduced if hypotension occurs during therapy.

Digoxin may be helpful and should be tried if symptoms persist after diuretics and vasodilator therapy. It is probably wise to begin with smaller than usual doses because digoxin precipitates or exaggerates arrhythmia in some patients. An initial maintenance dose of 5 μg/kg/day in two divided doses is appropriate, increasing to 8 to 10 μg/kg/day as needed and tolerated, to a maximum dose of 0.125 to 0.25 mg/day in adolescents. Digoxin is most useful if atrial fibrillation with rapid ventricular response is present.

The incidence of intracardiac thrombus formation is especially high in the presence of atrial fibrillation or severe congestive heart failure. Anticoagulation should be instituted in patients with an ejection fraction lower than 30 per cent unless there is some contraindication. Coumadin is the most commonly used anticoagulant. Prophylaxis against bacterial endocarditis is indicated in patients with mitral regurgitation.

Hypertrophic Cardiomyopathy

Hypertrophic cardiomyopathy is almost always primary and of unknown etiology and may be familial. A transient form occurs in newborns of diabetic mothers. There is abnormal thickening of the ventricular myocardium, usually most marked in the left ventricle but sometimes involving the right ventricle as well. The hypertrophy is commonly but not necessarily asymmetric, with the septum being much thicker than the left ventricular free wall. Consequently, the left ventricular cavity is small. There is often myocardial disarray microscopically. In some cases, there is left ventricular outflow tract obstruction, either at rest or inducible by various maneuvers or pharmacologic agents. Systolic function is normal, or even "super normal," contributing to left ventricular outflow tract obstruction. Diastolic function is abnormal, the left ventricle being less compliant than normal. Children with hypertrophic cardiomyopathy are often asymptomatic, and the diagnosis is frequently made during screening undertaken because of hypertrophic cardiomyopathy in a family member. Sporadic cases occur, but family members should always be screened by echocardiography to rule out subclinical familial disease. Although symptoms such as chest pain, dyspnea on exertion, and syncope are uncommon in children, sudden unexpected death may occur.

The treatment of hypertrophic cardiomyopathy is directed toward relief of symptoms and the prevention of sudden death. Heavy physical exertion should be discouraged and competitive sports forbidden because of the risk of sudden death. The pharmacologic treatment is difficult and potentially dangerous and does not prevent progression of the disease or sudden death. In general, treatment is reserved for symptomatic patients but is advocated by some if there is severe left ventricular outflow tract obstruction or ventricular ectopy or if there is a family history of hypertrophic cardiomyopathy and sudden death.

Therapeutic agents include beta-adrenergic agents, calcium channel blocking agents, and antiarrhythmics. Propranolol, a nonselective beta-blocker, is considered by most to be the first-line drug. Reduction of heart rate, decrease in myocardial oxygen demand, and decrease in left ventricular outflow tract obstruction may result in symptomatic improvement, but sudden death is not prevented. The usual starting dose is 1 to 2 mg/kg/day in three to four divided doses. The dose is gradually increased until effective beta-adrenergic blockade is signaled by a slowing of the resting heart rate. If propranolol is poorly tolerated, atenolol can be substituted in a dose 75 per cent of the daily propranolol dose, given once daily.

The calcium channel blocker verapamil has been shown to improve diastolic function in some individuals with hypertrophic cardiomyopathy. As with beta-adrenergic blockers, patients may improve symptomatically but sudden death still occurs. The usual dose in children is 5 mg/kg/day in three divided doses. The adolescent dose range is from 240 to 480 mg/day. Verapamil is dangerous in the presence of conduction abnormalities or very high left ventricular diastolic pressure and should be used very cautiously, if at all, in such patients.

Amiodarone is the drug of choice in patients with life-threatening ventricular arrhythmias, since other antiarrhythmic agents are usually ineffective. The loading dose is 10 mg/kg/day in two divided doses for 1 week, followed by a maintenance dose of 5 mg/kg/day in one dose. Amiodarone is potentially quite toxic, and the lowest effective dose should be sought. The onset of action is slow and the effect of a given dose level may not be apparent for 7 to 10 days.

One recent report suggests an early proarrhythmic effect in patients with a history of nonsustained ventricular tachycardia, with a consequent increase in the incidence of sudden death during the early months of therapy. Diuretics may be helpful in the presence of pulmonary congestion. Digoxin is contraindicated, since systolic function is normal or "super normal." Vasodilator therapy should not be employed in patients with hypertrophic cardiomyopathy because reduction in afterload may potentiate left ventricular outflow tract obstruction and result in hemodynamic deterioration. Surgery is reserved for those with severe left ventricular outflow tract obstruction (gradient > 75 mm Hg) whose symptoms are not controlled with medical therapy. Myotomy or myomectomy may improve symptoms but does not prevent sudden death. Prophylaxis in subacute bacterial endocarditis is indicated unless the mitral valve is normal and there is no left ventricular outflow tract obstruction.

Restrictive Cardiomyopathy

In a restrictive cardiomyopathy, systolic function is usually well preserved but diastolic function is abnormal. Fibrosis or deposits within the myocardium reduce compliance and result in high filling pressures. Diuretics may be tried cautiously if there are signs of systemic or pulmonary congestion. Digoxin is ineffective if there is normal systolic function, and vasodilators are potentially dangerous.

MYOCARDITIS

Acute myocarditis is not usually thought of as a cardiomyopathy but is considered here. The myocardial inflammatory process may be of infectious etiology, usually viral, but sometimes may be a hypersensitivity process, possibly induced by one of a variety of therapeutic drugs. If congestive heart failure is evident, diuretics are indicated. Digoxin may be tried, but in reduced dosage because of the risk of arrhythmia. Vasodilators may be poorly tolerated, but they also can be tried cautiously unless hypotension is present. The role of anti-inflammatory or immunosuppressive agents is still controversial, but most specialists agree that they are contraindicated in the very early stages or if the disease is mild or improving. If the clinical picture is severe, endomyocardial biopsy is useful in establishing the presence of acute inflammation or a hypersensitivity reaction. Under such circumstances, prednisone can be given in an initial dose of 1 to 2 mg/kg/day in two divided doses. The dose is tapered after several weeks to 0.3 mg/kg/day and maintained for several months. If steroids are ineffective or if the process recurs after discontinuation of the steroids, a course of azathioprine or cyclosporine should be considered.

HEART TRANSPLANTATION

Heart transplantation may be considered in children with cardiomyopathy who are very symptomatic and whose activities are severely limited in spite of optimum medical management. Patients with substantial elevation of pulmonary vascular resistance are not candidates for orthotopic heart transplantation but may be considered for heart-lung transplantation. The perioperative risk of heart transplantation is now low, but immunosuppressive therapy is required indefinitely. At present, cyclosporine is the major immunosuppressive agent and is usually supplemented with steroids and often with azathioprine. Major problems in the management of children undergoing heart transplantation include infection, chronic or episodic rejection with development of decreased myocardial function and/or coronary artery disease, reduced renal function, and systemic hypertension. A few centers are now using FK506, a more potent immunosuppressive agent having potentially fewer side effects than cyclosporine. Steroids can often be avoided if FK506 is used. Present results of heart transplantation in children are encouraging, and those who have undergone cardiac transplantation are often able to resume normal age-appropriate activities.

REFERENCES

Baron BJ: Cardiomyopathies. *In* Adams FH, Emmanouilides GC, Riemenschneider TA (eds): Heart Disease in Infants, Children, and Adolescents. Baltimore, Williams & Wilkins, 1989.

VanDohlen TW, Frank MJ: Current perspectives in hypertrophic cardiomyopathy: Diagnosis, clinical management, and prevention of disability and sudden cardiac death. Clin Cardiol 13:247–252, 1990.

Zuberbuhler JR, Fricker FJ, Griffith BP: Cardiac transplantation in children. Cardiol Clin 7:411–418, 1989.

SYSTEMIC HYPERTENSION

LEONARD G. FELD, M.D., PH.D.

Over the last decade, there has been an increasing interest in hypertension among pediatric health care providers. Clinical trials involving more than 40,000 adults have definitively shown that identification and treatment of patients with diastolic blood pressures (BPs) greater than 95 mm Hg prevent death and disability from cerebrovascular, cardiac, and renal disease. Despite the need to apply this information to the pediatric population, long-term data are not available to associate specific levels of blood pressure in children with future morbidity or mortality or to support treatment of childhood hypertension.

There is evidence to support the early identification and treatment of high blood pressure in children. Blood pressure tracking in childhood has shown a correlation of the blood pressure percentile at one examination with the percentile at a succeeding examination. This information supports the contention that essential or primary hypertension has its roots in childhood.

The traditional classification of childhood hypertension into primary and secondary forms is a useful approach for evaluation and treatment. It is estimated that 15 to 72 per cent of hypertensive children and adolescents have primary or obesity-related hypertension. Secondary hypertension in children is produced by renal parenchymal diseases, coarctation of aorta, renovascular lesions, endocrine disease, tumors, drug and toxins, and neurologic diseases. Eighty per cent of definable hypertension is related to renal parenchymal disease and 10 per cent to renovascular disease (see article on glomerulonephritis, p. 352).

The evaluation for primary and secondary hypertension is generally approached in phases, with screening studies aimed at finding the most common causes of secondary hypertension.

For a summary of these approaches, see the Task Force reference at the end of this article.

MANAGEMENT

Management strategies can be broadly divided into two interrelated categories, nonpharmacologic and pharmacologic. Selection of an appropriate therapeutic plan depends on clinical judgment based on the severity and duration of high blood pressure and on the presence of other diseases effected by hypertension. A healthy child with newly diagnosed mild to moderate hypertension may benefit from nonpharmacologic treatment and continued observation. A child with severe hypertension, end-organ damage, diabetes mellitus, hyperlipidemia, or underlying renal disease may require aggressive nonpharmacologic treatment and antihypertensive medications.

Nonpharmacologic Antihypertensive Therapy

Nondrug therapy is composed of two components: weight control with dietary modification and exercise. In an overweight child without a history of signs or symptoms related to a secondary form of hypertension and otherwise normal physical findings, an individualized weight control program should be the major focus of therapy. The goals of dietary intervention are reduction in body weight and in dietary intake of salt and fat. Reduction in weight and maintenance of ideal weight are often very difficult. We have found that the use of a 3-day dietary record analyzed by a computerized program is quite effective. If such a program is not available, a nutritional consult is helpful. The dietary analysis is discussed with the patient and compared with previous records. In this way, the patient along with the physician and dietitian sets dietary goals and objective information is used to assess progress.

The role of dietary sodium restriction is controversial. Because there are studies that link dietary sodium intake to elevation in blood pressure, sodium restriction is a potentially effective treatment for hypertension. The recommendation is to limit the use of salt in the preparation of meals and to restrict the consumption of foods containing high amounts of sodium when the patient is dining out.

The restriction of excessive dietary fat may prevent premature atherosclerosis and coronary heart disease. Recent studies have suggested that blood lipid abnormalities may have a detrimental effect in patients with renal disease. As stated above, the computer program is also used to assess dietary fat consumption and to evaluate the success of dietary intervention.

Dynamic exercise appears beneficial as an adjunct in many youngsters with primary hypertension. In fact, blood pressure has been shown to normalize in some adults and adolescents participating in such an exercise program. Thus, patients should be given a program of endurance exercise training. Guidelines are as follows:

1. The exercise uses a large amount of the patient's muscle mass (i.e., activities like swimming, running, and bicycling).
2. The activity must increase the heart rate to about 160 beats/minute (the patient should be shown how to monitor the pulse over 6 seconds and multiply by 10 to monitor it).
3. The activity should be done at least every other day, optimally five times per week.

Patients should be counseled to start off slowly and increase the pace.

In general, isometric exercise does not pose the risk to children and adolescents that it does in adults but guidelines are unclear.

Pharmacologic Antihypertensive Therapy

The major issues in managing childhood hypertension with medication include defining which groups of children require pharmacologic therapy, selecting appropriate agents, and designing an optimal follow-up care plan. The indications for pharmacologic intervention include:

1. Children with severe hypertension (BP > the 99th percentile for age and sex).
2. Children with significant hypertension (BP > the 95th percentile for age and sex) who are unresponsive to nonpharmacologic treatment.
3. Children with significant hypertension and associated end-organ damage or an irreversible cause of secondary hypertension.

When the decision is made to institute antihypertensive medication, the benefits of drug therapy must outweigh the risks. Compliance is a major problem with chronic drug administration. Adherence to antihypertensive therapy is optimized when the patient and family understand the indication for initiating therapy, how the medication works to reduce blood pressure, and the most common side effects of the drug.

The management of the hypertensive children and adolescents focuses on two main categories: hypertensive crises and chronic hypertension.

Hypertensive Crises

In general, the evaluation of childhood hypertension proceeds as a phased approach to determine the etiology and to initiate nonpharmacologic and/or pharmacologic therapy. Occasionally, hypertension can pose an immediate risk of devastating organ damage or death. In these circumstances, prompt and effective treatment is required, often before a specific cause for the elevated BP has been determined.

Hypertensive crises can be *emergency* or *urgency* situations. A hypertensive emergency is defined as a life-threatening circumstance in which the elevated BP must be lowered within 1 hour. Hypertensive urgency is a situation in which elevated BP should be reduced within 24 to 48 hours to eliminate potential patient risk. A BP level that exceeds age-related normal limits (or previous systolic and/or diastolic BP measurements) by 30 per cent (Table 1) requires immediate attention and hospitalization.

Hypertensive encephalopathy is a clinical syndrome that describes the association between marked hypertension and the presence of an acute, generalized cerebral dysfunction. The neurologic findings include severe headache, irritability, diminished alertness, impaired intellectual function, blindness, generalized seizures, or coma. In this entity, the central nervous system abnormalities cannot be explained by other processes, such as cerebrovascular accident, uremia, infection, and poisoning, or improvement in the clinical condition follows antihypertensive therapy.

Numerous antihypertensive medications are available for the treatment of hypertensive emergencies (Table 2). In most

TABLE 1. Hypertensive Crises: Blood Pressure Values by Age

Age (Years)	Hypertensive Crises (mm Hg)
<2	145/95
3–5	150/95
6–9	160/100
10–12	165/105
13–15	175/110
16–18	185/120

TABLE 2. Medications for Treatment of Hypertensive Crisis

Drug	Route	Dose	Maximum	Frequency
Sodium nitroprusside	IV	0.5 μg/kg/minute; *Neonate:* 0.3 μg/kg/minute	8.0 μg/kg/minute 6.0 μg/kg/minute	Continuous
Diazoxide	IV	1–3 mg/kg	10 mg/kg/day (600 mg/day)	Rapid push over 1–2 minutes
Labetalol	IV	0.2–0.4 mg/kg (1–3 mg/kg/hr)	3–4 mg/kg/day (300 mg/day)	Bolus (continuous)
Nifedipine	p.o./SL	0.25–0.50 mg/kg; <10 yr—2.5 mg 11–20 yr—5 mg; >20 yr—10 mg	20 mg/dose	30–60 minutes
Minoxidil	p.o.	0.1–0.2 mg/kg	0.5 mg/kg/day (40 mg/day)	2–6 hr
Clonidine	p.o.	0.05–0.10 mg	2.4 mg/day	1–2 hr
Hydralazine	IV/IM	0.2 mg/kg	0.6 mg/kg/dose (20 mg/dose)	2–6 hr
Phentolamine	IV	0.1–0.2 mg/kg (2–10 mg)	10 mg/dose	5–15 minutes
Adjunct drugs for hypertensive crisis (Diuretics)				
Furosemide	IV	1–6 mg/kg		If no response, repeat in 1 hr at higher dose
Ethacrynic acid	IV	0.5–1.5 mg/kg		If no response, repeat in 1 hr at higher dose

Abbreviations: IV, intravenous; IM, intramuscular; p.o., oral; SL, sublingual.

cases, intravenous medications are required. For hypertensive emergencies, the target level for BP within 1 hour is about a 25 per cent reduction, or a diastolic BP below 100 mm Hg. In urgent situations, BP should be gradually reduced by about 25 per cent over a 24- to 48-hour period.

Medications

NITROPRUSSIDE. Sodium nitroprusside is an instantly acting vasodilator and can be used in any type of hypertensive emergency, including the newborn period. The route of administration is by continuous intravenous infusion with simultaneous measurements of intra-arterial blood pressure. The contents of the 50-mg vial is dissolved in 1 liter of dextrose in water (50 μg/ml). The initial dose is 0.5 to 0.8 μg/kg/minute and titrated to a maximum dose of 8 μg/kg/minute, depending on the desired BP response. The onset of action is within minutes. Because the drug is not stable when exposed to light, the entire infusion solution should be freshly prepared and tubing should be covered with opaque material. If the infusion is continued for over 48 hours, plasma thiocyanate levels should be monitored. Patients with renal dysfunction are at risk for cyanide poisoning. The major side effects include hypotension, nausea, and vomiting. Contraindications include aortic coarctation and arteriovenous shunts (compensatory hypertension states). Adverse interactions with other medications include other antihypertensive agents, sympathomimetic bronchodilators, insulin, tricyclic antidepressants, and other antihypertensive agents.

DIAZOXIDE. Diazoxide is a vasodilator with salt-retaining properties. The major indication is hypertensive encephalopathy, including the newborn period. The contents of the vial is 300 mg/20 ml (15 mg/ml). Despite previous dosage recommendations of 5 to 10 mg/kg up to 150 to 300 mg, the preferred method is a minibolus of 1 to 3 mg/kg (up to 50 to 75 mg) given as a rapid intravenous bolus injection. The onset of action is within 5 minutes, although the duration of action may last from 4 to 24 hours. The dose may be repeated every 15 to 20 minutes until the desired response is achieved. Because controlled BP reduction is not ensured, the minibolus technique provides more precise reduction in BP. The major side effects include acute hypotension, hyperglycemia, angina, nausea, and fluid retention. In all cases of hypertensive crises, furosemide may be used as adjunctive therapy to prevent or treat fluid overload. Diazoxide should not be used in patients with aortic coarctation, arteriovenous shunts, intracerebral hemorrhage, acute pulmonary edema, and heart failure. Interaction with other medication include oral anticoagulants and other antihypertensive medications.

LABETALOL. Labetalol possesses both α- and β-adrenoceptor blocking activity. The major indications include hypertensive encephalopathy, cerebral infarction, intracerebral hemorrhage, and acute renal insufficiency. The preparation is 5 mg/ml in 20- or 40-ml vials. Despite the limited pediatric experience, labetalol may be given at an initial dose of 0.2 mg/kg (maximum 20 mg) by slow intravenous push. The dose may be increased to 0.4 mg/kg (maximum 40 to 60 mg) every 10 minutes up to a total dose of 3 to 4 mg/kg or 300 mg. A continuous infusion may also be used given at a rate of 2 ml/minute (200 mg in 160 ml of 5 per cent dextrose in water [D_5W]). The maximum hypotensive effect occurs within 5 to 15 minutes after injection. The major side effects include nausea, vomiting, scalp tingling, and hypotension. Because of the beta-blocking effect, labetalol is contraindicated in patients with congestive heart failure, asthma, or bradycardia. Interaction with other medication includes sympathomimetic bronchodilators, insulin, tricyclic antidepressants, and other antihypertensive agents.

NIFEDIPINE. Nifedipine is a calcium channel blocking agent. Indications include hypertensive encephalopathy, acute renal insufficiency, or pulmonary edema complicated by hypertension. The preparation is 10- or 20-mg capsules. The drug is given orally in a dose of 0.25 to 0.5 mg/kg (maximum 20 mg) and may be repeated in 30 to 60 minutes. The capsules may be punctured with a tuberculin needle and intentionally swallowed with water. If desired, sublingual administration may be used by puncturing or biting the capsule, releasing the liquid in the buccal mucosa. However, the onset of action is faster with oral dosing than with the sublingual route. The peak effect with the oral route is approximately 30 minutes. Major side effects include tachycardia, flushing, headaches, fluid retention, dizziness, lightheadedness, and nausea. Nifedipine should be used with caution in congestive heart failure. Interactions with other medications include beta-blockers, oral anticoagulants, cardiac glycosides, and other antihypertensive medications.

CLONIDINE. Clonidine is a central acting $alpha_2$-agonist.

Indications include acute renal insufficiency or pulmonary edema caused by hypertension and postoperative hypertension. The initial dose is 0.05 to 0.1 mg per dose (maximum 2.4 mg) orally. Because the effect is usually within 30 to 60 minutes with a peak effect within 2 to 4 hours, the dose can be repeated every 1 to 2 hours until the desired hypotensive response. The major side effects include drowsiness, dry mouth, sedation, and xerostomia. The contraindications include AV heart block and bradycardia. Owing to the central nervous system depressant effects, it should be avoided when continuous assessments of mental function are required (e.g., hypertensive encephalopathy). Interactions with other medications include sedatives, cardiac glycosides, beta-blockers, barbiturates, and other antihypertensive agents.

MINOXIDIL. When intravenous access is not possible, minoxidil is a reasonable alternative. The agent is an effective vasodilator and is given only by mouth. The initial dose is 0.1 to 0.2 mg/kg per dose (maximum 0.5 mg/kg per dose or 40 mg/day). The maximum effect is seen within 2 to 4 hours with a duration of 12 to 24 hours. The major side effects include edema, fluid retention, and electrocardiographic (EKG) T-wave changes. Contraindications are in patients with pheochromocytoma and congestive heart failure.

HYDRALAZINE. Hydralazine is a vasodilator and may be given as an intravenous bolus or intramuscular injection. The initial dose is 0.2 mg/kg per dose with a maximum of 0.6 mg/kg per dose. It may be given every hour until effective, then every 2 to 6 hours. The hypotensive response is usually within 10 to 20 minutes with a peak effect in 30 to 90 minutes. One of the major limitations of the drug is headache. Other side effects include tachycardia, nausea, fluid retention, and palpitations. Contraindications include myocardial ischemia and pulmonary edema. Interactions with other medications include monoamine oxidase inhibitors and other antihypertensive drugs. Despite a long pediatric experience with this drug, the availability of the newer agents, such as labetalol and nifedipine, has limited its use in acute situations.

PHENTOLAMINE. This agent is a peripheral α_1- and α_2-adrenergic blocker used to control hypertension during surgery for pheochromocytoma. The dose is 2 to 10 mg intravenously and may be repeated every 5 to 15 minutes. The onset of action is within 2 minutes, with a duration of up to 10 minutes. The major side effects include hypotension, tachycardia, headache, nausea, vomiting, and arrhythmias.

Conclusion

In summary, a variety of agents are available for hypertensive crises. In cases of hypertensive emergencies unresponsive to one or two doses of an intravenous or oral preparation, arrangements should be made to prepare and administer a sodium nitroprusside infusion.

Chronic Hypertension

The suggested "stepped care" approach to antihypertensive drug treatment for chronic hypertension is shown in Figure 1. To improve compliance, it is essential to familiarize the patient and family with the side effects of the medication and to select a medication that can be given only once or twice daily. Under each step of antihypertensive drug therapy, the medications are listed in order of preferred selection. As discussed below, some agents may offer distinct advantages to certain patients, despite an apparent deviation from the stepped approach. An example is the use of a clonidine cutaneous patch to increase compliance in an adolescent.

The goal of antihypertensive drug therapy is to lower systolic and diastolic blood pressure below the 95th percentile for age. The following guidelines are for primary hypertension (Table 3).

Approach to Antihypertensive Therapy: Step 1

DIURETICS. The diuretic agents include hydrochlorothiazide, chlorothiazide, and furosemide. The indications for initial therapy with diuretic therapy are Step 1, hypertensive care, fluid overload, and low renin essential hypertension. The medication is given once or twice daily. The side effects

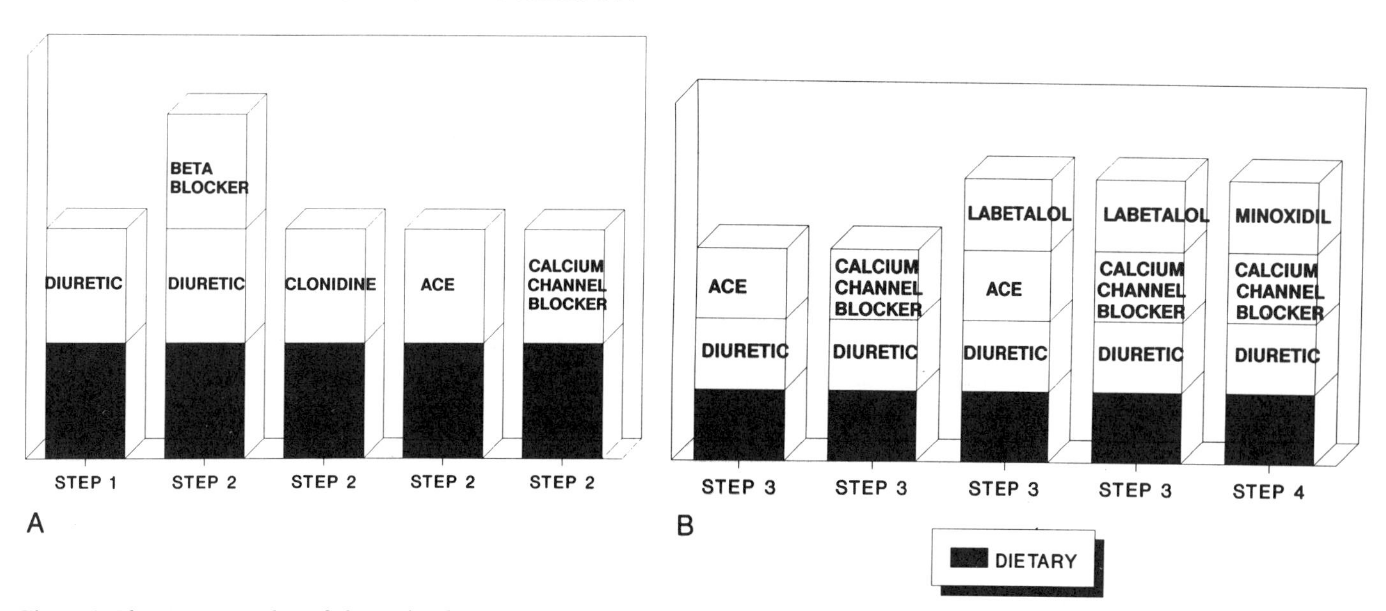

Figure 1. There are a number of alternative drug combinations in each step of antihypertensive management. Panel A and B include suggested approaches for Steps 2 and 3 antihypertensive drug therapy. The selection of a particular combination is based on the degree of blood pressure elevation, duration of disease, occurrence of end-organ damage, potential interference with other medications and lifestyle, and side effects limiting compliance.

TABLE 3. Medications for Treatment of Chronic Hypertension*

Drug	Initial Daily Dose	Maximum Daily Dose	Frequency	Available Formulations
Diuretics				
Hydrochlorothiazide	1.0 mg/kg (60 mg/m²)	100 mg	b.i.d.	50 mg/5 ml solution; 25, 50, 100 mg tablets
	3.0 mg/kg (<6 months of age)	37.5 mg	b.i.d.	
Chlorothiazide	20 mg/kg (600 mg/m²)	1000 mg	b.i.d.	250 mg/5 ml solution; 250, 500 mg tablets
	30 mg/kg (<6 months of age)	375 mg (up to 2 yrs)	b.i.d.	
Furosemide	1–2 mg/kg	320 mg or 4 mg/kg	b.i.d., q.d.	40 mg/5 ml, 10 mg/ml solution; 20, 40, 80 mg tablets
Potassium Sparing				
Spironolactone	1–3 mg/kg	6 mg/kg/24 hr	12–24 hr	25 mg
Triamterene	2–4 mg/kg	4 mg/kg/24 hr	12 hr	50, 100 mg
Metolazone	0.07–0.14 mg/kg	0.3 mg/kg/24 hr	24 hr	2.5, 5, 10 mg
β-Adrenergic Antagonists				
Nonselective				
Propranolol	1–2 mg/kg	8 mg/kg	b.i.d.	20 mg/5 ml solution; 10, 20, 40, 60, 80 mg tablets
Nadolol	40 mg†	640 mg	q.d.	20, 40, 80, 120 mg tablets
Selective				
Atenolol	50 mg†	100 mg	q.d.	25, 50, 100 mg tablets
Metoprolol	100–200 mg†	450 mg	q.d., b.i.d.	50, 100 mg tablets
Acebutolol	200–400 mg†	1200 mg	q.d.	200, 400 mg tablets
α-Adrenergic Antagonists				
Prazosin	1–2 mg	20 mg	b.i.d., t.i.d.	1, 2, 5 mg tablets
Complex Adrenergic Antagonists				
Labetalol	50–100 mg†	1200–2400 mg	b.i.d.	100, 200, 300 mg tablets
Central Sympatholytics				
α-Methyldopa	10 mg/kg (300 mg/m²)	65 mg/kg (2 g/m²)	b.i.d., t.i.d., q.i.d.	250 mg/5 ml solution; 125, 250, 500 mg tablets
Clonidine	0.05–0.1 mg tablet	2.4 mg by mouth	b.i.d., t.i.d.	0.1, 0.2, 0.3 mg tablets
	0.1 mg/day patch	0.6 mg by patch	q week	0.1, 0.2, 0.3 mg patches
Guanabenz	0.08–0.2 mg/kg (>12 yr)	64 mg	b.i.d.	4, 8 mg tablets
Direct Vasodilators				
Hydralazine	0.5–1.0 mg/kg (25 mg/m²)	4–8 mg/kg (200 mg)	t.i.d., q.i.d.	10, 25, 50 mg tablets
Minoxidil	0.1 mg/kg	1 mg/kg (50 mg)	b.i.d., q.d.	2.5, 10 mg tablets
Calcium Channel Blockers				
Nifedipine	0.25 mg/kg	1–2 mg/kg (180 mg)	t.i.d., q.i.d.	10, 20 mg capsules;
Extended Release		1–2 mg/kg (90 mg)	q.d.	30, 60, 90 mg tablets
Diltiazem	60–120 mg†	360 mg	b.i.d., q.d.	60, 90, 120 mg tablets
Verapamil	120–240 mg†	480 mg	b.i.d., q.d.	120, 240 mg tablets
Angiotensin-Converting Enzyme Inhibitors				
Captopril	0.05–0.1 mg/kg	4 mg/kg (200 mg)	b.i.d., t.i.d.	12.5, 25, 50, 100 mg tablets
Enalapril	1.25–2.5 mg†	40 mg	b.i.d., q.d.	2.5, 5, 10, 20 mg tablets
Lisinopril	2.5 mg†	20 mg	b.i.d., q.d.	5, 10, 20, 40 mg tablets

* Additional agents are available; however, not all are listed. The experience with the many new beta-blockers and converting enzyme inhibitors is limited in children.
† Pediatric dose is not established.

of thiazides include hypokalemia, weakness, hyponatremia, hypomagnesemia, hyperuricemia, hyperlipidemia, and glucose intolerance. Thiazide diuretics are ineffective if the glomerular filtration rate is less than 25 ml/minute × 1.73 m² (serum creatinine concentration > 1.5–2.0 mg/dl). Hydrochlorothiazide and chlorothiazide interact with corticosteroids, insulin, nonsteroidal anti-inflammatory agents, and cardiac glycosides and potentiate the hypotensive effect of other antihypertensive medications. The dose of chlorothiazide is fivefold to tenfold higher than the hydrochlorothiazide preparation. Both agents are available in a liquid preparation for infants.

Loop diuretics are used in patients with impaired renal function and in combination with other antihypertensive therapy. Studies have suggested that furosemide produces less hypokalemia compared with equivalent doses of hydrochlorothiazide. Most patients treated with furosemide have hypertension associated with renal insufficiency or cardiac disease. As with all diuretics, side effects include electrolyte disturbances, metabolic alkalosis, volume depletion, and hypotension. Furosemide also increases urinary calcium excretion resulting in nephrocalcinosis and bone demineralization. Interactions with other medications include nonsteroidal anti-inflammatory drugs, salicylates, aminoglycosides, cephalosporins, metolazone, digitalis, steroids, and ganglionic blocking agents.

Approach to Antihypertensive Therapy: Step 2

β-ADRENERGIC BLOCKERS. These drugs can be nonselective or selective. The selective agents have the theoretical clinical advantage of less β_2-receptor blockade and less side effects. The nonselective agents include propranolol, nadolol, timolol, and pindolol. Propranolol has enjoyed widespread use in pediatrics. The selective agents include atenolol, metoprolol, and acebutolol. The major effects of β-receptor blockade are the following: *β_1-receptor:* decreased heart rate, decreased conduction in the atria, AV node and ventricles, decreased renin secretion by the kidney, and decreased lipolysis; *β_2-receptor:* bronchoconstriction, arteriolar vasoconstriction, decreased gluconeogenesis, and decreased insulin secretion. Other side effects include fatigue, insomnia, hypertriglyceridemia, and masking symptoms of hypoglycemia. β-adrenergic blocking agents should not be prescribed in patients with congestive heart failure, reactive airway disease, heart block, or sick sinus syndrome. Most β-receptor blocking drugs include long-acting preparations to permit once-a-day dosing (Table 3). Drug interactions with these agents include insulin, catecholamine-depleting drugs, calcium channel blockers, cholestyramine, and cimetidine.

Approach to Antihypertensive Therapy: Step 3

COMPLEX ADRENERGIC ANTAGONISTS (LABETALOL). As discussed above, labetalol is a unique agent with α- and β-receptor blocking actions. It does not appear to affect exercise tolerance or alter blood lipid concentrations. Unfortunately, it only comes in 100-, 200-, and 300-mg tablets. Initial therapy in adults is 100 mg twice a day. In the young adolescent, a starting dose of 50 mg twice a day is appropriate. Indications for the use of labetalol include renal dysfunction, preoperative pheochromocytoma, acute withdrawal from beta-blocking drugs or central α-agonists (see below), and diabetic patients. The side effects include orthostatic hypotension, dizziness, fatigue, headache, nausea, dyspepsia, nasal stuffiness, giddiness, vomiting, and elevation of serum transaminases. Contraindications are similar to the β-receptor blocking agents.

α-ADRENERGIC AGONISTS. Clonidine, α-methyldopa, and guanabenz are agents in this category. Of these drugs, clonidine is the selection of choice. Clonidine is available in tablets and as a transdermal patch. As discussed above, the major side effects are drowsiness and nightmares. The initial dose is 0.05 to 0.10 mg given in two or three divided doses. In older children, the transdermal patch is very effective. The patch is available in 0.1-, 0.2-, and 0.3-mg strengths and is changed only once a week. The 0.1-mg patch is equivalent to 0.1 mg/day of the oral preparation. The advantages of the patch are the constant blood level within 2 to 3 days after applying the patch and improved compliance. In our experience, the patch is associated with fewer and milder side effects compared with the oral clonidine. If contact dermatitis develops, hydrocortisone is applied.

α-Methyldopa is still used at many centers. The dose is 5 to 10 mg/kg/day in two or three divided doses. With the large number of newer antihypertensive agents, our Center has selected other agents in situations where α-methyldopa was used in the past. The Coombs test is positive in up to 20 per cent of patients receiving chronic therapy. Other side effects are hemolysis and hepatic injury.

With all agents in this category, withdrawal can produce hypertensive crises and the drugs should be avoided in noncompliant individuals.

ANGIOTENSIN-CONVERTING ENZYME (ACE) INHIBITORS. The ACE inhibitors include captopril, enalapril, and lisinopril. Despite their inclusion as Step 3 therapeutic agents, many physicians use ACE inhibitors as first-line therapy (Step 1 or 2). Mechanisms of action of ACE inhibitors are to block the formation of angiotensin II and to prevent the degradation of vasodilatory prostaglandins and bradykinin. All three drugs reduce peripheral vascular resistance and are effective in low, normal, and high renin forms of hypertension.

Major side effects include skin rash, dysgeusia, dizziness, dry cough, headaches, neutropenia, hypotension, urticaria, and angioedema. With inhibition of renin-angiotensin-aldosterone axis, ACE inhibitors also cause natriuresis, diuresis, and elevation of the serum potassium concentration. In children with renal artery stenosis, particularly in bilateral disease, and with renal impairment, ACE inhibitors may cause renal failure. Any patient with renal impairment may have further compromise of renal function and increased proteinuria with this class of drugs.

Advantages of the ACE inhibitors include effective control of systemic blood pressure in children, lack of effect on blood lipids, and reduction in symptoms of congestive heart failure. There are major interactions with other antihypertensive agents (hypotension), nonsteroidal anti-inflammatory drugs, aspirin, and potassium-sparing agents. Based on the reported symptom of dry cough, ACE inhibitors should be cautiously used in patients with reactive airway disease. If the dosage of an ACE inhibitor has been maximized, addition of a thiazide diuretic may provide an additive effect to reduce blood pressure. As shown in Table 3, the recommended dosages for the three agents are quite different. If one of these drugs is added to an antihypertensive regimen, hypotension may occur. In cases of multiple drug therapy, some authors recommend starting ACE inhibitors at a very low dose, or reducing the dosages of the other antihypertensive medications by 30 to 50 per cent.

CALCIUM CHANNEL BLOCKING AGENTS. The agents in this group include nifedipine, diltiazem, and verapamil. The mechanism of action of all calcium channel blocking drugs is dilatation of peripheral arterioles. In comparison to many other antihypertensive agents, calcium channel blocking drugs have no effect on plasma lipid, glucose, potassium, or uric acid concentrations.

Nifedipine. Despite the apparent similarity of these agents, the clinical effect of nifedipine is different from that of verapamil and diltiazem. Nifedipine has two formulations: a capsule and a sustained-release tablet. The capsule has a peak effect in 30 to 60 minutes with a half-life of only 2 to 4 hours. As mentioned above, the capsule is bitten and swallowed in an acute emergency situation. Even though sublingual administration is widely used, the hypotensive effect is markedly improved when the capsule is bitten and swallowed with liquid. With the availability of a sustained-release tablet, the capsule is now reserved for acute rather than chronic therapy. The sustained-release formulation is the gastrointestinal therapeutic system (GITS). When the tablet is exposed to gastrointestinal fluid, it expands and releases a constant amount of nifedipine over a 24-hour period. This system permits once-a-day dosing. Because the tablet cannot be chewed and must be swallowed whole, it has limited use in a young pediatric patient. The tablet is available in 30-, 60-, and 90-mg strengths. Side effects include mild edema, slight increase in heart rate (not significant reflex tachycardia), dizziness, giddiness, lightheadedness, nausea, and myocardial infarction. All calcium channel blocking agents are contraindicated in patients with second-degree or third-degree heart block. Drug interactions include other antihypertensive agents, digoxin, cimetidine, and warfarin. There is an increased likelihood of congestive heart failure when used in combination with beta-blocking agents. Nifedipine may be used as monotherapy.

Verapamil and Diltiazem. These are both available in sustained-release preparations, although not the GITS formulation. The major side effect is constipation. Both drugs should be used with caution in patients with liver dysfunction, and are contraindicated in patients with AV conduction defects, Wolff-Parkinson-White syndrome, congestive heart failure, and sick sinus syndrome. There are no adverse effects on exercise tolerance (except in combination with a beta-blocking agent), or heart rate. Major drug interactions include beta-blocking agents, cyclosporine, digitalis, cimetidine, and other antihypertensive drugs. As with all sustained-release preparations of calcium channel blocking agents, the single dosing improves compliance and may be used in a wide spectrum of hypertensive patients.

OTHER VASODILATORS

Hydralazine. Hydralazine has been the mainstay in treating antihypertension in childhood for many years. However, the vast armamentarium of newer agents with fewer side effects has limited the use of hydralazine. The major side effects are reflex tachycardia, fluid retention, headaches, nausea, vomiting, palpitations, dizziness, postural hypotension, fatigue, and anxiety. This obligates combining a diuretic and beta-blocker with hydralazine resulting in triple-drug therapy. Contraindications include cerebrovascular disease, coronary artery disease, and mitral valve heart disorders. Hydralazine may also cause a systemic lupus erythematosus syndrome with positive serologic findings. Even though its use is limited, the variety of formulations (10, 25, and 50 mg) permits tablet scoring for use in infants and young children.

Minoxidil. Minoxidil is reserved for patients resistant (Step 4) to all other agents and combinations. It is extremely effective, but has a number of unpleasant side effects. Significant salt and water retention may develop and result in congestive heart failure, pericardial effusion, tachycardia, marked fall in blood pressure leading to cerebrovascular or cardiac ischemia, and hirsutism (on the forehead and other unusual areas). It must be used with extreme caution in patients who have recently been given other antihypertensive medications. Therapy should be started in a hospital setting to permit constant observation for a minimum of 24 hours. The dose should be 0.1 mg/kg given every 8 to 12 hours. The tablet may be scored to 1.25 mg for young children. In many cases, the initial dosage and frequency need to be reduced following a stable and sustained hypotensive response.

Refractory Hypertension

If combination therapy (Step 3) is ineffective in controlling systemic blood pressure, a re-evaluation of the patient is required. Four causes of refractory hypertension were included in the 1988 Report of the Joint National Committee on Detection, Evaluation, and Treatment of High Blood Pressure. They are:

1. *Noncompliance.* Failure to adhere to prescribed medical therapy is very difficult to resolve. Two approaches are 24-hour ambulatory monitoring and changing medications. If the expected decrease in blood pressure is not recorded following the "supposed" administration of a selected medication, in-center administration and monitoring may be necessary. In some situations, unpleasant side effects significantly reduce compliance and require a major change in the antihypertensive regimen.

2. *Secondary or associated conditions.* This category includes noncompliance with dietary instructions with continued or increasing obesity, renal parenchymal or renovascular disorders, or unrecognized secondary (endocrine, neurologic) causes of hypertension.

3. *Salt and water retention.* In this situation, the refractory hypertension may be related to inadequate diuretic therapy or side effects of vasodilator therapy (hydralazine), dietary noncompliance with sodium and fluid, or deterioration of renal function.

4. *Drug-related conditions.* Four areas require investigation to rule out a drug-related cause: (a) Are the prescribed doses too low? (b) Are inappropriate combinations being used (two agents in the same category—captopril and enalapril)? (c) Is there rapid inactivation of the medication (hydralazine, nifedipine)? and (d) What are the effects of other drugs (steroids, sympathomimetics, nasal decongestants, oral contraceptives, nonsteroidal anti-inflammatory drugs)?

SUMMARY

The approach to managing an infant or child with chronic hypertension is a team effort that includes the family, physician, and dietitian. A stepped approach is appropriate for the majority of children. However, the use of a long-acting preparation of an ACE inhibitor or a calcium channel blocker may increase compliance. Last, in most cases, therapy has to be individualized and close follow-up is required.

REFERENCES

Joint National Committee on Detection, Evaluation and Treatment of High Blood Pressure. (1988): Report. Arch Intern Med 148:1023, 1988.
Lauer RM, Clarke WR: Childhood risk factors for high adult blood pressure: The Muscatine Study. Pediatrics 84:633–641, 1989.
Portman RJ, Yetman RJ, West MS: Efficacy of 24-hour ambulatory blood pressure monitoring in children. J Pediatr 118:842–849, 1991.
Sinaiko AR, Gomez-Marin O, Prineas RJ: Prevalence of "significant" hypertension in junior high school–aged children: The Children and Adolescent Blood Pressure Program. J Pediatr 114:664–669, 1989.
Task Force on Blood Pressure Control in Children (1987): Report of the Second Task Force on Blood Pressure Control in Children. Pediatrics 79:1–25, 1987.

SYNCOPE AND HYPOTENSION

MICHELE MOSS, M.D.

Hypotension in the pediatric population most commonly accompanies shock but on rare occasion can occur with episodes of transient hemodynamic instability resulting in syncope. The threshold for a hypotensive blood pressure is determined by the age and activity of the patient. Syncope has a multitude of etiologic factors, not all of which are associated with hypotension. Syncope rarely occurs in the younger pediatric patient but is common in adolescents and older children.

HYPOTENSION

Hypotension is a serious sign in association with the severe hemodynamic instability of shock, but it can be an easily reversible and treatable symptom occurring with vasovagal or neurally mediated types of syncope (see text on syncope, p. 171). Shock can present without hypotension but always presents with evidence of decreased organ perfusion.

Shock is defined as an acute, life-threatening syndrome characterized by a deficient delivery of oxygen and other nutrients to the tissues. Delivery of oxygen to the tissues is defined as the product of cardiac output and content of oxygen in arterial blood. Cardiac output is determined by heart rate and stroke volume, which in turn is determined by preload, contractility, and afterload. Abnormalities of these determinants are the most common causes of shock.

Etiology and Diagnosis

Although there are multiple causes of shock, they can be of three types, defined by the major hemodynamic abnormality: hypovolemic, cardiogenic, and distributive (Table 1).

Defining which type of shock is present is easiest early in the course of the shock state; later, diagnosis becomes more difficult. As the shock becomes more severe, global lack of perfusion occurs with inability of the patient to compensate. Often, multiple hemodynamic abnormalities are present, and therefore the types of shock are harder to distinguish. The general diagnosis of shock itself is clinical, based mostly on physical examination with supporting evidence from laboratory evaluation. The specific type of shock is defined by the patient's history and distinctive physical and laboratory findings.

The physical examination of the patient in shock reveals evidence of decreased organ perfusion. Examination of perfusion to the extremities is the easiest to assess and is often the most revealing. Extremities are cool to the touch, with pale, cyanotic, or mottled color. Capillary refill of the toes or fingers is sluggish. The quality of the arterial pulsations in the radial, dorsalis pedis, and posterior tibial arteries is diminished, if not absent altogether. The assessment of the peripheral perfusion can be performed quickly and should be repeated frequently while the physician is managing a patient suspected of being in shock.

Perfusion to the kidneys is quickly evaluated by the quantity of urine output in patients with otherwise normal renal function. Central nervous system hypoperfusion produces a wide range of symptoms. Patients may be confused, irritable, or combative early in the course of shock but frequently progress to being comatose. Seizures can also occur owing to lack of cerebral perfusion. Infants may undergo subtle changes, such as inability to recognize or regard their parents. Decreased perfusion to the lungs results in cyanosis from ventilation-perfusion mismatching, even in the absence of pulmonary disease.

TABLE 1. Categories of Shock

I. *Hypovolemic*
   A. Hemorrhagic
   B. Nonhemorrhagic
      1. Extracorporeal loss
      2. Third-spacing

II. *Cardiogenic*
   A. Decreased contractility
   B. Arrhythmias
   C. Anatomic obstruction
   D. External obstruction

III. *Distributive*
   A. Anaphylaxis
   B. Sepsis
   C. Neurogenic
   D. Drugs

Hypovolemic Shock

Severe hypovolemia results in a lack of preload, and hence decreased cardiac filling, which in turn causes a fall in stroke volume and cardiac output. The hypovolemia may be due to hemorrhagic or nonhemorrhagic causes.

Hemorrhagic Hypovolemia. In the pediatric patient, trauma is the most common cause of hemorrhagic hypovolemia. In addition to the lack of cardiac output, hemorrhagic shock is associated with a lack of hemoglobin, which further impairs delivery of oxygen to the tissues. Usually, the diagnosis of trauma is obvious by history and physical examination; however, in cases of occult trauma such as child abuse, the history of trauma is unavailable or obscured. Careful examination for bruises, abrasions, burns, and other external signs of abuse must occur.

Nonhemorrhagic Hypovolemia. Nonhemorrhagic hypovolemia is most commonly caused by diarrhea in the pediatric patient, particularly in the small infant. The diarrhea results in a loss of noncellular intravascular volume. Other sources of fluid loss resulting in hypovolemia are other (nondiarrheal) gastrointestinal losses, urinary losses, excessive evaporative loss, and loss of fluid into the extravascular compartment ("third-spacing"). This leakage of fluid can occur with a variety of conditions, including burns, peritonitis, and pancreatitis. Third-spacing is also an integral part of distributive shock, especially sepsis (see below).

In addition to having the usual symptoms of shock, the patient with nonhemorrhagic shock will have evidence of dehydration on physical examination, including poor skin turgor with tenting of the skin, sunken fontanelle, sunken eyes, dry mouth, and lack of tears. Laboratory evaluation may reveal either hyponatremia or hypernatremia, elevated blood urea nitrogen (BUN), increased urinary specific gravity, and lactic acidosis.

Cardiogenic Shock

Cardiogenic shock is generally considered to be due to severe, acute dysfunction of the myocardium with poor contractility or "pump failure." Cardiogenic shock may also be due to extreme abnormalities of heart rate and to anatomic and external obstruction to cardiac output.

Decreased Contractility. Poor contractility can result from inflammation, as in viral myocarditis or rheumatic fever; from ischemia, as with birth asphyxia or abnormal coronary artery anatomy; or from toxins, such as gram-negative bacterial endotoxin. The history can help to distinguish the cause of the deterioration by suggesting recent viral or bacterial infection. Symptoms of angina, such as pallor, diaphoresis, and irritability, can be documented in infants with coronary artery abnormalities, particularly anomalous origin of the left coronary artery from the pulmonary artery. Physical examination reveals the usual symptoms and signs of shock; additionally, however, a displaced posterior myocardial infarction (PMI) or S_3 gallop will be noted on cardiac examination. The murmur of mitral regurgitation may be present. The chest x-ray (CXR) confirms the presence of cardiac enlargement, usually with pulmonary edema.

Arrhythmias. Tachyarrhythmias, most commonly supraventricular tachycardia in infants and children, can result in poor perfusion with shock. Severe bradyarrhythmias, such as complete heart block, can also present with hypotension and shock. Abnormalities of heart rate and rhythm are easily noted by physical examination and specifically diagnosed with an electrocardiogram (EKG).

Anatomic Obstruction. Obstruction to cardiac output is particularly common in the newborn infant with congenital heart disease. Infants with coarctation of the aorta, interruption of the aortic arch, hypoplastic left heart syndrome, and critical aortic stenosis frequently present in shock after closure of the ductus arteriosus owing to lack of systemic cardiac output. Differential quality of pulses and differential blood pressure are key physical findings in patients with coarctation or interruption of the aortic arch. The blood pressure is higher and the pulses are more easily palpable in the upper extremities than the lower extremities. All types of anatomic obstruction can be associated with severe metabolic acidosis. Respiratory distress and hepatomegaly are common. Cardiomegaly is present on CXR, frequently with increased pulmonary vascular markings and pulmonary edema. The specific anatomic diagnosis is made by echocardiogram.

External Obstruction. External compression of the heart due to cardiac tamponade or tension pneumothorax results in decreased cardiac filling and obstruction to cardiac output. In the pediatric patient, cardiac tamponade is usually due to pericardial fluid from viral, malignant, or autoimmune pericarditis; pus from bacterial pericarditis; or blood from chest trauma or cardiovascular surgery. Tension pneumothorax is usually due to chest trauma or severe pulmonary disease, especially in patients receiving positive pressure mechanical ventilation. Physical signs of tamponade and tension pneumothorax include pulsus paradoxus, distended jugular veins, and narrow pulse pressure with hypotension. Tension pneumothorax can also be noted by unilateral decreased breath sounds and deviation of the trachea away from that side. CXR confirms the diagnosis of tension pneumothorax but is helpful in cardiac tamponade only if cardiomegaly is present. The echocardiogram is helpful in diagnosing cardiac tamponade by confirming the presence of fluid, pus, or blood in the pericardial space.

Distributive Shock

Distributive shock is defined as defective distribution of cardiac output rather than as decreased cardiac output *per se*. The hallmark of distributive shock is massive vasodilation with pooling of blood in the venous system, often with capillary leak. When measured, cardiac output may be normal or even elevated. The major causes of distributive shock are anaphylaxis, septic shock, neurogenic shock, and certain drug ingestions.

Massive ingestions of medications, especially tricyclic antidepressives, barbiturates, antihypertensives, and phenothiazines, can result in the marked vasodilation of distributive shock. Trauma to the spinal cord above T-1 can also result in this type of shock. Other central nervous system injury can present with distributive shock, which may be difficult to differentiate from hemorrhagic shock in the trauma patient.

Anaphylaxis. Anaphylaxis is an IgE-mediated response to an antigen occurring in a previously sensitized patient. A wide variety of vasoactive mediators, including histamine and leukotrienes C_4 and D_4, are released, resulting in vasodilation with venous pooling and endothelial injury with leaking of intravascular fluid into the extravascular space. The history will reveal a sudden onset after exposure to an antigen, such as a drug or *Hymenoptera* sting. The symptoms include swelling, particularly of the lips and face, redness, airway obstruction with stridor or wheezing, and syncope due to profound hypotension. In contrast to patients with other types of shock, these patients have bounding pulses and warm extremities.

Sepsis. Septic shock is the most common cause of distributive shock and can occur at any age. Sepsis may occur in any pediatric patient but poses a greater risk to patients in the neonatal period, those with compromised immune systems either primarily or secondarily, and those with indwelling catheters and devices. Sepsis is most often due to bacterial infection but may be seen with infections from almost any organism, including viruses, rickettsiae, fungi, chlamydiae, or protozoa.

The clinical picture of septic shock frequently is biphasic. The *first phase* ("warm shock") is notable for marked vasodilation with bounding pulses and warm extremities with normal or increased cardiac output. However, patients also show evidence of poor organ perfusion with mild hypoxemia, mental status changes, and decreased urine output. Because of the apparent "good" perfusion to the extremities, warm shock is easily misdiagnosed. The *second phase* ("cold shock") features cool, pale extremities and poor arterial pulsations. Poor cardiac contractility with decreased cardiac output is usually present with cold shock. A patient with septic shock may progress from warm to cold shock but at the time of presentation may have either clinical picture. Patients with cold shock may be difficult to differentiate from those with other forms of shock. Infants may also present with subtle signs of sepsis, such as hypothermia, apnea, hypoglycemia, or hyperbilirubinemia, before progressing to shock.

Vasoactive mediators, thought to be responsible for the sepsis picture, are released as a result of the direct effects of the organism or from a toxin (e.g., endotoxin or exotoxin) produced by the infecting organism. The mediators most commonly implicated are tumor necrosis factor and interleukin-1 and interleukin-6, but more mediators and their role in sepsis are being described and investigated. Effects of these mediators include vasodilation and endothelial injury. In the septic patient, endothelial injury results in massive capillary leak, which significantly contributes to the inability to maintain blood pressure and organ perfusion during sepsis.

Evaluation and Monitoring of Shock

In all patients with shock, in addition to the history and physical examination, certain laboratory and radiographic evaluations are necessary to guide therapy. The arterial blood gas measurement allows direct assessment of the severity of arterial hypoxemia. The pH and P_{CO_2} will determine whether metabolic acidosis is present and, if so, how well the patient is compensating for the acidosis. Retention of carbon dioxide is an ominous finding because it indicates that the patient is unable to hyperventilate to maintain pH, suggesting that respiratory arrest may be imminent. Hematologic assessment should include a complete blood count, including platelet count. The level of hemoglobin is crucial not only in trauma patients but also in all patients with shock because of its importance in maintaining oxygen delivery. The white blood cell count may indicate that the cause of shock is infectious. The number of platelets can be decreased if disseminated intravascular coagulation is present. Accordingly, coagulation studies should also be performed, especially if there is difficulty controlling bleeding or if oozing occurs from minor trauma. Blood chemistries, including electrolytes, glucose, calcium, BUN, and creatinine, should be evaluated, since abnormalities are common. Because blood lactate reflects the extent of tissue hypoxia, observation of lactate levels during therapy helps to confirm clinical impressions of improvement or deterioration. Further laboratory assessments, such as blood and cerebrospinal fluid (CSF) cultures and liver function tests, may be needed, depending on the clinical scenario.

The chest radiograph is important in differentiating the types of shock. Evidence of pulmonary abnormalities, such as pulmonary edema, pneumonia or pneumothorax, should be sought. The presence of cardiomegaly indicates the likelihood of cardiogenic shock or septic shock with cardiac decompensation. Other radiographs and computed tomography (CT) may be indicated, especially in the trauma patient. The echocardiogram is imperative if structural cardiac abnormalities are suspected, but it is also useful in assessing left ventricular contractility.

Frequent assessment plus physical examination with close monitoring of vital signs of the patient is an integral part of therapy for shock. Each patient should be monitored with a continuous readout EKG (preferably with strip chart capabilities) in order to observe heart rate and arrhythmias. Blood pressure should be monitored closely. At initial presentation, an auscultory or Doppler determination of blood pressure should be performed. In the infant, the blood pressure should be measured in all four extremities. Oscillatory methods of blood pressure determination are useful because of the automated frequency of the reading; however, in the patient with poor perfusion or hypotension, these methods may not work.

As soon as possible, an intra-arterial catheter should be placed either percutaneously or by cutdown for continuous measurement of arterial blood pressure. The most common site of placement is the radial artery, but an arterial line may also be placed in the dorsalis pedis or posterior tibial artery. The femoral artery should be avoided because of risk to the perfusion to the leg, but it may be necessary to use it in patients with marked peripheral constriction. If the femoral artery is selected, a narrow-gauge catheter placed under sterile conditions is preferable.

In addition to monitoring blood pressure, the arterial catheter allows for frequent sampling of arterial blood for blood gas determination and other laboratory evaluations. Reassessment of pH and P_{CO_2} is necessary to monitor ventilation and acidosis. Oxygenation should be monitored closely not only because of the hypoxemia due to poor perfusion but also the risk of noncardiogenic (adult-type respiratory distress syndrome) or cardiogenic pulmonary edema. Pulse oximetry monitors oxygenation by continuously measuring the arterial per cent of oxyhemoglobin. Because good arterial pulsations are required to read the pulse oximeter, with poor perfusion the pulse oximeter may not be useful.

When perfusion does not return to normal with initial therapy (see next portion of text), measurement of the central venous pressure (CVP) may be indicated. The CVP reflects preload of the right ventricle, and when there is little pulmonary disease and a structurally normal heart, the CVP reflects left ventricular preload also. The CVP may be passed through the femoral, internal jugular, or subclavian vein. The tip of the catheter should be inside the thorax and above the diaphragm for accurate measurement of CVP. A thermodilution Swan-Ganz pulmonary artery catheter is necessary for direct measurement of cardiac output. Additionally, measurement of pulmonary arterial pressure and pulmonary capillary wedge pressure (PCWP) can be performed with the Swan-Ganz catheter. The PCWP reflects left ventricular preload more accurately than CVP, especially in patients with pulmonary disease and elevated pulmonary vascular resistance and in patients with severe, depressed left ventricular function. These catheters can be used in children, but skill in placement and experience in data interpretation are required.

A nasogastric tube should be placed and vented to prevent abdominal distention. Gastric secretions should be monitored every 4 to 8 hours for volume, pH, and presence of blood. A bladder catheter should be placed in any patient with hemodynamic instability. This enables close and accurate measurement of urine output. The urine should also be examined at least every 6 to 8 hours for specific gravity and presence of blood and glucose. Strict recording of all sources of fluid output as well as fluid input is necessary.

Therapy of Shock and Hypotension (Table 2)

Therapy centers around the maintenance of adequate oxygen delivery to the tissues. Therapy should be delivered aggressively and rapidly to prevent decompensation and irreversible organ and tissue damage. Frequent reassessment of the patient's response to therapy is imperative.

As in any unstable patient, attention to the airway with maintenance of oxygenation and ventilation is paramount. The patency of the airway should be ensured and increased concentrations of oxygen provided by mask. The amount of inspired oxygen delivered depends on the delivery system used but should be as high as possible until the arterial PO_2 can be measured. Endotracheal intubation should be performed if the patient appears to be tiring, experiences an altered level of consciousness, is profoundly hypotensive, or shows arterial blood gas values consistent with respiratory failure. Because pediatric patients in shock may deteriorate very rapidly to respiratory arrest, early endotracheal intubation should be performed.

After intubation, ventilation can be performed with either bag to tube ventilation or with mechanical ventilation. The patient should not be encouraged to do the work of breathing while still hemodynamically unstable. A significant amount of cardiac output may be diverted to the diaphragm and other muscles of respiration with spontaneous respirations. As much work as possible should be done by the ventilator. Often sedation and muscle paralysis are necessary but should be used with caution. Most sedatives can cause respiratory depression and can worsen hemodynamic instability or even cause hypotension in compensated patients. Muscle paralysis should be instituted only after a stable, adequate airway is in place.

The most commonly used intravenous sedatives are diazepam (0.04 to 0.2 mg/kg per dose every 2 to 4 hours); lorazepam (0.05 to 0.1 mg/kg per dose every 4 to 6 hours); morphine sulfate (0.05 to 0.1 mg/kg per dose every 1 to 4 hours); and midazolam (0.05 to 0.2 mg/kg per dose every 1 to 2 hours). Drugs used for muscle paralysis after the patient is placed on mechanical ventilation are pancuronium (0.1 mg/kg per dose) and vecuronium (0.1 mg/kg per dose). (Pancuronium has a longer half-life but frequently causes tachycardia and has been reported to lower blood pressure. Vecuronium has a shorter half-life but less hemodynamic effects, which often makes it preferable in patients in shock.)

Patients in shock need good intravascular access for infusion of large volumes of fluids and for infusion of medications, many of which are sclerosing. Initial placement of intravenous access may be difficult and time-consuming. Insertion of an intraosseous needle for infusion of fluid and medications may be necessary while intravenous access is being obtained.

A variety of needles have been used to obtain intraosseous access, including the Kormed-Jamshidi and Illinois bone marrow needles and 18- and 20-gauge spinal needles. Bone marrow needles designed specifically for intraosseous infusion are also available. The most common site of insertion is the proximal tibia on the flat anterior medial surface. The needle should be placed 1 to 3 cm distal to the tibial tuberosity and angled slightly away from the epiphysis. Other sites for placement include the distal tibia proximal to the midline of the medial malleolus and, in infants, the distal femur. When the needle is in place, bone marrow may be aspirated and fluids can be delivered without resistance. Essentially all medications and fluids that can be delivered intravenously may be given through an intraosseous route.

Because the intraosseous route is temporary, intravascular access should be obtained as soon as possible. Intravascular

TABLE 2. Medications for Hypotension and Shock

Infusion	Infusion Rate	Infusion	Infusion Rate
Inotropic Drugs		***Vasodilators***	
Dopamine		Nitroprusside	0.5–5.0 μg/kg/minute infusion
Dopaminergic	2.5–5.0 μg/kg/minute	Phentolamine	0.5–5.0 μg/kg/minute infusion
β-adrenergic	5–10 μg/kg/minute	Captopril	0.5–1.0 mg/kg/day divided every 8 hr enterically
β- and α-adrenergic	10–20 μg/kg/minute		
α-adrenergic	>20 μg/kg/minute	Hydralazine	0.1–0.5 mg/kg/dose every 4–6 hr IV
Dobutamine	2.5–20 μg/kg/minute		
Epinephrine	0.05–1.0 μg/kg/minute	Nitroglycerin	1–5 μg/kg/minute infusion
Norepinephrine	0.05–1.0 μg/kg/minute	***Maintenance of Ductus Arteriosus***	
Isoproterenol	0.05–1.0 μg/kg/minute		
Amrinone	Load: 7.5 mg/kg bolus Maintenance: 5–10 μg/kg/minute	Prostaglandin E_1	0.03–0.1 μg/kg/minute infusion

Drug	Dosage	Drug	Dosage
Volume Expanders		***Disseminated Intravascular Coagulopathy***	
Normal saline	20 ml/kg IV rapid push, repeat as needed; may use 5–10 ml/kg in cardiogenic shock	Fresh frozen plasma	10–20 ml/kg
Ringer's lactate		Cryoprecipitate	1 unit per 5 kg body weight to increase fibrinogen levels 75 mg/dl
Hetastarch			
5% Albumin			
Purified protein fraction (Plasmanate)		Heparin	Bolus: 50–100 units/kg, then Infusion: 10–25 units/kg/hr Use cautiously if active bleeding present
Acidosis Buffers			
$NaHCO_3$	1 mEq/kg IV (1 ml/kg of a 8.4% solution) *or* mEq $NaHCO_3$ = 0.3 × weight (kg) × base deficit	***Other Medications*** *Hypoglycemia* Glucose	0.25 g/kg IV bolus
THAM	mEq THAM = 0.25 × weight (kg) × base deficit	***Other Medications*** *Hyperglycemia* Regular insulin	0.1 unit/kg IV
Muscle Paralysis*			
Pancuronium	0.1 mg/kg/dose every 1 hr *or* as needed for movement	*Stress Ulcer Prevention* Ranitidine	1–2 mg/kg per 24 hr divided every 6–8 hr
Vecuronium	0.1 mg/kg/dose every 20–30 minutes *or* 0.1–0.3 mg/kg/hr infusion	Cimetidine	10–40 mg/kg/24 hr divided every 6–8 hr
Sedatives†		***Specific Therapy for Anaphylaxis***	
Benzodiazopines			
Diazepam	0.04–0.2 mg/kg/dose every 2–4 hr	Epinephrine	Bolus 5–20 μg/kg IV *or* Infusion 0.05–1.0 μg/kg/minute
Lorazepam	0.05–0.1 mg/kg/dose every 4–6 hr		
Midazolam	0.05–0.2 mg/kg/dose every 1–2 hr *or* 0.1–0.5 mg/kg/hr infusion	Diphenhydramine	1–2 mg/kg slow IV
		Dexamethasone	0.25–0.5 mg/kg IV
Narcotics		*or*	
Morphine sulfate	0.05–0.1 mg/kg/dose every 1–4 hr	Methylprednisolone	Load: 1–2 mg/kg Maintenance: 0.5 mg/kg/dose every 6 hr
Fentanyl	1–2 μg/kg/dose *or* as infusion 3 μg/kg/hr		

*Use only for intubation or after intubation is completed.
†Use cautiously in hemodynamically unstable patient, as all these drugs can worsen hypotension.

access may be obtained through percutaneous peripheral intravenous (IV) catheters, direct visualization of peripheral or central veins, or percutaneous IV catheter placement in the central venous circulation. Central venous access may be obtained through the femoral, internal jugular, or subclavian vein. Choice of location and method of insertion depend on the condition of the patient and the skill of the person performing the procedure. A minimum of two intravascular catheters are required to guarantee delivery of fluids and medications.

All patients in shock need optimal cardiac filling or preload. In patients with hypovolemic shock, increasing preload with intravascular volume expansion is often all that is needed for stabilization. Patients with septic shock and other forms of capillary leak may need massive infusions of fluid to maintain adequate preload because much intravascular fluid is lost in the extravascular tissues. Even patients with cardiogenic shock may need volume expansion because their preload demands are higher than normal because of the Frank-Starling mechanism.

Intravascular volume expansion can be provided using isotonic crystalloid solutions or colloid solutions. The isotonic crystalloid solutions are normal (0.9 per cent) saline and Ringer's lactate solution. The advantages of the crystalloid solutions are that they are readily available and inexpensive. Types of colloid solutions include 5 per cent albumin, Hetastarch, and fractionated protein solutions (Plasmanate). Blood products should be used aggressively in trauma patients. Blood should also be used to maintain hemoglobin concentrations at 13 to 15 g/dl in any form of shock.

The initial volume of fluid should be 20 ml/kg administered rapidly and repeated as necessary. Trauma patients may need continuous rapid blood replacement until bleeding is controlled. Septic patients and others with capillary leak syndrome may need vigorous, repeated boluses of fluid, often alternating crystalloid and colloid fluids. Patients with cardiogenic shock

TABLE 3. Inotropic Drugs

Drug	Dose	Effect	Adverse Effects
Dopamine	2.5–5.0 μg/kg/minute	Dopamine receptors; renal and mesenteric vasodilation	
	5.0–10 μg/kg/minute	β_1 increases heart rate	
	10–20 μg/kg/minute	β_2 and α	Tachycardia; arrhythmias
	>720 μg/kg/minute	α; vasoconstriction	
Dobutamine	2.5–20 μg/kg/minute	Predominantly β_1; increases contractility; mild heart rate; mild β_2 effects; vasodilation	Arrhythmias at higher doses
Epinephrine	0.05–1.0 μg/kg/minute	Predominantly β_1 and β_2; some α, especially at higher doses; higher doses may be needed	Arrhythmias; tachycardia; increases myocardial O_2 consumption
Isoproterenol	0.05–1.0 μg/kg/minute	β_1 and β_2; increases heart rate; is common bronchodilator as well as vasodilator	Arrhythmias; tachycardia; increases myocardial O_2 consumption
Norepinephrine	0.05–1.0 μg/kg/minute	Predominantly α; profound vasoconstriction; increases contractility	Decreases peripheral and renal perfusion
Amrinone	Load: 0.75 mg/kg/dose Maintenance: 5–10 μg/kg/minute Maximum: 15 mg/kg/day	Increases contractility; vasodilator	Thrombocytopenia; nausea

may be given small boluses of fluid, 5 to 10 ml/kg, if there is concern with pulmonary edema. Measurement of CVP may assist in guiding fluid therapy after initial resuscitative efforts. In the unstable patient, however, fluid resuscitation should not be delayed while one awaits placement of a central venous line.

Short-acting inotropic drugs are needed to support cardiac contractility, particularly in cardiogenic and septic shock. The most commonly used drugs—dopamine, dobutamine, and epinephrine—work by stimulating adrenergic receptors (Table 3).

Dopamine. Dopamine affects different receptors with different cardiovascular effects, depending on the dose. At low dose (2.5 to 5 μg/kg/minute), the predominant effect is that of renal and mesenteric vasodilation due to dopaminergic effects with mild positive inotropic effects. At moderate doses, 5 to 15 μg/kg/minute, the β_1-receptor is the predominant receptor affected; hence, positive inotropic effects are more apparent. Some increase in heart rate may also be seen. At higher doses, greater than 20 μg/kg/minute, predominantly α-receptor effects are seen with vasoconstriction, a direct increase in blood pressure being apparent. The dose of dopamine used depends on the severity of limitation of cardiac output. Usually, the drug is started at the lower dose range of 2.5 to 5.0 μg/kg/minute and increased until the desired improvement in perfusion is seen. The higher doses are used more commonly when there is significant hypotension despite aggressive fluid resuscitation. (See Table 4 for infusion formulations.)

Dobutamine. This drug works predominantly on the β_1-receptor located primarily in the heart resulting in positive inotropic effects and mild increases in heart rate. Mild peripheral vasodilation can be seen in some patients. A combination of dopamine and dobutamine at moderate doses is frequently used to improve contractility and maintain or improve renal blood flow.

Epinephrine. Epinephrine is added at doses of 0.05 to 1.0 μg/kg/minute when the response to these two drugs is not adequate. Epinephrine is the drug of choice in anaphylaxis. Because of its vasoconstrictive properties, epinephrine may be indicated primarily when there is severe hypotension secondary to sepsis or a drug ingestion.

Isoproterenol and Norepinephrine. Isoproterenol and norepinephrine also have some utilization in shock. Isoproterenol has β_1- and β_2-adrenergic properties and therefore improves contractility, increases heart rate and conduction through the atrioventricular (AV) node, and vasodilates peripheral vessels. Cardiac arrhythmias and marked sinus tachycardia occur commonly during isoproterenol administration, thereby reducing its usefulness. Norepinephrine, with mostly alpha adrenergic effects, is indicated when there is massive vasodilation and severe hypotension.

Amrinone. This is a phosphodiesterase inhibitor with positive inotropic and vasodilatory properties that has limited use in children. This drug is best used in cardiogenic shock when reduction of afterload as well as improved contractility is needed.

In addition to an emphasis on improving oxygen delivery, attention should be paid to minimizing oxygen utilization. Control of fever can decrease oxygen needs by as much as 30 per cent. Patients, especially infants, should be kept in a

TABLE 4. Formulation of Vasoactive Infusions

Drug	Action	Mixture Formula
Dopamine	Inotrope	6 × weight (kg) = mg in 100 ml of D_5W
Dobutamine	Inotrope	
Nitroprusside	Vasodilator	
Phentolamine	Vasodilator	1 ml/hr = 1 μg/kg/minute
Epinephrine	Inotrope	0.6 × weight (kg) = mg in 100 ml of D_5W
Norepinephrine	Inotrope	
Prostaglandin E_1	Ductus arteriosus dilator	1 ml/hr = 0.1 μg/kg/minute

Abbreviation: D_5W, 5 per cent dextrose in water.

neutral thermal environment to prevent excessive oxygen utilization to maintain core temperature. Shivering is particularly detrimental to patients with limited oxygen delivery because it can double tissue oxygen needs for the patient. As mentioned previously, sedation may be necessary to decrease agitation and work of breathing. Seizures should be controlled with anticonvulsants to decrease muscle work and, hence, the increased need for oxygen.

While working to improve oxygen delivery with volume expansion and inotropic support, the physician needs to treat problems secondary to decreased organ perfusion. Metabolic acidosis resulting from tissue anaerobic metabolism and production of lactic acid may need buffer therapy. Although the best treatment for lactic acidosis is improvement of tissue perfusion, sodium bicarbonate or tris(hydroxymethyl) aminomethane (THAM) may be needed. Sodium bicarbonate can be given either as a bolus of 1 mEq/kg IV (1 ml/kg of 8.4 per cent solution) or as a dose calculated to correct the base deficit noted on an arterial blood gas as follows:

$$\text{mEq NaHCO}_3 = 0.3 \times \text{weight (kg)} \times \text{base deficit}$$

Overdosage with sodium bicarbonate may produce hypernatremia, hyperosmolality, or metabolic alkalosis and therefore should be used with caution. Adequate ventilation must be present before sodium bicarbonate is used to prevent an increase in P_{CO_2}.

THAM can also be used to buffer metabolic acidosis as follows:

$$\text{mEq of THAM} = 0.25 \times \text{weight (kg)} \times \text{base deficit}$$

The advantages of THAM are it contains a lower amount of sodium and does not elevate CO_2 production. However, THAM can also cause hyperosmolality and metabolic alkalosis and usually requires a larger volume of fluid to correct a base deficit than $NaHCO_3$.

Disseminated intravascular coagulation (DIC) with widespread intravascular thrombosis and secondary fibrinolysis can be present in any patient in shock but is especially common in bacterial sepsis. Controversy exists as to the best means of treating DIC. Infusions of platelets and fresh frozen plasma may be needed to improve platelet and factor levels when bleeding is present despite concern that these infusions may promote further intravascular coagulation ("fuel the fire"). Treating low fibrinogen levels with infusions of cryoprecipitate (1 unit per 5 kg body weight to increase fibrinogen levels 75 mg/dl) have been used with limited success. Anticoagulation with heparin infusions to decrease intravascular clotting has also been advocated, especially in purpura fulminans; this therapy should be used with extreme caution in the presence of overt bleeding.

Glucose levels are frequently abnormal in pediatric shock patients. Infants may present with hypoglycemia because of limited glycogen stores and utilization. Hypoglycemia should be treated aggressively with 0.25 g/kg IV bolus (1 ml/kg of $D_{25}W$). Maintenance amounts of glucose should then be added to IV fluids. In other patients, stress hyperglycemia may be present and boluses of fluid for volume expansion in such individuals should never contain glucose. Hyperglycemia may result in a secondary glucose diuresis making volume resuscitation more difficult. Rarely, regular insulin (0.1 unit/kg IV) may be necessary to lower the serum glucose to decrease the diuresis.

Paralytic ileus and gastric paresis may occur during periods of decreased perfusion. Intermittent suction may be applied to the nasogastric tube if abdominal distention is excessive or impeding respiration but should be avoided to prevent injury and bleeding. Prevention of stress ulceration is recommended with the use of a histamine$_2$ blocker such as ranitidine (1 to 2 mg/kg every 24 hours divided every 6 to 8 hours) or cimetidine (10 to 40 mg/kg every 24 hours divided every 6 to 8 hours). Other antacids may also be used if needed.

Broad-spectrum antibiotics should be given to any patient suspected of having sepsis or any patient with shock of undetermined etiology. Antibiotics are chosen according to the age of the patient, presence of indwelling catheters, immune status, location of patient when sepsis developed (home or hospital), and other suspected sites of infection (e.g., urinary tract, central nervous system).

Patients with cardiogenic shock due to myocardial dysfunction may need adjustment of afterload to optimize contractility. In the presence of decreased contractility, increased afterload, usually due to peripheral vasoconstriction, will cause worsening of the cardiac output. After inotropic support has been initiated and blood pressure has stabilized, the use of vasodilating agents may be indicated. Prior to institution of these agents, it is imperative that the patient be adequately monitored, preferably with an arterial catheter and CVP or Swan-Ganz catheter. The agent used most commonly initially is nitroprusside (0.5 to 5.0 μg/kg/minute IV infusion) (Table 3). Nitroprusside is both an arteriolar and venous vasodilator with immediate onset of action and short half-life. Close attention to blood pressure is indicated because hypotension can occur quickly and at low doses in some patients. This can be reversed by either lowering the dose or giving fluids, depending on the CVP. Other vasodilators that have been used are captopril (0.5 to 1.0 mg/kg/day divided every 8 hours enterically), hydralazine (0.1 to 0.5 mg/kg per dose every 4 to 6 hours IV given as slow IV push no faster than 0.2 mg/kg/minute), and phentolamine (0.5 to 5 μg/kg/minute IV continuous infusion) (see Table 3).

In infants with anatomic obstruction to cardiac output opening the ductus arteriosus will be necessary to provide perfusion to the body below the site of obstruction. Prostaglandin E_1 (PGE_1) is infused in a dose of 0.03 to 0.1 μg/kg/minute to open the ductus (Table 3). PGE_1 can cause hypotension from vasodilation, which can be treated with volume expansion. Respiratory depression and apnea can also be a complication, especially at higher doses; thus, close monitoring of the airway and ventilation are necessary. The need for intubation and mechanical ventilation is not uncommon. PGE_1 may be used empirically in the infant younger than 2 weeks of age who presents in severe shock of undetermined etiology until an echocardiogram can definitively rule out obstructive congenital heart disease.

For external compression due to cardiac tamponade or tension pneumothorax, relief of the compression is the definitive therapy. A needle pericardiocentesis must be performed for cardiac tamponade. Surgical drainage or a pericardial window may then be needed to ensure that fluid does not reaccumulate. In the immediate postoperative cardiac surgical period, the sternum can be opened quickly at the bedside to relieve the pressure. Shock and cardiac arrest resulting from tamponade may not be manageable without drainage of the pericardium. Tension pneumothorax should initially be treated with needle thoracentesis, which can relieve "tension" and allow cardiac output to improve. A chest tube can then be inserted to protect from reaccumulation.

Anaphylaxis needs to be treated with epinephrine, as either a bolus (5 to 20 μg/kg IV, 0.1 ml/kg of 1:10,000 concentration) or an infusion (0.05 to 1.0 μg/kg/minute). Additionally, diphenhydramine (1 to 2 mg/kg IV over 5 minutes in a concentration of 10 to 50 mg/ml) should be given to antagonize the histamine release. Corticosteroids should also be administered (dexamethasone, 0.25 to 0.5 mg/kg given undiluted slow IV push, or methylprednisolone 1 to 2 mg/kg loading dose with 0.5 mg/kg per dose every 6 hours given IV slow push, maximum concentration of 125 mg/ml) if airway edema or bronchospasm is present.

SYNCOPE

Syncope can be a common and benign symptom in adolescent patients but may be life-threatening in certain patients. Even in patients with benign causes of syncope, the symptom may be very frightening to them or may significantly limit their lifestyle. The evaluation of syncope can be extensive and expensive; therefore, a careful history should be taken to guide the work-up. Most causes of syncope can be determined by history, physical examination, and an EKG.

Etiology and Diagnosis

Multiple causes of syncope exist, but they are usually cardiovascular or noncardiovascular (Table 5). Attempts should be made to try to distinguish the simple or "common faint" from other forms of syncope that are potentially more dangerous, such as primary cardiac syncope, arrhythmias, or seizures. Primary cardiac syncope includes severe acute obstruction to cardiac output, such as that seen with idiopathic hypertrophic subaortic stenosis or severe aortic stenosis. In patients with tetralogy of Fallot, syncope can also develop before surgical repair because of acute loss of pulmonary blood flow from increased subpulmonic and pulmonic stenosis.

Arrhythmias notoriously cause syncope—especially ventricular tachycardia and fibrillation, complete heart block or other severe bradycardias, and occasionally supraventricular rhythms. Patients with congenital heart disease, both before and after surgical intervention, can have arrhythmias; patients with structurally normal hearts may also experience arrhythmias. The presence of an accessory conduction pathway, as with Wolff-Parkinson-White syndrome, predisposes to supraventricular tachycardia (SVT). Although SVT uncommonly causes syncope, these patients may also develop atrial fibrillation and conduct rapidly down the accessory pathway, resulting in syncope. Some patients with SVT can become syncopal during the SVT, but some may lose consciousness if the SVT breaks into a slow sinus or AV block rhythm. Prolonged Q-T syndrome is a familial disease that predisposes the patient to ventricular fibrillation and disorganized ventricular tachycardia. These patients often have family members with a history of syncope or sudden death. The syndrome can be diagnosed by patient and family history in the presence of a prolonged corrected Q-T interval on EKG.

TABLE 5. Causes of Syncope

I. Cardiovascular
- A. Cardiac
  - 1. Primary cardiac
    - a. Obstruction to blood flow—obstructive hypertrophic cardiomyopathy
    - b. Aortic stenosis
    - c. Hypercyanotic episodes—tetralogy of Fallot
  - 2. Secondary cardiac—arrhythmias
    - a. Wolff-Parkinson-White syndrome
    - b. Prolonged Q-T syndrome with/without deafness
    - c. Arrhythmogenic right ventricular dysplasia with ventricular tachycardia
    - d. Congenital heart disease—operated and unoperated
  - 3. Drugs—cocaine, antiarrhythmics
- B. Vasovagal—the "common faint"
- C. Neurally mediated vascular
  - 1. Vagovagal syncope
  - 2. Orthostatic

II. Noncardiovascular
- A. Seizures
- B. Metabolic—hypoglycemia or hypoxia
- C. Hysteria
- D. Hyperventilation
- E. Vertigo
- F. Migraine
- G. Drugs—narcotics, barbiturates

The common faint (vasovagal syncope) frequently is associated with a prodrome lasting a few seconds to minutes. Pallor, lightheadedness, dizziness, diaphoresis, and nausea may be noted. The events surrounding the episode are often beneficial in diagnosing the common faint—standing in a hot church service or having blood drawn. Duration of the loss of consciousness is usually less than 1 minute, and occurrences are infrequent.

There are multiple noncardiovascular causes of syncope, including seizures and metabolic disturbances such as hypoglycemia. Hysteria and hyperventilation can result in presyncope or syncope. Drugs may cause syncope from cardiac reasons, cocaine with arrhythmias, or CNS effects, narcotics, or barbiturates.

Historical findings of concern would include the occurrence of syncope while the patient exercises or is supine. The presence of chest pain or palpitations may suggest cardiac syncope. Sudden loss of consciousness without a prodrome or aura is ominous. Frequent episodes or those lasting for more than 1 minute may not represent the simple faint. Symptoms and signs of seizure activity should be sought, including tonic posturing, loss of bowel or bladder control, prolonged loss of consciousness followed by sleepiness or confusion, and tendency for injury when falling. Vagovagal syncope is associated with strong vagal stimulation, such as passage of a nasogastric tube. Hysterical syncope rarely occurs without an audience and rarely results in injury.

The physical examination is often of little help unless the patient is unconscious. A complete cardiac and neurologic examination should be performed to rule out cardiac or neurologic causes. Blood pressure and heart rate should be determined with the patient both supine and standing to evaluate orthostatic changes. During the loss of consciousness, blood pressure, heart rate, and respiratory rate should be measured to detect hypotension, bradycardia, or both.

The laboratory evaluation should start with the EKG. Careful attention should be paid to the cardiac rhythm, presence or absence of chamber hypertrophy, and the measurement of intervals. The corrected Q-T interval should be calculated (Q-T divided by the square root of the R-R interval). The P-R interval should be measured to look for abnormalities of conduction. Blood chemistries that should be measured include glucose and calcium. The hemoglobin level should be measured to rule out occult blood loss and severe anemia.

Further testing will be indicated by the history and physical examination. A neurologic evaluation with an electroencephalogram (EEG) and a CNS imaging study may be performed. An exercise stress test to evaluate exercise-induced syncope can be performed in children usually older than 6 years old. A 24-hour ambulatory EKG may be needed if arrhythmias are suspected. Symptoms that occur infrequently may be evaluated with a transtelephonic EKG. Invasive evaluation with a cardiac catheterization and electrophysiologic study may be necessary in specific patients. The electrophysiologic study may uncover various tachycardias or abnormal sinus node function. Angiography can confirm coronary artery anatomy and can diagnose arrhythmogenic right ventricular dysplasia. The usefulness of these invasive tests in children and adolescents with syncope, however, is limited in contrast to that in adults.

Of some use in young patients with syncope, especially neurally mediated vascular syncope, is examination of the autonomic nervous system using the *tilt test.* The test is performed in various ways. However, the basic design starts with the patient lying supine and awake on a hydraulic table that is usually equipped with a footboard. Heart rate, blood pressure, and EKG activity are monitored frequently and, if possible, continuously. The patient is monitored supine, then elevated to 60 to 80 degrees. Vital signs are to be followed for up to 30 minutes after tilting or until syncope or presyncope develops. Infusions of isoproterenol have been used to promote symptoms.

The normal response to a tilt test is a transient decrease in blood pressure followed quickly by normotension. Heart rate should increase as the blood pressure recovers. Three abnormal responses have been described. The cardioinhibitory response is characterized by a marked decrease in heart rate at the onset of symptoms. Symptoms have also been noted in patients with a vasodepressor response—a significant fall in blood pressure associated with an increase in heart rate. The most common type of response in syncopal patients is a mixed response with both bradycardia and hypotension occurring.

Treatment

Therapy for syncope obviously depends on the cause. Pharmacologic treatment of arrhythmias and seizures is indicated. For patients with primary cardiac syncope due to structural heart disease, surgical palliation or repair is necessary. Syncope in patients with Wolff-Parkinson-White syndrome is an indication for surgical ligation or transcatheter ablation of the abnormal conduction pathway. Pacemaker insertion is indicated for patients with conduction blocks and bradyarrhythmias associated with syncope.

For neurally mediated vascular syncope and vasovagal syncope, the patient's disability caused by the syncope must be established. If a patient has rare episodes, further therapy is generally not warranted. For patients in whom episodes are frequent or that hinder their lifestyle, pharmacologic intervention may be indicated. Fludrocortisone acetate (Florinef) is used for patients with orthostatic hypotension and abnormal tilt test responses. A single daily dose of 0.1 mg is given orally to the adolescent patient. This drug causes fluid retention and maintenance of an increased intravascular volume. Hypertension can be an adverse effect of this medication. An increased salt diet can have a similar effect—the "potato chip and pickle diet." Drugs with negative inotropic effects such as β-receptor antagonists have also been used. Belladonna-type drugs with central anticholinergic effects have also been tried and have some success preventing bradycardia. The hemodynamic response to a tilt test does not clearly predict which medication will be of use preventing syncope.

PERIPHERAL VASCULAR DISEASE

WARREN G. GUNTHEROTH, M.D.
and D. EUGENE STRANDNESS, JR., M.D.

Clinically apparent blood flow obstruction occurs in both venous disorders and peripheral arterial disease. Particularly in children, arterial disease may be simply vasospastic. A thoughtful approach to both diagnosis and treatment is essential, since therapy may require simple clothing adjustment on one extreme to amputation on the other.

DISORDERS OF SMALL VESSELS (Frostbite)

If the extremity is still frozen or cold, moderately warm water (40° to 42°C) should be used promptly for fairly rapid rewarming. However, rewarming should not be attempted unless all danger of refreezing is eliminated. Thus, if the physician is being consulted by radio or telephone and the patient is remote from hospitalization, rewarming should be undertaken with great caution. The time for rewarming will depend on the depth to which the tissue is frozen; rewarming of deeper layers may require more than an hour if there has been through-and-through freezing.

After rewarming, subsequent care requires fastidious hygiene of the frostbitten extremity for a lengthy period of time. Surprising recovery is characteristic of frostbite injuries, so extirpation or amputation should be delayed. Daily care should include gentle cleansing, avoidance of pressure or even light contact, bed rest, and analgesics until the acute inflammation has subsided. Once the acute stage has resolved, physical therapy to restore full range of motion is essential. Whirlpool baths are an important adjunct.

DISORDERS OF PERIPHERAL ARTERIES

Vasoactive Disorders

Raynaud's Disease

Raynaud's phenomenon is a vasospastic disorder in which fingers and toes manifest a characteristic sequence of pallor, cyanosis, and rubor. The criteria for diagnosis of Raynaud's disease include provocation by cold or emotion, bilaterality, absence of gangrene, and absence of an underlying, primary disorder. If there is an underlying disorder, Raynaud's phenomenon is the appropriate term. The phenomenon may be secondary to certain serious associated problems, including one of the collagen diseases such as scleroderma, systemic lupus erythematosus, or mixed connective tissue disease. Raynaud's phenomenon may also be seen in hypothyroidism, in vasculitis, in hepatitis B antigenemia, and with a variety of obstructive arterial diseases. It can be related to the use of certain medications, including beta-blockers, cyclosporine, amphetamines, imipramine, vinblastine, and bleomycin. However, exhaustive work-ups are not routinely indicated in a child with good health and mild vasospastic complaints. Although primary Raynaud's is a benign disorder, the secondary form may lead to digital artery occlusion, fingertip ulcers, or even gangrene. Occlusion can be detected by measurement of the systolic pressures in the involved finger(s) using plethysmography or Doppler ultrasound. Finger pressures of less than 70 mm Hg, wrist-to-digit gradients greater than 30 mm Hg, and brachial artery-to-finger differences of greater than 40 mm Hg are consistent with occlusive disease in the hand or digits.

Therapy. The therapy of Raynaud's disease should be dictated by its generally favorable prognosis. Environmental changes may be all that is required. Thus, selection of a warm, dry climate may be helpful. Clothing that conserves body heat rather than just covering the extremities may lessen symptoms. Clothing should be both loose-fitting and yet wind-blocking (hard finished and tightly woven). Stocking caps may be quite helpful in lessening finger vasoconstriction. In addition, increased physical exercise may be helpful, especially in adolescent girls. Biofeedback may be successful to some degree in increasing digital temperature or aborting or lessening the severity of episodes.

Medication may be indicated in more severe cases. Presently, the calcium channel blocker nifedipine is the drug of choice, although there is not a specific approval for this indication by the Food and Drug Administration, despite mention of the agent's use for blocking contractile response of smooth muscle. While there has not been extensive pediatric use of nifedipine, the pediatric dose, based on an adult dose of 10 mg three times daily, is 0.2 mg/kg three times daily. Side effects, largely vasodilatation leading to lightheadedness, flushing, and headache, are usually tolerable. Subjective improvement occurs in 50 to 70 per cent of patients, though flow changes in the affected digits do not appear to occur. The new long-acting preparation of nifedipine has also been useful in Raynaud's disease. The alpha$_1$-blocker/vasodilator prazosin may also be effective, in an adult dose of 1 to 3 mg three times a day, or a pediatric dose of 0.01 to 0.05 mg/kg/day. Other agents, including the α-adrenoceptor blocker phenoxybenzamine (0.2 mg/kg twice daily), guanethidine (0.2 mg/kg daily) and reserpine (0.125 mg daily in an adult; 0.002 mg/kg in a child) have also been used. Recently, alternative drug therapy with the 5-HT2-receptor antagonist ketanserin (adult dose, 40 mg three times a day) has looked promising, although this agent is not yet available in the United States. Considering the side effects of many of these medications and the lack of improvement of actual digital blood flow, management without long-term drugs should be attempted.

Since studies of the mechanism of cold-induced Raynaud's phenomenon implicate α_2-adrenoceptors, specific blockers for this receptor may bring more effective therapy.

Chilblains (Pernio)

Chilblains involves itching, localized erythema, and sometimes blisters over the dorsum of the hand and proximal phalanges of fingers and toes and also over the heels and lower legs in response to cold. This is said to be a disorder of children in cool, damp climates. More of a nuisance than threat to life or limb, this disorder is treated acutely with antipruritics and soothing ointments in a lanolin-petrolatum base. Severe or persistent cases should be treated as outlined under Raynaud's phenomenon.

Acrocyanosis

This finding is more common than Raynaud's disease, but the overlap of acrocyanosis with the normal response to cold is greater. In acrocyanosis there is a more generalized response of the entire extremity in a glove or stocking pattern. There is generally only unremitting cyanosis, without the pallor and rubor phases seen in Raynaud's disease. Ulcerations are rare, and therapy is rarely needed unless for cosmetic reasons. When required, therapy is the same as for Raynaud's disease. Fortunately, this disorder is not secondary to collagen disorders, only primary.

Livedo Reticularis

Livedo reticularis and cutis marmorata are even milder peripheral vascular responses to cold, with net-like patterns of cyanosis in arms and legs. Therapy is generally not required.

Erythromelalgia

Erythromelalgia, which is rarer than Raynaud's disease, presents as a peripheral hyperreaction to heat, a counterpart to the reaction to cold seen in Raynaud's. Its symptoms may be debilitating, with distressingly hot, swollen, and tender hands and feet. Therapy should be directed toward both physical factors and medication. Cooling of the body in general as well as cool soaks to the affected extremities bring some degree of relief. Ephedrine may be effective in some instances (0.5 mg/kg every 4 to 6 hours, preferably with a tranquilizer or sedative). Aspirin should be used on a regular basis, not only for its analgesic effects but also because it appears that endogenous bradykinin may be involved in the pathogenesis of this disorder.

It has also been suggested that erythromelalgia is a type of "peripheral migraine" associated with serotonin release. Accordingly, antiserotonin agents, such as cyproheptadine (0.08 mg/kg per dose three times daily) has been suggested. In resistant cases, propranolol (1 to 2 mg/kg twice daily) has been tried.

Causalgia

Although a deep wound with injury to a nerve trunk leading to "major causalgia" is easily diagnosed, forms of minor causalgia may be hard to diagnose because they masquerade as primary vascular disorders. Thus, unilateral vascular disorders, particularly if associated with exquisite tenderness, swelling, and abnormal perspiration, should suggest post-traumatic sympathetic dystrophy, a form of minor causalgia. The vascular disorder is most often vasospastic but may occasionally resemble unilateral erythromelalgia.

Therapy. Therapy is the same regardless of the vascular disorder: paravertebral sympathetic blockade with injection of 1 per cent lidocaine. If the diagnosis is correct, subjective relief is striking and will last for several hours. Permanent improvement depends on vigorous physical therapy, starting at once under the effect of the block and continuing for days or weeks. This usually requires additional injections to permit relatively painless exercise of the limb in order to interrupt the cycle of pain and disuse. Sympathectomy is rarely indicated.

Obstructive Disorders

Trauma

The immediate goal of therapy for traumatic interruption of arterial flow is to prevent loss of tissue and limb. Continuity of the arteries must be restored, spasm relieved, intraluminal clots removed and prevented, and tissue edema managed so that the arterial lumen is not compromised.

Maintenance or restoration of adequate circulating blood volume is of primary importance, not only for the preservation of life but also for the intelligent assessment of the local circulation. Although actual gangrene is rare in children, a nonoperative approach to vascular injury prolonged beyond 6 to 8 hours may lead to subsequent limb weakness and atrophy. Thus, the ultimate function of the limb should govern acute management. Early intervention by a skilled surgeon may be truly conservative. Although arteriography may be helpful in locating the site and extent of obstruction, use of transcutaneous Doppler flowmeter is less traumatic and easily repeated at will.

Proper surgical technique includes scrupulous débridement; end-to-end anastomosis if adequate vessel length is available (avoiding tension), and autogenous vein graft replacement otherwise. Complete removal of distal clots is essential, as is relief of arterial spasm, fasciotomy to control the complications of associated edema and hematoma, and possible anticoagulation with heparin (see under thrombophlebitis).

Medical cannulation has become an increasingly frequent cause of arterial problems. Poor technique, or overly long cannulation, may lead to embolic problems as well as to frank occlusion. Left heart diagnostic studies via retrograde catheterization can produce subsequent leg shortening if the artery clots after the procedure. Instillation of heparin (100 units/kg) in the arterial catheter may be helpful. These patients should be observed closely for arterial pulses and long-term for leg growth.

Congenital Stenosis

Peripheral arterial stenosis rarely produces any definite signs or symptoms if congenital. Collateral circulation usually develops and prevents problems.

Arteritis

Inflammatory disease of arteries may occur either locally or as part of a widespread disorder, as in polyarteritis (See Section 11). When smaller arteries are involved, a muscle biopsy is the only means of sure diagnosis.

The most effective treatment is identification and removal of sensitizing drugs, infections or toxins, with steroids being used in severe, generalized arteritis. Major vessel arteritis obstructing blood flow can require bypass grafting, depending on the site and adequacy of collateral circulation.

Fistulas

Traumatic Fistulas

The most frequent cause of a traumatic peripheral vascular fistula in pediatric patients is likely related to needle puncture of the femoral vein by physicians. The treatment is obviously surgical, and care must be taken to be sure that closure of the fistulous connection does not compromise the arterial lumen.

Congenital Fistulas

Abnormal communications between small arteries and veins, especially if extensive, may be difficult to treat. As a result of the extensive and diffuse nature of congenital fistulas, surgical removal is rarely possible. Because edema and incompetence of superficial veins often develop, support stockings to prevent stasis changes are necessary.

DISORDERS OF PERIPHERAL VEINS (Thrombophlebitis)

Thrombophlebitis is rarely a pediatric problem, but its occurrence is attended by considerable risk to life if treatment is not prompt and effective. The aggressiveness and extent of therapy should be dictated by the extent of the thrombophlebitis. If it is progressing despite medical therapy or if pulmonary embolism has occurred, a more aggressive approach is mandatory. Search for coagulation markers, such as increased plasminogen activator inhibitor (PAI), and deficiencies of antithrombin II, protein C, or protein S should be considered.

Massive deep thrombophlebitis (phlegmasia cerulea dolens) involves the entire limb with edema as well as severe pain and cyanosis. The presence and quality of the pedal pulses depend on the systemic blood volume and pressure and on the degree of edema. In some cases, associated arterial spasm can also reduce arterial flow. In general, thrombectomy should not be attempted unless there is a strong question of limb viability. Venous ligation or plication is performed just below the renal vein but is indicated only in those patients with pulmonary embolism, which recurs while they are receiving adequate anticoagulant therapy. Similarly, the placement of an inferior vena caval filter (not removable during the life of the patient) should be considered only when all other options have failed. The use of fibrinolytic agents, such as streptokinase, urokinase, or recombinant human tissue-type plasminogen activator (rtPA), to promote clot lysis and resorption has been found useful in adults with massive deep vein thrombosis, but pediatric experience is extremely limited. Problems with bleeding may be substantial, and pediatric data are inadequate for clear recommendation of fibrinolytic therapy.

Venous thrombosis of the major deep veins is treated with bed rest, elevation, heat, and intravenous heparin. It is presently recommended that heparin be given by continous intravenous infusion to maintain either the whole blood clotting time at 2 to 2.5 times baseline values or the activated partial thromboplastin time at 50 to 80 seconds. A constant speed infusion pump is essential in order to avoid fluctuations in the rate of administration.

An oral anticoagulant, such as warfarin (Coumadin), is started when the status of the limb is satisfactory. The prothrombin time should be maintained at 1.2 to 1.5 times the normal control. Although there is no consensus about duration of therapy, it should be continued for at least 3 months when a major venous thrombosis has occurred. With pulmonary embolus, therapy should be continued for 3 to 6 months or even longer if the patient remains at risk.

If there is any edema in the affected limb with ambulation, it must be controlled, preferably with tailored, pressure gradient stockings from the level of the foot to the upper thigh.

REFERENCES

Coffman JD: Raynaud's phenomenon. New York, Oxford University Press, 1989.

Guntheroth WG, Morgan BC, Harbinson JA, Mullins GL: Raynaud's disease in children. Circulation 36:724–729, 1967.

Heijboer H, Brandjes DPM, Buller HR, et al: Deficiencies of coagulation-inhibiting and fibrinolytic proteins in outpatients with deep-vein thrombosis. N Engl J Med 323:1512–1516, 1990.

ACUTE RHEUMATIC FEVER

DAVID BAUM, M.D.

When a diagnosis of acute rheumatic fever is made, a patient should be hospitalized. With 2 or 3 days of evaluation, carditis and other manifestations of the disease can be assessed and therapy begun.

GROUP A STREPTOCOCCAL INFECTION

Because acute rheumatic fever is believed to be a poststreptococcal disorder, eradication of the organism should be accomplished as soon as the diagnosis is made. Treatment is recommended regardless of whether culture specimens of group A streptococci are obtained from the throat. The treatment of choice is intramuscular penicillin G (1,200,000 units for individuals weighing more than 60 pounds and 600,000 units for smaller children). Oral penicillin V (800,000 to 1,000,000 units/day in three or four divided doses), administered daily for 10 days, is an acceptable alternative. For individuals allergic to penicillin, a 10-day course of oral erythromycin (40 mg/kg/day divided into three or four doses) is recommended.

CARDITIS

Cardiac involvement in acute rheumatic fever is of utmost importance. If sufficiently severe, carditis may result in congestive heart failure and even death. If there is resulting extensive endomyocardial damage with mitral and aortic valvular deformity, the patient usually is disabled and life expectancy is shortened. Because carditis has become a more dominant feature of acute rheumatic fever in recent years, it is now a matter requiring even greater attention.

Patients with carditis should remain in the hospital, where their clinical course can be monitored closely and where laboratory support, such as chest radiography, electrocardiography, and echocardiography, is available. Echocardiography is particularly helpful in management because it allows sequential evaluations of myocardial function as well as assessment of mitral and aortic valve competence. In addition, echocardiography is an invaluable technique for differentiation of pericardial effusion from cardiomegaly and for monitoring their respective courses.

Management begins with bed rest. Restriction of activity is advised until carditis has subsided. Ambulation should always be gradual after an episode of carditis. The rate at which activity is increased must depend on the severity of the attack and the response of the patient.

Anti-inflammatory agents are useful in the treatment of carditis during attacks of rheumatic fever. Salicylates and corticosteroids are the drugs in current use. Although both are effective, steroids act more quickly and are more potent. Although steroids often bring carditis under control more quickly, there is no conclusive evidence of their superiority over salicylates in modifying residual cardiac abnormalities. Furthermore, because steroid side effects can be more troublesome, they are reserved for patients with more pronounced cardiac involvement.

With myocarditis and little or no cardiomegaly, treatment with salicylates is ordinarily sufficient. Aspirin, not sodium salicylate, should be used. The usual aspirin dose is between 70 and 100 mg/kg/day divided into four doses. Dosage adjustment should be made to maintain blood salicylate levels between 15 and 30 mg/dl. High doses of aspirin are continued until evidence of carditis has subsided and the sedimentation rate approaches normal. Then medication is withdrawn gradually over a 4- to 6-week period.

Steroid therapy is preferred in patients with carditis who become symptomatic or have moderate to marked cardiomegaly. In such patients, prednisone (1 to 2 mg/kg/day, divided into two or three doses) is administered. Antacids should be administered in conjunction with prednisone administration. Careful blood pressure monitoring is required, especially with development of aortic and mitral insufficiency, because hypertension may worsen the valvular incompetence. Steroids at these high doses are maintained until signs of cardiac inflammation have subsided and the sedimentation rate has returned to normal. Then, steroids should be tapered gradually over a 4- to 6-week period.

Individuals with carditis and congestive heart failure must be treated with steroids. Prednisone is used in the dosage regimen already described. Added measures are required because of the presence of heart failure. Diuretics, oxygen, and sodium restriction often are necessary. If digitalis is used, it should be given with extreme caution because the inflamed heart seems more sensitive to the drug. As in the case of patients who have other forms of myocarditis, afterload reduction with pharmacologic agents such as captopril is often helpful. The use of afterload reduction should prove particularly helpful when mitral and aortic valvular incompetence is present.

Rebound of the acute disease is not uncommon and frequently is observed a few weeks after drug therapy is stopped. Ordinarily, rebound is self-limited and subsides with a 3- to 4-week course of aspirin (60 to 75 mg/kg/day). To reduce the possibility of rebound in patients treated with steroids, aspirin in this medium dosage is given as prednisone is tapered. In such cases, the aspirin is continued for 2 to 4 weeks after the steroids have been stopped.

ARTHRITIS

Migratory polyarthritis involving the large joints of the body is the most common manifestation of acute rheumatic fever. Rheumatic joint inflammation in patients at bed rest ordinarily is responsive to salicylates in the dosage of 75 to 100/mg/kg/day. Overall improvement and a fall in sedimentation rate usually takes place with 1 to 2 weeks of treatment. It is then possible to reduce the salicylate dosage and begin ambulation. Provided that the child remains asymptomatic, salicylates can be withdrawn slowly in 1 to 2 weeks, while the child is carefully watched for a recurrence of symptoms. As soon as symptoms have gone, the patient may be discharged on no medications. If the individual remains asymptomatic over the next 6 weeks, a return to full activity follows. Careful observation for evidence of carditis is advised because cardiac involvement is frequently associated with rheumatic arthritis. If the patient has carditis, salicylate therapy must be guided by the cardiac abnormality.

CHOREA

Chorea is a late manifestation of rheumatic fever, appearing 3 to 6 months after known episodes of group A streptococcal infections. Symptoms may last from 2 to 6 months and frequently become a source of considerable emotional distress for the patient and the family. Unfortunately, no specific treatment is available. Efforts should be made to reduce physical and mental stress. It is particularly important to provide adequate protective measures to prevent injury when the uncontrolled choreiform movements become violent. One must remember to look for carditis when chorea is present, despite the long interval after streptococcal infection.

ERYTHEMA MARGINATUM

This uncommon manifestation of acute rheumatic fever is said to occur only when carditis is present. It is a nonpruritic rash for which no therapy is required.

SUBCUTANEOUS NODULES

These small, firm movable masses are found over extensor surfaces of the elbow, wrist, and knees but also may be suboccipital and along the spine. They are neither tender nor painful, and no treatment is necessary.

PROPHYLAXIS

Prevention of streptococcal infections is essential in persons who have had rheumatic fever because the disease has a tendency to recur. Many patients who have had an episode of rheumatic fever experience a second attack following untreated group A streptococcal pharyngitis. The most effective method of preventing streptococcal infections and subsequent rheumatic fever is by administering intramuscular benzathine penicillin G (1,200,000 units once per month). Oral penicillin V (200,000 to 400,000 units twice a day) is a less satisfactory alternative. For those individuals allergic to penicillin, oral sulfadiazine (1 g daily for those weighing more than 60 pounds and 0.5 g daily for smaller individuals) is recommended.

Prophylaxis should be continued until the fifth or sixth decade of life, especially if the patient's acute episode of rheumatic fever was associated with carditis and the individual has residual rheumatic heart disease. Adults with frequent exposure to children of school age or persons known to have frequent streptococcal infections should receive prophylaxis regardless of age.

INFECTIVE ENDOCARDITIS

Individuals with rheumatic heart disease are recommended for antibiotic prophylaxis for dental procedures, surgery of the upper respiratory tract, and gastrointestinal and genitourinary tract surgery and instrumentation. This antibiotic protection should be provided in addition to the prophylactic regimen used to prevent recurrence of streptococcal infections and acute rheumatic fever. Guidelines for antibiotic prophylaxis for infective endocarditis are periodically published by the American Heart Association.

MARFAN SYNDROME

RONALD V. LACRO, M.D.

Marfan syndrome is an autosomal dominant disorder of connective tissue affecting one in 10,000 individuals. The most important life-threatening complications include aneurysm of the aorta and aortic dissection. Recent genetic studies have identified abnormalities in the gene encoding for the connective tissue protein fibrillin. Mutations in the fibrillin gene exert a pleiotropic effect, producing multiple, seemingly unrelated phenotypic features that stem from a single genetic change. These features exhibit age dependency and extensive variability, not only between families but also within families. Although the gene responsible for Marfan syndrome has been identified, there currently is no readily available laboratory test to confirm or rule out this diagnosis. Rather, the diagnosis is made *clinically*, based on characteristic abnormalities of the musculoskeletal, ocular, and cardiovascular systems and a positive family history for the syndrome (Table 1). Early diagnosis is essential for optimal management, which focuses on recognizing abnormalities and altering the natural history of each clinical manifestation as early as possible.

The diagnosis, evaluation, and management of Marfan syndrome require coordinated, multidisciplinary skills. Patients and families are best served in Marfan syndrome clinics with demonstrated interest and expertise in heritable disorders of connective tissue. Multidisciplinary Marfan syndrome clinics are becoming more common; however, when these are unavailable to the family, the primary care physician may assume the responsibility of coordinating complex, multidisciplinary medical care. Even when a Marfan syndrome clinic is available, the pediatrician plays a number of important roles in the management of affected individuals. The primary physician should be familiar with the major features of the syndrome and must make the appropriate initial referrals for diagnosis. Once the diagnosis has been confirmed, the primary care physician can help to screen for age-dependent manifestations, particularly scoliosis. The pediatrician also provides ongoing support and advocacy for the family. Families, as well as clinicians caring for them, benefit greatly from the resources of the National Marfan Foundation.

NATURAL HISTORY AND MANAGEMENT

General guidelines for the management of patients with Marfan syndrome are given in Table 2. All patients should undergo a comprehensive medical evaluation at least annually, with more frequent examinations depending on severity of clinical manifestations.

Cardiac Features

Up to a third of patients have normal cardiac findings, yet nearly all affected individuals have abnormal echocardiograms, most often showing aortic root dilatation and mitral valve prolapse. Aortic dissection and rupture occur against a background of progressive aortic dilatation. A significant amount of dilatation may occur before any clinical symptoms or signs are evident, highlighting the need for early diagnosis of the syndrome, presymptomatic screening, and careful, long-term follow-up. The prevalence and degree of aortic regurgitation, as well as the risks for dissection and rupture, are proportional to the size of the aortic root. The presence of an aortic root of normal size does not exclude the syndrome completely but makes it less likely and rules out the main life-threatening complication of the disorder.

Individuals with Marfan syndrome should avoid contact sports (including basketball), isometric exercises, weight-lifting, and participation in physical activity to the point of exhaustion.

TABLE 1. Marfan Syndrome: Criteria for Diagnosis*

Skeletal
- Anterior chest deformity, especially asymmetric pectus excavatum/carinatum
- Dolichostenomelia (long arms and legs)
- Arachnodactyly (long fingers)
- Vertebral column deformity
  - Scoliosis
  - Thoracic lordosis
  - Reduced thoracic kyphosis ("straight back")
- Tall stature
- High, narrowly arched palate and dental crowding
- Protrusio acetabulae
- Abnormal joint mobility
  - Congenital flexion contractures
  - Hypermobility

Ocular
- Ectopia lentis (subluxation of the lens)†
- Flat cornea
- Elongated globe
- Retinal detachment (much more common after lens removal)
- Myopia

Cardiovascular
- Dilatation of the ascending aorta†
- Aortic dissection†
- Aortic regurgitation
- Mitral regurgitation due to mitral valve prolapse
- Calcification of the mitral annulus
- Mitral valve prolapse
- Abdominal aortic aneurysm
- Dysrhythmia
- Endocarditis

Pulmonary
- Spontaneous pneumothorax
- Apical bleb

Skin and Integument
- Striae distensae
- Inguinal hernia
- Other hernia (umbilical, diaphragmatic, incisional)

Central Nervous System
- Dural ectasia† (lumbosacral meningocele)
- Dilated cisterna magna
- Learning disability (verbal-performance discrepancy)
- Hyperactivity with or without attention deficit disorder

Genetics
- Autosomal dominant inheritance (25–30% of cases sporadic)

Requirements for Diagnosis
- In the absence of an unequivocally affected first-degree relative: involvement of the skeleton and at least two other systems; at least one major manifestation
- In the presence of at least one unequivocally affected first-degree relative: involvement of at least two systems; at least one major manifestation preferred, but this will depend somewhat on the family's phenotype
- Urine amino acid analysis in the absence of pyridoxine supplementation confirms absence of homocystinuria

Adapted from Beighton P, de Paepe A, Danks D, et al: International nosology of heritable disorders of connective tissue, Berlin, 1986. Am J Med Genet 29:581–594, 1988.

*Listed in approximate order of decreasing specificity.

†Major manifestation.

TABLE 2. Management of Patients with Marfan Syndrome

Regular examinations (at least annually)
  General medical
  Cardiologic, including echocardiography
  Ophthalmologic (more often for those with ectopia lentis or retinal detachment)
  Scoliosis screening until skeletal maturity
  Orthopedic (if indicated)
Examinations as needed
  Neurologic/behavioral
  Physical therapy
  Computed tomographic (CT) scanning or magnetic resonance imaging (MRI) of the aorta or the vertebral column (when aortic aneurysm distal to the root, chronic dissection, or dural ectasia is suspected)
Discussion with parents, patient, spouse, or significant other regarding psychosocial concerns, genetic counseling, and any new advances in treatment or research
Activity restriction, depending on age and cardiovascular features
Antibiotic prophylaxis for bacterial endocarditis (regardless of evident valve pathology)
Therapy with beta-blockers
Prophylactic composite graft repair of ascending aorta

Adapted from Pyeritz RE: The diagnosis and management of the Marfan syndrome. Am Fam Physician 34:83–94, 1986.

All patients should receive prophylaxis for subacute bacterial endocarditis, regardless of evident valve pathology.

Beta-blockers have been effective in slowing the rate of aortic root dilatation as well as in decreasing the incidence of aortic regurgitation and dissection. The objective of beta-blockade therapy is to reduce abruptness of ventricular ejection, thereby reducing the physiologic impact on the ascending aorta. Atenolol has the advantages of increased cardiac selectivity and once or twice daily dosing, but propranolol and other agents are also effective. Counting a patient's heart rate after several minutes of moderate exercise is an easy way to monitor drug efficacy and compliance. In older children, adolescents, and adults, heart rate during exercise should not exceed 100.

Composite graft operation, in which the aorta and aortic valve are replaced by a synthetic tube that has an artificial valve sewn into the proximal end, is recommended when aortic root diameter is about 6 cm.

Ophthalmologic Features

All patients should undergo an initial ophthalmologic examination with continued follow-up on at least a yearly basis, more frequently for those with ectopia lentis or retinal detachment. The latter complication is much more common in those who have undergone lens removal.

Skeletal Features

Scoliosis is common and may worsen rapidly during growth spurts. Scoliosis screening should be performed regularly until skeletal maturity has been achieved. Other skeletal findings that may necessitate orthopedic intervention include chest wall abnormalities, flat feet, and joint dislocations.

Neurologic and Behavioral Features

Learning disability and hyperactivity, with or without attention deficit disorder, may lead to school and behavioral difficulties. Methylphenidate HCl (Ritalin) therapy has been beneficial in some cases.

Counseling

Prudent management should include regular discussions with parents, patient, spouse, or significant other regarding psychosocial concerns, genetic counseling, and any new advances in treatment or research.

DIFFERENTIAL DIAGNOSIS

Conditions most often considered in the differential diagnosis include homocystinuria, familial or isolated mitral valve prolapse syndrome, familial or isolated annuloaortic ectasia (aortic dissection without clear features of Marfan syndrome), congenital contractural arachnodactyly, and Stickler syndrome.

Aortic root dilatation can be seen in a number of other syndromes, including other heritable connective tissue disorders: annuloaortic ectasia (aortic dissection without clear features of Marfan syndrome); Ehlers-Danlos syndrome, types I, II, III, and X; autosomal dominant cutis laxa syndrome; osteogenesis imperfecta, types I, III, and IV; and Larsen syndrome. In addition, aortic root dilatation is seen occasionally in Noonan syndrome and Turner syndrome. The natural history of the aortic manifestations in these other disorders is less well defined; however, the treatment is essentially the same as for Marfan syndrome.

KAWASAKI SYNDROME

ROBERT P. SUNDEL, M.D.
and JANE W. NEWBURGER, M.D., M.P.H.

Kawasaki syndrome (KS) is an idiopathic childhood vasculitis of small and medium-sized vessels that has become one of the leading causes of acquired heart disease in American children. The syndrome is characterized by fever, conjunctivitis, rash, mucosal inflammation, lymphadenopathy, and extremity changes; however, the major morbidity involves the heart. Coronary artery aneurysms or ectasia develops in approximately 15 to 25 per cent of untreated children with the disease and may lead to ischemic heart disease with angina, myocardial infarction, or sudden death. *Intravenous gamma globulin decreases the incidence of coronary artery aneurysms by threefold to fivefold if given within 10 days of disease onset.* Management of children with suspected KS, therefore, requires accurate and expeditious diagnosis and close monitoring of the cardiovascular system.

DIAGNOSIS

The diagnosis of KS rests on fulfilling at least five of six clinical criteria of mucocutaneous inflammation (Table 1). These criteria vary considerably in their frequency. Lymphadenopathy is most likely to be absent at diagnosis: As many as one half of children with KS (especially younger children) do not have lymphadenopathy at presentation. Fever, on the other hand, is a virtual *sine qua non* for the diagnosis. No laboratory values are included in the criteria for KS, but in ambiguous cases certain trends may be helpful. Early in the disease course, acute phase reactants (e.g., erythrocyte sedimentation rate, C-reactive protein) tend to be elevated, and there is often a leukocytosis and left shift in the white blood cell count. The hematocrit is frequently more than two standard deviations below normal, even early in the disease course. Urethritis, aseptic meningitis, and hepatitis are common features of the illness.

In two groups of children, KS may prove particularly difficult to diagnose. Some children in whom coronary artery abnormalities subsequently develop will not have fulfilled criteria (so-called atypical KS). Similarly, signs and symptoms

TABLE 1. Diagnostic Criteria for Kawasaki Disease

Fever lasting 5 days or more without any other explanation and at least four of the following criteria:

1. Bilateral conjunctival injection
2. Changes of the peripheral extremities, including the following:
   Erythema of palms or soles, edema of hands or feet (acute phase)
   Periungual desquamation (convalescent phase)
3. Mucous membrane changes, including the following:
   Injected or fissured lips
   Injected pharynx
   Strawberry tongue
4. Polymorphous rash
5. Acute nonpurulent cervical lymphadenopathy (at least one lymph node 1.5 cm or greater in diameter)

Adapted from MMWR 39 (No. RR-13): 17–18, 1990.

of KS are often obscure in infants younger than 12 months of age. The illnesses most likely to mimic KS are viral infections (measles, enteroviruses, adenovirus), toxin-mediated illnesses (toxic shock syndrome, beta-hemolytic streptococcal infection), and idiopathic immune or autoimmune diseases (drug reactions, juvenile rheumatoid arthritis). There is no definitive test for KS, but exclusion of alternatives will allow a presumptive diagnosis in most situations.

THERAPY

Aspirin

Aspirin was the first medication to be used for the treatment of KS because of its anti-inflammatory and antithrombotic effects. Experts vary in their dosage recommendations for treating KS, reflecting the paucity of objective data concerning an ideal regimen and different perceptions of theoretical and potential risks, such as Reye's syndrome. Additionally, aspirin-binding studies suggest that the hypoalbuminemia in children with KS predisposes them to toxic free-salicylate levels despite measured (bound) values within the therapeutic range. On the other hand, many clinicians have the impression that high-dose aspirin makes children less uncomfortable and benefits the associated arthritis seen in up to one third of cases of KS. Trials comparing high-dose and low-dose aspirin in KS are currently being conducted; until results are available, all dosing recommendations reflect an empiric compromise.

Typically, high aspirin doses (80 to 100 mg/kg/day divided four times a day) are employed during the inflammatory phase of illness; salicylate levels are monitored to avoid toxicity. Once the child has been afebrile for 2 or 3 days, aspirin may be decreased to antithrombotic doses of less than 5 mg/kg/day. If coronary arteries remain normal, salicylates may be discontinued approximately 7 weeks after the onset of fever. Following the acute inflammatory stage of KS, platelet counts may remain elevated for weeks, and coronary artery endothelium is thought to have diminished antiaggretory potential. Accordingly, low-dose aspirin is conventionally continued to provide some antithrombotic effects. Nonsteroidal anti-inflammatory agents other than salicylates are employed regularly in Japan. No differences in outcome have been noted with these agents, although occasional children with severe arthritis may obtain additional benefit.

Intravenous Gamma Globulin

Prospective, randomized, multicenter, controlled trials in Japan and the United States have demonstrated a significant decrease in coronary artery abnormalities when treatment is initiated within 10 days of onset of fever. Therapy with intravenous gamma globulin (IVGG) has additional benefits as well. Treatment results in a reduced prevalence of giant aneurysms (internal diameter at least 8 mm), the most serious form of coronary abnormality caused by the disease, and accelerates normalization of aberrant left ventricular systolic function and contractility. High-dose IVGG also reduces fever and laboratory indices of inflammation, suggesting a rapid, generalized anti-inflammatory effect. Standard treatment for KS has been four daily infusions of 400 mg/kg/day of IVGG. *Results of a recently concluded multicenter, randomized, controlled trial of 549 children with KS suggest that a single infusion of 2 g/kg over 10 hours is preferable.* Overall prevalence of coronary artery abnormalities was lower (12 of 260 versus 24 of 263 at 2 weeks of illness, $P = .042$) with the single-dose regimen than with four smaller daily doses. Furthermore, resolution of fever and systemic inflammation is faster, allowing earlier discharge from the hospital. The frequency of adverse effects is similar with the two treatment regimens; although fluid overload and development of congestive heart failure pose a theoretical concern, experience shows that these complications are quite rare.

Antithrombotic Therapy

The risk of coronary artery thrombosis is greatest during the subacute phase of the disease. At that point, usually beginning approximately 2 to 3 weeks after disease onset, smoldering coronary vasculitis coincides with marked thrombocytosis and hypercoagulability as a result of both endothelial and fluid-phase abnormalities. Low-dose aspirin (<5 mg/kg/day given as a single dose) is the mainstay of antithrombotic therapy in KS. Dipyridamole (3 to 6 mg/kg/day in three divided doses) may be substituted for aspirin when salicylates are contraindicated. For children without evidence of coronary artery ectasia or aneurysms, antiplatelet therapy is usually discontinued approximately 2 months after onset of illness once platelet count and ESR have normalized.

Children with coronary artery abnormalities require chronic antithrombotic therapy, usually with low-dose aspirin. Dipyridamole is sometimes added to aspirin therapy, although its value in this setting is controversial. The risk of coronary thrombosis and myocardial infarction is especially great in children with rapidly increasing coronary dimension or with giant aneurysms. In these children, treatment options include antiplatelet therapy (aspirin with or without dipyridamole), anticoagulation using warfarin (at doses adequate to achieve a 1.5-fold prolongation of the prothrombin time), or a combination of antiplatelet and anticoagulant therapy. No prospective data exist to guide the clinician in choosing an optimal regimen, and anecdotal reports suggest cases of thrombosis despite treatment with each of these drug combinations.

Thrombolytic Therapy

Despite the use of antithrombotic agents, myocardial infarction secondary to thrombotic occlusion of coronary aneurysms may develop in some children, especially those with giant aneurysms. In others, the presence of a coronary artery thrombus may be detected on serial two-dimensional echocardiography. Thrombolytic agents (e.g., urokinase or streptokinase), either intravenous or intracoronary, have been used with variable success. *Thrombolytic therapy for coronary artery thrombosis is most effective if begun within 3 to 4 hours of symptom onset.* Immediately following clot lysis, systemic heparin is begun in combination with aspirin. Maintenance of reperfusion then requires chronic oral antithrombotic therapy (for example, warfarin with dipyridamole), although the ideal regimen has not been established.

Surgical Management

Surgery in KS consists primarily of coronary artery bypass grafts (CABG) for obstructive lesions, although mitral valve replacement is occasionally necessary in children with papillary muscle dysfunction or valvulitis. The indications for CABG procedures in children have not been definitively established, but such surgery should be considered when progressive stenosis is demonstrated, the myocardium to be perfused through the graft is still viable, and no appreciable lesions are present in the artery peripheral to the planned graft site. *When these conditions are satisfied, surgery is an option if arteriography demonstrates critical stenosis of the left main coronary artery or if occlusions or progressive critical stenosis are present in two or more of the other coronary vessels.* Isolated stenotic lesions in the proximal left anterior descending artery or the right coronary artery are probably not an indication for bypass grafting. Optimal results are obtained with the use of internal mammary artery grafts, which increase in both diameter and length as the children grow.

Miscellaneous Treatment

Data are inadequate to allow firm recommendations concerning treatment of two groups of children: those who fail to respond to IVGG, and those who present with fever more than 10 days after the onset of KS. In both instances, aggressive management seems warranted in view of the association of prolonged fever with increased risk of developing coronary artery abnormalities. In children with persistent or recrudescent fever, we have reinfused IVGG, 1 to 2 g/kg, on the basis of the documented association of low post-infusion serum IgG levels with worse outcome. The risk of retreatment appears to be minimal, and many patients seem to improve promptly. However, assessment of the efficacy of IVGG retreatment awaits randomized, controlled studies. No other specific second-line therapy has been tested in patients for whom gamma globulin is ineffective; a potential role for corticosteroids is controversial. Similarly, there are no controlled trials of IVGG treatment in patients presenting after the 10th day of fever. Nonetheless, most clinicians with experience in KS treat such children with gamma globulin if they are still febrile or if they have coronary artery disease and any signs of active inflammation.

MONITORING

Coronary artery lesions resulting from KS change dynamically over time. The first echocardiogram and laboratory studies (especially complete blood count, platelet count, and ESR) are obtained upon admission for IVGG treatment. Follow-up studies and examinations are performed by a pediatric cardiologist approximately 2 and 4 weeks later unless evidence of a rapidly expanding aneurysm necessitates more frequent evaluations. Thereafter, the frequency of follow-up examinations is dictated by the severity of the coronary artery lesions. Despite IVGG therapy, 5 to 10 per cent of children will have echocardiographically demonstrable coronary artery abnormalities 2 weeks after the onset of fever. At least 50 per cent of these will regress within 12 to 24 months. Healing occurs by myointimal proliferation or organization of thrombus; in addition to histologic abnormalities, regressed aneurysmal segments show abnormalities of function. Because the long-term prognosis for children with regressed coronary abnormalities is unknown, we prefer to observe these children indefinitely at regular intervals. In general, any child with a coronary artery abnormality is seen by a pediatric cardiologist at least every 6 months and more often if clinically indicated.

If coronary arteries remain normal throughout the first month after acute KS, subsequent development of new lesions is extremely unusual. On the other hand, abnormalities in prostaglandin and lipid metabolism may persist for months after clinical resolution of the disease, suggesting long-term endothelial cell dysfunction. Therefore, follow-up cardiology evaluations should be obtained 1 year after onset of KS and then at intervals of 3 to 5 years. At these appointments, lipid profiles are also evaluated and prudent diet and exercise regimes discussed. From the purely clinical perspective, however, children without known cardiac sequelae during the first month of KS appear to return to their previous state of health without signs or symptoms of cardiac impairment and their overall prognosis appears to be excellent.

REFERENCES

Newburger JW, Takahashi M, Beiser AS, et al: A single intravenous infusion of gamma globulin as compared with four infusions in the treatment of acute Kawasaki syndrome. N Engl J Med 324:1633–1639, 1991.

MANAGEMENT OF INNOCENT MURMURS IN THE YOUNG

DAN G. McNAMARA, M.D.

PROBLEMS AND POTENTIAL SOLUTIONS

Rationale for This Topic

Having consulted on patients with "innocent" murmurs for some 35 years, the author has often heard about the logistical problems that pediatricians face in dealing with a "new" unexpected murmur in the midst of a busy day seeing well and sick young people. It takes more than a cursory listen to the heart to be reasonably sure that a murmur is innocent; however, pediatricians, accustomed to hearing these normal sounds, generally ignore those that are faint or transient—and rightly so. Probably there is no need to mention every innocent murmur to the parent any more than the many normal variants found in other organs and systems on routine physical examination of the developing individual.

But when a murmur is quite prominent or somewhat puzzling to the examiner, one has to decide at that time whether it indicates congenital or acquired heart disease or only a normal variant. The examiner must also decide whether the parents should be told about it before they are told by someone else. A prolonged and more-detailed-than-usual auscultation of the heart without some explanation is likely to alarm the parent who is accustomed to seeing only a fairly brief cardiac examination. If doctors inform a parent about an innocent murmur, they are obliged to explain the phenomenon, a simple enough thing to do except for the time involved to do it well.

It is for these reasons that a discussion of the management of innocent murmurs is timely and appropriate for this volume on therapy in pediatric practice.

Magnitude of the Problem

Innocent murmurs comprised 18.5 per cent (100 of 540 consecutive new patients under the age of 18 years in the first 4 months of 1990) referred to the cardiology service at Texas Children's Hospital, Houston, for known or possible congenital or acquired heart disease. It is certainly the single most frequent final diagnosis made in new patients beyond infancy in the outpatient clinic.

The author does not know the percentage of presumed healthy infants, children, or adolescents in whom pediatricians hear a new murmur that calls for a return visit, prompts the ordering of graphic tests, or necessitates a consultation with a pediatric cardiologist. Probably it is a daily problem in a busy practice.

Referring the patient for another opinion is a perfectly reasonable and certainly expedient way to handle a problematic innocent murmur, and aside from the time and expense and the possible parental anxiety in waiting for an appointment, there is no reason not to order a consultation.

Throughout the United States, pediatric cardiologists, including the author, have not really been discouraging these welcome referrals! Frankly, we enjoy seeing patients with a normal heart and innocent murmur. For one thing, such patients provide an excellent teaching opportunity for residents in pediatrics and fellows in a pediatric cardiology training program. Also, because parents bringing their child to a cardiology clinic for that first visit usually arrive fearing that there is important heart disease that might limit physical activity, require surgical repair, or shorten the child's life, it is professionally very satisfying to be able to give the good report that the heart is normal.

The ideal thing for all concerned is for pediatricians to manage innocent murmurs themselves. This can usually be achieved without graphic tests, and, by following some simple steps that require no more than a few extra minutes of time per week, one can learn to become expert at recognizing innocent murmurs. For a description of the four common innocent murmurs, see Table 1.

Many times, patients with innocent murmurs are referred by pediatricians who are reasonably certain, by physical examination alone, that a murmur is innocent; nevertheless, a parent insists on a second opinion. In discussing this matter with parents, the author has concluded that parents ask for another opinion when one of the following has occurred:

1. They have perceived, and may have been told, that the pediatrician is uncertain about the importance of the murmur.
2. The diagnosis is rendered after only a hurried and limited auscultation of the heart.
3. The physician recommends return visits to check the murmur again later.
4. The physician's explanation of innocent murmurs seems perfunctory to the parents or has been phrased in medical jargon.

Thus, an approach to management of innocent murmurs by pediatricians in the office is one that avoids management practices that unwittingly leave parents or teenaged patients feeling uneasy or confused.

Improving Management by Pediatricians Who Wish to Handle the Problem Themselves

Keeping the Ear Trained to Recognize Innocent Murmurs with Confidence

By the end of residency training, pediatricians have learned to recognize the several innocent murmurs peculiar to the young; some months or years after entering practice, however physicians may find that they have lost their once mastered skill of auscultation. Probably this can be largely avoided or rectified by taking advantage of the daily opportunity that a busy practice affords to refresh on hearing these normal variants of heart sounds which may appear transiently or may be elicited at one time or another in virtually all young people. A good time to search for innocent murmurs is on an occasion in which the patient has increased cardiac output, for example, immediately after vigorous exercise (enough to raise the heart rate to 120 to 130 beats per minute); in the infant shortly after a full feeding; when there is fever, infection, anxiety, or excitement; or with mild anemia. Each of these situations increases the intensity of latent or existing physiologic murmurs (as well as pathologic ones, for that matter).

One obstacle to a prompt and accurate evaluation of heart murmurs or unusual sounds is listening too long at only one valve area and with the subject placed in only one position. It is actually better to listen to only three to five cardiac cycles at each of the valve areas, moving back to the site where the murmur is loudest for a second brief listen if needed. This ought to be done with the child placed in each of the traditionally prescribed positions: supine, sitting, and standing, first at rest and then, when possible, immediately after exercise, which turns up the volume (intensity) of heart sounds and existing or latent murmurs.

In addition, it helps to note the effect of deep continuous, quiet, unforced respiration; the effect of deep held inspiration; and, finally, deep held expiration, with the patient supine. Of course, auscultation must be performed while the patient and the examining room are perfectly quiet, not always an easy thing to achieve in a busy office or with talkative onlookers. With practice, however, a complete auscultation can be accomplished in a quiet, cooperative patient in 2½ to 3 minutes.

This full cardiac examination is hardly practical and indeed unnecessary in every well child examined, but if one tries to elicit these murmurs once or twice per week, the examiner becomes and remains expert at it. The auscultatory skills developed in this way are then available when needed to evaluate a new unexpected murmur.

Gaining the Confidence of the Family and Patient

If the examiner has decided that a murmur is benign and tells the family about it, the diagnosis, which sometimes causes alarm, is far better accepted if the physician has performed a complete cardiovascular auscultation using the several maneuvers and putting the patient in the different positions cited above.

The topic described in this article pertains only to murmurs; a complete cardiovascular examination, of course, includes pulses, blood pressure, and palpation of the precordium—all too well known to most readers of this volume to itemize in detail.

Avoiding the Temptation to Make Return Appointments to Check on the Murmur

Once it has been determined by the primary care physician or the consultant that the murmur is innocent, it need not, and in fact, should not, be "checked on," at least ostensibly, at subsequent office visits. Parents are best advised that although the sound usually disappears as the patient matures, it need not disappear entirely in order to confirm that the sound is innocent. These murmurs often appear and disappear inexplicably. In fact, the two most common innocent murmurs (*Still's murmur* of childhood and *pulmonary valve flow murmur* of adolescence) are very likely to reappear intermittently or become louder whenever situations arise that increase cardiac output and when examining conditions are ideal (quiet, cooperative patient and quiet examining room).

Explaining Innocent Murmurs to the Family Orally and in Writing

The term murmur is so much a part of our medical vocabulary that physicians forget that many people do not know what the term means—let alone know the difference between an "innocent" and "pathologic" murmur. It helps family members to understand and accept the diagnosis if they have been informed on the elementary facts about innocent murmurs and how these sounds are produced, to some extent, in all individuals but heard more readily in

TABLE 1. Physicians' Guide to Normal Variants in Heart Sounds Often Heard in Young People and Some Common Pathologic Conditions That They May Resemble

1. Neonatal Pulmonary Artery Branch Murmur
- a. Age first heard: newborn to 6 weeks of age
- b. Age murmur disappears: 2–4 months
- c. Location: mid-axillary region and infraclavicular area; right or left side or both
- d. Patient position that amplifies murmur: supine.
- e. Character: soft, high pitched, short, and grade I–II/VI.
- f. Phase of cardiac cycle: mid-systole
- g. Confused with:
  - (1) Pathologic pulmonary artery branch stenosis, which produces a louder murmur
  - (2) Very mild pulmonary or aortic valve stenosis
- h. Murmur produced by: turbulence in pulmonary artery branches before maturation of pulmonary vascular bed

2. Venous Hum
- a. Age first heard: 2–3 years
- b. Age hum disappears: 7–8 years
- c. Location: right, left, or both infraclavicular areas near sternum and over manubrium sternum and base of neck over jugular veins
- d. Patient position that amplifies murmur: sitting or standing patient with head tilted up
- e. Patient position that obliterates venous hum: supine
- f. Character: soft, blowing grade I–III/VI
- g. Phase of cardiac cycle: continuous throughout systole and diastole
- h. Confused with: small patent ductus but PDA murmur persists and is often louder with patient supine; PDA murmur sharper and localized to pulmonary valve area
- i. Murmur produced by: turbulent flow of blood in jugular–left innominate vein and superior vena caval junction

3. Still's Aortic Valve Vibratory Murmur (the most common innocent murmur referred for cardiac consultation. Venous hum is more prevalent but seldom prompts referral)
- a. Age first heard: neonate, infant (uncommonly); 3–7 years (commonly)
- b. Age murmur disappears: early to mid-adolescence
- c. Location: sternal edge, third and fourth spaces with weak transmission to apex; murmur may transmit to right carotid artery
- d. Patient position that amplifies murmur: best heard in supine position during held expiration but may persist with standing position; murmur attenuated or obliterated by forced Valsalva maneuver or deep held inspiration
- e. Character: low-pitched, groaning, or musical; short, grade I–III
- f. Phase of cardiac cycle: mid-systole
- g. Confused with:
  - (1) Left ventricular false tendon; the inconsequential false tendon usually has less variation with change in body position and is heard over a wider area on the chest wall, including the apex
  - (2) Left ventricular HOCM with subaortic pressure gradient, but HOCM murmur persists with all positions
  - (3) MR murmur of acute rheumatic valvulitis but MR murmur is high-pitched and at the apex of the heart; it is unlikely to disappear entirely with erect position
  - (4) Small VSD; murmur of small VSD is actually not very similar to Still's murmur, but some patients are referred with a possible diagnosis of VSD; VSD murmur is long and harsh and persists in all patient positions
- h. Murmur produced by: aortic valve leaflet vibration during mid-systole

4. Pulmonary Valve Flow Murmur
- a. Age first heard: late childhood, early adolescence
- b. Age murmur disappears: early adult life; murmur may be heard in adult pregnant women or in adults with a thin chest wall and with increased cardiac output
- c. Location: left second intercostal space at sternal edge
- d. Patient position that amplifies murmur: murmur invariably heard best with patient supine, especially after exercise and during held expiration; murmur attenuated or obliterated by deep held inspiration and often simply with patient standing
- e. Character of murmur: high frequency, blowing, occasionally scratchy
- f. Phase of cardiac cycle: systole
- g. Murmur confused with:
  - (1) ASD of the secundum type, but ASD has wide splitting of S_2
  - (2) Mild pulmonary valve stenosis, but pulmonary stenosis is usually preceded by an ejection click and persists in all positions and with held inspiration

5. Normal Heart Sounds That May Prompt Referral for Cardiac Evaluation

Prominent Physiologic Splitting of S_2
- a. Age first heard: early to mid-childhood, rarely heard in young infants because heart rate is usually too fast to detect splitting
- b. Age sound disappears: S_2 splitting remains throughout life but is often hard to hear in adults with a thick chest wall
- c. Location: left second and third intercostal spaces and sternal edge
- d. Position which amplifies sound: S_2 splitting enhanced by supine position and during slow inspiration; S_2 splitting less prominent in standing position, during tachycardia, and during Valsalva maneuver held for 3–4 seconds
- e. Confused with: *fixed splitting* of S_2 found in ASD defect and with complete right bundle branch block. *Physiologic splitting* is very similar to pathologic fixed splitting, but in a cooperative child with a heart rate less than 120 beats/minute, lack of movement of S_2 is very clear when compared to normal splitting; in physiologic splitting, the "lub-dub" in expiration changes during slow inspiration to "lub-trrup"

Physiologic Splitting of S_1
- a. Age first heard: late childhood, adolescence, or an age that the heart rate slows to 60–80 beats/minute
- b. Age sound disappears: physiologic splitting remains throughout adult life but is harder to hear in obese or thick-chested individuals
- c. Location: left sternal border and third, fourth, and fifth spaces (tricuspid area); less prominent at apex
- d. Patient position that amplifies S_1 splitting: either supine or standing
- e. Sound attenuated or obliterated by: tachycardia 110–120 beats/minute or more
- f. Sound confused with:
  - (1) Mid-systolic click of mitral leaflet prolapse—the split sounds like "trrup′dub" and midsystolic click sounds like "lub-ip̆-dub"
  - (2) Aortic ejection click of bicuspid aortic valve; ejection click has a sharper, snappier sound than duller components of physiologically split first sound; ejection click best heard at apex with transmission to sternal edge

PDA, patent ductus arteriosus; HOCM, hypertrophic obstructive cardiomyopathy; MR, mitral regurgitation; VSD, ventricular septal defect; ASD, atrial septal defect.

children. They may not know that "normal" murmurs are prevalent in children because the chest wall is thinner and the heart relatively closer to the anterior chest wall than in the adult. Also, children are more likely than adults to experience events that increase the cardiac output (fever, infection, excitement, or anxiety in the doctor's office)—which makes the murmur louder.

It helps to name the particular murmur(s) found in the

patient. Naming the murmur adds credibility to the diagnosis and makes explanation easier. Also, parents are more readily convinced about innocent murmurs when they learn that research studies using intracardiac phonocardiography have shown that in healthy adults blood turbulence is created at the great vessel valves during the ejection phase of the cardiac cycle. This turbulence at the pulmonary valve can be heard as a pulmonary flow murmur and at the aortic valve as Still's aortic vibratory murmur under certain physiologic conditions. Similarly, turbulence in the jugular–superior vena caval junction in young children produces a venous hum. Pulmonary artery branch turbulence in the maturing neonate causes the neonatal transient murmur.

Because an oral explanation may take 15 to 20 minutes, not including time for questions, and because anxiety about a murmur on the part of parents may interfere with their paying full attention in the doctor's office, it has proved helpful, in the author's experience, to draft an explanation in lay terms for the family to take home to read and reread and share with family members who were not present at the doctor's office. The explanation used by several of the pediatric cardiologists at Texas Children's Hospital in Houston is presented under the heading "Information for Parents and Patients."

Allowing Normal Physical Activity (Including Competitive Sports and Avoiding Any Special Precautions for Handling Infection or Surgical Procedures)

Despite identification of the murmur as a purely innocent one, parents may nevertheless restrict the child from physical exertion or may worry needlessly if the child needs anesthesia unless they are informed that the only consequence of an innocent murmur is an inordinate concern about it.

Conclusion

If the pediatrician wishes to refer the patient with a troublesome, but most likely innocent, murmur to the pediatric cardiologist, this is a reasonable plan of management that is evidently in widespread use throughout this country, and, except for the time, expense, and possible anxiety for the parents and child associated with a visit to the consultant, this method of management can be quite satisfactory and definitive. For those physicians who prefer to handle these patients themselves in their office, the steps outlined in this article should provide the means to accomplish this successfully and expeditiously.

INFORMATION FOR PARENTS AND PATIENTS

Misconceptions about innocent murmurs in the young can cause a lot of unnecessary trouble and anxiety for the family. Some people are perfectly satisfied to accept a hurried dismissal of an innocent murmur: ". . . It's nothing. Forget about it." But others, despite full trust in their doctor, want more details. Although doctors certainly want to take the time to explain an innocent heart murmur, the demands of a busy practice sometimes make this impractical. This portion of the article can assist the physician in discussing a heart murmur with the family.

Heart Murmurs and Heart Sounds

What is the difference between a *heart murmur* and a *heart sound?* Usually, when the physician listens to the normal heart with a stethoscope, two heart sounds occur in each cardiac cycle and resemble something like "lub-dub." These two sounds occur with closure of the heart valves: the first sound, with closure of the valves between the upper and lower heart chambers (tricuspid valve on the right side and mitral valve on the left), and the second sound, with closure of the valves opening into the great vessels that leave the heart (pulmonary and aortic valves). Usually, while the heart pumps blood out and while it fills with blood, no sound is heard with a stethoscope, except in a high percentage of normal healthy young people, in whom prolonged sounds (called murmurs) may occur during the usually silent pumping phase of the heart cycle (*systole*) and sometimes also during the filling phase (*diastole*).

What makes the term murmur confusing is that some birth defects of the heart or acquired diseases also produce murmurs; thus, physicians must specifiy whether the murmur is either *innocent* (benign or functional), implying no recognizable abnormality or disease of the heart, or *organic,* indicating that the prolonged sound is caused by some abnormality of the heart or its blood vessels.

What is the importance of an innocent murmur? The only importance of an innocent murmur lies in the fact that it may be mistaken for an organic murmur. One or more of these insignificant noises can be heard at one time or another in most, but not all, young people. These murmurs usually disappear before adult life. They cause no harm, require no follow-up, call for no restriction of physical activity, and should be considered normal variants.

One reason that so many young people but few adults have these sounds emanating from the normal heart is that the thin chest wall of the child transmits sounds to the chest surface very readily. Also, the heart in the child is relatively close to the chest wall, which allows heart sounds as well as murmurs to be readily heard. The parent can borrow the doctor's stethoscope and listen to the heart of the fully grown adult and then to that of the infant, child, or adolescent. Even without medical training, the parent will realize how much louder the child's heart is.

Also, young people are often examined by the doctor when there is an increased rate of blood flow through the heart because of fever, infection, or simply the anxiety that goes with a visit to the doctor. This faster blood flow through the circulation brings out murmurs that may not be present at rest and makes existing murmurs louder.

Types of Innocent Murmurs

There are four common innocent murmurs and at least two variants of normal heart sounds that may sometimes lead to suspicion of an organic murmur or pathologic sound.

Neonatal Pulmonary Artery Murmur. In some newborns (perhaps 15 to 20 per cent) during the first few weeks of life, a short high-pitched murmur can be heard in the sides of the chest under the arms, in the front of the chest just below the collar bones or in the back between the "wings" (scapulae). These murmurs disappear within a few weeks and are unassociated with any enlargement of the heart or other sign of difficulty.

Still's Murmur (Aortic Valve Vibratory Murmur). Still's murmur (named for Dr. Still, the English physician who first described it) arises from normal aortic valve vibration produced by the rapid movement of the aortic valve leaflets when the heart pumps blood through the valve. The more rapidly blood moves through the valve during fever, exercise, or the anxiety associated with a doctor's examination, the greater the vibration and the more likely that the vibrations will be transmitted to the surface of the chest as a heart murmur.

Pulmonary Valve Flow Murmur. The production of this murmur, like that of Still's murmur, results from vibration of a valve, but at the pulmonary instead of the aortic valve.

Venous Hum. This is a continuous "whirring" sound heard in both phases of the cardiac cycle (systole and diastole). Venous hum occurs as blood flows through the large veins in the neck en route to the heart. In almost all young children, a venous hum can be brought out by sitting the child up and raising the chin.

Normal Variants of Heart Sound

The first heart sound is produced by closure of tricuspid and mitral valves, and the second heart sound is produced by closure of pulmonic and aortic valves. The valves close so nearly simultaneously that we often hear on two single sounds: "lub′-dub."

When the heart slows down with increasing age of the child, the tricuspid and mitral valve closure times separate slightly and we hear each valve closure separately; the lub′-dub becomes trrup′-dub. Although this is not a murmur, it can give the impression that it is either a murmur or an abnormal click of the mitral valve or the aortic valve.

MANAGEMENT OF INNOCENT MURMURS BY PHYSICIANS AND PARENTS

Once the physician determines that a heart murmur or an unusual sound is innocent, it is no longer necessary to check it; the child should not be restricted and no special precautions need be taken. Substituting the word "normal" for "innocent" may be the best way to think about it. That alone should guide the management of a young person who has one of these sounds, which can plague his or her life if not appropriately ignored.

6

Digestive Tract

DISEASES AND INJURIES OF THE ORAL REGION

JEFFREY I. RESNICK, M.D.
and HARVEY A. ZAREM, M.D.

CLEFT LIP AND PALATE

The spectrum of facial deformity in congenital clefts runs from the minimal microform cleft lip to the severe complete bilateral cleft lip and palate. Classification of these deformities takes into account the variable involvement of the lip and palate and whether unilateral or bilateral clefting is present.

The parents of a child born with a cleft lip and palate need a great deal of information that addresses both the immediate treatment as well as long-term expectations. Over the past two decades, multidisciplinary cleft palate teams have emerged in most major medical centers as a resource for treating the complex problems associated with cleft lip and palate. These teams include pediatricians, plastic surgeons, otolaryngologists, medical geneticists, speech and hearing therapists, dentists and orthodontists, and social workers. Although the primary pediatrician will assume care of the child with cleft lip and palate, the cleft palate team will provide guidance in ensuring that the proper interventions are carried out in a timely fashion. Whether or not a cleft palate team is available, the primary pediatrician needs to coordinate the care of the child with a cleft. The general sequence of events is outlined next.

In the newborn period, the evaluation of infant feeding and the search for other congenital anomalies take precedence. Associated defects are noted in approximately 15 per cent of involved infants. Feeding problems are associated with clefts of the palate, since many infants are unable to generate an adequate suck. The infant should not be discharged from the hospital until it is clear that he or she is feeding well. In the presence of a cleft palate, adequate feeding can be ensured with the use of a cross-cut nipple or a long, soft lamb's nipple, each of which empties by gravity. Breast-feeding, although not impossible, requires extraordinary effort by the mother to express milk in the absence of an adequate suck. By ensuring that the mother is feeding the infant well prior to hospital discharge, problems with failure to thrive should be minimized. However, close follow-up is necessary to ensure that weight gain is normal.

Timing of surgical repair of a cleft lip is somewhat variable, with lip repairs being done anywhere from the newborn period to 3 to 6 months of age. Most surgeons recommend repair of cleft lips at approximately 3 months of age, when the infant tolerates general anesthesia well and when the anatomic landmarks are better defined. The infant should be thriving, and a general guideline is the "rule of ten": weight over 10 pounds, hemoglobin over 10 g, age over 10 weeks. When a wide unilateral cleft lip is present, a preliminary lip adhesion procedure can be done at 4 to 6 weeks of age to align the lip segments better prior to definitive lip repair. However, this preliminary step is optional and is considered to be unnecessary by many surgeons.

Repair of cleft palate is necessary for proper development of speech. Speech pathologists would like to see restoration of normal anatomy as early as possible to maximize the chances for normal speech. *Most teams are now recommending repair of cleft palates at 1 year of age or earlier, assuming that no upper airway problems are present.* There are some theoretic concerns that early palate repair can lead to diminished growth potential for the maxilla, but the goal of normal speech outweighs these concerns.

Children with a cleft of the palate show an extremely high incidence of chronic otitis media. Many otologists have recommended that children with cleft palate undergo routine myringotomy with insertion of tubes to reduce the incidence of chronic otitis media with subsequent hearing loss. This is usually done at the same time as cleft palate repair when indicated. In any infant with cleft palate and a chronic middle ear effusion, ventilation tubes should be inserted. The family must be alerted to the incidence of otitis media to facilitate early diagnosis and treatment in order to minimize the chances of long-term scarring and hearing loss.

Parents of a child with cleft lip and palate will benefit from genetic counseling. Although most cases of cleft lip and palate are sporadic in nature, many syndromes and inheritance patterns may be present. A medical geneticist can best address the possible risks for future offspring as well as deal with the possible guilt associated with the present child.

By the age of 1 year, most children with clefts will have undergone repair of the lip and palate. Close attention must then be paid to speech development. Any speech delay must be investigated, with both receptive (hearing) and expressive components to be examined. An anatomic basis for poor speech can be present, with the most common problem being inadequate closure of the soft palate to the posterior and lateral pharyngeal walls. If this "velopharyngeal incompetence" is present, secondary surgery in the form of a pharyngoplasty or pharyngeal flap will be required if speech therapy alone does not correct the problem.

Residual palatal fistulas with communication between the oral and nasal cavities can result in problems. Large fistulas can cause escape of fluid or food particles through the nose and can, less frequently, affect speech. Small fistulas are rarely symptomatic. Closure of oral-nasal fistulas can often be combined with other revisional procedures in the child with a cleft.

Routine tonsillectomy and adenoidectomy should not be performed in the child who has undergone cleft palate repair. Frequently, the hypertrophic adenoids and tonsils aid in the occlusion of the velopharynx, improving speech quality by minimizing velopharyngeal incompetence. In some cases, a submucous cleft palate may become symptomatic after tonsillectomy and adenoidectomy. A submucous cleft may be recognized by a bifid uvula, the presence of a thin blue midline in the soft palate, and a notch in the posterior border of the hard palate in the midline. Before tonsillectomy and adenoidectomy are recommended, adequate soft palate length and function must be ascertained.

The child born with a unilateral or bilateral cleft lip and palate may expect a normal life pattern in view of the high quality of surgical, orthodontic, otologic, and speech therapy that has evolved. However, a significant number of developmental deformities will produce problems even with excellent surgical and dental care. Soft tissue problems, such as lip scars and soft tissue deficiency, will need to be addressed as the child grows. Bone grafting of alveolar clefts should proceed during the stage of mixed dentition to stabilize the maxilla. Orthognathic surgery may be required to optimize the dental occlusion in maxillary hypoplasia. One of the most difficult problems is correction of the associated nasal deformity that accompanies both unilateral and especially bilateral clefts. Multiple surgical procedures and orthodontics can be expected to achieve a satisfactory functional and aesthetic result into adolescence. Timing of these procedures will depend on the specific stage of development of the child as well as on the specific symptoms that arise.

RARE CRANIOFACIAL CLEFTS

As in the more common cleft lip and palate, rare craniofacial clefts may be quite subtle or may present with severe and often grotesque facial anomalies. (See the article on cranial malformations, Section 13, p. 429.) Involvement of the perioral region is often in the form of macrostomia or the presence of confluence of the oral cavity with the nasal cavity, maxillary sinus, or orbital region. Classification and treatment of these rare anomalies are beyond the scope of this text, but referral to a regional craniofacial team is indicated to optimize the complex care required.

MACROGLOSSIA

Macroglossia, or tongue enlargement, may be symmetric or asymmetric, with a unilateral form being the most common type. Primary macroglossia may be related to hyperthyroidism, glycogen storage disease, cretinism, or amyloidosis. A rare congenital cause is Beckwith-Wiedemann syndrome, associated with abdominal wall defects and hypoglycemia. Secondary causes include lymphangioma, hemangioma, neurofibroma, cystic lesions, and solid tumors. In the infant, the primary concern with macroglossia is the potential for mechanical airway obstruction. In the young child with significant macroglossia, an open bite and drooling are strong indications for partial tongue excision.

PIERRE ROBIN SEQUENCE

The primary problem in children with the Robin sequence is *retrognathia,* an underdeveloped mandible that is posteriorly displaced. This leads to glossoptosis, or inferior displacement of the tongue. Cleft palate is present in about half of the affected children. Children with Robin sequence often present with respiratory and feeding difficulties, manifested shortly after birth or as late as 1 to 2 months of age. Prone positioning of the infant usually improves both breathing and feeding. Frequent aspiration can accompany the Robin sequence. When the child is supine, upper airway obstruction from the tongue can cause asphyxiation. When the deformity is severe or when conservative positioning maneuvers fail, an operative procedure to secure the tongue forward (a tongue-lip adhesion) can be life-saving. This adhesion is temporary and may be reversed after the neonatal period, when the danger of respiratory obstruction has passed.

Many children with Robin sequence ultimately attain normal dental occlusal relationships, but close follow-up of mandibular growth is indicated. Cleft palate repair is usually delayed to about 18 months of age to allow for development of the upper airway.

TONGUE-TIE

Infants born with a short frenulum extending from the tongue to the central incisor area of the mandible are generally asymptomatic. If there are suspicions that a tongue-tie is leading to speech difficulties, evaluation by an experienced speech pathologist is warranted. Surgical release of the tongue with lengthening of the frenulum is a simple operative procedure that is effective in the rare symptomatic patient.

MACROSTOMIA

The diagnosis of macrostomia, or greatly exaggerated mouth width, is occasionally missed because it is associated with underdevelopment of the mandible. The distance between the midline of the upper or lower lip and the oral commissure is greater on the affected side than on the normal side (except in rare bilateral cases). Macrostomia is commonly associated with the first and second branchial arch syndrome (hemifacial microsomia), with variable hypoplasia of the entire half of the face, including the ear, temporal muscle, masseter muscle, parotid gland, zygoma, maxilla, and mandible. The macrostomia can be surgically corrected by Z-plasty. The management of the jaw and other related deformities is complex and best treated in a craniofacial center.

JAW DEFORMITIES

Micrognathia and Macrognathia

Micrognathia, or small jaw, may occur separately or in association with syndromes such as Pierre Robin sequence or hemifacial microsomia. Macrognathia, an enlargement of the mandible or mandibular prognathism, is characterized by an obtuse angle between the ramus of the mandible and the body of the mandible, often with an open bite deformity. A significant number of small and large mandibles occur as hereditary features and not necessarily as part of a specific syndrome. Unless jaw developmental deformities are extreme, they are usually not apparent until the child is 5 to 6 years of age. The child should be evaluated by an experienced orthodontist who is most capable of assessing dental and jaw development.

Treatment of the majority of children who require operative correction is deferred to the late teens, after full dental eruption. Severe facial deformities due to extreme jaw abnormalities are treated earlier, with treatment influenced by the dentition.

Bony Overgrowth of Jaws

A number of disorders with overgrowth of either the maxilla or mandible are not common but present a problem of diagnosis and treatment.

Arteriovenous Malformation

Overgrowth of the jaw may be the result of arteriovenous malformation, which is usually apparent by the increased prominence of the vessels; by a bruit in the external carotid and its branches to the involved area; and by increased warmth of the soft tissues. The management of an arteriovenous malformation involving the maxilla or mandible is difficult. The disease is invariably progressive and may be punctuated by bleeding episodes that require blood transfusions. Frequently it is necessary to ligate the external carotid artery to control the bleeding, but the ultimate treatment is radical excision of the involved parts. This decision is difficult because the surgery and resulting deformities can be extensive. However, once the diagnosis is established and the progressive risk of serious hemorrhage has been clarified, definitive treatment should be instituted.

Neurofibromatosis

The face may be involved in patients with *neurofibromatosis,* either local or diffuse (as in *von Recklinghausen's disease*). Overgrowth of the soft tissues and bones on the involved side of the face may be a consequence. There is increased bulk of the maxilla or mandible with gingival hypertrophy and displacement of the teeth. Management centers on the excision of offending tissues and sculpturing tissues to correct the deformity. To "cure" the disease with radical resection would entail an extensive operative procedure with removal of many normal structures and is never advisable. The course of this disease depends on the progression and age of onset of symptoms. The earlier the age of onset and the more rapid the course in youth, the worse the prognosis. Hemifacial hypertrophy, with enlargement of all the facial structures unilaterally (including jaws and teeth), presents a similar picture but lacks the soft tissue neurofibromas.

Fibrous Dysplasia

Fibrous dysplasia of the jaws is an unusual condition involving the mandible or maxilla, which is enlarged because of the fibrous and noncalcified tissue within the bone. Fibrous dysplasia is usually not evident until late childhood and is usually self-limited as the child passes puberty and growth ceases. This disorder must be recognized to avoid a radical excision of tissues. Conservative contouring of bone to reduce the deformity can be done to tide the child over until skeletal maturation occurs. In many instances, bony deformities will recur, requiring further operative intervention.

Infantile Cortical Hyperostosis

Infantile cortical hyperostosis *(Caffey's disease)* is a self-limiting disease of children seen with the onset of fever, soft tissue swelling, and periosteal new bone formation of the mandible. It occurs most commonly in the neonatal period (2 to 4 months of age) and may be mistaken for osteomyelitis of the mandible. The clavicles are often involved with overlying brawny induration of the soft tissues. The radiographic picture is one of increased density on the surface of the bone as a result of new bone formation.

In mild cases, no treatment is necessary except comfort measures. With severe involvement, treatment with corticosteroids is indicated. It is recommended that the steroids be continued over several months because exacerbations have occurred with early withdrawal of steroids.

Tumors

Tumors of the facial skeleton include benign and malignant odontogenic tumors (arising from primitive tooth elements) and osteogenic tumors. These tumors are uncommon in children. Treatment depends on the specific histologic diagnosis, with radical resections reserved for the malignant lesions.

TRAUMA

Most injuries about the oral region are minor, and hospitalization is not required. For the occasional severe injury, the most immediate concerns are control of the airway, ventilation, and control of major hemorrhage. Airway obstruction may be due to the tongue, laryngeal edema, or foreign material, including blood, vomitus, or teeth. Airway control may require tracheal intubation or emergency cricothyroidotomy. Most bleeding can be stopped by direct pressure. An adequate airway must be ensured, and a detailed search for other injuries, such as skull fracture, closed head injury, and cervical spine injury, must be undertaken. Evaluation of the thoracic cavity, abdomen, and extremities is mandatory before treatment of facial injuries is instituted.

Fractures

Fractures of the facial skeleton should be suspected in the presence of obvious deformity, asymmetry, bony instability or step-offs, tenderness or crepitance with palpation, dental malocclusion, intraoral lacerations, or visual disturbances. Definitive diagnosis of facial fractures in children will require x-ray evaluation. Plain radiographs, accompanied by panoramic films in selected cases, are most appropriate for the evaluation of the lower facial skeleton. A computed tomographic (CT) scan is essential for the detailed identification of fractures involving the midface and upper facial skeleton.

Fractures of the mandible in children are less common than in adults. Treatment of mandibular fractures in children depends on the site of the fracture as well as the state of the dentition, whether primary or mixed. Mandibular growth must be closely observed after a fracture, especially one involving the condylar and subcondylar regions.

Lacerations

Most lacerations around the mouth and face can be repaired using local anesthesia, often with the addition of mild sedation. Anesthesia in the face is accomplished by direct infiltration of lidocaine (Xylocaine), 1 per cent with epinephrine 1:100,000, or by regional nerve blocks. The entire upper lip can be anesthetized by injecting the infraorbital nerve bilaterally, and the entire lower lip can be anesthetized with bilateral mental nerve blocks. These simple nerve blocks are effective, and the child is usually cooperative once the area is anesthetized.

With the use of antibiotics, it is appropriate to close all facial wounds that are not overly contaminated, despite the fact that many hours have elapsed from the time of injury to the time of treatment. In animal bites or severe contamination, the use of tetanus toxoid, antibiotics, and judicious initial closure or delayed primary closure (within several days of injury) is indicated. An oral first-generation cephalosporin should be used in most instances. In selected cases, intramuscular or intravenous cephalosporins should be considered. It is rarely advisable to allow a wound of the face or oral region to heal secondarily because of the resulting scar deformity. If a wound is closed with the degree of contamination underestimated, close follow-up will allow for drainage of any resulting infection and prevent a serious consequence.

A large number of wounds seen in children in the emergency room are puncture wounds of the lower lip from the incisors. This "through-and-through" wound lacerates the mucosa, lower lip musculature, and skin. It is best cleansed with saline irrigation after local anesthesia and closed primarily. A two- or three-layer closure may be necessary, depending on the size of the wound.

Sutures on the face should be placed close to the edge of the wound and not tied overly tight to avoid suture marks. They should be removed approximately 4 to 5 days following the injury. The wound can be supported after suture removal with a porous adhesive tape, such as Steri-strips. These paper tape closures should remain on the skin for about 5 days.

When the laceration about the lip extends across the mucocutaneous junction (the white line between the vermilion of the mucosa and the skin), care must be taken to align the edges of the wound. This is best done with the aid of magnifying loupes by aligning the fine white "roll" that is apparent due to the thick sebaceous glands at the juncture. A small malalignment will be conspicuous. When there is significant loss of mucosa, it is often advisable to excise the wound in a V fashion and close the wound primarily. Other methods of addressing mucosal loss include rotation of an adjacent mucosal flap or harvesting a mucosal graft. Injuries in which there is a significant loss of lip tissue are difficult, and the reconstruction to restore mucosa, muscle, and skin is complex. Sometimes it is best to close the wounds in a simple fashion and defer extensive reconstructive procedures. When the immediate treating physician is not adequately experienced or if associated injuries prevent extensive primary surgery, it is always wisest to do a simple wound closure. Secondary procedures, which include mucosal flaps, cross-lip flaps, and tongue flaps, should be undertaken only by an experienced surgeon.

Lacerations of the tongue are usually a problem because of extensive bleeding. When necessary, bleeding can be controlled by large sutures encompassing a moderate amount of tongue tissue.

Injuries to Mucosa

In all significant injuries of the mucosa of the mouth, including lips, gingiva, tongue, soft palate, and pharynx, several steps have resulted in diminished infection and improved results. The child should be kept on a clear liquid diet for a minimum of 3 days. This prevents food particles from entering the wound as a nidus for infection. After resuming solid foods, it is wise to rinse the mouth after each meal with water or a mild salt solution (1 teaspoon of salt in a quart of water). Frequent washing of the mouth and irrigation of the wounds in this manner have resulted in excellent wound healing. Most surgeons agree that the use of an oral penicillin or first-generation cephalosporin for 5 days is safe and has resulted in a diminished incidence of wound infection and inflammation.

Injuries to the Parotid Duct

In all significant injuries about the mouth, the treating physician should be aware of possible injury to the parotid duct and facial nerve. Parotid duct injury, if not recognized, can result in parotid secretions into the tissues or in a parotid fistula, which is difficult to manage and often requires secondary procedures. If, on the other hand, the injury to the parotid duct is recognized at the time of injury, repair of the duct is simple and effective and is best accomplished with general anesthesia in the young child.

Injuries to Facial Musculature or Facial Nerve

Injuries to the facial musculature or to the facial nerve should be appreciated before treatment, especially prior to the administration of local anesthetics. The child should be asked to activate all of the muscles of facial expression, and asymmetry should be carefully noted. If injury to the facial nerve occurs anterior to a vertical line through the lateral canthus of the eye, the likelihood of recovery of function without surgical repair of the nerve is excellent. However, if the injury occurs proximal to this line, which is proximal to the anterior border of the masseter muscle, it is prudent to undertake nerve exploration. This must be done using general anesthesia with magnification and microsurgical repair.

Electrical Burns

Electrical burns of the mouth are unusual. They occur most commonly when a toddler places the juncture of an electrical appliance and an extension cord into the mouth. The saliva acts as a conductor and causes an electrical burn. Severe electrical burns can result in a loss of major portions of the upper and lower lip, with the most severe cases involving gingiva, tooth buds, and mandible. Fortunately, most of these injuries involve only the lips and oral commissure. Electrical injuries to the midportion of the upper and lower lip usually heal without severe deformity.

Immediately after the electrical burn, the degree of trauma is usually not evident. The child should be given sedation and antibiotics (oral penicillin or first-generation cephalosporin), and the family must watch the child carefully. *Late bleeding from the labial artery can be dramatic, and if it occurs, it does so 5 to 7 days following injury.* Parents are instructed to watch for bleeding and, if bleeding is present, to pinch the lip between the fingers and bring the child to the emergency room immediately.

Most surgeons prefer to treat electrical burns with antibiotic therapy and to allow secondary healing. This course is followed because it is often difficult to determine the extent of soft tissue loss in the early post-injury phase. By 3 weeks after the burn, demarcation has occurred and the degree of tissue loss is evident. If a late deformity occurs, reconstruction is undertaken electively.

SALIVARY GLAND TUMORS

DOUGLAS W. BELL, M.D.

Hemangiomas are the most common cause of parotid swelling in the newborn. Eighty per cent are present at birth, with the remainder discovered within the next 6 to 12 months. These benign lesions are diffuse, soft masses in the preauricular area and angle of mandible area. There may be a rapid growth for the first 6 months, but there is also regression because of vessel occlusion. There may be some redness of the overlying skin, but as the tumor regresses, the color subsides. The mass may increase in size with crying or straining. Only in a few cases in which the tumor continues to expand is surgery indicated. This involves a superficial parotidectomy, with identification and preservation of the facial nerve, which courses through the gland.

Lymphangiomas are benign congenital lesions of lymph vessels. More than 90 per cent occur in the cervical region, and many involve the parotid or submaxillary gland. These lesions do not undergo spontaneous regression. Thus, surgical dissection must be utilized to remove all the small cystic lesions.

Otherwise, there is a notable recurrence rate and multifocal lesions develop. Laser therapy may be used at times, and cryotherapy is helpful for intraoral lesions.

If the tumor mass develops later in childhood, the mass is usually firmer, more discrete, nontender, and of variable mobility. The most likely tumor is a benign mixed tumor containing both glandular and ductal elements. If such a mass persists, excisional biopsy with facial nerve protection is necessary.

Only 10 per cent of these masses are malignant. Such tumors expand rapidly and may be fixed to other tissues or may be tender. If there is facial paralysis, the tumor is assumed to be malignant. The most common malignant tumors of the parotid gland are mucoepidermoid carcinomas and sarcomas (rhabdomyosarcomas and undifferentiated tumors). Total parotidectomy with facial nerve preserved may be sufficient. If the nerve must be partially excised, immediate grafting techniques are used. Chemotherapy has made great advances and may be used as primary therapy. Radiation therapy is also part of the "triple attack" on these aggressive tumors. The exact protocol is determined by the cell type, rate of growth, and extent of tumor.

Submaxillary gland tumors are usually the benign mixed type and occur in older children. More rapid growth would signal a likely malignant potential. In either case, total removal of the submaxillary gland with sparing of the lingual nerve is the best treatment. Any further chemotherapy or irradiation would be decided based on the tumor cell type.

RECURRENT ACUTE PAROTITIS

ROBERT W. SEIBERT, M.D.

Recurrent acute parotitis (RAP) is an uncommon disease of early childhood to adolescence, with the majority of cases undergoing spontaneous resolution at around puberty. RAP refers to a clinical entity that, by definition, excludes other parotidites occurring as isolated events at the extremes of life: neonatal sialadenitis and acute suppurative parotitis-abscess in the debilitated elderly patient. Although the pathogenesis of adult parotitis may be related to localized lesions, such as Stenson's duct stricture or stones, in the majority of children there appears to be a strong association with pseudocystic dilatation of intralobular ducts or sialectasis. Stasis of ductal secretions leads to secondary bacterial infection with eventual fibrosis and acinar atrophy. The cause of sialectasis is unknown, although postviral inflammatory, autoimmune, and hereditary factors have been postulated. The most common bacterial pathogens isolated are coagulase-positive *Staphylococcus* and *Streptococcus viridans. Streptococcus pneumoniae, Escherichia coli,* and oral aerobic and anaerobic organisms are found less frequently.

CLINICAL PRESENTATION AND DIAGNOSIS

The typical presentation is painful, tender swelling of one or both parotid glands in a 4- to 10-year-old child. There may be low-grade fever and malaise with a slightly elevated white blood cell count and increase in neutrophils. Purulent secretions may be expressed from Stenson's duct orifice. Episodes recur at intervals of weeks to years.

Ultrasonography of the involved gland shows an enlarged, inflamed parotid, also ruling out mass lesions and stones. After resolution of an acute infection, ultrasound frequently shows a nonhomogeneous gland with multiple areas of hypoechogenicity and increased echogenicity, a finding that has been associated with sialectasis. Ultimate confirmation of sialectasis depends on contrast sialography, an invasive procedure that often requires heavy sedation or general anesthesia in a young child.

MANAGEMENT

Treatment may be both acute and prophylactic. Although mild infections apparently resolve without antimicrobial treatment, for most patients a penicillinase-resistant antibiotic is indicated until culture and sensitivity results are available. Amoxicillin–clavulanic acid (30 to 40 mg/kg in divided doses three times per day for 10 days) or erythromycin-sulfisoxazole (30 to 50 mg/kg four times per day) in the penicillin-allergic patient is usually effective as a first-line drug. Supportive measures, such as local heat, analgesics, and good hydration, by intravenous fluids if necessary, are important. Between acute episodes, treatment is directed toward reducing glandular stasis with massage, fluid intake, and sialogogues, such as lemon juice after meals. If bouts of infection occur with increasing frequency, a brief (2- to 3-month) course of a prophylactic antibiotic in a once a day dose might be considered.

Surgical intervention is reserved for cases that progress to complications such as parotid abscess, chronic fistulas, or severe recurrent infections that may be secondary to methicillin-resistant staphylococci. Total parotidectomy with facial nerve preservation is indicated in these rare instances.

DEVELOPMENTAL CYSTS OF THE NECK

STEVEN D. HANDLER, M.D.

BRANCHIAL ARCH CYSTS AND SINUSES

Branchial arch cysts and sinuses represent failure of obliteration of the embryologic branchial arch system. These lesions classically present as a smooth, round swelling at the anterior border of the sternocleidomastoid muscle. If an external opening is present, the diagnosis of branchial cleft sinus or fistula is obvious. (A branchial cleft sinus connects to the overlying skin, whereas a fistula communicates with both the overlying skin and the pharynx medially.) Ultrasound, computed tomography (CT), and magnetic resonance imaging (MRI) are often helpful in differentiating a cyst from a lymph node or other type of neck mass.

Surgical excision is the treatment of choice for these lesions. Sinus and fistula tracts drain continually and are a constant source of local irritation to the neck. Although small cysts may remain asymptomatic, they contain fluid and epithelial debris that have a potential to become infected. Infection of a branchial cleft cyst causes inflammation and scarring that can make surgical excision more difficult. If a lesion becomes infected, systemic antibiotics are administered until the infection subsides (usually 2 to 3 weeks) to permit surgical excision. Rarely, incision and drainage or needle aspiration of an acutely infected cyst may be required to control the infection prior to surgical excision.

Radiographic dye studies of the sinus or fistula tract are unnecessary and often misleading. The dye may not outline the full extent of the tract, or it may extravasate and give an inaccurate picture of the lesion. Similarly, injecting methylene blue into the tract prior to the procedure has the same drawbacks.

The operating surgeon must be familiar with the potential course and connections of the branchial arch anomaly and its relationship to adjacent structures. A second incision may be required to excise long tracts, which may enter the pharynx in the tonsillar fossa or piriform sinus. Any connection to the pharynx must be excised and the opening ligated securely. Incomplete excision of the lesion will result in recurrence of the anomaly.

A first branchial arch anomaly presents added difficulties, both in diagnosis and in management. These lesions present above the level of the hyoid bone and may course medially to the external auditory canal or the middle ear. If a first branchial arch anomaly is suspected, CT scanning is strongly recommended prior to surgical excision. Because these lesions often pass in close proximity to the branches of the facial nerve, the surgeon must begin the operation with a superficial parotidectomy and facial nerve dissection so that these neural elements can be protected during excision of the first branchial arch sinus tract.

THYROGLOSSAL DUCT CYSTS

Thyroglossal duct cysts are epithelial remnants of the embryologic descent of the thyroid gland. They may present anywhere along its course from the base of the tongue to the anterior neck. The typical appearance is that of a smooth, round mass in the midline of the neck at the level of the hyoid bone. The lesion usually moves with protrusion of the tongue and with swallowing. There is no opening to the skin unless the lesion has become infected and drained spontaneously or has been incised and drained.

The diagnosis of a thyroglossal duct cyst is usually obvious on clinical examination. Ultrasound, CT, or MRI may prove helpful in differentiating the lesion from other midline masses such as dermoid cysts or lymph nodes. Imaging of the thyroid gland is mandatory prior to surgical excision of a suspected thyroglossal duct cyst. This is to make sure that the lesion is not, in reality, ectopic thyroid or the child's only functioning thyroid tissue. *Although a thyroid scan has been the traditional imaging technique, we have found that ultrasonography of the neck can detect the thyroid gland in its normal position and has the advantage of avoiding radioactive isotopes.* The study can also be done on one visit to the hospital instead of the two visits required for a thyroid scan.

Surgical excision of a suspected thyroglossal duct cyst is the treatment of choice. Infection of a thyroglossal duct cyst causes inflammation and scarring that can make surgical excision more difficult. If a lesion becomes infected, systemic antibiotics are administered until the infection subsides (usually 2 to 3 weeks) to permit surgical excision. Rarely, incision and drainage or needle aspiration of an acutely infected cyst may be required to control the infection prior to surgical excision. Because the descent of the thyroid gland may leave epithelial remnants adjacent to, or within, the hyoid bone, the central portion of the hyoid bone is removed (Sistrunk procedure) with the surgical specimen. This does not create any disability in the child and decreases the chance of incomplete excision and subsequent recurrence of the lesion.

DISORDERS OF THE ESOPHAGUS

ARTHUR R. EULER, M.D.

Any classification of general esophageal disorders will not be entirely satisfactory because of the vast array of diseases that must be included. Although flawed in some aspects, a division into congenital and acquired lesions is used in this article because it is useful in the understanding of therapeutic approaches. These tend to be surgical for congenital disorders and medical and/or surgical for the acquired ones.

CONGENITAL ESOPHAGEAL DISORDERS

Congenital esophageal problems are usually associated with significant morbidity and occasional mortality. Clinical presentation usually involves swallowing difficulties, with the onset most often being soon after birth. If the clinical presentation is primarily one of a respiratory nature, it may not present until later and diagnosis is often delayed. For an optimal prognosis, these types of esophageal lesions require expert experienced pediatric surgical and medical specialists. Management should be undertaken in a neonatal or pediatric intensive care unit.

Esophageal Atresia with Tracheoesophageal Fistula

Approximately 85 per cent of congenital esophageal anomalies are characterized by a blind pouch, usually located in the upper half of the esophagus, plus a communication between a distal esophageal segment and the tracheobronchial tract. The gestational history is often associated with polyhydramnios, with the neonatal history being one of drooling, nasal drainage, and slight respiratory distress, followed by significant exacerbations of all these symptoms when the first oral feeding is taken.

Treatment is begun by elevating the head and upper thorax approximately 20 degrees and administering supplemental oxygen as required to maintain proper tissue oxygenation. The upper esophageal pouch is intubated, evacuated, and subsequently drained continuously with low-pressure suction. Hydration and nutrition are maintained with parenteral fluids until a gastrostomy tube is placed, which is usually done using local anesthesia soon after the diagnosis is made. Broad-spectrum antibiotics that cover the types of bacteria usually associated with aspiration pneumonia should be started. These measures lessen further pulmonary complications and provide necessary nutritional support until a definitive surgical repair is performed. This repair should not be undertaken until the neonate's condition is stable, particularly in regard to respiratory status.

Although some centers use a physiologic assessment approach that does not utilize weight, gestational age, or pulmonary condition as an absolute parameter, the most common determinants underlying choice of a surgical approach are the patient's weight and pulmonary status as initially defined in the classification system by Waterston. In group A, which contains neonates weighing above 2.5 kg who do not have aspiration pneumonitis or other abnormalities, an immediate single-stage approach via a right thoracotomy incision is appropriate. In group B are two separate clinical divisions: those who weigh between 1.8 and 2.5 kg and are well and those who weigh more but have moderate pulmonary disease and/or other moderately severe congenital anomalies. These patients are best managed by an initial period of gastrostomy feedings and medical therapy for their other problems before surgery is undertaken. In group C are those who are smaller (weighing less than 1.8 kg) and/or have severe pulmonary disease or congenital anomalies. These are best managed by fistula ligation and nutritional support, either parenterally or by gastrostomy, for several weeks before a definite esophageal repair is undertaken.

In very small neonates (weighing under 1.0 kg), some centers have recommended initial bonding of the gastroesophageal junction with gastrotomy. Definitive repair is undertaken when growth has occurred and lung function has improved. Other centers have reported excellent overall survival (90 per cent) with preliminary repair without gastrotomy.

One difficulty in correcting esophageal atresia is that a primary anastomosis of the proximal and distal segments may be impossible if the intervening gap is very great. Several surgical techniques have now been developed to elongate the two segments with the goal of eventually obtaining a primary anastomosis, thereby avoiding the necessity of a colonic or gastric tube interposition. End-to-side junctions are preferred because the incidence of side effects is less than with an end-to-end anastomosis.

Postoperatively gastrostomy feedings with glucose water are initiated when evidence of adequate gastric emptying is documented. Salivary secretions are continually and gently suctioned via a nasal catheter, which is usually placed at surgery just above the anastomotic site. Oral feedings are not initiated until 10 to 14 days postoperatively.

Leaks from the anastomotic site are the major and most serious postoperative complication. The most important pathogenetic factor underlying the development of such leaks is anastomotic tension determined by the distance between the esophageal pouches. An initial sign of an anastomotic leak is often saliva and/or feedings in the chest tube drainage. With extrapleural repairs, these leaks usually spontaneously remit so they are only followed expectantly with cessation of oral feedings and institution of parenteral nutrition. With transpleural repairs, serious empyema may occur; therefore, management consists of a cervical esophagostomy, distal esophageal closure, antibiotics, and chest tube drainage. Although anastomotic leaks occur in the early postoperative period, other problems, such as strictures at the anastomotic site, appear later. These are treated with repeated bougienage as necessary. *A significant factor in the development of these anastomotic strictures is gastroesophageal reflux, which is an almost universal finding. This may be treated with a histamine H_2 receptor antagonist, such as ranitidine (4 to 6 mg/kg/day in two divided doses) or cimetidine (1200 mg/1.7 m^2/day in four divided doses) and bethanechol (8.7 mg/m^2/day given in three divided doses);* often, however, esophagitis, stricture formation, and pulmonary disease still develop, with a Nissen fundoplication required. The severity of the complications induced by the gastroesophageal reflux is compounded by the abnormal esophageal peristaltic activity that all such patients have, particularly below the level of the anastomosis. There is no effective treatment for this. A less frequent postoperative complication is a recurrence of the tracheoesophageal fistula. This is treated by a second fistula ligation.

Being slow to feed, refusing meals, coughing and choking while eating, and vomiting are other common long-term postoperative medical problems, occurring in 50 per cent of children at age 7 years in one series. Hospital staff trained in nutrition and feeding disorders are invaluable, as are parent support groups in dealing with these problems.

Esophageal Atresia Without Tracheoesophageal Fistula

This type of atresia is present in fewer than 10 per cent of patients with these types of congenital esophagotracheobronchial anomalies. The approach is similar to that mentioned previously, with gastrostomy feeding being initiated along with measures to protect against further pulmonary aspiration by applying gentle suction to the proximal pouch. Any pulmonary disease is treated with appropriate antibiotics and oxygen as required. The definitive surgical approach is as for those with an associated tracheoesophageal fistula.

Tracheoesophageal Fistula Without Esophageal Atresia

This anomaly represents a smaller overall number, approximately 4 per cent, of these types of lesions. It is, however, the most difficult to diagnose because there is no abrupt and dramatic onset of symptomatology soon after birth. Rather, there is usually an insidious course of recurrent pulmonary problems resulting in a delay in proper diagnosis that may range from a few weeks to months. Any delay in surgery is usually due to delay in proper diagnosis rather than a delay in clinical presentation.

Esophagrams with barium infusion via a nasogastric tube into the esophageal lumen may be a more accurate diagnostic approach for this type of fistula than conventional radiographic methods. Bronchoscopy should be considered if the tube esophagram is negative. Most fistulas can be ligated by a cervical approach because most are located in the proximal esophagus; however, a thoracotomy is required for those located in the most distal esophagus.

Laryngotracheoesophageal Cleft

This anomaly results from nonfusion of the upper tracheoesophageal septum and cricoid primordium. In up to 20 per cent of patients, other anomalies such as esophageal atresia and tracheoesophageal fistula are present. The initial medical therapy for these infants is the same as for those with esophageal atresia and a tracheoesophageal fistula. These infants often have other severe congenital anomalies that require very skillful medical management. The mortality with laryngotracheoesophageal cleft alone is very high, often resulting from a delay in proper diagnosis. Endoscopic evaluation is very important, although the lesion may be confusing at endoscopy. The passage of an endotracheal tube into the larynx may be helpful because this placement often opens the cleft, confirming the diagnosis. Management can then be either by the endotracheal tube or by tracheostomy. Even with either of these in place, gastroesophageal reflux with aspiration still remains a problem. Maneuvers such as a double gastrostomy have been advocated to prevent this. Definitive early surgical repair should be undertaken as soon as the infant's overall condition permits.

Webs and Stenoses

Esophageal webs are composed of mucosa and submucosa but do not contain muscle. Congenital webs and stenoses are uncommon compared with strictures associated with gastroesophageal reflux. The clinical presentation of both these congenital lesions, however, is very similar to that seen with gastroesophageal reflux–induced strictures. This usually includes vomiting, dysphagia, and/or repeated pulmonary infections. These congenital lesions usually respond to bougienage, and surgical repair is rarely needed. Schatzki rings and other disorders associated with webs, such as the Plummer-Vinson syndrome, are covered in the text on acquired lesions.

Rings

Esophageal and tracheal compression can result from vascular anomalies, including a double aortic arch, an aberrant right subclavian artery, and a right aortic arch with a left ligamentum arteriosum. The resulting constriction may cause partial esophageal obstruction, resulting in dysphagia, vomiting, and/or respiratory distress, usually manifested by stridor. Diagnostic methods may include barium esophagram, bronchoscopy, computed tomography (CT), and angiography. Definitive vascular surgery is corrective; if symptoms are mild, however, surgery is often delayed until age 6 or 12 months, when the infant is larger.

Duplications

Duplications are usually cystic structures filled with fluid only; if they are of the neuroenteric type, there are always associated vertebral malformations. Clinical presentations may include gastrointestinal symptoms, such as vomiting or dysphagia, or respiratory ones, such as cough, wheezing, or dyspnea. With simple duplication cysts, excision via a thoracotomy is all that is required. Careful dissection is mandatory, for cysts may be multiple, may have a fine connection with the esophagus, and may be associated with extralobar pulmonary sequestration or diaphragmatic hernia. Magnetic resonance imaging (MRI) has been reported to be an accurate diagnostic method for evaluation of possible duplications, particularly cervical ones.

Diverticula

Rarely, congenital diverticula have been reported to be associated with tracheoesophageal fistula, but most occur alone. They are usually simple protrusions of mucosa and submucosa without any muscular component. Those immediately above the upper esophageal sphincter are called Zenker's diverticula, whereas those in the mid-esophagus or directly orad to the lower esophageal sphincter are called traction and epiphrenic diverticula, respectively. Zenker's diverticula are usually managed with a one-stage diverticulectomy. If the diverticulum is very small, some have advocated a cricomyotomy alone, which is intended to decrease esophageal pressure in the proximal esophagus. In patients with extremely large diverticula, one-stage diverticulectomy plus a cricopharyngeal myotomy may be considered.

Traction (mid-esophageal) diverticula are most often multiple and associated with an esophageal motor disorder. Unless they are extremely large, therapy is usually not indicated.

Epiphrenic diverticula are also thought to be associated with an esophageal motor disorder. Surgical therapy is directed at removing the diverticulum, and a myotomy is aimed at correcting the motor dysfunction, such as achalasia or diffuse esophageal spasm.

Sucking and Swallowing Problems

The coordination of sucking, swallowing, and breathing requires a high degree of neural sophistication. Many neonates and infants have only a mild motor dysfunction that requires a careful history and physical examination to exclude other disorders, plus instructions regarding feeding techniques and reassurance to the parents. In the case of a discrete lesion, such as a palatal cleft, that is interfering with the patient's ability to coordinate these activities, specific corrective therapy should be applied. These patients also benefit from being fed upright so that gravity can be used to prevent some nasopharyngeal reflux. If specific measures aimed at alleviating these problems are unsuccessful, a feeding gastrostomy should be considered. Unless such disorders are associated with other significant clinical abnormalities, most will improve with age so that most of these infants can eventually be returned to oral feedings. Such significant disorders include severe mental and physical impairments that result in swallowing incoordination. In these patients, a feeding gastrotomy placed in the gastric lesser curvature is often required. Whether an accompanying antireflux procedure should be done is a matter of some debate at present. In those with documented gastroesophageal reflux, this type of procedure should probably be undertaken when the gastrotomy is performed.

ACQUIRED DISORDERS OF THE ESOPHAGUS

Neuromuscular disorders of the esophagus can be either primary, as in cricopharyngeal dysfunction, or secondary, as in scleroderma.

Cricopharyngeal Dysfunction

This disorder, which involves abnormal upper esophageal sphincter relaxation, is also known as *cricopharyngeal achalasia* or *spasm.* Although usually primary in nature, cricopharyngeal dysfunction may be one of the manifestations of a systemic disorder, such as familial dysautonomia or generalized neural immaturity, as in a premature infant.

Pharmacologic therapy is not usually very helpful, although anticholinergics may decrease salivation somewhat, thereby reducing symptoms. Treatment is directed toward the primary systemic disease. Dilatation has been advocated and may be tried, although a large clinical trial assessing its efficacy has not been reported. Cricopharyngeal myotomy remains the definitive therapy. *Before this is undertaken, it is vital that the presence of a Zenker's diverticulum and the extremely rare occurrence of an organic lesion be excluded. If the dysfunction is secondary, treatment of the primary systemic disease is extremely important.*

Diffuse Esophageal Spasm

Diffuse esophageal spasm, which usually has a clinical presentation consisting of dysphagia and chest pain, has been associated with paroxysmal posturing, irritability, regurgitation, aspiration, and recurrent pneumonia in mentally retarded infants and children. Diagnosis is made by documenting tertiary contractions during an esophageal manometric study. Dilatations are not useful, nor does drug therapy give uniform clinical results. Long-acting nitrates in increasing doses have been reported to be helpful in some adult patients. Severe headaches are a serious side effect limiting their use. Calcium channel blocking agents, such as nifedipine, may eventually be shown to be the drug class of choice. In severe cases, a long esophageal myotomy may be considered.

Achalasia

Achalasia, or cardiospasm, is a disorder associated with failure of the lower esophageal sphincter to relax properly, with abnormal peristalsis in the smooth muscle portion of the esophagus and eventually often extreme dilatation of the esophageal body *(megaesophagus).* A familial history is rare, although sibling involvement without a history of consanguinity has been reported emphasizing the importance of good history taking. *With increasing immigration to the United States, the clinician should always be alert to the possibility of Chagas disease when achalasia occurs in children who have lived in Central or South America, particularly Brazil.*

The treatment of choice for most pediatric-age patients remains pneumatic dilatation or surgical myotomy of the lower esophageal sphincter. Simple bougienage is not effective. Pneumatic dilatation frequently gives sustained periods of relief in some children, but hospitalization is necessary because of the need for sedation and the risk of esophageal perforation. Endoscopic pneumodilatation has been reported, although it is not widely practiced at present. Dilatation may not be appropriate for younger children because of the increased risk of perforation. For these younger patients and older children who do not respond to dilatation or require frequent dilatation, a Heller myotomy is indicated.

If a long myotomy is required, an antireflux procedure such as a Nissen or Thal fundoplication should be considered. Because these antireflux procedures have been associated with severe, prolonged, postoperative dysphagia, however, they should be approached appropriately and performed only by pediatric surgeons experienced in treating achalasia.

Connective Disease Disorders

Esophageal dysfunction is found in a high percentage of patients with scleroderma, dermatomyositis, and mixed connective tissue disease and in a smaller percentage of those with systemic lupus erythematosus and periarteritis. It is also a significant gastrointestinal manifestation of diabetes mellitus; however, because this esophageal complication seems to occur only after the primary disease is present for many years, this type of esophageal dysfunction is very rare during the pediatric years. All of these diseases, when esophageal complications arise, are associated with abnormal peristaltic activity, low or absent lower esophageal sphincter pressure, and less often with a hypotensive upper esophageal sphincter. This pathophysiology results most often in gastroesophageal reflux, and subsequent complications, particularly strictures, are common. Therapy is directed at reducing the acid content of the refluxed material by intensive use of antacids or histamine H_2 receptor antagonists. Elevation of the head of the bed and fasting for a few hours before bedtime are also useful.

Metoclopramide (0.5 mg/kg/day) given in three divided doses has been used to enhance peristaltic activity and to increase lower esophageal sphincter pressure. Frequent bougienage may be required to treat strictures. In severe cases, a fundoplication may be needed to stop the gastroesophageal reflux and an interposition with colon or jejunum may be necessary to relieve the stricture.

Patients with chronic idiopathic intestinal pseudoobstruction syndrome may have a neurogenic, myogenic, or combined etiology for their disease and often have esophageal manometric abnormalities but rarely are symptomatic. Therapy is rarely needed; if it is, it should be directed at whatever esophageal abnormality exists. For example, if gastroesophageal reflux is the reason for the symptoms, the pharmacologic therapy discussed above should be considered.

Patients with cerebral palsy frequently experience vomiting and occasionally dysphagia. This usually results from abnormalities in lower esophageal sphincter pressure and peristalsis. Severe gastroesophageal reflux and stricture formation often occur. Therapy should be directed at decreasing the acid content of the refluxed material and increasing peristaltic activity with antacids or histamine H_2 receptor antagonists plus metoclopramide, respectively. Strictures should be treated with bougienage. Fundoplication may be required in cases that do not respond.

Esophageal abnormalities in patients with familial dysautonomia usually are similar to those in achalasia except that peristalsis is preserved. Neostigmine occasionally has been helpful. Measurements to prevent pulmonary aspiration, such as elevation of the head of the bed, fasting before bedtime, and sleeping prone, are important. A gastrostomy and fundoplication often are required.

Webs and Rings

Rings differ from webs in that they contain muscle in addition to mucosa and submucosa. The Plummer-Vinson or Paterson-Brown-Kelly syndrome consists of an upper esophageal web and iron-deficiency anemia. Abnormalities in gastric acid secretion and pernicious anemia may also occur. Treatment consists of bougienage and iron replacement. The risk of esophageal carcinoma is high; therefore, the importance of a surveillance program should be explained to the patient.

Schatzki rings are found in the distal esophagus and have been found at autopsy to mark the junction of esophageal and gastric epithelium, which is abnormally placed above the diaphragm. Often a simple explanation of the abnormal anatomic position of this junction plus instruction regarding the importance of chewing food slowly and the avoidance of swallowing large boluses is all that is required. If this is not sufficient, bougienage is indicated. Rarely is pneumatic dilatation required. Lower esophageal rings, if they can be distinguished from the more common Schatzki rings, should be treated with bougienage. These rings have been reported with the VACTERL syndrome (*v*ertebral, *a*nal, *c*ardiac, *t*racheal, *e*sophageal, *r*enal, and *l*imb anomalies).

Infectious Diseases

Thrush is the most common childhood candidal infection. With esophageal involvement, nystatin (Mycostatin, 250,000 units suspended in 10 ml of water every 2 hours) is indicated. Some have advocated suspending the drug in a viscous solution of 0.5 per cent methylcellulose and 0.7 per cent carboxymethylcellulose to improve adherence to the esophageal mucosa. With treatment failures, amphotericin, flucytosine, miconazole, and ketoconazole should be considered. Miconazole and ketoconazole are the least toxic of these therapeutic agents. The usual intravenous dosage for miconazole is 20 to 40 mg/kg/day, divided into three infusions given over 30 to 60 minutes. Ketoconazole is given as a once-daily oral dose of 3.3 to 6.6 mg/kg. Some studies suggest that a daily dosage of 7 to 10 mg/kg given two or three times a day may achieve better therapeutic serum concentrations.

Herpetic esophagitis often produces severe odynophagia, and although it is found most often in the debilitated host, it can also be documented in apparently immunologically competent patients. For this latter group, no specific treatment is usually warranted but symptomatic relief with cool liquid meals and viscous lidocaine is frequently helpful. In severe cases or with debilitated hosts, acyclovir (250 mg/m^2/day intravenously) may be considered.

Cytomegalovirus is the most frequently reported viral etiology of upper gastrointestinal disease in children. Herpes zoster-varicella virus has also been reported to cause esophagitis. Therapy for these viral causes of esophagitis is supportive and usually associated with a good prognosis.

Crohn's disease occasionally affects the esophagus. Except for the usual treatment regimen of sulfasalazine and corticosteroids, no specific therapy is available.

Graft-versus-host disease, although not a primary infectious disease of the esophagus, may involve the entire organ and can cause severe problems such as chest pain, dysphagia, and reflux symptoms. No specific therapy is available.

Mallory-Weiss Tears

Forceful vomiting or retching, particularly if recurrent and prolonged, can result in mucosal tears associated with hematemesis. Most of such bleeding remits without treatment; in recalcitrant cases, surgery should be undertaken, although some have advocated that a left gastric artery infusion of vasopressin be attempted first. Decisions regarding operative intervention should involve degree of blood loss and endoscopic appearance plus extent of the tear.

Perforation

Esophageal perforations may be *spontaneous,* as they frequently are during the neonatal period, or *induced,* as they most often are during childhood. The latter are usually caused by some instrumentation, usually of a blind nature; by chest trauma, such as that occurring in an automobile accident; or as a complication of caustic ingestion. Recently, there has been an increased association with endoscopy, particularly in neonates. The prognosis depends primarily on an early diagnosis and treatment. Surgery is the mainstay of therapy except perhaps in the case of a small cervical tear, in which a nonoperative approach consisting of antibiotics, parenteral nutrition, and close observation may be considered. The latter approach would be an exception.

Foreign Bodies

Foreign bodies can be removed from the esophagus in the most controlled and safe manner, with the child under general anesthesia and an endotracheal tube in place. In such a procedure, the most significant and serious complication occurring during foreign body removal from the esophagus—the aspiration of the foreign body into the tracheobronchial tree—can be avoided. *Because of this hazard, the removal of foreign bodies by means of a Foley catheter or while the child is receiving only parenteral sedation without an endotracheal tube in place should be avoided.* Most foreign bodies, regardless of shape or size, can be removed endoscopically. Recently the use of a magnetic tube to facilitate the removal of metallic objects, particularly button batteries, has been advocated. When these objects cannot be removed from the esophagus, an acceptable alternative is to dislodge them into the stomach, from which most foreign bodies pass without difficulty. If button batteries are dislodged into the stomach, attempts to remove them should continue because of possible bleeding, mercury poisoning, and mucosal burns if the battery were to rupture.

Another special case of an esophageal foreign body is a meat bolus that has become lodged in the esophageal lumen. Meat tenderizer may be considered to help resolve the obstruction. Papain (5 ml every 30 minutes for 4 to 6 hours) is given. Most often, the obstruction is relieved in 18 to 24 hours; if not, it can usually be relieved during subsequent endoscopy. Because meat tenderizer use has been associated with hypernatremia and erosions of the esophageal mucosa, close observation for the former and endoscopy for the latter are recommended.

Chemical Burns

The most commonly ingested chemicals are strong alkalis, usually the sodium or potassium hydroxide contained in drain cleaners. Most other alkalis and acids accidentally ingested by children are not usually associated with a high incidence or severity of esophageal damage. Suicide attempts with strong acids, such as concentrated hydrochloric or nitric acid, are, however, associated with severe injury. The presence or absence of oral injury is not predictive of esophageal lesions. Immediate first aid should consist of drinking a liquid, such as milk, to dilute the ingested substance to reduce further gastric damage and esophageal damage if reflux occurs. *Vomiting should not be induced.* Parenteral fluids should be started and a chest radiograph taken to exclude mediastinitis. Esophagoscopy should be performed within 24 hours and should be terminated as soon as an area of esophageal burn is encountered. If no lesions are found, the child is discharged without further treatment except for proper poison prevention instruction and psychiatric consultation if ingestion was a suicide gesture. In those with esophageal lesions, a broad-spectrum antibiotic is started. A special nasogastric tube, which serves as an intraesophageal stent, has been documented in a number of trials to be effective in preventing stricture formation. *Corticosteroid use has proved to be ineffective and is not indicated.* A tracheostomy may be required if laryngeal edema is present. A gastrostomy may also be placed at the time of the anesthesia for the endoscopy if severe lesions are seen. In severe cases, if a nasogastric tube intraluminal stent is not being utilized, a surgical thread is passed into the stomach as soon as the patient can swallow. This thread serves as the guide for future bougienage to relieve stricture formation; often, however, severe strictures that require an interposition of colon or jejunum still develop.

Because the risk for development of subsequent esophageal squamous cell carcinoma development in patients with severe lesions is high, a long-term prophylactic surveillance program should be undertaken. The most frequent time for such carcinoma formation is approximately 50 years after the ingestion, with the most common location being at the tracheal bifurcation.

Tumors

Most esophageal tumors encountered during childhood are benign, including leiomyomas, lipomas, inflammatory polyps, hemangiomas, hamartomas, and neurofibromas. In rare instances, leiomyosarcomas, lymphomas, squamous cell carcinomas, or some other type of gastric cancer may invade the esophagus. Clinical presentation usually involves one or more of the following: dysphagia, dyspnea, chest pain, or cough. Confusion with achalasia is frequent. Endoscopy with biopsy and cytologic examination is diagnostic. All of these tumors are treated by surgical resection. Leukemias are treated by radiation, parenteral chemotherapy, or a combination of both.

Varices

Hepatic disease–induced portal hypertension often results in severe gastrointestinal bleeding episodes. Patients presenting with this type of hemorrhage should be managed in an intensive care unit. Blood for typing and cross-matching of at least 2 units of blood (depending on the child's size) should be obtained, and both central venous and arterial blood pressure lines should be placed. In pediatric centers skilled in the technique, the primary approach is endoscopic sclerotherapy. In such centers, control of the bleeding and subsequent varix obliteration is achieved in the vast majority of cases. These objectives are accomplished by direct injection of a sclerosing agent into the varices. Although control of the hemorrhage is achieved most often with the initial injection, obliteration usually takes multiple subsequent injections. Complications of the technique include continued bleeding, retrosternal discomfort, esophageal ulcerations, stricture formation, and aspiration pneumonia. These problems can usually be treated conservatively. Recurrence of varices and hemorrhage usually occurs in fewer than 10 per cent of patients treated with sclerotherapy.

Another approach utilized in pediatric centers without the availability of endoscopic sclerotherapy is the placement of a pediatric Sengstaken-Blakemore tube and subsequent monitoring by personnel skilled in its use. The usual initial esophageal balloon pressure should range from 30 to 40 mm Hg up to the normal adult pressure of 40 to 60 mm Hg, depending on the child's size. Pulmonary aspiration is a significant complication arising from the use of this tube. Vasopressin should be given via a peripheral vein at a dose of 0.2 to 0.4 unit/1.73 m^2/minute. Side effects include water retention with subsequent hyponatremia, hypertension, cardiac arrhythmia, and seizure that results from the first two effects. If bleeding continues despite 24 hours of the above treatment or the patient's condition begins to deteriorate, surgery should be undertaken to decompress the portal vascular bed, as would be the case in patients whose bleeding fails to respond to sclerotherapy.

For patients who do cease bleeding after Sengstaken-Blakemore tube placement and vasopression administration, referral to a pediatric center skilled in sclerotherapy should be undertaken so that elective obliteration of the varices can be done. This usually requires repeated injections at 2- to 4-week intervals. *Somatostatin,* which has shown excellent results in stopping various types of gastrointestinal bleeding in adults, may assume an important role in the treatment of variceal hemorrhage, since it is associated with a low incidence of complications plus a higher efficacy rate than vasopressin.

Esophagitis and Strictures

These lesions are most often caused by prolonged repeated exposures of the esophageal mucosa to acidic gastric contents. If esophagitis is present, a regimen designed to reduce or neutralize the acidic content of the refluxed material and increase lower esophageal sphincter pressure plus enhance esophageal peristalsis should be undertaken. The former can be accomplished with antacids (30 ml/1.73 m^2/day in four divided doses), ranitidine (4 to 6 mg/kg/day in two divided doses), or cimetidine (1200 mg/1.73 m^2/day in four divided doses). Ranitidine has the advantages of less frequent dosing and little inhibitory effect on the hepatic cytochrome P_{450} isoenzyme system. The latter may be important when patients are taking other concomitant therapies such as theophylline. If an adequate response is not achieved after approximately 12 weeks of therapy, an agent to enhance esophageal peristalsis, such as bethanechol (8.7 mg/m^2/day), or metoclopramide (0.5 mg/kg/day), may be added to the regimen. Between these latter two drugs, metoclopramide is the drug of choice if delayed gastric emptying is also present because it increases this function better than bethanechol. Extrapyramidal symptoms occur with metoclopramide hydrochloride use, but these can be stopped with diphenhydramine hydrochloride. *Metoclopramide therapy should be terminated if these occur.* An alternative approach would be to increase the dose of the histamine H_2 receptor antagonist guided by its effect on 24-hour esophageal acid contact time (ACT). Although the exact reduction in ACT required to achieve healing is not known, a good objective is for the reduction to be less than 6 per cent per 24 hours.

In addition to the drug therapy listed above, postural therapy at an angle of 60 degrees should be maintained 24 hours a day in infants. Feedings should be thickened and given more frequently than normal, up to every 3 hours. In older patients, elevation of the head of the bed and fasting after the evening meal should be included along with cessation of smoking. With infants, these regimens should be continued until symptoms have been controlled and esophagitis is healed if it is present. With older children, therapy should probably be continued indefinitely, although studies supporting this position have not been done in this age group. In patients who do not respond to medical therapy over a period of 3 to 4 months and have severe disease, particularly if associated with Barrett's epithelium or a stricture, a fundoplication of either the Nissen or Thal type should be considered. If a stricture is present, bougienage is indicated at the initiation of the medical regimen and should be repeated as necessary until the stricture is relieved.

Repeated bougienage is often required in patients with chronic granulomatous disease and the dystrophic form of epidermolysis bullosa. In both diseases, dysphagia is often a major complaint, with patients with epidermolysis bullosa frequently also experiencing odynophagia. Some believe that dilatation is contraindicated in the latter patients, although some reports have indicated that skilled clinicians can accomplish successful dilatations with subsequent remissions lasting for a number of years. Corticosteroid therapy is also often helpful, with tapering of daily therapeutic dosages to maintenance levels being undertaken when relief of symptoms is achieved. Interposition surgery may be required in severe cases.

REFERENCES

Mahoney MJ, Migliavacca M, Milla PJ: Motor disorders of the esophagus in gastroesophageal reflux. Arch Dis Child 63:1333–1338, 1988.

Mayberry JF, Atkinson M: Achalasia and other diseases associated with disorders of gastrointestinal mobility. Hepatogastroenterology 33:206–207, 1986.

Milla PJ: Intestinal motility and its disorders. Clin Gastroenterol 15:121–136, 1986.

GASTROESOPHAGEAL REFLUX

JOHN J. HERBST, M.D.

Gastroesophageal reflux (GER) is one of the most common chronic gastrointestinal problems in children. Some amount of gastroesophageal reflux, especially after a meal, is common and physiologic in both children and adults.

The challenge to the physician is to identify which children are having significant problems and to treat them appropriately. In adults, heartburn is the most common symptom; in children, vomiting and respiratory symptoms are more common. The much greater occurrence of vomiting as a symptom of GER in children may be related to the fact that the reservoir capacity is only 6 ml in infants in contrast to 160 ml in adults; yet children ingest more than two times the volume on a weight basis than do adults. In infants, excessive spitting and vomiting usually improve as the size of the esophagus increases and an upright position is maintained at about 1 year of age. In the past, lower esophageal sphincter pressure was thought to be the prime determinant of GER. Pressure in the sphincter is not static, and reflux often occurs after brief spontaneous relaxation of the sphincter; however, many other factors, including increased abdominal pressure, gastric emptying, esophageal motility, salivation, swallowing, pharyngeal motor function, and central nervous system factors play a role in causing or altering the effects of GER. Hiatal hernia, position of the sphincter and angle of insertion of the esophagus into the stomach, and presence of a gastrostomy are anatomic factors that affect sphincter competence.

If esophageal motility is depressed, clearance of acid from the esophagus will be delayed, causing inflammation of the esophageal mucosa. Spontaneous salivation with swallowing washes the last traces of acid from the esophagus. Because salivation and frequency of swallowing are decreased during sleep, nighttime reflux is often prolonged and associated with severe esophagitis. If there is even minimal incoordination of the swallowing mechanism, there may be microaspiration and stimulation of chemoreceptors in the upper esophagus and pharynx following GER causing apnea or other symptoms of respiratory distress. Coughing, choking, wheezing, stridor, hyperextension of the neck, and/or tongue movements associated with refluxed material in the pharynx may be misinterpreted as signs of primary pulmonary disease, seizures or other central nervous system disorders rather than as symptoms of GER. Repeated expulsion of a large portion of refluxed material from the nares is suggestive of nasopharyngeal incompetence. Vomiting of large amounts of food may cause loss of weight or failure to thrive. It must be remembered that similar symptoms may be due to many other factors, including food intolerance, partial intestinal obstruction, reactive airway disease, and neurologic disorders.

DIAGNOSIS

Esophageal function and reflux may be evaluated with a variety of methods, including fluoroscopy, upper gastrointestinal scintigraphy, ultrasound, esophageal motility studies, prolonged esophageal pH monitoring, endoscopy, and biopsy of esophageal mucosa. Not all patients with symptoms of GER need to be studied, and all diagnostic methods are rarely needed to achieve a diagnosis. A careful history and physical examination can provide much valuable information and, for many patients, may be the only evaluation needed, especially in infants whose main problem is vomiting or spitting after meals. A more extensive evaluation is warranted if it is unclear whether the symptoms are caused by GER, if they are persisting despite medical therapy, if they are severe, or if surgery is being considered. Tests may confirm the presence of abnormal GER, rule out diseases that produce similar symptoms, or determine whether certain unusual symptoms are caused by GER. Because the tests must distinguish between normal physiologic reflux and an excessive amount, no test is infallible. An upper gastrointestinal (GI) series is almost universally available and generally provides valuable information. Although results of upper GI series will vary, 15 to 20 per cent of patients with GER will not be identified and at least a 25 per cent rate of false-positive results may be expected. More importantly, other conditions that may result in similar symptoms, such as duodenal bands, stenosis, volvulus, or other causes of partial intestinal obstruction can be detected. An upper GI series can also evaluate esophageal motility and the swallowing mechanism (especially if recorded on video tape).

Because some patients have severe vomiting with weight loss or failure to thrive as the major problem whereas others have major respiratory symptoms with minimal vomiting or spitting, it is obvious that superior esophageal sphincter function and pharyngeal clearance mechanisms are important in determining clinical symptoms. Unfortunately, present methods to study esophageal motility are not sophisticated enough to detect the subtle problems of pharyngeal clearance that are assuredly present. Thus, motility studies have limited clinical usefulness in evaluating patients with GER, although increased tertiary esophageal contractions and decreased lower esophageal sphincter tone commonly accompany severe reflux esophagitis.

Gastric scintiscan is simple, relatively noninvasive, and very sensitive in detecting reflux. Because some reflux is physiologic and scanning over the esophagus is relatively brief, it has limitations similar to a barium swallow. The test can provide evidence regarding gastric emptying, and reflux of the label into the lung field can document aspiration. Nevertheless, this has not been a very clinically helpful aspect of the test.

Flexible endoscopy and esophageal biopsy can evaluate esophagitis. Severe esophagitis with infiltration of eosinophils and polymorphonuclear leukocytes in esophageal biopsies may be noted without significant endoscopic changes. Milder changes are noted only on biopsy and include increased thickening of the basal layer and increased penetration of the dermal pegs into the stratified squamous epithelium. Such changes are noted in only about 15 per cent of patients without symptoms of GER but in approximately 95 per cent of patients with pathologic GER.

Prolonged pH monitoring is considered the "gold standard" by many, but it is an expensive, time-consuming test. Because sampling time is long, it is very good at separating pathologic from physiologic reflux. pH monitoring can document severity and frequency of reflux in infants who cannot communicate, and it can document reflux that occurs in the absence of obvious symptoms or during sleep. A causal relationship can be inferred if pH monitoring demonstrates that symptoms such as cough or apnea occur at the time of reflux.

TREATMENT

Treatment for patients with reflux may vary from simple postural therapy to major surgery, depending on severity of symptoms, and there is no universal agreement on the relative effectiveness of the different modes of therapy.

Diet Therapy

Avoidance of large meals and using small, frequent feedings with careful burping to remove the gastric bubble are important. In extreme cases, short-term use of constant gastric feedings or even transpyloric feeding to decrease the volume of stomach contents available for reflux is helpful. Formula thickening with cereal is recommended on the theory that reflux will be inhibited, but its effectiveness is related more to decreased volume of vomitus than frequency of reflux.

Positional Therapy

Placing the patient upright to prevent spillage of stomach contents into the esophagus is intuitive and time-honored in adults and children. Raising the head of the bed definitely improves heartburn in adults. In infants, the simplest approach is placement in the prone position. The additional benefit of raising the head by placing the child in a harness has recently been questioned but appears to be advisable if it can be conveniently accomplished. The supine position is the one most likely to enhance reflux.

Medical Therapy

If there is esophagitis, neutralizing gastric acid decreases the toxicity of gastric contents to the esophageal mucosa. Studies have shown that when esophagitis is healed, there is improved esophageal motility and clearance of refluxed material. A *milk* feeding in infants neutralizes gastric contents for approximately 45 minutes. *Antacids* (15 ml/m^2 of concentrated preparations) administered between feedings is effective but may cause diarrhea. *Cimetidine,* an H_2 blocker, is available as a syrup for infants; the usual dose is 20 to 40 mg/kg/day in four divided doses.

Although not as extensively studied in children, *ranitidine* is also available in liquid form for twice daily dosage, the usual dose being 2 to 4 mg/kg/day. Ranitidine and several other H_2 blockers available only in tablet form offer the advantages of a longer half-life and lack of an effect on the hepatic metabolism of other drugs, such as theophylline or anticonvulsants, that the child may be taking.

Omeprazol is extremely effective in inhibiting gastric acid secretion and works directly on the hydrogen ion pump. It is available only in sustained-release tablet form for once-a-day use. It is approved for treatment of severe esophagitis in adults but only for a 4-week course of therapy because of the occurrence of gastric carcinoid tumors with prolonged administration in rats.

Prokinetic agents such as *metaclopramide* (0.10 to 0.15 mg/kg per dose) or *bethanechol* (0.01 mg/kg four times a day before meals) has been shown to be helpful. In some studies, it has been difficult to show a decrease in reflux using pH monitoring but symptoms do improve. Some investigators have noted nervousness or irritability and tremors as side effects, but these problems are uncommon and respond to decreasing the dose. *Cisapride,* not yet available in America, has been shown to be effective in several studies.

Surgical Therapy

In patients with severe symptoms, in addition to use of drugs meticulous attention should be given to feeding, burping, and maintaining the head elevated position for as much of the day as possible. If significant improvement is not noted in 6 weeks, surgical intervention may be considered. Surgery should also be considered if there is a significant esophageal stricture secondary to esophagitis or if there are complications, such as apnea or gagging, not responding to medical therapy. Placing a gastrostomy increases the risk of abnormal reflux.

Because most patients being considered for a permanent gastrostomy have swallowing or central nervous system disorders in which GER is common, it is wise to evaluate such patients for GER and to consider doing a simultaneous antireflux procedure at the same time if the patient has significant GER.

There are several types of procedures, but a Nissen fundoplication or some variation is the most common. It is a safe procedure, with several series of more than 200 cases being reported without an operative mortality. Reflux is usually well controlled, but respiratory symptoms are controlled to the extent that the symptoms have been caused or aggravated by GER. As would be expected, basic motility problems are not cured and about a 25 per cent patients have some problems swallowing certain foods, such as vegetables, nuts, or meat. Varying degrees of gas bloat syndrome or an inability to belch or vomit occasionally occur but tend to improve with time. A rare but often fatal complication may occur in patients in whom distal obstruction from adhesions or other causes develops. If patients cannot burp or vomit, they may experience extremely tense abdominal distention with obstruction of blood flow leading to intestinal infarction.

Medical therapy, combined with expected improvement as the child develops, usually ensures a happy outcome. In a minority of infants with severe problems not responding to medical therapy, surgical intervention will regularly cure GER and complications are usually minor or rare.

NAUSEA AND VOMITING

LEWIS R. FIRST, M.D.

Vomiting, one of the most common symptoms in pediatrics, consists of the forceful expulsion of gastric contents through the mouth. It is a complex, coordinated process that is under control of the central nervous system. Nausea, frequently associated with vomiting, is a physical sensation that can be induced by visceral, vestibular, or emotional stimuli and may not necessarily progress to full emesis. It is characterized by a desire to vomit as well as by other autonomic symptoms such as salivation, pallor, diaphoresis, tachycardia, and anorexia.

MECHANISM AND SIGNIFICANCE

One cannot begin to consider the treatment of nausea and vomiting without an understanding of the mechanism by which vomiting occurs as well as the knowledge of the broad spectrum of diseases that can present with vomiting. Vomiting itself is controlled by two medullary areas in the midbrain. A variety of chemical agents and mediators send signals into the vomiting center (located in the region of the nucleus solitarius or adjacent portion of the lateral reticular formation) and the chemoreceptor trigger zone (in the area postrema of the floor of the left ventricle), resulting in emesis. Therefore, in order to control the act of vomiting, one therapeutic approach is to suppress medullary activity and, in turn, to gain motor control of vomiting.

Afferent stimuli to the medulla can arise from the posterior pharynx, abdomen, and other visceral organs, including the pleura, heart, urogenital, and biliary tracts in response to obstruction or infection. Metabolic factors, vestibular abnormalities, and certain medications (particularly morphine derivatives) may all affect the vomiting center as well, acting either directly or indirectly through the chemoreceptor trigger zone. In addition, impulses can be submitted either by vagal or sympathetic afferents to the vomiting center.

One might think of the clinical significance of vomiting as being a defense system that acts to identify and remove any accidentally ingested toxins before they can progress further into the gastrointestinal (GI) tract and result in worsening gastrointestinal symptoms. Nausea in itself may be a protective reflex, in that anorexia helps to prevent further ingestion of potentially toxic materials and the unpleasant sensations associated with nausea may create almost a behavioral aversion to an offending food or stimulus that would otherwise result in vomiting. The fact that vomiting can occur with some medications, such as chemotherapy, may again represent an appropriate physiologic protective response to the sensation of a toxin. Even the vomiting associated with gastrointestinal reflux may represent a defense system, in that the act of vomiting helps to remove refluxed gastric acid from inflaming the esophageal mucosa.

TREATMENT

An approach to the treatment of vomiting really begins with an assessment as to whether the vomiting is acute versus chronic in combination with the age of the child. When vomiting is the principal symptom, the history should focus on a description of the vomitus, its relationship to meals, and whether it is projectile or simply represents spitting or rumination. Associated symptoms and signs, such as headache, visual symptoms and vertigo, or other gastrointestinal symptoms, such as diarrhea, constipation, or jaundice, may be useful. The assessment of anorexia can also be important in sorting out an etiology. Family histories for migraine or ulcer disease can be extremely helpful. Vomiting without nausea may be a clue to a problem involving elevated intracranial pressure or mechanical obstruction within the GI tract or other viscera, since such vomiting is often very sudden and not preceded by nausea. If the child does not appear acutely ill, psychosocial issues that might contribute to poor feeding techniques should be pursued. An inability to gain weight in the setting of vomiting may suggest a more chronic underlying process.

Vomiting in Infancy

Vomiting in the newborn that is associated with abdominal distention or that is projectile, or that contains blood or bile is more worrisome and warrants immediate investigation, including the use of appropriate radiologic studies (described elsewhere in this text). Bilious vomiting should be considered a surgical emergency until proven otherwise. It is also worthwhile to consider sepsis, head trauma, narcotic withdrawal, peptic ulcer disease, and inborn errors of metabolism should vomiting be persistent in early infancy.

In the post-neonatal period, feeding problems as well as pyloric stenosis and viral and bacterial infectious disorders are most common. It is also possible that an infant with cow's milk protein allergy can also present with vomiting.

Vomiting in Older Children

In older children, acute vomiting is usually associated with abdominal pain and can represent obstruction or inflammation of an abdominal viscus. On the other hand, it may also be associated with congestion from upper respiratory infections, hepatitis, ingestions, pneumonia, or metabolic disorders such as diabetes. Persistent vomiting in an older age group makes one more concerned regarding elevated intracranial pressure, migraines, or peptic ulcer disease; in adolescents, anorexia nervosa and bulimia should be considered.

Once life-threatening obstructive or surgical disorders have been eliminated as possibilities, most vomiting, particularly in older children, usually results from some very common causes such as a viral gastroenteritis or food poisoning. In these cases, the vomiting usually resolves with 24 to 48 hours. If the vomiting is persistent or is associated with the use of chemotherapy or other medication, some pharmacologic attention to its treatment appears warranted. A psychogenic etiology for vomiting is often attributed to stress, which elevates adrenaline levels and in turn influences the chemoreceptive trigger zone. In the psychogenic setting, pharmacologic treatment may be warranted.

The cessation of vomiting is important for ensuring adequate hydration as well as avoiding Mallory-Weiss tears in the gastric mucosa, which can result in hematemesis. Vomiting occasionally results in episodes of aspiration and, in younger infants, failure to thrive. Dehydration and electrolyte abnormalities are the most worrisome aspects of persistent vomiting that warrant therapeutic attention. The entity of cyclic vomiting in older children (in which episodes of vomiting last a few hours to a few days) is often associated with dehydration, migraine, and/or stressful events. A therapeutic approach to this type of vomiting is certainly indicated, although often it is not very helpful.

Antiemetic Pharmacotherapy

For nausea and vomiting associated with a viral illness or an acute ingestion (assuming that the toxin has been appropriately treated), treatment is essentially supportive and consists of sips of clear fluids and a bland diet until the feelings of nausea and/or vomiting can pass (usually within 24 to 48 hours). If the vomiting persists and dehydration becomes a potential concern, antiemetic pharmacotherapy may be indicated, particularly in older children—in whom the benefits of such therapy will outweigh the side effects. Unfortunately, most antiemetics are oral agents, and these may not be useful if acute vomiting is occurring unless they can rapidly be absorbed from the mouth or stomach before emesis recurs.

TABLE 1. Drugs Useful for Control of Nausea and Vomiting

Drug	How Supplied	Principal Side Effects
Antihistamines		
Promethazine (Phenergan) Child: 1 mg/kg/dose q 4–6 hr p.o. or IM Adult: 25 mg p.o. or IM	Syrup: 6.25 mg/5 ml or 25 mg/5 ml Tablets: 12.5, 25, 50 mg Suppository: 12.5, 25, 50 mg Injection: 25 mg/1 ml	Headache Abdominal pain Urinary urgency Blood pressure changes Extrapyramidal and anticholinergic side effects
Dimenhydrinate (Dramamine) Child: 1.25 mg/kg/dose p.o. or IM, q.i.d. Adult: 50–100 mg/dose p.o. or IM q.i.d., 100 mg p.r. q.i.d.	Injection: 50 mg/ml Liquid: 12.5 mg/4 ml Tablets: 50 mg Suppository: 100 mg	Drowsiness Atropine-like effects
Dopamine Antagonists		
Metoclopramide (Reglan) Child: 0.1 mg/kg/dose p.o., IM, or IV q 6 hr Adult: 10 mg p.o. IM or IV q 6 hr	Injection: 5 mg/ml Syrup: 5 mg/ml Tablets: 10 mg	Extrapyramidal restlessness, sedation, lowered threshold to seizure
Thiethylperazine (Torecan) Child: 5 mg p.o. q.i.d. if $<$ 50 kg, 10 mg if $>$ 50 kg Adult: 10–30 mg p.o. q.i.d. 10 mg IM t.i.d.	Injection: 10 mg/2 ml Tablet: 10 mg Suppository: 10 mg	Extrapyramidal and anticholinergic effects
Perphenazine (Trilafon) Adult: 8–16 mg p.o. b.i.d.–q.i.d. 8–10 mg IV or IM q 6 hr or as continuous infusion	Tablets: 2, 4, 8, 16 mg Injection: 5 mg/ml	Extrapyramidal and anticholinergic effects
Prochlorperazine (Compazine) Child ($>$ 10 kg) 0.05 mg/kg IM q 6 hr or 0.1 mg/kg p.r. or p.o. q 6 hr Adult 5–10 mg/dose IM or p.o. 6 hr or 25 mg p.r. b.i.d.	Injection: 5 mg/ml Syrup: 5 mg/5 ml Oral concentrate: 10 mg/ml Suppository: 2.5, 5, 25 mg	Extrapyramidal more common than anticholinergic, sedation, dysphoria, orthostatic hypotension, lowered seizure threshold
Miscellaneous		
Phosphorated carbohydrate solution (Emetrol) Child: 1–2 tsp. q 15 minutes until nausea subsides Adult: 1–2 Tbsp. q 15 minutes until nausea subsides	Liquid: 1.87 g dextrose 1.87 g fructose 21.5 mg phosphoric acid/5 ml	Nontoxic
Lorazepam (Ativan) Usual dose 2–3 mg/day in divided doses	Tablets: 0.5, 1, 2 mg	For psychogenic vomiting
Diazepam (Valium) Child: 1–2½ mg, 3 or 4 times daily Adult: 2–10 mg, 3 or 4 times daily	Tablets: 2, 5, 10 mg	For psychogenic vomiting

Abbreviations: p.o., by mouth; IM, intramuscular; IV, intravenous; q, every; b.i.d., twice a day; q.i.d., four times a day; t.i.d., three times a day; p.r., per rectum.

Oral antiemetics may be more useful in the setting of anticipated vomiting, such as with chemotherapy or radiation therapy, or in the setting of persistent vomiting from hepatitis or psychogenic causes.

Most antiemetics work through the midbrain to influence central control of the sensations of nausea and vomiting. A complete list of antiemetics and their dosages appears in Table 1. The most common of these is metoclopramide, which blocks dopamine receptors in the chemoreceptor trigger zone and thus influences central control of vomiting. Unfortunately, it is associated with significant dystonic and dyskinetic reactions, including oculogyric crises, and therefore is not recommended for young children.

Phenothiazines are the drugs of choice for control of vomiting secondary to chemotherapy, with the most useful being thiethylperazine (Torecan) which can be given orally, intravenously, intramuscularly, or rectally. The dose is 10 mg for children 12 years of age or heavier than 50 kg; the dose is 5 mg in smaller children. Torecan provides prophylactic protection if given on a regular basis around the clock, being tapered to an individual's own need, rather than given on a general every-6-hour schedule. Other alternatives to Torecan include perphenazine (Trilafon), available for intravenous or oral administration; it can be given as a continuous infusion.

Prochlorperazine (Compazine) can be very useful in younger children for sedation and treatment of nausea but has less antiemetic effect than the two agents noted above. It is given at 0.5 mg/kg by mouth, per rectum, or intramuscularly (IM). Promethazine (Phenergan) works similarly to reduce the sensation of nausea and enhance sedation rather than to significantly decrease vomiting. Any child receiving a phenothiazine derivative, however, should be alerted to the possibility of extrapyramidal side effects (which can continue to occur for 48 hours after the drug is discontinued) but can easily be treated with the use of diphenhydramine or another antihistamine.

Antihistamines, such as dimenhydrinate, may be useful as prophalaxis against nausea and vomiting caused by motion sickness. Dimenhydrinate is not useful once the nausea and vomiting have started, however. Emetrol (a phosphated carbohydrate solution) may also be useful in children for relief of nausea associated with an upset stomach. It is not as efficacious in the cessation of vomiting once it occurs. Scopolamine patches placed over the mastoid are contraindicated for prevention of vomiting due to motion sickness. This is because the dosage on the patch may be too high and erratically absorbed in children, resulting in a variety of anticholinergic side effects.

If a psychogenic etiology is determined, with the precipitation of vomiting more of a factor than the actual effect, lorazepam or diazepam may be indicated. In the small infant, in whom phenothiazines may be contraindicated because their side effects outweigh their benefits, Phenergan might be tried first, with the addition of diphenhydramine for poor response or if toxicity occurs. In situations of cyclic vomiting or episodes of psychogenic etiology, techniques such as biofeedback and other behavior modification and psychotherapy modalities have been used successfully to decrease anticipatory nausea and vomiting cycles.

REFERENCES

Dodge JA: Vomiting and regurgitation. *In* Walker WA, Durie PR, Hamilton JR Walker-Smith JA Watkins JB (eds): Pediatric Gastrointestinal Disease. Philadelphia, BC Decker, 1991, pp 32–41.

CONSTIPATION AND ENCOPRESIS

MICHAEL J. PETTEI, M.D., Ph.D.
and MURRAY DAVIDSON, M.D.

The tendency to constipation is often hereditary. Firm stools and excessive stool size may develop in infants and children with this tendency, producing pain. This may lead to voluntary withholding with eventual onset of *encopresis* (involuntary stool passage), which constitutes a far greater problem than the original constipation. Therapy may need to be directed to (1) the tendency to constipation, (2) symptomatic constipation, or (3) stool withholding and eventual encopresis.

CONSTIPATION

The Tendency

Constipation is generally defined in comparative terms involving the degree of firmness, frequency of elimination, or difficulty with passage of stool. The greatest amount of objective data is available on stool frequency. Babies fed either at the breast or with the usual infant formulas may have bowel movements with each feeding (i.e., five to eight stools daily). Newborns on average have four bowel movements per day. Those who eliminate only one to two times per day during the first month of life are evidencing a tendency to constipation and constitute a disproportionate number of those in whom frank constipation develops. Between 4 and 6 months of age, infants commonly have only two to three movements per day while the infant with a tendency to constipation often begins to skip days. Although many babies get through this period without difficulty, some become symptomatic, for example, experiencing painful defecation, or with anal fissures developing.

Dietary therapy often forestalls later problems in the infant younger than 6 months of age with a tendency to constipation. Laxative fruits, such as apricots, prunes, and pineapple, added to infant pears, and the nonstarchy vegetables should be encouraged as well as an occasional water or juice bottle. It may be necessary to offer a difficult patient dark corn syrup or malt soup extract (dark Karo syrup or Maltsupex, 1 to 2 teaspoons from one to three times daily).

Although the resulting colonic fermentative process softens stools, it also increases gas in the intestinal tract. Occasionally this induces or worsens colic. For this situation, glycerin suppositories or rectal stimulation with a lubricated cotton swab may be used to induce a daily bowel movement until the child is 3 to 4 months old. Therapy should be sufficient to avoid uncomfortable bowel movements until the child is ready to cooperate in developing a regular daily bowel movement. Regularly timed evacuations may not be necessary for the general population, but during early childhood they ensure that the symptoms of difficult defecation, stool withholding, and eventual encopresis do not develop in the child with the tendency to constipate.

Symptomatic Constipation

It is during the first few months of life that organic causes for constipation most commonly present. Occasionally, underlying structural, endocrinologic, neurologic, or metabolic factors are the cause. These include partial obstructions, hypothyroidism, hypercalcemia, hypokalemia, spinal cord defects, hypotonia, and heavy-metal ingestions as well as the use of numerous medications. *The most frequently considered organic etiology for constipated infants is probably Hirschsprung's disease (congenital aganglionosis). Nevertheless, infants with functional constipation may pass less than one bowel movement daily from early on.*

As already mentioned, dietary therapy and fermentative stool softeners may not be helpful for constipation in young infants who may have a tendency to colic. Glycerin suppositories or rectal stimulation with a lubricated cotton swab may be used to induce a daily bowel movement. Once children are beyond 3 to 4 months of age and colicky episodes diminish, constipation may be treated with laxative fruits and juices, vegetables, and the addition of malt soup extract (Maltsupex, 1 to 2 teaspoons from one to three times daily). For many young infants, defecation is accompanied by considerable grimacing and grunting. Parents should be reassured that as long as the stools are of average frequency and consistency, no intervention is necessary.

In the latter part of the first year or in the second year of life, manifestations of constipation (straining, streaks of blood on the stool, small hard scybala, infrequent defecation) should not be approached with reassurances that the child will outgrow the problem. Although this is true in some instances, other youngsters experience increasing difficulties. Benign neglect at this age can result in a pattern of chronic constipation and stool-withholding behavior with eventual megarectum and encopresis. In the toddler, particular emphasis should be placed on the avoidance of excessive dairy products, especially to the exclusion of liberal water or juice intake. Maltsupex may be useful, laxative fruit snacks (prunes, apricots, raisins) may be substituted for sweets, and a number of different bran products (cereals, muffins) may be tolerated at this age. In some instances, limited amounts of a stimulant such as senna (Senokot or Castoria, 1 to 2 teaspoons daily) or lubricant (mineral oil, 1 to 2 tablespoons) may be necessary.

Voluntary Stool Withholding

Once children appreciate that they control their own bowel movements, they may voluntarily withhold stools to avoid painful movements. This behavior may begin before 1 year of age, but it is more usual in the middle to latter part of the second year of life. Another critical time for the development of stool withholding is during toilet training. Many toddlers develop an aversion to the toilet, resulting in withholding. When withholding becomes significant, training should usually be abandoned until regular, voluntary bowel movements have been re-established. Parents often mistake stool withholding for exaggerated attempts at defecation. It is often useful in this situation to compare the stiff, erect posturing of withholding to the natural squat position of defecation in explaining this behavior. In the toddler who presents with stool-withholding behavior of short duration and in whom significant megarectum has not occurred, short-term therapy may suffice. One to two hypertonic phosphate enemas (3 ml/kg) followed by forced daily evacuation for 2 to 3 weeks with mild laxative therapy (Senokot or milk of magnesia, 1 to 3 teaspoons per day, usually q.h.s.) is usually sufficient. Maintenance is achieved by dietary therapy as outlined above; bowel training; and, if required, mineral oil (1 to 2 tablespoons per day) or mild laxative therapy, depending on the age of the child.

ENCOPRESIS

With chronic stool withholding, the lower colonic segment gradually becomes distended with accumulated stool. The urge to defecate then becomes irregular, since a stretched wall seems to decrease rectal sensation. A vicious circle is thus set up. The retained material is difficult to pass, the patient refuses to try and then holds back, the rectum and sigmoid are distended, their walls gradually overstretch, and the urge is appreciated less frequently. When the rectum has become sufficiently distended, any additional stool that arrives from the more proximal colon cannot be accommodated and results in encopresis.

For children with chronic constipation in whom an enlarged rectum and encopresis have developed, treatment with a regimented program is useful. It is based on the premise that maintaining a relatively empty rectum devoid of retained stool over time results in a decrease in rectal size and an increase of rectal sensitivity to distention. Encopresis (overflow soiling) does not occur if rectal impactions are not permitted to accumulate. Thus, encouragement should be given to both the parents and the child that the most anxiety-provoking symptom—soiling—can usually be resolved quickly.

Treatment of Encopresis and Megarectum

The management of functional encopresis and megarectum consists of several steps. Before therapy is outlined, the family should be educated as to the usual natural history of encopresis with the removal of blame. After an explanation of the development of the megarectum and substantial stool retention, it should be pointed out that most soiling occurs involuntarily through an "overflow"-type mechanism without the control of the child.

Disimpaction

The initial phase of therapy involves disimpaction. The most effective, yet acceptable, method of achieving this is through the administration of hypertonic phosphate enemas (3 ml/kg) usually each morning and evening until the effluent is free of solid stool. On average, this entails two to four enemas (1 to 2 days). Because these enemas in overdosage can result in hyperphosphatemia or electrolyte abnormalities, they should not be utilized in those with significant medical problems (e.g., cardiac or renal failure) or in the very young child. No more than two enemas per day for 3 days should be advised without re-examination, which may include a serum chemistry profile and an abdominal film. Other regimens may include medicated suppositories; oral laxatives, such as bisacodyl or senna (Dulcolax or Senokot); or polyethylene glycol–electrolyte solutions.

Occasionally, the child presents with such long-standing megarectum and impaction that a "fecaloma" is present. This simply represents a hard, large, inspissated stool concretion occupying the entire cavity of the rectum. It can be ascertained either by noting the firmness of the stool on initial rectal examination or by the ineffectiveness of initial enema usage after re-examination. These impactions may be treated by a rigorous in-patient program, but they can usually be handled on an outpatient basis utilizing prolonged mineral oil enemas and mild oral laxative therapy in combination with conservative phosphate enema administration.

Preventing Reaccumulation of Stool and Stopping Stool-Withholding Behavior

The second phase of therapy is aimed at preventing the reaccumulation of stool and, if necessary, abolishing stool-withholding behavior. It should be pointed out that after catharsis the individual will not soil; however, if therapy is not initiated to prevent stool retention, the child will simply return to his or her former state after a given period of time. To "force" one or two stools daily, a sufficient, individually titrated dose of stimulant or osmotic laxative (senna, cascara, milk of magnesia, or lactulose) should be prescribed (e.g., Dulcolax or Senokot, one to three tablets, usually q.h.s.). Once the appropriate regimen is found and administered regularly, reaccumulation of impactions is rare. In those in whom impressive megarectum has developed over years, this regimen may need to be continued on a prolonged basis. *A high-*

dose mineral oil therapy (5 to 15 ml/kg twice a day) designed to achieve four to six daily bowel movements achieves a faster solution to the problem. However, this rigorous regimen has largely been abandoned because it is distasteful and difficult for most.

Establishing Regular Bowel Patterns

The final stage of treatment is directed at establishing a regular bowel pattern. Conditioning to at least daily bowel movements ensures softer stools and is reasonable in children old enough to cooperate (3 to 4 years old). The child must be encouraged to sit on the commode for 5 to 15 minutes at least once a day, usually after a meal (particularly breakfast). Young children should be encouraged to rest their feet on a footstool or other solid support to maintain mechanical leverage. For those taking stimulant laxatives and those with more normal-sized rectums, the dosage should be gradually decreased while a regular bowel habit is formed. Low-dose mineral oil therapy (30 to 60 ml q.h.s.) may be added upon laxative withdrawal to maintain the bowel training.

For those who do not voluntarily comply with the bowel-training program, more formalized behavior modification therapy may be of benefit. Manometric biofeedback may be useful for non-responders. The family should be cautioned that interruption of the normal routine (e.g., vacation, periods of illness) may give rise to acute constipation, which should be addressed promptly with enemas or laxatives to avoid recurrence of chronic problems. The rare child with chronic, voluntary fecal soiling without impaction or megarectum represents a significant behavioral problem and should be referred for psychiatric evaluation.

SUMMARY

As already mentioned, early recognition and anticipatory guidance with preventive dietary measures can help to avoid the establishment of chronic constipation and stool withholding. However, once established, stool withholding and encopresis rarely respond to diet alone. Adequate fluid ingestion, limited milk consumption, and dietary fiber should be advised, but major changes in diet are usually unattainable. Fiber in dietary form (breakfast cereals, bran muffins) or supplemental form (psyllium seed preparations) can be used in the older child with constipation.

ACUTE AND CHRONIC DIARRHEA IN INFANTS AND CHILDREN

JOEL W. ADELSON, M.D., Ph.D.
and KATHERINE B. FREEMAN, M.D.

ACUTE DIARRHEA

The acute onset of diarrhea in a previously well infant or child is a common occurrence in pediatric practice. Generally, there is an obvious increase in stool volume, a decrease in stool consistency, and an increase in the frequency of stooling. Most acute diarrheas are due to an infectious enteric pathogen. In some cases, the diarrhea will accompany infection at another locus, as in ear or urinary tract infections. In any acute diarrhea, the major clinical concerns, especially with infants, are the possibilities of dehydration, acidosis, and electrolyte imbalance—which, if left unchecked, can lead to shock, renal failure, and permanent damage to the central nervous system. Long-term sequelae may also include damage to the gastrointestinal tract, leading to chronic malabsorption and eventual failure to thrive.

Etiology and Diagnosis

In North America, the etiologic agent in acute diarrhea usually is one of a number of viral pathogens, most frequently rotavirus; fewer cases will feature a bacterial or parasitic etiology. The viral diarrheas tend to be characterized by watery stools, with less pain and rectal bleeding than in the bacterial types. Because the vast majority of diarrheal cases are self-limited and resolve in a few days, in most instances a search for the etiology is optional. On the basis of clinical judgment, the clinician may reserve the use of stool cultures, a search for ova and parasites, or a rapid assay for rotavirus for specific cases. Indications for work-up include a clinical presentation that is especially severe or atypical. Stool culture specimens should be obtained in children with persistent diarrhea, hospitalized patients, and those exposed to someone with an episode of bacterial diarrhea.

Treatment

Two methods of treatment are commonly employed for mild to moderate degrees of dehydration—oral and intravenous rehydration. Numerous trials have supported the efficacy of oral rehydration, which should be employed whenever possible. Fluid management consists of rehydration and maintenance phases. Both the American Academy of Pediatrics and the World Health Organization recommend that oral rehydration be accomplished with a higher sodium concentration (75 to 90 mEq/L) and a somewhat lower carbohydrate-to-sodium ratio (<2:1) than is contained in most of the common commercially available solutions (e.g., Pedialyte, Infalyte, Ricelyte). One commercial solution that meets initial rehydration standards is Rehydrate. However, for the average case of dehydration in children with acute gastroenteritis in the United States, the other currently available commercial products are probably acceptable.

Oral rehydration can also be accomplished in the vomiting child. This is best achieved by having the child take the solution slowly. In mild dehydration, rehydration should be accomplished over 4 hours using 50 ml/kg given slowly by mouth. In moderate dehydration, this should be accomplished with 100 ml/kg over 6 hours. Maintenance oral fluid (40 to 60 mEq Na/L) should then keep up with stool losses. This type of electrolyte solution is commonly available. Feeding should be reinstituted within 24 hours.

Whatever type of solution is used, parents should be informed that the diarrhea itself may be expected to continue briefly and that it is dehydration, not diarrhea, that is being treated or prevented. Because the diarrhea may be prolonged for several days, close follow-up is required to ensure that the patient does not become dehydrated again. In children who fail to respond to oral rehydration therapy or in those with severe dehydration, intravenous rehydration is appropriate. Guidelines for management are found in the article on parenteral fluid and electrolyte therapy, p. 410.

A common complication of many acute diarrheas, especially those due to the commonest pathogen, rotavirus, is a brief period (usually a few days, but occasionally up to 2 weeks) of intestinal villous damage leading to lactase deficiency. Thus, milk feeding (animal or human milk) may worsen the diarrhea by causing the retention of an osmotically active load of undigested lactose in the intestine. This usually is a minor problem, and in the case of the breast-fed infant, most physicians will reasonably elect to have the mother resume breast-feeding as early as possible after rehydration. In formula-fed infants, a brief changeover to a lactose-free formula will avoid problems from the transient period of lactose intolerance. For this purpose, a soy-based formula is usually selected. It is important for the physician to realize that the switch from a cow's milk-based formula to a soy-based formula is not being made because of the type of protein in the formula but because of the desire to avoid lactose for a brief period. The parent should not be told that the infant is "intolerant" or "allergic" to either cow's milk protein or lactose; the patient is simply temporarily deficient in lactase, and this deficiency should return to normal, usually within a few days. As soon as the formula is tolerated, the patient should resume a completely normal diet.

A second common pitfall usually encountered in older babies and children is the unnecessary and prolonged continuation (more than 1 to 2 days) of a limited diet, which is thought by some to be of value in treating acute gastroenteritis. One common form of limited diet, the so-called the "brat" diet, consists of *b*ananas, *r*ice, *a*pplesauce or *a*pple juice, and plain *t*oast. Too frequently the child is continued on this or on an even more restricted diet for several days in order to ensure that the stools are absolutely "normal" prior to resuming an unrestricted diet. Other infants are given excessive amounts of clear liquids or juices while waiting for the stools to normalize—which they may not do—given the lack of fiber in the diet and the high osmotic load present in the juices. This approach carries the further risk of precipitating or exacerbating general caloric and specific nutritional deficiencies and may contribute to frank failure to thrive if prolonged in an unnecessary fashion. In general, in both the infant and older child, a moderate increase in stool volume and frequency and a decrease in stool consistency is quite well tolerated, even if inconvenient, provided only that adequate hydration is maintained. The presence of a period of loose stools should not be the cause for great anxiety, and the parent should be carefully reassured about this.

In cases of severe acute diarrhea, often accompanied by fever and blood per rectum, a bacterial pathogen may be identified after appropriate culture specimens are obtained. Even in these cases, treatment with antibiotics is generally not indicated because the illness is usually self-limited, and treatment may prolong the carrier state for certain bacteria, such as *Salmonella,* and thereby create a greater risk of occurrence of the illness in family members and other contacts. Exceptions to this guideline include the very sick or debilitated child who may be poorly able to withstand the illness, infants younger than 3 months of age, and those with extraintestinal infection. Symptomatic patients with diarrhea caused by *Shigella* species should be treated with an appropriate antimicrobial agent. Antimotility agents may increase the risk of toxicity or complicate electrolyte losses and should be used very sparingly or not at all. If oral antibiotics have been given within 6 weeks prior to the diarrhea, pseudomembranous enterocolitis should be considered and *Clostridum difficile* stool culture and assay for toxins A and B obtained. In severe cases of diarrhea due to *C. difficile,* the treatment is oral vancomycin at 40 mg/kg/day, divided every 6 hours for 10 to 14 days. Metronidazole has been used for treatment in adult patients, and cholestyramine has been employed to suppress symptoms.

CHRONIC DIARRHEA

Etiology and Diagnosis

Diarrhea lasting several weeks or more almost invariably brings a worried patient and parent to medical attention. Frequently, the initial diagnosis may have been acute gastroenteritis, and the frustrated patient may arrive on a limited diet that is not relieving the symptoms and that, further, may lead to weight loss. The most important initial aspect to proper care of the patient will be to arrive at a diagnosis. In chronic diarrhea, the differential diagnosis is very extensive, encompassing a wide variety of causes that cannot be discussed here. Two of the more common possibilities are quite distinct and must be clearly differentiated from each other: *chronic nonspecific diarrhea,* and *intractable diarrhea.*

Chronic nonspecific diarrhea of infancy and childhood is a relatively harmless condition resulting from an unexplained inability to form solid stool. It appears to be due, at least in part, to some form of persistent derangement of intestinal motility. Characteristically, the children range in age from about 6 months to about 3 years, resulting in the common ailment "toddler's diarrhea." The clinical picture is generally that of a vigorous, well child, without vomiting or systemic signs or symptoms, who has been having several bouts of "muddy" or liquid stools daily for more than 4 weeks without pain or cramps, although there may be some distress just before and during stool passage. No bacterial, viral, or parasitic pathogen is found, nor are fecal leukocytes present. There is no evidence for weight loss (unless the diet has been restricted), nor does the stool exhibit a low pH or the presence of either reducing substances or occult blood.

Treatment

The best treatment, once more serious causes (see below) have been at least considered and, where warranted, carefully ruled out, is clear reassurance to the parent that the condition will eventually resolve, although months may elapse before resolution actually occurs. A serious effort should be made to ensure that the diet contains sufficient amounts of both fat and fiber to allow the intestine to achieve a normal motility pattern and to provide a gelatinous stool substrate. Treatment with psyllium (e.g., Metamucil, Per Diem, 2 to 3 g/day for 2 weeks) may be effective in thickening the stool. Other drugs, such as cholestyramine and metronidazole, have occasionally been used successfully, although they are not as widely advocated. Milk should not be avoided because lactose intolerance is not the problem. The child's continued growth should be ensured as well. In fact, some cases appear to resolve rapidly once a normal diet is reinstituted, although it is at times difficult to convince a frustrated and frightened parent to reinstitute a normal diet.

If the reinstitution of dairy products and normalization of the diet really does exacerbate the diarrhea, either lactose or sucrose malabsorption should be considered; in this case, reducing substances will be found in the stool after the ingestion of milk or sugared drinks and/or the stool pH should be low. (To detect sucrose malabsorption, the stool must be hydrolyzed before reducing substances are measured.) If available, a lactose or sucrose hydrogen breath test is a useful method of diagnosis of disaccharide malabsorption. If lactose is being malabsorbed, lactase enzyme–treated milk may be given; if sucrose is a problem in the diet, it may simply be avoided.

More serious problems with chronic diarrhea may be encountered in infants and babies, including a severe and long-lasting, postinfectious lactose intolerance or a chronic intractable diarrhea in which all disaccharides, including milk and table sugars, and even monosaccharides are not absorbed. In some cases, severe secretory diarrhea occurs. In such cases, a high stool output will continue, containing a relatively high sodium concentration, in spite of the patient not being fed by mouth. In some cases, damage to the intestine has been severe, leading to ongoing malabsorption, which results in further weight loss and malnutrition. As a consequence, there will be a partially debilitated immune system and a dysfunctional intestinal brush border with an impaired, slowly healing absorptive mucosa.

Such patients should be treated with a combination of enteral feeding, usually by continuous nasogastric infusion plus total parenteral nutrition (TPN). In the seriously ill patient, TPN provides the mainstay of calories while the gut itself is nourished by a constant nasogastric drip of a highly absorbable liquid diet composed of oligopeptides, glucose or glucose polymers, plus lipid in the form of medium-chain plus long-chain triglycerides. As recovery proceeds, the proportion of nasogastric feeding can be increased incrementally, the complexity of the diet gradually shifted toward more highly polymerized proteins, and the disaccharides sucrose and eventually lactose reintroduced. Further details on the complex management of chronic intractable diarrhea are not covered in this brief outline; the reader is referred to more complete texts on pediatric gastroenterology and nutrition.

Cow's milk protein intolerance is a common entity in which an otherwise well infant presents with blood in the stool; at times there may also be diarrhea and a protein-losing enteropathy. Such infants may benefit from a soy-based formula. However, about 25 per cent of infants who react to cow's milk protein are also sensitive to soy formulas and need to be given an elemental protein hydralysate formula. Cow's milk protein intolerance usually ameliorates at about 1 year of age, and milk and milk-containing foods may then be reintroduced.

Treatment for any form of chronic diarrhea must follow an exhaustive attempt to establish the specific etiology of the illness. Because the patient will frequently require prolonged hospitalization and invasive therapy such as TPN, it is of great importance that specific treatment of causes of prolonged diarrhea be instituted at the earliest possible time, so as not to rely on nutritional, fluid, and electrolyte repletion alone. Thus, bacterial overgrowth, celiac disease, inflammatory bowel disease, immune deficiency syndromes, Hirschsprung's disease, chronic bacterial or parasitic infections, cystic fibrosis and other causes of pancreatic insufficiency, congenital malabsorptive disorders, secretory tumors, and a variety of other entities should be vigorously sought while nutritional repletion is ongoing. Such a work-up is usually best completed at an academic center equipped to look for the multiplicity of causes that lead to severe chronic diarrhea and malabsorption. Treatment of these illnesses, of course, should be specific to the diagnosis.

RECURRENT ABDOMINAL PAIN

HELEN BUTLER CASTEEL, M.D.

Up to 10 per cent of children experience recurrent bouts of abdominal pain, which is defined as three or more episodes of pain that alter function over a 3-month period. Three categories of problems can be manifested as abdominal pain: organic, functional, and psychogenic; yet only 5 to 10 per cent of affected children appear to an have organic problem. Children may have pain simultaneously from more than one pain category, and all problems must be treated in order to alleviate symptoms.

ETIOLOGY AND DIAGNOSIS

The history and physical examinations are the most important aspects of the evaluation and care of the child with abdominal pain. The pain should be characterized insofar as the age of the child allows. Useful historical information includes (1) when the pain began; (2) location, duration, and character of the pain; (3) exacerbating symptoms; (4) medications; and (5) whether food relieves the pain. Approximately 60 per cent of patients report periumbilical pain regardless of the etiology, and 50 per cent have pain daily. The presence of associated symptoms, such as headache, vomiting, anorexia, diarrhea, constipation, pallor, fatigue, weight loss, mouth ulcers, urinary tract symptoms, menstrual cycle irregularities, sexual activity, perianal disease, and/or fever, should each be explored. The relationship of symptoms associated with the abdominal pain is also important. Bowel dysfunction and vomiting are the most common associated symptoms, occurring in 29 and 24 per cent of patients, respectively. Questions regarding social history should elicit the child's grade in school, school performance and attendance, school or home moves, who lives in the home, and recent changes in the home environment. The ages of the parents and siblings and their general health, as well as family history of inflammatory bowel disease, cancer, irritable bowel syndrome, and migraine headaches, should be determined.

A complete physical examination should be performed, with height and weight parameters and the general health and appearance of the child noted. A rectal or pelvic examination may be appropriate in some patients. The location of the pain or pain upon distraction, the presence of masses, rectal fissures, fistulas, or trauma may provide important clues as to the etiology of the complaints.

Certain symptoms suggest an organic basis for the abdominal pain. The younger preschool child is more likely to have organic pain than the school-aged child. Nausea, point tenderness, or pain in the right lower quadrant is relatively indicative of an organic disorder. An especially useful clue is nighttime awakening, as this symptom is infrequent in functional disorders. Organic causes of pain can involve multiple organ systems and include intestinal obstruction (such as volvulus or intussusception), inflammatory conditions (e.g., appendicitis, inflammatory bowel disease), hepatitis, cholecystitis, pancreatitis, and infections (e.g., giardiasis, bacterial pathogens).

Description of the pain as "continuous" typically denotes functional pain. Physical findings are often normal in patients with functional abdominal pain. The children appear healthy, and their growth is normal. The childhood equivalent of irritable bowel syndrome is the most common functional disorder causing abdominal pain. Synonyms are "chronic nonspecific diarrhea" and "toddler's diarrhea." Abdominal pain, constipation, and diarrhea are common features. The physiologic abnormality in irritable bowel syndrome is obscure. However, abnormalities in motility, abnormalities in prostaglandin concentrations in the rectum, and atypical effects from bile acids on the colon have all been postulated as causative. Providing reassurance to the parents and child that the pain is real and expressing a belief that the child is experiencing pain instills trust between the family and physician, permitting acceptance by the family of a diagnosis of functional pain. Although parents are advised that the pain is "real," they should also be informed that the pain may be enhanced by stress.

Rarely, the abdominal pain appears truly factitious. Chaotic home situations, depression, or emotional problems may present in this manner. Moreover, sexual abuse should be considered in a patient with abdominal pain that seems contrived.

In a healthy child with normal growth and no symptoms suggestive of organic disease, irritable bowel syndrome is the most likely cause and treatment can be initiated. If other disorders are suspected, however, diagnostic testing is indicated. Such studies may include a complete blood count (to look for anemia, high white blood cell count, or an increase in inflammatory cells), an erythrocyte sedimentation rate (to screen for inflammation), a liver transaminase (aspartate aminotransferase [AST] or alanine aminotransferase [ALT]), amylase, urinalysis and culture, and stool guaiac and ova and parasite examinations. Radiographic examination may include an upper gastrointestinal series with small-bowel follow-through (to look for Crohn's disease or malformations). An abdominal ultrasonogram may be indicated to examine the liver, spleen, pancreas, gallbladder, and kidneys. If peptic disease is strongly suspected, an upper intestinal tract endoscopy is the appropriate initial diagnostic test.

Hospitalization may be required for some patients in order to obtain nursing and physician observation of reported symptoms such as abdominal pain, vomiting, diarrhea, and fever. A brief hospital stay also "breaks the cycle" in functional or psychogenic pain by removing the child from a stressful environment.

TREATMENT

Treatment choices for chronic abdominal pain or organic origin are dependent on the diagnosis. Children with emotional disorders will likely need the assistance of a psychologist or psychiatrist trained in the management of children. Treatment modalities for irritable bowel syndrome include increasing dietary fiber, using bulk laxative agents (in both constipation and diarrhea), and instilling a better understanding of the condition on the part of the parents and the child. Relaxation training, behavioral modification, or psychologic care may be needed for unresponsive patients. Additionally, instructions for mandatory school attendance should be provided. A careful, complete history and physical examination and establishment of an atmosphere of trust and concern allow the physician to manage a patient with chronic abdominal pain most effectively.

REFERENCES

Gelber JR, Neustein S, Walker WA: Clinical aspects of recurrent abdominal pain in children. Adv Pediatr 37:31, 1908.

Olson A: Recurrent abdominal pain: An approach to diagnosis and management. Pediatr Ann 16:834, 1987.

PYLOROSPASM

GIULIO J. BARBERO, M.D.
and JOAN DiPALMA, M.D.

Pylorospasm is a descriptive term signifying that the pylorus closes more intensely than usual and suggests an abnormality in gastric motility and emptying. At best, pylorospasm is predominantly a clinical entity in which no tests or studies can readily confirm a definitive diagnosis.

There are two situations in which pylorospasm is suspected. First, pylorospasm is considered partially responsible for the vomiting and abdominal pain seen in peptic ulcer disease and duodenitis. In these cases, the inflammation and ulceration are documented by upper gastrointestinal radiography and/or endoscopy and biopsy. Proper treatment of these disorders with medical therapy usually manages the accompanying pylorospasm. Another situation is that of the infant younger than 3 months of age who presents with recurrent vomiting. Upper gastrointestinal radiography may demonstrate delayed gastric emptying. Investigations for gastroesophageal reflux, infection, and metabolic disease are negative.

The impact of pylorospasm in infancy is generally not profound. It is usually more of a nuisance, the vomitus frequently soiling all surrounding clothing and furniture. Fortunately, the degree of vomiting does not produce significant caloric deprivation to impair growth in most cases. Nevertheless, growth of the infant requires careful surveillance. Small, frequent feedings may be warranted. Changes of formula composition are of little value. An antispasmodic such as Donnatal Elixir (0.5 ml four times a day) or an atropine 1:1000 solution, one drop prior to each meal, may be helpful. Metoclopramide hydrochloride (0.1 mg/kg per dose) has been tried with variable success. Dealing directly with parental fears and concerns is also an important component to management. Environmental factors in the etiology of this uncertain entity are unclear. However, in examining such issues nonjudgmentally and supportively with the parents, a positive therapeutic alliance can frequently occur. Usually, the vomiting symptoms are limited in time and are not protracted. There is little evidence of this entity becoming chronic, but its relationship to other gastrointestinal disorders that may occur later in life is still of some interest.

PYLORIC STENOSIS

GIULIO J. BARBERO, M.D.
and JOAN DiPALMA, M.D.

Pyloric stenosis is a diagnosis that is reached after careful clinical, laboratory, and, at times, radiologic investigation. Diagnosis is based on the development of forceful, nonbilious vomiting usually 2 to 4 weeks after birth. The vomiting progresses in intensity, often with small and less frequent stools. Gastric waves pass across from left to right of the upper abdomen. The palpation of a pyloric "olive" confirms the diagnosis. Abdominal ultrasonography can be helpful in demonstrating the hypertrophied pylorus. Upper gastrointestinal series shows a dilated, poorly emptying stomach, with intensive contractions and a pyloric "string sign" indenting the antral lesser curvature of the stomach.

Once the diagnosis of pyloric stenosis has been made, there are three major components to therapy. First, the infant must be given required restorative care. Second, the hypertrophied pyloric muscle must be corrected surgically. Finally, the patient must be supported while being allowed to reach an adequate oral intake.

Infants with pyloric stenosis can present with clinical and metabolic derangements of varying severity. Some infants show little abnormality, particularly in the early part of the clinical process. These infants require minimal intervention and can proceed to the second phase of therapy. Other infants, because of intense vomiting and a decreased caloric intake, can present with dehydration, hypoglycemia, abdominal distention, or growth failure. The vomiting leads to a hypochloremic, hypokalemic alkalosis. If the vomiting is mild, it may be corrected by oral feedings every 3 hours with a 0.5 normal saline solution and 5 per cent glucose and added potassium chloride (KCl). More severe vomiting and dehydration require intravenous treatment with 0.25 to 0.5 normal saline with 5 per cent glucose at a rate of 125 to 150 ml/kg every 24 hours. After urination has been established, KCl can be added at 2 to 3 mEq/kg per 24 hours. With severe salt depletion, it may be necessary to increase the amount of sodium chloride by using a 0.75 to 1.0 normal saline solution. Serum electrolytes, as well as the infant's weight and hydration status, should be monitored carefully. Most infants will demonstrate a good response 12 to 48 hours into fluid and electrolyte correction. Occasional patients who show signs of recurrent hypoglycemia and poor nutrition may require parenteral hyperalimentation for several days. Marked abdominal distention can be managed with gastric lavage and gastric decompression via nasogastric suction. Once the infant has achieved an improved physical and metabolic state, the next therapeutic phase can be instituted.

Surgical intervention by Ramstedt pyloromyotomy is the procedure of choice for correction of pyloric stenosis. In this procedure, the hypertrophied pyloric and antral muscular layers are incised, leaving the mucosa intact. Two major complications that can arise are the incomplete division of the hypertrophied pyloric muscle and perforation of the duodenal mucosa. The latter is usually detected and repaired by the surgeon during the operative procedure. Both of these complications can become evident in the postoperative period. The procedure's mortality rate is less than 1 per cent. General anesthesia is required in most cases, and the patient should not be fed orally 8 to 12 hours prior to surgery.

Careful observation is imperative in the postoperative period. If the pyloromyotomy has been uncomplicated, nasogastric suction can be discontinued 4 hours after surgery. Two to three ounces of a glucose-electrolyte solution, such as Pedialyte or Ricelyte, or a 5 per cent glucose solution can be administered. Feedings can be advanced on the second day to breast milk or full-strength formula 2 to 3 ounces every 2 to 3 hours. Infants should be feeding liberally by the third postoperative day. Intermittent vomiting may occur in the first few days after surgery. On rare occasion, the emesis may be severe and continued intravenous replacement therapy and nasogastric suction may be required. If a perforation of the duodenal mucosa is suspected, feedings should be discontinued and nasogastric suction should be reinstituted for a 24-hour period. Oral feeds can then be resumed. If incomplete lysis of the hypertrophied pyloric muscle is suspected, it is best to stop feedings and start nasogastric suction and intravenous hyperalimentation. The infant will be able to feed orally in approximately 1 week. Repeat pyloromyotomy is rarely necessary. An upper gastrointestinal (GI) series is of little value at this point. Radiologic evidence of the pyloric abnormality may persist for months despite adequate surgical intervention.

With careful management during the preoperative and postoperative periods, an excellent outcome can be expected from the surgical approach to pyloric stenosis.

PEPTIC ULCER

DEBORAH A. GOLDMAN, M.D.

Peptic ulcer disease (PUD) has long been recognized in children. However, with the advent of newer diagnostic tools over the past two decades, the reports and documentation of PUD in children and adolescents has increased dramatically. Peptic ulcers are known to occur in an otherwise well child, the so-called *primary ulcer,* but also in association with an acute, stressful situation, such as a burn, sepsis, or with medications. These are known as *secondary ulcers.* Recently, there has been an explosion in understanding the pathophysiology and treatment of PUD. The advent of cimetidine and the subsequent histamine H_2 receptor antagonists has been followed by site protective agents such as sucralfate, prostaglandin analogues, new prokinetics agents, and the most recent H^+/K^+-ATPase inhibitor, all of which can provide treatment and/or prophylaxis for PUD.

PATHOPHYSIOLOGY

Our knowledge of the etiology of ulcer disease encompasses the imbalance between mucosal protective mechanisms and the aggressive forces presented to the mucosa. In addition, genetic factors, such as a positive family history, and possible infection with *Helicobacter pylori* also can play an important role. The dictum of "no acid–no ulcer" has steered most of the research; however, other aggressive forces are involved. For example, bile salts can break down the mucus layer, exposing the mucosa to acid and pepsin. It is the combination of acid and pepsin that is considered the major factor in ulcer formation.

The gastric mucosa also requires a defense mechanism—the mucus-bicarbonate barrier. Mucus acts as a physical barrier and as the unstirred layer that impedes the passage of hydrogen ion toward the mucosal cells. Bicarbonate secretion buffers the hydrogen ion. In addition, prostaglandins inhibit parietal cell function, stimulate gastric mucus secretion, and stimulate bicarbonate production. It is the interplay of these forces—the aggressive and protective mechanisms—that predisposes to most peptic injury.

PRIMARY PEPTIC ULCERS

Primary peptic ulcer can be a naturally recurring disease, and patients may require intermittent or continuous therapy. The ulcer often is seen in an otherwise well child with no precipitating factors. The presenting symptoms most often include abdominal pain and vomiting and, more rarely, melena and hematemesis. Lesions can be diagnosed by barium studies; however, the gold standard is endoscopy.

The first line of therapy for peptic ulcer disease is the inhibition of acid secretion by histamine H_2 receptor antagonists. Cimetidine, ranitidine, famotidine, and nizatidine are the most commonly used H_2 blockers; these H_2 blockers have different potencies and differing means of renal excretion. H_2 blockers are effective for duodenal, pyloric, and gastric ulcers in infants and children. Cimetidine is usually given in four equal doses (for neonates, 10 to 20 mg/kg/day; for older children, 20 to 40 mg/kg/day p.o.). Ranitidine can also be used in the pediatric population in a dose of 4 to 6 mg/kg/day divided two to three times daily.

H_2 blockers are generally well tolerated, and occurrence of adverse effects, such as hematologic abnormality, central nervous system toxicity, and cholestasis, should be monitored periodically. In addition, these agents, especially cimetidine, interact with other medications, such as theophylline, phenytoin, coumadin, and beta-blockers, because of metabolism by the hepatic P_{450} system. The recommended duration of therapy is 12 weeks of full dose and then institution of a maintenance dosage, often given as a single dose at night for 4 weeks and then discontinued if symptoms are resolved.

Another indication for H_2 blockers is the prevention of stress ulceration in a critically ill child. It is important to maintain a gastric pH greater than 4.0; if renal clearance is increased, a larger dose of H_2 blockers is required. Intravenous use, especially divided over 24 hours, is the most effective method; however, it can be given every 6 to 8 hours.

Another modality to treat peptic ulcer disease is the use of cytoprotective agents, which offer protection to the mucosa but do not affect gastric acidity. Agents such as bismuth compounds and sucralfate are in this category. Much of the work with bismuth compounds has centered on its bactericidal effect on *H. pylori.* It is also effective in healing ulcers and may in fact heal those resistant to H_2 antagonists. There are potential side effects, including possible neurotoxicity.

Sucralfate is effective in healing ulceration and is well tolerated. The dosage in children is variable, but the usual adult dose (1 g four times daily) is tailored to a corresponding lower dose in children. In general, a slurry of sucralfate can be made with 1 g in 15 ml of water. In younger children, 250 to 500 mg (5.0 to 7.5 ml) of the slurry four times daily is recommended. The main side effects include constipation and possible aluminum absorption. Sucralfate can affect the bioavailability of phenytoin (Dilantin), warfarin, and ciprofloxacin.

Omeprazole, the latest therapeutic modality, inhibits the parietal cell H^+/K^+-ATPase or proton pump and is the most potent inhibitor of acid secretion yet available. (I suggest in intractable esophagitis that a pediatric gastroenterologist be consulted.) Omeprazole is quite successful in healing ulcers; but because of elevated gastric levels and the possibility of hyperplasia of the gastric enterochromaffin-like cells, its use should be limited to short courses in treating peptic ulcer disease and reflux esophagitis. It is not yet approved for use in children; however, it has been used on occasion in the pediatric population with recalcitrant esophagitis and/or severe peptic ulcer disease unresponsive to other therapeutic modalities. This medication should be used only under the guidance of a pediatric gastroenterologist.

Antacids can provide symptomatic relief; however, they are not recommended as first-line therapy. Dosage in the pediatric population of the variety of over-the-counter preparations (including Maalox, Mylanta, and Alternagel) is 1 ml/kg four times daily in infants and 15 to 30 ml four times daily in older children or to keep pH greater than 4.0. They are effective in ulcer healing after 6 to 8 weeks of therapy and in the prevention of stress ulceration. The side effects of antacids depend on the type of antacid, dosage, and the duration of the treatment. Typically, one sees diarrhea after magnesium hydroxide and constipation with aluminum hydroxide preparations. In addition, the bioavailability of certain medications can be altered and thus one should be aware of concomitant medications and renal function.

With respect to management issues, the first line of therapy for peptic ulcer disease confirmed by upper gastrointestinal (UGI) series or esophagogastroduodenoscopy (EGD) is H_2 receptor antagonist for 8 to 12 weeks. If this fails, one may need to consider repeat EGD with biopsy to rule out *H. pylori* infection, which is treated with bismuth compound, ampicillin, and metronidazole (Flagyl) for 6 to 8 weeks. Another alternative to refractory peptic ulcer disease is omeprazole for a limited time.

Unfortunately, peptic ulcer disease in children can be difficult to treat and between 35 to 70 per cent of children have a recurrence. A large group will respond to further medical treatment, but a small number of patients require surgery because of pain, bleeding, perforation, or obstructive symptoms. The surgical procedures are numerous, the choice of which is largely dictated by side effects, complications, and recurrence rates.

SECONDARY PEPTIC ULCERS

Secondary peptic ulcers can occur in the setting of systemic illness or with certain medications, such as nonsteroidal anti-inflammatory drugs (NSAIDs), aspirin, and steroids. They often present in a more dramatic fashion. The signs and symptoms often include hematemesis, melena, perforation, and, rarely, abdominal pain.

The association of NSAIDs with peptic ulcer has not been conclusively established, and the mechanisms of such damage are not fully understood. However, there seems to be morbidity and mortality from peptic ulcer disease associated with the use of NSAIDs. The first step toward managing suspected NSAID-induced peptic lesions is stopping the medication or lowering the dose. H_2 receptor antagonists and sucralfate are effective for healing these lesions. However, misoprostol (prostaglandin E_1 analogue) is the drug of choice that has been shown to heal these ulcers, especially in the duodenum. This agent is also approved for prophylaxis of NSAID-associated gastric lesions; however, this should be used only for patients at high risk.

It is important to use prophylaxis in patients at risk for stress ulceration, especially those in the intensive care setting. Antacids given orally or through a nasogastric tube, with a magnesium-containing preparation often being alternated with an aluminum preparation to maintain a pH greater than 4, can be efficacious. H_2 blockers are given intravenously (either as continuous drip or every 6 to 8 hours). Sucralfate can also be effective given four times daily. If signs of bleeding become evident, endoscopy is indicated.

ACUTE GASTROINTESTINAL BLEED

With respect to management of acute GI bleeding, any bleeding sufficient to bring a patient to the hospital is a potential emergency. The presence of GI bleeding may not be obvious at first. If it is massive with hematemesis, hematochezia or shock, the first stage of management is to stabilize the patient, treat the shock, and restore the blood volume. One can then locate the source of the bleeding. One of the first diagnostic tests is to do nasogastric lavage. If the gastric lavage is heme-negative, the bleeding may have ceased or is distal to the pylorus. If bleeding persists, volume expansion and stabilization are crucial. Endoscopy can be performed and appropriate therapy instituted on the basis of the findings.

If the bleeding site cannot be identified, radiolabeled red blood cell scans or selective angiography may need to be performed. Rarely is laparotomy indicated unless bleeding is uncontrollable by medical means or if perforation is suspected. Angiography is indicated if bleeding persists at a rate of at least 0.5 ml/minute or greater. Pitressin (0.2 to 0.4 units/1.73 m^2/minute IV) may be required following the use of selective angiography. Mortality is correlated with initial hemoglobin, a large transfusion requirement, coexistence of another life-threatening condition, or the presence of a coagulopathy.

MALFORMATIONS OF THE INTESTINE

NANCY E. VINTON, M.D.

Congenital malformations of the intestinal tract can present the pediatrician with emergency situations at birth. Cautionary signs include polyhydramnios in the mother and bilious vomiting, abdominal distention, and failure to pass meconium in the neonate. Gastrointestinal bleeding and obstruction are more often the presenting signs in the older child. Prompt measures must be taken, prior to surgical intervention, to help prevent the high mortality rate still associated with congenital anomalies. Furthermore, the pediatrician may have to deal with sequelae from a surgical correction long after the malformation itself has ceased to be a problem.

MALFORMATIONS PRESENTING AS INTESTINAL OBSTRUCTION

Malformations leading to intestinal obstruction immediately after birth include duodenal web; annular pancreas; stenoses, atresias, or duplications anywhere along the intestinal tract; and malrotation with midgut volvulus. The higher the obstruction, the lesser the degree of abdominal distention but also the more rapid the onset of symptoms and the more urgent the need for intervention. Prompt treatment to relieve the distention from swallowed air and accumulating intestinal secretions avoids possible aspiration and respiratory compromise. Endotracheal intubation may be necessary to protect the infant's airway. Placement of a nasogastric or orogastric tube (No. 10 French Rapogle tube) effectively evacuates the stomach and prevents further abdominal distention. Only low intermittent suction is used because constant or high-pressure suction frequently results in gastric erosions in neonates. Intravenous ranitidine (2 to 4 mg/kg/day as a continuous or bolus infusion) should be started as additional prophylaxis against upper gastrointestinal hemorrhage and also for prevention of the gastric hypersecretion seen postoperatively if extensive bowel resection has taken place.

Correction of fluid and electrolyte imbalance due to loss of intestinal secretions must be undertaken preoperatively. Gastric outputs are replaced volume for volume with an intravenous solution of one-half normal saline and 30 mEq/L of potassium chloride, and maintenance fluids are given on an ongoing basis. If the malformation causing obstruction is malrotation with volvulus, severe acidosis secondary to bowel ischemia may need to be corrected intravenously with a 20 ml/kg bolus of normal saline or even with 1 mEq/kg of sodium bicarbonate. An associated congenital heart defect may be life-threatening and demand priority surgical intervention. In these cases, placement of a central venous catheter for total parenteral nutrition and continued gastric drainage allows deferral of intestinal surgery until it can be safely accomplished.

Surgical techniques to correct malformations causing intestinal obstruction are mentioned here briefly. The operation is performed using general endotracheal anesthesia. A right upper quadrant transverse incision (with extension to the left of the abdomen in cases of malrotation) is most often chosen because it yields ready access to the entire intestinal tract. Frequently, a gastrostomy tube is placed for chronic decompression of the bowel, protection of the anastomosis, and future enteral feeding attempts.

Duodenal webs are treated with duodenotomy and web excision. In annular pancreas, a bypass operation attaches proximal to distal duodenum so that the sequelae of invading pancreatic tissue are avoided (fistula or pseudocyst formation, peritonitis, and pancreatitis). Areas of stenosis or duplication, if small, are resected and a primary anastomosis is performed. In all of the above cases, a catheter must be passed through the bowel proximal and distal to the anastomosis to ensure that unsuspected webs are not present. Long tubular duplications may be unresectable without impairing the vasculature to the normal intestinal tract. In such cases, leaving the segment in place after complete mucosal stripping, with or without establishing drainage to the normal bowel, may be adequate therapy to prevent further obstruction or bleeding.

Complete atresia of the intestine (duodenal, jejunal, or ileal) may necessitate significant resection of the dilated proximal segment before primary anastomosis can be attempted. In cases of short-bowel syndrome, to salvage as much gut as possible, a tapering procedure along the antimesenteric border approximates the dilated proximal intestinal segment to the more normal caliber distal segment. Dilated, atonic proximal intestine may pose problems as a motility disorder in many children in subsequent years. Discordant motility patterns inherent to small and large bowel may give rise to a functional obstruction at the site of anastomosis between jejunum or ileum and colon. Conservative medical management (bowel rest with intravenous hydration and nutrition) during acute obstructive episodes is mandatory to minimize further intestinal resection. Later management includes use of motility agents, such as metaclopramide or cisapride, or further surgery to resect amotile segments.

In intestinal malrotation, obstruction occurs from midgut volvulus or from Ladd's bands lying across the duodenum that attach it to the displaced cecum found to the left of midline. With surgery, the bands are lysed and the volvulus is reduced by counterclockwise rotation of the gut around its mesentery. Recurrence of volvulus is rare, and no advantage has been noted with fixation of the mesentery. Intestinal malrotation should be looked for as a frequently associated malformation during surgery for duodenal and jejunoileal atresia. Malrotation presenting with volvulus can happen at any age, even in adulthood, and must always be included in the differential diagnosis of the patient with signs of upper intestinal obstruction, chronic or acute abdominal pain, and/or bilious vomiting.

MALFORMATIONS PRESENTING AS EVISCERATION

In the neonatal period, ruptured omphalocele and gastroschisis present an emergency situation that is unrelated to intestinal obstruction as discussed above. In these infants, initial management is aimed at protecting the eviscerated bowel from heat and fluid loss and from infection. Omphalocele with an intact peritoneal and amniotic sac, however, is not a surgical emergency because there is little risk of contamination, and the surrounding Wharton's jelly acts as insulation to prevent evaporative and heat losses. These infants do not require gastric drainage or intravenous therapy and are usually very stable. Nonoperative management of intact omphalocele is to induce granulation tissue to form over the sac with use of merbromin (Mercurochrome) or silver nitrate. This is a long and tedious process and can be circumvented by initial surgery to free up skin flaps that are then pulled over the omphalocele and sutured closed. In either case, the bowel is left as a ventral hernia until a staged closure of the defect can be arranged.

In gastroschisis and ruptured omphalocele, the exposed bowel must be dealt with immediately. With sterile gloves, exposed bowel should be situated centrally on the abdomen to prevent pulling against the vascular pedicle, which causes ischemia. The infant can then be placed up to the axillae inside a Lahey bag, if available. This is a sterile plastic bag with a cinch strap across the top used by abdominal surgeons to hold viscera exposed intraoperatively. The alternative is to cover exposed bowel with sterile saline-soaked gauze to prevent drying and then wrap the bowel with an abundant layer of sterile dry gauze to prevent heat loss. Use of an incubator also helps to maintain body temperature and prevent evaporative heat losses. A nasogastric or orogastric tube is placed to low intermittent suction to prevent abdominal distention with air both preoperatively and postoperatively. Ventilation by endotracheal tube may be necessary to stabilize the infant, but air leakage around the tube will also increase the probability of abdominal distention. Transcutaneous or peripheral arterial monitoring of oxygenation replaces the usual method of umbilical artery catheterization. Ampicillin and gentamicin are given intravenously to treat possible enteric sepsis. Intravenous access is mandatory prior to transport to another location for surgical intervention.

The aim of operative repair for these malformations presenting as evisceration is to create an internal cavity large enough to hold all of the abdominal viscera. Current techniques utilize polytef (Teflon) material sutured circumferentially to the abdominal musculature, forming a tubular structure around the exposed bowel. This is then managed either with a drawstring progressively drawn tighter or by sutures repeatedly opened and resutured to take up slack as the abdominal cavity enlarges to hold more intestine. After 7 to 10 days, the Teflon implant is removed because of an increasing risk of infection. Intravenous antibiotic coverage is continued and broadened to include staphylococcal organisms, and topical antibiotics are applied to the operative site throughout this time. The dangers of prematurely forcing the viscera into the small abdominal cavity include respiratory compromise and bowel ischemia.

Gastroschisis is often complicated by the presence of malrotation, intestinal atresia, and enteric fistulas. These complications may not be recognized at the time of initial surgery if the eviscerated bowel is densely adherent and may not become apparent until postoperatively when enteral feedings are attempted. A motility disorder of the remaining intestine also can delay enteral nutrition for months. Hence, in all of these infants, at the time of surgery a central venous catheter for total parenteral nutrition and a gastrostomy tube for later attempts at enteral feeding should be inserted. An infant with a ruptured omphalocele is not subject to these problems unless the exposed serosal surface of the bowel develops an infection.

OMPHALOMESENTERIC DUCT MALFORMATIONS

Malformations of the umbilicus that remain in continuity with the intestinal tract are the omphalomesenteric duct remnants—granuloma or polyp, sinus or fistula, Meckel's diverticulum or fibrous cord. These anomalies generally are not a problem in the neonatal period but may nonetheless cause life-threatening illness in the pediatric patient. A Meckel's diverticulum can present with massive gastrointestinal hemorrhage from ulceration due to ectopic gastric mucosa; as intestinal obstruction from volvulus, internal herniation, or intussusception; or as diverticulitis with or without perforation. After the child becomes hemodynamically stable, receiving intravenous fluids and antibiotics, abdominal surgery is performed to fully excise the lesion from its origin on the antimesenteric border of the distal ileum. Ileal resection may be necessary if the base of the diverticulum is wide or if there has been some compromise to the adjacent intestine. No sequelae result from this operation unless perforation has led to complications with peritonitis.

Umbilical granulomas may be treated with applications of silver nitrate. Polyps consist of intestinal mucosa, and local resection is required. Sinus tracts (ending blindly) or fistula tracts (in continuity with bowel and extruding feces) are treated with local antibiotics and débridement to facilitate drainage, but definitive therapy is complete excision through either an intraumbilical or an intra-abdominal approach. A fibrous cord remnant from an obliterated omphalomesenteric duct also should be excised, since it can be the lead point around which a volvulus or internal herniation of intestine may occur.

INTESTINAL MALFORMATIONS WITH LATER PRESENTATION

Internal hernias are defects in the mesentery in which small intestine can enter and become incarcerated. They can manifest at any age. During surgery the hernia is first reduced, which may require a further incision of the mesentery to release the incarcerated bowel. The mesenteric defect is then closed with sutures. Intestinal resection is dependent on the degree of damage from prior ischemia.

Umbilical hernia is an abdominal wall defect that occurs as a result of incomplete development or imperfect closure of the fascia of the umbilical ring. Most close spontaneously by 3 years of age. However, if they are greater than 1.5 cm in diameter at 2 years of age, they should be corrected surgically to prevent the risk of intestinal incarceration. This is accomplished easily by invagination and oversewing of the hernia sac, even as an outpatient procedure.

Mesenteric and *omental cysts* are usually intestinal lymphangiomas, the majority being mesenteric (70 per cent) and polycystic (85 per cent). They may be asymptomatic at birth but continue to grow in size so that by 5 years of age nearly 60 per cent are detected because of intestinal obstruction or mass effect. Complete resection without removing intestine is recommended but not always feasible if the cyst is too tightly adherent to bowel or too close to the mesenteric blood supply.

FOREIGN BODIES IN THE GASTROINTESTINAL TRACT

STEVEN L. WERLIN, M.D.

Ingested foreign bodies are a common occurrence in the pediatric population. Of those objects brought to medical attention, most (80 to 90 per cent) pass spontaneously, but 10 to 20 per cent require medical treatment such as endoscopic or surgical removal. An unknown number, perhaps even the majority, of children who ingest foreign bodies are never seen by a physician. Most foreign bodies that fail to pass lodge in the esophagus, primarily in areas of anatomic narrowing in the proximal esophagus. More than 90 per cent of foreign bodies that reach the stomach pass spontaneously. Foreign bodies that pass through the stomach may fail to pass other areas of acute angulation, for instance, at the cecum.

Because the ingestion of multiple foreign bodies is common, a thorough radiographic evaluation must be performed. In the case of acute ingestion, chest films (posteroanterior and lateral) will identify radiopaque foreign bodies in the esophagus. Care must be taken to include the neck (lateral neck) so that a foreign body in the proximal trachea or hypopharynx will be identified. Abdominal radiographs identify those radiopaque foreign bodies that have reached the stomach. A barium swallow will identify radiolucent foreign bodies in the esophagus. At times it may be difficult to determine whether a coin is lodged in the esophagus or in the trachea. In these cases, on lateral chest x-ray an esophageal foreign body always appears in the coronal plane (side on) whereas a tracheal foreign body is seen in the sagittal plane (face on).

ESOPHAGUS

All foreign bodies impacted in the hypopharynx or esophagus must be removed promptly. A variety of methods have been described. Endoscopic removal is the most popular method. Both rigid and flexible instruments have been used successfully. It is safer to use general anesthesia in order to protect the airway. Endoscopic removal is the only acceptable technique when the foreign body is sharp or has been present for more than 24 hours or when the child has had esophageal surgery or has a known anomaly of the esophagus. A rigid endoscope or a flexible endoscope with an overtube may be used for the removal of sharp foreign bodies.

Round foreign bodies impacted in the esophagus for less than 24 hours in a previously well child may be removed by the Foley catheter technique or pushed into the stomach with a bougie. Particular attention must always be paid to protection of the airway.

Impaction of food, particularly meat, occurs in children with congenital anomalies of the esophagus, acquired strictures, and achalasia. If the child cannot handle secretions, endoscopy is urgent. Early in the course, removal should be attempted; however, it may be easier to push fragments of food into the stomach in these circumstances. Papain is not recommended because its use has been associated with lethal complications.

Sharp and pointed foreign bodies can be difficult to manage. An open safety pin, with point upward, should be pushed into the stomach before removal. If the point is downward, the pin may be safely pulled into a rigid endoscope or removed with a flexible endoscope and an overtube. Razor blades, more commonly ingested by deranged adults than by children, are removed from the esophagus with a rigid endoscope or with a flexible endoscope and an overtube.

Disc batteries impacted in the esophagus must be removed with urgency because of the risk of caustic injury.

Foreign bodies that lodge at the pharynx or cricopharyngeus are best removed by an otolaryngologist using a rigid laryngoscope and a grasping clamp.

Complications of esophageal foreign bodies include perforation, stricture, tracheoesophageal fistula, and aspiration pneumonia.

STOMACH

Although the literature states that about 90 per cent of all foreign bodies that reach the stomach will pass spontaneously, this author has not removed a gastric foreign body in several years. When it is determined that a foreign body has reached the stomach, I give a single injection of metoclopramide (0.2 mg/kg). Most smooth foreign bodies will then pass the pylorus rapidly. I have used this technique successfully with objects as large as hair barrettes. Using this technique, I have seen no perforations. If the object does not pass with metoclopramide, a rare occurrence in my experience, I advise waiting at least several weeks before endoscopic removal of an asymptomatic foreign body is attempted. Patience is a virtue, and given enough time, most foreign bodies uneventfully pass through the pylorus.

Circular foreign bodies greater than 5 cm in circumference may not pass through the pylorus because of their large size. These large foreign bodies usually need to be removed endoscopically. Similarly, sharp foreign bodies, such as razor blades and open safety pins, should be removed. I allow straight pins to pass spontaneously. Alkaline button batteries should be removed if they remain in the stomach for longer than 24 hours.

Except for those found in newborn infants, gastric bezoars usually need to be removed surgically. In the newborn period, particularly in premature infants and those fed concentrated formula, lactobezoars may be formed from curdled milk. Treatment is simple. The infant should take nothing by mouth, and intravenous fluids administered. The bezoar generally dissolves spontaneously in 24 to 48 hours.

SMALL INTESTINE

Once the foreign body has passed the pylorus, eventual passage through the small and large intestine is virtually assured. Although the literature states that 15 to 30 per cent of objects eventually perforate the bowel, this has not been my experience. Even sharp or irregularly shaped objects usually pass through the intestinal tract uneventfully. When impaction occurs, it is usually at the C loop of the duodenum, the duodenojejunal junction, or the terminal ileum. Particular problems include patients with a Meckel's diverticulum in which button batteries can lodge or patients who have had prior intestinal surgery with anastomosis or adhesion formation with angulations, which can predispose to obstruction or perforation.

LARGE INTESTINE

Orally ingested foreign bodies that reach the colon will pass uneventfully. In contrast, rectally inserted foreign bodies should be removed promptly. Digital removal may be possible in situations such as a thermometer in an infant. A nasal or vaginal speculum can be very helpful in such cases. In older children, a rigid sigmoidoscope is usually used. A large variety of bizarre objects have been inserted and require removal. In the case of fragile objects, general anesthesia may be required.

INTUSSUSCEPTION

FREDERICK J. RESCORLA, M.D.
and JAY L. GROSFELD, M.D.

Intussusception is one of the more common acute abdominal conditions for which surgical intervention may be required in infancy and childhood. The term refers to a process in which one segment of bowel, usually the terminal ileum, invaginates into the cecum and continues to migrate distally, within the lumen of colon. The infant, typically a 6-month-old male, experiences intermittent episodes of abdominal pain that are frequently followed by nonbilious vomiting. As edema develops within the invaginated bowel, owing to compression of the veins and lymphatics of the intussuscepted mesentery, bleeding occurs with resultant passage of blood and mucus in the stool. If edema is allowed to progress, it worsens, eventually leading to mechanical bowel obstruction characterized by bilious emesis and abdominal distention. If the intussusception goes unrecognized, arterial compromise, perforation and its associated sequelae may occur.

CLINICAL PRESENTATION

Age and Sex Incidence

Intussusception represents the most common cause of intestinal obstruction in children from 1 month to 5 years of age. The highest incidence is observed in infants and children between the ages of 3 months and 2 years of age (80 per cent), with 65 to 70 per cent of patients younger than 1 year of age. Most series report a 2:1 male-to-female ratio. The presence of a seasonal incidence has been debated, with some reports noting an increased number of cases of intussusception presenting in late spring and summer with another peak in mid winter. Twenty per cent of cases occur following a previous upper respiratory infections and/or gastroenteritis.

Signs and Symptoms

The most common signs and symptoms associated with intussusception are abdominal pain, vomiting, and rectal bleeding. The pain is characterized by its intermittent but severe nature. A previously healthy child typically presents with intense pain, which causes the child to draw the knees up to the chest. The pain lasts for several minutes; as it resolves, the child returns to a previous activity or may lie quiet and prostrate. The intermittent nature of the pain is suggestive of this diagnosis but may also be noted in babies with gastroenteritis. The pain is often followed by nonbilious emesis early in the course. The vomiting at this point is reflex in nature and not due to obstruction. The presence of bilious emesis usually indicates a long-standing process that has progressed to a complete mechanical bowel obstruction.

Rectal bleeding is seen in most cases of intussusception and varies from occult blood to gross rectal bleeding. The most commonly observed pattern is generally described as "currant jelly" stool, reflecting passage per rectum of blood mixed with intestinal mucus. This often occurs several hours after the onset of pain and may be absent when the family initially brings the child to medical attention. The child may also continue to have one or two normal bowel movements after the onset of pain as the colon distal to the intususceptum is evacuated.

Physical Examination

The findings on physical examination vary, depending on the duration of the intussusception and the degree of bowel compromise. If seen early, the child appears fairly normal between episodes of pain. Later in the course, the child may appear lethargic and listless. Temperature elevation to approximately 38°C is commonly observed. In 65% of cases, the abdominal examination usually demonstrates a soft, nontender abdomen with a sausage-shaped mass positioned transversely in the upper right to mid abdomen. The mass itself may be tender to palpation. The right lower quadrant is often described as feeling "empty" as the lead point, usually the ileum (the intussusceptum), and the cecum (intussuscipiens) into which it invaginates, are drawn out of the right lower quadrant. Although in the typical case the mass is located in the mid upper abdomen, occasionally the intussusceptum continues distally to the rectum, where it is palpable on digital rectal examination or may even protrude from the anal orifice.

In cases that have progressed to complete obstruction, the distended loops of proximal small bowel lead to generalized abdominal distention and obscure the mass. Peritonitis usually indicates perforation and occurs as a late finding in neglected cases. If the child has not passed overtly bloody material per rectum, the initial digital examination may detect bloody mucus or may detect only *o*-toluidine (Hematest)-positive material. Occasionally the stool in the rectal vault will be Hematest-negative; if the remainder of the clinical evaluation is consistent with intussusception, absence of this one sign should not delay further diagnostic evaluation.

Associated Illness and Lead Points

Intussusception has been reported with increased frequency in children with hemophilia, Henoch-Schönlein purpura, B cell lymphoma, and cystic fibrosis. The presence of a pathologic lead point in cases of intussusception occurs in approximately 1 to 3 per cent of children younger than 5 years of age with the incidence as high as 18 to 25 per cent in children older than 5 years of age. Pathologic lead points may include a polyp (juvenile, Peutz-Jeghers), Meckel's diverticulum, intestinal duplication, papillary lymphoid hyperplasia, hemangioma, lymphoma, an appendiceal stump, or a suture line from a previous procedure.

DIAGNOSIS

A complete blood count is obtained and often demonstrates a leukocytosis (WBC > 10,000); however, this is a relatively nonspecific test. Plain abdominal roentgenograms are frequently nonspecific but may demonstrate an empty left colon and rectosigmoid. In cases that have progressed to complete obstruction, dilated small-bowel loops with air-fluid levels are noted proximal to the obstruction.

Although abdominal ultrasound and computed tomography (CT) have both been used to diagnose intussusception, these tests are rarely required. Ultrasonography may occasionally pick up the typical concentric rings of an intussusception when used to evaluate a child with an atypical presentation. Barium enema is the diagnostic procedure of choice. However, this study is also a mode of therapy which should be performed only after initial fluid resuscitation.

MANAGEMENT

Resuscitation

Initial management of a child with suspected intussusception includes intravenous fluid resuscitation on the basis of presence and severity of dehydration. If the process is of recent onset and either no or only mild dehydration is present, a bolus of 10 ml/kg of crystalloid (5 per cent dextrose in lactated Ringer's solution) is administered intravenously followed by maintenance fluids. If moderate to severe dehydration is present, we generally administer a bolus of 20 ml/kg of 5 per cent dextrose in lactated Ringer's solution and then infuse 0.45 per cent normal saline at twice normal maintenance. The stomach is decompressed with a nasogastric tube, and broad-spectrum antibiotics are administered to include both aerobic and anaerobic coverage. Our preference is either cefoxitin or a combination of ampicillin, gentamicin, and clindamycin. In addition, the operating room is notified to prepare for immediate laparotomy if attempted nonoperative reduction is unsuccessful or if a perforation occurs. An occasional child will require immediate surgical exploration. Indications for immediate exploration are perforation as evidenced by free intraperitoneal air on plain abdominal roentgenograms, peritonitis, or septic shock. Although a long-standing (>72 hours) intussusception may be less likely to decrease with a hydrostatic barium enema, a gentle diagnostic barium enema may be performed followed by an attempt at reduction.

Nonoperative Reduction

Before a hydrostatic reduction barium enema and after appropriate fluid resuscitation are attempted, the child is sedated with either morphine sulfate (0.1 mg/kg, if over 1 year of age) or secobarbital (Seconal, 1.0 mg/kg, with or without meperidine, 1.0 mg/kg, if younger than 1 year). In addition, one may use a combination of meperidine (1.0 mg/kg), promethazine (0.5 mg/kg), and chlorpromazine (0.5 mg/kg). A balloon catheter is inserted into the rectum and inflated, and the child's legs are then strapped together to prevent expulsion of the balloon. The bag of barium is raised 3 feet above the table. As the barium fills the colon, the diagnosis is confirmed by the appearance of the intussusceptum as a "coiled spring" intraluminal mass (Fig. 1). The 3 feet of hydrostatic pressure are allowed to reduce the intussusceptum under periodic fluoroscopic guidance. The procedure is discontinued if there is no proximal movement of the intussusceptum for a 5-minute period. The presence of barium dissecting along the intussusceptum proximally has been a sign of irreducibility. Although sporadic use of glucagon as a relaxant has been reported to enhance the success rate of barium reduction, this was not found efficacious in carefully randomized studies. Free reflux of barium from the cecum into a few loops of ileum with complete disappearance of the intussusceptum must be noted in a successful reduction. The reported success rate of hydrostatic barium reduction varies between 50 and 85 per cent. Patient groups associated with a low success rate include age younger than 3 months, prolonged duration of symptoms, an obstructive pattern on abdominal roentgenograms, and older children in whom the incidence of a pathologic lead point is higher.

Complications of attempted hydrostatic barium enema reduction include perforation with barium contamination of the peritoneal cavity as well as recurrence of the intussusception. Perforation rates of 0 to 2 per cent have been reported. This usually occurs in the setting of a complete mechanical bowel obstruction. The rate of recurrence of intussusception following hydrostatic reduction is 6 to 10 per cent in most series. Infants and children with more than two episodes of recurrence of intussusception are candidates for operative exploration.

An alternative form of enema reduction is hydrostatic reduction with saline under ultrasound guidance, which had

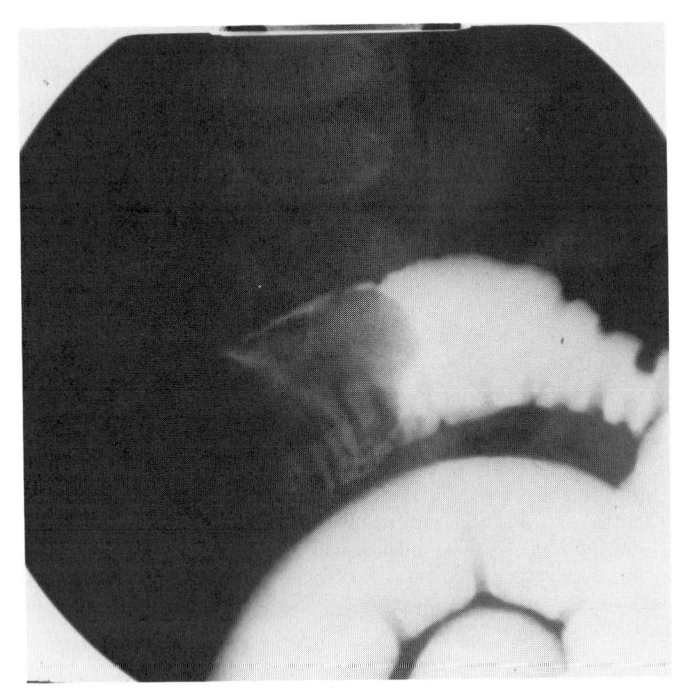

Figure 1. Barium enema demonstrates an intussusception within the transverse colon.

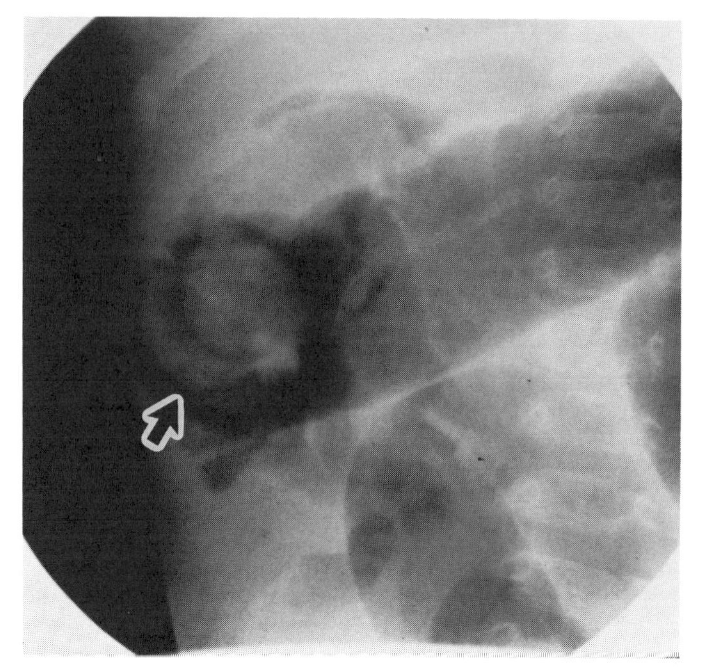

Figure 2. Radiography demonstrating an air enema reduction. Note the distended distal colon with the intraluminal intussusceptum *(arrows)*.

a success rate of 95 per cent in one series. An air enema reduction technique has also been reported with the use of air instilled per rectum at a pressure of 80 mm Hg in young infants and 110 mm Hg in older infants and children (Fig. 2). A success rate of 99 per cent was noted with this technique in a large series of patients from China. Of interest, 50 per cent of the patients in this series required a second reduction 2 to 3 hours after the first attempt. Recently, a study comparing barium and air reduction indicated that the latter technique was as efficient in reducing the intussusception and less dangerous in instances of perforation than the hydrostatic barium enema technique.

The management of the child successfully treated with nonoperative reduction has generally involved hospitalization for approximately 24 hours to allow restoration of normal diet and documentation of bowel function by observing passage of stool. We have cared for several patients who presented shortly after the onset of symptoms, who experienced prompt successful nonoperative reduction, and who were released after a relatively short (2 to 6 hours) observation period during which time diet was resumed, absence of recurrent pain was documented, and flatus was passed. The patient's families were counseled regarding the risk of recurrence following nonoperative reduction and were instructed to consult a physician if symptoms recurred.

Although reduction of an intussusception due to a pathologic lead point is unusual, if a pathologic lead point is identified in a child treated successfully with a reduction enema, a delayed laparotomy can be performed after an appropriate bowel preparation. This can be performed several days later to allow resolution of the edema associated with the intussusception. Infants and children who fail to respond to nonoperative reduction are promptly taken to the operating room for laparotomy, as noted next.

Operative Management

The stomach is completely emptied with a nasogastric tube. An "awake" intubation is performed to minimize the risk of aspiration. The abdomen is entered though a transverse right lower quadrant incision. The typical ileocecal intussusception is noted (Fig. 3). The colon just distal to the intussusceptum is identified, and the distal bowel is gently compressed between the surgeon's fingers and the intussusceptum is "milked back" to and subsequently through the ileocecal valve, totally reducing the intussusceptum (ileum) out of the intussuscipiens (colon and cecum). The peritoneal attachments (Jackson's veil) between the appendix and distal ileum are divided, and an appendectomy is performed.

Numerous lymph nodes are frequently seen in the distribution of the ileocolic vessels. No attempt at removal or biopsy is necessary. In addition, the site of the terminal ileum invagination (intussusceptum) is often edematous and thickened to manual palpation after reduction. This is not a pathologic finding. The bowel should not be opened unless

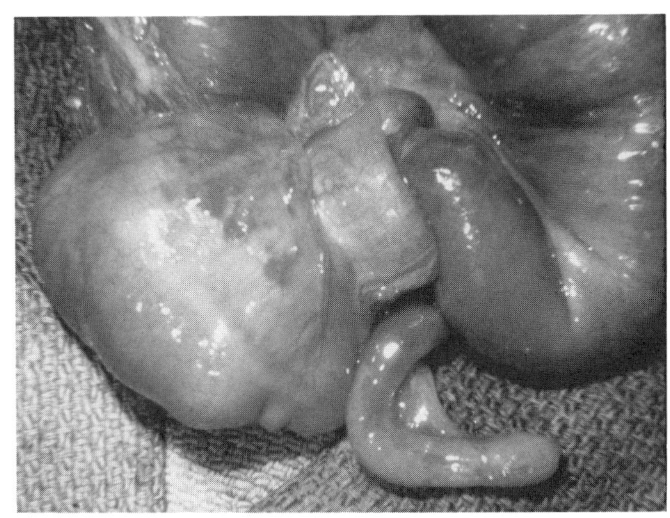

Figure 3. Operative photograph of a typical ileocecal intussusception.

an intraluminal pathologic lead point is noted. The diet is usually resumed within 24 hours of surgery, and the child is released when tolerating a regular diet.

If manual reduction is unsuccessful, resection with primary anastomosis between the ileum and colon is performed. A necrotic intussusceptum may be noted if a child has endured a long-standing process or has signs of peritonitis and/or sepsis preoperatively. In such cases, manual reduction is not attempted and resection with primary anastomosis is performed. There may be an occasional role for temporary ileostomy and delayed anastomosis in cases with perforation and diffuse contamination. Postoperative care in cases requiring resection includes intravenous fluids, antibiotics, and nasogastric decompression until bowel function returns, followed by restoration of regular diet.

Recurrence of intussusception after operative reduction has been reported in up to 6 per cent in some series. We have never seen a recurrence after surgical reduction.

SUMMARY

Intussusception is a common cause of abdominal pain in infancy and childhood requiring surgical intervention. Prompt diagnosis and intervention with either hydrostatic barium enema or air reduction allows nonoperative management of most cases. Nonoperative reduction failures require immediate operation and often may be manually reduced by the surgeon. Occasionally, in instances associated with delayed diagnosis, a bowel resection will be required. Careful and prompt attention to patient management can minimize morbidity and should eliminate any mortality.

HIRSCHSPRUNG'S DISEASE

THOMAS M. ROSSI, M.D.

Hirschsprung's disease (congenital aganglionic megacolon) is characterized by an absence of ganglion cells from the submucosal and intermuscular regions of the intestinal wall. The absence may occur from an arrest of the normal caudad migration of neural crest cells to the embryonic intestinal neural plexuses. An accumulation of extracellular matrix material, including components of the basal laminae of the muscularis mucosa, has recently been postulated to be the defect in the aganglionic tissue responsible for interference with migration of the neural crest cells.

In every case, therefore, a point exists distal to which ganglion cells cannot be identified. The junction between normally innervated intestine and the aganglionic segment is referred to as the "transition zone." *The disease is not necessarily limited to the colon, since some patients have aganglionic segments beginning in the proximal small intestine.* In 3 to 8 per cent of cases, either the entire colon or the colon as well as varying amounts of small bowel is affected. Confinement to the rectosigmoid area occurs in 80 per cent of patients. Since the migration of cells theoretically may be interrupted at even the most distal segment of the colon, the internal sphincter alone may be involved, i.e., ultra-short-segment Hirschsprung's disease.

The incidence of the disorder is 1 in 5000 live births. It is rare in low-birth-weight infants, and there is no known racial predilection. It is commonly assumed to be a sex-modified multifactorial trait. An increased sex ratio (4:1 male to female) and an elevated risk to siblings (4 per cent) exist, with the sex ratio decreasing and the recurrence risk to siblings increasing as the aganglionosis becomes more extensive. The percentage of affected girls with a positive family history is greater. There is also an association with Down syndrome and with Waardenburg syndrome.

SIGNS AND SYMPTOMS

Although most patients are recognized in early infancy, a small proportion may reach adolescence or adult life before the condition is diagnosed. Symptoms, therefore, vary according to the age of the patient. Hirschsprung's disease accounts for about one third of all cases of neonatal intestinal obstruction. Failure to pass meconium, anorexia, bilious emesis, and abdominal distention are frequent symptoms in the first few days of life. If neonatal symptoms are not as prominent, infants may present with symptoms of chronic constipation, abdominal distention, and failure to thrive. The onset of enterocolitis usually occurs within the first 3 months of life and may be heralded by unexplained fever and poor feeding. Abdominal distention, profuse diarrhea, and vomiting are the most prominent features. A protein-losing enteropathy may ensue. The etiology of enterocolitis in this situation has been attributed to *Clostridium difficile.*

Children with Hirschsprung's disease commonly seek medical attention for chronic constipation and abdominal distention. Fecal impaction, microcytic anemia, hypoproteinemia, and failure to thrive can be associated features. Intermittent episodes of intestinal obstruction secondary to fecal impactions may also occur. Encopresis is uncommon except in the rare instance of short-segment disease. The protuberant abdomen along with other signs of malnutrition simulate the malabsorptive syndromes.

DIAGNOSIS

The diagnosis of Hirschsprung's disease can be suspected on physical examination. In addition to the above-noted signs, rectal examination usually reveals a tight anal sphincter and empty rectal ampulla and, in infants, may yield a rush of fluid and gas following withdrawal of the digit. Exceptions to these findings exist for the short-segment disease, in which stool can be palpated in the rectum. Fecal masses are easily palpable on abdominal examination. In cases of enterocolitis, abdominal examination reveals signs of peritonitis and perhaps perforation. Perforation of the ileum, colon, or appendix may occur.

The radiographic features of Hirschsprung's disease include gaseous distention and absence of gas in the rectum when the patient is viewed in the prone position. An abrupt change in the caliber of the colon at the site of the transition zone can sometimes be identified on plain films. The barium enema, performed with the instillation of a small amount of radiopaque material just beyond the anal sphincter, classically reveals a distal narrowed zone representing the aganglionic segment; a transition zone; and a proximal dilated segment, representing the normal ganglion containing intestine. Newborns and infants with total colonic involvement may not exhibit these classic features. On the other hand, infants with Hirschsprung's disease fail to evacuate the barium completely over a 24-hour period whereas this sign is less helpful in older children.

Anorectal manometry offers a precise method of ruling out the disorder. A normal internal anal sphincter relaxes (as manifested by a decrease in pressure on the tracing recording) in response to balloon dilatation of the rectum. In Hirschsprung's disease, relaxation does not occur and often a pressure rise is demonstrated. The presence of the normal reflex rules out the disease. However, normal newborns and prematures may not exhibit the reflex because of delayed maturity of the neural plexuses. The distinctive anal reflex response provides a nonsurgical method for excluding the diagnosis. It also suggests that the severe constipation encountered in this disorder is related to the functional obstruction produced by an unyielding internal anal sphincter as well as by the failure of propulsive forces in the aganglionic rectum.

Rectal biopsy, by providing direct evidence of aganglionosis, is the definitive method of diagnosis. The absence of ganglion cells may be misleading in certain situations. *Because these cells are sparse in the distal colon and anal canal, care in interpretation of the histologic section is mandatory. Also, ganglion cells may be normally absent from the area 1 to 2 cm proximal to the anus. Biopsy specimens should be excluded from this zone in order to avoid confusion.* A help in distinguishing normal from aganglionic tissue has been offered by the availability of histochemical staining for acetylcholinesterase. Activity is high in aganglionic sections and may be more reliable than rectal manometry in the newborn and premature periods.

TREATMENT

Definitive treatment for Hirschsprung's disease is provided by resection of the aganglionic segment followed by a pull-through procedure of the normal intestine to the anal canal. An enterostomy, placed in the area of normal ganglionic intestine, is usually performed following establishment of the diagnosis. The definitive pull-through is made at a time when the infant is older, i.e., 6 to 12 months of age. In cases of ultra-short-segment disease, an internal sphincter myectomy (an extensive form of a full-thickness rectal biopsy) may be the only surgical therapy required.

Following enterostomy placement, in infants with Hirschsprung's disease extending to proximal intestinal segments, careful attention to fluid and electrolyte balance is important. *Hyponatremia, hypochloremia, and hypokalemia may occur if adequate replacement of stool losses are not attended to.* Electrolyte imbalance may be the cause of poor weight gain. Some infants may require more than 10 mEq/kg/day of sodium chloride to cover maintenance and abnormal losses. The concentration of stool electrolytes and the stool volume should be monitored frequently. As a guide, stool output greater than 10 to 20 ml/kg/day should be replaced with an appropriate electrolyte solution (based upon the concentration of stool electrolytes). If stool volumes are excessive, an overnight nasogastric or intravenous infusion of the electrolyte solution may be necessary. Periodic sampling of urine electrolytes is a useful method for determining whether adequate electrolytes are being provided. A low concentration of sodium and a high potassium concentration indicate inadequate replacement and a possibility of hyperaldosteronism. Adequate replacement is indicated by urine samples exhibiting more than 10 mEq/L of sodium in the absence of renal or adrenal disease or diuretics.

INFLAMMATORY BOWEL DISEASE

ALAN M. LEICHTNER

The term idiopathic inflammatory bowel disease refers to disorders characterized primarily by chronic intestinal inflammation of unknown cause. Although several variants have been described, the two major forms of inflammatory bowel disease (IBD) in children are *ulcerative colitis* and *Crohn's disease.* Determining the proper mode of therapy for a child with IBD requires that the specific diagnosis, the sites of the gastrointestinal tract affected by disease, and the disease severity be considered.

Ulcerative colitis involves only the colon and does so continuously. The rectum is always involved, and a varying extent of more proximal colon is affected. Fifteen per cent of children have only rectal involvement (ulcerative proctitis), 22 per cent have disease limited to the left colon, and the remainder have pancolitis. Crohn's disease, on the other hand, may affect any part of the gastrointestinal tract and may do so in a discontinuous fashion. About 50 per cent of affected children have both small- and large-intestinal involvement; 40 per cent have disease limited to the small intestine, with either diffuse involvement or only terminal ileitis; and 10 per cent have only colonic involvement and present with symptoms quite similar to those of children with ulcerative colitis. Upper gastrointestinal disease is often unappreciated in children with Crohn's disease and may occur in more than 30 per cent of patients. Not infrequently, clinical information may not permit the distinction between ulcerative colitis from Crohn's colitis in a given patient. The treatment of this so-called "indeterminate colitis" should be based on the general guidelines for the management of inflammatory bowel disease in children. Furthermore, several new forms of chronic IBD, including collagenous colitis, lymphocytic colitis, and pouchitis (occurring in the neorectum after ileoanal anastomosis) have been described, but detailed discussion of their therapy is beyond the scope of this review.

TREATMENT

Because the exact etiopathogenesis of ulcerative colitis and Crohn's disease remains unknown, no truly specific therapy exists. Current theories propose that intestinal inflammation results either from an appropriate response to an unidentified inciting environmental agent or as an inappropriate response to the normal environment because of an underlying structural abnormality or immune dysregulation. Virtually all modes of current therapy interfere with the inflammatory response at some point in the cascade. However, no agents have been demonstrated to prevent the initiation of this process.

Steroids

Corticosteroids are one of the earliest therapies for IBD and remain a cornerstone for the treatment of children with moderate to severe colitis of either type or with Crohn's disease affecting the esophagus, stomach, or small intestine. Clearly, children with severe systemic manifestations of their illness or possible surgical complications require admission for intravenous fluids, steroids, and observation. When used parenterally, 1 to 2 mg/kg/day (usual maximum 60 mg) of methylprednisolone or an equivalent dose of hydrocortisone is administered in two or more divided doses or occasionally as a constant intravenous infusion. Although no data exist in pediatric patients, a recent study in adults suggests that adrenocorticotropic hormone (ACTH) may be more effective than steroids if the patient has already received steroid therapy within the previous 30 days. Upon response to parenteral steroids (or initially for the less acutely ill patient), 1 to 2 mg/kg/day of prednisone is given orally, usually as a single morning dose, to minimize adrenal suppression. After 4 to 6 weeks, the daily dose is tapered by approximately 5 mg/week. Generally, to avoid adrenal insufficiency, children are maintained on a dose of prednisone equivalent to one-half the maintenance endogenous production of corticosteroids for about 1 month before discontinuation. Not infrequently, subsequent courses of steroid therapy are required or patients relapse during steroid taper. In the latter event, the dose can be tapered more slowly or the patient can be maintained with alternate-day steroids. However, there is no compelling evidence that alternate-day therapy is effective or that steroid therapy prevents recurrence of disease.

Steroids are also used topically in the treatment of disease limited to the left colon or rectum. For proctitis, hydrocortisone suppositories or foam can be administered once or twice daily and then tapered as disease activity is controlled. For disease extending proximally (up to the splenic flexure), hydrocortisone enemas are administered. Topical therapy may also be used as an adjunct in patients with even more extensive disease when symptoms referable to rectal involvement, such as urgency and tenesmus, are particularly severe.

The side effects of corticosteroid therapy are as follows. Acutely, fluid retention, hypertension, and hyperglycemia are concerns. The incidence of severe side effects, such as osteoporosis causing pathologic fractures, aseptic necrosis of bone, and cataracts, increases with the total daily dose and duration of therapy but not in a predictable fashion. The various negative cosmetic side effects, such as facial fullness, acne, and striae, can be of major import in young patients. Topically administered steroids can also be absorbed to an extent sufficient to result in adrenal suppression and systemic side effects. Newer agents for oral and topical use are being developed that, because of extensive first-pass metabolism or poor absorption, should cause less systemic toxicity.

Antibacterials (Sulfasalazine) (Table 1)

Sulfasalazine (SAS) is the mainstay of the treatment of chronic colitis in childhood. SAS consists of the active moiety 5-aminosalicylate (5-ASA) linked via an azo bond to sulfapyridine (SP). The parent compound is poorly absorbed and is delivered to the colon, where the flora split the bond to release the two components. Most of the 5-ASA remains in the lumen, whereas the SP is largely absorbed and may cause adverse effects.

SAS is used in the treatment of mild to moderate ulcerative colitis. It is also of benefit in Crohn's disease involving the large intestine. The dose is 50 to 70 mg/kg/day, up to a maximum of 4 to 6 g, in three or four divided doses, given orally. Some of the dose-related toxicity of the drug may be avoided by starting with a low dose and increasing it over 1 to 2 weeks. SAS has also been demonstrated to decrease the incidence of relapse when given to patients with ulcerative colitis in remission. The maintenance dose is approximately 50 per cent of the recommended therapeutic dose.

Adverse effects are reported in 10 to 45 per cent of children taking SAS. Dose-related toxicity includes nausea, vomiting, dyspepsia, headache, and hemolysis. Fever, rash, and hepatitis can occur as a result of idiosyncratic reactions. In adults, male infertility is a concern. Paradoxically, in a few individuals SAS may actually exacerbate the underlying colitis. Because of the potential of SAS to interfere with folate absorption, patients receiving the drug are usually instructed to take 1 mg of supplemental folate per day. Although desensitization to the drug is possible, the realization that many of the side effects are due to the SP moiety has prompted a search for ways of delivering the 5-ASA by itself.

Currently, a number of 5-ASA derivatives are undergoing testing and a few such agents are in use for treatment of inflammatory bowel disease in children. 5-ASA is absorbed from the upper gastrointestinal tract and, as a result, does not reach sufficient levels in the lumen of the colon for a significant therapeutic effect. However, both enema and suppository preparations have been used with excellent response for left-sided colitis and proctitis, respectively. Furthermore, olsalazine, which contains two 5-ASA moieties linked by an azo bond, has been approved as an oral agent for use in chronic colitis. Preliminary studies in children, however, have not yet demonstrated efficacy equal to that of SAS in the treatment of ulcerative colitis. A pH sensitive enteric-coated preparation of 5-ASA has been released but remains little tested in children. Future agents may permit delivery of 5-ASA to more proximal sites of the gastrointestinal tract and may be of potential use in the treatment of Crohn's disease of the small bowel.

Oral 5-ASA derivatives can generally be tolerated by 80 to 90 per cent of individuals who experience significant side effects from SAS. The most frequently reported 5-ASA side effects are nausea, headache, and diarrhea. Rarely, pericarditis or pancreatitis may occur. Topical agents have sometimes been associated with anal irritation and pruritus. As with SAS, 5-ASA derivatives may exacerbate colitis in certain individuals. Renal toxicity observed in some animal species has not been a clinical problem in humans.

TABLE 1. Drug Treatment of Inflammatory Bowel Disease

Drug	Dose
6-Mercaptopurine	1–1.5 mg/kg/day once daily
Metronidazole	10–15 mg/kg/day three or four times daily
Sulfasalazine	50–70 mg/kg/day three or four times daily

Immunosuppressants (Table 1)

Increasingly, the immunosuppressive agents 6-mercaptopurine (6-MP) and azathioprine (which is metabolized to 6-MP) are being prescribed for children with steroid-dependent or steroid-resistant inflammatory bowel disease.

6-MP

6-MP is a purine analogue that interferes with DNA synthesis and thus proliferation of cells of the immune system. Although data regarding pediatric patients are very limited, adult patients respond with proven efficacy to 6-MP used both in acute Crohn's disease and in the maintenance of remission. The response rate is highest for Crohn's disease of the colon and for fistulas. Controlled trials have also demonstrated utility of 6-MP in the treatment of ulcerative colitis, with a success rate in excess of 70 per cent for patients refractory to steroids and SAS. In steroid-dependent patients, use of 6-MP may permit reduction of the steroid dose. The mean time to response is approximately 3 months, although some patients take up to 9 months to respond. 6-MP is administered as a single daily dose of 1 to 1.5 mg/kg, with a usual maximum starting dose of 50 to 75 mg.

The side effects of 6-MP may be life-threatening, and therefore close monitoring is crucial. Short-term adverse reactions include nausea, hair loss, allergic reactions, hepatitis, pancreatitis, and bone marrow suppression. Leukopenia is fairly common, although reversible with decrease or *discontinuation* of the drug. Thus, complete blood counts, liver function tests, and serum amylase levels should be monitored weekly during the initiation of therapy. In long-term 6-MP use, increased susceptibility to infection and the possible late development of neoplasm become concerns. However, studies in adult patients with Crohn's disease have demonstrated the occurrence of only one unexpected malignancy in a group of approximately 400 patients. Nevertheless, the problem of potential malignancy is more ominous in pediatric patients.

Cyclosporine

More recently, cyclosporine has been used for treatment of IBD, although its use must still be considered investigational.

Preliminary data suggest that this agent may have a role in the treatment of fulminant colitis unresponsive to steroid therapy because, unlike 6-MP, cyclosporine seems to have a rapid onset of action. Cyclosporine also has been used in the treatment of chronic steroid-resistant Crohn's disease. Case reports of its use in children exist, but more study is required before it can be considered standard therapy.

Antibiotics

Broad-Spectrum Agents

Antibiotics are essential in the management of certain complications of IBD. Broad-spectrum parenteral antibiotics are indicated in the treatment of severe colitis, especially toxic megacolon, in which there is considerable risk of bowel perforation and resulting peritonitis, and in Crohn's disease complicated by abdominal or pelvic abscess formation. The standard combination of ampicillin, gentamicin, and clindamycin is often used, although equally efficacious alternatives are available. Ensuring adequate antibiotic coverage of bowel flora, especially anaerobes and enterococci, is critical.

Metronidazole (Table 1)

The antibiotic metronidazole has also been used as primary therapy for IBD, although whether its efficacy is the result of antibiotic action or some other mechanism is not known. Metronidazole has been shown to be effective in the treatment of Crohn's disease, particularly for colitis or for perianal involvement such as fistulas. Its role as adjunctive or remission maintenance therapy is less well established. Moreover, metronidazole seems to be of little benefit in the treatment of ulcerative colitis. The usual dose is 10 to 15 mg/kg/day divided in three or four doses. A beneficial response may not occur for up to 2 months. Generally, after improvement is noted, the drug is continued 3 or 4 months prior to tapering. The relapse rate can be as high as 70 per cent.

Common side effects include mild gastrointestinal disturbances and a metallic taste in the mouth. Patients should refrain from ingesting alcohol because metronidazole has a disulfiram (Antabuse)-like effect. The most striking side effect is a dose-dependent peripheral neuropathy that occurs in approximately 50 per cent of patients, but usually not until 6 months after the initiation of therapy. The neuropathy is reversible, although it may resolve slowly. To date, there have been no reports of oncogenicity or teratogenicity in humans as has been noted in laboratory animals.

Antispasmodics and Antidiarrheals

Symptomatic therapy with antispasmodic (e.g., tincture of belladonna, dicyclomine hydrochloride, propantheline bromide, and clinidium bromide) and antidiarrheal (e.g., diphenoxylate and loperamide) medications may be of help in patients with quiescent disease and persistent pain or loose stools. However, in the setting of active colitis, such drugs may precipitate an ileus and toxic dilatation of the colon.

Nutrition

Nutrition plays a critical role in the therapy of all children with IBD. Approximately 85 per cent of children with Crohn's disease and 70 per cent of children with ulcerative colitis exhibit weight loss at presentation. Furthermore, 30 per cent with Crohn's disease and up to 10 per cent with ulcerative colitis demonstrate growth failure.

Diet

The provision of a well-balanced diet, adequate in calories and protein, and the correction of specific nutrient deficiencies are of basic importance in the therapy of IBD. Patients with growth failure may require up to 150 per cent of the recommended daily allowance for calories. A protein intake of 2.4 to 3.0 g/kg/day may be necessary, especially if there is evidence of protein-losing enteropathy. Extensive involvement of the small intestine may result in lactose malabsorption, but it is important to restrict lactose only in truly intolerant patients so as not to compromise caloric intake unnecessarily. Similarly, restriction of dietary fiber should be reserved for patients with active colitis or potential obstruction, such as occurs with stricture formation.

Vitamin and mineral deficiencies occur not infrequently in children with IBD. Terminal ileal involvement may compromise vitamin B_{12} absorption. Folate deficiency should be especially considered in patients receiving sulfasalazine without vitamin supplementation. In addition, fat-soluble vitamin deficiency may occur in patients with significant fat malabsorption. Patients with IBD are also at risk for mineral deficiencies, especially of iron, zinc, calcium, magnesium, phosphate, and potassium.

Total Parenteral Nutrition

Although enteral routes for nutrition should generally be used whenever possible, total parenteral nutrition (TPN) is indicated in the management of acutely ill patients. In the absence of surgical complications, the role of strict bowel rest is controversial, although it is frequently prescribed. TPN is beneficial in severely malnourished patients, as part of preoperative and postoperative management, and in patients with short-bowel syndrome, high-volume fistulas, and certain other complications.

Enteral Nutrition As Primary Therapy

Not only is nutritional management a vital adjunct in the treatment of children with inflammatory bowel disease, but in patients with active Crohn's disease it has also been used as primary therapy. Enteral nutritional therapy, usually in the form of calorically dense formula administered via nasogastric tubes, has been as effective as steroids in some studies. Prolonged remission, however, is unusual. Especially dramatic results have been achieved in some prepubertal adolescent patients with growth failure. Nightly nasogastric feedings may be well tolerated by some children, but maintaining long-term compliance is difficult.

Surgery

Although the frequency of surgery in patients with IBD has decreased over the last several decades, many of the major therapeutic advances have been surgical. *In children with ulcerative colitis, proctocolectomy is curative.* The current indications for colectomy are fulminant colitis, including toxic megacolon; lack of response to medical therapy; chronic medical intractability; and dysplasia or carcinoma. The advent of the ileoanal pull-through procedure has permitted the restoration of continence in many children. This procedure involves anastomosis of a pouch (created from the terminal ileum) to the anus, after colectomy and rectal mucosectomy. Postoperatively, patients may have frequent stools and may need to defecate at night. Pouchitis, characterized by inflammation of the neorectum, may complicate this procedure and cause diarrhea and abdominal pain. This condition usually responds to treatment with metronidazole. The Kock pouch or continent ileostomy is less favored at present because of a high complication rate. For some patients, standard ileostomy remains a reasonable alternative.

Because any surgical procedure in a patient with Crohn's disease is unlikely to be curative and increases the likelihood that further procedures will be required, the best approach is a conservative one. Nevertheless, surgery is indicated in patients with fulminant colitis unresponsive to medical therapy; with disease unresponsive to medical and nutritional therapy, including growth failure in prepubertal children; or with intractable complications, such as fistulas, abscess formation, severe perianal disease, or strictures with resultant bowel obstruction. The recurrence rate in children after ileocolectomy approaches 50 per cent 5 to 10 years after surgery and correlates with the presence of residual disease evident on gross inspection of the bowel.

A major issue in the long-term management of children with ulcerative colitis is the greatly increased risk for carcinoma of the colon, especially in patients with pancolitis. This risk is low in the first 10 years after diagnosis but then increases by 0.5 to 1.0 per cent per year. Rather than recommend elective colectomy after an arbitrary time period, most gastroenterologists now perform surveillance colonoscopy at 1- to 2-year intervals, beginning at about 10 years after diagnosis. If dysplasia is found on biopsy, the risk of carcinoma is high and surgery is recommended. The risk of intestinal malignancy is also higher in patients with Crohn's disease than in healthy controls, but not to the same extent; and guidelines for surveillance have not be established.

SUMMARY

The management of children with IBD involves a delicately balanced combination of medications, nutritional support, and, in carefully defined circumstances, surgery. Corticosteroids and sulfasalazine remain the most frequent medications prescribed, although immunosuppressives and metronidazole have an established role in intractable disease and 5-ASA compounds may replace sulfasalazine for some patients. Future management will undoubtedly include new anti-inflammatory agents with fewer adverse effects and, it is hoped, therapy to effect a cure.

NECROTIZING ENTEROCOLITIS

ELIZABETH R. BROWN, M.D.

Necrotizing enterocolitis (NEC) occurs secondary to intestinal ischemia and bacterial overgrowth. NEC occurs in about 10 per cent of preterm infants weighing less than 1500 g at birth and in about 0.2 in 1000 term infants. The major risk factor for preterm infants is extremely low birth weight, and the onset of the disease tends to be during the first several weeks of life. In term infants, the onset is earlier (first week of life), and the associated risk factors include birth asphyxia, polycythemia, congenital heart disease, meningomyelocele and in utero cocaine exposure.

The diagnosis is based on the clinical symptoms of bilious vomiting, abdominal distention, and/or tenderness and bloody stools coupled with an abdominal radiograph showing air in the bowel wall (pneumatosis). The disease may progress to intestinal perforation in which air is seen in the biliary tree or free in the abdominal cavity.

DIAGNOSIS

It is difficult to differentiate NEC from feeding intolerance, particularly in the preterm infant. Infants who have abdominal distention, gastric residuals, dilated bowel loops, and guaiac-positive stools may have only feeding intolerance, but this constellation of findings may also be a prodrome of NEC. All infants exhibiting such findings should undergo a diagnostic evaluation and 24- to 48-hour "NEC watch." Such an infant should receive nothing by mouth (NPO), a nasogastric tube should be placed with intermittent suction, an evaluation for sepsis should be done, and an abdominal radiograph should be obtained. If no evidence for NEC is seen on the initial radiograph, the infant should be observed as just detailed for 24 to 48 hours. If the clinical findings resolve, careful feeding can be restarted.

TREATMENT

If the initial radiograph shows pneumatosis, if there is a fixed loop of bowel on serial abdominal radiographs, or if the clinical signs and symptoms become worse, more aggressive therapy is indicated. In addition to withholding feeding and placing a nasogastric tube, antibiotics should be started. The usual choice of antibiotics is broad-spectrum coverage with intravenous ampicillin and gentamicin in dosages recommended for septicemia. Particularly for extremely low-birth-weight infants in whom *Staphylococcus epidermidis* is a major cause of infection, vancomycin should be considered. Oral antibiotics have been tried to decrease gut flora but have not been shown to offer any advantage over intravenous (IV) antibiotics alone. Because of the concern about anaerobic organisms, clindamycin has been used in addition to a penicillin and an aminoglycoside. However, a recent report shows an increase in the development of later intestinal strictures with no improvement in acute outcome for those infants treated with clindamycin so that the ultimate usefulness of this agent for NEC is not clear. Because of immature renal function in the preterm infant and the association of ischemic renal damage in the term infant, serum aminoglycoside levels should be monitored and the dose adjusted accordingly.

Additional supportive therapy may be necessary for those infants with severe hypotension or disseminated intravascular coagulopathy. This includes the use of intravascular volume expansion pressors, and transfusions with platelets or fresh frozen plasma. Electrolyte disturbances are common as a result of third-space losses and nasogastric suctioning; thus, infants should undergo frequent monitoring of serum electrolyte levels and intravenous corrections of abnormalities as they occur.

The duration of therapy for infants in whom the diagnosis of NEC is confirmed radiographically should be prolonged for a minimum of 10 days. Factors influencing the duration of therapy should include severity of initial presentation, rapidity of response, return of bowel sounds indicating normal peristalsis, and clearing of blood from the stool. Infants with severe disease may need up to 3 weeks of NPO. During the period when feedings are withheld, adequate fluids and nutritional support are critical to recovery of the bowel. Intravenous alimentation is indicated with glucose, amino acids, and lipid emulsions sufficient to give at least 100 kcal/kg per 24 hours. This can be achieved with peripheral venous lines in most cases; however, if venous access is limiting nutritional support, placement of a central venous catheter should be considered.

SURGICAL INTERVENTION

There is some disagreement as to when surgical intervention is indicated. Most would agree that intestinal perforation would require surgery. Therefore, it is imperative to monitor all at-risk infants for this complication by obtaining serial abdominal radiographs every 4 to 6 hours during the acute phase of the illness with the infant positioned in such a way that free air in the abdomen would be readily visible (cross-table lateral or left lateral decubitus). Some surgeons believe that extensive pneumatosis, portal venous gas, a palpable mass (?abscess), particularly if associated with a red streak on the skin of the abdomen and/or laboratory evidence of intravascular coagulation, may be indications for operative intervention.

The operative procedure in the acute phase of NEC consists of resection of obviously necrotic bowel and creation of an ostomy. If there are substantial areas of bowel of questionable viability, a minimal resection is done with clinical follow-up. Occasional reoperation is necessary in the next 24 to 48 hours. This is preferable to removing questionable bowel at the initial surgery, as the most adverse outcome in surviving infants is the short-bowel syndrome. Effort should be made to preserve the ileocecal valve and distal ileum to decrease the long-term morbidity from extensive gut resection. Most clinicians believe that surgery should be avoided, if possible, in the acute phase of illness, even if this means later surgery for resection of intestinal strictures.

PROGNOSIS

After completion of 10 to 21 days of therapy, enteric feedings are reintroduced with great caution. Dilute standard infant formula should be begun in small volumes with slow increase in strength and volume. Although many clinicians begin feedings with an elemental formula, the advantage to this approach over standard formula has not been proven. NEC may recur, so that infants must be carefully evaluated during refeeding and any early signs of feeding intolerance should be acted on immediately. As refeeding progresses in increasing volume, some infants with strictures will show signs of intestinal obstruction that should be documented with the appropriate radiologic contrast study. Some of the strictures resolve spontaneously, whereas others require surgical resection; thus, several attempts at refeeding are indicated before surgery is indicated. More than 80 per cent of infants will survive NEC. However, a small fraction of survivors, particularly those with extensive surgical gut resection, will go on to have the short-bowel syndrome and will remain dependent on parenteral nutrition.

PERITONITIS

GAREY S. SIMMONDS, M.D.
JOSEPH T. ZERELLA, M.D.
and DENNIS W. SHERMETA, M.D.

Peritonitis can be an extremely grave illness in children with an estimated mortality rate of 1 to 2 per cent. Prompt diagnosis and appropriate treatment are required. Peritonitis is an inflammation of the semipermeable membranes that encompass the abdominal cavity. The two membranes are the visceral peritoneum, which covers the viscera, and the parietal peritoneum, which is the interiormost surface of the abdominal wall with some noted exceptions. Inflammation of the parietal areas can produce large cavitary shifts in fluid volume and intestinal dysfunction. There is significantly less pelvic space and less omentum in the infant than in the older child, which may account for peritonitis in the infant to tend to become generalized more rapidly. Because it is also difficult to recognize abdominal pain in the infant, one can see why peritonitis can overwhelm the infant very quickly.

CLASSIFICATION

Peritonitis can be divided into two major clinical categories: localized and generalized.

Localized peritonitis is classified as inflammation confined to a particular area of the abdomen, usually identified by the four quadrants of the abdomen. This form of peritonitis is a pathologic process, usually occurring in a visceral organ, which causes inflammation of the peritoneal covering of the organ. Older children usually perceive this process as a generalized pain because of the innervation of the visceral peritoneum. As the process progresses, the parietal peritoneum becomes involved. The efferent nerve fibers of the parietal layer allow for better localization of pain. This innervation enables the clinician to categorize the patient's pain to a given specific location on the basis of various muscular responses to stimulation of that area. The role of omentum in walling off the inflamed area in older patients helps to prevent the escalation of the disease to a generalized peritonitis.

In *generalized peritonitis,* the entire peritoneum or almost the entire peritoneum becomes inflamed. This is a much more serious event and may lead to shock and place the patient in extremis. The clinical manifestations of generalized versus localized peritonitis are quite different. In generalized peritonitis, the abdomen is extremely tender throughout and eventually becomes rigid. The abdomen is almost always devoid of bowel sounds in the generalized form; this is usually not the case in localized peritonitis. In the generalized form, there is a much greater fluid shift with consequent prostration and a markedly higher fever (39° to 41°C). The abdominal pain in generalized peritonitis can cause respiratory distress in the younger patient as a result of rapid and shallow breathing and impairment of diaphragmatic function. The white blood cell count is usually in excess of 15,000/mm^3 with a marked left shift.

ETIOLOGY

Appendicitis

Acute appendicitis is the most common cause of peritoneal inflammation seen in children. It occurs in all ages. We have seen acute appendicitis in a 2-week-old with erythema of the abdominal wall because of extension of the gangrenous tip of the appendix adherent to the undersurface of the abdominal wall. The child was being treated for necrotizing fasciitis of the abdominal wall and underwent an appendectomy with a rapid cure of the inflammation of the abdominal wall.

The diagnosis of peritonitis can be extremely difficult to make in very young patients. The young patient with appendicitis initially gives a history of poorly localized periumbilical or mid-abdominal pain. The pain is then usually localized to the right lower quadrant. This is a classic presentation of acute appendicitis. The appendix, however, may be in an abnormal position, such as in a retrocecal area, which may produce flank pain or upper abdominal pain. If the appendix is located in the pelvis, the pain may be deep and the patient may present with diarrhea secondary to sigmoid irritation from the direct contact of the tip of the appendix against the sigmoid colon. This is one of the reasons that a rectal examination is absolutely critical in any patient suspected of having appendicitis.

When evaluating a patient for the evidence of peritonitis, one must consider nonsurgical causes for abdominal pain. Gastrointestinal illness in a family member or social contacts can lead to a diagnosis of infectious gastroenteritis. Constipation, urinary tract infections, or lower lobe pneumonia can also present with abdominal pain. Mesenteric lymphadenitis frequently following upper respiratory tract infections can lead to a picture similar to that of peritonitis. *Yersinia* infection is especially known to produce peritoneal irritation similar to that in appendicitis. Appendicitis is uncommon in patients under the age of 2; however, idiopathic intussusception can occur in this age group presenting with a mass shaped something like an appendiceal abscess, easily palpable in the right lower quadrant.

A patient with a ruptured appendix presents with signs of generalized peritonitis. This occurs more frequently in younger children and infants because there is greater likelihood of a delay in the diagnosis or a delay in seeking treatment.

Primary Peritonitis

Primary peritonitis is a rare clinical entity that is usually secondary to blood-borne or lymph-borne bacterial infections. It is usually associated with ascites from whatever cause. Patients with nephrotic syndrome frequently present with pneumococcal primary peritonitis, which responds dramatically to rapid intravenous antibiotic therapy.

The diagnosis is made by paracentesis. In primary peritonitis, usually only one organism is isolated from culture specimens that are obtained. However, that is not always the case. The most common offending organisms are pneumococcal, group A *Streptococcus* and *Haemophilus* in younger children. Gram-negative infections are usually via the vagina. In female children aged 5 to 10 years, the vaginal environment is not acidic enough to protect against bacterial invasion; furthermore, the cervix is in an open position. The diagnosis may be difficult and is sometimes made at the time of laparotomy.

Treatment involves the use of appropriate antibiotics.

Gastrointestinal Perforations

Gastrointestinal perforations that produce peritonitis other than ruptured appendicitis are less common. Gastric perforations can be secondary to the erosion of a nasogastric tube or to hyperexpansion of the stomach while a patient is receiving mechanical ventilation.

Small-bowel and colon perforations are most often caused by necrotizing enterocolitis in the premature infant. The mortality from these perforations ranges from 20 to 50 per cent. The mortality is highest in premature neonates. Other causes of perforations are Meckel's diverticulum, gastroschisis, Hirschsprung's disease, small-bowel atresia, and meconium ileus.

Pancreatitis

The most common cause of pancreatitis in children is abdominal trauma. The pain is in the mid upper abdomen and may or may not radiate to the back. There is usually an elevated serum or urinary amylase level, but this is not always the case. In the case of a patient who has no history of trauma, abnormalities of the biliary tree or pancreatic ducts must be searched for as a cause for pancreatitis. Surgical intervention is usually not needed in the acute stages. If the patient deteriorates significantly, rapid surgical care may become necessary.

Peritonitis Secondary to Ventriculoperitoneal Shunt Infection

Pancreatitis secondary to ventriculoperitoneal shunts seems to be an increasingly common cause for localized abdominal pain and peritoneal signs. Resolution of the symptoms usually occurs promptly after tapping the shunt has revealed the specific organism at fault and appropriate antibiotic coverage has been initiated promptly. Surgical intervention is rarely indicated. However, large sequestered cysts can form. Such cysts occasionally cause bowel obstructions secondary to compression and may require surgical removal.

INITIAL MANAGEMENT

Peritonitis always causes third-space fluid losses that require prompt replacement. Patients should be hydrated with isotonic solutions at approximately 20 ml/kg over 30 minutes and continued until urine output is adequate and vital signs are stable. Electrolytes should be checked and abnormalities corrected appropriately. If a patient is hypotensive or requires fluid infusion of more than 30 ml/kg to effect changes in vital signs, a central venous catheter and arterial blood gases should be obtained to guide further fluid management. A child with an acute abdomen should receive broad-spectrum antibiotics, such as ampicillin (150 to 200 mg/kg/day), gentamicin (6 to 7.5 mg/kg/day), and clindamycin (30 mg/kg/day) or metronidazole (20 to 30 mg/kg/day). Triple therapy of ampicillin, gentamicin, and clindamycin is often given.

For primary peritonitis, the choice of antibiotics depends on the Gram stain of the fluid taken from paracentesis. Gram-positive organisms are most often recovered from primary peritonitis. After the diagnosis is made and a treatment plan formulated, the patient can be given pain medication. Morphine (0.1 mg/kg) can be administered every 2 to 3 hours intravenously. The child's fever should be controlled by a cooling blanket or acetaminophen (10 mg/kg/per dose per rectum). In a straightforward unruptured appendicitis with localized peritoneal signs, nasogastric decompression is probably not necessary. If generalized peritonitis is present or perforated viscus is suspected, nasogastric decompression is mandatory. If respiratory distress becomes a problem secondary to the massive abdominal distention, mechanical ventilation should be instituted. The patient should be placed rapidly in an intensive care unit in these circumstances. Detailed and sequential discussions with the parents of a child with peritonitis are important to keep parents attuned to the severity and favorable response to the various therapeutic modalities employed.

SURGICAL MANAGEMENT

Intraoperative Care

A patient with an unruptured appendicitis needs a simple appendectomy through an appropriate right lower quadrant incision. A ruptured appendix may be handled the same way, depending whether an abscess or generalized peritonitis is present. The abdomen should be thoroughly evacuated of as much purulent material as possible. If a localized abscess cavity continues to remain after removal of the appendix, drainage should be considered. Patients with the presentation of Meckel's diverticulitis should have a segmental resection of that portion of the ileum containing the diverticulum. Uncomplicated Meckel's can be simply resected and oversewn. Patients with necrotizing enterocolitis and bowel perforation can be handled in one of two ways—by either *primary anastomosis* or *exteriorization.* Primary anastomosis may be used in cases of localized small-bowel injury without any peritoneal contamination resection and exteriorization usually follows colonic involvement. There is considerable debate concerning timing and whether or not it is safe to do a primary anastomosis.

Postoperative Care

Children should take nothing by mouth for at least 24 hours after appendectomy and longer if clinical circumstances dictate. Patients with a ruptured appendix should receive intravenous antibiotics for at least 7 days postoperatively. Daily rectal examinations greatly aid in preventing the formation of loculations in the pelvis and the formation of pelvic abscesses. In the child with bowel perforations, nasogastric suction is necessary for several days postoperatively until normal bowel sounds and passage of gas and stools occur. Intravenous antibiotics should be continued for 7 to 10 days or until the patient is clinically improved. Stomas should be checked daily for viability with meticulous care to keep them moist and clean. A patient's postoperative diet should be started conservatively and advanced slowly.

POSTOPERATIVE COMPLICATIONS

One of the more frequent postoperative complications is atelectasis. This needs to be treated with an aggressive pulmonary toilet. Wound infections need to be opened and treated with frequent dressing changes. Intra-abdominal abscesses can be treated in several ways by conservative management with long-term antibiotics if the clinical situation is amenable or with percutaneous or open drainage. Stomal demise secondary to ongoing infection or lack of blood supply generally requires reoperation. Prompt surgical correction is also necessary for anastomotic leaks.

REFERENCES

Gorensek MJ, Lebel MH, Nelson JD: Peritonitis in children with nephrotic syndrome. Pediatrics 81:849–856, 1988.

Harken AH, Shochat SJ: Gram-positive peritonitis in children. Am J Surg 125:769–772, 1973.

UNCONJUGATED HYPERBILIRUBINEMIA

HASSAN H. A-KADER, M.D.
and WILLIAM F. BALISTRERI, M.D.

Although unconjugated hyperbilirubinemia is a common finding in neonates, the level of serum unconjugated bilirubin below which one can safely ensure that *kernicterus* (bilirubin-induced encephalopathy) will not develop is yet to be defined. Therefore, an understanding of the physiologic alterations and pathologic conditions that lead to unconjugated hyperbilirubinemia in the newborn is needed and early recognition, careful monitoring, and prompt management is essential in order to prevent long-term complications.

PHYSIOLOGIC JAUNDICE

It is very common to detect an elevated level of unconjugated hyperbilirubinemia during the neonatal period; because the elevation is most often related to dynamic perinatal changes in hepatic physiology, the term physiologic jaundice is applied. However, other causes of an elevation in the unconjugated bilirubin fraction, such as excessive hemolysis, certain drugs, and specific diseases, should be excluded before the diagnosis of physiologic jaundice is made. Typically, the serum bilirubin level peaks at the third day of life and declines within a few days, reaching normal level at the age of 7 to 10 days. Levels above 12 mg/dl in full-term babies and 15 mg/dl in prematures are atypical and may warrant further investigation. Treatment is rarely required.

Management

Phototherapy is an established and effective method that is widely used to control elevated serum levels of unconjugated bilirubin of any cause. Phototherapy is usually initiated in full-term infants at serum levels of unconjugated bilirubin higher than 15 mg/dl but at lower levels in the premature infant and in the presence of risk factors for kernicterus such as hypoxia, acidosis, hemolysis, and infection. The resultant bilirubin photoisomers are less toxic and more readily excretable in bile. The use of phototherapy is not without risks; therefore, phototherapy should be used conservatively. Because the most common side effect is increased insensible water loss leading to dehydration, fluid intake should be increased in patients under phototherapy. Loose stools may also result. The possibility of retinal damage necessitates protecting the eyes during phototherapy. Phototherapy should not be used in patients with conjugated hyperbilirubinemia because it may lead to hemolysis and skin bronzing.

Exchange transfusion has been effectively utilized to reduce markedly elevated levels of unconjugated hyperbilirubinemia unresponsive to phototherapy. It is indicated when the serum bilirubin level exceeds 20 mg/dl in babies weighing more than 2000 g, when the serum bilirubin level exceeds 10 to 20 mg/dl in those weighing between 1000 and 2000 g, or when the rise of serum bilirubin exceeds 0.5 mg/dl/hour.

BREAST MILK JAUNDICE

Breast milk feeding may be associated with unconjugated hyperbilirubinemia, which has been postulated to be due to either an increased enterohepatic circulation of bilirubin or inhibition of hepatic glucuronyl transferase. Bilirubin levels increase after the 4th day of life, peaking at the age of 2 weeks and decrease gradually. Less commonly, jaundice associated with breast feeding may manifest during the first 3 days of life. Although serum bilirubin levels may reach as high as 20 mg/dl, kernicterus has not been reported in association with breast-feeding alone. Interruption of breast-feeding results in rapid decline of the serum bilirubin level with either minimal or no increase following resumption. The condition is benign, and there is no documented need for phototherapy in the treatment of the disorder.

CRIGLER-NAJAAR SYNDROME

Crigler and Najaar described a severe form of unconjugated hyperbilirubinemia occurring in the absence of hemolysis and in patients with no liver disease. There are at least two phenotypes.

Type I is transmitted in an autosomal dominant fashion and typically presents soon after birth. The serum unconjugated bilirubin levels are markedly elevated (usually above 20 mg/dl). Kernicterus of some degree develops universally; therefore, early recognition and treatment are required. The marked hyperbilirubinemia is due to the complete absence of the enzyme bilirubin uridine diphosphate glucuronyl transferase in the liver.

The diagnosis may be made by the combined clinical and biochemical findings. The absence of bilirubin diglucuronide from bile is characteristic. Patients should be treated aggressively from early life; at a minimum phototherapy and exchange transfusion will be needed to control hyperbilirubinemia. As the patient matures, phototherapy becomes less effective; therefore, alternative management strategies, such as liver transplantation, should be an early consideration in these patients. In the future, gene or hepatocyte transfer may be utilized to supply the missing enzyme to affected patients.

Type II is usually a less severe clinical condition and is transmitted in an autosomal recessive pattern. Lower serum levels of unconjugated bilirubin (usually between 6 and 20 mg/dl) are found, and neurologic injury is less likely to occur. Bile contains predominantly bilirubin monoglucuronides. Phenobarbital decreases serum bilirubin levels in these patients through induction of hepatic glucuronyl transferase activity.

GILBERT SYNDROME

Gilbert syndrome is a mild, benign form of familial (possibly autosomal dominant) unconjugated hyperbilirubinemia affecting approximately 5 per cent of the population and manifesting after the neonatal period. The onset is usually after puberty. The incidence is highest in males. The total serum bilirubin level is usually less than 3 mg/dl; however, levels up to 6 mg/dl may be seen during periods of illness or stress. Patients with Gilbert syndrome excrete bilirubin monoglucuronide in bile, but there is reduced hepatic bilirubin glucuronyl transferase activity and a decreased amount of bilirubin diglucuronide in bile and serum. There is no risk for the development of kernicterus because the disorder typically becomes manifest after the neonatal period and serum bilirubin levels rarely reach extreme levels.

Although phenobarbital decreases serum bilirubin levels in patients with Gilbert syndrome, there is no need for treatment. Patients as well as their families should be alerted to the fact that visible icterus may occur during intercurrent infections and prolonged periods of fasting but should be reassured as to the benign nature of this finding.

CIRRHOSIS

JORGE A. BEZERRA, M.D.
and WILLIAM F. BALISTRERI, M.D.

Cirrhosis is an irreversible end stage of many forms of liver injury. Having established the diagnosis and confirmed the etiology, it may be possible in some cases to minimize liver damage by treating the cause. Galactosemia, fructosemia, cystic fibrosis, Wilson's disease, obstruction due to choledochal cyst, and total parenteral alimentation–associated hepatobiliary injury are examples of conditions potentially amenable to medical or surgical therapy if detected early. In many patients, however, the challenge is to deal with the long-term consequences of cirrhosis, such as undernutrition and the complications of portal hypertension (ascites, gastrointestinal hemorrhage, hepatic encephalopathy, and spontaneous bacterial peritonitis). The aim of treatment is to reduce discomfort, allow maximum growth, and control complications in anticipation of liver transplantation.

NUTRITION

The nutritional status of the patient with chronic liver disease should be precisely evaluated. In the absence of liver failure, a protein-rich (1.5 to 2 g/kg/day), low-fat, high-carbohydrate diet is advised. Steatorrhea often is minimized with the use of dietary formula or supplements containing medium-chain triglycerides. Supplementation with fat-soluble vitamins should include oral vitamin K (2 to 5 mg every other day), vitamin D (5000 to 8000 IU/day), vitamin E (50 to 400 IU/day as alpha-tocopherol), and vitamin A (10,000 to 15,000 IU/day as Aquasol A). Carefully monitoring for sufficiency (serum level of 25-hydroxy vitamin D, serum vitamin E to total lipid ratio) or toxicity will allow for adjustment of the dosage. Water-soluble vitamins should be given at twice the daily recommended allowances. Low serum iron levels may be seen and should be corrected. Finally, the balance of calcium, phosphorus, potassium, or magnesium may be altered and supplementation may be necessary.

ASCITES

Initially, sodium restriction of 1 to 2 mEq/kg/day is recommended. If this maneuver does not adequately address the ascites, spironolactone (2 to 4 mg/kg/day) should be added. Urinary electrolytes should be monitored; if the ratio of sodium to potassium does not increase, the dose of spironolactone may be increased up to 10 to 12 mg/kg/day. If the ascites remains poorly controlled, additional diuretics such as furosemide (1 to 2 mg/kg every other day to twice daily) may be helpful. Use of diuretics requires repeated measurement of serum and urine electrolytes, and serum urea and creatinine. Large-volume paracentesis of up to 20 ml/kg, followed by salt-free albumin infusion, may be useful in patients with tense ascites and respiratory difficulties.

GASTROINTESTINAL HEMORRHAGE

Lavage to the stomach should be performed when the patient with chronic liver disease and portal hypertension presents with hematemesis or melena. The presence of blood in the stomach is suggestive of esophageal varices. An upper endoscopy with sclerotherapy is the preferred approach in the hemodynamically stable patient. If blood volume is contracted, replacement should be infused continuously in order to avoid overtransfusion, which may suddenly increase the intravascular volume and precipitate further hemorrhage from esophageal varices. If bleeding continues, vasopressin (0.3 U/kg, maximum 20 U, diluted in 2 ml/kg of 5 per cent dextrose) should be administered over 20 minutes; this should be followed by 0.3 U/1.73 m^2/minute for 12 to 24 hours, then the dose should be tapered and discontinued. If the above measures fail, the use of a pediatric Sengstaken-Blakemore tube should be considered.

In patients with cirrhosis there is often an underlying bleeding diatheses (prolonged prothrombin time, thrombocytopenia); this should be sought and addressed. Cytomegalovirus (CMV)-negative fresh frozen plasma, cryoprecipitate, and platelets can be used as needed. After the acute hemorrhage is controlled, sclerotherapy seems to be an effective palliative measure and should be repeated at 1- to 4-week intervals. Shunting procedures are often unsatisfactory and may render eventual liver transplantation more difficult. (For another approach, see article on portal hypertension, p. 221.)

ENCEPHALOPATHY

Hepatic encephalopathy is a late complication seen in patients with cirrhosis. It may be precipitated by electrolyte imbalance (especially hypokalemia and metabolic alkalosis), the use of drugs (diuretics, sedatives), infection, and gastrointestinal hemorrhage. Therapy is focused on removal of precipitating factors and reducing ammonia production and absorption. Precipitating factors, such as hypokalemia and metabolic alkalosis, should be corrected, the drugs mentioned above should be discontinued if possible, and any infection must be treated.

Measures to stop bleeding and to remove enteric blood by aspiration and enema will reduce ammonia production. Additionally, protein restriction and oral neomycin, in a dosage of 100 mg/kg/day, will also reduce ammonia production and absorption. Lactulose (5 to 15 ml orally three to four times daily), a nonabsorbable synthetic disaccharide, is our preferred alternative to neomycin. Lactulose produces lactic and acetic acids, decreasing the pH in the colon and thereby reducing ammonia reabsorption.

Exchange transfusion, hemodialysis, peritoneal dialysis, and plasmapheresis have been utilized to treat both encephalopathy and coagulopathy; however, there are no data regarding their efficacy. Extracorporeal artificial support may offer hope in the future. Patients with hepatic encephalopathy are candidates for urgent liver transplantation; their transplant status should be upgraded to reflect their clinical condition.

SPONTANEOUS BACTERIAL PERITONITIS

Spontaneous bacterial peritonitis may occur in patients in whom cirrhosis is complicated by ascites. Symptoms and signs include fever, lethargy, poor feeding, vomiting, diarrhea, diffuse abdominal pain, abdominal distention and rigidity, and diffuse rebound tenderness. In up to 15 per cent of patients, however, the condition may be asymptomatic. Diagnostic paracenthesis is indicated in all suspected cases. The ascitic fluid should be assessed for cell count and differential, total protein, lactate, pH (with concomitant capillary or arterial pH), and microbiologic studies, including a Gram stain and both aerobic and anaerobic cultures. Antibiotic therapy should be initiated in all patients with an ascitic fluid polymorphonuclear leukocyte count of more than 500 cells/mm^3 or in any patient with signs of peritonitis and polymorphonuclear leukocytes of more than 250 cells/mm^3. Before sensitivity is known, ampicillin (200 mg/kg/day), gentamicin (7.5 mg/kg/day), and clindamycin (30 mg/kg/day) should be started. Decreased ascitic fluid pH and increased lactate may help in establishing the diagnosis; however, awareness of the condition remains the key to diagnosis.

LIVER TRANSPLANTATION

Unfortunately, in many patients with chronic liver disease and in hepatic failure, orthotopic liver transplantation may be the only remaining consideration. Poor prognostic signs indicative of the need for liver transplantation include (1) serum bilirubin greater than 10 to 15 mg/dl, (2) serum albumin less than 2.5 g/dl, (3) presence of hepatic encephalopathy, (4) prothrombin time greater than 5 seconds above control, (5) presence of the hepatorenal syndrome, (6) recurrent episodes of cholangitis, (7) spontaneous bacterial peritonitis or septicemia, (8) intractable ascites, and (9) the development of focal hepatocellular carcinoma. In the past, the requirement for a size-matched donor liver had contributed to the difficulty in obtaining organs for pediatric recipients. Currently, the use of segmental transplantation has increased the proportion of candidates transplanted and reduced the overall mortality.

TUMORS OF THE LIVER

SHUNZABURO IWATSUKI, M.D.
and THOMAS E. STARZL, M.D., Ph.D.

Increasing numbers of hepatic mass lesions are found incidentally by advanced imaging technology. Although most of these "incidental" tumors are histologically benign and do not require any therapy, they must be thoroughly investigated. Modern imaging technology is quite efficient in detecting small lesions but is not effective in producing pathognomonic findings of many hepatic lesions other than hemangiomas and cysts. Percutaneous needle biopsy often fails to establish a definitive diagnosis because of its limited sampling, and it can cause serious hemorrhage when unwisely performed for vascular lesions.

Major hepatic resections can now be performed with minimum operative risk (less than 5 per cent), but no surgeon should explore a hepatic mass without having the competence to perform all of the major resections, including a right and left trisegmentectomy.

BENIGN TUMORS

Most of the benign tumors of the liver are asymptomatic and are found incidentally during studies for other disorders or during abdominal operations. The general approach to a small incidental tumor (less than 3 cm in diameter) that is considered benign is close observation after "thorough" investigation. When the tumor changes its imaging characteristics or increases in size during close observation, it must be immediately excised. Larger incidental tumors, other than asymptomatic cavernous hemangiomas, deserve excisional therapy unless unequivocal benignity is confirmed.

Hemangiomas are the most common benign tumors of the liver. Giant cavernous hemangiomas should be treated by surgical excision, particularly when they are symptomatic (e.g., pain, mass-related complaints) or are found to have a necrotic center inside. The majority of giant cavernous hemangiomas require lobectomies or trisegmentectomies of the liver, but some located on the surface of the liver or pedunculated can be enucleated along pseudocapsular margins without significant loss of normal liver tissue. Ligation or embolization of the feeding hepatic artery and radiation therapy may be hazardous and do not have long-standing effects on the course of giant cavernous hemangiomas.

Infantile hemangioendotheliomas are most often seen in infants during the first 6 months of life and are distinct from cavernous hemangiomas. The lesions should be excised by anatomic hepatic resection whenever possible. Treatment with prednisone, diuretics, and digoxin can be used initially when the patient's condition prohibits surgery or the lesion is too extensive for resection. Response to prednisone may allow surgery to be performed safely in a few weeks. In extensive lesions, radiation to the liver may be used after pathologic diagnosis is confirmed. Favorable responses to steroids, radiation, and hepatic artery ligation or embolization have been reported. The treatment should be vigorous, because complete regression and cure are possible.

Other benign tumors include liver cell adenoma, focal nodular hyperplasia, hematoma, mesenchymoma, teratoma, and fibroma. Radiologic differentiation of these benign tumors from malignant tumors is unreliable. Pathologic confirmation of benign tumors is mandatory for each lesion. Large benign tumors should be treated by surgical excision, particularly when they are symptomatic. Adenoma has a tendency to rupture and cause life-threatening hemorrhage. Some adenomas cannot be easily differentiated from low-grade hepatocellular carcinoma by needle biopsies. If the diagnosis is uncertain, the lesion should be excised with an adequate margin without delay.

Congenital hepatic cysts are usually asymptomatic and do not require any therapy. Although aspiration, internal drainage, marsupialization, fenestration, and sclerotherapy have all been recommended for symptomatic congenital cysts, these approaches are no longer justifiable for the treatment of single or localized multiple cysts because hepatic resections can be performed quite safely now.

MALIGNANT TUMORS

The most common primary malignant tumor of the liver in children is hepatoblastoma. Hepatocellular carcinoma is the second most common and usually occurs in older children. Sarcomas of the liver, such as rhabdomyosarcoma and angiosarcoma, are rare. None of these has a favorable outlook, but fibrolamellar hepatocellular carcinoma, which is common in older children and young adults, has a better prognosis than other types of malignancy.

The treatment for all malignant liver tumors is complete surgical excision by anatomic hepatic resection. Hepatic resections of more than the right or left lobe of the liver can be performed quite safely. For example, a large tumor occupying the right lobe of the liver and the medial segment of the left lobe can be resected by right hepatic trisegmentectomy, leaving only the left lateral segment of the left lobe (to the left of the falciform ligament), or a large tumor occupying the left lobe and the anterior segment of the right lobe can be resected by left hepatic trisegmentectomy, leaving only the posterior segment of the right lobe (posterior to the right hepatic vein). These major hepatic resections can now be performed by experienced surgeons with less than a 5 per cent operative mortality.

We have found that computed tomography scan or magnetic resonance imaging is most useful in assessing the extent of the tumor, but findings can be misleading, particularly when a large tumor distorts normal anatomic boundaries. If the resectability is uncertain after extensive preoperative investigation, the patient should be referred to a surgeon who is experienced in major hepatic resection rather than undergo exploratory celiotomy by someone who is unprepared to undertake a definitive procedure.

After curative hepatic resection, we usually recommend that patients receive adjuvant chemotherapy for at least 1 year. We have been using combination chemotherapy with doxorubicin, dactinomycin, vincristine, and cyclophosphamide, and often mitomycin or cisplatin. The value of this approach has not been validated in randomized trials, but the patients who have received adjuvant chemotherapy after curative resections of large tumors have seemed to have longer tumor-free survival.

In general, liver transplantation (total hepatectomy and liver replacement) cannot offer good long-term results when applied to large malignant tumors that cannot be removed by subtotal hepatectomy. However, liver transplantation can result in a cure (more than 5-year survival) on more than isolated occasions. The most favorable lesions for transplantation, just as with resection, are the fibrolamellar hepatoma and epithelioid hemangioendothelial sarcoma. On the other hand, most of the patients who have received liver transplantation for other end-stage liver diseases, such as tyrosinemia and $alpha_1$-antitrypsin deficiency disease, and whose malignant tumors were small and incidental, survived tumor-free for several years.

The most common metastatic liver tumors in children are neuroblastoma and Wilms' tumor. Although chemotherapy and radiation therapy may be helpful in treating these metastatic tumors, the lesion should be excised whenever possible, particularly if it is localized to part of the liver. Hepatic resections for metastatic tumors are much safer than those for primary malignancy.

PORTAL HYPERTENSION

JOHN T. BOYLE, M.D.

Portal hypertension in childhood may be classified as *intrahepatic* or *extrahepatic*. Intrahepatic portal hypertension results from cirrhosis, which in the United States is most commonly caused by biliary atresia, chronic viral or autoimmune hepatitis, or $alpha_1$-antitrypsin deficiency. Extrahepatic portal hypertension is most commonly caused by portal vein thrombosis (cavernous transformation of the portal vein) or by hepatic venous or inferior vena caval obstruction (Budd-Chiari syndrome). The etiology in individual patients is usually suggested by real-time ultrasonography and Doppler flowmetry. Although anatomy of the portal circulation is best defined by angiography, information such as site of portal vein obstruction, distribution of collaterals, and dynamics of portal flow is of therapeutic importance only when shunt surgery is being contemplated.

Portal hypertension results in splenomegaly and esophageal varices. Clinical presentations include asymptomatic splenomegaly (with or without laboratory evidence of thrombocytopenia, anemia, or neutropenia), upper gastrointestinal (GI) bleeding from ruptured esophageal or gastric varices, or, rarely, ascites or bleeding hemorrhoids. In patients who present for the first time with upper GI bleeding, the possibility of bleeding esophageal varices is primarily suggested by a past history of jaundice, hepatitis, blood transfusion, sepsis, shock, chronic right-sided heart failure, pulmonary hypertension, exchange transfusion, omphalitis, or umbilical vein catheterization.

Because there are few reports in the pediatric literature regarding the management of variceal bleeding, therapy is based primarily on the adult experience. It is important to emphasize that there is no consensus on management policy in pediatric patients before, during, or after variceal bleeding.

TREATMENT

Management of Splenomegaly in Patients with Portal Hypertension

Every effort should be made to ensure that a child with portal hypertension leads as normal a life as possible. Normal school activity should be allowed with the exception of contact sports and physical education activities involving prolonged running or jumping. Oftentimes, education of school officials is required to explain signs and symptoms of bleeding.

Although hypersplenism is a common complication of splenomegaly in patients with portal hypertension, bleeding and infection related to thrombocytopenia and neutropenia are rare. Hypersplenism is not an indication for splenectomy in such patients. Nevertheless, the presence of fever in a patient with portal hypertension demands immediate and careful evaluation to identify a source of infection. It is my practice to recommend pneumococcal immunization to patients with cirrhosis and hypersplenism.

Prophylactic Management to Prevent the First Variceal Bleed

Patients should avoid nonsteroidal anti-inflammatory agents, which may cause GI inflammation or ulceration. Coughing associated with upper respiratory infections should be treated with antitussive agents.

The risk of first-time variceal bleeding in children with known portal hypertension is unknown. In adults, only 25 to 30 per cent of patients with esophageal varices will experience variceal hemorrhage. Therefore, the risk-benefit ratio is widely believed to be against the use of repeated sclerotherapy and shunt surgery as prophylactic therapy prior to the first variceal bleed. In adults, a number of randomized, double-blind trials have now reported a statistically significant reduction in the frequency of variceal bleeding for patients while on chronic beta-blocker therapy. Results have been best in patients with Child Class A or B (an index of liver dysfunction based on serum albumin, serum bilirubin, prothrombin time, and the presence of ascites and encephalopathy).

The main argument for prophylactic use of beta-blockade therapy is that there is little to lose. In the absence of cardiac decompensation, heart block, and reactive airway disease, propranolol appears to have a wide margin of safety in pediatric patients. It is imperative to remember that during acute bleeds propranolol may mask compensatory hemodynamic changes, a fact that must be taken into account during resuscitative efforts.

Patients with documented portal hypertension should undergo endoscopy at least every 2 years. In patients judged likely to be compliant, a decision to use prophylactic propranolol should be based on the etiology of the portal hypertension and the appearance of the esophageal varices and overlying esophageal mucosa at the time of diagnostic upper endoscopy. High-risk patients include those with cirrhosis, especially associated with bile duct damage, or those with tense varices that bulge into the esophageal lumen and have small cherry red spots, dilated blood vessels, or telangiectasia on top of the varices. The French have reported that approximately 80 per cent of such patients will go on to have bleeding episodes. In addition, gastric varices are more frequent in children who bleed. I begin propranolol at a dose of 1 mg/kg/day three times a day orally and increase the dose by 0.5 mg/kg/day up to 3 mg/kg/day to achieve a 20 to 25 per cent reduction in baseline heart rate. Side effects of weakness, lethargy, or depression may limit ability to increase dosage to achieve targeted reduction in heart rate.

Emergency Management of Acute Variceal Hemorrhage

Variceal hemorrhage usually results in hematemesis. Occasionally, however, a significant esophageal hemorrhage can present as melena without associated hematemesis. Any patient who presents with evidence of significant GI hemorrhage (hematemesis, hematochezia, or melena) should have a nasogastric tube passed and their stomach aspirated. Suspicion of bleeding esophageal varices is not a contraindication to pass a nasogastric tube. Not only is the presence of blood diagnostic of an upper GI bleed, but the color of the aspirate and response to lavage allows one to estimate the size of the bleed. Coffee-ground material in the lavage suggests a slow rate of bleeding that would not require immediate invasive measures to stop. Gastric lavage should be performed with normal saline at room temperature. The recommended volume for each infusion depends on age: 50 ml for infants, 100 to 200 ml for older children. There is no benefit to continuous lavage beyond 15 minutes if the return is not clearing. The tube can be left to gravity or low suction and irrigated every 15 minutes to assess the activity of bleeding.

The initial management of esophageal variceal hemorrhage is identical to that of massive upper GI bleeding from any source. The first priorities are to re-establish hemodynamic stability and protect the airway. Elective placement of an endotracheal tube is indicated in any patient with massive upper GI bleeding. Immediate resuscitation should be undertaken with crystalloid solutions (normal saline or Ringer's lactate) given as 20 ml/kg boluses until evidence of restoration of intravascular volume is observed, such as a rise in blood pressure or disappearance of physical signs of peripheral vasoconstriction. Colloid solutions, such as albumin or fresh frozen plasma, are used only when blood loss is massive and continuous and there is concern for a precipitous drop in plasma oncotic pressure (a risk factor for development of shock lung). Only rarely is low oxygen-carrying capacity of enough concern to require emergency transfusion of blood without complete cross-match methods. Patients with significant hemorrhage should be given nasal oxygen. Overexpansion of the intravascular volume is to be avoided because it may contribute to rebleeding. Following initial resuscitation, further intravenous volume replacement should be titrated to match continuing blood loss. Decision to begin transfusion at this point depends on the hematocrit value taken at the time of restoration of blood volume. Remember that the initial complete blood count drawn at the time of presentation does not reflect the severity of the GI bleed because of delay in hemodilution. Volume of transfused packed red blood cells should be calculated to correct the hematocrit to 30 volume per cent. In patients with suspected variceal bleeds, it is important to pay attention to the initial platelet count and prothrombin time, which may reflect the degree of hypersplenism or liver dysfunction. Platelet transfusion may be necessary for severe thrombocytopenia. Patients with increased prothrombin time should be given intravenous vitamin K and fresh frozen plasma. It is also important to look for precipitating factors in patients with suspected variceal bleeding. Because bleeding varices may be the presenting sign of sepsis in a patient with cirrhosis, any patient with fever should be started on broad-spectrum antibiotics pending result of blood cultures.

Emergency flexible endoscopy should be performed once the patient's vital signs have been stabilized. Actively bleeding esophageal varices or observation of a varix with an overlying clot confirms the site of variceal bleeding. Endoscopic detection of bleeding gastric varices or bleeding sites unrelated to portal hypertension (i.e., acute gastric erosions, peptic ulcer) will alter subsequent management. If active esophageal variceal bleeding is confirmed, the endoscopist has the option of performing emergency sclerotherapy to stop the hemorrhage. I prefer, however, to delay sclerotherapy until after the hemorrhaging has been controlled by pharmacologic agents or balloon tamponade if there is difficulty obtaining a clear field of vision. Sclerotherapy should not be considered a therapeutic option to control bleeding gastric varices.

Pharmacologic therapy of acute variceal hemorrhage employs the splanchnic arterial vasoconstrictor *vasopressin* to reduce portal blood flow and pressure. Vasopressin infusion may be initiated prior to diagnostic endoscopy if there is evidence of massive continuing hemorrhage (after initial nasogastric lavage) or recurrent bleeding. Vasopressin is given by continuous intravenous infusion through a large-bore peripheral catheter. I empirically begin by infusing 0.1 unit/minute and increase the dose by 0.05 unit/minute every 30 minutes up to a maximum of 0.2 units/minute in children younger than 5 years of age, 0.3 units/minute in children younger than 10 years, and 0.4 units/minutes in patients older than 10 years of age. The vasopressin is given in 5 per cent dextrose in water, the exact dilution being based on overall volumes of fluids being infused. Side effects, including myocardial ischemia, arrhythmia, cerebral and mesenteric ischemia, local tissue necrosis, activation of fibrinolysis, and water retention and hyponatremia, are potentially serious.

The concept that drugs which constrict the lower esophageal sphincter may decrease gastroesophageal collateral blood flow has recently been suggested by an adult study describing control of acute variceal bleeding following intravenous infusion of metoclopramide. Metoclopramide, 0.1 mg/kg IV every 4 hours, may be given in conjunction with vasopressin. Once bleeding has been temporarily controlled, vasopressin infusion should be continued at the dose that controls the bleeding for a minimum of 12 hours, preferably until elective sclerotherapy can be performed. Most patients with variceal bleeding are started on intravenous cimetidine or ranitidine following initial resuscitative efforts to decrease gastric acidity and secretions.

Balloon tamponade is reserved for patients in whom pharmacologic therapy has failed and the rate of bleeding precludes safe sclerotherapy. A four-lumen modified Sengstaken-Blakemore tube should be inserted only by a physician skilled in its use. A pediatric tube is used in children younger than 10 years; the adult tube is used in adolescents. In all patients the airway must be protected by an endotracheal tube. Passage through the nose is facilitated by pretreatment with Afrin nose drops and generous lubrication of the tube. Once the tube is in the stomach, 50 to 100 ml of air is infused into the gastric balloon and the tube is pulled back until resistance is encountered at the gastroesophageal junction. An emergency radiograph is obtained to ensure correct position. Additional air is infused into the gastric balloon (up to 150 ml in the pediatric balloon, 250 ml in the adult balloon), and the tube pulled taut and taped to a support structure outside the body (i.e., an orthopedic support bar, or face guard of a football helmet slipped over the child's head). In the vast majority of cases, only the gastric balloon needs to be inflated to control bleeding. Only if esophageal bleeding continues should the esophageal balloon be inflated. The volume of air in the esophageal balloon is determined by pressure in the balloon (measured by connecting the inflow tube to a sphygmomanometer), which should not exceed 40 mm Hg. If bleeding is controlled, balloon tamponade should be maintained for 12 to 24 hours, at which time elective sclerotherapy should be performed. Complications associated with Sengstaken-Blakemore tubes include rupture or erosion of the esophageal or fundic mucosa, occlusion of the airway by the balloon, or aspiration around the endotracheal tube because of inadequate drainage of oral secretions from the esophageal body.

If endoscopic sclerotherapy is not performed at the initial diagnostic endoscopy, it should be done on an elective basis within 6 to 24 hours after active bleeding has been controlled temporarily by pharmacologic therapy or balloon tamponade. Direct obliteration of large varices at the gastroesophageal junction is best achieved by intravariceal injections of a variety of sclerosing agents. The procedure may be repeated every 2 to 4 weeks until all varices at the location are obliterated. Major complications of sclerotherapy include sepsis, bleeding, mediastinitis, esophageal stricture, esophageal perforation, pleural effusion, and pericardial effusion. Minor complications include transient dysphagia, transient retrosternal discomfort, low-grade fever (<38.5°C for less than 24 hours), and esophageal mucosal ulcer. I prescribe sucralfate slurry (0.5 to 1.0 g in 1 ounce of water) for 5 days following sclerotherapy.

Emergency shunt surgery is indicated only if two attempts at sclerotherapy fail to control active bleeding. The exact type of shunt performed depends on the experience and individual preference of the surgeon. Emergency shunt should be considered the last resort because of the high operative mortality and unpredictable occurrence of postoperative encephalopathy. An alternative to emergency shunt surgery in patients with cirrhotic portal hypertension is esophageal transsection with or without devascularization.

Therapeutic Management After an Episode of Variceal Bleeding

In patients who have had variceal bleeding, the aim is to prevent recurrent bleeding. The treatment options in pediatrics are repeated injection sclerotherapy, long-term pharmacologic therapy with beta-blocking agents, portosystemic shunt surgery, and liver transplantation.

In patients with known untreatable progressive liver disease (particularly patients with biliary atresia with progressive biliary cirrhosis, or patients with alpha$_1$-antitrypsin deficiency that is progressing to cirrhosis), a significant variceal hemorrhage is an indication to list the patient for liver transplantation. Repeated sclerotherapy is the most widely practiced therapy prior to transplant in such patients. Experience with chronic pharmacologic therapy is limited. Every effort is made to avoid shunt surgery prior to transplantation, although shunt surgery is no longer considered an absolute contraindication to transplantation.

In patients with liver disorders without cirrhosis, such as congenital hepatic fibrosis, or with disorders amenable to specific medical therapy, such as chronic active hepatitis or Wilson's disease, repeated sclerotherapy should be the first-line treatment for prevention of subsequent bleeding episodes. In carefully selected patients with quiescent disease who experience recurrent bleeding despite sclerotherapy, shunt surgery is indicated.

There is no consensus on treatment to prevent further bleeding in patients with extrahepatic portal hypertension. Although long-term follow-up is limited, early reports indicate that the incidence of subsequent bleeding episodes is significantly reduced following repeated sclerotherapy. The rationale for repeated sclerotherapy is the natural history of childhood extrahepatic portal hypertension in which bleeding frequency dramatically decreases after adolescence, presumably because of the development of natural shunts. Even if shunt surgery is eventually required because of rebleeding from esophageal or gastric varices, sclerotherapy may serve as a temporizing measure until the patient is old enough to be a better candidate for shunt success. Long-term complications of sclerotherapy, described above, vary with the injection technique, the sclerosing solution used, and the length of follow-up. In reports to date, overall complication rates in the pediatric population have been acceptably low.

A number of difficulties have been reported following portosystemic shunts in children with extrahepatic portal hypertension, including a high incidence of rebleeding secondary to shunt thrombosis and development of mild hepatic encephalopathy. Most surgeons agree with Clatworthy's observation that shunts have a higher rate of long-term patency if they are constructed of veins larger than 1.0 cm in diameter. Angiographic evaluation or splenoportography is essential immediately prior to a shunting procedure to determine size of available portal tributaries. Theoretically, the selective distal splenorenal shunt of Warren and Zeppa, which preserves portal flow to the liver while shunting varices into the systemic venous circulation via the spleen and its distal vein, is the shunt procedure of choice to prevent encephalopathy. Although some studies have reported that other types of shunt surgery may result in minor developmental and/or learning disabilities in patients with extrahepatic portal hypertension and normal liver function, more recent studies have refuted these findings. Because of the young age of patients requiring shunt surgery and the variability of the anatomy and pathology of the portal tree in patients with extrahepatic portal hypertension, the first priority of surgery in this patient population must be long-term patency of the shunt. The surgeon, therefore, must decide which of a variety of shunt procedures is best for an individual patient.

CHRONIC ACTIVE HEPATITIS

BENJAMIN L. SHNEIDER, M.D.
and FREDERICK J. SUCHY, M.D.

ETIOLOGY AND DIAGNOSIS

Chronic active hepatitis (CAH) should be suspected in patients with persistently (>10 weeks) elevated transaminase levels (>3 times the upper limit of normal). Diagnosis is dependent on demonstrating portal inflammation and piecemeal necrosis by liver biopsy. CAH, which should be managed by pediatric gastroenterologists familiar with the spectrum of pediatric liver disease, can result from a variety of disorders, including Wilson's disease, alpha$_1$-antitrypsin deficiency, drug toxicity, and hepatitis B and C. Hereditary hemochromatosis has been infrequently reported to result in liver disease in children. In addition, autoimmune mechanisms may be responsible for the CAH referred to as "autoimmune" or "lupoid" hepatitis. Appropriate therapy of this diverse group of diseases requires accurate and timely diagnosis (Table 1).

TREATMENT

Wilson's Disease

The neuropsychiatric and hepatic manifestations of Wilson's disease can be managed with appropriate doses of penicillamine (10 to 20 mg/kg divided before meals). Blood counts and urinalysis should be observed for signs of toxicity.

Alpha$_1$-Antitrypsin Deficiency

Currently, medical therapies are not available for alpha$_1$-antitrypsin deficiency with the exception of symptomatic support. Protease inhibitor replacement therapy is not expected to ameliorate the hepatic aspects of this disease, which results from accumulation of the abnormal inhibitor in the liver. Liver transplantation can be very effective because the donor liver maintains its normal phenotype.

Hepatitis B and C

At present, most of the organized trials of immunomodulatory therapy in hepatitis B and C have been confined to adults. Alpha-interferon may be particularly helpful in adults with recently acquired and active hepatitis B. To date, trials in children have been disappointing, although proper patient selection may improve the results. In particular, patients with disease acquired after the perinatal period may show a better response to alpha-interferon. Early trials in hepatitis C appear promising, although significant problems with relapses exist. Further pediatric protocols for hepatitis B and C will need to be evaluated. Immunosuppressive therapy (e.g., prednisone) is not indicated in patients with chronic viral hepatitis and may result in enhanced viral replication and an increased mortality.

Autoimmune Hepatitis

Autoimmune hepatitis is a relatively common cause of CAH in children. Therapy is directed at preventing progression to cirrhosis and liver failure. Timely diagnosis may be critical, as demonstrated by the high incidence of cirrhosis in series in which a 6-month criterion was used to define chronicity. Autoimmune markers (liver-kidney-microsome, nuclear, and smooth muscle antibodies) are often present but not required for diagnosis. Some patients will only have elevated immunoglobulin levels. No prospective controlled trials of therapy in children have been performed, and thus regimens are based on adult studies and uncontrolled series in children. Immunosuppressive therapy usually results in biochemical and histologic remission of the hepatitis and prolongs survival in most patients with severe disease.

Initial therapy consists of prednisone (2 mg/kg up to 60 mg) given once daily for the first few weeks of therapy. If hepatic synthetic function is intact, transaminases can be used as a marker of disease activity. Once the alanine aminotransferase (ALT) is less than 2.5 times the upper limit of normal, the prednisone is tapered by 5 to 10 mg every 2 to 4 weeks. The goal is to reach the lowest dose of prednisone that will ensure biochemical remission for 12 to 24 months. Our experience with every-other-day dosing has been disappointing, and adult studies have shown that histologic remission may not be induced with this form of therapy.

If the maintenance steroid doses result in significant side effects, azathioprine (1.0 to 1.5 mg/kg up to 75 mg) is added as a steroid-sparing agent. Blood counts should be observed carefully. More than 75 per cent of patients can be expected to respond to therapy. Approximately 50 per cent of children can be completely weaned from immunosuppressive therapy once histologic remission is documented; relapse occurs in the others after a variable period of time. Antinuclear antibodies and a relatively short duration of illness prior to initiating therapy may be predictive of a successful attempt to wean from steroids. Recurrence defined by an increase in transaminases greater than five times the upper limit of normal should be re-treated, with a reasonable expectation for success in achieving remission. Patients who are weaned from immunosuppressive therapy should be monitored at least two times yearly for evidence of recurrence. Children who have advanced liver disease at the time of diagnosis or who progress in spite of immunosuppressive therapy have been successfully managed by liver transplantation.

TABLE 1. Diagnosis and Therapy in Chronic Active Hepatitis

Diagnosis	Laboratory Indicator	Therapy
Wilson's disease	Elevated urine copper; low ceruloplasmin	Penicillamine (10–20 mg/kg)
Alpha$_1$-antitrypsin deficiency	ZZ phenotype	Symptomatic Transplantation
Hepatitis B	sAg, cAb, eAg, eAb	Alpha interferon?
Hepatitis C	Hepatitis C Ab	Alpha interferon?
Autoimmune hepatitis	ANA, antiLKM, anti–smooth muscle, IgG	Prednisone (2 mg/kg) ± azathioprine

DISORDERS OF THE BILIARY TREE

MAUREEN JONAS, M.D.
and W. ALLAN WALKER, M.D.

BILIARY ATRESIA

Extrahepatic biliary atresia is the cause of about one third of all cases of neonatal cholestatic jaundice, with an incidence of approximately 1 in 10,000 to 15,000 live births in the Western world. In 10 per cent of cases, the atresia is of the correctable type, the patient having either a distal atresia with patent proximal hepatic ducts or cystic dilatation of the ducts at the porta hepatis. In these circumstances, correction is achieved by anastomosis of patent proximal extrahepatic duct remnants or the gallbladder to a Roux-en-Y jejunal loop. In the more common noncorrectable forms of atresia, there are no patent extrahepatic ducts and the gallbladder is usually absent or only a small remnant. In these lesions, correction is attempted by hepatoportoenterostomy (Kasai procedure), again using a Roux-en-Y jejunal limb brought up and attached to the porta hepatis after dissection and excision of the fibrous extrahepatic biliary tree remnants.

Success rates for this procedure in re-establishing bile flow and clearing jaundice are variable, depending on the series, but are reported in Japanese series as high as 70 to 80 per cent. In these patients, a 90 per cent chance of survival with reasonable quality of life to age 10 years is reported if the infant is operated on before 8 weeks of age. Success rates fall to 20 per cent or less if surgery is delayed beyond 3 months of age, probably owing to progression of intrahepatic disease. With the advent of orthotopic liver transplantation as a therapeutic option even in the young infant, some surgeons now advocate forgoing a Kasai procedure altogether in the patient diagnosed late (beyond 3 to 6 months of age) with biliary atresia. This is because the small chance of success at such a late age plus the difficulty and risks of reoperation in the right upper quadrant at a later time for transplantation may make liver transplantation the preferred primary therapy for the patient in these special circumstances. The untreated infant with atresia, however, faces a dismal mean survival of 11 months without transplantation.

Cholangitis After Portoenterostomy

Postoperative cholangitis is a major risk after portoenterostomy and, although often recurrent, even a single episode may contribute to a subsequent poor outcome in a patient who initially appeared to have a good surgical result with clearing of jaundice. The onset of cholangitis may be heralded by fever, leukocytosis with increased band count, and increase in sedimentation rate above the patient's baseline value. The patient may also demonstrate right upper quadrant tenderness, worsening liver function, and decreased bile flow with increasing serum bilirubin and clinical jaundice. However, any or all of these signs, symptoms, and laboratory assessments may be absent, normal, or unchanged from baseline in the post-Kasai infant. Therefore, fever alone, without an obvious source, merits prompt and thorough investigation. Given the significant and sometimes irreversible clinical deterioration experienced by some patients after an episode of cholangitis, some clinicians recommend admission to the hospital for all such post-Kasai patients with fever.

If preliminary investigations fail to reveal a source for the fever, a percutaneous liver biopsy may need to be performed for culture and sensitivity testing and for histologic examination in an attempt to diagnose active, acute cholangitis and isolate a pathogen with specific antibiotic sensitivities to thus guide appropriate therapy. Peripheral blood cultures alone are often inadequate for isolation of a specific pathogen.

In the absence of a specific bacterial isolate from liver or blood culture, broad-spectrum combination treatment with an aminoglycoside and cephalosporin as initial therapy takes advantage of the relatively good penetration by these drugs into bile. In our experience, use of gentamicin or tobramycin at 6 to 7.5 mg/kg/day in three divided doses with monitoring of serum levels and cephalothin (75 to 125 mg/kg/day in four divided doses) or cefoxitin (80 to 160 mg/kg/day in four divided doses) when broader coverage of anaerobic pathogens is desired, continued for 10 to 14 days, is adequate therapy in the majority of circumstances.

Fortunately, the incidence of cholangitis appears to decrease markedly by the end of the first year of life. However, until then, many physicians advocate the use of oral suppressive antibiotic therapy as prophylaxis against recurrent cholangitis, using trimethoprim-sulfamethoxazole (10 mg/kg/day of trimethoprim in two divided doses) or another appropriate oral antibiotic such as amoxicillin (40 mg/kg/day in three divided doses) or cefaclor (40 mg/kg/day in three or four divided doses). Cholangitis developing after the first year of life may indicate obstruction of the draining jejunal limb or development of large intrahepatic bile lakes with secondary infection or abscess formation and may require surgical treatment or percutaneous aspiration for drainage of infected intrahepatic fluid collections.

Nutritional Management

Nutritional therapy in the post-Kasai patient or the patient with chronic cholestasis of any cause is aimed at preventing or ameliorating the sequelae of lipid malabsorption due to decreased intraluminal concentrations of bile salts in the intestine. The use of infant formulas such as Portagen or Pregestimil (the latter having a higher percentage of essential fatty acids) that have a high percentage of their fat content as medium-chain triglycerides, which do not require micellar solubilization by bile salts, aids in providing more usable calories for weight gain and growth while still providing adequate amounts of essential long-chain fats. In the older child, a high-protein, low-fat diet is preferred, with medium-chain triglyceride oil supplementation as needed.

Prevention of fat-soluble vitamin deficiencies is achieved by oral supplementation with monitoring of levels to avoid toxicity. Vitamin A as Aquasol A should be given in a dosage of 10,000 to 25,000 IU/day. Vitamin D is administered as ergocalciferol (vitamin D_2) in a dosage of 5000 to 8000 IU/day or 3 to 5 μg/kg/day of 25-hydroxycholecalciferol, especially in the patient with signs of established rickets. Vitamin E is supplemented as oral alpha-tocopherol, as either the acetate or succinate ester, in dosages of 50 to 400 IU/day to start. It is not uncommon that adequate levels of vitamin E cannot be achieved by oral supplementation even with high doses of vitamin E (150 IU/kg/day or greater). A new oral preparation of vitamin E, alpha-tocopherol polyethylene glycol–1000 succinate (TPGS, 15 to 25 units/kg/day), has shown great promise in achieving adequate vitamin E levels in patients with chronic cholestasis and reversing some of the sequelae of chronic vitamin E deficiency in a small cohort study group. Finally, vitamin K is given orally in dosages of 2.5 to 5 mg/day but may need to be given intramuscularly if there is clinical bleeding or the prothrombin time remains significantly elevated, placing the patient at high risk for future bleeding.

Water-soluble vitamin supplementation is also necessary and should be given at twice the recommended daily dosage. Patients are also at risk for mineral deficiencies with chronic cholestasis, particularly calcium deficiency, which is exacerbated by the steatorrhea. While levels are being monitored, calcium intake should provide at least 50 to 200 mg/kg/day of elemental calcium as well as 25 to 50 mg/kg/day of elemental phosphorus. Zinc deficiency may be avoided by appropriate supplementation at 10 mg/day if needed. Finally, in the presence of ascites, dietary intake of salt may need to be restricted to prevent excess fluid retention.

Other Management Issues

Pruritus and xanthomas are particularly troublesome complications of chronic cholestasis. No truly satisfactory therapy exists for the severe, intractable pruritus that may occur in chronic cholestatic liver disease. Simple measures such as skin lubricants, topical corticosteroid or emollient creams, and trimming nails and covering hands are often inadequate. Some of the pharmacologic measures tried include phenobarbital (5 to 10 mg/kg/day), lipid-binding resins such as cholestyramine or cholestipol (0.5 g/kg/day), and antihistamines such as diphenhydramine (5 mg/kg/day) or hydroxyzine (2 mg/kg/day). Some centers have used carbamazepine (Tegretol) at doses of 20 mg/kg/day as well. Others have resorted to ultraviolet irradiation (UVB) of the skin, plasmapheresis, and even partial biliary diversion by externalized stoma to treat intractable pruritus. Ursodeoxycholic acid, currently approved in the United States only for dissolution of cholesterol gallstones in adults, is a polar bile salt that may have a role in improving bile flow and aiding in the clearance or dilution of toxic bile salts and thus ameliorating pruritus and other complications of chronic cholestatic liver disease.

Portal hypertension and its sequelae, including hypersplenism, ascites, and bleeding from esophageal varices, often accompany chronic, progressive liver disease and cirrhosis. (See article on portal hypertension, p. 221.) Bleeding varices are treated medically with intravenous vasopressin (Pitressin) in a dosage of 5 to 10 mU/kg/minute up to a maximum of 0.4 U/minute in 5 per cent dextrose. Complications include systemic hypertension and fluid overload. If this treatment is unsuccessful, the Sengstaken-Blakemore tube may be used with inflation only of the gastric balloon and never for more than 24 hours, with periodic deflation every 6 hours or so to prevent pressure necrosis. Chest radiography should always be done to confirm accurate placement of the tube. Endoscopic variceal sclerosis with various agents now has been used successfully and routinely to control acute variceal bleeding or to prevent recurrent bleeding after the patient has stabilized after an initial bleeding episode. No role currently exists for prophylactic sclerotherapy in children or adults with varices who have not had an initial bleeding episode. Conflicting evidence exists (all in adult studies) regarding the use of beta-adrenergic blocking agents, such as propranolol, for prevention of a first or subsequent variceal hemorrhage in patients with known varices. When used, a titrated dose is recommended to achieve a 20 to 25 per cent reduction in resting heart rate. Portosystemic shunting procedures in infants and young children are often technically difficult, and long-term results in terms of shunt patency are not promising. The shunts may also interfere with later attempts at liver transplantation and thus should be avoided unless acute intractable bleeding threatens the patient's immediate survival.

As mentioned above, liver transplantation has now become an accepted and widely available treatment of chronic liver failure limited mainly by donor organ availability, especially in the young infant.

DISEASES OF THE GALLBLADDER AND BILIARY TREE

Cholecystitis and Cholelithiasis

Cholelithiasis in children is often but not exclusively a complication of chronic hemolytic disease. With the increased use of ultrasonography, there has been an increased incidence reported of gallstones or biliary sludge, often in asymptomatic patients. Many of these patients are young infants who have been receiving total parenteral nutrition and may also have had ileal resection, another predisposing factor to cholelithiasis. Other infants whose neonatal course was complicated by prematurity, sepsis, diuretic use, and/or chronic parenteral nutrition have also been found to have stones, most often pigment stones. There is controversy as to whether asymptomatic large stones found incidentally warrant removal and cholecystectomy, since many stones, especially those found in infants, may subsequently resolve on their own. Since the natural history of these asymptomatic stones in children is not clear, many advocate expectant management in the asymptomatic, healthy patient. Clearly, the child who develops acute cholecystitis should be treated with antibiotics and undergo cholecystectomy. In the patient with cholesterol stones less than 2 cm and with any contraindication to surgery, such as patients with cystic fibrosis, oral medical therapy designed to dissolve gallstones with chenodeoxycholic acid or, more recently, ursodeoxycholic acid (10 mg/kg/day in two divided doses) may be an option. Data for use in young children are not available, and the recurrence rate may be as high as 50 per cent by 5 years.

Acute cholecystitis in the absence of stones is rare but has been described with typhus, typhoid fever, diphtheria, scarlet fever, shigellosis, viral infection of the gastrointestinal or respiratory tract, and infestation with *Giardia lamblia* or *Ascaris lumbricoides*. Malformations of the biliary tree, sphincter of Oddi spasm, and ectopic gastric mucosa in the gallbladder are also reported associated findings. Antibiotic therapy for 24 to 48 hours followed by elective cholecystectomy is the treatment of choice.

Hydrops of the Gallbladder

Hydrops of the gallbladder may be seen in a variety of infectious conditions, including upper respiratory infections, streptococcal disease, and *Pseudomonas* or *Salmonella* sepsis. It is a relatively common associated finding in Kawasaki disease and leptospirosis. It may also occur in relatively well infants who are taking nothing by mouth, possibly owing to poor peristalsis and stasis, and often resolves spontaneously after reinstitution of oral feeding. If hydrops of the gallbladder is associated with infection or sepsis, aggressive therapy with antibiotics is essential. If the patient is not toxic and serial ultrasonography shows a decrease or no increase in gallbladder size, the patient can continue to be observed and treated medically. If, however, the size continues to increase, then perforation is a clear risk and the patient should undergo cholecystectomy.

Choledochal Cyst

This is an uncommon, congenital biliary tract abnormality occurring in approximately 1 in 15,000 births and affecting females three to four times more often than males. The lesion may present in childhood as neonatal cholestasis but more commonly presents in later childhood with pain, variable jaundice. There are several variants ranging from a choledochocele at the ampulla of Vater to diffuse saccular dilatation of the common bile duct to the classic discrete cystic dilatation of a segment of the common bile duct. Complete excision of the cyst followed by choledocho–Roux-en-Y–jejunostomy is the preferred treatment. Simple aspiration of the cyst is unacceptable, as is choledochocystojejunostomy, as both involve an increased risk of cholangiocarcinoma of approximately 5 per cent in the retained cyst remnant. Untreated choledochal cysts may result in cholangitis, stone formation, or biliary cirrhosis with secondary portal hypertension. In spite of adequate excision of the extrahepatic cyst, later complications may ensue from associated intrahepatic ductal abnormalities.

Caroli's Disease

Caroli's disease is a disorder characterized by congenital, communicating ectasia and focal cystic dilatation of the intrahepatic biliary tree. It may be seen alone or in association with congenital hepatic fibrosis or choledochal cysts. One quarter of cases are associated with renal abnormalities, including cortical cysts and medullary sponge kidneys. Cystic disease of the pancreas is also reported. Recurrent episodes of cholangitis and stone formation due to stasis are common and require antibiotic treatment. In the rare instance of cystic abnormalities confined to one lobe or liver segment, hepatic lobectomy may be indicated.

Sclerosing Cholangitis

This disorder is most commonly seen in children in association with ulcerative colitis. However, recent reports describe its association in other disorders, including immunodeficiency syndromes and histiocytosis X. It may involve any or all areas of the intrahepatic or extrahepatic biliary tree, causing strictures, stasis, and subsequent stone formation. The only available treatment is to relieve biliary obstruction by T-tube external drainage, cholecystoduodenostomy or jejunostomy, or strictureplasty of lesions in the extrahepatic biliary tree. Corticosteroids usually offer only temporary relief, if any. Colectomy in patients with ulcerative colitis does not alter the course of this disease, which progresses from recurring cholangitis and obstruction to biliary cirrhosis, portal hypertension, and an increased risk of hepatic carcinoma. Liver transplantation is now a viable and more frequently used alternative, but recurrent disease in the graft has been reported in some adults.

Miscellaneous Disorders

In children, the most common tumors of the biliary tree are benign papillomas, adenomas, or fibromas and are treated by simple excision. The most common malignant tumor is sarcoma of the botryoid type. Simple rhabdomyosarcoma and cholangiocarcinoma also occur but are rare, and, despite excision and radiotherapy, long-term survival is poor.

Traumatic hemobilia and avulsion of bile ducts with late biliary stricture may be complications of abdominal trauma or child-battering. Avulsion of the bile ducts is treated by surgical drainage and operative repair of the tear. Traumatic hemobilia, resulting from rupture of blood-filled intrahepatic pseudocysts into the biliary tree, is also treated by surgical drainage and pseudocyst excision.

Intrahepatic cholestatic syndromes range from benign recurrent cholestasis to disorders characterized by paucity or hypoplasia of interlobular bile ducts. Those patients with duct paucity in syndromic association with other anomalies such as vertebral arch defects, peripheral pulmonic stenosis, and other findings that characterize the syndrome of arteriohepatic dysplasia seem to have an improved prognosis over those patients with isolated intrahepatic bile duct paucity. Treatment is supportive for the associated cholestasis, as described above for biliary atresia, and liver transplantation is also an option for patients with progressive chronic liver failure.

PANCREATIC DISEASES

KENNETH L. COX, M.D.

ACUTE PANCREATITIS

The general principles of treatment of acute pancreatitis are (1) to treat hypovolemia and electrolyte abnormalities, (2) to reduce pancreatic secretions, (3) to relieve pain, and (4) to remove the precipitating cause.

Correction of Fluid and Electrolytes

Correction of hypovolemia should begin immediately, utilizing a large-bore central venous catheter for fluid replacement and to monitor central venous pressure. Hypotension and low central venous pressure should be corrected as rapidly as possible with plasma, dextran, albumin, or whole blood. Shock is the main cause of death in acute pancreatitis. Shock is primarily a result of exudation of plasma into the retroperitoneal space and peripheral vasodilatation caused by increased kinin activity.

After hypovolemia has been corrected, the rate of intravenous infusions should be reduced so as to provide maintenance plus replacement of ongoing losses from nasogastric suctioning and exudation into the peritoneal and retroperitoneal spaces. Monitoring urine output and central venous pressure is a mechanism for assessing the adequacy of the fluid replacement. Major complications of treatment of severe acute pancreatitis are pulmonary edema and congestive heart failure; these usually occur 3 to 7 days after the onset of pancreatitis. Although in many cases the cause is unknown, in some cases fluid overload has occurred because of excessive fluid replacement. Thus, the amount of fluid replacement must be adjusted frequently for changes in intravascular volume.

Serum electrolytes, including calcium and magnesium, serum creatinine, and blood urea nitrogen determinations, will aid in selecting the appropriate electrolyte composition of intravenous solutions. Since between 2 and 17 per cent of patients with acute pancreatitis have renal failure, potassium should not be added to intravenous solutions until stable urine output has been established. In addition to maintenance sodium chloride and potassium chloride of 3 mEq/kg every 24 hours and 2 mEq/kg every 24 hours, respectively, losses from nasogastric suctioning should be replaced. Although 5 per cent dextrose solutions should be initiated, hyperglycemia and hypoglycemia occasionally seen in severe pancreatitis warrant careful monitoring of urinary reducing substances and blood glucose concentrations and changing the concentration of dextrose in the intravenous solution appropriately. Symptomatic hypocalcemia, i.e., tetany and seizures, should be treated with intravenous calcium gluconate, 0.1 to 0.2 g/kg/dose (not over 2 gm) as a 10 per cent solution administered slowly and stopped for bradycardia. For asymptomatic hypocalcemia, replacement may be accomplished by adding 10 ml or more of 10 per cent calcium gluconate to each 500 ml of intravenous solution. In severe pancreatitis, serum electrolytes, including calcium, should be measured at least daily so that adjustments in the electrolyte composition of intravenous solutions can be made if necessary.

Reduction of Pancreatic Secretions

Pancreatic exocrine secretions are reduced by fasting the patient. Usually feeding should not be reinstituted until abdominal pain and ileus have resolved and serum amylase, urinary diastase, and the amylase-creatinine clearance ratio have returned to normal. If oral alimentation cannot be taken within 5 days, then parenteral nutrition should be given. Since carbohydrate is less of a stimulant to pancreatic exocrine secretion than are protein and fat, the initial diet should consist of carbohydrates only. If the carbohydrate diet is tolerated without worsening or exacerbating symptoms, then a low-fat and protein diet may be given. Again, the diet should be discontinued if symptoms should recur.

Pain Relief

Nasogastric suctioning should be used to relieve nausea, vomiting, and abdominal pain. Since there is no evidence that gastric suctioning alters the clinical course of pancreatitis, it is not required in the treatment of mild-to-moderate pancreatitis. However, in severe pancreatitis or marked ileus, nasogastric suctioning should be used.

Relief of the severe abdominal pain associated with pancreatitis not only is important for patient comfort but also may reduce the cephalic phase of pancreatic secretion. Morphine sulfate should be avoided because it may worsen pancreatitis by causing sphincter of Oddi spasm. Meperidine hydrochloride (Demerol) may be administered intravenously or intramuscularly at 1 to 2 mg/kg every 3 to 4 hours for severe abdominal pain. If this does not reduce pain sufficiently, then the effect of Demerol can be potentiated by administering chlorpromazine (Thorazine) at 1 mg/kg intramuscularly simultaneously.

Other Therapies

Other therapies for acute pancreatitis remain controversial. Prophylactic antibiotics have not been shown to be beneficial. Secondary infection of the pancreas, usually by streptococci, coliforms, or staphylococci, occurs in 2 to 5 per cent of cases of pancreatitis. Identification of the infective organism(s) and the antibiotic sensitivities will allow selection of the appropriate antibiotics. If pancreatic abscess forms, surgical drainage is usually necessary. There is insufficient clinical evidence that suppressors of pancreatic exocrine secretion, such as anticholinergic drugs, glucagon, somatostatin, calcitonin, and tranquilizers, and inhibitors of pancreatic enzymes, such as aprotinin (Trasylol)* and epsilon-amino-caproic acid (EACA), are useful in the management of acute pancreatitis.

Persistence of abdominal pain and of elevation of serum amylase levels for 2 or more weeks after the onset of acute pancreatitis suggests the formation of a pseudocyst. Ultrasonography is an effective method of identifying pseudocysts, differentiating pseudocysts from inflammatory masses, and monitoring the size of pseudocysts. Many pseudocysts spontaneously resolve in 4 to 12 weeks. If the pseudocyst persists for 6 or more weeks or is enlarging, surgical internal drainage of the cyst into the stomach or upper small intestine has been the treatment of choice. More recently, ultrasonography has been used to guide percutaneous needle aspiration of the cysts and to place catheters for external drainage. This technique may be particularly useful in patients who are poor operative candidates.

Pancreatic fistulas most often occur following pancreatic trauma or drainage of pseudocysts. Most fistulas will spontaneously close. Those that have a high output or interfere with providing adequate oral alimentation often require prolonged periods of fasting and total parenteral nutrition (TPN). Intravenous lipids can be given as a part of TPN therapy because they do not appear to stimulate pancreatic secretion. Rarely, surgical closure of the fistula is necessary.

Chronic and recurrent forms of acute pancreatitis are rarely seen in children. Continued exposure to the precipitating cause, i.e., alcohol, cholelithiasis, child abuse, and so on, or familial pancreatitis must be considered. Hereditary pancreatitis is transmitted autosomal dominantly and is associated with lysinuria and cystinuria in some cases. Most cases of hereditary pancreatitis require total pancreatectomy for control of symptoms. Endoscopic retrograde cholangiopancreatography (ERCP) should be performed if etiology is unknown, since congenital papillary stenosis may be identified and treated by endoscopic papillotomy. ERCP may identify other obstructive abnormalities, such as gallstones, choledochal cysts, or duplication cysts, that can be surgically corrected. Malabsorption due to pancreatic exocrine insufficiency and, rarely, diabetes mellitus requiring insulin therapy are sequelae of chronic pancreatitis. Malabsorption should be treated with oral pancreatic enzyme replacement therapy. Severe chronic abdominal pain may necessitate prolonged fasting, using home parenteral nutrition or pancreatectomy. Chronic abdominal pain may be reduced by giving before each meal pancreatic enzyme extracts, which inhibit meal-stimulated pancreatic secretion.

PANCREATIC EXOCRINE INSUFFICIENCY

Cystic fibrosis, Shwachman-Diamond syndrome (pancreatic insufficiency and bone marrow hypoplasia), and chronic pancreatitis are main causes of pancreatic exocrine insufficiency in children.

Oral pancreatic enzyme extracts are the primary treatment, independent of the cause. The dose of pancreatic enzyme extract to be administered with meals depends on the severity of pancreatic exocrine insufficiency, the patient's age, the fat content of the diet, and the type of enzyme preparation. In general, dietary fat restriction is not necessary, and approximately 8000 lipase NF units (one Cotazym capsule or one Viokase tablet) should digest at least 15 g of dietary fat. Higher doses of enzymes may not improve digestion and may result in hyperuricemia. Ineffectiveness of oral pancreatic enzymes to completely correct malabsorption is in part due to the suboptimal pH of the stomach for enzyme activity. Reduction of gastric acidity with antacids or cimetidine or protection of preparations with enteric coating (Pancrease or Cotazym) has been reported to improve enzyme activity.

Deficiency of fat-soluble vitamins D, A, K, and E may occur with severe malabsorption. Clinical manifestations from vitamin deficiencies are rarely seen. Occasionally, bleeding diathesis due to hypoprothrombinemia from vitamin K deficiency and hemolytic anemia from vitamin E deficiency will occur. Prevention of vitamin deficiencies is usually accomplished by reducing malabsorption with oral pancreatic enzymes and by administering a multiple vitamin preparation at twice the minimum daily requirements. Additional supplementation with water-miscible vitamin E, 50 to 100 U daily, and with vitamin K, 0.5 to 5 mg daily, should be given to those who have severe malabsorption or laboratory evidence of deficiency in these vitamins.

Advising patients and families of the appropriate diet for age and dose of oral pancreatic enzymes will usually allow normal growth and development without significant malabsorptive symptoms. Occasionally, additional calories in the form of dietary supplements will be desired, or limited fat restrictions in the diet, i.e., a 15 to 20 per cent fat diet, will be necessary to control steatorrhea. Because elemental dietary supplements like medium-chain triglycerides and predigested protein are unpalatable, children will often refuse to take these preparations, especially for long periods of time. In these cases, nonelemental dietary supplements, such as Ensure, Sustacal, and Meritene, given with enzymes may be more acceptable.

ISOLATED PANCREATIC ENZYME DEFICIENCIES

Isolated pancreatic enzyme deficiencies are extremely rare. Diagnosis is made by pancreatic secretory studies revealing normal concentrations of pancreatic enzymes in duodenal aspirates except for the absence of a single enzyme.

Isolated lipase deficiency is an autosomal recessive disease that presents shortly after birth with oily diarrhea. Standard oral pancreatic enzyme preparations, as are used in cystic fibrosis, will correct the malabsorption.

Isolated amylase deficiency usually presents after 1 year of age. As starch becomes a larger part of the diet, watery diarrhea occurs. Analysis of the stool will reveal reducing substances (Clinitest positive at more than ¼ per cent) and an acid pH of less than 6.0. The diagnosis can be confirmed with a starch loading test, i.e., failure of blood glucose to rise following ingestion of 50 g of starch per square meter of body surface area. Treatment consists of starch elimination and supplementation with disaccharides.

Isolated trypsin or trypsinogen deficiency presents shortly after birth with diarrhea, anemia, hypoproteinemia, edema, and severe failure to thrive. Absence of trypsin or trypsinogen results in lack of proteolytic enzyme activity in duodenal secretions. Treatment consists of standard oral pancreatic enzyme preparations.

Isolated enterokinase deficiency is an autosomal recessive disease that also presents in the neonatal period with severe watery diarrhea, failure to thrive, anemia, hypoproteinemia, and edema. Enterokinase is produced in the brush border of the proximal small intestine. Since this enzyme is necessary for the activation of trypsin, duodenal aspirates lack proteolytic enzyme activity, which can be activated by adding enterokinase to the aspirate. Enterokinase can be assayed in the

*Aprotinin is an investigational drug and may not be available in the United States.

small-intestinal biopsy specimens. Standard oral pancreatic enzyme preparations are the required treatment.

CONGENITAL MALFORMATIONS

Annular pancreas is a ring of pancreatic tissue encircling the descending portion of the duodenum. Surgical intervention consists of a duodenoduodenostomy or duodenojejunostomy. The pancreas is left undivided so as to avoid formation of pancreatic fistulas. Pancreatic function is normal in these patients.

Approximately 2 per cent of the population have ectopic pancreatic tissue. Ninety per cent of these occur in the stomach, duodenum, or jejunum. Occasionally, the ectopic pancreas produces abdominal pain, gastrointestinal obstruction, bleeding, or intussusception. When these complications occur, the ectopic pancreatic tissue should be excised.

PANCREATIC TUMORS

Pancreatic tumors in children are very rare. Most are endocrine-secreting tumors, e.g., insulinoma, gastrinoma, VIPoma, and so on.

Ninety per cent of insulinomas are solitary tumors. Severe hypoglycemia often results in irreversible neurologic sequelae. Diazoxide, from 5 to 20 mg/kg every 24 hours, usually prevents hypoglycemia. Most children who have insulinomas during the first year of life will have remission before 5 to 6 years of age. Thus, surgical resection is not usually necessary in these younger children if hypoglycemia is prevented by diazoxide. Earlier surgery is indicated in children with localized tumors seen after 1 year of age or with hypoglycemia that is poorly controlled by diazoxide. Blind resections are often unsuccessful.

Twenty per cent of gastrinomas are solitary and benign. Gastrin secreted by the tumor stimulates gastric acid secretion, resulting in multiple gastric and duodenal ulcers and often diarrhea. Fasting serum gastrin levels may be only marginally elevated but will be markedly elevated (> 400 pg/ml) following intravenous secretin injection or calcium infusion. In adults, cimetidine, an H_2-receptor antagonist, has been shown to be an effective drug for controlling symptoms caused by the gastric hyperacidity. Those whose symptoms are not controlled by cimetidine usually require a total gastrectomy. Since the tumors are usually multiple and difficult to localize, surgical resection is often impossible.

Fortunately, carcinoma of the pancreas rarely occurs in children. However, recent reports from Japan indicate an increasing incidence in pancreatic carcinomas in children. Since clinical manifestations usually do not appear until extensive metastasis has occurred, prognosis of pancreatic carcinoma is poor, with a mean survival of 6 to 9 months after diagnosis in adults. Pancreaticoduodenectomy is recommended for the rare patient who has a small, localized lesion. In those with inoperable disease, supportive therapy consists of providing adequate nutrition and analgesia.

MALABSORPTIVE DISORDERS

ERIC S. MALLER, M.D.
and JOHN B. WATKINS, M.D.

The clinical presentation of malabsorptive disorders is extremely varied and may present with generalized disturbances in growth and loss of weight or may be more limited to the absorption of a specific substrate, such as vitamin B_{12} or lactose. Adequate treatment requires the establishment of the proper diagnosis, for example, the identification of the child with cystic fibrosis who presents with poor weight gain and large, foul-smelling stools, or the identification of excessive sorbitol ingestion in the child who presents with normal growth and intermittent abdominal pain and watery diarrhea.

Classically, a discussion of the treatment of malabsorptive conditions has focused on the malabsorption of specific classes of nutrients (e.g., carbohydrates, proteins, and fats). However, because many disorders affect the absorption of more than one nutrient, an alternative approach is to consider the treatment of malabsorptive disorders in terms of their pathophysiology. In this fashion, one can determine whether they arise from abnormalities of the intestinal intraluminal processes (i.e., maldigestion), intestinal mucosal function due to injury or loss of absorptive surface area following surgical resection, or, finally, from defects in the transport of absorbed nutrients from the enterocyte into the blood or lymphatics.

CARBOHYDRATE INTOLERANCE (Table 1)

Carbohydrate intolerance is a common presentation for malabsorptive disorders in children and may be due to the ingestion of poorly absorbed sugars or to disorders of both the intraluminal and the mucosal phase of digestion. Transient mucosal injury following a viral gastroenteritis or *Giardia* infestation commonly results in an acquired lactose intolerance. Symptoms may be short-lived, resolving over several days, or they may persist for several weeks or even months in the case of a resolving gluten-sensitive enteropathy *(celiac disease)*, depending on the extent of mucosal injury.

Treatment includes the short-term exclusion or decrease in the intake of lactose-containing foods. Alternatively, this may be achieved through the use of several newly developed formulations that contain glucose polymers derived from either corn or rice. These polymers have proved to be well tolerated in oral rehydration solutions and in infant formulas, providing both a reduced osmotic load and effective absorption. Late-onset lactase deficiency is the rule in most of the world's adult population occurring in childhood typically after 5 to 6 years of age in white children and after 3 to 5 years of age in other selected populations, including black and Asian children. A commercial lactase enzyme preparation may be added to milk or sprinkled on food, and this will typically result in a 70 to 90 per cent reduction in the lactose content. A pre-hydrolyzed, lactose-reduced milk is also commercially available. Individuals with lactose intolerance are often able to tolerate yogurt with active cultures without symptoms, as the bacteria in the yogurt produce an enzyme that survives passage through the stomach to remain active in the intestine.

Sucrase-isomaltase deficiency is present at birth, and mucosal function is otherwise normal. It may become apparent clinically later in infancy, coinciding with the introduction of sucrose-containing foods such as fruits and fruit juices. Restriction of sucrose results in an amelioration of symptoms, which also occurs with increasing age probably as a result in adaptation of the colonic bacterial flora and changes in colonic function.

In infancy and with toddlers who are growing well, the most common cause of carbohydrate intolerance is the ingestion of large amounts of the poorly absorbed or nonmetabolizable carbohydrates fructose, and sorbitol. Symptoms result from an osmotic diarrhea. These sugars are commonly used to sweeten many foods and soft drinks. They are commonly found in fruit juices, purées, and sugar-free gum. Treatment focuses on decreasing the intake of carbohydrate-containing beverages or substituting foods with lower quantities of the

TABLE 1. Treatment of Malabsorptive Disorders

Disorder	Treatment
Carbohydrate Intolerance	
Monosaccharide intolerance	
Congenital glucose-galactose malabsorption	Remove glucose and galactose from diet; substitute fructose
Sorbitol and fructose induced diarrhea	Remove offending carbohydrate from diet or substitute juices with lower sorbitol content
Disaccharide intolerance	
Lactase deficiency	Remove lactose from diet; add commercial lactase to milk; take commercial lactase tablets with meals containing lactose
Sucrase-isomaltase deficiency	Avoid sucrose in diet
Polysaccharide	
Amylase deficiency (congenital or secondary to pancreatic damage)	Avoid starch in diet
Fat Malabsorption	
Bile salt insufficiency (e.g., cholestasis, terminal ileal resection or dysfunction; primary bile acid malabsorption)	Low-fat diet; medium-chain triglyceride and fat-soluble vitamins A, D, E, K supplementation
Exocrine pancreatic insufficiency (e.g., cystic fibrosis, Shwachman syndrome, chronic pancreatitis)	Pancreatic enzyme replacement (enteric-coated and/or high lipase preparation) with H_2 blocker therapy; fat-soluble vitamins supplements; protein-calorie supplements
Intestinal lymphangiectasia	Medium-chain triglyceride and fat-soluble vitamin supplementation; low-fat diet
Abetalipoproteinemia	Treatment as for lymphangiectasia; vitamin E supplementation, parenterally or as oral alpha-tocopherol polyethylene glycol succinate–1000
Congenital lipase deficiency	Treatment as for exocrine pancreatic insufficiency
Selected Common Disorders Causing Mucosal Injury or Insufficient Absorptive Surface	
Celiac disease	Gluten-free diet; lactose-free diet until mucosal healing
Inflammatory bowel disease	Anti-inflammatory/immunosuppressive therapy; elemental enteral or possibly parenteral caloric supplementation
Short-bowel syndrome	Treat bacterial overgrowth with antibiotics; medium-chain triglycerides if extensive ileal resection; enteral or parenteral caloric supplementation
Bacterial overgrowth	Treat with appropriate antibiotics (e.g., trimethoprim-sulfamethoxazole, Neomycin)
Parasitic infestation (e.g., *Giardia*)	Treat with metronidazole or other antiprotozoal drug; lactose-free diet, if symptomatic
Specific Micronutrient Malabsorption	
Acrodermatitis enteropathica (zinc)	Zinc supplementation
Vitamin B_{12} malabsorption	Vitamin B_{12} supplementation usually parenteral; diagnose and treat any vitamin B_{12}-ingesting tapeworm (e.g., *Diphyllobothrium latum*)

offending sugar. Table 2 lists some common juices and their sorbitol and other carbohydrate content.

Glucose-galactose malabsorption and primary lactase deficiency are rare conditions but are of interest because they are due to congenital defects in specific transport and hydrolysis systems. These conditions are treated by removal of the specific sugar. Carbohydrate-free formulas are available for infants with profound carbohydrate intolerance and should never be used without providing a carbohydrate source, either orally or intravenously.

FAT MALABSORPTION (Table 1)

Fat malabsorption may occur in a wide variety of conditions, as fat digestion involves all phases of the digestive process: intraluminal, mucosal, and transport events. Intraluminal

TABLE 2. Carbohydrate Content and Osmolality of Fruit Juices

Juice	Carbohydrate (g/dl)				Osm/kg of Water
	Fructose	*Glucose*	*Sucrose*	*Sorbitol*	
Apple	6.2	2.7	1.2	0.5	638
Grape	7.5	7.1			1030
Pear	6.4	2.3	0.9	2.0	764
2% Sorbitol				2.0	142

From Hyams JS, Etienne NL, Leichtner AM, Theuer RC: Carbohydrate malabsorption following fruit juice ingestion in young children. Pediatrics 82:64–68, 1988.

causes of fat malabsorption characteristically affect lipolysis and the micellar solubilization of nutrient lipids. Examples of this type of abnormality include pancreatic insufficiency due to cystic fibrosis or, less commonly, recurrent pancreatitis and the Shwachman syndrome.

These disorders may be effectively treated with pancreatic enzyme replacement therapy. The efficacy of treatment may be improved by the use of enteric-coated microspheres and occasionally reduction of gastric acid secretion with H_2 receptor blockers. Decreased intraluminal bile acid concentration occurs with cholestatic liver disease and ileal resection. Loss of the ileocecal valve compounds the problem by often leading to bacterial overgrowth of the small bowel and deconjugation of the bile salts. These disorders often result in selective deficiencies of the lipid-soluble vitamins, A, D, E, and K. Children with these disorders and all others with significant fat malabsorption should receive fat-soluble vitamin supplementation.

Vitamin E replacement is often the most difficult and, when inadequate, leads to a syndrome of progressive neuromuscular dysfunction. Adequate vitamin E replacement therapy may be achieved by the use of a water-soluble preparation of vitamin E, alpha-tocopherol polyethylene glycol succinate–1000 (TPGS), 25 IU/kg/day.

The liquid preparation of *vitamin* D_2 (ergocalciferol) (1000 to 2000 units/day) is usually effective. If signs of vitamin D deficiency persist, the more potent 25- and 1,25-hydroxyvitamin D_3 products (calcifediol and calcitriol, respectively), may also be used.

Menadiol, a water-soluble preparation of vitamin K, is available in 5-mg tablets, and one-half tablet every other day with feeding is usually sufficient. Measurement of the prothrombin time can be utilized as an indicator of the adequacy of vitamin K replacement.

Vitamin A deficiency is the most difficult to recognize clinically, but it can be confirmed through the use of serum levels. Deficiencies are treated with replacement doses of 5000 to 10,000 units/day. To avoid toxicity, adequacy of therapy should be evaluated by obtaining serum levels.

An abnormal intraluminal environment due to bacterial overgrowth results in low bile acid concentrations caused by the deconjugation of bile acids, which may also produce a secondary intestinal mucosal injury. Treatment is aimed at identification of the bacterial etiologies and correction of any underlying motility disturbance or obstructed blind loop, which may have contributed to the overgrowth.

NET PROTEIN MALABSORPTION (Table 1)

Net protein malabsorption rarely, if ever, occurs in isolation. It may occur with fat malabsorption and disorders of pancreatic insufficiency. More commonly, it occurs in the setting of protein-losing enteropathy due to primary intestinal lymphangiectasia, small-intestinal mucosal injury secondary to a variety of causes, including celiac disease, extensive Crohn's disease, eosinophilic gastroenteropathy, or severe infectious enteritis, especially in the infant. Additionally, any disorder that increases vascular back pressure into the hepatic venous and, hence, the portal venous system draining the intestine (e.g., constrictive pericarditis, congestive heart failure (especially right-sided) or hepatic venous or inferior vena cava obstruction due to a congenital web or malignancy) can result in secondary intestinal lymphangiectasia and protein malabsorption and loss into the stool.

Therapy centers on treating and correcting the underlying heart disease or vascular obstructive lesion, if possible, or healing the mucosal injury by using anti-inflammatory and/or immunosuppressive therapy in Crohn's disease and a gluten-free diet in celiac disease. Supplementation of calories with use of a medium-chain triglyceride supplement and a diet low in long-chain fat in the case of primary or secondary lymphangiectasia bypasses the need for intact lacteal and lymphatic function and results in improved nutrition and immune function.

MALABSORPTION SECONDARY TO DECREASE IN INTESTINAL SURFACE AREA (Table 1)

Finally, the malabsorptive processes that arise from a decrease in intestinal surface area and injury to the mucosa, such as celiac disease, small-bowel resection, or extensive small-bowel involvement secondary to inflammatory processes (e.g., Crohn's disease), may result in insufficient intestinal surface area to permit effective nutrient absorption or the maintenance of adequate fluid and electrolyte homeostasis. Celiac disease, or gluten-sensitive enteropathy, is a condition resulting from an immune-mediated injury in response to the presence in the diet of the gliadin fraction of gluten. This fraction is found in grains such as wheat, barley, oats, and rye, and the disease is a specific diagnosis which requires a lifelong gluten-free diet. Many commercial substitutes for gluten containing foods are available as are cookbooks containing gluten-free recipes. Considerable knowledge and useful information may be obtained through national and local celiac disease organizations.

Inflammatory bowel disease, specifically Crohn's disease, requires targeted therapies to suppress the inflammatory response. These include immunosuppressant medications, such as prednisone, azathioprine, or cyclosporine and other agents, including sulfasalazine and the newer 5-aminosalicylate derivatives. Nutritional rehabilitation of the patient is an important adjunct to these medications and is often necessary to ensure adequate growth and to ameliorate the inflammatory process.

In some malabsorptive conditions, particularly when adequate oral intake cannot be maintained, or in patients with severe mucosal injury or reduced surface area as the result of small bowel resection, enteral feeding administered by a nasogastric or a gastrostomy tube is often an important adjunct to therapy. The selection of an appropriate formulation for the infant or child is based in part on the etiology of the malabsorptive condition. The normal progression is from blenderized to polymeric, and then chemically defined or modular, specialized formulas.

When normal growth is unable to be maintained by enteral feeding, total parenteral nutrition (TPN) may be necessary. Home parenteral nutrition is now an established form of treatment. A permanent central venous catheter can be surgically inserted and then used safely at home after a formal education and training program. The most effective care for children in home programs is achieved in conjunction with an experienced center able to provide adequate support services, including trained physicians, nurses, pharmacists, and nutritionists. The distribution of formulas, TPN solutions, and other supplies has been simplified by the emergence of a number of excellent national and regional companies. These companies may also be able to provide home evaluation and nursing support so that a number of children are able to receive their nutritional therapy at night and continue their regular activities during the day.

It should be noted that it is often possible to utilize enteral feeding administered continuously at night either by nasogastric or gastrostomy feeding. This method is recommended over parenteral feeding because it is associated with a lower risk of complications, is simpler to administer, and is less expensive.

DISORDERS OF THE ANUS AND RECTUM

BARRY SHANDLING, M.B., Ch.B., F.R.C.S.

ANAL STENOSIS

A congenital anal stricture is present, resulting in constipation, sometimes even prolapse, as the infant strains to evacuate. Simple dilation over the course of several weeks is all that is necessary. Dilation should not be discontinued too soon because stenosis may recur.

IMPERFORATE ANUS

The diagnosis of imperforate anus should be made at birth by careful inspection of the perineum. If doubt exists as to the patency of the anus, a thermometer may be used gently to probe the anus. There are several types of imperforate anus as a consequence of interference with the development of the hindgut and its separation from the urogenital portion of the primitive cloaca. The earlier the intrauterine development, the more complex the anomaly. Esophageal atresia often coexists.

Low Anorectal Malformations

In boys low anorectal malformation takes the form of a "covered" anus, with an anal occlusion resulting in a complete obstruction. This may also be incomplete with a tiny orifice appearing on the perineum anterior to the anus, even on the scrotum or undersurface of the penis. Between this orifice and the site of the anus, collections of meconium or clear mucus (perineal "pearls") may be seen. *In all cases of imperforate anus, no conclusions as to the type should be made until swallowed air reaches the rectum. This may take 24 hours.* The perineum should be inspected with a hand lens to look for a telltale green speck of meconium on the 2nd day of life. A relatively minor perineal operation is required to establish patency.

Girls with low anorectal malformation usually have an "ectopic" anus. The ectopic anus may be perineal, vestibular, or vaginal in location. For the first two types, dilation with or without a "cut-back" operation may be needed; for vaginal ectopic anus, posterior transplantation is needed. Both girls and boys with low malformations should be perfectly continent, provided that no foolish major surgical procedures are undertaken.

The levator ani muscle is what separates low from high varieties of imperforate anus.

High Anorectal Malformations

In boys with a blind-ending rectum above the levator ani, there is usually a fistulous connection between the rectum and the prostatic urethra. The diagnosis may be made with confidence by finding green staining of the diaper with voiding or by actually seeing a drop of meconium appearing at the tip of the urethra.

In a girl with a high anorectal malformation, the rectum is connected with the posterior vaginal fornix. This malformation is very rare. More commonly (with high varieties), there is a complex cloacal abnormality with a single cloacal opening onto the perineum. Within this cloacal tube, the urethra opens in front, the rectum opens behind, and the vagina opens above.

Both boys and girls with high varieties of imperforate anus require a colostomy in the neonatal period, followed by an operation at age 3 to 6 months to bring the bowel down to the perineum, where the anus should be.

PERIANAL AND ANAL LESIONS

Close observation of the perineum in infants and children (i.e., gently parting the buttocks with the thumbs as the parent keeps the child's hips acutely flexed and thighs abducted) is more useful than a rectal examination. A rectal examination, although more invasive, is essential, however, in all cases of chronic constipation.

ANAL FISSURE

An anal fissure is a tear or crack in the perianal skin at the mucocutaneous junction or even more distally in the anal skin. A fissure may result in blood in the stool or on the toilet paper. It is caused by the passage of a large, hard stool and causes intense discomfort with consequent inhibition of defecation. If the fissure is chronic, there may be infection with *Candida* or *Streptococcus.* I have known the condition to be perpetuated by cleansing the anus and surrounding skin with chemically impregnated paper, a very popular technique nowadays. Most fissures tend to heal if one can manage the invariably concomitant constipation. Operation is very rarely indicated. Scrupulous perineal hygiene, namely washing the perineum with soap and water in a bath after every stool, usually effects a cure.

PERIANAL ABSCESS AND FISTULA-IN-ANO

With any chronic perianal suppuration or inflammation, the coexistence of Crohn's disease must be looked for by appropriate radiologic and/or endoscopic studies.

In infancy a diaper rash may lead to a pustule and abscess formation. Alternately, infection may extend laterally from the anal crypts toward the ischiorectal fossa. A painful, tender nodule with redness of the overlying skin is enough of an indication for surgical drainage. One should not wait for fluctuation to develop. If the overlying skin is thin and transparent, no anesthetic is necessary. Parents must be warned, however, that in well over 50 per cent of cases a pustule will recur, will probably drain spontaneously, and will heal, only to recur again and again. This is the typical presentation of an anal fistula. The internal opening of such a fistula is radially opposite the external opening, on the pectinate line. Treatment consists of unroofing the fistula, thereby establishing drainage. Within 10 days the lesion should be healed. More complex types of fistulas (e.g., pelvirectal, which extend through the levator ani muscle) are virtually never seen in children.

HEMORRHOIDS AND PRURITUS ANI

Internal hemorrhoids, i.e., varicosities of the internal hemorrhoidal venous plexus, are not seen in children other than in association with portal hypertension. The latter must be treated if any success in managing the hemorrhoids is to be anticipated.

External hemorrhoids are really anal tags in association with an underlying fissure. Such tags may be itchy or may become inflamed. Treatment of the fissure usually results in resolution of the external hemorrhoid. Such hemorrhoids do not bleed. Any bleeding is from the underlying fissure. Bathing the perineum after defecation relieves any discomfort or pruritus. If scrupulous hygiene is practiced and constipation relieved, recurrence is not likely.

RECTAL PROLAPSE

Although rectal prolapse is alarming to parents, this condition is a benign one, with a strong likelihood of spontaneous resolution. The rectal mucosa may protrude several inches out from the anus. Usually found in toddlers and children up to 5 years of age, prolapse may be potentiated by straining at stool. Children with cystic fibrosis or those infected with parasites such as *Entamoeba histolytica* may present with rectal prolapse. Other factors include whooping cough, spinal cord lesions, rectal polyps, and malnutrition. Sweat chloride measurements should be obtained in all cases of rectal prolapse to rule out cystic fibrosis. Parents find that whereas in most cases the prolapsed rectum spontaneously retracts after defecation, occasionally the protruding bowel has to be manually reduced. The condition must be distinguished from a prolapsing rectal polyp and an intussusception presenting at the anus.

The vast majority of cases of rectal prolapse respond to simple measures, such as treatment of diarrhea or constipation; eradication of concomitant parasitic infections; and abandonment of the potty. This latter receptacle encourages the development of prolapse because the hips are acutely flexed with the thighs compressing the abdomen. The child should defecate on an adult toilet on a special seat that has a small hole so that accidental immersion is avoided. It is not my practice to recommend recumbent defecation or to tape the buttocks together. The simple measures described are successful in fully 90 per cent of cases. If not, the injection of a submucosal sclerosant (e.g., ethanolamine oleate) causes the mucosa to become "stuck down." If several series of injections fail to prevent prolapse, the insertion of a perianal suture—the Thiersch operation—will almost always result in a cure. Nothing more elaborate is necessary.

FECAL INCONTINENCE

True fecal incontinence is usually on a neurologic basis, found in patients with spinal dysraphism (spina bifida), tethered cord, and tumors and injuries of the spinal cord. The condition has been encountered in instances of sexual abuse. The anorectal muscle complex is lacking in tone, although the internal anal sphincter may have normal function. There should never be any reason to do a colostomy in such children because they may be perfectly managed satisfactorily with a daily large-volume (20 ml/kg of body weight) saline enema. Unless the patient can be given the enema in the knee-chest position, there will be reflux of the fluid out of the anus. Alternatively, using the enema continence catheter may render such incontinent children completely socially continent. The catheter has an inflatable tip so that the patients may be able to administer their own enemas without leakage and can become perfectly independent and socially acceptable.

ENCOPRESIS

Encopresis may be defined as the passage of fecal material into the clothing. It may occur with or without constipation.

Without Constipation. This is rare. There is no fecal retention and also no organic abnormality of either rectoanal sensation or of the muscles of continence. The causes are complex and emotional and are often related to sibling rivalry or an unsatisfactory relationship with parents. Treatment is difficult and best undertaken by a psychiatrist or psychologist.

With Constipation. There is usually a huge (almost impacted) fecal mass within the rectal ampulla. The anus becomes "taken up," like the cervix in parturition, and consequently patulous and incontinent. The large fecal bolus is too huge to transverse the anus, but fecal-stained mucus or liquid fecal material drains out around the mass, through the incompetent anus, and into the underwear. Children so afflicted often hide their clothing and appear to be oblivious to the foul miasma that invariably accompanies them. The findings on rectal examination are all too self-evident.

Treatment is difficult and will be of no avail unless and until the bowel is emptied. Phosphate enemas are inadequate. Digital disimpaction, with the patient under anesthesia if necessary, is needed. Of value is the use of sorbitol (2 mg/kg of a 70 per cent solution) followed by a diet rich in fiber, using natural wheat bran, cooked cereal, and bran bread plus plenty of fruit, vegetables, and salads coupled with a laxative. I find mineral oil messy, greasy, and ineffective. A small dose of sorbitol may be used on a regular basis. One should never let the child go more than 2 days without a stool, using a large-volume saline enema if 48 hours have elapsed without defecation. Regular contact with the parents is wise so that no regression ensues.

RECTAL POLYPS

Rectal polyps, also known as *juvenile polyps,* are probably not true tumors. They consist of cystic spaces and granulation tissue with an inflammatory cell infiltrate. Eighty per cent are single, and 80 per cent are located in the rectum. Painless rectal bleeding, sometimes with noticeable "slime" (mucus) in the stool, is the invariable presenting symptom. The blood may be on the surface of the stool if the polyp is in the distal rectal ampulla. It is mixed with the stool if more proximal. These polyps are neither malignant nor even premalignant. Many are self-curing, in that they outgrow their blood supply or twist off on their narrow stalks. Diagnosis is made by a skilled pediatric radiologist, who uses a double-contrast enema, followed by a sigmoidoscope to find and remove the polyp. Usually, a general anesthetic is required. Such polyps may be left alone for many years in the hope of effecting autoamputation. I would not wait until the child is beyond 10 years of age. The hemoglobin does not fall because the amount of blood loss, although alarming to the laity, is minimal.

COLIC

MARC WEISSBLUTH, M.D.

ETIOLOGY

Explanations of why healthy-appearing babies cry during the first few months of life may be grouped into four broad categories: (1) a developmental stage, (2) unmet biologic needs, (3) psychologic or emotional distress, and (4) medical problems. Published therapeutic interventions usually reflect the categorical bias of the clinical investigator, but an unbiased review of studies of infant crying leads to the conclusion that there is no single treatment of choice. There is no treatment that completely stops all colic symptoms. Some symptoms will always persist. Claims of treatment success are meaningless in the absence of clear entry criteria and explicit treatment outcome criteria. Exactly how much was the crying diminished and in what percentage of infants? Only when this information is available can a pediatrician or parent reasonably decide whether it is worthwhile to try a proposed treatment.

Many proposed so-called treatments are so simple that they probably will never be studied. These include the use of hot water bottles, noises from vacuum cleaners or hair dryers, different nipple shapes, heart beat or intrauterine recordings, and lamb's wool pads. *There is a subtle problem with encouraging parents to try using these seemingly benign items. When parents repeatedly engage in minitreatment trials with initial high hopes for success, the inevitable failure to eliminate colicky crying reinforces the parental perception that something is fundamentally very unhealthy in the child, themselves, or both.* This unwarranted perception of unhealthiness might persist long after the colic subsides and lead to beliefs and parenting practices that reinforce this false notion. The parents may be left with thoughts such as: my child is allergic; my child has a sensitive stomach; my child was ill the entire infancy and now needs special care; I could never calm my baby; I never had enough milk; he must have hated me then.

Category 1: A Developmental Stage

In a longitudinal study of infant crying that has been repeatedly cited in other studies of colic, infants were divided into three groups. The first group (51 per cent of the infants) was called "contented/mildly fussy" because they had paroxysms of unexplained irritability, fussiness, or crying less than 3 hours a day occurring less than 3 days in any one week. The second group (23 per cent of the infants) was called "fussy" because their paroxysms lasted more than 3 hours a day and occurred more than 3 days in any one week. The third group (26 per cent of the infants) was called "seriously fussy" or "colicky" because the spells continued for more than 3 weeks.

In the first two groups, there were prolonged periods of fussiness only in some infants. Even though there was less fussiness, irritability, or crying, studies have shown that some of these behaviors do occur in *all* babies. However, the behavior may appear as only fussiness, which is described by parents as an unsettled, agitated, *wakeful* state, and because sucking is soothing, the parents may report that there are times in the evening when the child has "difficulty feeding." The parents might not even call it "fussiness" during these fitful periods; however, crying occurred if the parents did not put forth extra efforts in rocking, carrying, or encouraging sucking.

The third group was originally labeled by British pediatricians as having "three months" colic or "evening" colic. The Chinese parents in my general pediatric practice call these behaviors "100 days of crying," the Vietnamese call it "3 months plus 10 days of crying," and the Japanese call it "evening crying." The Asian view is similar to that of Shakespeare's description of infant crying as merely the first act in the play of life. It appears, therefore, that some degree of unexplained irritability, fussiness, or crying is universal.

Further, most clinical researchers do not have data associating these behaviors with pathophysiologic mechanisms involving allergies or the gastrointestinal system. Additionally, there are no clear discontinuities in measurements of irritability, fussiness, or crying whether by direct observational studies in hospital nurseries, voice-activated tape recordings in homes, or parent-report diaries. Thus, grouping of infants or attaching labels based on these behaviors is completely arbitrary.

The ages of onset and termination for these behaviors are characteristic. They begin at about a few days after delivery or a few days after the expected date of delivery regardless of the degree of prematurity, and they end at about 12 to 16 weeks of age. Among those 26 per cent, or about one fourth of infants with the greatest amounts of crying, the crying begins in 80 per cent by the second week and an additional 10 per cent start by the third week. Only 2 per cent of infants start their crying attacks during the first week. In this infant group (26 per cent of infants), crying ceases in 60 per cent by the third month and in 100 per cent by the fourth month. Only 7 per cent of infants stop crying during their second month. The time course of experimentally induced crying by snapping a rubber band against the infant's leg or foot is similar: depressed reactivity during the first few days, then the crying increasing and markedly diminishing at 12 weeks of age.

The time of occurrence for these behaviors is also characteristic. Discrete periods appear to occur randomly during the first month; afterward, however, the periods occur predominantly in the evening hours. Among the one quarter of infants with the greatest amount of crying, 80 per cent start their spell between 5:00 P.M. and 8:00 P.M. and end by 12:00 P.M. and an additional 12 per cent start later, 7:00 P.M. to 10:00 P.M. and end later by 2:00 A.M. In only 8 per cent are the attacks randomly distributed throughout the day or night.

The state of the infant is also associated with these behaviors. Among the one fourth of infants with the greatest amount of crying, 84 per cent begin their crying spell when they are *awake* (8 per cent from a sleep state and 8 per cent variable), and when the crying spell ends, 83 per cent of the infants fall *asleep*.

Because the spells of unexplained irritability, fussiness, or crying are universal; the behaviors differ only in degree between infants; the behavior's onset and termination are locked to postconceptual age; and the behaviors exhibit state specificity and a circadian rhythm; it appears that these behaviors reflect normally maturing physiologic processes. The processes may involve the development of arousal-inhibitory or wake-sleep control mechanisms. Supporting this impression is the fact that consolidated night sleep organization occurs during the second month and the periodic organization of sleep and wake states occurs between 3 and 4 months of life. From this perspective, it makes no more sense to say that an infant "has" colic than it does to say that a teenager "has" adolescence.

However, colic is the popular term used by pediatricians to label infants in the top-quarter of irritability, fussiness, or crying. Studies in these particular infants using reproducible subject selection criteria (such as more than 3 hours/day, more than 3 days/week, more than 3 weeks) have shown that only about 3 per cent *usually* respond to rhythmic rocking motions or similar soothing interventions, 18 per cent *occasionally* respond, and 79 per cent *rarely* or *never* respond. Supplemental carrying or picking the child up more does not help these particular infants. Therefore, there is an element of inconsolability in this top-quarter group.

Treatment for the "contented/mildly fussy" infants (51 per cent) includes rhythmic rocking motions, swaddling, encouraging sucking, carrying the baby more even when there is no crying, and shortening the interval between feedings. Some parents report that music, lullabies, or rough mechanical sounds, such as a vacuum cleaner or running water, have a soothing effect. Treatment for the "fussy" infants (23 per cent) is similar, but these parents need to be told that often the paroxysms do not occur beyond 1 week in duration. Most parents will accept a watchful waiting approach if they know that the waiting period is brief. Placebo responses occur frequently in these two groups of infants because of the relatively brief duration of crying. Treatment for the "seriously fussy" or "colicky" infants (26 per cent) frustrates parents because no single soothing maneuver consistently helps to reduce the crying and sometimes nothing helps.

Treatment has progressed when parents know that their pediatrician is an ally, when they they know what is meant by colic, when they know not to waste their energy and upset their emotional stability on useless gimmicks, and when they feel that they are unlucky but not guilty. Parents have to be told repeatedly that the crying is not their fault.

In order to alleviate unnecessary guilt and prevent misdirected therapies focused on parental psychologic factors, parents should be informed that there is no sound scientific evidence to suggest that their inexperience, anxiety, or parenting practices are directly causing the colic. Self-doubt or feelings of inadequacy of parenting skills or failure to nurse well is a topic that should be openly discussed because all parents blame themselves for the infant's crying. Parents should also be told that treatments with sedatives, hypnotics, antiflatulents, antacids, antihistamines, alcohol, or gripe water are no better than a placebo. The physician should be patient, sympathetically supportive, and appropriately tentative when offering advice regarding remedies of questionable value, such as herbal teas or hot water bottles. The way in which the physician presents these therapies is important because overly encouraging home remedies or formula switching may only heighten parental anxiety when each of these items might eventually fail.

The major principle of management is not exactly what the physician recommends but how he or she does it. The physician should take the parents' complaint seriously and should perform a thorough examination. When colic is suspected, a thorough examination is diagnostic—and also therapeutic—because the thoroughness itself reassures the parents that their child is healthy and is being looked after by someone who really cares.

If the physician spends extra time in the office or on the phone, expressing optimism regarding the health of the child and emphasizing that this stressful period will soon end, this will help the parents to maintain their morale. Their increased optimism from reassurance might not only reduce parental anxiety but also cause the parents to handle their baby in a calmer fashion and thus actually reduce the crying. The major error in management is to trivialize the parents' complaint because colic is known to be a transitory condition with no known morbidity or complications.

Parents should be encouraged to take a break from their baby. They should use other people to help care for the baby when the crying is most severe. Even if this break is only a few hours or a few days a week, it sustains morale because it is a rest period that the parents can anticipate. It is important for the parents to learn to accept and love their baby despite the crying. Tell parents that it is true no one can care for their baby as well as they can, but during an inconsolable crying spell, the baby is probably unaware of who is doing the holding and rocking. Parents must understand that this break is for their pleasure and relaxation; it is not to do errands, chores, or housework. Parents need to be emphatically told that occasionally getting away from their crying baby is smart, not selfish. Taking care of themselves means that they will be better able to nurture their baby.

Category 2: Unmet Biologic Needs

Parents may attribute the crying to hunger or thirst and believe that their baby should be fed differently. For example, parents might try switching from breast to bottle, adding cereal to the formula, or offering juice or water. Usually, repeated examinations and documentation of good interval weight gain is sufficient to reassure the parents. Definitions of colic always include the notion of a healthy child who is gaining weight well. Therefore, a child who is crying because of hunger and poor weight gain would be diagnosed with failure to thrive, not colic.

Category 3: Psychologic or Emotional Distress

There are two older speculative ideas about causation and treatment of colic that have been supported and popularized by eminent physicians. These two nonempirical notions—"maternal anxiety" and "stimulus overload"—are really only guesswork. Maternal anxiety as the cause of colic has been described as the mother's "anxious overpermissiveness psychotoxically" disturbs the baby and parents overreact and the tension around the infant builds up. Neither description really addresses the issue of directionality of effects but merely assumes that the dominant causative factor is parental or maternal emotionality.

Treating the mother or parents would be the logical conclusion, but it should be clearly understood: there is no study meeting contemporary standards of clinical behavioral research investigating the effects parents and children have on each other that supports this conclusion. In fact, contemporary research suggests that specific parenting patterns do not result from or cause colic. Also, when parents were observed to be trying many different ways to calm their colicky baby, it was assumed by older psychoanalytically inclined writers that parents were causing the colic in the first place by something called stimulus overload. This notion also has no basis in fact. Sensitivity to external stimulation may be a recognizable trait in some post-colicky infants, but the stimulus overload speculation does not fit well with the fact that paroxysmal colicky spells often occur in dark rooms only in the quiet evening hours. Treatment strategies built around the unsupported and, I think, erroneous notion that parents cause colic usually create unnecessary parental guilt, which lowers their self-esteem. If parents can accept the fact that they have a difficult temporary situation that is not their fault, they are better able to avoid feelings of helplessness or hopelessness. When they stop overintellectualizing or practicing self-analysis, they can better carry out simple treatment strategies. Pediatricians should explicitly and repeatedly address this issue of parental nonculpability as part of the treatment process.

Category 4: Medical Problems

Some infants may have a specific medical problem that causes these crying behaviors and requires specific treatment. These infants then are diagnosed as having that particular problem (e.g., lactose intolerance); they are not diagnosed as having colic. Colic is the term used in the absence of diagnosable medical problems. Therefore, because the concept of colicky behaviors carries the exclusion of a diagnosable medical problem, there is not a specific medical treatment for colic.

Recent research has focused on gastrointestinal reactions to components of cow's milk found in infant formulas or in the breast milk of nursing mothers who are drinking cow's milk. However, even when changing formulas appears to reduce the crying in some infants, it would be a mistake to generalize these results and conclude that about 26 per cent of infants cry excessively as a result of components of cow's milk in their diet.

A careful history and physical examination are usually sufficient to establish the diagnosis of infantile colic. The physical examination, or repeated examinations, should be considered as a sufficient diagnostic test. Laboratory tests or radiographic examinations, sometimes including hospitalization, are usually unnecessary if the child is gaining weight normally and has a normal physical examination. Tests such as blood counts or urine cultures are sometimes performed to create the impression of professional thoroughness in order to reduce parental anxiety. Under the guise of a laboratory work-up, physicians may hope to better convince the family (and sometimes themselves) that there is no organic disease. Thus, after winning their trust and confidence in his or her professional judgment, the pediatrician can better support the parents as they wait out the 3 or 4 months of colic. However, one potential problem of doing laboratory tests performed with the intent to reduce parental anxiety rather than on the basis of clinical suspicions is that a somewhat abnormal result may occur. Obviously, the slightly abnormal test result does not necessarily signify pathology. Nevertheless, one abnormal test could lead to further unneeded tests in a fruitless search to eliminate some uncommon or obscure condition. Another disadvantage in performing laboratory tests is that the performance of the tests themselves or hospitalizing the infant might reinforce the parents' belief that something must be medically wrong with their child. After all, they may think, why else would the doctor do these tests if he or she did not truly suspect something might be wrong with my baby? With this attitude, the discovery of a few normal results might only cause parents to request additional tests, studies, or consultations.

On the other hand, if the physician does not perform tests, this might lead to heightened anxiety or parental dissatisfaction based on a perception of a lack of thoroughness and may cause the parents to change pediatricians. There is enormous variability among families and pediatricians in how they handle the stresses caused by a colicky infant. Sensitivity to this variability of how both the parents and the pediatrician are affected should encourage a highly individualized approach to working up and treating an infant who might have colic.

The method that the physician uses to explain the reason for the tests might make a great difference. Some parents might feel much more relaxed when the physician tells them that he or she honestly does not think the test will show anything abnormal but that it will be done so that they can stop worrying. Other parents find this approach unacceptable.

POST-COLIC PROBLEMS

Parents inevitably want to know whether the constant attention will spoil the child, that is, create a crying habit. Data are available to support the contrary conclusion that consistent and prompt parental responsiveness to crying in early infancy tends to reduce, not increase, crying at age 1 year. On the other hand, recent research suggests that although most parents can learn to distinguish between mild, non-distress, fussy vocalizations and intense, need-based crying, some parents respond to both types indiscriminately. Then, over several months, the frequency of crying may increase, but if they selectively ignore mild vocalizations and only respond promptly to severe crying, overall crying with fussing may decrease. Parents of "contented/mildly fussy" infants (51 per cent) and some "fussy" infants (23 per cent) may successfully practice this differential responsiveness under 3 to 4 months of age. But parents of "colicky" infants (26 per cent) might not be as able to respond differentially and/or these infants might not be self-soothing until after 3 to 4 months of age. Therefore, one potential post-colic problem is indiscriminate parental responsiveness to every type of cry sound, which leads to more infant crying. In addition to not responding to mild, fussy vocalization, parents can learn to ignore crying caused by the baby's being overtired.

After about 6 weeks of age, for some "contented/mildly fussy" or "fussy" babies, when they begin to exhibit specific social smiling, they might benefit from less attention when overly tired. The soothing parental efforts might be so socially pleasurable to these infants that they fight sleep to enjoy the parents' company. The end result is fatigue-driven fussiness. However, for "colicky" babies, because they are so irregular regarding sleep-wake transitions, it is difficult for parents to distinguish between colicky crying and fatigue-driven crying until the infant is about 3 to 4 months old. At this age, for "colicky" babies, the evening crying spells have diminished and most parents should now be encouraged to give the child less attention when they think that the child is tired and needs to sleep. After 3 to 4 months, most parents are better able to differentiate the child's need to sleep from the desire to play.

The failure of parents to shift their strategies after the child is about 3 to 4 months of age, in response to the child's increasing social maturity, often causes severe post-colic sleep problems. Thus, after the colic passes, the older child is never left alone at sleep times and is deprived of the opportunity to develop self-soothing skills. These children never learn to fall asleep unassisted. The resultant sleep fragmentation/sleep deprivation in the child driven by intermittent positive parental reinforcement, leads to fatigue-driven fussiness long after colic is resolved. Letting the child "cry it out" probably helps no one when the child is under several weeks of age. However, letting the child "learn to sleep" after 3 to 4 months helps produce a calmer, less fussy baby. Parents should be told that they should allow their child to learn the self-soothing skill of falling asleep unassisted, and they should be reassured that they are not hurting the child. Learning to be alone to develop self-soothing skills is a developmental healthy habit for the child, and pediatricians can guide parents' behavior, which helps or hinders its evolution.

7

Blood

ANEMIA AND CHRONIC DISEASE

A. KIM RITCHEY, M.D.

The traditional definition of the anemia of chronic disease is a mild to moderate hypoproliferative anemia associated with a spectrum of chronic disorders, including various renal diseases, infections, rheumatic diseases, cancer, and others. Laboratory characteristics of this anemia include (1) normochromic, normocytic or (especially in children) hypochromic, microcytic red blood cells, (2) a low reticulocyte count relative to the degree of anemia, (3) low serum iron and total iron-binding capacity, (4) normal to low per cent transferrin saturation, and (5) normal to increased ferritin.

The etiology of the anemia of chronic disease has been attributed to a combination of factors, including (1) a block in the utilization of adequate iron stores, (2) shortened red blood cell survival, and (3) inadequate erythropoietin production and/or utilization. Treatment has emphasized appropriate management of the underlying disease with few specific recommendations regarding the anemia *per se* other than ruling out other treatable causes of anemia and general supportive care.

The modern treatment of anemia associated with chronic diseases must be more disease specific. Knowledge of the relative importance of different pathogenetic mechanisms leading to the anemia and the availability of hematopoietic growth factors (especially erythropoietin) dictate this change in approach, as outlined for several conditions in the text that follows.

ANEMIA WITH RENAL DISEASE

The degree of anemia associated with renal disease varies from mild to severe. In general, the severity of the anemia parallels the degree of renal compromise. Although mild to moderate anemia associated with non-uremic inflammatory kidney disease is probably a result of the mechanisms described above, most of the information regarding anemia and kidney disease deals with the anemia of chronic renal failure.

The pathogenesis of the anemia of renal failure is multifactorial: (1) decreased erythropoietin production, (2) shortened red blood cell life span, (3) inhibition of erythroid proliferation by uremic "toxins," (4) depletion of iron or folate, (5) blood loss, and (6) aluminum toxicity. The most important factor in this list is the lack of erythropoietin.

Traditional treatment of the anemia of renal failure has included transfusions when clinically indicated, androgens (primarily in adults), and hematinics for proven nutritional deficiencies. However, the recent release of recombinant human erythropoietin (rHuEpo) has dramatically changed the treatment of this anemia and the lives of patients with kidney diseases. This hematopoietic hormone has been shown to correct anemia in virtually all patients and to improve their sense of well-being and quality of life while not exacerbating the underlying disease. In general, rHuEpo is very well tolerated but problematic side effects include hypertension (new or exacerbation of pre-existing hypertension), seizures, and thrombosis (of arteriovenous shunt or artificial kidney).

Most of the studies of rHuEpo have been performed in adults, and there are limited data regarding its use in children with renal failure. Guidelines for the use of rHuEpo in children with renal failure are evolving, and treatment with it should be initiated only under the auspices of an experienced pediatric nephrologist. Children with hematocrit values less than 30 per cent (probably closer to 20 per cent) are candidates for rHuEpo therapy. Prior to treatment, blood pressure should be under control, iron status documented, and any iron deficiency treated. During treatment with rHuEpo, blood pressure and iron status should be monitored closely and therapy should be promptly instituted for either hypertension or evolving iron deficiency. Although the ideal dose of rHuEpo has not been determined, one recommendation is to start with 50 units/kg IV or SC (range 25 to 100 units) two or three times per week with the goal of achieving a hematocrit of 26 to 30 per cent. The dose of rHuEpo may have to be adjusted upward, but changes should be initiated slowly. Once the ideal hematocrit level has been attained, the dose or frequency of rHuEpo should be adjusted down to maintain this level. Reasons for failure of rHuEpo include (1) iron deficiency, (2) osteitis fibrosa cystica, (3) inflammation or infection, (4) blood loss, and (5) aluminum toxicity.

ANEMIA WITH CHRONIC INFECTION OR INFLAMMATION

The pathogenesis of the anemia associated with chronic infection or inflammatory states, such as juvenile rheumatoid arthritis (JRA), includes the traditional factors mentioned in the introduction. However, erythropoietin deficiency is much less prominent than in the anemia of chronic renal failure; and there is new evidence that cytokines such as tumor necrosis factor (TNF) from activated macrophages may directly suppress the proliferative capacity of the marrow.

Chronic Infection

As a result of improved antimicrobial treatment, anemia associated with chronic infections, such as tuberculosis, chronic osteomyelitis, and the like, is infrequently seen. However, there currently is no curative therapy for human immunodeficiency virus (HIV) infection. In fact, anemia is the most common hematologic side effect seen in acquired immunodeficiency syndrome (AIDS). The anemia may be secondary to the disease itself or to treatment with zidovudine (AZT). Treatment of the anemia associated with AIDS consists of excluding other treatable causes of anemia (e.g., nutritional deficiency or blood loss) and administering transfusions when clinically indicated. A trial of rHuEpo in adults with AIDS on AZT has shown that for patients with low endogenous erythropoietin levels, rHuEpo was effective in reducing transfusion requirements and increasing hematocrit values. The role of rHuEpo in the management of children with AIDS has not been studied, but treatment with it should be considered for children with moderate to severe anemia and low erythropoietin levels.

Rheumatic Diseases (Juvenile Rheumatoid Arthritis, Systemic Lupus Erythematosus)

Anemia is the most common hematologic finding in children with rheumatic disorders. Fifty to 60 per cent of children with systemic JRA have anemia, and the severity of the anemia correlates with the disease activity. The primary causes for the anemia include the traditional mechanisms outlined for the anemia of chronic disease and iron deficiency. The high incidence of iron deficiency seen in this population is likely due to chronic gastrointestinal blood loss secondary to aspirin-induced gastritis and impaired intestinal absorption of iron. It may be difficult to distinguish between the anemia of chronic disease and iron deficiency because of overlapping laboratory abnormalities. A trial of iron should be instituted for those children who have either a low ferritin level or a lower than expected hematocrit level or mean corpuscular volume for age and disease activity (even in the face of normal or elevated ferritin levels). rHuEpo has been given to a few adults with rheumatoid arthritis, resulting in a significant rise in hematocrit. The role that rHuEPo will play in the treatment of children with rheumatic disorders is unclear.

ANEMIA WITH CHILDHOOD CANCER

The risk of anemia is high with most childhood neoplasms. Unlike the other chronic diseases discussed, the pathogenesis of the anemia may vary throughout the disease course. This high risk for anemia of varying etiology usually ends when treatment is completed.

The likely causes of anemia depend on the stage of treatment of the cancer. At diagnosis, the anemia is likely to be secondary to effects of the disease itself such as (1) marrow replacement (leukemia, neuroblastoma), (2) immune hemolytic anemia (lymphoma), (3) blood loss (thrombocytopenia), and/or (4) anemia of chronic disease (cancers presenting with a more chronic course, e.g., Ewing's sarcoma). Chemotherapy or radiation therapy may also cause anemia by producing marrow suppression, decreasing red blood cell survival (e.g., cisplatin), or producing folate deficiency (e.g., methotrexate). Other causes of anemia during treatment include infections that may lead to hemolysis (e.g., disseminated intravascular coagulation) or red blood cell aplasia (e.g., human parvovirus).

Treatment of the anemia associated with cancer depends on the etiology. At diagnosis, correction of severe anemia with transfusions and prompt induction of remission are the goals. During treatment of the cancer, a mild to moderate degree of anemia is usually tolerated, with transfusions being given only as clinically indicated. Preliminary studies of rHuEpo in adults with cancer and anemia indicate a possible role for this hormone; however, studies in children have not been performed to date.

ANEMIA OF IRON DEFICIENCY

JAMES A. STOCKMAN III, M.D.

Iron-deficiency anemia is defined as anemia caused by an inadequate availability of iron to sustain bone marrow erythropoiesis. It should be noted that iron deficiency and iron-deficiency anemia are not the same. Symptoms related solely to iron deficiency may occur in the absence of anemia and yet are responsive to iron treatment. For this reason, it is important to prevent the progression of iron deficiency to the later stages that result in anemia.

ETIOLOGY

There are a number of causes of iron-deficiency anemia. This state results from an imbalance between the amount of iron that must be absorbed from the diet, offsetting losses of iron that may occur from normal or abnormal processes. Although blood loss is the most common cause of iron deficiency in adults, this may not be true in children, in whom dietary iron deficiency or failure to absorb iron during periods of recurrent infection is much more prevalent.

DIAGNOSIS

The diagnosis should be made on the basis of (1) a careful history and physical examination to determine whether or not diet or blood loss is the cause of iron deficiency; (2) the performance of certain diagnostic tests or trials of iron to define whether or not the patient is truly iron-deficient; and (3) determination of the specific cause if iron deficiency is found.

Iron deficiency leads to a progression of laboratory abnormalities. The first finding is a fall in serum ferritin levels, followed shortly thereafter by a decline in serum iron and a rise in serum iron-binding capacity. Concomitant with this are a rise in free erythrocyte protoporphyrin levels in the blood and a decline in mean corpuscular volume (MCV) of the red blood cell. Finally, anemia develops. Laboratory tests for iron deficiency are based on these serially evolving abnormalities. Nonetheless, a clinical trial of therapeutic doses of iron constitutes both correct treatment as well as a diagnostic test for iron-deficiency anemia.

FOOD IRON

Term infants should have an intake of 1 mg/kg of iron per day throughout the first year of life. It is additionally recommended that premature infants receive twice this quantity of iron during this period. Thereafter, the average requirement per day for iron from all food sources in the diet should be approximately 10 to 15 mg/day. This amount should be approximately doubled in girls following the onset of menstruation.

The form of iron in the diet influences the percentage of iron that is assimilated. The range of iron absorption from the diet varies between 5 and 15 per cent in most instances. On average, however, 50 per cent of the iron in breast milk is absorbed in contrast to much less than 10 per cent of the iron in cow's milk. In iron-fortified formulas containing 12 mg of iron per liter, the average iron absorption ranges from 3 to 4 per cent. The latter amount of iron is sufficient to prevent iron deficiency in infants who receive formulas with iron. Since 1972, an electrolytically reduced form of small-particle iron has been added to dry infant cereals in the United States. It is estimated that 4 per cent of this iron will be absorbed by normal infants. These dry cereals contain 0.45 mg of iron per gram of dry cereal. Thus, there is approximately 1 mg of iron per tablespoon of such foodstuffs. The ingestion of 12 tablespoons of dry cereal per day should provide the infant with sufficient iron to prevent the development of iron deficiency, even if no other sources of iron are available. Because cow's milk is a poor source of iron, the use of cow's milk feeding during the first 6 to 12 months of life should be avoided. Cow's milk compromises the absorption of both food iron and medicinal iron and may contribute to the genesis of iron deficiency by inducing occult gastrointestinal blood loss. It should be noted that the absorption of iron from breast milk can be significantly inhibited by solid foods given near the time of breast-feeding. Vegetarians should be advised to eat ascorbic acid–containing vegetables or to supplement their meals with ascorbic acid, which markedly enhances iron absorption. On the other hand, the common beverage tea markedly inhibits iron absorption.

BLOOD LOSS

Iron-deficiency anemia can be caused by blood loss from a number of different sources, the most common being the gastrointestinal tract. Remarkable quantities of iron can be lost into the urine as hemosiderin. Intravascular hemolysis can cause the deposition of hemosiderin in renal tubular cells, which are then shed into the urine, causing hemosiderinuria. Paroxysmal nocturnal hemoglobinuria may also result in iron deficiency. Internal bleeding within soft tissues may sequester iron, preventing its recycling for new blood formation. In addition, any child with unexplained iron-deficiency anemia should be potentially considered to have idiopathic pulmonary hemosiderosis, a rare cause of iron deficiency.

The most frequent causes of gastrointestinal blood loss include early introduction of cow's milk into the diet of an infant, infectious or inflammatory bowel disease, ulcer disease, or Meckel's diverticulum.

Treatment of iron-deficiency anemia resulting from blood loss may be in the form of iron replacement therapy as noted below, assuming that the rate of blood loss does not exceed the availability of therapeutic iron to keep pace with increased rates of erythropoiesis. In such situations, if there is cardiovascular compromise, blood transfusions may be necessary. For most patients who are normovolemic, a simple booster transfusion with packed red blood cells (15 ml/kg) is sufficient to raise the hemoglobin 3 to 5 g/dl. If cardiac decompensation has occurred in the face of severe iron-deficiency anemia, it may be necessary to manage the patient with a partial exchange transfusion with packed red blood cells.

IRON REPLACEMENT

The standard treatment for iron-deficiency anemia is the administration of oral iron salts. The available iron salts are ferrous sulfate, ferrous gluconate, and ferrous fumarate. The commonly available iron preparations are in the form of ferrous sulfate. These preparations are all given orally.

The dose of iron that seems to be capable of producing an adequate rise in hemoglobin concentration with the least side effects in most children is 1.5 to 2 mg/kg of elemental iron administered three times daily between meals. This amount, assuming average bioavailability of 20 per cent, provides sufficient iron to permit a daily rise in hemoglobin of more than 0.4 g/dl. The rise in hemoglobin actually observed in any particular patient depends on the initial level of hemoglobin and the duration of observation period. The lower the hemoglobin concentration, the greater the rise per day. The shorter the observation period, the greater the calculated hemoglobin rise per day. If the initial hemoglobin is low, the rise in hemoglobin may start at 0.3 to 0.4 g/dl or more for the first week of treatment and then fall off gradually to 0.1 g/dl toward the end of treatment. A verification of the adequacy of treatment can be noted by the prompt onset of reticulocytosis beginning at 2 to 3 days and peaking at 7 to 10 days after initiation of treatment. Alternatively, the hemoglobin may be rechecked in 2 to 4 weeks when maximal therapeutic response and return to normal should have occurred.

The maximal dose of elemental iron necessary for most children is 180 mg/day. For infants and small children, a calibrated dropper with a solution containing 15 mg of elemental iron per 0.6 ml can be used. Toddlers can take syrup or elixir containing 30 or 45 mg of elemental iron per 5 ml, and older children can be given tablets or capsules containing 40 or 60 mg of elemental iron. Absorption is twice as effective when the medication is given on an empty stomach and markedly enhanced in the presence of ascorbic acid.

The side effects of oral iron therapy generally occur only with high doses of medicinal iron. These side effects have been reported to include constipation, abdominal cramps, and nausea. These effects can be minimized if iron is given with a meal, although the inhibition of iron absorption associated concomitant food intake may offset the advantage of this approach. With oral iron therapy, all stools will soon become black, but medicinal iron does not cause guaiac positivity on stool examination. If liquid iron preparations are used, there is a risk of staining of the teeth. Such dark staining is not permanent and may be minimized by administration of the medication at the back of the tongue or allowing the child to take the medication through a straw. Rinsing the mouth and brushing the teeth immediately after administration of the drug may also minimize this side effect.

Intramuscular administration of iron is indicated only if it is not possible to achieve compliance with the use of oral iron or under the unusual circumstance in which iron malabsorption occurs. Various iron preparations have been used for the parenteral treatment of iron deficiency. In these preparations, iron is bound to a substance that stabilizes the iron in a complex. Substances such as saccharose, dextrin, dextran, or modified dextran have been used as stabilizers. All of these iron preparations are of high molecular weight. Recently, low-molecular-weight iron complexes or iron–sorbitol–gluconic acid preparations have been investigated. Iron dextran (Imferon) is the most widely used product in the United States. Iron dextran contains 50 mg/ml of elemental iron. The calculation for the volume of iron dextran required, based on an average blood volume of 75 ml/kg, additional iron replacement of 50 per cent for replenishment of iron stores, and the fact that 1 g of hemoglobin (Hb) contains 3.5 mg of iron, is as follows:

$$\text{ml of iron dextran} = \text{wt (kg)} \times \text{desired rise in Hb (g/dl)} \times 0.076$$

Children younger than 1 year of age should not receive more than 2 ml of iron dextran at one time. Between the ages 1 and 2 years, 3 ml is the maximal dose. No more than 2 ml should be given in one site. It may be necessary to give the total calculated dose over several days. Imferon, if improperly given, can tatoo the skin. On rare occasions, potentially fatal anaphylactic reactions may occur. Parenteral administration of iron can also cause vomiting, chills, fevers, arthralgia, and urticaria.

FAILURE TO RESPOND TO IRON TREATMENT

Oral iron therapy occasionally fails to correct iron deficiency. In these instances, one should determine whether the diagnosis is correct. Other causes of failure to respond to iron therapy include the presence of mixed nutritional deficiencies, especially folic acid deficiency; failure of compliance; improper administration of iron; improper dosage; malabsorption of iron; and poor iron utilization. The latter generally results from chronic disease states. Iron deficiency associated with sideroblastic anemia or in the presence of lead poisoning may fail to respond to treatment. Unsuspected, continued blood losses may not respond to iron therapy. As noted, noncompliance and failure to absorb iron may be indications for iron dextran administration.

For every child treated for iron deficiency, a return to normal hemoglobin levels should be confirmed. Once this has occurred, if oral iron therapy has been used for treatment, it should be given for an additional 2 to 3 months to replenish iron stores. If it cannot be determined that iron deficiency is simply due to dietary causes, further surveillance for occult blood loss may be necessary, even though there is a therapeutic response to medicinal iron.

REFERENCES

Dallman PR: Iron deficiency: Does it matter? J Intern Med 226:367–372, 1989.
Dallman PR, et al: Diagnosis of iron deficiency: The limitations of laboratory tests in predicting response to iron treatment in 1-year-old infants. J Pediatr 99:376, 1981.
Dienard AS, Schwartz S, Yip R: Developmental changes in serum ferritin and erythrocyte protoporphyrin in normal (nonanemic) children. Am J Clin Nutr 38:71, 1983.
Lozoff B: Behavioral alterations in iron deficiency. Adv Pediatr 35:331–359, 1988.
Monzon CM: Anemia in infancy and childhood: A systematic approach to evaluation. Postgrad Med 78:275, 1985.
Newhouse IJ, Clement DB: Iron status in athletes: An update. Sports Med 5:337–352, 1988.
Oski FA, Stockman JA III: Anemia due to inadequate iron sources or poor iron utilization. Pediatr Clin North Am 27:237, 1980.
Seshadri S, Gopaldas T: Impact of iron supplementation on cognitive functions in preschool and school-aged children: The Indian experience. Am J Clin Nutr 50:675–684, 1989.
Siimes MA, Järvenpää AL: Prevention of anemia and iron deficiency in very low birth weight infants. J Pediatr 101:277, 1982.
Soewondo S, Husaini M, Pollitt E: Effects of iron deficiency on attention and learning processes in preschool children: Bandung, Indonesia. Am J Clin Nutr 50:667–673, 1989.

APLASTIC ANEMIA

BRUCE CAMITTA, M.D.

Aplastic anemia is a group of diseases in which decreased or defective hematopoietic stem cells result in a hypoplastic bone marrow and peripheral blood cytopenias. Marrow toxins may damage stem cells directly. Alternatively, aplastic anemia may be caused by activation of the immune system or damage to the marrow microenvironment. In a minority of patients, the disease is heritable. Despite extensive testing, the etiology of marrow aplasia is unknown in 50 per cent of cases.

Prognosis in aplastic anemia depends on the severity of the disease. Severe aplastic anemia has been defined as the presence of two or three peripheral blood criteria (neutrophils $< 0.5 \times 10^9/L$, platelets $< 20 \times 10^9/L$, and reticulocytes < 1 per cent after correction for hematocrit), a hypocellular marrow, and the absence of marrow fibrosis or malignancy. Without specific therapy, 80 per cent of patients with severe aplastic anemia die from infection, hemorrhage, or other complications.

INITIAL EVALUATION

Marrow biopsy is most accurate for evaluation of marrow cellularity and fibrosis. Hematologic malignancy should be excluded by morphologic and chromosome analyses of a marrow aspirate. If Fanconi's anemia is suspected, the sensitivity of chromosomes to breakage by diepoxybutane should be tested. Other diagnostic tests include Ham or sugar water test (paroxysmal nocturnal hemoglobinuria), liver enzymes and hepatitis serologic studies (especially hepatitis C), Epstein-Barr virus studies (mononucleosis, X-linked lymphoproliferative syndrome), and bone films (Fanconi's anemia, osteopetrosis). Histocompatibility typing (HLA-A,B,DR) should be performed on the patient, parents, and all full or half siblings.

SUPPORTIVE CARE

Previous medications should be stopped and new ones used sparingly. Certain restrictions should be imposed in view of neutropenia (limit interpersonal exposures, no rectal drugs or manipulations) and thrombocytopenia (decrease straining, no aspirin, no intramuscular [IM] injections). Oral hygiene should be gentle and may be maintained by brushing with a toothette and use of a chlorhexidine mouth wash. Prophylactic antibiotics are not indicated.

Transfusions should be given only when necessary. Red blood cells are indicated for symptomatic anemia and massive acute hemorrhage. In the absence of trauma, most patients tolerate platelet counts as low as $10 \times 10^9/L$ without significant bleeding. When needed, one unit per 6 to 10 kg raises the platelet count by $50 \times 10^9/L$. Granulocyte transfusions should be reserved for gram-negative bacterial septicemia or soft tissue infection refractory to antibiotics alone. Sensitization to histocompatibility antigens can be decreased by using single donors and washed, filtered, or ultraviolet irradiated blood products. Family members should not donate blood products for any child who might eventually receive a marrow transplant from a family member. Cytomegalovirus (CMV)-seronegative patients should receive CMV-negative blood products.

MILD APLASTIC ANEMIA

No treatment has been shown to change the long-term course of mild aplastic anemia. If blood counts are stable and transfusions are not required, the patient should be observed. Androgens (oxymetholone, 3 to 5 mg/kg/day orally; nandrolone decanoate, 3 to 5 mg/kg/week IM) may cause improvement in some patients. Potential benefits of androgens must be weighed against toxicities incurred with long-term use (virilization, hepatic dysfunction, or tumors). Androgens may be helpful for several years in patients with Fanconi's anemia. Patients in whom marrow aplasia becomes severe should be treated as described below.

SEVERE APLASTIC ANEMIA

Bone Marrow Transplantation

Bone marrow transplantation from a histocompatible sibling is the treatment of choice for severe aplastic anemia. In untransfused patients, long-term, disease-free survival of 85 per cent is possible. In transfused patients, a success rate of 70 per cent may be achieved, albeit at the expense of increased regimen-related toxicities. As a result of decreasing family size, only 25 to 35 per cent of patients have a matched sibling donor. Recent data suggest that partially matched related or unrelated individuals can be used as marrow donors. Again, the 50 per cent success rate is achieved at the risk of increased regimen-related toxicities.

Immunosuppressive Therapy

In approximately 50 per cent of patients with aplastic anemia, there is laboratory evidence for anti–bone marrow autoimmunity. Similarly, about 50 per cent of patients experience complete or partial improvement in blood counts after treatment with antilymphocyte or antithymocyte globulin (ALG or ATG). However, there is poor correlation of in vitro tests with patient responses. Responses are usually incomplete, late relapse (or progression to other hematologic disease) occurs in 25 per cent of patients, and the mechanism of action is not known (monoclonal anti–T cell antibody is not effective). ALG (Upjohn) is most commonly used in the United States (20 mg/kg/day for 7 to 10 days). Concomitant low-dose (2 mg/kg/day of prednisone or its equivalent) or higher-dose steroid therapy does not improve the response rate but may decrease serum sickness or bleeding. High-dose steroid therapy alone is generally ineffective.

Initial uncontrolled trials of cyclosporin A showed widely varying (0 to 50 per cent) response rates. In a recent randomized study, adding cyclosporin A (6 to 12 mg/kg/day) to ALG plus methylprednisolone increased responses from 62 to 82 per cent. Once again, most responses were incomplete; long-term follow-up is not yet available. Cyclosporin A blood levels should be monitored to limit potential renal, hepatic, neurologic, and vascular complications.

Colony-Stimulating Factors

Hematopoiesis is regulated by a series of interacting glycoproteins. Many of these agents have been cloned and are being tested in patients with hematopoietic disorders. Both granulocyte colony-stimulating factor (G-CSF) and granulocyte-macrophage colony-stimulating factor (GM-CSF) increase neutrophils in some patients with aplastic anemia (especially those with milder disease). However, responses of red blood cells or platelets have been uncommon. Factors, which are more likely to produce trilineage hematopoietic responses (interleukin 3, stem cell factor), are now being tested.

RECOMMENDATIONS

Bone marrow transplantation from a matched sibling is the treatment of choice for patients with severe aplastic anemia. For patients without a matched sibling, ALG or ATG (with or without cyclosporin A) should be tried. While one is awaiting response to ALG, a search for a partially matched related or unrelated donor should progress. Locating such a donor often requires 3 to 4 months. Ninety per cent of patients who improve after ALG begin to respond within 3 to 4 months. If there is no response to ALG by that time, bone marrow transplantation using a partially matched donor or treatment with colony-stimulating factors should be considered. These newer therapies should be reserved for patients on closely monitored protocols.

Families of patients with aplastic anemia may obtain information and support from the Aplastic Anemia Foundation of America (Telephone: 301–955–2083).

MEGALOBLASTIC ANEMIA

PHILIP LANZKOWSKY, M.D.

ETIOLOGY

Megaloblastic anemias in children are relatively uncommon and usually are due to folate or, more rarely, vitamin B_{12} deficiency. The causes of folate deficiency include (1) inadequate diet, (2) malabsorption (which may be congenital or acquired, e.g., gluten-induced enteropathy, sprue, pancreatic insufficiency, short-gut syndrome), (3) drug-induced inhibition of dietary folate absorption (phenytoin, phenobarbital), (4) increased folate utilization (growth, increased metabolic rate, e.g., fever, thyrotoxicosis, malignant disease, hemolytic anemias), and (5) drug-induced inhibition of folate metabolism (methotrexate, pyrimethamine, trimethoprim).

The causes of vitamin B_{12} deficiency include (1) dietary insufficiency (rare), (2) absence or abnormality of gastric intrinsic factor, (3) abnormal absorption of the vitamin B_{12} intrinsic factor complex as a result of previous small-intestinal surgery or lack of intestinal receptors (rare), and (4) inherited abnormalities of vitamin B_{12} transport protein.

Rarer metabolic causes of a macrocytic anemia (e.g., thiamine deficiency) have occurred in offspring of consanguineous marriages who have presented with neurologic abnormalities. The anemia was responsive to 25 mg of thiamine daily.

The metabolism of folic acid and vitamin B_{12} is interrelated, and this must be considered when therapy is instituted. Large doses of vitamin B_{12} may correct the hematologic problems that are due to folate deficiency. Conversely, large doses of folate may correct the hematologic disturbances that are due to lack of vitamin B_{12}. Folate, however, does not correct the neurologic problem associated with vitamin B_{12} deficiency, and large doses of folate should not be given until vitamin B_{12} deficiency has been excluded.

TREATMENT

Folic Acid Deficiency

Successful treatment of patients with folate deficiency involves (1) correction of the folate deficiency; (2) amelioration of the underlying disorder, if possible; (3) improvement of the diet by increased folate intake; and (4) follow-up evaluations at intervals to monitor the patient's clinical status.

The most recent recommended daily allowance (RDA) of folic acid for men and women aged 25 to 50 years is 200 μg/day and 180 μg/day, respectively, reflecting an allowance of 3 μg/kg/day. For infants from birth to age 1 year, it is 3.6 μg/kg/day. During pregnancy, the RDA is 400 μg/day. For lactating women, the RDA is 280 μg/day the first 6 months and 260 μg/day for the second 6 months. Rich sources of folate include liver, kidney, wheat bran, yeast, spinach, asparagus, black-eyed peas, lentils, and lima and navy beans. Green leafy vegetables, most whole grains, beef, almonds and peanuts, corn, beets, potatoes, turnip greens, and broccoli contain good amounts of folic acid. The vitamin is ubiquitous in foods.

In cases of a suspected folate deficiency, a therapeutic trial can be instituted with 50 to 100 μg of folate per day orally. This dose produces a prompt reticulocytosis in cases of folate deficiency but is without effect in patients with vitamin B_{12} deficiency. An optimal response occurs in most patients with 100 to 200 μg folic acid daily. Nevertheless, it is usual to treat deficient patients with 0.5 to 1.0 mg daily orally. Commercially available preparations include tablets (0.25, 0.4, 0.8, 1.0 mg) and an elixir (1.0 mg/ml). To reduce the folate content would not significantly reduce the cost, and because pteroylmonoglutamic acid does not produce side effects except in patients with vitamin B_{12} deficiency, there is little reason to reduce the dose. Further, a smaller oral dose might not always be effective in patients with folate malabsorption. In most patients, 5 mg of folic acid given orally daily for 7 to 14 days induces a maximal hematologic response and significant replenishment of body stores. This may be given orally because, even in those with severe malabsorption, sufficient folate is absorbed from this dose to replenish stores. Before folic acid is given (in these large doses), it is always necessary to ensure that vitamin B_{12} deficiency is not present.

Response to Treatment

The clinical and hematologic response to folic acid is prompt. Within 1 to 2 days, the patient's appetite improves (often becoming voracious) and a sense of well-being returns, with increased energy and interest in surroundings. There is a fall in serum iron (often to low levels) in 24 to 48 hours and a rise in reticulocytes in 2 to 4 days which reaches a peak at 4 to 7 days; hemoglobin levels return to normal in 2 to 6 weeks. The leukocytes and platelets increase with the reticulocytes, and the megaloblastic changes in the marrow diminish within 24 to 48 hours; however, large myelocytes, metamyelocytes, and band forms may be present for several days.

Duration of Therapy

The duration of therapy depends on the underlying pathology, but usually folic acid is given for several months until a new population of red blood cells has been formed. It is often possible to correct the cause of the deficiency and prevent its recurrence (e.g., by an improved diet, a gluten-free diet in celiac disease, or treatment of an inflammatory disease, such as tuberculosis or Crohn's disease). In these cases, there is no need to continue folic acid for life. In other situations, however, it is advisable to give folic acid continually to prevent recurrence of the deficiency (e.g., chronic hemolytic anemia, such as thalassemia) or in patients with malabsorption who do not respond to a gluten-free diet.

Megaloblastic anemia occasionally develops in patients receiving drugs that are folic acid antagonists (methotrexate, pyrimethamine, trimethoprim). These drugs inhibit the enzyme that reduces dihydrofolate to tetrahydrofolate. In some cases, folate deficiency can be severe, especially in patients with marginal or depleted folate stores. In these cases, the antagonism can be overcome by folinic acid, one 5-mg tablet daily.

In cases of a functional deficiency of folate or cobalamin, such as in an inborn error of metabolism or transport, only massive doses of vitamin may be helpful. Diagnosis is made only by appropriate biochemical tests, often on cultured fibroblasts obtained by skin biopsy. Inborn errors are rare, and patients often show mental deficiency, aminoacidemia, and growth failure rather than presenting as simple cases of anemia.

Vitamin B_{12} Deficiency

In conditions in which a patient is at risk for vitamin B_{12} deficiency (e.g., total gastrectomy or ileal resection), prophylactic administration of vitamin B_{12} should be prescribed.

Patients with suspected vitamin B_{12} deficiency are given a therapeutic trial with 25 to 100 μg of vitamin B_{12}. This dose corrects the hematologic problem caused by this vitamin deficiency but does not correct the defect in folate-deficient patients. The reticulocyte response to this therapy is similar to that noted in folate deficiency.

Optimal doses for children are not as well defined as those for adults. When the diagnosis is firmly established, several daily doses of 25 to 100 μg may be used to initiate therapy. Alternatively, in view of the ability of the body to store vitamin B_{12} for long periods, maintenance therapy can be started with monthly intramuscular injections in doses between 200 and 1000 μg. Most patients with vitamin B_{12} deficiency require treatment throughout life.

Patients with defects affecting the intestinal absorption of vitamin B_{12}, because of either abnormalities of intrinsic factor or ileal uptake, respond to parenteral vitamin B_{12}. Such a therapeutic maneuver completely bypasses the defective step and is the chief means by which these two groups of patients are managed currently.

Patients with complete transcobalamin II deficiency respond only to large amounts of B_{12} (1 mg intramuscularly twice or three times weekly). The exact mechanism of this response remains to be defined.

Patients with methylmalonic aciduria with defects in the synthesis of vitamin B_{12} coenzymes are likely to be benefited by massive doses of vitamin B_{12} (1 to 2 mg vitamin B_{12} parenterally daily). However, not all patients in this group are benefited by vitamin B_{12}.

In vitamin B_{12}-responsive megaloblastic anemia, the reticulocytes begin to increase on the 3rd to 4th day, rise to a maximum on the 6th to 8th day, and fall gradually to normal on about the 20th day. The height of the reticulocyte count is inversely proportional to the degree of anemia. Beginning bone marrow reversal from megaloblastic to normoblastic cells is obvious within 6 hours and is completely normoblastic in 72 hours.

Prompt hematologic responses are also obtained with the use of oral folic acid. Folic acid, however, is contraindicated because it has no effect on neurologic manifestations and has been known to precipitate or accelerate their development. Indeed, megaloblastic anemia should never be treated before a serum folic acid or vitamin B_{12} assay has determined the precise cause so that correct treatment can be administered. Iron is occasionally required when a generally inadequate diet has been given that is deficient in this mineral.

HEMOLYTIC ANEMIA

ROBERT W. WARREN, M.D., PH.D.
and KENNETH L. MCCLAIN, M.D., PH.D.

Hemolytic anemias may be caused by defects inside the red blood cell membrane, such as molecular enzymatic or hemoglobin defects, or problems within or at the membrane resulting in lysis of the red blood cells and release of hemoglobin. The membrane-associated problems include intrinsic protein abnormalities and structural, vascular, or autoimmune phenomena that result in hemolysis. The nature of the defect must be defined so that appropriate preventative and therapeutic interventions will be successful.

Characteristic findings in all forms of hemolytic anemia include decreased hemoglobin level for age, reticulocytosis, elevated serum indirect bilirubin level, low haptoglobin level (useful only after 6 months of age), elevated serum lactate dehydrogenase (LDH) level, hemoglobinuria, and hemoglobinemia. The last three are characteristically found when red blood cells are destroyed in the vascular space.

There are a few general caveats for treatment of hemolytic anemia. *Folic acid is a basic need for all patients with chronic hemolytic anemia.* Supplementation with 1 mg daily maintains the necessary amounts of carbon atoms for DNA and RNA synthesis.

Second, transfusion of packed red blood cells should be done only when there is physiologic reason (e.g., pulse and respirations above the norm for age or anemia-associated growth disturbance). The patient with extremely low hemoglobin levels (<5 g/dl) should receive 5 ml/kg of packed red blood cells over several hours to prevent further cardiac problems. A transfusion may not be indicated if the reticulocytosis is compensating for the anemia. Diagnostic studies must be done prior to transfusion to avoid confusion about etiology of the process, which heterologous red blood cells may generate.

Third, if a splenectomy is indicated for treatment of a hemolytic anemia, the patient should be immunized against pneumococcal, meningococcal, and *Haemophilus* type B bacteria. After the splenectomy, prophylactic treatment with penicillin twice a day is necessary to minimize the chance of overwhelming sepsis.

RED BLOOD CELL MEMBRANE ABNORMALITIES

The most frequent membrane abnormality causing hemolytic anemia in childhood is *hereditary spherocytosis* (HS). Infants may have spherocytosis and anemia associated with Rh or ABO incompatibility, thus making the diagnosis of HS more difficult. HS should be considered in a child older than 1 month of age who is newly jaundiced, with a high reticulocyte count and many spherocytes on peripheral blood smear. Antibody-mediated hemolytic anemias also cause spherocytosis but usually there is a positive Coombs' test. An osmotic fragility test is necessary to confirm the diagnosis of HS. The clinical presentation of HS is quite variable, with a majority of patients having only slight anemia. Nevertheless, any HS patient may have dangerous "aplastic" crises associated with viral infections and heralded by decreased exercise tolerance, pallor, decreased hematocrit values, and reticulocytes. Besides folic acid and transfusions when indicated, splenectomy is the only therapy for HS and is appropriate for those patients with profound anemia and hemolysis. If possible, splenectomy should be delayed until the patient is at least 6 years old and has been properly immunized.

Hereditary elliptocytosis (HE) is said to be less frequent than HS, but prevalence studies suggest that it may occur in 1 out of every 2000 people. Generally, HE is associated with mild to moderate hemolysis. Some infants with the homozygous form or a variant (known as *hereditary pyropoikilocytosis*) have severe hemolysis. Red blood cells show budding fragments, bizarre poikilocytes, and some spherocytes. The therapy for these patients is similar to that for those with HS.

Other causes of hemolysis from membrane defects can be tentatively identified by inspecting the morphology of the red blood cells and conducting appropriate diagnostic studies. Mechanical injury from fibrin strands causes very bizarre red blood cell fragments. This may occur (1) when disseminated intravascular coagulopathy (DIC) complicates sepsis, (2) as a result of cardiac valves, or (3) from other vascular prostheses. Severe hypophosphatemia (<0.1 to 0.3 mg/dl) has been shown to deplete red blood cell adenosine triphosphate (ATP) and cause hemolysis. Thermal injury, bacterial toxins (*Clostridium* sp.), and venoms from snakes or spiders have also been implicated in hemolytic anemias.

The presence of spiculated red blood cells and hemolytic anemia can suggest either membrane or intrinsic red blood cell problems. Echinocytes are found within uremia, in glycolytic pathway defects, in stored blood, or in microangiopathic anemias. Acanthocytes are seen in patients with severe liver disease, abetalipoproteinemia, the McLeod blood group, and anorexia nervosa and in infants with vitamin E deficiency or severe glucose-6-phosphate dehydrogenase (G-6-PD) deficiency.

ENZYME DEFICIENCIES

The only energy source available for red blood cells to maintain the integrity of water, ions, hemoglobin shape, and membrane stability is through the glycolytic pathway and production of ATP. Thus, abnormalities in glycolysis and the pentose shunt may cause hemolytic anemias.

Deficiency in the structure or amount of G-6-PD results in decreased life span of the red blood cells, which may not be significant until there is an oxidant stress, such as infection, drug administration, or diabetic ketoacidosis. The drugs most often associated with hemolysis include acetylsalicylic acid, ascorbic acid, methylene blue, antimalarials, chloramphenicol, nalidixic acid, nitrofurantoin, sulfonamides, naphthalene, and benzene. Usually, hemolysis occurs several hours after exposure to the inciting agent. Ten per cent of black males and 3 per cent of black females in the United States have the Gd^{A-} form of G-6-PD deficiency; their anemia is moderate, usually with hemoglobin level greater than 6 g/dl, but hemoglobinuria and jaundice occur with hemolytic crisis. Individuals with the Mediterranean form of G-6-PD deficiency have lower enzyme levels in the red blood cells and thus may have life-threatening hemolysis with exposure to drugs. They also have constant hemoglobinuria and jaundice. The acute therapy for these patients in heart failure is transfusion of packed red blood cells, but of course avoidance of the inciting agents is most important. High-dose oral vitamin E has been reported to improve red blood cell survival in patients with the Mediterranean type of G-6-PD deficiency who are not splenectomized.

Pyruvate kinase deficiency is the second most common cause of congenital nonspherocytic hemolytic anemia. Infants present with hyperbilirubinemia and may require an exchange transfusion. For severely affected individuals, a chronic transfusion program may be necessary. Gallstones are a common problem. High doses of salicylates should be avoided in these patients.

UNSTABLE HEMOGLOBINS

Because sickle cell anemia and thalassemia are covered in another article (see p. 245), this discussion is limited to the congenital Heinz body hemolytic anemias. Patients have nonspherocytic hemolytic anemia with jaundice, splenomegaly, and hemoglobinuria or bilirubinuria. Multiple types of unstable hemoglobins result from single amino acid substitutions, which prevent proper globin to heme linkage. Dissociation of the globin molecules from heme results in aggregates of globin and heme called *Heinz bodies,* which are stained by supravital stains, such as methyl violet. The patient presents in childhood with hemolytic anemia, jaundice, and splenomegaly. Sometimes there may be hypochromia and prominent basophilic stippling. These children rarely need blood transfusions but should receive folic acid and avoid oxidant drugs, as do those with G-6-PD deficiency. Splenectomy may be of benefit for those with severe hemolysis.

IMMUNE HEMOLYTIC ANEMIA

The red blood cells are coated with immunoglobulin and/or complement and are lysed intravascularly or engulfed by reticuloendothelial cells. This immune reaction can be directed against native red blood cell constituents, producing a true autoimmune hemolytic anemia, or it may be directed against altered or foreign molecules in the red blood cell membrane.

The direct Coombs' test is the diagnostic study for immune hemolytic anemia (IHA). In this test, reagent antisera, which contain antibodies against human immunoglobulins and complement, are incubated with the patient's red blood cells. If these red blood cells are coated with immunoglobulin, complement, or both, they are agglutinated by the reagent antisera and the test is positive. On the other hand, IgM usually disassociates from red blood cells and therefore is not directly detectable by this method. The direct Coombs' test differs from an indirect antiglobulin test, which measures the ability of the patient's serum to agglutinate red blood cells from other individuals. This antibody screening test is typically a less sensitive indicator for IHA and may be negative when the direct Coombs' test is positive.

There are two types of IHA, defined by whether the etiologic antibodies react best at warm or cold temperatures. Warm and cold types differ in their etiology, immunologic and pathophysiologic mechanism, course, and therapy of disease.

Warm Type Immune Hemolytic Anemia

Warm type IHA is produced by IgG antibodies, which bind best at 37°C and which are directed against proteins in the red blood cell membrane, such as the Rh blood group. Warm type IHA is the most common form of IHA in children. In almost all of these children, the course of anemia is chronic; the anemia is generally attributable to an underlying disease, such as malignancy, immunodeficiency, or collagen vascular disease. Drug-induced IHA, such as that following alterations in the red blood cell membrane with penicillin, are less common in children but also produce an IgG-mediated warm type IHA.

In warm type IHA, hemolysis occurs by two major mechanisms. In the first, reticuloendothelial cells recognize the Fc portion of IgG_3 (or to a lesser extent IgG_1 and IgG_2), and phagocytose red blood cells coated with these immunoglobulins. Hemolysis is extravascular and occurs predominantly in the spleen. Intravascular hemolysis of red blood cells is the second major mechanism and is complement-dependent. This is a less likely form of hemolysis in warm type IHA because IgG antibodies generally react with protein antigens in the red blood cell membrane, which are too far apart for complement fixation. Nevertheless, in some cases of warm type IHA, this does occur and hemolysis may be rapid and dramatic.

The most important therapy for warm type IHA depends on successful treatment of the underlying disease, but IHA itself is also treated symptomatically. In fact, the great majority of children with warm type IHA respond to a few days of steroid therapy. In this case, steroids are typically given as 1 to 2 mg/kg of prednisone in divided doses or as equivalent amounts of other steroid preparations intravenously. Some authors have also advocated large pulse doses of steroids, when more typical steroid doses are ineffective.

Because hemolysis is generally extravascular and in the spleen in warm type IHA, reduction of splenic clearance of IgG-coated red blood cells may be necessary in a crisis. The administration of intravenous immunoglobulin following protocols typical for the acute treatment of idiopathic thrombocytopenic purpura may at least temporarily reduce splenic clearance of IgG-coated cells and help to stabilize hematocrit values. In addition, splenectomy remains an element of therapy for the child with extremely severe IHA, mediated by extravascular hemolysis, that is unresponsive to other therapeutic intervention. As with any other form of IHA, transfusion of red blood cells is necessary if the child is hemodynamically unstable. If required, transfusions should be given slowly and monitored carefully and in the minimal amount to stabilize the cardiovascular system.

Cold Type Immune Hemolytic Anemia

Cold type IHA is mediated by antibodies that react best at low temperatures. These typically follow viral infection or immunizations. Important infectious agents include *Mycoplasma pneumoniae,* Epstein-Barr virus, mumps, cytomegalovirus, herpes zoster, and rubeola. Cold type IHA occurring following infection is usually acute and self-limited, rarely lasting more than days to weeks.

Cold type IHA is usually mediated by IgM antibody, but one form of cold type IHA is mediated by an IgG called the Donath-Landsteiner antibody. In cold type IHA, the direct Coombs' test is positive with an anticomplement reagent but generally will not show the presence of immunoglobulin. However, it is possible to do a specific test for the Donath-Landsteiner antibody. In addition, the anti-P specificity of the Donath-Landsteiner antibody, as opposed to the more typical anti-I specificity of an IgM cold type antibody, can often be demonstrated. Cold type antibodies bind to red blood cells at relatively low temperatures, such as are found near skin surfaces. Both the typical IgM and also the special IgG Donath-Landsteiner antibody fix complement efficiently. Thus, complement-mediated reactions continue to occur on the red blood cell membrane, long after the inciting antibody has eluted off, as the red blood cell returns to the central circulation. Complement-mediated intravascular hemolysis may then occur; this is typical of paroxysmal cold hemoglobinuria, the form of cold type IHA produced by the Donath-Landsteiner antibody. On the other hand, C3b-coated red blood cells may bind to C3b receptors on macrophages, such as those in the liver. Therefore, it is also possible for red blood cells to be extravascularly hemolyzed in cold type IHA.

The mainstay of treatment for cold type IHA in children involves maintaining patient warmth. Body surfaces should be covered with blankets or clothing, and only warm food and liquids should be administered to children who have acute and severe hemolysis.

Steroids are generally not effective for cold type IHA, since their ability to affect complement-mediated lysis is limited at best. On the other hand, if hemolysis is occurring extravascularly, steroids may be of some benefit because they do inhibit monocyte-macrophage function effectively. Extremely high doses of steroids (such as intravenous methylprednisolone at a dose of 30 mg/kg/day to a maximum of 1 g) may perhaps be effective in cold type IHA because they may inhibit complement activation as well as monocyte and macrophage function.

Neither intravenous immunoglobulin nor splenectomy has any role in the treatment of cold type IHA.

A number of cytotoxic drugs have been tried for the treatment of chronic cold type IHA, such as may occur in some children with lymphoreticular malignancy. Such treatments have generally proved to be unsuccessful. On the other hand, in the patient with cold type IHA in extremis, it is theoretically possible that plasma exchange would be effective because the hemolytic antibodies might be removed by this technique.

Finally, as in the case of warm type IHA, blood transfusions should be given only if the patient is hemodynamically unstable or hypoxic. Because cold-reacting antibodies generally bind to common red blood cell antigens, antibody screen–negative donor red blood cells are usually impossible to find. *Therefore, if it is necessary to transfuse, it is imperative that a blood warmer be applied on the infusion line, as close to the patient as possible;* it is also important that the packed red blood cells be washed to remove any plasma that might serve as an additional source of complement.

REFERENCES

Bunn HF. Human hemoglobins: normal and abnormal. *In* Nathan DG, Oski FA (eds): Hematology of Infancy and Childhood, 3rd ed. Philadelphia, WB Saunders Co, 1987, pp 613–640.

Lux SE. Hemolytic anemia. *In* Nathan DG, Oski FA (eds): Hematology of Infancy and Childhood, 3rd ed. Philadelphia, WB Saunders Co, 1987, pp 443–544.

Mentzer WC Jr. Pyruvate kinase deficiency and disorders of glycolysis. *In* Nathan DG, Oski FA (eds): Hematology of Infancy and Childhood, 3rd ed., Philadelphia, WB Saunders Co, 1987, pp 545–582.

Piomelli S. G6PD Deficiency and related disorders of the pentose pathway. *In* Nathan DG, Oski FA (eds): Hematology of Infancy and Childhood, 3rd ed., Philadelphia, WB Saunders Co, 1987, pp 583–612.

Report of the Committee on Infectious Diseases. American Academy of Pediatrics, 21st ed. Evanston, Ill, 1988, pp 46–48.
Warren RW, Collins ML. Immune hemolytic anemia in children. CRC Crit Rev Oncol Hematol 8:65–73, 1988.

THALASSEMIA

HELEN S. MAURER, M.D.

THALASSEMIA MAJOR

The thalassemias are hereditary anemias resulting from reduced or absent synthesis of the alpha or beta globin chains. In severe beta thalassemia, the erythroid precursors are destroyed in the bone marrow, contributing to a transfusion-dependent anemia. The treatment consists of a regular blood transfusion program and chelation therapy to prevent iron overload.

Transfusion Therapy

Regular blood transfusions are given to maintain the hemoglobin level between 10 and 14 gm/dl. The purpose is twofold: to suppress endogenous ineffective erythropoiesis and to prevent complications of chronic hypoxia.

In general, 10 to 15 ml/kg of leukocyte-poor packed red blood cells are infused at a rate of 5 ml/kg/hour every 3 to 5 weeks. Removal of the leukocytes by a simple bedside filter can minimize fever and the urticarial reactions resulting from alloimmunization to leukocyte antigens. For patients who have experienced reactions in the past, pretreatment with acetaminophen and diphenhydramine hydrochloride can prevent recurrence of symptoms.

Transfusion therapy is initiated in infancy on the basis of the clinical symptomatology of the patient. Indications include poor appetite and a decrease in growth rate and activity level despite the hemoglobin level. If the hemoglobin drops below 8 g/dl and is associated with increasing spleen size, transfusions are also initiated. On an adequate transfusion program, one can expect that the growth rate would be normal until the patient is 8 to 10 years of age. Maintaining the hemoglobin level above 10 g/dl prevents the expansion of the bone marrow with the associated cosmetic deformities and pathologic fractures that were seen in the thalassemia patients in the past. Hypersplenism from splenomegaly secondary to extramedullary hematopoiesis can be delayed and sometimes prevented by early appropriate transfusion therapy. Dietary iron absorption from the gastrointestinal tract is reduced when the hemoglobin levels are normal or near normal.

One of the most common serious complications of transfusion therapy is the possibility of transmission of viral infections. Currently, blood is routinely tested for hepatitis A, B, and C and human immunodeficiency virus (HIV). Hepatitis B vaccine is given to all nonimmune patients prior to institution of transfusion therapy. Since most non-A and non-B transfusion-related hepatitis is believed to be caused by hepatitis C, effective screening of donors for hepatitis C should reduce the incidence of cirrhosis.

Management of Chronic Iron Overload

Repeated transfusions lead to a large quantity of iron accumulation and result in dysfunction of the liver, heart, and endocrine organs. Currently, the most effective available method to remove excess iron is daily subcutaneous infusions of deferoxamine. The goal of this therapy is to maintain iron balance without causing serious toxicity.

A regular chelation program begins when the child is about 3 years of age, when the serum ferritin level is between 1000 to 1500 ng/ml. Growth failure, bone dysplasia, sensorineural hearing loss, and retinal damage are associated with high-dose chelation therapy administered to young patients with minimal iron burdens. Ideally, deferoxamine should begin well prior to the development of irreversible organ damage. When one begins chelation at age 3 years and monitors the patient carefully for toxicity, serious complications can usually be avoided. The deferoxamine is given at 25 to 50 mg/kg diluted into sterile water to a concentration of 200 mg/ml. A 27-gauge butterfly needle is inserted into the subcutaneous tissue of the abdomen or thigh. The medication is infused slowly over 10 to 12 hours by means of a portable, battery-operated syringe infusion pump. The pump is strapped to the leg or with a belt around the waist. Skin irritation can be lessened by adding 5 to 10 mg of hydrocortisone to the medication and by frequently rotating the infusion sites.

One of the common problems with this management is poor compliance in adolescents and young adults. In order to maintain iron balance, chelation must be done for a minimum of 10 hours a night for at least 5 days/week. Experience has shown that compliance is better when the patients are instructed to treat themselves 7 days/week.

Patients with severe iron overload who have not received chelation therapy in early childhood may benefit by high-dose deferoxamine intravenous infusions at a maximum concentration of 15 mg/kg/hour at the time of the blood transfusion and, if possible, for 48 hours or longer each month.

A low-iron diet with a limitation of red meats and avoidance of tea with meals may assist in reducing the iron absorption from food sources.

Splenectomy

Some patients with thalassemia major experience hypersplenism as blood transfusion requirements increase. When the packed red blood cell requirement exceeds 250 ml/kg/year, most patients cannot maintain iron balance with the usual deferoxamine chelation program. Splenectomy reduces the blood transfusion requirement and restores iron balance. Prior to splenectomy, the patient should receive pneumococcal vaccine. After splenectomy, penicillin (250 mg twice daily) should be administered to reduce the incidence of pneumococcal sepsis. Splenectomy is not recommended for children younger than 2 years of age because of the increased risk of overwhelming sepsis in these patients. On an intensive transfusion regimen, hypersplenism usually does not develop until later in childhood or early adolescence.

Complications of Iron Overload

Cardiac Complications

The primary causes of death in patients with thalassemia is chronic congestive heart failure and cardiac arrhythmias. Studies have shown that these complications are largely prevented by a consistent chelation program instituted before the child reaches 10 years of age. Cardiac death occurs primarily in noncompliant adolescents and young adults.

Endocrine Abnormalities

Growth Retardation. With a good transfusion program, children grow normally until 8 to 10 years of age and then the growth rate begins to fall. This occurs even in children who began iron chelation at 3 years of age and have maintained iron balance with serum ferritin levels below 1000 ng/ml.

Abnormal Pubertal Development. Delayed onset of puberty is still common in children who began chelation at 6 to 7 years of age. Hormone replacement can be administered to allow development of normal secondary sex characteristics.

Diabetes Mellitis. This complication is now seen in the older patients who are noncompliant with respect to chelation therapy. They are insulin-dependent, and the diabetes is often difficult to control.

Hypoparathyroidism. This complication usually presents with symptoms of hypocalcemia. Treatment consists of calcium supplements and vitamin D.

Bone Marrow Transplantation

Thalassemia can be cured with a successful bone marrow transplant utilizing a human leukocyte antigen (HLA)–matched sibling donor. The 2-year, event-free survival is approximately 75 per cent in large treatment centers in Italy and Greece. The prognosis is best in children younger than 16 years of age without significant hepatomegaly or hepatic fibrosis.

Because of the 25 per cent early mortality and the concern about possible malignancies in the long-term survivors, bone marrow transplantation is less commonly recommended in the centers in the United States.

Oral Iron Chelators

Considerable research effort is being directed toward developing safe, effective oral iron-chelating agents. One compound which is now in clinical trials and shows some early promise is 1,2-dimethyl,3-hydroxypyrid,4-one(L-1). Urinary iron excretion is similar to that with subcutaneous deferoxamine, but stool iron is considerably less. Despite the good iron excretion, ferritin levels did not fall significantly in patients during the initial 15 months of the therapeutic trial. Longer trials need to be done before the safety and efficacy of this agent can be determined.

Prevention of Thalassemia Major

The use of genetic counseling and antenatal diagnosis has reduced the number of new cases of thalassemia to less than 10 per cent of the number expected in some regions of Cyprus and Italy. By the use of chorionic villous biopsy specimens or fetal blood sampling, an accurate diagnosis can be made at 8 to 14 weeks of gestation in many cases.

THALASSEMIA INTERMEDIA

Thalassemia intermedia refers to a disorder in patients with homozygous or heterozygous beta thalassemia who are able to maintain a hemoglobin of 6 to 9 g/dl without regular transfusions. Symptoms of chronic hypoxia or skeletal changes due to marrow expansion may be indications for utilizing a transfusion program.

Because of chronic anemia, iron absorption from the gastrointestinal tract may be increased. Low-iron diets should be prescribed and serum ferritin levels monitored in all patients. Even those patients not requiring regular transfusions may need intermittent deferoxamine chelation therapy to maintain iron balance.

THALASSEMIA MINOR

Thalassemia minor (or trait) may result in a mild hypochromic microcytic anemia. The patients are usually asymptomatic and require no specific therapy. However, an accurate diagnosis is still important in order to provide genetic counseling to prospective parents. In addition, thalassemia trait must be distinguished from iron-deficiency anemia. Toxicity from iron overload has been reported in patients with thalassemia trait as a result of chronic iron administration.

ADVERSE REACTIONS TO BLOOD TRANSFUSION

MARTIN T. FOSBURG, M.D.

Although concern among physicians and the general population about the safety of blood transfusion is at its zenith, transfusion therapy is measurably safer now than at any time in the past as a result of a series of recent scientific and technologic breakthroughs, including (1) the discovery of the hepatitis C virus, (2) the introduction of rigorous donor screening procedures, and (3) the development of low-cost filters that permit bedside leukocyte depletion of blood products. Despite these advances, transfusion therapy continues to be associated with serious and rarely fatal side effects.

The best way to prevent side effects of transfusion therapy is to avoid or minimize transfusion. *Transfusion should never be used to correct a laboratory value: it should be used only to prevent or reverse specific clinical problems resulting from lack of one or more elements of blood.* Because each component of banked blood (red blood cells, white blood cells, platelets, plasma, and citrate anticoagulant) is associated with potential side effects, patients should be transfused only with the needed component. The appropriate use of blood products is covered in other articles in this book. It is perhaps a sign of the times that confrontation with a frightened patient or irate parent may be the first adverse consequence of ordering a blood product.

TRANSFUSION REACTIONS

About 5 per cent of transfusions are associated with some form of reaction. There are several categories: hemolytic, febrile nonhemolytic, and urticarial; however, there is considerable overlap among them in etiology, symptoms, and therapy.

Hemolytic Reactions

Hemolysis results from the interaction between antibodies in the recipient plasma and antigens on the surface of transfused red blood cells. These antibodies have two sources. Naturally occurring antibodies are developed in response to exposure to bacterial antigens. Antibodies to blood groups A and B are in this category. After infancy, immunocompetent individuals will have sufficient titers of anti-A or B to provoke intravascular hemolysis with transfusion of ABO-incompatible blood. Alternatively, antibodies may develop in response to transfusion of red blood cells with antigens not found in the recipient. Up to 15 per cent of chronically transfused patients may develop antibodies to "minor" blood group antigens.

To prevent hemolytic transfusion reactions, the blood bank performs several laboratory tests: ABO and Rh typing of donor and recipient red blood cells, screening donor and recipient plasma for red blood cell antibodies, and, finally, cross-matching (i.e., mixing recipient serum and donor red blood cells). These tests are sufficiently sensitive that when hemolytic reactions do occur, they almost invariably result from a clerical error: either improperly labeling patient or donor specimens or giving a properly labeled blood product to the wrong patient. Clerical errors are rare owing to rigid rules regarding handling specimens in the blood bank and patient identification prior to blood administration. Most instances of blood going to the wrong patient happen in settings like the operating suite, where persons unfamiliar with the patient may be called in to assist in an emergency situation.

The clinical signs of an acute hemolytic reaction may include fever, chills, nausea, emesis, abdominal and back pain, tachycardia, hypotension, shock, and anuria. The symptoms are due to antibody-antigen interaction with consequent complement activation. Because the diagnosis of hemolysis is usually not immediately apparent from the clinical symptoms, laboratory confirmation is essential. The differential diagnosis includes another type of transfusion reaction (see below), coincidental sepsis, and transfusion of blood contaminated with bacteria. Laboratory findings confirming hemolysis include anemia, spherocytosis, hemoglobinemia, hemoglobinuria, a positive Coombs' test, and, in some cases, hypofibrinoginemia.

Therapy is aimed at preventing or reversing shock and establishing urine flow (see below). Consumption coagulopathy is treated by stopping the transfusion, thereby removing the precipitating factor. Fresh frozen plasma, cryoprecipitate (for fibrinogen), and platelet concentrates are administered as needed to correct coagulation abnormalities. Heparin (bolus of 100 units/kg followed by an infusion of 10 to 15 units/kg/hour) should be reserved for patients who have persistent bleeding despite blood product support or who otherwise deteriorate with supportive care alone.

Delayed hemolytic reactions are seen only in multiply transfused and multiparous patients. A patient previously sensitized to minor red blood cell antigens may have antibody titers below the level necessary for detection if there has been a sufficiently long interval since the transfusion. Following a subsequent transfusion, an anamnestic response occurs. In 3 to 14 days sufficient antibody is produced to cause hemolysis. The clinical signs and symptoms associated with an immediate reaction are usually absent. The presenting symptom is unexplained anemia. The diagnosis is confirmed by a positive Coombs' test and identification of a new red blood cell antibody. The only way to make the diagnosis is to be aware of this entity and order a repeat Coombs' test when unexplained anemia develops in a multiply transfused or multiparous patient 3 to 14 days after transfusion. Frequently, delayed hemolytic reactions occur in patients with concurrent infection.

Febrile Nonhemolytic Reactions

The occurrence of fever, chills, and diaphoresis within minutes to hours following a transfusion is most often caused by a reaction between antibodies in the host and leukocyte (and, less often, platelet or plasma protein) antigens in the blood product. Because the formation of these antibodies requires prior exposure, only multiply transfused (and multiparous) patients are at risk. Such reactions are common with platelet transfusion and almost universal with granulocyte transfusion. In many patients chronically transfused with packed red blood cells, febrile reactions will also develop. *Febrile, nonhemolytic reactions can be entirely prevented or lessened in severity by administering white blood cell–depleted red blood cell products and platelet concentrates.*

Washing red blood cells dilutes the plasma 1:600 but leaves 10 per cent of the original white blood cells. Frozen, deglycerolized red blood cells retain only 1 in 1×10^6 of the original plasma and <1 per cent of the white blood cells. *Leukofiltration removes more than 99 per cent of the white blood cells from red blood cell products and about 75 per cent of the white blood cells from platelets (at a cost of a 10 per cent loss of platelets).* The newly developed filters allow for leukocyte depletion at the bedside. Platelets may also be leukocyte-depleted by differential centrifugation. Of the available methods for leukocyte removal, filtration is the simplest and least expensive.

The symptoms of febrile reactions range from a minor elevation in temperature to a syndrome of high fever, rigors, pain, dyspnea, and hypotension. The severity is a function of the number of white blood cells transfused and the rate of transfusion. A severe and sometimes fatal form of white blood cell reaction can be seen with granulocyte and, rarely, platelet transfusions. It is characterized by dyspnea, chest pain, hypoxemia, and pulmonary infiltrates on x-ray.

Granulocyte transfusions are associated with such a high incidence of moderate to severe febrile reactions that pretreatment with narcotics, acetominophen, and steroids is routine in many centers. Granulocytes obtained by apheresis are less likely to cause febrile reactions than those collected via filtration. Granulocyte transfusions must be given slowly and patients very closely monitored.

Urticarial Reactions

Urticaria can be seen with the first transfusion a patient receives. Allergy to a protein in the donor plasma is often suspected but rarely proven. Reactions are seen with fresh frozen plasma, intravenous (IV) gamma globulin, less often with cryoprecipitate, and rarely with factor concentrates. Reactions to albumin are extraordinarily rare. These reactions vary in severity from a single, small wheal to life-threatening urticaria or anaphylaxis. Fever and rigors can be seen with these reactions. When possible (i.e., with red blood cell transfusion), such reactions can be prevented by the use of plasma-poor products.

Patients with anaphylactic reactions to plasma or plasma products should be tested for IgA deficiency. About 1 in 650 persons either lack IgA or have antibody of limited specificity and thus form anti-IgA when exposed to plasma or IgA-containing plasma products, such as IV gamma globulin.

TREATMENT OF TRANSFUSION REACTIONS

The initial treatment of all transfusion reactions is symptomatic and directed to the specific symptoms present and their severity. In all cases, the transfusion should be stopped immediately. In patients with *minimal symptoms* (e.g., a slight fever or appearance of one wheal), the transfusion may be resumed after the physician has examined the patient, reviewed the situation (including the patient's previous transfusion history), determined that a serious reaction is not occurring, and administered appropriate therapy. Even then, the patient should be carefully observed and the transfusion re-started at a very slow rate.

If symptoms are *moderate or severe*, the transfusion is stopped and the blood product, along with freshly drawn patient blood and urine specimens plus a written description of the incident, are returned to the blood bank. (If facilities are available at the bedside, a urine dipstick is sampled for blood, a spun hematocrit value is obtained, and the supernatant plasma is examined for evidence of hemolysis.) With these samples, the blood bank can quickly determine (1) that this was the correct unit for the patient, (2) whether hemolysis has occurred, and (3) whether there is a new antibody in the patients serum or coating the red blood cells, thereby identifying hemolytic reactions.

Patients with *mild febrile reactions* may require no treatment, or they may respond to acetominophen orally or per rectum. Moderate or severe reactions with fever, rigors, and pain respond to a combination of acetominophen and opiates. Morphine (0.1 mg/kg IV over 3 to 5 minutes) or other opiate is the treatment of choice to reverse or prevent rigors. Opiates should not be used if urticaria or hypotension is present. Pulmonary reactions due to leukoagglutinins may be lessened in severity or prevented by pretreatment with low-dose steroids (e.g., hydrocortisone 1 mg/kg IV).

Mild to moderate urticarial symptoms are best treated with oral or intravenous benadryl (1.25 mg/kg) or other H_1 blocker. If symptoms are more severe, methylprednisolone (2 mg/kg IV) is added. Patients with persistent symptoms 1 hour or more after treatment with parenteral H_1 blockers and steroids may benefit from the addition of an H_2 blocker, e.g., ranitidine (1 mg/kg given by slow [5-minute] IV infusion). Patients with recurrent urticaria with transfusion can be pretreated with these agents. Because steroids have a delayed onset of action, premedication should be given 45 to 60 minutes prior to transfusion.

Life-threatening urticarial and anaphylactic reactions with upper airway obstruction, bronchospasm or shock require emergency treatment. Epinephrine (1:1000, 0.01 ml/kg, maximum 0.5 ml, SC or IM) is given immediately and may be repeated 5 to 10 minutes later. Methylprednisolone (2 mg/kg IV push) should be given with or immediately after the first dose of epinephrine. If there is good response, an aqueous suspension of long-acting epinephrine (Sus-Phrine, 1:200, 0.005 ml/kg, maximum 0.3 ml, SC) is then given. If bronchospasm persists aminophylline (6 mg/kg IV over 15 minutes) is administered. In life-threatening allergic reactions, antihistamines play a subsidiary role and may be administered for persistent urticarial symptoms only after epinephrine, steroids, and aminophylline. Early treatment with epinephrine is the key to stopping these reactions before secondary complications develop.

Severe reactions characterized by hypotension and some combination of fever, rigors, urticaria, pain, nausea, and emesis may be due to intravascular hemolysis, severe allergic reactions, or sepsis from transfusion of contaminated blood. The initial treatment is aimed at restoring the circulation, preventing shock, and maintaining urine output.

If there is any symptom suggesting urticaria or anaphylaxis, epinephrine is administered as described above. Normal saline (20 ml/kg over 3 to 5 minutes) is given for hypotension and may be repeated once if there is no response. Methylprednisolone (2 mg/kg IV) is administered simultaneously.

If hypotension persists, a central venous catheter is essential for guiding further therapy. If the central venous pressure (CVP) is less than 4 to 6 mm Hg, further volume repletion with crystalloid, colloid, or red blood cells is necessary before administration of pressors or diuretics. When venous pressure is restored, dopamine (5 μg/kg/minute) or other pressor can be started.

If the arterial pressure and CVP are adequate but the patient has not voided, a single dose of mannitol (200 mg/kg IV over 3 to 5 minutes) or furosemide (1 mg/kg IV push) may be used to induce diuresis. (Renal failure in this setting is due to shock and/or complement activation, both resulting in decreased renal perfusion.) If anuria persists despite restoration of the circulation and diuretic therapy, dialysis may be needed.

In patients who demonstrate *high fevers* with rigors during or immediately following transfusion, blood culture specimens should be obtained and broad-spectrum antibiotics administered (e.g., vancomycin, 50 mg/kg, and ceftazidime, 50 mg/kg both IV) within a maximum of 15 minutes unless there is a compelling reason not to do so (such as patients with a history of repeated similar reactions). Delay in initiating antibiotics can make the difference between an uneventful recovery and shock, multiple organ failure, and death in patients with bacterial sepsis from contaminated blood or other causes (see text below).

In all settings where transfusions are administered, the above medications and materials must be immediately at hand (including antibiotics) and personnel should be trained so that drugs can be located and drawn up without delay. A chart listing all of the medications with their doses and kept with the medications can be invaluable to staff called on to treat the patient.

BACTERIAL CONTAMINATION

Blood products may be contaminated by bacteria introduced at the time of collection (from an inadequately sterilized venipuncture site) or during subsequent handling and preparation of components. The usual pathogens are *Pseudomonas* and other gram-negative organisms that can grow in the cold and utilize citrate as a carbon source. Gram-positive organisms are occasionally responsible. Platelet concentrates, because they must be stored at room temperature and are prepared in an "open" system, are a particular risk. The symptoms, including fever, rigors, pain, emesis, and hypotension, usually appear after a latent period of about 30 minutes. Transfusion of blood through an infected indwelling central venous catheter, particularly if it has been capped prior to the transfusion, produces symptoms identical to those found with transfusion of an infected blood product.

Treatment is described above. The diagnosis is confirmed by Gram stain of a centrifuged specimen from the suspected unit and from culture of the unit and patient.

CITRATE TOXICITY

Blood products are anticoagulated by the addition of citrate, which prevents clotting by binding calcium. *When infused rapidly, citrate may cause acute hypocalcemia.* Products that contain the most plasma (whole blood, fresh frozen plasma, and platelet concentrates) are associated with the highest risk of producing toxicity. Citrate toxicity is most often seen in patients already prone to hypocalcemia (from small size, shock, or hepatic or renal failure) who receive large amounts of citrate-containing blood products. Examples are exchange transfusion in neonates and massive transfusion of whole blood or plasma for shock. The symptom complex of citrate intoxication in children is acute abdominal pain, emesis, and pallor followed in minutes by hypotension and bradycardia. In anesthetized and critically ill children, hypotension and bradycardia may be the initial symptoms. The diagnosis is made by finding an ionized calcium level depressed by more than 25 per cent. (Total calcium, in contrast, will be normal or elevated.)

Treatment is a slow (3- to 5-minute) infusion of calcium chloride (100 mg/ml 10 per cent, 0.3 ml/kg) or calcium gluconate (100 mg/ml, 10 per cent, 1.0 ml/kg) with close monitoring of pulse and blood pressure. (Too-rapid administration of calcium can cause abdominal pain, hypertension, and reflex bradycardia.) The calcium should be administered through a separate, secure IV line. Patients receiving large amounts of citrate-containing blood products, particularly those who are prone to hypocalcemia, should be carefully observed by serial determinations of ionized calcium.

VOLUME OVERLOAD

Circulatory overload and congestive heart failure may result from rapid administration of blood products, particularly in patients with volume intolerance from cardiac or renal compromise. Common settings include patients with profound anemia (e.g., sickle cell patients during an aplastic crisis) and critically ill patients with renal failure and consumption coagulopathy. Patients with profound anemia can receive packed red blood cells very slowly (1 to 2 ml/kg/hour) with close monitoring, including serial measurements of central venous pressure. A diuretic (e.g., furosemide, 1 mg/kg) may be administered if signs of congestive failure (respiratory distress, hypoxemia) develop. This method may not be appropriate for plasma products, with which more rapid transfusion is often necessary. An alternative is to give either red blood cell or plasma products by exchange transfusion. A partial exchange, replacing aliquots of patient blood with packed red blood cells can rapidly raise the hematocrit level. Plasmapheresis allows for the delivery of a virtually unlimited amount of red blood cell or plasma products rapidly without risk of volume overload.

ALLOIMMUNIZATION

Multiply transfused patients may become sensitized to human leukocyle antigen (HLA) and other antigens found on leukocytes and platelets. HLA sensitization may preclude solid organ or bone marrow transplantation. In addition, sensitization may make patients refractory to platelet transfusions. This may lead to lethal bleeding complications in patients requiring prolonged platelet support for intensive chemotherapy or bone marrow transplantation. All such patients should receive leukocyte-depleted blood products from the time of diagnosis.

TRANSFUSION-ASSOCIATED GRAFT-VERSUS-HOST DISEASE

Transfusion of more than 1 × 10^7/kg viable lymphocytes to an immunodeficient patient can cause graft-versus-host disease. Susceptible patients include premature infants, those with inherited disorders of the immune system, patients undergoing intensive chemotherapy or total nodal irradiation, patients with acquired immunodeficiency syndrome (AIDS) and those receiving post-transplant immunosuppression. Graft-versus-host disease can develop if immunocompetent patients receive a sufficient dose of lymphocytes from HLA identical or closely matched donors, such as parents or siblings. All blood products except fresh frozen plasma can cause graft-versus-host disease; once the disease is acquired, fatalities approach 100 per cent. There is no therapy. It can be prevented by irradiating blood products at a dose of 1500 to 5000 cGy.

PROBLEMS ASSOCIATED WITH MASSIVE TRANSFUSION

Replacement of more than one blood volume is associated with several problems.

Citrate Toxicity

See aforementioned discussion.

Alkalosis and Hypokalemia

During massive transfusion, alkalosis may develop from metabolism of citrate to bicarbonate. Each unit of whole blood generates 22.8 mEq of bicarbonate. In response to alkalosis, potassium moves into cells in exchange for hydrogen. It may be difficult to correct hypokalemia while the patient is alkalotic.

Dilutional Coagulopathy

A moderate drop in the platelet count is frequently associated with massive transfusion. Platelet transfusion may be indicated if the count falls below 50,000 mm^3 in patients at high risk for bleeding. Stored whole blood is deficient in factors V, VIII, and XI. Massive transfusion with such blood may cause depletion of these factors.

Pulmonary Dysfunction

Microaggregates, composed of leukocyte and platelet debris, accumulate during storage of whole blood. Depending on the age and type of blood product transfused, a variable number of microaggregates are administered. These settle in the pulmonary capillary bed and may cause hypoxemia via alterations in pulmonary blood flow. *This is easily avoided by transfusing through a microaggregate filter.*

Hyperkalemia

The plasma potassium level of whole blood increases to higher than 20 mEq/L by day 28 of storage. Massive transfusion of aged blood may produce acute hyperkalemia sufficient to cause cardiac arrest. Use of whole blood stored less than 7 days or packed red blood cells and fresh frozen plasma instead of whole blood can prevent this problem.

Hypernatremia

Fresh frozen plasma obtained from whole blood anticoagulated with CPD* has a sodium concentration of about 165 mEq/L. ACD† plasma, obtained via apheresis, has a sodium of about 150 mEq/L. Massive transfusion with CPD plasma (as occurs in intensive plasma exchange) can cause hypernatremia. The label on the plasma bag will indicate the type of anticoagulant. Provision of an adequate amount of free water will ameliorate this problem.

Hypothermia

Massive transfusion of inadequately warmed blood products can cause hypothermia, particularly in neonates and other patients with temperature instability. Symptoms include bradycardia and hypotension. Use of a calibrated blood warmer will prevent this problem. Warming blood in hot water is not recommended because it can easily overheat or underheat the blood.

AIR EMBOLUS

Air embolus has been a rare problem since collapsible plastic bags were substituted for glass bottles. In a seriously ill patient, as little as 10 ml of air can cause symptoms of acute chest pain and dyspnea. Treatment consists of clamping the IV line and placing the patient in a head-down, feet-up position on the left side. Careful attention to the IV apparatus and the use of infusion pumps with pressure-sensitive alarms and automatic shut-offs can prevent accidental infusion of air.

INFECTION

Transmission of viral infection remains the most common lethal side effect of transfusion therapy. Post-transfusion hepatitis, AIDS, and cytomegalovirus (CMV) are responsible for most serious transfusion-related infections in developed countries.

Post-transfusion Hepatitis

Hepatitis B. Until a generation ago, up to 30 per cent of transfusions led to hepatitis B. The elimination of paid donors and the introduction of screening tests for hepatitis B viral antigens have reduced the incidence to about 1 in 1000 transfusions. It is still possible to transmit hepatitis B if an infected person donates during the incubation phase. Ten to 15 per cent of infected persons develop chronic active or persistent hepatitis, which may end in cirrhosis and liver failure. Chronic infection with hepatitis B increases the risk of hepatocellular carcinoma. As a result of these serious sequelae, all patients scheduled to receive chronic transfusions should receive hepatitis B vaccine.

Hepatitis C. Previously known as "transfusion associated non-A, non-B hepatitis," hepatitis C has occurred with an incidence of 6 to 8 per cent. Initially asymptomatic in 70 per cent of cases, in 50 per cent of patients hepatitis C progresses to chronic hepatitis and in 25 per cent to cirrhosis, portal hypertension, and liver failure. Hepatitis C has been a major

*CPD, citrate-phosphase-dextrose.
†ACD, acid-citrate-dextrose.

cause of chronic liver disease in the United States and by far is the most serious adverse consequence of blood transfusion. The virus responsible for hepatitis C was isolated in 1989, and an effective screening test was introduced at the same time. All blood for transfusion has been screened since 1990. Studies in the United States and Europe have shown the incidence of the disease has decreased by more than 90 per cent as a result of screening for hepatitis C. It is hoped that with more experience and the development of more sensitive screening tests, the risk will be reduced still further.

AIDS

Human immunodeficiency virus (HIV) can be transmitted by any blood product except for certain plasma products processed by heat treatment. The risk of acquiring AIDS via transfusion peaked between 1976 and 1983. Two major strategies were developed to deal with this problem. Comprehensive donor screening was introduced to eliminate those at high risk for the disease from the donor population. In 1983 a screening test for antibodies to HIV was introduced. AIDS can still be transmitted by blood that has tested negative for HIV antibody if it is donated during the incubation phase of the disease. *The current risk of acquiring HIV by screened blood in the United States is estimated to be between 1 in 80,000 to 1 in 150,000.* The future is uncertain. The introduction of more sensitive tests for HIV antibody and antigen will no doubt detect infected units and eliminate them from the donor pool. However, if the disease spreads widely into the general heterosexual population, current donor screening procedures, which focus on "high-risk groups," will not be as effective.

Directed donation, in which recipients bring in friends and family members to serve as their donors, was accepted by the blood bank community in response to pressure from a public understandably frightened by this lethal illness. *To date, studies have shown the incidence of HIV positivity in directed donors to be equivalent to or higher than that of the general donor population. In contrast, programs such as advance donation (pre-donation) prior to elective surgery or intraoperative red blood cell salvage actually decrease the risk of acquiring AIDS or other infections.*

Human T Cell Lymphotrophic Virus Type 1

This retrovirus causes a degenerative neurologic syndrome and T cell lymphoma and leukemia. Actual instances of acquiring the disease as a result of transfusion are very rare. All blood for transfusion is screened for HTLV-1.

Cytomegalovirus

Cytomegalovirus does not pose a significant threat to immunocompetent individuals. It can lead to lethal systemic infections in immunodeficient patients, such as neonates and transplant recipients. *Because CMV is carried in and transmitted by lymphocytes, patients may be protected by either receiving white blood cell–depleted blood products or any blood product from a CMV antibody-negative donor.*

Malaria

Because malaria is readily transmitted by red blood cells from infected individuals, blood banks do not accept donors who have resided in or traveled to areas where malaria is endemic. Isolated outbreaks of malaria from transfused blood result from blood donors who are unaware that they are carrying the disease. The presenting symptom is usually fever of unknown origin. The illness may be difficult to diagnose because it is rarely considered in the differential diagnosis in areas where malaria is not endemic.

Other Infections

Epstein-Barr virus, syphilis, Chagas disease, filariasis, brucellosis, and babesiosis are potentially transmissible via transfusion.

PROBLEMS ASSOCIATED WITH CHRONIC RED BLOOD CELL TRANSFUSIONS

Iron Overload

Iron causes dose-related damage to the skin, liver, various endocrine organs, and heart. Each milliliter of packed red blood cells contains 1 mg of iron. Chronically transfused patients show signs of organ damage (skin darkening, liver damage) at iron accumulations of 400 to 600 mg/kg. This is followed by insulin-dependent diabetes, pubertal failure, and growth failure. Patients die from congestive heart failure or arrhythmias at iron accumulations of greater than 1000 mg/kg. Laboratory signs of iron overload are elevated serum ferritin and fully saturated transferrin. Chelation therapy with daily 12 hour infusions of desferioxamine can prevent serious organ damage if initiated early and may partially reverse organ damage in affected patients. Because this therapy is cumbersome and expensive, alternatives to chronic red blood cell transfusion (erythropoietin, renal transplant, bone marrow transplant) should be pursued.

Hypersplenism

Chronic red blood cell transfusions lead to hypersplenism in some proportion of patients. The mechanism is not fully defined. Hypersplenism may lead to a shortened survival of transfused red blood cells, thus increasing transfusion requirements as well as causing leukopenia and thrombocytopenia. Splenectomy may be needed to normalize transfusion requirements or, rarely, to correct symptomatic cytopenias.

MEASURES TO AVOID REACTIONS

With currently available technology, many transfusion-related adverse effects can be prevented or minimized. In general, transfusions should be avoided or their number reduced, when possible. If transfusion is necessary, autotransfusion via pre-donation, intraoperative salvage, or hemodilution should be used if possible. When banked blood is needed, the patient should receive only the needed component(s). Medical and nursing staff should be educated in the diagnosis and treatment of transfusion reactions. Patients receiving blood products should be closely observed and the transfusion stopped and appropriate therapy administered at the first sign of a reaction. Leukocyte-depleted blood products should be used for all chronically transfused patients. Appropriate precautions, as outlined above, should be taken when blood products are given to immunosuppressed patients and during massive transfusion.

DISSEMINATED INTRAVASCULAR COAGULATION

HARVEY J. COHEN, M.D., PH.D.

Disseminated intravascular coagulation (DIC) is a syndrome and not a disease. It is the result of an acquired failure of hemostasis characterized by poorly controlled protease activity in the blood, resulting in an increase in fibrin formation and fibrinolysis. It is always triggered by an underlying disease process. DIC can be caused by tissue injury, obstetric complications, cancer, overwhelming infections, cardiovascular disease, immunologic phenomena, liver disease, pancreatitis, pulmonary disease, neurologic disease, and certain toxins, such as snake venoms. The term purpura fulminans is used to describe DIC associated with widespread arterial and venous thrombosis. The most common clinical manifestations of purpura fulminans include skin necrosis, gangrene of the digits, and hemorrhagic adrenal infarction. Purpura fulminans is most commonly seen in children following streptococcal or meningococcal infections.

PATHOGENESIS

DIC is manifested by a decrease in clotting factors, an increase in fibrin split products, and a decrease in platelet count. A microangiopathic hemolytic anemia may also be part of this syndrome. It is important to keep in mind that DIC is not an exaggerated version of normal clot formation and clot lysis; rather, it occurs when the intricate balanced interplay among clotting factors and inhibitors is overcome. DIC may be initiated by exposure of blood to tissue factor or to any of a wide variety of proteolytic enzymes. This may lead to destruction of clotting factors, fibrinolysis, or a neutralization of natural anticoagulants, such as antithrombin III or antiplasmin. Most patients with acute DIC have no pathologic evidence of stable fibrin clot formation despite having greatly increased fibrin activity and soluble fibrin in their blood. Thus, thrombosis, although sometimes seen in DIC, is often not a problem. Solid fibrin clot formation may also be limited by rapid fibrinolysis, depletion of fibrinogen, and inhibition of fibrin polymerization by circulating fibrin split products.

DIAGNOSIS

The diagnosis of clinically significant DIC is not usually difficult. If a patient with an underlying disorder has an elevated prothrombin time (PT) or partial thromboplastin time (PTT) associated with a decrease in fibrinogen and an increase in fibrin split products together with thrombocytopenia, the diagnosis can be made with reasonable certainty. *The presence of liver failure causes the most difficulty in diagnosing DIC, since it can produce similar abnormalities.* Determining factor VIII activity may be helpful in distinguishing the two phenomena, since factor VIII is consumed in DIC but is made normally in liver failure. The PT provides a rough indication of the degree to which components of the extrinsic pathway have been depleted, whereas the PTT provides a rough indication of the degree to which components of the intrinsic pathway have been depleted.

THERAPY

Success in the treatment of DIC is dependent on the ability both to diagnose and treat adequately the underlying disease. High-grade DIC that persists once such treatment has been given is an ominous sign. The mortality rate in severe DIC is high, exceeding 80 per cent in some series. Death, however, usually results from progression of the underlying disease rather than the DIC itself. Because it is not possible to accomplish the reversal of the underlying disease process rapidly enough in some instances, it is important to attempt to reverse the coagulopathy of patients with DIC; such steps may be life-saving.

Treatment Options

Two treatment options are available for the reversal of DIC: replacement of clotting factors and platelets, and use of pharmacologic inhibitors of coagulation or fibrinolysis. It must be kept in mind that the treatment is designed not to reverse or correct clotting abnormalities but to correct and prevent bleeding or, rarely, excessive clot formation.

Replacement Therapy

Clotting factors and coagulation inhibitors may be replaced by giving fresh frozen plasma. Although theoretically the use of fresh frozen plasma might be construed as adding "fuel to the fire" and exacerbating the DIC, this does not occur. This may be due to the fact that fresh frozen plasma contains not only coagulation factors but also regulators of coagulation that are deficient in DIC. In patients with DIC, there is also increased fibrinolysis and, therefore, a disproportionate consumption of fibrinogen may be occurring. This can be detected and followed by the quantitative fibrinogen assay. If this occurs, cryoprecipitate, which contains five to ten times more fibrinogen than whole plasma, can also be utilized. Thrombocytopenia in DIC is often not severe unless accompanied by other disorders associated with decreased platelet production. When needed, however, platelets can be given as part of the therapeutic regimen. The potential for volume overload and transmission of blood-borne viral infections must be kept in mind whenever blood products are given.

General guidelines for replacement therapy are to give fresh frozen plasma (approximately 10 to 15 ml/kg) to achieve a PT within 2 to 3 seconds of the control value. Cryoprecipitate (approximately 1 bag per 5 kg) is given for a fibrinogen level of less than 100 mg/dl; and platelet transfusions (1 to 3 units per 10 kg) are given for a platelet count of less than 20,000/ml or, if there is major bleeding, with a platelet count of less than 50,000/ml.

Antithrombin III concentrates have been shown to affect experimental DIC, but clinical experience with this product is limited. It is important to keep in mind that patients with DIC are at risk for vitamin K and folate deficiency. Thus, if DIC is prolonged, the use of vitamin K (5 to 10 mg/day) and folic acid (1 mg/day) should be considered.

Inhibitors of Coagulation and Fibrinolysis

The use of heparin and antifibrinolytic agents in DIC is still controversial. Treatment with these agents has never been shown conclusively to improve survival in DIC, and is associated with the risk of either exaggerating bleeding (heparin) or increasing thrombosis (antifibrinolytic agents). Nonetheless, these agents need to be considered on an individual basis.

Heparin is particularly likely to help patients with DIC associated with certain cancers, especially acute promyelocytic leukemia, and chronic DIC disorders, such as those due to vascular diseases and retained dead fetus. It is also rational to give heparin to patients with evidence of purpura fulminans. If heparin is used, a dose of 5 to 10 units/kg/hour, significantly lower than that normally used for anticoagulation, is recommended. Heparin should be given by continuous intravenous infusion whenever possible. When heparin is used in the treatment of DIC, the dose should be sufficient to prolong the partial thromboplastin time to approximately 1.5 times control, similar to what is done in patients with deep venous thrombosis. ϵ-aminocaproic acid and tranexamic acid are lysine analogues that inhibit fibrinolysis. These drugs may reduce bleeding and fibrinogen consumption in patients with increased fibrinolysis. However, they run the risk of converting a bleeding disorder into a thrombotic condition. They should, therefore, be used with great caution. When used to treat DIC, these antifibrinolytic drugs are usually given in conjunction with heparin to minimize the potential for thrombosis. Antifibrinolytic agents, together with heparin, have been useful in treating the coagulopathy associated with acute promyelocytic leukemia and antifibrinolytic agents alone have been beneficial in patients with the Kasabach-Merritt syndrome. If ϵ-aminocaproic acid is used, it should be given at a dose of 3 g/m² over 1 hour as a loading dose, followed by 1 g/m² every hour by continuous infusion.

Other Therapies

Other therapeutic modalities that have been used in the treatment of DIC include antiplatelet agents, dextrans, alpha-adrenergic blocking agents, and protease inhibitors. A genetically engineered protease inhibitor, $alpha_1$-antitrypsin Pittsburgh, has been shown to inhibit thrombin and other clotting factor protease activities and has attenuated DIC and improved survival in experimental DIC. These and other experimental agents have not as yet been approved for therapeutic use. It is hoped that the development of specific coagulation factors may offer promise in the future.

SICKLE CELL DISEASES

SHARADA A. SARNAIK, M.D.

Despite significant advances in the understanding of the pathophysiology, clinical features and molecular biology of sickle cell disease (SCD), treatment remains at a somewhat primitive level of symptomatic and supportive care. The disease is characterized by tremendously variable severity, between patients as well as within individuals over time. Approximately 90 per cent of all hospital admissions are accounted for by only 10 per cent of a given patient population.

The sickling disorders include:

1. SS, homozygous S (sickle cell anemia).
2. SC, double heterozygosity for hemoglobin (Hb) S and Hb C.
3. Sickle–beta thalassemia, double heterozygosity for Hb S and beta thalassemia, which includes S beta-O (no Hb A), or S beta+ thalassemia (small amount of Hb A).

PATHOPHYSIOLOGY OF SICKLING

Valine in position 6 of the beta globin chain instead of glutamic acid causes profound insolubility of Hb when deoxygenated. Polymer accumulates, and red blood cells sickle and become rigid. This decreases flow properties and causes vaso-occlusion, which sets up a vicious circle of stasis, low Po_2, high acidity, increased viscosity, further polymer formation, and more vaso-occlusion to perpetuate the cycle.

CLINICAL FEATURES

Decreased Red Blood Cell Survival

Membrane damage shortens red blood cell survival and results in *hemolytic anemia* with pallor, jaundice, fatigue, gallstones, and poor growth. The shortened red blood cell survival also causes *aplastic crises* in which a temporary decrease in erythropoiesis leads to life-threatening decrease in hemoglobin levels from viral infections.

Vascular Obstruction

Vascular obstruction from sickling leads to episodic, variable, unpredictable, and disabling musculoskeletal pain. Specific areas of obstruction include:

1. *Bone infarction,* which is common at all ages. (*Dactylitis* or hand-foot syndrome, is an early childhood symptom.)
2. *Splenic sequestration crisis,* a life-threatening and recurrent syndrome of childhood; sudden pooling of blood in the spleen results in hypovolemic shock.
3. *Stroke,* occurring after a sudden obstruction in cerebral blood vessels, results in central nervous system infarction or hemorrhage. (Accompanying neurologic symptoms include focal paresis, aphasia, and visual or cranial nerve deficits.)
4. *Acute chest syndrome,* from pulmonary infarction and/or pneumonia, a frequent reason for hospitalization. (If the syndrome is severe, patients experience "white-out" of their lungs, become hypoxic, and may even require mechanical ventilation.)
5. *Recurrent splenic infarction,* leading to loss of splenic function and *overwhelming bacterial infections,* which are a common cause of death.
6. *Renovascular obstruction,* causing loss of urine concentration capacity, hematuria and glomerular nephropathy. (Nephrotic syndrome progressing to end-stage kidney failure is infrequent but devastating.)

Sickle Cell Trait

Sickle cell trait is a benign carrier state with an incidence of 10 per cent in blacks in the United States. It can cause hematuria, loss of urine concentration, and problems with strenuous exercise at high altitudes or during flights in unpressurized aircraft.

MANAGEMENT

Ambulatory (Outpatient) Care

It is recognized that most patients with sickle cell disease will have long periods of freedom from serious medical symptoms. The role of outpatient management is thus critical and should be the focus of attention. The mortality rate in young children is still very high; however, good *health care maintenance* with anticipatory guidance for potential complications has been shown to lower mortality rates.

Universal *newborn screening* should be routine, and children diagnosed with any of the sickling diseases should be observed closely for routine pediatric care, including childhood immunizations and well-baby visits.

In addition to standard immunizations, 23-valent *pneumococcal vaccine* should be given at 2 years of age, with boosters at 5 and 10 years of age. Influenza virus vaccine is beneficial, but optional. Hepatitis B vaccine is usually given only to patients who are receiving chronic transfusions. *Prophylaxis with oral Penicillin VK* (125 mg twice a day) is started at the age of 2 months and continued until 4 years of age. Patients with penicillin sensitivity are treated with erythromycin. Suggested follow-up visits are scheduled at 2-month intervals, until the patient reaches 2 years of age, and then every 3 months thereafter.

Laboratory investigations at each visit should include a complete blood count and reticulocyte count to establish steady-state values. Iron and folate supplements are given only for documented laboratory evidence of deficiency.

Mild to moderate pain episodes are best managed at home. Prevention should be stressed. This includes recognition and avoidance of known precipitating factors, such as exposure to cold, lack of adequate oral fluids (dehydration occurs easily due to loss of urine concentration capacity), overexertion to the point of exhaustion, overindulgence in alcohol, and exercise at a high altitude. Once pain occurs, specific guidelines for fluid intake are given: 150 ml/kg per 24 hours or 3 to 4 liters per 24 hours for adults. Local application of moist heat increases comfort. Acetaminophen or ibuprofen is used for mild pain.

Moderate pain is treated at home with codeine (1 mg/kg per dose every 4 hours). An antispasmodic such as dicyclomine (Bentyl, 10 mg per dose every 6 hours) is added for codeine-associated nausea in children over 10 years. The use of more potent narcotics, such as hydromorphone (Dilaudid) or meperidine, for the outpatient management of pain should be avoided.

Chronic and frequent pain results in a significant disruption of life. Patients feel a loss of control, and are often anxious and depressed. Psychosocial factors can interfere with pain management, and some patients are perceived to exhibit drug-seeking behavior. This scenario is challenging and requires skillful and time-consuming teamwork, often not practical in the usual pediatric office. Such patients should be referred to a center with support services, such as psychologists, social workers, and rehabilitative specialists. Nonsteroidal anti-inflammatory drugs daily for several weeks are useful for chronic hip pain from avascular femoral head necrosis or back pain from infarction of vertebral bodies. Chronic transfusions to interrupt pain cycles are rarely used and should be considered only as a stopgap measure. Repeated transfusions can result in serious long-term morbidity from iron toxicity, hepatitis, and alloimmunization and cannot be recommended for a non–life-threatening problem such as pain.

Inpatient Management of Complications

Severe pain episodes warrant symptomatic and supportive care with potent narcotic analgesics, hydration, and correction of hypoxia or acidosis. *Febrile episodes* are treated aggressively with intravenous antibiotics until culture results are obtained, covering patients younger than 10 years of age for *Haemophilus influenzae* and *Pneumococcus* and older patients for enteric organisms.

Acute chest syndrome (pulmonary infiltrate with/without effusion) is managed with antibiotics (pneumonia is clinically indistinguishable from infarction) and supplemental oxygen with transfusion if there is respiratory distress.

Right upper quadrant syndrome (RUQ pain, hepatomegaly, jaundice, fever, nausea and vomiting) is treated symptomatically with antibiotics and hydration. A differential diagnosis of this symptomatology includes cholecystitis, hepatitis, hepatic vaso-occlusion, or lower right rib infarction. Acute cholecystitis is an indication for elective cholecystectomy once acute inflammation has subsided.

Preparation for major surgery should include *preoperative transfusion* to avoid the well-described increased risks of general anesthesia in sickle cell disease. Although there are no data to substantiate these criteria, patients are transfused 2 weeks before surgery to bring sickle cell hemoglobin (Hb S) values to less than 30 per cent.

Priapism lasting longer than 8 hours is treated with transfusions, warm soaks, analgesics, and hydration. The bladder should be kept empty. The role of surgical procedures for priapism in children is controversial. There have been no studies to support the need for surgical intervention, nor have there been data showing a high incidence of later impotence in children who are managed by transfusion alone.

Stroke should be managed with immediate transfusion to reduce Hb S concentration to below 30 per cent. This is achieved by three serial partial exchange transfusions 12 hours apart, when 5 ml/kg of phlebotomy is followed by 12 ml/kg of adsol-preserved packed cell transfusion. Automated red blood cell pheresis, if available, is quicker, but it exposes patients to more donor units. The hematocrit level should be monitored closely and kept below 35 per cent to avoid problems with increased viscosity in the face of high levels of Hb S. Diagnostic procedures include computed tomography (CT) scanning with contrast and cerebral angiography, both of which are performed after the Hb S level is below 30 per cent, to avoid the known risks of contrast media in sickle cell disease.

Splenic sequestration and aplastic crises are both emergencies that require immediate blood transfusions and monitoring for shock.

TABLE 1. Indications for Transfusion in Sickle Cell Disease

Acute
1. Hemoglobin <5 g/dl (aplastic and splenic crises)
2. Priapism, stroke, sepsis
3. Chest syndrome with hypoxia
4. Before general anesthesia
Chronic
1. Stroke
2. Splenic sequestration
3. Leg ulcer (?)
4. Pregnancy (?)

Indications for Blood Transfusions (Table 1)

Transfusions are used judiciously for (1) severe anemia with hemoglobin levels below 5 g/dl (usually seen with aplastic or splenic crises), (2) strokes, (3) pneumonia with respiratory distress, (4) priapism, (5) severe sepsis, and (6) before general anesthesia. *Chronic transfusion regimens,* in which Hb S levels are kept below 30% are reserved for situations that are both life-threatening as well as highly recurrent. Currently, stroke and splenic sequestration fit these criteria. Patients are transfused with 1 or 2 units every 3 to 4 weeks to suppress endogenous Hb S production. This has been shown to prevent sickle-related symptoms.

Future Strategies

Future techniques are the subject of current research and include specific anti-sickling agents, such as membrane-active drugs, drugs to increase fetal hemoglobin (hydroxyurea), gene therapy, and bone marrow transplantation.

Sickle Cell Trait

Management of sickle cell trait involves genetic counseling along with reassurance regarding its benign nature. Hematuria should be investigated to exclude additional etiologic factors, such as infection, polyps, or other urologic problems. If the etiology is attributed to the trait, management is conservative, with increased fluids and rest until it resolves.

SUMMARY

Although there is no curative approach to sickle cell disease, much can be done to improve the quality of life of patients; not the least among these is consistent and comprehensive care from a knowledgeable team of physicians, nurses, and social workers. Health education to promote self-determination can and does have a positive impact on the prognosis of the sickling disorders.

LEUKOPENIA, NEUTROPENIA, AND AGRANULOCYTOSIS

PHILIP A. PIZZO, M.D.

Children with low white blood cell counts share in common an increased risk of serious infection. The incidence of these infections is directly related to the depth and duration of the neutropenia and inversely related to the degree of preservation of other phagocytic host defenses. Neutropenias may be transient (such as those associated with drug-induced bone marrow suppression, viral infections, or immune-mediated events) or prolonged in duration (such as those associated with congenital deficiencies of myelopoiesis or acquired bone marrow failure states). Less frequently, neutropenias can be cyclic and intermittent.

One of the major difficulties in the management of the neutropenic patient is the inability to distinguish a fever that portends a potentially life-threatening infection from a less serious complication. In the prospective assessment of 300 neutropenic children in whom fever developed, we were unable to ascertain any clinical or laboratory parameters that could distinguish a patient with a bacteremia from one whose culture specimens were entirely negative. Thus, when faced with a neutropenic child who has become febrile, we must assume a potentially life-threatening infection until proven otherwise. For this reason, children with a neutrophil count of less than 500/mm^3 who become febrile (we have defined fever as a single oral temperature elevation above 38.5°C or three oral temperatures above 38.0°C during a 24-hour period) require admission to the hospital for examination, a chest radiograph, urinalysis, cultures of throat and urine, and at least two preantibiotic blood cultures. The initial evaluation should be performed promptly and expeditiously, and as soon as possible after its completion (ideally within 2 to 3 hours after the onset of fever) the patient should be started on an empiric antimicrobial regimen.

EMPIRICAL ANTIBIOTIC THERAPY

The goal of empiric antibiotic therapy is to prevent rapid clinical deterioration and early mortality related to an undiagnosed and untreated bacterial infection. Because both gram-positive and gram-negative bacteria can cause such infections, it is imperative that the empiric antimicrobial regimen instituted effectively cover the predominant potential pathogens at a particular institution. *In approximately 10 per cent of cases, bacteremias may be polymicrobial, which further underscores the need for effective broad-spectrum coverage.* Indeed, perhaps more than any other aspect of management, the practice of promptly instituting empiric broad-spectrum antimicrobial coverage when the granulocytopenic patient becomes febrile has accounted for a significant reduction in the incidence of fatal infectious complications. Until recently, it has been possible to achieve such broad-spectrum coverage only by the use of combination antimicrobial therapy. In most centers, this has included the combination of a beta-lactam (e.g., a cephalosporin or antipseudomonal penicillin) with an aminoglycoside. A variety of two- and three-drug combinations have been effectively utilized, and since no particular regimen has shown itself to be singularly effective, the choice of agents should be based upon the pattern of infection observed at a given treatment center. When an aminoglycoside is included in the drug regimen, it is imperative that serum levels be monitored within 24 hours after the start of therapy and then serially to ensure that effective drug levels are being obtained and that potential ototoxicity and nephrotoxicity are minimized.

During the last decade, a number of new beta-lactam antibiotics have been introduced, particularly the third-generation cephalosporins and the ureidopenicillin and piperazine penicillins. The third-generation cephalosporins are unique in having a very broad spectrum of activity that in some cases (e.g., ceftazidime, cefoperazone) includes not only the enterobacteriaceae but also *Pseudomonas aeruginosa*, gram-positive isolates, and anaerobes. The extended-spectrum penicillins offer increased effectiveness against *P. aeruginosa*, *Klebsiella* sp., and a variety of anaerobes. Additional new agents include the carbapenems (which have perhaps the broadest spectrum of activity of any antibiotic), the monobactams, and the quinolones. The role that each of these new antibiotics will play in the management of the neutropenic cancer patient is evolving. Antibiotic combinations (e.g., a third-generation cephalosporin plus an aminoglycoside or a third-generation cephalosporin plus an extended-spectrum penicillin) are the regimens most frequently used. On the other hand, the unique spectrum of some of the third-generation cephalosporins and carbapenems raises the possibility that one of these drugs might be used as monotherapy for the initial empiric management of the febrile neutropenic patient. Several studies have evaluated monotherapy and suggest that it is a viable option, particularly during the initial treatment of the neutropenic patient who becomes febrile. Regardless of whether a single broad-spectrum antibiotic or a combination of antibiotics is employed, it is imperative that patients be closely monitored. Indeed, neutropenic patients are subject to infections or even multiple infectious complications. In particular, patients with prolonged granulocytopenia (i.e., more than 7 days) or whose preantibiotic evaluation revealed a clinically or microbiologically defined site of infection (see below) are likely to require additions to or modifications of the initial empiric regimen. These may include the addition of other antibiotics as well as antifungal, antiviral, or antiparasitic agents. Such additions or modifications of the initial antibiotic regimen can best be viewed as adjuncts that help to ensure the successful treatment and survival of the patient.

It is also notable that the changing pattern of infection has led to the reintroduction of an older antibiotic, vancomycin. This drug is particularly effective in the treatment of infections by coagulase-negative staphylococci, methicillin-resistant *Staphylococcus aureus*, and the multiply resistant JK-corynebacteria. Indeed, vancomycin is increasingly used in centers where indwelling intravenous catheters are employed and also has been advocated by some investigators as a component of the initial empiric regimen. Even though gram-positive organisms have increased in prevalence, they are generally less virulent than gram-negative organisms and, in most centers, vancomycin can be withheld until there is microbiologic confirmation of a gram-positive infection. Exceptions to this are centers with a high incidence of methicillin-resistant *S. aureus*.

Because its spectrum of activity is restricted solely to gram-negative aerobes, aztreonam cannot be used alone in the febrile neutropenic patient. However, it does offer, for the first time, a bactericidal antibiotic that can be employed in the penicillin- or cephalosporin-allergic patient, particularly if combined with an agent with activity against gram-positive aerobes (e.g., vancomycin).

Although the quinolones represent a promising new class of antibiotics and offer the prospect of agents that can be administered orally, they are not yet available for children younger than 18 years of age. They do, however, deserve careful study to assess their potential safety for pediatric patients.

MANAGEMENT OF NEUTROPENIC PATIENTS WITH DEFINED SITES OF INFECTION

Following the initial evaluation and institution of empiric antibiotic therapy, clinical and microbiologic findings that clarify the etiology of the child's fever may become available. Under any circumstance, it is imperative that each patient be examined daily until the resolution of the granulocytopenic episode, since both evolving infections and the emergence of second or superinfections are not infrequent. Additions to or modifications of the initial empiric regimen are frequently necessary, particularly in patients who remain neutropenic for protracted periods. Some examples are considered in the following paragraphs.

Bacteremia. Positive blood cultures are surprisingly infrequent in the granulocytopenic patient with cancer, accounting for only 10 to 20 per cent of the infectious complications. This low incidence may reflect the fact that patients are evaluated and treated early (the improved survival of these patients justifies this approach to management). When the initial preantibiotic blood cultures are positive, it may be necessary to modify the antimicrobial regimen. When coagulase-negative staphylococci are isolated, the addition of vancomycin (40 mg/kg/day in four divided doses) is usually necessary, since these organisms are frequently resistant to beta-lactam antibiotics. Although it has usually been considered to be necessary to remove a foreign body when a site of infection has been defined, nearly 90 per cent of catheter-associated bacteremias (particularly with *Staphylococcus epidermidis*) can be effectively treated with antibiotics alone, without catheter removal. However, if the patient remains bacteremic after 48 hours of appropriate therapy, or if the infection recurs when the antibiotic course is completed (generally 10 to 14 days), catheter removal is necessary. Similarly, if the infection is due to *Bacillus* species or *Candida* or if there is evidence of a tunnel infection, catheter removal is virtually always necessary.

Another question that commonly arises when a gram-positive organism has been isolated is whether the spectrum of the antimicrobial regimen can be narrowed to control the pathogen specifically. The results from a retrospective analysis suggested that patients remaining neutropenic for longer than a week had an increased risk for a subsequent infection with gram-negative bacteria when they were treated with a narrow-spectrum antibiotic (e.g., oxacillin, nafcillin). In a prospective study, however, it appears that a narrow spectrum of therapy can be effective as long as the clinician is cognizant that second infections or superinfections might arise during the course of treatment.

The current standard of practice for treating gram-negative bacillary infections in granulocytopenic patients is to utilize a two-drug combination. When such therapy is instituted early, current data suggest that nearly 90 per cent of granulocytopenic patients will survive the episode. The duration of therapy is generally 10 to 14 days. However, if the patient remains neutropenic when treatment is completed (even though all sites of infection have cleared), recurrent infection may occur and the patient should be appropriately monitored. Should a residual focus of infection remain in the neutropenic patient, even at the completion of a standard 14-day trial of therapy, antibiotics should be continued until either the resolution of the granulocytopenia or the disappearance of all signs of infection.

In addition to antibiotics, adjunctive therapies are frequently considered in the neutropenic patient who has a positive blood culture. Foremost among these have been white blood cell transfusions. While this mode of therapy was popularly employed during the mid-1970s, current data suggest that leukocyte transfusions are largely ineffective in the supportive management of granulocytopenic patients, even when patients have a documented gram-negative bacteremia. Most probably, this reflects the inability to transfuse adequate numbers of qualitatively normal neutrophils to overcome the quantitative impairment. At present, leukocyte transfusions seem best restricted to neonates with sepsis and perhaps to patients with chronic granulomatous disease. As an alternative to cell component therapy, consideration has been given to antibody replacement by passive immunization. Observations have suggested that patients receiving cytotoxic therapy may have decreased titers of antibody to the core glycolipid of the Enterobacteriaceae. Studies have shown that the passive infusion of antisera with increased core glycolipid titers (so-called J5 antisera) may decrease mortality in patients with proven or putative sepsis. However, our studies with both J5 antisera and pooled immunoglobulins have failed to demonstrate a reduction in the incidence of fever or infection in patients becoming neutropenic. Nor does their administration change the patterns or outcome of secondary infections in patients with persistent neutropenia. Although recent studies with human monoclonal antibodies against J5 (i.e., HA-IA) appear to reduce mortality in patients with documented gram-negative bacteremia, no significant benefit has been shown for patients who do not have a microbiologically confirmed bacteremia. Further, no studies to date have shown any benefit from these preparations in patients who were neutropenic.

Head and Neck Infections. The oral cavity is a frequent site of primary or secondary infection in the neutropenic patient. Aphthous ulcers frequently occur when the neutrophil count is lowered (e.g., in cyclic neutropenia). Drug-induced stomatotoxicity can result in ulcerations that become secondarily infected by endogenous oral bacteria, thus providing a nidus for local infection and a portal to systemic invasion. We have observed that approximately 20 per cent of patients who receive antibiotics while neutropenic develop a marginal gingivitis characterized by a red periapical line of gingival necrosis. The addition of a specific antianaerobic antibiotic (e.g., clindamycin, 30 mg/kg/day in four divided doses) has appeared to improve this process and can result in the defervescence of the patient who had been febrile on standard antibiotic therapy.

Infection of the oral cavity with *Candida* sp. is common and is characterized by the presence of white mucosal plaques. The diagnosis can be confirmed by scraping and examining the material under wet mount for pseudohyphae and budding yeasts or by culture. Although many centers routinely utilize nystatin for both prophylaxis and therapy, our experience has been that this agent is relatively ineffective. Alternatively, clotrimazole oral troches can be effective. Ketoconazole and fluconazole have been shown to be effective for the oral thrush that occurs in patients with acquired immunodeficiency syndrome (AIDS), but we have found that children with oral mucositis frequently have difficulty in swallowing the tablets. If the mucositis due to *Candida* becomes particularly severe, a short course of intravenous amphotericin B (0.1 to 0.5 mg/kg/day for 5 days) has the highest likelihood of success.

Gingivostomatitis can also be the result of infection with *Herpes simplex,* and a severe necrotizing mucositis may ensue. This infection can be treated with parenteral acyclovir (750 $mg/m^2/day$ in three divided doses). In particularly high-risk groups (patients undergoing intensive chemotherapy or bone marrow transplantation), prophylactic administration of acyclovir may prevent herpetic gingivostomatitis.

While sinus infection in the neutropenic child might be due to aerobic or anaerobic bacteria, consideration should be given to the possibility that the process might be fungal (particularly *Aspergillus* or *Mucor*). Fungal sinusitis may result in the rhinocerebral syndrome with subsequent invasion of the cranial vault. Diagnosis requires histologic demonstration of invading hyphae, and treatment includes both surgical débridement and parenteral amphotericin B (1.0 to 1.5 mg/kg/day). These infections may require protracted courses of amphotericin, usually over 2 or more months. Patients developing the rhinocerebral syndrome should also be carefully monitored for the development of pulmonary aspergillosis, which worsens the clinical outlook.

It is also important to note that middle ear infections in the neutropenic child may be due to gram-negative bacteria as well as to the usual respiratory pathogens. Hence, we institute broad-spectrum antibiotic therapy for neutropenic children who develop otitis media, particularly if a specific diagnosis cannot be made by tympanocentesis.

Respiratory Tract Infections. The lung is the single most common site of infection in the granulocytopenic patient. Presumably, the majority of these infections are the result of aspiration, although they may also occur as part of a hematogenous infection. Indeed, when a gram-negative bacteremia occurs in concert with a pneumonitis, the prognosis is particularly ominous. It should be underscored that the usual signs and symptoms and even the radiographic manifestations of pneumonia may be muted in the granulocytopenic patient. It is, therefore, imperative to monitor serially and even to repeat chest radiographs in neutropenic patients who have persistent fever, since an infiltrate may not be apparent at the time of initial evaluation but may become evident later in the treatment course. A particular difficulty posed by pulmonary infections is their general inaccessibility to direct microbiologic evaluation. Sputum is usually not a reliable diagnostic specimen and is rarely produced in children anyway. Because these patients are not infrequently thrombocytopenic as well, the performance of more direct diagnostic procedures is often fraught with danger.

For the child who presents with a localized pneumonic process and who is febrile and neutropenic, gram-negative pneumonia must be assumed, although gram-positive bacteria, legionellae, mycoplasmas, viruses, and even drugs must also be considered. Our general policy is to start the neutropenic patient who has a localized pulmonary infiltrate on broad-spectrum antibiotics, following standard preantibiotic evaluation as outlined earlier. The patient is carefully monitored, and if improvement is observed within 48 to 72 hours after the initiation of antibiotics, a full course of therapy (at least 2 weeks) is administered. If, however, the patient has failed to improve or is deteriorating after an adequate 48- to 72-hour antibiotic trial, attempts to make a more specific diagnosis by bronchoscopy or open lung biopsy are then pursued.

Another perplexing problem is the finding of a new pulmonary infiltrate in the patient already receiving antibiotics. This is not an uncommon problem, since nearly one third of all the pulmonary infiltrates we have observed in pediatric granulocytopenic patients have occurred in this setting. We have observed that when the infiltrate occurred together with a rise in the patient's granulocyte count, the outcome was nearly always favorable and the infiltrate probably reflected the "lighting up" of a prior site of infection by the recovering neutrophils. However, when the infiltrate occurred in a patient who was persistently granulocytopenic, and particularly when it progressed over 2 or 3 days, the most likely diagnosis was a fungal pneumonia (particularly *Aspergillus* or *Candida*). Ideally, it is preferable to establish a microbiologic diagnosis in these patients so that the need for and duration of antifungal therapy can be clearly delineated. Studies suggest that the finding of *Aspergillus* in sputum or bronchoalveolar lavage (BAL) fluid in a febrile neutropenic patient with a new or evolving pulmonary infiltrate is highly associated with *Aspergillus* pneumonia. If the patient's clinical course prohibits the performance of an appropriate diagnostic procedure (such as an open lung biopsy) even if sputum or BAL cultures are nondiagnostic, empiric antifungal therapy with amphotericin B should be promptly instituted.

Diffuse interstitial infiltrates are not unique to the granulocytopenic patient. When they occur in patients receiving immunosuppressive therapy (particularly steroids), *Pneumocystis carinii* pneumonia should be considered. However, bacteria, fungi, and viruses can also present as interstitial infiltrates, raising the question of how aggressively the diagnosis should be pursued. Numerous investigations suggest that the open lung biopsy is the most reliable diagnostic technique, although not without hazard in the patient who is neutropenic and thrombocytopenic. Recent experience with bronchoalveolar lavage suggests that this procedure may have a role in the diagnostic repertoire, but further evaluation is clearly necessary. Alternatively, a trial of antimicrobial therapy might be adequate. We observed in a randomized trial that empiric antibiotic therapy with trimethoprim-sulfamethoxazole and erythromycin was an effective alternative to an invasive diagnostic procedure in non-neutropenic cancer patients with diffuse pulmonary infiltrates, although improvement was not observed for 4 to 5 days. It is not yet established whether similar recommendations can be drawn for neutropenic patients, but if empiric antimicrobial therapy is to be utilized in the neutropenic patient with diffuse infiltrates, it is important to include broad-spectrum antibiotics in addition to coverage for *Pneumocystis* and *Legionella*. Moreover, if the patient is already receiving antibiotic therapy at the time of onset of the pulmonary lesions, the addition of antifungal therapy appears warranted.

Cardiovascular Infections. Primary or secondary cardiovascular infections are surprisingly infrequent in the neutropenic child. Although endocarditis has been described with gram-negative as well as gram-positive bacteria and fungi, this is a rare complication, even in patients who have had bacteremias and fungemias. Thus, unless there is evidence of persistent bacteremia in the patient on antibiotic therapy, we do not recommend protracted courses of antibiotics. Myocardial abscesses can occur with bacteria as well as fungi, and myocarditis may be a manifestation of toxoplasmosis in the compromised host.

Gastrointestinal Infections. The onset of retrosternal burning pain aggravated by swallowing in the patient who is already receiving broad-spectrum antibiotics suggests the presence of esophagitis. Although esophagitis can rarely be due to bacteria, it is more likely the result of infection with *Candida* or *Herpes simplex*. Since esophagoscopy can be associated with bleeding or a bacteremia in neutropenic patients, we prefer to establish a tentative diagnosis by looking for cobblestoning with a barium swallow. If evident, either oral clotrimazole or a short course of amphotericin B is initiated with the expectation that if the process is due to *Candida* sp. symptomatic improvement should be observed within 48 hours. If improvement does not occur, the addition of acyclovir or esophagoscopy and biopsy should be considered.

Although the gastrointestinal tract is a major reservoir of potential pathogens, primary gastrointestinal sites of infection are less common in neutropenic patients. A syndrome worthy of note is *typhlitis*. Patients generally present with right lower quadrant abdominal pain and rebound, mimicking an acute abdomen or a perforated appendicitis. Patients are usually already receiving broad-spectrum antibiotics. Although it is possible that some patients may be treated with supportive care alone, several reports suggest that surgical intervention and removal of the necrotic cecum is essential for effective control.

Diarrhea in the neutropenic patient, particularly when there has been exposure to antibiotics or chemotherapeutic agents, may be due to *Clostridium difficile*. The diagnosis can be established by examining the stool for cytotoxins. The presence of toxin-associated diarrhea warrants the initiation of either oral vancomycin or metronidazole.

Hepatitis due to type B virus has decreased in recent years, but infection with type C virus continues to be a problem for patients receiving cytotoxic therapy and blood transfusions. Using abdominal computed tomography scanning or ultrasonography, we have recently observed a series of neutropenic patients who developed "bull's-eye" lesions in their livers; these have been shown by biopsy to be due to hepatic candidiasis. This process has required protracted courses of amphotericin B therapy. Indeed, our most recent experience suggests that the best response is likely to occur with the combination of amphotericin B and 5-fluorocytosine.

The incidence of perianal cellulitis in neutropenic patients has decreased during the last decade, perhaps because of the more aggressive and earlier use of antibiotics in these patients. Although it is commonly assumed that the major cause of perianal cellulitis is gram-negative bacilli, our review of patients treated at the National Cancer Institute suggests that mixed infections (i.e., gram-negative rods and anaerobes) are most common. Whether patients with developing evidence of perianal cellulitis should be managed conservatively or treated with surgical débridement remains controversial. We have observed that the early addition of a specific antianaerobic antibiotic (e.g., clindamycin or metronidazole) to standard gram-negative coverage when the patient first begins complaining of perianal tenderness may avoid the need for an invasive surgical procedure.

Genitourinary Tract. Except in patients with primary genitourinary malignancies or those who have indwelling catheters, infections of the genitourinary tract are infrequent, even in neutropenic cancer patients.

Rarely, the syndrome of bladder thrush may occur, hallmarked by the presence of *Candida* in urine cultures and cytoscopic evidence of superficial invasion. Treatment of this process generally requires the instillation of amphotericin B into the bladder on a daily basis or a trial of systemically administered amphotericin B.

Central Nervous System Infections. Surprisingly, bacterial meningitis remains uncommon in the neutropenic patient, even in patients with bacteremia. When evidence of meningitis is present, particularly in children with leukemia, careful examination of the cerebrospinal fluid for gram-positive rods should be made, since *Listeria monocytogenes* can be a noteworthy pathogen in this patient population.

UNEXPLAINED FEVER IN NEUTROPENIC PATIENTS

Nearly two thirds of the children who present with fever and neutropenia fail to have a clinically or microbiologically defined site of infection. Nonetheless, it is probable that many of these children have an occult site of infection and that the diagnosis has simply been masked by the early institution of empiric antimicrobial therapy. In the absence of overt infection, however, the duration of antibiotic treatment can be a real problem. We have found that patients can be stratified into low- and high-risk groups. Low-risk patients with unexplained fever have periods of neutropenia lasting a week or less. When the antibiotics are continued in these patients until the resolution of granulocytopenia and then are stopped, the patients appear to do quite well. Similarly, patients whose blood counts are rising and whose bone marrow is recovering can also be treated with abbreviated courses of antibiotics. On the other hand, high-risk patients have neutropenia for longer than a week. Stopping antibiotics in these patients while they remain neutropenic, particularly if they are also still febrile, appears to be associated with recrudescent infection and in some cases with clinical deterioration. Our studies suggest that patients with prolonged granulocytopenia who defervesce after the initiation of empiric antibiotic therapy should be treated for 2 weeks unless the granulocytopenia resolves before then. While stopping antibiotics at 2 weeks in the persistently neutropenic patient is still associated with recurrent fever in one third of patients, careful and expectant observation can usually prevent serious sequelae. However, stopping antibiotics in patients who are persistently febrile and neutropenic is associated with serious sequelae in more than half. Simply continuing antibiotics alone is not a solution, since many of these patients develop evidence of invasive fungal disease. Therefore, our recommendation for patients with persistent fever and neutropenia is that they continue the broad-spectrum antibiotics and that an antifungal agent be added until the eventual resolution of the granulocytopenia.

While these cases are challenging, it is clear that a high degree of success can be achieved in the management of infectious complications in granulocytopenic patients if treatment is started early and appropriate additions to and modifications of therapy are carefully employed.

CONGENITAL AND ACQUIRED BLEEDING DISORDERS

GERALD S. GILCHRIST, M.D.

PLASMA COAGULATION FACTOR DEFICIENCIES

Inherited Disorders

General Principles of Management

The hemophilias and other inherited disorders of blood coagulation are characterized by an inherited inability to produce one of the plasma factors needed for normal hemostasis or by the inheritance of an abnormal molecule with reduced functional activity.* The tendency to "spontaneous" bleeding into joints and muscles, particularly in those with severe deficiencies (<1 per cent of normal), can produce serious physical, economic, and psychosocial problems. Thus, the treatment of patients with hemophilia requires a multidisciplinary team approach of which only one component is replacement of the missing factor by transfusion of material harvested from normal human plasma or in vivo stimulation of production or release of the deficient protein. Awareness of the fact that blood products have been responsible for transmission of a variety of viral diseases, including acquired immunodeficiency syndrome (AIDS) and hepatitis, has led to the development of increasingly more purified products derived from human plasma and production of various coagulation factors in vitro using recombinant DNA technology. These purified products can still contribute to the development of circulating inhibitors to the missing factor, but development of immune-complex disease related to the repeated infusion of plasma proteins from large pools of blood donors is less of a problem. Another approach to elevating factor

*With the exception of fibrinogen, which is usually measured in mg/dl of plasma, standard assay systems for other coagulation factors are based on the ability of the patient's plasma to correct the clotting time of factor-deficient plasma. The value is then expressed as a percentage of the correction produced by plasma from a normal pool of donors. Thus, the usual range of normal values is from 50 to 150 per cent of normal but is sometimes expressed as 50 to 100 units/dl of activity.

VIII levels is to exploit the ability of DDAVP [1-(3-mercaptopropionic acid)-8-D-arginine vasopressin, desmopressin acetate] to stimulate the release of preformed factor VIII from endothelial cells. This is effective only in patients with relatively mild hemophilia A or type 1 von Willebrand's disease.

The interdisciplinary approach to the management of patients with hemophilia and other inherited disorders of blood coagulation has resulted in the designation of Comprehensive Hemophilia Diagnostic and Treatment Centers in the United States and Canada. These Centers have the resources and expertise to provide a complete range of services to the affected patient and the family. In larger metropolitan areas, patients may receive their primary and ongoing care at the Centers, but in rural and less densely populated areas, it is essential that primary care physicians outside the center participate actively in the development and execution of appropriate management programs designed to meet individual needs. We recommend periodic in-depth evaluations at a Center to monitor the appropriateness of the replacement therapy program, to detect significant complications of the disease or its treatment, and to ensure that the patient is given every opportunity to participate appropriately in the mainstream of society. At these sessions, patients are evaluated by a pediatric hematologist, orthopedic surgeon, specialist in physical medicine, dental surgeon, geneticist, and social service consultant. We screen for an inhibitor, for evidence of liver and kidney disease, and for evidence of impairment of immune function.

After this multidisciplinary evaluation, the program for the upcoming year is reviewed with the patient, and, if necessary, appropriate modifications are made. This includes a replacement therapy plan, exercise programs to maintain or restore joint function, and communication with primary physicians, schools, employers, and appropriate community, regional, and state agencies. Plans are also developed for surgical or medical consultation or treatment of other problems identified during the evaluation. More frequent evaluations may be necessary. For example, it is now recommended that asymptomatic patients with evidence of exposure to human immunodeficiency virus (HIV) be evaluated at least every 6 months. Between visits to the Center, patients are expected to submit monthly reports documenting the site and frequency of bleeding, its nature, and the response to therapy. This is of particular importance for patients on home treatment programs. These records are reviewed by the Center personnel, and appropriate contacts are made with the patient, family, and primary physician regarding any recommended changes in treatment. This type of contact is greatly facilitated by hemophilia nurse specialists and social workers experienced in dealing with hemophilia patients and their problems. All patients and potentially affected family members should be made aware of the availability of complementary DNA (cDNA) probing techniques for carrier detection and prenatal testing.

Even patients with mild to moderately severe hemophilia experience musculoskeletal hemorrhage and are sometimes more seriously affected by many of the psychosocial complications that result from restrictions placed on a young child's participation in normal day-to-day activities. From both a physical and psychologic viewpoint, we prefer to have children participate in physical education programs and most normal peer group activities to the extent that they are able. Contact sports should be avoided. Early entry in a competitive swimming program is recommended, for swimming provides an excellent physical and psychologic outlet for the patient. Table 1 indicates sports in which the physical, social, and psychologic benefits often outweigh the risks. For each individual, the risk-benefit ratio must be evaluated. Attempting to isolate or overprotect the hemophiliac from all types of potentially dangerous activity can produce psychologic problems that ultimately may prove more devastating than the physical crippling. The physician has the ultimate responsibility of advising appropriate restrictions for individual patients, taking all these factors into consideration.

TABLE 1. Physical Activities for Hemophiliac Patients

Recommended Sports	Risks Outweigh Benefits
Golf	Boxing
Swimming	Football
Benefits Can Outweigh Risks	Hockey
Baseball	Motorcycling
Basketball	Racquetball
Bicycling	Skateboarding
Bowling	Wrestling
Frisbee	
Gymnastics	
Horseback riding	
Ice skating	
Roller skating	
Running and jogging	
Skiing	
Soccer	
Tennis	
Volleyball	
Waterskiing	
Weightlifting	

Adapted from "Hemophilia and Sports" published by the American Red Cross and the National Hemophilia Foundation, 1984.

Replacement Therapy

The prevention and treatment of hemorrhage and musculoskeletal deformities rank high in the list of priorities for the patient with hemophilia. At present, material for replacement therapy is still extracted from normal human plasma. *There is limited indication for the use of single donor products, such as fresh frozen plasma (FFP) or cryoprecipitate, because neither product can undergo viral inactivation by heat or other means.** If no concentrated product is available, FFP remains the only means of supplying the missing procoagulant (e.g., factors V and XI). Cryoprecipitate remains an important source of fibrinogen and is also useful in supplying the factor VIII needs of infants and young children, in whom a stockpile of units can be obtained by repeated pheresis of a single donor. Highly purified concentrates of factor VIII are produced by an extraction process using monoclonal antibodies. Subsequent to cloning of genes for a variety of clotting factors, products containing pure human factor VIII have been produced using recombinant DNA technology. Two such products have been evaluated in the United States and await review and approval by the Food and Drug Administration (FDA). All blood-derived factor concentrates are subjected to various procedures aimed at viral inactivation. *Heat and/or solvent-detergent treatment of concentrates has effectively eliminated HIV as a contam-*

*We are 100 per cent certain that heat treatment eliminates HIV. In the United States we remain more concerned about the risks for hepatitis, both for heat-treated and non–heat-treated products. In countries where the incidence of HIV infection is much higher and the ability to screen donors is limited, the situation is very different. In all cases, however, one has to weigh the potential benefits of transfusion against the potential risks. In the United States, those treating hemophilia and similar conditions are convinced that the risk for transmission of HIV is minimal to nonexistent even with fresh frozen plasma and cryoprecipitate. The only exception is the high-risk donor who does not fill out the blood bank questionnaire truthfully and who might have been exposed to HIV but has not yet undergone seroconversion.

inant. Pasteurization and/or monoclonal-antibody purification seem to be effective against hepatitis B and C.

In developing a rational replacement therapy program, one must have a knowledge of the potency of the various therapeutic products available for replacement therapy, an awareness of the levels of the missing factor needed for hemostasis in the particular clinical situation, and the approximate infusion half-life of the missing factor.

Table 2 lists the various products licensed for the treatment of coagulation deficiencies. The potency of the lyophilized concentrates varies considerably, but each vial has the number of units of activity listed on the product label. Table 3 lists the equivalent volumes of products containing factor VIII or factor IX that contain 100 factor VIII or factor IX units, respectively. Table 4 lists the approximate half-disappearance times of various coagulation factors following infusion. The decay patterns are complex, but for practical purposes these figures reflect the approximate time for the initial peak increments to decrease by 50 per cent.

The in vivo recovery of the missing factor depends on its molecular weight and whether or not it is evenly distributed within the intravascular and extravascular spaces. For example, after infusion of a given quantity of factor VIII, almost all of it is measurable in the circulation and approximately 1 unit of factor VIII/kg of body weight will elevate the in vivo factor VIII level by approximately 2 per cent. On the other hand, when compared with factor VIII, factor IX is a smaller molecule and, since it is distributed extravascularly, produces only 25 to 50 per cent of the increment after infusion. These figures are approximations but are of practical value in day-to-day patient management.

Pharmacologic Approaches

A number of naturally occurring and synthetic hormones can elevate plasma levels of factor VIII and von Willebrand factor (VWF). These include estrogen, which stimulates increased synthesis, and DDAVP, which causes release of factor VIII/VWF from endothelial cells and has been widely used to treat patients with relatively mild hemophilia A (factor VIII >5 per cent of normal) and with mild to moderately severe type I von Willebrand's disease (VWD). Following an IV infusion of 0.3 μg/kg, peak levels are seen within 15 to 30 minutes with the expected half-life of about 12 hours. The increment in factor VIII/VWF levels is variable but reasonably consistent within families. Because the baseline level may increase anywhere from 1.5 to sixfold, each patient should have a trial dose with factor VIII/VWF assays to document

TABLE 2. Products Used in Coagulation Deficiencies

Method of Viral Inactivation	Product	Manufacturer	Hepatitis Risk	Clinical Use
		Factor VIII Products		
a. Solvent detergent + dry heat				
1. TNBP cholate 6 hr ≥ 24°C	Factor VIII-SD	NY Blood Center	Low	Hemophilia A
2. TNBP polysorbate 80 6 hr, 27°C	Koate-HP	Cutter	High	Hemophilia A
TNBP polysorbate 80 6 hr, 27°C	Profilate OSD	Alpha	High	Hemophilia A
b. Monoclonal antibody purified				
1. Pasteurized (10 hr, 60°C)	Monoclate-P	Armour	Low	Hemophilia A
2. Solvent-detergent TNBP/ Triton X-100 (pasteurized, ≥ 10 hr, ≥ 25°C)	Hemofil M	Baxter-Hyland	Low	Hemophilia A
Solvent-detergent TNBP/ Triton X-100 (pasteurized, ≥ 10 hr, ≥ 25°C)	AHF-M	American Red Cross	Low	Hemophilia A
c. Heated in aqueous solution (pasteurized, 10 hr, 60°C)	Humate P	Behringwerke (distributed by Armour)	Low	von Willebrand
Heated in aqueous solution (pasteurized, 10 hr, 60°C)	Koate HS	Cutter	Low	von Willebrand
d. Porcine VIII purified by ion exchange chromatography	Hyate:C	Porton (distributed by Armour)	Low	Factor VIII inhibitors
		Factor IX Products		
a. Dry heat (72 hr, 68°C)	Konyne HT	Cutter	High	Hemophilia B, Factor II, VII, IX, and X deficiency, factor VIII inhibitors
Dry heat (72 hr, 80°C)	Konyne 80	Cutter	?Low	Hemophilia B, Factor II, VII, IX, and X deficiency, factor VIII inhibitors
Dry heat (144 hr, 68°C)	Proplex T	Hyland	High	Factor II, VII, IX, X deficiency
Dry heat (144 hr, 68°C)	Autoplex	Hyland	High	Factor VIII inhibitors
b. Suspension heated in an organic solvent (20 hr, 60°C)	Profilnine HT	Alpha	Low	Hemophilia B
Suspension heated in an organic solvent (20 hr, 60°C)	Alfanine*	Alpha	Low	Hemophilia B
Vapor heated (10 hr, 60°C, + 1 hr 80°C)	FEIBA	Immuno	? Low	Factor VIII inhibitors

Adapted from National Hemophilia Foundation Recommendations, 1991.
*Low thrombogenic risk.
Note: This listing does not include Recombinate, licensed 12/10/92 and manufactured by Baxter.
Abbreviation: TNBP, tri-n-butyl phosphate.

TABLE 3. Equivalent Volume Containing 100 Units* of Activity

Product (ml)	Factors II, VII, IX, X	Factors VIII
Reference plasma	100	100
Fresh frozen plasma	125	110
Cryoprecipitate†	—	15–25
Factor VIII concentrate	—	0.5–2.0‡
Prothrombin complex concentrate	4	—

*One unit is defined as the amount of coagulant activity present in 1 ml of plasma having 100 per cent activity.
†The factor VIII content of individual bags is variable. The average bag of cryoprecipitate contains 100 factor VIII units with a range of 50 to 200 units.
‡Preferred product.

the magnitude of the rise. If the peak level is considered suboptimal, supplemental replacement therapy will be necessary. It should also be appreciated that in most (but not all) patients tachyphylaxis occurs, resulting in decreasing responsiveness if the drug is given more frequently than every 24 to 48 hours. Side effects of DDAVP, such as flushing, changes in blood pressure, tachycardia, and water retention, can be avoided by diluting the dose in 50 ml normal saline and administering over 30 minutes.

DDAVP can be used alone to control bleeding episodes and to cover dental extractions and even major surgery. An intranasal formulation of DDAVP has been developed in Sweden and has been found effective in clinical trials in the United States. A request for FDA approval has been submitted. This product delivers 150 μg per activation. The effective dose in children is 150 μg and in adults 300 μg.

Factor VIII Deficiency (Hemophilia A, Classic Hemophilia). One factor VIII unit/kg elevates the plasma level by 2 per cent. To achieve a 50 per cent level in a child weighing 20 kg, 500 units of factor VIII are given by rapid infusion. This requires approximately five bags of cryoprecipitate, ±700 ml of plasma or 2.5 to 10 ml of concentrate. After ±12 hours, the level will have dropped to 25 per cent; to maintain levels above 25 per cent over a period of time, infusions will have to be repeated every 12 hours using a dose calculated to produce a 25 per cent increment in plasma factor VIII level. The potency, in vivo recovery, and half-disappearance time are quite variable, so that levels of factor VIII may have to be monitored by specific assay. *This is not usually necessary in the treatment of isolated joint or muscle hemorrhage, but it is critical in the management of intracranial hemorrhage or in patients undergoing major surgery.* This is most effectively done by measuring factor VIII before and 30 minutes after an infusion and repeating it 8 to 12 hours later. This provides an indication of the lowest level prior to infusion, the increment following infusion, and the decay rate. This information allows the dose to be adjusted when it is essential that minimum plasma levels be maintained. For patients undergoing major surgery, continuous infusion of factor VIII avoids the wide variations in plasma levels and reduces the number of assays needed to monitor therapy. A protocol for continuous infusion of factor VIII is detailed in Table 5.

Specific regimens are outlined for certain conditions later in this chapter.

Factor IX Deficiency (Hemophilia B, Christmas Disease.) The in vivo recovery of factor IX is lower than that of factor VIII. One factor IX unit/kg elevates the circulating plasma level by only about 1 per cent. Thus, in order to achieve a peak post-infusion increment of 50 per cent, 50 units/kg would have to be administered. A child weighing 20 kg requires 1000 to 2000 ml if fresh frozen plasma is used. Concentrates contain ±500 factor IX units in 20 ml so that 1000 units of activity can be administered in a volume of 40 ml. Because of the longer biologic half-life of factor IX, the infusions can be given less frequently. However, *it should be appreciated that the first phase of factor IX disappearance is rapid; if high hemostatic levels are needed over a prolonged period of time, the frequency of infusions may approach that used in factor VIII replacement.* In potentially life-threatening situations or to cover surgical procedures, laboratory monitoring of plasma factor levels is critical.

Although we have the impression that lower levels of factor IX may be adequate to produce hemostasis in various clinical situations, we use the same general guidelines as are used for factor VIII–deficient patients. This means that most severely affected hemophilia B patients will have to be treated routinely using concentrates. With milder deficiencies, we attempt to control minor bleeding with fresh frozen plasma, but major trauma or surgery usually necessitates the use of concentrates. The new, more purified factor IX preparations appear to be associated with a reduced hepatitis risk than the earlier products (see Table 2). DDAVP has no effect on factor IX levels.

Von Willebrand's Disease. VWD is characterized by a deficiency of a plasma factor (VWF) that is necessary for the promotion of normal platelet adhesiveness and the synthesis of factor VIII coagulant activity. A number of subtypes have been recognized. Some (e.g., *type I*) are characterized by reduced production of normal VWF, whereas in others (e.g., *type II*) there is production of an abnormal molecule. *Type III* refers to almost complete absence of VWF in plasma. Both sexes are equally affected. Bleeding tends to be mucosal and cutaneous, although hemarthroses can occur in patients with extremely low factor VIII levels. Epistaxis is common in childhood and is often aggravated by local lesions in the nose and, during the winter months, by reduced humidity. Thrombin-soaked nasal packs and cauterization are sometimes needed and may require replacement therapy. Menorrhagia can be severe but can usually be controlled with cyclic oral contraceptive therapy, in part because exogenously administered estrogen also stimulates increased synthesis of VWF and factor VIII in mild to moderately affected individuals.

Infusion of normal (and even hemophilic) plasma stimulates exaggerated in vivo production of coagulant factor VIII

TABLE 4. Approximate Biologic Half-Life of Coagulation Factors After Infusion

Factor VII	4–6 hr
Factor VIII	12 hr
Factor V	20 hr
Factor IX	24 hr
Factor X	30 hr
Factor XI	48 hr
Fibrinogen	72 hr
Factor II	72 hr
Factor XIII	10+ days

TABLE 5. Guidelines for Continuous Infusion of Factor VIII Concentrates

1. Infuse bolus to increase to desired level (1 unit/kg elevates level by 2%).
2. Maintain 25%: 1 units/kg/hr.
   50%: 2 units/kg/hr.
   75%: 3 units/kg/hr.
3. Dispense factor VIII in batches for 12-hour infusions mixed in 500 or 1000 ml of normal saline.
4. Assay factor VIII levels once daily to ensure that appropriate level is maintained.

activity, which may be sustained at hemostatic levels for 72 hours or longer. The secondary rise in circulating factor VIII occurs over a 10- to 24-hour period. Thus, to prepare a patient for elective surgery an infusion of plasma (10 to 15 ml/kg), cryoprecipitate (one bag/10 kg), or one of the wet heat-treated concentrates (Humate P or Hemofil M) (see Table 2) is given 8 to 24 hours earlier. In an emergency, enough material should be given to produce an immediate rise in factor VIII coagulant activity to 50 per cent. This provides adequate coverage during the period of in vivo synthesis. The decision to provide further therapy is determined by monitoring the plasma factor VIII level. We aim to maintain the circulating factor VIII above 50 per cent and VWF level at 25 to 50 per cent for 10 days after a major operation.

The bleeding time is often shortened 2 to 4 hours after infusion but rarely to normal levels. In our experience, hemostasis has been satisfactory in spite of failure to correct the bleeding time.

Factor XI Deficiency (Hemophilia C, Plasma Thromboplastin Antecedent Deficiency). Very little factor XI enters the extravascular space so that one can apply the same dosage calculations as for factor VIII. No concentrates are available, but satisfactory hemostasis can be maintained because the biologic half-life is from 40 to 48 hours. A series of three plasma transfusions in a dose of 10 ml/kg every 6 to 8 hours produces a peak rise in factor XI of about 50 per cent, and levels above 25 per cent can be maintained easily with daily transfusions of 10 ml/kg or less. In an emergency, partial exchange transfusion may be necessary if circulatory overload is a concern.

Factor XII Deficiency (Hageman's Disease). Deficiency of factor XII is not associated with abnormal hemostasis. No particular precautions or replacement therapy is needed in spite of the markedly prolonged in vitro coagulation times.

Factor XIII Deficiency. Deficiency of fibrin-stabilizing factor is easily treated. A single infusion of plasma (2 to 3 ml/kg) is sufficient to obtain normal hemostasis and correct the abnormal in vitro clot solubility. To reduce exposure to plasma from multiple donors, a single, healthy compatible donor can be identified for periodic plasmapheresis, since most patients will require only 250 to 500 ml of plasma every 2 to 4 weeks.

Congenital Afibrinogenemia, Hypofibrinogenemia, and Dysfibrinogenemia. To maintain normal hemostasis, plasma levels must be 80 to 100 mg/dl. These can be readily achieved with single-donor cryoprecipitate, which contains about 250 mg per bag. After infusion, fibrinogen enters the extravascular space. Two to four bags of cryoprecipitate per 10 kg of body weight will elevate plasma fibrinogen by 50 to 100 mg/dl. This can be administered over an 8- to 12-hour period to minimize volume overload, depending on the volume of cryoprecipitate in each bag. Adequate circulating levels can be maintained by daily infusion of 0.6 to one bag of cryoprecipitate per 10 kg of body weight. Lyophilized factor concentrates are virtually fibrinogen-free.

Deficiencies of Factors II, VII, or X. These rare inherited disorders do not respond to vitamin K therapy. Their in vivo recovery is similar to that of factor IX, although their biologic half-lives vary (see Table 4). The same principles for the use of plasma or prothrombin complex concentrates apply. Even moderately severe deficiency of factor VII may result in very little bleeding. We have successfully operated on patients with as little as 20 per cent of normal factor VII without factor replacement.

Factor V Deficiency. Factor V is extremely labile, and only fresh or fresh frozen plasma should be used for replacement therapy. The in vivo recovery and biologic half-life are similar to those for factor IX, and the same general principles apply. Factor V is not a vitamin K–dependent factor and is not present in cryoprecipitate or other concentrates.

Special Treatment Situations

Musculoskeletal Hemorrhage. We stress prompt recognition and treatment of hemarthrosis or intramuscular bleeds, particularly those involving the gastrocnemius muscle or if nerve compression is suspected. All patients or parents should be made aware of the early signs or symptoms of hemarthrosis and the need for early treatment, which should be made readily available on an outpatient basis if the patient is not on a home treatment program. If treatment is given in an emergency room, clinic, or doctor's office, an outline of the patient's treatment program should be kept on file as an ongoing prescription for replacement therapy. Physician evaluation is not necessary for patients who are known to the facility and have demonstrated a working knowledge of hemophilia and its treatment. Naturally, if the well-informed patient or parent requests it, intervention by a physician is certainly indicated.

A smooth-flowing system is essential to the success of an outpatient treatment program. Traditionally, when the need for replacement therapy had to be evaluated with each bleed, treatment was inevitably delayed because the average physician in an emergency room was usually less well informed about hemophilia than the patient.

Our procedure is to have the patient's treatment program on record in the emergency room, blood bank, or any other treatment facility. In addition, we advise the patient to carry a copy of the program at all times. At the earliest sign of bleeding into an area that would require replacement therapy, a phone call is made to the treatment facility with a request that the appropriate number of vials or bags of materials be prepared for infusion at the time the patient anticipates arriving there. Occasionally, less responsible patients fail to keep these appointments, to the chagrin of hospital personnel, but this is a rare occurrence in our experience and should alert one to re-evaluate whether that particular patient's treatment program is appropriate. Table 6 lists the principles for outpatient or home therapy for the treatment of musculoskeletal bleeding. Joint aspiration is rarely indicated and then only to relieve pressure symptoms in a markedly swollen joint.

Specific factor assays need not be monitored unless the clinical response is considered unsatisfactory. If assay is indicated and the increment in factor level is not consistent with the dose infused, the possibility of an inhibitor or some deterioration in the potency of the infusion material has to be considered.

The presence of synovitis with hypervascular friable synovium should be suspected in patients who have repeated episodes of bleeding into a single joint with documented satisfactory increments in plasma procoagulant levels. The inflamed synovium sets the stage for recurrent hemorrhage. In order to break this vicious circle, we initially prescribe short 4- to 5-day courses of prednisone (40 mg/m²/day in

TABLE 6. Guidelines for Replacement Therapy After Joint or Muscle Hemorrhage

1. Treat at *earliest* sign of hemarthrosis or intramuscular bleeding.
2. Increase factor VIII or IX level to ±40 per cent of normal.*
3. Repeat dose at 24 hours if no response.
4. Evaluate if patient is still symptomatic at 48 hours.
5. Maintain mobility unless pain or swelling is severe.

*It is often possible to produce hemostasis with lower levels if the treatment is instituted very early.

three divided doses) to be administered in conjunction with replacement therapy. If this fails to have the desired effect after 6 to 8 weeks of observation, a longer course of prednisone (3 to 4 weeks) is considered. Alternatively, a prophylactic infusion program aimed at maintaining factor VIII or IX levels above 5 per cent can be effective and should be continued for at least 3 months. In selected instances, surgical synovectomy should be considered in a joint that is the site of recurrent hemorrhage with synovial thickening but before radiographic evidence of hemophilic arthropathy has developed. Nonsurgical synovectomy utilizing colloidal ^{32}P chromic phosphate has been employed successfully in Canada but must still be considered investigational. In older patients, joint replacement has successfully eliminated painful, crippling deformities in weight-bearing and upper extremity joints.

Dental Management. Preventive dental care should be part of the hemophiliac's overall treatment plan. Most routine dental procedures can often be performed without replacement therapy, particularly if regional anesthesia is avoided. We advise local infiltration of the affected tooth if local anesthesia is needed. Loss of deciduous teeth is not usually associated with significant bleeding, but if oozing is persistent, it can usually be controlled with thrombin-soaked gauze. Extraction of permanent teeth requires appropriate replacement therapy or DDAVP with the aim of achieving a 50 per cent level of the missing factor immediately prior to the procedure. Epsilon-aminocaproic acid (EACA, Amicar) or tranexamic acid (Cyklokapron) is given to inhibit fibrinolytic activity in the oral cavity. This prevents the fibrin clot in the tooth socket from dissolving. Clot formation is also enhanced by packing the socket with thrombin-soaked oxidized cellulose.* The dose of EACA is 100 mg/kg given orally or intravenously immediately before the procedure and every 6 hours for 7 to 10 days thereafter. It is most easily administered as a 25 per cent syrup, which contains 1.25 g in each 5 ml, but is also available in tablet form. Tranexamic acid is also an effective antifibrinolytic agent (25 mg/kg every 8 hours orally or intravenously). These drugs should not be used in the presence of hematuria or if there is evidence of active intravascular coagulation. With a single infusion of replacement therapy or DDAVP and adequate consolidation of the clot, no further replacement therapy is usually necessary unless the clot is dislodged from the tooth socket.

Epistaxis and Intraoral Hemorrhage. Epistaxis is more common in patients with VWD than in those with hemophilia. Packing with thrombin-soaked oxidized cellulose (see Dental Management above) is helpful if other local measures fail. Replacement therapy or DDAVP may be necessary, particularly if the oozing is generalized without an identifiable bleeding point to cauterize.

The toddler with hemophilia tends to have problems with intraoral bleeding as a result of trauma to the tongue, lips, frenulum, or oral mucosa. Because it is impossible to "immobilize" these areas, the clot is easily dislodged, leading to recurrent bleeding and the need for repeated doses of replacement therapy. This series of events can be modified by prompt replacement therapy aimed at elevating factor levels to 50 per cent, local application of thrombin-soaked oxidized cellulose, and oral EACA or tranexamic acid as recommended for dental procedures.

Pain Control. One of the goals of early control of bleeding is to reduce the need for analgesia. Particularly in older patients with established hemophiliac arthropathy, drug abuse and addiction can be serious problems. In addition, aspirin and aspirin-containing drugs should not be used because of their action on platelet function and their ability to aggravate the pre-existing hemostatic defect. A list of aspirin-containing drugs is available from the National Hemophilia Foundation. Although other nonsteroidal anti-inflammatory drugs (NSAIDs), such as ibuprofen (Motrin) or indomethacin, affect platelet function, the effect is rapidly reversed when treatment is discontinued. In contrast, the effect of aspirin persists for the life span of the exposed platelet. *Thus NSAIDs deserve a trial in patients with symptoms suggestive of arthritis in joints which have been the site of recurrent hemorrhage in the past.* We prefer to use nonacetylated salicylates in the form of choline magnesium trisalicylate (Trilisate) or salicysalicylic acid (salsalate, Disalcid, 500 to 1000 mg twice a day), which does not affect platelet function but does exert an anti-inflammatory effect. Although the effects of phenylbutazone, phenothiazides, and phenacetin on platelet function are less well defined, they should be avoided in patients with bleeding disorders.

Hematuria. Hematuria is often unresponsive to replacement therapy in spite of hemostatic blood levels being attained. Bed rest for 24 to 48 hours seems to be advantageous in some patients. Prednisone (40 to 60 mg/m^2 per 24 hours) in divided doses, usually causes the hematuria to subside in 48 hours, after which time the dose should be tapered and stopped over the next 3 days. EACA is contraindicated in the management of hematuria and can produce thrombosis in the urinary tract.

Inhibitors. Approximately 10 per cent of those with severe hemophilia A develop inhibitors that are capable of neutralizing infused factor VIII. The frequency of inhibitor formation is much lower in hemophilia B. Some patients have low titers of inhibitor (<5 Bethesda units) and do not have an anamnestic rise in inhibitor level after an infusion. These inhibitors can often be overcome by treating with larger and more frequent doses of the missing factor. In patients with more potent inhibitors, a number of therapeutic approaches have been tried. Some investigators have recommended withholding replacement therapy, hoping that the inhibitor titer will drop, but in our experience this rarely happens and usually leads to increasing disability resulting from untreated musculoskeletal hemorrhages. Various trials of immunosuppressive therapy have not met with success in hemophiliacs with inhibitors. In life-threatening situations, exchange transfusion utilizing the continuous-flow centrifuge has been effective in replacing the patient's inhibitor-containing plasma with normal plasma. The beneficial effect is temporary because the antigenic stimulus invariably produces an anamnestic antibody response and even higher levels of inhibitor within 5 to 7 days.

A number of other approaches have been developed for management of "high responders." These include the use of activated and nonactivated prothrombin complexes to "bypass" the need for factor VIII, highly purified porcine factor VIII, induction of immune tolerance using varying doses, and schedules of factor VIII and immunoabsorbence of IgG antibodies during plasmapheresis. Two newly developed ribosomal DNA (rDNA) products—factor VIIa and tissue factor—are currently being evaluated.

The high-responding patient should ideally be managed by a Center having all the resources to treat and monitor bleeding episodes.

Head Injury. Any significant injury to the head in a patient with an inherited disorder of blood coagulation deserves immediate replacement therapy prior to careful neurologic evaluation. Similarly, a patient with hemophilia should receive replacement therapy if a headache lasts for more than 6 to 8 hours. We instruct patients to immediately infuse sufficient material to elevate the factor level to 100 per cent. Surgical

*Oxycel or Surgicel saturated with a solution of powdered thrombin dissolved in 0.5 per cent sodium bicarbonate.

evacuation of intracranial accumulations of blood ideally should be undertaken in Hemophilia Centers, where facilities are available for careful monitoring of blood levels.

Nerve Compression. Compression of peripheral nerves can occur whenever there is bleeding in a closed fibromuscular compartment. Hemorrhage into the iliopsoas sheath can lead to permanent femoral nerve palsy. Early recognition and prompt replacement therapy are essential. On occasion, surgical decompression is necessary if there is danger of permanent loss of neuromuscular function.

Major Surgery. Elective surgical procedures should be undertaken only in hospitals with facilities to monitor coagulation factor levels and only after it has been established that there is no evidence of an inhibitor in the patient. Factor levels above 30 per cent must be maintained for 7 to 10 days after major procedures by either intermittent or continuous infusion of the missing factor.

Emergency surgical procedures should be performed after administering enough of the missing factor to produce a blood level of 100 per cent. If specific factor assays cannot be done, normalization of the partial thromboplastin time (PTT) can be accepted as reasonable indirect evidence of satisfactory response; however, the patient should be transferred to a Hemophilia Center as soon as possible if such transfer is considered safe on clinical grounds.

Immunizations. All children should receive routine immunizations that can all be given subcutaneously. In addition, hepatitis B vaccine should be given to all patients who are likely to have been exposed to blood products. The child who is HIV-positive or who lives in a household with an HIV-infected parent or sibling should receive killed polio (Salk) vaccine to prevent passage of live virus in the household.

Home Infusion Therapy

Home therapy should be considered if the patient requires reasonably frequent factor infusions or DDAVP and after careful psychosocial evaluation of the patient and the family. Formal training in infusion procedures and intravenous technique is mandatory, and it is the responsibility of the supervising physician to ensure that the patient and family are completely familiar with the indications for treatment and the signs and symptoms that would mandate physician evaluation.

Home treatment has obvious psychologic and economic advantages for both the patient and the family. In addition to making early treatment more available, home therapy also means that, for the first time, many of the patients have some control over their lives and the management of their disease. Home infusion is not without hazards, however. These include lack of medical supervision, increased danger of hepatitis in relatives, poor intravenous technique, overutilization of material, product deterioration, and illegal use of intravenous equipment. Although many people have expressed concern about poor intravenous technique at home, we have not encountered any serious problems. We insist that the patient and family keep detailed records, and, as with the outpatient treatment program, we advise that they check with the physician if more than two successive daily infusions are needed for control of a single bleeding episode. Furthermore, each patient in the home infusion program must return at least once a year for evaluation of the total management program. A number of studies have shown that there is increased use of replacement therapy initially, but this eventually levels off. However, even if replacement therapy utilization remains high, this is usually balanced by the reduced cost to the patient and the improvement in school and work attendance. To guard against product deterioration, it is essential that the patient have adequate instructions and facilities for storage. To ensure that patients who are traveling in other areas receive prompt and appropriate therapy, each patient is provided with a card outlining the diagnosis and the dose of replacement therapy. This is also useful in protecting patients who have to account to law enforcement authorities for venipuncture marks and the possession of venipuncture equipment.

The institution dispensing the infusion material has an obligation to guard against abuse and sale of venipuncture equipment through illegal channels. To monitor this, we insist that all materials be returned to the clinic after their use, and spot checks are made to ensure that used syringes, needles, and other equipment are returned. Patients are encouraged to restock their supply when they have enough material left for only one infusion. Ordinarily, we supply enough for four infusions at a time, and this can be done through the mail. We have increasingly taken advantage of home service companies that arrange for shipment of therapeutic materials, arrange to bill third-party payers, and keep the Hemophilia Center updated on each patient's product utilization.

Prophylactic Replacement Therapy

Although it is now possible to provide satisfactory prophylaxis, it is not a practical consideration for most patients. However, it may be indicated in selected situations as, for example, in patients who have had repeated central nervous system (CNS) hemorrhage or in the control of repeated hemarthrosis into a single joint (see above). Prophylaxis is also required during periods of intensive physical therapy.

Dose schedules must be individualized. For factor VIII, we generally advise infusions every 2 to 3 days, with doses calculated to raise the factor VIII level to 40 to 50 per cent. Lower doses and less frequent treatment often can produce the desired effect by maintaining factor VIII levels above 2 to 3 per cent of normal.

Educational Resources

A wide variety of educational materials are available.* These include informative brochures suitable for patients, physicians, teachers, nurses, and other individuals who deal with the hemophilic patient and family. The brochures cover subjects such as pain control, dental care, physical therapy, financial counseling, teaching home therapy, sports, and so on. In addition, the National Hemophilia Foundation publishes a directory of Hemophilia Treatment Centers and descriptions of state and federal programs for assisting the hemophiliac and the family. An international list of Hemophilia Centers is also available.†

Acquired Disorders

Vitamin K Deficiency

Hemorrhagic Disease of the Newborn

PREVENTION. In healthy full-term infants, the problem of hemorrhagic disease of the newborn has been virtually eliminated by the administration of vitamin K at or soon after delivery. The naturally occurring compound—vitamin K_1 oxide (phytonadione)—is the preferred form because synthetic vitamin K analogues can produce hemolysis. Neonatal hemolysis and the risk of kernicterus are a particular problem in the presence of a deficiency of red blood cell glucose-6-phosphate dehydrogenase (G-6-PD). It has been well estab-

*National Hemophilia Foundation, The SoHo Building, 110 Greene Street, Suite 406, New York, NY 10012.

†The World Federation of Hemophilia, 4616 St. Catherine Street West, Montreal, Quebec, Canada H3Z 1S3, publishes *Guide for Traveling Hemophiliacs*, which lists hemophilia centers located in 68 countries.

lished that as little as 0.025 mg of vitamin K_1 can prevent the deficiencies of the vitamin K-dependent factors in a neonate with reasonably mature liver function. Thus, the recommended dose (0.5 to 1.0 mg intramuscularly or subcutaneously or 1 to 2 mg orally) is already far in excess of the neonate's physiologic needs and higher doses have no added beneficial effect. Particularly with the water-soluble analogues, higher doses increase the risk of kernicterus.

Infants of mothers being treated with phenytoin (Dilantin) or phenobarbital are occasionally found immediately after birth to have hemorrhage secondary to depletion of vitamin K–dependent factors. This is in contrast to the usual case of hemorrhagic disease of the newborn in whom the various clotting factors are transferred transplacentally and symptoms become manifest only beyond the first 24 hours of age. Some recommend the administration of vitamin K during labor to the mother who is on anticonvulsant therapy, to prevent bleeding secondary to the trauma of delivery.

TREATMENT. Premature infants, particularly those with complications such as hypoxia, acidosis, or infections, do not respond to the administration of vitamin K as well as do healthy term infants. When hemorrhagic manifestations prove to be due exclusively or in large part to a deficiency of vitamin K–dependent factors, the clinician has to resort to the use of replacement therapy with fresh or fresh frozen plasma if the patient is not responsive to vitamin K. The amount of procoagulant that can be safely administered to the newborn in this fashion is limited by the relatively low concentrations of procoagulants in whole plasma. On an average, plasma contains 1 unit of procoagulant activity in each milliliter and an infusion of 10 mg/kg will produce an elevation of only about 10 per cent in the circulating level of factor IX and the other vitamin K–dependent factors. Because of concern for volume overload, central venous pressure should be constantly monitored, particularly if an umbilical vein catheter is already in place for other reasons. As a practical approach, 10 ml of fresh frozen plasma per kilogram can be administered every 12 hours, and this should provide hemostatic levels of the missing factors, although the levels of each procoagulant will vary because of variations in in vivo recovery and intravascular biologic half-life. For example, factor VII, although stable in stored plasma, has a short in vivo half-life of 4 to 6 hours. In contrast, 50 per cent of infused prothrombin (factor II) is still present 72 hours later.

Prothrombin complex concentrates are commercially available. In these concentrates, the vitamin K–dependent factors are concentrated in approximately 1/25 the volume, compared with plasma. However, because of the increased risk of hepatitis, these concentrates should not be used unless it has been impossible to provide satisfactory hemostatic levels with single-donor plasma.

High-risk neonates should continue to receive supplemental parenteral or oral vitamin K, particularly if they are receiving broad-spectrum antibiotics or total parenteral nutrition.

Impaired Intestinal Absorption. Vitamin K deficiency can develop as a result of fat malabsorption and after prolonged administration of broad-spectrum antibiotics. Thus, patients with conditions in which vitamin K deficiency might be anticipated should receive the water-soluble form of the vitamin prophylactically. For treatment of bleeding in these situations, intramuscular or intravenous vitamin K_1 should be given. Replacement therapy with blood products is rarely necessary.

Liver Disease. In advanced liver disease, there is defective synthesis of the vitamin K–dependent clotting factors and treatment with vitamin K is often ineffective. If there is overt bleeding or if the patient is being prepared for surgery, plasma infusions may be necessary. If possible, prothrombin complex concentrates should be avoided because of the added risk of hepatitis in the face of pre-existing liver dysfunction. Thrombosis is another recognized complication of treatment with prothrombin-complex concentrates, and this hazard may be increased in the patient with liver disease who is unable to clear activated coagulation factors from the circulation.

Coumarin Anticoagulants. The coumarin anticoagulants are rarely used therapeutically in pediatric practice, but they can cross the placenta, producing neonatal bleeding. More commonly, accidental ingestion of medication or rat poison can produce severe depletion of vitamin K–dependent factors. Intravenous administration of 5 mg of vitamin K_1 normalizes the prothrombin time within 6 to 12 hours, regardless of how much dicumarol is taken. The synthetic water-soluble analogues are less effective than the naturally occurring compound.

Circulating Anticoagulants. Circulating inhibitors of coagulation can develop in children without pre-existing coagulation factor deficiency. They may be directed against specific coagulation factors but are usually nonspecific and appear to be directed against the prothrombinase complex. They are rarely associated with abnormal hemostasis, in spite of significant in vitro abnormalities. Treatment is directed at the underlying disease as, for example, in systemic lupus erythematosus. We have not encountered problems at renal biopsy, even when significant in vitro inhibition is present. Many of these inhibitors, particularly those detected during "preoperative screening," seem to be related to viral infections and gradually disappear over weeks or months without specific therapy.

PLATELET DISORDERS

Thrombocytopenia

Treatment varies with the severity of the thrombocytopenia and the pathophysiologic basis for the reduction in platelet count. In general, patients with levels of normally functioning platelets above 50,000/mm^3 have normal hemostasis. In the presence of platelet dysfunction, however, hemostasis is defective in spite of normal levels of circulating platelets. At the other end of the spectrum, children with conditions such as immunologic or so-called idiopathic thrombocytopenic purpura (ITP), characterized by shortened platelet survival and maximal compensatory production of platelets, may have reasonably normal hemostasis and normal bleeding times even with platelet counts as low as 10,000/mm^3.

Impaired Platelet Production (Leukemia, Aplastic Anemia)

Reduced production of platelets is usually the underlying mechanism for the thrombocytopenia complicating *aplastic anemia, acute leukemia,* and other conditions characterized by *bone marrow failure.* However, intravascular coagulation and fibrinolysis precipitated by complicating infection or by the disease process itself can aggravate the degree of thrombocytopenia. Platelet transfusions may be needed in acute leukemia during the period of induction of remission, at times of drug-induced pancytopenia, or at relapse. Because of the increase in the use of bone marrow transplantation, platelet transfusion should be used sparingly, particularly in patients with aplastic anemia. The use of "prophylactic platelet transfusions," particularly from family members, appears to be contraindicated in any patient who may be a candidate for bone marrow transplantation in the future. Children with documented immune deficiency or those who are to receive intensive immunosuppressive therapy are at risk for graft-versus-host disease related to the infusion of viable donor lymphocytes. This problem is obviated by irradiating all blood products prior to administration.

Obviously, in the presence of active or potentially life-threatening hemorrhage, platelet replacement using random unrelated donors should not be withheld. Ultimately, however, restoration of normal platelet count can be expected only when the underlying disease process is brought under control.

Immune Thrombocytopenia

In so-called *idiopathic thrombocytopenic purpura* (ITP), one of the most common causes of thrombocytopenia in children, the reduced platelet count results from the production of autoantibodies directed against the patient's platelets, usually following a relatively mild viral infection. Splenic sequestration of antibody-coated platelets is enhanced, and the degree of thrombocytopenia depends on the ability of the bone marrow to compensate for varying degrees of shortened platelet survival. Underlying disorders, such as *systemic lupus erythematosus* or *lymphoma,* must be sought and, if present, treated appropriately.

The treatment of acute ITP has been the subject of controversy for many years. A number of studies have demonstrated that corticosteroid therapy shortens the time from diagnosis to *normalization* of platelet count. However, the natural history of the disease is such that hemorrhagic manifestations usually clear within a week or two of onset whether or not corticosteroids are given and in spite of persistently low platelet counts. It is during this period that normalization of the bleeding time can be documented in the absence of an increase in platelet count. Thus, *clinical* improvement does not necessarily depend on a rise or normalization of the platelet count. In addition, the use of corticosteroids has not reduced the incidence of chronic cases.

One of the major concerns of clinicians caring for these patients is the risk of intracranial hemorrhage, but this is a very rare complication and usually occurs within the first few days of illness, often before treatment can be instituted or expected to exert a therapeutic effect. Thus, in the presence of mild clinical bleeding confined to the skin or mucous membranes, it has been our policy to hospitalize the patient for a few days of observation. Within 3 to 7 days, the hemorrhagic manifestations have usually subsided and the patient can be discharged to home care, where the parents are advised to take reasonable precautions against significant trauma. We advise against bicycle riding, tree climbing, skating, sledding, and contact sports, but in older children who can take reasonable precautions, there is no contraindication to returning to a normal classroom situation.

The effectiveness of intravenous gamma globulin (IVIG) in elevating the platelet count has added to the controversy over the treatment of acute ITP. Although on average, the rate of rise in platelet count induced by IVIG is not much more rapid than that produced by prednisone, the proportion of very rapid responders (i.e., those with normal platelet counts within 24 to 48 hours) is much higher. This has led to the use of IVIG in the acute situation if there is active bleeding or if it is apparent that it would be difficult to restrict the patient's physical activities.

Although IVIG is still very expensive, it can significantly shorten or eliminate the period of observation in the hospital, thus balancing out the costs of treatment. The original recommended dosage schedule provided for administration of 400 mg/kg/day for 5 days. Similar results can be obtained using 1 g/kg/day for 2 days, thus further reducing treatment costs. If after approximately 6 months the platelet count has not risen above 50,000/mm^3, a trial of corticosteroid therapy is indicated. Prednisone (40 to 60 mg/m^2 every 24 hours in three divided doses) is administered for 1 to 4 weeks. Whether or not there has been a response, the dose should be tapered over 4 to 6 weeks. By monitoring the platelet count during drug withdrawal, it is possible to define a minimal dose level at which an adequate platelet level might be maintained. Even in the absence of proven long-term benefits from corticosteroid therapy, it seems prudent to treat patients with fulminating hemorrhage or intracranial bleeding at the time of diagnosis. Although platelet transfusions are not considered appropriate as routine therapy in patients with ITP, transient hemostasis may be achieved that could be critical in a life-threatening situation.

Prolonged corticosteroid therapy is usually unacceptable to teenagers, who become very concerned about the cosmetic effects of corticosteroids, even for these relatively short treatment periods. Under these circumstances and when platelet counts above 50,000 cannot be maintained without treatment, IVIG should be considered. IVIG produces a satisfactory increment in platelet count in most patients with chronic ITP, but thrombocytopenia generally recurs within 1 to 4 weeks and booster doses are necessary. The major role of IVIG in chronic ITP seems to be to avoid or postpone splenectomy, particularly in very young children, or to produce rapid elevation in platelet count in the face of active bleeding or in anticipation of a surgical procedure. The recommended dosage schedule is 1 g/kg/day for 2 consecutive days.

Splenectomy is still a very effective treatment for chronic ITP in spite of concerns about post-splenectomy infection. Presplenectomy immunization against *Streptococcus pneumoniae, Neisseria meningitidis* and *Haemophilus influenzae* B enhance the safety of the procedure. Permanent benefit can be anticipated in well over half the patients subjected to splenectomy. In patients who have previously had a response to prednisone therapy, the drug should be administered during the week prior to surgery in order to achieve and maintain hemostatic platelet levels. However, it should be stressed that even with severe thrombocytopenia it is rare to encounter excessive bleeding at splenectomy in these patients. We usually have platelet concentrates available in the blood bank to be administered only if the surgeon encounters excessive oozing during the operative procedure. To my recollection, we have never had to administer platelets under these circumstances, and their effect, in any event, would be short-lived because infused platelets are rapidly cleared from the circulation as they become coated with antibody. Even in patients who have not previously responded to therapy, corticosteroid coverage is essential during the perioperative period to protect against the effects of adrenal insufficiency.

Relapse after splenectomy-induced remission should alert the clinician to search for an accessory spleen by ^{99m}technetium scanning. If the accessory spleen is present, its removal usually results in a second remission. In many cases, relapses are transient and, like the initial episode, are often provoked by a minor viral infection. These patients are considered to have a "compensated thrombolytic state," and relapse is precipitated either by an increase in the rate of platelet destruction or by a decrease in platelet production. Patients usually recover within a week or two but are often given corticosteroids or IVIG, which, in my experience, does not alter the natural history of the condition in this rare but troublesome group of patients.

Approximately 5 per cent of patients fail to achieve remission after an appropriate period of observation followed by an adequate trial of prednisone, IVIG, and/or splenectomy. In these cases, immunosuppressive therapy with cyclophosphamide or azathioprine has been used with variable success. Vincristine sulfate, which has some immunosuppressive qualities and has a positive effect on platelet production, has brought about remissions in adults with ITP. Vinblastine-treated random donor platelets have been transfused to adults with ITP with the intent of delivering a "cytotoxic" agent to the areas of platelet sequestration. At present, all these immunotherapeutic approaches must be considered investigational. Their use should be considered only after the risks of such therapy have been carefully weighed against the hazards of chronic thrombocytopenia in a particular patient.

Neonatal Thrombocytopenia

Thrombocytopenia in the high-risk neonate is most commonly related to intrauterine or postnatal infection. Treatment is usually directed against the underlying disease process. Less frequently, neonatal thrombocytopenic purpura develops as a result of transplacental passage of platelet antibodies from either a mother with active or "compensated" autoimmune thrombocytopenia or one who is isoimmunized by her infant's platelets. Isoimmunization occurs when the mother lacks antigens present on the infant's platelets, and the mother becomes immunized against fetal platelets in much the same way as the erythrocytes are affected in hemolytic disease of the newborn. There is then passive transfer of maternal antibodies across the placenta, which react with antigens on the fetal platelets. The PLA-1 antigen has been most frequently incriminated in isoimmune neonatal thrombocytopenia.

In symptomatic newborn infants with platelet counts below 20,000 to 30,000/mm^3, prompt therapy is indicated. The ideal form of therapy in isoimmune thrombocytopenia is the transfusion of platelets that lack the antigen against which the antibody is directed. These nonreactive platelets can be obtained from the mother and washed free of antibody before the infant undergoes transfusion. If previous infants have been affected, maternal platelets can be harvested by plateletpheresis prior to delivery so that they can be available for transfusion soon after birth if the infant is affected. Alternatively, if the offending antigen has been identified with a previously affected infant, an unrelated donor lacking the antigen could be used as a source of platelet concentrate for the affected infant. If compatible platelets are not available, as is true in most cases of maternal autoimmune thrombocytopenia, we recommend proceeding with exchange transfusion using freshly drawn whole blood (<24 hours from donation) from a random donor. This has the effect of removing circulating antibody from the infant's circulation while providing at least temporary correction of the thrombocytopenia with donor platelets. Subsequent platelet transfusion may be necessary if the platelet count is not sustained at hemostatic levels.

Although they are frequently recommended, corticosteroids have not been proved to be of benefit in neonatal thrombocytopenia. Without specific therapy, recovery can be anticipated in 4 to 6 weeks, by which time most of the maternal antibody would have been cleared from the fetal circulation.

Preliminary studies have produced evidence to suggest that administration of corticosteroids or IVIG to mothers prior to labor can elevate the fetal platelet count. The risk for neonatal thrombocytopenia is highest in those with maternal autoimmune thrombocytopenia. Some have recommended that subsequent infants born to the mothers of infants with neonatal thrombocytopenia be delivered by cesarean section. We make this recommendation only if neonatal thrombocytopenia is documented by cordocentesis or by fetal scalp sampling. The rationale for advising cesarean section is to avoid trauma to the head during vaginal delivery.

Disorders of Platelet Function

An increasing number of congenital and acquired disorders are now recognized and should be suspected in any patient having a normal platelet count with a prolonged bleeding time and normal levels of VWF.

Inherited Disorders

Glanzmann's Thrombasthenia, Bernard-Soulier Syndrome, "Storage Pool Disease." For the increasing number of inherited disorders of platelet function now recognized, no specific therapy is usually available to correct the basic platelet defect so that transfusion of normal platelets is required to cover serious bleeding episodes or major surgical procedures. Because these patients are not on any form of immunosuppressive therapy, there is a strong likelihood that they will develop antibodies directed against donor platelets. This problem can be circumvented by identifying donors who are compatible with respect to HLA antigens. This reduces the possibility of developing resistance to future transfusions, and transfusions from these donors are often effective when the patient has become resistant to transfusion from random donors. DDAVP can also normalize the bleeding time in patients with storage pool disease. Results are unpredictable, but a trial of DDAVP would be reasonable in patients with unexplained prolonged bleeding times or with various congenital or acquired qualitative platelet defects other than Glanzmann's thrombasthenia.

Congenital Afibrinogenemia. Congenital afibrinogenemia is associated with platelet dysfunction, presumably as a result of the lack of fibrinogen on the platelet surface. Transfusion of plasma or cryoprecipitate corrects both the prolonged bleeding time and the in vitro platelet abnormalities.

Type I Glycogen Storage Disease. Patients with type I glycogen storage disease have abnormalities of platelet function; the hemorrhagic tendency is mild, although it does tend to become more severe with advancing age. Correction of the underlying metabolic disturbances results in correction of the platelet abnormalities, but this often takes up to a week, so that careful preparation is needed prior to major surgical procedures in this group of patients.

Acquired Disorders

Uremia. Abnormal bleeding in patients with chronic uremia is often associated with abnormal platelet function, related in part to elevated levels of serum guanidinosuccinic acid. Hemodialysis or successful renal transplant corrects both the bleeding time and the in vitro abnormalities of platelet function. The administration of DDAVP or cryoprecipitate has been shown to correct the bleeding time in this group of patients, although the mechanism by which they exert this effect is not clear. The chronically uremic patient with a bleeding diathesis who fails to respond to DDAVP or cryoprecipitate may require hemodialysis to achieve hemostasis.

Drug-Induced Platelet Dysfunction. A number of commonly used drugs have been shown to produce abnormal platelet function. Aspirin is the most widely used of these agents, but antihistamines, antidepressants, tranquilizers, α-adrenergic blocking agents, local anesthetics, and non-aspirin analgesics (like phenylbutazone and indomethacin) may have similar effects. In general, few of these agents produce symptomatic bleeding unless there is an underlying hemostatic defect. Discontinuing the particular medication results in a return to normal of platelet function; the in vitro abnormalities may persist for up to a week after aspirin administration, but the effect is more transient after exposure to other NSAIDs.

Platelet Transfusions

To minimize the hazard of volume overload in the pediatric patient and to improve utilization of blood components in general, platelets are administered in the form of platelet concentrates through 170 μ blood filters. Although there is significant risk of spontaneous and life-threatening hemorrhage at platelet counts below 10,000/mm³, many patients are able to maintain adequate hemostasis under resting conditions so that the platelet count should not be used as the sole indication for transfusion. This is particularly true in patients who have thrombocytopenia characterized by increased platelet turnover. Platelet transfusions, however, should be considered in the severely thrombocytopenic patient with leukemia or marrow aplasia with evidence of active hemorrhage, even if only in the form of spontaneous petechial eruptions. Patients with platelet counts between 10,000 and 50,000/mm³ are at risk from hemorrhage related to varying degrees of trauma; platelet transfusions aimed at raising and maintaining the platelet count above 50,000/mm³ would be necessary to cover minor or major surgical procedures. Patients with platelet counts above 50,000/mm³ are usually able to maintain normal hemostasis if platelet function is normal and if there is no associated coagulation defect.

Although most blood banks can provide sufficient quantities of platelet concentrate to meet the needs of the thrombocytopenic patient, current routine blood bank procedures do not test for compatibility of platelets for transfusion. Thus, there is significant risk of platelet antibodies developing after transfusion of platelets from random donors, resulting in unresponsiveness to future platelet transfusions. This is a particular concern in patients with aplastic anemia because immunosuppressive therapy is usually not part of their treatment program. Thus, before a platelet transfusion program for an individual patient is initiated, the risk of hemorrhage at the time of transfusion has to be carefully weighed against the future needs of the patient, the likelihood of antibody production, and the potential for marrow graft rejection caused by transfusion of foreign lymphocytes.

Patients with qualitative platelet disorders or those with aplastic anemia who are not candidates for bone marrow transplantation and in whom long-term platelet transfusion programs are anticipated should be typed with respect to the HLA antigens, since these seem to relate closely to platelet antigens. If HLA-compatible donors can be identified, transfusion from these donors has proved very effective for long periods of time in patients who have developed resistance to transfusion of platelets from random donors.

The dose of platelet concentrate can be calculated based on observations that platelets derived from 1 unit of whole blood produce an average increment in platelet count of 13,000/mm³/m² body surface. The administration of plasma concentrate (6 units/m²) produces an increment in platelet count of 50,000/mm³ or above in the majority of recipients. If hemorrhage continues in spite of an adequate increment in platelet count, a search should be made for a local lesion to account for the continued bleeding. Febrile patients with or without documented sepsis responded less well to platelet transfusions, as measured by increment in platelet count; even with a less than satisfactory rise in the platelet count, however, hemostasis can often be achieved and maintained.

To evaluate response to a platelet transfusion, the platelet count should be obtained prior to the transfusion, 1 hour after its completion, and again the next morning. *On an average, 50 percent of the infused platelets will have disappeared from the circulation after 24 hours, so that it is often necessary to repeat the transfusion every 2 to 3 days.*

Fresh platelet concentrates have a limited shelf life. To maintain adequate inventories of blood components, it is extremely helpful to the blood bank for the clinician to attempt to anticipate the patient's platelet transfusion requirements as far in advance as possible. Methods for long-term platelet cryopreservation are being actively explored. When the techniques are perfected and become more generally available, it will be possible to stockpile platelet concentrates from selected donors or from the patients themselves, while they are in remission, for use at some future time.

TREATMENT OF ACUTE LEUKEMIA IN CHILDREN

AMY LOUISE BILLETT, M.D.
and STEPHEN E. SALLAN, M.D.

Acute leukemia is the most common childhood malignancy. There are approximately 2500 new cases diagnosed each year in United States children under the age of 15. Acute lymphoblastic leukemia (ALL) accounts for 75 to 80 per cent of cases, and acute myelogenous leukemia (AML) accounts for 20 to 25 per cent of cases. Although acute leukemia in childhood was once incurable, now 65 to 70 per cent of children with ALL and 45 to 50 per cent of children with AML can be cured. The cure rate has improved significantly in recent decades because of improvements in chemotherapy and supportive care for all patients and the advent of bone marrow transplantation for patients with AML and recurrent ALL.

Patients with a suspected diagnosis of acute leukemia should be referred to a tertiary care pediatric treatment center for initial evaluation and treatment under the guidance of an experienced pediatric hematology-oncology staff. Because acute leukemia is a rare disease and each patient can contribute to the development of more effective and less morbid future treatments, we always recommend treatment on a research protocol. Before specific therapy can be instituted, however, a clear diagnosis must be made by performing a bone marrow aspiration. Although initial treatment plans can be developed using only morphologic study and cytochemical stains, cell surface immunophenotyping and cytogenetics are critical to further characterize a leukemia and its appropriate therapy.

SUPPORTIVE CARE

Supportive care is an important determinant of outcome in children with acute leukemia. When the diagnosis of acute leukemia is suspected, we recommend immediate institution of hydration, alkalinization, and allopurinol as described below. Initial management and supportive care to stabilize the patient must be carried out before the initiation of specific antileukemia therapy.

Metabolic Disorders

Metabolic problems can occur in all patients but are more common in patients with a white blood cell count greater than 100,000/μl. Initial metabolic assessment includes measurements of serum electrolyte, creatinine, uric acid, calcium, magnesium, and phosphate levels. Metabolic parameters must be followed carefully during the first several days because abnormalities may worsen when specific antileukemia therapy is instituted and cell lysis occurs. Prevention of uric acid nephropathy requires hydration with twice-maintenance fluid, alkalinization with sodium bicarbonate to achieve a urine pH

>6.0, and allopurinol (100 mg/m^2 every 8 hours) to decrease uric acid production. We use 5 per cent dextrose with one-half normal sodium bicarbonate at 3000 ml/m^2/day without potassium. Although mild elevations in creatinine can occur during tumor lysis, dialysis is rarely needed.

Emergencies

In addition to serious infections, bleeding, and metabolic disorders, there are two rare but important emergency situations. Children with T cell ALL can present with an anterior mediastinal mass causing airway compression or superior vena cava syndrome that requires immediate treatment with radiation therapy or intravenous steroids. Children with a white blood cell count greater than 100,000/μl at the time of diagnosis may have leukostasis, which is manifested by signs and symptoms of central nervous system (CNS) and pulmonary hypoperfusion from sludging. Immediate treatment with hydration and either leukapheresis or exchange transfusion is indicated for symptomatic patients.

Blood Component Support

Hematologic abnormalities are common in children with acute leukemia. Platelet transfusions are indicated for bleeding or a platelet count less than 20,000/μl. Symptomatic anemia or a hematocrit value under 25 per cent requires transfusion with packed red blood cells. If the presenting hematocrit level is extremely low, exchange transfusion or pheresis may be required to allow increasing it without causing significant volume overload. To prevent complications, all blood products should be cytomegalovirus (CMV)-negative, irradiated to prevent graft-versus-host disease, and white blood cell–filtered to prevent sensitization and subsequent transfusion reactions. Use of single-donor, pheresis-pack platelet transfusions prevents sensitization from exposure to multiple donors. Human leukocyte antigen (HLA)–matched platelet transfusions are rarely necessary. Coagulation parameters should be assessed at presentation of all children with a suspected diagnosis of acute leukemia. Coagulation disorders are most common with acute promyelocytic leukemia (M3), and the use of low-dose heparin therapy in this setting is recommended by some experts.

Infection

Infection can be a significant problem in children with acute leukemia both at presentation and during therapy. Not only are patients at increased risk of infection because of neutropenia, immunosuppression, mucosal damage, and indwelling foreign bodies, but neutropenia and steroid therapy can mask signs and symptoms of infection. Fever in the setting of neutropenia requires a thorough physical examination (including careful attention to all mucocutaneous surfaces, culture of blood and urine, and cerebrospinal fluid as indicated) and immediate institution of broad-spectrum antibiotics to treat both gram-positive and gram-negative organisms. Initial antibiotic choices are dependent on the usual pathogens and sensitivities at an individual institution. We use a combination of a semisynthetic penicillin and an aminoglycoside.

Treatment for possible fungal infection is indicated for patients with prolonged neutropenia who remain persistently febrile while receiving broad spectrum antibacterial coverage. Fungal infections are more common in patients receiving more intensive therapy. White blood cell transfusions are recommended for patients with proven bacterial sepsis that is not responding to appropriate antibiotics when there is expected recovery from neutropenia within 7 to 10 days. Most centers use prophylactic trimethoprim-sulfamethoxazole to prevent *Pneumocystis carinii* infections, although myelosuppression from this drug can be problematic in the patient receiving chemotherapy.

Hematologic growth factors (G-CSF and GM-CSF) are now commercially available. Although there are preliminary data that the use of growth factors can decrease the duration of neutropenia and the severity of infection in patients receiving chemotherapy, it is too early to provide guidelines for their general use. Concerns pertaining to the effects of growth factors on leukemic cells remain unanswered.

Gastrointestinal complications, including mucositis and infection, are common in children receiving therapy for acute leukemia and especially dangerous is *typhlitis* (inflammation of the cecum).

Varicella-zoster infections can be life-threatening in a child with leukemia. It is extremely important to assess titers at presentation to determine any previous immunity. In a nonimmune patient, varicella-zoster immunoglobulin prophylaxis should be given within 72 hours of an exposure. In addition, acyclovir is indicated when primary disease or disseminated zoster infection develops. Measles is a growing problem in many communities and thus a potential problem for children with leukemia. Susceptible patients who are exposed to measles should receive 200 to 400 mg/kg of gamma globulin for prevention.

Psychosocial Support

Psychosocial support of the child and family is very important during treatment for acute leukemia. Not only do all patients need a primary physician and nurse, but social workers and psychologists need to be available to the patient and family.

ACUTE LYMPHOBLASTIC LEUKEMIA

Diagnosis and Treatment Factors

Once the specific diagnosis of acute lymphoblastic leukemia has been established, treatment should be initiated using a research protocol. It is important to identify factors at the time of diagnosis that can guide treatment decisions. Once called "prognostic factors," "treatment factors" is the more appropriate term, since intensive therapy can change outcome. The most important adverse factors that indicate the need for more intensive therapy include high initial white blood cell count (>20,000/mm^3); age under 2 years or above 9 years, T cell immunophenotype, CNS disease at diagnosis, and the presence of the Philadelphia chromosome translocation, t(9;22).

Remission Induction

The treatment of ALL involves four phases: remission induction, central nervous system (CNS) treatment, intensification, and continuation. Treatment begins with intensive remission induction, designed to eradicate all measurable disease and to achieve complete remission. *Complete remission* is defined as return of normal hematopoiesis and no evidence of leukemia in the bone marrow (<5 per cent blasts) or any other extramedullary site. There is significant, although unmeasurable, residual leukemia present when complete remission is first achieved. The 1-month induction period involves the use of vincristine and prednisone and one or more of the following agents: an anthracycline (doxorubicin or daunorubicin), asparaginase, and methotrexate as well as intrathecal chemotherapy. We believe that early intensive therapy is important for all patients, regardless of treatment factors. Greater than 90 per cent of children with ALL achieve complete remission, and approximately 3 per cent can be expected to die of toxicity during induction.

CNS Treatment

Specific central nervous system (CNS) therapy is required because all patients have leukemic invasion of the meninges at diagnosis, although only 3 per cent have measurable blasts in the cerebrospinal fluid. Because many antileukemic drugs administered systemically have little or no CNS penetration, specific CNS therapy should be instituted during remission induction, and more intensive CNS treatment added once complete bone marrow remission is achieved. Although cranial radiation therapy and concurrent intrathecal chemotherapy are highly effective, the combination has been associated with long-term neuroendocrine and neuropsychiatric sequelae. Therefore, most investigators try to reduce toxicity and withhold cranial radiation from some patients.

Intensification and Continuation

Intensification, also called "consolidation," is systemic treatment to eliminate unmeasurable but known residual disease. Cycles of multiple drugs to prevent the emergence of resistant clones can be administered continuously for many months or at regular intervals throughout the treatment program. Intensification therapy often begins concurrent with CNS treatment.

Continuation therapy, once called "maintenance therapy," is less intensive treatment intended to kill any residual leukemic cells. Therapy is continued until the patient has been in continuous complete remission for 24 months. Methotrexate and 6-mercaptopurine are the mainstays of continuation therapy in most programs, but we believe that additional drugs are important. Ongoing research to identify minimal residual disease in patients in complete remission will be used in the future to tailor the duration of individual patient therapy.

Several general principles are important during ALL treatment. Once complete remission is achieved, maximal amounts of drugs should be used with dose adjustments to achieve an absolute neutrophil count nadir from 750 to 1,000/μl and platelet nadir from 75,000 to 100,000/μl. Toxicity should be monitored and treated. During this period, it is also important to monitor the child's entire picture, including growth, nutrition, psychosocial issues, and family support.

Treatment Protocol (Dana-Farber Cancer Institute Program)

Drugs commonly used to treat ALL are shown in Table 1. The specific drugs used to treat ALL vary within institutions and with different treatment factors. Our program from the current Dana-Farber Cancer Institute Leukemia Treatment Consortium is presented as an illustration of a current treatment protocol. This article represents only a general discussion and should *not* be used to treat an individual patient.

We emphasize early treatment intensity during remission induction and therefore use five systemic drugs (prednisone, vincristine, doxorubicin, asparaginase, methotrexate) and intrathecal therapy. After complete remission is obtained, CNS therapy and intensification begin concurrently. Patients with no high-risk treatment factors receive intrathecal cytarabine and methotrexate four times in 2 weeks. If there is any high-risk treatment factor, 1800 cGy of radiation to the cranium is administered concurrently with intrathecal therapy. Intensification chemotherapy for all patients includes weekly intramuscular *Escherichia coli* asparaginase. If an allergic reaction occurs, we substitute alternative asparaginase preparations, either polyethylene glycosylated (PEG) *E. coli* asparaginase or *Erwinia* asparaginase.

In patients with no high-risk treatment factors, intensification therapy includes 20 weekly doses of asparaginase with a concurrent 3-week cycle, including pulses of prednisone and vincristine, 2 weeks of 6-mercaptopurine, and weekly parenteral methotrexate. Patients with any high-risk treatment factor receive the above regimen plus doxorubicin (30 mg/m^2 every 3 weeks) until a total cumulative dose of 360 mg/m^2 is achieved. Asparaginase is given and methotrexate held until completion of doxorubicin therapy.

Continuation therapy for all patients consists of cycles of prednisone, vincristine, mercaptopurine and methotrexate. Parenteral therapy during continuation prevents problems with drug absorption and patient compliance. In addition, all patients receive intrathecal cytarabine and methotrexate every 18 weeks throughout the 2 years of treatment in remission.

B Cell Acute Lymphoblastic Leukemia

The natural history of mature B cell ALL, also known as L3 or Burkitt's leukemia, mimics that of Burkitt's lymphoma. We treat these rare patients on protocols for disseminated Burkitt's lymphoma.

Bone Marrow Transplantation

Because two thirds of children with ALL can be cured with chemotherapy, we do not recommend bone marrow transplantation in first remission, except for patients with the Philadelphia chromosome translocation, t(9;22). These patients have an extremely high risk for relapse with chemotherapy alone, and allogeneic transplantation is recommended.

TABLE 1. Systemic Drugs Used in Treatment of Acute Lymphoblastic Leukemia

Drug	Dosage	Route	Principal Side Effects
Prednisone	40–120 mg/m^2 daily × 5	p.o.	Immunosuppression, hypertension, hyperglycemia, obesity, mood changes
Vincristine	1.5–2.0 mg/m^2 q 1–3 weeks (2.0 mg maximum)	IV	Peripheral neuropathy, obstipation, alopecia
Doxorubicin or Daunorubicin	30 mg/m^2 q 3 weeks	IV	Myelosuppression, emesis, alopecia, cardiac damage, mucositis
Asparaginase*	25,000 IU/m^2 weekly	IM	Allergic reactions, pancreatitis, coagulopathy, hepatitis, encephalopathy
Methotrexate	30–40 mg/m^2 weekly	IV/IM	Myelosuppression, hepatitis, mucositis
	1 g/m^2 over 24 hours†	IV	
	4 g/m^2 over 1 hour†	IV	
6-Mercaptopurine	50 mg/m^2 daily	p.o.	Myelosuppression, hepatitis, mucositis
	1 g/m^2 over 4–8 hours	IV	

*Alternative preparations (polyethylene glycocylated [PEG] and *Erwinia*) are available from the National Cancer Institute as a substitute for patients with allergic reactions to native *Escherichia coli.*

†Leucovorin rescue required.

TABLE 2. Systemic Drugs Used in Treatment of Acute Myelogenous Leukemia

Drug	Dosage	Route	Principal Side Effects
Cytarabine	100 mg/m^2 daily by continuous infusion × 3–7 days or 1–3 g/m^2 q 12 hrs × 4–8 doses	IV	Myelosuppression, alopecia, emesis, mucositis, fever, diarrhea, conjunctivitis, cerebellar dysfunction
Daunorubicin	45 mg/m^2 daily × 2–3 doses	IV	Myelosuppression, alopecia, emesis, mucositis, cardiac damage
6-Thioguanine	100–200 mg/m^2 daily × 4–7 days	p.o.	Myelosuppression, hepatitis, alopecia, mucositis, immunosuppression
Etoposide (VP-16)	100–250 mg/m^2 daily × 1–3 days	IV	Myelosuppression, alopecia, hypotension, allergic reactions
Azacitidine	100–300 mg/m^2 daily × 2–5 days	IV	Myelosuppression, emesis, rash

Relapsed Acute Lymphoblastic Leukemia

Relapsed ALL is currently the sixth most common childhood malignancy. Adverse prognostic factors include short duration of initial remission (< 24 months), bone marrow involvement at relapse, and intensive initial therapy. As initial therapy has become more intensive, reinduction rates have fallen to 75 per cent. If a child with relapsed ALL achieves second remission, continued chemotherapy cures fewer than 30 per cent of patients in most reported series. We therefore recommend matched allogeneic bone marrow transplantation, which is curative in approximately 50 per cent of patients. Deaths after allogeneic transplantation are usually caused by infection or graft-versus-host disease. For the 85 per cent of patients without a matched sibling donor, we recommend autologous bone marrow transplantation with in vitro purging of the marrow. In reports from two centers, approximately 35 to 40 per cent of patients can be cured with this treatment.

Of note, relapse is the most significant cause of failure in this patient population. There are few published reports regarding the efficacy of matched unrelated donor transplantation.

ACUTE MYELOGENOUS LEUKEMIA

Advances in therapy of AML in the past 20 years have resulted in complete remission rates of approximately 80 per cent, with 40 to 50 per cent of patients remaining in continuous complete remission. The treatment of AML differs in a number of ways from that of ALL. Because AML is a stem cell disease, treatment involves more myelosuppressive therapy with different drugs and often more toxicity. If complete remission is achieved, matched allogeneic bone marrow transplantation is recommended because such therapy has resulted in more long-term cures.

Induction

Induction therapy involves a combination of daunorubicin and cytarabine in most successful regimens. Because single-arm studies suggest that a third agent may increase the complete remission rate, a third drug (such as thioguanine or etoposide) is often added. We currently use a regimen including cytarabine as a 7-day continuous infusion, daunorubicin in three daily bolus doses, and daily thioguanine. Since 5 to 10 per cent of patients die of complications, such as infection or hemorrhage, careful attention to toxicity and supportive care is required.

CNS Therapy

CNS therapy usually consists of intrathecal drug at regular intervals during induction and subsequent therapy. Although 20 per cent of patients have CNS disease at diagnosis, this has not been an adverse prognostic factor. Without specific CNS therapy, however, approximately 20 per cent of patients in hematologic complete remission will relapse in the CNS.

Continuation

Although there is presumed residual disease at the end of induction chemotherapy, the optimal duration of continuation therapy in AML is unknown. Most continuation therapy regimens use drugs such as cytarabine, etoposide, 6-thioguanine, daunorubicin and 5-azacitidine in varying combinations and doses (Table 2). The most intensive chemotherapy regimens have provided long-term, continuous, complete remission rates of 45 per cent.

Bone Marrow Transplantation

Because chemotherapy is curative in fewer than 50 per cent of patients with AML, allogeneic bone marrow transplantation in first complete remission has become the treatment of choice. Leukemia-free survival can be expected in 60 to 80 per cent of children with AML after allogeneic bone marrow transplantation in first remission. The major causes of morbidity and mortality after transplantation are graft-versus-host disease and infection, although toxicity is usually less severe in children than in adults. Unfortunately, only 15 per cent patients have a matched sibling donor. The role of autologous bone marrow transplantation is under active investigation. Current protocols randomize children without an allogeneic donor to receive either a short course of chemotherapy or autologous bone marrow transplantation with in vitro purging of the marrow. The indications for transplantation from a matched unrelated donor for children with AML in first remission have not been established.

Relapsed Acute Myelogenous Leukemia

The prognosis in relapsed AML is extremely poor. Not only is it extremely difficult to obtain a second complete remission, but such remissions tend to be extremely short-lived. Bone marrow transplantation is recommended if the patient achieves a complete or near complete remission. For those few patients who experience relapse after initial chemotherapy, achieve second complete remission, and undergo bone marrow transplantation, survival ranges from 30 to 40 per cent. Of note, bone marrow transplantation in early relapse can be as effective as transplantation in second remission.

MANAGEMENT OF THE CHILD CURED OF CANCER

DANIEL C. PLUNKET, M.D.

The majority of children with cancer now survive with no evidence of disease. They represent a growing group of children and young adults who need special health assessment for an indefinite period, indeed for the rest of their lives.

Management of these fortunate children and their families can be considered in three categories: (1) the expected changes in the child and family, (2) the potential late effects of anticancer therapy, and (3) the possibility of development of a second cancer.

EXPECTED CHANGES

After cancer treatment is discontinued, parents and health professionals alike are often amazed at the child's increase in activity, weight gain, and overall improved sense of well-being. Some of this improvement can be explained by the emotional boost of being free of medication, but much of it is somatic. Hair grows, laboratory abnormalities normalize, and the child begins to act and look like what society says is normal. The child and the parents are tremendously gratified. Siblings reassert themselves as they begin to feel free of the restrictions that the disease has imposed. There is good evidence that most siblings will resolve their feelings of jealousy and being "left out." Parents, whose relationship will probably have been severely strained by the disease and its treatment, will need to re-examine their communication. Cancer is often economically devastating, a devastation that persists beyond cessation of therapy.

Parental concerns remain and may be appropriate, as is concern about recurrence of disease. Some concerns are based on misconception, such as concern for continued increased risk of infection, which was present during treatment. Some concerns are indicative of abnormal parenting, such as over-concern for the child, now considered "vulnerable." Studies support full reintegration of the child into the normal school system. Child and parents alike may be frightened by such a "full" return after 2 to 4 years of academic compromise. Routine follow-up tests may be resisted, partly from denial and partly from a real concern that the child remains a "test patient" in a study protocol of some oncology group, a probable situation. By means of the prognostic profiles furnished by the cancer therapists (see below), the child can usually be promptly reintegrated into the normal environment. Immunizations with live virus vaccines can be safely resumed within 6 months of cessation of therapy. Physicians must clearly demonstrate that their interest is in the child and the family and not just the disease the child has survived; at the same time, they must press for acceptance on the part of the child and family of indefinite follow-up for possible late effects (including second cancer) of the successful treatment of the malignancy.

LATE EFFECTS OF THERAPY

The late effects of anticancer therapy are becoming better understood as more children survive their disease.

Surgery leaves obvious and generally predictable ill effects. Intestinal obstruction secondary to abdominal surgery, locomotor problems secondary to musculoskeletal resection, pulmonary problems arising from thoracic surgery, central nervous system dysfunction as a consequence of intracranial or intraspinal surgery, and head and neck abnormalities secondary to regional surgery are late effects that are common but not as predictable. Surgical sequelae, therefore, must be specially considered in long-term evaluation. Every patient should receive a functional prognosis given by the oncologic surgeon for use in follow-up management.

Radiation and chemotherapy produce late effects that may be additive and hard to separate, although, overall, radiation seems the more potentially damaging. Growth problems are most commonly secondary to epiphyseal radiation damage. Growth hormone deficiency, thyroid dysfunction, and premature sexual maturation are more common in those treated with irradiation for brain tumors (and, with the thyroid, for head and neck tumors). Deficiencies in cognition, learning, and thus school performance are to be expected with brain irradiation of 2400 cGy or greater, as given to brain tumor patients, and, until recently, as prophylaxis (combined with intrathecal methotrexate) for acute lymphoblastic leukemia and non-Hodgkin's lymphoma. Gonadal irradiation in excess of 1800 cGy may (uncommonly) castrate and may be expected to produce deficient sperm production in both prepubertal and postpubertal males. Chemotherapy with alkylating agents (especially cyclophosphamide) may prevent sperm production. This effect is related to the total cumulative dose and is more likely to occur when therapy was given during or after puberty. The ovaries are more resistant, though ovarian failure is common with radiation doses over 4000 cGy. Late pulmonary fibrosis has been described with the use of busulfan, BCNU (carmustine), cyclophosphamide, mercaptopurine, bleomycin, and methotrexate, especially if radiation to the lung also occurred. Clinically significant liver damage is uncommon and, when seen, is usually secondary to fibrosis as a result of methotrexate and/or irradiation. Renovascular hypertension is an uncommon late complication of radiation to the kidney and/or chemotherapy for Wilms' tumor or neuroblastoma. Cisplatin may be expected to cause glomerular damage, usually mild, as well as sensorineural deafness, often profound. Ifosfamide may cause renal tubular dysfunction, and its cousin, cyclophosphamide, frequently induces angiomatous changes of the bladder wall which may lead to hematuria. Methyl CCNU (lomustine) is associated with long-term renal damage, resulting in renal insufficiency. The anthracyclines doxorubicin and daunorubicin regularly cause permanent, though not necessarily clinically significant, myocardial damage that is cumulative dose–related, more common in young children and often not manifested for years after therapy. Radiation to the heart increases the risk of damage at a lower cumulative dose of anthracycline. Periodic pre- and post-exercise echocardiographic studies are indicated indefinitely for anyone who received these agents, especially those receiving cumulative doses in excess of 450 mg/m^2. Permanent skin damage is now uncommon but was frequent with orthovoltage irradiation used in the past. Abdominal irradiation (commonly for Wilms' tumor) increases the risk for spontaneous abortion, infertility, and, to a minor extent, the chance for a low-birth-weight infant. There is no sound evidence to suggest an increased risk of birth defects after irradiation and/or chemotherapy. There is an increased chance for early menopause after abdominal irradiation.

As with surgery, every patient at cessation of therapy should receive a functional prognosis given by the radiotherapist and the pediatric oncologist for reference in follow-up management.

There is an increased incidence of psychologic difficulties in children cured of cancer compared with those in sibling controls, but in the main they are not severe. Survivors often perceive themselves as different from their peers as a consequence of their ordeal. Often this difference is perceived as an advantage, not a deficiency. Psychologic evaluation is best directed toward assessing the coping quality of the child and the family. School performance is the best indicator of the patient's ability to deal with the trauma of the past. Conferences with parents should be periodic. Group encounter sessions involving several parents of children with cancer who have completed therapy can be organized through support groups of the oncology center, hospital, or church. The adolescent needs special support as the desire for autonomy becomes more realistic. A psychologic assessment of the patient and family should be made at the end of therapy and periodically updated. This assessment should include psychometric testing, evaluation of coping mechanisms and their quality, assessment of quality of life and evidence of behavioral disturbances manifested as poor school performance, depression, anxiety, and chemical dependency.

RISK OF SECOND CANCER

Children cured of cancer are at increased risk for a second cancer, usually several years later. The type of the cured cancer, the way it was treated, the family history, and perhaps the age of the child when first treated are variables that influence this risk. Risk assessment information is changing as more and more data are available. Several studies have estimated an overall second cancer cumulative risk of 3 to 4 per cent at 15 to 20 years after the original cancer diagnosis. This contrasts with an estimated risk of a first cancer in a person 8 to 35 years of age—which is only 1 in 1000. Retinoblastoma and Hodgkin's disease have been treated successfully longer than other cancers and are thus overrepresented in published studies of second cancers; these two tumors are associated with a higher incidence of second primary cancer than most others, thereby further confounding large studies grouping all children surviving cancer. Certain syndromes (e.g., neurofibromatosis and multiple endocrine adenomatosis) increase the risk. Radiation, particularly orthovoltage, increases the risk of cancer in the irradiated field as well as leukemia, usually acute nonlymphocytic leukemia. Use of alkylating agents has been related to increased later risk of acute leukemia, with Ewing's sarcoma and Hodgkin's disease being primary diagnoses most highly correlated. More recently, the anthracyclines have been linked to a subsequent increased risk of leukemia. There is an increased risk of brain tumors in children given prophylactic cranial irradiation, often with concomitant intrathecal chemotherapy, in acute leukemia or lymphoma.

Such epidemiologic information is being combined with a growing body of information on families at increased risk of cancer to allow increasingly more valuable information to use in counseling the patient and family. Such information is already being used to justify alternative methods for treating a given cancer. Examples include nonalkylating agent therapy for Hodgkin's disease and no radiotherapy for Wilms' tumor or cranial radiation prophylaxis in leukemics.

Part of the prognostic information that should be developed for each child whose primary cancer treatment is ending must include second cancer risk. A detailed review of the current literature on types and risk of second neoplasms in child cancer survivors appears in the references.

The physician caring for a child cured of cancer should plan periodic follow-up indefinitely in order to assess (1) the child's and family's return to a more normal state of living, (2) evidence of development of organ or psychologic dysfunction, and (3) signs or symptoms to suggest relapse of the first cancer or a second malignancy. Management should also include provision of counseling about risk of late effects and interventions to treat social, behavioral and physical problems—problems that will indefinitely be assumed to be related to the first cancer and its treatment until proven otherwise. Finally, all the concerns related to the child cured of cancer are present and of even more concern in the survivor of a bone marrow transplant.

REFERENCES

Cullen JW: Second malignant neoplasms in survivors of childhood cancer. Pediatrician 18:82–89, 1991.

Green DM, D'Angio GJ: Late Effects of Treatment of Childhood Cancer. New York. Wiley-Liss, 1992.

8

Spleen and Lymphatic System

POST-SPLENECTOMY SEPSIS

FOUAD HAJJAR, M.D.
and HOWARD A. PEARSON, M.D.

Among its many functions, the spleen plays a major role in protection of the host against bacteria when the blood is infected. This role has been well documented since the first report on post-splenectomy sepsis in 1952 by King and Shumacker.

The anatomy of the spleen is unique. The spleen facilitates filtering foreign elements, such as bacteria, from the blood by phagocytosis; it also initiates the production of opsonic antibody by splenic lymphocytes.

Both the liver and spleen participate in filtration and phagocytosis. Efficient hepatic phagocytosis is opsonin-dependent and requires the presence of preformed specific antibodies (IgM or IgG) and complement. The spleen, in contrast, can clear organisms effectively in the absence of specific antibody. In the nonimmune host, therefore, the spleen performs most of the filtration and phagocytic activity; in its absence, bacteria cannot be cleared effectively from the blood. As a result, overwhelming bacteremia ensues.

Severe or fatal sepsis with disseminated intravascular coagulation (DIC) in patients with functional or anatomic asplenia (post-splenectomy infection, PSI) is a well-recognized phenomenon. Although the risk of PSI is lifelong, risk is greatest in young children in the first year following surgery, probably as a result of the paucity of naturally acquired antibodies. The reason for splenectomy is another important determinant of risk. The incidence of infection is greater in patients splenectomized for an underlying hematologic or oncologic disease than in patients splenectomized for trauma. The increased risk is especially high if there is a concomitant immunologic abnormality.

The organisms responsible for PSI are, in most cases, encapsulated bacteria. *Streptococcus pneumoniae,* irrespective of serotype, causes more than half of such infections. Implicated next most often are *Haemophilus influenzae* type b (HIB) and *Neisseria meningitidis. Escherichia coli, Pseudomonas aeruginosa, Staphylococcus aureus,* and group B streptococci have caused PSI in small numbers of patients. Increased severity of malaria and of babesiosis have been described also in splenectomized patients.

IMMUNIZATION

Since *S. pneumoniae* and *H. influenzae* type b cause the majority of cases of PSI and because polysaccharide vaccines are available, immunization against infection with these organisms should be performed prior to elective splenectomy or immediately thereafter in cases of emergency splenectomy. These polysaccharide antigens stimulate the formation of circulating antibodies in the immunologically mature asplenic patient, although their immunogenicity in unconjugated form in infants and young children may be sharply limited. A polyvalent pneumococcal vaccine composed of the unconjugated capsular polysaccharides of the 23 capsular types responsible for approximately 90 per cent of invasive pneumococcal infections is available. Children under 2 years of age may respond poorly to this vaccine. If a child is vaccinated before 2 to 3 years of age, revaccination may be desirable at age 6 to 8 years, although definitive evidence supporting this practice is lacking. Rarely, severe local reaction may follow revaccination of adults, but such reactions do not appear to be a problem in children.

The newly available conjugate HIB vaccine to prevent infection with *H. influenzae* type b is immunogenic in infants as young as 2 to 3 months of age. It is especially important that it be administered to asplenic children younger than 2 years of age. A booster dose of vaccine should be given at age 5.

A tetravalent meningococcal polysaccharide vaccine to prevent infection with organisms of serogroups A, C, Y, and W-135 is available (in the United States). Most of these polysaccharides are not predictably immunogenic in children younger than 2 years of age. The vaccine is recommended for asplenic patients 2 years of age and older.

It should be emphasized that there are no studies demonstrating conclusively the efficacy of these vaccines in preventing PSI. However, vaccination against the encapsulated bacteria is recommended because the vaccines are safe and the infections they are designed to prevent are often fatal.

PROPHYLACTIC ANTIBIOTICS

Prophylactic penicillin, used in patients younger than 4 years of age with the functional hyposplenism from sickle cell disease, decreases the incidence of pneumococcal sepsis by 85 per cent. Penicillin prophylaxis is indicated for all young asplenic patients. The recommended dosage for infants younger than 6 months is 62.5 mg of Penicillin VK orally, twice daily; 125 mg orally twice daily for those between 6 months and 2 years; and for those over the age of 2 years, 250 mg orally twice daily.. Erythromycin may be substituted for penicillin in allergic patients.

Some authorities recommend indefinite penicillin prophylaxis in all asplenic patients. Others do not use it in children older than 6 years of age. A study currently in progress should determine whether or not prophylactic penicillin can be stopped safely in children with sickle cell disease at 6 years of age.

It is very important to apprise asplenic patients and their families about the role of the spleen and to instruct them to seek immediate medical attention for any significant febrile illnesses (temperature > 102°F). Health care providers should also be aware of possible serious significance of fever in asplenic patients.

TREATMENT OF SUSPECTED SEPSIS

Any significant febrile illness (temperature > 102°F), or lower grades of fever if the patient has chills, in a splenectomized patient should be taken seriously. Blood culture specimens should be obtained. *Appropriate intravenous antibiotic therapy should be instituted immediately, even before culture reports are available.* Antibiotics should be selected based on the most common pathogens and certainly should be active against pneumococci and *H. influenzae.* We recommend intravenous (IV) cefuroxime (150 mg/kg/day divided in three doses IV) or ceftriaxone (50 mg/kg/day in a single dose IV).

When the patient appears ill, hospitalization is indicated. Even if not admitted, febrile patients should be closely observed for several hours after the institution of antibiotic therapy.

SPLENECTOMY, CONSERVATIVE MANAGEMENT

Splenectomies should be performed only when absolutely indicated, and, when possible, an attempt should be made to defer splenectomy in infants and younger children until a later age (older than 6 years). Pediatric surgeons have become more conservative in the management of splenic trauma and splenic rupture. It is often possible to manage these patients nonoperatively. Splenic repair, partial splenectomy, and peritoneal implantation (induction of splenosis) have also been advocated.

INDICATIONS FOR SPLENECTOMY

FOUAD HAJJAR, M.D.
and HOWARD A. PEARSON, M.D.

There are a number of indications for splenectomy. However, because of the recognition of the syndrome of overwhelming post-splenectomy sepsis (PSI), patients should be evaluated individually in decisions regarding the necessity and timing of the operation. Because the incidence of PSI is highest in infancy and early childhood, whenever possible the operation should be deferred until the child is at least 6 years of age.

The indications for splenectomy can be divided into medical and surgical categories.

MEDICAL INDICATIONS

Congenital Hemolytic Anemias

Hereditary spherocytosis and hemolytic elliptocytosis are related to abnormalities of spectrin, an important constituent of the red blood cell membrane. These diseases are manifested as chronic hemolytic anemias, and many patients with well-compensated hemolysis are totally asymptomatic. Removal of the spleen completely corrects the hemolysis, although the membrane defect persists. Early splenectomy (before age 6 years) should be considered only in children with severe anemia that affects growth and activity. Splenectomy may prevent cholelithiases and the rare aplastic crises.

Certain severe, nonspherocytic hemolytic anemias (pyruvate kinase deficiency) are improved—although not usually cured—by splenectomy.

Immunohematologic Disorders

Splenectomy may be indicated for children with very severe or chronic immunohematologic disorders—notably idiopathic thrombocytopenia purpura (ITP) and autoimmune hemolytic anemia (AIHA).

In childhood, ITP is usually self-limited, more than 90 per cent of patients recovering within 9 to 12 months. Chronic (> 1 year's duration) cases are usually cured or substantially improved by splenectomy. However, rare causes of chronic thrombocytopenia—especially the Wiskott-Aldrich syndrome—must be considered and excluded before one recommends the operation in young males.

Most cases of AIHA are very acute but self-limited. Chronic cases may benefit from splenectomy. In multiply transfused patients (e.g., those with refractory anemias, Cooley's anemia) a state of accelerated destruction of transfused red blood cells often develops. Splenectomy usually corrects this, even when the spleen is not greatly enlarged.

Staging for Hodgkin's Disease

Staging laparotomy and splenectomy are still advised for patients with stage I and II Hodgkin's disease for whom radiation therapy is the treatment of choice. Partial splenectomy is not advocated. More extensive disease (stage III and IV) is treated primarily with systemic chemotherapy, and staging laparotomy and splenectomy are not generally employed.

Hypersplenism

The term hypersplenism is used when four elements are present: (1) peripheral cytopenia, (2) normal or increased marrow production of the affected cell line, (3) significant splenomegaly, and (4) cure after splenectomy. Obviously, a diagnosis of hypersplenism is often entertained even when all of these criteria are not met.

Patients with massive splenomegaly, as in lipidoses, especially Gaucher's disease, often have low white blood cell and/or platelet counts. Such "cytopenias" may reflect increased dilution in an enlarged splenic pool rather than accelerated destruction. Therefore, splenectomy may not be indicated unless infection or bleeding is occurring. However, in massive splenomegaly, splenectomy may be indicated in order to relieve the considerable mechanical burden of a greatly enlarged organ.

SURGICAL INDICATIONS

Splenic Cysts

Splenic pseudocysts result from liquefaction of intrasplenic hemorrhage and most often are a result of splenic trauma. Splenic pseudocysts and rare "true cysts" may necessitate splenectomy because of their large size. Ultrasonography is diagnostic. Splenic malignancies other than those of reticuloendothelial origin are very rare.

Traumatic Rupture of the Spleen

Long considered an absolute indication for emergency splenectomy, traumatic injury of the spleen is now approached more selectively. Most instances of acute splenic injury can be managed nonoperatively if the patient and the hematocrit value are stable. Serial imaging studies show spontaneous repair of the lacerated spleen within 1 to 2 months. If the patient is hemodynamically unstable, splenorrhaphy or other techniques to surgically repair the spleen may obviate the need for total excision.

The risk of PSI infection after removal of the spleen because of trauma is low, especially in children older than 6 years of age. Splenosis subsequently develops in about 50 per cent of children undergoing splenectomy for trauma, but the protective effect of splenosis is uncertain.

LYMPH NODE INFECTIONS

BASIL J. ZITELLI, M.D.

Lymph node infections in children are common and usually affect toddlers and older children to a greater extent than neonates. Lymph nodes are normally palpable in children, with the anterior cervical and inguinal nodes most easily palpable. Anterior cervical nodes are abnormally enlarged if they measure greater than 1.0 cm, and inguinal lymph nodes are enlarged if they are larger than 1.5 cm in diameter. Lymph node enlargement is caused by several different pathologic processes but generally is secondary to either expansion of existing cellular elements such as lymphocytes and histiocytes, or invasion by cells extrinsic to lymph nodes, such as malignant cells or polymorphonuclear leukocytes, during bacterial infection. The evaluation of lymph nodes should include location, size, shape, consistency, mobility, inflammation, suppuration, and skin discoloration as well as examination for noncontiguous adenopathy and evidence for systemic disease.

ACUTE ADENITIS

Acute suppurative lymphadenitis in children is generally thought to be due to invasion of the lymph node by infectious agents from some distal site. Knowledge of regional lymph node drainage areas may help the clinician to find the primary infectious site. Cervical lymphadenitis is most common in children and must be distinguished from infected congenital lesions such as thyroglossal duct cyst, branchial cleft cyst, and cystic hygroma. Reactive lymphadenopathy from common viral infections usually produces bilateral, mildly enlarged, minimally tender, discrete nodes whose changes generally parallel the course of the respiratory infection. Rubella, erythema infectiosum, roseola infantum, and other common childhood viral illnesses may be associated with posterior auricular and occipital lymph node enlargement. Epstein-Barr virus, cytomegalovirus, and human immunodeficiency virus (HIV) infections may cause generalized lymphadenopathy associated with a clinical picture of infectious mononucleosis. Kawasaki syndrome features unilateral cervical lymph node enlargement as part of its diagnostic criteria; however, cervical adenopathy may be the least consistent clinical finding, especially among white patients. Viral infections are usually self-limited, and generally no specific therapy is required.

The child with acute, suppurative cervical lymphadenitis may present with fever, toxicity, and rapid enlargement of a tender, erythematous mass, usually in the lateral neck. A prodrome of an upper respiratory infection may have preceded the onset of adenitis by 2 to 3 days. Leukocytosis with a left shift is common. A careful examination of the ears, pharynx, and tonsils as well as a meticulous dental examination may yield the source of the primary infection. Because up to 80 per cent of acute unilateral suppurative cervical lymphadenitis is caused by *Staphylococcus aureus* or group A beta-hemolytic *Streptococcus*, needle aspiration generally is not recommended if the node is not fluctuant.

Therapy can be initiated with a semisynthetic penicillin or cephalosporin to cover both staphylococci and streptococci. Dicloxacillin sodium (50 to 100 mg/kg/day in four divided doses) or cephalexin (50 to 100 mg/kg/day in four divided doses) continued for 10 days may be adequate oral therapy. If oral therapy fails, intravenous therapy with a beta-lactamase–resistant semisynthetic penicillin (e.g., nafcillin, 100 mg/kg/day in four divided doses) should be initiated.

Young infants up to 7 weeks of age may have acute lymphadenitis associated with otitis media, poor feeding, and bacteremia. In addition to the usual pathogens mentioned above, group B *Streptococcus* has been implicated as a major pathogen. These infants should be admitted and given intravenous therapy for presumed sepsis with nafcillin (100 mg/kg/day) *and* gentamicin (7.5 mg/kg/day in three divided doses). When group B streptococcus has been identified nafcillin can be discontinued and penicillin 100,000 units to 200,000 units/kg/day in four divided doses may be substituted. Rarely, isolated anaerobic infections, *Haemophilus influenzae,* and fungi may cause suppurative lymphadenitis.

Diagnostic aspiration of a lymph node generally is not necessary in the usual patient, but it may aid in the specific bacteriologic diagnosis in patients not responding to therapy or in immunocompromised hosts in whom opportunistic infections can occur. If the node softens and becomes fluctuant, incision and drainage should be performed. A drain should be placed in the abscess, and material should be obtained for culture and Gram's stain. Anaerobic, acid-fast, and fungal specimens for culture should be obtained. The drain may be removed when there is adequate saucerization of the wound.

SUBACUTE ADENITIS

Subacute or chronic infections of lymph nodes are commonly caused by cat-scratch disease (CSD) or mycobacterial infection. CSD follows contact with a cat, a cat scratch or a cat lick on an open skin wound. (See article in Section 18.) CSD generally is benign, and lymph nodes often will regress spontaneously over several months. Excision of the involved node is generally curative. Although no results from double-blinded, comparative antibiotic trials have been published, a variety of antibiotics have been tried. In children, intravenous gentamicin (5 mg/kg/day in three divided doses) for 10 to 14 days was associated with clinical improvement in systemic CSD. Oral trimethoprim-sulfamethoxazole (40 mg/kg/day in two divided doses) for 7 days also was associated with improvement of regional lymph node infections in children. Ciprofloxacin has been used to treat adults with CSD lymphadenitis; however, this antibiotic is not recommended for use in children. Therapy is not recommended in patients with uncomplicated local infections.

Tuberculous lymphadenitis is relatively uncommon with most mycobacterial lymph node infections due to *Mycobacterium scrofulaceum* or *Mycobacterium avium–intracellulare.* Therapy of *M. tuberculosis* adenitis is the same as for pulmonary tuberculosis. Atypical mycobacterial infections may spontaneously suppurate and drain. Antibiotic therapy for atypical mycobacterial disease is generally not indicated or necessary.

Spontaneous resolution may occur over several months, or excision of the involved nodes may hasten cure.

UNCOMMON CAUSES OF LYMPHADENITIS

Less common lymph node infections are caused by *Yersinia pestis* (plague), *Francisella tularensis* (tularemia), and *Chlamydia trachomatis* (lymphogranuloma venereum). Humans may become infected with *Y. pestis* through domestic animals that have had contact with infected wildlife. High fever, malaise, weakness, chills, and development of large, fixed, exquisitely tender regional lymph nodes are typical of bubonic plague. Therapy for children under 8 years of age consists of streptomycin (30 mg/kg/day in two divided doses) or chloramphenicol sodium succinate (50 mg/kg/day in four divided doses) for 10 days. Children older than 8 years may receive tetracycline (25 to 50 mg/kg/day in four divided doses).

Tularemia is most frequently contracted by contact with infected animals or their carcasses, producing fever, headache, malaise, vomiting, and, in one form, development of tender, swollen axillary or inguinal lymph nodes. A portal of entry sometimes can be seen as an ulcerated papule distal to the regional adenopathy. Therapy consists of gentamicin (6 mg/kg/day in three divided doses) or streptomycin (30 mg/kg/day in two divided doses) for 7 to 10 days. The streptomycin dose may be reduced to 15 mg/kg/day after 3 days.

Lymphogranuloma venereum is a sexually transmitted infection. Primary lesions of small, multiple tender papules or ulcers are seldom seen. Bilateral inguinal adenopathy with rectal bleeding and ulceration is a more common finding. In patients older than 8 years of age, tetracycline (40 mg/kg/day in four divided doses) is given orally for 21 days. Effective therapy includes oral doxycycline (4 mg/kg/day, maximum dose 200 mg, divided in two doses). Erythromycin and sulfisoxazole are also probably effective and are indicated in children younger than 8 years.

LYMPHEDEMA

JAMES M. LEWIS, M.D.

Lymphedema is defined as chronic swelling of a body part due to the accumulation of lymph in interstitial tissues. This imbalance in lymph formation and transport may be due to maldevelopment or dysfunction of lymphatic vessels, lymph node obstruction, or chronic venous stasis.

Lymphedema is broadly classified as either primary (idiopathic) or secondary. *Secondary lymphedemas* are caused by processes that destroy or obstruct the lymphatic vessels and nodes: neoplasm (primary or metastatic), recurrent lymphangitis or cellulitis, parasitic infestation, excisional surgery, trauma, and irradiation. Although the etiology of *primary lymphedema* is unknown, evidence points to an underlying developmental insufficiency that may be triggered by environmental factors. The continuum of primary lymphedemas is further subdivided by age of onset into congenital, praecox (3 months to 35 years), and tarda (greater than 35 years). *Milroy's disease* is strictly defined as familial congenital lymphedema, whereas *Meige's disease* represents familial lymphedema praecox. Primary lymphedema may be present in several genetic disorders, including Turner syndrome, Noonan syndrome, distichiasis-lymphedema syndrome, intestinal lymphangiectasis, and yellow nail syndrome.

DIAGNOSIS

The diagnosis of lymphedema is made clinically by careful history and physical examination. Lymphedema praecox most commonly presents as insidious, painless swelling in the lower extremity of an adolescent girl. Lymphoscintigraphy with technetium-99m (^{99m}Tc)–labeled antimony-sulfur colloid may be helpful in questionable cases both to diagnose lymphedema and to differentiate primary from secondary causes. *Lymphangiograms, venograms, and biopsy are not indicated.*

TREATMENT

The treatment of secondary lymphedemas is directed toward the underlying etiologic agent. *Filariasis,* a common cause of lymphedema in tropical countries, may be treated early with diethylcarbamazine to decrease lymphangitis and prevent fibrosis. In later stages, lymph nodovenous shunting procedures may be performed to create alternate pathways for lymphatic drainage. Severe lymphedema or elephantiasis with extreme disfigurement, decreased mobility, and recurrent lymphangitis may require subcutaneous excisional procedures, such as the Charles operation.

The treatment of idiopathic primary lymphedema consists primarily of supportive measures to decrease tissue fluid, improve existing lymphatic flow, and prevent further subcutaneous fibrosis. Lymphedema, however, is a chronic disease with no therapeutic regimen available to completely restore the extremity to a normal appearance. Although diuretics have been effective in reducing edema in adults, they are not recommended for pediatric patients. The affected lower extremity should be elevated by raising the foot of the bed 6 to 12 inches at night and maintaining a horizontal position during the day as often as possible. Exercise may improve lymphatic flow by the extrinsic compression of lymph vessels by muscle contractions and arterial pulsations. The external support of a carefully fitted, high-pressure elastic stocking (Jobst) will augment this effect and prevent further accumulation of fluid. Intermittent, sequential compression of the limb by a programmable pneumatic pump (Jobst, Wright Linear, Lympha-Press) in a daily regimen (used at night) combined with elastic hose has provided dramatic improvement in selected patients. Progressive injury to lymphatics causing worsening of the edema may be prevented by the avoidance of trauma, careful hygiene of the skin and nails, and prophylaxis or vigorous treatment of bacterial or fungal infections.

Cellulitis and lymphangitis secondary to group A streptococci or coagulase-positive staphylococci are frequent complications of lymphedema. Typically, chills and fever develop and patients may appear toxic with lethargy, headache, nausea and vomiting. Local signs include erythema, induration, tenderness, enlargement of the extremity or lymph nodes, and red streaking. Therapy should include intravenous antibiotics, bed rest, moist heat, and analgesics. Lymphangiosarcoma is a rare, late but dreaded complication of lymphedema. The development of a violaceous lesion, especially if accompanied by ulceration or necrosis, necessitates prompt diagnosis by multiple, deep biopsy specimens followed by aggressive medical and surgical therapy.

Surgical treatment of lymphedema is reserved for patients with severe, progressive disease with complications who do not respond to intensive medical therapy. Because of the unpredictable course of primary lymphedema, surgery should be postponed until the full extent of the swelling is apparent or the child is older than 2 years of age. Procedures to debulk genital lymphedema, however, may be the exception to this rule. All surgical options are associated with a low success rate along with frequent complications, persistent disproportion, and residual scarring.

The chronic, progressive nature of lymphedema often causes considerable family, social, and emotional problems, particularly for adolescents. Patients and parents can benefit from thorough explanations, genetic counseling if appropriate, and opportunities to express feelings and participate in therapeutic decisions.

REFERENCES

Klein MJ, Alexander MA, Wright JM, et al: Treatment of adult lower extremity lymphedema with the Wright Linear Pump: Statistical analysis of a clinical trial. Arch Phys Med Rehabil 69:202–206, 1988.

Lewis JM, Wald ER: Lymphedema praecox. J Pediatr 104:641–648, 1984.

Smeltzer DM, Stickler GB, Schirger A: Primary lymphedema in children and adolescents: A follow-up study and review. Pediatrics 76:206–218, 1985.

LYMPHANGIOMA

WILLIAM J. POKORNY, M.D.

Lymphangiomas are tumors of the lymphatic system that result from obstruction of developing anomalous lymphatic vessels. The lymphatic system arises from five primitive lymphatic sacs: the paired jugular sacs in the neck, a single sac at the root of the mesentery, and paired posterior sacs in relationship to sciatic veins. The peripheral lymphatic vessels form as outbuddings from these five sacs.

CLASSIFICATION

Lymphangiomas have been classified into three macroscopic forms: (1) lymphangioma simplex, or capillary lymphangioma; (2) cavernous lymphangiomas, which consist of dilated lymphatic channels; and (3) cystic lymphangiomas, or cystic hygroma, which consist of large lymphatic "lakes" measuring 1 to 5 cm in diameter. These lakes are typically multiple and may or may not communicate. Lesions are frequently mixed in character.

During childhood lymphangiomas most commonly take the form of cystic hygroma and typically occur in or about the neck as a result of sequestration or obstruction of one of the jugular lymphatic sacs in the neck. Mesenteric or omental cysts result from obstruction of the developing lymphatics from the sac at the root of the mesentery. Congenital lymphedema and intestinal lymphangiectasia may represent variations of these malformations caused by congenital lymphatic obstruction.

DIAGNOSIS

Routine antenatal ultrasonographic evaluation has significantly contributed to our understanding of this anomaly. It is now known that cervical lymphangiomas detected by ultrasonography during the second trimester of fetal development differ from those diagnosed at, or shortly after, birth and treated by the pediatric surgeon. Cervical lymphangiomas are divided into two distinct types: (1) the *posterior, bilateral form,* which is diagnosed by antenatal ultrasound, and (2) the *anterior, unilateral form,* which may develop during the first 2 years of life. Each carries a very different prognosis, although both result from a failure of the cisterna chyli to communicate with the jugular vein.

Posterior Lesions

The posterior and more common type of cervical lymphangioma is recognized during the second trimester of fetal development. These lymphangiomas occur as bilateral swellings of the jugular lymphatic sacs. Approximately 78 per cent of affected fetuses have chromosomal anomalies. The majority of these are 45X karyotype or 45X/46XX mosaicism. The remainder are autosomal trisomies and, less commonly, various chromosomal structural anomalies. The 45X fetuses typically have an association of posterior cervical cystic hygroma, generalized subcutaneous edema, and a preductal coarctation. *The thickened, webbed neck seen in patients with Turner syndrome is the end result of this localized lymphatic obstruction.* The majority of fetuses with normal karyotypes are found to have other anomalies, so that the posterior cystic hygroma may be only one manifestation of a broader pattern of malformations, including autosomal recessive disorders and possible teratogenic exposure. *Recent reports of cases of posterior cervical lymphangiomas suggest that chances that a pregnancy will produce a healthy child is less than 1 in 10. Because of this poor prognosis, most couples now opt for pregnancy termination.* To aid in genetic counseling, an antenatal cytogenetic analysis should be performed at the time of ultrasonographic detection, particularly if the karyotype is normal. An autopsy is essential in all nonsurvivors to define the anomalies and aid in genetic counseling of the family.

Anterior Lesions

In contrast to the posterior lesion, the anterior cervical lymphangioma is usually unilateral; it is an isolated lesion present at birth in 50 to 60 per cent of patients, or it becomes apparent during the next 2 to 3 years. The differential diagnosis of these lesions includes teratoma, sarcoma, hemangioma, neuroblastoma, and goiter. Although growth of the lesion is unpredictable, rapid growth may occur in intermittent periods. Transient enlargement typically occurs with upper respiratory tract infection. Spontaneous regression occurs but is quite uncommon. These tumors may become quite large and present a mechanical obstacle to birth and may actually require a cesarean section. Anterior cervical tumors may also obstruct the airway of the developing fetus requiring immediate intubation or tracheostomy. For this reason, the obstetrician must work closely with the pediatrician and pediatric surgeon, who should be immediately available at delivery. Cystic hygromas diagnosed after birth typically consist of thin-walled, multiloculated cysts that contain clear lymph fluid. Despite the fact that these are benign lesions, the cysts may invade tissue planes and appear to infiltrate normal tissue. The majority are asymptomatic and present as soft, fluid-filled masses in the subcutaneous tissue of the posterior triangle of the neck and axilla. However, depending on their location within the developing fetus and infant, they may be symptomatic and life-threatening. Involvement of the tongue, pharynx, or larynx may result in airway obstruction, and pressure on the periodontal tissue may result in a loss of teeth and deformity of the mandible.

TREATMENT

Surgical excision is the treatment of choice. Because of the potential growth with extension into previously uninvolved areas and the hazard of infection, particularly following upper respiratory infections, delay in surgical treatment is unwarranted. However, the surgeon must keep in mind that these are not malignant lesions and, although total excision is ideal, one should not damage or sacrifice normal structures or disfigure the child. If the tumor is totally excised, recurrence is uncommon. On the other hand, if small amounts of cystic tumor are left, the recurrence rate is 10 to 15 per cent. Various sclerosing agents have been used to destroy the lining of any remaining cysts.

Mesenteric cysts may become huge, presenting as a distended, nontender abdomen and may be confused with ascites. They also result from obstructed lymphatics and are typically filled with clear or milky lymphatic fluid. Ultrasonography is usually diagnostic, and the treatment is surgical excision.

Intestinal lymphangiectasia results from congenital lymphatic obstruction of the peripheral lymphatics. The dilated lymphatics involve the lamina propria, submucosa, and serosa. These patients typically present with malabsorption caused by loss of protein into the gut and, if they remain untreated, malnutrition, growth retardation, anemia, hypoproteinemia, and lymphocytopenia will develop. Chylous ascites may also be associated with intestinal lymphangiectasia. Typical roentgenographic findings of the gastrointestinal tract include thickening of the jejunal folds, flocculation of the barium within the lumen of the gut, and dilatation of the small bowel. Duodenal or jejunal biopsy will confirm the diagnosis. Treatment consists of a high-protein, medium-chain triglyceride diet. Intractable chylous ascites may be treated with a peritoneal-venous shunt.

Congenital lymphedema most commonly involves the lower extremity, particularly the dorsum of the foot. The amount of swelling typically lessens during the first 2 years of life, and for this reason therapy should be directed at protecting the extremity from injury and infection. Operative intervention should be reserved only for patients with severe congenital lymphedema that persists beyond 3 years of life.

(See preceding article on lymphedema.)

MALIGNANT LYMPHOMA

WILLIAM L. CARROLL, M.D.

Childhood lymphomas are diseases of the lymphoreticular system and are broadly classified into *Hodgkin's disease* and *non-Hodgkin's lymphoma* (NHL). Although NHL originates in developing B cells and thymocytes, the cell of origin in Hodgkin's disease remains uncertain. In general, the natural history of Hodgkin's disease in children is similar to that in adults. Disease usually spreads from one lymph node area to a contiguous group. In contrast, many cases of NHL are disseminated at diagnosis even though only limited organ involvement may be appreciated on clinical examination. These biologic differences are apparent in the treatment philosophy guiding clinicians in the care of these patients. In addition to eradicating disease, attention needs to be given to minimizing the side effects of treatment on the developing child.

HODGKIN'S DISEASE

The successful treatment of children with Hodgkin's disease continues to evolve. The major issue today is not whether cure can be achieved but what is the safest modality to use in the developing child. Greater emphasis is being placed on avoiding the long-term complications of treatment.

Staging

Accurate staging of Hodgkin's disease is essential in planning appropriate therapy, determining prognosis, and comparing newer treatment strategies designed to minimize side effects of therapy. The Ann Arbor staging system is universally accepted and is shown in Table 1.

TABLE 1. Ann Arbor Clinical Staging Classification for Hodgkin's Disease

Stage I*	Involvement of a single lymph node region (I) or single extralymphatic organ or site (Ie).
Stage II	Involvement of two or more lymph node regions on the same side of the diaphragm (II) or localized involvement of an extralymphatic organ or site and one or more lymph node regions on the same side of the diaphragm (IIe).
Stage III	Involvement of lymph node regions on both sides of the diaphragm (III), which may be associated with splenic involvement (IIIs) or by localized involvement of an extralymphatic organ or site (IIIe) or both (IIIse).
Stage IV	Diffuse or disseminated involvement of one or more extralymphatic organs or tissues, with or without associated lymph node involvement.

*The absence or presence of fever, night sweats, or unexplained loss of greater than 10 per cent body weight in the preceding 6 months is denoted by the suffix letters A or B, respectively.

In addition to a careful history and physical examination with particular attention to lymph node size and character, the laboratory evaluation includes a complete blood count, liver and renal profile, erythrocyte sedimentation rate, and alkaline phosphatase and serum copper levels. Although the latter tests are frequently used in adults to monitor disease activity, findings may be falsely elevated in the growing child or may be associated with acute inflammation. Radiographic assessment to identify all sites of disease usually includes chest radiography and computed tomography (CT) of the chest, abdomen, and pelvis. Additional information may be provided by magnetic resonance imaging (MRI), and serial radionuclide scans with gallium-67 may be useful to assess residual disease activity in nodal groups that remain enlarged despite an initial response to treatment. Radiographic assessment of the retroperitoneum and spleen is often problematic in younger children. Bipedal lymphangiography is an excellent test to evaluate potential disease in iliac and lower para-aortic lymph nodes but may be technically difficult in the younger child. A bone marrow aspirate and biopsy are routinely performed to evaluate potential disease in this organ.

The role of staging laparotomy, which typically includes splenectomy, liver biopsy, and sampling of subdiaphragmatic nodal groups, is controversial. One third of patients with clinical stages I and II as determined by clinical and radiographic assessment are found to have subdiaphragmatic disease when surgical staging is performed. Therefore, surgical staging is beneficial in planning radiation therapy and is mandatory for patients being treated with this modality alone. Additionally, in girls an oophoropexy can be performed to remove these structures from the radiation field in patients with pelvic disease. Surgical staging, however, is currently being performed much less frequently for childhood Hodgkin's disease. Few children are being treated with radiation therapy alone. More effective regimens of systemic chemotherapy are likely to eliminate radiographically inapparent disease in most patients, thus rendering a staging laparotomy unnecessary. The surgery itself may be associated with complications such as post-splenectomy sepsis.

Treatment

Remarkable cure rates for Hodgkin's disease have been achieved with radiation therapy, chemotherapy, or a combination of both modalities. In general, children and adolescents enjoy a better prognosis than older adults, with 10-year, relapse-free survival rates approaching 90 per cent. With such excellent results, particular attention must be given to minimizing the long-term side effects of therapy on children undergoing active growth and development. Stage I and IIe patients without large mediastinal masses may be treated with radiation therapy alone. Doses of 35 to 40 Gy to clinically involved areas and adjacent lymph node groups (extended field) are curative in 60 to 90 per cent of cases. A select group of stage I patients with disease confined to the upper neck can be treated with radiation therapy limited to the involved nodal group alone (involved field). However, a significant amount of soft tissue deformity and impaired bone growth may be seen in younger children who receive such high-dose radiation therapy. In an effort to avoid such side effects, investigators have previously used combined modality therapy employing both low-dose (15 to 25 Gy) involved field radiation therapy and chemotherapy. Increasing concern about the long-term side effects of radiation therapy, such as delayed bone growth and the development of second malignancies, has led to the diminished use of this modality. Few children are currently treated with radiation therapy alone. Greater reliance on effective chemotherapy has eliminated the use of radiation therapy in many protocols.

MOPP (nitrogen mustard (M), Oncovin [vincristine] (O), procarbazine (P), prednisone (P)), was the first highly successful drug combination in the treatment of Hodgkin's disease (Table 2). Six cycles is a standard duration of treatment for most patients. Newer combinations, including CVPP (cyclophosphamide, vinblastine, procarbazine, prednisone) and COPP (cyclophosphamide, vincristine, procarbazine, prednisone), have not been found to be significantly superior to MOPP. The major acute side effects of this therapy include vomiting, alopecia, and pancytopenia. Of more concern are the long-term complications of sterility and second malignancies. ABVD (doxorubicin [Adriamycin], bleomycin, vinblastine, dacarbazine) (Table 2), an alternative combination containing non–cross-resistant drugs, appears to be as effective and perhaps somewhat superior to MOPP. It is also effective in patients who fail to respond to MOPP. However, it can be associated with pulmonary fibrosis and cardiomyopathy owing to bleomycin and Adriamycin, respectively. Since all such complications are dose-related, many current protocols utilize alternating cycles of MOPP-ABVD, thereby limiting the total doses of each regimen.

Children with advanced-stage disease are treated primarily with chemotherapy. In general, six to 12 courses of therapy are given. The prognosis for these patients is also excellent: up to 77 per cent of patients with stage IVB disease are free of tumor at 5 years when treated with 12 cycles of alternating MOPP-ABVD. Studies have shown that patients who receive significantly less than the prescribed doses of these medications do less well; thus, it is important that therapy be delivered on schedule without decreasing doses unless significant toxicities develop. Again, radiation therapy may be used in conjunction with chemotherapy but is often reserved for sites of initial bulky disease or targeted to sites of incomplete regression.

Therapy for Relapse

Patients who fail to improve after receiving radiation therapy alone have an excellent outcome when treated with chemotherapy. In fact, the chance of achieving cure is identical to that for previously untreated patients of the same stage.

Therapy for patients who experience relapse after chemotherapy is more problematic. Patients relapsing after MOPP frequently achieve a second remission with these same drugs. Response is especially favorable in patients who had an initial clinical remission that lasted longer than 12 months. ABVD or a combination of ABVD-MOPP may also be used with equally good results. Patients who relapse after MOPP-ABVD combination therapy may achieve a second clinical remission, but rarely is this result durable. These patients may experience multiple relapses over a prolonged time period but eventually succumb to their disease. Newer drug combinations, such as APE (cytarabine, cisplatin, etoposide) appear promising, but longer follow-up is needed. High-dose chemotherapy followed by autologous bone marrow transplantation is a treatment option, with one third of patients remaining free of disease after such therapy.

Late Effects

The successful therapy for Hodgkin's disease has led to the recognition of the late effects of radiotherapy and chemotherapy in children. The most serious of all side effects is the development of a second malignant tumor. This risk approaches 10 per cent at 15 years. The risk for leukemia and NHL is greatest 5 to 10 years after completion of therapy and is related to the use of alkylating agents. The incidence of solid tumors continues to rise over time, and these appear to be associated with the use of radiation therapy.

Sterility is another serious side effect. Girls who receive pelvic irradiation face a high risk for ovarian failure, and therefore ovarian transposition preceding treatment is required. Most girls treated for Hodgkin's disease without pelvic irradiation maintain fertility. Male sterility is a more significant problem, with azoospermia developing in the majority of males after six cycles of MOPP. ABVD carries a lower risk of this problem, with azoospermia developing in less than a third of patients. However, a small portion of patients may recover testicular function many years later.

Thyroid dysfunction is commonly seen after radiotherapy, and patients should be followed up with regular thyroid function tests. The cardiomyopathy associated with doxorubicin may be enhanced in patients receiving mediastinal irradiation. Children should be followed up with echocardiography or cardiac nuclear gated angiography. Pulmonary

TABLE 2. Treatment Regimens for Hodgkin's Disease

	Dose (mg/m²)	Route	Days
MOPP*			
Mechlorethamine (nitrogen mustard)	6	IV	1, 8
Oncovin (vincristine)	1.4 (maximum dose 2 mg)	IV	1, 8
Procarbazine	100	p.o.	1 to 14
Prednisone	40	p.o.	1 to 14
ABVD*			
Adriamycin (doxorubicin)	25	IV	1, 15
Bleomycin	10	IV	1, 15
Vinblastine	6	IV	1, 15
Dacarbazine	375	IV	1, 15

*Cycles repeated every 28 days.

function tests should also be performed in patients who have received bleomycin because up to 40 per cent of children may display abnormalities. These side effects emphasize the price of cure for the patient with Hodgkin's disease. The current challenge is to minimize their occurrence without sacrificing the gratifying results achieved with modern treatment.

NON-HODGKIN'S LYMPHOMA

The non-Hodgkin's lymphomas of childhood are distinctly different from those that occur in adults. Almost all of these tumors bear diffuse architecture and display high-grade aggressive behavior. Low-grade follicular lymphomas are distinctly rare in children. Childhood NHL is a somewhat heterogeneous group of diseases that can be classified on the basis of clinical characteristics, histopathology, immune phenotype, and cytogenetic features. Most pediatric cases of NHL can be classified histologically into three major groups that differ in response to various treatment modalities: (1) lymphoblastic lymphoma, (2) diffuse, small, non–cleaved cell lymphoma (Burkitt and non-Burkitt type), and (3) large cell lymphoma.

Staging and Diagnostic Evaluation

The clinical staging system useful in childhood NHL considers both extent of disease and tumor burden (Table 3). Imaging procedures should include chest radiograph (CT if abnormal), abdominal and pelvic CT or ultrasound, and bone scan. Up to 20 per cent of patients have bone marrow involvement, necessitating bone marrow aspirate and biopsy in all patients. Cerebrospinal fluid analysis for malignant cells is also essential. In addition to a complete blood count and liver profile, measurements of tumor lysis, such as uric acid, potassium, phosphorus, and calcium levels, are essential. Assessment of the associated complications of renal failure (blood urea nitrogen, creatinine, urine output) is important prior to initiation of therapy. Serum lactate dehydrogenase (LDH) is a measure of tumor burden and may be prognostically important. Because these tumors must be considered to be disseminated at diagnosis, a staging laparotomy and lymphangiography are not part of the routine management.

Treatment (Initial Management)

Many tumors are rapidly proliferating and are associated with concomitant metabolic alterations. Acute tumor lysis syndrome manifested by elevated uric acid levels, hyperkalemia, hyperphosphatemia, and hypocalcemia is a major concern at presentation, especially in patients with Burkitt's lymphoma. The associated acute renal failure may necessitate the application of dialysis in some patients. These metabolic derangements need to be corrected prior to the institution of chemotherapy. Vigorous hydration with fluid (3L/m^2/day), alkalinization to increase the solubility of uric acid, and the administration of allopurinol should be routine in all patients. Hyperphosphatemia may become more of a problem after the first few days of therapy, and at this point alkalinization should be discontinued. Patients with mediastinal masses may present with severe respiratory distress and should be treated promptly. Chemotherapy usually results in rapid tumor shrinkage, but low-dose radiation therapy may need to be given emergently in some cases.

TABLE 3. St. Jude Children's Research Hospital Staging Classification for Childhood Non-Hodgkin's Lymphoma

Stage I	A single tumor (extranodal) or single anatomic area (nodal) excluding the mediastinum or abdomen.
Stage II	A single tumor (extranodal) with regional lymph node involvement. Two or more lymph node areas on the same side of the diaphragm. Two single (extranodal) tumors with or without regional lymph node involvement, on the same side of the diaphragm. A primary gastrointestinal tumor with or without involvement of associated mesenteric nodes.
Stage III	Two single tumors (extranodal) or two or more nodal areas above and below the diaphragm. All primary intrathoracic tumors (mediastinal, pleural, thymic), all extensive primary intra-abdominal disease, all paraspinal or epidural tumors regardless of other tumor sites.
Stage IV	Any of the above with initial central nervous system involvement or bone marrow involvement.*

*Greater than 25 per cent abnormal cells is classified as leukemia.

Therapy

The successful therapy for childhood NHL was largely accomplished by the recognition that these tumors are usually disseminated at diagnosis and aggressive chemotherapy can be curative. The application of treatment principles developed in the treatment of acute lymphoblastic leukemia led to the encouraging results seen with modern chemotherapy.

Localized Disease

Patients with localized disease (stages I and II) of all histologic classifications respond well to a shortened course of combination chemotherapy lasting 8 months or less. The most successful of these regimens is shown in Table 4. Radiotherapy can be safely omitted in these children, and central nervous system (CNS) prophylaxis with methotrexate is reserved for patients with head and neck tumors only. Currently, studies are under way to determine whether maintenance chemotherapy is necessary after remission is achieved with multiagent initial chemotherapy.

Advanced Disease

The cornerstone of treatment for advanced disease is combination chemotherapy. Although earlier protocols also relied on radiation therapy to involved areas or bulky disease at diagnosis, this modality is generally deleted in most current protocols. Specific therapy is dependent on tumor histology. Patients with lymphoblastic lymphoma respond to intensive chemotherapy regimens initially designed for patients with ALL. The most successful of these is the ten-drug LSA_2L_2 protocol, which was one of the first highly intensive protocols to be developed (Table 4). Many current programs are modified versions of this plan. Duration of therapy generally lasts 18 to 24 months. These children are at high risk for CNS dissemination, and intrathecal chemoprophylaxis is mandatory. Patients with CNS disease at diagnosis require craniospinal irradiation. Overall, results are encouraging, with relapse-free survival rates ranging from 60 to 80 per cent at 2 years.

The optimal therapy for patients with large cell lymphoma has not clearly been established. The APO regimen (doxorubicin, prednisone, vincristine) (Table 4) has been used in a limited number of patients with excellent results—76 per cent disease-free survival at 4 years. More recently, a 12-week chemotherapy MACOP-B regimen is being used in children with encouraging results (Table 4); these patients are at a much lower risk for CNS disease, and many may not require prophylaxis.

Until very recently, children with small non–cleaved cell lymphoma fared poorly. The development of highly intense chemotherapy and improved supportive care during periods

TABLE 4. Treatment Regimens for Childhood Non-Hodgkin's Lymphoma

Regimen	Induction	Consolidation	Maintenance	CNS Prophylaxis	Duration	Indications
Localized lymphoma	Cyclophosphamide Doxorubicin Vincristine Prednisone	Cyclophosphamide Doxorubicin Vincristine Prednisone	6-Mercaptopurine Methotrexate	Methotrexate*	8 months	All histologies
LSA_2L_2	Cyclophosphamide Vincristine Methotrexate Doxorubicin Prednisone	Cytarabine 6-Thioguanine L-Asparaginase Carmustine	6-Thioguanine/cyclophosphamide Hydroxyurea/daunorubicin Methotrexate/carmustine Cytarabine/vincristine	Methotrexate	18 months	Lymphoblastic
APO	Vincristine Doxorubicin Prednisone	Doxorubicin Vincristine Prednisone 6-Mercaptopurine L-Asparaginase	Vincristine Doxorubicin Prednisone 6-Mercaptopurine Methotrexate	Methotrexate +/− XRT	2 years	Lymphoblastic Large cell
COMP	Cyclophosphamide Vincristine Methotrexate Prednisone		Cyclophosphamide Vincristine Methotrexate Prednisone	Methotrexate	18 months (6 months localized disease)	SNCC† Large cell
MACOP-B	Methotrexate Doxorubicin Cyclophosphamide	Vincristine Bleomycin Prednisone	Myelosuppressive and nonmyelosuppressive agents given on alternating weeks	Methotrexate (+/−)	3 months	Large cell
POG 8617	Cyclophosphamide Doxorubicin Vincristine	Methotrexate Cytarabine	Induction and consolidation repeated 3 times	Methotrexate Cytarabine	6 months	SNCC

*For head and neck tumors only.
†Small non–cleaved cell.
Abbreviations: XRT, cranial irradiation; CNS, central nervous system.

of associated bone marrow aplasia has dramatically improved the outlook for these children. Most current regimens rely heavily on high-dose, fractionated therapy with an alkylating agent (cyclophosphamide). The COMP regimen (cyclophosphamide, vincristine, methotrexate, prednisone) was first shown to be effective for patients with small non–cleaved cell lymphomas with a 60 per cent long-term survival in contrast to the limited effectiveness of this treatment plan in patients with lymphoblastic lymphoma. These patients are also at risk for CNS dissemination, and all treatment plans incorporate some form of prophylaxis to this site. Newer-generation protocols incorporating doxorubicin and methotrexate-cytarabine have reported an 80 per cent disease-free survival (Table 4). Even patients with significant bone marrow involvement are curable with such therapy, although patients with CNS disease at diagnosis continue to do poorly.

Many of the above treatment plans for advanced disease employ intensive pulse therapy with rotating drug combinations. These protocols result in severe bone marrow aplasia, and the biggest challenge for clinicians caring for such patients is the provision of supportive care through these episodes. Fever during neutropenic periods (absolute neutrophil count $< 500/mm^3$) mandates admission to the hospital and broad-spectrum antibiotic coverage after culture specimens are obtained. The availability of cytokines such as G-CSF and GM-CSF may limit these episodes and associated infections. These patients may be at risk for serious bleeding, and prophylactic platelet transfusions for patients whose platelet count falls below $20,000/mm^3$ may be necessary.

Late Effects

Many of the late effects associated with chemotherapy summarized in the text on Hodgkin's disease are applicable to long-term survivors of NHL. Alkylating agents (and potentially epipodophyllotoxins) are associated with the risk of a second malignant tumor and sterility primarily in males. The risk of doxorubicin-associated cardiomyopathy merits periodic evaluation of patients with electrocardiography, echocardiography, and/or radionuclide angiography.

In contrast to patients with Hodgkin's disease, those with advanced NHL require CNS prophylaxis with chemotherapy and possibly radiation therapy. The studies of long-term impact on neuropsychologic performance have yielded diverse results. Radiation therapy to the CNS has been associated with intelligence quotient (IQ) drops of 10 points or more in many patients. The incidence of disability increases in patients treated for active CNS disease, those treated at an early age (younger than 5 years), and those requiring high doses of intrathecal methotrexate in addition to radiation therapy. Patients at risk should be seen regularly with particular attention paid to school performance. Formal neuropsychologic testing may be indicated in patients, and additional educational needs may be addressed with supplemental programs.

BURKITT'S LYMPHOMA

WILLIAM S. FERGUSON, M.D.

Burkitt's lymphoma is a rapidly growing malignant neoplasm of B-lymphocyte origin. Burkitt's lymphoma is currently considered a subtype of diffuse undifferentiated lymphoma (DUL). The division between Burkitt's and non-Burkitt's DUL is made on the basis of histologic appearance; however, there appears to be little difference between the two subtypes in terms of biology or response to treatment. The rapid rate of growth that is characteristic of DUL makes prompt recognition, evaluation, and treatment imperative. Furthermore, the rapid cell turnover can cause significant metabolic derangements ("tumor lysis syndrome") even prior to the initiation of cytoreductive therapy. Thus, the care of patients with suspected DUL is best handled in centers familiar with the diagnosis and treatment of childhood cancers and capable of providing intensive medical support.

EPIDEMIOLOGY AND CLINICAL PRESENTATION

Burkitt's lymphoma is quite common in equatorial Africa, where it comprises about half of all childhood neoplasms. The jaw is the most frequent site of presentation among African patients, particularly among younger patients; the abdomen is a common site among older children. Bone marrow involvement is uncommon, and the central nervous system (CNS) is involved at the time of presentation in about 20 per cent of children. Pain and constitutional symptoms are also relatively uncommon among African patients.

The diffuse undifferentiated lymphomas are much less common in North America, where they account for about half of non-Hodgkin's lymphomas and fewer than 5 per cent of all childhood cancers. The median age of American patients is about 12 years; the male-to-female ratio is about 2.5:1. By far the most common site among North American patients is the abdomen, and many patients will present with bulky and/or multifocal disease. At the time of presentation, about 20 per cent will have bone marrow involvement and more than 10 per cent will have CNS disease. Constitutional symptoms, such as fever or weight loss, are relatively common among American patients.

Metabolic disturbances, such as elevated serum potassium, phosphate, and uric acid levels, are frequently present, particularly among patients with a large tumor burden; at times there will be overt renal failure. Serum lactic dehydrogenase (LDH) levels are invariably elevated, occasionally to extremely high levels.

EVALUATION

Patients suspected of having DUL should undergo prompt and complete staging to evaluate the extent of tumor. Computed tomography (CT) of the chest and abdomen (the latter performed with oral and intravenous contrast) is usually best for delineating the extent of disease in those areas. Ultrasound may be equal to CT for detecting abdominal disease, particularly in young patients who have minimal retroperitoneal fat and who would require sedation in order for an adequate CT scan to be performed. A bone marrow aspiration with biopsy is mandatory, as is a lumbar puncture to look for CNS disease. A bone scan should be considered to reveal bony involvement, which is present in about 10 per cent of cases. Although routine gallium scans have been advocated by many authors in the evaluation of non-Hodgkin's lymphomas, they probably contribute little to the evaluation of patients in whom CT scans can be easily obtained.

A complete blood count, together with determination of serum electrolyte, creatinine, phosphorus, uric acid, and LDH levels, should be performed in all patients.

Definitive diagnosis of non-Hodgkin's lymphomas depends on obtaining tissue for histologic and biochemical examination. Because prompt initiation of chemotherapy is the standard therapy for these tumors, surgical biopsy should usually be directed to the most accessible and easily resected site of tumor.

TREATMENT

Metabolic Management

Some degree of tumor lysis syndrome is often present even before antineoplastic chemotherapy is begun, and the massive tumor cell death that results from the initiation of therapy can lead to severe metabolic derangements. Supportive care measures should be started immediately, even for patients awaiting transfer to a tertiary care center for definitive evaluation and therapy.

All patients should start allopurinol (50 to 100 mg three times a day) and intravenous hydration at 1½ to two times maintenance with fluid containing sufficient sodium bicarbonate to raise the urine pH ≥ 7 (usually 40 to 70 mEq/L). Urine output should be closely monitored; placement of a Foley catheter may be prudent, particularly because there may be sufficient urinary crystals to cause urinary obstruction. Hyperkalemia should be treated with sodium polystyrene sulfonate (Kayexalate), and oral aluminum hydroxide antacids are given to control hyperphosphatemia. Serum electrolyte, uric acid, calcium, phosphorus, and creatinine levels should be monitored frequently. Dialysis may be necessary because of renal failure or severe metabolic disturbances.

Surgery

Although complete surgical removal of tumor can result in improved prognosis, most patients will have disease that is multifocal or sufficiently bulky that complete resection is impossible. Thus, surgical excision should be reserved for patients in whom more than 90 per cent removal of tumor can be achieved with modest operative morbidity (such as patients with limited disease of the small intestine). Heroic attempts at "debulking" are *not* indicated; because of the tremendous growth rate of DUL, the tumor mass may exceed that at presentation by the time the patient has recovered sufficiently to start chemotherapy.

Radiation

Radiation therapy provides little additional benefit to most patients who receive adequate chemotherapy. Significant neurologic deficits resulting from bulk disease (e.g., an extradural mass causing spinal cord compression) may be most expeditiously treated with radiation, although steroids and systemic chemotherapy may also lead to rapid diminution in tumor size.

Chemotherapy

Chemotherapy can provide cure even for patients with advanced disease. Cyclophosphamide is the single most active agent against DUL and is part of all successful chemotherapeutic regimens. Indeed, among African patients with Burkitt's lymphoma, there have been documented cures following treatment with cyclophosphamide alone. Many other antineoplastic agents also show activity against these tumors.

Although there was some success in treating DUL with the treatment plans useful in the treatment of leukemia and lymphoblastic lymphoma (such as the Sloan-Kettering LSA_2L_2 and Dana-Farber APO* regimens), protocols involving periodic cycles of intensive chemotherapy have demonstrated better disease-free survival. Examples include the COMP* regimen used by the Children's Cancer Study Group, and the St. Jude's "Total B" regimen (fractionated cyclophosphamide plus vincristine and doxorubicin, alternating with high-dose methotrexate and Ara-C). Although it has been traditional to give chemotherapy for 12 to 18 months, it has now become apparent that shorter courses of treatment (6 months or less) are equally effective, especially among patients with limited disease.

Although only a minority of patients present with CNS disease, the CNS is a common site of relapse unless some form of specific prophylactic therapy is given. Accordingly, intrathecal ara-C and/or methotrexate have been incorporated into current treatment regimens and appear to be successful in preventing CNS recurrences.

*APO = vincristine, doxorubicin, prednisone.

*COMP = cyclophosphamide, vincristine, methotrexate, prednisone.

PROGNOSIS

About 90 per cent of patients with limited (stage I or II) disease can expect to be cured. Among patients with stage III disease, 60 to 80 per cent will be long-term survivors. Among patients with CNS or bone marrow involvement (stage IV), cure rates have generally been 40 per cent or less, although somewhat better results are now being seen in patients treated with exceptionally aggressive measures.

The majority of patients who experience relapse do so within about 8 months; those who remain free of disease for 1 year can be considered "cured," since late relapses are rare among American patients.

TREATMENT OF RECURRENT DISEASE

Some patients with recurrent disease have responded to intensive, myeloablative chemotherapy, usually followed by bone marrow transplant. However, as the intensity of front-line treatment has increased, it has become increasingly difficult to induce second remissions among those patients who fail to improve with standard therapy. Thus, at this time the outlook for the majority of patients who relapse is dismal.

FUTURE TRENDS

The improved survival for most patients with DUL has been achieved at the price of significant toxicity; considerable morbidity and mortality result from the current treatment regimens. Thus, the current thrust of research is to reduce morbidity for the majority of patients while trying to improve survival for those with stage IV disease.

Decreasing the duration of therapy from 12 to 18 months to approximately 6 months has not significantly altered survival, and further shortening of therapy may be possible. Advances in supportive care, particularly in terms of preventing infection, will also be important in decreasing treatment-related mortality and morbidity. Of particular current interest is the role to be played by hematopoietic growth factors (G-CSF and GM-CSF). By reducing the period of profound granulocytopenia that follows chemotherapy, they may decrease the incidence of severe infection. Alternatively, such bone marrow support may allow dose intensification among patients at high risk of recurrence and thus improve their chances of survival.

9

Endocrine System

HYPOPITUITARISM AND GROWTH HORMONE THERAPY

DENNIS M. STYNE, M.D.

Growth hormone (GH) was originally extracted and purified from human pituitary glands donated post mortem. For more than 25 years, it was suggested that the limited source of GH be used to treat classic GH-deficient patients. In 1983, the possibility arose that the use of human pituitary–derived GH carried the risk of infection with the prions (slow virus) of Creutzfeldt-Jakob disease, which was found to have an increased incidence among patients previously treated with human GH. At that time, recombinant DNA–derived GH was in clinical trials, and owing to the elimination of the use of human pituitary–derived GH, all patients in the United States were switched to recombinant DNA–derived GH. Because recombinant DNA–derived GH supplies are theoretically unlimited, new pressures arose to treat children with disorders other than GH deficiency.

DIAGNOSIS

Despite decades of study, it remains difficult to determine who is GH deficient. The classic patient demonstrating poor growth rate (below the 5th percentile or under 4 cm/year between ages 5 and 10 years), cherubic appearance, proportionate short stature, increased subcutaneous adiposity, low GH on secretagogue testing, and low spontaneous secretion of GH is not difficult to diagnose. However, many patients vary from this classic description, including those with late-onset growth failure due to a tumor or central nervous system irradiation. This article refers only to evaluation of GH secretion.

Deciding which patient has inadequate GH secretion is difficult for several reasons. Random GH determinations are useless because GH concentrations are low for most of the day in both normal and GH-deficient patients. Thus, stimulated GH concentrations must be considered. However, standards are difficult to determine because most "normal" GH secretion reported in clinical studies is based on analysis of children who are statistically short, the only subjects who are likely to undergo testing for GH deficiency. Furthermore, the radioimmunoassay employed has significant influence. For example, a GH level of slightly higher than 10 ng/ml, which would be considered normal in most laboratories, may be reported as a value of 7 ng/ml or less by a different laboratory. These differences appear to be due to the choice of antibody used in the assay.

Two tests of GH secretion are necessary to determine sufficiency or deficiency, because any normal child has a 10 to 20 per cent chance of failing to respond to one secretagogue during one test. For secretagogue testing, peak GH concentrations are measured 10 minutes after 10 minutes of vigorous exercise, or 30, 60, and 90 minutes after the start of a 30-minute intravenous infusion of 0.5 g/kg of arginine (maximum of 20 g) or an oral dose of L-dopa (125 mg for body weight up to 15 kg, 250 mg up to 35 kg, and 500 mg over 35 kg; usually causes nusea) or clonidine (0.1 to 0.15 mg/m^2; causes drowsiness and possibly hypotension or bradycardia). Insulin-induced hypoglycemia by the intravenous infusion of a 0.1-unit/kg push is effective but dangerous. This insulin tolerance test requires confirmation of a normal basal glucose before infusion of insulin and the maintenance of an available intravenous line for 25 per cent dextrose infusion if the blood glucose drops too far and precipitates coma or seizure. GH-releasing hormone has just become commercially available for testing but, although theoretically preferable, has not yet shown improved results over the use of the older agents.

Alternative methods of testing for GH deficiency are proposed but may not add much to diagnostic possibilities. For instance, the integrated GH concentration in the patient over a 24-hour period may be obtained by frequent blood sampling through an indwelling catheter over that period. Alternatively, some investigators believe that frequent sampling over only the nighttime sleep period is equally informative. In fact, these integrated concentrations of GH do not appear to add much to the diagnosis of GH deficiency.

Serum insulin-like growth factor 1 (IGF-1) concentrations are related to GH secretory status but also to age and nutritional status. Thus, although IGF-1 levels are diagnostically low in an older child with classic GH deficiency, they may be ambiguous in a more subtle case. The combination of serum IGF-1 and IGF-2 determinations increases the accuracy of diagnosis, but there are patients with normal values of both factors who may still benefit from GH therapy. The measurement of IGF-binding protein 3 (IGFBP-3), a high-molecular-weight protein that varies directly with GH secretory status, is a new addition to the diagnostic armamentarium; IGFBP-3 is said to differentiate GH deficiency better in the newborn and in infancy than does IGF-1, but IGFBP-3 also is sensitive to nutritional status.

Thus, the diagnosis of patients with conditions other than classic GH deficiency remains problematic. Studies of children who are significantly short (height > 3.5 SD below the mean for age) or growing poorly (below the 3rd percentile growth velocity for age), with a significantly delayed bone age but normal GH secretion, show no more than a 50 per cent chance of responding to GH with an increase in growth velocity. Most short children are not as severely affected and stand a lesser chance to respond to GH.

It appears that one way to determine whether a severely short child with no endocrine, systemic, nutritional, or psychosocial condition to explain decreased growth could benefit from GH is to attempt a 3- to 6-month trial period of the medication with exacting measurements for 3 to 6 months before therapy and during treatment. Unfortunately, short-term observation of such patients does not answer the question of whether such therapy will increase their final height. Controlled studies are under way to answer that question.

TREATMENT

At present, GH is administered almost solely by pediatric endocrinologists. Before therapy is initiated, possible side effects are discussed with the family. Although elevation of blood glucose, increased incidence of slipped capital epiphysis, and, of course, potential local infection at the injection site are theoretic side effects more than observed complications, they must be considered. Furthermore, worldwide there are a few children and young adults previously treated with GH who have developed leukemia without any predisposing cause such as chromosomal breakage syndromes, previous tumors, or irradiation. The incidence of such cases is so low that at present it cannot be determined whether such cases occur as a result of chance or are due to a predilection of GH to induce leukemia. It is known, however, that GH therapy adds no statistical increase in the incidence of recurrence of tumors.

Recombinant DNA–derived GH is administered by injection with various possible doses and regimens. Although classically given intramuscularly, subcutaneous injection has proved to be efficacious and easier and is therefore preferable. Originally given three times per week, dosing daily or six times per week improves growth rate when the total weekly dose is maintained constant. Initially, a weekly dose of 0.3 mg/kg of methionyl GH and 0.18 mg/kg of recombinant DNA–derived GH was recommended; however, doses of up to double this are now used in some cases. The percentage gain in growth rate is less than the percentage increase in dose, and higher doses are therefore considerably more expensive for height achieved.

Growth hormone therapy in GH deficiency exerts greater effects in patients with younger bone ages. Thus, in the first decade of life, doubling of the growth rate is often seen (e.g., 4 cm/year increasing to 8 to 9 cm/year), whereas during the teenage years, therapy may add only 2 cm/year to the pretherapy rate. Furthermore, growth is greater in the first year of therapy compared with that in the later periods. Thus, long-term studies of patients treated in past decades demonstrate final heights below that expected for genetic potential; this is probably due to the combination of limited supply of GH and periods without therapy plus older ages at time of diagnosis and onset of therapy. Nonetheless, it appears likely that if GH therapy is started in the first years after birth and is administered consistently, the GH-deficient patient is likely to reach a height close to the genetic potential.

SHORT STATURE

JUDITH L. ROSS, M.D.

GROWTH HORMONE DEFICIENCY

Growth hormone (GH) deficiency and treatment are described in detail in the article on hypopituitarism and growth hormone therapy (p. 284) and thus are discussed only briefly here. GH deficiency is most commonly diagnosed on the basis of diminished release of GH in response to one or two provocative tests such as L-dopa, clonidine, insulin-hypoglycemia, or propranolol-glucagon. The normal GH response to these tests has been defined as a peak GH response of 6 to 10 ng/ml.

Treatment of GH deficiency involves administration of synthetic recombinant GH three to seven times weekly as a subcutaneous or intramuscular (IM) injection. The dose of GH is 0.06 to 0.1 mg/kg three times weekly or 0.03 to 0.05 mg/kg/day. At present, there is no uniformly accepted initial starting dose or dosage schedule. Side effects from GH administered to GH-deficient children are minimal or absent. Questions have been raised about an increased incidence of slipped capital femoral epiphysis in association with GH treatment, but the controversy about this finding is not resolved. The incidence of antibody formation in response to synthetic GH is low, and the antibodies are not associated with attenuation of growth.

CONSTITUTIONAL GROWTH DELAY

Children with constitutional growth delay are commonly evaluated for short stature, usually in the second decade of life. They are also frequently evaluated for delayed puberty. The past history of these children is characterized by a normal birth weight and length with a fall off to 1 to 2 standard deviations (SD) below the mean in the first 1 to 3 years of life and a further growth deceleration to 2 to 3 SD below the mean in early adolescence, when puberty and the pubertal growth spurt would normally be commencing (95 per cent confidence limits, 9 to 13 and 9.5 to 13.5 for girls, and 10 to 14 and 11.5 to 15.5 for boys). Height is frequently below the 5th percentile on the growth curve when these children are evaluated in their early teens. Skeletal or bone age is usually 1 to 3 years delayed in these children and corresponds to the height age. Boys present for evaluation more frequently than girls. This may represent a referral bias, in which short boys are referred more often than short girls for medical attention.

Often, a positive family history of delayed puberty in one parent can be elicited. Menarche may have commenced after age 15 to 16 years in the mother, or the father may recall still growing during the late teenage years.

Treatment options include the following:

1. *Supportive care.* Because the natural history of this condition is that, ultimately, attainment of normal puberty and normal adult height occur, the child and family can be reassured that no pharmacologic intervention is necessary. Ongoing individual and family psychologic support may still be required.
2. *Testosterone.* Alternatively, if the child is suffering significant psychologic distress secondary to concern about short stature and/or the pubertal delay and has reached the age of 14 years, a short course of testosterone enanthate can be initiated (50 to 100 mg intramuscular dose per month for 3 to 6 months). This type of regimen has been found to result in a temporary increase in growth velocity, an increase in virilization, and an improvement in self-esteem, with no seri-

ous side effects or significant increase or decrease in final adult height.

As mentioned, girls with constitutional delay of growth and puberty with no other diagnosis to explain the findings are evaluated considerably less often than boys. The concern in these girls is generally the delayed puberty rather than the short stature.

Treatment options include careful reassurance and follow-up or, alternatively, initiation of treatment with low doses of ethinyl estradiol (50 to 100 ng/kg/day), which is a growth-promoting dose of estrogen that is accompanied by some minimal breast development. The dosage of ethinyl estradiol can gradually be increased to complete pubertal development.

Studies are also currently being performed to evaluate the safety and efficacy of GH treatment in children with constitutional growth delay. The routine use of GH cannot be recommended in these children until the results of such studies are available.

TURNER SYNDROME

The diagnosis of Turner syndrome should be considered in a newborn with lymphedema and webbed neck and in a female child presenting with short stature and/or delayed sexual maturation. Children younger than 9 or 10 years of age often have normal levels of luteinizing hormone and follicle-stimulating hormone. Karyotypes should be sent. Only after age 10 years do levels of these gonadotropins rise to the castrate range. Children diagnosed with Turner syndrome should also be screened via renal ultrasonography and cardiac echocardiography and for thyroid hormone levels because of the increased incidence of renal, cardiac, and thyroid abnormalities.

Short stature is a very common feature in girls with Turner syndrome. Their mean final adult height ranges from 142.6 to 147.3 cm. In general, the children are born small for gestational age (birth weight and length, on average, 1 SD below mean), grow at a decreased rate during childhood, and lack a pubertal growth spurt. The final height of these children is significantly correlated with midparental height. The etiology of the short stature does not seem to be related to GH deficiency or abnormalities in adrenal or gonadal hormones. Serum insulin-like growth factor 1 levels are commonly decreased.

Treatment options for the short stature include oxandrolone, GH, and low-dose estrogen, alone and in combination, which have been used to stimulate growth. These hormone interventions have increased growth rates for 1 to 3 years in girls with Turner syndrome. The increase in growth velocity with these interventions is usually maximal in the first year and wanes with time. Androgen (oxandrolone) side effects can include weight gain, hirsutism, clitoromegaly, and changes in liver enzyme levels. Low-dose estrogen side effects can include early, minimal breast development. GH treatment in girls with Turner syndrome has been associated with increased insulin levels without accompanying hyperglycemia. Whether the later incidence of diabetes or cardiovascular disease in growth hormone–mediated Turner syndrome patients will be increased is unknown. There has been no growth treatment to date that is associated with a significant increase in final adult height of women with Turner syndrome. Studies are currently being performed that will evaluate the long-term safety and efficacy of GH, GH and oxandrolone, and GH and low-dose estrogen. The results of these studies should form a sounder basis from which to make recommendations to promote growth of girls with Turner syndrome.

OTHER CONDITIONS ASSOCIATED WITH SHORT STATURE

Intrauterine Growth Retardation

Intrauterine growth retardation (IUGR) (full-term infant, $<$ 2500 g and $<$ 48 cm) occurs secondary to significant illness or infection in the mother or fetus; exposure to toxins, including cocaine and ethanol; chromosomal abnormalities; multiple gestation; and unknown etiologic factors. Children who are part of multiple gestations or children with IUGR of unknown etiology without congenital malformations or perinatal complications are more likely to demonstrate catch-up growth. This catch-up growth generally occurs in the first 2 years of life. The growth failure in the remainder of children with IUGR does not appear to occur on the basis of GH or thyroid hormone deficiency, malnutrition, or any other identifiable metabolic abnormality.

Small series of patients have been treated with GH, with some children responding with increases in growth velocity. Recommendation for treatment with GH in these children cannot be made until the results of long-term safety and efficacy studies are known.

Achondroplasia and Hypochondroplasia

Short stature is a common manifestation of achondroplasia and hypochondroplasia, which are the most common skeletal dysplasias and are inherited in an autosomal dominant fashion. The growth failure predominantly affecting the limbs may be obvious in infancy or may become apparent in childhood and adolescence. These children have no identifiable endocrine abnormality, and, in particular, they are not GH or thyroid hormone deficient.

Preliminary, short-term studies have demonstrated an increase in growth velocity in some children with achondroplasia or hypochondroplasia treated with GH. These results are encouraging, but long-term safety and efficacy studies are required before GH therapy can be recommended for these children.

Additional Etiologies

A variety of systemic disorders are also associated with short stature, including major chromosomal anomalies, chronic renal failure, and congenital heart disease. Management of these conditions is discussed elsewhere.

TALL STATURE

MITCHELL E. GEFFNER, M.D.

The "definition" of tall stature depends on cultural background, sex, and family height patterns. In the United States, it is rare for boys to seek evaluation for isolated tall stature. With greater acceptance of tall females in our society, referrals for evaluation of tall girls are dwindling. In clinical practice, girls are considered to be tall if their adult height projects to greater than 183 cm (72 inches). Analogous to the role of short parental heights in contributing to a short adult height of a child, tall parental stature plays a pivotal role in leading to tall stature of a child. Before one concludes that tall stature is due to familial factors, however, certain organic disorders associated with excessive and/or rapid height growth should be considered, at least on clinical grounds. Excessive height frequently occurs in boys with Klinefelter syndrome and may occur in either sex in association with Marfan syndrome or homocystinuria. Rapid growth, reflected by crossing of height percentiles and advancement of bone age, prior to age 10 years occurs in association with sexual precocity, untreated thyrotoxicosis, and perhaps exogenous obesity.

ESTROGEN THERAPY FOR GIRLS

The only effective pharmacologic therapy for girls with familial tall stature is high-dose estrogen. Sex steroids promote rapid osseous maturation, during which time height growth per year is less than expected for each year of bone age advancement. Although administration of estrogens to limit the height of tall girls has been practiced for many years, its current use has been limited because of concern about serious side effects as well as greater acceptance of tall women in our society. Various forms of estrogen have been employed and at various dosing schedules. These include ethinyl estradiol, 0.06 to 0.5 mg/day; Premarin (conjugated estrogens), 10 mg/day; and estradiol valerate, 6 to 8 mg/day. In some studies, the estrogen was given on days 1 to 23 of each month and combined with a progestational agent (such as Provera, 5 to 10 mg) from day 10 or 14 to day 23 of each month. The addition of the progestational agent is reserved for those girls who are at least 1 year into puberty to provide cyclic withdrawal bleeding, which markedly diminishes the likelihood of estrogen-induced uterine neoplasia. Initiation of menses in younger subjects would not be appropriate for psychodevelopmental reasons.

In most females, the greatest efficacy of estrogen treatment is seen when begun between 10 and 12 years of age and continued until growth ceases (bone age 15 years). It has been confirmed in a controlled study that followed tall girls until growth cessation that ethinyl estradiol at a dose of 0.1 mg/day was as effective as a dose of 0.3 mg/day, in both cases resulting in approximately a 40 per cent decrement in predicted remaining adult height. This occurred regardless of whether the initial bone age was less than or greater than 12.5 years. However, the estrogen resulted in a diminution in adult height prediction, which, in absolute terms, was greater in those girls with younger bone age (7.4 cm, or about 3 inches) than in those girls with older bone age (3.6 cm, or about 1.5 inches).

Because the doses of estrogen employed for height reduction are at least three times the normal "replacement" dose and the dosage may be employed for as long as 5 years, concern about untoward effects must be registered. The actual risk of estrogen-mediated side effects, such as suppression of the hypothalamic-pituitary-ovarian axis, endometrial carcinoma, thrombophlebitis, and hypertension, is unknown. Clinical but mostly anecdotal experience suggests that side effects are minimal or transient and usually consist of nausea, weight gain, and anemia secondary to excessive uterine bleeding. Use of progestational withdrawal should prevent development of endometrial neoplasia and hypermenorrhagia.

Although I am reluctant to prescribe estrogen, some endocrinologists may consider estrogen use for the girl who, by analysis of growth velocity and bone age, is likely to exceed 183 cm in adult height and who, along with her parents, has significant psychosocial concerns about this prediction. Initiation of treatment as early as age 10 years appears most efficacious and is not associated with untimely pubertal development. Ethinyl estradiol at a dose of 0.1 mg/day for 1 year, followed by cycling with Provera beginning in the second year, appears both efficacious and reasonably safe. Treatment efficacy should be evaluated by measurement of height, weight, and blood pressure every 3 months, with semiannual determination of bone age and hepatic function.

TESTOSTERONE TREATMENT FOR BOYS

Analogous to the use of estrogens to limit growth of the tall female child, high-dose testosterone has been employed in boys whose adult heights project to greater than 200 cm (79 inches). As already mentioned, it is extremely rare that any pharmacologic approach is requested by male patients. However, if there are overriding psychosocial concerns, treatment may be indicated. The regimen that is most commonly recommended is a long-acting (oil-based) testosterone ester (e.g., enanthate) given at a dose of 500 mg/m^2 as monthly intramuscular injections. This dose extrapolates to greater than four times the normal adult testosterone production rate when viewed on a daily basis. Its use should be restricted to boys who are at least 1 year into puberty. As with high-dose estrogens, the efficacy of testosterone is best in boys in whom treatment is commenced relatively early. For boys started between the bone ages of 12 and 14, greater than 14 to 15, and greater than 15 years, the adult height predictions are reduced by approximately 8 cm (slightly greater than 3 inches), 5.7 cm (slightly greater than 2 inches), and 3 cm (slightly greater than 1 inch), respectively (mean duration of treatment, 1 to 2 years). However, a recent study suggests a similar reduction in projected adult height with only a 6-month course of testosterone enanthate given as 50 mg intramuscularly every 2 weeks.

An increased risk of side effects needs to be considered with such supraphysiologic doses of testosterone. These include suppression of the hypothalamic-pituitary-testicular axis, which occurs frequently, as manifested by decreased testicular size. Such suppression appears fully reversible but may take more than 1 year from the time of discontinuation of treatment. Sperm counts also normalize in this time frame. Advancement of pubertal changes also occurs, but no other significant side effects have been noted during follow-up.

OTHER APPROACHES

Low-dose estrogens have been employed on occasion to treat tall males, with at least short-term success. It has recently been noted that tall adolescents have mild elevations in serum growth hormone (GH) concentrations and paradoxically increased responses of the serum GH concentration following stimulation with thyrotropin-releasing hormone and/or oral glucose. This has led to trials of bromocriptine therapy, analogous to its use in some patients with acromegaly. Reported results, using daily doses as high as 7.5 mg for up to 8 months, have been variable, although most studies suggest a reduction in predicted adult height similar to that seen with high-dose sex steroid therapy. Cholinergic muscarinic blockers, under experimental conditions, have been used to induce partial suppression of GH secretion in tall children, but without significantly reducing short-term height velocity.

The newest experimental approach has involved administration of octreotide, a long-acting analogue of somatostatin, to suppress GH secretion. Given as once-daily or twice-daily subcutaneous injections for 6 to 12 months to adolescent boys and girls with constitutional tall stature, immediate reductions in growth rate occurred in most subjects along with reductions in their predicted adult height by 4.9 cm (approximately 2 inches) on average in one study.

Development of other similarly acting but more efficacious drugs may add to our pharmacologic armamentarium to treat familial tall stature.

REFERENCES

Bartsch O, Weschke B, Weber B: Oestrogen treatment of constitutionally tall girls with 0.1 mg/day ethinyl oestradiol. Eur J Pediatr 147:59–63, 1988.

Brämswig JH, Lengerke HJV, Schmidt H, Schellong G: The results of short-term (6 months) high-dose testosterone treatment on bone age and adult height in boys of excessively tall stature. Eur J Pediatr 148:104–106, 1988.

Tauber MT, Tauber JP, Vigoni F, Harris AG, Rochicchioli P: Effect of the long-acting somatostatin analogue SMS 201-995 on growth rate and reduction of predicted adult height in ten tall adolescents. Acta Paediatr Scand 79:176–181, 1990.

TREATMENT OF THYROID DISORDERS IN CHILDREN

BORIS SENIOR, M.D.
and AB SADEGHI-NEJAD, M.D.

Management of thyroid disorders has advanced, not from the discovery of more potent or specific new medications but from the development of more sensitive and accurate methods of hormonal assay. These methods permit earlier and more exact diagnosis and enable one to monitor and regulate therapy with greater precision. These advances are particularly relevant in the case of the newborn.

CONGENITAL HYPOTHYROIDISM

Before screening programs were introduced, diagnosis was often delayed for 2 months or more. The longer the delay in initiating treatment, the greater the harm to cognitive function. Regional screening programs now identify children with congenital hypothyroidism within 2 or 3 weeks of birth. Prompt therapy may allow unimpaired mental development. Accordingly, once a diagnosis has been made through the screening program, no time should be lost in initiating therapy after obtaining a confirmatory blood sample and performing a technetium scan to locate the thyroid. A sublingual position confirms permanent hypothyroidism, whereas failure to demonstrate a thyroid gland, in most cases, indicates agenesis. More rarely, maternally transmitted thyrotropin receptor blocking antibodies may impair the scan and simulate the picture of agenesis. In such cases, the hypothyroidism may be temporary, and once the patient is about 3 years old, therapy should be withheld for a trial period of a month to test the effect.

In other cases, prematurity or intercurrent illness can affect the screening tests, leaving the diagnosis in doubt. In these cases, too, it seems best not to delay therapy but, rather, to re-evaluate the diagnosis by stopping treatment when the patient is 3 years old. Increased uptake of tracer with an enlarged gland indicates an enzymatic block in the synthesis of hormone, almost always as a result of autosomal recessive transmission. One should also be alert to the possibility that a low serum level of thyroxine (T_4) without an elevated thyroid-stimulating hormone (TSH) level may result from a deficiency of T_4 binding globulin or because of hypopituitarism.

However brought about, congenital hypothyroidism is treated the same—namely, with immediate replacement therapy using L-thyroxine. The aim is to attain a serum level of T_4 of between 12 and 16 μ/dl. This range, which is higher than that present in normal children, is needed to reduce TSH secretion. To achieve this level, a dose of L-thyroxine of 10 to 15 μg/kg once daily is required. Because L-thyroxine comes as 25-μg tablets, the dose, in practice, turns out to be either 37.5 or 50 μg once daily. We instruct parents to crush the tablets in a small quantity of formula or applesauce. Not all of the medication may be taken if given in a full bottle. A careful explanation to the parents of the nature of the disorder and of the need to administer the medication regularly is an important component of management.

At subsequent visits, the levels of T_4 and TSH should be used to monitor adequacy of dosage. These visits should be reasonably frequent during the first year: at 1 month and then at intervals of 2 months. The intervals are increased to 3 months during the second year and then twice yearly thereafter.

The initially elevated TSH should show a steady decline but, despite adequate replacement of L-thyroxine, may take months to fall into the normal range. If, at subsequent visits, the TSH fails to fall or actually rises, the dose may be inadequate or the patient may not be receiving the medication as prescribed. A discussion with the parents, avoiding any element of accusation, will usually clarify and rectify the situation.

As the patient grows, the dose of L-thyroxine is gradually increased, usually in increments of 25 μg, such that the teenager receives between 0.075 and 0.15 mg/day or about 2 to 3 μg/kg/day. The size of the patient and the level of TSH are guides to increasing the dose. The TSH level, if suppressed below the normal range, is also a sensitive indicator of an excessively high dose of L-thyroxine.

HYPOTHYROIDISM DURING CHILDHOOD AND ADOLESCENCE

There is not the same sense of urgency associated with treating a hypothyroid child or adolescent as with congenital hypothyroidism. In these patients, the disorder, almost always caused by autoimmune factors, tends to be long-standing. Adverse effects, both at the time of diagnosis and over the long term, usually involve growth. Effective treatment requires daily L-thyroxine in a dose of 2 to 3 μg/kg. In most cases, this works out to between 0.075 and 0.15 mg/day. One should be aware that children and particularly adolescents will often forget to take any form of daily medication and/or neglect to refill a prescription. Supervision by the parents as well as by the physician is needed.

The disorder, as with other autoimmune conditions, may fluctuate in severity or even undergo remission. Some believe that greater secretion of TSH generates increased release of the thyroid antigen responsible for provoking the autoantibody response in the first place. Thus, the use of L-thyroxine not only restores a euthyroid state but also, by suppressing TSH, even may have a beneficial effect on the basic illness. Although in most cases the hypothyroidism is permanent and treatment lifelong, some patients do experience remission and restoration of normal thyroid function. The patients who are more likely to undergo remission are those with lesser degrees of hypothyroidism; T_4 and triiodothyronine (T_3) levels within the normal range; and only mild elevation of the TSH. After a year of replacement treatment in such patients, it can be determined whether the hypothyroidism is permanent by stopping therapy for a month.

Patients with Down syndrome are at high risk for hypothyroidism and, on testing thyroid function, often have a modest increase in the level of TSH as the sole abnormality. Other conditions, such as cystinosis and various forms of end-stage renal disease, are associated with hypothyroidism. The same approach of a period of replacement therapy and then stopping treatment for a month will enable one to distinguish between those who require long-term treatment and those in whom treatment can be withheld.

CONGENITAL HYPERTHYROIDISM

This disorder results from the transplacental passage of maternally derived thyroid-stimulating immunoglobulins. The mother either is being treated or has been treated in the past for hyperthyroidism. If the mother is under treatment during pregnancy, the fetus will be exposed to the thyroid-stimulating immunoglobulins as well as to the antithyroid medication prescribed for the mother up to the time of delivery. This often delays the appearance of hyperthyroidism in the newborn for some days, until the effect of the medication has diminished and the more persistent stimulatory action of the immunoglobulins can become manifest. The hyperthyroidism is of limited duration, rarely lasting for longer than 3 months, but is usually severe and may be life-threatening. Once it is recognized, treatment should not be delayed.

The thiourea derivatives, propylthiouracil or methimazole (Tapazole), are the agents of choice. Propylthiouracil is prescribed in a dose of 5 to 15 mg/kg per 24 hours given in equally divided doses at 8-hour intervals (three times per day). This usually works out to 10 to 15 mg every 8 hours. If methimazole is used, the dose is 0.5 to 1.0 mg/kg every 12 hours. Because of its prompt although temporary inhibitory effect, iodide can be added in the form of Lugol's iodine, 1 drop every 8 hours. If the hyperthyroidism is particularly severe, a β-adrenergic blocking agent such as propranolol, 2 mg/kg every 24 hours divided into three to four equal doses, may be given.

The response to this combined therapy is fairly rapid. The heart rate falls in hours with propranolol, and hormone levels decrease within days, particularly if iodine is a component of the treatment. Careful monitoring of treatment is essential in order to reduce the drugs gradually and prevent hypothyroidism. Because the hyperthyroidism results from maternally transmitted thyroid-stimulating immunoglobulins, there should be no recurrence once remission is achieved.

HYPERTHYROIDISM IN CHILDHOOD AND ADOLESCENCE

There are three forms of therapy for hyperthyroidism in children. All are effective. Surgery in skilled and experienced hands, in most cases, gives good results, but excision of too little or too much gland will leave the patient still thyrotoxic or permanently hypothyroid. Of greater concern is the possibility of serious surgical complications, such as section of the recurrent laryngeal nerve or hypoparathyroidism. For these reasons, few select surgery as the first choice; as a result, ever fewer surgeons acquire the requisite skill and experience.

Radioiodine works well. The treatment is simple and inexpensive, and the result is predictable. Hypothyroidism follows soon after or, in some, at a later date. However, because hypothyroidism is a common end result of hyperthyroidism, no matter which therapy is given, its appearance in radioiodine-treated patients is not viewed as a major deterrent. Radioiodine has now been administered for many years without the appearance of any serious long-term sequelae. Carefully conducted studies have failed to reveal any increased incidence of local or distant malignancies or any damage to the offspring of treated subjects. Even though only pregnancy remains as a contraindication to the use of radioiodine, both physicians and parents are reluctant to employ radioiodine as a first choice in children.

Accordingly, most turn to antithyroid medication as the initial treatment, selecting either propylthiouracil or methimazole. Overall, using either agent, one expects to achieve a long-term remission rate of greater than 50 per cent. Side effects occur in 3 to 4 per cent of recipients. A transient urticarial rash is the most common adverse reaction. More serious potential ill effects include a lupus-like reaction with joint and serous membrane involvement and agranulocytosis. In most cases, prompt cessation of treatment aborts these reactions. It is therefore important that the patient and families have a clear understanding of the potential risks of treatment and of the need to contact the treating physician promptly should any untoward effect be suspected. If a reaction necessitates stopping treatment, one can switch to the other agent. If that also provokes a toxic effect, one must choose between surgery and radioiodine. Our choice has been the latter.

Propylthiouracil and methimazole are functionally similar and appear to be equally effective in controlling hyperthyroidism, but there are certain significant differences. Propylthiouracil is in large measure protein-bound. Therefore, less of it crosses the placenta, making it the agent of choice for the treatment of pregnant hyperthyroid women. The effect of methimazole lasts longer. It is necessary to give propylthiouracil every 8 hours, whereas methimazole needs to be given only twice daily, and in milder cases will prove effective when taken only once daily. Because treatment continues for months, patients find that having to take any medication three times a day is onerous and they frequently fail to adhere to the prescribed schedule. We find that compliance has improved since we have changed to methimazole.

An additional problem affecting compliance is that the ravenous appetite associated with hyperthyroidism persists during treatment. Therefore, unless the patient understands and adheres to a carefully planned dietary program, weight gain, often of a degree that is unacceptable to the patient, will occur once the hypermetabolism is controlled. The patient tends to blame the medication for the weight gain, and compliance suffers. The initial dose of propylthiouracil is 5 to 10 mg/kg every 24 hours given in three equally divided doses at 8-hour intervals. Progress is followed by the clinical state, particularly gain in weight and reduction in heart rate, and by the levels of T_4, T_3, and TSH. Relying on the T_4 level alone can be misleading, as it may fall to a normal level when the T_3 level is still elevated and the TSH level is suppressed. The best index of euthyroidism is a return of the TSH level to a normal range. When this occurs, the dose of propylthiouracil is reduced. At this stage, L-thyroxine may be added, between 0.05 and 0.1 mg/day, depending on the size of the patient. The introduction of L-thyroxine suppresses TSH and reduces the release of thyroid antigens. This should diminish the generation of antibodies and aid in inducing a remission.

Depending on how hyperthyroid the patient is, the dose of methimazole is 15 to 20 mg once or twice daily. As the hyperthyroidism is brought under control, the dose is decreased to once daily and reduced in total amount. L-Thyroxine may then be added as for propylthiouracil.

In hyperthyroid children, β-adrenergic blockers rarely need to be used. However, if the hyperthyroidism is particularly severe, propranolol may be prescribed in a dose of 2 to 4 mg/kg/day in three to four equally divided doses.

Severe ophthalmopathy is unusual in children. If the eyelids do not close completely, an artificial lubricant and patching at night will prevent dryness and irritation. For milder forms of the disorder, no specific treatment is needed.

OTHER THYROID DISORDERS

Hashitoxicosis

One subgroup of children presenting with the clinical and biochemical findings of hyperthyroidism rapidly becomes and remains hypothyroid soon after treatment is started. This particular variant of autoimmune thyroid disease that mimics hyperthyroidism is sometimes referred to as hashitoxicosis. The initial hyperthyroid presentation results from the release of preformed thyroid hormone, and the natural progression of the disease is to hypothyroidism, with or without treatment. A distinguishing feature in these patients, if tested, is a low uptake of radioiodine as opposed to the high uptake present in hyperthyroidism. One should be careful not to persist with antithyroid medication in this group.

Thyroiditis

Replacement therapy with L-thyroxine is the mainstay of treatment for this viral inflammatory disease. Fever, if present, should respond to nonsteroidal anti-inflammatory medication. In more severely affected patients, a short course of a corticosteroid such as prednisone (2 mg/kg once daily) should be effective.

Thyroid Nodules

If the initial studies, including ultrasonography and radionuclide scan, have not clarified the nature of the nodule, a suppressive dose of L-thyroxine for 3 to 6 months may be prescribed as a therapeutic trial, or an excisional biopsy may be performed. Should L-thyroxine cause the nodule to become smaller or disappear, treatment would continue indefinitely. If biopsy shows the nodule to be a component of a multinodular goiter, the treatment consists of long-term L-thyroxine. Over time, the goiter should slowly diminish in size. Treatment remains lifelong. If biopsy shows that the nodule is a simple adenoma, the operation would be curative and no further measures would be needed.

The treatment of a papillary, follicular, or combined papillary-follicular carcinoma remains controversial in terms of which patients should receive ablative amounts of radioiodine and when. Surgery consists of removal of the tumor-containing hemithyroid. Whatever the final decision regarding radioiodine, because these tumors are thyrotropin-dependent, long-term replacement therapy with L-thyroxine in amounts that suppress TSH should be instituted.

REFERENCES

Delange F, Fisher DA, Malvaux P: Pediatric Thyroidology. Basel, S Karger AG, 1985.

New England Congenital Hypothyroidism Collaborative: Characteristics of infantile hypothyroidism discovered on neonatal screening. J Pediatr 104:539, 1984.

PARATHYROID DISEASE

THOMAS O. CARPENTER, M.D.

The classic endocrine function of the parathyroids is to maintain normal concentrations of extracellular calcium. Therapy of parathyroid disorders is directed toward maintenance of adequate calcium and phosphate concentrations when normal regulation of parathyroid hormone (PTH) secretion is disrupted. This article therefore outlines principles of management of parathyroid-related hypocalcemia and hypercalcemia.

HYPOCALCEMIA

Acute

Hypocalcemia occurs in hypoparathyroidism, pseudohypoparathyroidism, and uncompensated secondary hyperparathyroidism. Acute, symptomatic, severe hypocalcemia should be treated with intravenous calcium, preferably calcium gluconate (which contains 9 per cent elemental calcium). A bolus injection of 10 to 20 mg elemental calcium per kilogram of body weight is given as initial therapy over 2 to 3 minutes. Cardiac monitoring should be performed. As calcium can be toxic to tissues, it should never be administered intramuscularly. Although it has been recommended that up to four total bolus injections may be given in a 24-hour period, we prefer to institute a continuous calcium infusion if repetitive doses are required. The calcium load presented to the kidneys is significantly less for the effect ultimately achieved. We recommend elemental calcium up to 60 mg/kg per 24 hours as a constant infusion. The dose can be adjusted within this range, to a total serum calcium greater than 7.0 mg/dl and alleviation of signs and symptoms or to the normal range of serum calcium.

Chronic

Chronic management of primary hypoparathyroidism or pseudohypoparathyroidism usually involves vitamin D therapy (Table 1). Recent experience in the United States suggests that calcitriol, or $1,25(OH)_2D_3$, is an effective, if costly, means of therapy for hypoparathyroidism. This active vitamin D metabolite has a relatively short half-life (6 to 12 hours in the circulation) and therefore has the advantage of a more rapid escape from toxic effects, if encountered, than the less polar metabolites, vitamin D or calcidiol (25-OHD). Calcitriol is available in 0.25- and 0.5-μg capsules. The calcitriol is in an oil-based solution within the capsule. When it is essential to give small infants this medication, an 18-gauge needle can be used to withdraw the viscous oil into a 1-ml syringe. After removal of the needle, the oil can be administered orally, directly to the infant. Doses smaller than 0.25 μg may be administered by this manipulation if necessary. Calcitriol is very potent, and we elect to start small children with 0.25 to 0.50 μg/day in one to two daily doses. This dose can be increased as necessary to maintain adequate serum calcium; we have rarely required a total daily dose in children as high as 1.5 μg, and we have not administered greater than 2.0 μg/day to children.

Alternatively, other vitamin D metabolites may be used. Vitamin D in large doses is effective in maintaining serum calcium, but arriving at a therapeutic yet nontoxic dose is more difficult. This compound is successively hydroxylated in liver and kidney to yield the much more potent $1,25(OH)_2D$. Because of significant storage of vitamin D in adipose tissue, its effects may persist months after toxicity is recognized and administration has ceased. This material is available as an oral solution (8000 units/ml) or as a tablet containing 50,000 units. We have used vitamin D in doses of 10,000 to 150,000 units/day in certain individuals with pseudohypoparathyroidism. Usually, doses between 50,000 and 100,000 units/day will maintain a normal serum calcium. The major advantage to this form of therapy is its relatively low cost.

Also available is 25-OHD, an intermediate in the synthesis of the more active $1,25(OH)_2D$. It is more expensive than vitamin D and still requires renal 1α-hydroxylation for activation. Toxic effects persist for days to weeks after discontinuation of the medication. There does not seem to be a significant advantage for the use of this compound in the

TABLE 1. Summary of Drugs Used in Parathyroid Disease

Calcitonin
Calcium (as salts of carbonate, citrate, gluconate)
Diphosphonates
Furosemide
Hydrochlorothiazide
Magnesium (as salts of chloride, citrate, gluconate, sulfate)
Prednisone
Vitamin D (ergocalciferol, cholecalciferol)
Vitamin D metabolites
25-Hydroxyvitamin D (calcidiol)
1,25-Dihydroxyvitamin D (calcitriol)
Dihydrotachysterol (DHT)
1α-Hydroxyvitamin D

treatment of parathyroid disorders; however, it may prove to be a useful vitamin D metabolite when metabolic bone disease accompanies the electrolyte disturbance. This compound is available in 20- and 50-μg capsules and is used in doses of 3 to 6 μg/kg/day.

Dihydrotachysterol is a synthetic vitamin D metabolite that does not require 1α-hydroxylation for activation. This is because the A-ring of the molecule is rotated 180 degrees, thereby placing the hydroxyl moiety at the 3-carbon in a position that stereometrically resembles the 1-hydroxyl group in the native activated hormone. This compound was widely used prior to the availability of $1,25(OH)_2D_3$, but is now comparable in cost and offers no distinct advantage over $1,25(OH)_2D_3$. We have previously used dihydrotachysterol in doses up to 2.5 mg/day; it is available in 0.125-, 0.2-, and 0.4-mg tablets and as a 0.2-mg/ml solution.

In Europe and Canada, 1α-OHD is used in doses up to 3.0 μg/day, with the similar advantages of $1,25(OH)_2D_3$.

In addition to vitamin D metabolites, added calcium can be helpful in patients with inadequate PTH or PTH action. We suggest that patients be on a total oral intake of at least 30 to 50 mg/kg/day of elemental calcium, including that derived from dietary sources. In some cases, we have introduced as much as 1000 to 1500 mg elemental calcium as a daily dietary supplement. Supplementary calcium may be given to small children conveniently as calcium glubionate (Neo-Calglucon, Sandoz). This preparation contains 115 mg calcium per 5 ml of syrup. Tablet preparations include calcium gluconate and calcium carbonate (e.g., Tums, Rolaids). The selected agent is usually given in three to four doses per day.

When serum calcium is too low and serum phosphate is persistently greater than 8.0 mg/dl, one tendency is to increase calcium supplementation, because calcium, particularly when given with meals, will serve in part as a phosphate-binding agent. An increase in vitamin D dosage in this situation may tend to increase serum phosphate as well as calcium, thereby increasing the calculated product of serum calcium concentration × serum phosphate concentration (calcium-phosphate product), which is correlated with an increased risk of soft tissue calcification.

Serum calcium is monitored twice weekly for 1 to 2 weeks until levels are stable and then no less frequently than every 3 months. In the event that hypercalcemia is encountered, all forms of vitamin D and supplemental calcium should be immediately discontinued.

A urinary calcium-to-creatinine ratio is worth monitoring, as hypercalciuria may precede hypercalcemia. (The normal range of this ratio is from 0.05 to 0.19; symptomatic hypercalciuria is >0.35.) This is particularly true in the management of hypoparathyroidism (i.e., in the absence of PTH). In hypoparathyroidism, the normal calcium-retaining effect of PTH in the distal renal tubule is absent, so that at comparable serum calcium levels the hypoparathyroid individual is likely to excrete a greater quantity of urinary calcium than the individual with intact parathyroid function. For this reason, we do not necessarily aim to correct serum calcium to normal levels but, rather, to maintain a level at which the patient is asymptomatic; this usually results in keeping the total serum calcium between 8 and 9 mg/dl. In the extreme situation in which serum calcium is below 7.5 mg/dl and symptomatic hypercalciuria (urine calcium-to-creatinine ratio > 0.35, and hematuria or dysuria) is present, the addition of thiazide diuretics may be useful. We have not used thiazides in infants younger than 2 years of age, in part because of the relatively high calcium-to-creatinine ratios seen in normal infants. In older children, hydrochlorothiazide can initially be administered in two divided doses of 25 mg/day. Dosage should not exceed the lesser of 0.5 mg/kg/day or 100 mg total daily dose. In pseudohypoparathyroidism, hypercalciuria is generally not a problem, even during therapy. Despite resistance to PTH-induced phosphaturia in the proximal renal tubule, the elevated PTH levels seen in this condition effect significant calcium retention. This phenomenon eliminates the need to follow urinary calcium excretion carefully in most cases of pseudohypoparathyroidism.

Special Considerations

Functional hypoparathyroidism may exist in magnesium deficiency. Patients with magnesium deficiency may be refractory to treatment with calcium or with vitamin D but respond well to magnesium replacement. Infants with hypomagnesemic tetany can be treated with 5 to 10 mg elemental magnesium/kg with a 50 per cent solution of $MgSO_4 \cdot 7H_2O$, either intravenously or intramuscularly. This dose should be administered slowly with cardiac monitoring and can be repeated every 12 to 24 hours. In older children, elemental magnesium (2.4 mg/kg, maximum 180 mg) can be given intravenously over 10 minutes. For oral maintenance, we use elemental magnesium (12 to 36 mg/kg/day) as magnesium citrate, diluted in water. Chloride and gluconate salts are also available.

We have recently observed that, in several patients with DiGeorge syndrome, vitamin D supplementation was not necessary to maintain normal serum calcium levels after the first month of life. Some of these patients did not require calcium supplementation above that in the diet. Interestingly, previously undetectable PTH levels during hypocalcemia were subsequently measured in the normal range during normocalcemia. These observations suggest that many patients with DiGeorge syndrome have partial hypoparathyroidism and, at least when dietary intake is normal, can maintain normal serum calcium levels. This phenomenon may be more likely to be seen when vitamin D therapy has been withheld, given the known suppressive effects of $1,25(OH)_2D$ on PTH synthesis. Future recommendations for the treatment of this syndrome may warrant management with calcium alone until the possibility of transient or partial hypoparathyroidism has been excluded.

Infants born to mothers with hyperparathyroidism are at risk for transient hypoparathyroidism. The duration of this complication may be several months. The use of low-phosphate formula, such as Similac PM 60/40, may reduce the risk of hypocalcemic tetany and is recommended in such cases.

HYPERCALCEMIA

Acute management of severe hypercalcemia is usually accomplished by administration of fluids and furosemide (Lasix). We suggest fluid administration of 1½ times normal maintenance of normal saline (NS) with appropriate added potassium. Furosemide (1 mg/kg) can be given intravenously every 6 hours as necessary. Calcium and vitamin D intake is eliminated. Once this effect is maximized, other therapy can be instituted.

If hypercalcemia is due to increased bone resorption, as in hyperparathyroidism, subcutaneous calcitonin (2 units/kg every 4 hours) may be tried. Diphosphonate compounds are currently being used in adults in clinical trials and are likely to be used in children with such problems. Glucocorticoids are usually not helpful in managing hypercalcemia resulting from hyperparathyroidism or humoral hypercalcemia of malignancy.

Hypercalcemia due to increased intestinal absorption of calcium is treated with glucocorticoids (up to 2 mg/kg/day of prednisone). In addition, dietary calcium and vitamin D should be reduced or eliminated.

Ultimately, therapy for severe infantile hyperparathyroidism will warrant parathyroidectomy. Finally, it is important to be aware of benign elevations in serum calcium, such as in familial hypocalciuric hypercalcemia, so that inappropriate treatments are not instituted.

DISORDERS OF THE ADRENAL GLAND

MARIA I. NEW, M.D.
LEFKE P. KARAVITI, M.D., Ph.D.
and CHRISTOPHER CRAWFORD

The adrenal cortex produces numerous steroid products, both precursors and active hormones, which are categorized into three types: mineralocorticoids, glucocorticoids, and sex steroids. Two cortical hormones are fundamental to normal physiologic function, and, by the controlled secretion of these hormones, the adrenal cortex is an element in two systems:

1. The hypothalamic-pituitary-adrenal (HPA) axis, which modulates adrenal synthesis of *cortisol* via the stimulatory peptide factor adrenocorticotropic hormone (ACTH). The HPA axis maintains the plasma cortisol concentration according to systemic demand. Cortisol supports normal glucose provision and utilization (glucocorticoid action) but is also a key component in many other metabolic processes. The necessary cortisol level has basal and circadian cyclic components, and the requirement increases under stress (physical or emotional stress, febrile illness, trauma, or surgery).
2. The adrenal hormone *aldosterone* ensures maintenance of normal plasma volume and electrolyte balance. Adrenal synthesis of aldosterone is stimulated by angiotensin II and by serum potassium. Aldosterone stimulates exchange transport of sodium ions across epithelium (mineralocorticoid action); the principal effect is increased sodium reabsorption and potassium excretion in the renal distal tubule. High serum potassium induces aldosterone secretion and promotes kaliuresis directly. The renin-angiotensin-aldosterone (RAA) system, by being responsive to plasma perfusion and distal tubular delivery of sodium in the kidney, provides feedback to increase vasopressor tone acutely and to promote aldosterone-dependent positive sodium balance, thereby adjusting the plasma volume relative to the total intravascular space.

Total absence of glucocorticoid and mineralocorticoid function is incompatible with life. Isolated case reports of infants with adrenal aplasia describe death as occurring within a few days of birth. Different types of hypoplasia of the adrenal cortex occur but are rare. Adrenal hemorrhage associated with trauma at delivery has been reported rarely. Adrenal insufficiency presenting in infancy will most often be caused by one of the forms of congenital adrenal hyperplasia (CAH), which results from inborn steroidogenic enzymatic defects. For this reason, the CAH syndromes are presented first and all other forms of adrenal insufficiency are considered in the subsequent text.

Errors in steroid synthesis from the enzymatic defects causing CAH also involve sex hormone production and, depending on the genetic sex, may affect the development of the sex phenotype. As a consequence, patients with CAH often present as infants with genital ambiguity or pseudohermaphroditism rather than with adrenal insufficiency. Undiagnosed or sex-misassigned children are at risk for adrenal crisis.

OVERVIEW OF THERAPEUTIC APPROACH

Therapy in all forms of adrenal insufficiency involves hormonal replacement. Maintenance therapy aims to provide essential glucocorticoid or mineralocorticoid in doses and scheduling approximating physiologic requirements. In addition, when there is steroid hormonal excess (affecting sex phenotype or electrolyte and volume status), administered steroids should suppress endogenous overproduction.

Acute states are considered in a later portion of this article. Adrenal crisis requires immediate correction of metabolic parameters as well as increased hormonal replacement consistent with the degree of stress, to be subsequently tapered to maintenance. Medical procedures (surgery and immunization) and other stress situations require increased steroid coverage.

Assessment of hyperadrenalism requires detailed endocrine evaluation supported by pharmacologic and imaging tests, and treatment is dictated by the specific diagnosis. The standard approach in many of the forms of hyperadrenalism is surgical. Radiotherapy may be indicated in recurrence of central (pituitary-hypothalamic) Cushing syndrome. Medical management has been interim (reducing hyperglucocorticoid effects before surgery or before pituitary ablation in Cushing syndrome) or palliative (in adrenocortical carcinoma); but other therapies have been tried in atypical cases or are being investigated for routine treatment in Cushing syndrome.

CONGENITAL ADRENAL HYPERPLASIA

CAH is based in inborn metabolic errors occurring at any step in cellular biosynthesis of cortisol from cholesterol in the adrenal cortex, causing reduced efficiency of cortisol production. Release of the stimulatory peptide ACTH from the anterior pituitary into the plasma is increased in the effort to maintain circulating cortisol homeostatically, which in turn increases the index of activity of the adrenocortical cells. Hyperplasia of the adrenal cortex develops as a consequence in all cases, whereas for each enzyme block, specific steroid precursors are generated and secreted in excess and others are underproduced according to the position(s) of the enzyme in the biosynthetic pathways. Hormonal effects of these steroid imbalances result in distinct clinical syndromes for each of the enzyme defects.

In the greatest number of cases by far, CAH is due to defects in the enzyme *steroid 21-hydroxylase;* defects in the enzymes *steroid 11β-hydroxylase* and *3β-hydroxysteroid dehydrogenase* account for almost all other cases. Blocks at the positions controlled by these three enzymes promote androgenic steroid synthesis relative to cortisol production. The adrenal 21-hydroxylase and 11β-hydroxylase defects result in production of potent androgens that can cause complete external virilization of genetic females and are called virilizing forms. Complete 3β-hydroxysteroid dehydrogenase defects (this enzyme is also active in the gonads) restrict androgen production to weekly hormonal precursors only, which, although causing incomplete masculinization of genetic males, may still induce androgenizing effects in females by peripheral conversion of inactive androgens to active ones.

Defects of either of the two remaining enzymes in cortisol synthesis, *steroid 17α-hydroxylase/17,20-lyase* or *cholesterol desmolase* (side-chain cleavage enzyme), which are both also gonadal enzymes, limit sex steroid synthesis and therefore cause incomplete development of genetic males. These forms of CAH are extremely rare.

Genital Ambiguity and Its Therapy

In the preponderance of cases of classic CAH (whether the salt-losing or simple virilizing form of the 21-hydroxylase defect, or 11β-hydroxylase or 3β-hydroxysteroid dehydrogenase deficiency), clitoromegaly is the presenting sign in females at birth. In some cases, an only mildly enlarged clitoris may be limited from further enlargement by steroid treatment and may become hidden by the labia majora as the child grows. Most cases, however, will require surgical correction. Previously, clitoral resection (removal) was standard. Now, a modified approach involves reduction of erectile tissue mass with preservation of the sexually sensitive glans clitoridis. This procedure, called *clitoral recession*, can be performed by age 1 year and is now generally advised. Posterior labial fusion also occurs, which, with increasing degrees of prenatal virilization (specific to the 21-hydroxylase and 11β-hydroxylase deficiency forms), progresses to the formation of a urogenital sinus or, in the most extreme cases, a phallic urethra. Clitorovaginoplasty allows recession of the clitoris and correction of labial fusion in a single stage. Vaginoplasty for correction of introital stricture (which may also require continuing use of mechanical dilators) should await the end of sexual maturation for the best reconstructive result, but optimal timing of surgery is uncertain. Consultation with an experienced psychoendocrinologist to ensure a good psychosocial outcome for the adolescent girl is advisable.

Genital development occurring in genetic males affected with any of the forms associated with defective testosterone synthesis (3β-hydroxysteroid dehydrogenase, 17α-hydroxylase/17,20-lyase, and cholesterol desmolase defects) may be so incomplete that a female sex assignment may offer better prospects for the child to undergo normal phenotypic development and achieve adult sexual function. An informed decision as to sex of rearing and the corrective surgical procedures to be performed is made by the family and pediatric endocrinologist with the participation of a urologist, gynecologist, surgeon, and psychoendocrinologist. Sex hormone replacement conforming with the sex of assignment is necessary to induce and maintain secondary sex characteristics at puberty in boys and in the 46,XY or 46,XX girl.

Hormonal Replacement

Treatment of all forms of CAH first consists of glucocorticoid replacement. This not only corrects metabolic imbalance from lack of cortisol in overt insufficiency states but also inhibits ACTH release and reduces adrenal stimulation, thereby suppressing endogenous production of other steroids. In classic 21-hydroxylase deficiency CAH, the lowering of serum androgen levels averts further virilization and prevents the inappropriate advance of bone age, allowing normal growth and puberty to occur. In steroid 11β-hydroxylase deficiency, the same suppression of androgens occurs; in addition, the suppression of sodium-retaining steroids controls hypertension. In genetic females with 3β-hydroxysteroid dehydrogenase deficiency, elevated levels of androgen precursors (Δ^5-steroids) are brought down, which limits production of stronger androgens by peripheral conversion, thus reducing virilizing effects.

Of the several steroids available, hydrocortisone is preferred as the direct replacement of the physiologic hormone. Synthetic steroids, which must be used in smaller amounts for equivalent potency to hydrocortisone, make effective dose determination more difficult in young children. Dose adjustment is especially important in children because of the negative effects of glucocorticoids on growth; thus, the synthetic compounds are more commonly used for adolescents and adults. The hydrocortisone dose varies quite widely with the individual child. An average requirement is 15 to 20 mg/m^2/day in two or three divided doses.

In forms of CAH in which sodium cannot adequately be retained—namely, salt-wasting 21-hydroxylase deficiency, 3β-hydroxysteroid dehydrogenase deficiency, and cholesterol desmolase deficiency—mineralocorticoid replacement is also necessary. Florinef (9α-fluorohydrocortisone, or fludrocortisone) is the most commonly used replacement, and the usual dose is 0.05 to 0.1 mg/day. Administration of mineralocorticoid to 21-hydroxylase deficiency patients without overt salt wasting ("simple virilizers") with high plasma renin activity (PRA) has also been found to be beneficial. PRA closely correlates with the ACTH level, and, at a given glucocorticoid dose, normalization of PRA can further decrease ACTH and thus improve androgen suppression. Hormonal control without increased glucocorticoid dosing results in improved statural growth.

Sodium chloride tablets are used for oral sodium supplementation in infants. These tablets, which come unscored in 1-g size (providing 17.5 mEq of sodium), can be divided in half when crushed for dissolving to allow dosing in 0.5-g amounts in water or the infant's feeding formula.

Therapy should be regulated by clinical and biochemical parameters. Clinically, it is important to monitor the child's growth and pubertal development. Biochemically, sensitive measurements of control are serum 17α-hydroxyprogesterone (17-OHP) and Δ^4-androstenedione (Δ^4-A). In females and prepubertal males, serum testosterone is also useful but not in newborn males or pubertal males.

PRA is also a helpful index of therapeutic control in the other forms of CAH. In the other mineralocorticoid-deficient forms (3β-hydroxysteroid dehydrogenase deficiency and cholesterol desmolase deficiency), as in salt-wasting 21-hydroxylase deficiency, negative sodium balance causes PRA to be elevated, and normalization of PRA indicates that good control has been established. In those forms of CAH with mineralocorticoid excess (11β-hydroxylase deficiency and 17α-hydroxylase deficiency), PRA is suppressed; therefore, the recovery (↑) of PRA will be an index of adequate treatment.

Follow-up visits should be at 3-month intervals. In addition to monitoring of the parameters mentioned, the growth velocity must be reckoned carefully on each of these occasions and a bone age should be obtained at least yearly.

Nonclassic or Late-Onset Forms: Steroid 21-Hydroxylase and 3β-Hydroxysteroid Dehydrogenase Deficiencies

Partial defects of the 21-hydroxylase and 3β-hydroxysteroid dehydrogenase enzymes exist, which are reflected in changes in levels of serum androgens intermediate between normal values and the extreme abnormal values seen in the classic congenital disorders. These nonclassic forms occur very frequently and show increased prevalence in certain ethnic populations (Table 1).

Changes in adrenal secretion and serum concentrations of specific steroid precursors occur that may be identified in the baseline but, in any case, are clearly evoked by a standard Cortrosyn stimulation test. Random baseline serum cortisol and ACTH values are normal, and diurnal cortisol is usually normal; however, androgenic steroids are increased. Clinical expression of hyperandrogenism in these nonclassic deficien-

TABLE 1. Nonclassic Steroid 21-Hydroxylase Enzyme Defects

Defective Allele(s)	Population	Disease Frequency
95+% B14-positive	Ashkenazic Jews	1/27
70% B14-positive	Hispanic	1/40
All B14-negative	Yugoslav	1/50
Uncharacterized	Italian	1/300
Heterogeneous	Overall	1/1000

cies is a function of individual hormonal sensitivities and variations in peripheral steroid metabolism. Thus, the same changes in hormonal values produced by a given partial defect can in different individuals produce a range of symptoms varying in degree of severity and age of appearance. Although some cases may be asymptomatic at the time of identification by biochemical or genetic studies, longitudinal observation has shown that the hyperandrogenemia can rapidly become symptomatic and that symptoms can wax and wane throughout life.

The spectrum of signs and symptoms by which these nonclassic forms of CAH manifest include (1) in childhood, the premature appearance of pubic hair, or precocious puberty or pseudopuberty (clitoromegaly is usually seen only in the classic forms); (2) peripubertally and in adulthood, menstrual disturbance, oily skin or acne often exacerbated by stress, and hirsutism or temporal balding; and (3) in adulthood, infertility and height less than that genetically predicted.

Treatment of nonclassic adrenal enzyme defects in adolescents and adults consists of glucocorticoid replacement generally with long-acting synthetic dexamethasone at a lower dose or in the same doses as for the classic congenital forms, using 17-OHP and Δ^4-A levels to monitor control.

OTHER FORMS OF ADRENAL INSUFFICIENCY

The other causes of adrenal insufficiency are primary adrenal insufficiency, secondary insufficient production of adrenal hormones (panhypopituitarism, isolated low ACTH production), and defects of hormone action (adrenal unresponsiveness to ACTH, peripheral steroid resistance).

The symptoms of adrenocortical insufficiency include malaise and easy fatiguability; gastrointestinal symptoms, such as gastric intolerance (refusal of food, vomiting) or diarrhea; hypoglycemia; acidosis; and dehydration, with the reduced intravascular fluid volume causing lowered blood pressure and azotemia and leading to cardiovascular collapse, shock, or death.

Primary Adrenocortical Insufficiency (Addison's Disease)

Addison's disease may stem from congenital adrenal *hypoplasia* or from destruction of the glandular tissue by autoimmune process or infection. Autoimmune adrenalitis is at present the most likely cause, occurring alone or often as part of a number of polyglandular autoimmune syndromes. In the past, many cases (most of those originally observed by Addison) developed from tuberculosis, but this cause is now infrequent. Fungal infections (e.g., histoplasmosis, coccidioidomycosis, blastomycosis, torulosis) can cause development of chronic adrenal insufficiency. Hemorrhage may occur in certain septicemias, among which an important type is fulminating meningococcemia (Waterhouse-Friderichsen syndrome). Other causes of loss of function include amyloidosis, hemochromatosis, and invasion by metastatic neoplasm. Adrenal failure has been reported in acquired immunodeficiency syndrome (AIDS).

In cases in which progression of the underlying disease is slow, the gradual diminution of steroid output over time may delay diagnosis. This is potentially serious. A helpful sign is hyperpigmentation, often presenting as failure to lose suntan in whites.

Treatment

Adrenocortical insufficiency warrants continuous replacement with glucocorticoid and mineralocorticoid hormones. The usual maintenance dose of hydrocortisone ranges from 12 to 20 mg/m^2/day in two or three divided doses, and Florinef from 0.05 to 0.1 mg/day.

Important parameters to monitor treatment include growth, blood pressure, serum electrolytes, and PRA. If Addison's disease has an underlying infectious etiology (e.g., tuberculosis, histoplasmosis), it is important to treat the infection concomitantly.

Secondary Adrenal Insufficiency (ACTH Insufficiency)

In contrast to primary adrenal insufficiency, secondary adrenal insufficiency is characterized by insufficient glucocorticoid but normal mineralocorticoid levels, because the production of the latter by the zona glomerulosa of the adrenal cortex is under the control of other trophic factors (angiotensin II and potassium concentration). This occurs in hypopituitary conditions resulting from hypophysectomy or suppressed secretion of ACTH consequent to exogenous steroids. Glucocorticoid replacement therapy is the same as that described for primary adrenal insufficiency.

ACTH Unresponsiveness

Therapy is the same as for secondary adrenal insufficiency.

Glucocorticoid Resistance

This rare familial condition appears to involve occurrence in kindreds of different mutations affecting functionality of the glucocorticoid receptor. Pituitary cortisol resistance, arising from the same receptor abnormality, results in increased ACTH secretion and adrenal cortisol production, thus compensating for the generalized tissue resistance. Clinical manifestations of this condition arise from ACTH elevations or increased ACTH-dependent adrenal activity. Elevated levels of glucocorticoid increase steroid binding to the mineralocorticoid receptor, and thus cause excess mineralocorticoid effect. Furthermore, ACTH stimulation of the adrenal also produces elevations of adrenal androgens. Symptoms, therefore, are hyperpigmentation, hypertension and/or hypokalemic alkalosis, or any syndrome of androgen excess such as hirsutism, polycystic ovarian disease, oligo-ovulation or anovulation, or precocious puberty. Treatment consists of a long-acting, glucocorticoid receptor–specific agent such as dexamethasone.

EMERGENCY TREATMENT

It is prudent for the patient with adrenal insufficiency or on steroid replacement/suppressive therapy to wear a Medic-Alert bracelet, medallion, or card and to be trained by health care staff in the self-administration of hydrocortisone.

Adrenal Crisis

Acute adrenal insufficiency requires prompt medical recognition and treatment. It may be precipitated in any hypofunctional adrenal condition (Addison's disease, congenital CAH), when patients are not yet diagnosed, are noncompliant with therapy, or are under unusual stress and medication has not been adjusted. Stresses may be psychologic or emotional, from physical exertion, or secondary to immunization, infection, trauma, or surgery.

In an adrenal crisis, there may be significant hyponatremia, marked hyperkalemia, hypoglycemia, and dehydration with shock. Therapy consists of volume expansion, correction of electrolyte imbalance, restoration of plasma glucose, and increased steroid replacement.

Initially, 10 to 20 ml/kg of normal saline should be given intravenously over 30 minutes to 1 hour. Alternatively, plasma volume expanders (e.g., Plasmanate) should be used at 10 to 20 ml/kg if the patient is in shock. Following the fluid bolus, volume replacement should be started, using normal saline with 5 per cent dextrose in children and with 10 per cent dextrose in infants. One half of the total estimated fluid deficit (in severe dehydration, about 10 per cent of body weight) can be replaced over the first 8 hours, and the rest can be replaced over the next 16 hours.

Hydrocortisone sodium succinate (Solu-Cortef) should be administered immediately in a dose of 100 mg/m^2 (i.e., 25 mg for an infant, 50 mg for a small child, and 100 to 150 mg for a larger child or adolescent) intravenously or intramuscularly. Hydrocortisone or Solu-Cortef should be continued at the rate of 100 mg/m^2/day divided in four doses and given every 6 hours either intravenously or by intramuscular injection.

Correction of hyponatremia may then be addressed directly by making a more precise determination of the patient's body sodium deficit. This is done by the following calculation:

$$\text{Na deficit [mEq]} = (\text{serum } [\text{Na}^+]_{\text{normal}} - [\text{Na}^+]_{\text{observed}}) \text{ [mEq/L]} \times (0.6 \times \text{euvolemic weight}) \text{ [kg]}$$

One half of the sodium deficit may be administered in the first 8 hours with intravenous fluids (over and above maintenance sodium), and the second half over the next 16 hours. Persistence of hyperkalemia may necessitate a Kayexalate enema. Rarely are other measures needed.

Mineralocorticoid replacement should be determined by the patient's electrolytes. The crisis is well managed acutely by the initial dose of hydrocortisone and saline infusion. Florinef may be started at the maintenance dose (0.05 to 0.1 mg/m^2/day) as soon as the patient can tolerate oral treatment.

It is important not to overtreat the child, as overtreatment may lead to hypokalemia and muscle weakness and to sodium and fluid retention with resulting hypertension, hypernatremia, edema, and congestive heart failure. The patient's clinical condition, including weight, fluid and electrolyte input and output, blood pressure, electrocardiogram, and serum electrolytes, must be monitored closely.

As the patient recovers and is able to tolerate oral liquids, intravenous fluids may be progressively discontinued. If hydrocortisone was given in acute-stage dose for less than 3 days, it may be reduced to maintenance without tapering. At this stage, a definitive cause of the adrenal insufficiency must be established. If the problem was entirely acute, such as septic shock occurring in the context of limited adrenal reserve, glucocorticoids provided in the acute stage have ensured the maintenance of vascular responsiveness to tonic amines and no further treatment is necessary. If the problem is one of chronic insufficiency, continued steroid replacement at maintenance doses is required. The oral dose of hydrocortisone may vary from 12.5 to 25 mg/m^2/day in two or three divided doses, and Florinef from 0.05 to 0.15 mg/day.

Perioperative Management of Patients with Addison's Disease and CAH

When a patient with chronic adrenal insufficiency is stressed (e.g., during a febrile illness or surgery), the oral dose of hydrocortisone must be doubled or tripled, depending on the degree of stress and the condition of the patient. For patients undergoing immunization, the dose should be doubled. If in the particular stress situation oral dosing would not be tolerated, parenteral administration must again be instituted. The stress dose of parenteral hydrocortisone is 40 to 60 mg/m^2/day in three or four divided doses. If the stress is a febrile illness, the increase should be continued for the duration of the illness and then maintenance therapy resumed. If the stress is surgery, either intravenous or intramuscular hydrocortisone should be administered in a dose of 40 to 60 mg/m^2/day starting 24 hours before surgery. While on call to the operating room on the day of surgery, intravenous or intramuscular Solu-Cortef should be administered, 25 mg if under 6 months of age, 50 mg if 6 months to 2 years, or 100 mg if over 2 years. During surgery, Solu-Cortef should be administered by continuous infusion, 2 mg/hour if under 2 years of age or 4 mg/hour if over 2 years. When back from surgery, Solu-Cortef or hydrocortisone should be administered at 80 mg/m^2/day by intravenous injection divided every 6 hours or every 8 hours for the first day postoperatively, continuing for 3 to 5 days depending on the procedure and the patient's condition, after which time the dose may be reduced to maintenance regimen.

For emergency surgery, a larger dose of hydrocortisone intravenously or intramuscularly should be administered (50 mg for a small child or 100 mg for a larger child or adolescent), and management continued as previously outlined.

If there is any suspicion of a suppressed adrenal state in otherwise adrenally competent patients because of a period of glucocorticoid administration at any time in the preceding 12 months, the protocol just described should also be followed to cover any major stress such as surgery.

CUSHING'S DISEASE AND CUSHING SYNDROME

Chronic hypercortisolemic states result in a wide range of symptoms. Clinical expression of any or all of these is termed Cushing syndrome. The name Cushing's disease is properly reserved for those cases caused by the presence of an ACTH-producing adenoma of the anterior pituitary gland. Treatment of Cushing syndrome follows from the specific cause, which is investigated by a number of diagnostic procedures. Note that although the etiology in many cases may clearly be established, there are examples of atypical responses in every form of Cushing syndrome, and no one test, including the most recent protocols, is 100 per cent definitive.

Lack of cortisol suppression on low-dose dexamethasone testing identifies an abnormality in the HPA axis. High-dose dexamethasone testing is then done to distinguish the following: In Cushing's disease proper, that is, pituitary micro- or macroadenoma, the adrenal cortex is driven to overproduce cortisol (and becomes hyperplastic) owing to excess stimulation by ACTH from tumorous pituitary tissue. Pituitary evaluation by magnetic resonance imaging (MRI) or computed tomography (CT) scan will provide confirmation of Cushing's disease. In the case of microadenomas not detected on CT scan, lateralization of ACTH oversecretion may be possible by inferior petrosal sinus sampling after corticotropin-releasing factor (CRF) stimulation, permitting hemihypophysectomy to be performed. Excess ACTH unresponsiveness to serum cortisol inhibitory feedback can also originate from neoplasms with neuroendocrine characteristics occurring at other sites; Cushing syndrome of this cause is called ectopic ACTH syndrome. Ectopic ACTH syndrome exhibits the most marked elevations of plasma ACTH; these are unaffected by high-dose dexamethasone testing. This syndrome is extremely rare in children. When it does occur, it may be due to adrenal rest tumors, thymoma, Wilms' tumor, or pancreatic neoplasm. When ACTH is suppressed by high-dose dexamethasone testing, a central (i.e., hypothalamic-pituitary) abnormality is excluded, and presence of adrenal tumor may be revealed by adrenal CT scan.

Iatrogenic Hypercorticoidism

Symptoms of Cushing syndrome may develop as a result of sustained exogenous steroid administration. This may be hypercortisolism from administration of excess hydrocortisone or from excess of some other potently acting synthetic glucocorticoid. This may be an unavoidable side effect of therapy necessary in serious autoimmune or neoplastic conditions or for protection against graft rejection. In other cases, such as bronchial asthma, management of cushingoid signs may be possible by adjustment of steroid dosage. In all such cases, the HPA axis will be suppressed, and tapering of doses will be necessary, with a significant post-period during which steroids may have to be increased for stress cover.

Treatment of Cushing Syndrome

Several treatment options are available for Cushing's disease. Recent advances in surgical techniques include selective surgical removal of the pituitary microadenoma(s) by the transsphenoidal route or the use of the gamma-knife. Postoperatively, adrenal insufficiency secondary to insufficient ACTH production results. This requires glucocorticoid replacement therapy, which may be tapered and discontinued in the case of a return of normal pituitary-adrenal function. When ACTH overproduction is well lateralized, hemihypophysectomy can be performed, which avoids permanent pituitary insufficiency from complete removal of the gland. Ablation of the ACTH-producing tumor, alternatively, may be achieved by radiotherapy. Exposure of the hypothalamus (which is observed to be very radiation sensitive) and reduced hypothalamic function after pituitary irradiation provide a possible explanation for the longer period before the return of circadian rhythm following this treatment. A pituitary tumor may recur a number of years after pituitary resection, most likely because the tumor results from overstimulation of the pituitary by the hypothalamic-releasing hormone (CRF). Total bilateral adrenalectomy is no longer regarded as an option because of two major disadvantages: need for lifelong steroid replacement therapy and risk of Nelson syndrome (postoperative development of ACTH-producing pituitary tumor).

In Cushing syndrome due to an adrenal tumor, surgical resection is the treatment of choice. When an autonomously functional unilateral adrenal adenoma is removed, as is usually the case, the remaining adrenal gland is often atrophic. Therefore, these patients should be supplemented with glucocorticoid therapy before, during, and after surgery until the remaining gland returns to normal, which may take many months depending on the duration of pituitary-adrenal suppression from the tumor glucocorticoid production. If bilateral tumors are present, total adrenalectomy is indicated and the patient is then committed to lifelong glucocorticoid and mineralocorticoid treatment in the doses outlined for primary adrenal insufficiency. In the case of a nonresectable adrenal carcinoma, the following drugs have been of some efficacy as palliative agents: *o,p'*-DDD, or mitotane (Lysodren), an adrenocorticolytic; metyrapone (Metopirone), a steroidogenic inhibitor at the 11β-hydroxylating step; cyproheptadine hydrochloride, a serotonin antagonist that acts centrally to inhibit ACTH secretion by the anterior pituitary; and aminoglutethimide, also an inhibitor of steroidogenesis, in this case blocking the cholesterol desmolase (cholesterol to Δ^5-pregnenolone) step. These agents, however, are not without side effects, and the results of their use with children, for which there is only limited experience, are disappointing.

When the syndrome is secondary to a nonpituitary source of ACTH (that is, ectopic ACTH), the underlying disease is treated.

VIRILIZING, FEMINIZING, AND NONFUNCTIONAL ADRENOCORTICAL TUMORS

Surgical removal of these tumors is the treatment of choice when possible. If a tumor also produces cortisol, there will be suppression of normal adrenal cortex, requiring glucocorticoid replacement until function is restored.

ADRENAL MEDULLA: PHEOCHROMOCYTOMA

Pheochromocytoma generally arises from the adrenal medulla, but it may be found anywhere along the sympathetic chain. Definitive treatment consists of surgical excision, which in these cases entails removal of the entire adrenal capsule. In children, pheochromocytoma may occur bilaterally, requiring subsequent lifelong glucocorticoid and mineralocorticoid hormonal replacement.

Two serious complications may occur during surgery: severe hypertension and cardiac tachyarrhythmia, or hypotension. Episodes of the former, which are extremely dangerous, occur when surgical manipulation of the tumor causes massive discharge of catecholamines into the circulation. On the other hand, an abrupt fall in blood pressure can occur upon removal of the source of excess catecholamines, with hypovolemic shock ensuing. Appropriate preoperative and operative management of the patient is crucial in preventing these complications.

Preparation usually begins 1 to 3 weeks before surgery. To be protected against catecholamine release, the patient is placed on α-adrenergic blockade with or without β-adrenergic blocking agents. The most commonly used α-blocker is phenoxybenzamine hydrochloride (Dibenzyline), which has a long half-life and can be given at 12-hour intervals. The usual starting dose is 5 mg every 12 hours, but must be adjusted to the patient individually in the hospital. Phentolamine (Regitine) is less satisfactory for prolonged use because of its shorter half-life, but it is equally effective in α-blockade and is particularly useful in the management of acute hypertensive episodes occurring spontaneously, provoked by a radiographic procedure, or during surgery. The emergency dose of phentolamine is 1 mg intravenously or intramuscularly.

Blockade of β-adrenergic receptors may be indicated when α-blockade alone fails to lower blood pressure or when tachyarrhythmias develop. As myocardial depressants, beta-blockers may precipitate congestive heart failure in patients with hypertensive cardiomyopathy. Propranolol (Inderal) is the most commonly used beta-blocker. Dosage calculation for this drug in children should be on the basis of body weight rather than surface area. The usual dose is 5 to 10 mg orally every 6 to 8 hours, but, again, the dose must be adjusted to the needs and response of the individual patient. Emergency dose for tachyarrhythmia is 1 mg administered intravenously over 1 minute. Most recently, metyrosine (Demser), a tyrosine hydroxylase inhibitor (therefore reducing catecholamine production) has been used in conjunction with adrenergic blockade. The usual starting dose is 5 to 10 mg/kg/day orally every 6 hours, adjusting for the individual.

Close intraoperative monitoring of the pheochromocytoma patient should include central venous and arterial pressures. There should be adequate administration of intravenous fluids during surgery to prevent hypovolemic shock following resection of the tumor. Preoperative administration of extra phenoxybenzamine may also be helpful in increasing peripheral intravascular volume expansion.

Hypertension developing during surgery can be controlled with either phentolamine or sodium nitroprusside intravenously. Supraventricular tachyarrhythmias can be treated with propranolol intravenously, and ventricular arrhythmias with lidocaine. It should be reiterated that hydrocortisone should be available for start of continuous intravenous infusion as soon as bilateral adrenalectomy has been performed, should this be necessary.

Persistence of hypertension after surgery for more than 48 hours is reason to suspect a remaining tumor(s). The importance of complete abdominal exploration at surgery should be emphasized. Also, patients may be normotensive and asymptomatic postoperatively but still have residual tumor; thus, it is important to document return of plasma and/or urinary catecholamines to normal.

Pheochromocytoma patients and their families should be followed for many years, both because of the risk of recurrence of this type of neoplasm and because of its association with conditions such as multiple endocrine adenomatosis, neurofibromatosis, and von Hippel–Lindau disease.

ENDOCRINE DISORDERS OF THE TESTIS (HYPOANDROGENISM)

ROBERT L. ROSENFIELD, M.D.

INDICATIONS FOR ANDROGEN THERAPY

Microphallus

Microphallus occurs as part of the spectrum of intersex (with hypospadias) if intrauterine hypoandrogenism is severe, or it occurs as an isolated phenomenon (with a penile urethra) if the androgen deficiency is less severe. Microphallus may occur as part of the congenital hypopituitarism syndrome in association with hypoglycemia or hyperbilirubinemia or both. It must be distinguished from pseudomicrophallus. The latter may be congenital, caused by abnormal scrotal or perineal development, or acquired, from obesity in which the penile shaft is buried in the suprapubic fat pad.

Androgen therapy is indicated to facilitate hypospadias repair or for psychologic reasons. Low-dose testosterone stimulates growth of the penis, provided that the child does not have androgen resistance. The optimum age for treatment is within the first 6 months of life, when the minipuberty of the newborn normally stimulates a surge in testosterone secretion and penile growth. However, there is no evidence that the ultimate size of the penis will become normal. A 3-month course of topical testosterone or depot testosterone (25 mg IM every 3 weeks four times) will stimulate penile growth without virilizing the child. A second or third course of treatment as the child grows tends to normalize penis size for age. Reassurance as to the adequacy of a small penis for sexual satisfaction of the partner is usually indicated. Extreme microphallus is an indication for sex reversal in early infancy.

Sexual Infantilism

In patients in whom the diagnosis of primary or secondary hypogonadism can be established early (as when gonadotropins are elevated or anorchia or anosmia are present), physiologic androgen replacement therapy can be begun at about 12 years of age. Typically, the bone age is 11 to 12 years and the linear growth rate begins to fall at this time. In such cases, therapy can commence with an anabolic dose of depot testosterone (50 mg/m^2 IM monthly for 1 year). In the long-term treatment of hypogonadal boys, we advise subsequently advancing virilization with depot testosterone (100 mg IM monthly for 1 year, followed by 200 mg monthly for 1 year, followed by the adult maintenance dose of 200 mg every 2 weeks). If short stature is a major problem, we advise advancing these doses according to a slower schedule.

Once clinical virilization is complete in the late teenage years, oral androgen analogues may be substituted for testosterone injections. In hypogonadal patients, associated hormone deficiencies, particularly those of thyroid or growth hormone, should be concurrently replaced in order for the full expression of the androgen treatment to be manifest. The underlying disease that may be the cause of the hypogonadism should be treated appropriately. Hypogonadal patients can be reassured that they will experience normal sexual development and sexual function in response to androgen therapy, without compromising growth potential. Patients with infertility often have feelings of "incompleteness" about not being able to father children, and these feelings must be recognized and discussed when they surface. In patients with anorchia, testicular prostheses can be placed surgically during mid childhood and larger ones can be implanted in the teenage years if desired.

Klinefelter Syndrome

Approximately half of the patients with Klinefelter syndrome are mildly hypoandrogenic. Androgen replacement therapy is indicated for these patients. Gynecomastia may be aggravated by virilizing doses of testosterone. When gynecomastia is severe, reduction mammoplasty is the only available treatment. The infertility in Klinefelter syndrome is irreversible.

ANDROGENS AND ANABOLIC AGENTS

Topical Androgens

Crystalline testosterone in 1 per cent hydrophilic petrolatum (nonformulary) may be prescribed with thin application twice daily as one to three 3-month courses for microphallus.

Parenteral Androgens

Depot forms of testosterone are the preferable agents to induce full sexual development in sexually infantile males. Intramuscular injection of depot forms of testosterone results in peak blood levels within a few days, which decline to baseline levels by approximately 3 weeks. The depot forms of testosterone available for intramuscular use are the cypionate (Depo-Testosterone) and enanthate (Delatestryl) esters in cottonseed and sesame oil, respectively. The former is available in a concentration of 100 mg/ml, and both are available in concentrations of 200 mg/ml in 10-ml containers.

Oral Androgens

Methyltestosterone (17α-methyltestosterone) is short-acting, with a half-life of about 2.5 hours. The usual oral dose for maintaining secondary sexual characteristics in hypoandrogenic patients is 5 to 20 mg twice a day. This agent is available generically in 10- and 25-mg tablets.

Fluoxymesterone (9α-fluoro-11β-hydroxy-17α-methyltestosterone [Halotestin]) has a half-life of about 10 hours. The usual dose for maintenance of secondary sexual characteristics in hypogonadal males is 10 to 20 mg/day. It is available in tablets of 2, 5, and 10 mg.

Anabolic Steroids

Anabolic steroids are synthetic modifications of the testosterone molecule, which have been claimed to exhibit partial separation of anabolic from androgenic effects according to bioassays in animals. They are used for the treatment of short stature, which is associated with hypogonadism syndromes. The most widely used for this purpose is oxandrolone (17α-methyl-2-oxo-dihydrotestosterone [Anavar]). The usual dose for growth stimulation in boys is 0.1 mg/kg/day. It is available in 2.5-mg tablets and is given in one to two daily doses. It is available as an orphan drug from Gynex, Vernon Hills, Illinois.

Gonadotropin Therapy

Gonadotropin therapy has no place in the treatment of hypogonadal teenagers. Human chorionic gonadotropin has a place only as a diagnostic agent. Gonadotropin or pulsatile gonadotropin-releasing hormone therapy is indicated only in hypogonadotropin patients at an age when they desire spermatogenesis for fertility in adult life. The gonadotropin effect on spermatogenesis continues for only as long as the treatment is given.

ADVERSE EFFECTS OF ANDROGENS

Androgen treatment of children carries the risk of compromising adult height through premature epiphyseal closure. This is a time- and dose-related effect. The risk can be avoided by use of the physiologic treatment regimen previously outlined. Androgen therapy is not generally appropriate until a bone age of approximately 11 years has been achieved. Height prediction should be made from an evaluation of height and bone age before treatment and at 6-month intervals during treatment.

The parenteral (depot) forms of testosterone have several advantages over orally active androgens. They provide the natural form of testosterone itself. This is the only form of androgen available that is potent enough to bring about full virilization. Furthermore, the 17α-methyl–substituted steroids are unique in their ability to cause intrahepatic cholestasis (causing nausea, often in the absence of jaundice, and usually reversible when the drug is discontinued), hepatic cellular carcinoma, and peliosis hepatis.

Acne and gynecomastia are side effects of all androgens. If a full androgen replacement is begun suddenly in eunuchoid individuals, the frequency of erections may be very disturbing psychologically. Sodium and fluid retention is an inherent effect of androgens and may present problems in patients with a pre-existent tendency to the development of edema.

GYNECOMASTIA

JOSEPH I. WOLFSDORF, M.B., B.Ch.

Gynecomastia refers to breast enlargement in the male, and in pediatric medicine it occurs in three age groups—neonatal, prepubertal, and pubertal.

Neonatal

Many newborn infants have palpable breast tissue that increases in size in the first few days of life. Neonatal gynecomastia results from transplacental passage of maternal estrogen to the fetus and can be expected to resolve spontaneously within a few weeks or, in occasional cases, a few months. No investigation or therapy is required. Gynecomastia may be accompanied by galactorrhea ("witch's milk"), and it is important to instruct parents not to manipulate the infant's breasts in an attempt to discharge the milk because this can lead to infection.

Prepubertal

Gynecomastia before puberty is rare and warrants a thorough search for a possible source of exogenous estrogens, such as ingestion of contraceptive pills, use of an estrogen-containing cream, or consumption of milk, meat, or poultry that contains estrogens. The breast is exquisitely sensitive to estrogen, and gynecomastia can develop in boys exposed to trace amounts of estrogens in foods, making it difficult or impossible to identify the source. Furthermore, gynecomastia may persist after the exposure to estrogen has ceased; consequently, at the time of evaluation, the causative pharmacologic or environmental factor may no longer be present. Other causes of prepubertal gynecomastia should be assiduously sought by endocrinologic investigation and appropriate imaging techniques; ultrasonography of the testes may be valuable in identifying an impalpable testicular tumor, and computed tomography (CT) and magnetic resonance imaging (MRI) of the abdomen in identifying adrenal tumors. Other causes include estrogen-secreting adrenal or testicular tumors, congenital adrenal hyperplasia (especially 11β-hydroxylase deficiency), and trophoblastic (human chorionic gonadotropin [hCG]–secreting) tumors. The virilization of sexual precocity may be associated with gynecomastia, as it would in normal adolescent development (see later).

Treatment of the underlying disorder will stop progression of the gynecomastia. If the work-up is negative, the patient may be said to have idiopathic prepubertal gynecomastia, for which there is no specific therapy, and the gynecomastia can be expected to resolve spontaneously within a few years.

Pubertal

A firm disc of subareolar breast tissue, often slightly tender, is common in healthy adolescent boys (occurring in approximately 40 per cent) and may be accompanied by elevation of the areola. This is usually most evident at about 14 years of age, corresponding to Tanner stages III to IV of pubertal development, and the diameter of the breast usually does not exceed 4 cm. The breasts are typically unequal in size, and the discrepancy can be marked. The patient and his parents should be reassured that this is a normal developmental phenomenon related to the production of sex hormones and does not signify pathology. The condition can be expected to regress spontaneously within 24 months and does not warrant treatment. Extremely prominent breast enlargement can occur as an expression of pubertal gynecomastia (pubertal macromastia), but before one ascribes it to this cause, it is appropriate to undertake a thorough search to rule out an estrogen-secreting tumor of the adrenal gland or testis or a trophoblastic (hCG-secreting) tumor. Other pathologic causes of gynecomastia are drug exposure, liver disease, Graves' disease, and disorders characterized by testicular deficiency (e.g., Klinefelter syndrome.) Drugs that may cause gynecomastia include spironolactone, digitalis, methyldopa, cimetidine, phenothiazines, tricyclic antidepressants, isoniazid, ketoconazole, and marijuana. The presence of galactorrhea warrants testing for a prolactinoma. The testes should be carefully examined for the presence of a tumor and their size determined as accurately as possible. A testicular volume exceeding 4 ml or length greater than 2.5 cm excludes Klinefelter syndrome from further consideration. Differentiation of mammary tissue from adipose tissue by palpation may be difficult in obese youths in whom the appearance of gynecomastia (pseudogynecomastia) is usually principally the result of accumulation of adipose tissue in the area of the breast. Weight loss will reduce the size of breasts, largely composed of adipose tissue. Gynecomastia must also be differentiated from rare tumors that may present as breast enlargement, such as lipoma, neurofibroma, and breast cancer.

Severe physiologic gynecomastia with more than 5 cm breast tissue and pronounced areolar changes seldom resolves spontaneously, or, if it does, will take several years to occur. Because pronounced gynecomastia is difficult to conceal and is a source of extreme embarrassment to the afflicted youth, a reduction mammoplasty, using a circumareolar incision, is recommended sooner rather than later to spare the patient further embarrassment and any possibility of confusion about his sexual identity. Modern surgical techniques can be expected to result in a barely noticeable hairline scar.

Testosterone therapy is contraindicated in adolescent gynecomastia and will actually increase the size of the breasts. Testosterone therapy may be indicated in patients with Klinefelter syndrome with subnormal testosterone levels; however, its effect on gynecomastia is not consistently beneficial.

Various drug regimens have been reported to be effective for the treatment of gynecomastia; however, the studies have not been well controlled nor have the beneficial effects of these medications been widely confirmed. They include dihydrotestosterone heptanoate, which cannot be aromatized to estrogen; testolactone, which inhibits steroid aromatase activity and decreases estrogen synthesis; and the antiestrogens tamoxifen and clomiphene.

AMBIGUOUS GENITALIA

SELVA S. SCHENKMAN, M.D.
and EDNA H. SOBEL, M.D.

The assignment of gender usually occurs in the delivery room. The case of a newborn with ambiguous genitalia represents a medical and social emergency. Designation of sex must await expeditious and rational investigation to establish the sex of rearing. *During this period, the infant must be monitored for the emergence of a metabolic problem: hypoglycemia or hyponatremia.* The family will require support; explanation that the sex structures of the child developed incompletely during fetal life is needed. Diagrams of fetal sexual differentiation will be helpful to show the similarities of external genital appearance of boys and girls at the 3rd month of gestation.

A good history is required to differentiate exogenous (maternal) from endogenous (fetal) causes of ambiguity. A family history of unexpected neonatal death will direct attention to the possibility of an adrenal enzyme defect.

Useful details in physical examination include the presence of palpable gonads and perineal malformations. Rectal examination is helpful because the cervix of an infant girl is often palpable. The presence of internal feminine structure may be revealed by pressure on the uterus, which may cause mucus to be extruded from a urogenital sinus. Ultrasonography is usually not definitive because there is little fat to provide contrast.

Laboratory procedures should be chosen on the basis of probable etiology. Those usually selected are karyotype, which is much more reliable than a buccal smear, and 17-OH progesterone, 11-deoxycortisol, and testosterone.

Spot urine check for sodium (Na^+) and potassium (K^+) ratio can be useful because abnormal salt balance will become evident in the urine before it is reflected in the plasma. By the 5th day of life, plasma renin, Na^+, and K^+ will identify the infant with salt-wasting congenital adrenal hyperplasia (CAH). Other procedures, such as adrenocorticotropic hormone (ACTH) stimulation and gonadotropin stimulation, will come later, if needed.

It is useful to design the investigation in accordance with knowledge of normal sex differentiation. Sex differentiation is sequential and involves several phases from the moment of conception. The genetic sex is determined at fertilization. The gonadal sex is determined by the chromosomes. The function of the gonadal axis determines the internal and external phenotype. Finally, gender identity is acquired postnatally by the individual through lived experiences, environment, and personal hormonal milieu.

The fetal ovary does not secrete testosterone or müllerian-inhibiting factor (MIF). The normal female is born without male differentiation of the external genitalia and without müllerian repression (with uterus and fallopian tubes). The fetal testis does secrete testosterone and MIF. Fetal androgens cause stimulation of the wolffian ducts, posterior migration of the labioscrotal folds, so that the phallus lies anterior to the scrotum, elongation of the genital tubercle, midline fusion of the genital folds and swellings to form the penis and scrotal sacs. In the male, the source of androgen is the fetal testis. In a female fetus, any source of androgen will cause complete or partial male differentiation of external genitalia. Failure to secrete enough androgen results in various degrees of male pseudohermaphroditism.

There are four pathophysiologic categories of sexual ambiguity:

1. Virilization of an ovary-bearing 46,XX female *(female pseudohermaphroditism)*. Such a child has normal internal müllerian structures and is potentially fertile. The etiology is fetal or transplacental. In the fetus, increased androgen production occurs because of an enzyme block that interferes with cortisol production and leads to increased ACTH secretion. In 90 per cent, the error is 21-OH deficiency, and in 10 per cent is 11-OH or 3-BOH dehydrogenase deficiency. All are inherited as autosomal recessive traits.

Leydig cell tissue in a 46,XX fetus with dysgenetic testes produces androgen, which masculinizes the genitalia. Such testes usually do not produce MIF, so the müllerian structures are preserved.

Androgen may reach the fetus in the first trimester from a maternal virilizing disorder or because of androgen treatment of the mother. One must remember that androgens can be ingested by "accident" (e.g., use of geriatric vitamin preparations).

2. Gonads palpable and incomplete masculinization of the testis-bearing 46,XY male *(male pseudohermaphroditism)*.

The etiology includes hypothalamic-hypophyseal abnormality, whereby the fetal testis does not receive stimulation to produce testosterone. Such infants may become hypoglycemic because of insufficient growth hormone or ACTH. Androgen synthesis may be defective in adrenal and testis 20,22-desmolase deficiency; 17,20-desmolase deficiency; or 17-OH dehydrogenase deficiency. A human chorionic gonadotropin (hCG) stimulation test may be useful during infancy to clarify testicular capacity to produce androgen.

Abnormalities in testosterone metabolism are another possible cause: 5α-reductase deficiency, abnormality of testosterone receptors, or a post-receptor defect. If one testis is defective, müllerian structures may persist on that side.

Androgen insensitivity comes into question only if a normal-appearing girl has an inguinal hernia. The sex of rearing must be feminine in such a child.

3. *True hermaphroditism.* In this case, the infant has both ovarian and testicular tissues with abnormal internal and external genital structures. In 80 per cent, karyotype is 46,XX; in 10 per cent, 46,XY; in 10 per cent, mosaicism (5 per cent have female genitalia and 45,X/XY).

The gonad distribution most frequently encountered is ovary/testis or ovatestis/ovary. In the management of patients with no palpable gonads, exploratory laparotomy is almost always included. If the gonad is dysgenetic or streak, it should be removed. If there are functional ovaries and female external appearance, the testicular tissue should be removed. If there is a testis in an abnormal position and male gender can be assigned, the testis should be exteriorized and any müllerian remnants or streak gonad removed. hCG stimulation and accurate hormonal evaluation should be carried out before laparotomy.

4. Anatomic disruption of normal female or male structures. In these disorders, defects of embryogenesis are included. The mechanism is neither hormonal nor chromosomal. The endocrinologist as a subspecialist should be involved for the clarification and management of sex reversal or for hormone replacement therapy in the case of gonadal reversal.

Sex assignment in infants with sexual ambiguity must involve all these points, but will mainly be dictated by the external genital appearance and the capacity of potential full function at the time of puberty and adulthood. In virilized female infants with CAH, the female gender should always be assigned, as these patients have normal internal müllerian structures and fertile ovaries.

Reconstructive surgery should be performed before age 3 years, when the toddler is first aware of his or her sex identity. Cases of hypogonadism with micropenis or hypopituitarism with associated growth hormone deficiency will require evaluation and replacement treatment. Dysgenetic tissue (gonads) should be resected, as the potential for malignancy increases with age. In cases of complete androgen insensitivity (testicular feminization), the testes should remain in place until after puberty, as they allow feminization at puberty and their potential for malignancy is very low.

Once an infant is given a sex of rearing, the family should have a clear understanding and no doubts in their minds. Psychologic support and therapy should be made available when necessary for the family and child.

REFERENCES

Drucker S, New MI: Disorders of adrenal steroidogenesis. Pediatr Clin North Am 34:1055–1066, 1987.

Money J: Psychologic counseling: Hermaphroditism. *In* Gardner LI (ed): Endocrine and Genetic Diseases in Childhood and Adolescence, 2nd ed. Philadelphia, WB Saunders Co, 1975, pp 609–618.

Saenger P: Abnormal sexual differentiation. J Pediatr 104:1–17, 1984.

Styne DM: Ambiguous genitalia. *In* Fitzgerald PA (ed): Handbook of Clinical Endocrinology. Greenbrae, Calif, Jones Medical Publications, 1986, pp 65–79.

PRECOCIOUS AND DELAYED PUBERTY

JAMES P. GUTAI, M.D.

Precocious puberty may be defined in girls as the development of breast tissue and pubic hair prior to 8 years of age. It must be distinguished from *premature thelarche,* which is the early development of breasts only, and *premature adrenarche,* which is the early development of pubic hair only. In boys, the enlargement of testes from a 3-ml volume to a 4-ml volume and the development of pubic hair before 9 years of age define precocious puberty. Because the gonads in boys are easy to palpate, the differential between central precocious puberty and peripheral precocity is easier. In true precocious puberty, the testes are enlarged by the stimulation of the pituitary gonadotropins. *A significant percentage of boys with central precocious puberty have brain tumors.* A negative central nervous system work-up should be repeated 6 months after the initial evaluation. In girls, there is not an increased incidence of central nervous system tumors. Rather, precocious puberty represents an early desensitization of the normal feedback control of gonadotropin secretion.

Peripheral precocious puberty implies either an extrapituitary source of gonadotropins or a gonadotropin-independent secretion from either the testes or the ovary. This may be associated with hepatomas that secrete chorionic gonadotropins or with primary testicular or ovarian disorders. Virilizing adrenal hyperplasia is associated with rapid growth, phallic enlargement, and the early development of pubic hair. However, the testes remain small.

Normal puberty is characterized by a growth acceleration and subsequent epiphyseal fusion. As puberty begins, approximately 75 per cent of final height is attained. Thus, a feature of precocious puberty is the early attainment of final height, which results in short stature. The child with precocious puberty may be the object of teasing by other children and also have difficulty with secondary sex characteristics, such as pubic hair, breast enlargement, or frequent erections. Many girls have emotional difficulties when menarche occurs before age 9. The goals of management should be to establish the correct diagnosis, reverse the secondary sex characteristics, preserve as much adult height as possible, and prevent long-term psychologic consequences of early development.

CENTRAL PRECOCIOUS PUBERTY

At present, no drug is marketed with an indication for the treatment of precocious puberty. The long-acting gonadotropin-releasing hormone (GnRH) agonists provide the physiologic treatment of choice because they alter the early activation of the pituitary hypothalamic system. Until recently, either daily subcutaneous injection or multiple daily intranasal administration of these drugs was required. This made compliance problematic. However, use of these drugs in studies showed a significant decrease in sex steroid concentrations and height velocities and an increase in the predicted adult height. *Currently, pediatric endocrinologists (using informed consent protocol) are using the depot form of leuprolide acetate in varying intramuscular doses from 0.3 mg/kg per dose to a total monthly dose of 7.5 mg or greater.* The goals of such therapy should be to decrease the sex steroid concentrations to achieve a prepubertal response to intravenous GnRH.

These patients require close follow-up and should be managed only by a pediatric endocrinologist. Prior to the availability of the GnRH agonists, medroxyprogesterone acetate, a progestational agent that blocks gonadotropin secretion, was the only drug available for the treatment of central precocious puberty. Although it was effective in lowering sex steroid concentrations, halting the progression of secondary sexual characteristics, and delaying menarche, there appeared to be little effect on skeletal maturation and final adult height. A significant side effect has been increased body weight, which is associated with its glucocorticoid potency. Currently, medroxyprogesterone acetate (50 to 200 mg every 2 to 4 months) is used to halt menses in severely impaired adolescents for whom menses may be a significant hygiene problem.

PERIPHERAL PRECOCIOUS PUBERTY

Because the sex steroid production is independent of pituitary gonadotropin secretion, the GnRH agonists have no role in the treatment of this heterogeneous group of conditions. It is vitally important that the proper diagnosis be made. If a tumor of the ovaries, testes, or adrenal is the basis of the increased sex steroid hormone concentrations, the treatment is surgical. In boys, non–salt-losing adrenal hyperplasia may cause a peripheral precocious puberty and is treated with appropriate doses of glucocorticoid. Ketoconazole, an antifungal agent, used in doses of 400 to 600 mg/day, has been used successfully to treat many cases of gonadotropin-independent testosterone excess. This agent inhibits testosterone biosynthesis but is potentially hepatotoxic. Moreover, adrenal function was significantly impaired.

The aromatase inhibitor testolactone has been used in the treatment of children with McCune-Albright syndrome, sexual precocity, café au lait spots, and fibrous dysplasia of bone. When administered orally in divided doses of 20 to 40 mg/kg/day, testolactone results in a suppression of estradiol concentrations and a cessation of menses. The antiandrogen cyproterone acetate in doses of 70 to 150 mg/m^2/day has been used to lower serum testosterone in some cases of the idiopathic testosterone hypersecretion, but adrenal function was significantly impaired.

The needs of the child with precocious puberty are often ignored. The physician must spend time with the family explaining that this is the early activation of a normal process. The parents should be encouraged to talk with their child to reinforce this concept. Children with sexual precocity rarely have increased libido. They may be confused and frightened about the changes occurring in their bodies. Because they are taller than their peers, they are often assumed to be older and thus have an increased degree of social maturity. All of these factors can result in withdrawal and social isolation. The physician should always ascertain how the child is functioning at home and with peers and should be prepared to recommend professional counseling as the situation indicates.

DELAYED PUBERTY

Puberty in girls is considered to be delayed if there is neither pubic hair development nor breast budding by age 13. The lack of testicular enlargement (3-ml volume to 4-ml volume) or pubic hair development in boys by age 14 signals the need for an evaluation. Puberty is characterized by an increase in both the amplitude and the frequency of pituitary luteinizing hormone (LH) pulses, which is in response to the activation of the hypothalamic pulse generator.

Alterations in the time of onset of puberty may be caused by chronic illnesses, nutrition, extreme exercise, hypothyroidism, genetic defects (gonadal dysgenesis, Klinefelter syndrome), hypothalamic hypogonadism, or constitutional delay. A much higher percentage of girls are found to have a specific etiology for the delay, whereas the majority of boys are found to have constitutional delay. Differentiation between hypothalamic hypogonadism and constitutional delay is difficult. In many cases, the correct diagnosis is made only by time and the response to therapy. As many more children with neoplastic diseases are surviving into adolescence and adulthood, the effect of both chemotherapy and radiation on puberty must be recognized.

Girls

The girl with short stature and delayed puberty must have a karyotype to rule out gonadal dysgenesis (Turner syndrome or mosaicism). Adolescents with gonadal dysgenesis may not have the classic physical findings of gonadal dysgenesis, but rather only delayed puberty and short stature. *Current therapy of children with Turner syndrome is human growth hormone with or without a weak androgen such as oxandrolone.* The time of introduction of estrogen is based on the bone age, height prediction, and psychologic needs of the adolescent. We have usually delayed replacement therapy until the bone age is at least 13 years.

Treatment regimens vary and include the use of conjugated estrogens or ethinyl estradiol by mouth or injections of depot estrogen. A daily oral dose of 0.3 mg conjugated estrogen or 5 μg ethinyl estradiol or a monthly injection of 0.5 mg depot estradiol (estradiol cypionate) will stimulate breast development, preserve adult height, and not initiate menstrual flow. In girls with primary gonadal failure that is not caused by gonadal dysgenesis, or in girls with hypothalamic dysfunction, usual replacement is over a 2- to 3-year period. The timing is based on bone age and psychologic needs.

With the use of oral conjugated estrogens (Premarin, 0.3 mg/day) or ethinyl estradiol (20 μg every other day), some breast budding is achieved. The dose of estrogen is increased at 3- to 4-month intervals until the full adult replacement of 1.25 mg/day conjugated estrogen or 50 μg ethinyl estradiol is reached. When vaginal spotting occurs, cyclic estrogen therapy on days 1 through 21 of the cycle should be used. After 1 to 2 years of cyclic estrogen withdrawal bleeding, oral progesterone (Provera, 10 mg/day) may be used on days 17 to 22 of the cycle. Once full adult height is reached, most girls prefer to take oral contraceptives. The contraceptive pill that contains the lowest dose of estrogen is preferable. Other regimens using intramuscular depot estrogen have been used. Current trials are under way using transdermal estrogen patches. The advantage of the transdermal route is that it avoids the first passage of the estrogen through the liver and the effect on liver proteins.

When delayed puberty is secondary to elevated prolactin, the response to bromocriptine mesylate should be assessed. A starting dose of 1.25 mg at bedtime will minimize significant side effects of nausea. This dose should be gradually increased until full replacement of 2.5 mg two to three times a day is achieved.

Psychogenic amenorrhea, athletic amenorrhea, and anorexia nervosa may be part of a spectrum. Both caloric restriction and weight loss may cause an arrest of pubertal development. In such cases, both the family and the adolescent will require counseling regarding the role of nutrition in the lack of pubertal development. Obesity as well as undernutrition may be responsible for delays in pubertal maturation.

Boys

A wide variety of conditions may delay puberty in boys. Constitutional delay is the most common reason, but this must be differentiated from hypothalamic hypogonadism. Systemic diseases associated with malnutrition, weight loss, stress, and malabsorption may result in delayed puberty. As in girls, hyperprolactinemia and hypothyroidism may result in pubertal delay. Poorly controlled diabetes may also cause growth failure, delayed puberty, and hepatomegaly (Mauriac syndrome). Pharmacologic doses of glucocorticoids for a variety of conditions can result in delayed puberty. It is important that the primary disease be treated before therapy for delayed puberty.

Primary testicular defects are associated with elevated gonadotropins and low concentrations of testosterone. A partial list of etiologic factors includes absent testes, irradiation, chemotherapy, infection (mumps, coxsackievirus), Klinefelter syndrome, sickle cell disease, and bilateral testicular torsion. These children will require lifelong replacement with testosterone. The start of therapy should be dependent on the bone age, height, and psychologic needs. Most treatment protocols use a depot form, either testosterone cypionate or enanthate. The oral testosterone preparations having a methyl group at the 17 position have been implicated in nausea, cholestasis, and a risk of hepatocellular carcinoma.

It is desirable to attempt to duplicate the normal pubertal time span of 3 to 4 years. An initial starting dose of 50 mg intramuscularly monthly may be increased at 3- to 4-month intervals until adult replacement doses of 200 mg every 2 weeks are achieved. Men receiving a single monthly dose of

400 mg of testosterone may describe a waning of the testosterone effect with a loss of libido. It is important to teach the adolescent how to give his own injections. This described regimen will cause normal pubertal progression and adult sexual function. When spermatogenesis is a goal, pulsatile GnRH has been successful. Prior treatment with sex steroids does not preclude the later use of pulsatile GnRH.

As mentioned, constitutional delay is the most common cause of late puberty in boys. It is associated with short stature, delayed bone age, and delayed puberty. Constitutional delay can be difficult to distinguish from hypogonadism, but overnight frequent sampling of gonadotropins and GnRH testing may be of some aid. The association of anosmia and hypothalamic hypogonadism is Kallmann syndrome. However, patients with hypothalamic hypogonadism may have a normal sense of smell. Usual treatment protocols recommend initial starting doses of 50 to 150 mg depot testosterone monthly for 3 to 6 months. This should not be used until skeletal age is greater than 12.5 years. With this limited time span and dose, there does not appear to be any compromise in adult height.

At the end of the specific treatment protocol, testicular size should be evaluated. If there has been an increase in testicular size, hypothalamic hypogonadism is unlikely. In any case, pubertal maturation should be followed at 3- to 4-month intervals. A spontaneous progression of pubertal development confirms the diagnosis of constitutional delay of puberty. These boys need reassurance that they will continue to grow after other boys have stopped and that they are a variant of normal. If there is not a spontaneous progression of puberty and there is no change in either testosterone concentration or response to GnRH, a second cycle of testosterone therapy for 4 to 6 months is indicated. A lack of pubertal progression 6 months after the end of the second treatment cycle may indicate hypothalamic hypogonadism.

10

Metabolic Disorders

INFANTS BORN TO DIABETIC MOTHERS

JOHN P. CLOHERTY, M.D.

The recent reduction in perinatal mortality and morbidity in infants of diabetic mothers (IDMs) has been due to improvements in medical and obstetric care of mothers and advances in the care of the newborn. A major cause of this improvement has been the prolongation of pregnancy; furthermore, the ability to assess pulmonary maturity in the fetus has reduced the incidence of respiratory distress syndrome (RDS) in IDMs. Infants of mothers with severe renal and vascular disease are often delivered early because of maternal problems (hypertension, renal failure) or fetal distress. These infants are more likely to have complications such as asphyxia, respiratory distress syndrome, jaundice, and poor feeding. Before the delivery of the IDM there should be clear communication between specialists in medicine, obstetrics, and pediatrics so that problems can be anticipated.

CLASSIFICATION

Mothers with diabetes are classified according to White's classification (Table 1). There is a relationship between perinatal outcome and White's class. The risk of complications is minimal in gestational diabetes. Macrosomia and neonatal hypoglycemia are sometimes seen. The most difficult maternal, fetal, and neonatal problems occur in women with renal, cardiac, or retinal disease. Class F disease (renal) has an adverse affect on fetal outcome. It is associated with the necessity for early delivery. Class H (cardiac disease) is associated with maternal death. Retinopathy may progress during pregnancy.

MATERNAL-FETAL PROBLEMS

Fertility

Diabetic women appear to have normal fertility.

Abortions

There is no increase in the spontaneous abortion rate in early pregnancy in *well-controlled* diabetic pregnancies as compared with nondiabetic pregnancies. The spontaneous abortion rate in nondiabetic pregnancy is 16 per cent. Women with poor diabetic control in pregnancy have a significantly increased incidence of spontaneous abortion.

Problems During Pregnancy and Delivery

In the first half of pregnancy, hypoglycemia and ketonuria are common. The nausea and vomiting seen in any pregnancy may make control difficult. Moderate hypoglycemia not associated with hypotension may not be harmful to the fetus.

In the second trimester, the *insulin requirement* increases. This increased requirement is sometimes associated with *ketoacidosis,* which may result in fetal mortality.

In the third trimester, a major problem is *sudden, unexpected fetal death.* Such deaths are sometimes associated with ketoacidosis, pre-eclampsia, or maternal vascular disease of the decidua and myometrium, but many are unexplained. The incidence of this problem has decreased during the past 20

TABLE 1. White's Classification of Maternal Diabetes (Revised)

Gestational diabetes (GD)	Diabetes not known to be present before pregnancy Abnormal glucose tolerance test in pregnancy
GD diet	Euglycemia maintained by diet alone
GD insulin	Diet alone insufficient—insulin required
Class A	Chemical diabetes: glucose intolerance prior to pregnancy; treated by diet alone; rarely seen
Class B	Insulin-dependent: onset after 20 years of age; duration less than 10 years
Class C	C_1: Onset between 10 and 19 years of age C_2: Duration 10 to 19 years
Class D	D_1: Onset before 10 years of age D_2: Duration 20 years or more D_3: Benign retinopathy (microvascular disease) D_4: Hypertension (not pre-eclampsia)
Class F	Nephropathy with over 500 mg/day of proteinuria
Class R	Proliferative retinopathy or vitreous hemorrhage
Class RF	Criteria for both classes R and F coexist
Class H	Clinical evidence of arteriosclerotic heart disease
Class T	Prior renal transplantation

All classes below A require insulin. Classes R, F, RF, H, and T have no criteria for age of onset or duration of disease but usually occur in long-term diabetes.

Thanks to Michael F. Greene of the Brigham and Women's Hospital, Department of Obstetrics and Gynaecology, for review of the obstetric text.

years with the use of tests of fetal well-being, but it still occurs occasionally.

In the third trimester, class F mothers may have anemia, hypertension, and decreased renal function. Women with class H disease have a great risk of myocardial failure with infarction. Women with class R disease have a risk of neovascularization, vitreous hemorrhage, or retinal detachment; their infants are usually delivered by cesarean section.

Fetal macrosomia and enlargement of the cord and placenta may be seen in gestational diabetics and in classes A, B, C, and some D diabetic pregnancies. Macrosomia increases the potential for difficult delivery, obstetric trauma, or primary cesarean section.

In diabetic women with vascular disease (especially class F), there is an increased risk of in utero growth retardation (20 per cent). This growth retardation is associated with a small infarcted placenta, decreased uteroplacental perfusion, abnormal results in tests of fetal well-being, such as non–stress test (NST) and oxytocin challenge test (OCT), and increased incidence of in utero fetal death, fetal distress, neonatal complications, and poor outcome. Hypertension in pregnancy is the largest cause of premature delivery and thus of RDS in our patient population.

Many diabetic pregnancies are associated with *polyhydramnios.* Although this is usually not a sign of significant fetal anomaly (as it is in the nondiabetic pregnancy), it may be associated with premature rupture of membranes, cord prolapse, abruptio placentae, or early delivery because of maternal distress. Women with the best metabolic control have the least polyhydramnios.

PREGNANCY MANAGEMENT

Diabetic women should be educated about the need to gain metabolic control of their diabetes *before* conception. This control will decrease the incidence of major congenital anomalies. Good control throughout the pregnancy improves the perinatal outcome. If the patient has gestational diabetes (GD) or class A diabetes, she should be managed by diet to keep the fasting plasma glucose below 105 and the postprandial plasma glucose below 120 mg/dl. If these goals are not reached by dietary therapy, then insulin should be used. Oral agents should not be used, since they cross the placenta and may be associated with severe neonatal hypoglycemia if used near the time of birth. Gestational diabetics who can maintain fasting plasma glucose under 105 mg/dl and 2-hour postprandial blood glucose levels under 120 mg/dl on a diabetic diet should be observed with daily home capillary glucose monitoring because 50 per cent of them eventually require insulin in pregnancy. If they are maintained on diet alone, the fetus does not appear to be at risk for stillbirth. If the mother develops an insulin requirement, has required insulin in the past, or has pre-eclampsia or a history of stillbirth, she should be treated as any other insulin-requiring diabetic. Diabetics who require insulin should maintain fasting plasma glucose levels as in gestational diabetes. Hemoglobin A_1 (HbA_1) is measured to assess control over a longer period of time.

At the first prenatal visit, a thorough medical history and physical examination are done. The estimated date of confinement is determined by history of last menstrual period and ultrasonography if necessary. Besides the usual prenatal tests, the following studies are done: glycosylated hemoglobin (HbA_{1c}), thyroid function studies, urinalysis, serum creatinine, and an ophthalmologic evaluation. The mother should begin a comprehensive diabetes education program stressing the importance of good glycemic control to reduce perinatal morbidity and mortality. Mothers with poor metabolic control at this visit or at any time should be admitted for regulation.

At the next visit, the mother's situation is reviewed and her diabetic control assessed. She is informed about the risks of congenital malformations in diabetic women in relationship to her glycemic control as measured by her level of glycosylated hemoglobin.

In the second trimester, an increasing insulin requirement is anticipated to avoid ketoacidosis, which is associated with fetal death. Maternal serum alpha-fetoprotein (AFP) is measured at 16 to 18 weeks. Diabetic pregnancies are associated with a lower maternal serum AFP level than nondiabetic pregnancies. Fetal ultrasonography is done at 18 weeks to rule out anomalies and to confirm the duration of the pregnancy. This examination, when performed by experienced personnel, leads to diagnosis of most (95 per cent) major anomalies of the central nervous system, heart, skeleton, gastrointestinal tract, and urinary tract. Hematocrit, renal function, blood pressure, diabetic control, and fetal growth are monitored.

In the third trimester, there is usually a rise in insulin requirement until 34 to 36 weeks. The problems in this trimester are fetal demise, premature delivery, and macrosomia. The mother must be monitored for glycemic control, polyhydramnios, pre-eclampsia, premature labor, and decreasing renal function. The fetus must be monitored for well-being, size, and pulmonary maturity. Ultrasonography is repeated at 26 to 28 weeks, and weekly NSTs are started. Mothers with problems may need to start this monitoring at 26 weeks. Before 30 weeks, the oxytocin challenge test is probably more reliable than the NST. In the Joslin Pregnancy Clinic, with careful maternal care and fetal monitoring, there have been only two unexplained, unanticipated fetal deaths after a normal NST or OCT since 1976 (about 1000 patients). This is still a significant problem, and results such as these can be obtained only with much meticulous effort.

Amniocentesis is performed at 38 weeks for measurement of the lecithin-sphingomyelin (L/S) ratio and saturated phosphatidylcholine (SPC) level, unless there are fetal or maternal reasons to accomplish delivery earlier. In our laboratory, in nondiabetic pregnancies with an L/S ratio greater than 2:1, there is a 5 per cent incidence of RDS; with an SPC greater than 500 μg/dl, there is a 1 per cent incidence. The levels of L/S and SPC considered "mature" in an IDM should depend on the experience of the local laboratory. In our hospital, 10 per cent of IDMs with L/S between 2.0 and 3.5:1.0 have RDS and 1 per cent of IDMs with L/S greater than 3.5:1.0 have RDS. An SPC of 500 μg/dl is usually considered mature in non-IDMs; in our hospital, 11 per cent of IDMs with SPC between 501 and 1000 had RDS, and 0.3 per cent of IDMs with SPC over 1000 had RDS. In the 255 diabetic pregnancies from which these data are taken, none had RDS if the SPC was greater than 1000 μg/dl and the L/S was over 3.5:1.0. We thus consider a fetus of a diabetic mother to have mature indices when the L/S is over 3.5 and the SPC is over 1000. Tables 2 and 3 give the risk of RDS so that the risks of a premature delivery can be evaluated.

Diabetic pregnancies requiring insulin should continue to 38 to 39 weeks as long as (1) there are no maternal contraindications and (2) there is evidence of fetal growth and well-being. This practice will result in more vaginal deliveries, more mature babies, and a lower perinatal mortality and morbidity, because the increased incidence of RDS in IDMs is not seen at term but rather in premature births. The time of delivery is decided in each case by an assessment of maternal health and of the relative fetal and neonatal risks as judged by gestational age, pulmonary maturity, and tests of fetal growth and well-being. Mothers with vascular complications (e.g., White's class F) who have proteinuria of more than

TABLE 2. Lecithin-Sphingomyelin Ratio, Saturated Phosphatidylcholine, and Respiratory Distress Syndrome in Infants of Diabetic Mothers at the Boston Hospital for Women 1977–1980

SPC μg/dl	<2.0:1.0	2.0–3.4:1.0	≥3.5:1.0	Mild, Moderate, or Severe RDS/Total
Not done	0/1	0/12	0/13	0/26 (0%)
≤500	6/6	1/9	1/2	8/17 (47%)
501–1000	0/2	3/20	1/15	4/37 (11%)
>1000	0/0	2/22	0/142	2/164 (1.2%)
Total (RDS)	6/9 (67%)	6/63 (10%)	2/172 (1/2%)	14/244 (5.7%)

Abbreviations: SPC, saturated phosphatidylcholine; RDS, respiratory distress syndrome.

400 mg/day without a urinary tract infection in the first half of pregnancy and who have elevated blood pressure and a creatinine clearance of less than 90 ml/minute often require hospitalization at 26 weeks' gestation for bed rest and antihypertensive medication. They are the group at greatest risk for uncontrollable hypertension and decreasing renal function and are most likely to have fetuses with intrauterine growth retardation and fetal distress, leading to early delivery. The perinatal survival (after 24 weeks' gestation) in this group is about 85 to 90 per cent. More recent data (after 24 weeks' gestation) from the Joslin Clinic show no increased mortality but more prematurity and low birth weight. There are still fetal losses in the second trimester. These mothers with vascular disease have an increased risk of intrapartum fetal distress, cesarean section, perinatal asphyxia, and RDS.

Emergency delivery may be necessary even in the face of pulmonary immaturity because of maternal problems such as hypertension, decreasing renal function, and pre-eclampsia or because of poor fetal growth or evidence of fetal distress. Because of the difficulty in controlling the maternal diabetes while waiting for an effect, we usually do not use steroids to accelerate fetal pulmonary maturity unless the L/S ratio is less than 2:1 and the SPC is less than 500 μg/dl and the patient is at very high risk for delivery in the following 7 days. This policy is usually followed at Brigham and Women's Hospital, but other centers may not follow it. The route of delivery selected is based on the usual obstetric indications. If the infant appears large on the basis of clinical and ultrasonographic examination (greater than 4000 g), cesarean section is usually indicated because of the risk of shoulder dystocia. Prolongation of gestation beyond 38 weeks does not increase the incidence of dystocia and birth trauma. In labor the maternal blood glucose is kept below 120 mg/dl, and fetal well-being is assessed by electronic monitoring and measurement of fetal scalp pH. About 25 per cent of diabetic women undergo primary cesarean section because of fetal distress in labor. Because of failure of induction, dystocia, or fetal distress in labor in our insulin-requiring diabetics, 47 per cent undergo primary cesarean section. Twenty-five per cent undergo subsequent cesarean section, and 28 per cent undergo vaginal delivery.

TABLE 3. Lecithin:Sphingomyelin (L/S) Ratio and Saturated Phosphatidylcholine (SPC) and Respiratory Distress Syndrome (RDS) in Infants of Mothers with Insulin-Requiring Diabetes Mellitus Antedating Pregnancy at the Brigham and Women's Hospital, Jan. 1, 1983, to June 30, 1988

Insulin-Dependent Diabetics L/S to Delivery Internal ≤ 72 Hours					
L/S		SPC	No RDS	RDS	%
≥3.5		≥1000	255	0	0
—		≥1000	288	1	0.3
≥3.5		—	285	1	0.3
2.0–3.4	and	≥1000	31	1	3.1
2.0–3.4	and	500–999	25	4	13.8
—		500–999	52	7	11.9
2.0–3.4		—	57	5	8.1

From Green MF, Torday J, Wilson M, Richardson D: Abstract presented at the Meeting of the Society of Perinatal Obstetricians, New Orleans, February 1989.

Samples were all obtained within 72 hours of delivery.

EVALUATION OF THE INFANT

The evaluation of the infant in the delivery room begins prior to the actual delivery. Immediately before opening the amniotic sac at the time of cesarean section, the obstetrician can obtain a sterile sample of amniotic fluid for culture, Gram's stain, L/S ratio, shake test, or SPC when indicated.

Once the baby has been delivered, a careful assessment made on the basis of the Apgar score should indicate the need for any resuscitative efforts. The infant should be dried well and placed under a heat source, with careful attention paid to clearing the airway of mucus. The stomach is not suctioned at this point, because of the risk of reflex bradycardia and apnea with pharyngeal stimulation. In the delivery room, a screening physical examination for major congenital anomalies should be performed and the placenta should also be examined. A specimen of cord blood should be obtained for glucose determination in anticipation of the reactive hypoglycemia associated with hyperglycemia at delivery. Cord pH may also be measured.

In the nursery, the initial care involves the simultaneous provision of what is needed to support the baby and continuous evaluation of the infant. This includes providing warmth, suction, and oxygen as needed, while checking vital signs (heart rate, temperature, respiratory rate, perfusion, color, and blood pressure). The presence of cyanosis should make one consider cardiac disease, RDS, transient tachypnea of the newborn (TTN), or polycythemia. A careful examination should be done for the presence of anomalies because of the 6 to 9 per cent incidence of major congenital anomalies in IDMs. Special attention should be paid to the brain, heart, kidneys, and skeletal system. Reports indicate that IDMs have a 35 per cent risk of significant hypoglycemia, a 22 per cent risk of hypocalcemia, a 19 per cent risk of hyperbilirubinemia, and a 34 per cent risk of polycythemia; therefore, the following studies are performed:

1. *Blood glucose* levels are checked at 1, 2, 3, 6, 12, 24, 36, and 48 hours.
2. *Hematocrit* levels are checked at 1 hour and 24 hours.
3. *Calcium* levels are checked if the baby appears jittery or is sick for any reason.
4. *Bilirubin* levels are checked if the baby appears jaundiced.

The baby is fed oral or intravenous glucose by 1 hour of age (see Hypoglycemia below). Every effort is made to involve the parents in the care of the baby as soon as possible.

SPECIFIC PROBLEMS FREQUENTLY OBSERVED IN IDMs

Respiratory Distress

In studies from the 1960s, IDMs had an approximately sixfold increased risk of RDS in contrast to that in infants of nondiabetic mothers of the same gestational age, independent of the method of delivery. With changes in the management of pregnant diabetics resulting in longer gestations and more vaginal deliveries, the incidence of RDS in IDMs has fallen from 28 per cent in 1950–1960 to 8 per cent in 1975–1976 to 5.7 per cent in 1983–1984. Since the major difference in the incidence of RDS between diabetics and nondiabetics is in infants before 37 weeks of gestation, the longer gestations allowed by better in utero surveillance and the more accurate prediction of pulmonary maturity have had a marked influence on the reduction of RDS in the IDM. Most of the deaths from RDS are in infants under 37 weeks' gestation who were delivered by cesarean section because of fetal distress or maternal indications. Delayed lung maturation in IDMs occurs because hyperinsulinemia may block cortisol induction of lung maturation. Other causes of respiratory distress that may be present in IDM are cardiac or pulmonary anomalies (4 per cent), hypertrophic cardiomyopathy (1 per cent), transient tachypnea of the newborn, and polycythemia. Pneumonia, pneumothorax, meconium aspiration, and diaphragmatic hernia should be considered in the differential diagnosis. The following studies should be done in infants with respiratory distress.

Gastric aspirate should be obtained during the first hour of life, after the baby has been stabilized. The gastric aspirate may be used for *Gram's stain* for polymorphonuclear leukocytes and bacteria, and *gastric aspirate shake test* may be used to assess the amount of pulmonary surfactant in the newborn's lungs if prenatal studies of pulmonary maturity were not performed. *Chest roentgenogram, blood gases, electrocardiogram,* and blood pressure measurements should be done. If hypertrophic cardiomyopathy or a cardiac anomaly is thought to be present, an *echocardiogram* should be done. *Blood culture specimens* should be obtained. Spinal fluid examination and culture should be included if the infant's condition allows and if infection is suspected. The differential diagnosis and management of respiratory disorders are discussed elsewhere in this book.

Hypoglycemia

Hypoglycemia is defined as a blood glucose level less than 30 mg/dl in any infant, regardless of gestational age and whether associated with symptoms or not.

Incidence. The incidence of hypoglycemia in IDMs is 30 to 40 per cent. The onset is frequently within 1 to 2 hours of birth and is most common in macrosomic infants.

Pathogenesis. The pathogenesis of the neonatal hypoglycemia of the IDM is explained by the maternal hyperglycemia-fetal hyperinsulinism hypothesis of Pederson. The correlation between fetal macrosomia, elevated HbA_1 in maternal and cord blood and neonatal hypoglycemia, and also between elevated cord blood C-peptide or immunoreactive insulin levels and hypoglycemia, suggests that control of maternal blood glucose in the last trimester may decrease the incidence of neonatal hypoglycemia in IDMs. Some studies have shown less neonatal hypoglycemia if the maternal blood glucose is in the normal range at delivery. Mothers should not receive large doses of glucose before or at delivery because this may stimulate an insulin response in the hyperinsulinemic offspring. We attempt to keep the maternal blood glucose at delivery below 120 mg/dl. Hypoglycemia in small-for-gestational-age infants born to mothers with vascular disease may be due to inadequate glycogen stores; it may present later (e.g., 12 to 24 hours of age). Other factors that may cause hypoglycemia in IDMs are decreased catecholamine and glycogen secretion as well as inadequate substrate mobilization (diminished hepatic glucose production and decreased oxygenation of fatty acids).

Symptoms. If IDMs have symptoms from hypoglycemia, they usually are quiet and lethargic rather than jittery. Other symptoms such as apnea, tachypnea, respiratory distress, hypotonia, shock, cyanosis, and seizures may occur. Symptomatic infants are probably at greater risk for sequelae than if they are asymptomatic. The significance of hypoglycemia without symptoms is unclear, but management to maintain the blood sugar in the normal range appears to be indicated.

Diagnosis. Blood glucose is measured at birth and at 1, 2, 3, 6, 12, 24, 36, and 48 hours. It is measured more often if the infant is symptomatic and has had low blood glucose and to check the response to therapy.

Treatment

ASYMPTOMATIC INFANTS WITH NORMAL BLOOD GLUCOSE. In our nursery, we begin to feed "well" IDMs by bottle or gavage with dextrose 10 per cent (5 ml/kg body weight) at or before 1 hour of age. Infants weighing less than 2 kg should not be given oral feedings; they should have parenteral dextrose starting in the first hour of life. Larger infants can be fed hourly for three or four feedings until the blood glucose level is stable. The feedings can then be given every 2 hours and later every 3 hours; as the interval between feedings increases, the volume is increased.

If the infant feeds successfully by 12 hours of age and the blood glucose is normal, he or she should be given 20 cal/30 ml formula, with extra dextrose added as needed. This method of rapid oral feeding prevents or corrects the hypoglycemia in most "well" IDMs.

If by 2 hours of age the blood glucose is low (under 30 mg/dl) in spite of feeding or if feedings are not tolerated, as indicated by large volumes retained in the stomach, parenteral treatment is warranted to raise the blood glucose.

SYMPTOMATIC INFANTS. *This group includes infants with low blood glucose after an enteral feed, sick infants, and infants less than 2 kg in weight.* The basic element in treatment is *intravenous glucose administration.* This must be done through a reliable route.

Administration of intravenous glucose is usually by peripheral vein. These sites have fewer infectious and thrombotic complications than those seen with central catheters. Peripheral lines may be difficult to place in obese IDMs, and sudden interruption of the infusion may cause a reactive hypoglycemia in these hyperinsulinemic infants. In emergency situations with symptomatic babies, we have utilized umbilical venous catheters placed in the inferior vena cava until a stable peripheral line is placed.

Specific treatment is determined by the baby's condition. If the infant is in distress (e.g., seizure or respiratory compromise), 0.5 to 1 g of glucose/kg is given by an IV push of 2 to 4 ml/kg of 25 per cent dextrose in water (D/W) at a rate of 1 ml/minute. For example, a 4-kg infant would receive 8 to 16 ml of 25 per cent D/W over 8 to 16 minutes. This is followed by a continuous infusion of dextrose at a rate of 4 to 8 mg/kg/minute of glucose.

The concentration of dextrose in the intravenous fluid depends on the total daily fluid requirement. For example, on day 1 the usual fluid intake is 65 ml/kg, or 0.045 ml/kg/minute. Therefore, 10 per cent D/W would provide 4.5 mg/kg/minute of glucose, and 15 per cent D/W would provide 6.75 mg/kg/minute. In other words, 10 per cent D/W at a standard intravenous fluid maintenance rate usually supplies sufficient glucose to raise the blood glucose level above 30 mg/dl. The concentration of dextrose and the infusion rates, however, are increased as necessary to maintain the blood glucose in the normal range.

Another method is to give 200 mg/kg of glucose (2 ml/kg of 10 per cent dextrose) over 2 to 3 minutes. This is followed by a maintenance drip of 6 to 8 mg/kg/minute of glucose (10 per cent dextrose at 80 to 120 ml/kg/day).

If the infant does not have symptoms but has a blood glucose level in the hypoglycemic range, an initial push of concentrated sugar should not be given. (This is to avoid a hyperinsulinemic response.) Rather, an initial infusion of 5 to 10 ml of 10 per cent D/W at 1 ml/minute is followed by the continuous infusion of glucose at 4 to 8 mg/kg/minute. Blood glucose levels must be carefully monitored at frequent intervals after intravenous glucose infusions are initiated to be certain of adequate treatment of the hypoglycemia as well as to avoid hyperglycemia and the risk of osmotic diuresis and dehydration.

Giving glucose through an umbilical artery line may result in normal glucose levels in the feet while there are still low levels in the rest of the body. If glucose is given to a hyperinsulinemic infant through a high umbilical artery line, the pancreas may be stimulated to release excess insulin. Repositioning the line to a low line will resolve this.

Parenteral sugar should never be abruptly discontinued because of the risk of a reactive hypoglycemia. As oral feeding progresses, the rate of the infusion can be decreased gradually and the concentration of glucose infused can be reduced by using 5 per cent D/W. It is particularly important to measure blood glucose levels during this process of tapering the intravenous infusion.

Since the hypoglycemia of most IDMs responds to the above treatment, unresponsiveness or persistence (over 96 hours) should make one consider the other problems (e.g., infection, islet cell tumor). Hydrocortisone (5 mg/kg/day IM in two divided doses) has occasionally been helpful. In our experience, other drugs (epinephrine, diazoxide, or growth hormone) have not been necessary in the treatment of the hypoglycemia of IDMs.

In a hypoglycemic infant, if difficulty is experienced in achieving vascular access, we administer crystalline glycogen intramuscularly (IM) or subcutaneously (SC) (300 μg/kg to a maximum dose of 1.0 mg). This is ten times the dose used in non-IDMs. This causes a rapid rise in blood glucose in large IDMs who have good glycogen stores, although it is not reliable in the smaller infants of maternal classes D, E, and F. This rise in blood glucose may last 2 to 3 hours and is useful until parenteral glucose can be administered.

Hypocalcemia

Hypocalcemia (calcium less than 7 mg/dl) is found in 22 per cent of IDMs. It is not related to hypoglycemia. Hypocalcemia may be caused by a delay in the usual postnatal rise of parathyroid hormone (PTH). Other factors in IDMs may be vitamin D antagonism at the intestine from elevated cortisol and hyperphosphatemia from tissue catabolism. There is no evidence of elevated serum calcitonin concentration in these infants in the absence of prematurity or asphyxia. Other causes of hypocalcemia, such as asphyxia and prematurity, may be seen in IDMs. The nadir in calcium levels occurs between 24 and 72 hours, and 30 to 50 per cent of IDMs become hypocalcemic as defined by a total serum calcium under 7 mg/dl. Hypocalcemia in "well" IDMs usually resolves without treatment. We do not routinely measure serum calcium in "well" asymptomatic IDMs. If an infant is sick for any reason, such as prematurity, asphyxia, infection, or respiratory distress, or if there are symptoms of lethargy, jitteriness, or seizures, serum calcium levels should be measured. If the infant has symptoms that coexist with a low calcium level, has an illness that will delay onset of calcium regulation, or is unable to feed, treatment with calcium may be necessary. Hypomagnesemia should be considered as a cause of hypocalcemia in IDMs, since the hypocalcemia may not respond until the hypomagnesemia is treated.

Polycythemia

Polycythemia is common in IDMs. In infants who are small for gestational age, polycythemia may be related to placental insufficiency, causing hypoxia and increased erythropoietin. In IDMs it may also be due to reduced oxygen delivery secondary to elevated glycosylated hemoglobin in both maternal and fetal serum. If there was fetal distress, there may be a shift of blood from the placenta to the fetus. There is a positive correlation between elevated hematocrit values in IDMs and poor glycemic control as measured by maternal HbA_1 in the third trimester.

Jaundice

Hyperbilirubinemia (bilirubin greater than 15) is seen with increased frequency in IDMs. Bilirubin levels over 16 were seen in 19 per cent of IDMs at Boston Hospital for Women (now Brigham Women's). Bilirubin production is increased in IDMs in contrast to that in infants of nondiabetic mothers. When measurement of carboxyhemoglobin production is used as an indicator of increased heme turnover, IDMs are found to have increased production compared with controls. There may be decreased red blood cell life span because of less deformable red blood cell membranes, possibly related to glycosylation of the red blood cell membrane. Other factors that may account for the increased jaundice are prematurity, impairment of the hepatic conjugation of bilirubin, and an increased enterohepatic circulation of bilirubin. Infants born to well-controlled diabetic mothers have less hyperbilirubinemia. The increasing gestational age of IDMs at delivery has contributed to the decreased incidence of hyperbilirubinemia. Hyperbilirubinemia in IDMs is diagnosed and treated as in any other infant.

Congenital Anomalies

Congenital anomalies are found more frequently in IDMs than in infants of nondiabetic mothers.

Incidence. In a series of 150 IDMs in 1976 and 1977 from the Boston Hospital for Women, 9 per cent had major anomalies, and anomalies accounted for 50 per cent of the perinatal mortality. As mortality from other causes, such as prematurity, stillbirth, asphyxia, and RDS falls, malformations become the major cause of perinatal mortality in the IDMs. Infants of diabetic fathers showed the same incidence of anomalies as the normal population; consequently, the maternal environment may be the important factor. Most studies show a 6 to 9 per cent incidence of major anomalies in IDMs. The usual major anomaly rate for the general population is 2 per cent. Anomalies seen in IDMs are central nervous system (anencephaly, meningocele syndrome, holoprosencephaly), cardiac, vertebral, skeletal, and renal, as well as situs inversus and the caudal regression syndrome (sacral agenesis). The central nervous system and cardiac anomalies make up two thirds of the malformations seen in IDMs. Although there is a general increase in the anomaly rate in IDMs, no anomaly is specific for IDMs, although half of all cases of caudal regression syndrome are seen in IDMs.

Pathophysiology. In a study of 116 IDMs at Boston Hospital for Women in 1981, there was a positive correlation between poor control of diabetes in early pregnancy (as measured by maternal HbA_{1c} levels) and major congenital anomalies in offspring of these pregnancies. This finding suggests that good metabolic control before conception and in the first 3 months of pregnancy may decrease the incidence of major congenital anomalies. There have been several other studies correlating good metabolic control of diabetes, as measured by maternal glycohemoglobin values in early pregnancy, with decreased incidence of anomalies in offspring. A multicenter study of IDMs compared outcomes in 347 diabetics who were full participants in a rigid control program from early pregnancy, 279 diabetics coming for care in late pregnancy, and 389 nondiabetic pregnancies. Major malformation rates were 4.9 per cent in the full participants, 9.0 per cent in the late entrants, and 2.1 per cent in the controls. There were no significant differences in the home glucose results from weeks 5 to 12 in the mothers of the malformed and normal infants, nor were there any significant differences in levels of glycosylated hemoglobin or frequency of hypoglycemic episodes in the mothers of the malformed and normal infants. Of note, diabetic women coming for early care had fewer infants with malformations than those coming late for care. This study could not show a correlation between hyperglycemia, elevated glycosylated hemoglobin levels, and malformations in women who prospectively opted for rigorous control of diabetes. The authors believed that some, but not all, malformations can be prevented by good control of blood sugar and that more subtle means are needed to identify the teratogenic mechanisms in IDMs. There were only a few diabetic women in both the full participant and late entry groups who had glycosylated hemoglobin levels as high as those seen in the earlier studies. Thus, most of the women in this study had rather good control of diabetes in pregnancy.

A more recent study at the Brigham and Women's Hospital/Joslin Clinic measured the relationship between hemoglobin A_1 in the first trimester and spontaneous abortions and major malformations in 303 insulin-requiring diabetics. The range of diabetic control was broader than in the above study. The risk for spontaneous abortion was 12.4 per cent with first trimester Hb_{A1} under 9.3 per cent and 37.5 with Hb_{A1} over 14.3 per cent. The risk for major malformations was 3 per cent with Hb_{A1} under 9.3 per cent and 40 per cent with Hb_{A1} over 14.4 per cent. The risks were high with poor control in the first trimester but reasonable (4 per cent) with "acceptable control."

Detection. Because of the high incidence of malformations in IDMs, ultrasonography should be performed in early pregnancy. Maternal AFP should also be measured. The newborn should undergo a careful physical examination for diagnosis of any anomalies that were missed by intrauterine surveillance.

Poor Feeding

Poor feeding is a major problem in these infants. It occurred in 37 per cent of a series of 150 IDMs at the Boston Hospital for Women. Sometimes poor feeding is related to prematurity, respiratory distress, or other problems; however, it often occurs in the absence of other problems. In our experience (unpublished), it was found in 17 per cent of classes B to D IDMs and in 31 per cent of class F. Infants born to class F diabetic mothers are often premature. There was no difference in the incidence of poor feeding in large-for-gestational-age infants versus appropriate-for-gestational-age infants and no relation to polyhydramnios. Poor feeding is a major reason for prolongation of hospital stay and parent-infant separation.

Macrosomia

Macrosomia, defined as a birth weight over the 90th percentile or over 4000 g, may be associated with an increased incidence of primary cesarean section or obstetric trauma such as fractured clavicle, Erb's palsy, or phrenic nerve palsy due to shoulder dystocia. There was a 28 per cent incidence of macrosomia (over 4000 g) in IDMs at the Brigham and Women's Hospital between 1983 and 1984. An association was found between elevated maternal blood glucose levels in the last trimester and macrosomia. There also was an association between hyperinsulinemia in IDMs and macrosomia and between macrosomia and hypoglycemia. Macrosomia is not usually seen in infants born to mothers with class F diabetes. Better control of maternal diabetes in the third trimester should be associated with less macrosomia, resulting in less trauma and a lower primary cesarean section rate.

Myocardial Dysfunction

Transient hypertrophic subaortic stenosis resulting from ventricular septal hypertrophy in IDMs has been frequently reported. The infants may present with congestive heart failure, poor cardiac output, and cardiomegaly. This cardiomyopathy may complicate the management of other illnesses such as RDS. The diagnosis is made by echocardiography, which shows hypertrophy of the ventricular septum, the right ventricular anterior wall, and the left ventricular posterior wall in the absence of chamber dilation. Cardiac output decreases with increasing septal thickness.

Most symptoms resolve by 2 weeks of age. The septal hypertrophy resolves by 4 months of age. Most infants respond to supportive care. Digitalis and other inotropic drugs are contraindicated unless myocardial dysfunction is seen on echocardiography. Propranolol is the most useful drug.

The differential diagnosis of myocardial dysfunction due to diabetic cardiomyopathy of the newborn includes (1) postasphyxial cardiomyopathy, (2) myocarditis, (3) endocardial fibroelastosis, (4) glycogen storage disease of the heart, and (5) aberrant left coronary artery coming off the pulmonary artery. There is some evidence that good control of diabetes in pregnancy may reduce the severity of hypertrophic cardiomyopathy.

Renal Vein Thrombosis

Renal vein thrombosis may occur in utero or post partum. Intrauterine and postnatal diagnosis may be made by ultrasonography. Postnatal presentation may be as hematuria, flank mass, hypertension, or embolic phenomena. Most renal vein thrombosis can be managed conservatively (nonsurgically) with fluid and electrolyte therapy as well as heparin, allowing preservation of renal tissue.

Small Left Colon Syndrome

Small left colon syndrome presents as generalized abdominal distention because of inability to pass meconium. Meconium is obtained by passage of a rectal catheter. An enema performed with meglumine diatrizoate (Gastrografin) is diagnostic and often results in evacuation of the colon. The infant should be well hydrated before Gastrografin is used. The infant may have some problems with passage of a stool in the first week of life, but this usually resolves after treatment with half-normal saline enemas (5 ml/kg) and glycerine suppositories.

Perinatal Survival

Despite all these problems, the diabetic woman has a 95 per cent chance of having a healthy child if she is willing to participate in a program of pregnancy management and surveillance in a modern perinatal center. In 147 IDMs over 24 weeks of gestation born to mothers who required insulin at the Boston Hospital for Women in 1976 and 1977, the perinatal mortality was 34 per 1000. Between 1977 and 1980 at the same center the perinatal mortality of infants born to women with class B, C, D, H, or R diabetes was 20 per 1000. In the earlier series 24 infants born to class F diabetic women had a perinatal mortality of 125 per 1000. More recent data at the Brigham and Women's Hospital do not show an increased perinatal mortality in pregnancies complicated by class F diabetes as compared with other insulin-requiring diabetics. However, there is increased morbidity.

In a series of 215 IDMs at the Brigham and Women's Hospital from 1983 to 1984, the total perinatal mortality from 24 weeks of gestation to 28 days post partum was 28 per 1000. There was one intrauterine demise of a singleton near term. Thus, perinatal survival is encouragingly good and results from advances in medical, obstetric, and neonatal treatment. More infants are born healthy than ever before, and, if ill, more survive.

Risk of Insulin-Dependent Diabetes in Offspring of Diabetic Parents

Infants born to an insulin-dependent diabetic father have a 6 per cent risk of having insulin-dependent diabetes by age 20. In infants born to an insulin-dependent mother, the risk is 1.3 per cent. This difference may be due to some effect on the fetal immune system that makes the offspring of the diabetic mother more resistant to the development of diabetes.

REFERENCES

Cloherty JP, Stark AR: Manual of Neonatal Care, 3rd ed. Boston, Little, Brown & Co, 1991.

Greene MF, Hare JW, Cloherty JP, et al: First-trimester hemoglobin A_1 and risk for major malformation and spontaneous abortion in diabetic pregnancy. Teratology 39:225–231, 1989.

Hare JW: Diabetes Complicating Pregnancy. New York, Alan R. Liss, 1989.

Kitzmiller JL, Cloherty JP, Graham CA: Management of diabetes in pregnancy. *In* Kozak GP (ed): Clinical Diabetes Mellitus. Philadelphia, WB Saunders Co, 1982.

Mills JL, Knopp RH, Simpson JL: Lack of relation of increased malformation rates in infants of diabetic mothers to glycemic control during organogenesis. N Engl J Med 318:671–676, 1988.

POLYCYTHEMIA

SHELLY C. BERNSTEIN, M.D., Ph.D.

During the first week of life, hemoglobin values above 22.0 g/dl or hematocrit (Hct) values of more than 65 per cent should be considered evidence of polycythemia. In childhood and adolescence, hemoglobin values above 17.0 g/dl or hematocrit values of more than 50 per cent are significantly elevated. The diagnosis of polycythemia should be verified by venipuncture; capillary blood samples should not be used. Hemoconcentration due to dehydration must be excluded as a cause.

NEONATAL POLYCYTHEMIA

Polycythemia in the neonate may be due to twin-to-twin transfusion, maternal-fetal transfusion, delayed cord clamping, placental insufficiency, congenital adrenal hyperplasia, maternal diabetes mellitus, Down syndrome, or Beckwith syndrome. The signs and symptoms may consist of lethargy, plethora, cyanosis, jaundice, respiratory distress, congestive heart failure, seizures, priapism, thrombocytopenia, renal vein thrombosis, necrotizing enterocolitis, hypoglycemia, and hypocalcemia. Many infants with polycythemia are, however, asymptomatic.

Prophylactic treatment is not recommended. However, all infants with polycythemia should be monitored carefully, and at the first sign of symptoms, treatment should be instituted. Treatment should be designed to reduce the venous hematocrit value to approximately 60 per cent, accomplished by partial exchange transfusion, using fresh frozen plasma to reduce the hematocrit value while maintaining the blood volume. The volume of exchange may be estimated from the following formula:

$$\text{volume of exchange (ml)} = \frac{\text{blood volume} \times (\text{observed Hct} - \text{desired Hct})}{\text{observed Hct}}$$

The infant's blood should be removed in volumes of 10 ml for full-term (and smaller volumes for low-birth-weight) infants and replaced with an equal volume of fresh frozen plasma. A blood volume of 80 ml/kg may be estimated for newborn infants. The procedure is usually performed through an umbilical venous line. Simple phlebotomy should not be performed unless the infant is hypervolemic.

CHILDHOOD POLYCYTHEMIA

Primary Polycythemia

Polycythemia Vera. This disorder consists of an increase in red blood cell mass of unknown etiology, often accompanied by thrombocytosis, and is rarely seen in childhood. The Polycythemia Vera Study Group recommends phlebotomy for patients under the age of 40 years. Erythrocytapheresis with isovolemic exchange of saline or 5 per cent albumin, rather than simple phlebotomy, should be performed to maintain the hematocrit value between 40 and 45 per cent. Patients with complications (such as massive splenomegaly, vascular obstruction, or symptoms associated with hypermetabolism) or with extreme thrombocytosis (platelet counts greater than 1×10^{12}/L) should be treated with myelosuppressive agents. Hydroxyurea (30 mg/kg, orally in three divided doses per day) is given until the platelet count falls to 1.1×10^{11}/L. At that time, busulfan (0.12 mg/kg, maximum dose of 6 mg orally per day for 7 days) is given. This dose may be repeated for another 7 days if significant myelosuppression does not occur. Periodic pulses of busulfan may be required to control thrombocytosis and may need to be performed on a regular basis. Repeated erythrocytapheresis will lead to iron deficiency, causing an increase in whole blood viscosity related to decreased erythrocyte deformability, as well as thrombocytosis. Therefore, iron deficiency should be avoided by oral iron supplementation.

Benign Familial Polycythemia. This term is used to describe familial cases with increased red blood cell mass that are otherwise normal, with no other recognizable etiology. Therapy is not required unless the patient has symptoms related to hyperviscosity. Erythrocytapheresis or phlebotomy may then afford symptomatic relief.

Secondary Polycythemia

This condition refers to an increase in red blood cell mass secondary to a recognizable cause and may result from tissue hypoxia, leading to a compensatory response of erythropoietin, or from increased production of erythropoietin despite normal tissue oxygenation.

Cyanotic Congenital Heart Disease. In children with cyanotic congenital heart disease with a right-to-left shunt, polycythemia develops in response to chronic systemic arterial desaturation. Symptoms are headaches, irritability, anorexia, and dyspnea. In addition, polycythemia, when accompanied by iron deficiency, may be associated with an increased incidence of intravascular thrombosis and a consumptive coagulopathy. Arterial saturation should be surgically corrected, if possible. If the patient has symptoms, reduction of hematocrit values should be attempted cautiously by partial exchange transfusion or erythrocytapheresis. Since acute phlebotomy in these patients may result in vascular collapse, cyanotic spells, cerebrovascular accidents, or seizures, sudden hemodynamic alterations should be avoided. Erythrocytapheresis should be performed, during which time the volume of red blood cells removed is continuously replaced by infusion of equal volumes of saline or 5 per cent albumin, estimating the total exchange volume from the above formula. The hematocrit should be reduced to 60 to 65 per cent over 30 to 60 minutes. Strict adherence to critical blood volume maintenance must be made. On the average, Coulter hematocrit values are 4 to 5 per cent lower than spun hematocrit values in patients with cyanotic congenital heart disease. Thus, the degree of polycythemia may be seriously underestimated with the former. Because of the complications associated with iron deficiency and polycythemia, iron deficiency should always be corrected. These measures have led to reduced coagulation abnormalities, decreased operative mortality, and symptomatic improvement in polycythemic patients with cyanotic congenital heart disease.

Abnormal Hemoglobins. A number of hemoglobin variants have been described with a marked increase in oxygen affinity and compensatory polycythemia via increased production of erythropoietin. Other than erythrocytosis, affected individuals have minimal clinical manifestations, with the exception of one reported family with Hb Malmö, the children of whom were reported to have cardiovascular symptoms. Hematocrit values rarely are high enough to necessitate treatment.

Congenital methemoglobinemia due to NADH-diaphorase I deficiency and acquired methemoglobinemia due to exposure to various agents capable of oxidizing heme iron to the ferric state may produce cyanosis and polycythemia. Treatment of methemoglobinemia, regardless of the etiology, is dictated by the severity of the hypoxia. Most patients with hereditary disease require no therapy. Severe methemoglobinemia can be treated initially by methylene blue (1 to 2 mg/kg administered intravenously as a 1 per cent solution). Further treatment is accomplished with daily oral doses of methylene blue (1 to 2 mg/kg).

Inappropriate Erythrocytosis. Polycythemia has been associated with a number of tumors in which erythropoietin secretion is elevated, such as Wilms' tumor, hepatoma, cerebellar hemangioblastoma, and benign lesions of the kidney, such as cysts and hydronephrosis. Endocrine disorders, such as pheochromocytomas, aldosterone-producing adenomas, and Cushing's syndrome, as well as exogenous administration of testosterone or growth hormone may also cause increased red blood cell mass. Correction of the underlying condition results in elimination of the polycythemia.

INSULIN-DEPENDENT DIABETES MELLITUS

ROBERT KAYE, M.D.

The diagnosis of insulin-dependent diabetes mellitus (IDDM) is usually made by the presence of polyuria, polydipsia, and ketonuria together with a random blood glucose concentration exceeding 200 mg/dl. Recurrence of enuresis, weight loss, and vulval moniliasis and rapid changes in visual acuity may also be present at onset.

In asymptomatic individuals, diagnosis is based on fasting capillary or venous whole blood glucose ≥ 120 mg/dl and a 2-hour value ≥ 180 mg/dl (venous whole blood) or ≥ 200 mg/dl (capillary whole blood) during an oral glucose tolerance test. (Glucose dose is 1.75 g/kg up to a maximum of 75 g.)

DIET THERAPY

Dietary recommendations for the diabetic child do not differ significantly from those appropriate for other children. Restrictions of the intake of total fat, particularly saturated fats and cholesterol, may be appropriate for all children but should be routine for diabetic children in view of the accelerated atherosclerosis that complicates the disease. *A polyunsaturated:saturated fat ratio of 1.2:1.0 rather than the usual 0.3:1.0 is a reasonable goal.* This can be accomplished by reducing the intake of fat of animal origin, substituting margarine for butter, ingesting low-fat milk, using vegetable oils in cooking, and limiting egg yolk consumption.

The probable relationship of hyperglycemia to diabetic complications warrants limitation of concentrated, simple carbohydrates in the diet and supports the utilization of complex, slowly absorbed carbohydrates, especially fiber-containing breads, vegetables, and fruits.

Diabetes related dietary principles include:

1. A daily meal plan relatively consistent in caloric intake.
2. Provision for changes in physical activity with extra food for increased activity and additional insulin for extra food.
3. Avoidance of hypoglycemia by reasonably consistent meal timing and provision of snacks.

Food preferences of individual patients should be considered in developing the meal plan. The *exchange system,* which divides foods into seven categories—each with comparable composition and caloric value, is useful in this regard and provides for variety in meal planning.*

We recommend a caloric distribution of 50 to 55 per cent carbohydrate, 15 to 20 per cent protein, and 25 to 30 per cent fat.

Caloric intake is estimated from the formula

$$\text{caloric intake} = 1000 + 100 \times \text{age (in years)}$$

Since children vary in caloric requirement to maintain normal growth and weight gain, the calculation should be considered an approximation, with a variance of ± 20 per cent among individuals. As children grow, caloric intake, of course, must be increased. For the non-obese child, appetite should determine its magnitude. Children with excessive weight gain will need some behavioral deterrent on intake, and there should be a ceiling on caloric intake prescribed.

The distribution of the caloric intake for meals and snacks will differ between younger and older children but should approximate 10 per cent of total calories for each snack. Younger children usually have a mid-morning, mid-afternoon, and bedtime snack. These serve the purpose of satisfying hunger as well as protecting against insulin-induced hypoglycemia. Older children usually prefer to omit the mid-morning snack, as do their nondiabetic peers. The balance of calories (70 to 80 per cent) are distributed at the major meals.

INSULIN THERAPY

At the time of diagnosis, the diabetic child will have little or no endogenous insulin secretory capacity and will be dependent on exogenous insulin for metabolic maintenance. Currently, insulins are available from several manufacturers; they are derived from animal and biosynthetic sources and are present in preparations with varying durations of action. Removal of contaminants from animal-derived materials has lessened the incidence of subcutaneous tissue atrophy, insulin allergy, and resistance secondary to antibody formation.

The most widely used preparations are regular insulin and Semilente for rapid onset and brief duration of activity; neutral protamine Hagedorn (NPH) insulin and Lente for intermediate action; and Ultralente for more prolonged

*"Exchange Lists for Meal Planning" is available for $1.75 from the American Diabetes Association, 1660 Duke Street, Alexandria, VA 22134.

TABLE 1. Features of Insulin

Type of Preparation*	Onset (Hours)	Peak (Hours)	Duration at Peak	Intensity
Rapid-acting				
Regular P-B, P, B	½	2–4	6–8	Marked
Semilente P-B	½	2–4	10–12	Marked
Intermediate-acting				
NPH P-B, P, B	2	8–10	18–24	Moderate
Lente P-B, P, B	2	8–12	20–26	Moderate
Long-acting				
Ultralente P-B	6	18–24	36+	Mild

*Preparations available from Eli Lilly and Company.
Abbreviations: P-B, pork beef mixture; P, pork only; B, beef only; NPH, neutral protamine Hagedorn (insulin).

and slowest onset of effect. These characteristics are listed in Table 1.

The preparations in Table 1 are also available as Humulin of recombinant DNA origin and differ from the other types by a more rapid onset and somewhat shorter duration of action.

Pure pork and synthetic insulins are less antigenic than those derived from beef and are useful in patients developing insulin resistance as a result of insulin antibody formation.

Insulin action is modified by the site of injection and exercise of the injected area. Peak concentrations are most rapidly achieved with abdominal injection and slowest from the anterior thigh. Concentrations are highest after deltoid and lowest after buttock administration.

INITIAL TREATMENT OF NEWLY DIAGNOSED PATIENTS

At the time of diagnosis, most patients will not be significantly dehydrated or acidotic and will be able to take oral feedings without vomiting. An estimate of insulin requirements can best be made by administering regular insulin before the major meals and NPH insulin prior to the bedtime snacks. The first dose is 0.2 units/kg, which is adjusted upward or downward by 1 or 2 units on the basis of blood glucose concentration determined prior to the next meal or bedtime snack. Self-monitoring of blood glucose by the patient or parent is standard procedure and is discussed later. The adjustments in dosage are made in an effort to bring the glucose concentration within the approximate range of 80 to 180 mg/dl. Ideally, this process should be continued for 4 to 5 days until this level of glycemia has been attained and the patient has entered the "honeymoon phase" of decreasing insulin requirements. In reality, this rather leisurely schedule of adjustment may not be available because of constraints placed on length of stay by hospital utilization committees and third-party payers.

The total of the four-times-daily regular insulin administrations provide an estimate of the insulin requirements in a once- or twice-daily schedule of injections. When the total of the four daily insulin injections is less than 20 units, a single pre-breakfast dosage of a mixture of regular and NPH insulins given 30 to 40 minutes before breakfast may be adequate to achieve glucose control in the target range of 80 to 180 mg/dl. The quantity of regular insulin in the mixture is based on the previous day's pre-breakfast insulin dosage. The amount of the NPH insulin is based on the sum of the three injections given before lunch, dinner, and the bedtime snack on the previous day. Because of the likelihood that insulin requirements are in a declining phase (honeymoon period), it is prudent to reduce these estimates by 20 per cent to avoid hypoglycemia.

Patients requiring more than a total of 20 units of insulin in the four-times-daily injection phase of the estimate of insulin requirements should be placed on a twice-daily regimen of regular and NPH insulin before breakfast and the evening meal. The quantitative guides for this transition are as follows: A.M. regular insulin based on the pre-breakfast regular insulin dosage of the previous day; A.M. NPH insulin based on the pre-lunch regular insulin dosage; and P.M. regular insulin and NPH insulin based on the previous day's pre-supper and bedtime snack dosages, respectively. An example is given in Table 2. For the reasons cited above, each of the dosages in Table 2 should be reduced about 20 per cent.

The preceding plan of insulin treatment may fall short of achieving the target glycemic goals (80 to 180 mg/dl) but should restore the patient to an asymptomatic status, a sense of well-being, and a physiologic gain in weight. At follow-up visits and via telephone communication, further adjustments can be made with the goal of achieving near-normal glycemia.

First priority is given to bringing the pre-breakfast glucose concentration into the target range by increasing the pre-breakfast NPH insulin in patients on a once-daily regimen and the evening NPH insulin in those receiving two daily injections. This is based on the fact that lowering the starting point of the day's glycemic excursions will be reflected throughout the balance of the day. If blood glucose levels before lunch are too high, the pre-breakfast regular insulin dose should be increased. The glucose concentration in the late afternoon is the guide for adjustment of the pre-breakfast NPH dosage, and the glucose value before the bedtime snack determines adjustments in the evening regular insulin dosage.

For patients receiving one injection of a mixture of regular and NPH insulins in the morning, the latter is relied on to control the blood glucose level from afternoon to the following morning.

Adjustments in insulin dosage should approximate 1 unit in patients receiving a daily dosage of less than 20 units and in increments or decrements of 2 units for those requiring larger quantities.

Since about 80 per cent of diabetic children ultimately require two doses of insulin daily to achieve reasonable control of blood glucose, the criteria for the transition from a one- to a two-dosage regimen are described.

NPH insulin exerts its peak blood sugar–lowering effect in the mid to late afternoon. The upper limit on the morning NPH insulin dosage is reached when the blood glucose concentration at that time is in the target range. Therefore, elevated blood glucose values noted in the evening and the following morning indicate the need for a second injection of insulin at bedtime. This injection should include both regular and NPH insulins if both the bedtime and the pre-breakfast levels are elevated. If only the latter measurement is too high, NPH insulin alone is indicated. An example is given in Table 3.

The quantity of the second injection in Table 3 conforms

TABLE 2. Example of Insulin Requirement in Patients Requiring More Than 20 Units

Previous Day's Dosage			
Before breakfast	*Lunch*	*Supper*	*Bedtime*
10 regular	6 regular	4 regular	8 NPH
Twice-Daily Insulin Regimen			
Before breakfast		*Before supper*	
10 regular/6 NPH		4 regular	8 NPH

Abbreviation: NPH, neutral protamine Hagedorn (insulin).

TABLE 3. Example of a Second Injection of Insulin for Elevated Blood Glucose (8 Regular/18 NPH on Once-Daily Regimen)

Glucose Concentration (mg/dl)			
Pre-breakfast	*Pre-lunch*	*Pre-supper*	*Bedtime*
280	110	120	260
Transition to Two Doses			
Pre-breakfast		*Pre-supper*	
6 regular/16 NPH		2 regular/ 2 NPH	
Result Glucose Concentration (mg/dl)			
Pre-breakfast	*Pre-lunch*	*Pre-supper*	*Bedtime*
140	105	115	150

Abbreviation: NPH, neutral protamine Hagedorn (insulin).

to the recommendation for dosage increments given above. Reduction in the A.M. dose was made because of the anticipated reduction in the pre-breakfast blood glucose concentration resulting from the additional insulin given before supper and the probability that the levels before lunch and dinner, which were in a relatively low range, might be reduced further to hypoglycemic levels.

The interpretation of the basis for elevated fasting glucose levels may be erroneous. The *Somogyi effect* (e.g., hyperglycemia occurring as an exaggerated response of the counterregulatory hormones to prior hypoglycemia) is often invoked. Studies in which hypoglycemia has been induced by insulin in the early morning hours reveal only modest subsequent elevations of blood glucose rather than levels above 250 mg/dl that are often encountered.

Another influence on the level of fasting blood glucose is the "dawn phenomenon." This refers to the normal course of diurnal glucose variations in which a nadir is reached at approximately 3:00 A.M. with a gradual rise subsequently. This phenomenon should be taken into account because it suggests that a concentration of blood glucose of 70 mg/dl at 7:00 A.M. is likely to have been preceded by one of about 30 mg/dl or less at 3:00 A.M.. Therefore, it is prudent to regard a fasting blood glucose level above the lower limit of the target range of 80 to 180 mg/dl as a therapeutic goal.

Markedly elevated fasting glucose concentrations are most often due to inadequate insulin action during the night and are indicative of a need to increase the evening dosage of NPH insulin. Measurements of blood glucose concentrations at about 3:00 A.M. will clarify the situation and may eliminate consideration of reactive hyperglycemia as the cause of elevations of fasting blood glucose.

The approximate insulin requirements over time can be predicted and are useful in reassuring parents who may become concerned as insulin dosages increase with growth and puberty. *Unusually high daily levels* suggest insulin resistance, which may result from excessive insulin antibody formation, stimulation of the counterregulatory hormones (glucagon, epinephrine, and growth hormone) resulting from overtreatment with insulin, excessive caloric intake, and prolonged emotional arousal.

Unusually low levels of insulin may be encountered in patients who factitiously report satisfactory glucose measurements. Such patients usually fail to gain weight, and they have elevated glycosylated hemoglobin values and persistent ketonuria.

Patients with reduced counterregulatory hormone secretion, particularly growth hormone deficiency, and those with significant residual beta cell function (demonstrated by C-peptide responses to a mixed meal) have lower than average insulin requirements.

During the first week or 10 days of insulin therapy, a fall in insulin requirement (the honeymoon period) usually occurs. This phenomenon is probably the result of a reversal of the hormonal milieu of the untreated diabetic state in which noncarbohydrate fuels provided the major energy source facilitated by activation of the counterregulatory hormones. Partial recovery of beta cell function may also be contributory. The decline in insulin requirement usually continues for 2 to 3 months, when a nadir is reached. Over the following 18 months, a gradual rise occurs to approximately 0.4 and 0.5 to 0.7 units per pound of body weight in the prepubertal and adolescent patient, respectively. After completion of growth, a reduction of about 30 per cent in insulin requirement is usual.

MANAGEMENT OF INTERCURRENT EVENTS

Adjustments in caloric intake and an in insulin dosage may be required with strenuous exercise, illness, surgery, or excessive fluctuations in glucose concentration. In regard to these situations, it is reasonable, when one is adjusting insulin dosage, to place major emphasis on avoidance of hypoglycemia with its potential for neurologic injury. This position is supported by the progressive loss of counterregulatory hormone response to hypoglycemia with increased duration of diabetes: initially that of glucagon and later of catecholamines. As a consequence, some patients may become "hypoglycemia-unresponsive," lacking the warning symptoms of pallor, anxiety, and jitteriness attributable to catecholamine stimulation. When a hypoglycemic event occurs that is not explained by a missed or delayed meal or unusual exertion, a 10 per cent reduction in insulin dosage should be made. The reduction should be made in the component of the insulin prescription, exhibiting maximal glucose-lowering effect at the time of the reaction.

When glucose concentrations are found to be excessively high during routine testing—about 250 to 300 mg/dl—supplementary, regular insulin is indicated. An appropriate amount is about 10 per cent of the total daily dosage.

Extreme variations in physical activity may be managed, if anticipated beforehand, by a 10 per cent reduction of the insulin dose, with maximal action during the exercise period. Alternatively, ingestion of 5 to 10 per cent of the daily caloric allotment in a concentrated carbohydrate form may be given before the activity.

Surgical procedures entailing general anesthesia alter the usual balance between insulin, caloric intake, and energy expenditure. These may be compensated for by a reduction in insulin dosage by administering half of the usual daily amount as NPH insulin prior to the procedure. Maintenance quantities of intravenous fluids are supplied by a 0.2 per cent sodium chloride in 5 per cent glucose solution until oral feedings are resumed. Glucose levels are determined at 2- to 4-hour intervals, and the glucose content of the infusate is adjusted to maintain plasma concentrations at about 200 mg/dl. If hyperglycemia occurs in the postoperative period, supplements of regular insulin equivalent to 10 per cent of the usual daily dosage should be administered at 4- to 6-hour intervals.

Gastroenteritis with vomiting is a common situation confronting the caretakers of the diabetic child. Insulin should be administered at about 80 per cent of the usual dosage because of the anticipated reduction in caloric intake. Carbohydrate must be provided to avoid hypoglycemia and to support oxidation of ketone bodies. Sugar-containing carbonated beverages and fruit juices, which are approximately 10 per cent carbohydrate solutions, are administered in volumes sufficient to supply maintenance requirements for water. This quantity is divided into 24 aliquots and administered hourly. Most episodes of vomiting terminate spontaneously in 6 to 8 hours. Persistence of gastroenteritis beyond this time usually necessitates glucose-containing fluids administered by the parenteral route.

Monitoring Glycemic Control

All patients and/or parents should be thoroughly instructed in use of the techniques for self-monitoring of blood glucose. Proper use makes reasonable the goal of achievement of nearly normal glucose concentrations for most patients. The technique should replace urine testing for glucose as a guide to the adjustment of insulin dosage. Tests of urine for ketone bodies remain useful at times of metabolic derangement during illness. Discrepancies between simultaneous glucose determinations in blood and urine have been demonstrated and establish the superiority of the former. Obtaining capillary blood samples for testing has been facilitated by the development of spring-driven lancets that pierce the skin of the finger tip with minor discomfort. A number of these devices are available, including Autolet, Penlet, Glucolet, and Soft Touch. Reflectance meters that utilize glucose oxidase–impregnated strips are capable of providing reasonably accurate estimates of capillary blood glucose concentration. They are available at modest cost. Among those in wide use are Accu-Chek II, Glucometer 3, and Life Scan One Touch Meter. The frequency of blood testing recommended to patients should be flexible, taking into account age, metabolic stability, and intensity of treatment goals. In the early months of treatment, when insulin requirements undergo more rapid change, testing four times daily—before meals and at bedtime—is desirable. Later on, alternate-day testing may be a reasonable compromise. In any case, a sampling of blood glucose excursions throughout the day should be obtained at least 2 to 3 days weekly. Schoolchildren usually prefer to perform the pre-lunch test on weekends.

The determination of glycosylated hemoglobin (HbA_1 or HbA_{1C}) is extremely useful in evaluating and documenting the quality of glycemic control. The measurement is based on a nonenzymatic, irreversible reaction that occurs between glucose and hemoglobin, resulting in the glycosylation of the latter, the extent of which varies directly with the patient's average glucose concentration. In our laboratory, normal individuals have 5 to 6 per cent of their total hemoglobin as the glycosylated derivative. HbA_{1C} values reflect the average blood glucose concentration of the previous 6 to 8 weeks as the irreversible glycosylation remains for the life of the affected red blood cell. Glycosylation of other body proteins occurs and may cause functional and structural alterations of importance in the development of diabetic complications.

The measurement provides patients with a quantitative measure of their quality of glycemic control; when this value is elevated, it can serve as an incentive for improvement in attention to diet and other aspects of management. Among diabetic children, levels of 6.5 to 7.5 per cent are achievable in those with meticulous attention to management parameters. Less dedicated patients are likely to test in the 9 to 12 per cent range. Test frequency at about twice yearly is reasonable.

Intensive Treatment Regimens

In the normal individual, circulating insulin concentrations rise with nutrient intake and subside to basal levels during the postabsorptive period, which permits utilization of liver glycogen stores and alternate fuels. This pattern can be best mimicked by giving regular insulin before meals and an intermediate-acting insulin (NPH) or Lente before bedtime. In some intensive treatment regimens, Ultralente is given once or twice daily to provide basal concentrations of insulin. Insulin pumps can be programmed to deliver boluses prior to meals and basal quantities throughout the balance of the day. Intensive treatment regimens are capable of achieving nearly normal glycemia and glycosylated hemoglobin values when combined with strict uniformity of caloric intake and exercise and with adjustments in insulin dosages based on frequent blood glucose testing. Only rare individuals in the pediatric age group can be expected to adhere to the very considerable demands of such a treatment program.

Diabetic Ketoacidosis

Diabetic ketoacidosis (DKA) can be viewed as the culmination of essentially total deficiency of insulin. In the absence of insulin, hepatic glucose production is increased threefold to fourfold over its usual postabsorptive level of about 15 g/hour. Glucose uptake by insulin-responsive tissues, which normally equals glucose production, is reduced to one third of the physiologic level. Lipolysis is uncontrolled and results in overproduction and accumulation of ketone bodies. The latter are strongly acidic substances that can severely deplete the bicarbonate-buffering system with the development of metabolic acidosis. Because the maximum rate of ketogenesis in human liver approximates 50 mEq/hour, it is apparent that the body's buffering mechanisms may be overpowered.

Hyperglycemia raises serum osmolality, leading to withdrawal of water from the intracellular into the extracellular compartment. The transfer of water helps to maintain intravascular volume and partially protects against peripheral circulatory failure. With increasing hyperglycemia, the renal threshold for glucose is exceeded and a solute diuresis is induced. The electrolyte composition of the urinary losses approximates a hypotonic solution containing 75 mEq/L of sodium chloride and 15 to 30 mEq/L of potassium chloride. As continued losses of water and electrolyte exceed intake, dehydration supervenes. Reduced whole body and renal perfusion adversely affect organ system function. The kidney's capacity to excrete hydrogen, sulfate, and phosphate ions is reduced with augmentation of the acidosis initially caused by ketone accumulation.

In severe DKA, body water deficits approximate 10 per cent of body weight. As mentioned above, the water and electrolyte losses are consequent to the solute diuresis and are hypotonic with respect to extracellular fluid. Their replacement should be accomplished by administering intravenous fluids with an average sodium concentration of 75 mEq/L.

Initial fluid therapy is directed at expanding blood volume and improving tissue perfusion and therefore should provide a sodium concentration approximating that of plasma (e.g., normal saline). Because extracellular and plasma volumes are partially maintained by the osmotic effects of hyperglycemia, they will be reduced as insulin treatment lowers glucose concentration. The resulting shift of water from the vascular to the intracellular space mandates the need to expand blood volume before this occurs in order to avoid further deterioration of the circulation and the development of shock. Water moves into cells, which in the central nervous system may result in fatal cerebral edema. Maintaining a modest elevation in glucose concentration at about 200 to 250 mg/dl for the first 12 to 18 hours of treatment and avoidance of hyponatremia should prevent this complication.

Fluid therapy in DKA should provide maintenance and deficit repair and quantities of water, sodium, potassium, chloride, and phosphate as presented in Table 4. As previously mentioned, the deficit of 100 ml/kg represents a loss of 10 per cent of body weight. The sodium deficit of 7 mEq/kg in a water deficit of 100 ml/kg is equivalent to 70 mEq in each

TABLE 4. Fluid and Electrolyte Requirements in Diabetic Ketoacidosis

	Maintenance/m²	Deficit Repair/kg
Water	1500 ml	100 ml
Sodium	60 mEq	7–10 mEq
Potassium	50 mEq	5–10 mEq
Chloride	40 mEq	5 mEq
Phosphate	10 mEq	3 mEq

liter of water or a solution of approximately half the concentration of physiologic saline.

Phosphate losses in the urine may lead to significant deficits and should be replaced by administering one half of the potassium as the phosphate salt and the remainder as the chloride.

Therapy is initiated by the administration of physiologic saline (20 ml/kg/hour) until brisk urine flow occurs. The rate is then reduced to 10 ml/kg/hour. When glucose falls to 250 mg/dl, the fluids are changed to 5 per cent glucose in one-half normal saline and infused at approximately 5 ml/kg/hour. A brisk urine output is indicative of adequate renal perfusion consequent to re-establishment of a relatively adequate intravascular volume.

The quantities of insulin recommended for treatment of DKA have been markedly reduced in the past decade. This change has been referred to as "low-dose insulin therapy." A more appropriate designation would be "physiologic-dose therapy."

Normal individuals who have been made hyperglycemic by intravenous infusion of glucose develop insulin levels of about 150 microunits per milliliter (μ units/ml). Gluconeogenesis and lipolysis are effectively suppressed at concentrations of approximately 40 (μ units/ml). Uncontrolled lipolysis and gluconeogenesis are the major factors responsible for the metabolic derangements of DKA. Glucose uptake by muscle progressively increases with insulin concentrations up to 300 μ units/ml. The quantities of insulin employed in "low-dose" insulin therapy yield concentrations in the maximally effective to high-physiologic range (100 to 200 μ units/ml) and can be achieved by intravenous administration of a loading dose of 0.1 units/kg followed by 0.1 units/kg/hour.

Subcutaneously injected insulin suffers from the disadvantage that it may be poorly absorbed during the early phases of treatment, when peripheral circulation is impaired. With this route, there is also some risk of late hypoglycemia because large amounts of insulin may be absorbed from subcutaneous depots when peripheral circulation is restored. Both of these problems are avoided by continuous intravenous administration of insulin.

After 12 to 18 hours of continuous intravenous therapy, improvement in the patient's metabolic status, as evidenced by partial correction of dehydration, restoration of mental alertness, and nearly normal acid-base status, usually permits further insulin treatment to be accomplished by the subcutaneous route. The insulin dosage then employed is about 0.2 units/kg every 4 to 6 hours.

Minor disadvantages of the intravenous route for the treatment of DKA are the requirement that insulin delivery be controlled by a pump rather than by gravity. As insulin binds to plastic tubing, the infusion apparatus must be pre-rinsed with the insulin solution in order to saturate its binding sites. In the rare patient with high titers of anti-insulin antibodies, the initial period of insulin infusion may merely accomplish titration of the antibodies rather than correction of the metabolic derangement. It is mandatory to ascertain the effectiveness of the insulin-fluid regimen by determining that a fall in blood glucose of approximately 75 to 100 mg/dl has occurred in the first hour of treatment. If this has not been accomplished, the rate of insulin infusion should be increased by 50 to 100 per cent. Because the half-life of intravenous insulin is only a few minutes, interruption of the infusion may lead to rapid decompensation. In contrast to the subcutaneous and intramuscular routes of administration, the intravenous method provides no depot of insulin.

It should be mentioned that the fall of blood glucose concentration in the initial period of treatment of DKA is primarily the result of dilution, since extracellular fluid volume is expanded combined with increased renal glucose excretion as renal perfusion is restored, rather than the result of insulin-mediated glucose utilization.

Potassium

Potassium administration should be delayed until urine flow is well established. Prolonged anuria is unusual even in the severely dehydrated child with DKA. It is also important to delay administration of potassium intravenously until there is laboratory confirmation that hyperkalemia is not present. Increased potassium concentration in serum is common as potassium shifts from intracellular to extracellular fluid as a consequence of acidemia. The shift of water from the intracellular to the extracellular compartment in response to the osmotic effects of hyperglycemia often masks an elevation of serum potassium concentration. The potassium deficit will require several days or longer for complete correction because its uptake into cells is limited by the uphill concentration gradient between the potassium concentration of extracellular and intracellular water.

Potassium is administered in a dosage of 3.5 mEq/kg, with half as chloride and half as phosphate. This quantity is an approximation and may have to be increased as indicated by the results of biochemical monitoring. It is not unusual for potassium levels to fall to about 3.1 mEq/L after 18 to 24 hours of treatment.

Bicarbonate Therapy

In occasional patients with DKA, acidosis may be sufficiently severe as to constitute a threat to survival. At pH values of about 7.0 and below, myocardial and respiratory center functions are depressed. The lower limit of acidemia that can be tolerated by humans for short periods is approximately 6.85. Because sudden large shifts of pH toward normal following administration of sodium bicarbonate solutions can have adverse effects, its use should be limited to situations in which acidosis *per se* constitutes a threat to life. Arterial pH values below 7.1 or serum bicarbonate concentration of about 5 mEq/L are indications for administration of bicarbonate to supply needed buffers and promptly raise pH to a safer level. Minute volume of respiration increases only slightly as pH falls from 7.4 to 7.2. With further declines to about 7.05, there is a marked increase in ventilation. As pH decreases further, depression of the ventilatory response to acidosis occurs. This is accomplished by a rise in P_{CO_2} and may lead to a catastrophic fall in pH. Less severe degrees of acidemia can be tolerated by the patient and will be corrected as accumulated ketone bodies are metabolized to bicarbonate with insulin therapy.

Abrupt increase in blood pH should be avoided because it will be accompanied by a decrease in the release of oxygen from oxyhemoglobin. With acidosis, the oxygen dissociation curve is shifted to the right, facilitating release and delivery of oxygen to tissues. This beneficial adjustment compensates somewhat for the impaired tissue perfusion consequent to hypovolemia. This effect is offset by a shift in the opposite direction resulting from depletion of 2,3-diphosphoglycerate (2,3-DPG) in the red blood cells. This compound is a major red cell metabolite of glucose and is diminished by both acidosis and phosphate depletion. Initially, these opposing effects on the oxyhemoglobin dissociation curve tend to balance each other. Rapid correction of acidosis by administration of bicarbonate removes the beneficial shift to the right and unmasks the adverse effects of 2,3-DPG depletion. This is especially harmful if it occurs before intravascular volume has been restored by intravenous fluid administration.

When sodium bicarbonate administration is indicated, a dosage of 2.5 mEq/kg infused in about 1 hour is appropriate. Assuming a volume of distribution for sodium of 50 per cent of body weight, this quantity should increase serum bicarbonate concentration by approximately 5 mEq/L and restore buffering capacity to a more physiologic level.

Other therapeutic measures may also be indicated. Cyanotic patients should be given oxygen. In the unconscious patient, it is advisable to remove gastric contents by suction to minimize the danger of aspiration with vomiting. Bladder catheterization should be limited to anuric patients. The optic discs should be examined for evidence of increased intracranial pressure indicative of cerebral edema. If this complication is suspected, reduction of excess brain water should be attempted by increasing the blood glucose concentration and by administration of mannitol. Inducing hyperventilation will decrease cerebral blood flow and may be particularly helpful in this situation.

GENERAL ASPECTS OF TREATMENT

In many medical centers, the physician's treatment efforts are greatly enhanced by the availability of a team of professionals who can effectively address the various aspects of diabetes care. Included are a nutritionist as a resource for dietary issues and a diabetes treatment nurse to participate in instructions concerning the pathophysiology of diabetes, techniques of insulin administration, blood glucose monitoring, and insulin dosage adjustments. An individual with skills in counseling parents concerning developmental and adjustment problems is a major resource for the parents and the treating physician.

When such a team is not available for group management of patients, the physician must assume most of the educational role with assistance from appropriate colleagues in the community.

Doctors who treat diabetic patients soon become aware of their limitations in achieving appropriate therapeutic goals, as the roles of the patient and parents in the outcome are so large. The quality of the educational program provided to a family during the initial period of treatment is critical to the success of the treatment program. The instruction should include the physiology of fuel metabolism and how it is affected by insulin; how diet and exercise influence day-to-day management; recognition and treatment of hypoglycemia; the technique of insulin injection; the natural history of diabetes, including expected changes in insulin dosage with time; and some insight into prognosis. It is appropriate to stress the prospect that modern methods of achieving metabolic control, particularly glucose self-monitoring, may improve the outcome of the disease as well as the expectation that ongoing research efforts may lead to major therapeutic advances.

In the early period of treatment, patients should be seen by the physician at 3-month intervals. Many parents of diabetic children find the visits comforting because of the reassurance derived from learning that their child is developing well and is remaining free of overt complications. The treatment team or individual physician should be available to the patient and family by telephone on an around-the-clock basis.

There are support groups for patients and their families sponsored by the American Diabetes Association and the Juvenile Diabetes Foundation. In addition, many children are helped by association with other patients in camps for diabetic children.

In the effort to assist patients in achieving optimum control, one should avoid making the demands of the treatment regimen so onerous as to contribute to its rejection by the patient. Patients should be informed, in an age-appropriate manner, about the rationale for the treatment program with the hope of securing their compliance. Allowing youngsters to assume developmentally reasonable responsibility for self-care assists them in the transition to greater autonomy. This transition is fostered by seeing the adolescent patient separately from the parent, developing a direct relationship with the patient, and attempting to separate diabetes from the other issues involving the adolescent's need for "distancing" from the parents.

Parents should be advised to moderate overt expressions of their unhappiness about the occurrence of the disease. These displays add to patients' negative feelings about the disease and themselves as the cause of the parent's unhappiness.

It is worth repeating that the diet prescribed for the diabetic child should be sufficient to provide satiety. Non-obese children have demonstrated adequate endogenous controls matching caloric intake with the requirements for energy and growth. The obese patient should be urged to adhere to a diet designed to reduce or limit gain in weight. The diabetic child should be extended freedom to participate in activities acceptable to the family for their nondiabetic children. Unnecessary restrictions are likely to increase resentment against the disease and thus prove counterproductive.

A not uncommon counterproductive attitude is exhibited by parents who express a form of denial of the realities of diabetes by being overly casual in their supervision of diet and blood glucose monitoring. Problems may surface that indicate a need for special attention to the patient's emotional status, including deteriorating school performance, truancy, faking test results, omitting insulin injections, and the occurrence of repeated episodes of ketoacidosis.

Diabetes offers many opportunities for counterproductive patient behavior: patients may deliberately omit insulin doses; others have covertly injected unprescribed amounts of insulin, causing hypoglycemic reactions in spite of marked reductions in prescribed insulin dosage; and some patients defeat attempts to achieve a reasonable level of control by capricious food ingestion.

In a small minority of patients, emotional stress can result in metabolic decompensation. These patients often require frequent hospitalizations for the treatment of diabetic ketoacidosis. It has been possible to reproduce the decompensation in glucose and ketone hemostasis by subjecting such children to interviews designed to simulate their individual emotional stresses. Emotional distress elicited during the stress interview was shown to be accompanied by increased blood levels of growth hormone cortisol and urinary catecholamines. The metabolic responses to the stress could be blunted by prior administration of a beta-blocking agent, suggesting that increased catecholamines were most responsible for the observed metabolic changes. Resolution of the problem could most often be achieved by family psychiatric therapy designed to assist the patient to verbally vent feelings of distress rather than to repress them.

Experimental Treatment Developments

An extensive research effort is focused on efforts to improve the outcome and management strategies of insulin-dependent diabetes. Insulin pumps implanted subcutaneously and powered telemetrically that deliver insulin intraperitoneally via catheter are under promising trial. The device obviates the need for injections except for periodic filling of its insulin reservoir.

A convincing body of evidence supports an autoimmune etiology of IDDM. A variety of interventions of value in other autoimmune disease have been tried with some evidence of benefit. Intravenous corticosteroid pulses and gamma globulin have yielded minimal effects. Immunosuppressive agents, particularly cyclosporine A, have been more effective in obviating the need for exogenous insulin. Trials of this agent in newly diagnosed patients have achieved a success rate of about 40 per cent. Toxic effects, particularly in the kidney, preclude further trials in patients. Newer, less harmful immunosuppressive agents may be developed and may achieve a place in suppressing the manifestations of the disease. In an animal model, a monoclonal antibody against the T cells exerting a cytotoxic effect on the pancreatic beta cell has been successful in reversing the immunologically mediated process.

Pancreas transplantation, which requires lifelong immunosuppression to avoid rejection, has an established therapeutic role when combined with kidney transplantation in the diabetic patient with end-stage renal disease. Recent results document a 1-year functional outcome of 62 per cent, declining, to 36 per cent after 3 years. The results of pancreas transplantation alone are less favorable. Until less toxic methods of immunosuppression are developed and more prolonged graft survival is achieved, pancreas transplantation is not an acceptable option for the diabetic child.

Beta cell transplantation has not yet achieved reversal of the disease. However, it does have a number of promising attributes, including the possibility of in vitro manipulations to minimize graft antigenicity and the relative simplicity of introducing beta cells by injection rather than by a surgical procedure required for transplantation of the entire or hemipancreas.

Research is also identifying some of the factors responsible for diabetic complications. The progress of diabetic renal disease can be slowed by improved glycemic control, antihypertensive treatment, and, probably, restriction of dietary protein intake.

It is reasonable to predict that the outcome for today's properly treated diabetic children will be more favorable than for those treated in the past. The results of the Diabetes Control and Complications Trial currently in process may establish the efficacy of near normalization of blood glucose in delay and prevention of diabetic complications.

REFERENCES

Dahlquist G: Epidemiological studies of childhood insulin-dependent diabetes. Acta Paediatr Scand 80:583–589, 1991.

Ellis EN: Concepts of fluid therapy in diabetic ketoacidosis and hyperosmolar hyperglycemic nonketotic coma. Pediatr Clin North Am 37:313–321, 1990.

Johnson AB, Taylor R: Diabetes mellitus. Postgrad Med J 66:1010–1024, 1990.

HYPOGLYCEMIA IN METABOLIC DISORDERS

ROBERT SCHWARTZ, M.D.

DIAGNOSIS

The diagnosis of hypoglycemia may be approached from several perspectives: (1) statistical, (2) hormonal responsiveness (i.e., epinephrine release with associated symptoms), (3) neurophysiologic responses (i.e., BAER [brainstem auditory evoked responses]), and/or (4) neurobehavioral long-term follow-up.[1]

Symptomatic Hypoglycemia

Symptomatic hypoglycemia requires immediate treatment to avoid an adverse neurobehavioral outcome. As in insulin-dependent diabetes, mild hypoglycemia may be treated in one of two ways:

1. Orally with fruit juice and added sucrose (to a total of 15 per cent carbohydrates). Thus, orange juice, which contains 10 per cent carbohydrate, may have 5 g of sucrose (1 teaspoonful) added to 3 ounces (90 ml).
2. With glucagon (30 to 50 μg/kg IM not to exceed 1 mg).

For severe symptomatic hypoglycemia, intravenous dextrose (0.5 g/kg as a 15 to 25 per cent solution) is required. The latter should not be used alone but should be followed immediately by further carbohydrate, either parenterally or orally. This is best accomplished with a continuous infusion of dextrose at a basal rate of 4 to 6 mg/kg/minute in young infants, 2 to 4 mg/kg/minute in older infants and children, or the adult rate of 1 to 2 mg/kg/minute in adolescents. Continued carbohydrate administration is indicated to avoid reactive hypoglycemia. Therapy is continued until the patient is stabilized and a normal plasma (or blood) glucose level has been documented by a laboratory chemical analysis. Further therapy is dependent on defining a specific etiology.

Because symptoms of hypoglycemia are nonspecific and may be attributed to discharge of the sympathetic-parasympathetic nervous system, a blood determination for glucose analysis (not by reagent test strips, which are unreliable) must be obtained. Determination of the etiology may depend on analysis of hormones, such as insulin or growth hormone; substrates, such as lactate or beta-hydroxybutyrate; amino acids; or abnormal metabolites, such as urinary organic acids.

Asymptomatic (Incidental) Hypoglycemia

Asymptomatic, or incidental, hypoglycemia presents a different problem. First, it must be documented by a reliable chemical determination. Second, the reference for normal values must be reliably established. For term infants and older infants and children, normal plasma glucose concentration is greater than or equal to 40 mg/dl (2.2 mM). For preterm infants, the older criteria of Cornblath and Schwartz[1] are acceptable. Thus, hypoglycemia is considered at a plasma glucose concentration below 25 mg/dl (1.39 mM) for the first 2 days of life. Infants and children with values below these recommended limits should be treated orally. It is prudent not to ignore documented hypoglycemia even though no long-term adverse outcome has been reported. No long-term effects of asymptomatic hypoglycemia during the initial days after birth have been demonstrated in infants of diabetic mothers. An association between hypoglycemia (plasma glucose <47 mg/dl [2.6 mM]) and later (2 or more years) neurobehavioral dysfunction has been reported. However, this study was not designed originally to answer the question of the significance of hypoglycemia in preterm infants and has been criticized as inadequate.[2] Thus, vigorous therapy for asymptomatic infants is presently unwarranted.

Specific diagnoses will determine further therapy. Thus, a young infant or adolescent (but not usually a child) may have hyperinsulinemic hypoglycemia due to beta cell dysfunction in the former or islet cell adenoma in the latter. Persistent, intractable hypoglycemia may necessitate parenteral dextrose at very high rates (above 12–14 mg/kg/minute up to 24–26 mg/kg/minute) given as a 25 per cent solution via a central catheter. When such extraordinary rates of dextrose are required, further medical therapy with diazoxide, which suppresses insulin secretion, at 5 to 25 mg/kg/day in three equally divided oral doses is indicated. Failing stabilization of the blood glucose concentration, control may be achieved with somatostatin at 8 μg/kg/hour intravenously for 1 to 7 days and adjunct support with glucagon at 100 μg/kg IV or IM every 2 to 3 hours. These latter therapies are expedient and temporizing. They are particularly useful in preparation for surgical intervention. The sooner the latter can be accomplished, the better the outcome. *Near-total (99 per cent) pancreatectomy is the recommended procedure for severe, intractable, or recurrent symptomatic hypoglycemia.*

Neonatal Hypoglycemia

Neonatal hypoglycemia may occur in association with midline facial defects, septo-optic-pituitary dysplasia, or isolated growth hormone or multiple pituitary deficiencies. Once it has been documented, treatment with human growth hormone (0.025 mg/kg/day SC once daily) plus maintenance cortisol acetate (12 to 16 mg/m²/day) will prevent recurrence of hypoglycemia.

ASSOCIATED DISORDERS

Glycogen Storage Disease

A variety of genetic metabolic disorders are associated with hypoglycemia. Of the various types of glycogen storage diseases, hypoglycemia is *not* associated with type II (Pompe's disease), type IV (Andersen's disease), type V (McCardle's disease), or type VII (Tarui's disease). The remaining types present with hypoglycemia of varying severity and symptoms.

Type Ia Disease

The most striking is type Ia *(von Gierke's disease)* which is due to absence of microsomal glucose-6-phosphatase, the gatekeeper of hepatic glucose release. Any brief fast or acceleration of glucose utilization results in a fall in plasma glucose concentration to unmeasurable levels in association with severe lactic acidosis. Ketonuria is not a usual feature. These patients, if untreated, are often asymptomatic, presumably because of alternate substrate (lactate) utilization by the brain.

Initial parenteral therapy includes dextrose bolus (0.25 g/kg as a 25 per cent solution) followed by a continuous rate at two to three times maintenance (i.e., 8 to 10 mg/kg/minute with 75 mEq/L of sodium bicarbonate) until stabilization and oral intake are achieved. Thereafter, enteral nutrition must be provided continuously (as by nighttime nasogastric feeds) or intermittently by frequent feeds (every 3 to 4 hours) around the clock. *The recent recognition of the effectiveness of oral raw corn or tapioca starch has been a major contribution to the management of this disorder.* It is consistently effective in children over 2 years of age and sometimes in younger ones. Thus, around-the-clock plasma glucose determinations every 3 to 4 hours are necessary to evaluate its effectiveness and duration. Doses of 2 to 3.5 g/kg may be required to sustain normoglycemia for up to 5–6 hours. Smaller doses are not usually effective. Once a patient has been metabolically stabilized for several months, cerebral responsiveness to hypoglycemia may recur. Thus, it is prudent to alert families to the potential consequences of omitting a feed. Although type Ib is due to a different defect, glucose-6-phosphate translocase, the metabolic consequences are similar to those in type Ia and therefore are treated similarly.

Types III and IV Disease

The other types of glycogen storage diseases are milder in regard to hypoglycemia. Thus, type III (debrancher, amylo-1,6-glucosidase) and type VI complex (phosphorylase or phosphorylase kinase) impair glycogenolysis. Hypoglycemia does not usually occur after a brief fast, as in type I disease, but does occur after a prolonged fast (i.e., overnight or longer). Normally, gluconeogenesis would prevent the occurrence of hypoglycemia after a prolonged fast. Why this is less effective in these patients is unclear. Treatment involves avoiding long fasts or hypercatabolic states, consuming a high-protein diet, and possibly taking a raw cornstarch feed at bed time (vide supra).

Other Disorders of Carbohydrate Metabolism

Other disorders of carbohydrate metabolism include *hereditary fructose intolerance* (fructose-1-aldolase B deficiency), in which symptomatic hypoglycemia occurs within 30 minutes of ingestion. This disorder is best managed by preventative therapy directed at rigid restriction of dietary fructose and fructose-containing polysaccharides, i.e., sucrose. Inadvertent fructose ingestion requires parenteral dextrose therapy (0.25 to 0.5 g/kg) as a bolus. Glucagon is ineffective and is contraindicated. Hypoglycemia has been described in association with galactosemia but is very rare and likely due to the associated hepatitis rather than to a metabolic disorder. No unusual therapy is indicated.

Defects in the enzymes of gluconeogenesis involve pyruvate carboxylase, phosphoenolpyruvate carboxykinase, and fructose-1,6-diphosphatase. These very rare genetic disorders present with symptomatic hypoglycemia after fasting. Provision of gluconeogenic substrates (alanine, lactate, pyruvate) does not prevent hypoglycemia in the former two, but glycerol may. In contrast, no gluconeogenic substrates are effective in fructose-1,6-diphosphatase deficiency. Symptomatic hypoglycemia is treated with parenteral dextrose (see earlier). Fasting and hypercatabolic states should be avoided. Frequent feedings of a high-carbohydrate diet with supplemental raw cornstarch at bedtime may prevent early morning hypoglycemia.

Defects in Amino Acid Metabolism

Defects in amino acid metabolism (especially the branch-chain amino acids) or in fatty acid metabolism (involving carnitine transport or specific dehydrogenases) have been recognized in the past two decades as causes of hypoinsulinemic, hypoketonemic hypoglycemia.[3] Although the mechanisms have not been clearly proven, two events are likely in several of these disorders:

1. Following a fast, glycogen stores are depleted and hepatic glucose production declines. If ketones cannot be produced, alternate substrate for brain metabolism is limited and symptomatic hypoglycemia supervenes.
2. In addition, if the metabolic block specifically limits formation of acetyl CoA, an activator of pyruvate carboxylase, gluconeogenesis cannot be initiated.

Irrespective of the specific metabolic block, hypoglycemia is treated with parenteral dextrose acutely and continuously until the abnormal metabolic situation is stabilized. Prevention of hypoglycemia depends on identification of the specific metabolic block and devising strategies to minimize the effects. Thus, 3-hydroxy,3-methyl glutaryl CoA lyase deficiency is associated with a severe metabolic organic acidosis and hypoglycemia. Limiting leucine intake to minimum amounts compatible with normal protein anabolism diminishes the risk of these complications unless a hypercatabolic state, as with an intercurrent infection, supervenes. Home blood glucose monitoring may be beneficial in anticipating significant, symptomatic hypoglycemia. A similar approach is indicated in the disorders of fatty acid metabolism.

NUTRITIONAL THERAPY

Nutritional management should be an important aspect of the treatment of disorders of carbohydrate metabolism. The advice of a skilled, well-trained nutritionist is essential. Therapy may be *primary* and *preventative,* as in the recommendations to avoid fruits containing fructose, table sugar containing sucrose, and processed foods containing sugar fillers in the management of hereditary fructose intolerance. Alternatively, therapy may be *secondary* and *adjunctive,* as in the recommendation to avoid galactose (lactose) and fructose (and sucrose) in type I glycogen storage disease. Each disorder must be carefully assessed for optimal nutrient intake.

SUMMARY

In conclusion, hypoglycemia should be viewed as a disease complex of multiple, diverse etiologic factors. When hypoglycemia is symptomatic, prompt parenteral therapy is indicated to prevent acute and long-term cerebral dysfunction. Optimal long-term management must be individualized and depends on precise knowledge of the basis for the metabolic derangement. With effective expectant therapy, prognosis is often favorable.

REFERENCES

1. Cornblath M, Schwartz R (eds): Disorders of Carbohydrate Metabolism in Infancy, 3rd ed. Cambridge, Blackwell Scientific Publications, Inc, 1991.
2. Cornblath M, Schwartz R, Aynsley-Green A, Lloyd J: Hypoglycemia in infancy: The need for a rational definition. Pediatrics 85:834–837, 1990.
3. Stanley CA: New genetic defects in mitochondrial fatty acid oxidation and carnitine deficiency. Adv Pediatr 34:59–88, 1987.

DIABETES INSIPIDUS

LOUIS J. MUGLIA, M.D.
and JOSEPH A. MAJZOUB, M.D.

ETIOLOGY

Diabetes insipidus (DI) exists when, in the presence of plasma hyperosmolality, an appropriately concentrated urine is not formed. This defect stems from either insufficient secretion of vasopressin (*hypothalamic* or *central DI*) or renal unresponsiveness to vasopressin *(nephrogenic DI).*

Hypothalamic Diabetes Insipidus

Hypothalamic DI occurs most frequently in association with tumors involving the hypothalamus or following their resection (craniopharyngioma, germinoma). Because the magnocellular neurons of the hypothalamic paraventricular and supraoptic nuclei, which synthesize vasopressin destined for release from the posterior pituitary, are distant from the pituitary, substantial suprasellar extension of anterior pituitary tumors must develop prior to the occurrence of DI. DI, however, develops in approximately 20 per cent of patients following the surgical removal of anterior pituitary tumors, particularly when associated with high transection of the pituitary stalk. Infiltrative malignancies (leukemia, lymphoma) and systemic diseases (histiocytosis, sarcoidosis, Whipple's disease) may cause substantial destruction of vasopressin containing neurons with little mass effect. Nonsurgical trauma, vascular lesions, infection, and pituitary infarction associated with parturition are less common causes.

Idiopathic hypothalamic DI comprises a relatively common subgroup of patients. Pedigrees exhibiting an autosomal dominant mode of inheritance have been described, but the majority of these cases are not familial.

Nephrogenic Diabetes Insipidus

Nephrogenic DI most commonly results from acquired defects, such as chronic tubulointerstitial renal disease, obstructive uropathy, hypercalcemia, hypokalemia, or drug effects (e.g., lithium). A congenital X-linked recessive form has also been defined.

CLINICAL FEATURES

Thirst, polyuria, and polydipsia are the hallmarks of DI. Urine output in general exceeds 3 L/m^2/day, with nocturia (and sometimes enuresis) a common feature. The urine is often colorless, even upon the first morning voiding. A marked preference for cold liquids is expressed by most patients, with drinking occurring through the night. In infants, failure to thrive or recurrent fever of unknown origin may be the primary complaints.

To screen for DI, it is useful to obtain a serum sample and second-voided urine sample after a defined fast. The duration of the fast should be determined by the usual length the patient can abstain from fluids to avoid excessive dehydration. A serum osmolality of greater than 295 mOsm/kg of water (H_2O) with a urine osmolality less than 295 mOsm/kg H_2O establishes the diagnosis. If the serum osmolality is less than 295 mOsm/kg H_2O and the urine osmolality is less than 600 mOsm/kg H_2O, a water deprivation test is needed to establish the diagnosis. Hourly serum and urine electrolytes and osmolality, as well as weight, are measured beginning at 4 hours of fasting until the serum osmolality rises above 295 mOsm/kg H_2O or the urine osmolality exceeds 600 mOsm/kg H_2O. Blood pressure and pulse should be monitored hourly to guard against the development of clinically important hypovolemia.

THERAPY

Postoperative Management

Water balance is normally regulated by vasopressin and thirst. The potential for significant problems arises when both of these components are compromised, as in postoperative situations in which intravenous fluids are used and damage to the hypothalamus or posterior pituitary has occurred. Patients in this setting should be monitored and stabilized in an intensive care unit. During the postoperative period, DI can develop in many patients undergoing craniotomy and manipulation of the hypothalamic-pituitary region. The classic "triphasic" response may develop in cases of pituitary stalk transection, in which, after an initial 1 to 3 days of DI, inappropriate vasopressin secretion develops that may last for several days before the subsequent return of DI.

Because of this lability in neuroendocrine function, it is often best to manage acute postoperative DI *in children* with fluids alone, avoiding the use of vasopressin therapy. This method consists of matching input and output hourly within the range of 1 to 3 L/m^2/day (40 to 120 ml/m^2/hour). These limits are derived assuming an obligate daily solute excretion of approximately 500 mOsm/m^2 and normal renal function without an excess of extrarenal water loss (due to vomiting, diarrhea, diaphoresis, and so on). When intravenous fluids are used, the basal 40 ml/m^2/hour should be given as D_5 ¼ normal saline (NS) and the remainder, depending on the urine output, as 5 per cent dextrose in water (D_5W). Potassium chloride (40 mEq/L) may be added if oral intake is to be delayed for several days. For hourly urine volumes under 40 ml/m^2/hour, no additional fluid should be administered. For hourly urine volumes in excess of 40 ml/m^2/hour, the excess volume should be replaced with D_5W up to a total maximum replacement of 120 ml/m^2/hour. For example, in a child with a surface area of 1 m^2 (approximately 30 kg), the minimal infusion rate would be 1 m^2 times 40 ml/m^2/hour = 40 ml/hour of D_5 ¼ NS. If an hourly urine output was 60 ml, an additional 20 ml/hour D_5W would be given, for a total infusion rate of 60 ml/hour. This may result in a serum sodium in the 150 mEq/L range, and a mildly volume contracted state, should DI be present. Patients may also become mildly hyperglycemic on this regimen, particularly if they are also receiving postoperative glucocorticoid therapy. This fluid management protocol, because it does not employ vasopressin administration, prevents any chance of hyponatremia.

Alternatively, a vasopressin infusion (Pitressin) may be started at 1.5 mU/kg/hour with fluids restricted to 1 L/m^2/day. However, whenever exogenous vasopressin is administered along with intravenous fluids, thirst, and vasopressin regulatory mechanisms are bypassed, providing a setting in which serious complications associated with water intoxication may occur. When this protocol is used, great care must be taken to avoid iatrogenic hyponatremia. With either protocol, patients may be switched from intravenous to oral fluids as soon as possible to facilitate their management.

Chronic Diabetes Insipidus

Therapy for patients with chronic DI must be individualized. In infants with continued DI, formula is continued at 3 L/m^2/day without vasopressin replacement. Institution of exogenous vasopressin therapy in this age group would require fluid restriction to a degree that would jeopardize adequate growth. For children and adolescents with an intact thirst mechanism, intranasal desamino-D-arginine vasopressin (DDAVP) is begun as a single nighttime dose of 2.5 to 10 μg, with a usual duration of action of 12 to 24 hours. A second dose may be given in the morning if adequate antidiuresis is not maintained. Patients are instructed to alternate nares to minimize mucosal edema and irritation, which can reduce absorption, as can rhinorrhea and congestion. Excessive doses may cause mild abdominal cramping or diarrhea. All patients should be allowed a period of at least 1 to 2 hours daily when escape from the effects of DDAVP occurs so that any excess water accumulated may be excreted. This minimizes the chance of water intoxication.

Partial Vasopressin Deficiency

In patients with partial vasopressin deficiency states, chlorpropamide (4 mg/kg/day) has been found to augment residual vasopressin action. Hypoglycemia is the primary complication of this therapy.

REFERENCES

Bartter FJ, Detea CS: Diabetes insipidus, its nature and diagnosis. Lab Management 20:23, 1982.

Coggins CH, Leaf A: Diabetes insipidus. Am J Med 42:807, 1967.

Harris AS: Clinical experience with desmopression: Efficiency and safety in central diabetes insipidus and other conditions. J Pediatr 114:711–718, 1989.

Knoers M, Monnens LA: Amiloride-hydrochlorothiazide vs indomethacin-hydrochlorothiazide in the treatment of nephrogenic diabetes insipidus. J Pediatr 117:499–502, 1990.

RICKETS

CRAIG B. LANGMAN, M.D.

Rickets is an inherited or acquired disease of bone in growing children that results in the undermineralization of newly formed osteoid; it is called *osteomalacia* in the adult. The majority of diseases that result in rickets may be directly related to a disturbance in the normal metabolic pathway for vitamin D.

VITAMIN D PHYSIOLOGY

Vitamin D is synthesized in the skin from a common steroid precursor, 7-dehydrocholesterol, which undergoes several photoisomerization reactions leading to the production of the parent compound, *cholecalciferol* (vitamin D_3). Cholecalciferol made in the skin or ingested in the diet is transported by an alpha$_2$-globulin, vitamin D–binding protein, to the liver where the parent compound undergoes hydroxylation by a P_{450} mixed-function oxidase, producing 25-hydroxycholecalciferol, or 25-hydroxyvitamin D, *calcidiol,* 25(OH)D.

25(OH)D is the major circulating substrate of the vitamin D endocrine system and serves as a measure of the vitamin D status of a child. Produced in the liver, 25(OH)D is transported by the vitamin D–binding protein to the proximal tubule of the kidney, where an intramitochondrial P_{450} enzyme complex hydroxylates the number one position carbon, producing 1,25-dihydroxycholecalciferol, or 1,25-dihydroxyvitamin D, *calcitriol,* 1,25$(OH)_2$D.

1,25$(OH)_2$D is the active metabolite of the vitamin D endocrine system. Its classic target organs include the intestine, where it increases the transcellular transport of calcium and phosphorus and regulates the gene expression of specific calcium-binding proteins called *calbindins,* and the osteoblast, where it regulates osteocalcin gene transcription and is associated with calcium mobilization and osteoid mineralization. In its classic target organs, 1,25$(OH)_2$D acts by binding to a high-affinity receptor that shares a structural homology to other steroid hormone receptors. Thus, 1,25$(OH)_2$D may directly affect gene transcription through its interaction with the vitamin D receptor protein. Similar vitamin D receptor proteins have been found in a myriad of cell types not thought to play a critical role in calcium homeostasis, the classic function of vitamin D.

Rachitic diseases may involve abnormalities at any point in the vitamin D metabolic pathway, including at the level of the vitamin D receptor (see below). The possibility that some of these latter diseases may have alterations of the vitamin D receptor in nonclassic target organs associated with the rachitic condition and lead to other cellular dysfunctions is an active area of clinical investigation.

Table 1 lists the usual circulating levels of 25(OH)D and 1,25$(OH)_2$D in neonates, infants, and children. The discussion of disturbances of vitamin D metabolism follows from the pathway described above; the therapy of rachitic disorders may be rationally based in a similar manner.

NUTRITIONAL DISORDERS

Simple nutritional absence of sufficient quantities of vitamin D (deprivational rickets) is not uncommon in the United States in the 1990s and is related largely to poor socioeconomic conditions and insufficient exposure to adequate levels of sunlight throughout the year. The Recommended Daily Allowance (RDA) for vitamin D for infants and children is 400 IU daily, and intakes substantially below this result in vitamin

TABLE 1. Normal Levels of Vitamin D in the Blood

Age Group	25(OH)D (Calcidiol, ng/ml)	1,25$(OH)_2$D (Calcitriol, pg/ml)
Neonate (0–30 days)	5–15	15–150
Infant (1–12 months)	15–40	20–65
Child (1–12 years)	15–40	20–60
Adolescent (12–16 years)	15–45	20–80

D deficiency. Deprivational rickets is seen most commonly in the first 18 months of life in children. Although the bony changes of rickets may be appreciated in the skull and upper extremity, deprivational rickets most commonly becomes clinically apparent when the exaggerated bowing of the lower extremities is seen (Table 2).

The blood biochemical profile of deprivational rickets reveals modest hypocalcemia, hypophosphatemia for age, secondary hyperparathyroidism, serum levels of $25(OH)D_3$ at the lower limit of assay detection or undetectable, and low to low-normal levels of $1,25(OH)_2D$ (Table 3). Urinary calcium is generally absent, and marked phosphaturia is present so that the tubular reabsorption of phosphorus is reduced below normal (<85 per cent).

Deprivational rickets heals quite nicely with 2000 to 4000 IU vitamin D daily for approximately 3 months. (See Table 4 for pharmacologic preparations of vitamin D and its metabolites.) Several notes of caution apply to this therapy. Profound and symptomatic hypocalcemia may develop with severe, long-standing deprivational rickets during the first several days of therapy from the "hungry bone syndrome," in which calcium is deposited preferentially in bone at the expense of the extracellular fluid. Supplemental oral calcium therapy may offset this tendency toward worsening hypocalcemia. Vitamin D intoxication may occur with prolonged use of this amount of the drug and in the absence of usual follow-up examinations and blood biochemistry profiles. It is recommended that children with deprivational rickets have monthly determinations of serum biochemistries and that therapy be shortened if serum intact parathyroid hormone (PTH) levels normalize sooner than the expected 3 months' duration of treatment.

INTESTINAL DISEASES

Vitamin D obtained from dietary intake is absorbed in the proximal small bowel, and diseases that affect this process may produce a clinical picture not dissimilar from that of deprivational rickets. These include, but are not limited to, surgical resection of small intestine, celiac disease, and cystic fibrosis or other disorders of pancreatic exocrine insufficiency. A careful history, physical examination, and thoughtful laboratory evaluation will uncover those intestinal diseases in which rickets occurs.

The treatment in rickets associated with intestinal diseases utilizes the parent vitamin D compound, but generally with a higher dosage (4000 to 10,000 IU daily) than for deprivational rickets. It is recommended that initial therapy be tailored by subsequent monitoring, at least monthly, of blood levels of calcium, phosphorus, intact PTH, and levels of 25(OH)D and $1,25(OH)_2D$. The length of such treatment is highly dependent on the activity or acuity of the underlying disease process.

TABLE 2. Manifestations of Rickets: Physical Examination

1. Overproduction of cartilage at metaphyses, producing hard, fusiform, painless swellings at the wrist, knees, and costochondral junction
2. Proximal myopathy, especially of the hips and shoulder
3. Frontal bossing and flattening of the skull
4. Chest wall deformities: Harrison sulcus, rachitic rosary
5. Valgus or varus deformities of the knee
6. Anterior tibial bowing
7. Specific findings of systemic or metabolic diseases in which rickets occurs
8. Positive Chvostek and/or Trousseau sign
9. Tetany, laryngospasm, or cardiac dysrhythmia

HEPATIC DYSFUNCTION

The use of anticonvulsant medications, which increase the activity of hepatic P_{450} mixed-function oxidases with subsequent deficiency of 25(OH)D, may be associated with the development of rickets. It remains controversial whether medication use alone can produce clinical disease or whether some component of lack of sunlight exposure or intestinal disease must coexist for frank rachitic bone changes to be present. Nevertheless, up to a third of children taking anticonvulsant medication may have subnormal levels of 25(OH)D.

In those children receiving anticonvulsants who have a reduced serum level of 25(OH)D, therapy with the parent compound (2000 to 4000 IU daily) has proved successful in normalization of the reduced levels. In distinction to deprivational rickets, the period of time to normalization may be lengthier, ranging from 6 to 12 months.

Patients with a reduction in hepatic mass from any cause (e.g., cirrhosis, biliary atresia) may acquire vitamin D deficiency from an inability to produce adequate amounts of substrate, 25(OH)D from the parent vitamin D compound. Although substantially higher levels of the parent compound vitamin D (10,000 to 50,000 IU daily) may be employed, it is easier to simply bypass the defect in synthesis of 25(OH)D by provision of exogenous $25(OH)D_3$ at a dosage of 1 to 2 μg/kg daily. It is strongly recommended that frequent determinations of blood levels of calcium, phosphorus, intact PTH, and of both 25(OH)D and $1,25(OH)_2D$ be performed to guarantee safety of therapy no matter which vitamin D compound or metabolite is chosen.

KIDNEY DISORDERS

Congenital absence of the renal proximal tubule enzyme complex which produces the active metabolite $1,25(OH)_2D$ is termed *vitamin D–dependent rickets, type I,* and is inherited as an autosomal recessive trait. Severe hypocalcemia with rickets is commonly present in the first 6 to 9 months of life.

Therapy with the missing and active metabolite is recommended for safety and efficacy and may be accomplished with an initial dosage of 0.01 μg/kg daily in two divided doses. Subsequent monitoring of serum levels of minerals, intact PTH, and $1,25(OH)_2D$ will determine the expected dosage increases as the child grows.

Specific defects in the ability of the kidney to reclaim filtered phosphorus appropriately and to increase the synthesis of $1,25(OH)_2D$ adequately in response to the resulting hypophosphatemia is associated with rickets and is termed *vitamin D–resistant* or *X-linked hypophosphatemic* rickets (which describes its inheritance pattern). The biochemical profile is worth noting, since it is one of the few rachitic disorders associated with normocalcemia and lack of secondary hyperparathyroidism (see Table 3). It is associated with abnormalities of dental development that lead to caries formation and pulp abscesses.

Therapy of this disorder is complex and controversial but generally consists of the administration of substantial and frequent amounts of phosphate salts (Neutrophos, 50 to 100 mg/kg daily up to a maximum of 4 to 6 g) and exogenous $1,25(OH)_2D_3$ (25 to 100 ng/kg) twice daily. It remains unclear whether the dental problems remit with this pharmacologic therapy. Toxicity from the therapy includes the development of hypercalcemia, secondary hyperparathyroidism, and, perhaps, nephrocalcinosis and related renal glomerular or tubular dysfunction. It is strongly recommended that therapy be tailored to an individual patient, that frequent biochemical follow-up be performed, and that an expert in pediatric bone and mineral disorders be consulted in the long-term care of such patients.

TABLE 3. Biochemical Profile of Common Rachitic Disorders

Disorder	Ca^{2+}	PO_4^{3-}	PTH	25(OH)D	$1,25(OH)_2D$	Additional Comments
Deprivational rickets	↓/↓↓	↓	↑	↓ or Absent	↓ or Normal	↓ TRP
Malabsorption	↓ or Normal	↓ or Normal	↑	↓ or Absent	↓	
Anticonvulsants	↓ or Normal	↓	↑	↓	↓ or Normal	
Reduces hepatic mass	↓	↓	↑	↓ or Absent	↓	
Vitamin D–dependent rickets, type I	↓↓	↓	↑	Normal or ↑	0	Autosomal recessive
Fanconi syndrome	↓	↓↓	↑	Normal	↓	
Vitamin D–resistant (X-linked) rickets	Normal	↓↓	Normal	Normal	Normal or ↑	
Chronic renal insufficiency	Normal	↑	↑↑	Normal	↓	
Vitamin D–dependent rickets, type II	↓↓	↓↓	↑↑	Normal or ↓	↑↑	

Abbreviations: Ca^{2+}, blood ionized calcium; PO_4^{3-}, serum phosphorus; PTH, intact parathyroid hormone; TRP, tubular reabsorption of phosphorus.
Key: ↓, value decreased below normal; ↓↓, value markedly decreased below normal; ↑, value increased above normal; ↑↑, value markedly increased above normal.

Complex disturbances of renal proximal tubular dysfunction in which acidosis occurs and in which most filtered substances are reabsorbed in less than normal amounts is termed *Fanconi syndrome.* The disorder may be isolated or may be part of other systemic or metabolic defects. A complete evaluation of the patient should be undertaken to uncover these latter possibilities. Rickets is seen commonly in Fanconi syndrome irrespective of cause.

Therapy of the rachitic component of Fanconi syndrome includes provision of adequate phosphate, calcium, and exogenous $25(OH)D_3$(1 to 2 μg/kg daily) or $1,25(OH)_2D_3$ (0.025 to 0.05 μg/kg daily) in addition to correction of the acidosis with supplemental alkali therapy.

Chronic renal insufficiency with reduction in functioning nephron mass is associated with a bone disease termed *renal osteodystrophy,* and this includes rickets. The pathogenesis of the disturbance is complex, but there is an inability to synthesize adequate amounts of $1,25(OH)_2D$. This defect arises presumably through suppression of synthesis by phosphate desensitization to the stimulatory effects of PTH, suppression from chronic metabolic acidosis, or lack of sufficient mass of functional renal tissue. Other forms of bone disease occur and may coexist with the rickets.

Therapy is directed toward limitation of phosphate intake and suppression of secondary hyperparathyroidism (to high normal levels of intact PTH) with $1,25(OH)_2D_3$ (0.25 to 1.5 μg daily). Careful attention to follow-up determinations of serum calcium, phosphorus and intact PTH levels is mandatory. Occasionally, deprivational rickets coexists in children with chronic renal insufficiency and responds nicely to the therapy discussed above for that condition.

TABLE 4. Selected Vitamin D Pharmacopoeia

Compound	Preparation
Ergocalciferol (vitamin D_2)	8000 IU/ml
	25,000 IU/tab
	50,000 IU/tab
$25(OH)D_3$ (25-hydroxyvitamin D_3)	20 μg/tab
	50 μg/tab
$1,25(OH)_2D_3$ (1,25-dihydroxyvitamin D_3)	0.25 μg/tab
	0.50 μg/tab
	1.0 μg/ml
	2.0 μg/ml
Dihydrotachysterol	0.125 mg/tab
	0.2 mg/tab
	0.4 mg/tab
	0.2 mg/ml

One IU = 0.025 μg = 65 pmoles vitamin D.

VITAMIN D RECEPTOR DEFECTS

Florid rickets occurs in children with specific gene defects that result in a mutated vitamin D receptor protein, termed *vitamin D–dependent rickets, type II.* The disorder is quite uncommon, often familial, and may be associated with alopecia totalis. No specific recommendation can be made for treatment of such patients. However, varying suprapharmacologic dosages of $1,25(OH)_2D_3$ have been employed in the past; some children do not respond at all without the institution of another renally produced vitamin D metabolite, 24, 25-dihydroxyvitamin D_3.

RICKETS OF PREMATURITY

Calcium transfer and subsequent fetal bone mineralization occur mostly in the third trimester of pregnancy. Disruption of that process induced by a premature birth often results in lack of normal bone mass accretion in the premature neonate; this is termed *osteopenia.* Osteopenia of prematurity has been confused frequently with inadequate mineralization of newly formed osteoid, which is termed "rickets."

Therapy of osteopenia of prematurity is best made with provision of supplemental calcium and phosphorus intakes to approximate those of transplacental transfer rates. Under these circumstances, provision of adequate levels of vitamin D is essential. Generally, 400 to 1200 IU daily is given. Larger amounts of supplemental vitamin D or the use of the more potent metabolites—$25(OH)D_3$ or $1,25(OH)_2D_3$—are usually not advantageous and are often associated with serious toxicities. Premature neonates in whom frank rickets is manifested may have differing biochemical profiles, depending on the step in the normal pathway of vitamin D metabolism, that are affected by coexisting medical problems. Those problems include intestinal malabsorption, hepatic dysfunction, acidosis, and mineral deprivation. The therapy needed for the premature infant with rickets must be tailored to specific circumstances.

HYPERALIMENTATION

The usefulness of total parenteral alimentation cannot be denied as life-saving for children with the inability to ingest adequate caloric loads enterally. Unfortunately, metabolic bone disease has been a not infrequent occurrence in such children. The factors that underlie it are varied, but include chronic acidosis and perhaps the accumulation of aluminum at the mineralization surface of bone. Children are normocalcemic or mildly hypercalcemic and have low-normal or low concentrations of serum phosphorus; hypercalciuria is prominent. Circulating levels of 25(OH)D are normal, and levels of $1,25(OH)_2D$ are in the low-normal range.

Therapy with vitamin D or its metabolites has been largely unsuccessful in reversing the rachitic disease and is generally associated with serious toxicities.

REFERENCES

DeLuca HF: The vitamin D story: A collaborative effort of basic science and clinical medicine. FASEB J 2:224, 1988.

HYPOCALCEMIA AND TETANY

JOHN T. HERRIN, M.B.B.S.

Tetany is a condition of neuromuscular irritability resulting from hypocalcemia and/or hypomagnesemia. This hyperexcitable state of the peripheral and central nervous system is manifest as a sustained contracture or "paralytic" state in which the muscles of hands and feet assume a characteristic position of toes down and increased arch while the hand shows extension of the fingers with thumb tightly adducted into the palm (Trousseau sign). Hyperexcitability of facial muscles results in a positive Chvostek sign. Occasional patients will demonstrate "grand mal" seizures or focal seizure activity. These characteristic changes are common outside the neonatal period and, in fact, may be provoked by handling the infant or tapping the muscle, as in an attempt to elicit muscle reflexes.

Tetany-associated laryngospasm and even laryngeal closure with respiratory difficulty may be seen spontaneously in some patients, whereas tight adduction of the cords may be precipitated by attempts at endotracheal intubation.

Although rational or chronic treatment necessitates provision of calcium and/or magnesium and correction of an acid-base disturbance, empiric correction may be required in acute tetany. Hypocalcemia and hypomagnesemia are the result of a number of underlying disease processes. Knowledge of potential causes will thus allow rapid clinical evaluation of the tetanic state, and after empiric correction adjustments may be made on the basis of clinical response and chemical monitoring.

Tables 1 and 2 provide guidelines to further investigation after symptomatic relief has occurred. Stabilization and repletion are performed concurrently.

THERAPEUTIC SCHEME

Hypocalcemia—Emergency Therapy

Emergency therapy consists of returning the serum ionized calcium level to normal, if possible, by correction of pathophysiologic processes. For example, in hyperventilation tetany, control can be gained by repairing the acid-base deficit by rebreathing into a paper or plastic bag; this sufficiently elevates the partial pressure of carbon dioxide to allow pH adjustment to normal and correction of the tetany.

In a symptomatic patient with tetany and especially seizure activity, calcium is provided at 10 mg/kg (0.5 mEq/kg) as elemental calcium by a slow and steady intravenous infusion (10 to 20 minutes) under electrocardiographic (EKG) control to ensure that cardiotoxicity (manifested by bradycardia and QRS changes) does not occur. This initial dose is followed by a further infusion of 10 mg/kg of elemental calcium intravenously (IV) over a period of 4 to 6 hours with monitoring of plasma ionized calcium levels. The aim is to restore serum total calcium to 7 mg/dl in the premature neonate or 8 mg/dl in the full term neonate or infant. Values for ionized calcium below 3.5 mg/dl (0.88 mmol/L) represent hypocalcemia. Calcium is added to the supplemental intravenous infusion to provide 20 to 40 mg/kg/day or oral supplements at 60 to 100 mg/kg/day. If the calcium requirement remains elevated, vitamin D as 1,25-dihydroxycholecalciferol intravenously as Calcijex (0.01 μg/kg) or orally as Rocaltrol (0.125 to 0.25 μg) may be provided to assist the absorption of calcium from the gut. Depending on the underlying condition, longer-term calcium supplementation may be necessary (e.g., in the patient

TABLE 1. Etiology of Hypocalcemia

I. **Neonatal Period**
   A. Early
      1. Postnatal calcitonin surge (prematurity)
      2. Delayed PTH response (IDM)
      3. Perinatal anoxia and prematurity
      4. Infant of mother with hyperparathyroidism
   B. Late (5–10 Days of Age)
      1. Vitamin D deficiency
      2. Elevated serum phosphate-phosphate loading
      3. Hypomagnesemia
      4. Parathyroid agenesis

II. **Beyond Neonatal Period (Several Weeks to Months)**
   - Vitamin D deficiency
   - Hypophosphatemia
   - Premature infants
   - Parathyroid hypoplasia (DiGeorge syndrome)
   - Transient hypoparathyroidism
   - Acquired idiopathic hypoparathyroidism
   - Polyglandular autoimmune disease
   - Surgical
     - Thyroidectomy
     - Parathyroidectomy
   - Radioiodine administration
   - Renal tubular disease
     - Galactosemia
     - Wilson's disease
     - Cystinosis
     - Liver disease
   - Pseudohypoparathyroidism
     - Type I
     - Type II
   - Transient hypocalcemia secondary to increased complexing
     - Transfusion with citrated blood products
     - Albumin infusion in nephrotic syndrome
     - Phosphate loading—oral or intravenous
   - Acute pancreatitis
   - Hyperventiliation syndrome with tetany
   - Renal failure

Abbreviations: PTH, parathyroid hormone; IDM, infant of diabetic mother.

TABLE 2. Etiology of Hypomagnesemia

- Neonatal
  - Often associated with hypocalcemia
  - Small for gestational age
- Chronic bowel disease, or short-gut syndrome
- Primary hypoparathyroidism
- Maternal hyperparathyroidism
- Primary hyperaldosteronism
- Hypomagnesemia associated with hypokalemia
  - Aminoglycoside
  - Cisplatin
  - Cyclosporine
- Renal wasting and tubular magnesium-losing states
  - Fanconi syndrome
  - Chronic interstitial nephritis
  - Renal tubular acidosis
- Diuretic therapy
- Bartter syndrome

TABLE 3. Calcium and Magnesium Supplementation in Hypocalcemia and Tetany

Supplement	Dosage
Calcium carbonate (40% elemental calcium)	500 mg tab = 200 mg calcium
Calcium chloride 10%	IV 100 mg/kg per dose, 200–500 mg/kg/day IV
	p.o. Infant: 400–800 mg/kg/day q 6 hr
	Child: 200–500 mg/kg/day q 6 hr
	1.36 mEq elemental Ca/ml
	IV 20 mg/kg per dose
Calcium gluconate 10%	0.45 mEq elemental calcium/ml
Dihydrotachysterol	0.025–0.05 mg/kg/day
25-Hydroxyvitamin D_3	0.7–2.8 mg/kg/day
1,25-Dihydroxyvitamin D_3	20–50 mg/kg/day
Calcium-enriched milk	Add 400–800 mg elemental calcium to 1 L breast milk or Similac PM 60/40
Magnesium sulfate 10%	100 mg/ml = 0.8 mEq/ml
Magnesium sulfate 50%	500 mg/ml = 4.0 mEq/ml
Magnesium gluconate tablets	500 mg = 4 mEq
Magnesium gluconate syrup	54 mg/5 ml

with chronic renal failure or endocrine abnormalities such as pseudohypoparathyroidism).

Hypomagnesemia

If serum magnesium levels are low and stores are markedly depleted with ongoing (magnesium) losses, it will be difficult to correct the calcium levels without concurrent correction of the magnesium deficit. Although magnesium can be given intravenously in an emergency, slow adjustment of intracellular stores is necessary. Rapid change in extracellular magnesium, as in attempted rapid replacement, may produce toxicity with somnolence, hypotension, and marked sedation with respiratory compromise. Monitoring of both plasma magnesium levels and clinical status, including neurologic activity, is necessary to ensure that such toxicity (hypermagnesemia) does not occur. If hypomagnesemic seizures are present, 0.4 to 0.8 mEq/kg (50 to 100 mg/kg) of elemental magnesium per dose IV or (IM) as 50 per cent magnesium sulfate (4 mEq/ml) should be administered.

Hypomagnesemia may be seen clinically in the small-for-gestational-age neonate or in association with prolonged gastrointestinal losses (diarrhea), diuretic therapy, or renal tubular magnesium losses associated with aminoglycoside therapy, cyclosporine administration, or anticancer therapy, particularly cisplatin. If magnesium depletion is marked, parenteral replacement will be necessary. Magnesium sulfate, 25 to 50 mg/kg (0.2 to 0.4 mEq/kg/day) may be added to the IV fluids, or the dose may be administered intramuscularly each 12 hours for three to four doses and then every other day until adequate oral supplementation can be attained. In the patient with thrombocytopenia, such intramuscular injection for supplementation is contraindicated and magnesium should be added to the IV fluid (25 to 50 mg/kg/day) or oral supplements used (100 to 200 mg/kg every 6 to 8 hours in three or four divided doses). Oral magnesium supplements are given in small and multiple doses throughout the day to avoid the cathartic and laxative properties of magnesium salts. Such diarrheal losses both decrease absorption and may further increase body losses. Magnesium gluconate appears to be well tolerated. Practical doses as elemental magnesium are 10 mg three times a day in infants, 25 mg three times a day in children 6 to 12 years of age, and 500 mg tablets two to three times per day for adolescents.

Magnesium oxide may also be used three or four times daily to provide 20 to 40 mg/kg/day as alternative oral supplementation. In long-term cancer therapy or aminoglycoside therapy, magnesium supplementation to intravenous fluids may be necessary in addition to the oral supplement to sustain adequate serum levels while total body stores are being repleted. Table 3 shows available calcium and magnesium supplements with appropriate dosage.

Calcium and magnesium ions are important in regulation of vascular tone and maintenance of membrane potentials. Changes in their homeostasis in disease states and acid-base disorders can produce painful and uncontrolled muscular contraction, cardiac arrhythmia, or respiratory or locomotor difficulties. Acute empiric management should provide sufficient control to allow investigation and institution of rational long-term therapy.

IDIOPATHIC HYPERCALCEMIA

BARBARA POBER, M.D.

Idiopathic hypercalcemia is defined as an elevation in total serum calcium above 11.0 mg/dl, diagnosed after the exclusion of other known causes of hypercalcemia. Hypercalcemia may be mild (11.0 to 13.0 mg/dl) with little symptomatology or more severe (>13.0 mg/dl), generally accompanied by failure to thrive, abdominal pain, vomiting, constipation, muscle weakness, polydipsia, and polyuria. A complication of longstanding hypercalcemia can be nephrocalcinosis.

One of the most common causes of hypercalcemia in childhood is *Williams syndrome.* This syndrome is a rare (1 in 20,000) congenital condition that can include transient hypercalcemia and/or hypercalciuria, cardiovascular abnormalities (most commonly supravalvar aortic stenosis), extreme irritability during infancy, slow physical growth, characteristic facial appearance, learning difficulties, and/or mental retardation.

The cause, true frequency, and natural history of idiopathic hypercalcemia, especially in Williams syndrome, remains unknown. The hypercalcemia may be secondary to excess absorption from the gastrointestinal tract. There have been no consistent abnormalities detected in levels of parathyroid hormone, calcitonin, and vitamin D.

THERAPY

Treatment of persistent mild hypercalcemia consists of dietary restriction of calcium (to < 400 mg/day which is less than half the Recommended Daily Allowance [RDA]), elimination of vitamin D supplementation, and avoidance of excess sunlight. Corticosteroids (prednisone, 1 to 2 mg/kg/day) will also gradually reverse hypercalcemia as a result of increased intestinal absorption of calcium, but long-term steroid treatment is not indicated because of possible adverse effects. Given the fact that hypercalcemia is typically transient, long-term therapy of any modality is generally not indicated and attempts to discontinue therapy should be made on a regular basis. Individuals with Williams syndrome, even those who are normocalcemic, should avoid markedly excess dietary calcium, as hypercalcemia has recurred under such circumstances.

Extremely severe hypercalcemia (>15.0 mg/dl) should be treated with intravenous fluids and furosemide (1 mg/kg every 6 hours), as needed. Hypercalcemia secondary to excess bone resorption can be treated with calcitonin (salmon calcitonin, 4 IU/kg every 12 hours IM or SC).

Familial hypocalciuric hypercalcemia occurs secondary to decreased calcium clearance in the kidneys. This is a benign autosomal dominant disorder, and no treatment is required.

WILSON'S DISEASE*

JANNA C. COLLINS, M.D.
and I. HERBERT SCHEINBERG, M.D.

GENETICS AND PATHOGENESIS

Wilson's disease (WD) occurs only in individuals with a pair of abnormal genes that have been localized to chromosome 13q14-q21. The worldwide prevalence of such individuals (abnormal homozygotes) is about 1 in 30,000; prevalence of the heterozygous carrier, in whom the disease never develops, is 1 in 90.

The genetic defect, located in the liver, impairs the normal hepatic excretion of dietary copper. Soon after birth, the resultant accumulations of the metal sequentially induce fatty changes, inflammation, necrosis, and fibrosis—all culminating in cirrhosis generally by the onset of adolescence. The evolving or end stages of this pathologic progress may be clinically manifested as self-limited or fulminant hepatitis or as portal hypertension and hepatic insufficiency. Suddenly (causing hemolysis) or gradually, copper diffuses from copper-saturated hepatocytes into the blood stream and then into the brain with disastrous toxic effects.

Although neither hepatic nor cerebral symptomatology has ever been reported in children under the age of 5 years, about 80 per cent of patients with WD have become ill or died of the disorder by the age of 21.

Because the outcome of untreated WD is serious illness and early death and since timely appropriate treatment can prevent both, a pediatrician should suspect, and unequivocally confirm or rule out, the diagnosis in any child with a family history of the disease; unexplained hepatic, neurologic, or psychiatric disease; corneal copper deposits (Kayser-Fleischer rings); or unexplained deficiency of ceruloplasmin. To avoid an untreated fatal outcome, specific treatment must be instituted immediately following the establishment of a firm diagnosis in any symptomatic or asymptomatic individual over the age of 1 year. Because therapy of WD is not without risk, neither heterozygous carriers of one WD gene nor individuals with an unconfirmed diagnosis of WD should be treated.

The criteria that are necessary to confirm the diagnosis of WD vary with the mode of presentation to the physician and are given in Table 1. Procurement and preparation of serum and tissue and the quantitative determinations of serum ceruloplasmin and hepatic copper should be performed by appropriately trained personnel in facilities where they are routinely and reliably done. The presence or absence of Kayser-Fleischer rings should be certified by slit-lamp ophthalmologic examination. Rarely, when the diagnosis of WD is suspected despite a normal ceruloplasmin level, determination of 24-hour urinary copper excretion or of the rate of incorporation of radio-copper into ceruloplasmin may be necessary to establish or exclude the diagnosis of WD.

TABLE 1. Sufficient Criteria for a Confirmed Diagnosis of Wilson's Disease (WD) in the Various Modes of Clinical Presentation

	C	KF	H or KF
1. Asymptomatic (~10% of Patients)			
a. Siblings, children, or first cousins of a WD patient	+		+
b. Deficiency of serum ceruloplasmin			+
c. Kayser-Fleischer rings detected on ophthalmologic examination	+		
2. Hepatic (~45% of Patients)			
a. Acute or chronic active hepatitis	+		+
b. Fulminant hepatitis, with Coombs'-negative hemolysis	+	+	
c. Cirrhosis, with or without chronic active hepatitis	+		+
d. Amenorrhea; irregular menses	+		+
3. Cerebral (~45% of Patients)			
a. *Neurologic* (movement disorder complex of dystonia, dysarthria, drooling or tremors, incoordination, athetosis and scanned speech; or any combination)	+		
b. *Psychiatric* (sudden onset of socially inappropriate behavior; depression; deterioration of performance in school; obsessive, manic-depressive, or schizophrenic symptomatology)	+		

Abbreviations: C, serum ceruloplasmin < 20 mg/dl; KF, presence of Kayser-Fleischer corneal rings; H, hepatic copper concentration > 250 μg/g dry liver.

TREATMENT

The principal specific medications used are penicillamine (β, β-dimethyl cysteine); trientine (triethylene tetramine dihydrochloride); BAL (British anti-lewisite; 2,3-dimercaprol); and zinc salts (Table 2). With drug treatment, foods rich in copper (e.g., liver, chocolate, nuts, mushrooms, shellfish) should be eaten only in moderation. Medical treatment must be lifelong.

Orthotopic liver transplantation is the only generally accepted therapy for fulminant hepatitis due to Wilson's disease, in which medical treatment is almost always ineffective.

Penicillamine

Penicillamine (Cuprimine, Merck, Sharp and Dohme; Depen, Carter-Wallace), approved by the Food and Drug Ad-

TABLE 2. Medications Used in Treatment of Wilson's Disease

Drug	Form	Dosage
Penicillamine	250 mg tablets	0.25 g/kg/day p.o. b.i.d.—q.i.d. 30 minutes a.c. or 2 hours p.c.
Trientine	250 mg tablets	Alternative drug, same dosage schedule
Pyridoxine	10–25 mg/day p.o.	Supplement during penicillamine
BAL	3 ml IM	Additional drug for refractory neurologic symptoms
Zinc gluconate	Tablets	2 mg/kg/day p.o. b.i.d.–t.i.d.

Abbreviations: BAL, British anti-lewisite (dimercaprol); p.o., orally; b.i.d., twice a day; t.i.d., three times a day; q.i.d., four times a day; a.c., before meals; p.c., after meals; IM, intramuscularly.

*From the National Center for the Study of Wilson's Disease, Inc.

ministration (FDA) for the treatment of WD in 1963, is the drug of choice. Penicillamine promotes urinary excretion of copper and detoxifies excess copper remaining in the liver. It is given orally at an initial total daily dose of 0.02 g/kg to a maximum of 1 g. The total dose should be rounded to a multiple of 250 mg, the size of the capsules or tablets available. Two to four divided doses are administered on an empty stomach 30 minutes before—or 2 hours after—eating. Because of penicillamine's antipyridoxine activity, about 10 to 25 mg of pyridoxine daily should be added to the diet.

Complete blood counts, a liver chemistry profile, and routine urinalysis should precede institution of penicillamine treatment. During the first month of treatment, parents and child should be alert for the development of fever and rash, sometimes accompanied by lymphadenopathy. Blood counts are required twice weekly to detect leukopenia or thrombocytopenia. With any of these reactions, penicillamine should be discontinued. After subsidence of fever or rash, penicillamine can usually be successfully reinstituted by gradually increasing to a full dose over a 2- to 3-week period, with concomitant low-dose prednisone. The latter can be gradually tapered soon after the full dose of penicillamine has been uneventfully reached.

If leukopenia or thrombocytopenia that is significantly below the baseline value develops, generally trientine must be substituted for penicillamine.

Late adverse reactions to penicillamine are described in the package circular. The most common serious one that requires substituting trientine for penicillamine is the development of proteinuria of greater than 1 g in 24 hours. A casual urine specimen should be qualitatively tested, by dipstick, at monthly intervals, during the first year, and every 3 months thereafter.

The patient's progress should be evaluated at 1- to 2-month intervals for the first year of therapy. Improvement in cerebral symptoms and signs and in hepatic symptoms and chemistries and the fading of Kayser-Fleischer rings are, of course, the best indicators of success.

Reduction in the level of free, toxic copper in serum (which equals total serum copper − ceruloplasmin copper) to less than 10 μg/dl indicates that dosage of penicillamine and compliance of the patient are ideal. In contrast, a free serum copper greater than 20 μg/dl strongly suggests inadequate dosage or noncompliance, particularly if clinical response is poor and Kayser-Fleischer rings persist. Measurement of urinary copper excretion, though occasionally of diagnostic value, is of little help in evaluating therapeutic progress.

The tremors or dystonia in about 10 per cent of patients with neurologically manifest WD will worsen—usually transiently—during the first weeks of penicillamine therapy. If worsening persists or if improvement in neurologic symptomatology has not occurred after 6 months of penicillamine therapy, the addition of BAL to the regimen should be considered.

Trientine

Trientine (Syprine, Merck Sharp and Dohme), the only other drug approved (in 1985) by the FDA for WD, is used primarily for patients with a life-threatening reaction to penicillamine. It is administered in two to four divided doses, also at 0.02 g/kg/day to a maximum of 1 g/day. In the 20 years since its introduction by Walshe, it has apparently proved to be equally effective therapeutically to penicillamine, although it has been used in far fewer patients than has the latter.

The only adverse reaction to trientine has been a sideroblastic anemia, similar to the anemia of copper deficiency, in two patients who received 2 g or more of trientine daily. About half of patients receiving 1 g daily exhibit a moderate number of circulating siderocytes and an increase in the red blood cell distribution width (RDW), without anemia.

BAL

BAL (Dimercaprol Injection, USP, BAL in oil, Hynson, Westcott & Dunning) has proved of value in patients with severe tremors or with athetotic movements that have not responded optimally to penicillamine or trientine. BAL, the first specific drug for WD, introduced in 1948 by Cumings, is an uncharged molecule that may, therefore, be capable of diffusing across the blood-brain barrier more readily than the ionic penicillamine or trientine molecules.

A minimum of 20 deep intramuscular injections, each of an ampule containing 300 mg dimercaprol in 3 ml of peanut oil, should be given, following an initial injection of 0.3 ml to detect sensitivity. Five injections a week is an optimal frequency, with sites of successive injections as follows: beginning at the upper outer quadrant of the right buttock, alternate to left and right with the third injection about an inch below the first; the fourth, an inch below the second and so on. Before injecting close to the sciatic nerve, the pediatrician begins the second series of injections an inch lateral to the first injection, and so on. A rise in blood pressure, accompanied by tachycardia, is the most common adverse reaction.

Zinc

Zinc gluconate and other zinc salts in a dosage providing 2 mg/kg elemental zinc daily, have proved effective in ameliorating—and preventing the progression of—hepatic dysfunction in patients who have previously undergone decoppering therapy by penicillamine or trientine.

Dietary supplements of zinc can cause the sideroblastic anemia of copper deficiency in normal individuals and has apparently done so in at least one patient with WD.

Orthotopic hepatic transplantation is indicated for wilsonian acute fulminant hepatic failure and for some patients with decompensated and progressive cirrhosis that has not responded to pharmacologic agents. Transplantation cures the genetic defect causative of hepatic copper toxicosis and leads to normal balance of dietary copper. But clear evidence of reversal of cerebral symptomatology is lacking.

REFERENCES

Scheinberg IH, Sternlieb I. Wilson's Disease. Vol 23. Major Problems in Internal Medicine. Philadelphia, WB Saunders Co, 1984.

THE HYPERPHENYLALANINEMIAS

MARK S. KORSON, M.D.
FRANCES J. ROHR, M.S., R.D.
and SHARON GRAY, M.P.H., R.D.

PHENYLKETONURIA

The hyperphenylalaninemias are a heterogeneous group of metabolic disorders, resulting from a defect in the hydroxylation of phenylalanine to tyrosine. In most cases, this defect occurs because of a mutation or deletion in the phenylalanine hydroxylase (PAH) gene itself and is known as phenylketonuria (PKU) in its more severe phenotype. The wide range of abnormal phenylalanine levels in untreated PKU probably results from compound heterozygosity of multiple allelic mutations. A classification of persistent hyperphenylalaninemia is found in Table 1.

TABLE 1. Classification of Persistent Hyperphenylalaninemia

Disorder	Blood Phenylalanine (mg/dl) (μmol/L)	Therapy
Classic phenylketonuria	>20 (>1200)	Dietary
Atypical phenylketonuria	12–20 (720–1200)	Dietary
Mild hyperphenylalaninemia	2–12 (120–720)	None
Pterin defects	6–30 (360–1800)	Combination of neurotransmitter, tetrahydrobiopterin, and folinic acid supplementation, with phenylalanine restriction in some cases

The incidence of PKU (i.e., PAH deficiency requiring dietary therapy) varies widely with ethnic background, but approximates 1 in 10,000 to 15,000 newborn infants in the United States. The incidence of mild hyperphenylalaninemia, or PAH deficiency not requiring treatment, is estimated at about half this number. PAH deficiency is most common in the populations of northern Europe (particularly Ireland, Scotland, Belgium, and West Germany) and among Jews of Yemenite origin.

In nearly all cases, the diagnosis of hyperphenylalaninemia is made through newborn screening using the semiquantitative Guthrie bacterial inhibition assay. Subsequent confirmation is then advised by more precise fluorometric or high-performance liquid chromatography (HPLC) blood amino acid analysis. The persistent elevation in phenylalanine is not associated with other amino acid abnormalities, except occasionally for a diminished level of tyrosine. Urine amino acid analysis is unreliable for neonatal PKU screening. Similarly, although ferric chloride testing typically demonstrates the presence of urinary phenylketones, this method is associated with many false-negative results in the newborn period and is therefore not suitable for routine PKU screening. Transient phenylalanine elevations may be seen in prematurity, in liver disease from metabolic and other causes, and in situations in which maternal phenylalanine levels are high. In still other cases, initial elevations may spontaneously drop to normal during the newborn period.

When successful implementation of newborn screening for phenylketonuria (PKU) occurs within a health care system that adequately supports patients on dietary therapy, the clinical symptoms of the untreated state, namely psychomotor retardation, seizures, and eczema in a fair-complexioned individual, are rarely seen. A new set of concerns has arisen, however, regarding those individuals in whom dietary therapy ended during childhood, following what used to be accepted protocol in several metabolic clinics at one time. Many of these patients, now adults, are showing evidence of cognitive deterioration as well as emotional difficulties such as depression, anxiety, thought disorder, and agoraphobia. Reinstitution of therapy in those individuals, as well as in never-treated individuals, may be helpful in clearing or alleviating the severity of some of these symptoms.

PAH deficiency is inherited in an autosomal recessive fashion. Carrier testing exists for PAH deficiency, either by quantitative measurement and calculation of the fasting phenylalanine-tyrosine ratio or, more accurately, with restriction fragment length polymorphism analysis and, increasingly, with PAH mutation-specific oligonucleotide probes. In a majority of families, prenatal DNA diagnosis is also possible using these latter techniques.

Principles of Nutritional Management

Since excessive phenylalanine intake might compromise long-term development, the primary goal of treatment for PKU is the safe restriction of dietary phenylalanine to the minimum required for normal growth. Phenylalanine is an essential amino acid and occurs naturally in all protein food sources. Therefore, dietary restriction requires that such foods as milk, cheese, fish, meat, poultry, eggs, legumes, and nuts be eliminated from the diet. Because the degree of natural protein restriction needed to maintain phenylalanine levels within a therapeutic range would result in negative nitrogen balance and therefore be inadequate to support normal growth, medical foods are an integral part of the PKU diet. These are specialized, highly nutritious formula preparations that help to ensure complete and balanced nutrition in the PKU diet.

Given the variability of biochemical expression of the hyperphenylalaninemias, dietary treatment is tailored to individual need. Growth rate, age, and the degree of residual PAH activity are all factors that determine an individual's tolerance for phenylalanine (i.e., the amount of phenylalanine that can be ingested in order to maintain a blood level of phenylalanine within the therapeutic range). Although individuals with PKU may show a wide range of tolerance to phenylalanine, a typical PKU diet usually contains less than one-tenth the amount of phenylalanine found in an unrestricted diet. Changing rates of growth may lead to fluctuations in blood phenylalanine levels, and frequent dietary adjustments may be required, particularly during infancy.

The therapeutic range for blood phenylalanine is generally considered to be 2 to 8 mg/dl (120 to 480 μmol/L). Blood tyrosine levels should be maintained between 0.6 and 1.8 mg/dl (35 to 100 μmol/L) to avoid a tyrosine deficiency state. Excessive restriction of dietary phenylalanine with prolonged blood levels under 2 mg/dl (120 μmol/L) can lead to dermatitis, poor growth, brain damage, and even death. Prolonged blood level elevations (i.e., greater than 10 mg/dl or 600 μmol/L) due to excessive dietary phenylalanine intake and/or chronic medical food refusal may result in neurodevelopmental complications and require appropriate dietary counseling and intervention. Transient blood phenylalanine elevations, however, secondary to protein catabolic states during brief illnesses or to a short period of refusal of medical food are thought not to be clinically significant, and no dietary changes are required.

Other nutrient needs for individuals with PKU, including energy and protein, are thought to be similar to those of normal infants and children. Despite significant dietary restrictions, infants and children with treated PKU show normal growth patterns.

Components of the PKU Diet

Medical Foods

A medical food is a protein source that is formulated to be low in or devoid of a particular amino acid, in this case phenylalanine; it contains vitamins, minerals, and, in some cases, carbohydrates and fat. The medical food is the primary source of nutrition for infants and children with PKU, providing approximately 80 per cent of protein, vitamin, and mineral requirements. Sold in powder form, it is usually prepared as a liquid and consumed as a formula in infancy and as a milk substitute thereafter. The various medical foods available for different age groups are presented in Table 2; they are similar in that all are used as a protein substitute. Only Lofenalac contains a small but significant amount of phenylalanine that must be considered when calculating the total daily phenylalanine intake.

TABLE 2. Medical Foods Used in the Treatment of Phenylketonuria in the United States

Medical Food	Intended Age for Use	Energy-Yielding Nutrients (% of Total Calories)
Analog XP*	Infancy	L-amino acids (11%), fat (39%), carbohydrate (50%)
Lofenalac†	Infancy, childhood	Casein hydrolysate (13%), fat (35%), carbohydrate (52%)
PKU-1†	Infancy	L-amino acids (28%), carbohydrate (72%)
Maxamaid XP*	1–8 years	L-amino acids (71%), carbohydrate (29%)
Maxamum XP*	8+ years, pregnancy	L-amino acids (46%), carbohydrate (54%)
Phenyl Free†	2+ years, pregnancy	L-amino acids (20%), fat (15%), carbohydrate (65%)
PKU-2†	Childhood	L-amino acids (90%), carbohydrate (10%)
PKU-3†	Adolescence, pregnancy	L-amino acids (95%), carbohydrate (5%)

*Ross Laboratories, Columbus, Ohio.
†Mead-Johnson, Evansville, Indiana.

The various medical foods differ with respect to the amount of carbohydrate and fat they contain, so that energy content varies with the preparation used. Those medical foods with low or no carbohydrate and no fat are relatively low in energy, allowing greater flexibility in dietary planning for older children. Infants or toddlers with normally higher energy requirements may require supplementation of fat and carbohydrate. The vitamin and mineral composition of the medical foods vary as well, making some more appropriate for infancy, others for childhood, and still others for pregnancy and adulthood.

Protein in the form of L-amino acids or casein hydrolysate renders a characteristic flavor to the medical foods that is different from regular infant formula. When this is introduced within the first few months of life, the infant grows accustomed to the flavor and accepts it readily. If introduced later (e.g., in late-diagnosed PKU or for diet reinitiation in adults with PKU), the taste is not as easily accepted. Some of the medical foods can be purchased already flavored for better acceptance.

The particular type of medical food used, then, depends on the age of the individual with PKU, dietary likes and dislikes, and the cost and availability of the medical foods. The cost of medical foods for a young child approximates $3000 to $4000 yearly and may be covered by insurance or public health programs. In some states, public health departments provide the medical food but also determine which brand is used.

Natural Protein

Since phenylalanine is an essential amino acid, a small amount is needed in the diet to meet growth requirements. In infancy, phenylalanine is provided as part of the medical food, from standard infant formula or from breast milk. When the child is about 4 to 6 months of age, solid foods are introduced but are limited to measured amounts of cereals, fruits, and vegetables. Phenylalanine is measured in milligram amounts or by an equivalent (or exchange) system; comprehensive lists are available that show the phenylalanine content of most foods. As the child's appetite grows and interest in solid foods develops, increasing amounts of solid food are incorporated into the diet and the percentage of dietary phenylalanine from formula or breast milk diminishes. Eventually, all phenylalanine intake comes from solid food. High-protein foods remain forbidden at any age.

Specialty Low-Protein Products

Special manufactured products, such as breads, pastas, cookies, and low-protein flour for baking, can be ordered from a few commercial distributors. These products contain flours that are modified to lower their protein content compared with regular wheat or rice flours. This modification also changes the structure of the protein, however, and the specialty products have a texture different from that of their natural counterparts. Recipes using the low-protein flours are available. Low-protein products are useful in providing variety and energy to the diet. The earlier these foods are introduced, the greater the likelihood of acceptance and long-term compliance.

Free Foods

"Free foods" contain little or no phenylalanine and are therefore either pure carbohydrate or fat. Examples include fruits and fruit juice, sugar candies, and non-diet soft drinks. They are used primarily to provide extra calories to the diet and are often necessary to prevent hunger and promote normal growth.

Issues in Diet Management

Neonatal Management and Breast-Feeding

Once the diagnosis of PKU has been made, the blood phenylalanine level should be brought down to within the therapeutic range as quickly as possible. This requires the use of a PKU medical food product. However, a small amount of natural protein is necessary and is provided as part of the medical food or as standard infant formula or breast milk. If formula or breast milk is used, a phenylalanine-free medical food (such as Analog XP or PKU-1) is prescribed. It is important to consider that the phenylalanine content of breast milk varies from mother to mother and that breast milk generally contains less phenylalanine than standard infant formula or cow's milk, with concentrations highest in colostrum, declining with the duration of lactation.

Irrespective of the dietary approach, stabilization of the phenylalanine level may take several weeks and frequent monitoring is essential in order to ensure a safe drop in the level as well as determine the child's phenylalanine tolerance. If breast-feeding is allowed, tolerance can be calculated by analyzing the phenylalanine content of breast milk and determining an infant's average weight gain during feedings. This approach, however, requires a very motivated mother. A simpler alternative involves specifying the number of breast-feedings to be allowed within a 24-hour period (generally two to four feedings), with phenylalanine-free formula given at all other feedings.

The phenylalanine levels of breast-fed infants can be as easily controlled as those of bottle-fed ones. The importance of regular blood level monitoring, with dietary adjustments as needed, cannot be overstated. A guide is currently available for mothers wishing to breast-feed.

Medical Food Refusal

The large majority of children with PKU who are on a special diet take their medical food willingly. Chronic refusal, however, can lead to weight loss, lethargy, and other serious nutritional, medical, and neurodevelopmental sequelae. Elevated blood phenylalanine levels may occur because of protein catabolism. The reasons vary for medical food refusal and depend on age. In toddlers, it is often due to assertion of autonomy. School-aged children may refuse when they begin to eat lunch at school for the first time. Rejection of authority or of matters important to close authority figures may be fundamental in adolescent compliance problems. In most cases, allowing the child to make choices, such as which brand of formula is bought, how it is flavored, and at what times it is taken, helps to alleviate these problems. In some cases, however, behavioral or psychologic intervention is indicated.

Aspartame

Aspartame, marketed as NutraSweet, is an artificial sweetener composed of phenylalanine and aspartic acid and is found in many foods and drugs. Aspartame should be avoided by individuals with PKU who are maintaining a phenylalanine-restricted diet. However, for those who are no longer adhering to the diet and for carriers of PKU, the amount of phenylalanine from aspartame ingestion is small relative to high-protein foods and moderate use will not alter blood phenylalanine levels.

Monitoring the Diet

Blood Phenylalanine

Blood phenylalanine levels should be monitored regularly, at least once a week in infancy until levels fall to within the therapeutic range. The frequency and method of blood monitoring vary from clinic to clinic. Amino acid HPLC and fluorometric analyzers provide quantitative phenylalanine levels; such precision is necessary for optimal monitoring in a PKU treatment center. Supplemental home monitoring requires the parents to obtain either a blood filter paper specimen for Guthrie testing (the PKU newborn screening method) or a capillary tube specimen used for fluorometric quantitation.

Growth

Length and weight are followed regularly in all children on a medical diet; in infants and young children, head circumference is monitored as well.

Nutrient Intake at Home

It is recommended that intermittent 3-day food records of a child's total diet be completed by parents and submitted to the clinic nutritionist for analysis. With adequate consumption of medical food and careful diet planning, intakes of energy, protein, vitamins, and minerals should meet or exceed requirements for growth. As a rule, supplemental vitamins and minerals are not necessary as long as the medical food is consumed in recommended quantities.

Nutritional Status

Amino acid profiles, iron indices, albumin, and trace metals (when possible) are good indicators of nutritional status on a phenylalanine-restricted diet. Subclinical deficiencies of trace metals have been reported in some studies of children with PKU and have resulted in newer formulations for medical foods. Iron is potentially a problem in adolescence, but this depends on the type and quantity of medical food consumed.

Maternal PKU

Infants born to mothers with PKU who do not adhere to a low-phenylalanine diet during pregnancy are at risk for microcephaly, low birth weight, and congenital heart disease. These children are also at very high risk for mental retardation; for women with classic PKU, this risk exceeds 90 per cent. The maternal PKU syndrome presumably results from a teratogenic effect of high maternal blood phenylalanine on the developing fetus and is unrelated to whether or not the infant is born with PKU.

Because the phenylalanine-restricted diet has been helpful in preventing mental retardation in children with PKU, it is hypothesized that maintaining the maternal phenylalanine level within the therapeutic range before conception and throughout pregnancy may prevent the adverse effects of maternal PKU. The National Maternal PKU Collaborative Study is evaluating this premise. To date, only 15 per cent of the study population began the PKU diet prior to conceiving, and many came to attention during the first 4 weeks of gestation. Preliminary results indicate that women whose blood phenylalanine levels have been tightly controlled (i.e., 2 to 6 mg/dl, 120 to 360 μmol/L) prior to conception and during pregnancy have had infants born with normal weight, length, and head circumference measurements when compared with controls and established norms. These data reinforce the need for both education about the risks of maternal PKU and the importance for adults (especially women) to maintain a well-controlled diet throughout life.

THE PTERIN DEFECTS

Rarely, hyperphenylalaninemia is caused by a defect in the metabolism of tetrahydrobiopterin, the cofactor for PAH, resulting from an inborn error of biopterin synthesis or a deficiency of the tetrahydrobiopterin recycling enzyme, dihydropteridine reductase (DHPR). The biopterin synthesis disorders include guanosine triphosphate cyclohydrolase (GTC) deficiency and 6-pyruvoyltetrahydrobiopterin synthase (PTS) deficiency. These metabolic errors interfere with the normal hydroxylation of phenylalanine, tyrosine, and tryptophan and lead to the deficient synthesis of the monoamine neurotransmitters dopamine, norepinephrine, and serotonin. Such an abnormal metabolic state is believed to be deleterious for the developing brain.

Compared with PKU, the pterin disorders are usually associated with much milder neonatal elevations of phenylalanine. However, they result in more severe and often earlier symptoms in the untreated state. Affected infants usually show a progressive neurodegenerative course that may include altered muscle tone and hyperreflexia, movement disorder, sleep disturbance, seizures, mental retardation, and hyperthermia. These occur despite adequate dietary control of the hyperphenylalaninemia. PTS deficiency is more heterogeneous in its phenotype, with central, peripheral, and transient forms being described.

Evaluation

It is recommended that all hyperphenylalaninemic newborns be screened during their initial metabolic evaluations with a blood filter paper for DHPR deficiency and a urine filter paper to measure the relative concentrations of neopterin and biopterin, the principal pterin metabolites. In normal infants and in infants with PKU, the concentrations of neopterin and biopterin are roughly equal. The concentrations of both metabolites are extremely low in GTC deficiency. In patients with PTS deficiency, neopterin is present in excessive amounts and biopterin concentrations are very low; in DHPR deficiency, it is biopterin that is present in greater concentrations relative to neopterin. An assay of enzyme activity in a blood filter paper specimen provides the most reliable method for ruling out DHPR deficiency.

Abnormal pterin results demand subsequent analysis of monoamine neurotransmitter metabolites in the cerebrospinal fluid (CSF) to determine whether and how significantly they are reduced. In PTS deficiency, low metabolite concentrations confirm the presence of a central defect whereas normal or elevated concentrations suggest that the defect may be only peripheral in nature; in these cases, neurotransmitter therapy may not be indicated. In some cases, clarification of the type of PTS deficiency necessitates tetrahydrobiopterin loading and a formal assessment of phenylalanine tolerance.

Therapy

The treatment of generalized pterin defects combines dietary phenylalanine restriction (when phenylalanine levels exceed 10 to 12 mg/dl or 600 to 720 μmol/L) with neurotransmitter replacement therapy. The latter involves combination L-dopa (1 to 16 mg/kg/day), 5-hydroxytryptophan (1 to 20 mg/kg/day), and carbidopa (0.2 to 2 mg/kg/day). Tetrahydrobiopterin supplementation (1 to 20 mg/kg/day) is prescribed in cases of infants with biopterin synthetic defects. In DHPR deficiency, in which folate deficiency may occur, folinic acid (12.5 to 37.5 mg/day) is the preferred form of the vitamin for supplementation.

Therapeutic efficacy can be measured by clinical observation and, ideally, by measuring CSF neurotransmitter metabolites after therapy has begun, allowing potential titration of drug dosages. Monitoring of such a therapeutic regimen also necessitates close observation for potential adverse side effects. Despite the theoretical rationale behind these therapies and reasonable outcomes in certain cases, the long-term prognosis for affected individuals remains variable. This may reflect, however, the paucity of cases available for study and a bias of reporting toward late-diagnosed cases that show discouraging results. Regardless, it would appear that in generalized pterin deficiencies, combination therapy is indicated once a diagnosis is made (with appropriate follow-up monitoring) in order to provide an affected infant with the best possible chance for a satisfactory clinical outcome.

The incidence of the pterin defects is estimated at 1 to 3 per cent of infants with persistent hyperphenylalaninemia. Like PKU, disorders of tetrahydrobiopterin metabolism are inherited in an autosomal recessive fashion. Carrier testing and prenatal diagnosis (enzyme assay in amniocytes and chorionic villi) are possible for DHPR deficiency. Heterozygotes for GTC deficiency can be determined by enzyme assay, and prenatal diagnosis is available for the biopterin synthesis disorders by measurement of pterin metabolites in amniotic fluid (GTC and PTS deficiencies) and fetal erythrocyte enzyme assay (PTS deficiency).

AMINO ACID DISORDERS

VIVIAN E. SHIH, M.D.

Amino acid disorders are, with a few exceptions, autosomal recessive traits. Clinical manifestations are usually nonspecific, and developmental delay is a frequent complaint. Some disorders are associated with acute metabolic crisis, appearing as early as the first few days of life. Lethargy, seizures, or ataxia during these episodes is caused by metabolic ketoacidosis and/or hyperammonemia. Early treatment may be life-saving and may prevent brain damage.

PRINCIPLES OF TREATMENT

The principles of treatment of amino acid disorders are to correct the amino acid imbalance and to remove accumulated toxic metabolites. Management includes long-term therapy with special diet, vitamins and other medications, and aggressive therapy for acute metabolic decompensation. Enzyme replacement by organ transplantation for inborn errors of amino acid metabolism is a recent development and has been used with encouraging results in patients with tyrosinemia type I and with ornithine carbamyl transferase (OCT) deficiency.

Long-term therapy of amino acid disorders is based largely on diet manipulation to reduce the accumulated abnormal metabolites and to supply the deficient amino acid. This is especially true for diseases in which one or more of the essential amino acids accumulate. Essential amino acids are present in all forms of food protein. The intake of these amino acids can be regulated by restriction of the total amount of dietary protein in combination with the use of a semisynthetic medical food that provides the basic nitrogen requirement for these patients. These medical foods are commercially available from several manufacturers, and their dispensing requires a prescription.

A calculated amount of regular infant formula is prescribed to meet the requirements for the essential amino acids that have been omitted from the semisynthetic formula. Solids may be introduced into the diet in the usual manner but are limited to foods with a low-protein content. An older patient is given a low-protein diet, and, if necessary, the diet is supplemented with the appropriate essential amino acid mixture to ensure nutritional adequacy. Parents and/or patients are instructed to keep a diary and to calculate intake using food value books or an exchange list similar to a system used by diabetic patients.

The essential amino acid requirements in normal infants vary considerably with age and growth rate. The requirements for patients with a metabolic disorder are usually lower than those recommended for normal infants, and the "tolerance" limit to the amino acids varies from patient to patient, depending on the severity of the enzyme deficiency. Insufficient caloric intake often leads to a catabolic state and, consequently, an increase in blood levels of the affected amino acids. Infection or surgery can have the same adverse effects. Thus, starvation should be avoided and infection treated promptly.

A number of enzyme reactions in amino acid metabolism require a cofactor, often a derivative of a vitamin, most commonly that of B_1 (thiamine), B_2 (riboflavin), B_6 (pyridoxine), B_{12} (cobalamin), and C (ascorbic acid). An enzyme deficiency can be due to a defect in its coenzyme synthesis or to an altered enzyme-coenzyme interaction. Megavitamin therapy has been used to enhance enzyme activity and has been shown to be beneficial in certain patients. All newly diagnosed patients should be given a 2- to 4-week trial therapy of the appropriate vitamin to determine their biochemical response. The dosage is somewhat arbitrary but is usually between 10 to 100 times the daily requirement. Although water-soluble vitamins are low in toxicity, side effects of extremely high doses of pyridoxine (B_6) have been reported.

The treatment of several amino acid disorders is described next to illustrate the various aspects of management.

SPECIFIC TREATMENT

Homocystinuria Due to Cystathionine β-Synthase Deficiency

Homocystinuria due to cystathionine β-synthase (CS) deficiency is among the most frequent of treatable amino acid disorders. In addition to homocystine accumulation, methionine is frequently increased and plasma cystine is always low as a result of reduced synthesis caused by the enzyme block.

Homocystinuria is a multisystem disease. In the untreated state, developmental delay, skeletal abnormalities, osteoporosis, and dislocated lenses gradually appear during childhood. Vascular pathology in this disorder is reminiscent of that seen in arteriosclerotic diseases, and a thromboembolic event, such as stroke or heart attack, is often the cause of death. Early treatment from infancy can minimize brain damage and reduce the risk of vascular complications; however, dislocation of the ocular lenses and osteoporosis are recalcitrant to therapy.

A therapeutic trial of pyridoxine may be given at a daily dose between 25 mg and 300 mg in combination with 0.5 to 1.0 mg folic acid. If no change in methionine and homocystine levels is observed in 2 weeks, the patient may be considered pyridoxine-nonresponsive. For pyridoxine-responsive patients, pyridoxine administration in combination with a moderate restriction of food protein intake is often adequate. The minimum effective dose of pyridoxine should be determined by titration. In some patients, the dose could be as low as 5 mg a day.

Dietary therapy is designed to limit the intake of methionine, which is the only dietary source of homocystine, and to supplement cystine, which is an essential amino acid in CS-deficient patients. In general, vegetable foods are lower in protein—and particularly in methionine—than are animal products and are suitable for homocystinuric patients.

There is enough evidence to indicate that accumulation of homocystine rather than methionine causes vascular pathology and its complications. Other measures to lower homocystine accumulation have been tried, particularly in patients resistant to dietary treatment. Betaine promotes the conversion of homocysteine to methionine and is a new drug under investigation. It is particularly useful for patients diagnosed belatedly who are unable to comply with diet restriction. Aspirin and dipyridamole have been used to reduce the thrombotic tendency in homocystinuria but are without definitive benefit.

Stressful situations, such as pregnancy and surgery, are risk factors for vascular complications. The maintenance of proper treatment and hydration before, during, and after surgery are thought to reduce the risks. It is notable that, in contrast to the children of mothers with phenylketonuria (PKU), the children of homocystinuric women are usually normal.

Maple Syrup Urine Disease

Maple syrup urine disease (MSUD) is a disorder in the metabolism of the branched chain amino acids (BCAA), namely leucine, isoleucine, and valine. Oxidative decarboxylation of the ketoacids of these amino acids is impaired. As a result, the BCAAs and their keto acids accumulate and clinically recurrent ketoacidosis and brain damage develop. Untreated patients die in infancy or suffer from severe neurologic disabilities. Early treatment greatly improves the prognosis.

Typically, an affected newborn gradually experiences lethargy and poor feeding toward the end of the first week of life. As the disease progresses, the baby appears "septic" and is ketotic and dehydrated. Rigorous intravenous treatment to correct the fluid and electrolyte imbalance and to provide high caloric intake is essential. Peritoneal dialysis facilitates the removal of toxic metabolites and is recommended as an initial treatment for neonates. Oral or nasogastric tube feeding should be initiated as soon as possible. Maintaining high caloric intake and balanced nutrition parenterally can be achieved by intravenous administration of glucose with or without insulin, lipid, and a special amino acid solution. This amino acid mixture contains no BCAA and is designed to maintain balanced parenteral nutrition in MSUD patients during the period when oral feeding cannot be established.

Treatment for recurrent ketoacidosis in older children can follow the same principles except that the more conservative intravenous therapy regimen should be tried first unless the patient's neurologic status is severe enough to require immediate correction of the metabolic abnormalities by dialysis.

For long-term dietotherapy, a BCAA-free semisynthetic formula is used in combination with a regular formula and/or low-protein foods. For thiamine-responsive patients, thiamine is given in pharmacologic doses. Frequent monitoring by plasma amino acid analysis is necessary.

When there is fever or other early signs of intercurrent illness, the protein intake should be reduced and the caloric intake maintained by encouraging carbohydrate- and fat-containing foods. Because of the importance of early detection of acute complications, parents are usually instructed to perform a urine test for ketones and/or for ketoacids at home when there are behavioral changes, dietary indiscretion, or illness that may precipitate metabolic imbalance. A preparation of citrate/sodium citrate may be given as a temporary measure to alleviate the metabolic acidosis. Although the frequency and severity of metabolic crisis decrease with age, lifelong dietotherapy is necessary.

Urea Cycle Disorders and Hyperammonemic Syndromes

There are six urea cycle enzymopathies. Most severely affected patients experience a fulminating and often fatal neonatal course. Severe brain damage often occurs in infants presenting with intolerance to feeding, failure to thrive, and developmental delay. Episodic lethargy, ataxia, and coma are symptoms of acute hyperammonemia. The main goal of treatment for urea cycle disorders (UCDs) is to prevent ammonia intoxication.

Neonatal onset of hyperammonemia is a medical emergency that requires aggressive therapy to remove ammonia and prevent catabolism. In addition to intravenous administration of glucose and electrolytes, a mixture of sodium benzoate and phenylacetate (Ucephan) and arginine is given. Benzoate/phenylacetate facilitates the removal of ammonia (in the form of amino acids) by an alternate route bypassing the urea cycle. Two amino acids, glycine and glutamine, conjugate with these drugs and are excreted as hippurate and phenylacetylglutamine, respectively. Arginine is an essential amino acid in patients with all the UCDs except arginase deficiency. Intravenous lipid may be used to supply the necessary additional calories.

Hemodialysis is an efficient way to remove ammonia and should be started as soon as possible in neonates with hyperammonemic coma. The duration of hyperammonemia in the newborn stage is inversely related to the intellectual outcome of these patients. In older children, hemodialysis may be necessary when the intravenous therapeutic regimen fails to make progress.

A protein-restricted feeding regimen should be given as soon as oral feeding is tolerated. The protein allowance depends on the severity of the defect. An intake of 1.2 to 1.5 g protein/kg/day in the first 6 months of life is usually adequate for growth. In the severely affected patients, especially boys with the X-linked OCT deficiency, it may be necessary to give less, with one-half the nitrogen requirement in the form of an essential amino acid mixture and one-half in the form of natural food protein. Benzoate/phenylacetate and arginine or citrulline are indicated in some patients. Any infection should be treated vigorously and elective surgery postponed to minimize the risk of metabolic decompensation. Liver transplantation as a form of enzyme therapy should be considered in difficult cases and should be performed as early as feasible to prevent brain damage.

Because UCDs with a neonatal onset are associated with a grave prognosis, it is important to initiate treatment at birth for patients diagnosed prenatally. Prospective treatment has also been instituted in neonates at risk while results of diagnostic tests are being awaited. There have been no apparent adverse effects from this prospective treatment in unaffected infants.

Organic Acid Disorders

Many of the organic acid disorders are enzyme defects in the intermediary metabolism of amino acids, in particular the branched chain amino acids. The clinical manifestations are similar to those seen in MSUD and include recurrent ketoacidosis with or without the association of hyperammonemia, protein intolerance, failure to thrive, and developmental delay.

The treatment regimen also follows the same principles. In addition, carnitine supplement has been of value in the treatment of some of these disorders, such as methylmalonic acidemia, propionic acidemia, and glutaric acidemia. Carnitine is a semiessential nutrient and plays an important role in transporting fatty acids into mitochondria for oxidation. It binds with the excess amounts of acyl-CoAs in these disorders and removes them by renal excretion, thus depleting the free carnitine and causing secondary carnitine deficiency. In the case of isovaleric acidemia, glycine has a similar role facilitating the excretion of isovaleric acid as isovalerylglycine.

Fatty Acid Oxidation Defects

The major symptoms of fatty acid oxidation defects are vomiting, lethargy, and seizures in association with hypoketotic hypoglycemia and increased serum free fatty acids. Transient hepatomegaly is a common finding, especially in long-chain acyl CoA dehydrogenase deficiency. These disorders, particularly the medium-chain acyl-CoA dehydrogenase deficiency (MCADD) have been found in a number of infants who died suddenly. Hypoglycemic attacks are often precipitated by an extended period of fasting or by an infection, and patients are normal between these episodes.

Treatment is relatively simple. Frequent feeding and avoidance of fasting beyond 10 hours are the most important measures to prevent hypoglycemia. Moderate restriction of fat intake and carnitine supplement to facilitate the removal of the abnormal acyl-CoAs are adjunctive treatments.

HYPERLIPOPROTEINEMIA

JOSEPH LOSCALZO, M.D., Ph.D.

CLASSIFICATION OF DYSLIPIDEMIAS

Childhood dyslipidemias may be operationally categorized by plasma or serum lipid measurements as hypertriglyceridemia, elevated low-density lipoprotein (LDL) cholesterol, low high-density lipoprotein (HDL) cholesterol (hypoalphalipoproteinemia), or a combination of these abnormalities (Table 1). Dyslipidemias in childhood affect principally two organ systems: the pancreas and the vasculature. Markedly elevated levels of triglycerides (>400 mg/dl) are associated with an increased risk of acute pancreatitis. Elevated total or LDL cholesterol, decreased HDL cholesterol, or both (as reflected in an elevated total-to-HDL cholesterol ratio) are associated with an increased risk of atherosclerosis. Population values for total cholesterol, LDL and HDL cholesterol, triglycerides, and the total-to-HDL cholesterol ratio are given in Tables 2 and 3.

Atherosclerotic vascular disease is a process that begins in childhood, continues throughout life, and becomes clinically apparent (with rare exception, such as in homozygous familial hypercholesterolemia or type IIA hyperlipoproteinemia) only in middle age or later. The decision to treat dyslipidemic disorders in children or adolescents that are manifested by atherogenic lipoprotein profiles must be predicated on evidence supporting the views that these disorders (1) are associated with (preclinical) atherosclerotic disease in childhood, (2) track from childhood into adulthood, and (3), when diagnosed in childhood, predict the development of clinical atherosclerotic disease in adulthood.

Recent epidemiologic evidence supports the first two views. In the Bogalusa Heart Trial, serum total cholesterol and LDL cholesterol levels were associated with the size and number of aortic fatty streaks. Longitudinal clinical tracking studies (Muscatine) indicate that approximately two thirds of children with total cholesterols above the 90th percentile remained above the 75th percentile in adulthood. Inferential evidence exists in support of the view that children with a genetically determined atherogenic lipoprotein profile develop atherosclerotic coronary heart disease in adulthood.

TABLE 1. Operational Diagnostic Categories of Pediatric Dyslipidemias

I.	Hypertriglyceridemia
II.	Elevated low-density lipoprotein cholesterol
III.	Decreased high-density lipoprotein cholesterol
IV.	Combinations of above disorders

POPULATION SCREENING

The decision about which population of children to screen for atherogenic lipid profiles is currently controversial. Recent recommendations by the National Cholesterol Education Program suggest screening children and adolescents if a parent or grandparent has had premature cardiovascular disease or if a parent has an elevated total cholesterol level (>240 mg/dl). *If these recommendations were to be routinely adopted, approximately 25 per cent of children in the United States would be screened and approximately 50 per cent of these (or 14 million) would be candidates for therapy (Table 4), which, in the majority, would involve changes in diet.*

TREATMENT

Dietary Management

Dietary modification remains the first approach and mainstay of therapy for children with dyslipidemias. As a general principle of dietary management, the physician should seek to achieve the ideal body weight with normal growth velocities in these children, to reduce total fat intake to less than 30 per cent of total calories, and to reduce cholesterol intake to less than 75 mg/kg/day. Of the less than 30 per cent of dietary calories as fat, 7 per cent or less should be derived from saturated fats, 14 per cent from monounsaturates, and 9 per cent from polyunsaturates. The diet should also contain the recommended dietary allowances of total calories, protein, minerals, and vitamins. Children 2 years of age and younger should be excluded from these dietary modifications because of the importance of dietary fat in neural growth and development.

The goal of dietary therapy should be to reduce LDL cholesterol below 160 mg/dl and the ratio of total-to-HDL cholesterol below 6. Should these goals fail to be achieved, pharmacologic therapy should be considered in high-risk patients, namely, those with very marked elevations of LDL cholesterol; those with very marked elevations in total-to-HDL cholesterol; or those with moderately elevated LDL cholesterol, total-to-HDL cholesterol, normal triglycerides, and two other childhood risk factors (Table 5).

TABLE 2. Range of Lipid Values in Children and Adolescents

	Total Cholesterol (mg/dl)			LDL Cholesterol (mg/dl)			HDL Cholesterol (mg/dl)			Triglycerides (mg/dl)		
	5th Percentile	*Mean*	*95th Percentile*	*5th Percentile*	*Mean*	*95th Percentile*	*5th Percentile*	*Mean*	*95th Percentile*	*5th Percentile*	*Mean*	*95th Percentile*
Age 0–4												
Males	114	155	203							29	56	99
Females	112	156	200							34	64	112
Age 5–9												
Males	121	160	203	63	93	129	38	56	75	30	56	101
Females	126	164	205	68	100	140	36	53	73	32	60	105
Age 10–14												
Males	119	158	202	64	97	133	37	55	74	32	66	125
Female	124	160	201	68	97	136	37	52	70	37	75	131
Age 15–19												
Males	113	150	197	62	94	130	30	46	63	37	78	148
Females	120	158	203	59	96	137	35	52	64	39	75	132

Data from Lipid Research Clinics Population Studies Data Book.

Pharmacotherapy

Among the lipid-lowering agents currently available, the bile acid sequestrants or binding resins are the best studied and most commonly used in children. Resins administered at 0.3 to 0.4 g/kg/day will lead to an additional 10 to 30 per cent reduction in total and LDL cholesterol beyond the effect of diet alone. Notwithstanding the potential these agents have to produce fat malabsorption, no changes in levels of vitamins A, D, E, or K have been detected with their use. *Folate levels are, however, significantly reduced, for which reason children treated with resins should receive folate supplementation 1 hour before or 2 hours after treatment.*

Nicotinic acid also effects a further reduction in total and LDL cholesterol beyond that produced by diet and bile acid sequestrants, with the additional benefit of an increase in HDL cholesterol. Hydroxymethylglutaryl CoA reductase inhibitors (lovastatin, provastatin, simvastatin) are very effective in lowering total and LDL cholesterol as well, but their long-term safety has yet to be determined. The unknown safety features of these latter agents with long-term use and their potentially adverse effects on cholesterol synthesis in the central nervous system, adrenal glands, and gonads preclude the general application of their use in children and adolescents—with the exception of those rare individuals with homozygous familial hypercholesterolemia (see below). Fibric acid derivatives (gemfibrozil, clofibrate) may also prove useful in selected cases, but, again, their safety with long-term administration has not yet been determined in the pediatric population.

TABLE 3. Range of Total-to-HDL Cholesterol Ratio in Children and Adolescents

	5th Percentile	Mean	95th Percentile
Age 5–9			
Males	2.1	2.8	4.2
Females	2.2	3.5	4.8
Age 10–14			
Males	2.2	2.9	4.3
Females	2.3	3.0	4.2
Age 15–19			
Males	2.2	3.4	5.2
Females	2.1	3.0	4.7

Data from Lipid Research Clinics Population Studies Data Book.

Other General Therapeutic Considerations

In addition to these general pharmacotherapeutic principles, individuals with atherogenic lipid profiles should also be instructed in other aspects of risk factor modification. Appropriate attention should be paid to nonlipid factors that may have an indirect impact on lipid metabolism, including physical activity, smoking cessation, and blood pressure control. Other secondary causes for dyslipidemias should also be considered and treated when appropriate, including hypothyroidism, diabetes mellitus, nephrotic syndrome, autoimmune diseases (especially systemic lupus erythematosus), and renal failure.

Specific Treatment of Selected Dyslipidemias

Selected disorders that may necessitate special therapeutic considerations include marked hypertriglyceridemia, particularly hyperchylomicronemia, and familial hypercholesterolemia.

Hyperchylomicronemia

Hyperchylomicronemia (Fredrickson type I hyperlipoproteinemia) is a consequence of deficient lipoprotein lipase activity that is a rare (<1 in 100,000) autosomal recessive disorder, the hallmarks of which are marked elevations in triglycerides (>1000 mg/dl), eruptive xanthomata, and recurrent pancreatitis. Two types of molecular abnormalities have been found to produce this phenotype: apoprotein CII defi-

TABLE 4. General Therapeutic Options in Pediatric Dyslipidemias

Treatment	Lipid Abnormality ↑ *TG*	↑ *LDL-C*	↓ *HDL-C*
Dietary modification	+	+	+
Bile acid sequestrants	–	+	–
Nicotinic acid*	+	+	+
HMG CoA reductase inhibitors*	–	+	±
Fibric acid derivatives*	+	±	+

*Use only in selected cases as discussed in text.
Abbreviations: TG, triglycerides; LDL-C, low-density lipoprotein cholesterol; HDL-C, high-density lipoprotein cholesterol; HMG, hydroxymethylglutaryl.

TABLE 5. Characteristics of High Risk Patients in Whom Pharmacologic Therapy May Be Considered

1. Very marked elevations of LDL cholesterol
2. Very marked elevations of total-to-HDL cholesterol
3. LDL cholesterol ≥ 160 mg/dl or ≥ 95th percentile for age
   a. Plus total-to-HDL cholesterol ≥ 6
   b. Plus two other childhood risk factors

Abbreviations: LDL, low-density lipoprotein; HDL, high-density lipoprotein.

ciency and circulating inhibitor(s) of lipoprotein lipase. Treatment is best effected with a very low total dietary fat intake and the use of medium-chain triglycerides in cooking to improve dietary palatability. Severely symptomatic individuals with apoprotein CII deficiency may benefit from plasma transfusion. Avoidance of estrogen and alcohol use in adolescence should also be advised.

Secondary Hypertriglyceridemia

Secondary severe hypertriglyceridemia from hypothyroidism, diabetes mellitus, systemic lupus erythematosus, and renal failure is generally less than 1000 mg/dl. Treating the underlying condition is of paramount importance as an initial approach, with additional benefit derived from fat restriction and weight reduction. Rarely, nicotinic acid or fibric agents (e.g., gemfibrozil) may be required for optimal treatment, but the use of these agents should be restricted to those individuals with triglycerides between 400 to 1000 mg/dl who fail to respond to alternate conservative measures and continue to suffer episodes of pancreatitis.

Familial Hypercholesterolemia

Familial hypercholesterolemia is a rare disorder (1 in 1,000,000) caused by an abnormality in the function or a true absence of the LDL (apo B/E) receptor. This disorder is marked by the development of accelerated atherosclerosis and consequent myocardial infarction or stroke in the first two decades of life. For this reason, aggressive treatment directed toward reducing LDL cholesterol should be prescribed. Hydroxymethylglutaryl CoA reductase inhibitors, at the very least, should be considered in all such patients, and in selected cases more aggressive therapeutic options may be required, including plasmapheresis, LDL-apheresis, portacaval anastamosis, partial ileal bypass, and liver transplantation.

Heterozygous familial hypercholesterolemia is much more prevalent than the homozygous form (1 in 500) and is a milder disorder, the hallmarks of which are tendinous xanthomata, LDL cholesterol higher than the 99th percentile and usually at twice the mean value for any given age range, and a family history suggesting monogenic transmission (three generations affected with xanthomata, premature atherosclerotic coronary heart disease, or isolated LDL cholesterol elevations with normal triglycerides levels). Treatment with hydroxymethylglutaryl CoA reductase inhibitors may be required in late adolescence in affected individuals.

Hypoalphalipoproteinemia

The treatment of severely depressed HDL cholesterol (marked hypoalphalipoproteinemia) is generally more difficult than that for the disorders discussed thus far. Aerobic exercise, avoidance of tobacco use, and achievement of ideal body weight may lead to a 5 to 10 mg/dl increase in HDL cholesterol in selected individuals.

GALACTOSEMIA

GILBERT N. JONES III, M.D.

Classic galactosemia results from a deficiency of the enzyme galactose-1-phosphate uridyl transferase, which catalyzes the second step in the metabolic pathway that converts the hexose sugar galactose to glucose-1-phosphate. An important product of transferase activity is uridine diphosphate (UDP) galactose, the donor molecule for the synthesis of galactose-containing glycoproteins, glycolipids, and glycosaminoglycans. Clinical diseases resulting from deficiency of galactokinase, the first step of galactose metabolism, and UDP galactose-4-epimerase, the third step of galactose metabolism, are also known. When normal metabolism of galactose is impaired, alternate metabolic pathways become activated and galactose is converted to galactitol and galactonate. In galactokinase and transferase deficiencies, galactitol synthesis within the lens appears to cause cataract formation by pulling water into the lens with consequent tearing of zonula fibers. Galactose-1-phosphate accumulates in many organs in transferase deficiency and is thought to be responsible for the clinical abnormalities of the infant acutely ill with galactosemia.

These abnormalities, which include vomiting, diarrhea, hepatic and renal dysfunction, altered consciousness, impaired immune function, and cataracts, are prevented or reversed by exclusion of all galactose from the diet. Supportive therapy includes resolution of dehydration and electrolyte abnormalities. Bacterial infections, most commonly due to gram-negative organisms, are treated with the appropriate antibiotics. Hepatocellular dysfunction usually resolves rapidly, but hypoalbuminemia may necessitate albumin replacement if ascites or anasarca is present. In jaundice, exchange transfusion may be required if indirect bilirubin reaches neurotoxic levels. Neither exchange transfusion nor dialysis is indicated for removal of toxic galactose metabolites. All infants and children diagnosed as having galactosemia should be evaluated by an ophthalmologist when the diagnosis is made and at least yearly thereafter. Approximately half of cataracts present in infancy resolve with early initiation of dietary galactose exclusion. Cataracts may progress in poorly controlled children or may be irreversible in those with late initiation of therapy.

DIET THERAPY

The fundamental component of therapy is the elimination of galactose from the diet. The primary source of galactose is the disaccharide lactose, found in milk and milk products. In the first year of life, a soy protein–based formula is substituted for animal milk–based formulas or human milk. A casein hydrolysate (Nutramagen or Alimentum) may be used as an alternative. Cereals, vegetables, fruits, and meats may be added to the diet at the appropriate times. Beans and peas contain oligosaccharides in which galactose is present, but since free galactose is not derived from these polymerized sugars, no restriction of their intake is necessary. Obvious sources of galactose include cheese, ice cream, yogurt, puddings, and breads. Many prepared foods also contain galactose. These include, but are not limited to, baked goods, confections, and some frozen foods. Certain drug preparations contain lactose as a filler. The involvement of a dietitian in the management of these individuals is encouraged. The dietitian can educate the family regarding potentially harmful foodstuffs, provide the family with recipes of foods that can be prepared at home using galactose-free milk substitutes, and assess the patient's diet to ensure adequate intake of calories, protein, vitamins, and minerals such as calcium.

Some authorities allow limited liberalization of the diet as children with galactosemia enter school. Milk and milk products remain a lifetime prohibition. Recent data comparing the long-term complication rates in galactosemic individuals who maintained a diet completely free of all galactose and those who only avoided all milk and milk products showed no differences in intelligence quotient (IQ) scores. Although these data suggest that limited loosening of the diet is acceptable, it must be emphasized that individuals who included some milk-containing foods in their diet had significantly lower IQ scores. Patients and their families must be informed that no increased tolerance for galactose occurs with advancing age. Liberalization of the diet must be viewed as a compromise to prevent larger dietary infractions, not as a routine progression of therapy.

Children with galactosemia who have experienced delay in initiation of dietary treatment usually have severe intellectual impairment. Routine newborn screening for galactose-1-phosphate uridyl transferase deficiency identifies affected infants prior to onset of the acute toxicity syndrome in order to prevent permanent mental retardation. In infants with a positive screen, dietary restriction of galactose should begin immediately while results of confirmatory enzyme studies are awaited.

LONG-TERM COMPLICATIONS

Although early initiation of a galactose-free diet is essential in preventing the more severe intellectual impairment seen in this disorder, it is now clear that even in optimally treated children with galactosemia, intellectual impairment and other problems may develop. A recent long-term survey of 350 children with galactosemia revealed that 45 per cent had developmental delay. Moreover, IQ or developmental quotient (DQ) appears to decline with increased age, despite adequate dietary control. Speech problems were present in 50 per cent of children over the age of 3 years. Eighteen per cent had problems with coordination, gait, balance, fine motor tremors, and severe ataxia. Formal testing of development and speech should be performed at yearly, or biennial intervals. Treatment of learning or speech disorders is determined by the results obtained.

Hypergonadotrophic hypogonadism, irregular menses, and decreased fertility develop in most adolescent or adult women with classic galactosemia. Women with these symptoms may require treatment by a reproductive endocrinologist. Testicular function is normal in galactosemic men. Growth is often severely delayed in childhood and adolescence but continues during the late teen years so that the final height is usually normal.

Concern that deficiency of UDP-galactose may contribute to the long-term complications of galactosemia has stimulated interest in the hypothesis that uridine administration, which increases UDP galactose in galactosemic cells in vitro, may ameliorate these problems. Uridine should be given only in the setting of well-controlled, closely monitored clinical trials, which are under way.

The recurrence risk of galactosemia to a couple who have had a child with galactosemia is 1 in 4 with each pregnancy. Prenatal diagnosis is available by biochemical testing of amniocytes or chorionic villi or by analysis of DNA obtained from these tissues. Eliminating galactose in the diet of women pregnant with a potentially galactosemic fetus is controversial. There are no data to support severe restriction of maternal galactose ingestion in this setting.

Variant forms of the transferase enzyme possess diminished catalytic activity. For example, individuals with one Duarte gene and one classic galactosemia gene have 25 per cent of normal activity. These individuals will be ascertained as having galactosemia by newborn screening techniques, but do not need to restrict galactose intake. Identification of variants is achieved by quantitative measurement of red blood cell enzyme activity and by starch-gel protein electrophoresis.

Individuals with galactokinase deficiency develop cataracts, but not the other toxic symptoms seen in classic galactosemia. Restriction of dietary galactose prevents progression of the cataracts.

Most individuals found to lack UDP galactose-4-epimerase activity in red blood cells have been clinically normal. The rare individuals with symptomatic epimerase deficiency have improved with dietary galactose restriction. Unlike the situation in classic galactosemia, however, small amounts of galactose in the diet appear necessary for UDP galactose synthesis to occur.

REFERENCES

Segal S: Disorders of galactose metabolism. *In* Scriver CR, *et al* (eds): The Metabolic Basis of Inherited Disease. New York, McGraw-Hill, 1989, pp 453–480.

Waggoner DD, Buist NRM, Donnell GN: Long-term prognosis in galactosemia: Results of a survey of 350 cases. J Inher Metab Dis 13:802–818, 1990

Ng WG, Xu YK, Kaufman FR, Donnell GN: Deficit of uridine diphosphate galactose in galactosemia. J Inher Metab Dis 12:257–266, 1989.

DISORDERS OF PORPHYRIN, PURINE, AND PYRIMIDINE METABOLISM

RUSSELL W. CHESNEY, M.D.
and THOMAS McC. CHESNEY, M.D.

The porphyrias are a family of diseases related to inherited defects of the various enzymes involved in the synthetic pathway for heme in red blood cell precursors and hepatocytes. For each specific enzyme deficiency, there is a fairly specific symptom complex and an increase in the concentration of the substrate compound for that enzyme, with increased excretion of that substrate compound in urine and/or feces. Those porphyrias that are predominantly manifested in erythroid precursors are associated with hemolytic anemia and skin manifestations because porphyrin rings present in great excess in the red blood cells and skin absorb light with the consequent production of singlet oxygen and free radicals in the tissues with cellular and tissue damage. Hydrogen peroxide and lipid peroxides are generated that damage cellular and lysosomal membranes with autodigestion of the cutaneous tissues. Those porphyrias that predominantly manifest in the liver will have skin manifestations if porphyrin rings are overproduced (the enzyme defect is distal to porphobilinogen [PBG] deaminase) but will not if only porphyrin precursors (PBG, delta-aminolevulinic acid synthetase [d-ALA]) are overproduced. The hepatic porphyrias may manifest as crises combining abdominal pain, nausea, autonomic neuropathy with hypertension and tachycardia, peripheral neuropathy, and central nervous system presentations including seizures, paralysis, or coma. Therapy of the porphyrias is thus directed against cutaneous photosensitivity, hemolysis, and the prevention or improvement of visceral crises. Effective therapy is predicated upon accurate diagnosis, which in turn has implications for family screening in these genetic disorders.

The rate-limiting step in porphyrin synthesis is at the first enzyme d-ALA synthetase which catalyzes the synthesis of succinyl CoA and glycine to form d-ALA. This enzyme is under feedback inhibition by heme (by repression/depression of messenger RNA for d-ALA synthetase) such that an enzyme deficiency anywhere along the heme synthetic pathway will result in increased d-ALA synthetase activity, forcing more precursors into the pathway. This has led to attempts to suppress d-ALA synthetase and disease activity by hypertransfusion and by intravenous (IV) administration of heme. In addition, hormones and certain lipid-soluble, slowly metabolized drugs that require biotransformation by the hepatic cytochrome P_{450} system bring about acute attacks in the hepatic porphyrias, and avoidance of these drugs in such patients is a mainstay of patient management. The list of offending drugs includes such major components of the pediatric pharmacopoeia as barbiturates, carbamazepine, chloramphenicol, ethchlorvynol, griseofulvin, halothane, hydantoins, imipramine, phenytoin, primidone, sulfonamides, and theophylline. Patients with hepatic porphyrias should receive only carefully selected drugs, should not purchase or use over-the-counter medications, and should wear a MedicAlert bracelet identifying them as having a porphyria.

Clinically manifest porphyrias are rare in childhood but certainly do occur. The autosomal recessively inherited forms—congenital erythropoietic porphyria (CEP), PBG synthase deficiency, and hepatoerythropoietic porphyria (HEP)—manifest in infancy or early childhood; dominantly inherited acute intermittent porphyria (AIP) typically manifests in the third decade; and porphyria cutanea tarda (PCT) occasionally presents in childhood. Hereditary coproporphyria (HCP) and variegate porphyria (VP), which combines the features of AIP with those of PCT, are basically postpubertal disorders, emphasizing the role of sex steroids in the pathogenesis of these disorders. Acute attacks of the hepatic porphyrias are also often related to the menstrual cycle, and latent PCT may be brought out by oral contraceptives or estrogen replacement therapy in older women.

CONGENITAL ERYTHROPOIETIC PORPHYRIA

Congenital erythropoietic porphyria (CEP), also known as congenital porphyria, erythropoietic porphyria, or Gunther's disease, is a very rare autosomal recessive disorder that manifests early in life and displays mutilating photosensitivity with blistering and cutaneous infections leading to disfiguring scarring of the sun-exposed skin. The enzyme defect is in uroporphyrinogen III cosynthetase, which allows overproduction of isomer I porphyrinogens that are unable to be metabolized to heme. Large amounts of uroporphyrin are excreted in the urine, which is red to burgundy, and the disease may first be suspected by pink to red-brown staining of the infant's diaper by porphyrin-laden urine or stool. Photoprotection is a major component of the management of the cutaneous aspects of this disease. Because conventional sunscreens are most effective in the ultraviolet spectrum (280 to 320 nM) and porphyrins absorb maximally in the Soret band (400 to 410 nM), they are of little benefit. Barrier-type sunscreens, such as zinc oxide paste or the newer titanium dioxide-based agents, must be used in addition to broad-brimmed hats and long sleeves. Clothing of darker colors and tighter weaves may be important, since considerable light passes through thin white fabrics. The hemolytic anemia of this condition (photohemolysis) may be improved by splenectomy, especially if splenomegaly is present, and periodic red blood cell transfusions to maintain the hematocrit level around 40 per cent may suppress bone marrow activity and porphyrin production. There are, of course, dangers attendant to repeated transfusion therapy, including infectious diseases and iron overload; however, this method has provided prolonged disease suppression in selected patients. Finally, activated charcoal in large doses by mouth has been used to complex with porphyrins in the gut and remove them from the enterohepatic circulation.

CONGENITAL ERYTHROPOIETIC PROTOPORPHYRIA

Congenital erythropoietic protoporphyria (EPP) is a disease of childhood photosensitivity also known as solar urticaria. Patients experience an acute sunburn-like reaction with stinging, burning, reddening, and edema of the skin after only a few minutes of exposure to sunlight. The enzyme deficiency is in ferrochelatase, the ultimate enzyme in the heme synthetic scheme that inserts an iron atom into the protoporphyrin ring. Protoporphyrin is increased in the stool and red blood cells contain elevated free protoporphyrin levels and fluoresce (fluorocytes). The skin manifestations are improved by avoidance of direct sunlight and by photoprotective measures as outlined above under CEP. In addition, patients with EPP have demonstrated increased light tolerance with the prolonged oral administration of beta carotene (30 to 150 mg/day) to maintain the serum beta carotene level at 600 to 800 μg/dl. Effective doses turn the skin a slight yellow color and improve symptoms by functioning as an oxygen and free radical quencher in the tissues. Hemolytic anemia may also be a problem in EPP and may be associated with gallstones; these may require splenectomy and cholecystectomy. Protoporphyrin crystals are deposited in hepatocytes; in rare instances patients experience hepatic failure and a shriveled, dark brown-black liver and are candidates for liver transplantation.

CONGENITAL HEPATOERYTHROPOIETIC PORPHYRIA

Congenital hepatoerythropoietic porphyria (HEP) is a very rare condition affecting individuals who inherit a porphyria cutanea tarda gene from both parents. There is markedly decreased red blood cell uroporphyrinogen decarboxylase activity, elevated urinary uroporphyrins, and elevated red blood cell protoporphyrin. Vesicles, bullae, and erosions of the skin appear before age 2, followed by scleroderma-like skin changes, mutilation, and hypertrichosis. Treatment is unsatisfactory, with only rigorous photoprotection available.

PORPHOBILINOGEN SYNTHETASE DEFICIENCY

PBG synthetase deficiency is exceedingly rare and displays increased urinary PBG without ALA (the two are always elevated together in other disorders). There are acute attacks (see acute intermittent porphyria) in this recessive disorder but no skin changes.

PORPHYRIA CUTANEA TARDA

The most common form of porphyria, PCT usually becomes clinically apparent in adult life, as the name implies, but occasionally manifests in childhood. There are two forms, familial and sporadic, the latter representing a latent enzyme defect which is brought out by the development of chronic liver disease (often due to alcohol) and/or iron overload or exposure to certain drugs or sex steroids. The enzyme defect in PCT is in uroporphyrinogen decarboxylase, and there is massive excretion of urinary uroporphyrins. Skin manifestations include increased skin fragility, blistering, development of tiny milia cysts, and sclerodermatoid changes of the dorsa of the hands and fingers, and hyperpigmentation and hypertrichosis, particularly around the eyes and lateral forehead. In adults, the mainstay of therapy, in addition to local skin treatments, is phlebotomy in an effort to reduce hepatic iron stores, as well as removal of offending drugs and alcohol. In children, PCT has been successfully controlled with oral S-adenosyl-l-methionine (12 mg/kg/day for 3 weeks) combined with oral chloroquine (100 mg twice weekly). The adenosylmethionine increases glutathione while the chloroquine increases urinary porphyrin excretion until it returns to normal; cutaneous manifestations disappear. Oral charcoal as an adsorbent has also been used as experimental therapy in PCT.

ACUTE INTERMITTENT PORPHYRIA

Also known as Swedish porphyria, AIP is an autosomal dominant disorder in which the enzyme defect is in PBG deaminase and is the prototype of the hepatic porphyrias in which acute visceral attacks occur. Patients with AIP may, under the influence of the menstrual cycle or in response to drugs, experience attacks of acute abdominal pain with nausea, vomiting, leukocytosis, and fever that may precipitate surgical intervention. Alternately, or concomitantly, there may be highly variable neurologic symptoms with neuropathies, seizures, altered mentation, loss of consciousness, paresis, and even respiratory paralysis. Patients with acute attacks are managed in hospital under observation, with respiratory support if necessary.

Initial treatment is with large amounts of oral or hypertonic glucose and careful fluid and electrolyte management as inappropriate secretion of antidiuretic hormone (ADH) and hyponatremia occur. If the attack resists these measures, intravenous hemin (Panhematin, Abbott Laboratories) is administered at a dose of 1 to 4 mg/kg/day given over 10 to 15 minutes through a large intravenous line from a freshly reconstituted vial. This is repeated daily for 3 to 14 days, depending on clinical response. Administration of intravenous hemin, a heme compound processed from blood and containing ferric iron, may be complicated by phlebitis and a transient coagulopathy with prolongation of the prothrombin time (PT) and partial thromboplastin time (PTT) and thrombocytopenia. These complications may be reduced with the availability of heme arginate, a less toxic heme product used in Europe (Normosang). In acute attacks of AIP, large amounts of ALA and PBG are excreted in the urine; it is important to remember that these metabolites are always elevated in these patients, just much more so with acute attacks. In postpubertal women with acute attacks brought on by the menstrual cycle, luteinizing hormone–releasing hormone (LHRH) antagonistic analogues are being used to suppress ovulation and porphyric attacks. Although this treatment is still experimental, it may be available with an Investigational New Drug (IND) certificate.

VARIEGATE PORPHYRIA

Variegate porphyria (VP) has been most extensively studied in South Africa and is sometimes known as South African porphyria. It combines the clinical features of AIP with those of PCT, although in VP the skin fragility and sclerodermatoid changes may be even more pronounced than in typical PCT. VP is a postpubertal dominantly inherited disease of variable expressivity with the enzyme defect at the level of protoporphyrinogen oxidase and with overexcretion of protoporphyrin in the stool and coproporphyrin in the urine. In acute attacks there is superimposed hyperexcretion of ALA, PBG, and urinary uroporphyrins as with AIP.

Treatment essentially combines that for acute attacks outlined under AIP and photoprotective measures, including avoidance of trauma to the skin and prompt antibiotic therapy for any cutaneous infections that may arise. Beta carotene or canthaxanin, a synthetic carotene analogue, may be tried, but phlebotomy is ineffective in this disorder.

HEREDITARY COPROPORPHYRIA

Hereditary coproporphyria is a rare autosomal dominant disorder in which coproporphrinogen oxidase deficiency is associated with markedly increased excretion of coproporphyrins in the feces and urine between and during acute attacks and in which photosensitivity and blistering are occasionally seen. Treatment is as for AIP with glucose and hemin infusions and avoidance of inducing drugs.

HYPERURICEMIA

Uric acid stones do not occur in most mammals other than man because the enzyme uricase converts relatively insoluble uric acid to allantoin. In man, uric acid is the end product of purine metabolism arising from endogenous nucleic acids and nucleotides as well as ingested nucleoproteins and oligonucleotides. Uric acid is excreted in the urine, and the final urinary concentration is the difference between the rate of renal tubular secretion and reabsorption. Uric acid solubility increases from 150 mg/L at pH 5.0 to 2000 mg/L at pH 7.0, but urine is often supersaturated regarding uric acid.

Whereas hyperuricemia leads to gout in adults, uric acid stones are the main result in children. Uric acid stones usually occur under the following circumstances: uric acid overproduction, low urinary volume, or persistently low urine pH. Uric acid overproduction of endogenous origin arises in gout, other enzyme defects (Lesch-Nyhan syndrome), myeloproliferative or lymphoproliferative disorders, and polycythemia. Exogenous purine ingestion can occur after massive sweetbread gluttony. Both chronic diarrhea and persistent ileostomy drainage can also result in uric acid nephrolithiasis. With a uric acid excretion in excess of 1000 mg daily associated with a urine pH of 5.0, stones will develop in fully 50 per cent of subjects.

By far the most common cause of uric acid nephropathy in children is the *tumor lysis syndrome*. In children with leukemia, lymphoma, and Burkitt cell lymphoma, there is rapid cell turnover and breakdown of nucleic acids, particularly following chemotherapy. The therapeutic approach to the tumor lysis syndrome includes hydration, alkalinization of the urine, and the use of agents that reduce uric acid synthesis from xanthine, mainly allopurinol, the xanthine oxidase inhibitor. Pretreatment with high doses of intravenous fluids (1 to 3 liters per day according to weight and size of the child), oral bicarbonate (2 to 6 g every 24 hours) or sodium citrate (20 to 60 ml every 24 hours) and allopurinol at 10 to 20 mg/kg every 24 hours should begin 24 to 72 hours prior to the initiation of chemotherapy. In some children, hyperuricemia occurs spontaneously prior to the initiation of chemotherapy and may result in acute uric acid nephropathy. In these cases, hydration and the use of allopurinol along with Shohl's solution or Polycitra (neutral sodium-potassium citrate) are indicated, providing the patient does not have oliguric renal failure. In this instance, either hemodialysis or peritoneal dialysis may be required.

Allopurinol is an effective agent in reducing both hyperuricemia and urinary uric acid excretion. A dose of 5 to 10 mg/kg/day reduces the formation of the three main end products of purine metabolism—xanthine, hypoxanthine, and uric acid. The product of the enzymatic oxidation of allopurinol is the xanthine analogue oxopurinol, which itself can inhibit xanthine oxidase. In patients with moderate renal failure, the concentrations of oxopurinol will rise and necessitate reduction of allopurinol dosage by one third. Among other side effects of allopurinol are skin rashes, drowsiness, headache, diarrhea, nausea, and vertigo. Rarely agranulocytosis, granulomatous hepatitis, and exfoliative dermatitis may occur. A syndrome of maculopapular rash, eosinophilia, fever, and elevated liver function studies have been described in children with renal failure; this syndrome disappears with adjustment of dosage.

Childhood gout should be treated with fluids, citrate, and allopurinol in the doses indicated above; the elimination of purine-rich foods, such as organ meats (liver, sweetbreads, kidney, sardines, anchovies, wild game) is indicated. Fortunately, these foods are uncommon in a child's diet.

LESCH-NYHAN SYNDROME

Deficiency of hypoxanthine-guanine phosphoribosyl transferase in this recessive disorder leads to uric acid overproduction associated with self-mutilation, choreoathetosis, and mental retardation. Patients demonstrate biting of fingers and lips and may require physical restraints to diminish this behavior. Hyperuricosuria and urate gravel, which appears before 1 year of age, as well as urate stones are treated with fluids, alkalinization, and allopurinol at 100 to 300 mg every 24 hours. Therapy should be individualized with the aim of normalizing serum urate levels and urinary urate excretion.

The neurologic manifestations and self-mutilation of Lesch-Nyhan syndrome are not influenced by allopurinol therapy. Physical restraints are used to prevent both self-mutilating behavior and aggressive attacks on attendants. Extraction of teeth can reduce lip biting. Nondestructive behavior deserves positive reinforcement, which is preferable to punishment in controlling self-destructive or aggressive behavior.

When acute attacks of gout develop in these patients, treatment with colchicine can be used at 0.5 to 1.0 mg/kg every 24 hours. This dose is usually associated with diarrhea.

XANTHINURIA

Xanthine may accumulate with deficiency of xanthine oxidase, the enzyme responsible for the conversion of xanthine to uric acid. Large amounts of xanthine are excreted into the urine. This condition is characterized by a low serum uric acid concentration and xanthinuria. Xanthinuria is treated by promoting the solubilization of xanthine in the urine with increased fluid intake and oral citrate therapy.

OROTIC ACIDURIA

Orotic aciduria is the main inherited disorder of pyrimidine metabolism. Characterized by megaloblastic anemia, it cannot be reversed by folate, ascorbic acid, or vitamin B_{12}. Leukopenia, growth delay, and blue sclerae occur. Orotic acid crystals are present in the urine because of reduced activity of two enzymes of pyrimidine metabolism—orotidylic acid decarboxylase and orotidylic pyrophosphorylase.

Therapy of orotic aciduria consists of replacement of the pyrimidine nucleotides, citylic acid, and uridylic acid at 150 mg/kg every 24 hours. An improved hematologic picture along with diminished urinary orotic acid excretion then ensues. High fluid volumes are also recommended to reduce orotic acid crystalluria.

REFERENCES

Kappas A, Sassa S, Galbraith RA, Nordmann Y: The porphyrias. *In* Scriver CR, Beaudet AL, Sly WS, Valle D (eds): The Metabolic Basis of Inherited Disease. Vol II. New York, McGraw-Hill, Inc, 1989, pp 1305–1366.

Rieselbach RE: Urolithiasis: Uric acid stones. *In* Glassock RJ (ed): Current Therapy in Nephrology and Hypertension. Vol 2. Philadelphia, BC Decker, Inc, 1987, pp 73–77.

LYSOSOMAL STORAGE DISEASES

JOHN W. BELMONT, M.D., Ph.D.
and ARTHUR L. BEAUDET, M.D.

The lysosomal storage diseases are due to the genetic deficiency or dysfunction of one or more lysosomal enzymes. This group of disorders includes the lipid storage diseases, the mucopolysaccharidoses, the mucolipidoses, glycoprotein storage diseases, and type II glycogen storage disease (Table 1). The pattern of organ involvement depends on the site of degradation of the accumulating macromolecules. Almost all the disorders are autosomal recessive defects, although a few are X-linked. Although these diseases are heterogeneous and often have infantile, juvenile, and adult forms associated with the same enzyme defect, the disorders regularly exhibit a progressive course. An enzyme-specific diagnosis is a prerequisite for optimal management.

TREATMENT

Medical and surgical management of patients with these diseases is largely symptomatic and supportive, but a few specific forms of intervention are important. Hypersplenism develops frequently in adult Gaucher disease,* and splenectomy is indicated for correction of significant hematologic abnormalities. Myringotomy and pressure equalization tubes (tympanostomy) to prevent recurrent ear infections are very important in the mucopolysaccharidoses, mucolipidoses, and similar phenotypes such as mannosidosis. Hearing can be preserved in intellectually normal patients; recurrent episodes of fever, irritability, and family stress can be avoided in profoundly impaired children.

It should be noted that many of these patients require "routine" surgery (e.g., herniorrhaphy, tympanostomy). The risks of general anesthesia for these procedures are increased secondary to airway difficulties (particularly for mucopolysaccharidoses and related phenotypes) and coexisting chronic heart disease. Preoperative cardiac evaluation consisting of electrocardiogram (EKG) and echocardiogram is recommended for patients in whom chronic upper airway obstruction may have led to right ventricular dysfunction, for patients with significant valvular dysfunction, and for those in whom ischemic cardiomyopathy is advanced. Cardiac and respiratory failure occur in type II glycogen storage disease and are managed symptomatically as for any cardiac and skeletal myopathy.

Orthopedic Measures

Judicious use of corrective orthopedic procedures is appropriate, particularly for the mucopolysaccharidoses such as mild Hunter, Morquio, and Maroteaux-Lamy diseases, in which intellectual impairment is minimal or absent. The Morquio phenotype is associated with odontoid hypoplasia

*Gaucher disease includes three clinically distinct genetic entities involving the storage of glucosylceramide (glucocerebroside).[1]

TABLE 1. Lysosomal Storage Diseases

G_{M1} gangliosidosis	Sialadenosis
G_{M2} gangliosidosis, Tay-Sachs	Aspartylglycosaminuria
G_{M2} gangliosidosis, Sandhoff	Hurler, MPS IH*
Krabbe leukodystrophy	Scheie, MPS IS
Metachromatic leukodystrophy	Hunter, MPS II
Niemann-Pick disease	Sanfilippo A, MPS IIIA
Gaucher disease	Sanfilippo B, MPS IIIB
Fabry disease	Sanfilippo C, MPS IIIC
Wolman disease	Sanfilippo D, MPS IIID
Cholesteryl ester storage disease	Morquio, MPS IV
Farber lipogranulomatosis	Maroteaux-Lamy, MPS VI
Pompe disease, glycogenosis type II	β-Glucuronidase deficiency, MSP VII
Acid phosphatase deficiency	Multiple sulfatase deficiency
Fucosidosis	Mucolipidosis II, I-cell disease
Mannosidosis	Mucolipidosis III
	Mucolipidosis IV

*MPS, mucopolysaccharidosis.

with instability at the atlantoaxial joint. This joint should be evaluated carefully, even in the absence of symptoms. Prophylactic cervical fusion is indicated during the first decade if instability is significant, since acute and chronic cervical cord damage is likely.

Renal Transplants

Patients with Fabry disease* have progressive renal impairment, and renal transplantation and dialysis should be considered according to usual criteria. Renal involvement is usually severe enough to require such intervention in adult hemizygous males but not in heterozygous females. Painful neuropathy occurs in males and females with Fabry disease, and symptomatic relief often can be obtained with phenytoin (Dilantin) in usual therapeutic dosage (4 to 7 mg/kg/day).

Family Support

Many of the disorders cause intellectual impairment, and special educational and training support is indicated. At times the possibility of progressive dementia exists, but the child should be given special educational support, since prognosis is never certain. Unfortunately, many children with these diseases experience progressive and, ultimately, severe neurologic impairment.

Proper emotional and social support for the family is very important. Some of the lysosomal storage diseases are among the most tragic and burdensome conditions occurring in pediatrics. The family should be encouraged to explore local resources for respite care. This can be of value in the event of family illness and can allow the family vacation time. A decision on eventual long-term institutional care should be left to the discretion of the family. Assistance can be provided with some medical problems. Seizures occur in many of the disorders and can be treated routinely. Constipation is common and can be managed with stool softeners, laxatives, and enemas. Feeding difficulties will progress and may require blenderized or liquid diets.

Behavioral abnormalities, including emotional outbursts, crying out as if in pain, and failure to sleep at night, are extremely burdensome for the family. Sedative medications may assist a family in managing a child at home, but erratic responses to drugs are not unusual in the face of brain damage. Chloral hydrate (50 mg/kg per dose) or a long-acting benzodiazepine (e.g., lorazepam, 0.02 to 0.05 mg/kg per dose) can be effective. Nonsteroidal anti-inflammatory agents may be helpful in the management of joint pain. Behavioral difficulties are particularly severe in the Sanfilippo mucopolysaccharidoses but occur with other juvenile disorders. Major tranquilizers, such as thioridazine HCl (Mellaril,† in doses up to 3 mg/kg/day), may be quite helpful.

Finally, there may be many difficult ethical decisions to be made late in the course of the disease. When endless hours are required for each feeding, nasogastric tube feeding or gastrostomy may be indicated. Discussions with the family should be held prior to beginning artificial feeding, since these techniques may prolong the life of a helpless child, a result that may or may not be desired by the family. The family should be involved in deciding when to hospitalize and how to manage pneumonias in terminally ill children.

*Fabry disease is caused by the deficiency of α-galactosidase activity, which is responsible for the degradation of α-galactosyl terminal glycolipids. The main storage product is trihexosylceramide, formed from the action of β-hexosaminidase on globoside, the major red blood cell glycosphingolipid.[2]

†*Manufacturer's precaution:* Mellaril is not recommended for children under 2 years of age.

Enzyme Therapy

Specific correction of the enzyme defects in these diseases is a subject of active research. Although prenatal diagnosis and other reproductive options can prevent the disease in subsequent siblings, these diseases will continue to occur unless heterozygote screening, as applied to Tay-Sachs disease, can be extended to other disorders. For the present, effective therapy is a major need. Enzyme replacement is one modality. Enzyme activity can be delivered to some organs, such as the liver and spleen. There might be cause for optimism that certain non–central nervous system (CNS) manifestations could be treatable by enzyme infusion. To be effective in treating CNS damage, enzyme replacement must overcome the additional obstacle of the blood-brain barrier. A mannose-modified human placental glucocerebrosidase preparation (Ceredase) has been approved by the Food and Drug Administration (FDA) for the treatment of type I Gaucher disease. Early clinical results indicate that this therapy can alleviate the anemia, bone disease, and hepatosplenomegaly associated with the condition. The recommended starting regimen is 60 units/kg IV every 2 weeks. Therapy with Ceredase is extraordinarily expensive, and the indications for its use are the subject of current research.

Bone Marrow Transplants

Recent reports have revived interest in bone marrow transplantation as a mode of therapy. Bone marrow transplantation has been performed for a wide variety of these disorders. Success in either halting or slowing the progression of peripheral complications has been demonstrated in Hurler, Maroteaux-Lamy, and Gaucher diseases. Some families may wish to explore the opportunities for their children to participate in human studies, but treatment or prevention of CNS symptoms is uncertain at present. For a few patients with Hurler disease and metachromatic leukodystrophy, the progression of CNS deterioration was reported to be slowed following transplant, but long-term follow-up will be necessary.

Bone marrow transplantation remains in the category of a research therapy used in a small fraction of patients. Many variables are relevant to the decision whether or not to explore transplantation, including exact diagnosis, age at diagnosis, attitude of the family, and availability of a human leukocyte antigen (HLA)-matched, unaffected sibling donor.

Gene Replacement

The hope of replacing the defective gene itself *(somatic gene therapy)* is still quite uncertain, although considerably more realistic than at the time of the last edition of this book. Numerous complementary DNAs (cDNAs) for genes encoding lysosomal enzymes have been cloned. Strategies for gene therapy are being formulated, and human trials are under way for adenosine deaminase deficiency. Because alternative treatment is so limited, lysosomal storage diseases are attracting research interest. On the other hand, there are potential drawbacks, such as the possible need to target genetic material to the CNS. Considerable obstacles still remain, and the feasibility of such therapy remains in question.

Counseling

The final aspect of management of the lysosomal storage diseases is concerned with the family and prevention of future cases. The first step is complete *genetic counseling,* including a discussion of the risk of the disease, the burden of the disease, and reproductive options. In autosomal recessive conditions, the major risk is for subsequent pregnancies of the parents of the propositus. Occasionally, a sibling of the mother will marry a sibling of the father, creating a high-risk situation. Genetic counseling must be extended to maternal relatives in the case of X-linked diseases. Heterozygote detection is feasible for most of the diseases in question and can be offered to aunts, uncles, and unaffected siblings of the parents with autosomal recessive disorders. For reliable heterozygote detection, however, a laboratory should have substantial experience in assaying normal controls and obligate heterozygotes. Samples from the obligate heterozygote parents of the propositus should be assayed simultaneously to assist in family-specific interpretation of unusual laboratory data which may result from rare alleles (mutant forms of the gene) in a family. Heterozygote testing of relatives is most important in disorders in which the carrier frequency is great, such as for Gaucher or Tay-Sachs disease in the Ashkenazi Jewish population. Mass screening for heterozygotes has been applied for the prevention of Tay-Sachs disease but has not been used significantly for other lysosomal storage diseases to date.

As part of the genetic counseling process, contraception, sterilization, adoption, and artificial insemination should be discussed as alternative methods for reducing the risk of disease. Prenatal diagnosis has been accomplished for almost all the lysosomal storage diseases. The enzyme defects routinely are demonstrable in cultured fibroblasts and amniotic fluid cells. The newer diagnostic procedure of *chorionic villus biopsy* is proving reliable for most or all lysosomal storage diseases. This earlier prenatal test is attractive to many families with these high genetic risks. The vast majority of biochemical prenatal diagnoses in the last decade has involved the lysosomal storage diseases, with Tay-Sachs disease, type II glycogen storage disease, Krabbe leukodystrophy, metachromatic leukodystrophy, and Hurler disease among the most frequently tested.

REFERENCES

1. Behrman RE, Vaughan VC III: Nelson Textbook of Pediatrics, 13th ed. Philadelphia, WB Saunders Co, 1987, p 333.
2. *Ibid.*, p. 332.

11

Connective Tissue

JUVENILE RHEUMATOID ARTHRITIS

ILONA S. SZER, M.D.

The rheumatic diseases are a diverse group of conditions characterized by inflammation of the connective tissues. Manifestations of this chronic inflammation may include arthritis, fever, and rash as well as evidence of specific extra-articular organ inflammation, such as nephritis, carditis, and uveitis.

To control the often crippling, and sometimes fatal, sequelae of inflammation, the management of rheumatic diseases in children calls for a coordinated, interdisciplinary approach that not only addresses specific disease manifestations but also ensures normal function for both child and family at home, at school, and in the local community.

A high level of expertise is required from professionals experienced in dealing with children and skilled in pediatric rheumatology, nursing, physical and occupational therapy, nutrition, social services, ophthalmology, and orthopedics. Ideally, this team of experts should be available each and every time the child is seen at the tertiary pediatric rheumatology center to avoid fragmentation of care, miscommunication, and multiple visits.

At the level of the local community, a similar team of consistent providers led by the pediatrician should be identified. All of the health providers must have knowledge of the federal and state education laws regarding special services for chronically ill children. Through education, the parents become child advocates and, as such, members of the management team. Yearly school meetings should be encouraged and, whenever possible, attended by a member of the health care team to outline the specific education plan for the child and ensure optimal function in the classroom.

JUVENILE RHEUMATOID ARTHRITIS

The principles of therapy for children with various types of juvenile rheumatoid arthritis (JRA) are largely the same whether the onset of disease was pauciarticular (four or less joints involved), systemic, or polyarticular (five or more joints involved), even though these onset subtypes represent distinct clinical entities with the common feature of chronic joint inflammation. The overall prognosis for children with JRA is good, although children with pauciarticular onset juvenile rheumatoid arthritis carry a more favorable prognosis regarding long-term joint function than do children who have multiple joint involvement. Because rapid bony destruction is less common in children than adults and many will achieve remission prior to adulthood, maintenance of proper joint function and strength is critical. This is accomplished by anti-inflammatory drugs and physical and/or occupational therapy.

The goal of initial drug therapy is to reduce inflammation, which produces pain, swelling, warmth, and tenderness. Once pain control is achieved, children are able to tolerate an individualized exercise program aimed at maintaining normal ambulation, joint range of motion, muscle strength, and at reducing and preventing flexion contractures and muscle atrophy. With daily physical and occupational therapy, most children with arthritis are fit to participate in normal recreation and play and to be independent in activities of daily living, including unassisted ambulation. The use of wheelchairs, buggies, and crutches should never be encouraged. These and other assistive devices should be deferred for as long as possible. Above all, a positive attitude toward an independent and productive future should be encouraged and practiced.

Drug Therapy

Control of inflammation is the goal of the medical therapy for children with chronic arthritis. In general, the milder the disease, the less medicine will be required to achieve control. Approximately 5 per cent of children with JRA may not require drug treatment because they do not experience pain, stiffness, or limitation of motion. Mild, painless swelling that does not interfere with function may be left untreated unless there is muscle atrophy from even minimal favoring or leg length discrepancy resulting from accelerated local growth.

Nonsteroidal Anti-inflammatory Drugs (NSAIDs)

Salicylates. In some centers, salicylates remain the mainstay of treatment for children with JRA. Salicylates come in a variety of sizes and preparations requiring different dosing regimens (Table 1). In general, an anti-inflammatory serum level of approximately 20 mg/dl or 200 mg/L can be achieved within 10 days of initiating salicylates at 70 to 100 mg/kg/day for children weighing less than 25 kg and 50 to 70 mg/kg/day for children whose weight exceeds 25 kg. The dose for all patients should be titrated to the desired clinical response, as some children respond to a lower dose whereas others may require a much higher amount. For example, children with systemic-onset JRA often benefit from salicylate doses above 120 mg/kg/day to achieve the required anti-inflammatory level and subsequent control of symptoms.

Unfortunately, the rate of intolerance rises when the sali-

TABLE 1. Drug Therapy for Chronic Childhood Arthritis

	Size (mg/tab)	Schedule	Dose (mg/kg/day)	Maximum Amount (mg/day)
Nonsteroidal Anti-inflammatory Drugs (NSAIDs)				
Salicylate preparations				
Acetylsalicylate (aspirin)	81,325	q.i.d.	60–100 to achieve serum level of 20–25 mg/dl	
ZORprin	800	b.i.d.		
Choline Mg (Trilisate)	500*	t.i.d.		
Choline Salicylate (Arthropan)	650*	t.i.d.		
Nonsalicylate NSAIDs approved for children				
Tolmetin sodium (Tolectin)	200,400	t.i.d.	15–30	2000
Naproxen (Naprosyn)	250,375,500	b.i.d.	10–20	750
Naproxen liquid	125*	b.i.d. or t.i.d.	10–15	750
NSAIDs not approved for use in children				
Indomethacin (Indocin)	25, 75SR	bid, t.i.d., or q.i.d.	1–3	200
Ibuprofen (Motrin, Advil)	200,300,400	q.i.d.	30–70	2400
Fenoprofen Calcium (Nalfon)	200,300,600	q.i.d.	40–50	3200
Meclofenamate Sodium (Meclomen)	50,100	t.i.d.	4–6	300
Sulindac (Clinoril)†	150,200	b.i.d.	4–6	400
Piroxicam (Feldene)†	10,20	o.d.	0.5	20
Diclofenac (Voltaren)†	25,50,75	b.i.d.	2–3	100–200
Slow-Acting Antirheumatic Drugs (SAARDs)				
Gold salts				
Myochrysine, Salgenol	3	Every week (IM)	0.5–1‡	25–50§
Auranofin (Ridaura)		o.d.	0.1	
Hydroxychloroquine (Plaquenil)	200	o.d.	7.0	300
Methotrexate	2.5	Every week (IM or p.o.)	0.1–0.3‡	20-25§

*mg/5 ml.
†Not tested in children.
‡mg/kg/week.
§per week.
Abbreviations: o.d., once a day; b.i.d., twice a day; t.i.d., three times a day; q.i.d., four times a day; IM, intramuscularly; Mg, magnesium.

cylate level approaches 25 to 30 mg/dl. The most commonly encountered side effects in young children are irritability and personality changes, with concomitant rise in hepatic transaminase levels. These abnormalities are usually dose-related and resolve when the drug is reduced or stopped. Nausea, vomiting, and rapid, heavy breathing, indicating metabolic acidosis, are clear indicators of salicylism and call for prompt discontinuation of the drug. The risk of Reye syndrome, associated with salicylate intake, has recently been emphasized. Fortunately, only a handful of case reports describe an association of high-dose, chronic salicylate use with Reye syndrome. In our clinic, we recommend stopping aspirin temporarily for children with chickenpox or flu-like syndrome with vomiting. In addition, we recommend flu vaccines for children receiving salicylates. During the last several years, other NSAIDs (see below) have replaced salicylates in many clinics, largely because of their less frequent (and thus easier) dosing regimens and less frequent liver toxicity.

Nonsalicylated NSAIDs. Tolmetin sodium (Tolectin) and naproxen (Naprosyn) are the only other NSAIDs labeled by the Food and Drug Administration (FDA) for use in children with chronic arthritis (Table 1). At a dose of 20 to 30 mg/kg/day, tolmetin can be the initial agent tried or may substitute for aspirin in children who either do not respond to salicylates or cannot tolerate a dose required to achieve control. Tolmetin is usually well tolerated, but its effectiveness may not be as great as that of salicylates or naproxen. A 1-month trial is probably sufficient, although 3 months may be needed before the treatment is switched to another agent. Gastrointestinal irritation and, rarely, headaches may limit the utility of tolmetin administration and necessitate change to another drug.

Naproxen is the most recently approved agent for the treatment of childhood arthritis. This drug is preferred because of its easier, twice-daily dosing schedule. It is also available in liquid form appropriate for young children. As with tolmetin, naproxen may take weeks to control symptoms; however, it is well tolerated and safe. Rarely, gastrointestinal intolerance, headache, and drowsiness necessitate discontinuation. A recent report found an association between naproxen and a distinctive photodermatitis, termed Naprosyn-induced pseudo-porphyria, particularly in children who are blond and have fair skin. In several clinics, children have been identified who developed scarring after minor trauma on sun-exposed areas, such as the nose and cheeks. Naproxen has been discontinued in these youngsters.

Ibuprofen has recently been approved for children to treat fever and minor aches and pain, but the indication for arthritis is still pending.

Over the last decade, many additional NSAIDs have become available for adults with arthritis; some of these have been tested in children through collaborative multicenter trials. Dosing, efficacy, and side effects are known, but there is no approval from the FDA for use in children. These include fenoprofen, meclofenamate sodium, and indomethacin (Table 1). In our clinic, we usually start with naproxen, followed by tolmetin or salicylates. If any of the approved agents or combinations fails to control inflammation sufficiently, we try an NSAID not approved for children but one that has been studied for both safety and efficacy in a pediatric setting. All anti-inflammatory medications should be taken with milk or after a meal. It may also be appropriate to prescribe antacids such as Maalox, Mylanta, or Tums. Sucralfate may also be used prophylactically.

The total length of treatment varies for each patient. Generally, anti-inflammatory therapy is required for as long as there is active inflammation. For most children with pauciarticular onset JRA, therapy is continued for 1 to 2 years using as parameters the clinical signs and symptoms and weaning the medicine 3 to 4 months after signs of inflammation have subsided. Blood tests may not be of value in assessing the activity of the disease but may be used for those patients whose test findings were abnormal at the onset of the disease. The antinuclear antibody, often positive in children with arthritis, particularly if complicated by iritis, may remain in the serum for many years and does not serve as a guide to drug management.

Children with polyarticular and systemic-onset JRA require treatment for prolonged periods of time, often marked by times of lesser disease activity during which lower doses, or no medicine, may be given. The principle of the least medicine sufficient to control inflammation that interferes with normal function applies at all times.

Second-Line Agents

The slow-acting, antirheumatic drugs (SAARDs), also known as disease-modifying or remittive agents, are reserved for those children with aggressive, multijoint disease who are at risk for crippling and disability. These children are adversely affected despite proper use of NSAIDs and are threatened with poor function such as nonambulation. Administration of SAARDs, which include gold salts, penicillamine, hydroxychloroquine, and sulfasalazine, must be carried out in a pediatric rheumatology setting because of the high risk of side effects and the absolute need for close follow-up. Gold salts, previously available only in the form of intramuscular injection (Myochrysine or Salgenol), are now available in pill form (Auranofin). Both preparations have been studied in children and are only mildly effective but quite toxic. Up to 30 per cent of children do not tolerate intramuscular gold, necessitating its withdrawal. The incidence of side effects as well as efficacy is somewhat less with the oral preparation. Reasons for discontinuation include allergic rashes and itching, mouth sores, diarrhea, proteinuria, and eosinophilia. Children with systemic-onset JRA are at a serious, albeit small additional risk for the development of life-threatening disseminated intravascular coagulation (DIC) reported after the second injection of intramuscular gold. This complication has not been reported following administration of Auranofin, although it has been seen in children with systemic-onset JRA who did not receive IM gold. Although the potential for inducing remission exists with gold therapy, this event is exceedingly rare. More commonly, there seems to be a modification of disease activity with improved function, less pain and stiffness, and more endurance. It may take up to 6 months for clinically appreciable change to occur, but a positive effect may be noted after the 2nd month. A 6-month trial of one or the other form of gold is usually attempted for selective patients.

Hydroxychloroquine (Plaquenil) is commonly used for adults with arthritis. This agent, the mechanism of action of which is not understood, has been studied in children and found no more effective than placebo. However, because of its relative short-term safety, it may be tried for 3 to 6 months if the disease is not too aggressive and if time is of no issue. Long-term toxicity of hydroxychloroquine is limited to the eyes and secondary to accumulation of the drug in the macula. We recommend twice yearly ophthalmologic evaluations and discontinue the drug if there is interference with color or peripheral vision.

D-Penicillamine, often helpful in adult rheumatoid arthritis, has not been found effective in children when compared with placebo. The rate of side effects is high, making this agent of limited, if any, use in the pediatric rheumatology setting.

Sulfasalazine (Azulfidine), a combination of salicylate and sulfa, effective in controlling symptoms of inflammatory bowel disease, has been studied in adults with arthritis and used anecdotally in children. It appears to be safe and efficacious in treating arthritis. Controlled studies in children with arthritis are needed, but in the meantime the drug has been used safely and effectively, particularly in adolescents with spondyloarthropathies.

Corticosteroids

Systemic and local steroids have a limited, but important, role in the treatment of JRA. Their use should be restricted to the pediatric rheumatology clinic and avoided at all costs. There are, however, several specific criteria for their use.

First, systemic steroids are often needed to control extra-articular manifestations of systemic-onset JRA, such as hectic fever, anemia, and pericarditis. Steroids should be weaned and gradually discontinued as soon as control of these signs and symptoms is achieved. Although the initial indication for corticosteroids is not arthritis, joint inflammation responds exceedingly well to steroids and tapering may result in severe flare of arthritis. Small doses of prednisone (1 to 5 mg daily or every other day) may enable an otherwise bedridden child to function independently.

Second, a local steroid injection into an inflamed or contracted joint may significantly improve functioning in a child with monoarticular disease that is unresponsive to medical and physical therapy. Some pediatric rheumatologists advocate repeated injections and have shown that some children thus treated undergo remission and do not require further intervention. The use of steroid drops in the treatment of eye inflammation is reviewed elsewhere.

Although steroids are potent anti-inflammatory agents and offer rapid relief of symptoms, the many risks associated with their administration—in addition to osteoporosis, avascular necrosis of bone, and muscle atrophy—should absolutely discourage their use in children with chronic joint inflammation.

Third-Line Agents

Cytotoxic drugs, which include methotrexate, cyclophosphamide (Cytoxan), azathioprine (Imuran), chlorambucil (Leukeran), and cyclosporin A, are reserved for those children whose disease is crippling and unresponsive to conventional therapies.

However, methotrexate is now used earlier in children at risk and appears both safe and extremely efficacious in preventing joint destruction. A multicenter methotrexate trial has been completed and documents significant improvement in children who received methotrexate compared with those receiving placebo; there were no serious side effects noted during a 6-month trial. Thus, this agent is effective while not posing a high risk of side effects. As with adult trials, methotrexate was effective in 70 per cent of pediatric patients in contrast to 20 per cent receiving placebo. Most patients who respond, however, may not enter true remission. Recent data from studies of adult patients suggest that the dose may need to be increased with time and that discontinuation of the drug may result in severe, hard-to-control exacerbations. These considerations in children are all the more potent, since we may be committing our young patients to a lifetime of cytotoxic therapy. Side effects may include bone marrow, liver, and, rarely, renal and gonadal toxicity.

Azathioprine, cyclophosphamide, chlorambucil, and cyclosporine A have not been studied in children with JRA.

Physical Management

Physical and occupational therapy form a cornerstone in the management of chronic childhood arthritis. Because the potential for remission exists for many children, it is imperative to preserve joint integrity. Tendon and ligament shortening and muscle atrophy are common in JRA. The goal of a physical therapy program, including passive, active, and resistive exercises, is to preserve full range of motion and muscle strength. This is accomplished by a daily exercise program carried out at home by the parent, at school by a school therapist, or in a hospital or health club setting. Normal play and recreation are always encouraged.

The goal of occupational therapy is to preserve independence in activities of daily living and age-appropriate function, often curtailed by arthritis of the small joints of the hands and wrists. Daily exercise in addition to specific training in various tasks is prescribed and monitored by the occupational therapist.

Nighttime use of splinting devices and braces should be limited to persistent contractures only. The most frequent use of splinting is in wrist arthritis to arrest progressive loss of wrist dorsiflexion (extension) or ulnar deviation and to prevent hand weakness. Splints are fabricated to encourage as much dorsiflexion and position of function as possible. We do not prescribe resting or day splints unless children report hand fatigue while writing. Air splints may sometimes be used for children with elbow flexion contractures or small children with knee contractures, at night only. Bivalve knee braces are used during sleep for children with flexion contractures. Small lifts are frequently placed inside shoes or over the soles for children with leg length discrepancy. This is particularly common in youngsters with pauciarticular-onset JRA with one knee or ankle inflammation. Leg lengths must be monitored regularly because with time the discrepancy diminishes and the lift should be removed.

Complications (Iridocyclitis)

One of the most important and potentially devastating extra-articular complications of JRA is inflammation of the anterior uveal tract. Iritis or iridocyclitis is asymptomatic, but it can be diagnosed easily by a slit-lamp examination, which reveals cells and flare in the anterior chamber of the eye. Children with pauciarticular-onset JRA are at the highest risk for the development of this complication, which may result in blindness if it remains unrecognized. Ophthalmologic evaluations must be performed quarterly for children with pauciarticular-onset JRA and once or twice per year for all other children with chronic arthritis. The need for slit-lamp examination continues for several years after the arthritis has remitted.

Treatment is highly successful if initiated early before any scarring takes place. Management consists of local steroid eye drops, often given in conjunction with mydriatic drops. Unfortunately, long-term side effects of local steroid application include cataract formation and, rarely, glaucoma.

SYSTEMIC-ONSET JUVENILE RHEUMATOID ARTHRITIS

Extra-articular manifestations of systemic-onset JRA often overshadow the arthritis and necessitate special management. Control of fever may sometimes be accomplished with salicylates alone or with tolmetin, naproxen, or ibuprofen. As already mentioned, rather high doses of salicylate may be needed, presumably as a result of malabsorption, increasing the risk of toxicity as the child improves and begins to absorb the drug. When the illness is complicated by severe anemia and/or pericarditis, systemic steroids are usually required for control. The dose of 1 to 2 mg/kg/day achieves response in virtually all children. Because steroids may lower the serum salicylate level, aspirin levels must be monitored carefully and the dose adjusted appropriately. As steroids are decreased, salicylate levels may rise again.

Pericarditis, if present, is often complicated by a pericardial effusion, which may warrant surgical drainage. The procedure can be done in the cardiac catheterization laboratory, and the drain is left in place for 24 to 48 hours. By this time, systemic steroids usually take effect and drains may be removed. Once control is achieved, steroids are tapered to an alternate-day regimen and slowly discontinued while salicylates or other NSAIDs are maintained. Because systemic manifestations abate in the majority of children within 6 to 12 months, long-term management focuses on arthritis and is identical to that discussed previously.

SPONDYLOARTHROPATHY SYNDROMES

Adolescents with spondyloarthritis are treated similarly to youngsters with other forms of chronic arthritis, with additional attention to lumbosacral spine flexibility and chest expansion. The physical therapy program focuses on both range of motion and strengthening of low back and respiratory muscles. It is generally believed that spondyloarthritis responds better to tolmetin and naproxen than to salicylates. Similarly, gold is thought not helpful for this form of arthritis; however, in the occasional patient with severe peripheral joint involvement, it may be of benefit. Gold or other SAARDs have not been studied in patients with spondyloarthritis, neither is there any experience with methotrexate. Sulfasalazine has been shown to benefit adult patients with spondyloarthropathies, and we have used it as well as methotrexate successfully in adolescent males. Eye involvement in spondyloarthritis is usually symptomatic and responds well to local steroid drops.

DERMATOMYOSITIS

The treatment of children with dermatomyositis varies from center to center (see also Section 14, p. 480). Although all pediatric rheumatologists treat this disease with steroids and physical therapy, dosing schedules vary greatly.

In our clinic, the approach to dermatomyositis is aggressive and results have been encouraging. The course of treatment can be summarized as induction and maintenance therapy, which is completed over a 2-year period in most children. The initial dose of prednisone is between 2 to 3 mg/kg/day using a split regimen. Physical therapy is initiated early and prescribed twice daily to improve strength and mobility. Stretching of Achilles tendons and hamstrings is imperative. Children are seen weekly or admitted to the hospital if there is any compromise of the palatal or respiratory muscles.

Once muscle enzymes return to normal (2 to 8 weeks), the dose is consolidated to once daily and maintained until muscle strength reaches near normal level (2 to 3 months). At this time, follow-up can be adjusted to monthly visits and the dose tapered every month by 10 per cent, provided that muscle enzymes remain normal and muscle strength continues to improve.

Within 12 to 18 months, the daily dose is usually weaned to 5 mg/day, where it is maintained for another 6 to 8 months and then slowly discontinued. With this protocol, many children are functioning well within 2 to 3 months and are at less risk for late complications of poorly controlled disease, such as muscle contractures, persistent weakness, and calcinosis. We do not use alternate-day steroid therapy for dermatomyositis, but others do.

The rate of complications, except for commonly encountered cushingoid appearance, weight gain, and temporary growth arrest, has been low in our patients. Occasionally, however, the prednisone cannot be tapered because of recurrence of weakness. For those patients, cytotoxic therapy, usually given in the form of methotrexate, either orally or through intramuscular injections at 1 mg/kg/week (usually not exceeding 20 to 25 mg weekly), is prescribed. Following the addition of methotrexate, prednisone can usually be tapered to 5 mg/day followed by cautious and gradual methotrexate elimination.

Treatment of Skin Manifestations

The rash of dermatomyositis usually begins to fade as muscle strength improves and does not require special treatment. In some children, however, severe cutaneous manifestations develop. Sunscreens and other devices protecting skin from ultraviolet light should be tried. Steroid creams usually do not help. Hydroxychloroquine may be of use in some cases. The dose is the same as that for arthritis (Table 1).

Vasculitic ulcers are common early signs in dermatomyositis. These respond to corticosteroid treatment but often become super-infected with skin flora and require local hygiene, frequent soaking, and systemic antibiotics.

SYSTEMIC LUPUS ERYTHEMATOSUS

BALU H. ATHREYA, M.D.

Systemic lupus erythematosus (SLE) is a multisystem disease with protean manifestations. The natural history of the disease is characterized by exacerbations and remissions, and the variability of manifestations between individuals makes it difficult to conduct controlled clinical trials of available forms of therapy. There are also differences of approach in defining what constitutes activity of the disease and what constitutes a flare. Consequently, treatment of SLE is largely empirical, even in 1993, and should be managed in conjunction with a pediatric rheumatologist experienced in the care of these patients.

GENERAL MANAGEMENT PRINCIPLES

General principles of management of SLE in children should include:

1. Individualizing treatment according to the organ system(s) involved and the severity of the involvement.
2. Preventing major flares to the extent possible by avoidance of precipitating factors, such as sun exposure, certain drugs, and emotional stress.
3. Detecting and managing flares early.
4. Minimizing the toxicity related to therapeutic modalities.
5. Recognizing and treating secondary problems, such as bacteremia, pneumonitis, and hypertension promptly.
6. Planning for the child's growth and psychosocial development—not just for the disease.

Careful attention should be paid to the following general measures: (1) education of the child and the family; (2) counseling on nutrition, exercise, and precipitating factors, such as exposure to sun and medications; (3) stress reduction; (4) discussions concerning sex education, including use of birth control methods and risks of pregnancy; (5) discussions about the effects of disease and drugs on growth and development; and (6) discussions that involve educational and vocational counseling.

PHARMACOLOGIC THERAPY

The rash of SLE with or without mild systemic symptoms, such as fever, malaise, and arthralgia, is best treated with an antimalarial drug (hydroxychloroquine) starting at 7 mg/kg/day for 2 months, then reduced to 5 mg/kg/day, with the maximum daily dose not to exceed 400 mg. Topical steroids may also be used for limited cutaneous involvement, with care taken not to induce cutaneous atrophy (especially facial).

For more resistant dermatitis (e.g., lupus profundus), dapsone may be tried in an experimental protocol. It is important to test for glucose-6-phosphate dehydrogenase (G-6-PD) deficiency before using hydroxychloroquine and dapsone.

Nonsteroidal anti-inflammatory drugs (NSAIDs), for example, salicylates, tolmetin, indomethacin, and naproxen, may be beneficial for children with low-grade fever, arthritis, and mild pleuropericarditis with or without the addition of small doses of prednisone (0.25 mg/kg/day). However, NSAIDs are known to cause hepatotoxicity (particularly with salicylates) and, infrequently, serious nephrotoxicity. Therefore, careful monitoring is indicated. *Because ibuprofen has been associated with an aseptic meningitis syndrome in SLE, this is not a preferred NSAID for patients with SLE.* Salicylsalicylic acid, choline-magnesium salicylate, and sulindac may be safer nonsteroidal drugs for use in patients with SLE, although they have not been approved for use in children.

Prednisone (0.5 to 1 mg/kg/day in divided doses) is indicated for moderate systemic disease, including high fever, myositis, mild pleuropericarditis, arthritis, weight loss, and lymphadenopathy. For more severe disease characterized by high fever, pleuropericarditis, or myocarditis, hemolytic anemia, thrombocytopenia, most neurologic problems, and glomerulonephritis, high-dose oral prednisone (2 mg/kg/day in divided doses) is used for 4 to 6 weeks followed by gradual tapering after stabilization of the activity of the disease. Although the benefits of intravenous (IV) bolus methylprednisolone ("pulse steroid" therapy) are not well established in conditions other than rapidly progressive renal disease, one may use this form of therapy in acutely ill children with rapidly progressive multisystem disease. Caution is indicated in the use of "pulse steroid therapy" in the presence of an infection, hypertension, electrolyte abnormalities, or myocarditis. The dose is usually given as 30 mg/kg of methylprednisolone (maximum dose: 1000 mg) suspended in 50 to 100 ml of 5 per cent dextrose in water (D_5W) over 45 to 60 minutes with careful, frequent monitoring of cardiac status and blood pressure. In children with hypertension, it may be safer to administer the calculated dose slowly over 1 to 2 hours.

Recent studies have established the value of IV cyclophosphamide for severe renal disease in adults. In a recent multicenter trial involving children and adolescents with SLE, IV cyclophosphamide was used only in children who had failed to establish a satisfactory response to optimal steroid treatment. In the presence of rapidly progressive renal disease (particularly diffuse proliferative glomerulonephritis), one may elect to use IV cyclophosphamide as follows after informed parental consent: 750 to 1000 mg/m^2 body surface once a month for 6 months; some centers continue this therapy once every 2 to 3 months for 1 to 2 more years. A nadir white blood cell (WBC) count should be done 10 to 14 days after each dose and the dose adjusted to maintain the WBC count in the 3000 to 4000/mm^3 range. Recent reports indicate that this therapy is not curative; indeed, the disease tends to flare when the treatment is stopped. One hopes, however, to achieve a satisfactory delay in the progression of the renal lesion. This form of therapy reduces the bladder toxicity of oral cyclophosphamide (hemorrhagic cystitis), but the long-term effects on fertility and oncogenicity are of concern.

Once the disease is brought under control, the aim of further therapy should be to reduce the dose of prednisone to the lowest possible level consistent with control of activity, preferably given every other day. Azathioprine, methotrexate, and hydroxychloroquine may be used as steroid-sparing agents to achieve this goal, depending on the organ system involved and the severity of the disease.

One other treatment of value is intravenous human gamma-immunoglobulin; this is particularly useful for the treatment of the thrombocytopenia in SLE and, to a lesser extent, for the treatment of hemolytic anemia. The dose is 1 g/kg to be given on two consecutive days. For severe rapidly progressive disease with multisystem involvement, the use of plasmapheresis in combination with IV cyclophosphamide is justifiable.

FOLLOW-UP

Serologic abnormalities (anti-ds DNA antibodies, complement) alone without evidence of increasing disease activity do not necessitate treatment. In children already taking steroids or immunosuppressive agents for established organ system involvement, some authorities believe that serologic abnormalities should be normalized as nearly as possible to avoid irreversible renal disease. However, such a goal of therapy may lead to the use of unacceptable doses of steroids for prolonged periods, subjecting the child to the other drug-related morbidities of SLE—opportunistic infections, aseptic necrosis, premature atherosclerosis, and early myocardial infarction. Therefore, I do not try to normalize serology—if the patient is clinically well. However, I use serologic tests to help me decide how rapidly to withdraw steroids.

The prognosis for childhood SLE has improved considerably with a 10-year survival rate of over 95 per cent. However, data on long-term effects of the disease (chronic renal failure, organic brain disease) and treatment (growth failure, sterility, atherosclerosis, myocardial infarction, and malignancy) are not available or only now becoming recognized. Future studies on these very important clinical issues and on the use of biologic or pharmacologic agents with more precise immunomodulatory effects are expected to improve the treatment and outcome of children with SLE.

12

Genitourinary Tract

RENAL HYPOPLASIA AND DYSPLASIA

ELLIS D. AVNER, M.D.

Renal hypoplasia and dysplasia are developmental abnormalities of the kidney that result in a reduced number of complete nephrons or abnormal parenchymal differentiation, respectively. Renal hypoplasia is the consequence of failed inductive interaction of ureteral bud and metanephric blastema, whereas renal dysplasia results from abnormal inductive interaction of these renal anlagen at any time during nephrogenesis (mid first to mid third trimester of gestation). Although each has a precise histopathologic definition, hypoplasia and dysplasia often coexist in the same kidney and can be difficult to differentiate clinically and radiographically. Both hypoplasia and dysplasia can be unilateral or bilateral, and diffuse or focal. These patterns of renal involvement give rise to distinct clinical syndromes with sets of signs, symptoms, and disease associations that mandate specific monitoring and management strategies.

BILATERAL HYPOPLASIA AND DYSPLASIA

Both hypoplasia and dysplasia may occur as isolated abnormalities or in association with central nervous system malformations and certain genetically determined syndromes (Meckel, Jeune, Zellweger, branchio-oto-renal, Beckwith-Wiedemann, Laurence-Moon-Biedl, oral-facial-digital I). Bilateral renal hypoplasia and dysplasia are commonly associated with obstructive abnormalities of the ureters or lower urinary tract. The clinical manifestations and renal prognosis of bilateral hypoplasia or dysplasia are based on the volume of functioning renal parenchyma present. In their most severe forms, in which embryonic dysgenesis at an early stage of renal formation leads to minute kidneys or totally disorganized renal parenchyma with little if any functioning renal mass, severe oligohydramnios leads to the neonatally lethal pulmonary hypoplasia of Potter syndrome. Although chronic renal failure can be treated from birth even in small premature infants, there is currently no effective long-term therapy for the pulmonary insufficiency associated with inadequate lung development. More commonly, infants with bilateral hypoplasia or dysplasia survive the neonatal period and, as infants or young children, present with small kidneys and decreased renal function. Even with a relatively well preserved glomerular filtration rate, tubular sodium wasting and an inability to concentrate the urine maximally are common clinical features. Affected individuals are thus particularly susceptible to severe volume depletion with common childhood illnesses that produce fever, vomiting, or diarrhea. In addition, tubular acidosis may lead to chronic failure to thrive and osteodystrophy.

Because of the strong association of renal dysplasia with obstructive uropathy and vesicoureteral reflux, infants and children with bilaterally small kidneys should undergo ultrasonography, with further evaluation (i.e., voiding cystourethrography) as indicated. Overall management includes genetic counseling for parents because, in cases of severe bilateral dysgenesis, the risk of having another affected child is 3.5 to 4.4 per cent (>200 times the normal prevalence rate). In addition, parents of severely affected infants and their unaffected children have an increased risk of having silent genitourinary malformations. Specific management includes sodium and free water supplementation based on measured urinary losses, and alkali supplementation to maintain serum bicarbonate levels between 22 and 26 mEq/L. Suppressive antibiotics are indicated if vesicoureteral reflux is present. Although data are sparse, infants and children with bilateral hypoplasia or dysplasia may be at some increased risk of hypertension, renal infection, and nephrolithiasis. Periodic monitoring for such complications, therefore, is recommended. As detailed in other articles in this section, chronic renal failure is treated with aggressive nutritional support, dietary phosphate binders, 1,25-dihydroxyvitamin D, erythropoietin, and dialysis, as indicated.

UNILATERAL HYPOPLASIA AND DYSPLASIA

Single small kidneys are not uncommonly detected by routine abdominal ultrasonography in asymptomatic infants and children. In most instances, such kidneys have histopathologic elements of both hypoplasia and dysplasia and are commonly associated with ipsilateral ureteral obstructive abnormalities or vesicoureteral reflux. Unilateral hypoplasia and dysplasia have been associated with a small but statistically significant increased risk of hypertension, and patients should be monitored accordingly. In the presence of obstruction or vesicoureteral reflux, nephrolithiasis and pyelonephritis may occur and require specific therapy.

A particular clinical syndrome of unilateral hypoplasia is segmental hypoplasia, or the Ask-Upmark kidney. Patients with segmental hypoplasia often present with severe hypertension, and the ensuing evaluation reveals a small kidney with diminished lobulation and deep transverse grooves on its cortical surface. Although previously believed to be a unique type of hypoplasia in which nephrogenesis has been arrested in one or a few renal lobules after the formation of juxtamedullary nephrons, recent evidence supports the view that the Ask-Upmark kidney is an acquired lesion secondary to vesicoureteral reflux and renal infection. Initial management is directed toward control of hypertension, which is generally associated with an activated renin-angiotensin system and which responds well to angiotensin-converting enzyme inhibitors. Additional evaluation and therapy are directed toward vesicoureteral reflux, if present, and long-term control of infection. In cases of intractable hypertension or infection, nephrectomy or partial nephrectomy may be indicated.

Unilateral multicystic dysplasia represents a unique clinical presentation of unilateral renal dysplasia. Infants and children commonly present with an enlarged cystic abdominal mass of nonfunctioning, dysplastic renal tissue associated with ipsilateral ureteral atresia. Although usually sporadic, unilateral multicystic dysplasia may rarely be familial or associated with ventricular septal defect, tracheoesophageal fistula, trisomy 21, or lumbar myelomeningocele. Radiographic evaluation with ultrasonography, voiding cystourethrography, and radionuclide scanning, recommended in all cases, reveals contralateral renal abnormalities in 30 per cent of cases. Such abnormalities include ureteropelvic junction obstruction, ureterovesicular junction obstruction, and vesicoureteral reflux and require prompt evaluation and therapy to preserve long-term renal function. Traditionally, multicystic dysplastic kidneys have been surgically removed to confirm diagnosis and prevent the reported complications of hypertension, infection, and malignant degeneration. However, in most instances of multicystic dysplastic kidney, ultrasonography, with confirmation, if needed, by radionuclide or computed tomography scanning, is diagnostic and obviates the need for tissue analysis. Furthermore, critical analysis reveals that the reported complications of multicystic dysplasia are rare and, in the case of hypertension and infection, poorly documented. Because most multicystic dysplastic kidneys involute over time, current recommended management includes only serial sonographic evaluations and monitoring for hypertension and infection. Nephrectomy is reserved for cases with atypical sonographic features, failure of involution, or documented infection or hypertension.

All unilateral renal lesions that significantly compromise functioning renal parenchyma lead to contralateral renal hypertrophy. Such findings, coupled with evidence in experimental models that hypertrophy may lead to progressive glomerular hypertension and sclerosis, have led some investigators to recommend low-protein diets or pharmacologic agents that decrease intraglomerular pressure (such as angiotensin-converting enzyme inhibitors) for patients with unilateral renal lesions. There are currently no convincing data that infants or children with unilateral hypoplasia or dysplasia are at significant long-term risk for progressive glomerular sclerosis. Furthermore, to date, results of controlled studies of dietary therapy in children with decreased renal functional mass have not demonstrated any beneficial effects of low-protein diets on preservation of renal function. Thus, low-protein diets (which are unpalatable and may adversely affect growth) and specific therapy with pharmacologic agents, such as angiotensin-converting enzyme inhibitors (with known side effects and unknown long-term effects on the growing child), cannot currently be recommended for infants and children with unilateral renal hypoplasia or dysplasia. However, patients and their parents should be advised of the potential risk of trauma to a hypertrophied unilateral kidney through participation in contact sports.

REFERENCES

Bernstein J, Gilbert-Barness E: Congenital malformations of the kidney. *In* Tisher CC, Brenner BM (eds): Renal Pathology. Philadelphia, JB Lippincott, 1989, p 1278.

HYDRONEPHROSIS AND DISORDERS OF THE URETER

JOHN T. HERRIN, M.D.

Hydronephrosis is a condition in which the renal pelvis is dilated. "Hydroureter" or megaureter indicates the presence of a dilated ureter. In patients with hydronephrosis and significant obstruction, there may be associated caliceal dilatation, renal parenchymal atrophy, and thinning. However, the belief that all hydronephrosis is due to obstruction and requires operative intervention is no longer tenable. Present evidence suggests that in many cases dilatation of the ureter is not associated with obstruction and progressive loss of renal function or parenchyma. Nonobstructive dilatation of the ureter may occur as a primary isolated condition or as a secondary phenomenon (e.g., with prune-belly syndrome, diabetes insipidus, marked concentrating defects following vesicoureteral reflux, or neurogenic bladder).

Hydronephrosis still occurs predominantly as a result of obstruction to the ureteropelvic junction or ureterovesical junction of the ureter. This may result from (1) intrinsic ureteral lesions—adynamic segment or fibrosis; (2) extrinsic obstruction secondary to surrounding fibrous bands, crossing vessel, or localized scarring; or (3) intraluminal obstruction. In the infant and child, intraluminal obstruction is rarely a cause of hydronephrosis but may occur in association with calculus, blood clot, or mechanical obstruction from a "fungus ball." Ureteral polyp and intraureteral tumor are extremely rare.

PRESENTING SYMPTOMS

Most symptomatic cases are demonstrated in the course of investigation of hematuria, urinary tract infection, pain, or enuresis.

A significant number of asymptomatic patients are now found via antenatal ultrasonography or incidentally in the investigation of other congenital anomalies, congenital heart disease, or abdominal pain.

CLASSIFICATION AND GENERAL FEATURES

1. *Obstructive hydronephrosis* (Table 1). This may occur with either intrinsic or extrinsic lesions and is associated with progression. Increasing degrees of dilatation of the pelvis with caliceal dilatation and progressive parenchymal loss with associated loss of renal function follow obstruction.

2. *Nonobstructing hydronephrosis* (Tables 1 and 2). Under certain conditions, there will be partial obstruction or a non-

TABLE 1. Hydronephrosis

Type
Dilated nonobstructive hydronephrosis
True obstruction
Differential Diagnosis
Multicystic kidney disease
Coexisting reflux and hydronephrosis
Abnormalities of rotation/position
Indications for Surgery
Progressive hydronephrosis or renal damage*
Symptomatic disease
Painful hydronephrosis
Recurrent hematuria

*Renal damage as measured by serial studies, radionuclide washout scan, perfusion pressure-flow studies.

TABLE 2. Megaureter*

- **Obstructed**
  - Primary
    - Intrinsic
      - Amuscular segment
      - Atresia
      - Stenosis
      - Ectopic ureter
    - Extrinsic
      - Crossing vessel
      - Fibrous bands
  - Secondary
    - Prune-belly syndrome
    - Neurogenic bladder
    - Megacystis
      - Megaureter syndrome
- **Refluxing**
  - Primary
    - Vesicoureteral reflux
    - Ectopic ureter
  - Secondary
    - Neurogenic bladder
    - Ureterocele
    - Prune-belly syndrome
    - Bladder outlet obstruction
- **Nonobstructed** (Dilated)
  - Nonrefluxing
  - Spontaneous cure reflux
  - Polyuric syndromes
    - Nephrogenic diabetes insipidus
    - Concentrating defects
  - Idiopathic

*In primary obstructed or refluxing megaureter, radiologic anatomy of bladder and urethra is normal. Classification as secondary megaureter or hydronephrosis implies an abnormality in bladder, urethra, or ureter.

progressive lesion. After an initial dilatation of the renal pelvis, stabilization may occur and there is no further loss of renal parenchyma or renal function. Persisting dilatation of the ureter may occur after spontaneous resolution of vesicoureteral reflux.

3. *Prenatal hydronephrosis* (Figs. 1 and 2). The practice of antenatal ultrasonographic examination has led to the demonstration of a group of infants with dilated renal tracts. At present, intrauterine surgery is experimental. Approximately 30 per cent of these lesions will clear spontaneously; thus, reevaluation postnatally at 4 to 10 days is recommended and further action is taken based on the result. Earlier evaluation (days 1 to 2) is recommended if posterior urethral obstruction is suspected from antenatal evaluation.

4. Hydronephrosis and hydroureter *associated with vesicoureteral reflux.*

5. *Transient or intermittent symptomatic hydronephrosis* may produce flank pain, colic, or hematuria of sufficient degree to necessitate therapy. Investigation in this group is required during a symptomatic episode if interval investigation (ultrasonography, intravenous pyelography) fails to demonstrate a lesion.

6. *Intraluminal obstruction* with hydronephrosis. The treatment group involves removal of the intraluminal lesion or nephrostomy and/or stent drainage to bypass the obstructing lesion (e.g., in postoperative edema until the anastomosis and edema clear, leaving an unobstructed ureter).

7. *Ectopic ureter and ureteroceles* may both be associated with obstruction, infection, interference with bladder function, and/or drainage from ipsilateral or contralateral ureters. These anomalies are often associated with duplex systems and, if obstruction is present, antenatally significant dysplasia.

TREATMENT

Treatment depends on associated conditions as well as on the hydronephrosis. Surgical intervention is mandatory in patients with hematuria and/or pain secondary to significant obstruction or rupture after trauma.

In the patient with hydronephrosis found incidentally during antenatal ultrasonography or during investigation for an unrelated condition, objective evaluation should be performed to determine the functional significance (i.e., if the dilated renal pelvis is associated with obstruction that, if left untreated, will lead to progressive loss of renal parenchyma and function) (Table 3).

Standard radiologic methods of anatomic review demonstrate the presence of a dilated system but do not provide an adequate appraisal of degree of obstruction; the magnitude of pelvicaliceal dilatation is not a reliable guide to presence of obstruction. However, sequential review to document degree and progression of obvious damage is best accomplished by standard radiologic tests. In an endeavor to attain treatment before parenchymal loss is present, (1) radionuclide diuretic "washout" scanning and/or (2) pelvic perfusion and pressure studies are performed.

The loss of renal parenchyma is proportional to the *magnitude* and *duration* of raised intrapelvic pressure. The intrapelvic pressure depends on the urine flow rate and the duration of diuresis as well as the degree of obstruction. An elastic dilated system may, in fact, provide partial protection from transmitting pressure to the nephron. Full evaluation and close follow-up are necessary to protect renal function (Table 4). Ureteropelvic systems that are dilated but not obstructed are defined by lack of rise in intrapelvic pressure even under maximal diuresis and thus do not pose a risk for progressive renal damage.

Two major groups of investigations currently used are (1) radionuclide evaluation with a diuretic washout and (2) pressure measurement under perfusion conditions, that is, Whitaker testing or pelvimetrics. There are advantages and drawbacks to each technique because neither directly measures intrarenal pressure.

The diuretic-augmented renal scan is a "noninvasive" isotope study. Prolonged retention of radionuclide in a dilated, unobstructed collecting system results from a reservoir effect. When urine flow is augmented, urine containing tracer leaves the unobstructed system and is replaced by tracer-free urine, providing a washout effect (Table 4).

The pressure perfusion study, on the other hand, is invasive, requiring percutaneous puncture of the renal pelvic collecting system. Sedation and/or general anesthesia may be required. The interpretation of the study rests on the observation that an unobstructed ureter transports fluid at 10 ml/minute with only a mild rise in intrapelvic pressure. A mild to severe obstruction leads to a marked rise in pressure even at lower flow rates.

These techniques measure different parts of the spectrum of obstructions, so differences in results obtained require skilled interpretation to guide therapy. If the techniques are standardized in an institution and if the interpretation is

TABLE 3. Determinants of Progression of Hydronephrosis

1. Parenchymal mass—growth, volume
2. Urine output
3. Urine flow rate
4. Level of intrapelvic pressure
5. Duration of increased intrapelvic pressure
6. Compliance of renal pelvis
7. Outflow restriction

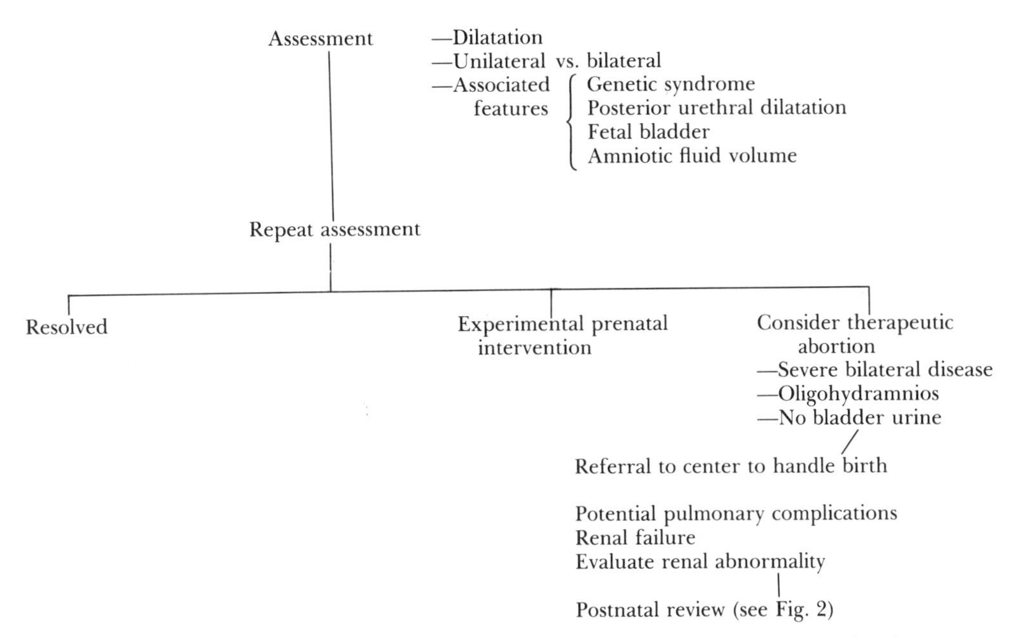

Figure 1. Algorithm for the evaluation and treatment of the patient with hydronephrosis.

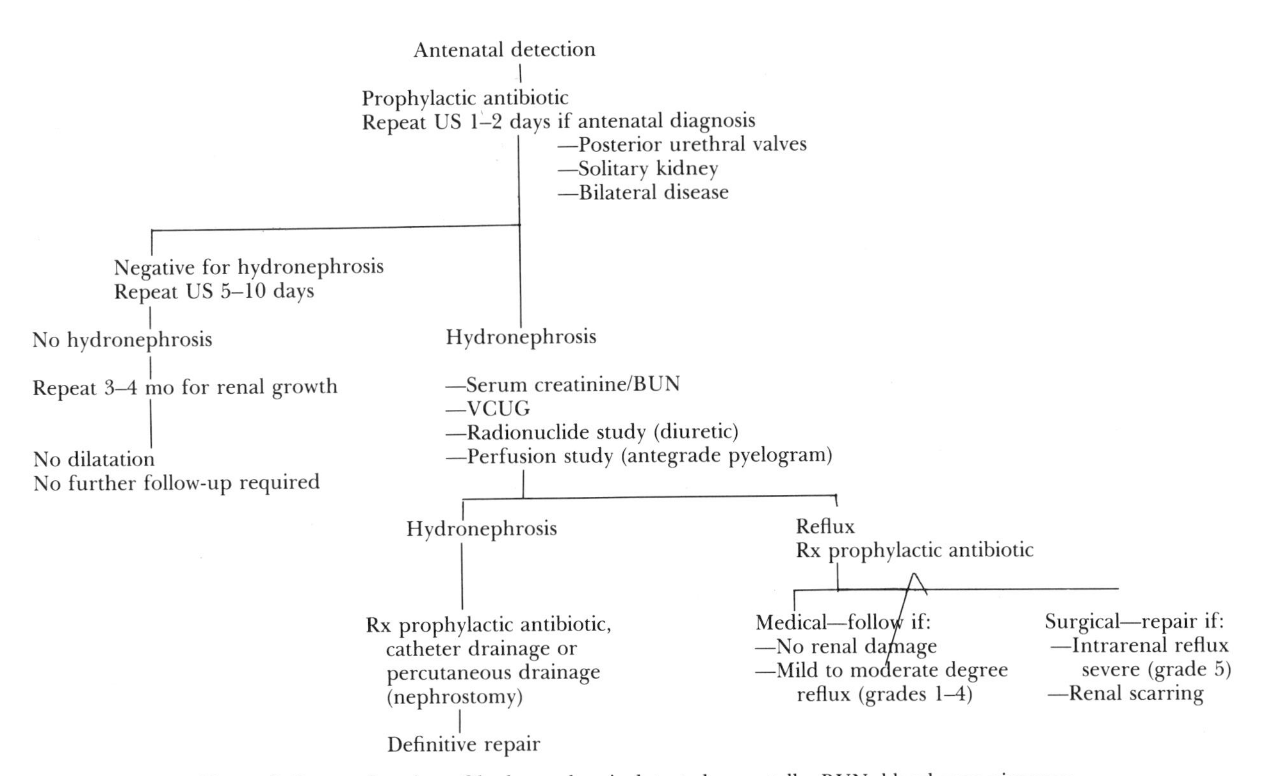

Figure 2. Postnatal review of hydronephrosis detected prenatally. BUN, blood urea nitrogen; VCUG, voiding cystourethrogram; US, ultrasound.

TABLE 4. Diagnosis and Treatment of Hydronephrosis

Study	Group 1 *Potential Obstruction*	Group 2 *Equivocal or Incidental*	Group 3 *Probable*	Group 4 *Symptomatic*
Clinical	Asymptomatic			Symptomatic
Conventional radiology	← Dilated system →			
Diuretic-augmented radionuclide scan	Normal clearance tracer; residual function in hydronephrotic kidney	Increase time to clear 15–20 minutes	Unequivocal increase time to clear compared to normal	
Reflux study			Reflux + obstruction (repeat with bladder catheter)	
Perfusion study			Positive; treat with nephrostomy drainage	
Sequential study	Repeat scan 6 mo then each 12 mo	Repeat scan 3 mo while patient stable or improving	Repeat function study in 2 wk	
Treatment	Observe while patient stable (5% deteriorate and need surgery)	Observe while patient stable or improving; surgery if patient deteriorates	Attempt salvage; trial of drainage for renal function; if <10%, consider nephrectomy	

performed with regularity, the results of radionuclide washout and perfusion studies, taken together, provide an excellent guide to differentiate patients with potentially progressive hydronephrosis from those with nonobstructive dilatation.

In patients with ureterovesical junction obstruction, urine culture, voiding cystourethrogram, and urodynamic study may be needed to exclude secondary causes (severe urinary infection, vesicoureteral reflux, neurogenic bladder, or dysfunctional voiding).

Treatment of Defined Abnormalities

The selection of methods to assess and correct hydronephrosis and dilated ureters reflects institutional preferences based on availability and expertise of radiologic and surgical personnel.

When objective evidence confirms the presence of urinary tract obstruction, the treatment is surgical. Periodic ultrasonography and renal scan (diuretic augmented) should be performed in children with a dilated but nonobstructed ureter to ensure that asymptomatic renal damage does not occur. We suggest ultrasonography at 4 months, 18 months, and 3 and 5 years to define anatomic change, together with a renal scan at 4 months and at 3 years if the ultrasonogram is stable. Further studies are necessary in the case of progressive abnormalities seen on ultrasonogram. Various abnormalities include the following.

Ureteropelvic Junction Obstruction

The ureteropelvic junction is the most common site of obstruction, and the most common corrective procedure is a dismembered Anderson-Hynes pyeloplasty. The abnormal ureteropelvic junction is excised, and the normal ureter and pelvis spatulated and reanastomosed. Aberrant blood vessels or bands causing angulation of the ureteropelvic junction are corrected during the same operation. Management of such extrinsic abnormalities alone rarely relieves the obstruction.

Ureterovesical Junction Obstruction (Primary)

The treatment of primary ureterovesical junction obstruction requires excision of the abnormal ureteral segment and reimplantation into the bladder. If the ureter is significantly dilated, some remodeling of the ureter may be necessary to attain a proper ratio of ureteral diameter to length of submucosal tunnel to prevent vesicoureteral reflux. Various methods of tapering, folding, or plication of the ureter are used, depending largely on institutional preference.

Secondary Ureterovesical Junction Obstruction

Treatment of the primary cause is usually followed by improvement or clearing of the obstruction. Thus, vigorous treatment of urinary infection, suppressant antibiotic therapy for the patient with vesicoureteral reflux, intermittent catheterization for drainage, and consideration of pharmacologic detrusor or sphincter blockade or stimulation may be necessary.

Ectopic Ureter and Ureterocele

After suitable hydration and antibiotic therapy lead to stabilization, urinary drainage by nephrostomy is established, if necessary, prior to definitive repair. Definitive correction may be complex and requires an individualized approach. If the obstructed segment is dysplastic or nonfunctional, heminephrectomy or excision of the dysplastic cap is appropriate.

Drainage of a duplex system by ureteroureterostomy or ureteropyelostomy may be a practical way to drain functioning renal parenchyma. The final decision is made at surgery. Because attempted salvage of a hydronephrotic kidney is associated with little risk, attempts at drainage and re-evaluation of renal function are common.

Removal of the lower ureter (i.e., segment in the patient with ureterocele or ectopic ureter) depends on the position of the ureter and related structures (e.g., bladder neck and the presence or absence of vesicoureteral reflux). A period of review may be necessary after attaining drainage of the distal ureteral stump before definitive repair. Reflux or obstruction in the ipsilateral or contralateral ureter may resolve after drainage of the ureterocele. Initial repair of the affected ureter is then observed closely over 6 to 12 months, and definitive repair is then undertaken.

Prenatal Diagnosis of Hydronephrosis

At present, diagnostic criteria for intrauterine obstruction are being defined in experimental animals. The most efficient use of prenatal diagnosis is to identify those infants with an anomaly who will derive the most benefit from early postnatal evaluation. A scheme for follow-up is outlined in Figures 1 and 2. The detection of hydronephrosis in the perinatal period provides a new challenge to pediatricians and pediatric urologists to determine the significance of the underlying lesion and its relationship to renal and pulmonary function (see Figs. 1 and 2). This will allow for future intrauterine intervention on an experimental basis, planned delivery of the fetus, and expectant therapy for the early hours to days after birth. Early evaluation and therapy for potentially serious obstructive lesions before infection occurs provide protection from the rapid loss of renal parenchyma that can result from the combination of obstruction and infection.

Associated Intraluminal Pathology

In patients who show hydronephrosis secondary to intraluminal obstruction or in whom vesicoureteral reflux is associated with hydronephrosis and hydroureter, the treatment and evaluation is that of the underlying lesion. Testing determines the relative contributions of reflux or hydronephrosis to the defined anatomic lesion and provides guidelines for therapy.

Delayed Deterioration in Renal Function

A number of patients will show progressive, slow deterioration in renal function or decompensation of apparently well maintained renal function for some years, with the onset of hypertension and proteinuria and the development of focal glomerulosclerosis with progression to end-stage renal disease.

In the patient with a dilated ureter or hydronephrosis, careful evaluation of renal and ureteral anatomy and function is necessary to plan rational therapy. Careful long-term follow-up is necessary to protect remaining renal function after relief of obstruction. In patients with dilated nonobstructed urinary tracts, close long-term monitoring should be instituted to prevent progressive asymptomatic deterioration in renal function.

MALIGNANT TUMORS OF THE KIDNEY

PERRY D. NISEN, M.D., Ph.D.

Wilms' tumor (nephroblastoma) is the most common malignant tumor of the kidney in childhood, with an incidence of 7 in 1,000,000. Males and females are affected equally, with a median age at diagnosis of 2 to 3 years. Wilms' tumor most commonly presents as an abdominal mass detected by the parent. In about 20 per cent of cases, there is associated malaise, abdominal pain, microscopic or gross hematuria, hypertension, anemia, or fever. The differential diagnosis includes neuroblastoma, rhabdoid tumor of the kidney, clear cell sarcoma of the kidney (CCSK), renal cell carcinoma, mesoblastic nephroma, carbuncle, hamartoma, multicystic kidney, multilocular cystic nephroma, rhabdomyosarcoma, primitive neuroectodermal tumor, hepatoblastoma, and lymphoma. Neuroblastoma, in contrast to Wilms' tumor, tends to be calcified, does not displace the collecting system, and is suprarenal or paravertebral. Rhabdoid tumor and CCSK were previously thought to be variants of Wilms' tumor but are now recognized as distinct entities associated with a poor prognosis. Renal cell carcinoma, which is the most common malignant renal tumor of adults, is very rare in childhood and is also associated with a poor prognosis. Mesoblastic nephroma occurs in infancy, is histopathologically benign, and is treated by surgical excision alone.

Wilms' tumor can occur in association with congenital anomalies, including hemihypertrophy, aniridia, and genitourinary (GU) anomalies. Patients with hemihypertrophy or aniridia should be regularly screened for the development of Wilms' tumor by abdominal ultrasonography. Syndromes associated with an increased incidence of Wilms' tumor include WAGR complex (*W*ilms' tumor, *a*niridia, *g*enitourinary (GU) anomalies, mental *r*etardation), Beckwith-Weidemann syndrome, Drash syndrome, Perlman syndrome, and neurofibromatosis.

Wilms' tumor has been the subject of intense investigation by molecular geneticists. The tumors frequently demonstrate deletion of chromosomal DNA sequences (loss of heterozygosity) at 11p13 (WAGR patients have an inherited deletion in this region) or 11p15 (Beckwith-Weidemann syndrome). A putative tumor suppressor gene (WT1) has been isolated from 11p13, which may be involved in the pathogenesis of Wilms' tumor. The N-*myc* oncogene is overexpressed in these tumors as well.

Wilms' tumor tends to spread locally to the pseudocapsule, renal sinus, blood vessels, and lymphatics. Sites of distal metastases (which can be present at diagnosis) include lung, lymph nodes, liver, bone, and brain. The diagnostic work-up for the patient with Wilms' tumor includes a physical examination (looking for hemihypertrophy, aniridia, and GU anomalies), complete blood count, and urinalysis. Imaging studies include intravenous pyelogram, abdominal sonogram, chest radiograph, computed tomography (CT) scan or magnetic resonance imaging (MRI) of the chest and abdomen, and possibly bone scan, skeletal survey, and CT scan or MRI of the head (for metastatic disease).

TABLE 1. National Wilms' Tumor Study—4 Staging Criteria

Stage	Criteria
I	Tumor limited to the kidney and completely excised. The surface of the renal capsule is intact. The tumor was not ruptured before or during removal. There is no residual tumor apparent beyond the margins of excision.
II	Tumor extends beyond the kidney but is completely excised (i.e., penetration through the outer surface of the renal capsule into the perirenal soft tissue). Vessels outside the kidney substance are infiltrated or contain tumor thrombus. The tumor may have been biopsied or there has been local spillage of tumor confined to the flank. There is no residual tumor apparent at or beyond the margins of excision.
III	Residual nonhematogenous tumor confined to the abdomen. Any of the following may occur: (a) lymph nodes on biopsy are found to be involved in the hilus, the periaortic chains, or beyond; (b) there has been diffuse peritoneal contamination by the tumor, such as by spillage of tumor beyond the flank before or during surgery, or by tumor growth that has penetrated through the peritoneal surface; (c) implants are found on the peritoneal surfaces; (d) the tumor extends beyond the surgical margins either microscopically or grossly; (e) the tumor is not completely resectable because of local infiltration into vital structures.
IV	Hematogenous metastases. Deposits beyond stage III (e.g., lung, liver, bone, and brain).
	Bilateral renal involvement at diagnosis. An attempt should be made to stage each side according to the above criteria on the basis of extent of disease prior to biopsy.

From D'Angio GJ, Breslow N, Beckwith JB, et al: Treatment of Wilms' tumor: Results of the Third National Wilms' Tumor Study. Cancer 64:349—360, 1989.

TABLE 2. National Wilms' Tumor Study—Treatment Protocols for Various Stages

Stage/ Pathology	Surgery	Radiation Therapy 1080 cGy	Chemotherapy
I/FH, I/UH	+	−	Actinomycin D + vincristine (24 wk) vs. pulsed, intensive (18 wk)
II/FH	+	−	Actinomycin D + vincristine (22 wk vs. 65 wk) vs. pulsed, intensive (18 wk vs. 60 wk)
III/FH IV/FH CCSK	+	+	Actinomycin D + vincristine + doxorubicin (26 wk vs. 65 wk) vs. pulsed, intensive (24 wk vs. 54 wk)
II–IV/UH	+	+	Actinomycin D + vincristine + doxorubicin (+/− cyclophosphamide) (65 wk)

Abbreviations: FH, favorable histology; UH, unfavorable histology (anaplastic); CCSK, clear cell sarcoma of the kidney; RT, radiation therapy.

Histopathologically, Wilms' tumors are typically triphasic, with blastemal, epithelial, and stromal components; however, any one of the cell types can predominate. An important prognostic factor is whether the tumor has histologically favorable (minimal cellular abnormalities) features (overall survival ~90 per cent) or unfavorable (anaplastic) features (overall survival ~50 per cent). The prognosis for affected patients depends on the stage and histology of the tumor. The current staging criteria used by the National Wilms' Tumor Study (NWTS) is summarized in Table 1. Therapy also depends on the stage and histology of the tumor. The current success in treatment of Wilms' tumor is based, in large part, on the analysis of patients treated according to previous NWTS protocols. The current NWTS protocols (NWTS-4) are designed to determine if pulsed, intensive actinomycin D therapy is as effective as standard 5-day treatment (all stages); if treatment can be shortened from 15 months to 5 months (stages II to IV, favorable histology [FH]); and if the addition of cyclophosphamide improves outcome in stages II to IV, unfavorable histology (UH). The NWTS-4 therapeutic protocols are outlined in Table 2. Overall 4-year survival rates of patients in the NWTS-3 study were 96.5 per cent (stage I, FH); 92 per cent (stage II, FH); 87 per cent (stage III, FH); 73 per cent (stage IV, all UH). A challenge for future NWTS studies will be to determine optimal therapy for bilateral Wilms' tumor, relapse, CCSK, and rhabdoid tumors of the kidney.

MANAGEMENT OF ACUTE AND CHRONIC GLOMERULONEPHRITIS

SHERMINE DABBAGH, M.D.
LARRY E. FLEISCHMANN, M.D.
and ALAN B. GRUSKIN, M.D.

Glomerulonephritis is said to be *acute* (e.g., postinfectious acute glomerulonephritis, systemic lupus erythematosus [SLE], Henoch-Schönlein purpura) if the disease presents abruptly, irrespective of the cause. The major features of acute glomerulonephritis include hematuria, proteinuria, hypertension, and edema; it may or may not progress to renal failure. *Chronic* glomerulonephritis is the clinical presentation of a number of glomerulopathies characterized by slow, progressive decrease in renal mass leading to end-stage renal disease. We first describe the general principles of management of various problems in acute and chronic glomerulonephritis and subsequently consider disease-specific treatments (Table 1).

PRINCIPLES OF MANAGEMENT

Electrolyte Abnormalities

Sodium and Fluids

Sodium and water overload occurs in two settings in children with glomerulonephritis. First, decreased glomerular filtration rate (GFR) leads to fluid retention. Second, the increased vascular volume leads to moderate edema with resultant pulmonary congestion and hypertension. Therapy with loop diuretics (e.g., furosemide, 1 to 3 mg/kg/day) produces an effective loss of salt and water in most children. In those in whom a severely decreased GFR makes this therapy ineffective, peritoneal dialysis and hemodialysis may be necessary. Long-term management of salt and water balance is accomplished by careful monitoring of intake and output, limitation of dietary sodium with replacement of only that amount of sodium excreted, and judicious use of diuretic agents.

When chronic nephritis is accompanied by nephrotic syndrome, the resulting edema is often moderate to severe but without accompanying vascular engorgement or hypertension. Sodium limitation and therapy designed to alleviate the underlying condition (Table 1) are the mainstays of treatment. The assistance of a nutritionist knowledgeable in renal dietetics is invaluable for long-term planning of and compliance with palatable sodium-restricted diets, which can either prevent the formation of edema or reduce its severity.

Potassium

Hyperkalemia is a serious, life-threatening complication of glomerulonephritis. It occurs when renal failure impedes the kidney's ability to excrete potassium, and it arises more quickly in acute nephritides than in chronic progressive renal failure. In the latter, the colon adapts by increasing potassium excretion. Less life-threatening effects of hyperkalemia include muscle weakness and flaccid paralysis. The most serious effects of hyperkalemia are on the heart. As serum potassium increases, the resting transmembrane potential is lowered toward the excitation threshold. These depolarization changes lead to elevated tented T waves followed by flattening of the P wave, widening of the QRS segment, and the eventual appearance of a sine wave pattern, ventricular fibrillation, asystole, and death. Therapy must be immediate if changes beyond elevated T waves are present, and it is urgent if serum potassium concentration exceeds 6.5 mEq/L.

Therapy consists of rapid initiation of several steps that can be performed simultaneously (Table 2). Calcium counteracts the membrane effects of hyperkalemia, and its onset of action is within seconds to minutes. Sodium bicarbonate fosters the transfer of potassium into the intracellular fluid; in addition, it corrects hyponatremia, which often accompanies hyperkalemia and accentuates its effects. Although bicarbonate administration is of greatest value when acidosis accompanies hyperkalemia, it lowers serum potassium concentrations even when pH is normal. Insulin promotes the entry of potassium into cells. It should be administered with glucose, both to foster the further release of endogenous insulin and to protect the patient from hypoglycemia.

The preceding steps shift potassium into cells, yet they fail to remove potassium from the body. Potassium removal is accomplished by the rectal (preferred) or oral administration of sodium-potassium exchange resin (Kayexalate), which re-

TABLE 1. Mnemonic Classification of Glomerulonephritis and Disease-Specific Therapy

Disease (RICH)	Progression to CRF	Treatment
*R*apidly progressive GN		
Goodpasture syndrome	Yes	Plasmapheresis, combined with azathioprine or cyclophosphamide (1–2 mg/kg/day) and prednisone (2 mg/kg/day)
Wegener's granulomatosis	Yes	Prednisone (1 mg/kg/day) and cyclophosphamide (2 mg/kg/day)
Idiopathic diffuse crescentic GN	Yes	Pulse methylprednisolone IV (10 mg/kg/day for 3 doses q.d. or q.o.d.) followed by oral prednisone ± cyclophosphamide ± plasmapheresis
*I*mmunologic		
Membranoproliferative GN	Slow	Alternate-day prednisone (2 mg/kg/day; max., 80 mg)
Membranous nephropathy	Slow	Same as for membranoproliferative GN
*I*gA nephropathy (Berger's disease)	Occasional	Symptomatic
*I*nfectious		
Postinfectious acute GN	Rare	Symptomatic
"Shunt" nephritis	Rare	Treat the underlying infection
Subacute bacterial endocarditis	Rare	Treat the underlying infection
*C*ollagen vascular diseases		
Systemic lupus erythematosus	Yes	Prednisone (2 mg/kg/day, p.o.) ± cyclophosphamide (500–1000 mg/m², IV, every 1–3 months)
Scleroderma	Yes	Angiotensin converting enzyme
Polyarteritis nodosa	Yes	Prednisone (2 mg/day, p.o.), cyclophosphamide (2 mg/kg/day, p.o.)
*H*ematologic		
Sickle cell glomerulonephropathy	Yes	Prednisone; but results are poor
Tumor-related glomerulonephropathy	Variable	Treat the underlying tumor
*H*ereditary nephritis	Yes	Symptomatic
*H*enoch-Schönlein purpura	Occasional	Symptomatic

Abbreviations: CRF, chronic renal failure; GN, glomerulonephritis; q., every; q.o.d., every other day; IgA, immunoglobulin A; p.o., by mouth.

moves 1 mEq of potassium for each mEq of sodium released. To ensure retention of the resin enema, it may be necessary to raise the child's hips, insert a ballooned rectal catheter, or tape the buttocks shut. Hemodialysis and/or peritoneal dialysis are necessary when the GFR is markedly reduced and the preceding measures fail. Although loop diuretics produce significant potassium losses in normal patients, they are of little value in most cases of hyperkalemia associated with acute oliguric renal failure. If urine output is present, however, the administration of furosemide may be of supplemental benefit.

Spurious hyperkalemia, due to the release of potassium from intracellular fluid into the serum because of hemolysis or clot formation, may be encountered when blood is drawn through too small a needle or is roughly handled during specimen preparation, or in the presence of marked leukocytosis (e.g., leukemia with white blood cell counts in excess of 100,000) or thrombocytosis. Determination of plasma potassium, rather than serum potassium, is indicated when severe leukocytosis or thrombocytosis is present.

Hypokalemia, although usually not a problem in acute glomerulonephritis, may complicate therapy of chronic glomerulonephritis when long-term use of diuretics is prescribed. The cardiac effects of hypokalemia include the appearance of ventricular ectopic beats, S-T segment depression, biphasic T waves, and a U wave. These changes must be differentiated from the "strain pattern" of left ventricular hypertrophy. Hypokalemia, when prolonged, produces decreased peripheral vascular resistance and lowers blood pressure. Constipation, ileus, muscle weakness, and, in some cases, rhabdomyolysis may occur with severe or prolonged hypokalemia. Life-threatening digitalis toxicity may occur in hypokalemic patients who are receiving these agents.

Therapy of hypokalemia can be accomplished in a more conservative fashion than can that of hyperkalemia. Oral supplementation with a number of commercially available potassium chloride preparations (3 to 5 mEq/kg/day) are often therapeutically effective. When rapid correction is indicated, intravenous supplementation is advised. Concentrations of potassium in the intravenous fluids should not exceed 40 mEq/L, unless the patient is monitored continuously. Concentrations in excess of 60 mEq/L are seldom indicated. In special situations, higher concentrations of potassium may be delivered at a rate not to exceed 0.5 mEq/kg/hour (maximum, 30 to 40 mEq/hour).

Acid-Base Balance

Acidosis occurs in both acute and chronic glomerulonephritis. Its correction should not be attempted until hypocalcemia

TABLE 2. Treatment of Hyperkalemia

Agent	Action	Dose
Calcium gluconate (10%)	Counteracts the cardiac effects of potassium	100–200 mg/kg per dose over 30–60 minute
Sodium bicarbonate	Shifts potassium intracellularly	1 mEq/kg per dose over 30–60 minute
Glucose and insulin	Shifts potassium intracellularly	0.5 g/kg of glucose with 0.3 U regular insulin per gram of glucose over 2 hr
Kayexalate	Exchanges potassium for sodium in the gut	1–2 g/kg/day, divided q 6 hr in 70% sorbitol solution (3 ml/g resin) p.o. or nasogastric tube; or as a retention enema in 20% sorbitol solution (5 ml/g resin)

has been treated, lest tetany occur. The magnitude of the bicarbonate requirement may be estimated from the following formula:

$$\text{mEq of } HCO_3^- \text{ needed} = \text{mass [kg]} \times 0.6 \times (\text{desired} - \text{actual } HCO_3)$$

At most, half of the required bicarbonate should be administered over the first 12 hours; rapid bicarbonate infusions are indicated only for emergency treatment of hyperkalemia. Oral therapy with bicarbonate or citrate (Shohl's solution [Bicitra], 1 to 3 mEq/kg/day) usually corrects the acidosis.

Divalent Ion Metabolism in Glomerulonephritis

Acute Glomerulonephritis

Hypocalcemia and *hyperphosphatemia* often complicate the course of acute glomerulonephritis. Hypocalcemia is thought to be caused by direct complexation of calcium with increased amounts of phosphate. The latter is retained because of decreased filtration, particularly when the GFR is less than 25 ml/minute/1.73 m^2. The propensity to develop hyperphosphatemia is compounded by the fact that many patients are catabolic, having a resultant breakdown of tissues and phosphorus release. Hypocalcemia may result in tetany or seizures, which can be precipitated by aggressive correction of metabolic acidosis in the presence of low serum calcium concentrations. If hypocalcemia is severe (calcium <7 mg/dl) and/or the patient is unable to tolerate oral supplementation of calcium, correction is achieved by the infusion of 100 to 200 mg/kg per dose of 10 per cent calcium gluconate over 1 to 2 hours. If the patient is asymptomatic, he or she can be supplemented orally with 25 to 50 mg of elemental calcium/kg/day in divided doses in the form of calcium carbonate or calcium glubionate (Neo-Calglucon).

Hyperphosphatemia is treated with dietary restriction of phosphorus and phosphate binders. Calcium carbonate (63 to 125 mg/kg/day) given with meals can be an effective phosphate binder. Aluminum hydroxide should be avoided, particularly in infants and patients with reduced renal function, because of its potential to accumulate in bone and brain.

Chronic Glomerulonephritis

Treatment of calcium and phosphorus imbalance with the renal insufficiency of chronic glomerulonephritis is directed toward the prevention of renal osteodystrophy. Thus, the intake of dairy products is limited to restrict phosphorus intake. Calcium-containing phosphate binders, such as calcium carbonate or calcium acetate, are prescribed with meals to treat hyperphosphatemia (25 to 50 mg elemental calcium/kg/day in three to four divided doses). Aluminum hydroxide gels are generally avoided, except when hypercalcemia and hyperphosphatemia coexist. Because $1,25[OH]_2D$ levels are decreased in renal failure for various reasons, including hyperphosphatemia, patients are supplemented with $1,25[OH]_2D$ (Rocaltrol) orally (15 to 30 ng/kg/day). In children unable to swallow capsules, a suspension of $1.25[OH]_2D$ in corn oil (0.05 to 0.1 μg/ml) can be used. This suspension is stored in brown bottles and is safe for 1 week only.

Nutritional Aspects of Glomerulonephritis

Acute Glomerulonephritis

Nutritional support in acute glomerulonephritis seldom is a problem in children who maintain normal renal function. In children who develop azotemia with or without oliguria, it is necessary to impose dietary restrictions. Thus, the prescription of calories and protein in patients with acute renal failure due to acute glomerulonephritis depends on whether dialysis is required. Because oliguria is often short-lived and self-limited, the objectives in the early stages are to prevent starvation and ketoacidosis and to minimize endogenous tissue breakdown. These can be accomplished by providing carbohydrates orally (in the form of hard candy or its equivalent) or intravenously (as dextrose in water) to supply 20 to 25 per cent of the total energy requirements. Additional calories given as carbohydrate or fat do not appreciably prevent additional endogenous protein breakdown. This regimen can generally be safely used for 24 to 48 hours.

With the persistence of renal dysfunction, there is a decrease in protein synthesis, which tends to occur after 48 hours and warrants more aggressive nutritional support. If endogenous tissue proteins are to be spared, the intake of protein of high biologic value should be 0.5 to 1.0 g/kg/day with caloric intakes that approach requirements for age and weight. If peritoneal dialysis is initiated, protein intake should be 1.5 to 2.0 g/kg/day to compensate for the obligatory losses of protein in the dialysate. Such increased needs are not required in hemodialysis. Central hyperalimentation is rarely required. The dietary manipulations of mono- and divalent ions in patients with acute renal insufficiency were described previously.

Chronic Glomerulonephritis

No adjustments in dietary intake are required in chronic glomerulonephritis with normal renal function. With the development of renal insufficiency, proper nutrition necessary for linear growth and weight gain must be balanced with the need to restrict protein intake to prevent possible hyperfiltration injury and control uremic symptoms. Protein intakes of 1.8 to 2.5 g/kg/day are needed to promote growth, particularly in prepubertal children. Calorie intakes close to requirements for weight are recommended to prevent endogenous protein catabolism and supply amino acids for gluconeogenesis.

Children with decreased creatinine clearances have decreased food intake secondary to multiple factors, which include anorexia of chronic disease, accumulation of "uremic toxins," altered taste acuity, and increased water intake. It may become necessary to provide aggressive nutritional support by supplementing diets with carbohydrates (e.g., Polycose), fat (e.g., medium-chain triglyceride oil), or proprietary formulas (e.g., Osmolite, Travasorb Renal). Feeding via nasogastric or gastrostomy tubes may be necessary.

Hypertension (see also p. 158)

Hypertension is a common and occasionally life-threatening association of both acute and chronic glomerulonephritis. Therapy is directed toward either reducing extracellular volume (diuretics) or lowering peripheral vascular resistance (antihypertensive drugs). Available drugs, dosing data, and major toxicities are summarized in the article on systemic hypertension, Section 5. Therapy is initiated at the lowest recommended dose and is gradually increased until an appropriate effect is obtained, no further response can be expected, or an unacceptable toxicity occurs. When combinations of drugs are used, agents with different mechanisms of actions should be used. Appropriate clinical and laboratory monitoring to ensure safety and efficacy is indicated. Safety and efficacy for many blood pressure agents have not been established in children.

Diuretics

Acute Hypertension. Acute hypertension occurs most commonly in children who develop postinfectious glomerulonephritis. It also occurs in children with other glomerular disorders in which a rapid decrease in GFR occurs and in children with chronic hypertension secondary to chronic glomerulonephropathies.

Diuretics alone, particularly intravenously administered loop diuretics, by decreasing extracellular volume, may control the hypertension of acute nephritis. Their use is also indicated to control the sodium retention that occurs when vasodilatory antihypertensive agents are used either acutely or chronically. When one treats severe hypertension, it is best to administer diuretics intravenously initially; subsequently, orally administered agents can be used. Life-threatening events, such as encephalopathy and heart failure, should initially be treated with a combination of vasodilators and diuretics. The simplest method to evaluate the response to diuretic therapy is to monitor changes in weight; the computation of fluid balance (output minus input, including an estimate for insensible losses) may also be used in monitoring.

Chronic Hypertension. Diuretics alone infrequently normalize the hypertension associated with chronic glomerulonephropathies. Most commonly, diuretics are used in conjunction with antihypertensive drugs. A low-sodium diet is also indicated in treating chronic hypertension, except in patients with salt-losing nephropathies. Diuretics acting within the proximal tubule or loop of Henle are usually needed, particularly when the GFR is significantly depressed.

PSYCHOSOCIAL ISSUES

Acute Glomerulonephritis

The acute nephritic syndrome, particularly when severe, causes fear and anxiety in both parents and child. Explanations should be provided about the natural history of the disease, particularly the development of renal failure requiring dialysis and transplantation. Life-threatening events should be anticipated and explained. Indicated procedures such as renal biopsy and dialysis should be discussed with both parents and child.

Chronic Glomerulonephritis

Acceptance of the diagnosis and its implications is the major psychologic goal for patients with progressive renal failure. An understanding of the impact of progressive renal failure on growth and the need to prepare for the multidisciplinary approach to the treatment of end-stage renal disease should occur early. Regular visits to pediatric end-stage renal disease programs may maximize growth potential and may better enable families to cope and prepare for the rigors of dialysis and transplantation.

DISEASE-SPECIFIC THERAPY

Rapidly Progressive Glomerulonephritis

Rapidly progressive glomerulonephritis (RPGN) refers to a clinical syndrome of a rapid and progressive decline in renal function associated with hematuria and proteinuria, which in most patients, if not treated early, leads to end-stage renal failure in weeks or months. The prognosis for *idiopathic diffuse crescentic glomerulonephritis* is poor unless treatment is instituted early. Intravenous "pulse" methylprednisolone administered daily or every other day for three to four doses, followed by oral prednisone daily or every other day for several weeks, may prove beneficial. Pulse steroid therapy is usually combined with the administration of cytotoxic agents such as cyclophosphamide or azathioprine. Dialytic therapy may be required until remission is achieved.

Patients with *Goodpasture syndrome* may respond to pulse methylprednisolone therapy and cytotoxic drugs. However, the most dramatic improvement occurs after plasmapheresis. Initial therapy with daily 3- to 4-L plasma exchanges combined with 1 to 2 mg/kg/day of azathioprine or cyclophosphamide, plus 2 mg/kg/day of prednisone, has been recommended. Renal and pulmonary function tests are monitored. Anti-GBM (glomerular basement membrane) antibodies are followed. Generally, therapy with cytotoxic drugs should not exceed 2 months. Bilateral nephrectomy is indicated in the very rare presence of uncontrollable hypertension or pulmonary hemorrhage.

The dismal outlook for patients with *Wegener's granulomatosis* has been altered by the use of steroids and cytotoxic medications. Long-term therapy with cyclophosphamide (2 mg/kg/day) and prednisone (1 mg/kg/day for 3 to 4 weeks; then convert to 1 mg/kg on alternate days) results in remission of the disease even in patients with apparent end-stage renal failure. Relapses may occur when azathioprine is substituted for cyclophosphamide, especially when anti-neutrophil cytoplasmic autoantibodies (a marker for many vasculitides, including Wegener's granulomatosis) are still present.

The treatment of *polyarteritis nodosa* includes the aggressive treatment of hypertension as previously described. Pulse methylprednisolone therapy and the use of cytotoxic drugs (azathioprine and/or cyclophosphamide) have improved the prognosis of the disease. The added benefit of plasmapheresis is debatable.

Acute Glomerulonephritis Due to Infectious Causes

The treatment of *postinfectious acute glomerulonephritis* is symptomatic. Prolonged bed rest does not affect the long-term prognosis. All patients should be assessed for the presence of hypertension, fluid retention, electrolyte imbalance, and reduced renal function. Although hospitalization is not required in the absence of such signs, patients need to be monitored for the possible development of edema, hypertension, and oliguria. This can be assessed by frequent office visits and specific instructions to the parents to call the physician should edema, weight gain, reduced urine output, or headache develop.

Should oliguria and edema develop, the patient's fluids are restricted to 300 to 400 ml/m^2 (30 ml/100 kcal/day) and sodium intake is limited to 1 to 2 mEq/kg/day. Diuretics (e.g., furosemide) are usually helpful if significant edema is present. Because the response to diuretics depends on the degree of renal insufficiency, the dose of furosemide varies between 1 and 5 mg/kg/day. Thiazides, such as hydrochlorothiazide, are helpful if the creatinine clearance is greater than 30 cc/minute/1.73 m^2. Metolazone (Zaroxolyn, 0.07 to 0.14 mg/kg/day orally) is useful as adjunct therapy in cases of severe edema with partial response to furosemide. When edema is related to hypoalbuminemia, patients may require an infusion of 25 per cent albumin (0.3 to 1 g/kg per dose) followed by furosemide (1 to 2 mg/kg per dose) intravenously every 6 to 12 hours to control the edema.

The addition of antihypertensive medications may be required to control the hypertension (see previously). Electrolyte and divalent ion disturbances are handled as they develop (see previously).

Few patients require dialysis (peritoneal or hemodialysis) or hemofiltration to control azotemia, fluid overload, and electrolyte imbalance. Rarely, patients may have a clinical course similar to RPGN and require the administration of intravenous pulse methylprednisolone and cytotoxic agents. Most patients with uncomplicated disease undergo a diuresis in 7 to 10 days. Gross hematuria usually disappears in 2 weeks, hypertension in 1 month, and proteinuria in 3 months. Microscopic hematuria may persist over 2 to 3 years in the presence of normal renal function.

Therapy for *"shunt" nephritis* and *nephritis associated with subacute bacterial endocarditis* is mainly supportive, with emphasis on treating the underlying infection. Infected shunts need to be removed and cardiac valves may need to be replaced.

Immunologic Diseases

Almost 50 per cent of patients with *membranoproliferative glomerulonephritis* (MPGN) present with a well-defined nephrotic syndrome; 30 per cent have asymptomatic proteinuria associated with recurrent gross or microscopic hematuria and features of acute nephritic syndrome or various degrees of renal insufficiency. The treatment of MPGN remains controversial. Generally, improvement in the prognosis has been observed with the use of oral alternate-day prednisone, particularly in MPGN type I. Encouraging results have been reported with the use of anticoagulants and inhibitors of platelet aggregation in adults; there is little experience with the use of these agents in children. Such agents should be used with caution because of possible bleeding complications. MPGN type II is usually unresponsive to treatment.

Membranous glomerulonephritis presents as a nephrotic syndrome, or chronic renal failure, and can be associated with other underlying diseases, including hepatitis B, syphilis, SLE, various carcinomas, sickle cell disease, and various medications (e.g., D-penicillamine, captopril, probenecid). When specific therapy for the underlying cause is possible, membranous nephropathy usually resolves. Of children with idiopathic membranous nephropathy, fewer than 5 per cent progress to renal failure within 5 years of diagnosis. The majority of children achieve a complete remission within 5 years; frequently, these remissions have been spontaneous. Nonspecific treatment to control edema is indicated. Alternate-day prednisone has been used in patients with severe proteinuria with variable results. The role of cytotoxic agents (cyclophosphamide, 1 to 2 mg/kg/day; and chlorambucil, 0.1 to 0.2 mg/kg/day) is uncertain. Such agents may decrease the severity of the proteinuria and maintain renal function when used in conjunction with oral prednisone or intravenous pulse methylprednisolone.

Collagen-Vascular Diseases

The effects of steroids on the extrarenal manifestations of *SLE* are dramatic and well described. Most renal lesions respond to daily oral prednisone treatment (1 to 2 mg/kg/day). This can be combined with oral cytotoxic agents, such as cyclophosphamide or azathioprine (1 to 2 mg/kg/day), which also spares the patient the prolonged use of high-dose prednisone. The serious prognosis of diffuse proliferative lupus glomerulonephritis, with its tendency to progress to renal failure, warrants the initial use of steroids and cytotoxic agents. We initiate treatment of diffuse proliferative lupus nephritis with prednisone (2 mg/kg/day) and pulse intravenous cyclophosphamide (500 to 1000 mg/m^2; maximum, 1000 mg) every 1 to 3 months. In the presence of renal failure, pulse methylprednisolone (10 mg/kg/day IV for three to four doses), followed by oral prednisone (2 mg/kg/day; maximum, 80 mg) for 1 to 2 months is used in conjunction with intravenous pulse cyclophosphamide. This therapeutic approach has resulted in improved renal function and pathology. In addition, patients can be maintained on low-dose oral prednisone, thus minimizing its complications. Hemorrhagic cystitis and bladder carcinomas are known complications of cyclophosphamide; sodium 2-mercaptoethanesulfonate (MESNA), which has been used to prevent cyclophosphamide-induced bladder toxicity during cancer chemotherapy, may prove beneficial in lupus patients receiving pulse cyclophosphamide. MESNA is given as an intravenous bolus injection in a dose equal to 20 per cent of the cyclophosphamide dose (weight-per-weight) just before cyclophosphamide administration and at 4 and 8 hours after the dose. The total daily dose of MESNA is 60 per cent of the total cyclophosphamide dose.

The role of plasmapheresis in treating lupus nephritis remains controversial. Preliminary data on the use of cyclosporine in lupus nephritis in uncontrolled trials have been encouraging; however, the risks and benefits of this potentially nephrotoxic medication need further study prior to its broad use.

The aggressive treatment of *scleroderma* with angiotensin–converting enzyme inhibitors has altered its poor prognosis. Angiotensin-converting enzyme inhibitors can forestall the progression of the disease and decrease skin hardening. Minoxidil has been used to control the malignant hypertension. Calcium channel blockers have been successfully used to control Raynaud's phenomenon, and D-penicillamine softens the skin and halts progression of the disease in internal organs. Steroids, antiplatelet agents, and cytotoxic drugs are ineffective in controlling the renal disease. The role of plasmapheresis is doubtful.

Patients with *mixed connective tissue disease* present with features resembling SLE, scleroderma, and polymyositis. The renal response to prednisone is usually favorable.

Glomerulonephritis in Hematologic Diseases

In addition to the tubular defects that characterize *sickle cell anemia,* affected patients may develop lesions that resemble membranoproliferative glomerulonephritis, focal segmental glomerulosclerosis, membranous nephropathy, and minimal change nephrotic syndrome. The course of these glomerulopathies is generally one of persistent and progressive proteinuria and ultimate development of end-stage renal disease. Treatment with prednisone and/or cytotoxic agents has been disappointing. Symptomatic therapy of the various renal syndromes is indicated.

Nephrotic syndrome and other forms of glomerulonephritis have been reported in association with many *neoplasms.* In addition to amyloidosis, membranous nephropathy and minimal change nephrotic syndrome have been widely reported. Generally, these glomerulonephritides respond to treatment of the underlying neoplasm. Response to steroids and cytotoxic agents is poor. Progression to renal failure is variable.

Immunoglobulin A Nephropathy (Berger's Disease)

Treatment of immunoglobulin A (IgA) nephropathy is supportive. Trials with steroids, cytotoxic drugs, anticoagulants, antiplatelet agents, cyclosporine, and phenytoin have yielded variable results. It is estimated that approximately 1 to 2 per cent of patients with Berger's disease progress to renal failure each year. Spontaneous complete remissions are rare and occur after the fourth year of diagnosis.

Henoch-Schönlein Purpura

Patients with renal involvement present with microscopic hematuria, nephritic syndrome, or nephritic-nephrotic syndrome. The renal disease can be associated with reduced GFR, hypertension, RPGN, and progressive renal failure.

In view of the high frequency of spontaneous remissions, the favorable course, and the lack of progression of the renal focal lesions, aggressive treatment (other than symptomatic) is not indicated in Henoch-Schönlein purpura. Patients with progressive and complicated renal disease (crescents on biopsy associated with reduced GFR and/or severe nephrosis) have been treated with a combination of steroids, cytotoxic medications, anticoagulants, or intensive plasmapheresis. Results have not been consistent. Steroids provide temporary relief for abdominal pain but have little effect on the renal disease.

Hereditary Nephritis

The natural history of hereditary nephritis (Alport syndrome) is progression to renal failure before the fifth decade in males; females usually experience a more benign course. Treatment is symptomatic.

NEPHROTIC SYNDROME

JOSE R. SALCEDO, M.D.
and JAMES C.M. CHAN, M.D.

Nephrotic syndrome results from proteinuria that is sufficiently severe to cause hypoalbuminemia, hyperlipidemia, and massive sodium and water retention. Edema is the cardinal clinical feature and the major presenting symptom of nephrotic syndrome. Pleural effusion and ascites also frequently occur.

Two factors contribute to the fluid retention in this condition: (1) diminished transcapillary oncotic pressure gradient, promoting fluid movement from the vascular space into the interstitium, which is most prominent when the serum albumin concentration is less than 2 g/dl; and (2) sodium retention by the kidneys, which sense the diminished vascular volume as indication of fluid depletion.

There are three major categories of nephrotic syndrome in childhood:

1. Primary idiopathic nephrotic syndrome, synonymously known as childhood nephrosis, lipoid nephrosis, minimal change nephrotic syndrome, nil disease, or foot process disease.
2. Secondary nephrotic syndrome.
3. Congenital nephrotic syndrome.

The combined results of three major studies reviewing the histopathologic distribution among children with idiopathic nephrotic syndrome is shown in Figure 1. Most children, if biopsied, show minimal change histology at presentation. Therapy with steroids for these patients, particularly for those younger than 6 years of age, is almost always considered before further intervention.

Figure 2 depicts the association of age with histopathologic lesions other than minimal change. Whereas minimal change histology entails a favorable clinical outcome, other histopathology on renal biopsy is usually associated with a more unfavorable prognosis.

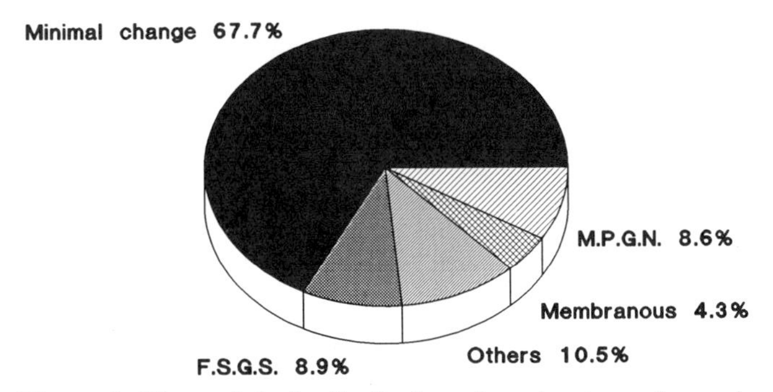

Figure 1. Histopathologic distribution of nephrotic syndrome in children. F.S.G.S., focal segmental glomerulosclerosis; M.P.G.N., membranoproliferative glomerulonephritis. (Data from A report of the International Study of Kidney Disease in Children. J Pediatr 98:561, 1981; White et al: Lancet 1:1353, 1970; and Habib et al: Pathol Annu 6:417, 1971.)

TREATMENT

Prednisone is the drug of choice for the treatment of idiopathic nephrotic syndrome of childhood. Initially, 2 mg/kg/day (60 mg/m²/day) is given in two daily doses (maximum 80 mg/day). This regimen is maintained for 4 weeks. Prednisone is then tapered to a single morning dose given every other day for an additional 4 weeks. The tapering, alternate-day dose consists of a progressive decrease in weekly intervals (40, 30, 20, and 10 mg/m²/day [1.3, 1.0, 0.7, and 0.3 mg/kg/day]) and, finally, cessation of drug therapy.

According to the International Study of Kidney Disease in Children,[1] prednisone therapy (60 mg/m²/day for 1 month) leads to remission in 93 per cent of newly diagnosed patients. After 2 months of prednisone therapy, 36 per cent of patients remain in remission and another 18 per cent manifest infrequent relapses (i.e., one or two relapses in a 5-year period). The remainder have more frequent relapses.

The first relapse, defined as the reappearance of proteinuria for 3 to 4 consecutive days, is treated with a similar drug regimen, beginning with 2 mg/kg in two divided doses until remission occurs; that is, when the urine becomes protein-free for three consecutive days, subsequent treatment for four additional weeks follows the same pattern as the initial induction. The primary objectives of this therapy are not only to minimize the frequency of relapses and their complications but also to avoid drug-related side effects.

Monitoring the drug treatment and the clinical expression of the disease is essential to successful outcome. The child should be weighed, and the urinary protein should be tested with a dipstick every morning. A flow sheet or a calendar should be employed for daily recording of the child's weight, the dipstick-detected proteinuria level, and the prednisone dosage. This monitoring provides essential data concerning the status of the disease and its response to treatment.

Intercurrent illness (e.g., viral syndromes) can be associated with significant proteinuria, which alone does not necessarily indicate a relapse. The possibility of a relapse should be strongly considered if marked (3+ or 4+) proteinuria persists for 3 to 4 days, particularly when it is associated with moderate to severe weight gain and periorbital edema. Otherwise, careful observation and mild salt dietary restriction for a few days may be sufficient.

The therapeutic response and the incidence of side effects associated with the "standard" prednisone therapy may vary widely owing to differences in the severity of the disease, frequency of relapses, and, occasionally, idiosyncratic reaction to the drug. Prednisone is biologically inactive. In the liver, it is converted by 11-β-hydroxysteroid dehydrogenase to its active metabolite, prednisolone, by reduction at the 11-keto position. A trial of prednisolone or methylprednisolone (Medrol), should be considered for a child demonstrating unresponsiveness to the standard prednisone therapy.

The criteria for percutaneous renal biopsy include (1) frequent relapses (i.e., more than two relapses in a 6-month period) and (2) failure to undergo remission in response to the initial prednisone therapy, as occurs in approximately 7 per cent of newly diagnosed children with primary idiopathic nephrotic syndrome.

Treatment with alkylating drugs should be reserved for patients whose renal biopsy demonstrates minimal change histology and who manifest substantial side effects of the disease or the steroid therapy. The two most common alkylating drugs used are cyclophosphamide (Cytoxan, 2 mg/kg/day for 10 weeks) and chlorambucil (Leukeran, 0.2 mg/kg/day for 8 weeks). Cyclophosphamide should be administered in the morning and, ideally, while maintaining a good urine flow to decrease the risk of hemorrhagic cystitis which is a

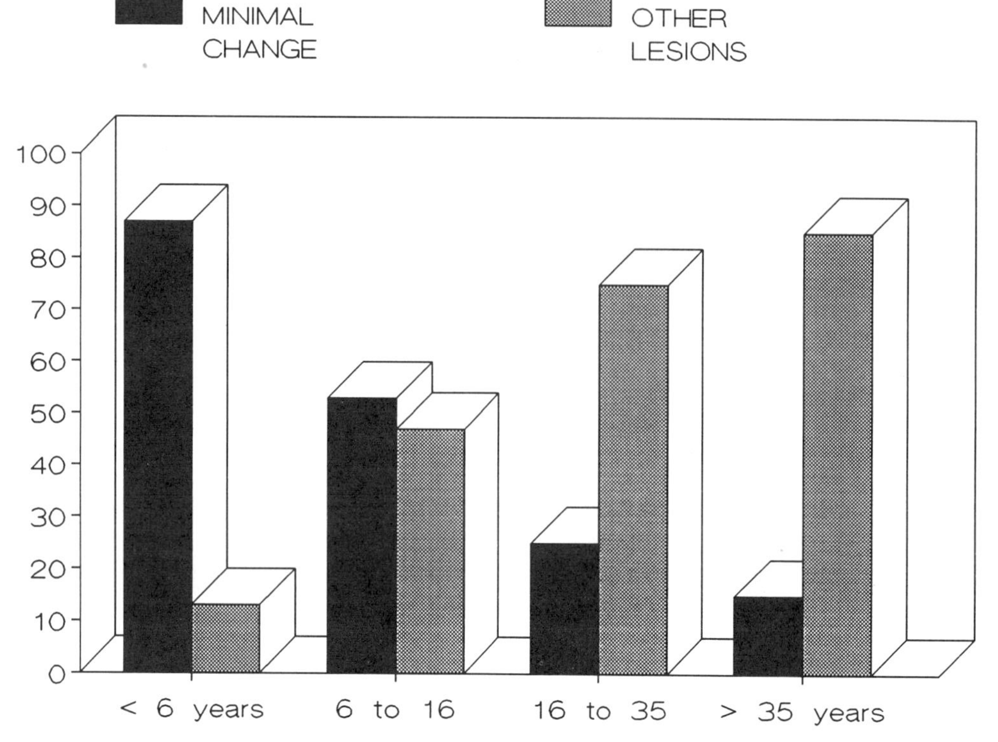

Figure 2. Age and the prevalence of minimal change disease. (Combined data from the International Study of Kidney Disease in Children: J Pediatr 98:561, 1981; and Glassock RJ: Management of the idiopathic nephrotic syndrome. Contrib Nephrol 23:158, 1980.)

known complication of this drug. Both drugs are administered concomitantly with prednisone (60 mg/m^2/day) given every other day. This therapeutic regimen can induce prolonged remissions. Complete blood counts should be performed every 2 weeks during this drug treatment because both medications can cause neutropenia and increase susceptibility to infections.

Patients who are steroid-resistant from the outset may not respond fully to any form of therapy. However, they may manifest a significant reduction in proteinuria in response to cytotoxic drugs. The guarded prognosis associated with persistent nephrotic syndrome has led to drug trials that include intermittent pulses of methylprednisolone, intravenous nitrogen mustard, levamisole, and, more recently, cyclosporine A. The results of these investigations have been inconclusive.

The withdrawal of steroids and cytotoxic drugs is recommended after 4 to 6 months for refractory patients who fail to experience remissions.

The edema of nephrotic syndrome is treated with salt and water restriction; failure to restrict fluids can result in hyponatremia. The use of diuretics is reserved for patients with massive edema. In this context, the use of converting enzyme (ACE) inhibitors may reduce proteinuria and elevate serum albumin, thus reducing the tendency for edema formation.[2]

Patients with anasarca, massive scrotal or labial edema, or pleural or pericardial effusions should be given an intravenous infusion of "furosemide-albumin complex,"[3] which is prepared by mixing albumin and furosemide before it is infused. The recommended doses are albumin at 25 per cent concentration (1 g/kg) mixed with (or followed by) 1 to 2 mg/kg furosemide infused over 2 to 4 hours, followed by a single oral dose of 2.5 mg metolazone at the end of the infusion. This combination is very effective in most patients. However, caution should be exercised during the furosemide-albumin infusion because of the potential risk of inducing fluid depletion or electrolyte disturbances. Potassium-rich food should be offered during chronic diuretic therapy. Once a target weight has been achieved, the judicious use of a single morning dose of 0.5 mg/kg may maintain a good fluid balance until the patient becomes protein-free or achieves an arbitrarily dry weight, at which point diuretics can be temporarily discontinued.

INFECTIOUS COMPLICATIONS

Infection remains one of the most common causes of morbidity and mortality in nephrotic syndrome. The high doses of steroids and cytotoxic drugs contribute to the susceptibility and increased risk of infection. Moreover, the nephrotic patient demonstrates (1) hypogammaglobulinemia as a result of urinary losses and changes in immunoglobulin metabolism; (2) decreased immunoregulatory functions, which alter lymphocyte function; and (3) decreased bacterial opsonization. Gram-positive and gram-negative encapsulated organisms (e.g., *Streptococcus pneumoniae, Escherichia coli,* and *Haemophilus influenzae*) pose substantial risks to nephrotic patients. Spontaneous peritonitis can present as the initial manifestation of a relapse or as a complication of severe anasarca, particularly when the patient is on steroid therapy. Peritonitis should be suspected, even in the absence of fever, because steroid can occasionally mask the febrile reaction. Thus, abdominal discomfort and positive abdominal findings should prompt one to obtain a peritoneal tap and blood cultures. Gram-negative and gram-positive antibiotic coverage should be administered until culture results are available. Appropriate antibiotics should be used when cultures are positive and the sensitivity of the organism is determined. Many nephrologists believe that polyvalent pneumococcal vaccine should be administered to all patients 2 to 3 weeks after the last dose of steroids.

HYPERCOAGULABILITY AND THROMBOEMBOLIC COMPLICATIONS

Thromboembolism is a serious complication of nephrotic syndrome. It can affect the arterial and venous vascular beds. The renal vein and deep veins of the lower extremities are the major sites of thrombus formation and the potential grounds for pulmonary emboli. Numerous defects in the coagulation cascade have been described in nephrotic syndrome. In fact, nephrotic syndrome is marked by a hypercoagulable state, which can be aggravated by thrombocytosis and increased blood viscosity resulting from hemoconcentration.

The treatment is focused on the prevention of this complication by

1. The judicious use of diuretics and avoidance of fluid depletion.
2. Slow administration of albumin infusion without diuretics to reduce hemoconcentration and blood viscosity in the mildly edematous patient.
3. The use of platelet adhesion inhibitor drugs (i.e., acetylsalicylic acid, 1 grain every other day, or dipyridamole).
4. Avoidance of immobilization and femoral venipunctures.

The systemic administration of urokinase or heparin may be indicated in the event of thromboembolic complications; this therapy is usually followed by a course of sodium warfarin (Coumadin) for a minimum of 6 months.

CALCIUM AND VITAMIN D

Hypocalcemia has long been recognized in nephrotic patients. It was initially ascribed to a reduction of protein-bound calcium, caused by hypoalbuminemia. It is now established that not only total plasma calcium but also plasma ionized calcium is low in the nephrotic state. The lower plasma calcium results from a reduction of 25-hydroxyvitamin D, 24-25-dihyroxyvitamin D, and, particularly, 1,25-dihydroxyvitamin D due to urinary losses of vitamin D protein carrier complex. The lower circulating level of vitamin D results in decreased gastrointestinal calcium absorption. Symptomatic hypocalcemia is rare in nephrotic children; however, muscle cramps or twitching and occasional symptoms can be documented. Greater risks for children with frequent relapses are bone demineralization and osteomalacia. Vitamin D therapy should be given to patients with protracted nephrotic syndrome, in particular, and to those showing signs of bone demineralization.

IMMUNIZATIONS (VACCINATIONS)

Live viral vaccines are contraindicated for nephrotic patients receiving either corticosteroids or immunosuppressive drugs. Inactivated bacterial vaccines can be administered to these patients while they are receiving treatment; however, the efficacy of these vaccines may be compromised. The ability to develop a normal immunologic response usually returns 3 to 12 months after immunosuppressive therapy is discontinued. Because nephrotic patients are susceptible to infectious complications (see earlier), vaccination with influenza and pneumococcal polysaccharide vaccine (Pneumovax) is recommended. If feasible, specific serum antibody titers or other immunologic responses should be determined after immunization to assess immune function and guide future management of exposures. An occasional relapse may occur following immunization.

SECONDARY NEPHROTIC SYNDROME

Secondary nephrotic syndrome is relatively uncommon during childhood. Systemic lupus erythematosus, severe poststreptococcal glomerulonephritis, and Henoch-Schönlein purpura are the conditions most likely to be associated with nephrotic syndrome. Other diseases that may present with nephropathy and nephrotic syndrome include (1) human immunodeficiency virus (HIV)–associated nephropathy, (2) sickle cell anemia, (3) congenital heart disease, and (4) systemic viral and bacterial infections such as quartan malaria, subacute bacterial endocarditis, infected ventriculoatrial shunts *(Staphylococcus albus)*, hepatitis B, varicella, and syphilis. The treatment for secondary nephrotic syndrome should focus on the primary disease.

CONGENITAL NEPHROTIC SYNDROME

Congenital nephrotic syndrome of the Finnish type is a rare autosomal recessive disease. Originally observed in Finland, familial and sporadic cases have now been described in many countries and in a variety of ethnic groups. The syndrome is characterized by in utero proteinuria that can be detected as elevated α-fetoprotein, a large placenta, and nephrotic syndrome immediately after birth. Affected patients tend to have extremely low serum gamma globulin concentrations and are very susceptible to infections and vascular complications. They are candidates for renal transplantation. Steroids or cytotoxic drugs in this disease are ineffective and predispose patients to severe infections. Preparation for transplantation includes (1) biweekly or monthly intravenous gamma globulin infusions (500 mg/kg); (2) home infusion of albumin (1 g/kg over several hours); and (3) adequate nutrition to sustain growth and achieve a weight of 6 to 8 kg. Bilateral nephrectomies and the institution of continuous cycling peritoneal dialysis may be indicated even in early infancy. If these measures are effective, the patient may be sustained until early transplantation.

REFERENCES

1. Nephrotic syndrome in children: Prediction of histopathology from clinical and laboratory characteristics at the time of diagnosis. A report of the International Study of Kidney Disease in Children. Kidney Int 13:159–165, 1978.
2. Heeg JE, DeJong PE, Van Der Hem GK, et al: Efficacy and variability of the antiproteinuric effect of ACE inhibition by lisinopril. Kidney Int 36:272–279, 1989.
3. Inoue M, Okajima K, Itoh K, et al: Mechanism of furosemide resistance in analbuminemic rats and hypoalbuminemic patients. Kidney Int 32:198–203, 1987.

RENAL VENOUS THROMBOSIS

BERNARD GAUTHIER, M.B., B.S., F.R.A.C.P.

Renal venous thrombosis (RVT) is most commonly a problem of infants, with 75 per cent of cases occurring in the neonatal period and only 7 per cent after the first year of life. It presents with gross hematuria in most cases and is associated with renal enlargement, renal insufficiency, and evidence of disseminated intravascular coagulation. RVT occurs most often in infants who have suffered perinatal asphyxia or dehydration or who have been born to diabetic mothers. RVT has occurred less frequently for some years.

The recommendations offered in this article are based on an extensive review of the literature and on personal experience. However, reports on the treatment of RVT are derived from uncontrolled studies and from anecdotal data, often involving very small numbers of patients and sometimes single patients. Thus, in the absence of systematic studies, recommendations about the treatment of RVT can be only tentative.

Retrospective reviews of 83 infants with RVT have shown that the condition is associated with a mortality rate of 16 per cent. Among the survivors, many had received only supportive therapy and available data provide no evidence that a more aggressive approach might have been more effective. In particular, it is now recognized that there is no place in the acute phase for surgical treatment. Moreover, therapy with thrombolytic agents or anticoagulation is of unproven benefit and carries definite risks, especially in infants with a birth weight below 1500 g, who are particularly susceptible to intracranial hemorrhages. For these reasons, supportive therapy is the preferred form of treatment in uncomplicated cases.

SUPPORTIVE TREATMENT

The following problems may need to be treated or corrected:

- Dehydration, hyperosmotic state
- Electrolyte abnormalities, acidosis
- Acute renal failure
- Hypertension
- Disseminated intravascular coagulation

Thrombolytic Therapy

Rapid relief of acute renal failure with restoration of renal blood flow by thrombolytic therapy has been reported in adults and in one child with bilateral RVT or thrombosis of the renal vein of a single kidney. Thrombolytic therapy may therefore have a place in patients who experience bilateral RVT (or RVT in a single kidney) with severe acute renal failure. Because thrombolytic therapy is effective if started within 7 days of thrombosis, its use may be deferred until it is clear that no clinical improvement is occurring spontaneously.

Both streptokinase and urokinase have been used in the treatment of RVT. Urokinase may be preferable because it is less likely to cause allergic reaction. Moreover, in a report of the treatment of occlusive arterial disease in adults, urokinase proved to be much more effective than streptokinase. Smaller than usual doses of thrombolytic agents (urokinase, 3000 units/kg initially over 1 hour, followed by 3500 units/kg/hour and 1400 units/kg/hour after the first 24 hours) have been used effectively by infusion into the arteries of affected kidneys. Even smaller doses (streptokinase 50 to 100 units/kg/hour, equivalent to 1/15 to 1/30 of the usual dose) have been used successfully by infusion directly into the area of thrombosis in a few infants with vascular, mostly arterial, thrombosis.

Anticoagulation

The place of anticoagulation in the management of children with RVT is even harder to define than the place of thrombolytic therapy. Anticoagulation does not remove thrombi already present. It can only limit extension of a thrombotic process and offer some protection against pulmonary embolism. In the treatment of RVT, anticoagulation has been recommended to limit extension of RVT itself and its spread to the contralateral kidney. However, such extension has not been demonstrated in infants and children.

Anticoagulation is indicated when RVT occurs as part of a diffuse thromboembolic disorder or when there is evidence of pulmonary embolization, which is seldom the case in infants. Anticoagulation should be considered in steroid-resistant nephrotic states associated with proven thrombosis.

Surgery

Surgical treatment has little to offer for children with RVT. Thrombectomy cannot restore blood flow because the thrombosis usually starts in the small intrarenal veins, predominantly the interlobular and arcuate veins. If hypertension develops later, removal of an atrophic kidney may be curative but should be reserved for children whose contralateral kidney is intact, as demonstrated by a normal technetium 99m dimercaptosuccinic acid (^{99m}Tc DMSA) scan.

Patients with progressive glomerulopathies associated with nephrotic syndrome who are still nephrotic at the time of transplantation are at risk for post-transplant RVT of the graft. In these patients, bilateral native nephrectomy a few weeks before the transplant should be considered to allow correction of the hypercoagulable state associated with the nephrotic syndrome.

Specific Treatment

RVT may occur as a complication of various systemic disorders. Maintenance anticoagulation or supplying the deficient factor(s) may be indicated in RVT associated with antithrombin III deficiency, protein C and protein S deficiency, and familial defective plasminogen function.

LONG-TERM PROGNOSIS

Three recent studies reported follow-up data on 26 children who had had RVT in the neonatal period. Imaging studies at follow-up showed atrophy, scarring, or nephrocalcinosis of one or both kidneys in 83 per cent of cases. A decreased concentrating capacity was shown in 47 per cent, hypertension in 31 per cent, and a decreased glomerular filtration rate in 27 per cent. Renal tubular acidosis and hyperphosphaturia have also been reported as long-term sequellae of RVT.

FOLLOW-UP

In the acute phase, sonography is the method of choice to follow the resolution of the thrombosis and the return of the affected kidney(s) to a normal or subnormal size.

After recovery, children who have had an episode of neonatal RVT should be followed indefinitely with the following:

- ^{99m}Tc DMSA scan when aged 6 months to 1 year
- Yearly height and blood pressure measurement
- Yearly urinalysis, serum creatinine, and estimation of glomerular filtration rate, serum electrolytes, inorganic phosphorus, and alkaline phosphatase

CHRONIC RENAL FAILURE

THOMAS E. NEVINS, M.D.

Chronic loss of kidney function in children arises from a reduced renal mass secondary to congenital malformation or acquired renal disease. Whatever the cause, the progression of chronic renal failure (CRF) is frequently silent and may be recognized only after another event reveals the problem.

To assess and follow children with CRF practically, it is helpful to have a measure of renal function that is more sensitive than a simple serum creatinine test. Classic creatinine clearance is such a measure, but is cumbersome because it requires an accurately timed urine collection. For children older than 2 years of age, the creatinine clearance expressed in ml/minute/1.73 m^2 may be estimated from the formula

$$\text{patient height [cm]} \times 0.55/\text{serum creatinine [mg/dl]}$$

In children younger than 1 year of age, the same equation may be used but with the constant factor 0.45, a reflection of the infant's reduced muscle mass. Although these equations do not give precise measures of glomerular filtration, they do provide a clinically useful gauge of the residual renal function and help in tracking the course of CRF in growing children.

The goal of conservative CRF therapy is the maintenance of optimal growth, development, and function in the affected child. Ultimately, most of these children become candidates for renal replacement therapy—transplantation or dialysis. In the short term, the primary care physician needs to be aware of potential acute problems as well as the techniques commonly employed for chronic management.

ACUTE PROBLEMS

Although CRF is often insidious, it may present abruptly, posing life-threatening problems in children just as in adults. In at least two circumstances—hyperkalemia and severe hypertension—prompt recognition and urgent clinical interventions are required to minimize patient morbidity and mortality.

Hyperkalemia

Because 98 per cent of the total body pool of potassium is intracellular, small shifts in its distribution may produce profound alterations in serum potassium. Normally, such shifts or increases in intake are moderated by renal excretion of excess potassium. In CRF, however, this excretory capacity is limited, and the situation may be further aggravated by acidosis, renal bicarbonate wasting, or volume depletion.

When hyperkalemia is suspected, the patient should have prompt laboratory and electrocardiographic (EKG) confirmation. If EKG changes (high peaked T waves or widened QRS) are present, treatment should begin immediately (Table 1). In this acute clinical setting, continuous EKG monitoring provides instantaneous feedback to guide further therapy. However, these acute treatments are temporizing, and their use signals the immediate need to correct the underlying cause or to initiate dialysis.

Hypertension

When the reduced capacity of the kidney to excrete excess salt and water is overwhelmed, the result is often serious hypertension, risking the integrity of the cerebral vasculature and producing systemic symptoms. Because normal blood pressure in children extends over a relatively wide range, the absolute level of blood pressure associated with these risks varies; however, patients with serious problems generally have diastolic pressures above 100 mm Hg. Hypertensive symptoms (headaches, disturbed vision, seizures, heart failure) vary with the severity of the pressure elevation but are most dramatic in patients with recent or abrupt onset of hypertension. The goal of acute treatment is to reduce blood pressure to less dangerous levels but not necessarily to normal. Hypertensive emergencies require the immediate initiation of therapy (Table 2) both to alleviate symptoms and to minimize the risk of intracranial hemorrhage.

Once blood pressure is acutely under control, a program of sodium reduction and chronic medication (see article on hypertension, p. 158) should be instituted. In a few patients with CRF, blood pressure will not be adequately controlled even by aggressive multidrug regimens; for these children, the initiation of dialysis, with or without nephrectomy, may be necessary.

CHRONIC PROBLEMS

Apart from the emergencies just described, chronic complications are regularly the most important sequelae of reduced renal function. The subtlety of these problems and the length of time that the children are at risk permit rather profound aberrations of growth, bone metabolism, bone marrow production, and neural function to arise.

Growth and Nutrition

The major "work" of childhood is growth. Uremia impairs normal growth, and many children are first diagnosed with CRF during an evaluation for "failure to thrive." A goal of successful CRF treatment is the maintenance of reasonable growth velocities with a height, weight, and head size in the normal range.

Many children with CRF are initially seen with a history of very poor intake. The first approach is to improve the quality and quantity of their diet, emphasizing protein with high biologic value and adequate calories while stressing potassium and phosphorus restriction.

Of equal importance is the issue of appropriate fluid intake. The diet of adults with renal failure routinely includes salt and water restrictions as a means of minimizing fluid overload and improving blood pressure control. However, many children with CRF have kidneys that "waste" salt and water. This means that restricting intake will regularly lead to intravascular volume depletion, hypernatremia, and hypotension. When a child with CRF is recognized, a careful assessment of hydration, diet, volume status, and blood pressure is required. These clinical observations, coupled with the urinary sodium excretion, should allow the physician to make a reasoned judgment about the need for dietary sodium and water restrictions. For example, a child with good urine volumes who has a high urinary sodium level and is normotensive without medication probably needs no restriction. Actually, restricting intake in such a patient often leads to decreased renal perfusion and a rising creatinine level.

TABLE 1. Treatment of Hyperkalemia

Drug	Dose-Route	Comments
Calcium gluconate	100 mg/kg IV	Given slowly over several minutes with monitoring for bradycardia. Infiltration will cause severe local tissue injury.
Sodium bicarbonate	1–2 mEq/kg IV	Given over several minutes; may cause tetany if given before IV calcium. Infiltration will cause severe local tissue injury.
Glucose	1–2 g/kg IV	Given as 20 to 50% dextrose; may administer exogenous insulin as needed for significant hyperglycemia.
"K-Cocktail"	1–2 ml/kg/hr IV	Composed of Calcium gluconate, 3 g Sodium lactate, 200 mEq Regular insulin, 30 units All mixed in 500 ml of 20 or 30% dextrose in water.
Sodium polystyrene sulfonate resin	1–2 g/kg p.o. or p.r.	Administered in 3–5 ml of 20% sorbitol/g of resin. May require several hours to have an effect. Administration both orally and rectally adds to efficacy.

TABLE 2. Treatment of Hypertension

Drug	Dose-Route	Comments
Hydralazine	0.1–0.4 mg/kg IV or IM	Dose may be increased and repeated in 10–15 minutes, minimal acute toxicity, less effective as a chronic medication.
Nifedipine	0.25–0.5 mg/kg p.o. or sublingually	Effective orally, but awkward to use because the smallest dosage size is a 10-mg capsule.
Diazoxide	3–5 mg/kg IV	May be given as a bolus (smaller doses) or slow infusion (over 15–20 minutes) to "titrate" blood pressure reduction. Cannot be given as a bolus through a central catheter (arrhythmia risk). Repeated dosing may lead to hyperglycemia.
Labetalol	0.5–3 mg/kg IV	After an initial dose, the blood pressure may be adjusted by a slower continuous infusion.
Sodium nitroprusside	Continuous IV infusion at 0.5–8.0 μg/kg/hr (50 mg in 1000 ml of D_5W = 50 μg/ml)	May cause profound, abrupt hypotension; requires continuous careful monitoring. Thiocyanate accumulation may occur and produce toxicity.

In addition to dietary or fluid restrictions, other barriers to adequate nutrition exist in children with CRF. Most patients experience anorexia, the etiology of which is unknown. Especially in younger children, gastroesophageal reflux with vomiting is common and may significantly complicate the struggle to maximize oral intake. Previously, efforts directed at supplementing children's daily caloric intake to the level of 100 per cent of the recommended daily allowance (RDA) for calories resulted in improvements in weight and serum protein values but less regularly in accelerated growth. To achieve these dietary goals, feeding tubes or gastrostomies may be required. At the same time, chronic overfeeding should be avoided because it primarily leads to obesity.

The dietary therapy of adult CRF has refocused attention on the role of diet in the progression of renal disease and has emphasized the potential importance of reduced dietary protein in slowing the decline of adult renal function. However, at present, there are no published trials in childhood CRF to provide guidelines for modifying dietary protein, especially while attempting to maintain nutrition and growth. On the other hand, studies of infants managed with meticulous attention to nutritional therapy, before dialysis became necessary, indicate that growth is possible but requires an adequate diet, maintenance of near-normal fluid and electrolyte balance, and significant residual renal function. Similarly, in older nondialyzed children with CRF, careful conservative management can yield sustained growth, although the rates are often in the low normal range.

At present, a balanced approach to CRF is to provide 100 per cent of the dietary RDA for size while continuing to monitor height, weight, head size, and renal function carefully. If growth failure persists, nonrenal causes (syndromes, endocrine problems) should be sought. Finally, if growth failure persists, the physician needs to consider proceeding to transplantation or dialysis.

Recombinant human growth hormone (r-hGH) is now available and offers a potential approach to growth retardation in CRF. To the degree that growth delays in CRF result from end-organ unresponsiveness or circulating inhibitors, the administration of additional exogenous r-hGH could improve growth. Preliminary studies indicate that uremic patients do respond to supplemental r-hGH. At present, the experimental use of r-hGH in CRF seems best restricted to defined protocols until the optimal dosing, potential risks (glucose dysmetabolism, slipped epiphyses, malignancy) and benefits (improved protein utilization, nutrition and growth) are more clearly defined.

Osteodystrophy

As renal tubular function declines, there is simultaneously a reduced excretory capacity for phosphorus, resulting in dietary phosphorus retention and secondary stimulation of parathyroid gland activity. There is simultaneously a reduction in the conversion of 25-hydroxyvitamin D to the active 1,25-dihydroxy-metabolite. These primary derangements in normal phosphorus and calcium metabolism lead to reduced bone mineralization and renal osteodystrophy. The best laboratory test to document these events is the serum level of parathormone (parathyroid hormone, PTH). But, in CRF, inactive fragments of PTH accumulate, so the appropriate PTH assay should measure primarily the active ("intact" or "N-terminal") portion of the hormone. Alkaline phosphatase can also serve as a rough surrogate for PTH, but it is often elevated in growing children or patients who also have liver disease.

To minimize parathyroid gland stimulation, serum phosphorus levels should be maintained normal for age, and serum calcium levels should be at the upper limits of normal. If serum proteins are low, it may be necessary to measure the ionized calcium to gauge the level of physiologically active calcium accurately.

Because the initiating event in hyperparathyroidism is decreased phosphorus excretion, the primary approach to therapy is to restrict the dietary burden of phosphate. For infants, this is accomplished by choosing the formula with the lowest phosphorus content. Older children should be instructed in a low-phosphorus diet and in the avoidance of dairy products. In addition, it is usually necessary to prescribe an oral phosphate-binding compound. Previously, aluminum-containing antacids were used; however, the recognition of aluminum accumulation and toxicity has led to a relative prohibition on any aluminum-containing medications. At present, calcium carbonate is the most widely used phosphate-binding agent in children. Patient acceptance is generally good, but the use of high doses may be complicated by hypercalcemia. Calcium carbonate is 40 per cent elemental calcium by weight; the usual initial dose is equivalent to the RDA for age (600 to 1200 mg/day elemental calcium) divided and given at meals.

The availability of the bioactive form of vitamin D for either oral (Rocaltrol) or intravenous (Calcijex) administration has significantly improved the prevention and treatment of renal osteodystrophy. The smallest available oral dose size is a 0.25-μg capsule, and the usual beginning dose for older children and adults is 0.25 μg/day. In younger children, smaller doses may be obtained by aspirating the capsule contents (0.25 μg

Rocaltrol/0.17 ml of liquid in each capsule) and giving a fraction of that material orally. Again, the dosage needs to be individualized according to the patient's response.

Use of the intravenous vitamin D preparation in hospitalized or hemodialysis patients avoids questions of compliance or absorption and achieves higher blood levels of vitamin D. This approach may be particularly useful for initiating treatment in patients with severe secondary hyperparathyroidism.

During osteodystrophy treatment, the "calcium-phosphorus product" (Ca [mg/dl] × PO_4[mg/dl]) should be maintained at 70 or lower. Higher values involve risk of metastatic calcification, tissue injury, and further decline in renal function. Serum calcium levels should be observed frequently (every 1 to 2 weeks) as treatment is initiated or changed. If hypercalcemia occurs, both the calcium supplement and the vitamin D may be withheld. In a few days, after documenting reduced serum calcium levels, drug doses can be adjusted and treatment resumed.

Anemia

Decreased erythropoietin (EPO) production in diseased kidneys, coupled with the shortened half-life of red blood cells in uremia, regularly produces anemia. Without transfusion support, most uremic children maintain their hemoglobin level at only 4 to 6 g/dl. This anemia is a major factor in their decreased exercise tolerance and may also have an impact on their sense of well-being, appetite, and growth.

Recombinant human EPO is now available and is effective in adults and children. The major benefit of EPO treatment in children is the avoidance of random blood transfusions, which simultaneously carry the risks of hypervolemia, infection, iron overload, and sensitization to HLA antigens. Most patients benefit from maintaining a hematocrit value in the range of 27 to 30 per cent and experience relatively few problems. After adequate iron stores are documented (serum ferritin ≥100 ng/ml or iron/total iron binding capacity ≥30 per cent), CRF patients may begin EPO therapy (25 to 50 units/kg subcutaneously once or twice weekly). Patients on hemodialysis may receive intravenous EPO with each dialysis treatment.

An increase in reticulocytes is usually noted within 2 weeks of starting EPO. A gradual hematocrit rise of 3 to 5 per cent per month is generally well tolerated, whereas increases greater than 8 per cent per month are usually an indication to withhold or reduce the EPO dose. Dosage must be individualized to reach the target hematocrit value; typical adjustments are about 25 units/kg per dose. Once the hematocrit goal is achieved, less frequent or smaller doses are usually required for maintenance. Regular monitoring of the iron stores is necessary to avoid development of occult iron deficiency, and dialysis patients should receive supplemental folic acid.

Several complications, including hypertension, seizures, and thromboses, have also appeared in patients treated with EPO. Increased red blood cell mass is regularly associated with increasing blood pressure. In uremic children, who may already have neurologic problems, the occurrence of seizures may be temporally associated with rapidly rising hematocrit values and blood pressure. Such patients receiving EPO need careful follow-up and strict attention to blood pressure control. Finally, several reports have noted an increased incidence of thrombosis (especially occurring in arteriovenous fistulas) in adult patients on EPO. In pediatric hemodialysis patients, this complication may be more likely in a poorly functioning fistula and might require adjustment in heparin use on hemodialysis.

Bleeding Diathesis

It has long been recognized that uremic patients have a clinically significant coagulopathy. This is characterized primarily by platelet dysfunction, which is signaled by easy bruising and a prolonged bleeding time. The exact cause of this problem is unclear, but it is thought to result from the accumulation of uremic toxins with advancing CRF. Usually, symptoms are noted when the creatinine level exceeds 6 to 7 mg/dl. Patients receiving regular dialysis generally demonstrate improved or normal bleeding times. Similarly, patients with higher hematocrit values (≥30 per cent) experience fewer clinical bleeding problems. Recently, it has also been shown that treatment with DDAVP (deamino-8-D-arginine vasopressin) improves uremic platelet adhesiveness by releasing endogenous stores of von Willebrand factor. Alternatively, administration of cryoprecipitate also increases circulating von Willebrand factor and improves platelet function.

To minimize bleeding problems, all patients with CRF should be advised to avoid aspirin and aspirin-containing products, which further impair platelet function. Additionally, an effort should be made to keep the hematocrit of patients with CRF, around 30 per cent, primarily by administering EPO (see earlier). The institution of regular dialysis treatments at an appropriate stage also lessens the chances of serious hemorrhage. For elective surgery or significant clinical bleeding, DDAVP may be acutely administered (0.3 μg/kg IV over 10 to 15 minutes). The peak effect of vasopressin is seen at 30 minutes and is largely lost by 90 minutes. If further therapy is needed, the dose may be repeated and additional von Willebrand factor may be supplied by giving cryoprecipitate.

Neurology

It appears that the nervous system is the primary "target organ" in CRF. Indeed, patients with untreated, advancing uremia exhibit progressive neurologic hypofunction and changes on electroencephalogram (EEG) and die in coma. Less dramatically, adults or children with CRF have impaired intelligence quotient (IQ) testing, lethargy, and somnolence and also experience progressive peripheral and autonomic neuropathy. The cause of this neural impairment is unknown, but, again, it is thought to be due to the accumulation of uremic toxins. Adequate dialysis or transplantation reverses EEG changes, improves activity level, and stabilizes or reverses the neuropathies.

In the rapidly growing brains of younger children, additional problems appear. Infants with significant uremia from birth are subject to acquired microcephaly, developmental delays, and, in the most severely affected, seizures and chorea. Aluminum accumulation, malnutrition, and uremia may all be synergistic factors leading to these problems in the developing infant brain.

In recognition of this potential group of complications, children should undergo careful neurodevelopmental assessments, EEG examination when appropriate, and a thorough evaluation for any paroxysmal neurologic activity that is noted. At present, no specific therapy is known, but avoiding aluminum intake (monitoring of blood aluminum levels), aggressive nutritional support, and early institution of renal replacement therapy all seem to be prudent approaches to CRF in infancy.

Medications

In CRF, altered protein binding, glomerular filtration rate, and tubular secretion combine to affect the kinetics of most drugs. Therefore, the diagnosis of CRF in a child requires a re-examination of all medications to be sure that the dosage is appropriate for the level of renal function. Certain medications should simply be prohibited in CRF, including aspirin (see earlier), as well as magnesium, potassium, and aluminum salts (toxic accumulation). Recognized nephrotoxic drugs (e.g., aminoglycosides, amphotericin) should be used only when an effective nontoxic agent is unavailable. If nephrotoxic drugs are required, ongoing scrutiny of serum drug and creatinine levels is appropriate to avoid drug accumulation and further renal impairment.

The general principles for drug therapy in CRF are as follows:

1. Minimize drug exposure, using only indicated drugs at the smallest effective dose.
2. The initial drug dose is usually unchanged; use measured drug levels whenever possible to guide subsequent dosing.
3. Consult a reference work for guidance with specific drugs (see References).

CONCLUSION

Thirty years ago, childhood CRF was a uniformly fatal disease. Today, the outlook is quite different. Renal transplantation is an established therapy available to all children. Rehabilitation after transplantation has been remarkable, with the children growing, attending school, and living essentially normal lives for years. Dialysis also plays a crucial role, serving as a bridge between the time when renal replacement therapy is required and the time when a functioning renal transplant is available.

Currently, the meticulous care of children with CRF is repaid with a minimum of long-term handicaps and many gratifying patient outcomes.

REFERENCES

Bennett WM, Aronoff GR, Golper TA, et al: Drug Prescribing in Renal Failure, 2nd ed. Philadelphia: American College of Physicians 1991.

Trompeter RS: A review of drug prescribing in children with end-stage renal failure. Pediatr Nephrol 1:183–194, 1987.

PERITONEAL DIALYSIS

STEVEN R. ALEXANDER, M.D.

The peritoneal cavity has been used in the treatment of children's disorders for at least 70 years. In 1918, Blackfan and Maxcy described the successful treatment of severely dehydrated infants using intraperitoneal injections of saline solution, a technique that is still used today in rural areas of some developing countries. Peritoneal dialysis was first used to treat children with acute renal failure more than 40 years ago, and since the 1960s, it has widely been considered to be the dialytic treatment of choice for acute renal failure in infants and young children, primarily because the technique is intrinsically simple, safe, and easily adapted for use in patients of all ages and sizes. The technique has been adapted even for infants weighing as little as 350 g.

Renal replacement therapy for pediatric patients was once limited to peritoneal dialysis in all but the most highly specialized pediatric centers. Many more pediatric nephrology programs can now routinely offer hemodialysis and hemoperfusion in patients weighing as little as 5 kg, and the recent development of *continuous arteriovenous hemofiltration* (CAVH) has added another valuable renal replacement technique to the arsenal of the pediatric nephrologist. However, peritoneal dialysis remains the most frequently employed pediatric renal replacement therapy worldwide for both acute and chronic renal failure.

INDICATIONS FOR DIALYSIS

Acute Renal Failure

In general, the indications for renal replacement therapy in children with acute renal failure (see also p. 428) may be summarized as follows:

1. Circulatory overload, usually manifest by congestive heart failure, hypertension, or pulmonary edema.
2. Intractable metabolic acidosis.
3. Hyperkalemia.
4. Severe hyponatremia or hypernatremia in the oligoanuric patient.
5. Uremic encephalopathy, usually associated with very high or rapidly rising serum urea nitrogen concentrations.
6. Bleeding, if due to uremia.
7. The need to remove fluid so that optimal nutrition, transfusions, and other therapies can be given to the oligoanuric patient.

For children with acute renal failure, the choice among the available therapeutic modalities (hemodialysis, peritoneal dialysis, or CAVH) should take into account the degree of expertise of the facility as well as the patient's size, clinical condition, and prognosis for recovery of renal function. Severe, life-threatening hyperkalemia or acidosis is most effectively treated with hemodialysis, although peritoneal dialysis may be preferred in some centers because of the rapidity with which it can be instituted. The hemodynamically unstable patient will tolerate hemodialysis poorly and should be treated with peritoneal dialysis or CAVH. Hemodialysis or hemoperfusion is preferred for treatment of poisonings.

Chronic Renal Failure

Chronic maintenance dialysis is required when the creatinine clearance falls below 5 to 10 ml/minute/1.73 m^2. Dialysis is often instituted at higher clearances in infants and young children when growth is poor, especially if head circumference falls below normal. The decision to begin chronic dialysis must always be individualized, but every effort must be made to begin dialysis soon enough to avoid any potentially severe or life-threatening consequences of renal failure, such as circulatory overload or hyperkalemia. Dialysis is often begun while the child is being prepared for renal transplantation, although nearly 25 per cent of North American children now receive transplants without any prior dialysis.

Today, the chronic dialytic therapy of choice for most young pediatric patients (those younger than 10 years of age) in North America is continuous peritoneal dialysis, which can be performed in the home. Either continuous ambulatory peritoneal dialysis (CAPD) or continuous cycling peritoneal dialysis (CCPD) may be used in children of any age, and both offer distinct advantages over hemodialysis as maintenance renal replacement therapy: near steady-state biochemical and fluid control, no disequilibrium syndrome, greatly reduced dietary restrictions, freedom from repeated dialysis needle punctures, improved control of hypertension, and a reduced requirement for blood transfusions. Most important, the simplicity and safety of CAPD and CCPD allow performance in the home by all but the most disrupted families, thereby returning the child with end-stage renal disease to regular school attendance and allowing family vacations and other normal childhood activities. During CAPD, the child (most children assume responsibility for some, if not all, of their own CAPD or CCPD home care after age 11 or 12 years) or the parent exchanges the dialysis solution four or five times in each 24 hours, using plastic containers commercially available in several different volumes and dextrose concentrations. In CCPD, an automated cycler is employed to perform the fluid exchanges during the 9 to 12 hours that the infant or child is in bed each night. CCPD has several advantages over CAPD in convenience for the child and the family, making it the current favorite in many large pediatric dialysis centers in the United States.

CONTRAINDICATIONS TO PERITONEAL DIALYSIS

There are few absolute contraindications to peritoneal dialysis in pediatric patients. The absence of an adequate peritoneal cavity, as in infants with omphalocele, diaphragmatic hernia, or gastroschisis, is an obvious contraindication. Recent abdominal surgery is only a relative contraindication, as long as there are no draining abdominal wounds. Patients with urinary tract diversions, such as vesicostomies or ureterostomies, and with bilateral polycystic kidneys, colostomies, gastrostomies, and prune-belly syndrome have all been successfully treated with peritoneal dialysis. Following renal transplantation, peritoneal dialysis is routinely used to treat acute renal allograft dysfunction or severe rejection episodes when the allograft has been placed in an extraperitoneal location. Extensive intra-abdominal adhesions may prevent successful peritoneal dialysis in some patients. The presence of a ventriculoperitoneal shunt in hydrocephalic children or the presence of a severe infection of the abdominal wall may also be a relative contraindication, although, again, the decision to begin peritoneal dialysis must be individualized, weighing risks against the availability of an alternative dialytic method.

PHYSIOLOGIC PRINCIPLES

The physiology of peritoneal dialysis has been extensively studied in adult subjects, but relatively few studies have been done with children. The peritoneum functions as a semipermeable membrane that permits the passage of water and solutes by the processes of diffusion and convection. Anatomic studies have shown that the surface area of the peritoneum is proportional to that of the body surface area in both children and adults. Thus, the peritoneal membrane in the child is larger, relative to body weight, than in the adult, and this property may be reflected by an increased ability to transfer solutes and water across the peritoneum of younger patients. Available data on this subject remain sparse and inconclusive, however. What is known is that the child's peritoneum allows passage of glucose into the blood from the dialysate and the transfer of proteins out of the blood into the dialysate more rapidly than is seen in adults. Removal of fluid (ultrafiltration) from children, especially infants, may be difficult using long-dwell exchanges (e.g., >2 hours) because the relatively rapid absorption of dextrose from the dialysate results in a more rapid decline in the osmolar gradient between blood and dialysate. Higher concentrations of dextrose in the dialysate and shorter dwell times are commonly employed in infants to offset these problems. Recent studies have suggested that the subdiaphragmatic lymphatic absorption of dialysate is greater in children than in adults, providing yet another reason why ultrafiltration may be difficult in some children.

CATHETER PLACEMENT

Access to the peritoneal cavity may be readily achieved using a temporary (percutaneous) catheter, although after about 72 hours the incidence of peritonitis rises sharply when the same temporary catheter is used. Surgical placement of a chronic peritoneal catheter, even in the setting of acute renal failure, has the obvious advantages of ensuring good immediate function and indefinite catheter life span. These advantages must be weighed in the individual patient against the risks and delays associated with an operative procedure that may require general anesthesia.

Percutaneous placement of a temporary peritoneal catheter in children is a simple procedure requiring great care and attention to detail. This procedure has been associated with all of the serious complications one might expect to see in cases of penetrating abdominal trauma, from massive hemorrhage to bowel perforation. Disposable catheters appropriate for use in children are widely available. Traditional techniques employ a trocar to perforate the peritoneum, which is distended at the time of catheter placement. This method has been replaced in some centers by the use of a modified Seldinger technique, which eliminates the trocar. The Seldinger technique requires the puncture of the only mildly distended peritoneal cavity with an 18-gauge needle, through which a guide wire is inserted into the peritoneal cavity; the needle is then withdrawn. The hole in the abdominal wall and peritoneum is then enlarged with dilators of increasing size inserted over the guide wire until the peritoneal catheter is itself inserted over the guide wire, and the guide wire is then withdrawn.

Although the Seldinger (guide wire) method is gaining popularity, the trocar technique is still widely used and many of the technical "pearls" are common to both methods. The trocar technique is described in detail next.

TROCAR CATHETER INSERTION

The catheter is inserted as follows:

1. Empty the bladder with a small sterile feeding tube (8 French). This tube is removed after successful placement of the peritoneal catheter to reduce the risk of urinary tract infection.
2. Ensure adequate sedation of older infants and children. Adults can be instructed to perform a Valsalva maneuver at the moment of trocar insertion, but children are rarely able to cooperate to this degree. Good sedation may increase the intraperitoneal priming volume required to safely perforate the now-relaxed child's peritoneum. Careful attention must be given to cardiorespiratory status throughout the procedure to prevent respiratory embarrassment caused by a large priming volume.
3. Scrub the skin of the lower abdomen with a surgical skin cleaner, followed by the application of an appropriate antiseptic, such as povidone-iodine.
4. Inject a local anesthetic subcutaneously and carry down to the peritoneum at a point in the midline that is two-thirds the distance up from the symphysis to the umbilicus.
5. Use a 16-gauge polyethylene over-the-needle catheter (e.g., Intracath) to infuse dialysate to distend the abdomen. Smaller needles (18 to 21 gauge) may be used without polyethylene catheters, but inflow is slower and subcutaneous dialysate infusion may go unrecognized for some time. The Intracath (with needle in place) is attached to the dialysate inflow line and inserted below the skin surface; an assistant then opens the clamp on the inflow line. By watching the drip chamber in the inflow line, one can see dialysate pass drop by drop into the subcutaneous tissue. The Intracath is then advanced until a steady stream of dialysate is observed in the drip chamber, demonstrating free flow of dialysate into the peritoneal cavity. The needle catheter is then advanced a bit farther, with the inflow line momentarily detached while the steel needle is withdrawn, the line reattached, and the remaining plastic catheter advanced until it is well within the peritoneal cavity. At least 30 ml/kg of *warmed* dialysate is

TABLE 1. Peritoneal Dialysis Solution Containing Bicarbonate

	ml	Na^+ (mEq)	Cl^- (mEq)	Mg^{++} (mEq)	SO_4^- (mEq)	HCO_3^- (mEq)	Hydrous Dextrose (g)
NaCl (0.45%)	896.0	69	69				
NaCl (2.5 mEq/ml)	12.0	30	30				
$NaHCO_3$ (1.0 mEq/ml)	40.0	40				40	
$MgSO_4$ (10%)	1.8			1.5	1.5		
$D_{50}W$	50.0						25
	999.8	139	99	1.5	1.5	40	25

Modified from Nash MA, Russo JC. Neonatal lactic acidosis and renal failure: The role of peritoneal dialysis. J Pediatr 91:101–105, 1977.
Calculated osmolality = 423 mOsm/kg H_2O.

infused while close attention is given to the vital signs of the child. Neonates may require additional ventilatory and/or circulatory support at this stage. When adequately filled, the abdomen will be fully distended and the abdominal wall taut enough to provide firm resistance to insertion of the dialysis trocar catheter. Large priming volumes may be required; the absolute limit in each case is determined by the point at which the inflow stream begins to fluctuate with respiration.

6. After removing the Intracath, make a small stab wound with a No. 11 blade at the site of the puncture, with care taken not to enter the peritoneum proper.

7. Trim the dialysis catheter, if necessary, for smaller infants. "Ideal" intraperitoneal catheter length may be estimated as 1 cm less than the distance from xiphoid to umbilicus; this ensures that the first fenestrations of the catheter will reside at least 3 cm inside the peritoneal cavity. Generally, short catheters perform better than long ones. The cut edges of a trimmed catheter should be beveled with iris scissors to reduce the risk of injury to abdominal viscera.

8. Insert the catheter and trocar together (the catheter "riding" the trocar into the peritoneal cavity) using a rotating motion and steady pressure directed at right angles to the plane of the abdominal wall at the insertion site. Considerable force may be needed to puncture the peritoneum; if the abdominal wall can be depressed substantially without penetrating the peritoneum, additional distending fluid is needed. Once the peritoneum has been penetrated, the trocar and catheter are directed toward the right or left lower quadrant. The catheter is advanced as the trocar is withdrawn.

9. When good in-and-out flow of dialysate has been demonstrated, trim the extra-abdominal portion of the catheter so that only 4 to 6 cm extend above the abdominal wall. The catheter is secured with a silk pursestring suture and water-resistant tape.

10. Should initial in-and-out exchanges yield cloudy or persistently bloody fluid or result in the appearance of diarrhea or polyuria (the high dextrose concentration of dialysate quickly resolves any question about the origin of the diarrhea or polyuria), remove the catheter immediately and replace it. Poor catheter drainage is a much more frequently encountered problem at this stage and is usually due to omental envelopment or obstruction of the temporary catheter. When this occurs, it is probably best to replace the temporary catheter with a surgically placed chronic catheter.

11. When a percutaneously placed catheter is used, initial exchange volumes are usually 20 to 30 ml/kg, with a gradual increase to 40 to 50 ml/kg over the first 24 hours of dialysis. When surgically placed catheters are used, a smaller exchange volume (20 ml/kg) is necessary during the initial 24 hours of dialysis to reduce the likelihood of dialysate leakage at the insertion site.

12. Warm the dialysate to body temperature to prevent hypothermia and enhance diffusion of small solutes.

PRESCRIPTION IN ACUTE RENAL FAILURE

The initial peritoneal dialysis prescription for the child with acute renal failure should reflect the clinical status of the patient and the goals of dialytic therapy. In the severely uremic child with hyperkalemia and acidosis, frequent exchanges are used during the initial stabilization on dialysis. With dialysate that contains 2.5 per cent dextrose, the exchange volume is infused over 5 to 10 minutes, allowed to dwell for 15 to 35 minutes, and allowed to drain for 5 to 15 minutes. More than two complete exchanges per hour can be accomplished but are rarely worthwhile. The amount of ultrafiltration required is determined by the fluid status of the child. Relatively euvolemic children may be dialyzed with 1.5 per cent dextrose solutions, although adequate fluid removal to allow intravenous alimentation, transfusions, and other therapies often necessitate 2.5 per cent dextrose solutions. The most hypertonic solution (4.25 per cent dextrose) is reserved for patients who are fluid overloaded. Hyperglycemia, hypernatremia, and hypovolemia are common complications associated with prolonged use of 4.25 per cent dextrose solutions. Heparin (500 units/L) is routinely added to the dialysate during the first 24 hours of treatment and during episodes of peritonitis.

Some critically ill infants are unable to tolerate the lactate that is absorbed from commercially available dialysis solutions because absorbed lactate worsens the lactic acidosis in these patients. Dialysate can be reformulated to contain bicarbonate instead of lactate, as shown in Table 1. Note that calcium must be supplemented intravenously when bicarbonate-containing dialysate is used.

Initial stabilization on peritoneal dialysis often requires 24 to 48 hours of frequent exchanges (30 to 60 minutes each, depending on catheter function and nursing staff resources) to remove accumulated solutes and excess fluid and to correct acidosis and hypertension. Once the patient is stabilized, if a permanent catheter is in place, peritoneal dialysis may be continued indefinitely while the return of renal function is awaited. By gradual extension of dwell periods and increase in exchange volumes, a typical maintenance CAPD regimen (e.g., 35 to 40 ml/kg per exchange, four to six exchanges per

TABLE 2. Empiric Intraperitoneal Antibiotic Dosages for Suspected CAPD or CCPD Peritonitis

	Loading Dose	Maintenance Dose
Cephalothin*	25 mg/kg (in a single exchange)	250 mg/L
plus		
Tobramycin*	1.7 mg/kg (in a single exchange)	4 to 6 mg/L

*May be mixed in dialysis fluid without affecting potency.
Abbreviations: CAPD, continuous ambulatory peritoneal dialysis; CCPD, continuous cycling peritoneal dialysis.

TABLE 3. Antibiotic Dosing Guidelines for the Treatment of Peritonitis in Pediatric Patients Receiving Continuous Peritoneal Dialysis*

	Half-Life			Dose‡		
				Initial		Maintenance
	Normal	ESRD	CAPD	mg/kg	mg/L of Dialysate	mg/L of Dialysate
Aminoglycosides						
Amikacin†	1.6	39	ND	5.0–7.5 IV/IP	—	6–7.5
Gentamicin†	2.2	53	32	1.5–1.7 IV/IP	—	4–6
Netilmicin†	2.1	42	ND	1.5–2.0 IV/IP	—	4–6
Tobramycin†	2.5	58	36	1.5–1.7 IV/IP	—	4–6
Cephalosporins						
Cefamandole	1.0	10	8.0	—	500	ND
Cefazolin	2.2	28	27	—	250–500	125–250
Cefoperazone	1.8	2.3	2.2	—	1000	500
Cefotaxime	0.9	2.5	2.4		1000	250
Cefoxitin	0.8	20	15	—	500	100
Ceftazidime	1.8	26	16	—	500	125
Ceftizoxime	1.6	28	11	—	500	125
Ceftriaxone	8.0	15	13	—	500	ND
Cefuroxime	1.3	18	15	—	750	250
Cephalothin	0.2	3.7	ND	—	1000	250
Moxalactam	2.2	20	16	—	500	ND
Cephradine	0.9	12	ND	—	250	125–250
Cephalexin	0.8	19	9	12.5 p.o.	—	12.5 mg/kg per dose q 8 hr p.o.
Penicillins						
Ampicillin	1.2	15	ND	—	250	50
Azlocillin	0.9	5.1	ND	—	250	250
Ticarcillin	1.2	15	ND	75 IV	—	75 mg/kg per dose q 12 hr IV
Vancomycin and others						
Vancomycin†	6.9	161	83	15 IV/IP	—	25–30
Clindamycin	2.8	2.8	ND	—	150	150

*Continuous peritoneal dialysis — CAPD or CCPD.
†Blood levels should be obtained periodically to avoid toxicity.
‡Current recommendations are adapted from the adult literature and are subject to change as/if new information on pediatric dosage becomes available.
Abbreviations: ESRD, end-stage renal disease; CAPD, continuous ambulatory peritoneal dialysis; IV/IP, intravenously/intraperitoneally; q, every; p.o., by mouth; ND, no data.

24 hours) may be reached in a few days. Continuous, prolonged-dwell peritoneal dialysis (either CAPD or CCPD) has become the standard approach to the treatment of acute renal failure in our center, once the child has been stabilized with an appropriate period of frequent exchanges to correct fluid and electrolyte disturbances and to lower the blood urea nitrogen (BUN). The near steady-state biochemical and fluid control achievable with CAPD and CCPD may be of particular benefit to critically ill children with acute renal failure whose cardiovascular status may be precarious.

PERITONITIS

The most common complication of both acute and chronic peritoneal dialysis is peritonitis. Sixty-five per cent of children treated with CAPD or CCPD for end-stage renal disease have at least one episode of peritonitis before they have completed the first 12 months of therapy. The most frequently cultured pathogens are *Staphylococcus epidermidis* and *S. aureus,* although gram-negative organisms and *Candida* sp. account for 20 to 30 per cent of peritonitis episodes. Antimicrobial agents should not be administered prophylactically but, rather, should be started empirically before culture results are available when patients show signs and symptoms of peritonitis. Peritonitis usually presents with cloudy peritoneal effluent in a mildly febrile child who may also have abdominal pain and tenderness. The peritoneal effluent will usually contain more than 100 white blood cells/mm^3, more than 50 per cent of which are polymorphonuclear neutrophils. Gram stain of the effluent demonstrates organisms in only 25 per cent of cases that eventually show positive cultures. When signs and symptoms of peritonitis are present, a sample for bacterial culture is obtained and antibiotic therapy begun immediately, using the intraperitoneal route.

Most authorities now recommend beginning intraperitoneal therapy with a first-generation cephalosporin in combination with an aminoglycoside until bacteriologic identification of the organism has been accomplished. Dosages for initial (empiric) intraperitoneal cephalothin and tobramycin are shown in Table 2. Currently recommended dosages and routes for many antimicrobials commonly used to treat peritonitis are shown in Table 3.

HEMODIALYSIS

ANTONIA C. NOVELLO, M.D., M.P.H.

Pediatric nephrologists consider renal transplantation the optimal therapeutic modality for children with renal failure; i.e., a successful transplant provides the best opportunity for normal growth and development and for alleviating the psychologic distress of chronic renal failure. However, prolonged dialysis may be needed in some children.

Dialysis is a technique for removing metabolites and toxins and for maintaining a satisfactory equilibrium of electrolytes and fluid volume in patients with disordered excretory capabilities. Hemodialysis, simply stated, is a diffusive process in which blood comes into contact with a balanced salt solution (dialysate) across a semipermeable membrane and solutes pass by diffusion along a concentration gradient, their rate of removal being determined by their physicochemical properties. Isotonic fluid removal is achieved by applying a hydrostatic pressure gradient on the membrane.

Hemodialysis has been performed in children since the early 1960s. The technique has been utilized in preparation for renal transplant during the search for a suitable donor, after a failed renal transplant, and for the treatment of life-threatening clinical complications. Nevertheless, there seems to be limited experience with long-term (longer than 5 years) hemodialysis in children. Despite this, the overall survival is good, with one report indicating a 5-year actuarial patient survival rate of 95 per cent. Several other options for the treatment of children with chronic renal failure (CRF) have become available during the past decade: continuous ambulatory peritoneal dialysis (CAPD), continuous cycling peritoneal dialysis (CCPD), and chronic intermittent peritoneal dialysis (IPD).

The number of patients in the pediatric age group with end-stage renal disease (ESRD) reportedly varies from 1 to 3.5 per million population per year. Prior to the widespread availability of hemodialysis and the newer peritoneal dialysis techniques (CAPD, CCPD, and IPD), definite treatment was not initiated until severe uremic complications were apparent. Currently, hemodialysis is begun before severe symptomatology occurs. Absolute indications for dialysis are uncontrollable hypertension with hypertensive encephalopathy or congestive heart failure, congestive heart failure unresponsive to loop diuretics, pericarditis, peripheral neuropathy, renal osteodystrophy, and bone marrow depression with either severe anemia, leukopenia, or thrombocytopenia.

In most instances, symptoms arising from involvement of a single organ system predominate and dictate the need for dialysis. In the child without such absolute indications, the decision to institute dialysis should be based on his or her ability to perform usual daily activities. In these cases, derangements in biochemical parameters can be useful indicators for starting dialysis, i.e., blood urea nitrogen (BUN) greater than 150 mg/dl, carbon dioxide content less than 12 mEq/L, potassium level greater than 6.0 mEq/L, falling hematocrit (less than 20 per cent, necessitating transfusion in the face of hyperkalemia and volume overload), and severe hypocalcemia (calcium level < 7.0 mg/dl). These biochemical abnormalities in combination with a glomerular filtration rate of less than 5 ml/minute/1.73 m^2 indicate the imminent need for dialysis.

Two other situations may require emergency initiation of hemodialysis: accidental poisoning and acute renal failure. As alternatives, hemoperfusion and peritoneal dialysis, respectively, might be considered in such cases. Peritoneal dialysis is widely available and has the advantage of not requiring heparinization.

DIALYSIS PRESCRIPTION FOR CHILDREN

Vascular Access

Patients undergoing hemodialysis require a vascular access that permits high blood flow rates. Three types of access are commonly used: shunts, fistulas, and temporary access. The Thomas femoral shunt is the preferred access for children weighing less than 15 kg or younger than 5 years of age who require hemodialysis. With any type of vascular access, the goal is to use the largest cannula that fits comfortably without compromising the intima of the vessel in which it is inserted. Disadvantages of the shunt include infections, clotting episodes, and, in some children, inhibition of normal activity and anxiety because of the presence of the external cannula. Ischemic damage to the leg where a groin shunt was placed has been reported as a rare complication.

In children with ESRD who will undergo long-term dialysis and whose weight is more than 15 kg, an arteriovenous fistula—a forearm vein anastomosed to a radial artery—is preferred. Fistulas differ from shunts in requiring "maturation." They must be constructed at least 3 weeks before utilization is anticipated. When the anastomosis provides insufficient blood flow, an alternate internal arteriovenous fistula can be created using either a bovine graft or synthetic material. Recently, microsurgical techniques in infants weighing less than 5 kg have been described. A detrimental effect, as with the use of shunts, is thrombosis. At times, the high fistula flow demands an excessively high cardiac output, resulting in eventual systolic hypertension and heart failure.

For temporary vascular access, percutaneous catheters have been used via femoral, subclavian, or internal jugular veins, even in children weighing as little as 6 kg.

Dialyzers

Because of the low cardiac output and the small vascular volume in children, the extracorporeal volume of the dialyzers, blood flow rates, and blood lines must be kept to a minimum. The ideal is to fill both the dialyzer and the blood tubing with less than 10 per cent of the child's blood volume (10 ml/kg body weight). Hollow fiber dialyzers are preferable to flat or coil dialyzers because their blood compartment is relatively small and rigid.

Three types of dialyzers are available today: parallel plate, hollow fiber, and coil. Children are usually dialyzed with parallel plate or hollow fiber dialyzers. The main consideration in choosing a dialyzer is its ultrafiltration coefficient and blood compartment volume. Pediatric dialyzers are generally designed for children in either the 10 to 20 kg (0.5 to 0.6 m^2) or the 20 to 40 kg (1.0 m^2) weight range. Children weighing more than 40 kg (1.3 to 1.6 m^2) can usually be treated using adult dialyzers. Children weighing less than 10 kg require a 0.25 m^2 dialyzer.

Delivery System

No special modifications of existing delivery systems are required for pediatric patients. The usual dialysate solution has the following composition: calcium, 3.5 mEq/L; potassium, 1.0 or 2.0 mEq/L; sodium, 135 mEq/L; chloride, 100 mEq/L; magnesium, 1.6 mEq/L; acetate, 38 mEq/L; and glucose, 0 to 250 mg/dl. If the child demonstrates intolerance (nausea, vomiting, hypotension) to acetate, as may occur with high-efficiency dialyzers, bicarbonate can be substituted for acetate in the bath. Likewise, the use of dialyzers with inappropriately high clearance values should be avoided in children. Several techniques, such as intravenous infusion of saline, human albumin, vasopressors, or mannitol, can be used to minimize ultrafiltration-induced hypotension. Separate filtration followed by isovolemic hemodialysis may also be employed. In order to minimize the need for these interventions, the ultrafiltration rate should be calculated to remove the desired quantity of fluid evenly during the course of dialysis.

Prescription

Many schemes have been proposed to determine the optimal frequency, duration, and clearance of dialysis in pediatric patients. The most commonly used method to determine the adequacy of dialysis is kinetic modeling. This technique employs urea as a marker of uremic toxicity and allows for the development of treatment options permitting maintenance of BUN within predetermined limits. The goal is to keep a time-averaged concentration of urea within the range of 60 to 70 mg/dl (predialysis BUN level of about 80 to 100 mg/dl and post-dialysis level of about 20 to 30 mg/dl).

The dialysis index, which compares and relates dialyzer surface area × weekly hours of dialysis ÷ body surface area, has been formulated according to values derived from adult experiences. In most pediatric centers, the initial prescriptions of dialyzer clearance and time schedule depend on the child's weight (surface area), fluid accumulation between dialysis treatments, and the pre-dialysis level of BUN. In most centers, dialysis is usually prescribed three times a week for periods ranging from 4 to 6 hours, utilizing standard priming and heparinization techniques described in the literature.

Ultrafiltration

During ultrafiltration, fluid removed from the plasma is replaced with fluid equilibrated from the expanded interstitial space. The degree of ultrafiltration varies according to the desired weight loss. Excessive ultrafiltration (greater than 3 kg for adolescents or 2 kg for younger children) is frequently necessary. This can cause hypotension, nausea, vomiting, headaches, and cramps. When hypoalbuminemia (less than 3 g/dl) is present and ultrafiltration is required, the albumin level must be raised to improve tolerance of ultrafiltration. Although equilibration is rapid, signs of plasma volume depletion occur at times. In this event, separate ultrafiltration for 1 hour prior to the initiation of dialysis will aid in the removal of fluid without concomitant hypotension.

Nutrition and Diet in Dialyzed Children

Since growth failure and nutritional energy deficiencies are commonly recognized in dialyzed children with ESRD, an effort should be made to maximize the number of calories ingested. This is difficult, inasmuch as caloric intake must be kept high while sodium, potassium, phosphorus, protein, and fluids must be limited. Today, the goal is to strike a fair balance among these needs. The energy and protein content of the diet must be supplemented and not limited, and dietary restrictions must not produce nutrient deficiencies, even if this means a greater dialytic requirement. The goal is to provide 80 to 100 per cent of the recommended daily allowance energy requirements for these children. Daily dietary recommendations are: calories, 2000/m^2; protein, 1.5 to 2.5 g/kg, or 3 to 4 g/kg in small children (less than 10 to 16 kg); sodium, 40 mEq/m^2; potassium, 30 mEq/m^2; and fluids, 500 ml/m^2 plus an amount equal to urine volume. B complex vitamins and folic acid, 1 mg daily, are also supplemented. Phosphate-binding gels (preferably without aluminum), 1 to 3 capsules three times a day with meals, or calcium carbonate is given to reduce the serum phosphorus level.

In general, therefore, the dietary intake of dialyzed children should include a balanced energy intake and a protein intake of approximately 2 g/kg/day.

COMPLICATIONS OF HEMODIALYSIS

Hypertension. Virtually all patients undergoing hemodialysis have periods of hypertension. The usual mechanism is volume expansion, which generally responds to dietary fluid and salt restriction. Ultrafiltration to dry weight also controls hypertension in more than 90 per cent of patients. Occasional hypertension episodes are not controlled by dialysis, and these patients may require hypertensive medication. Occasionally, hypertensive medications are ineffective and bilateral nephrectomy is necessary for blood pressure control. This is rare, however, with the availability of captopril and minoxidil. Most of these cases are associated with high levels of renin. Post-nephrectomy hypertension is mostly volume-related. If hypertension persists after nephrectomy, it may be due to changes in peripheral resistance or to vasoactive substances produced outside the kidney. Nevertheless, blood pressure control during hemodialysis generally improves once the patient is well dialyzed.

Anemia. Children with CRF have a normochromic, normocytic anemia secondary to deficient erythropoiesis. When they undergo dialysis, this state is complicated by a continuing loss of blood, mostly in the dialyzer and because of frequent sampling for laboratory determinations. Increased hemolysis due to the mechanical trauma of the extracorporeal circulation is a minor additional factor. If the patient has undergone bilateral nephrectomy, the anemia worsens. Most children need transfusions to maintain the hematocrit level above 20 per cent. Complications from frequent transfusion procedures include infection with hepatitis B antigen, tissue iron deposition, and sensitization to HLA antigens. If patients fail to respond to iron (e.g., adolescents with fused epiphyses), benefit may be obtained from nandrolone phenpropionate* (Durabolin, 50 to 100 mg IM every week for boys and every 2 weeks for girls). This is helpful in stimulating erythropoiesis. This treatment should not be used in patients with unfused epiphyses.

Osteodystrophy. Chronic dialysis usually stabilizes existing renal osteodystrophy. Two types of lesions have been recognized by x-ray examination: rickets-like lesions (osteomalacia) and subperiosteal bone resorption (secondary hyperparathyroidism or osteitis fibrosa). Meticulous control of acidosis and calcium and phosphorus balance by pharmacologic agents or dietary maneuvers may alleviate these problems. Controlling secondary hyperparathyroidism prior to dialysis is also important. During dialysis, the dialysate calcium should be high (7.0 mg/dl) to allow the ionized calcium to be transferred to the patient. Parathyroid hyperplasia, however, rarely involutes with the use of a high calcium-containing dialysate alone. Vitamin D analogues and supplemental calcium result in a more dramatic response. Dihydrotachysterol (0.2 or 0.4 mg daily) and supplemental calcium carbonate (500 to 2000 mg daily) have been advocated. If hypocalcemia persists, 1,25-dihydroxycholecalciferol (Rocaltrol, 0.25 μg once or twice daily) should be used instead.

Despite dietary restrictions, most children are also hyperphosphatemic, requiring aggressive therapy to maintain serum phosphorus between 4 and 5 mg/dl. This should be accomplished with phosphate-binding gels (not containing aluminum) or calcium carbonate. If by x-ray examination the lesions of hyperparathyroidism fail to show evidence of healing, or if they worsen despite correction of calcium and phosphorus parameters, parathyroid gland extirpation (3½) may be indicated. In the presence of rickets, however, parathyroidectomy is not beneficial. Chronic aluminum loading may cause rickets, as is evident on bone biopsy. Aluminum can be chelated by weekly infusions of desferrioxamine.

Cardiovascular Alterations. Left ventricular performance, as measured by systolic time intervals, may be depressed by uremia; this effect has been reported on echocardiography. In children, hemodialysis results in improvement in left ventricular function. Pericarditis develops in 2 to 19 per cent of patients on dialysis—in some, years after the initiation of dialysis and, in others, within the first 3 months. Echocardiography appears to be the most helpful method for assessment of patients with pericarditis. Major hemodynamic complica-

*This use is not listed by the manufacturer.

tions occur as a result of cardiac tamponade and constrictive pericarditis. In patients with dialysis-associated pericarditis, intensive dialysis alone (3 to 4 weeks) is usually curative. Heparin dosage in these individuals should be reduced and carefully monitored because hemorrhage may cause cardiac tamponade. Other treatment modalities are peritoneal dialysis, charcoal hemoperfusion, systemic or intrapericardial steroids, and pericardial stripping. Furthermore, hypertriglyceridemia is frequently found in children on dialysis. Hypercholesterolemia and an increased fraction of low-density lipoproteins can also occur.

Psychosocial Problems. In children, dialytic treatments are time-consuming, medical complications are common, and loss of schooling is frequent, often leading to poor peer-group interactions. Associated complications are loss of self-esteem, social isolation, and lack of independence. The treatment goal is to allow patients as much responsibility as possible for their daily care; the ultimate goal is rehabilitation and community integration.

Seizures. In most instances, a specific cause cannot be identified, and thus the seizure is attributed to the disequilibrium syndrome. Patients with high BUN, especially those during their first or second dialysis treatment, are at greater risk. Disequilibrium is prevented by using a relatively high dialysate sodium concentration (140 to 145 mEq/L), by decreasing the efficiency of urea clearance to 1.0 to 1.5 ml/minute/kg, or by infusing 25 per cent mannitol (1 g/kg), over the course of dialysis, in order to maintain extracellular fluid osmolality. In some cases, prophylactic phenobarbital prior to and/or during dialysis has been advocated.

Hepatitis. Evidence supports the conclusion that infection with hepatitis B virus increases morbidity and mortality. The incidence of hepatitis in children treated with chronic hemodialysis is approximately 10 per cent. Blood parameters to be followed monthly as a precaution are serum glutamic-oxalic transaminase (SGOT), serum glutamic-pyruvic transaminase (SGPT), bilirubin, and hepatitis B antigen levels. Elevation of SGOT and SGPT in the absence of hepatitis B antigen may be due to hepatitis A or hepatitis C. Methods established to decrease the incidence of HBsAG-positive hepatitis among patients and staff of hemodialysis units include the provision of gowns and gloves, use of disposable equipment, routine screening for hepatitis B virus, dialysis of HBsAg-positive patients in isolation, and possibly utilization of home dialysis. To contain or prevent an epidemic, hyperimmune serum may be given to ESRD patients and staff members recently exposed to hepatitis virus. Hepatitis B vaccine is also an effective prophylaxis. There is a significant incidence of "e" antigenemia in children with persistent hepatitis antigenemia, indicating infectivity of these patients.

RENAL TRANSPLANTATION IN CHILDREN

TERESITA L. MELOCOTON, M.D.
and ROBERT B. ETTENGER, M.D.

Successful renal transplantation continues to be the optimal therapeutic modality in children with end-stage renal disease (ESRD). Advances in immunosuppressive management, histocompatibility matching, perioperative and postoperative care, and the diagnosis and treatment of acute rejection have all contributed to improved patient survival and graft outcome in pediatric patients. However, there are a number of technical, metabolic, immunologic, and psychologic factors that make pediatric renal transplant patients different from adults.

INCIDENCE AND ETIOLOGY OF END-STAGE RENAL DISEASE IN CHILDREN

The United States Renal Data System reported that, in 1988, 11 patients per million total population (pmtp) aged 0 to 19 years began ESRD therapy. The majority of children presenting with ESRD are between 11 and 15 years of age. In infants younger than 1 year of age, the incidence approaches 0.2 pmtp.

The causes of ESRD in children differ from those in adults, with an increased incidence of congenital and hereditary diseases in the pediatric age group. In the 1991 North American Pediatric Renal Transplant Cooperative Study (NAPRTCS) report for the calendar years 1987 to 1990, there were 1560 patients registered who were 18 years of age or younger. The five most frequent diagnoses were: aplastic/hypoplastic/dysplastic kidneys (18 per cent), obstructive uropathy (16 per cent), focal segmental glomerulosclerosis (12 per cent), reflux nephropathy (5 per cent), and systemic immunologic disease (5 per cent).

PATIENT AND ALLOGRAFT SURVIVAL RATES

Patient and allograft survival rates have been steadily improving in children and adolescents, although, in many cases, the outcomes still do not match those observed in adults. According to current NAPRTCS data, actuarial graft survival rates (± standard errors) in recipients of living donor grafts are 89 ± 1.3 per cent, 82 ± 1.7 per cent, and 79.5 ± 2.1 per cent at 1, 2, and 3 years, respectively. For cadaver donor grafts, the results are 74 ± 1.6 per cent, 67 ± 1.9 per cent, and 62 ± 2.3 per cent at 1, 2, and 3 years, respectively. In the United States over the last 4 years, living related donor grafts were used in approximately 43 per cent of the transplantations performed.

There are relatively scarce data on long-term (i.e., ≥ 10 years) outcome in pediatric renal transplant patients. The few studies available report overall patient survival rates of 45 to 68 per cent at 20 years after transplantation. Cadaver donor graft survival rates at 15 to 20 years are approximately 20 per cent; living related donor graft survival rates are slightly better at 20 years—35 per cent.

CRITERIA FOR ACCEPTABILITY FOR RENAL TRANSPLANTATION

Generally, almost all children with ESRD are candidates for renal transplantation. However, a number of factors must be considered when one evaluates these children for transplantation.

Mental and Neurologic Status

Psychosis and developmental delay are not by themselves contraindications to dialysis and transplantation. The child with psychosis or developmental delay presenting for ESRD care requires a careful evaluation to determine whether the psychologic illness is long-standing or is closely related temporally to the onset of uremia. The uremic state may cause depression and developmental delay in children. Initiation of dialysis often improves the uremic symptomatology and allows progression to transplantation in situations in which it may have been predicted to be unfeasible. On the other hand, severely retarded children respond poorly to the imposed constraints of ESRD care. A child with a very low intelligence quotient (IQ) (e.g., < 40) cannot comprehend the need for procedures that are often painful. In this situation, the family must be involved and supported in the decision whether to pursue definitive ESRD care.

Psychosocial Factors

Psychosocial and emotional problems in children and adolescents undergoing ESRD therapy frequently are manifested as noncompliance with the therapeutic regimen. More than 50 per cent of all pediatric renal transplant recipients are noncompliant with at least one of the immunosuppressive medications; this figure rises to almost 65 per cent when only adolescents are considered. *Because noncompliance invariably leads to graft rejection, it is crucial to identify the potentially noncompliant patient during dialysis, if possible.* In general, it is unwise to place a child or adolescent on a waiting list when there is a strong conviction by the transplant team that noncompliance is highly likely. Behavior modification programs, securing family support, and working with the pre-illness personality traits of the child are the keys to obtaining post-transplant compliance.

Pre-existing Malignancy

Wilms' tumor is the most common malignancy requiring ESRD care in childhood. Transplantation in children with Wilms' tumor should be deferred for at least 1 year following treatment of the tumor in order to detect presence of malignancy and avoid the risk of overwhelming sepsis following transplantation.

Urologic Abnormality

The presence of significant reflux in native kidneys is often associated with recurrent infection. If these infections cannot be controlled with antibiotic prophylaxis, native nephrectomy may be required.

The presence of an abnormal lower urinary tract is not a contraindication to transplantation. If the bladder has been defunctionized because of a prior diversion procedure, vigorous attempts can be made to use it. In recipients with abnormal bladders, there is an increased incidence of post-transplant urologic complications and urinary tract infections. Although some centers have noted relatively poor graft outcome in children with obstructive uropathy, graft outcome in these children has been identical to that in children with normal lower urinary tracts at the University of California, Los Angeles (UCLA). If the bladder is not usable, a diversion, such as a continent ileal loop or bladder augmentation, can be created prior to transplantation.

In a child with a neurogenic bladder, self-catheterization can be employed successfully and safely after transplantation. Problems may include urinary tract infection when catheterization technique is poor and renal dysfunction from partial obstruction if the patient is noncompliant with catheterization.

Generalized Infection

Before transplantation is considered, it is important to treat any infection. If unrecognized, infections can disseminate when transplant immunosuppression is started.

Transplantation in the Child on Peritoneal Dialysis

In many centers, peritoneal dialysis rather than hemodialysis is the favored mode of dialysis therapy in children and adolescents. Although at one time this was a controversial issue, it is now agreed that children on continuous ambulatory peritoneal dialysis (CAPD) or continuous cycling peritoneal dialysis (CCPD) show graft and patient survival rates comparable to those of children receiving hemodialysis.

In the absence of infection, the peritoneal dialysis catheter is left in place until good graft function has been established for 4 to 8 weeks. The catheter may then be removed.

Extraperitoneal placement of the transplant allows use of the peritoneum for dialysis during episodes of acute tubular necrosis or severe rejection. The catheter may also be used to drain post-transplant ascites, a complication occasionally seen in children who were on CCPD or CAPD prior to transplantation.

A recent episode of peritonitis does not disqualify a patient for transplantation if he or she has been infection-free and the peritoneal fluid specimens for culture have been negative for at least 2 weeks (i.e., after a full course of treatment for peritonitis). The incidence of post-transplant infectious complications in CAPD and CCPD patients has been low. Infections such as peritonitis, exit-site infection, and tunnel infections respond to appropriate antibiotic therapy; catheter removal is needed in severe exit-site and tunnel infections.

Primary Renal Disease

In children, recurrence of the primary disease following renal transplantation may account for from 5 to 10 per cent of graft loss. The two main disease categories that can potentially involve the graft are (1) inherited metabolic diseases and (2) primary glomerulonephritis.

Inherited Metabolic Diseases

Inherited metabolic diseases that can involve the graft include diabetes mellitus, cystinosis, oxalosis, Fabry's disease, and sickle cell anemia. In pediatrics, cystinosis and oxalosis are of major significance.

Cystinosis. In nephropathic cystinosis, recurrence of Fanconi syndrome has not been described despite the accumulation of cystine crystals in the graft interstitium. Interestingly, there is no accumulation of cystine in the tubular or glomerular epithelial cells, as is seen in native cystinotic kidneys; instead, the interstitial cystine appears to result from the elevated cystine content of host leukocytes that transit the transplanted kidney. The major post-transplant consequences of cystinosis are extrarenal manifestations (e.g., loss of vision, photophobia, and hypothyroidism), and these continue to progress after transplantation.

Oxalosis (Primary Hyperoxaluria Type I). The results of kidney transplantation are poor in oxalosis because of recurrence. Complications such as infection, acute tubular necrosis, and rejection can promote oxalate deposition in the kidney. Recent reports suggest that successful transplantation in patients with primary hyperoxaluria is possible. These reports stress the importance of vigorous preoperative reduction of serum oxalate levels with daily hemodialysis, immediate postoperative diuresis, and post-transplant management with pyridoxine, neutral phosphate, magnesium, and noncalciuric diuretic therapy. Nevertheless, even with this regimen, the rate of recurrence is still high. Preliminary reports suggest that combined liver and kidney transplantation may result in improved outcome, because the liver serves as a source of the deficient enzyme, thereby sparing the transplanted kidney from the toxic effects of oxalate deposition.

Glomerulonephritis

Focal Segmental Glomerulosclerosis (FSGS). FSGS is one of the most common glomerular diseases leading to ESRD in children and has one of the highest potentials for recurrence in the allograft. The recurrence rate ranges from 30 to 43 per cent, and half of these patients may lose the graft because of the recurrence. Risk factors implicated in the development of FSGS recurrence are (1) short history of nephrotic syndrome (<3 years between onset of nephrotic syndrome and development of renal failure); (2) presence of mesangial cell proliferation in the native kidney; (3) children older than 6 years of age at onset of the original nephrotic syndrome; and (4) recurrence in a previous transplant.

Proteinuria and slow graft failure are the hallmarks of recurrent FSGS. Proteinuria may be massive and often occurs within hours to days after transplantation; it can also recur insidiously weeks or months later. Graft failure is not predictable; often, there is a moderately long course of graft function punctuated by the clinical problems associated with nephrotic syndrome.

There is no definitive treatment for recurrence. There have been attempts at reversal using cyclophosphamide, plasmapheresis, and/or cyclosporin A (CsA) with variable success. We have had success in inducing remission with early plasmapheresis and high-dose CsA, but results are still preliminary.

Despite the potential for recurrence of FSGS, children with this disease should not be excluded from transplantation. Most centers, however, prefer using cadaver donor grafts rather than living related donor grafts in children who are at high risk for recurrence.

Immunoglobulin A Nephropathy and Henoch-Schönlein Purpura (HSP). Histologic recurrence of immunoglobulin A (IgA) nephropathy and HSP occurs frequently, but graft failure is rare. Occasionally, recurrence of these diseases can be clinically significant, with nephrotic syndrome, crescents, and graft failure. It is recommended that transplantation be delayed until 6 to 12 months after HSP has abated.

Hemolytic-Uremic Syndrome (HUS). HUS is the most common cause of primary renal failure in children. It has been suggested that HUS recurs in more than 50 per cent of cases, although this is not a universal experience. Transplantation is deferred until all clinical manifestations of HUS have completely abated. HUS can be classified into different subtypes, and it is likely that these subtypes vary in their propensity to recur.

CsA has been associated with recurrence of HUS. At UCLA, we have used low-dose CsA in selected patients with HUS without clinically significant recurrence. If there has been a rapid recurrence of HUS in a first-use CsA-treated graft, its reuse should be avoided.

Membranoproliferative Glomerulonephritis (MPGN). Histologic evidence of recurrence regularly occurs in patients with MPGN type II, and to a lesser extent in patients with MPGN type 1. The clinical impact of MPGN is usually benign. Graft failure from recurrence appears to supervene in no more than 10 to 15 per cent of patients with MPGN.

Alport Syndrome (Hereditary Nephritis). This entity is characterized by the absence of a specific glomerular basement membrane antigen. Although, strictly speaking, recurrence does not occur, a small number of patients generate an antibody to the glomerular basement membrane antigen of the transplanted kidney. This can produce a clinical picture of extracapillary proliferative glomerulonephritis and rapidly progressive graft failure. Plasmapheresis and substitution of cyclophosphamide for azathioprine are occasionally effective in blunting the process, but graft failure is the usual outcome.

FACTORS AFFECTING RENAL TRANSPLANT OUTCOME

Recipient Age

In general, recipients younger than 6 years of age have a lower graft survival rate than older recipients. This is particularly true of recipients of cadaver donor allografts. Primary graft nonfunction and vascular thrombosis occur more frequently in children younger than 6 years of age. Children younger than 2 years of age are particularly vulnerable to graft loss. According to NAPRTCS data, the 1-year graft survival rate for cadaver donor transplant recipients who are 2 years old or younger is only 50 per cent, compared with approximately 70 per cent in older age groups. Living related donor transplant recipients who are 2 years old or younger have a survival rate of 73 per cent, compared with 86 to 94 per cent in older age groups. Graft survival in children from 2 to 6 years of age has improved dramatically over the past few years as a result of a better understanding of immunosuppression in children (see later) and improvement in transplant surgical techniques. At UCLA, the 1-year graft survival rate in children younger than 6 years of age is 93 per cent.

Donor Age

It has traditionally been assumed that young children should receive cadaver kidneys from young donors. However, for children, the optimal age for cadaver kidney donors appears to be between 6 and 50 years. Kidneys from very young donors (younger than 1½ years of age) often fail because of graft thrombosis and primary nonfunction. Similarly, almost all studies document relatively poor outcome in pediatric transplant recipients receiving grafts from donors younger than 4 to 6 years of age.

Human Leukocyte Antigen (HLA) Matching

Renal transplants from HLA-identical sibling donors have the highest rates of success, with 1-year graft survival rates usually exceeding 90 per cent. Children receiving transplants from parents or haploidentical siblings generally have better allograft survival than those receiving cadaver donor transplants.

Optimally matched HLA-B and -DR cadaver donor grafts have a calculated half-life (i.e., the number of years to the time when half the graft is lost) of approximately 12 years, in contrast to a half-life of only 5 to 7 years for less well matched grafts. However, the value of sharing cadaver donor transplants over long distances on the basis of HLA matching continues to be controversial. This is because the prolonged storage time needed to facilitate long-distance sharing may predispose to early renal dysfunction, acute tubular necrosis, and consequent diminished graft survival. Current evidence suggests that it is appropriate to attempt to secure fully HLA-matched cadaver allografts, even over long distances. Fully matched kidneys have a 1-year cumulative graft survival rate of 90 per cent compared with a 79 per cent graft survival rate in a control (nontransported) group that was not well matched.

WORK-UP OF THE POTENTIAL DONOR

Many centers prefer living-related to cadaver donor transplantation. Generally, living donor transplantation produces more favorable results because of better histocompatibility matching. Moreover, the operation can be planned and scheduled to meet the needs of the family. Finally, the supply of cadaver organs is limited; therefore, it is more expeditious to use a living donor transplant rather than wait for a compatible cadaver donor.

Best results are seen with an HLA-identical sibling; however, excellent results can also be obtained with a haploidentical relative, and many centers have reported good results with totally unmatched relatives and/or living nonrelated donors. Most living donors are highly motivated immediate family members. All donors must be ABO blood group–compatible and should be in excellent medical condition with normal renal function. Recipient sera should be devoid of antibodies to donor HLA-A, -B, -C, and -DR antigens (i.e., there should be a negative lymphocyte cross-match). See Table 1 for evaluation of the potential living donor.

Excellent graft outcome can also be obtained using a cadaver donor. See Table 2 for the criteria used when screening

TABLE 1. Evaluation of the Potential Living Donor

1. History, physical examination, repeated BP determinations.
2. ABO blood group, tissue typing, lymphocyte cross-match, mixed lymphocyte culture.
3. CBC, platelet count, BUN, creatinine, glucose, cholesterol, triglycerides, calcium, phosphorus, uric acid, prothrombin time, creatinine clearance, HIV and hepatitis B, C surface antigen, CMV titer, VDRL, SGOT, SGPT, bilirubin, alkaline phosphatase, pregnancy tests in females.
4. Urinalysis, urine c/s, 24-hr urine protein.
5. Chest x-ray, EKG.
6. Renal ultrasound or IVP, renal angiogram.
7. Psychiatric evaluation.

Abbreviations: BP, blood pressure; CBC, complete blood count; BUN, blood urea nitrogen; HIV, human immunodeficiency virus; CMV, cytomegalovirus; SGOT, serum glutamic-oxaloacetic transaminase; SGPT, serum glutamic-pyruvic transaminase; EKG, electrocardiogram; IVP, intravenous pyelogram; c/s, culture and sensitivity.

potential cadaver donors. All donors must be ABO blood group–compatible, and HLA matching should be as close as is practical to minimize acute rejection and optimize long-term graft outcome. The lymphocyte cross-match must be negative to avoid hyperacute rejection.

WORK-UP OF THE RECIPIENT

Prior to transplantation, the recipient should be evaluated thoroughly, as outlined in Table 3.

IMMUNOSUPPRESSION

The immunosuppressive agents used in pediatric transplantation are CsA, corticosteroids, azathioprine, and antilymphocyte preparations.

Prior to the cyclosporine era, corticosteroids and azathioprine were the mainstays of maintenance immunosuppression. Short- and medium-term results were quite inferior to what can be achieved today (see later), and higher maintenance doses of corticosteroids were necessary.

TABLE 2. Criteria for Screening Potential Cadaver Donors

1. Minimum age 3 years (preferably 6 years), maximum 65 years (preferably 50 years or younger), with no history of hypertension, primary renal disease, diabetes mellitus, or malignancy other than primary nonmetastasized CNS or skin cancer.
2. Absence of generalized bacterial infection; if infection documented, donor is usable if receiving appropriate antimicrobial therapy for at least 24 hours.
3. Viral infection.
   a. Negative HIV antibody and hepatitis B, C surface antigen studies.
   b. If donor is CMV seropositive, recipient should be seropositive as well, unless recipient receives CMV prophylaxis.
4. Normal urinalysis and preterminal hourly urine output of at least 0.5 ml/kg.
5. Normal serum urea nitrogen and creatinine—may be elevated if donor is kept dry; i.e., prerenal azotemia is present.
6. Cold ischemia time less than 48 hours, preferably less than 36 hours.
7. Declaration of brain death by the patient's physician.
8. ABO compatibility with recipient.
9. Negative complement-dependent cytotoxicity cross-match using donor T lymphocytes and recipient serum from the day of transplant.

Abbreviations: CNS, central nervous system; HIV, human immunodeficiency virus; CMV, cytomegalovirus.

TABLE 3. Evaluation of the Renal Transplant Recipient

1. HLA typing and periodic testing for anti-HLA antibodies; antibody testing 2 to 4 weeks after every transfusion.
2. Chest X-ray, EKG, and echocardiogram.
3. Identify and treat infection adequately (urinary tract, peritoneum, etc.).
4. Screen for HIV, hepatitis B and C, CMV antibody, and TB.
5. Urologic evaluation with cystoscopy, VCUG, and urodynamic studies (when indicated); if massive reflux and treatment-resistant infection, consider nephrectomy, otherwise avoid.
6. Control hypertension with adequate dialysis, antihypertensive agents, or, as last resort, bilateral nephrectomy.
7. Diagnose and treat bone disease (hyperparathyroidism, necrosis); parathyroidectomy prior to transplant if hyperparathyroidism uncontrollable.
8. Remove rejected transplanted kidneys if symptomatic.
9. Control nephrotic syndrome.
10. If neutropenia and/or thrombocytopenia present, control hypersplenism (partial splenectomy or embolization).
11. Establish patterns of medication compliance; psychiatric evaluation.
12. Control of seizures with drugs that are not hepatic p-450 enzyme inducers, if possible.
13. Identify any drugs the patient is on that can interfere with prednisone, azathioprine, cyclosporine (i.e., Rifampin, Tegretol, Allopurinol).
14. Evaluate hepatic function; abnormalities may affect metabolism of immunosuppressive agents.

Abbreviations: EKG, electrocardiogram; HIV, human immunodeficiency virus; CMV, cytomegalovirus; TB, tuberculosis; VCUG, voiding cystourethrogram.

The adverse effects of *corticosteroids* include obesity, cushingoid facies, hyperlipidemia, aseptic necrosis of bone, acne, hypertension, and, most significantly in children, growth retardation. Growth suppression occurs with doses of prednisone exceeding 8.5 mg/m^2/day, or 0.25 mg/kg/day. Because of the growth-suppressive effects of corticosteroids, the concept of alternate-day steroid therapy was introduced. In general, growth velocity has been improved by alternate-day therapy and side effects have been reduced. However, some have expressed concern that the use of alternate-day therapy has been associated with a concomitant increase in the incidence of rejection.

As an alternative to alternate-day therapy, some centers have adopted a low-dose daily prednisone regimen. If prednisone can be reduced to less than 0.25 mg/kg/day, young recipients of well-functioning grafts grow well. Others have advocated discontinuation of corticosteroids altogether. Unfortunately, only one third to one half of children can be maintained rejection-free off prednisone. In many instances, there is a permanent decrease in renal function that is sustained during a rejection episode when steroid withdrawal is attempted. Because growth is dependent on renal function (see later) as well as steroid dose, any attempt at steroid withdrawal must be carefully considered, and, if attempted, close observation is mandatory to detect rejection before significant or permanent renal dysfunction supervenes.

Azathioprine is now considered an adjunct to prednisone and CsA in a "triple therapy" regimen, allowing for use of lower doses of the other two agents. The main adverse effects of azathioprine are neutropenia and hepatic enzyme elevations. Some centers have electively converted recipients from CsA to azathioprine to prevent CsA toxicity or because of financial concerns. However, conversion involves a high incidence of acute rejection.

CsA has become the standard maintenance immunosuppressive agent in renal transplantation because of its efficacy in preventing rejection. CsA is more difficult to use in children than in adults. Because the intestinal absorption of CsA is directly proportional to the length of a person's small bowel, young children absorb CsA less well than do adults. Moreover, children metabolize cyclosporine more rapidly than do adults. The half-life of cyclosporine is age-dependent, so that young children metabolize cyclosporine much more rapidly than do older children. Hence, certain children may require higher doses and/or more frequent dosing schedules to achieve therapeutic blood levels. Finally, CsA is nephrotoxic, especially during early graft dysfunction. The technical challenges of transplantation in children make long vascular anastomosis times and resultant early graft dysfunction more likely. For this reason, many centers avoid intravenous CsA during the early postoperative period.

At UCLA, we use a "sequential" immunosuppressive protocol (Table 4) that was modified for use in pediatric cadaver transplantation. In a sequential program, CsA is withheld initially and an antilymphocyte preparation is instituted to forestall rejection; the antilymphocyte preparation is continued until graft function begins to normalize. Doses of CsA (mg/kg) are frequently higher in children than in adults to achieve appropriate CsA blood levels, as shown in Table 5.

With the sequential protocol and the therapeutic guidelines in Table 5, primary cadaver actuarial graft outcome has been 94 per cent at 1 year and 80 per cent at 5 years. In pediatric retransplant recipients, the actuarial graft survival rate has been 84 per cent at 1 year and 70 per cent at 3 years.

Adverse effects of CsA include acute (reversible) and chronic (irreversible) nephrotoxicity, hepatotoxicity, hypertrichosis, gingival hyperplasia, hypomagnesemia, hypertension, coarsening of facial features, and tremors. CsA blood levels can be raised by a number of drugs, such as erythromycin, verapamil, diltiazem, metaclopramide, and ketoconazole. CsA blood levels can also be decreased by a number of drugs, such as carbamazipine, phenobarbital, dilantin, and rifampin. If such drugs are necessary, CsA blood levels must be carefully monitored and CsA doses adjusted if the levels move from the therapeutic ranges (Table 5).

TABLE 4. "Sequential" Immunosuppression Protocol in Pediatric Cadaveric Transplantation

I. Six to 12 hours Prior to Transplantation

CsA (10 mg/kg p.o.) is given if the antithymocyte preparation to be used for induction therapy is Atgam (Upjohn). If OKT3 (Ortho-Biotech) is to be used for induction therapy, the preoperative CsA dose is lowered to 4 mg/kg.

II. Induction Therapy

A. Anti-thymocyte globulin (15 mg/kg) or OKT3 (2.5 mg if body weight <30 kg, or 5 mg if body weight >30 kg); use daily until serum creatinine ≤2 mg/dl, or for total of 10 days.

B. Azathioprine (1 to 2 mg/kg/day).

C. Prednisone (0.5 mg/kg/day initially; minimum, 20 mg/day). The first dose of corticosteroid is given intraoperatively as Solu-Medrol (Upjohn) (10 mg/kg IV).

III. Maintenance (Serum Creatinine ≤ 2 mg/dl)

A. Cyclosporine (12 mg/kg/day p.o. divided b.i.d.; divide it t.i.d. if the child is a rapid metabolizer). For children 6 years of age or younger, cyclosporine dose is 500 mg/m²/day p.o. divided b.i.d. or t.i.d. Overlap cyclosporine and antithymocyte preparation for 1 to 3 days to allow achievement of an appropriate 12-hour CsA trough level.

B. If serum creatinine has not fallen to 2 mg/dl or lower by day 10 of antilymphocyte preparation, start cyclosporine at a reduced dose of 6 to 8 mg/kg/day to achieve 12-hour through serum level of 100 to 150 ng/ml.

C. Azathioprine (1 to 2 mg/kg/day).

D. Prednisone (taper to 0.15 to 0.18 mg/kg/day by 6 months after transplantation).

Abbreviations: CsA, cyclosporin A; p.o., by mouth; b.i.d., twice a day; t.i.d., three times a day.

REVERSAL OF ACUTE REJECTION EPISODES IN CHILDREN

Impaired graft function is the hallmark of an acute rejection episode (ARE). Prior to the introduction of CsA, AREs were routinely manifested by a symptom complex consisting of graft pain and swelling, fever, decreased urine output, weight gain, hypertension, and an increase in the serum creatinine level. Because CsA dramatically attenuates the rejection process, today AREs are frequently manifested only by elevations of serum creatinine or blood pressure. Although rejection is the most common cause of renal dysfunction, urologic obstruction, CsA nephrotoxicity, renal artery stenosis, and infection can also result in impaired graft function.

The first-line treatment for ARE in children is the administration of intravenous pulses of methylprednisolone without altering basal maintenance immunosuppression. Methylprednisolone doses range from 5 to 10 mg/kg/day given daily or on alternate days for a total of three to five doses. An alternative approach is to use an oral prednisolone pulse, wherein large doses (i.e., 100 to 300 mg) are used for 3 days and then tapered off in 3 to 4 days to baseline maintenance immunosuppression. In 10 to 25 per cent of patients, renal function fails to return to baseline or continues to worsen after completion of high-dose steroid therapy. In this situation, percutaneous allograft biopsy is indicated to establish the diagnosis and prognosis of the allograft.

OKT3, a murine monoclonal antibody that targets the T cell receptor antigen complex, has also been used as a potent antirejection therapy in children. Table 6 summarizes the OKT3 treatment protocol for children. OKT3 is successful in reversing or stabilizing acute rejection in 90 per cent of children treated for acute rejection. The side effects of OKT3 include fever, diarrhea, vomiting, headache, pulmonary edema, and conjunctivitis. Viral infections occur in as many as 25 per cent of children treated with OKT3; infections with viruses from the herpes group, especially cytomegalovirus (CMV), is common.

COMPLICATIONS

Infections

Infection is the major complication of immunosuppression. The cause of infection may be bacterial, viral, fungal, or parasitic. Bacterial infections of the lungs and urinary tract are common in the first few weeks after transplantation. Opportunistic infections are usually not manifest until 1 to 2 months after transplantation. Infections with viruses from the herpes group (CMV, *Herpesvirus hominis*, varicella-zoster virus, Epstein-Barr virus) are of particular concern in children. Children have often not acquired immunity to these agents prior to transplantation, and primary infections with these viruses are usually the most severe. The use of prophylactic intravenous immunoglobulin (either standard or hyperimmune) or oral acyclovir (800 mg/m² four times a day, with modification for impaired kidney function) is effective in reducing the severity of CMV in transplant recipients.

Fungal and protozoan infections, once common in the renal transplant setting, are dramatically less common today. This is in part due to current practices that limit maintenance and antirejection immunosuppression. Many centers use trimethoprim-sulfamethoxazole prophylactically for the first few months after transplantation against *Pneumocystis carinii* pneumonia; this agent also decreases the incidence and severity of urinary tract infections.

TABLE 5. Therapeutic "Targets" for Immunosuppression

	Weeks After Transplantation				
	0–4	*4–8*	*8–12*	*12–16*	*16–36*
12-hr CsA whole blood trough TDX (ng/ml)	500–750	350–500	300–450	250–350	175–300
12-hr CsA whole blood trough high-pressure liquid chromatography	150–200	125–175	100–150	75–175	50–100
Prednisone dosage (mg/kg)	0.5	0.33	0.25	0.18–0.20	0.15–0.18
Azathioprine dosage (mg/kg)	2	2	2	2	2

Abbreviations: CsA, cyclosporin A; TDX, Therapeutic Drug Analyzer System, fluorescence polarization immunoassay.

Hypertension

Hypertension occurs in more than 75 per cent of patients after renal transplantation. In the immediate post-transplant period, hypertension is usually related to hypervolemia, especially when there is acute tubular necrosis and decreased urinary output. It is also a frequent finding in acute rejection and resolves with reversal of the ARE. The etiology of persistent post-transplant hypertension includes chronic rejection (60 per cent), renal artery stenosis (20 per cent), effects of the native kidney (5 per cent), recurrence of the primary renal disease (5 per cent), and unknown (10 per cent). In addition, both corticosteroids and CsA contribute significantly to post-transplant hypertension. As one of its major nephrotoxic side effects, cyclosporine reduces renal blood flow, which, in turn, leads to increased renal sodium reabsorption and consequent hypertension. Calcium-entry blockers are useful in controlling post-transplant hypertension because they may improve blood flow in cyclosporine-treated patients. Diuretics should be used with caution in combination with cyclosporine because of their propensity to induce some degree of prerenal azotemia.

Growth Retardation

Uremic children awaiting transplantation are usually 2 to 5 standard deviation scores (SDSs) for height below the median for normal controls. Although growth after renal transplantation is most often superior to growth during dialysis, a normal growth pattern is not always attained. Factors affecting growth after transplantation include age at transplant, allograft function, and corticosteroid use.

In general, the younger the child, the better the rate of post-transplant growth. According to NARPTCS data, recipients younger than 5 years of age exhibit an immediate increase in height of about one third SDS in the first 6 months after transplant. Once a patient attains a bone age of 12 years, further growth is disappointing, although there are studies that report some significant growth in the adolescent recipient. Expedited transplantation in the young appears to be justified in an attempt to normalize stature.

TABLE 6. Treatment Protocol for Children Receiving OKT3

A. **Before Initiating Therapy**
   Chest x-ray
   If weight is more than 3% above dry weight, start dialysis
   Discontinue cyclosporine; continue azathioprine and prednisone unchanged

B. **Prior to First and Second Doses of OKT3**
   Tylenol (acetaminophen), 10–15 mg/kg p.o. or p.r.
   Benadryl (diphenhydramine hydrochloride), 0.5–1.0 mg/kg IV
   Methylprednisolone, 10 mg/kg

C. **Dose of OKT3**
   Body weight <30 kg = 2.5 mg OKT3
   Body weight >30 kg = 5.0 mg OKT3

An allograft glomerular filtration rate (GFR) less than or equal to 60 ml/minute/1.73 m^2 is associated with poor growth and low somatomedin levels. Most growth improvement is observed when the GFR is at least 90 ml/minute/1.73 m^2.

The exact mechanism by which corticosteroids impair growth is unknown. They may act to suppress growth and delay puberty by a blunting of both growth hormone and gonadotropin secretion, by increasing somatomedin inhibitors, or by directly impairing growth cartilage. The degree of growth impairment is directly related to the steroid dose. Some centers have attempted to withdraw corticosteroid therapy in post-transplant children receiving CsA. Children successfully maintained without prednisone show significant catch-up growth. Unfortunately, if corticosteroid withdrawal cannot be successfully maintained, allograft rejection often occurs, with a resultant decrease in GFR.

Improved growth velocity has been observed in both prepubertal and pubertal children with renal transplants treated with recombinant human growth hormone (rhGH) for 6 to 36 months. Most experience suggests that renal function is well preserved during rhGH treatment. However, some studies have indicated that rhGH treatment may be associated with an increased rate of GFR deterioration in some patients.

Delayed Sexual Maturation

It has been thought that successful renal transplantation improved pubertal development. However, recent observations suggest that in the post-transplant adolescent, there is a delay in the appearance of secondary sexual characteristics associated with an appreciable blunting of gonadotropin pulsability. It is likely that long-term steroid treatment interferes with the onset and progression of puberty and the pubertal growth spurt.

In female pubertal recipients, menses usually return within 6 months to 1 year after transplantation. Adolescent patients should be given appropriate contraceptive information. Oral contraceptives are effective. However, patients need to be monitored closely for adverse effects such as hypertension, abnormal coagulability, and increase in CsA levels. New agents with very low hormone dosages appear to be the appropriate oral agents.

REHABILITATION

Within 1 year after transplantation, more than 90 per cent of children attend school and only approximately 8 per cent are not involved in any vocational or educational programs. In long-term survivors (older than 10 years of age), the overwhelming majority of patients perceive an average or above-average quality of life in respect to family, social life, sexual life, professional life, and overall health. The most common medical complications include warts, skin cancer, mild cataracts, hypertension, atherosclerotic vascular disease, and various musculoskeletal complaints. Adolescent female transplant recipients as well as adolescent male transplant recipients can successfully produce children without any consistent pattern of abnormalities reported in the offspring. However, approximately 50 per cent of the newborns were small for gestational age. Deterioration of renal function during pregnancy occurs in about 12 per cent of patients, being more frequent in those with pre-existing impaired renal function. The renal impairment may reverse after delivery in some patients.

HEMOLYTIC-UREMIC SYNDROME

JOSEPH R. SHERBOTIE, M.D.
and BERNARD S. KAPLAN, M.B., B.Ch.

The hemolytic-uremic syndrome (HUS) is defined by acute hemolytic anemia (with fragmented erythrocytes), thrombocytopenia, and acute renal injury (azotemia, abnormal urinary sediment). It is the most frequent cause of acute renal failure in children and is an important cause of end-stage renal failure. There are many causes of HUS (Table 1). The typical form of the syndrome is usually preceded by a prodrome of gastroenteritis with bloody stools, is designated as the D+ or postdiarrheal form, and is often associated with infection by enteropathogenic organisms that produce Shiga-like toxins (verotoxins). The toxins damage endothelial cells, mainly in the kidneys, and produce a cascade of biologic effects (Table 2). Seasonal and geographic variations in numbers of cases are common, and epidemics have occurred. Young children and infants are usually affected, but HUS can occur in older children and adults. There is a slight preponderance of females in some series. The syndrome rarely occurs in black children.

The phenotype of HUS without antecedent diarrhea (D−; atypical HUS) can occur sporadically and in families. Both autosomal recessive and dominant patterns of inheritance are described. The prognosis of these forms of HUS is poor; recurrent episodes may occur, and no causative agents have been implicated. Thrombotic thrombocytopenic purpura (TTP) is a related syndrome that is uncommon in children.

CLINICAL PRESENTATION

As mentioned, typical HUS usually begins with gastroenteritis and bloody diarrhea. Within several days, signs of anemia, thrombocytopenia, and renal insufficiency of variable severity develop. Severe, anuric acute renal failure is not uncommon. Central nervous system involvement occurs in as many as one third of patients and may be manifest with seizures, obtundation and focal neurologic deficits. Life-threatening gastrointestinal complications include bowel infarction, bleeding, and obstruction. Less frequent but severe problems can occur as consequences of myocardial, pulmonary, pancreatic, or hepatic involvement.

TABLE 1. Classification of Hemolytic-Uremic Syndrome (HUS)

Idiopathic HUS
Secondary HUS
- Infections
  - Verotoxin (Shiga-like toxin)—*Escherichia coli* 0157:H7
  - *Shigella dysenteriae*
  - *Streptococcus pneumoniae*
- Inherited forms of HUS
  - Autosomal Recessive HUS
  - Autosomal Dominant HUS
- Drug-associated HUS
  - Cyclosporin A
  - Mitomycin-C
  - Oral contraceptives
- Pregnancy-associated HUS
- Transplant-associated HUS
- Cancer-associated HUS

From Kaplan BS: Hemolytic-uremic syndrome and thrombotic thrombocytopenic purpura. *In* Jacobson HR, Striker GE, Klahr S (eds): The Principles and Practice of Nephrology. Philadelphia, BC Decker, 1991, pp 324–329.

TABLE 2. A Theoretic Succession of Interrelated, Overlapping, Synchronous, and Asynchronous Events

1. *Escherichia coli* infection
   - Colonic injury
   - Entry to circulation of SLT
   - Gb3 receptor on endothelial cells
   - Inhibition of endothelial cell protein synthesis by SLT
2. Possible access of LPS
   - LPS stimulation of production of TNF and IL-1
   - Synergistic injury to endothelial cells
3. LPS stimulation of leukocytes
   - Release of proteases
4. Activation of platelets
   - Local procoagulant state
5. Endothelial cell injury
   - Perturbed endothelial cell function—prostacyclin, vWF, tPA
   - Exposure of collagen
   - Endothelial cell swelling
   - Narrow lumen, reduced GFR

From Kaplan BS, Cleary TG, Obrig TG: Recent advances in understanding the pathogenesis of the hemolytic uremic syndromes. Pediatr Nephrol 4:276–283, 1990.

Abbreviations: SLT, Shiga-like toxin; Gb3, glycolipid globotriaosyl ceramide; LPS, lipopolysaccharide; TNF, tumor necrosis factor; IL-1, interleukin 1; vWF, von Willebrand factor; tPA, tissue plasminogen activator; GFR, glomerular filtration rate.

DIAGNOSIS

The fully developed syndrome is easy to diagnose. Involvement of additional organs or milder disease with less renal involvement may be confounding. The differential diagnosis includes TTP, disseminated intravascular coagulation, and hemorrhagic shock and encephalopathy syndrome. Putative causes of HUS are shown in Table 1.

The peripheral blood smear must be examined for fragmented erythrocytes. The white blood cell count is often elevated in the typical form of HUS. Very high counts may portend serious problems, such as an intra-abdominal catastrophe. At diagnosis, bloody diarrhea is often seen and some patients have rectal prolapse. Fever is not uncommon. Bruising, petechiae, and mild jaundice are sometimes seen. The patient may be dehydrated; on the other hand, volume overload and hypoalbuminemia, secondary to loss of protein through the kidneys or intestine, can cause edema. Hypertension occurs mainly as a result of volume expansion. Irritability, drowsiness, twitching, and even seizures may occur. The nutritional status can deteriorate acutely.

Laboratory evaluations should include a complete blood count, reticulocyte count, peripheral smear, and Coombs' test. Serum chemistry profiles should be used to assess electrolytes, calcium, phosphorus, renal function, acid-base status, hepatic and pancreatic functions, and lipids. Blood cultures are indicated in febrile patients. Stool should be cultured for *Escherichia coli* 0157:H7. Specimens from urine culture should be examined for red blood cells, protein, casts, and specific gravity. The patient's intake and output (urine volume, stool, vomitus), weight, and blood pressure should be followed closely. Hemoglobin concentration; white blood cell and platelet counts; serum sodium, potassium, and carbon dioxide; and creatinine concentrations should be monitored serially until recovery. Imaging studies and renal biopsy are not done routinely.

MANAGEMENT

With improvements in supportive care, particularly acute peritoneal dialysis and hemodialysis, and control of hypertension, the acute mortality rate has decreased to less than 15 per cent. The management of HUS remains primarily supportive.

It is important to weigh the patient, to measure the blood pressure, and to determine whether there is urine in the bladder before starting treatment. The assessment of volume status is critical. Dehydration must be carefully and appropriately managed. In many cases, the diagnosis of HUS may not be apparent or suspected at presentation. Therefore, it is not uncommon to overhydrate such a patient and produce hyponatremia, hypertension, and edema. Failure to produce urine after adequate rehydration, development of edema, increasing pallor, a falling serum sodium level, and an increasing serum creatinine concentration are indications that the diagnosis may not be uncomplicated gastroenteritis. Rehydration must always be effected, with careful monitoring to avoid volume overload. If there is anuria despite expansion of the intravascular volume, the patient can be challenged with furosemide (3 to 4 mg/kg IV). This can be repeated if required.

Electrolyte imbalances are corrected as indicated. Hyponatremia is often present and is usually dilutional as a result of volume overload. Despite the presence of acute renal failure, hyperkalemia is rarely a problem early on in HUS. Hyperkalemia can be treated with glucose and insulin infusions, bicarbonate administration, and calcium infusions. Potassium can be removed with a sodium polystyrene sulfonate resin (1 g/kg per dose as often as every 6 hours orally or rectally in a slurry containing sorbitol to avoid impaction), which exchanges potassium for sodium. The resin must be removed in a reasonable period and care must be taken in a volume-overloaded patient, to avoid worsening sodium overload, and in a patient with a friable intestinal mucosa. Severe metabolic acidosis can be treated with oral bicarbonate equivalents or with intravenous acetate or bicarbonate to maintain an acceptable serum bicarbonate level. Hypokalemia may be seen at the time of presentation even with renal failure. Caution must be exercised when administering potassium to patients with renal insufficiency; mild hypokalemia (3 to 3.5 mEq/L) is best left untreated.

Indications for dialysis are the same as those in acute renal failure from any cause. Although it has become traditional to start dialysis as early as possible after onset of anuria in HUS, there is no absolute evidence that delaying this procedure has any untoward effects on outcome, provided that there are no specific indications for dialysis. Specific indications include volume overload resistant to diuretics, intractable metabolic acidosis, neurologic sequelae of uremia, and hyperkalemia. Relative indications for dialysis include the need to administer large amounts of fluid such as blood and intravenous nutrition in a patient with oligoanuric renal failure. Severe hyperphosphatemia with concomitant hypocalcemia can also be treated with dialysis.

In young children, peritoneal dialysis is simpler technically than hemodialysis. It is continuous, obviates the need for anticoagulation, and provides additional calories in the form of dextrose absorbed from the dialysate. Despite thrombocytopenia and a prolonged bleeding time, insertion of the dialysis catheter rarely causes much blood loss. Catheters designed for acute peritoneal dialysis are easier to insert and function well, but their life span is limited because of infection. Dialysis can be started with this type of catheter and continued for 48 to 72 hours to improve fluid balance and metabolic status. If it is thought that dialysis will be needed for several weeks, a Tenckhoff catheter with a Dacron cuff can be inserted at the outset. Hemodialysis or hemofiltration is effective in treating the acute renal failure of HUS and is indicated in patients who have had recent abdominal surgery or in those with massive volume overload. Dialysis should be done only by physicians who have had experience using this treatment in children.

Anemia should be treated with transfusion(s) of washed packed red blood cells. Transfusions are initiated when the hemoglobin level reaches 6 g/dl or less. It is rarely necessary to raise the hemoglobin to above 8 to 10 g/dl because increasing the hemoglobin too much may cause or exacerbate hypertension. Platelet infusions are discouraged unless there is significant active bleeding. Exogenous platelets are rapidly consumed or destroyed in HUS.

Hypertension is managed by maintaining euvolemia, by avoiding overtransfusion, and by the judicious use of antihypertensive agents such as hydralazine (0.15 to 0.5 mg/kg per dose IV every 4 to 6 hours), captopril (0.15 to 2 mg/kg per dose orally every 8 hours), or nifedipine (0.15 to 0.5 mg/kg per dose orally every 6 hours). Other antihypertensive agents are also effective. Maintaining the blood pressure at or below the 90th percentile for age and size is a reasonable goal. It is advisable to avoid using medications that may interfere with the neurologic examination (e.g., methyldopa).

Nutrition should provide at least the age-appropriate recommended daily allowance (RDA) for calories. This may necessitate dialysis in oligoanuric patients. With dialysis or adequate renal function, the RDA for protein should also be given. Most patients with HUS have hyperlipidemia, and this should be considered when administering calories as intralipid. Patients unable to tolerate enteral feedings may require total parenteral nutrition via a centrally placed venous catheter.

Anticoagulation, thrombolytic therapy, antiplatelet agents, prostacyclin, corticosteroids, infusions of immunoglobulin G or fresh frozen plasma, and plasmapheresis have not been proven to benefit typical HUS. Anecdotal reports suggest that plasma infusions and plasma exchange may be of value in atypical HUS and TTP and in patients with significant central nervous system involvement. Plasma infusion is contraindicated in *pneumococcus*-associated HUS, which is often Coombs' test–positive.

PROGNOSIS

With appropriate supportive care, including timely dialysis, more than 90 per cent of patients with typical HUS survive. End-stage renal failure occurs in about 15 per cent. Recurrences almost never occur in typical cases and suggest another form of the syndrome. The prognosis of HUS inherited as an autosomal recessive or dominant disorder is poor. There may be recurrent episodes, renal failure, thrombotic events, and recurrence after renal transplantation. Clues to the diagnosis of atypical forms include the absence of bloody diarrhea, unusual age of onset, family history, and a relentless, insidious course. With typical HUS, multiple children of different ages in a family may be simultaneously affected, as one would suspect in an infection. We recommend that every sibling of the affected patient be examined. For older patients, patients with very high white blood cell counts, and patients with protracted renal failure, the prognosis may be worse. There is no evidence that dehydration initiates the renal injury. Some patients who recover may remain well for many years before progressing to end-stage renal failure. Renal histology early in the course may provide prognostic information in typical HUS but will not affect acute management; renal biopsy is therefore not essential in every patient. The diagnosis and therefore the prognosis of patients with atypical HUS may be confirmed by a renal biopsy. Occasionally, patients have neurologic sequelae, and diabetes mellitus has developed in a few.

PERINEPHRIC AND INTRANEPHRIC ABSCESS

STEPHEN R. SHAPIRO, M.D.
and RAYMOND D. ADELMAN, M.D.

Intranephric and perinephric abscess formation in children is rare. In most cases, early antibiotic therapy probably aborts the process. When suppuration and necrosis have occurred, an abscess is formed. A renal carbuncle represents coalescence of multiple abscesses into a multiloculated cavity. A perirenal abscess occurs when the infection extends beyond the renal capsule but is confined by Gerota's fascia. A pararenal abscess is present if the infection extends beyond Gerota's fascia.

In currently reported series, *Staphylococcus* is still the cause of most renal abscesses in children. *Escherichia coli* is the organism cultured next most frequently. Other organisms reported include *Proteus, Pseudomonas,* and *Candida albicans.*

Recent abdominal or urologic surgery is common in children with perinephric abscess. These operations include appendectomy, nephrectomy, bowel resections, and pyeloplasty. Renal abscesses can also occur in otherwise healthy children. Occasionally, with *Staphylococcus,* a minor remote focus, such as a cutaneous, respiratory, or dental site, is identified as a source of infection. An underlying urinary tract abnormality may exist, particularly with gram-negative organisms, such as vesicoureteral reflux, obstructive uropathy, renal vein thrombosis, renal calculi, or renal trauma. Occasionally, abscesses have been associated with congenital heart disease involving *Staphylococcus* or *Streptococcus viridans.* Children with an abnormal host response to infection, such as chronic granulomatous disease, diabetes mellitus, or leukemia, or those treated with immunosuppressive drugs, such as transplant recipients, are predisposed to renal abscesses. Recent or concomitant infections may be found in these children, including endocarditis, carbuncle, psoas abscess, and necrotizing enterocolitis.

Blood and urine culture specimens must be obtained after confirmation of the diagnosis by radiographic techniques. Urine organisms predict the perinephric abscess organism in up to 20 per cent of cases. Blood cultures are usually negative. Appropriate parenteral doses of antibiotics must be started as soon as cultures have been obtained. Since it may be difficult to distinguish an abscess radiographically from other lesions (Wilms' tumor in the infant and child, renal cell carcinoma in the teenager, renal hamartoma, and lymphoma), and since pathogens isolated from abscess cultures do not always correlate with those from the urine, we recommend fine-needle aspiration and percutaneous drainage of the abscess unless contraindications exist. The aspirated material should be cultured aerobically and anaerobically, and fungal cultures should also be done. Negative cultures are obtained in 5 to 10 per cent of cases, possibly owing to inadequate culture techniques. A Gram stain should also be performed. If necessary, special stains for the various fungi and acid-fast bacilli can be obtained.

Since a spectrum of renal parenchymal inflammatory disease exists, from acute cellulitis to perinephric abscess, if the condition of the child permits, a trial of intensive antibiotic treatment may be warranted before determining a need for percutaneous aspiration and/or surgical drainage.

Currently, percutaneous catheter drainage offers an attractive alternative to open surgical drainage for patients with a renal or perirenal abscess. After needle aspiration of the purulent material, a catheter or multiple catheters can be inserted into the abscess cavity or cavities. In addition, percutaneous drainage of the urine from the kidney can also simultaneously be accomplished if indicated by obstructive uropathy (ureteropelvic junction obstruction, ureteral calculi). The abscess cavity can then be irrigated with antibiotic solution, or, in some cases, the catheter may be left indwelling without irrigation, combined with antibiotic therapy. Resolution of the abscess occurs in several days to 4 to 6 weeks. Percutaneous abscess drainage duplicates surgical treatment in providing decompression, continual drainage, and evacuation. In most reported cases, adequate drainage of the abscess cavity has been accomplished with a catheter size as small as 8.3 French using the pigtail variety of catheter.

Indications for removal of the catheter include resolution of fever, cessation of drainage, return of the white blood cell count to normal, and a sinogram showing nearly complete closure of the abscess cavity. Following removal of the catheter, the drainage tract will rapidly close if all infected material has been adequately removed.

Percutaneous drainage of the abscess will fail if the cavity is inadequately drained, if there are multiple pockets of pus that are not recognized, or if there is continuous drainage despite adequate catheter placement. The last situation might suggest enteric fistula from erosion of the abscess into the second portion of the duodenum on the right side or the descending colon on the left side. Percutaneous techniques have now proved suitable even for the small infant or neonate, in whom renal abscesses are, fortunately, extremely rare.

Some patients may require operation without percutaneous drainage or subsequent to it. The decision to perform surgery should be based on the patient's general condition, associated pathologic findings, and the condition of the involved kidney. For example, poorly functioning or nonfunctioning kidneys, particularly those with multiple abscesses, would mandate surgical treatment, probably by nephrectomy and drainage. The clinical response is also critical. Percutaneous drainage of an abscess should result in defervescence within 48 to 72 hours. Failure of such a response may suggest inadequate drainage.

Initial antibiotic therapy must include gram-negative coverage (for *E. coli, Proteus,* and *Pseudomonas*) and coverage for *Staphylococcus.* Accordingly, an aminoglycoside and an antistaphylococcal agent in combination will be necessary. Tobramycin (6.0 to 7.5 mg/kg/day*) is recommended, since there has been an increasing resistance of *Pseudomonas* to gentamicin in recent years. Ceftazidime (100 to 150 mg/kg/day*) may be substituted for tobramycin. Intravenous doses of cefazolin (100 mg/kg/day) or nafcillin (100 to 150 mg/kg/day*) continue to provide the best coverage for *Staphylococcus.* In patients allergic to penicillin, vancomycin (45 to 60 mg/kg/day*) should be substituted. Antibiotic doses should be lowered for neonates. *Candida* infections will require amphotericin B. Although documentation in the literature does not exist, it is assumed that parenteral therapy should be continued for 14 days, to be followed by oral therapy for an additional 2 to 4 weeks, as indicated by the clinical condition.

*Not to exceed recommended adult dosages.

URINARY TRACT INFECTIONS IN CHILDREN

LAMIA F. ELERIAN, M.D.
and RAYMOND D. ADELMAN, M.D.

Urinary tract infections (UTIs) are common, occurring in as many as 5 per cent of females and 1 to 2 per cent of males during childhood. UTIs may be conveniently divided into two clinical categories: uncomplicated (lower tract infection or cystitis) and complicated (upper tract infection or pyelonephritis). *Prompt diagnosis and appropriate management of UTIs is important, especially in infancy and early childhood, to prevent serious renal damage.* Fortunately, most cases of UTI resolve without any sequelae. However, parenchymal scarring occurs in 10 to 15 per cent of children with UTIs; of these, 10 per cent develop hypertension, and a smaller number develop renal insufficiency.

A diagnosis of UTI is made when a child has a properly obtained, clean-voided, mid-stream urine culture growing 10^5 colonies or more per milliliter of a single organism, a catheterized urine culture growing 10^3 colonies or more per milliliter, or a suprapubic tap growing any number of colonies. Clinical experience and data in adults suggest that some symptomatic patients may have UTIs with even lower colony counts.

In newborn infants, UTIs may be associated with septicemia. There may be hematogenous seeding of renal parenchyma during septicemia or, conversely, an invasion of the blood stream from the urinary tract. Beyond the neonatal period, most infections are believed to be secondary to the ascent of bacteria from the periurethral area. There has been recent progress in the understanding of the pathogenic bacterial mechanisms underlying UTIs. Bacteria adhere to glycolipid receptors on the uroepithelial cells by receptor-specific fimbriae, allowing the bacteria to ascend the urinary tract in association with decreased ureteral motility. A relationship exists between adherence and both the incidence and the severity of pyelonephritis. When bacteria reach the kidneys, they activate complement, which stimulates chemotaxis and inflammation, ultimately leading to injury of the renal parenchyma and scarring. Host factors that influence the development of a UTI include age, gender, local defense mechanisms, presence of urinary tract abnormalities, circumcision, sexual activity (especially in adolescent females), and instrumentation of the urinary tract.

Gram-negative enteric bacteria are the most common organisms causing UTIs, with *Escherichia coli* causing about 80 per cent of infections. Other organisms causing acute infection include *Klebsiella, Enterobacter* sp., and, occasionally, enterococci. Coagulase-negative *Staphylococcus* is a common cause of infection in adolescent girls, and group B *Streptococcus* in newborns. Chronic infections or infections in patients receiving antimicrobial suppression are frequently caused by *Proteus, Pseudomonas,* or *Candida.* Uncommon causes of UTI in ambulatory children include *Haemophilus influenzae* and adenovirus, which causes acute hemorrhagic cystitis.

The incidence of UTI varies with age and sex. Male predominance is evident only for the first 2 or 3 months of life. Children at increased risk for UTI include premature infants; children with systemic or immunologic disease; children with urinary tract abnormalities, renal calculi, or constipation; children with a family history of UTI or renal anomalies; and females younger than 5 years of age with a previous history of UTI.

Obstruction and urinary stasis, whether anatomic or functional, predispose to infection. An example is incomplete bladder emptying with neurogenic bladder, voiding dysfunction in otherwise neurologically normal children (bladder-sphincter dyssynergia), and vesicoureteral reflux (VUR) or large bladder diverticula (aberrant micturition).

Vesicoureteral reflux is found in 30 to 50 per cent of children with UTI. Reflux predisposes to incomplete bladder emptying, facilitates ascent of infected urine to the kidneys, and is associated with increased risk of pyelonephritis and renal scarring. Pyelonephritis can, however, occur in the absence of reflux. *Most damage to the kidneys occurs during infancy and early childhood, a time when UTI is, unfortunately, frequently underdiagnosed.*

TREATMENT

The main objectives in the management of UTI are to identify and treat children with UTI, to prevent the serious sequelae of UTI, and to identify children with urinary tract abnormalities who are at risk for repeated UTI and its sequelae.

The approach to treatment of symptomatic UTI in children depends on the age of the patient, the clinical severity of the UTI, the presumed site of infection, the presence of structural abnormalities, and the patient's compliance. Immediate treatment of a UTI, especially in infants and young children with VUR or other urinary tract abnormalities, is of crucial importance because delay increases the risk of renal parenchymal scarring. In one study, the incidence of scarring was 17 per cent in children inadequately treated compared with 4.5 per cent in those treated promptly.

Most patients with a UTI can be treated in the outpatient setting. Controversy exists about the need for antibiotic therapy for asymptomatic bacteriuria. Treatment may have no effect on the emergence of symptoms, clearance of VUR, kidney function, kidney growth, or progression of kidney scars; eradication of organisms of low virulence may be followed by recolonization by more virulent organisms and precipitate acute pyelonephritis; drug side effects may occur. Relative indications for treatment of asymptomatic bacteriuria include age younger than 5 years, a urinary tract abnormality, or development of symptomatic UTI. The antibiotics and duration of therapy are similar to those used in treating symptomatic uncomplicated UTIs and are listed in Table 1.

In neonates and young infants, UTIs are frequently associated with sepsis and significant mortality and morbidity; thus, treatment should include parenteral antibiotics following a complete sepsis work-up. The antibiotics usually used are a combination of ampicillin and an aminoglycoside (Table 2). Parenteral therapy for neonates is continued for 7 to 10 days; for infants, therapy is continued until clinical improvement occurs and follow-up urine and blood cultures are sterile at 24 to 48 hours after the start of antibiotics. If the patient shows delayed improvement or is suspected of having pyelonephritis on clinical or radiologic grounds, or if there is obstruction of the urinary tract, parenteral therapy may have to be continued for 7 days or longer. The antibiotics available include the aminopenicillins, the cephalosporins, and the sulfonamides in older infants. The choice of an oral antibiotic is dependent on the susceptibility of the causative organism. It is important that compliance by the parents be assured before an oral antibiotic is substituted.

In older infants and children with clinical evidence of acute pyelonephritis and in those with upper tract infection associated with urologic abnormalities and/or surgical procedures, hospitalization and intravenous antibiotic therapy are frequently indicated. Antibiotics used include a combination of an aminoglycoside and ampicillin or, alternatively, a third-generation cephalosporin (Table 2). The antipseudomonas and extended-spectrum penicillins, such as piperacillin and azlocillin, are active against *Pseudomonas* and have been used successfully as a single-agent therapy for severe and complicated UTI. Aminoquilolones are not recommended for prepubertal children and should be used only in cases of multiple resistant *Pseudomonas*. Once the antimicrobial susceptibility of the bacteria causing the infection is known, antimicrobial therapy should be adjusted so that treatment is directed more specifically against the organism. When there is evidence of clinical improvement and urine and blood cultures are sterile, therapy can be given orally to complete a minimum of 10 to 14 days. Shorter-duration therapy can result in relapses. Some patients with pyelonephritis can be successfully treated in an outpatient setting with daily ceftriaxone (Table 2).

In children with lower tract infection with or without reflux, oral therapy with amoxicillin, sulfisoxazole, trimethoprim-sulfamethoxazole, nitrofurantoin, or a cephalosporin can be used (see Table 1). Selection of the antibiotic should be made on the basis of presumed antimicrobial coverage, safety, side effects, and cost. Uncomplicated UTI and asymptomatic bacteriuria usually respond to treatment within 24 to 48 hours, as evidenced by clinical improvement, a negative Gram stain of the urine specimen, and a sterile urine culture. Failure of the patient to respond to treatment suggests noncompliance, poor absorption of the drug, bacterial resistance, or presence of an underlying structural abnormality and indicates the need for prompt radiologic evaluation.

Patients are usually treated for 7 to 10 days. Although successful treatment with shorter courses, 1 day, 3 days, or a single dose, has been reported, controversy exists regarding its use in children. This mode of therapy should be reserved for selected patients with asymptomatic bacteriuria and older girls with a clinical picture of cystitis, a documented normal genitourinary tract, and poor compliance.

Other therapeutic measures that should be included in the management of any case of UTI are an increase in fluid intake, correction of constipation, frequent and complete emptying of the bladder, and proper hygiene. Children should be counseled about "holding" urine and about self-induced trauma due to exploration, masturbation, and foreign objects (e.g., dolls, toys) in the diaper.

Because mild to moderate reflux usually disappears with increasing age, surgery is not indicated if subsequent urine cultures are sterile, long-term prophylactic therapy can be maintained, and sonograms every 1 to 2 years document adequate renal growth without progressive scarring. Patients should be referred to an experienced pediatric urologist for ureteral reimplantation if there is severe VUR, increased VUR, uncontrolled infection, progressive scarring, renal growth arrest, or medical noncompliance. Whether ureteral reimplantation has a beneficial effect in preserving renal function, improving renal growth, or altering the course of chronic renal deterioration, especially when decreased renal function is already present, is still unclear.

Follow-up

Appropriate management necessitates follow-up cultures. A urine culture specimen by dipslide or calibrated loop should be assessed 3 to 7 days after completion of therapy to exclude relapse. Relapses usually occur within 1 week of therapy completion, are caused by the same bacteria, and often signify pyelonephritis. Recurrences usually occur weeks to months after an infection and are usually caused by different organisms. Every patient who has had a documented UTI should have two to three follow-up cultures per year to detect recurrence.

TABLE 1. Oral Antimicrobial Therapy for Urinary Tract Infections (UTIs) in Children

Indication	Antibiotic	Dose
Asymptomatic bacteriuria or uncomplicated UTI (cystitis)	Amoxicillin	40–50 mg/kg/day p.o. in 3 divided doses
	or	
	Sulfisoxazole	120–150 mg/kg/day p.o. in 4 divided doses
	or	
	TMP/SMX	TMP 10 mg/kg/day + SMX 50 mg/kg/day p.o. in 2 divided doses
	or	
	Cephalexin	50 mg/kg/day p.o. in 4 divided doses
	or	
	Cefixime	3 mg/kg/day p.o. given once daily
Chemoprophylaxis	TMP/SMX	TMP 2 mg/kg/day + SMX 10 mg/kg/day p.o. every 1–2 days at bedtime
	or	
	Nitrofurantoin	1–2 mg/kg/day p.o. every day at bedtime

Prophylactic Therapy

The indications for chemoprophylaxis of UTI are based on the functional status of the urinary tract and on the frequency of recurrences. Usually, three documented infections in 1 year indicate the need for prophylactic therapy. Prophylaxis is also recommended for all children younger than 5 years of age with VUR or other urinary tract abnormalities. TMP/SMX given nightly or on alternate nights or nitrofurantoin given nightly is highly effective in preventing recurrences, and each has few side effects (see Table 1). Prophylactic therapy should be continued for 6 months to 2 years, or longer if indicated. Breakthrough urinary infections commonly occur in children who are receiving chemoprophylaxis. These infections are usually caused by enterococci, *Proteus*, and *P. aeruginosa*.

TABLE 2. Intravenous Therapy for Complicated Urinary Tract Infections

Indication	Antibiotic	Dose
Neonates* and young infants	Ampicillin	75–100 mg/kg/day IV in 4 divided doses
	plus	
	Gentamicin†	7.5 mg/kg/day IV in 3 divided doses × 10–14 days
Complicated UTI‡ (pyelonephritis) in older infants and children	Ampicillin	100–200 mg/kg/day IV in 4 divided doses
	plus	
	Gentamicin†	6–7.5 mg/kg/day IV in 3 doses
	or	
	Cefotaxime	100–200 mg/kg/day IV in 3 divided doses
	or	
	Ceftriaxone	50–75 mg/kg/day IV or IM in a single or 2 divided doses

*Doses must be adjusted for neonates younger than 1 week old.
†Optimal management requires monitoring of serum concentrations.
‡See text for antibiotic therapy for *Pseudomonas* and multiply resistant organisms.

A radiologic evaluation of the urinary tract in children with UTI is indicated in order to identify those patients with VUR, obstruction, or other urinary tract abnormalities. In about 50 per cent of children with the first proven occurrence of symptomatic UTI, a structural abnormality is found. Radiologic evaluation is indicated in the following patients: (1) all children younger than 3 to 5 years of age with the first episode of UTI, (2) all male patients of any age with the first episode of UTI, (3) all female patients with recurrent UTI or with clinical pyelonephritis, and (4) all children with an abnormal voiding pattern, poor growth, hypertension, suprapubic mass, an elevated blood urea nitrogen or creatinine concentration, or a family history of urinary tract abnormalities.

The choice of a particular examination depends on the clinical picture, the facilities available, and the experience and skills of the radiologist. Both voiding cystourethrography and renal sonography are the initial studies. If both tests are normal, no further radiologic evaluation is indicated. If VUR is detected, evaluation of both upper tract structure and function is recommended. If morphologic changes are identified by ultrasonography in the absence of reflux, a search for urinary tract abnormalities such as anatomic obstruction, ureterocele, ectopic kidney, or duplicated system should be performed. The intravenous urogram (IVU) can be used in this search in most instances, but quantitative scintigraphy with Tc-99m DMSA, Tc-99m DTPA, Tc-99m glucoheptonate, or I-123 or I-131 iodohippurate (Hippuran) is preferable for neonates and patients in whom poor renal function is anticipated. Moreover, recent studies have suggested that Tc-99m DMSA scan may be superior to IVU in detecting early renal scars, especially in young children.

UROLITHIASIS

F. BRUDER STAPLETON, M.D.

Urolithiasis is being recognized with increasing frequency in children, particularly in high-risk groups—those with neurogenic bladder, bronchopulmonary dysplasia, steatorrhea, or those receiving corticosteroid therapy, hyperalimentation, or antineoplastic chemotherapy. Pediatricians must have a high sensitivity to the possibility of urolithiasis because the classic symptom of incapacitating renal colic is unusual in children. Abdominal or flank pain occurs in approximately 50 per cent of children with urolithiasis. Either microscopic or macroscopic hematuria heralds urinary stones in greater than 90 per cent of pediatric patients. Urinary infection is a common complication.

DIAGNOSIS

Preventive medical therapies should be directed toward specific causes of urolithiasis. Whenever possible, evaluation of urolithiasis should begin with analysis of the mineral composition of the stones. In the case of struvite (infection-related), cystine, or urate stones, specific diagnoses can be determined through stone analysis, and the diagnostic evaluation can be narrowly directed. In the majority of patients, however, the stone is composed of calcium oxalate and further extensive metabolic studies are warranted. Additional diagnostic studies should be deferred until the stone episode has resolved and the urinary infection has been eradicated. For patients with calcium oxalate or calcium phosphate stones or when a stone is not recovered, a 24-hour urine sample is collected while the patient is eating a customary diet. The urine is analyzed for calcium, oxalate, uric acid, citrate, and cystine. Normal values are given in Table 1. An abnormal value should be confirmed with a second collection. When hypercalciuria is discovered, serum concentrations of parathyroid hormone, calcium, phosphorus, and bicarbonate should be determined. Urinary tract infection should always be excluded in children with urolithiasis.

Further characterization of the pathogenesis of confirmed hypercalciuria is warranted. After 2 weeks of dietary calcium and sodium restriction, 24-hour urine calcium excretion is measured. Persistent hypercalciuria without hypercalcemia suggests a renal tubular defect, primary hypercalciuria, or renal tubular acidosis. When dietary calcium and sodium restriction results in normalization of urinary calcium excretion, the diagnosis of "absorptive" idiopathic hypercalciuria is assigned.

MEDICAL THERAPY

Therapies for urolithiasis consist of preventive medical management and acute intervention of obstructive calculi. General management includes hypotonic diuresis with water loading and, when appropriate, antibiotic therapy for urinary infection and/or analgesics.

Hypercalciuria accounts for approximately 40 per cent of all pediatric cases of urolithiasis. In addition to increased water intake, a "no added salt" and low-oxalate diet is recommended. For children with absorptive hypercalciuria, a reduction in dietary calcium intake (400 to 600 mg/day) is recommended. If urinary calcium excretion does not decline to the normal range with such dietary management, hydrochlorothiazide (1 to 2 mg/kg/day) is used as an additional anticalciuric measure. All children receiving diuretic therapy should be advised to ingest a diet rich in potassium, and serum potassium concentrations should be monitored. Alkali therapy (2 to 4 mEq/kg) is given to patients with renal tubular acidosis in four divided doses. Citrate therapy (potassium citrate) is helpful in patients with reduced urinary citrate excretion and hypercalciuria.

Primary hyperoxaluria requires aggressive medical therapy and dietary oxalate restriction. Urinary calcium excretion is reduced by hydrochlorothiazide diuretic therapy (2 mg/kg/day) and large doses of inorganic phosphates. Pyridoxine is administered in an attempt to reduce oxalate production in patients with type I hyperoxaluria. The starting dose (10 mg/kg/day) may be increased gradually (to a total of 500 mg/day). Finally, magnesium hydroxide is given to increase the solubility of calcium oxalate. Hyperoxaluria secondary to gastrointestinal disease requires therapy for the primary malabsorptive disorder.

Therapy for uric acid stones includes efforts to alkalinize the urine and to maintain a high urine flow rate. Diagnostic studies should determine whether a treatable cause of hyperproduction of uric acid is present. When uric acid production is increased, as in Lesch-Nyhan syndrome, allopurinol therapy (5 to 10 mg/kg) is warranted. Therapy with potassium citrate is useful in decreasing the risk of urinary urate crystallization by alkalization of the urine.

Cystinuria also necessitates aggressive urinary alkalinization

TABLE 1. Normal Values for Urinary Excretion

Calcium	<4 mg/kg/day
Uric acid	<0.57 mg/dl GFR
Oxalate	<50 mg/1.73 m^2 BSA
Citrate	>400 mg/g creatinine
Cystine	<60 mg/1.73 m^2 BSA

Abbreviations: GFR, glomerular filtration rate; BSA, body surface area.

and a large fluid intake to produce a hypotonic diuresis. When recurrent stones persist despite these measures, D-penicillamine is helpful in reducing the risk of urolithiasis. Penicillamine combines with cystine to form a more soluble cysteine disulfide complex. Unfortunately, D-penicillamine has a large number of adverse effects, including gastrointestinal discomfort, loss of taste perception, bone marrow depression, proteinuria, membranous glomerulopathy, optic neuritis, myasthenia gravis, and trace metal deficiencies. Potentially less toxic agents, mercaptopropionylglycine (MPG) and captopril, have been suggested as alternatives to D-penicillamine; however, neither drug has been approved as therapy for cystinuria in children.

SURGICAL THERAPY

Approximately 40 per cent of urinary stones are passed spontaneously in children. A number of surgical procedures are available for the removal of calculi within the urinary tract. Surgical management of urinary stones in children ranges from surgical lithotomy to extracorporeal shock-wave lithotripsy. Traditional surgical lithotomies are often required when nephrolithiasis is associated with congenital obstruction, which can be corrected simultaneously. Because many stones in children are discovered in the lower ureter, cystoscopic manipulation and basket extraction are commonly used. The success of cystoscopic extraction depends on the size of the calculus. This technique of stone removal is indicated only for urinary stones in the lower third of the ureter. Laser lithotripsy, which utilizes flexible uteroscopy, offers promise for fragmenting higher ureteral stones.

Percutaneous nephrolithotomy has been used in children with upper tract stones. The advantage of this technique is the ability to avoid general anesthesia and major surgical trauma. Unfortunately, small children require general anesthesia during the procedure and the large size of the surgical instruments relative to the smaller pediatric renal mass has limited the widespread application of this approach. As smaller instruments are developed and greater experience with this technique is gained, percutaneous treatments may be used in greater numbers of children.

Extracorporeal shock-wave lithotripsy has been used effectively for the dissolution of upper tract calculi in children. This therapy is difficult to apply to infants because of the requirement for immersion. Children are positioned in a large immersion tank while seated on a harness platform. Styrofoam padding is used to position the child and to shield the lung fields from pulmonary contusion. General anesthesia is required to ensure immobility and to provide adequate analgesia. Upper tract stones less than 2 cm in diameter are particularly amenable to shock-wave lithotripsy, but lower tract stones and staghorn calculi are not responsive. Cystine stones often respond poorly to shock-wave lithotripsy.

A major problem with the use of extracorporeal shock-wave lithotripsy in children is that of adjusting the port and gantry to fit small pediatric patients. Complications of lithotripsy include entry-site ecchymosis, pain, ureteral obstruction, subcapsular renal hematuria, branchial nerve palsy, cardiac arrhythmia, and pancreatitis. Shock-wave lithotripsy is contraindicated in children with hemorrhagic diatheses. Most recently, a new piezoelectric lithotriptor has been developed. This method localizes the stone with ultrasound, and neither immersion nor, in most cases, anesthesia is required. Hematuria following the procedure is less common than with shock-wave lithotripsy, and no radiation exposure is required.

VESICOURETERAL REFLUX

BILLY S. ARANT, JR., M.D.

Renal scarring associated with vesicoureteral reflux (VUR) is the most common cause of hypertension and chronic renal insufficiency in patients younger than 30 years of age. The variables determining the severity of renal injury from VUR are age, infection, and pressure. Younger patients, especially those younger than 5 years of age, are considered at greater risk for renal injury; however, new scars have been identified even in adolescents. When the urine is infected, particularly with P-fimbriated *Escherichia coli,* renal scarring is more likely. Finally, the pressure within the collecting system is a major determinant not only of renal injury but also of the grade of VUR. When intravesical pressure is high, as in anatomic or functional obstruction of the bladder outlet, renal damage is observed more often, even in the absence of infection.

Primary VUR is found in 30 to 50 per cent of infants and children (boys and girls) studied by voiding cystourethrography (VCUG) following the first urinary tract infection (UTI). Moreover, 30 to 40 per cent of asymptomatic siblings will also have VUR. Diagnostic ultrasound examination is recommended widely in the evaluation of patients with VUR and for screening those at risk. Unfortunately, ultrasonography is limited to detecting only severe distortions in the urinary tract associated with VUR, such as a dilated collecting system or gross renal scarring. Although VUR is more common in infants than in children, it should never be considered a normal developmental finding. VUR is observed rarely in otherwise normal urinary tracts that have never been infected.

Some reference sources have recommended that VCUG be done only at 4 to 6 weeks after acute UTI to minimize finding transient VUR, which may be present only when the bladder mucosa is inflamed. This practice is not based on appropriate clinical evidence. In fact, the reported incidence of VUR in patients with UTI studied by VCUG after 6 weeks was not different from those studied after 1 week. The only contraindication to VCUG at any time is untreated UTI. VUR that occurs during VCUG may be under higher pressure; if the infected urine is forced retrograde into the papillary collecting ducts, the risk of acute pyelonephritis is greater. Furthermore, 80 per cent of girls with UTI will experience a recurrence, which may occur in the interval between completing a 10-day course of treatment and the time VCUG is done. The risk of renal injury increases with the number of UTIs.

The clinical grade assigned to VUR depends on either the pressure generated within the collecting system during the study or previous injury to the collecting system from chronic VUR and UTI. In the normal urinary tract, VUR is limited by the relative competency of the ureterovesical junction, diuresis, antegrade peristalsis, and ureteral caliber, which is determined mainly by smooth muscle tone and elasticity. The technique used for VCUG in cooperating patients is for the bladder to be filled gradually at a pressure of 70 cm H_2O until the patient can no longer suppress bladder contractions. At the same intravesical pressure, higher grades of VUR may be seen in neonates and young infants because formation of ureteral smooth muscle and elastic fibers is not completed until several months after birth at term. Contrast material is often infused into an infant's bladder by syringe during fluoroscopic observation. *When the operator is inexperienced or impatient, the bladder may not relax immediately and intravesical pressure may increase to more than 70 cm* H_2O. *What may have been only grade I or II VUR may be changed to grade IV VUR in these very compliant collecting systems.* If damage has been caused by previous VUR, pressure, and infection, an inelastic collecting system will appear dilated even when intravesical pressure is low. Grade IV VUR resulting from acute distention can be distinguished from chronic dilation by intravenous urography—in acute distention, the collecting system will be normal. The treatment plan for a patient with VUR should not be decided only by the grade of VUR on a single study.

CLINICAL MANAGEMENT

Medical

Conservative treatment includes maintaining the urine sterile and the intravesical pressure low for as long as VUR persists. There is no increased morbidity in conservatively treated patients whose VUR does not resolve even after more than 10 years. There is increased risk when patients are not compliant with treatment, which consists not only of taking a single dose of antibiotic daily but also of maintaining a voiding schedule such that the bladder is emptied completely every 2 to 3 hours during the day. The antibiotic is given as a single bedtime dose so that the drug will be excreted promptly into the urine, where it will remain until morning; this is the interval when bladder bacteria are not being washed out by frequent micturition. A different schedule may be necessary for patients not yet toilet-trained or for those with nocturnal enuresis. Antibiotic prophylaxis is accomplished most reliably and with the least side effects by trimethaprim (1 to 2 mg/kg) alone or in combination with sulfamethoxazole (4 to 5 mg/kg), or with nitrofurantoin (1 to 2 mg/kg), which is tolerated best if given with food. These drugs alter bowel flora less than other antibiotics and have proved effective and safe in long-term studies. Antibiotic prophylaxis should be maintained until VUR has resolved.

Because no individual antibiotic is more than 85 per cent successful at preventing UTI, surveillance for bacteriuria must be routine even for patients on prophylaxis. Urine specimens for culture should be obtained every 2 to 3 months and any time urinary symptoms or unexplained fever occurs. Breakthrough UTI should be treated for 10 days, according to drug sensitivities, with an antibiotic other than the one given for prophylaxis. Increasing the dose of the same drug is naive unless one suspects that the patient is noncompliant with daily prophylaxis. Prophylaxis can resume with the same antibiotic previously used once the UTI has been eliminated. If antibiotic prophylaxis cannot be maintained for any reason, urinary surveillance for bacteriuria must be performed even more methodically. Routine culture specimens can be analyzed and the urine monitored twice weekly at home by dipstix that can detect bacteria (nitrite) and pyuria (leukocyte esterase).

Adjunctive measures should include careful attention to bowel habits because constipation can be associated with infrequent or incomplete bladder emptying, residual bladder urine, and recurrent UTI. Hygiene is also important. The perineum and periurethral tissue of girls and the prepuce of boys must be kept clean. The incidence of UTI in uncircumcised male infants is 20 times higher than in circumcised infants. Circumcision as a measure to prevent UTI has been debated but, to date, not recommended.

With the medical treatment just described, VUR can be expected to resolve, on average, in 10 to 15 per cent of ureters annually. Spontaneous resolution is more likely in grades I to II VUR than in grade III or higher but occurs even in grade IV VUR. In patients with VUR who exhibit no VUR on single VCUG during follow-up, 10 to 15 per cent will exhibit VUR on a subsequent study. Thus, VUR should be considered resolved when two consecutive VCUG studies 6 to 12 months apart are normal.

Surgical

VUR can be corrected surgically by one of several techniques for ureteral reimplantation. When performed by an experienced pediatric urologist, surgical correction is very successful. Complications to reimplanting a ureter include failure to eliminate VUR completely, which is observed more commonly in dilated collecting systems, and ureterovesical junction obstruction. Therefore, a postoperative examination of the collecting systems by ultrasonography and VCUG is essential to ensure successful surgical treatment. Consideration should be given to reimplanting both ureters even when VUR has been observed on only one side. One reason for doing this is that a refluxing ureter decompresses bladder pressure during micturition. If that ureterovesical junction is rendered suddenly competent, the higher intravesical pressure may be sufficient to cause VUR to occur on the opposite, unoperated side. Surveillance for bacteriuria must be continued for at least 6 months after surgical correction, and some surgeons prescribe antibiotic prophylaxis during this postoperative period.

The clinical management of VUR, therefore, can be either conservative (medical) or surgical. Preference for surgical treatment is usually based on higher grades of VUR, presence of renal scarring, recurrent infection, and failure of VUR to resolve before puberty (after which girls are at greater risk of developing UTI once sexual activity has begun). When patients were allocated randomly to medical or surgical treatment in two prospective clinical trials, however, no advantage of one treatment over the other was found. The preliminary conclusion of one of the studies was that the occurrence of UTI was similar between treatment groups but that febrile episodes of UTI, or clinical pyelonephritis, were observed less often in patients treated surgically; the other study reported no differences between treatment groups. Moreover, the occurrence of new renal scars or the progression of old scars was the same regardless of treatment. Renal scarring was the same in each group. Therefore, either treatment can be supported. The risks of repeated radiographic studies, urinary surveillance for bacteriuria, and antibiotic therapy must be measured against the risks of surgical and anesthetic complications. An argument can be made that surgical correction is less expensive than medical therapy in the long-term follow-up of children with VUR.

Another treatment recommended in the past and still performed frequently in females is urethral dilatation. This procedure was shown in three different prospective studies performed more than 20 years ago to have no benefit on the clinical course of UTI or VUR. Moreover, it involves the needless risk of anesthesia, added expense, and needless anxiety. A relatively new procedure used widely in Europe but only by licensed investigators in the United States, where it is still considered experimental, is the "sting" operation, whereby polytetrafluoroethylene paste is injected by needle under the intramural portion of the distal ureter during cystoscopy to render the ureterovesical junction more competent. Collagen may be used with less risk in the future. This procedure has the potential for eliminating reflux, but it has not been studied in randomized trials to prove its merit over either conservative medical management or traditional surgical correction.

PROGNOSIS

Even though VUR may resolve spontaneously or be corrected surgically, patients should be observed systematically through adolescence, the rationale being that renal injury from VUR sustained early in life may not manifest as radiographically apparent renal scars for up to 6 years or longer.

It is not that scarring takes so long to develop but, rather, that the relatively thin renal cortex of the normal infant kidney may not contract sufficiently to be obviously scarred on early intravenous pyelography. As the cortex adjacent to the scar grows normally or hypertrophies, the scar is identified more easily. The Tc-99m DMSA renal scan can detect areas of photon deficiency that represent either acute inflammation or scarring. If no scarring is obvious by Tc-99m DMSA scan 2 years after VUR has resolved, the likelihood of finding scarring at a later date is small.

After a single episode of UTI or after recurrent infections, as many as 30 per cent of children have identifiable renal scarring on subsequent examination. In half of those with scarring, hypertension develops and in 1 in 100 chronic renal insufficiency occurs before age 30. If there is one or more renal scars in either kidney, the patient should be monitored at regular intervals for increasing blood pressure, even into adult life. Resection of a single polar scar or nephrectomy may cure hypertension if the contralateral kidney is absolutely normal. If scarring is bilateral or in a solitary kidney, renal function should be assessed regularly throughout adolescence, but unilateral nephrectomy is never indicated to treat hypertension. In some females with renal scarring, hypertension or deterioration of renal function occurs during pregnancy.

One should not hesitate to identify VUR in infants and children. VCUG should be performed in patients at risk: infants and children with UTI and their prepubertal siblings. Once identified, patients with VUR should be observed regularly to minimize the risk of further renal injury. Renal injury from VUR is, in theory, preventable. Why not make every reasonable effort to reduce the risk?

REFERENCES

Arant BS Jr: Vesicoureteric reflux and renal injury. Am J Kidney Dis 17:491–511, 1991.

NEUROGENIC BLADDER IN CHILDREN

CRISTINE FROEMMING, M.D.
and RICARDO GONZALEZ, M.D.

The most common cause of neurogenic bladder in children is myelodysplasia. Less common causes are sacral agenesis, cerebral palsy, spinal cord injury, and acquired neurologic disorders (neoplasms, demyelinating diseases, inflammatory disorders, pelvic surgery, and trauma). The cause is usually obvious, but some children may present for assessment of urinary incontinence, recurrent urinary tract infections, unexplained detrusor trabeculation, vesicoureteral reflux, or hydronephrosis.

The consequences of neurogenic bladder dysfunction are urinary incontinence, deterioration of renal function, and urinary tract infections. The evaluation of the child with congenital neurogenic bladder should start shortly after birth. Detrusor function and bladder compliance, sphincter mechanisms, interaction between the sphincters and the detrusor, anatomy of the bladder and kidneys, and renal function should all be assessed. This information can be obtained by cystometrography, electromyography of the external sphincter, voiding cystourethrography, renal and bladder ultrasonography, and other tests as needed.

Bladder dysfunction may be variable. The bladder may be atonic, hyperreflexic, compliant, or noncompliant. The external sphincter may be innervated or partially or totally denervated. If contractile, the sphincter may relax during detrusor activity or may fail to relax or contract when the detrusor contracts (dyssynergia). The bladder may empty completely at low or high pressure or may fail to empty and only overflow. Upper tract damage results from high intravesical pressure resulting from dyssynergia or low bladder compliance, which leads to detrusor hypertrophy and thickening, vesicoureteral reflux, hydronephrosis, urinary tract infection, and renal scarring. Incontinence results from failure to store urine as a result of incompetence of the sphincters or poor bladder capacity due to hyperreflexia or low compliance. Incontinence may be a manifestation of overflow in cases of an atonic detrusor with a partially innervated sphincter.

TREATMENT OF THE NEWBORN

The goal of treatment in the first few years of life is the preservation of renal function. The newborn is considered at low risk for kidney damage if there is no hydronephrosis, vesicoureteral reflux, or detrusor trabeculation and if the intravesical pressure is low (<30 cm H_2O) and the sphincter is denervated or relaxes in synergy with the detrusor contraction. The bladder may empty spontaneously, or there may be retention and overflow. If urinary retention is significant and causes infection or hydronephrosis, clean intermittent catheterization should be performed four or five times a day with a 5 French infant feeding tube. The need for intermittent catheterization in such newborns is often temporary and results from the spinal shock that may follow the operation to close the spinal defect.

The use of suprapubic pressure (Credé's maneuver) is contraindicated because the high pressures generated may be transmitted to the kidneys, since the urethral sphincter may contract in response to increased intra-abdominal pressure.

On the other hand, if the sphincter does not relax when the bladder contracts (dyssynergia) or if the detrusor is noncompliant, the intravesical pressure will be high and vesicoureteral reflux, hydronephrosis, and detrusor trabeculation will be present at birth or will develop later. This high-risk newborn requires bladder drainage by clean intermittent catheterization and anticholinergic medications to relax the detrusor. Oxybutynin (Ditropan, 0.2 mg/kg/day in two doses) is usually well tolerated; however, because side effects may occur, the parents must be well versed in the possible symptoms of atropine intoxication. If intermittent catheterization or oxybutynin is not tolerated (or follow-up cystometrography fails to show a decrease in intravesical pressures in response to the treatment), a temporary, tubeless cutaneous vesicostomy effectively decompresses the bladder and protects the upper tracts. In the infant without reflux, an alternative to vesicostomy is close observation for infection, bladder thickening, appearance of new reflux, or hydronephrosis. When vesicoureteral reflux is present, catheterization is done with sterile disposable catheters (in contrast to clean catheters in other cases) and antibacterials at reduced dose are given for prophylaxis. The commonly used drugs for antibacterial prophylaxis are sulfamethoxazole and trimethoprim in combination (Bactrim, Septra) or nitrofurantoin at one-third the normal therapeutic dose. Others prefer a low dose of amoxicillin in the first few months of life, but it is less effective in our experience.

There must be close follow-up of the infant with neurogenic bladder because the neurologic status may change as a result of growth of the lower vertebral column, with tethering and stretching of affected nerve segments. We advocate repeating serum creatinine, renal ultrasonography, radionuclide cystography, and urodynamic studies every 3 to 4 months in the first year of life for the child at high risk or with vesicoureteral reflux. Renal growth is an important parameter, although it is well established that the kidney size in a patient with myelodysplasia is smaller when compared to standards for age. In the infant at low risk, urodynamic evaluation is repeated in 3 months; if the situation is unchanged, follow-up every 6 months and eventually yearly is sufficient.

VESICOURETERAL REFLUX

Vesicoureteral reflux is the predominant mechanism by which renal damage occurs. The principal therapeutic measures are to maintain urine sterility and to decrease the intravesical pressure as described previously. Reflux associated with high intravesical pressure may resolve with anticholinergic medications and intermittent catheterization in a substantial number of patients. The urine should be kept sterile, and cultures should be monitored at frequent intervals. If the bladder pressure decreases but either reflux persists or urine cultures are positive, antireflux surgery should be performed. Ureteral reimplantation in such children is associated with an excellent success rate. In contrast, if bladder pressure remains high despite appropriate treatment, antireflux operations are likely to fail. When bladder pressures remain high, a temporary cutaneous vesicostomy will protect the upper tracts until more definitive measures can be taken.

In older children, antireflux surgery and enterocystoplasty to augment the bladder capacity and reduce intravesical pressure is very effective. A child with a bladder augmentation is best catheterized with a 10 French or larger catheter because of the presence of mucus in the urine. Thus, the youngest age at which an enterocystoplasty can be performed is determined by the caliber of the urethra and, in general, is lower in females than in males. If vesicoureteral reflux is present, a ureteral reimplantation is performed at the time of the enterocystoplasty. For bladder augmentation in children with neurogenic bladder, the small intestine or left colon is preferred over the cecum. Exclusion of the right colon and the ileocecal valve from the intestinal tract may lead to acceleration of the intestinal transit and fecal incontinence.

Children with bladder augmentation depend on intermittent catheterization for emptying for the rest of their lives. The urine is usually colonized with bacteria; however, in the absence of reflux or symptoms, no treatment is indicated. Recurrent symptomatic infections can be prevented with oral antibacterials or bladder irrigations with nonabsorbable antibiotics. Follow-up of the child with a bladder augmentation should include monitoring the upper urinary tracts and ruling out bladder lithiasis, which occurs in about 5 per cent. The risk of neoplasms may be increased; however, as in the case of ureterosigmoidostomies, a long latency period of more than 7 years is likely to exist. A unique complication observed in patients after enterocystoplasty is spontaneous bladder rupture, which presents with abdominal pain and sepsis. The risk is higher in patients with high urethral resistance who comply inadequately with the prescribed regimen of intermittent catheterization.

URINARY INCONTINENCE

The age at which to initiate treatment for urinary incontinence varies with the child's psychologic development and social circumstances. In most cases, we prefer to start taking steps to achieve continence by the time the child is in the first grade. Urinary incontinence caused by overflow when the bladder is compliant is best treated by intermittent catheterization every 4 hours. This can be done by the caregiver until the child shows sufficient motivation and skill to perform self-catheterization.

Because intermittent catheterization is at the core of most other measures to achieve continence, it is always the initial step taken. If the child fails to be dry between catheterization done at reasonable intervals, the cause may be decreased bladder compliance, hyperreflexia, or low urethral resistance.

The treatment of high intravesical pressure has been discussed previously. The treatment of low outlet resistance is always surgical. When the incontinence is caused only by a denervated sphincter and the bladder is capacious and compliant, implantation of an inflatable artificial sphincter around the bladder neck has a high success rate and offers the possibility of spontaneous voiding without the need for intermittent catheterization. Many children require anticholinergic medications to improve the bladder storage capacity, and about 50 per cent need intermittent catheterization to facilitate emptying. Approximately one third of patients with low urethral resistance also require an enterocystoplasty to improve bladder compliance. The need for the enterocystoplasty may be obvious prior to the implantation of the artificial sphincter or may become apparent later when the child fails to gain continence despite a successful operation. We advise caution in performing bladder augmentations in children with sphincter denervation and small bladder capacity because, in many, the bladder will expand after outlet resistance is increased. Children with artificial sphincters need lifelong follow-up to detect possible changes in detrusor function that may lead to recurrent incontinence or hydronephrosis.

Other methods to increase outlet resistance, such as bladder neck tubularization operations, invariably require bladder augmentation and intermittent catheterization, and we consider them inferior to the artificial sphincter. Urethral fascial slings increase outlet resistance without decreasing the bladder capacity, but long-term results in large series of patients have not been reported.

If the urethra cannot be catheterized or if other anti-incontinence procedures have failed, a continent abdominal urinary stoma constructed with bowel or the cecal appendix is indicated.

With the treatment methods currently available, loss of renal function in children with neurogenic bladder dysfunction should not occur, and 85 per cent of children with myelomeningocele should achieve continence by the time they reach the first or second grade.

EXSTROPHY OF THE BLADDER

JAMES MANDELL, M.D.

Bladder exstrophy is generally characterized by a defect in the anterior abdominal wall, with the inner surface of the bladder and urethra exposed. On close inspection, one can see the ureteral orifices at the bladder trigone and the posterior aspect of the bladder neck. The rectus muscle and fascia and the symphysis pubis are widely separated. The rectum is anteriorly placed, and inguinal hernias are commonly present. In males, there is a spade-like glans and a dorsal urethral groove, and the prostate, verumontanum, and ejaculatory ducts are visible. Affected females have a bifid clitoris and an anteriorly placed vagina. The bladder varies in size and compliance. In some cases, the bladder can easily be indented with the examiner's finger; in others, there is a fibrotic plate.

The functional problems associated with bladder exstrophy include urinary incontinence, a foreshortened, dorsally curved phallus with complete epispadias, and vesicoureteral reflux. The difficulties in achieving ultimate post-repair continence involve bladder capacity and the lack of a continence mechanism. The bladder capacity may not be sufficiently large to accommodate socially acceptable voiding intervals because of anatomic or functional deficiencies. There is also complete absence of a continence mechanism at both the bladder neck and the urogenital diaphragm. The presence of the dorsally curved, short phallus (chordee) is caused by the attachment of the corporal bodies to the inferior aspect of the pubic ramus, which is widely separated. Although the upper urinary tracts are invariably normal at birth in infants with exstrophy, the ureters enter the bladder nonobliquely; thus vesicoureteral reflux occurs once the bladder is closed. There is little or no functional defect in gait associated with the widened pubis or rotated pelvic bones.

TREATMENT

Management of the child with bladder exstrophy is not simple, consistent, or universally successful. Currently, if a newborn is recognized with this defect, immediate referral to a pediatric institution is recommended. Prior to transfer and to surgery, the bladder should be covered with cellophane (Saran) wrap. Vaseline gauze should be avoided. An initial renal ultrasound examination is performed and is almost always normal. We favor an immediate (within 72 hours) closure of the bladder. The surgical technique involves mobilization of the bladder and closure of the bladder, the bladder neck, and the posterior urethra. No attempt is made at this time to tighten the bladder neck to achieve continence. The closure also includes dissection of the prostate gland off the urethral plate, creation of short paraexstrophic skin flaps, and penile lengthening by mobilization of the corpora cavernosa. The pubis is approximated with sutures and held in place for 3 weeks postoperatively with lower extremity traction and internal rotation of the hips. During this initial postoperative period, ureteral stents and a suprapubic bladder catheter are left in place. Complications commonly seen following this initial procedure are wound dehiscence and bladder prolapse through the newly created bladder neck. Helpful surgical hints include using a complete lower-body skin preparation and draping to enable good manual approximation of the symphysis; using a posterior or anterior pelvic osteotomy if the child is out of the immediate neonatal period; anchoring the closed bladder to the abdominal or retroperitoneal fascia; and using absorbable sutures to approximate the pubis.

If the bladder is too small to close primarily, delayed closure is recommended, either along with an initial urinary diversion or with a simultaneous bladder augmentation. Pelvic osteotomy is mandatory in this setting. Correction of the epispadias is usually performed when the child is between 2 and 4 years of age. In the female, repair of the bifid clitoris is also done. If the bladder capacity is less than 60 ml, the urethral repair is performed first. If the bladder is of good size, the urethral repair can be done simultaneously with the bladder neck reconstruction and ureteral reimplants. The latter is done using the crossed trigonal method. Techniques for achieving continence include bladder neck reconstruction using part of the native bladder and surrounding tissues, or, failing this, insertion of an artificial sphincter. Ureterosigmoidostomy has been used for many years with some success, but we no longer consider this a primary form of treatment.

Long-term issues involving continence, sexual and psychologic health, and performance cannot be overlooked. Children with exstrophy of the bladder must be vigilantly monitored for urinary tract infection, and renal function must be followed closely. These children will need surgical input well into adult life, and perfection is never achieved.

PATENT URACHUS AND URACHAL CYSTS

ANTHONY ATALA, M.D.
and ALAN B. RETIK, M.D.

The allantois appears around day 16 of gestation as an outpouching from the caudal wall of the yolk sac. As the bladder enlarges, the allantois involutes to form a thick tube called the urachus. The urachus allows free communication between the urinary bladder and the umbilicus in the abdominal wall. After birth, the urachus becomes a fibrous cord called the median umbilical ligament. The lumen in the inferior portion of the urachus remains patent approximately one third of the time. The abnormalities associated with the umbilicus are usually due to embryologic abnormalities of the urachus.

PATENT URACHUS

Failure of the urachus to regress completely results in a patent urachus: a communication between the bladder and the umbilicus. The usual presenting sign is a discharge of fluid from the umbilicus, which increases with voiding. Urethral obstruction may be present. Umbilical swelling, due to an associated umbilical hernia or urachal vascular engorgement, and skin discoloration may be present.

A voiding cystourethrogram may show the patent urachus and may also rule out the presence of a lower urinary tract obstruction. Analysis of fluid from the umbilicus for blood urea nitrogen and creatinine may be helpful. Injection of methylene blue transurethrally may confirm the communication. Treatment consists of identification and extraperitoneal excision of the urachal tract with a bladder cuff.

EXTERNAL URACHAL SINUS

Persistence of the distal urachus with an opening at the umbilicus results in an external urachal sinus. This may become symptomatic at any age but usually during childhood. Drainage, fever, paraumbilical tenderness, and inflammation may be present. A voiding cystourethrogram should be obtained to rule out a patent urachus and the presence of lower urinary tract obstruction. Sinography may aid in the diagnosis.

Treatment consists of excision of the sinus. Concomitant removal of any attached intraperitoneal structures is necessary if omphalomesenteric duct remnants are present.

URACHAL CYSTS

A urachal cyst occurs when both ends of the urachus are closed and only the central portion of the canal remains patent. The central lumen may enlarge from epithelial desquamation and degeneration. These cysts are usually asymptomatic until they attain a considerable size or become infected. Lower abdominal pain is the most frequent presenting complaint and may be associated with fever, voiding symptoms, gastrointestinal upset, and a palpable mass. Peritoneal irritation may give rise to symptoms that mimic an acute abdomen. Rupture of the cyst into the bladder, umbilicus, or peritoneal cavity may occur. Diagnostic studies should include a voiding cystourethrogram in the lateral position to demonstrate the compressive effect on the bladder, and an ultrasonogram.

Treatment consists of removal of the cyst if it is uninfected and drainage and marsupialization if an abscess is present. An alternative is first to drain the cyst percutaneously with ultrasound guidance and then to perform a surgical excision at a later date.

DISORDERS OF THE BLADDER AND URETHRA

JOHN W. DUCKETT, M.D.

MALIGNANT TUMORS

Uroepithelial Tumors

Uroepithelial tumors are universally of low grade and stage, and seldom do they recur. They are rare in the second decade of life and even rarer in the first but have occurred as early as 5 years of age. Uroepithelial tumors may be resected transurethrally, fulgurating the base. Periodic endoscopic reevaluation is needed for several years, but then the course is benign.

Rhabdomyosarcoma

Genitourinary rhabdomyosarcomas compose 27 per cent of all rhabdomyosarcomas; the incidence is approximately 1.2 in 100,000 children per year. There is a 3:1 male to female predominance. Approximately one third of pelvic rhabdomyosarcomas arise in the prostate and bladder, whereas another 25 per cent arise in the uterus and vagina. The remainder arise from the pelvis and grow intraperitoneally as a mass lesion with no specific site of origin.

The most common cell type by far is the *embryonal rhabdomyosarcoma.* The *botryoid sarcoma* is a subtype of the embryonal rhabdomyosarcoma that lies submucosally and has a papillary component. It is commonly found in the bladder. The *alveolar* type is more common in the older child and is associated with a poor prognosis; it is decidedly more rare than the embryonal type. The *pleomorphic* type is exceedingly rare in children.

In the past, the prognosis for these tumors was discouraging and radical extirpation was the primary treatment. In recent years, there has been a more encouraging response to vincristine, actinomycin D, and cyclosphosphamide treatment, and primary ablative surgery is postponed.

Currently, a tissue diagnosis is made and the patient is treated with chemotherapy for approximately 2 months. Response of the tumor is monitored. Radiation therapy is added later if the chemotherapeutic response is not satisfactory. Extirpative surgery is used to control local tumor, but it is hoped that such surgery is performed before distant metastasis has occurred.

Under this regimen, there is an approximately 75 per cent tumor-free survival rate; however, maintenance of the bladder occurs in only 35 per cent of cases.

BENIGN TUMORS

The two benign tumors of the bladder are *hemangiomas* and *neurofibromas.* They usually coexist with similar tumors in adjacent organs and may be controlled with local excision if symptomatic; otherwise, they should be left alone.

Polyps of the urethra are seen as hamartomatous growths arising from the verumontanum in boys. They may protrude down the urethra and cause symptoms of outlet obstruction. The polyps may, in addition, float freely into the bladder as a mass lesion. They may be excised with transurethral manipulation or removed through the bladder. Recurrence has not been reported.

BLADDER DIVERTICULA

Diverticula of the bladder are usually congenital anomalies. Most occur at the hiatus of the ureter as *paraureteral diverticula* associated with vesicoureteral reflux, involving a weak musculature adjacent to the hiatus. Resolution of reflux in this situation is unlikely but has been reported.

Other diverticula may occur in the posterior wall and up to the dome. These may be multiple, and generally excision is required. They are associated with infection and hematuria. If left until adulthood, these diverticula are prone to evolve into malignancy of a transitional cell type. Bladder diverticula are also associated with outlet obstructions, such as posterior and anterior urethral valves.

DYSFUNCTIONAL VOIDING

With the benefit of more common application of urodynamic studies in children, a new class of voiding abnormalities is being identified and appropriately treated. Urge syndrome and urge incontinence, fractionated voiding, staccato voiding, and lazy bladder syndrome are varieties of treatable conditions. Vesicoureteral reflux is more common in this group and will resolve if the child relearns proper voiding habits. Some of these children go on to experience true destruction of the urinary tract—the Hinman syndrome. Referral to a dysfunctional voiding center is worthwhile in terms of enhancing outcome.

POSTERIOR URETHRAL VALVES

This is the most common severe obstruction in males. Most instances of posterior urethral valves are now being detected in the neonatal period as prenatal ultrasonography becomes prevalent.

Bilateral hydronephrosis with a distended bladder is the typical appearance on ultrasonography. If the fetus does not demonstrate oligohydramnios, there are no indications for intervention in the prenatal period. In the face of oligohydramnios, poor renal development is likely and bilateral pulmonary hypoplasia will prevail. These fetuses have little chance of surviving. Intervention has been accomplished as early as 21 weeks of gestation without altering the ultimate course. Currently, there is very rarely a need for prenatal drainage procedures or early delivery.

Newborns with posterior urethral valves may have a weak urinary stream or abdominal masses, especially an enlarged bladder. Urinary ascites may be the presenting problem with respiratory distress. If the diagnosis is delayed, the infants present with azotemia, acidosis, and failure to thrive. Infection may occur with rapid dehydration and deterioration.

A stabilization period follows diagnosis. This entails drainage of the bladder with either a suprapubic cystocatheter or a No. 8 feeding tube through the urethra, control of infection with parenteral antibiotics, correction of acidosis, and electrolyte stabilization.

The valves should be destroyed either by transurethral electrocautery using miniature instruments or by treating a temporary vesicostomy to divert the urine through a vent in the bladder. The vesicostomy decompresses the upper tracts quite nicely, and it is not necessary to perform high ureterostomies in most cases. At a later date, the valves can be ablated and the vesicostomy closed.

If there is still renal failure following either drainage of the bladder or relief of the obstruction in the urethra, it is appropriate to perform a renal biopsy and a high ureterostomy if there is evidence of inadequate decompression. This is a rare occurrence these days.

This child is then observed carefully with a "wait and see" program. Reimplanting ureters and correcting reflux have been shown to complicate the situation more than improve it. These procedures may be needed but are better done at a later date and for very specific reasons.

The long-term prognosis with valve patients depends on

how much damage has been done to the kidneys in utero. If, at the time of diagnosis, the creatinine level drops to below 0.8 mg/dl, the prognosis is generally satisfactory. This represents about 50 per cent of glomerular filtration rate corrected for age.

The long-term prognosis of patients with posterior urethral valves who sustained severe kidney damage in utero is discouraging despite optimal care in the neonatal period; in later life, a significant number will experience chronic renal failure and will need dialysis and transplant. The outcome for many of these children can be predicted at an early age, and the parents can be well prepared for what lies ahead.

There are other subtle and symptomatic problems associated with posterior urethral valves, such as wetting. This incontinence is not uncommon in the years prior to puberty; however, after puberty, prostatic growth appears to control it satisfactorily. Inadequate bladder emptying is occasionally a problem and may necessitate intermittent catheterization or other means of improving voiding. Some children carry a full bladder that obstructs the upper tracts, requiring double and triple voiding at least twice daily to empty their entire systems. The bladder function must be optimal before a transplant is attempted.

About 20 per cent of patients have a functionless kidney that refluxes, requiring a nephrectomy. Bilateral reflux carries a worse prognosis than unilateral reflux or no reflux.

ANTERIOR URETHRAL VALVES

The disorder known as anterior urethral valves is more appropriately called a diverticulum of the anterior urethra. This is a defect of the spongiosum that creates a valve-like lip of the diverticulum. Excision or transurethral ablation of the lip is required. Some affected children undergo severe upper tract changes.

Congenital Urethral Membrane

This is a variable obstruction in the membranous proximal bulb that acts as a diaphragmatic obstruction. The etiology of the disorder is different from that of posterior urethral valves. It may be considered a congenital urethral stricture, but this term should be abolished. Males with this condition experience severe upper tract changes.

Prominent Urethral Folds

These are normal folds coming from the verumontanum that may be quite prominent in little boys. They are similar to urethral valves but do not form a fusion anteriorly with an obstructing web. They should not be considered obstructing "mini valves."

Megalourethra

Megalourethra is a rare lesion most often associated with prune-belly syndrome. There are two types:

1. The *scaphoid* type is a deficiency of the corpus spongiosum that allows ballooning of the urethra during voiding and may be repaired with techniques used for the correction of hypospadias.
2. The *fusiform* type involves a deficiency of the corpora cavernosa, as well as the spongiosum, that results in an elongated flaccid penis with redundant skin. This is usually seen in severe forms of the prune-belly syndrome and may be repaired if the patient survives.

HYPOSPADIAS

Hypospadias is an anomaly that occurs in 1 in 300 boys in a wide spectrum of presentations. There are two basic problems: the first is the lack of completion of the urethral folding up to the tip of the penis; the second is congenital curvature, or a bending of the penis due to a deficiency on the ventrum with a fibrous replacement. The more severe the defect, the more likely it is that chordee is present.

Classification should be based on the location of the meatus after the chordee is released. Under these criteria, 65 per cent of hypospadias cases are subcoronal and can be managed with a simple meatal advancement and glanuloplasty (MAGPI). Another 10 per cent occur on the penis and may be repaired with a more extensive extension of the urethra to the tip. The other 25 per cent are penoscrotal and more proximal, and these require much more extensive reconstruction.

Management

Numerous techniques are available for repair of hypospadias. One of the most modern is the MAGPI technique (see earlier). For the more proximally placed urethra, an onlay preputial island flap may be utilized for those without chordee. Finally, the more severe types may be managed with a transverse preputial island flap, with vascularized tissue creating the neourethra. Free skin grafts have also been used for this purpose but are associated with more complications.

Complications

A complication rate of about 10 to 15 per cent should be expected for more severe conditions, with an overall rate of 5 per cent. Problems include urethral cutaneous fistulas and strictures that require secondary surgical techniques. Other complications are infections, diverticula, and residual chordee.

The currently accepted techniques are one-stage procedures that may be done on an outpatient basis. Six to 18 months of age is the preferred time for surgery. Microscopic and optical magnification methods with fine, delicate instruments are essential.

OTHER DISORDERS OF THE URETHRA

Urethral Strictures

A midbulbar urethral stricture is most commonly associated with trauma due to instrumentation or a straddle injury. "Congenital urethral strictures" are not a specific entity. Urethral dilation for such a diagnosis is inappropriate. A narrowing of the bulbar urethra should not be considered a congenital stricture; there is a common bulbar spasm during voiding cystourethrography that gives the appearance of a stricture.

Meatal Stenosis

Males. A narrowed urethral meatus is very common in the circumcised male, and meatotomy is not required. A tight web on the ventrum deflects the urinary stream upward, and a meatotomy is indicated for improvement in stream direction. Very few meatal stenoses create significant obstruction. These are usually an inflammatory replacement of the meatus with balanitis xerotica obliterans.

Meatal Stenosis

Females. "Lyon's ring" is a collagenous area just inside the meatus that is the narrowest spot in the female urethra. For many years, it was considered an obstructing problem and dilation and fracture were recommended. There are occasional meatal stenoses that require enlargement, but this condition is much rarer than was previously thought.

Prolapse of the Urethra

Urethral prolapse occurs predominantly in black girls and causes irritation and bleeding. There is a circumferential eversion of urethral mucosa, which becomes inflamed and should be carefully excised. This condition rarely recurs. Differential diagnoses to be considered are ectopic ureterocele and botryoid sarcoma.

Accessory Urethra

Urethral duplications in boys are usually asymptomatic and appear on the dorsum as an epispadiac extra urethra. More complex channels may be present, and it is necessary to excise the accessory channel to correct chordee or troublesome double voiding. Girls may have an accessory urethra in the clitoris with a posteriorly displaced urogenital sinus.

UNDESCENDED TESTES

MARTIN A. KOYLE, M.D.
and RONALD R. PFISTER, M.D.

Cryptorchidism represents the single most common disorder of sexual differentiation in males. The cause is uncertain but is probably multifactorial and dependent on hormonal and mechanical factors. Although in the past surgical therapy for an undescended testis in a young boy was recommended at age 5 to 7 years or even as late as puberty, this is probably an unreasonable delay.

EPIDEMIOLOGY

The incidence rate of cryptorchidism in term male infants is between 3 and 4 per cent. By 9 months of age, the majority of such testes will have descended spontaneously into the scrotum, leaving approximately 1 per cent of boys with an empty scrotum. Histologic data have demonstrated a reduced number of germ cells in the truly undescended testis by age 1 year, with a marked diminution in number of cells by age 2 years. Thus, fertility may be threatened if the testis is not treated and brought down at an early date. On the other hand, no current data unequivocally support the concept that early orchiopexy improves fertility. The Leydig cells do appear normal at virtually any age at which orchiopexy is performed, and thus testosterone production should not be affected by delayed surgical therapy. Although carcinoma of the testis, particularly in the intra-abdominal testis, is a potential complication of cryptorchidism, there is no evidence that earlier orchiopexy reduces the risk. However, orchiopexy places the testis into such a position that it can be palpated with ease by the patient for lifelong monitoring for any change. Treatment of the undescended testis also allows for repair of the omnipresent accompanying hernia and minimizes the risk of torsion, which reportedly occurs more commonly with cryptorchid testis.

DIAGNOSIS

In managing the unilaterally undescended testis, one must differentiate a true cryptorchid testis from the more common retractile testis. Repeated examinations by the physician, as well as parental examinations while the child is in a warm bath, are often necessary to differentiate the two entities. Histologically and functionally, retractile testes are normal and do not warrant surgery. In rare instances, however, such testes can be "trapped" in an ectopic position, in which case orchiopexy should be considered.

Approximately 20 per cent of children with cryptorchidism have impalpable testes. We have found ultrasonography to be helpful in locating only those testes that already may be palpated by hand; thus, ultrasonography does not appear to be valuable in identifying testes preoperatively. Computed tomography, magnetic resonance imaging, gonadal venography, and herniography have been used with varying degrees of success in locating the nonpalpable undescended testes but are invasive, expensive, and time-consuming studies that necessitate sedation, anesthesia, and/or radiation. At present, our approach to the child with the unilateral undescended testis is to proceed to direct inguinal exploration because most nonpalpable testes are indeed canalicular or lie just above the internal ring. Alternatively, we offer laparoscopy in an attempt to locate the impalpable testis, to identify the gonadal vessels entering an open internal ring, or to define a blind-ending intra-abdominal spermatic cord. Laparoscopy is done at the same operative sitting but precedes open surgical exploration.

Special attention must be directed to the child with bilateral impalpable testes. Even in a newborn without overt genitourinary anomalies, such as hypospadias, it is important to rule out an intersex state (see also articles on hypospadias and intersex, Sections 9 & 12). Thus, appropriate chromosomal studies, endocrinologic data, and radiologic investigation may be indicated in such a child to exclude adrenogenital syndrome and other intersex abnormalities. If such an infant is found to be an otherwise normal karyotypic and phenotypic male, we wait until the child's first birthday before further evaluation. At that age, if testes are not present, because of the negative feedback loop involving the hypothalamic-pituitary-gonadal axis, serum follicle-stimulating hormone (FSH) and luteinizing hormone (LH) levels should be abnormally high. If serum testosterone, FSH, and LH levels are all normal or slightly depressed, we perform a human chorionic gonadotropin (hCG) stimulation study (2000 IU IM every other day for 5 doses). A serum testosterone level ten times that of prestimulation levels indicates that at least one testis is present. In the anorchid state, basal gonadotropin levels are markedly elevated and there is no response in testosterone levels to exogenous hCG administration.

TREATMENT

At this time, there are insufficient data to indicate a role for the use of hCG or gonadotropin-releasing hormone (GnRH) to induce testicular descent in the truly undescended testis. A critical review of the literature suggests that hormonal stimulation will probably promote descent of the retractile testis but will not be associated with descent of the cryptorchid testis. Thus, we use hormonal stimulation in equivocal cases or in those with bilateral cryptorchidism. Some investigators have found that preoperative stimulation will also enlarge a nonpalpable testis, making it palpably obvious so that the need for laparoscopy can be determined.

We usually suggest surgical correction of an undescended testis near the time of the first birthday because of the previously mentioned histologic data. Palpable testes are best approached via a standard inguinal incision. In the majority of patients, such surgery is performed in the outpatient setting. The location of nonpalpable testes can be confirmed by preoperative laparoscopy, as mentioned previously. This ensures the proper location of incision and allows the surgeon to select the best surgical option.

If the testes are not seen at the internal ring or have been identified by laparoscopy to be intra-abdominal, the peritoneum is opened. Although the testes begin their descent from a higher lumbar level, it is unusual to locate the impalpable testis as high as the kidney. The surgeon must make an appropriate decision regarding the best technique for bringing the intra-abdominal or high undescended testis into the scrotum without disturbing the collateral blood supply to the testis. The spermatic cord can be divided (as described by Fowler and Stephens), relying on vascular supply via collaterals, particularly the vasal artery; however, long-term studies have demonstrated the viability of such testes to be only 60 to 70 per cent.

As an alternative to the Fowler-Stephens approach, a two-stage procedure might be chosen, with preliminary clipping of the gonadal vessels through the laparoscope or by surgically bringing the testis as far into the inguinal canal as possible and then wrapping it in Silastic. Secondary re-exploration and orchiopexy are planned for 6 to 12 months later.

Some groups have found success with autotransplantation of the testes and microvascular reanastomosis of the spermatic vessels to the inferior epigastric vessels. This procedure can be accomplished in conjunction with the Fowler-Stephens technique in an attempt to increase the chances for success. This approach is indeed tedious and probably not worthwhile in a child with a normally descended contralateral testis. Primary orchiectomy is preferable in such a patient. The diagnosis of vanishing or absent testis cannot be made, and thus surgical exploration is not complete unless blind-ending gonadal vessels are encountered. A blind vas or an empty inguinal canal is not sufficient by itself. In our opinion, a testicular prosthesis should be offered for psychologic reasons in such cases when the testis is absent or removed, even in the young child.

There has been much debate regarding the optimal therapy for the postpubertal male with an undescended testis. If orchiopexy is performed in the male beyond puberty, a biopsy is performed to identify carcinoma in situ, an entity that may portend the development of malignancy. We discuss the available options with the family—that is, no surgery versus orchiopexy versus orchiectomy.

In general, for the high nonpalpable or intra-abdominal testes, we recommend exploration, orchiectomy, and placement of a prosthesis if the contralateral testis is normally descended. Such testes usually demonstrate severe, if not complete, germinal atrophy and absent spermatogenesis. Until the age of 32 years, the risks of such surgery are less than the risks of developing cancer; thus, surgery appears to be justified. Beyond this age, however, recent data argue against surgery, even orchiectomy. However, the patient beyond this age has to weigh the facts appropriately and make the decision himself. In intersex states, in which the testes may be dysgenetic (mixed gonadal dysgenesis, testicular feminization) and prone to malignant degeneration (gonadoblastoma and seminoma), primary orchiectomy should be considered early.

SUMMARY

Early diagnosis and management of the undescended testis should be pursued. Such a practice may lead to attainment of maximal fertility potential. Although such early intervention probably does not reduce the risk of carcinogenesis, it at least places such a testis in a location where it can be readily palpated.

REFERENCE

Fowler R, Stephens FD: The role of testicular vascular anatomy in salvage of high undescended testes. Aust NZ J Surg 29:92, 1959.

PENIS, SPERMATIC CORD, AND TESTIS

JAMES MANDELL, M.D.

PENIS

Care of the child's normal penis has been a focus of concern and controversy for some time. The uncircumcised penis is covered by a relatively adherent foreskin for the first few years of life. Thereafter, the foreskin may be easily or not so easily retracted for proper hygiene. The only statement agreed upon is that good hygiene is important for health commencing with puberty. The possible problems associated with an intact foreskin include phimosis, paraphimosis, balanoposthitis, and urinary tract infection.

Phimosis is the inability to retract the foreskin, and *paraphimosis* is the inability to pull the foreskin back over the glans after first retracting it. *Balanoposthitis* is infection or inflammation of the prepuce and/or shaft skin due to trauma or poor hygiene. Removal of the material produced by the subcoronal glands *(smegma)* is the main hygiene issue.

Urinary tract infections in male neonates are much more common in those who are uncircumcised. Disadvantages associated with the circumcised phallus are the cost of the procedure, the potential surgical complications, and the longer-term risk of meatal stenosis.

Hypospadias

The hypospadiac penis is a relatively common problem (1 in 300) that is usually easily diagnosed in the nursery. The urethral meatus does not reach the end of the glans and may be seen anywhere from near the tip of the penis all the way down to the perineum. There is an absence of the ventral prepuce, which gives the appearance of a "dorsal hood." Ventral curvature of the phallus (chordee) is often present.

Hypospadias is usually an isolated defect, but, when it is associated with other findings such as undescended testes, one must consider an intersex syndrome. This is critical because a female with salt-losing congenital adrenal syndrome can appear exactly as a male with severe hypospadias and nonpalpable gonads. It is important for the obstetrician and pediatrician to realize that a child with even the mildest form of hypospadias must not be circumcised. Not only can injury to the urethra occur if circumcision is performed but the foreskin is needed for the repair.

The repair of this anomaly is currently performed when the child is between 6 and 12 months of age. In most cases, a single-stage repair can be performed by experienced surgeons. With the severest forms, a second stage may be necessary. Complications requiring additional surgery occur in about 5 to 20 per cent of cases, depending on the complexity of the procedure.

Epispadias

Isolated epispadias (without bladder exstrophy) is much less common than hypospadias. It also can range in severity from distal (glanular) to very proximal (penopubic). Dorsal chordee is common. With the severest forms, urinary incontinence may also be present due to deficient formation of the bladder neck and urethral sphincter.

Timing of repair of epispadias is similar to that of hypospadias if incontinence is not present. If it is present, primary attention is directed toward bladder neck reconstruction, which involves many more potential complications and deviations from a straightforward course.

Other Congenital Penile Problems

Several other congenital anomalies requiring surgical intervention may occur. *Chordee* without hypospadias may create potential future problems with sexual function. *Penile web* or torsion may also be unsightly or functionally significant. *Micropenis* is a very difficult problem to address because a phallus shorter than 2 cm in stretched length will probably not allow the child to function well later in an adult male sexual role. *Megalourethra* (an elongated, tortuous phallus with outpouching of the urethra) may be an isolated finding, but its presence should alert the clinician to look for the other stigmata of prune-belly syndrome.

Acquired Penile Problems

Acquired penile problems include *priapism,* which is a persistent erection that is not physiologic in nature. In children, it can be associated with hematologic abnormalities such as sickle cell disease or leukemia. Treatment is variable, and its effectiveness debatable.

Another problem is *meatal stenosis,* a narrowing of the urethral meatus due to chronic irritation. This is found almost exclusively in circumcised males.

SPERMATIC CORD AND TESTES

Torsion of the Testicle

The "acute scrotum" is one of the most common and potentially significant genital problems in childhood. The differential diagnoses include torsion of the testicle, torsion of the appendages of the testicle or epididymis, incarcerated hernia, epididymitis, orchitis, allergic reaction, and trauma. Torsion is certainly the most common of these diagnoses and one of the most important to recognize.

Torsion of the testicle occurs in a bimodal pattern, first in the immediate postnatal period and later near puberty. Neonatal torsion has been thought to have a different anatomic and clinical presentation than the childhood form. This may not be entirely true, however, as we have seen at least six cases of bilateral neonatal torsion, both synchronous and asynchronous, implying that the risk of acquired anorchia exists in both groups. The childhood presentation may be more easily confused with an inflammatory condition, but the rule is: *Presentation of an acutely painful, swollen hemiscrotum is torsion of the testicle until proven otherwise.*

The treatment, if the torsion is seen early enough (<8 hours), is immediate surgical exploration; detorsion of the affected side, if salvageable; and, if not, orchiectomy. Septopexy (fixation to the scrotal septum) of the other testicle is mandatory.

Torsion of the Appendix Testis or Epididymis

Torsion of the appendix testis or epididymis is also very common but involves none of the same risks; however, it is not always possible to differentiate from torsion of the testicle. In terms of the other possible differential diagnoses, a careful examination usually allows one to distinguish between them. Although viral epididymo-orchitis is seen in childhood, the diagnosis of epididymitis due to bacterial source is one of exclusion. If the latter is definitively diagnosed, urologic evaluation is indicated.

Testis Tumors

Testis tumors are relatively rare in childhood but can be quite aggressive, especially postpubertally. The diagnosis is usually made on the basis of the physical findings of a painless, firm mass in the testicle. Laboratory studies include α-fetoprotein and β unit of human chorionic gonadotropin. An inguinal approach with radical orchiectomy is standard. The need for retroperitoneal lymphadenectomy and/or chemotherapy is determined on the basis of the age at presentation and the histology. In early childhood, the teratomas or granulosa cell tumors are more likely to behave benignly if completely excised. Postpubertally, however, most tumors are managed as in the adult.

Varicocele

Varicocele of the scrotum is a collection of dilated veins draining the testis. It is much more common on the left side and may occur in as many as 10 per cent of adolescent males. The importance of this finding is related to the fact that males presenting with infertility have a high incidence of varicoceles, and ligation of the varicocele has been said to improve sperm count and fertility. It has also been shown that the testicle associated with moderate- to large-sized varicocele is often smaller and softer than its corresponding mate. Whether this means that spermatic vein ligation will ultimately change the incidence of fertility in these adolescents is unknown at this time.

Spermatocele and Hydrocele

The other lesions of the spermatic cord include spermatocele and hydrocele. Spermatocele is unusual, is unlikely to be symptomatic, and rarely warrants surgical intervention. Hydrocele of the cord is sometimes difficult to differentiate from a communicating hydrocele and often results in the need for surgical intervention.

REFERENCES

King L: Urologic disorders. Curr Sci 2:359, 1990.

Rozenman J, Hertz M, Boichis H: Radiological findings of the urinary tract in hypospadias: A report of 110 cases. Clin Radiol 30:471, 1979.

HERNIAS AND HYDROCELES

DONALD H. NGUYEN, M.D.
and MICHAEL E. MITCHELL, M.D.

PATHOGENESIS

During the 3rd month of gestation, the processus vaginalis develops from the peritoneal lining as an outpouching into the internal inguinal ring. As the testes begin to descend into the scrotum at the 7th week, the processus vaginalis extends into the inguinal canal. Upon completion of testicular descent, the processus vaginalis spontaneously closes sometime after birth. The exact time of closure is not known, but the incidence of patent processus vaginalis at birth varies between 15 and 37 per cent and can be as high as 57 per cent. The processus vaginalis may remain patent for several months after birth and then close, but it stays patent throughout life in approximately 20 per cent of cases. A *hydrocele* occurs when fluid fills the processus vaginalis between the parietal and visceral tunica vaginalis. If the patent processus communicates with the abdominal cavity and contains abdominal contents, such as fluid, a loop of bowel, or an ovary, it becomes an *indirect inguinal hernia.*

HERNIAS

The incidence 'of indirect inguinal hernia in the pediatric population is 3.5 to 5.5 per cent in full-term newborns and 9 to 30 per cent in preterm newborns. Males are affected six to nine times more often than girls. The right side is affected twice as commonly as the left side in both sexes. *Bilateral hernias* tend to occur more commonly in premature newborns (44 to 55 per cent), compared with 8 to 10 per cent in full-term infants. The incidence of hernia is slightly higher in twins and in individuals from the same family (11.5 per cent).

On examination, an inguinal hernia presents as a bulge or smooth mass in the inguinal region that may extend from the internal inguinal ring laterally, down past the pubic tubercle and into the scrotum. Increased abdominal pressure, such as occurs during crying, coughing, or the Valsalva maneuver, may cause the mass to increase in size. *A helpful maneuver to increase intra-abdominal pressure is to hold the child with the arms outstretched and legs extended to induce struggling.*

During periods of relaxation, the hernia may reduce spontaneously. A hernia that cannot be reduced is termed *incarcerated.* Nonreducible or incarcerated hernias in children result in ischemia of the sac content and can rapidly develop into a *strangulated hernia* with infarction of the hernia sac contents. This condition represents a surgical emergency. If the hernia is readily reducible, the inguinal swelling may not be apparent on physical examination and the diagnosis is made on the basis of the history. In the younger child, a coexisting undescended testis may be palpated as being the hernia. Therefore, it is important to identify and note the position of the ipsilateral testis in relation to the hernia. If the testis is undescended, it will need to be brought down into the scrotum as part of the hernia repair. Transillumination of the mass may reveal a mixed-fluid-filled structure. Occasionally, bowel sounds can be heard on auscultation. A radiographic study to demonstrate air in the loop of bowel in the scrotum is rarely needed.

In a *sliding hernia,* part of the hernia wall is made up of an intra-abdominal structure such as bowel, appendix, fallopian tube, or bladder. *Direct inguinal hernia* occurs very rarely in the pediatric population. It results from a weakness in the inguinal canal *medial* to the inferior epigastric vessels and therefore medial to the normal path of descent of the testis. In children, it is often a complication following repair of an indirect hernia.

Femoral hernia is extremely rare (< 0.2 per cent) in children and represents a defect inferior to the inguinal ligament. It occurs in females twice as often as in males.

Management

More than half of pediatric hernias occur in children younger than 1 year of age. In young infants who present with *incarcerated hernias,* surgical repair can be performed 24 to 48 hours after the hernia has been reduced. Most repairs are performed on an elective outpatient basis, except for those in the very young infant (younger than 6 months) or premature infant, who need overnight monitoring for possible postanesthesia apnea and bradycardia. Generally, endotracheal intubation is recommended for the very young child, and masked general anesthesia is sufficient in the older. Spinal anesthesia can be used and may be less inducive to postoperative apnea.

Postoperative pain control can be achieved with plain acetaminophen in most infants younger than 6 months of age. In older children, acetaminophen with codeine may be required. No preoperative or postoperative antibiotic is needed routinely. Bathing is resumed at 48 hours, and heavy activity can usually be allowed at the second postoperative week. Postoperative scrotal swelling or hydrocele represents fluid accumulation in the distal hernia sac, which resolves spontaneously in most cases. Scrotal hematoma is rare and is usually associated with complete resection of the scrotal component of the hernia sac.

Hernias in Girls

Girls are less affected with hernias than boys, with sex ratios ranging from 1:3 to 1:10. Girls tend to have a slightly higher rate of incarcerated hernias than boys (39 versus 22 per cent). Not uncommonly, there is a fallopian tube or an ovary in the hernia sac. Incarceration associated with an ovary is not an indication for immediate surgical exploration because vascular compromise is rarely seen.

Prepubertal inguinal hernia is the most common presentation of *complete testicular feminization.* This form of male pseudohermaphroditism (46,XY) is characterized by a phenotypic female caused by an androgen receptor defect, resulting in a lack of virilization of the external genitalia and no internal sexual organs except for the presence of gonads. If the vagina is short and blind-ending or absent, ultrasonography of the pelvis should be performed to confirm the absence of the uterus.

Contralateral Exploration

Controversy remains to date regarding whether the contralateral side should be explored in *unilateral inguinal hernia* in children. The presence of a patent processus vaginalis can be demonstrated in 48 to 85 per cent of cases on the contralateral side. However, in unilateral hernia repairs, the incidence of subsequent hernia development on the opposite side is only 14 to 16 per cent in long-term follow-up. Until the controversy is resolved, the following may serve as a guide: *In children younger than 1 year of age, unilateral repair with contralateral exploration should be performed. In children older than 1 year of age, the opposite side should be explored only if clinically indicated (i.e., a thickened cord or history).* Another reasonable approach is to perform a diagnostic test (such as the pneumoperitoneum or Goldstein test) intraoperatively. If the test result is positive (presence of air or crepitus in the contralateral groin or scrotum), the opposite side should be explored and repaired.

HYDROCELES

Hydroceles present most frequently in infancy. On examination, they appear as painless swellings of the scrotum that transilluminate brightly. Typically, hydroceles surround the testes, but occasionally they are situated above the testis; careful palpation during transillumination reveals the testis displaced inferiorly and posteriorly. When diagnosed at birth, hydroceles tend to be bilateral; they are almost always associated with a patent processus vaginalis. The diagnosis is made by history, physical examination, and transillumination. Diagnostic aspiration of the hydrocele should never be attempted, as occasionally fluid-filled bowel trapped in a hernia may transilluminate and give a false diagnosis of hydrocele. Furthermore, aspiration may introduce infections into the processus vaginalis that then spread to the peritoneal cavity, causing peritonitis.

Communicating hydrocele is associated with an incompletely closed processus vaginalis. Parents give the history of a "coming and going" swelling of the scrotum, and on physical examination the fluid in the hydrocele may be forced back into the peritoneal cavity. When peritoneal fluid travels in only one direction (one-way valve) down into the scrotum, the communicating hydrocele may present as a tense and enlarging transilluminating mass.

Hydrocele of the spermatic cord results from incomplete closure of the lower end of the processus vaginalis, with the mid and upper portion remaining patent. Occasionally, a hydrocele is not detected clinically until events that increase the intraperitoneal pressure and/or fluid occur. Such situations are reported in patients in whom ascites or mesenteric adenitis developed or who have undergone ventriculoperitoneal shunting or peritoneal dialysis.

Abdominoscrotal hydrocele has been reported only rarely. The exact cause is unknown, but it is thought to occur when the scrotal component of the hydrocele extends past the inguinal canal and into the abdominal cavity. Hydroceles that develop in the postpubertal adolescent boy are similar to those in the adult and are usually associated with an imbalance of serous fluid secretion and absorption by the tunica vaginalis.

Worthy of mention is the *hydrocele associated with testicular tumor* in children. As many as 50 per cent of pediatric testicular tumors are associated with a reactive hydrocele. It is therefore important to locate, identify, and palpate the testis carefully through the hydrocele sac in every patient.

Management

In most children, the processus vaginalis closes spontaneously during the 1st year of life and the hydrocele fluid is reabsorbed. Thus, therapy consists of observation during the 1st year and high ligation of the processus vaginalis via an *inguinal approach* if the hydrocele persists after 1 year of age or if there is evidence of a concomitant hernia. The distal processus is left open, and no attempt at removal of the entire tunica vaginalis is made. Sclerosing therapy is to be avoided in the pediatric population. This therapy is very painful, and the sclerosing agents can reflux back into the peritoneal cavity and cause chemical peritonitis.

Treatment of postpubertal hydroceles is based on their size and the degree or severity of symptomatology (usually pain) and is similar to treatment of hydroceles in the adult. Hydrocelectomy is performed via a *scrotal* incision.

VULVA AND VAGINA

DAVID MURAM, M.D.

DEVELOPMENTAL DISORDERS

Minor differences in the contour or size of vulvar structures are not unusual. There is often considerable variation in the distance between the posterior fourchette and the anus or between the urethra and the clitoris, giving the vulva different appearances. In muscular girls, the perineal body may be exceptionally thick and wide; the vulva situated deeply between the bulging sides of the perineum, forming a "vulva retroussé." Rare anomalies of the vulva include a caudal appendage, which resembles a tail, and variations in the insertion of the bulbocavernosus muscle, which may alter the appearance of the labia majora and, at times, obliterate the fossa navicularis. Duplication of the vulva is an extremely rare anomaly that may be associated with duplication of the urinary and intestinal tracts.

There is commonly considerable variation in the size and shape of the labia minora. One labium may be quite larger than the other, or both labia may be unusually large. Labial enlargement and asymmetry have been wrongly assumed by some to be the result of masturbation. The patient can be assured that these differences are simple minor variations that usually require no treatment. If the asymmetry is significant or if the labia are pulled into the vagina during sexual intercourse, the large labia may be trimmed surgically.

Ambiguous Genitalia

"Ambiguous genitalia" denotes partial or incomplete virilization of the external genitalia. Ambiguous genitalia may therefore be seen in genetic females who were virilized in utero, in undervirilized males, or in true hermaphrodites. In general, exposure to androgens after 12 weeks of gestation leads only to clitoral hypertrophy. Examination of the genitalia shows an enlarged clitoris but a normal vestibule, urethra, and vagina. The labia majora are altered by redundancy, wrinkling, and skin pigmentation. Exposure to androgens at progressively earlier stages of embryologic development also leads to clitoral hypertrophy but, in addition, to retention of the urogenital sinus and fusion of the labioscrotal folds. In these severely virilized individuals, the labia are fused in the midline to form a median raphe. The area of fusion may be partial or may extend the entire distance from the perineum to the phallus. When virilization is extensive, the fused labia form a wrinkled, pouch-like structure that resembles the scrotum in a cryptorchid male. The vaginal opening is absent. Instead, a single opening is present that extends to a common passage connecting the urethra and vagina. Müllerian and gonadal development remains unaffected because neither is androgen-dependent.

Treatment

The surgical correction of genital ambiguity should be done only after the completion of the medical evaluation. Reconstruction of the female external genitalia is best accomplished in two stages. The first stage, done prior to the infant's discharge from the hospital, consists of clitoral reduction. The purpose of the surgical reduction is to attain female appearance to the external genitalia. When a reduction clitoroplasty is done, the surgeon should attempt to preserve the neurovascular connections to the glans; in this manner, a functional clitoris of normal size can be created. Removal of the entire clitoris is rarely indicated.

The second stage, vaginal reconstruction, should be delayed until after pubertal development. In general, if only labial fusion is present, division of the labia is all that is required. Minor degrees of narrowing of the vaginal introitus can be easily corrected. When a significant narrowing is present, enlargement of the introitus may require the use of rotated skin flaps or a split-thickness skin graft.

Other Causes of Clitoral Enlargement

Enlargement of the clitoris caused by a benign neoplasm has been observed in a few infants. Von Recklinghausen's disease (neurofibromatosis), lymphangiomas, and fibromas may involve the clitoris and cause enlargement. Therapy consists of excision of the neoplasm and thereby reduction of the clitoris to normal size.

Clitoral Agenesis or Duplication

Clitoral agenesis is a very rare condition. Splitting or duplication of the clitoris is caused by failure of the corpora to fuse in the midline. Bifid clitoris usually occurs in conjunction with bladder exstrophy, epispadias, and absence or cleavage of the symphysis pubis. The labia majora are widely separated, and the labia minora are separated anteriorly but can be traced posteriorly around the vaginal orifice. The vaginal orifice is narrow, and the vagina is shortened and rotated anteriorly. The pelvic floor is incomplete, and uterine prolapse is often observed in these patients. Other congenital anomalies may be present (e.g., spina bifida). At puberty, pubic hair growth is absent over the midline.

Anomalies of the Hymen

Variations in the appearance of the hymen are extremely common. The orifice may vary in diameter from very small to very large. There may be one or more small orifices. A thick median ridge separating two lateral hymenal orifices may suggest a septate vagina. The hymenal diaphragm may be a thin membrane or may be a thickened and fibrous one, forming a firm partition. Occasionally, what initially appears to be an imperforate hymen is found to have one or more tiny openings and is called a *microperforate hymen.* Although most of these variants are of no clinical significance, hymenal anomalies require surgical correction if they block the escape of vaginal secretions or menstrual fluid, interfere with intercourse, or prevent an indicated vaginoscopy and treatment of a vaginal disorder.

An *imperforate hymen* occurs when the hymen forms a solid membrane without an aperture. It is assumed that an imperforate hymen represents a persistent portion of the urogenital membrane and occurs when the mesoderm of the primitive streak abnormally invades the urogenital portion of the cloacal membrane. Demonstration of vaginal patency should be part of the examination of the genitalia of the newborn, and therefore imperforate hymen should be diagnosed at birth. When the vagina is obstructed, accumulation of vaginal secretions may distend the vagina, a condition called *mucocolpos* or *hydrocolpos.* When this condition occurs, the thin hymenal membrane is stretched out and forms a bulging, shiny, thin protuberance. Unless a mucocolpos is diagnosed and the fluid drained, the distended vagina forms a large mass that may interfere with urination and, at times, be mistaken for an abdominal tumor. If the diagnosis of an imperforate hymen is not established during childhood, the condition is suspected when an adolescent girl presents with primary amenorrhea and recurrent lower abdominal pain. Menstrual flow fills the vagina *(hematocolpos)* and then the uterus *(hematometra)* and may spill through the tubes into the peritoneal cavity. Inspection of the vulva generally reveals a dome-shaped, purplish-red hymenal membrane bulging outward in response to the collection of blood above it. On rectal examination, the distended vagina is palpable as a large cystic mass.

To relieve the obstruction, the central portion of the membrane is excised to provide a large aperture. Sutures are usually not necessary. In postmenarcheal girls, follow-up evaluation of the vagina and pelvis should be deferred for 4 to 6 weeks to reduce the risk of introducing infection. Endometriosis and vaginal adenosis are known, but not inevitable, complications in such patients.

Anomalies of the Vagina

Failure of Vertical Fusion

Transverse vaginal septa are the result of faulty canalization of the embryonic vagina. These septa may be without an opening (complete or obstructive), or they may have a small central aperture (incomplete or nonobstructive). They are usually found in the mid vagina but may occur at any level. When the septum is located in the upper vagina, it is more likely to be patent *(incomplete);* if the septum is located in the lower part of the vagina, it is often *complete.*

An incomplete septum is usually asymptomatic, and therefore correction during childhood or early adolescence is not required. The central aperture allows for vaginal secretions and menstrual flow to egress from the vagina. However, a complete septum results in signs and symptoms similar to those of an imperforate hymen. Unfortunately, the diagnosis of a transverse vaginal septum is often delayed until after menarche, when menstrual blood is trapped behind an obstructing membrane. If the diagnosis of a complete septum is established prior to menarche, it should be incised, creating an aperture to allow discharge. Incision of a complete septum should be done only when the upper vagina is distended and the membrane is bulging. The distention confirms the presence of an upper vaginal segment, facilitates the procedure, and reduces the risk of injury to adjacent structures.

Failure of Longitudinal Fusion

Duplication of the vagina is an extremely rare condition that is often associated with duplication of the vulva, bladder, and uterus. Each part of the vagina is encircled with a separate muscular layer. A more common anomaly is the vagina divided by a longitudinal septum, with both parts encircled by the same muscular layer. These longitudinal septa occur when the distal ends of the müllerian ducts fail to fuse properly. If there are no symptoms, longitudinal septa warrant no treatment. Division of the septum is indicated when dyspareunia is present, when obstruction of drainage from one half of the vagina is noted, or when the physician suspects that a septum would interfere with a vaginal delivery.

Vaginal Agenesis

Individuals with the Rokitansky sequence are genetic females. They develop normally in adolescence and have all of the usual feminine attributes; because the müllerian ducts fail to form, however, the uterus and vagina do not develop. However, the external genitalia are normal. A ruffled ridge of tissue represents the hymen, inside which there is an indentation marking the spot where the introitus would normally be found.

In many patients, other developmental defects are present as well, affecting the urinary tract (45 to 50 per cent), the spine (10 per cent), and, less frequently, the middle ear and other mesodermal structures. Therefore, at some time during childhood, in any child with vaginal agenesis, there should be an evaluation of the urinary tract, the spine, and hearing. In addition, a chromosome analysis should be obtained to rule out the rare instances in which vaginal agenesis represents the effects of testicular activity. An exploratory laparotomy is not indicated in these patients, and the absence of the uterus can be confirmed by a pelvic sonogram.

Treatment

Creation of a satisfactory vagina is the objective in treatment of vaginal agenesis, and this should be deferred until the girl is contemplating an active sexual life. Several techniques have been utilized. A nonoperative creation of a vagina using graduated vaginal dilators has been described. The technique is relatively risk-free but motivation and patient cooperation are required. The area that the vagina should occupy is a potential space filled with comparatively loose connective tissue that is capable of considerable indentation. The patient is given a series of dilators of graduated sizes and lengths and is taught to place them against the vaginal dimple and to apply constant pressure. This maneuver is repeated daily for 20 to 30 minutes with wider and longer dilators. The procedure takes a few months to complete, and persistence and patience are necessary.

If the procedure fails, the vaginal space can be developed surgically, between the urethra and the bladder anteriorly and the perineal body and the rectum posteriorly. This cavity is then lined by a split-thickness skin graft overlying a plastic or soft silicone mold. An alternative procedure is the Williams vulvovaginoplasty, which utilizes the labia majora to construct a coital pouch.

Partial Vaginal Agenesis

Vaginal agenesis may be limited to only a segment of the vagina. The lower vagina is not canalized and is replaced by a soft mass of tissue. Absence of the distal vagina is identified when only the upper vagina, cervix, and uterus are seen on pelvic sonogram. If the uterus has developed normally, the upper part of the vagina will fill with blood when menstruation begins. The symptoms are similar to those associated with a transverse vaginal septum. Whereas vulvar inspection reveals findings identical with those of vaginal agenesis, the rectoabdominal palpation reveals a large, boggy pelvic mass. Sonographic evaluation confirms the diagnosis. In these patients, the obstruction to menstrual flow must be removed. In some, drainage of the uterus can be achieved through a reconstructed vagina. In others, particularly when the uterus is rudimentary, consideration may be given to hysterectomy.

INFECTIONS AND SKIN DISORDERS OF THE GENITALIA

Vulvovaginitis

Vulvovaginitis is the most common gynecologic disorder in children. The young child is susceptible to infections for the following reasons:

1. Lack of estrogen.
2. Contamination by stool and other debris.
3. Impaired immune mechanisms of the vagina.

In young children, perineal hygiene is often less than adequate and contamination by stool and other debris is common. The vaginal mucosa is thin and atrophic because of the lack of estrogen and is less resistant to infections.

Vulvovaginitis can be divided into three major etiologic groups:

1. *Nonspecific vulvovaginitis.* Polymicrobial infection associated with disturbed local homeostasis (e.g., poor perineal hygiene, foreign body).
2. *Secondary inoculation.* Vaginal infection resulting from inoculation of the vagina with pathogens affecting other areas of the body by transfer through contact or by blood-borne transfer (e.g., urinary tract infections).
3. *Specific infections.* Specific primary vaginal infection, most commonly sexually transmitted (e.g., gonorrhea).

The symptoms of vulvovaginitis vary from minor discomfort to relatively intense perineal pruritus, a sensation of burning accompanied by a foul-smelling discharge. Vaginal discharge may vary from minimal to copious. The irritating discharge inflames the vulva and often causes the child to scratch the area to the point of bleeding. Acute vulvovaginitis may denude the thin vulvar or vaginal mucosa, but bleeding is usually minimal; as a rule, the mucopurulent or purulent discharge is little more than blood-stained. Inspection of the vagina reveals an area of redness and soreness that may be minimal or that may extend laterally to the thighs and posteriorly to the anus. Evaluation of the vaginal secretions should include:

1. Smears for Gram stain
2. Bacterial cultures
3. Cultures for mycotic organisms
4. Wet mount for
   a. Mycotic organisms
   b. White and red blood cells
   c. Vaginal epithelium (estrogen effect)
   d. Trichomonads
   e. Parasitic ova

Nonspecific Vulvovaginitis

The child complains of vaginal discharge and vulvar itch. The discharge can be scant or copious. It is observed by the parent on the child's underclothing and may be yellow-white, green, or tan in color. The odor is a source of great concern to the older child and always to the parent. Vulvar skin changes, such as excoriation due to scratching, erythema, edema, and maceration, and denudation of epithelium may be seen. The wet mount will show a mixture of white blood cells, bacteria, and other debris. Vaginal cultures may assist the clinician in identifying an offending organism.

Improvement of perineal hygiene is important to relieve the symptoms and to prevent recurrences. The child is instructed to sit in the tub, open her thighs, and wash the vulvar area with warm water and soap. There is no need to put soap in the vagina. Following the bath, the child is told to pat dry the vulvar area. On occasion, the mother may wish to apply a small quantity of baby powder to the vulva to ensure that the area is kept dry. Loosely fitting white cotton undergarments are worn. Bubble baths and detergent washing of underpants should be avoided.

Antimicrobial therapy would be expected to contribute to clinical improvement. Amoxicillin (20 to 40 mg/kg/day in three divided doses) is effective against a variety of potentially pathogenic organisms in nonspecific vulvovaginitis.

When the infection is severe and extensive mucosal damage is seen, a short course of topical estrogen cream is given to promote healing of vulval and vaginal tissues. When irritation is intense, hydrocortisone cream may be necessary to alleviate the itch.

In children in whom an infection is documented for the first time, vaginoscopy can be delayed. Vaginoscopy is necessary to exclude a foreign body or tumor in girls with recurrent vaginal infections if the infection is refractory to treatment or when a foul-smelling, bloody discharge is present.

Foreign bodies in the vagina induce an intense inflammatory reaction and result in a blood-stained, foul-smelling discharge. Usually the child does not recall inserting the foreign object or will not admit to it. The most commonly found foreign bodies are rolled pieces of toilet paper, which appear as amorphous conglomerates of grayish material. They are usually found on the posterior vaginal wall. Because many foreign bodies are not radiopaque, radiographs are of little value. Vaginoscopy is essential, not only to discover and remove objects situated in the vagina but also to exclude other causes of the bleeding. Although a foreign body that is situated in the lower third of the vagina can be washed out with warm saline, vaginoscopy is still indicated to confirm that no other foreign bodies are present in the upper vagina.

Specific Infections

Sexually transmitted diseases (STDs) should be treated according to the Centers for Disease Control (CDC) guidelines. The specific therapy to be used depends on the organism and the prevalence of resistant organisms within a given community. Some states require that all STDs in children be reported to the child protective services agency.

Gonococcal Infections. Whereas gonococcal infection causes cervicitis, endometritis, and salpingitis in an adolescent, the predominant presentation in the prepubertal child is vaginal discharge, vaginitis, and secondary vulvitis. Erythema, inflammation, and signs of scratching are commonly noted. The hymen, anus, and vagina should be examined for evidence of penetrating injury. Vaginal cultures are extremely helpful to obtain objective laboratory data if allegations of sexual abuse are present. *Chlamydia* culture can also be done, as this pathogen can accompany gonococcal infection. Rectal and pharyngeal cultures are helpful for documenting coexistent infection.

A saline wet mount is used to examine for other vaginal pathogens (trichomonads, clue cells).

Because of the increasing prevalence of penicillinase-producing *Neisseria gonorrhoeae* (PPNG) in the community, alternative therapies are now recommended in documented infection. The CDC currently recommends treatment of gonorrhea in adolescents and adults with ceftriaxone in areas hyperendemic for PPNG (single-dose ceftriaxone, 125 mg IM for children weighing <45 kg and 250 mg IM for children >45 kg). In adolescents and adults, it is recommended to continue therapy with doxycycline (100 mg twice daily for 14 days). Follow-up culture is required at the completion of therapy to identify patients with persistent infections.

Chlamydial Infections. Chlamydial vulvovaginitis in children causes a green, yellow, or brown discharge and signs of secondary vulvitis. Vaginal specimens for *Chlamydia* should be obtained for culture. In adolescent and adult women, chlamydial antigen testing is commonly employed to avoid the expense and time delay associated with culture. In prepubertal children, however, the endocervical columnar cells cannot be sampled and cultures are recommended to accurately determine the presence of the organism.

Erythromycin is the safest and most effective agent for *Chlamydia* in children—50 mg/kg/day orally in four doses for 10 days is the usual dose for children weighing less than 45 kg. Doxycyline (100 mg orally twice daily for 10 days) can be used in children weighing more than 45 kg and in adolescents. Treatment efficacy should be evaluated with a subsequent culture.

Trichomonas vaginalis. *Trichomonas vaginalis* is a motile protozoan that is a very common cause of vulvovaginitis in adolescent and adult women. Trichomoniasis is relatively rare in childhood. Patients present with vaginal discharge and vulvar pruritus. The discharge can range from scant to profuse and is usually malodorous. The color can be yellow, green, or gray. Vulvar inflammation is common. The diagnosis is confirmed by microscopic examination of the wet mount when motile, flagellated organisms are seen.

Treatment consists of local vulvar care and antibiotic therapy. Metronidazole (Flagyl) is currently recommended. The pharmacokinetics of metronidazole in children are similar to those in adults. Based on these data, the currently recommended dose is 15 mg/kg/day in three doses for 7 days.

Candidiasis. Candidal vulvovaginitis is common in adolescents and adults. The patient with candidal vulvovaginitis complains of severe vulvar pruritus and dysuria. There may be a small amount of white or yellow curd-like discharge. Examination reveals diffuse erythema and hyperemia of the vulva. Inflammation may extend inferiorally to the perianal region or laterally toward the inner thighs. Excoriation and desquamated areas are seen. White plaques or satellite candida lesions may be identified. The dermatologic appearance can sometimes be confused with lichen sclerosus. The diagnosis is made by examination of the fungal hyphae and buds with the saline or potassium hydroxide wet mount. Culture specimens can be analyzed if the diagnosis is in doubt.

Treatment of candidal vulvovaginitis in children is limited by the difficulty in administering intravaginal topical therapy. Options include topical vulvar therapy with an anticandidal cream (miconazole, buconazole, clotrimazole) with a corticosteroid preparation. Intravaginal tablets (clotrimazole) can be used in adolescents. Oral nystatin for recurrent infections has been helpful in some cases but has not been well studied in children.

Genital Herpes. Single or multiple vesicles occurring anywhere on the genitalia may rupture spontaneously to form shallow, painful ulcers. The incubation period of primary infections is 2 to 7 days. The diagnosis is usually confirmed by obtaining viral cultures. Tingling or itching may be present a day or two before the vesicles appear. Urinary symptoms often develop, including dysuria or even urinary retention, which may require continuous bladder drainage. Patients who have mild episodes respond to treatment with analgesics, sitz baths, local hygiene, and treatment of secondary infection. Local anesthetics may be useful in patients with severe dysuria. Recurrent infections are usually milder, with a duration of 4 to 5 days. Adult patients are advised to avoid transmission by abstinence from intercourse until crusts disappear and skin has healed.

In primary infections, oral acyclovir (200 mg five times daily for 10 to 14 days) decreases viral shedding, healing time, and number of new lesions. Treatment of recurrent episodes is less effective. For severe disease, acyclovir is recommended (5 mg/kg IV every 8 hours for 5 to 7 days) until clinical resolution occurs. Continuous daily suppressive therapy with acyclovir (200 mg two to three times a day) reduces the frequency of recurrences by at least 75 per cent. Safety and efficacy have been clearly documented with treatment up to 3 years.

Condyloma Acuminatum. This is the most common STD of viral origin, with increasing incidence among adolescents. The human papilloma virus (HPV), types 16, 18, and 31, is strongly associated with the development of genital dysplasia and carcinoma. The disease is highly infectious, presenting clinically as single or multiple soft, fleshy, papillary or sessile, often painless growths. The incubation period is 6 weeks to 8 months.

The lesions respond to treatment with cryotherapy with liquid nitrogen or cryoprobe. Podophyllin (10 to 25 per cent) in compound tincture of benzoin is applied weekly to small areas and thoroughly washed off in 1 to 4 hours. Normal skin should be protected with petroleum jelly. Trichloroacetic acid (80 to 90 per cent) may be applied to the warts with repeated applications at weekly intervals. Extensive lesions may require electrodesiccation, cryotherapy, laser therapy, or surgical excision under anesthesia.

Diaper Rash

Acute diaper rash may be treated with wet compresses of water, saline, or Burow's solution. The dermatitis usually responds to a 1 per cent hydrocortisone cream or lotion. Nystatin powder is applied to the skin when dry to treat monilial infection.

Lichen Sclerosus

Vulvar pruritus may be caused by any of several vulvar or perineal dermatologic disorders. These conditions are often not limited to the vulva but, rather, affect other body areas as well. Lichen sclerosus of the vulva is a hypotrophic dystrophy. Although it mainly affects women in the postmenopausal age group, it is occasionally seen affecting young children. The symptoms consist of vulvar irritation, dysuria, and pruritus.

Examination of the vulva shows flat, ivory-colored papules that may coalesce into plaques and, in extreme cases, may involve the entire vulvar skin. The lesion does not extend laterally beyond the middle of the labia major nor does it encroach into the vagina. The clitoris, posterior fourchette, and anorectal area are frequently affected. Affected areas are predominantly white, but some have pronounced vascular markings. The lesions tend to bruise easily, forming bloody blisters that are susceptible to secondary infections. Histologically, the skin shows flattening of the rete pegs, hyalinization of the subdermal tissues, and keratinization. In children, hypoplastic lichen sclerosus has no known malignant potential.

Treatment consists of improved local hygiene, reduction of trauma, and the short-term use of hydrocortisone creams to alleviate the pruritus. Treatment may be repeated when exacerbations occur.

Marked improvement in symptoms and appearance of the skin lesions following puberty is described. Review of the literature suggests that up to 50 per cent of affected children improve significantly or recover during puberty.

Labial Adhesions

The presence of labial adhesions in prepubertal children is believed to be a relatively common finding. It occurs most frequently in girls age 2 to 6 years. Labial adhesions are usually asymptomatic and thus unreported in many youngsters. The cause is not known but is probably related to the low levels of estrogen in the prepubertal child. It is suggested that the thin skin covering the labia may be denuded as a result of local irritation and scratching. The labia then adhere in the midline, stick to each other, and, as re-epithelialization occurs on both sides, remain fused in the midline. A recent study showed that labial adhesions were more prevalent in prepubertal girls who were sexually abused.

Most children with small degrees of labial adhesion are asymptomatic. When symptoms do occur, they usually relate to interference with urination or to the accumulation of urine behind the obstructing membrane. Dysuria and recurrent vulvar or vaginal infections are the cardinal symptoms. On rare occasions when complete occlusion is present, urinary retention may occur.

If the patient is asymptomatic, no treatment is needed for a minimal to moderate degree of labial fusion. When the degree of fusion is significant or the child is symptomatic, a short course of treatment with estrogen (Premarin) cream (applied twice daily for 7 to 10 days) may separate the labia. When such medical treatment fails or if severe urinary symptoms exist, surgical division of the fused labia is indicated.

Recurrence of labial adhesions is common because the estrogen-deficient state exists until puberty. Following puberty, the condition resolves spontaneously. Improved perineal hygiene and removal of irritants from the vulva may prevent recurrences.

URETHRAL PROLAPSE

The urethral mucosa is an estrogen-dependent tissue. During childhood, it is thin and atrophic. Occasionally, the urethral mucosa prolapses through the urethral meatus. Because of venous obstruction, the prolapsed tissue becomes swollen and occasionally undergoes necrosis. It forms a hemorrhagic, very sensitive vulvar mass that bleeds quite easily. The urethral orifice can be identified in the center of the mass, which is separated from the vagina.

When the lesion is small and urination is unimpaired, a short course of therapy using estrogen cream (small amount applied twice daily for 5 to 7 days) is beneficial. The use of broad-spectrum antibiotic therapy has been employed by some investigators. Resection of the prolapsed tissue should be considered if urinary retention is present, the lesion is large and necrotic, or the child is examined under anesthesia.

GENITAL TRAUMA

Most injuries to the genitalia during childhood are accidental, but some are the result of child abuse. The physician must determine how the child sustained the injury because abused children must be removed from an unsafe environment. Many genital injuries are of minor significance, but a few are life-threatening and require major surgical procedures. With severe trauma or very young children, it may be necessary to perform the examination using general anesthesia.

Because the perineum and vulva are extremely vascular and the subcutaneous tissues are loosely arranged, an injury may cause blood vessels underneath the perineal skin to rupture. Blood accumulates under the skin and forms a hematoma, producing a rounded, tense, and tender swelling, the size of which depends on the amount of bleeding. A contusion of the vulva does not typically require treatment. A small vulvar hematoma can usually be controlled by pressure with an ice pack. A large hematoma, or one that continues to increase in size, should be incised, the clotted blood removed, and bleeding points ligated. If the source of the bleeding cannot be found, the cavity should be packed with gauze and a pressure dressing applied. The pack is removed in 24 hours. Prophylactic broad-spectrum antibiotics may be advisable. The vulva should be kept clean and dry. When the urethra is obstructed by the hematoma, it is necessary to insert a suprapubic catheter. Pelvic radiographs may be necessary in some patients to rule out a fracture of the pelvis.

Most vaginal injuries occur when an object penetrates the vagina through the hymenal opening. Such penetration results in a laceration or a tear of the hymenal ring. There is usually very little bleeding from a hymenal injury, but bleeding indicates vaginal penetration and thus the possibility of additional vaginal injuries. Therefore, a detailed examination is necessary to exclude injuries to the upper vagina. When a vaginal laceration extends to the vaginal vault, a laparotomy is indicated to exclude extension of the tear into the broad ligament or the peritoneal cavity. Bladder and bowel integrity must also be confirmed. Vaginal wounds involve the lateral walls. Generally, there will be relatively little blood loss and the child will not have much pain if the damage is only mucosal. The child will complain of intense pain when a lacerated blood vessel retracts underneath the vaginal mucosa and forms a hematoma. If the torn vessel is small, bleeding may stop spontaneously. Larger vessels may form large, tense hematomas that may distend the vagina. Evacuation and ligation of the bleeding vessel is necessary.

NEOPLASMS OF THE VULVA AND VAGINA

Although uncommon, genital tumors must be considered whenever a girl is found to have a chronic genital ulcer, a nontraumatic swelling of the external genitalia, tissue protruding from the vagina, foul-smelling bloody discharge, abdominal pain or enlargement, virilization, or premature sexual maturation. Despite their rarity, virtually every type of genital neoplasm reported in adults has also been found in girls under 14 years and about half of these have been malignant.

Benign Tumors

Most benign tumors of the vagina in children are unilocular cystic remnants of the mesonephric duct. Other benign neoplasms include teratomas, hemangiomas, simple cysts of the hymen, retention cysts of the paraurethral ducts, benign granulomas of the perineum, and condylomata acuminata. Small cysts of the mesonephric (Gartner's) duct do not require surgery when asymptomatic. Large cysts may interfere with urination or vaginal drainage and must be treated surgically. The cyst is opened, most of the accessible cyst wall is removed, and the edges are marsupialized to prevent reaccumulation of fluid. Obstruction of a paraurethral duct may form a relatively large cyst, distorting the urethral orifice. Marsupialization or excision is the recommended treatment.

Teratomas usually present as cystic masses arising from the midline of the perineum. Although a teratoma in this area may be benign, local recurrence may be a problem. Therefore, a generous margin of healthy tissue should be excised about the teratoma's periphery.

Capillary hemangiomas usually disappear as the child grows older, and no therapy is needed. In contrast, *cavernous hemangiomas* are composed of vessels of considerable size and injury to them may cause serious hemorrhage. For this reason, cavernous hemangiomas are best treated surgically.

Invasive Tumors

Embryonal carcinoma of the vagina *(botryoid sarcoma)* is seen most commonly in the very young age group (younger than 3 years old). In a younger child, the tumor is often situated in the lower vagina; in an older child, the tumor more often affects the upper vagina or the cervix. The tumors arise in the submucosal tissues and spread rapidly beneath an intact vaginal epithelium. The vaginal mucosa then bulges into a series of polypoid growths that may protrude through the vaginal orifice. The diagnosis is confirmed by histologic examination of a biopsy specimen.

Combination chemotherapy regimen (often vincristine, actinomycin D, and cyclophosphamide) has been employed in recent years with success. Following the course of chemotherapy, the tumor is re-examined and resubmitted for biopsy. If the tumor is resectable, radical hysterectomy and vaginectomy are performed but the ovaries are preserved. Exenteration is not recommended. If the tumor is still unresectable following chemotherapy, radiotherapy is employed to further assist in shrinking and controlling tumor growth.

Vaginal adenosis is the presence of glandular epithelium resembling that of the endocervix and associated with transverse cervical and vaginal ridges. Such changes are encountered in about two thirds of females exposed in utero to maternally administered diethylstilbestrol (DES) and related synthetic compounds. It is estimated that the risk of *clear cell carcinoma* in these individuals is 0.14 to 1.4 in 1000. Clear cell carcinoma has not been described in prepubertal girls or in those younger than 14 years of age. Thus, the American College of Obstetrics and Gynecology recommends that a thorough gynecologic evaluation, including colposcopy, be performed on all DES-exposed females at menarche or by age 14, whichever comes first. Vaginal adenosis is often asymptomatic, necessitating no therapy.

Treatment of clear cell adenocarcinoma involves radical surgical excision, as the lesion is invasive. Early staging to determine the extent of spread helps in selecting the appropriate procedure. Vaginectomy, hysterectomy, extensive lymph node dissection, adjunctive chemotherapy, and radiation therapy may all be indicated.

UTERUS, FALLOPIAN TUBES, AND OVARIES

MARGARET POLANECZKY, M.D.

Many common gynecologic disorders can be evaluated and treated completely by the pediatrician. Whenever possible, a thorough pelvic examination should precede the institution of any therapy. If performed in a sensitive manner by an experienced clinician, the examination need not be a traumatic experience for the patient. In the patient deemed unsuitable for speculum examination, a careful bimanual and rectal examination, supplemented by ultrasonography if necessary, can often provide enough information to allow further evaluation and treatment to proceed.

COMMON MENSTRUAL DISORDERS

The average age of menarche in the United States is 12.8 years, with a range of 9 to 16 years. Menarche usually occurs within 2 to 2.5 years after breast budding and 1 year after the growth spurt. Up to 50 per cent of young women do not ovulate during their first few menstrual cycles. As a result, menses in the young adolescent may be irregular and are often prolonged or heavy.

Normally, young women should begin to have regular, ovulatory cycles by 1 to 2 years after menarche. Normal cycle length ranges from 21 to 45 days, with menstrual flow lasting 2 to 7 days. The average blood loss during a normal menstrual period is 30 to 40 ml, or up to four well-soaked pads or tampons per day. On the first and second days, flow may be slightly heavier.

Primary Amenorrhea

Primary amenorrhea is defined as any one of the following: (1) the absence of menarche by age 16 years in the otherwise normal pubertal female; (2) the absence of menarche by age 14 years in the young woman who lacks breast and pubic hair development; or (3) the failure of menarche to appear within 2 years of completed sexual maturation.

The diagnostic evaluation of primary amenorrhea is summarized in Figure 1. The work-up begins with a complete history and physical examination, after which the patient may be classified into one of four diagnostic groups based on the presence or absence of breast development and internal female genitalia. Follicle-stimulating hormone (FSH) levels, testosterone levels, and/or karyotype are then performed selectively to arrive at a final diagnosis. Treatment is best undertaken in conjunction with an endocrinologist or adolescent gynecologist. Although prognosis will vary according to diagnosis, treatment should be designed to achieve, whenever possible, the following goals:

1. Successful gender identification.
2. Normal height and breast development.
3. Normal sexual function.
4. Cyclic menstrual bleeding.
5. Preservation of reproductive function.
6. Protection from bone and cardiovascular consequences of estrogen deficiency.
7. Prevention of future malignancy.

Hypogonadotropic Hypogonadism

These individuals have primary amenorrhea accompanied by sexual immaturity; pelvic examination reveals the presence of a normal vagina and uterus. FSH levels are low, indicating that the primary defect lies in either the pituitary or the

TABLE 1. Suggested Estrogen Replacement Regimens

- Conjugated estrogens (Premarin) 0.625–1.25 mg on days 1–25
  plus
  Medroxyprogesterone acetate (Provera) 5–10 mg on days 14–25
  or
- 17β-estradiol (Estrace) 1–2 mg on days 1–25
  plus
  Medroxyprogesterone acetate (Provera) 5–10 mg on days 14–25
  or
- Oral contraceptive (30–35 μg estrogen with nonandrogenic progestin)

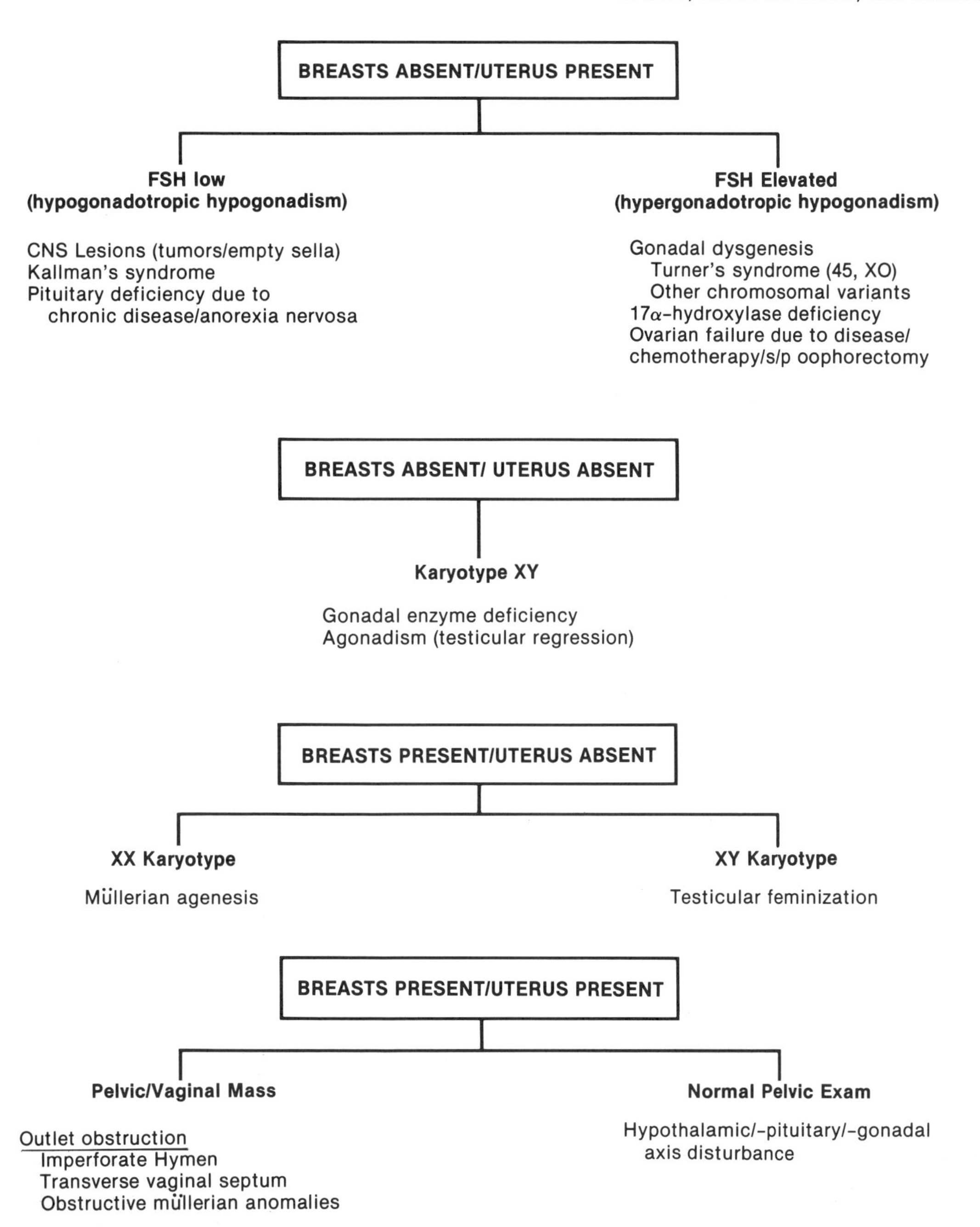

Figure 1. Diagnostic approach to patients with primary amenorrhea. FSH, follicle-stimulating hormone; CNS, central nervous system. (Adapted from Maschak CA, et al: Clinical and laboratory evaluation of patients with primary amenorrhea. Obstet Gynecol 57:719, 1981. Reprinted with permission from the American College of Obstetricians and Gynecologists.)

hypothalamus. Careful central nervous system (CNS) evaluation should be performed to rule out the presence of a craniopharyngioma or other CNS lesion.

A typical individual in this category is the young woman who has permanent deficits of pituitary hormones as a result of irradiation or surgery for a brain tumor. Others include those with the empty sella syndrome and Kallman syndrome. In addition, individuals with severe early-onset anorexia nervosa or certain chronic diseases, such as thalassemia major, often experience hypogonadotropic primary amenorrhea as a result of hypothalamic-pituitary dysfunction.

All of these patients require estrogen replacement therapy to induce sexual maturation, prevent bone loss, and allow for normal menstrual function and vaginal lubrication. In patients with pituitary insufficiency, therapy may also include growth hormone, thyroid hormone, and adrenal replacement.

Estrogen replacement typically begins with low-dose conjugated estrogens (Premarin, 0.3 to 0.625 mg daily on days 1 to 25), with medroxyprogesterone acetate (Provera, 5 to 10 mg added on days 14 to 25). An alternative regimen for the younger adolescent is to begin with estrogen alone, in order to induce breast development, adding cyclic progestin once menses ensue. In either case, it is usually necessary to increase the estrogen dose to 1.25 mg over 1 to 2 years in order to complete breast development.

Suggested long-term estrogen replacement regimens are summarized in Table 1. Because recent evidence suggests that the duration of progestin is more important than the dose in preventing the development of uterine malignancy due to unopposed estrogen, 12 days of progestin therapy is now recommended rather than the traditional 10 days of therapy. Micronized 17β-estradiol (Estrace), in doses of 1 to 2 mg, is an alternative to conjugated estrogens. Another long-term treatment option is to use an oral contraceptive. This is often easier for the patient than taking two different medications. Because oral contraceptive therapy will be continued indefinitely, pills containing high doses of the more atherogenic progestin, levonorgestrel, should be avoided. Oral contraceptive therapy should not be used until breast development is complete because there has been some concern that their use before then may lead to tubular breast formation.

It is important to remember that the ovaries and internal genitalia of these patients, although unstimulated, are otherwise normal. The patient and her parents should be advised that future pregnancy is possible. This is usually accomplished by combining estrogen replacement with induction of ovulation using human menopausal gonadotropins (hMG).

Hypergonadotropic Hypogonadism

Patients with hypergonadotropic hypogonadism present with sexual immaturity and amenorrhea; pelvic examination reveals the presence of a vagina and uterus. FSH levels are elevated, revealing the primary defect to be in the ovary. Karyotype should be performed, which most commonly will reveal the diagnosis to be gonadal dysgenesis due to Turner syndrome (XO karyotype). Less common are other X chromosomal variants. Even rarer are primary defects in ovarian steroid production due to 17α-hydroxylase deficiency or ovarian failure secondary to ataxia-telangiectasia, galactosemia, or myotonic dystrophy.

If karyotype reveals the presence of any portion of a Y chromosome, surgical removal of the gonadal streak must be performed to avoid malignant degeneration. Gonadectomy is usually performed before puberty because the gonad is nonfunctional.

Lifelong hormonal replacement, in the form of cyclic estrogen and progesterone, should be initiated in early adolescence. In patients with gonadal dysgenesis in whom short stature is of concern, lower doses of estrogen are used initially to avoid premature epiphyseal closure. One suggested plan for patients with Turner syndrome is to begin with prepubertal daily low-dose estrogen, such as 0.3 mg conjugated estrogens or 5 μg of ethinyl estradiol. (A short course of anabolic steroids is often added at this point to stimulate bone growth. The use of growth hormone is currently under investigation as an alternative adjunct to increase final height in these patients.) The estrogen dose can be doubled every 6 to 12 months. Once menses ensue, cyclic progestin is added because the prolonged use of estrogen alone carries a risk of endometrial cancer as a result of unopposed stimulation of endometrial growth. When final height is achieved, estrogen treatment regimens are the same as those discussed earlier (Table 1).

The patient and her parents should be advised that, because of recent advances in reproductive technology, future childbearing may be possible using oocyte donation.

Testicular Regression and Testicular Enzyme Deficiencies

Individuals with this rare form of hypergonadotropic hypogonadism are genetic males who lack testosterone because of a gonadal enzyme deficiency or early gonadal regression ("vanishing testes"). They appear female and present with sexual immaturity and primary amenorrhea; however, pelvic examination reveals a blind vaginal pouch and absent uterus. FSH levels are elevated, and XY karyotype confirms the diagnosis.

Treatment includes surgical removal of the intra-abdominal gonad and estrogen replacement therapy as outlined previously. Obviously, one needs to be judicious in counseling these patients in order to avoid gender confusion. Classic practice has been to tell the patient that her reproductive organs never developed and to avoid discussion of genetic sex. However, this may not be appropriate for all patients, and discussion must therefore be tailored to the individual.

Testicular Feminization (Androgen Insensitivity)

Individuals with this disorder are chromosomal males who have normal internal male gonads but lack normal androgen receptor function. As a result, despite circulating male levels of testosterone, the wolffian ducts fail to develop and the external genitalia develop as female. Because of normal gonadal production of müllerian-inhibiting factor (MIF), the müllerian system regresses during development, leaving only fibrous remnants of internal genitalia.

At puberty, a normal growth spurt occurs and breasts develop as a result of low levels of estrogens, which are produced directly by the gonad and made peripherally from androgen conversion. Because puberty appears to be progressing normally, these individuals do not usually present until late in adolescence, when the expected menses never arrive. Physical examination at that time reveals a young woman of normal height with absent or sparse axillary and pubic hair and an absent or shortened vagina. Confirmatory laboratory studies include XY karyotype and male testosterone levels.

Consultation with a gynecologist should be made at this point to plan for gonadectomy and long-term estrogen replacement. The male gonads, which may be either intra-abdominal or inguinal, carry a 20 per cent risk of malignant degeneration and should be removed. Classic teaching has been that gonadectomy be deferred until after full height and breast development have occurred. However, a number of patients have now been described with incomplete forms of testicular feminization who become virilized during puberty. For this reason, gonadectomy is now recommended at the time of diagnosis, regardless of the pubertal status of the patient. Once the gonads have been removed, long-term estrogen replacement should begin. Typical treatment regimens are 0.625 to 1.25 mg conjugated estrogens or 1 to 2 mg 17β-estradiol daily. Because no uterus is present, cyclic progestin need not be added. Patients should be counseled that future pregnancy will not be possible. The decision to discuss genetic sex is best made on an individual basis and is usually deferred until after adolescence.

Müllerian Agenesis (Rokitansky-Kuster-Hauser Syndrome)

This is a fairly common disorder, found in 15 per cent of patients presenting with primary amenorrhea. Affected individuals are genetic females who have normal functioning ovaries but lack a vagina and uterus as a result of anomalous development of the müllerian system. They classically present either in late adolescence with primary amenorrhea or in early adulthood after unsuccessfully attempting intercourse. On examination, these young women are of normal height and exhibit normal breast and axillary hair development. Although the external genitalia are normal, the vagina either is absent or forms a short blind pouch. Karyotype confirms a normal XX chromosomal complement and excludes rare forms of incomplete androgen insensitivity or pseudohermaphroditism.

Once the diagnosis is made, intravenous pyelography should be performed because of the 15 to 40 per cent incidence of associated renal abnormalities in this disorder.

Cardiac and skeletal examination detects associated disorders in as many as 12 per cent of patients.

Careful counseling is key to helping these young women maintain self-esteem and a healthy body image. Rather than telling them they were "born without a vagina," they should be told that their vagina is "not completely developed." A gynecologic specialist should be consulted early in the course of the evaluation to plan for the creation of a functioning vagina once the patient has achieved full growth and is psychologically prepared. The classic operation has been the *McIndoe split-thickness graft*. However, the *Williams procedure*, which combines a very simple surgical procedure with postoperative dilators, is now the usual first-line surgical approach. The nonsurgical *Frank procedure* involves the use of progressively larger surgical dilators to create a functioning vagina. A racing bicycle seat with attached dilators works well for many patients. The long-term success of either method depends on patient involvement in learning how to maintain the created vagina.

Because these patients have normal functioning ovaries, hormonal replacement is not necessary. Although individuals with müllerian agenesis cannot carry a pregnancy or give birth, they should be counseled that genetic offspring may be possible through ovum retrieval, in vitro fertilization, and embryo transfer to the uterus of a volunteer surrogate.

Outlet Obstruction

This category includes young women with imperforate hymen, transverse vaginal septum, or other genital tract anomalies that lead to obstruction of menstrual effluent. These patients often present with a history of normal Tanner development, amenorrhea, and cyclic pelvic pain. Pelvic examination and/or ultrasonography reveal a pelvic mass, usually a distended vagina or hematocolpos.

Treatment of a transverse vaginal septum or imperforate hymen involves simple surgical excision of the obstructing membrane. If the obstruction occurs as a result of cervical agenesis or other anomalies, such as bicornuate uterus with a blind horn, repair is more complicated. The surgery should be performed by a gynecologist or surgeon with expertise in the repair of congenital genital anomalies.

The coexistence of renal and müllerian anomalies should prompt a thorough evaluation of the urinary tract in patients with obstruction due to anomalous genital tract development. Future pregnancy rates vary, depending on the nature of the obstruction and repair, ranging from 25 to 100 per cent.

Abnormalities of the Hypothalamic-Pituitary Axis

When pubertal development and pelvic anatomy are normal yet menses has not occurred, there is usually a disturbance in the hypothalamic-pituitary axis. Possible causes include systemic disease, pituitary adenomas, constitutional delay, exercise-induced amenorrhea, and anorexia nervosa. The management of these patients is identical to that of patients with secondary amenorrhea.

Secondary Amenorrhea and Oligomenorrhea

Secondary amenorrhea is defined as the absence of menstruation for at least three cycles or at least 6 months in females who have already experienced regular menstruation. Oligomenorrhea is defined as four or fewer menses per year. Although menses are often irregular in young adolescents, they should stabilize within 1 to 2 years from the time of menarche. Amenorrhea or oligomenorrhea occurring more than 2 years after menarche should be considered abnormal and warrants investigation and treatment. Oligomenorrhea or amenorrhea accompanied by galactorrhea or hirsutism should be investigated regardless of how much time has passed since menarche.

The diagnostic evaluation of secondary amenorrhea is summarized in Figure 2. After one excludes pregnancy, a thyroid-stimulating hormone (TSH) and prolactin level should be obtained to rule out thyroid disease and pituitary adenoma. Androgen levels are also indicated if the patient is hirsute. If the initial TSH level is elevated, the patient should be referred for thyroid replacement therapy. Normal menses should resume once the patient becomes euthyroid. Hirsute patients with elevated dehydroepiandrosterone sulfate (DHEAS) or testosterone levels need further evaluation to rule out ovarian or adrenal tumors, congenital adrenal hyperplasia, and Cushing syndrome. Consultation with a pediatric endocrinologist or gynecologist is recommended at this point.

If TSH and prolactin levels are normal, a progestational challenge is performed to evaluate estrogen status. One frequently used regimen for this test is medroxyprogesterone acetate (Provera, 5 to 10 mg for 10 days). This regimen results in a withdrawal bleeding in the patient with an estrogen-primed uterus, establishing the diagnosis of anovulation, usually due to *polycystic ovary (PCO) syndrome* (also PCOS). Absence of a withdrawal bleed mandates determining an FSH level to distinguish patients with hypothalamic dysfunction from those with ovarian failure. If withdrawal bleeding does not occur and there is a history of previous uterine curettage, a combined estrogen-progestin regimen should be given (conjugated estrogens, 2.5 mg daily for 25 days, with medroxyprogesterone acetate, 5 to 10 mg, on days 14 to 25). Failure to bleed after this is indicative of Asherman syndrome, and the patient should be referred to a gynecologist for further evaluation and therapy.

Pregnancy

The young woman who presents with amenorrhea must be considered pregnant until proven otherwise. It is best to have a low threshold of suspicion for ordering pregnancy testing because the menstrual history may be unreliable in the adolescent patient. The possibility of an ectopic gestation should be considered in any pregnant patient who gives a history of spotting or pelvic pain, however minimal, or if examination of the pregnant patient reveals a normal-sized uterus, adnexal mass, or adnexal tenderness. If an ectopic pregnancy is suspected, immediate referral to a gynecologist or emergency room can be life-saving.

If pregnancy is diagnosed, sensitive, nondirective counseling should take place immediately and appropriate referrals made. The teenager should be encouraged, when possible, to inform her parents. For many reasons, teenagers frequently delay obtaining prenatal care or do not obtain care at all; those who desire pregnancy termination often delay until it is too late. Judicious and persistent follow-up is important in ensuring that the teenager actually keeps her referral appointments.

Polycystic Ovarian Syndrome

The most common cause of anovulation in the postmenarchal adolescent is PCO syndrome. This disorder is characterized by oligomenorrhea, hirsutism, infertility, and, often, obesity. When spontaneous menses do occur in PCO syndrome, they are often prolonged or heavy (dysfunctional uterine bleeding [DUB]).

PCO syndrome occurs as a result of inappropriate signals along the hypothalamic-pituitary-ovarian axis. This is reflected in the high luteinizing hormone (LH)-to-FSH ratio often found in these patients. Elevated LH levels lead to increased ovarian androgen production with resultant hirsutism. Per-

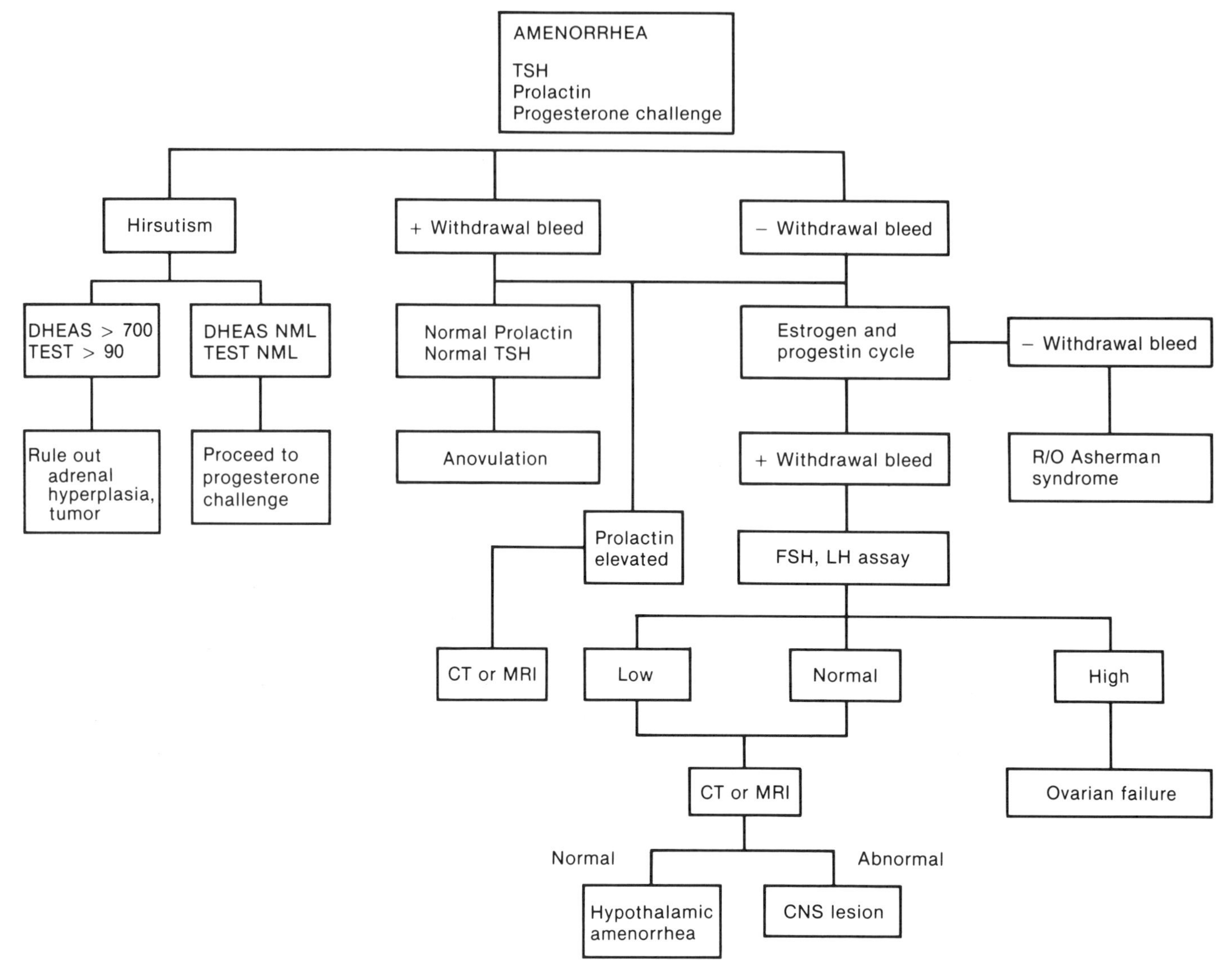

Figure 2. Evaluation of secondary amenorrhea. TSH, thyroid-stimulating hormone; DHEAS, dehydroepiandrosterone sulfate; FSH, follicle-stimulating hormone; LH, luteinizing hormone; R/O, rule out; CT, computed tomography; MRI, magnetic resonance imaging; CNS, central nervous system; NML, normal. (Modified from Speroff L, et al: Clinical Gynecologic Endocrinology and Infertility, 4th ed. Baltimore, Williams & Wilkins, 1989, p 178.)

sistent anovulation results in prolonged periods of unopposed estrogen stimulation of the uterine endometrium, leading to breakthrough bleeding, prolonged and heavy menses, and long-term risk for endometrial hyperplasia and malignancy.

Treatment of PCO syndrome with oral contraceptives attempts to interrupt this cycle. Oral contraceptives work by suppressing pituitary FSH and LH production, essentially placing the ovary into quiescence, thus decreasing ovarian estrogen and androgen production. In addition, the progestin in the contraceptive counteracts the effects of prolonged endogenous estrogen on the uterine endometrium and, over time, will result in lighter, shorter, more regular menses. A low-dose (30 to 35 μg) pill is preferred. In patients with DUB, a 50-μg pill such as Ovral or Demulen 1/50, which also contains a strong progestin, will be initially useful in controlling the bleeding. Once menses are lighter and regular, a less androgenic low-dose pill can be used for long-term therapy. Hirsute patients with PCO syndrome may benefit from long-term therapy with a nonandrogenic pill such as Ovcon 35. These patients may also be optimal candidates for use of the new triphasic gestodene- and norgestimate-containing oral contraceptives, which are expected to be approved by the Food and Drug Administration (FDA) by 1993. These two new compounds are highly potent progestins with little or no androgenic activity.

Teenagers with PCO syndrome who are not sexually active or who prefer not to take an oral contraceptive can be treated with cyclic progestin to induce menses and protect against the long-term risk of endometrial hyperplasia. This can be done one of two ways. For the first 10 days of each month, 10 mg of medroxyprogesterone acetate can be administered to induce regular menses. Alternatively, 10 days of medroxyprogesterone acetate can be administered every 3 months in the absence of spontaneous menses. This latter regimen has the advantage of allowing for the return of normal menses, which will occur in 60 to 70 per cent of patients who present in early adolescence with amenorrhea due to immaturity of the hypothalamic-pituitary-ovarian axis.

Although patients with PCOS may experience infertility, the overall prognosis for a future successful pregnancy is good. A small but significant percentage will conceive spontaneously. Approximately 75 per cent of remaining patients will ovulate after treatment with clomiphene citrate (Clomid).

Hyperprolactinemia

It is estimated that 5 to 10 per cent of patients with both amenorrhea and elevated serum prolactin and 25 per cent of those with amenorrhea, galactorrhea, and high prolactin levels have pituitary adenomas. Therefore, all patients with elevated prolactin should undergo CNS imaging of the pituitary either by computed tomography (CT) scan or magnetic resonance imaging (MRI). Prolactinomas are classified as either microadenomas (<1 cm) or macroadenomas (>1 cm). Less than 5 per cent of microadenomas progress to macroadenomas. Other causes of hyperprolactinemia include medications, stress, breast stimulation, hypothyroidism, and renal failure. Psychotropic medications, in particular, are a common cause of drug-induced hyperprolactinemia and galactorrhea.

Hyperprolactinemia from any cause results in hypoestrogenemia, and these patients are at real risk for osteoporosis if not treated. Treatment has several goals: normalization of prolactin levels, return of normal estrogen levels, resumption of normal menses, and preservation of fertility.

Primary treatment of pituitary adenomas used to be surgical—namely, transsphenoidal resection. Rates of response were as high as 80 per cent. However, "cure" rates were only 10 to 40 per cent because tumor regrowth and recurrence of hyperprolactinemia were common. As a result, medical therapy with bromocriptine (Parlodel) is generally recommended for all microadenomas. Recent evidence suggests that bromocriptine therapy alone is probably appropriate for most macroadenomas and should be attempted for at least 6 months prior to consideration of surgical resection.

Bromocriptine is a dopamine agonist that inhibits prolactin release by the pituitary, resulting in the shrinkage of pituitary lactotrophs. Approximately 80 to 90 per cent of patients with microadenomas respond to bromocriptine therapy. Side effects of this therapy include nausea, headache, and orthostatic hypotension. Therefore, therapy is begun with low doses (1.25 mg), which are taken only at bedtime. If this is tolerated, the dose is gradually increased over several weeks until appropriate reduction in prolactin levels occurs. Final therapeutic doses range from 2.5 to 15 mg daily, usually taken in two divided doses. Prolactin levels should be measured frequently, and the patient should be maintained on the lowest dose that will produce normal prolactin levels. Menses usually resume in 6 to 8 weeks; suppression of galactorrhea may not occur for several months. Some patients require estrogen replacement therapy along with bromocriptine in order for menses to occur. It should be remembered that once prolactin levels normalize, ovulation will usually return and contraception will be necessary. The decision whether and when to stop therapy is individualized and controversial; tumor regrowth will occur in the majority of cases.

There is a subgroup of patients with hyperprolactinemia and amenorrhea who have no visible tumor on CT scan or MRI. These young women with functional hyperprolactinemia are still at risk for osteoporosis secondary to hypoestrogenemia. Treatment is either bromocriptine, as detailed previously, or estrogen replacement therapy if bromocriptine is not used. Most of these patients respond to very low doses of bromocriptine, such as 1.25 mg daily. If the patient elects not to take any medication, close observation with periodic bone mass measurements and calcium supplementation is indicated.

Prognosis for future pregnancy in patients with hyperprolactinemia is good. Bromocriptine therapy usually results in ovulation. The decision to continue bromocriptine therapy during pregnancy depends on the size of the adenoma, visual field measurements, and the presence or absence of associated symptoms such as headache.

Ovarian Failure (Hypergonadotropic Amenorrhea)

A typical patient in this category is the young woman who has had her ovaries removed as a result of malignancy or who has experienced ovarian failure secondary to cancer chemotherapy or radiation therapy for Hodgkin's disease. In the absence of such a history, patients with premature ovarian failure should have a karyotype, since premature ovarian failure in adolescence may be due to variants of gonadal dysgenesis or Turner's mosaicism. If any portion of a Y chromosome is present, gonadectomy should be performed. Patients with normal chromosomes should be referred for further evaluation to rule out autoimmune and multiple endocrine disorders.

Treatment consists of lifelong estrogen replacement. A typical regimen is 0.625 to 1.25 mg conjugated estrogens on days 1 to 25 with 5 to 10 mg medroxyprogesterone acetate added on days 12 to 25. Note that 12 days a month of progestin therapy is now being recommended rather than the traditional 10 days as a result of recent evidence that longer duration of progestin offers better protection against endometrial cancer. An oral contraceptive is an alternative estrogen replacement regimen and, for many teenagers, is simpler to take. Periodic bone density measurements taken during the first several years of therapy ensures the adequacy of estrogen replacement.

Because pregnancy may occur in as many as 10 per cent of patients with premature ovarian failure, contraception is advised for those not taking an oral contraceptive. Prognosis for future fertility is poor; it is probably highest for patients who elect to undergo oocyte donation with embryo transfer to their intact uterus. Rare pregnancies have been reported after high-dose estrogen in combination with exogenous gonadotropins has been given to patients with ovarian failure and intact ovaries.

Exercise-Induced Amenorrhea

As many as 50 per cent of teens involved in competitive athletics experience hypothalamic amenorrhea. Ballet dancers also commonly experience this form of amenorrhea. Although the etiology of this disorder is not well understood, it may result from a complex interplay of low body fat percentage and psychologic stress. Elevated prolactin levels are often found in these individuals and may contribute as well. Whatever the cause, young women with this disorder are estrogen-deficient and should therefore be treated.

The simplest way to treat exercise-induced amenorrhea is to decrease the amount of exercise. If amenorrhea persists or if the patient is unwilling to curtail her training, estrogen replacement therapy should be begun because these women are hypoestrogenic and at risk for osteoporosis. Compliance with estrogen replacement therapy can be a problem in the serious athlete, and fractures in such individuals have been reported. Periodic bone density measurements documenting bone loss may help to persuade such individuals to comply with treatment. All patients with exercise-induced amenorrhea should be encouraged to increase their calcium intake, either by diet or by supplements, to 1500 mg daily. However, one must emphasize to the patient that unless estrogen therapy is added, the use of calcium alone probably does nothing to help maintain bone mass.

Anorexia Nervosa

Anorexia nervosa is a potentially life-threatening disorder characterized by abnormal eating habits, severe weight loss, and distorted body image. Although the exact nature of the hypothalamic amenorrhea that occurs in most patients with anorexia nervosa is unclear, these patients are almost always estrogen-deficient.

The complex medical and psychologic problems associated with anorexia nervosa mandate a team approach to management of patients with this disorder, employing psychiatric counseling, close medical supervision, nutritional consultation, and estrogen replacement therapy. Estrogen replacement can be given as conjugated estrogens (0.625 to 1.25 mg on days 1 to 25, with the addition of 10 mg medroxyprogesterone acetate on days 12 to 25). Alternatively, an oral contraceptive can be used. Menses will usually return spontaneously once normal weight is achieved. Chronic estrogen replacement, calcium supplementation, and periodic bone density measurements are indicated for the young woman whose anorexia persists for more than a year.

Dysmenorrhea

Dysmenorrhea, or painful menstruation, is the most common gynecologic problem in the adolescent female and the leading cause of school absenteeism in this population. *Primary dysmenorrhea* is defined as painful menses with no identifiable pelvic pathology. *Secondary dysmenorrhea* refers to painful menses resulting from a pelvic abnormality such as endometriosis or pelvic inflammatory disease (PID). A careful pelvic examination, including rectovaginal examination, should be performed in the adolescent presenting with dysmenorrhea to exclude pelvic pathology prior to initiating therapy for primary dysmenorrhea. Failure of treatment for presumed primary dysmenorrhea warrants repeated evaluation for pelvic pathology and referral to a gynecologist.

Most dysmenorrhea during adolescence is primary. Because it occurs almost exclusively in ovulatory cycles, it typically begins several months after menarche and may worsen gradually as ovulatory cycles become established. Although the etiology of dysmenorrhea is not completely understood, almost all of the symptoms of primary dysmenorrhea can be explained by the action of uterine prostaglandins. For this reason, therapy of primary dysmenorrhea aims to decrease prostaglandin production by the endometrium.

Prostaglandin synthetase inhibitors (PGIs) are the first-line treatment for mild dysmenorrhea in the adolescent who is not sexually active. These medications work by blocking the production of prostaglandins within the endometrium. A wide range of PGIs are available, although not all classes are suitable for treatment of dysmenorrhea. Most patients experience significant relief with the fenamate and propionic acid derivatives without untoward side effects. Some of the more commonly used regimens are outlined in Table 2. Because of side effects, indomethacin, phenylbutazone, and oxyphenylbutazone should be avoided. Aspirin has been shown to be no more effective than placebo in relieving dysmenorrhea.

Treatment with a PGI should be initiated at the onset of the menstrual flow and continued for the duration of symptoms. Because most of the newer PGIs have a rapid onset of action, there is no need to begin treatment before the onset of menses. If there is no response, the initial dose can be increased. Switching to a different class of PGI may also be effective. If this fails, the oral contraceptive should be considered.

The oral contraceptive is effective in more than 90 per cent of patients with primary dysmenorrhea and is the treatment of choice for the sexually active teenager. It acts by preventing ovarian stimulation of endometrial prostaglandins and by decreasing the total amount of endometrium available for prostaglandin production. Any low-dose (30 to 35 μg) pill can be used. Because the reduction in prostaglandin production is cumulative over time, the maximal effect of the oral contraceptive may not be seen for several months. If symptoms persist after several months, a PGI can be added. Failure of medical treatment at this point warrants referral to a gynecologist for further evaluation and possible laparoscopy. Consideration should also be given to the possibility that psychologic factors may be involved in the etiology of the patient's pain.

TABLE 2. Prostaglandin Synthetase Inhibitors Effective in the Treatment of Primary Dysmenorrhea

Drug	Dose
Fenamates	
Meclofenamate sodium (Meclomen)	100 mg t.i.d.
Mefanamic acid (Ponstel)	500 mg initially, then 250 mg t.i.d.
Propionic Acid Derivatives	
Ibuprofen (Advil, Motrin)	400 mg q.i.d.
Naproxyn sodium (Anaprox DS)	550 mg t.i.d.
Naproxyn (Naprosyn)	500 mg initially, then 250 mg q.i.d.
Ketoprofen (Orudis)	25–50 mg q.i.d.

Abbreviations: t.i.d., three times a day; q.i.d., four times a day.

Transcutaneous electrical nerve stimulation (TENS) is currently undergoing investigation as a treatment for dysmenorrhea. TENS most likely works as a pure analgesic without directly affecting the activity or production of endometrial prostaglandins. Although still experimental, TENS has few reported side effects, and may be an alternative therapy for those patients with dysmenorrhea who for some reason are unable or unwilling to take oral contraceptives or PGIs.

Dysfunctional Uterine Bleeding

DUB is defined as abnormal endometrial bleeding occurring in the absence of structural pelvic pathology. In the adolescent, DUB is usually the result of anovulation secondary to immaturity of the hypothalamic-pituitary-ovarian axis. Prolonged periods of anovulation lead to an overestrogenized endometrium lacking the progesterone-induced stability and control of sloughing that normally occurs with ovulatory menses. The clinical presentation is that of prolonged periods of amenorrhea interspersed with prolonged heavy menses. Over time, bleeding may begin to occur every 1 to 2 weeks and can be life-threatening.

DUB is a diagnosis of exclusion. Therefore, all patients presenting with abnormal vaginal bleeding should have a careful history and thorough pelvic examination (including a Papanicolaou [Pap] smear, wet mount and cultures for *N. gonorrhoeae* and *Chlamydia*) to rule out pelvic pathology, such as trauma, genital tract malignancy, vaginitis, cervicitis, and PID. Pregnancy should always be considered in the differential diagnosis of abnormal vaginal bleeding. Bleeding disorders (e.g., von Willebrand's disease and idiopathic thrombocytopenic purpura) should be ruled out when DUB presents at menarche or is associated with significant hemorrhage or anemia.

The management of the patient with DUB depends on the severity of the bleeding and the level of anemia and is summarized in Table 3.

Mild DUB

DUB presenting without acute hemorrhage or anemia may be managed with observation and reassurance only. However,

TABLE 3. Management of Dysfunctional Uterine Bleeding

Mild DUB: inconvenient, unpredictable bleeding/Hb > 12 g/dl
- Reassurance
- Fe supplementation
- Consider oral contraceptive
- Reevaluate every 3–6 months

Moderate DUB: irregular, prolonged, heavy bleeding/Hb > 10 g/dl
- Hormonal therapy:
  - Provera (10 mg daily for 5–7 days every 35–40 days)
  - *or*
  - Oral contraceptives
- Fe supplementation
- Menstrual calendar
- Reevaluate in 1–2 months

Severe DUB: irregular, heavy prolonged bleeding/Hb < 10 g/dl
- Not actively bleeding
  - Oral contraceptive
  - Fe supplementation
  - Reevaluate in 1–3 months
- Active mild to moderate bleeding
  - Ovral, 1 tablet every 6 hr for 24–48 hr, tapered over the following week to 1 tablet daily
  - Fe supplementation
  - Reevaluate in 1 week, then in 1–3 months
- Active heavy bleeding
  - Hospitalize
  - Transfuse if necessary
  - Hormonal therapy:
    - Ovral, 1 tablet every 6 hr for 24–48 hr, tapered over the week to 1 tablet daily *or* Premarin (20–25 mg IV every 4 hr) for maximum 6 doses with concurrent Ovral (1 tablet every 6 hr, tapered over the following week to 1 tablet daily)
    - *followed by*
    - Oral contraceptive for 6 to 12 months (consider continuous regimen, i.e., without placebos, until Hb normalizes)
    - D & C if hormonal therapy fails
    - Re-evaluate 1–2 weeks and 1 month after discharge, then in 1–3 months until menstrual pattern and Hb stable

Adapted from Muram D. Vaginal bleeding in childhood and adolescence. *In* Menstrual Cycle Disorders. Obstet Gynecol Clin North Am 17:405, 1990.

Abbreviations: DUB, dysfunctional uterine bleeding; Hb, hemoglobin; Fe, iron; D & C, dilatation and curettage.

most adolescents and their parents would prefer some form of treatment given the inconvenience and anxiety accompanying unpredictable menses. These patients can be offered the regimen described next for patients with DUB.

Moderate DUB

This category includes patients presenting with mild anemia (hemoglobin [Hgb] >12 g/dl) but no acute bleeding. If the patient is sexually active, an oral contraceptive is the treatment of choice and should be prescribed in the routine fashion. A pill with high progestational activity (e.g., Nordette, Demulen 1/35, or Lo/Ovral) should be used initially to attain a stable decidualized endometrium. Once lighter flow is established, any low-dose pill can be used.

An alternative to oral contraceptive therapy is the use of cyclic progestin in the teenager who is not sexually active. Medroxyprogesterone acetate (10 mg) is given for 5 to 7 days every 35 to 40 days in the absence of spontaneous menses. This regimen allows for the recognition of the return of ovulatory menses. However, progestin alone may not halt DUB if it has been prolonged; estrogen is often needed as well to restore endometrial tissue where severe desquamation has occurred. An oral contraceptive therefore provides the best treatment in such situations. Iron therapy should be added to either regimen, and the patient should be reevaluated frequently.

Severe DUB

Patients who present with Hgb levels lower than 10 g/dl but who are not actively bleeding should be placed on an oral contraceptive and given iron supplementation. Because prolonged bleeding may result in little residual endometrial tissue on which progestin may exert its organizational effect, a high-estrogen–high-progestin oral contraceptive (e.g., Ovral, Demulen 1/50) should be used. The patient should be reevaluated frequently to ensure the efficacy of treatment.

Patients presenting with mild to moderate bleeding and anemia can usually be managed as outpatients with intensive oral contraceptive therapy. A high-estrogen–high-progestin oral contraceptive can be given (one tablet every 6 hours for 24 to 48 hours). Bleeding should diminish or stop within 12 to 24 hours on this regimen. The patient should be warned that this regimen may cause nausea, and appropriate antiemetics should be prescribed when necessary. Over the next week, the dose can be gradually tapered to one tablet daily for the next several months, followed by a low-dose (30 to 35 μg) pill for another 3 to 6 months. At this point, if the patient does not require contraception, the oral contraceptive can be discontinued and bleeding reassessed.

Patients presenting with life-threatening bleeding or severe anemia require hospitalization, possible transfusion, and high-dose estrogen therapy. Premarin (20 to 25 mg) can be given intravenously every 4 hours for a maximum of six doses. Because the endometrium resulting from such therapy is inherently fragile, concurrent high-dose progestin must be given. This can be in the form of a high-progestin oral contraceptive (e.g., Ovral, one tablet every 6 hours for 24 to 48 hours), which is then tapered gradually to once a day dosage. Alternatively, medroxyprogesterone acetate (10 mg every 12 hours) can be used initially and replaced with an oral contraceptive in 24 to 48 hours, which is then tapered gradually to once a day. Bleeding that does not respond to intravenous estrogen requires immediate dilatation and curettage (D & C).

The first menses following hormonal therapy for DUB is usually heavy and may worsen a pre-existing anemia. In the patient with a low hemoglobin level whose bleeding has stopped, the oral contraceptive can be given in a continuous fashion (i.e., without placebos) to prevent withdrawal bleeding. Once the hemoglobin level is increased, the patient can be allowed to cycle regularly on the oral contraceptive.

DUB persists for up to 2 years in 60 per cent of patients, 4 years in 50 per cent, and 10 years in 30 per cent. Most patients with a prolonged history of DUB have PCO syndrome and should be maintained on either cyclic progestin or an oral contraceptive.

GONORRHEA, CHLAMYDIAL INFECTION, AND PELVIC INFLAMMATORY DISEASE

Gonorrhea and chlamydial infections are occurring in epidemic proportions in adolescents, most likely as a result of increasing sexual activity in this population. The serious sequelae of these infections, if untreated, include PID, infertility, Fitz-Hugh–Curtis syndrome, ectopic pregnancy, and pelvic adhesions.

Gonorrhea

The majority of reported cases of infection with *Neisseria gonorrhoeae* occur in adolescent females. Overall, 3 to 7 per cent of teenage females attending family planning clinics test positive for gonorrhea; the rate among indigent black teenagers has been reported to be as high as 10 per cent.

Symptoms suggestive of gonorrheal infection include vaginal discharge, dysuria, and vaginal burning or irritation. However, the majority of gonorrheal infections in the adolescent female are asymptomatic, and therefore screening for gonorrhea is recommended on a twice-yearly basis for all sexually active teenagers. Suggestive physical findings include mucopurulent cervical discharge, cervical friability, and inflammation of the endocervical glands. Specimens should be taken from both the endocervix and the rectum because rectal culture increases the yield of detection by 5 per cent. Pharyngeal cultures probably do not add significantly to the detection rate but should be performed if the history or physical examination is suggestive.

Treatment for uncomplicated gonorrheal infection should be given to any adolescent female with a positive screening culture. Patients with a history or physical findings suggestive of gonorrheal infection, or who report sexual contact with an individual with suspected urethritis, should be cultured *and* treated at the same visit. Patients who present with PID should be cultured and hospitalized for intravenous antibiotic therapy.

Table 4 summarizes the current Centers for Disease Control (CDC) recommendations for the treatment of uncomplicated gonorrheal infection. These recommendations have undergone major changes in the past decade as a result of the emergence of antibiotic-resistant organisms. Most large urban centers now report endemic levels of penicillinase-producing *N. gonorrhoeae* (PPNG), tetracycline-resistant *N. gonorrhoeae* (TRNG), and organisms with chromosomally mediated resistance to multiple antibiotics (CMRNG). For this reason, the CDC now recommends ceftriaxone as first-line therapy for uncomplicated gonorrheal cervicitis. This regimen has the added advantage of being effective against incubating syphilis. Spectinomycin is a second-line treatment reserved for allergic patients, except where spectinomycin-resistant organisms are endemic. Penicillin may be used only in areas with low incidence of antibiotic resistance and, even then, only when the organism can be proven to be penicillin-sensitive. All cases of gonorrhea must be reported to the state for contact tracking and notification.

Depending on the geographic location, the incidence of concomitant infection with *Chlamydia* can be as high as 60 per cent. *For this reason, all patients undergoing treatment for gonorrhea must receive treatment for chlamydial infection as well, even when only gonorrhea is isolated.*

Ciprofloxin, a quinalone antibiotic, has recently been introduced in the United States as a single-agent therapy for combined gonorrhea and chlamydial infections. At present, this drug is contraindicated in patients under 17 years of age because of reported cases of drug-associated arthropathy.

All adolescent patients receiving treatment for gonorrhea should be screened for syphilis and counseled regarding human immunodeficiency virus (HIV) risks, HIV testing, and condom use. As a result of the association of hepatitis B infection with high-risk sexual activity, consideration should be given for screening and/or vaccination for hepatitis B in these adolescents as well. The patient should be told to notify her partner(s), who should also receive prompt treatment. She should be advised to refrain from sexual activity until both she and her partner have been treated and both have a proven negative test of cure. Although treatment failures with ceftriaxone are rare, reinfection is common. Repeat cultures performed 14 days to 1 month after treatment will detect both reinfection and treatment failures. The addition of a rectal culture at this time increases the detection rate by as much as 5 per cent.

Chlamydia

Chlamydia trachomatis is the most common sexually transmitted organisms in the United States. Among sexually active adolescent females, the incidence of chlamydial cervicitis ranges from 8 to 33 per cent and is highest among inner-city black and Hispanic teens attending family planning clinics. Risk factors for chlamydial infection other than young age and race include multiple sexual partners, history of gonorrhea, oral contraceptive use, and a history of a partner with urethritis. In addition, the finding of purulent cervical discharge associated with cervical friability—so-called "mucopurulent cervicitis"—is highly predictive of a positive culture for *C. trachomatis*. Most infections with *Chlamydia* in the female are asymptomatic, including *Chlamydia*-associated PID, which is notorious for being a "silent" infection.

All sexually active adolescent females should be screened for chlamydial cervicitis twice yearly, and treatment should be given to any teenager with a positive screening test. Rapid screening tests, utilizing immunofluorescence and DNA hybridization technology, are now widely available and provide a less expensive, faster alternative to culture. Care must be taken, however, to use proper technique in obtaining specimens for culture or screening; if endocervical cells are not present in the specimen, a false-negative result may be obtained. Therefore, if chlamydial cervicitis is highly suspected on the basis of either history or the presence of mucopurulent cervicitis, treatment should be given regardless of screening test results. Patients with diagnosed *Chlamydia* need not be treated for concomitant gonorrhea unless the culture for *N. gonorrhoeae* is positive. Any teenager who reports contact with a partner suspected or found to have either gonorrheal or chlamydial urethritis should be cultured and treated at the same visit for both *N. gonorrhoeae* and *Chlamydia*.

Current recommendations for treatment of *Chlamydia* are outlined in Table 4. Because of increased patient compliance, the doxycycline regimen is preferred in adolescents, despite its higher cost. Tetracycline derivatives are contraindicated in pregnancy; therefore, a negative pregnancy test may be obtained prior to initiating therapy for *Chlamydia* in the adolescent female if doing so does not delay treatment. If pregnancy is of concern, the erythromycin regimen can be used. A disadvantage of the erythromycin regimen is its associated gastrointestinal upset, particularly in the pregnant teenager. In this situation, a liquid preparation may be better tolerated. A single-dose, long-acting azolide antibiotic (Azithromycin) has been approved by the FDA for treatment of uncomplicated *Chlamydia* cervicitis. To date, it has not yet been studied in adolescents or approved by the CDC. The use of oral and intracervical clindamycin preparations for the treatment of chlamydial cervicitis is currently under investigation and may provide an alternative to erythromycin in the pregnant adolescent.

Because of the prolonged life cycle of *Chlamydia,* test of cure cultures may still be positive 3 to 6 weeks after treatment. This fact must be counterbalanced with the need for early follow-up in the adolescent to ensure compliance with the treatment regimen. A compromise plan might be to see the patient in follow-up in 2 weeks to ensure completion of therapy and again 1 month later for a test of cure. If history at the 2-week visit reveals suboptimal antibiotic ingestion, the patient can be re-treated. This visit is also a good time to reinforce contraceptive and condom use. The patient's partner should receive prompt evaluation and treatment for exposure to *Chlamydia.* The patient should be advised to refrain from intercourse until both she and her partner have had a negative test of cure.

About 15 per cent of patients with *Chlamydia* are infected

TABLE 4. Treatment of Gonorrhea and *Chlamydia* Infections

Uncomplicated Gonorrheal Infection

- Preferred regimen
  Ceftriaxone 250 mg IM
  plus
  Doxycycline 100 mg orally b.i.d. for 7 days
  (effective against incubating syphilis)
- Preferred alternative regimen
  Spectinomycin 2 g IM
  plus
  Doxycycline 100 mg orally b.i.d. for 7 days
- In areas with < 3% incidence resistant organisms *and* when penicillin sensitivity is proven:
  Amoxicillin 3.0 g orally
  or
  Ampicillin 3.5 g orally
  or
  Aqueous procaine penicillin G 4.8 million units IM
  (all of the above with probenecid 1 g orally)
  plus
  Doxycycline 100 g orally b.i.d. for 7 days
- In children weighing < 45 kg:
  Ceftriaxone 125 g IM once
  or
  Spectinomycin 40 mg/kg IM once

Uncomplicated Chlamydial Infection

- First-line therapy:
  Doxycycline 100 mg orally b.i.d. for 7 days
  or
  Tetracycline hydrochloride 500 mg q.i.d. for 7 days
- If tetracyclines contraindicated or not tolerated:
  Erythromycin base or stearate (500 mg orally q.i.d. for 7 days)
  Erythromycin ethylsuccinate (800 mg orally q.i.d. for 7 days)

only in the urethra and not the cervix. These patients may present with the so-called "acute urethral syndrome," defined as dysuria and urinary frequency accompanied by sterile pyuria. Because specimens of *Chlamydia* from the urethra are often of low yield, these patients should receive presumptive treatment for *Chlamydia,* using the same treatment regimens as for chlamydial cervicitis.

Pelvic Inflammatory Disease

PID refers to ascending infection of the uterus, fallopian tubes, and ovaries, most often as a consequence of gonorrheal or chlamydial cervicitis. It is one of the most serious gynecologic disorders of adolescence and, in 1980, was responsible for 45,000 hospital admissions in young women aged 15 to 19 years. Long-term sequelae of PID include infertility, ectopic pregnancy, pelvic adhesions, and chronic pelvic pain.

Risk factors for PID include multiple sexual partners, young age at first intercourse, prior history of *N. gonorrhoeae* or *Chlamydia,* and lack of any contraceptive use. The risk of acquiring PID for the sexually active 15-year-old female is estimated to be as high as 1 in 8.

The diagnosis of PID can sometimes be difficult and has been shown to be inaccurate as often as 35 per cent of the time. Use of the following diagnostic criteria, however, may increase the accuracy of the diagnosis in an emergency room setting to as high as 90 per cent:

1. Abdominal tenderness, with or without rebound, *plus*
2. Cervical motion tenderness, *plus*
3. Adnexal tenderness, *plus*
4. One or more of the following: fever of 38°C, leukocyte count of 10,000 or more, elevated erythrocyte sedimentation rate, purulent cervical discharge, or pelvic abscess on ultrasonographic or bimanual examination.
5. Negative pregnancy test.

Approximately 20 per cent of adolescents with acute PID have concomitant tubo-ovarian abscesses. Because as many as 70 per cent of these may be missed on initial examination by the pediatrician, *use of pelvic ultrasonography should be routine whenever an adolescent female is diagnosed with acute PID in the pediatric setting.*

Treatment of PID in the adolescent female mandates hospitalization for intravenous antibiotic therapy; there is no place for ambulatory treatment in this population, for a number of reasons. Teenagers typically present later in the course of infection than older patients with PID and thus tend to have more serious infection. In addition, adolescents have high rates of noncompliance with outpatient regimens as well as with timely follow-up. Finally, earlier, aggressive management may be associated with lower rates of serious sequelae, such as ectopic pregnancy and infertility.

Antibiotic therapy should include broad-spectrum coverage aimed at eradicating *N. gonorrhoeae* and *Chlamydia,* as well as gram-negative bacilli, aerobic streptococci, and anaerobes. Current CDC recommendations for the treatment of PID are given in Table 5. Clindamycin is only about 90 per cent effective against *Chlamydia.* Therefore, if chlamydial infection is strongly suspected, it is probably best to use the doxycycline-containing regimen. Intravenous antibiotic therapy should be continued for at least 4 days *and* until the patient has been afebrile for at least 48 hours. Failure of the patient to clinically improve within 24 to 48 hours of hospitalization mandates consultation with a gynecologist and consideration of laparoscopy in order to ensure definitive diagnosis and treatment.

The presence of right upper quadrant pain in the setting of acute PID suggests perihepatic involvement, the so-called Fitz-Hugh–Curtis syndrome. These patients are treated in a similar fashion to those with uncomplicated PID. However, failure of clinical improvement mandates right upper quadrant ultrasonographic examination to rule out the presence

TABLE 5. Recommended Antibiotic Regimens for Treatment of Pelvic Inflammatory Disease

- Cefoxitin (2.0 g IV every 6 hr) *or* Cefotetan (2.0 g IV every 12 hr)
  plus
  Doxycycline (100 mg IV or p.o. every 12 hr)

Continue treatment for a total of 4 days *and* until the patient is afebrile for at least 48 hr. The patient is then discharged on doxycycline (100 mg p.o. b.i.d.) to complete 10–14 days of therapy.

This regimen provides optimal coverage of both *Neisseria gonorrhoeae,* including penicillinase-producing *N. gonorrhoeae,* and *Chlamydia trachomatis.* It may not provide optimum anaerobic coverage for patients with tubo-ovarian abscess or IUD-associated PID.

or

- Clindamycin (900 mg IV every 8 hr)
  plus
  Gentamicin (2.0 mg/kg loading dose IV, then 1.5 mg/kg IV every 8 hr)

Continue treatment for a total of 4 days *and* until the patient is afebrile for at least 48 hr. The patient is then discharged on either clindamycin (450 mg p.o. q.i.d.) or doxycycline (100 mg p.o. b.i.d.) to complete 10–14 days of therapy.

This regimen provides excellent coverage of anaerobes and gram-negative organisms. Although it may theoretically be suboptimal for treatment of *C. trachomatis* and *N. gonorrhoeae,* a recent study has shown this regimen to be equivalent to the cefoxitin-doxycycline regimen in eradicating *N. gonorrhoeae* and *C. trachomatis.*

Abbreviations: p.o., by mouth; b.i.d., twice a day; IUD, intrauterine device; PID, pelvic inflammatory disease; q.i.d., four times a day.

of a perihepatic abscess. If significant right upper quadrant findings persist after resolution of PID, consideration should be given to other reasons for the pain, such as hepatitis or gallbladder disease.

While the patient is in the hospital, she should be well hydrated with intravenous fluids and given appropriate pain medication. Bed rest in the semi-Fowler position is recommended because it is the most comfortable for the patient with abdominal pain and because it will facilitate drainage of purulent material into the cul-de-sac. Screening for syphilis should be performed, and testing for human immunodeficiency virus (HIV) done with the patient's consent after appropriate pretest counseling. HIV testing is especially important because recent studies have suggested that the prevalence of HIV infection in patients presenting with PID is higher than in similar control populations. Screening and/or vaccination for hepatitis B is also appropriate in these patients. The time in the hospital should be utilized to educate the patient about sexually transmitted diseases and birth control. If the patient is not using birth control, she can be offered a prescription for an oral contraceptive at this time. Condom use should be reinforced. The patient's sexual partner(s) should be contacted and treated. When possible, parental involvement should be sought and encouraged, especially in the very young adolescent.

At discharge, the patient is given a prescription for oral doxycycline to complete 14 days of therapy. She can be seen for follow-up in 1 to 2 weeks, at which time pelvic examination and specimens for *N. gonorrhoeae* are obtained for culture. The addition of a rectal swab for gonorrhea will increase detection of resistant organisms. Test of cure for *Chlamydia* is performed at 1 month after discharge.

When pelvic abscess is suspected based on physical or ultrasonographic examination, the clindamycin-containing treatment regimen will provide broader anaerobic coverage. Alternatively, clindamycin or metronidazole can be added to the doxycycline-containing regimen if chlamydial coverage is of chief concern. The duration of antibiotic therapy in this situation is controversial. Intravenous antibiotic coverage should be continued, at minimum, for 5 to 7 days and until the patient has been afebrile for at least 48 to 72 hours, the white blood cell count has normalized, and the patient's abdominal examination is completely benign. At this time, follow-up and ultrasonographic examination should show the abscess to be either stable or decreased in size. If this has not occurred, a gynecologist should be consulted. If ultrasonographic examination shows the abscess to be resolving, the patient may be discharged on oral doxycycline to complete 14 days of therapy. Some clinicians will also continue oral anaerobic coverage, although this has not been well studied. The patient should be seen in an outpatient setting at 1 week, 4 weeks, and 8 weeks after discharge. Failure to note either complete or near-complete resolution of the pelvic abscess by ultrasonography at 6 to 8 weeks after discharge mandates referral to a gynecologist for appropriate surgical management. Occasionally, pelvic masses such as endometriomas or ovarian neoplasms may be misdiagnosed as tubo-ovarian abscesses in the setting of acute PID.

Brief mention should be made of the use of other antibiotic regimens for the treatment of PID. Recent studies have been done evaluating the effectiveness of some of the newer penicillins, multigeneration cephalosporins, and quinalones, either alone or in combination with other drugs, in the treatment of PID. Until further data are available on these regimens, it is recommended that the CDC guidelines be followed in treating the adolescent female with PID.

Gonorrhea and Chlamydial Infections in Children

Gonorrhea and chlamydial infections can occur in prepubertal females as a result of sexual abuse, although the prevalence is low. *Chlamydia* is seen more often than *N. gonorrhoeae* in these circumstances. Upper genital tract infection in children is rare, and most infections with *Chlamydia* and *N. gonorrhoeae* are confined to the vagina and/or extragenital sites. Vaginal, rectal, and pharyngeal specimens must be obtained for culture in all children in whom sexual abuse is suspected, since their history of assault may be incomplete. Treatment is given only if infection has been documented and is similar to that of adults with uncomplicated infection, although dosages may need to be adjusted for children weighing under 45 kg.

CERVICAL CYTOLOGY

Regular cervical Pap smears should be obtained in all females beginning at age 18 years or at the onset of sexual activity. From 10 to 14 per cent of sexually active teenagers have abnormal Pap smear findings on routine screening. The sexually active young adolescent, given her young age at first intercourse and likelihood of multiple partners over her lifetime, is at high risk for cervical cancer and should be advised to have at least yearly Pap smears for the rest of her life.

Human papilloma virus (HPV) disease, sometimes manifested as venereal warts, accounts for the majority of abnormal Pap smears in the adolescent population. HPV disease is occurring in epidemic proportions in young sexually active women; as many as 50 per cent of university students show evidence of HPV infection by DNA analysis of cervical and vulvar smears. Young women with external genital warts are 3.8 times more likely to develop cervical carcinoma in situ than young women without warts; they therefore constitute a particularly high risk subgroup of teenagers.

Pap smear classification was changed in 1988 in an attempt to make the diagnostic categories more meaningful in terms of malignancy risk and treatment. The numerical "class" system has been replaced by a system based on the presence of squamous intraepithelial lesions (SIL) of low malignant potential (HPV changes and mild dysplasia); high malignant potential (moderate dysplasia, severe dysplasia, and carcinoma in situ); or invasive carcinoma. The suggested management of these Pap smear categories is summarized in Table 6. Referral to a gynecologist for any abnormal Pap test is appropriate if the practitioner has any question regarding management.

Mention should be made about the management of those patients with grossly visible lesions on the cervix. These patients should be referred immediately to a gynecologist for colposcopy and cervical biopsy. It is not appropriate merely to perform a Pap smear and manage on the basis of the Pap smear alone.

PELVIC MASSES

Most abdominal-pelvic masses in the prepubertal female are ovarian in origin. Prior to 3 years of age, the most common cause of ovarian enlargement is a physiologic ovarian cyst. After 5 years of age, most ovarian masses in the prepubertal child are teratomas, and as many as 30 per cent of these may be malignant. Germ cell tumors, such as dysgerminomas, endodermal sinus tumors, embryonal carcinoma, and gonadoblastomas, also tend to present in childhood and adolescence. Therefore, pelvic masses in the pediatric age group are aggressively evaluated and treated by excision. Chemo-

TABLE 6. Management of Papanicolaou Smear Abnormalities As Reported Under the 1988 Bethesda System

Report	Recommended Action
Specimen adequacy	
Satisfactory	No further action.
Unsatisfactory or less than satisfactory	Repeat smear.
Descriptive diagnoses	
Inflammation	R/O vaginitis, cervicitis. Otherwise, follow Pap routinely.
Cervical cytology	
Within normal limits	No further action.
Atypical squamous cells of undetermined significance	Evaluate for vaginitis or cervicitis; treat if present and repeat smear in 4 to 6 weeks. If no evidence of vaginitis or cervicitis, refer to gynecologist for further evaluation.
Low-Grade Squamous Intraepithelial Lesion (SIL)	
Cellular changes associated with HPV	If no history or clinical evidence of condyloma, or prior history of abnormal Pap smear, repeat Pap smear in 3 months. If second Pap smear shows persistent HPV changes, refer to gynecologist for evaluation. If history of condyloma or visible condyloma present, refer to gynecologist for evaluation and/or treatment.
Mild dysplasia/CIN	Referral for colposcopy and biopsy.
High-Grade Squamous Intraepithelial Lesion (SIL)	
Moderate dysplasia, CIN 2	Referral to gynecologist for colposcopy and biopsy.
Severe dysplasia, CIN 3	
Carcinoma in situ, CIN 3	
Squamous cell carcinoma	

Abbreviations: R/O, rule out; HPV, human papilloma virus; CIN, cervical intraepithelial neoplasia.

therapy may also be given for certain tumors. When possible, attempt is made to preserve ovarian tissue and function.

After puberty, the most common pelvic mass is an enlarged pregnant uterus. The possibility of an ectopic pregnancy must always be considered as well, especially if there is pain or a prior history of PID. The association of pain, amenorrhea, and a pelvic mass suggests obstruction of menstrual effluent due to müllerian abnormalities.

Most ovarian masses in the adolescent age group are either follicular or hemorrhagic cysts. Ten to 20 per cent are benign cystadenomas. Less common are germ cell tumors, including dysgerminomas, embryonal cell tumors, endodermal sinus tumors, granulosa-theca cell tumors, and gonadoblastomas.

Ovarian enlargement can result in torsion of the adnexa. Ovarian torsion often presents with a history of intermittent pain associated with nausea and vomiting. The patient's pain, which can be severe, will often seem out of proportion to the findings on abdominal examination. Ovarian torsion is an emergency because compromise to the ovarian blood supply can lead to loss of the ovary as a result of gangrene. Rapid diagnosis and immediate surgery may allow for preservation of the involved adnexa.

In the adolescent patient, asymptomatic ovarian enlargement of less than 5 cm noted on routine examination can be followed clinically. If ovarian enlargement persists over two cycles, ultrasonography is indicated. If a sonogram shows the cyst to be clear and unilocular, the most likely diagnosis is a benign functional cyst. The traditional management of these patients has been to prescribe an oral contraceptive (35 or 50 μg pill) in order to suppress ovarian function and decrease cyst size. The patient is then reassessed either by pelvic or ultrasonographic examination after 4 to 6 weeks. If the cyst is decreasing in size, the patient can be maintained on the oral contraceptive and evaluated again in 4 to 6 weeks. At this point, most cysts will have resolved, and the patient can then be followed routinely. If the cyst is the same size or larger, the patient should be referred to a gynecologist for possible surgical management.

Recent data suggest that the rate of disappearance of functional ovarian cysts is not affected by therapy with oral contraceptives. In a controlled, randomized study, two groups of patients with unilocular ovarian cysts were treated with either oral contraceptives or expectant management. Both groups had similar rates of cyst resolution, and all cysts that had not resolved by 9 weeks were found at surgery to be pathologic.

If the initial sonogram shows the cyst to be complex in nature, the possibility of pregnancy or a tubo-ovarian abscess should be ruled out. If there is a history of dysmenorrhea or findings on examination suggestive of endometriosis, adnexal enlargement may be due to an endometrioma; referral for possible laparoscopy or excision should be made. Occasionally, ultrasonographic findings may suggest a dermoid cyst; MRI at this point can be diagnostic, and referral to a gynecologist is appropriate. The possibility of ovarian malignancy must always be considered in the differential diagnosis of a complex ovarian mass. However, most complex ovarian cysts in the adolescent age group are hemorrhagic corpus luteal cysts that usually resolve spontaneously. These patients can be managed expectantly with re-evaluation in 6 to 8 weeks, at which point the cyst should be either resolved or significantly decreased in size. Depending on the size of the cyst, vigorous exercise may be proscribed in the interval in order to minimize the risk of rupture or torsion. Mild analgesics can be given if necessary, although the presence of anything other than minimal discomfort warrants referral to rule out torsion or rupture. Persistence or enlargement of the cyst after 6 to 8 weeks warrants referral for surgical management.

If the sonogram shows the mass to be larger than 5 cm, a gynecologist should be consulted. Depending on the patient's symptoms and medical status and the radiographic appearance of the ovary, larger masses may occasionally be managed expectantly but should be done so only in consultation with a gynecologist. If the sonogram shows the ovary to contain a solid mass or to be suspicious of malignancy, immediate referral for surgical management should be made.

PREMENSTRUAL SYNDROME

Premenstrual syndrome (PMS) refers to a constellation of symptoms, such as bloating, mood swings, depression, headache, and cramps, which occur 7 to 14 days before the menses and usually resolve at some point after menstrual flow has begun. Studies have shown a consistently high prevalence of premenstrual symptomatology in adolescent females, ranging from 73 to 96 per cent of young women studied.

The cause of PMS is unknown, although numerous theories exist. Most presume that the symptoms are hormonally mediated; however, no consistent hormonal abnormalities have as yet been found in patients with PMS. A variety of medications have been used to treat PMS, including oral contraceptives, diuretics, vitamin supplements, and progesterone suppositories. No single treatment has withstood the test of a well-controlled, double-blind placebo trial, although in a given patient any one of these therapies may provide symptomatic relief.

For the adolescent patient with premenstrual symptoms, first-line therapy includes education, reassurance, a well-balanced diet, and restriction of salt, sugar, and caffeine. Regular aerobic exercise may increase well-being and alleviate mild depressive symptoms. If dysmenorrhea is significant, PGIs or the oral contraceptive can be used. Caution should be used in prescribing diuretics in the adolescent patient, particularly those with eating disorders. However, a trial of a mild diuretic (such as spironolactone, 25 mg daily during the week preceding the menses) may alleviate breast tenderness and bloating in some individuals. Progesterone suppositories should be reserved for severe cases and prescribed in consultation with a gynecologist. The use of gonadotropin-releasing hormone agonists is currently under study and holds promise for the older female with severe PMS; it is probably not a suitable therapy for the adolescent patient.

CHRONIC PELVIC PAIN

The management of chronic or recurrent pelvic pain in the adolescent depends on the history and nature of the pain and the extent of the prior diagnostic evaluation. Many times, a careful history reveals the pain to be cyclic in nature, suggesting the diagnosis of dysmenorrhea. A trial of PGIs or oral contraceptives may offer significant relief in addition to confirming the diagnosis. Pain that is cyclic and related to ovulation *(mittelschmerz)* may also respond to oral contraceptive therapy.

The evaluation of noncyclic pain includes a thorough pelvic examination with screening for pregnancy, urinary tract infection, sexually transmitted diseases, and occult blood. Associated gastrointestinal symptoms suggest pathology of the gastrointestinal tract; radiologic or endoscopic evaluation may be indicated. Thickening or nodularity of the uterosacral ligaments in association with dysmenorrhea suggests a diagnosis of endometriosis. A history of sexually transmitted disease, PID, or abdominal surgery suggests either subclinical PID or pain from pelvic adhesions. Psychologic factors may play a role in some adolescents with chronic pelvic pain and should be considered early in the diagnostic work-up. Recent studies have shown that an approach that combines psychologic evaluation with medical diagnostic evaluation and therapy has the most success in resolving chronic pelvic pain.

Laparoscopy should be reserved for those adolescents with abnormal findings on pelvic examination or whose diagnosis remains elusive despite persistent symptoms that compromise normal activity. Approximately 30 per cent of young women undergoing laparoscopy for chronic pelvic pain have normal findings at surgery. Of the remainder, PID and endometriosis are the most frequent pathologic diagnoses.

FLUID AND ELECTROLYTE THERAPY

AIDA YARED, M.D.
and IEKUNI ICHIKAWA, M.D.

In the pediatric age group, fluid and electrolyte requirements are relatively high and disorders common owing to several factors: (1) fluid losses are proportional to body surface area (BSA), which is larger per body weight (BWt) in children; (2) renal ability to concentrate urine and conserve sodium is limited in infants; (3) access of infants to fluids may be limited, as they cannot talk or walk; and (4) children are more likely to have anorexia or vomiting accompanying diarrhea and therefore may be more at risk of dehydration.

BACKGROUND PHYSIOLOGY

Body Fluid Compartments

In the average child, total body water (TBW) constitutes 60 per cent of BWt. There is less TBW in the obese child (little water is associated with fat), and more in the severely malnourished or young infant (as much as 80 per cent in the premature infant). Of this TBW, one third (20 per cent of BWt) is intracellular fluid (ICF), and two thirds (40 per cent of BWt) is extracellular fluid (ECF). ECF is further divided, one third being intravascular (~7 per cent of BWt), and two thirds being in between cells (interstitial, transcellular; 13 per cent of BWt).

Clinical Relevance

The percentage of BWt as TBW is often used in calculating replacement therapy for dehydration, especially in correcting hyponatremia. Although this is practically useful, note that sodium (Na^+) is not distributed evenly into TBW (see later).

As mentioned, intravascular fluid is estimated as 7 per cent of BWt, or 70 ml/kg. This figure can be used to calculate blood volume (e.g., in the context of hemorrhage, administration of blood products, or exchange transfusion). A higher figure (80 ml/kg) is used for newborns.

Of all the compartments of TBW, intravascular fluid is the most clinically relevant in discussions of dehydration and shock.

Ions in Body Fluids

The ionic compositions of ECF and ICF differ markedly. In ECF (as reflected by serum chemistries), Na^+ is the principal cation (140 mEq/L); small amounts of potassium (K^+; ~4 mEq/L), calcium (Ca^{++}), and magnesium (Mg^{++}) are also present. Chloride (Cl^-; 100 mEq/L) and bicarbonate (HCO_3^-; 22 to 25 mEq/L) are the major anions. In ICF, the principal cation is K^+ (~150 mEq/L), whereas Na^+ concentration is very low (~10 mEq/L) (i.e., the opposite of serum values; and the anions are mostly phosphates, sulfates, and HCO_3^-). The contrast between Na^+ and K^+ in ECF and ICF is due to the presence on cell membranes of Na^+/K^+ exchangers, which actively extrude Na^+ from cells and pump K^+ into cells.

Because there is virtually no Na^+ or Cl^- in the ICF, cell membranes can be considered "functionally" impermeable to Na^+ and Cl^-. Hence, NaCl is the determinant of the partition of body water between ECF and ICF.

There is also a transcellular hydrogen H^+/K^+ exchange.

The composition of intravascular fluid and the rest of ECF is similar, except for minor differences (Donnan's effect) having no clinical relevance that are dictated by the presence of proteins (6 to 7 g/dl) in the intravascular compartment only.

Clinical Relevance

Most of the body's K^+ is intracellular. With cell destruction, a large K^+ load can be released (e.g., rhabdomyolysis or tumor lysis), involving the risk of hyperkalemia. Packed red blood cell transfusion, when cells are hemolyzed, may be a source of exogenous K^+.

As mentioned, there is a transcellular H^+/K^+ exchange; thus, in the presence of acidosis, K^+ may come out of the cells as excess H^+ is taken in; conversely, during alkalosis, K^+ may be sequestered intracellularly.

Insulin leads to intracellular uptake of K^+, accompanying glucose. This can be used in the acute treatment of hyperkalemia. Rapid intravenous glucose administration (e.g., total parenteral nutrition [TPN]) may lead to hypokalemia unless K^+ intake is commensurately increased; conversely, abrupt discontinuation of intravenous glucose at high concentration involves the risk (in addition to hypoglycemia) of hyperkalemia.

Partition of Body Fluids

Boundary Between ICF and ECF

The osmolalities across the cell membrane determine the fluid partition between ICF and ECF.

Clinical Relevance. If a child has an increase in osmolality as a result of a nonpermeable solute (e.g., glucose in the absence of insulin during diabetic ketoacidosis), the high osmolality in ECF will lead to the movement of water from ICF to ECF, and the ICF will shrink at the expense of the ECF. Peripheral perfusion, at the same degree of fluid losses, is likely to be better in a hypernatremic child than in a hyponatremic child.

Fluid shifts across plasma membranes (ICF to ECF) can be induced pharmacologically with a cell-impermeant solute (e.g., mannitol, used to dehydrate cells during increase in intracranial pressure).

Boundary Between Intravascular Space and Rest of ECF

Starling's forces across capillaries determine the partition between intravascular versus extravascular spaces. Of the four Starling forces (hydraulic and oncotic pressures inside and outside a vessel wall), only two are clinically relevant: intraluminal hydraulic pressure (dependent on systemic arterial pressure or venous pressure) and oncotic pressure (dependent, under physiologic circumstances, on plasma protein concentration).

Clinical Relevance. In hypertension, a small amount of fluid is expected to exit the intravascular space because of the increase in Starling's forces; the same occurs in congestive heart failure because of the increase in venous pressure, partly accounting for the peripheral edema.

Conversely, in hypoproteinemic states such as nephrotic syndrome, oncotic pressure decreases and fluid exits from the intravascular space to the interstitium.

Intravascular volume can be increased pharmacologically by administering a solute intravenously that does not cross blood vessels, such as albumin (used as a "plasma expander").

These considerations are important in deciding whether to give colloid or normal saline. If a normal child is given 1 L of plasma, it will stay within the intravascular space. If given 1 L of normal saline, it will be distributed equally into all ECF (i.e., only one third will go into the intravascular space); thus, the degree of intravascular repletion is not equivalent when a child is given, for resuscitation, 10 ml/kg of colloid (plasma or albumin solution) versus the same volume of a crystalloid solution (normal saline or lactated Ringer's solution). In a child with compromised cardiac function, for example, colloid will carry a higher risk of circulatory overload and congestive heart failure and should be used with caution.

If a child is hypoproteinemic (nephrotic syndrome or liver disease), the plasma osmotic pressure is low. If given 1 L of normal saline, more than two thirds will go to the interstitial space, and it may be readily anticipated that such an intervention will lead to more "edema" than "intravascular expansion."

Regulation of Osmolality and Volume

Water and Na^+ balance is regulated largely independently. Regulation of osmolality is made primarily by adjusting water; regulation of volume, by adjusting Na^+.

The central nervous system (CNS)–renal axis regulates water balance by sensing plasma osmolality. A water deficit (e.g., excessive sweating, high salt intake) results in an increase in serum osmolality. This activates hypothalamic receptors in the brain, resulting in release of antidiuretic hormone (ADH), stimulation of thirst, and, hence, intake and conservation of water, restoring serum Na^+ to normal. Na^+ balance is not affected in this scheme.

Conversely, if water intake is excessive, a slight decrease in serum osmolality will result, shutting off ADH and leading to elaboration of a dilute urine, thus allowing free water loss and return of serum Na^+ to normal.

Regulation of volume depends on Na^+ handling. In the presence of renal hypoperfusion or hypotension, specialized cells in the kidney are stimulated to release renin. Renin, a proteolytic enzyme, converts renin substrate to angiotensin I, which, in turn, is cleaved by angiotensin-converting enzyme into angiotensin II. Angiotensin II has two actions: it is a vasoconstrictor, thus restoring blood pressure, and it releases aldosterone from the adrenals, promoting renal Na^+ retention and, hence, restoration of volume.

Under conditions of extreme hypotension or volume depletion, ADH is also activated; in this case, volume conservation takes priority over serum Na^+ or osmolality.

Clinical Relevance

A child in shock who may need 1 L of normal saline (NS) would require 2 L of $\frac{1}{2}$ NS or 4 L of $\frac{1}{4}$ NS because the amount of NaCl administered is the critical determinant of volume status rather than the volume of water administered.

PARENTERAL FLUID AND ELECTROLYTE THERAPY

Two important points need to be kept in mind:

1. Parenteral fluid and electrolyte therapy is *better avoided* unless necessary. Thus, in the treatment of severe gastroenteritis, oral hydration is increasingly recognized as a valid alternative.
2. In the presence of normal homeostatic mechanism (CNS, adrenal and kidney function), the body can maintain adequate volume and electrolyte concentrations over a wide range of administered fluids and electrolytes.

In general, parenteral fluid therapy is *intravenous*. The peritoneal membrane is very effective in fluid and electrolyte transfer. Thus, in the child on acute or chronic *peritoneal* dialysis, adjustment of dialysate K^+ level can be used to correct serum K^+ level. Glucose in the peritoneal dialysate is absorbed, and its concentration can be increased to provide a source of calories; peritoneal dialysis can be used to treat severe hypernatremia and hyperkalemia. *Intraosseous* fluid administration is very effective; although fallen in disuse for a long time, it is now regaining favor as a rapid and effective way of administering fluids, electrolytes, and medications under extreme emergency situations. Thus, the practicing pediatrician should be familiar with intraosseous fluid administration technique.

Parenteral fluid administration serves three purposes:

1. *Maintenance* when the child is unable to take oral fluids because of gastrointestinal indications, risk of aspiration, or anticipated surgery.
2. *Correction* of losses or deficits that have already occurred.
3. *Replacement* of ongoing losses.

TABLE 1. Estimation of Body Surface Area from Weight

Weight (kg)	Factor × Weight	+ Factor	Example
0–5	0.05	0.05	2 kg, BSA = 0.05 × 2 + 0.05 = 0.15 m^2
5–10	0.04	0.10	9 kg, BSA = 0.04 × 9 + 0.10 = 0.46 m^2
10–20	0.03	0.20	14 kg, BSA = 0.03 × 14 + 0.20 = 0.66 m^2
20–40	0.02	0.40	37 kg, BSA = 0.02 × 37 + 0.40 = 1.14 m^2

Abbreviations: BSA, body surface area.

Table 1 shows the calculation of BSA (m^2) from weight alone. Alternatively, normograms can be used to find BSA from height and weight. It has become customary, for convenience, to base calculations on BWt (or estimated BWt). Calculation per BSA should be used, however, when body composition markedly deviates from normal (e.g., extreme obesity), when BWt is likely to fluctuate (e.g., edema), or when extreme accuracy is required (e.g., acute renal failure).

Maintenance Therapy

There are obligatory losses from sweat, stool, and a portion of the urine (for excreting solutes) that need to be replaced every day. Strictly, the daily fluids needed by a child would be the sum of these losses. Practically, "maintenance fluids" and "maintenance electrolytes" have become widely used as the amounts needed in the otherwise normal child who can take nothing by mouth (NPO). Under most other circumstances, these estimates are generous.

Fluid Requirements. Fluid requirements are directly linked to metabolic rate and energy expenditure (1 ml water/cal); caloric expenditure, in turn, depends on BSA, and thus proportionately decreases with increasing body size. In the average child, caloric and, hence, fluid requirements (ml/day) can be estimated using BWt (kg) from Table 2. Note that, calculated this way, the fluid requirement in the small infant is 100 ml/kg (i.e., 10 per cent of BWt) whereas in the 40-kg child, it is 1900 ml (~5 per cent of BWt).

Sodium Requirement. The requirement is very small, and the mature kidney is able to reabsorb all filtered Na^+ (i.e., achieve a urine Na^+ concentration close to nil) during Na^+ deprivation. However, this capability may be limited in infants, involving the risk of hyponatremia. Maintenance Na^+ is 2 to 3 mEq/kg. Note, however, that a normal child can tolerate much higher Na^+ intake (~10 mEq/kg/day).

Potassium Requirement. Maintenance K^+ is 2 to 3 mEq/kg BWt. In the normal child, a K^+ concentration of 20 mEq/L in intravenous fluids is appropriate and safe. In severe hypokalemia, 40 mEq/L can be given, and, under extreme conditions, 60 mEq/L, provided that the access line is very good (extravasation can lead to severe tissue necrosis) and that its tip is away from the heart (risk of arrhythmias). It is always safer to run the risk of hypokalemia rather than hyperkalemia, as the latter may be fatal. Hypokalemia is not as life-threatening as hyperkalemia, except in the child on digitalis.

Alkali. There are no alkali requirements. However, the daily acid production is 1 to 2 mEq/kg/day. This is the amount that needs to be neutralized in a child with no renal function.

The anion used in intravenous fluids is usually Cl^-. In the presence of acidosis, acetate can be substituted for part or all of Cl^-. Although a weak acid itself, it is metabolized to HCO_3^- in the liver; its use should be avoided in the presence of liver dysfunction. Adequate volume expansion (reversal of shock) cannot be achieved with $NaHCO_3$ but, rather, requires NaCl.

Customarily, maintenance intravenous solutions are given as 5 per cent dextrose with 35 mEq/L NaCl + 20 mEq/L KCl. Note that 5 per cent dextrose is added to any hypotonic solution to prevent hemolysis as well as to provide calories.

A volume of fluid below maintenance should be administered to any child with either (1) impaired ability to dilute the urine (e.g., syndrome of inappropriate ADH [SIADH], heart failure, nephrotic syndrome, or liver cirrhosis) or (2) a low glomerular filtration rate (e.g., renal failure with oliguria or anuria). A higher fluid volume should be administered to a child with high fever (+12 per cent for each degree Celsius above 37°C).

TABLE 2. Calculation of Caloric Expenditure and Maintenance Fluid Requirement Based on Body Weight

Body Weight (kg)	Caloric Expenditure (kcal) and Fluid Requirement (ml)
Up to 10	100 × weight
10–20	1000 + 50 × (weight − 10)
Over 20	1500 + 20 × (weight − 20)

Correction Therapy

Management of dehydration starts with knowledge of (1) the *severity* of dehydration and (2) the *type* of dehydration.

The severity of dehydration, expressed as percentage of BWt lost, is best determined from current and baseline weights. If this information is lacking, the degree of dehydration can be approximated as 5 per cent (the child has a history of losses and may be thirsty, but his or her examination is normal); 10 per cent (the child has clinical signs of dehydration: decreased skin turgor, sunken eyeballs, depressed fontanelle, dry mucous membranes, decreased tearing, decreased urine output; vital signs may show tachycardia, but blood pressure is normal); or 15 per cent (shock, i.e., low blood pressure with signs of peripheral low perfusion: decreased pulses, cyanotic cold extremities, change in consciousness, (oliguria or anuria). The severity of symptoms is also related to how rapidly the losses occurred.

Laboratory tests that are helpful are blood urea nitrogen, serum creatinine and electrolytes, and urinalysis.

Dehydration is classically divided into *hypernatremic* (Na^+ >145 mEq/L), *normonatremic*, and *hyponatremic* (Na^+ <135 mEq/L).

All body fluids that are likely to be lost in large amounts in the otherwise normal child—namely, in stool, urine, and sweat—have a Na^+ concentration below that of plasma (Table 3). Thus, any excessive losses are expected to lead to hypernatremia. However, most replacement fluids that are given orally to children have a low Na^+ concentration (Table 4). Thus, repletion of the child with fluids leads, depending on its degree, to normonatremia or hyponatremia. Hypernatremia is more likely to occur in young infants because of their limited ability to concentrate the urine and their more frequent inability to take fluids orally. The physician should keep in mind that, in the three forms of dehydration, deficits in both water and sodium do exist but in different proportions. Therefore, replacement therapies differ. Additionally, some

TABLE 3. Electrolyte Content of Major Body Fluids

Fluid	Na (mEq/L)	K (mEq/L)	Cl (mEq/L)
Gastric	20–80	5–20	100–150
Pancreas, small intestine, bile	120–140	5–15	80–130
Ileum	45–135	3–15	20–115
Diarrhea	10–90	10–80	10–110
Sweat, normal	10–30	3–10	10–35
Sweat, cystic	50–130	5–25	50–110

Abbreviations: Na, sodium; K, potassium; Cl, chloride.

specific problems accompany hyponatremia and hypernatremia.

If the type of dehydration is not known, it is safest to begin normal saline because this will start to correct all three types of dehydration.

Acidosis. Metabolic acidosis often accompanies dehydration. It is due to a combination of (1) alkali loss (high HCO_3^- content in small intestinal fluid), (2) the starvation ketoacidosis that often accompanies dehydration, (3) lactic acid production if there is peripheral hypoperfusion, and (4) in severe cases, renal hypoperfusion and inability to excrete acid. Acidosis usually does not need correction unless the child is in shock, is tired of respiratory effort (constant crying), or has persistent and severe ongoing losses. In such cases, 1 to 2 mEq/kg HCO_3^- can be given either as a slow intravenous push (0.5 mEq/ml solution) or added to the intravenous fluids. HCO_3^- "space" is ECF, and total HCO_3^- (tCO_2) deficit is estimated as

$$(\text{Normal } tCO_2 - \text{current } tCO_2) \times 0.4 \times \text{BWt}$$

Alkalosis. Alkalosis may be present when vomiting has been predominant and severe (e.g., pyloric stenosis). If the child's intake has been poor for several hours, there may be starvation *ketosis* (detectable by smell or urinalysis). Urine glucose should be negative; otherwise, diabetes mellitus has to be ruled out.

Shock. Shock is an emergency. Rapid restoration of intravascular fluid takes precedence over diagnostic studies. The initial management of shock is similar in all forms of dehydration and consists of first giving 10 to 20 ml/kg of a colloid solution (plasma, dextran, or 5 per cent albumin) over 30 to 60 minutes. Alternatively, lactated Ringer's or saline solution can be used, but the volume required to achieve the same volume expansion would be larger. *Colloid solutions are favored over crystalloid in younger infants, in the presence of hypernatremia, and in more seriously sick children.*

The percentage of dehydration indicates the volume of fluids needed. Thus, 5 per cent corresponds to 50 ml/kg, which has to be given to the child in addition to maintenance fluid. In the child with a lesser degree of dehydration, the decision to give intravenous versus oral fluids depends largely on his or her condition, the cause of the illness, the reliability of caregivers, and the availability of close follow-up. Intravenous fluid is certainly necessary (1) in shock, (2) in smaller infants, (3) in children with uncontrollable vomiting, (4) in a fatigued child, and (5) with CNS changes. When fluids are given intravenously, the deficit is calculated and added to maintenance; half is given over 8 hours and half over the following 16 hours. The amount of the fluid target is the same orally as intravenously.

TABLE 4. Electrolyte Composition of Some Commonly Used Oral Solutions

	Na	K	Cl	Base (mEq/L)
Water	0	0	0	0
Cow's milk	25	35	30	
Breast milk/formula	7	15–20	12	
Carbonated soft drinks	0–10	0–15	0–15	0–15
Kool-Aid	0	0	0	
Apple juice	2	25	0	
Orange juice	0	50	0	50
Pedialyte	45	20	35	
Ricelyte	50	25	45	
Rehydrate	75	20	65	
Gatorade	21	2.5	17	
WHO solution	90	20	80	30

Abbreviations: WHO, World Health Organization.

Normonatremia. A 5 per cent dextrose solution with Na^+ (40 to 60 mEq/L) is given.

Hyponatremia. The child should be given Na^+ (60 to 100 mEq/L) in intravenous fluid. Na^+ concentration can be decreased as soon as the serum Na^+ is within a normal range because ongoing losses are likely to contain no more than 30 to 40 mEq/L Na^+.

Alternatively, Na^+ deficit can be estimated as

$$(\text{Desired } Na^+ - \text{current } Na^+) \times 0.6 \times \text{BWt}$$

This amount is added to maintenance requirements. Again, half of the calculated fluid and electrolytes is given over 8 hours and half is given over the following 16 hours.

Hypertonic (2 or 3 per cent) NaCl is rarely needed and is reserved for the child with symptomatic hyponatremia (seizures). If seizures are present, the amount of Na^+ should be calculated to bring serum Na^+ to 120 mEq/L acutely (seizures are unusual above this value and, if present, raise the possibility of diagnoses such as meningitis with SIADH), or up by 5 mEq/L. This is calculated as

$$Na^+ \text{ deficit (mEq/L)} = [120 - Na^+] \times 0.6 \times \text{BWt}$$

One ml of 3 per cent saline provides 0.5 mEq Na^+. The calculated volume can be given over 15 to 30 minutes and should be stopped as soon as the child's neurologic status improves. The rest of the Na^+ replacement should be calculated in the same way to increase serum Na^+ by no more than 20 mEq/day; otherwise, the patient will face the risk of osmotic demyelination (a dramatic irreversible CNS disorder). Severe hyponatremia must neither be corrected too rapidly nor overcorrected.

In the usual uncomplicated case, intravenous fluid Na^+ concentration should be decreased as soon as serum Na^+ is normal.

Hypernatremia. Although textbooks classically report that the skin is typically "doughy" in hypernatremia, this is an unreliable sign. Rapid correction of hypernatremia, especially if it has developed slowly (over 2 to 3 days), involves the risk of creating an osmotic gradient across the cell membranes and, hence, rapid water shift into cells, the serious effect of which is brain edema. Therefore, after initial resuscitation (with colloid if needed), replacement and maintenance fluids for 2 days are estimated and given at a constant rate over 48 hours. The choice of solution is variable. If the hypernatremia has developed very slowly, normal saline is preferable. Na^+ in a concentration of up to 70 mEq/L is safe in the more acutely ill child. As the serum Na^+ improves, the concentration of Na^+ in the fluid can gradually be decreased to 30 to 40 mEq/L.

Hypernatremic dehydration should be differentiated from salt poisoning, in which case there are obviously no deficits. If doubt exists, a urine Na^+ is informative ($<$20 mEq/L with depletion; high in salt poisoning).

Two special problems accompany hypernatremia: hyperglycemia (which usually resolves spontaneously) and the risk of hypocalcemia as hypernatremia corrects. To avoid these problems, 1 ampule of 10 per cent calcium gluconate can be added to each 500 ml of fluids, and serum Ca^{++} should be monitored.

Potassium Replacement. Although the dehydrated child likely has K^+ deficits, there is no extreme urgency in replacing K^+ because (1) the accompanying acidosis often leads to maintenance of serum K^+ level (transcellular H^+/K^+ exchange), and (2) in the presence of a contracted intravascular volume and decreased renal perfusion, there is risk of hyperkalemia. Thus, K^+ replacement can be delayed until the child achieves urine output.

As soon as the child is able to take fluids by mouth, an oral electrolyte solution should be started (Table 4) and the intravenous fluids appropriately curtailed.

Replacement Therapy

Replacement fluid should have the same volume and composition as the fluid being lost. Composition can be estimated (Table 3), or an actual sample of fluid can be sent to the laboratory for measurement of electrolytes.

SPECIFIC ELECTROLYTE DISORDERS

Disorders of Sodium Concentration

Hyponatremia

When an unexpectedly low serum Na^+ value (<135 mEq/L) is obtained on a blood test, a serum osmolality value will differentiate the following:

1. *Normal osmolality,* or *pseudohyponatremia.* This is an artifact when plasma lipids are high (nephrotic syndrome, hypothyroidism, familial hyperlipidemia). It does not require correction.
2. *High osmolality.* Excess osmoles other than Na^+ are in the plasma that shift water from ICF to ECF, thus diluting Na^+. These osmoles can be endogenous (glucose) or exogenous (mannitol).
3. *Low osmolality.* This is true hyponatremia. Clinical manifestations of hyponatremia are neurologic: lethargy, apathy, and disorientation, culminating in seizures and coma.

There are four causes of true hyponatremia:

1. *Water intoxication,* which is due to excessive water intake. In the normal individual, the ability of the kidney to excrete water is very good. Thus, hyponatremia due to water excess occurs only if the intake is enormous or the glomerular filtration rate is limited—namely, in infants and children with renal disease. Excess water intake can occur in infants on diluted formula, infants force-fed water, and infants given swimming lessons. Treatment is by withholding water and treating associated problems, as well as by educating the parents.
2. *Hyponatremic dehydration.* Discussed previously.
3. *Hyponatremia with edema.* The most common causes are heart failure (low cardiac output), nephrotic syndrome, and liver cirrhosis (low serum proteins). Water and Na^+ are retained, but more water than Na^+. Typically, there is edema and third-spacing (pleural effusion, ascites). The diagnosis is reached by history and physical examination. Attempts to correct the hyponatremia with Na^+ only worsen the edema. Treatment is restriction of Na^+ as well as water, together with judicious use of diuretics.
4. *SIADH.* This is the most common cause of hyponatremia in hospitalized children. SIADH should be suspected in any child with CNS pathology (meningitis, encephalitis, hypoxia, trauma) or respiratory pathology (infection, assisted ventilation). This syndrome is so common during meningitis (occurring in 35 to 50 per cent of patients) that it is customary to restrict fluids to approximately 65 per cent of maintenance. However, it is very important to observe serum Na^+ and urine specific gravity closely. If serum Na^+ is decreasing and urine specific gravity is very high, use of normal saline solution or diuretics (furosemide) may be indicated. Hypertonic saline is rarely needed.

The four forms of hyponatremia can easily be distinguished by history, physical examination, and laboratory data (Table 5).

Hypernatremia

Clinical manifestations of hypernatremia (Na^+ >145 mEq/L) are also neurologic: lethargy, seizures, intracranial hemorrhage, and coma. In hypernatremic dehydration, the signs and symptoms are those of the underlying disorder (e.g., enteritis) and the dehydration. Chronic hypernatremia can present with failure to thrive and developmental delay.

The causes of hypernatremia can be divided into (1) too much Na^+ (salt poisoning) and (2) too little water (hypernatremic dehydration) from low intake or excessive losses.

Salt poisoning occurs particularly in infants (from mistakes in food preparation or intentional child poisoning) and when large amounts of $NaHCO_3$ are given intravenously during cardiopulmonary resuscitation. It is treated with hypotonic saline in children with normal kidney function. In the acute event, administering diuretics (furosemide) while replacing urine output with 5 per cent dextrose has been advocated.

Hypernatremic dehydration is more common and is a result of too little water intake or excessive water loss.

It is very difficult to become hypernatremic if the thirst mechanism and water intake are intact. Thus, hypernatremia is more common when there is inability either to express thirst verbally (infant, unconscious patient) or to seek or obtain water actively (infant, bedridden patient), or in the unusual situation when no fresh water is available. Young infants are particularly at risk, especially those who are breast-fed (when intake cannot be quantitated) and those with diarrhea and fever (especially in a hot, dry environment). This risk is compounded by the fact that insensible water losses are higher in the younger child. Less common causes of decreased intake are central lesions that impair the thirst mechanism (adipsia).

Excessive losses can be gastrointestinal (discussed earlier) or renal, that is, diabetes insipidus (DI). DI is the inability to concentrate urine; hence, the affected individual has a continuously high urine output (polyuria) with excessive drinking (polydipsia).

DI can be *central,* in which there is absent or insufficient ADH; however, the child shows a good response to exogenous ADH. More than one third of cases are idiopathic, some are familial, and others are secondary to a CNS lesion.

DI can be *nephrogenic,* in which the kidney does not respond to ADH. If ADH administration during the water deprivation test suggests a renal origin for DI, drug intake, renal disease, and sickle cell trait should be ruled out.

Treatment of hypernatremic dehydration depends on whether the child has lost only water (DI) or water and electrolytes (diarrhea). In the case of pure water loss, give hypotonic saline. Otherwise, it is safest to start a high Na^+ concentration fluid (NS or $\frac{1}{2}$ NS) and then gradually decrease Na^+ concentration.

In chronic hypernatremia, serum Na^+ should not be decreased faster than 10 mEq/L/day to avoid the risk of cerebral edema.

Central to the long-term treatment of DI is the education of parents and child about the need for fluid, especially in hot weather, with fever, or with gastroenteritis. Central DI can be treated with ADH or its analogues (desmopressin

TABLE 5. Laboratory Data and Treatment of the Four Types of Hyponatremia

	Laboratory Data	Treatment
Water intoxication	Low sp. gr., low UNa, low BUN	Restrict water
Dehydration	High sp. gr., low UNa, high BUN	Give water and Na^+
HypoNa with edema	High sp. gr., low UNa, ± high BUN	Restrict Na^+ (and water)
SIADH	High sp. gr., high UNa, low BUN	Restrict water

Abbreviations: sp. gr., urine specific gravity; UNa, urine Na^+ concentration; BUN, blood urea nitrogen; SIADH, syndrome of inappropriate antidiuretic hormone.

acetate [DDAVP] intranasally is the most convenient form). Nephrogenic DI can be treated with thiazides (e.g., hydrochlorothiazide) or nonsteroidal anti-inflammatory agents (e.g., ibuprofen).

Potassium Disorders

Hyperkalemia

There are several causes of spurious hyperkalemia, such as hemolysis upon drawing blood and thrombocytosis (platelets >500,000/mm³). The most direct way to document whether hyperkalemia is significant (while one awaits a second value) is to obtain an electrocardiogram (EKG). The earliest sign is tenting of the T waves. Obviously, in high-risk settings (cell breakdown or acute renal failure), hyperkalemia should be addressed immediately, as it is life-threatening.

Causes. The causes of hyperkalemia are

1. Hemolysis, high platelet count (spurious).
2. Transcellular shift (acidosis).
3. Cell breakdown.
3. Increased intake (salt substitutes).
4. Decreased excretion (renal failure, adrenal insufficiency, K^+-sparing diuretics).

Symptoms. These include weakness, paralysis, and cardiac arrythmias. Hyperkalemia can lead to cardiac arrest. K^+ should not be added to the intravenous fluids of a dehydrated child before establishing that the child is producing an adequate volume of urine. It is important to anticipate hyperkalemia (e.g., in any child at risk of decrease in renal function) and to take steps to prevent it by removing K^+ from intravenous fluids, avoiding K^+-containing medications, and washing packed red blood cells prior to transfusion.

Treatment. Hyperkalemia can be treated by

1. Antagonizing its membrane effects with Ca^{++} (1 to 2 ml/kg 10 per cent calcium gluconate IV slowly under EKG monitoring).
2. Sequestering K^+ intracellularly with HCO_3^- (1 to 2 ml/kg $NaHCO_3$ 0.5 mEq/ml over 1 hour), dextrose (0.2 to 0.4 g/kg), and insulin (0.2 units/kg).
3. Removing K^+ from the body via the gastrointestinal tract (Kayexalate, 1 g/kg orally or rectally, will decrease serum K^+ by ~1 mEq/L) or via urine (furosemide, 1 mg/kg).
4. Dialysis as a last resort.

Hypokalemia

Hypokalemia can be due to (1) hiding K^+ in cells (transcellular shifts) or (2) true deficit.

Transcellular shifts can occur with alkalosis, insulin and glucose (e.g., TPN), or sympathomimetics (e.g., treatment of asthma). Treatment is not needed except for the underlying disorder.

A true deficit can occur when K^+ is lost into the gastrointestinal tract (gastroenteritis) or urine as a result of diuretics (including glucose or drugs), exogenous steroids (as in nephrotics, asthmatics, chemotherapy), or endogenous steroids (adrenal abnormality, usually with hypertension and other symptoms). A rare disorder is Bartter syndrome (hypokalemic metabolic alkalosis).

Hypokalemia presents with ileus, hypotonia, decreased reflexes, as well as impaired urine concentration. EKG can show prominent U waves. Hypokalemia is a serious concern in the child taking digitalis, as it potentiates digitalis toxicity.

Treatment depends on the cause. Losses should be replaced, preferably orally, and the total daily dose should be divided into three or four doses. K^+ can be added to intravenous fluids. There is no place for rapid intravenous K^+ administration.

Acid-Base Disorders

Acid-base balance is maintained by the kidneys and the lungs; therefore, knowledge of the respiratory status of the patient is essential in interpreting a plasma HCO_3^- level. In the child with respiratory problems, determining blood gas levels may be essential, at least during initial evaluation. Treatment of respiratory acidosis or alkalosis consists of correcting the underlying respiratory problem.

Metabolic Alkalosis

Three questions need to be asked:

1. Did the patient receive an exogenous alkali? (Usually HCO_3^-; however, lactate and citrate are weak acids and common anions in TPN, metabolized by the liver into HCO_3^-.)
2. Did the patient lose H^+ (via gastric suction, vomiting)?
3. Is the patient deficient in Cl^-? (Cl^- can be lost in the sweat [cystic fibrosis], intestine [congenital Cl^- diarrhea], and urine [diuretics, steroids].)

In addition, in patients with respiratory problems, CO_2 retention can lead to renal HCO_3^- retention; this can lag behind adjustment of respiratory status, leading to a transient metabolic alkalosis. Obviously, no treatment is needed in this case, as the kidneys will excrete the excess alkali if given time.

The treatment of metabolic alkalosis consists of (1) correcting the underlying cause (e.g., gastric suction, pyloric stenosis); (2) replacing the Cl^- deficits (adding Cl^- to intravenous fluids, substituting Cl^- for lactate or citrate in TPN); and (3) replacing K^+ deficits if any (usually with KCl). Ammonium chloride or a carbonic anhydrase inhibitor (acetazolamide, 5 mg/kg/day) may be used. Specific causes (steroid excess, Bartter syndrome) should be addressed.

Metabolic Acidosis

The patient with acidosis presents with lethargy and decreased cardiac contractility. The child tries to compensate by hyperventilating, and breathing will be rapid and deep (Kussmaul's breathing); the infant may be crying in a prolonged, unconsolable pattern.

Metabolic acidosis can be due to (1) loss of alkali or inability to excrete normal daily acid produced or (2) gain of "foreign" acids not normally present in the circulation. These two forms can be distinguished by calculating the anion gap (AG):

$$AG = Na^+ - (Cl^- + tCO_2)$$

Normal Anion Gap (<15 mEq/L) Acidosis. Alkali can be lost in the gastrointestinal tract, and acidosis often accompanies diarrhea (small intestinal fluid is rich in HCO_3^-). Such losses are the most common cause of acute acidosis. The kidneys can also have an impaired ability to maintain acid-base balance (renal tubular acidosis). Rarely, renal HCO_3^- loss can be iatrogenic (acetazolamide, a carbonic anhydrase inhibitor). In all these forms of acidosis, the serum Cl^- is typically high, as a cation to accompany Na^+ and maintain electroneutrality.

High Anion Gap Acidosis. A high anion gap (>15 mEq/L) indicates that an unusual acid has been added to the plasma. These acids can be exogenous (salicylate) or endogenous. The most common endogenous acids are lactate (it increases with hypoxia, hypoperfusion), ketoacids (in diabetes mellitus), and various acids in advanced chronic renal failure. Rare causes are congenital metabolic disorders (type I glycogen storage disease and organic acidemias).

Metabolic acidosis, particularly if the serum pH is greater than 7.25, should be allowed to correct spontaneously while the underlying cause (dehydration, hypoxia, insulin deficiency) is treated. Potential risks of correction include an acute increase in carbonic acid, hence, in CO_2 gas. CO_2 rapidly crosses the blood-brain barrier, where it can lead to cerebrospinal fluid acidosis, increase in intracranial pressure, and brain edema.

Alkali is rarely given if the plasma pH is greater than 7.25. Conditions in which alkali is given are severe acidosis, threatening hyperkalemia (because of H^+/K^+ shifts), or deficient defense mechanisms (severe intractable diarrhea, renal tubular acidosis, renal failure). Daily acid production is 1 to 2 mEq/kg/day; correction is given over 24 to 48 hours. A push of 1 to 2 mEq/kg may be given acutely if necessary, with an adequately dilute (0.5 mEq/ml) HCO_3^- solution.

MALIGNANT HYPERTHERMIA

ROBERT C. PASCUCCI, M.D.

Malignant hyperthermia (MH) is a syndrome characterized by the acute onset of a hypermetabolic state in skeletal muscle, usually in response to the administration of anesthetic agents, particularly halothane (and other potent inhalation anesthetics) and succinylcholine. Susceptibility to MH is thought to be inherited, with some recent evidence indicating that the genetic abnormality is located on chromosome 19. The precise pathophysiology of the syndrome is still under investigation but appears to involve an aberrancy in intracellular movement of calcium (Ca) through the sarcoplasmic reticulum, such that Ca^{2+} accumulates in the cytosol, inducing sustained muscle contracture and resulting in excessive production of heat, carbon dioxide (CO_2), and lactate. Prior to the availability of specific therapy, the full-blown syndrome involved a mortality rate greater than 50 per cent. With early recognition and prompt administration of dantrolene (see later), the mortality rate has declined to less than 10 per cent.

DIAGNOSIS

Early recognition of MH depends on the anesthesiologist's vigilance in continuously monitoring patients during their operative course. MH is largely a clinical diagnosis: Early signs include unexplained tachycardia, hypertension, and tachypnea, with evidence of increased CO_2 production (an increased end-tidal or arterial P_{CO_2} despite adequate or increased minute ventilation). As the syndrome develops, acidosis (both metabolic and respiratory), peripheral mottling and cyanosis, ventricular dysrhythmias, and generalized muscle rigidity appear. Fever, despite the syndrome's name, is a relatively late sign; body temperature can easily rise above 40°C. The syndrome does not always appear in its most malignant state, however, and accurate diagnosis of more temperate cases is sometimes difficult. Not all signs may be present, and some may be masked by the anesthetic technique employed. *Although most cases develop within the first few hours of anesthesia, it is possible for the syndrome to appear in the immediate postoperative period as well. The pediatrician must therefore include MH in the forefront of the differential diagnosis of postoperative fever.*

TREATMENT

Initial and immediate treatment of MH includes discontinuation of all possible triggering drugs, *hyperventilation with 100 per cent oxygen, and prompt administration of the specific therapeutic agent, dantrolene.* Dantrolene, a direct-acting skeletal muscle relaxant, appears to slow calcium release by the sarcoplasmic reticulum, effectively reversing the MH aberrancy. The drug is highly effective for this indication, and the intravenous preparation should be available wherever potent inhalation anesthetics are administered. Dantrolene is commonly administered in 1 mg/kg increments, given as quickly as possible, until the syndrome is controlled. The usual dose required is 2.5 mg/kg, but occasional patients will require as much as 10 mg/kg as a single dose. Intravenous dantrolene is supplied in a lyophilized form and must be reconstituted with preservative-free *sterile water* before administration; no other diluent can be used. This requires some foresight because 60 ml of sterile water is needed for each 20 mg of drug; a large volume of sterile water for injection must be readily available.

Ongoing therapy is directed toward other manifestations of the syndrome and should be provided in an intensive care setting. Acidosis is treated with hyperventilation and bicarbonate, as necessary. Hyperthermia may necessitate administration of iced intravenous solutions, surface cooling, and irrigation of the stomach, rectum, and (if available) peritoneal or pleural cavities with cold saline. Hyperkalemia is not uncommon and may be severe enough to justify use of a glucose-and-insulin infusion to shift some potassium back into the intracellular compartment. Ventricular dysrhythmias may resolve spontaneously or in response to dantrolene, which has some antiarrhythmic effect. Procainamide is theoretically better than lidocaine in this setting, as the latter has been found to trigger MH under experimental conditions. However, there have been no reports of such triggering in clinical use, and many physicians would not hesitate to administer lidocaine if otherwise indicated. Cardiovascular collapse is possible and is treated in conventional fashion with fluids, pressors or other cardioactive medications, and ventilatory support.

The child experiencing an MH episode should be closely monitored afterward; arterial blood gases, serum electrolytes and creatine phosphokinase (CK), urine output, and urine myoglobin content should be measured on a regular basis. An elevated CK level (often well into the thousands of units) is common, peaking 8 to 12 hours postoperatively, and lends confirmation to the diagnosis. Myoglobinuria and acute tubular necrosis are possible renal complications, requiring surveillance and possible treatment with osmotic diuretics or other appropriate management. Additional doses of dantrolene are given every 6 hours for approximately 24 hours after symptoms subside, as recrudescence may occur.

PREVENTION

As with any disease, prevention is better than cure. Because MH is an inherited condition, a careful preoperative review of the family history for "anesthetic reactions," muscle difficulties (marked cramping or soreness, particularly if occurring after exercise), or episodes of sudden unexplained death may alert the anesthesiologist and pediatrician to potential trouble. Unfortunately, at present, the only definitive test for MH susceptibility is in vitro caffeine-halothane contracture testing, in which muscle strips freshly obtained from the patient by biopsy are tested for abnormal contractile response to increasing concentrations of halothane and caffeine. The test not only is invasive (biopsy) but also must be performed in close enough proximity to a testing center to allow rapid transport of the fresh muscle specimen to the laboratory. It is recommended that children experiencing a clinical episode suggestive of MH be biopsied, if possible, to confirm or refute the diagnosis. Patients found to be "MH susceptible" should be given a MedicAlert (or similar) bracelet and provided suitable counseling. If the testing has not or cannot be performed, prudence should guide the choice of a "nontriggering" anesthetic technique for patients with a personal or family history of a suspicious episode.

Efforts continue to find a reliable, less invasive, and more widely available test for the disease. Recent evidence suggests that magnetic resonance imaging analysis of muscle phosphate patterns may hold some promise. It should be emphasized that a "safe" anesthetic can be provided to these patients even if MH susceptibility has been confirmed. However, special preparations are necessary, and early consultation with an anesthesiologist is essential. Although there is some rationale for administering dantrolene prophylactically to susceptible patients, the incidence of adverse side effects (gastrointestinal discomfort, significant weakness, sedation) is quite high. Expectant management, using only anesthetic agents known to be nontriggering and administering dantrolene only if evidence of the syndrome appears, is more often thought to be the proper course of action.

REFERENCES

Flewellen EH, Nelson TE, Jones WP, et al: Dantrolene dose response in awake man: Implications for management of malignant hyperthermia. Anesthesiology 59:275, 1983.

Heffron JJ, McCarthy TV: Current views of the molecular basis of the malignant hyperthermia syndrome. Acta Anaesthesiol Belgica 41:73–78, 1990.

HEAT-RELATED ILLNESSES

ROBERT C. PASCUCCI, M.D.

Temperature regulation in humans represents a constant balance, under active hypothalamic control, between heat loss and heat gain. The heat-related illnesses discussed here are incurred because of an inability to maintain that balance. In these illnesses, although the hypothalamic regulatory mechanism is functioning well (at least at the outset) and attempts to maintain a normal temperature, heat gain or production occurs in excess of the body's ability to compensate by increasing heat loss, resulting in an excessive rise in body temperature.

Infants and children are particularly at risk for heat-related illnesses; they have a relatively large surface area–to–body mass ratio, predisposing them to rapid warming from the environment. More important, they may lack the simplest but perhaps most effective method of responding to changes in temperature: the ability to move to a different environment. The classic, and tragic, example of this is the infant, perhaps too heavily dressed, who is left sleeping in a car seat in an automobile while "a few errands" are run by the caretaker.

COMMON SYNDROMES

The common syndromes seen are referred to as *heat cramp, heat exhaustion,* and *heat stroke.*

Heat Cramp

Heat cramp refers to the sudden onset of severe cramping pain in muscle. Commonly seen in athletes, even those conditioned to heat and exercise, these cramps probably represent a syndrome of adequate fluid replacement without sufficient electrolyte replacement; hyponatremia and hypochloremia are common.

Rest, cooling, and electrolyte replacement, either orally or intravenously, are usually sufficient to effect relief.

Heat Exhaustion and Heat Stroke

Heat exhaustion and *heat stroke* are progressively more severe forms of heat illness. Both are characterized by water (and sometimes electrolyte) depletion, hemoconcentration, and central nervous system (CNS) disturbances. Distinction between the two illnesses may be made in several ways. Patients with heat exhaustion, the more benign of the two, rarely have a temperature in excess of 39°C; they may be profusely diaphoretic on examination, and CNS dysfunction is moderately severe (headache, disorientation, paresthesias, lethargy/agitation, vomiting). Heat stroke is characterized by temperatures in excess of 41°C. The ability to sweat has often been lost, resulting in hot, dry, pale or pink skin. Normal thermoregulatory controls have been obliterated. CNS dysfunction is profound, and coma, seizures, pupillary changes, and other evidence of severe CNS insult are often present. Heat stroke represents a true medical emergency, with a mortality rate as high as 70 per cent, depending on age, general health, and the severity and duration of heat stress that has been experienced.

Treatment

The management of heat exhaustion is straightforward. The patient is moved to a cool environment, and rehydration is accomplished gradually—orally in milder cases and intravenously in more severe cases and in those with significant CNS dysfunction. Initial rapid rehydration with 10 to 20 ml/kg normal saline over the first 15 to 20 minutes may be followed by more gradual rehydration over the next 12 to 24 hours. If serum electrolytes document salt depletion, extra sodium (Na^+) may be given in this gradual rehydration. A typical calculation of Na^+ deficit may be made using the formula:

$$Na^+ \text{ deficit (mEq)} = (135 - S_{Na}) \times \text{TBW (L)}$$

where S_{Na} = measured serum Na^+ and TBW = total body water, estimated at 50 to 60 per cent of body weight. If seizures or severe muscle cramps are present, 3 per cent saline (a hypertonic solution) may be administered, with an initial dose of 5 ml/kg given over 10 minutes. Serum and urine electrolytes should be measured frequently to guide further therapy; adequate Na^+ replacement should result in a rise in urine Na^+ concentration.

Patients with heat stroke are often very ill, presenting with complete cardiopulmonary collapse. Initial priorities therefore include the standard ABCs of resuscitation as well as the rapid reduction of body temperature. Issues relating to cardiopulmonary resuscitation are beyond the scope of this article; essentially, one must guarantee an airway and ventilatory support and restore the circulation, which will likely require infusion of a large volume of isotonic fluids in addition to other therapy.

Severe hyperthermia is in itself a direct cellular toxin, and thus rapid reduction of body temperature is essential to reduce morbidity and mortality. Multiple modalities must often be used simultaneously to remove heat from the patient as quickly as possible, invoking the classic mechanisms of *evaporation, conduction, convection,* and *radiation* to induce these losses. Clothing should be removed, and the patient should be placed in a cool room, which allows free radiation of heat from the patient to the environment. Vigorous surface cooling (especially of the head and scalp), with application of ice bags, cold-water wetting, and fanning induces heat loss by conduction, convection, and evaporation. Infusion of cool intravenous fluids or, if possible, direct blood cooling through an extracorporeal circuit allows heat removal by conduction.

Much of the efficacy of the surface techniques depends on maintaining good skin blood flow, a feature often quite compromised in these hypovolemic patients. Generous volume administration and the judicious use of chlorpromazine (0.05 mg/kg IV) will maintain or restore skin blood flow; chlorpromazine will also inhibit the shivering response, which in this situation would be counterproductive. There is little benefit to be gained by administration of conventional antipyretics (aspirin, acetaminophen); dantrolene has been investigated and, in general, found to be ineffective.

The many details of the care of these patients may best be reviewed in a systems-oriented fashion as follows.

Respiratory. Adequate ventilatory support will ensure good oxygenation and relieve any respiratory component of acidosis. Adult respiratory distress syndrome (ARDS) has been reported in patients with heat stroke and may require management with increased distending airway pressures, fluid restriction (once intravascular volume has been restored), diuresis, and other therapy directed toward respiratory failure.

Cardiovascular. Careful restoration of circulating volume is aided by direct measurement of arterial and central venous pressures. Inotropic support is often required, as a supranormal cardiac output is required and there may have been direct myocardial damage secondary to heat. It is very reasonable to consider drugs that increase myocardial contractility without undue increase (or, better, actual decrease) in peripheral vascular resistance. Dobutamine, isoproterenol, and amrinone are possibilities; extreme care must be taken with their administration to avoid excessive vasodilation in the setting of volume depletion.

Fluid/Renal Considerations. Blood urea nitrogen, creatinine, serum and urine electrolytes, calcium, glucose, serum creatine kinase and lactic dehydrogenase (to assess muscle breakdown), urine myoglobin, and hourly urine output should all be assessed regularly. Renal dysfunction, either secondary to myoglobinuria or to acute tubular necrosis following a period of circulatory insufficiency, is a common complication of severe heat injury. Diuretics (furosemide or mannitol) should be administered to maintain adequate urine flow, but only after ensuring adequate intravascular volume. If actual renal failure intervenes, standard renal failure regimens, with consideration of dialysis by usual criteria, should be followed.

Hematologic. Hemoconcentration secondary to water and plasma losses (third-spacing) should be noted and treated accordingly. Direct platelet activation and hyperaggregability by heat have been shown to occur experimentally; platelet dysfunction, alone or in combination with generalized disseminated intravascular coagulation, is often present. There is some experimental evidence (but no clinical data) that aspirin may ameliorate the platelet hyperaggregability if given early in the course of treatment. There are also anecdotal reports of improved survival with exchange transfusion and low-dose heparin administration.

Neurologic. Severe CNS dysfunction may result from direct thermal injury to the brain or from cerebral edema secondary to hypoxic-ischemic injury and to the fluid shifts occurring during resuscitation. Seizures are not uncommon. The management of these complications follows standard guidelines, with aggressive anticonvulsant therapy and control of intracranial hypertension with modest dehydration. Consideration should be given to direct measurement of intracranial pressure and further therapy (barbiturates, paralysis, and the like) if the situation warrants.

Prognosis

The prognosis for intact recovery from severe heat stroke, as mentioned earlier, is guarded. As most cases of heat injury are preventable, pediatricians should educate parents and others to be aware of situations in which such injury can occur in children (while overdressed, left in a closed vehicle, or engaged in vigorous sports activities in hot, humid weather). Children with cystic fibrosis, cardiopulmonary compromise, or congenital skin abnormalities are at increased risk for heat-related illnesses. Providing generous fluid and electrolyte replacement and appropriate rest periods in a cool environment and recognizing developing heat illness early will aid in reducing the morbidity and mortality of these conditions.

REFERENCES

Brink LW: Abnormalities in temperature regulation. *In* Levin DL, Morriss FC (eds): Essentials of Pediatric Intensive Care. St. Louis, Quality Medical Publishing, 1990, pp 175–185.

Squire DL. Heat illness. Fluid and electrolyte issues for pediatric and adolescent athletes. Pediatr Clin North Am 37:1085–1089, 1990.

Thompson AE: Environmental emergencies: Environmental and exertional heat. *In* Fleisher GR, Ludwig S (eds): Textbook of Pediatric Emergency Medicine, 2nd ed. Baltimore, Williams & Wilkins, 1988, pp 607–612.

HEMATURIA AND PROTEINURIA

EILEEN D. BREWER, M.D.

When a child is diagnosed with hematuria or proteinuria or both, optimal management mandates a detailed medical history and further laboratory evaluation to determine the underlying cause so that specific therapy can be initiated. A list of etiologic possibilities by category is given in Table 1. A guide to laboratory management is presented in Table 2.

HEMATURIA

Hematuria is usually defined as greater than 5 red blood cells per high-powered field (RBC/hpf) in a centrifuged urine sediment. Because urinary tract infection is the most common cause of hematuria, the first step in the management is a urine culture and sensitivities.

Urinary Tract Infection

If a urinary tract infection is present, appropriate antibiotic therapy should be instituted (see article on urinary tract

TABLE 1. Probable Causes of Hematuria and Proteinuria

Hematuria	Proteinuria	Hematuria and Proteinuria
Urinary tract infection	Transient	Glomerulonephritis
Drugs	Orthostatic	Acute poststreptococcal
Antibiotics	Glomerulonephritis	Membranoproliferative
Anticoagulants	Minimal change disease	Mesangial proliferative
Cyclophosphamide	Focal segmental glomerulosclerosis	Focal segmental glomerulosclerosis
Trauma	Diffuse mesangial proliferative	Membranous nephritis
Glomerulonephritis	IgM nephropathy	Lupus nephritis
IgA nephropathy	Membranoproliferative	IgA nephropathy
Membranoproliferative	Membranous nephritis	Henoch-Schönlein purpura
Lupus nephritis	Lupus nephritis	Hereditary nephritis (Alport syndrome)
Henoch-Schönlein purpura	Interstitial nephritis	Hemolytic uremic syndrome
Acute poststreptococcal	Diabetic nephropathy	Renal vein thrombosis
Sickle cell disease/trait	Reflux nephropathy	
Hereditary nephritis (Alport syndrome)	Obstructive uropathy	
Benign familial hematuria		
Polycystic kidney disease		
Renal vein/artery thrombosis		
Hydronephrosis/hydroureter		
Tumor		
Wilms'		
Hemangioma		
Rhabdomyosarcoma		
Carcinoma, papilloma		
Bladder diverticulum		
Foreign body in bladder/urethra		
Hemorrhagic urethritis		
Nephrocalcinosis/urolithiasis		
Hypercalciuria		
Benign hematuria		

Abbreviations: IgA, immunoglobulin A; IgM, immunoglobulin M.

infection, p. 379) and a follow-up urinalysis obtained after therapy is complete. No further evaluation is necessary if hematuria is absent on follow-up. If the urine culture is negative or if the hematuria persists in two of three specimens obtained on different days, further evaluation is mandatory.

Drugs

A careful history will reveal whether the patient has received a hematuria-causing drug, including antibiotics such as methicillin, anticoagulants, or cyclophosphamide. If possible, the drug should be discontinued or an appropriate substitution made with an agent that does not cause hematuria. *When large doses of cyclophosphamide are anticipated for chemotherapy of cancer, preventive therapy is usually attempted with 2-mercaptoethanesulfonate (mesna), given as 30 to 60 per cent of the cyclophosphamide dose in divided doses just before chemotherapy and every 3 to 4 hours after for four doses. The timing is critical because, to prevent damage, mesna must bind acrolein, the toxic metabolite of cyclophosphamide, before it has a chance to come into contact with the uroepithelium.*

When hemorrhagic cystitis does occur, bleeding is often brisk with many clots, which can be obstructive to drainage of the upper urinary tracts. An affected patient should be treated with an indwelling, multiple-hole, large-lumen catheter in the bladder to allow evacuation of clots and continuous irrigation with saline. If bleeding persists or blood transfusion is required, bladder instillation of chemical cauterizing agents, such as silver nitrate, alum, and formalin, is necessary. A 0.5 to 1.0 per cent solution of silver nitrate in sterile water can be instilled for 10 to 20 minutes intermittently. Multiple instillations may be required, and success may be short-lived.

Alum appears to be a simpler and more successful form of therapy. A 1.0 per cent solution of either the ammonium or the potassium salt of aluminum in sterile water can be given as a continuous bladder irrigation until bleeding stops (average, 21 hours). Alum acts as an astringent to cause protein precipitation over the bleeding surface. Although bladder absorption of aluminum from topical alum is minimal, rare cases of increased serum aluminum levels and encephalopathy have been reported. If alum therapy is used in a child with renal failure, careful monitoring of serum aluminum levels is important. Occasionally, patients have had an allergic reaction to alum that resolves after discontinuing irrigation.

Because formalin is the most effective chemical agent but not the safest, it should be used only if hemorrhage is intractable. Formalin acts by hydrolyzing proteins and coagulating the superficial bladder mucosa and submucosa. It is contraindicated in the patient with vesicoureteral reflux because of the risk of renal injury. Even in a patient without reflux, the reverse Trendelenburg position should be used during instillation to minimize any chance of formalin reflux into the kidneys. Formalin therapy is painful, and general anesthesia is necessary. A variety of concentrations of solution and instillation times have been used. One per cent formalin, although safe, is rarely effective. Ten per cent formalin has been associated with severe complications, including renal failure, papillary necrosis, and ureteral fibrosis if reflux occurs; bladder fibrosis and ureterovesical obstruction; and peritonitis or delayed fistula formation if bladder extravasation occurs. A 2.5 to 4 per cent solution instilled for 15 to 30 minutes may be best. The procedure can be repeated multiple times if unsuccessful at first. If bleeding is still not controlled, surgical intervention may be necessary; however, every attempt should be made to preserve the bladder.

Trauma

If a recent history of blunt trauma to the abdomen is obtained and there is either gross hematuria alone or microscopic hematuria in the presence of hypotension, an intravenous pyelogram (IVP) or computed tomography (CT) scan (if multiple viscera are suspected to be involved) should be obtained to evaluate for renal contusions, lacerations, pedicle injuries, or bladder rupture. If abnormalities are present, urologic consultation should be obtained to determine the need for further surgical management versus bed rest and careful follow-up. In the child who has sustained penetrating trauma (gunshot, stab wound) and has greater than 5 RBC/hpf on urinalysis, radiographic contrast studies are mandatory to direct therapy, as the likelihood of a urinary tract injury is high.

Glomerulonephritis

Gross or microscopic hematuria that occurs concomitantly with a febrile illness is typical of a variety of chronic glomerulonephritides, including immunoglobulin A (IgA) nephropathy, membranoproliferative glomerulonephritis, and lupus nephritis. If hematuria occurs 1 to 3 weeks after an upper respiratory infection or skin infection, acute poststreptococcal glomerulonephritis is more likely. In the child with a history of a typical, albeit evanescent rash of Henoch-Schönlein purpura or lupus, the nephritis of one of these diseases is likely the cause of the hematuria. In all cases, further laboratory investigation should include assessment of renal function (blood urea nitrogen [BUN] and serum creatinine) and serum complement (C_3 and C_4) and antinuclear antibody (ANA) levels. If poststreptococcal glomerulonephritis is suspected, antistreptolysin O, antihyaluronidase, and antideoxyribonuclease B titers should be obtained. When the diagnosis cannot be determined clinically, a renal biopsy is needed. Percutaneous needle biopsy under conscious sedation is preferred. Once a diagnosis is made, supportive or specific therapy can be instituted (see article on glomerulonephritis, p. 352).

Sickle Cell Disease or Trait

The patient with sickle cell disease or trait may have hematuria from a urinary tract infection, papillary necrosis, or just sickling of RBCs in the renal medulla with sludging within the renal arterioles, resulting in extravasation of blood into the tubular urine. If gross hematuria occurs, an IVP should be obtained to determine if papillary necrosis is present or has caused obstruction. The patient should then be treated with oral hydration and bed rest until the bleeding remits, usually in less than a week. If the hemoglobin is less than 10 g/dl, transfusion with packed RBCs to raise the proportion of nonsickling cells is desirable. In the patient with microscopic hematuria only and a negative urine culture, no further therapy is necessary.

Hereditary Nephritis (Alport Syndrome); Benign Familial Hematuria

A family history of hematuria, sensorineural deafness, or males requiring dialysis or transplantation will direct management toward familial forms of hematuria. If the family history is negative but the parents have never been tested, a screening urinalysis on the parents should be done. An audiogram on the patient may identify hereditary nephritis. A renal biopsy with electron microscopic examination of the glomerular basement membrane is often necessary to make the diagnosis. The most affected family member, either the child or an adult relative, should be chosen for biopsy.

No specific therapy currently exists to stop the progression of hereditary nephritis to end-stage renal disease. Most hereditary nephritis is X-linked and an affected male will eventually experience end-stage renal failure in the second to fourth decade of life. Boys should undergo close follow-up of renal function and blood pressure to allow intervention early with supportive therapy (see article on chronic renal failure, p. 360). An affected female is unlikely to develop chronic renal failure but will be a genetic carrier of the disease. At an appropriate age, she should be counseled about her potential to pass the disease on to her sons and daughters.

Benign familial hematuria is autosomal dominant and not associated with proteinuria, renal failure, or deafness. Affected patients do not need long-term follow-up. A letter stating that the patient has benign familial hematuria may be useful to the family so that further medical evaluation is avoided when screening urinalyses are required for school, employment, camp, or athletic physical examinations.

Other

If the medical history and physical examination do not provide a guide to further management, anatomic evaluation of the urinary tract by a screening renal ultrasonographic examination should be done. This imaging test may disclose *polycystic kidney disease, renal vein or artery thrombosis, hydronephrosis or hydroureter,* or *Wilms' tumor* as the source of hematuria; specific therapy can be initiated as described in other articles in this section.

The bladder may not be well visualized by ultrasonography, and cystography may be necessary to diagnose a *bladder hemangioma, rhabdomyosarcoma or carcinoma, bladder diverticulum,* or *foreign body in the bladder or urethra.* Cystoscopy is rarely indicated in the management of hematuria in childhood because bladder tumors are extremely rare and can almost always be found by cystography. *Hemorrhagic posterior urethritis* may be identified by cystoscopy, but therapy, which is reassurance and watchful neglect, is not changed by cystoscopic

TABLE 2. Laboratory Management of Hematuria and Proteinuria

Hematuria	Proteinuria	Hematuria and Proteinuria
Urine culture	24-hour urine protein and creatinine (or spot urine prot/Cr)	BUN, serum creatinine
CBC, platelet count	BUN, serum creatinine	Serum albumin, total protein, cholesterol
PT, PTT, bleeding time if coagulopathy	Serum albumin, total protein, cholesterol	Serum C_3 and C_4, ANA
Sickle cell screen in blacks	Blood glucose	Renal ultrasound
BUN, serum creatinine	Serum C_3 and C_4, ANA	CBC, platelets, PT, PTT, bleeding time
Serum C_3 and C_4, ANA	Renal biopsy if suspect GN	Renal biopsy
ASOT, AHT, anti-DNase B	Renal ultrasound	
Renal biopsy if suspect GN	VCUG for suspected VU reflux	
Renal ultrasound/IVP/VCUG		
24-hour urine calcium and creatinine (or spot urine Ca/Cr)		

Abbreviatons: prot, protein; Cr, creatinine; CBC, complete blood count; PT, prothrombin time; PTT, partial thromboplastin time; BUN, blood urea nitrogen; C_3 and C_4, complement; ANA, antinuclear antibody; ASOT, antistreptolysin O titer; AHT, antihyaluronidase titer; anti-DNase B, antideoxyribonuclease B; GN, glomerulonephritis; IVP, intravenous pyelogram; VCUG, voiding cystourethrogram; VU, vesicoureteral; Ca, calcium.

findings. When bright-red gross hematuria persists or recurs, cystoscopy may be helpful at the time of active bleeding to localize blood to one or both ureteral orifices or to the bladder or urethra.

Nephrocalcinosis; Urolithiasis

Nephrocalcinosis from a variety of causes can result in persistent microscopic and, occasionally, gross hematuria. Nephrocalcinosis is best diagnosed by renal ultrasonographic examination. If the underlying cause is distal renal tubular acidosis, oral bicarbonate supplements will correct the acidosis (see article on renal tubular disorders, p. 381) but significant nephrocalcinosis will not resolve; thus, microscopic hematuria may continue. Nephrocalcinosis can be caused by furosemide therapy in the premature newborn. If possible, discontinue furosemide. Hematuria may persist until the nephrocalcinosis resolves, either spontaneously or with oral chlorothiazide therapy (20 to 30 mg/kg/day divided every 12 hours).

Kidney and bladder stones are uncommon in non–Third World children, but, when they occur, they often cause gross or microscopic hematuria. An underlying disorder, such as oxalosis, hypercalciuria, or a congenital anomaly of the urinary tract with infection, should be sought so that the appropriate specific therapy can be instituted (see article on urolithiasis, p. 381).

Hypercalciuria

Gross or microscopic hematuria may be caused by hypercalciuria in the absence of identifiable urolithiasis. Any child with unexplained hematuria should have a 24-hour urine collection for calcium excretion (normal, <4 mg/kg/day). To ensure adequacy of the collection, creatinine excretion should also be measured (normal, 15 to 25 mg/kg/day). If a 24-hour urine cannot be reliably collected, as in the child with enuresis, screening with a first morning, fasting spot urine specimen for calcium-to-creatinine ratio (normal, <0.21) may be useful, although less reliable diagnostically.

All affected children should be treated preventively with a large daily fluid intake of one and a half to two times the recommended maintenance fluid intake for size, and a reduction in dietary sodium intake to less than 3 g daily. Moderate restriction of calcium intake to no more than 600 mg daily and avoidance of supplemental vitamin D are suggested if the child has absorptive hypercalciuria.

Whether long-term thiazide therapy should be initiated for hypercalciuria without urolithiasis is uncertain. An increased risk of developing urolithiasis exists in affected children, but it is difficult to predict which 15 to 20 per cent may develop stones. Older children with gross hematuria at presentation and a family history of urolithiasis are at greatest risk, but even these parameters are not sensitive enough predictors to recommend that thiazide therapy always be given to this group. The risk-to-benefit ratio of thiazide therapy in children with hematuria and hypercalciuria is still poorly characterized. Long-term thiazide therapy in other children involves the well-known risk of serum electrolyte and other biochemical disturbances. In general, if the child has recurrent gross hematuria and a strong family history of urolithiasis, at least 1 year of oral chlorothiazide (10 to 20 mg/kg/day divided every 12 hours) seems warranted. The decision to continue therapy should be made by individual case.

Any child with hematuria and hypercalciuria should have yearly follow-up to assess the degree of hypercalciuria and the persistence of hematuria. Yearly ultrasonographic examinations have proved to be of little value.

Benign Hematuria

When the entire history, physical, and laboratory evaluation is normal, the patient may be designated as having benign hematuria. Because benign hematuria is a diagnosis of exclusion, long-term follow-up is necessary to affirm this diagnosis. An exact regimen for follow-up is uncertain. Because one would not want to misdiagnose a potentially treatable problem, it may be safe to adopt a 3-month follow-up for the 1st year, every 6 months for the 2nd year, and then annually. Minimum annual follow-up should include a history and physical examination, blood pressure determination, urinalysis, and serum creatinine measurement. The occurrence of poor growth, hypertension, proteinuria, RBC casts, or decreased renal function should prompt extensive re-evaluation.

PROTEINURIA

The character and amount of proteinuria must be determined before appropriate therapy can be instituted. The majority of patients will have glomerular proteinuria. However, patients with renal tubular disorders, such as cystinosis and Lowe's syndrome, may have tubular proteinuria, which is characterized by the predominance of low-molecular-weight (MW) species such as lysozyme (MW 15,000 daltons) and β_2-microglobulin (MW 11,800 daltons). Proteins less than or equal to the MW of albumin (40,000 daltons) are normally filtered by the glomerulus and then reabsorbed and catabolized in the proximal tubule. Patients with tubular disorders or tubular toxicity from drugs such as the aminoglycosides may have 1 to 3+ albuminuria by dipstick but do not need an evaluation for glomerular disease. Therapy should be directed to the specific tubular disorder (see article on renal tubular disorders, p. 422).

Glomerular proteinuria is predominantly albumin or higher-molecular-weight proteins. In the asymptomatic child, urine protein of 1+ (30 mg/dl) by dipstick or greater than 100 mg/m^2 per 24 hours is considered significant and needs further laboratory evaluation. Proteinuria greater than 1000 mg/m^2 per 24 hours (or >40 mg/m^2/hour) is considered to be in the nephrotic range, and the management should be geared toward supportive care and specific therapy of the underlying glomerulonephritis (see article on nephrotic syndrome, p. 357).

Transient Proteinuria

Transient proteinuria usually does not exceed 2+ (100 mg/dl) by dipstick. A variety of causes, including fever, pneumonia, exposure to cold, adrenalin administration, recent seizure, emotional stress, and congestive heart failure, may give rise to transient proteinuria. If transient proteinuria is suspected, the approach to management should be to obtain a follow-up urinalysis in 10 to 14 days. If proteinuria persists after 2 weeks, another cause should be suspected.

Orthostatic Proteinuria

Orthostatic proteinuria is more common in adolescents and rarely occurs before the age of 6 years. The amount of proteinuria usually does not exceed a total of 1000 mg in 24 hours. After quantitating the 24-hour urine protein excretion (checking for adequacy of collection with creatinine excretion), a convenient way to test for orthostatic proteinuria is by home evaluation of urine specimens obtained immediately upon rising in the morning (it is critical that the patient void before going to bed) and after physical activity in the afternoon on several different days. If the urine is consistently negative in the morning and positive in the afternoon, orthostatic proteinuria is likely, and no further evaluation or therapy is needed. If the serial urine dipstick evaluations are equivocal, a split 24-hour urine collection should be collected to compare the protein excretion in 8 to 10 hours of recumbency overnight with 14 to 16 waking hours when upright. If the nighttime recumbent protein excretion is less than 6 mg/m^2/hour and the daytime upright protein excretion is greater than 6 mg/m^2/hour, the patient has orthostatic proteinuria. If there is little difference in the nighttime and daytime protein excretion, the patient has constant proteinuria and another cause should be sought. If the diagnosis of orthostatic proteinuria is made, no therapy is necessary.

Physical activity should not be restricted. Annual or semiannual follow-up, during which blood pressure, urinalysis, and, periodically, serum creatinine are assessed, is necessary to prevent the possibility of missing another renal disease masked initially by the orthostatic character of the proteinuria.

Glomerulonephritis

Persistent, nonorthostatic proteinuria (arbitrarily >6 months or >1000 mg/m^2/day) or the presence of hypertension, impaired renal function, reduced C_3 or C_4, or a positive ANA titer is suggestive of chronic glomerulonephritis and requires a renal biopsy for diagnosis. A variety of forms of chronic glomerulonephritis (see Table 1) may present with isolated proteinuria as the only sign of disease. If proteinuria is in the nephrotic range, patients are initially treated with oral prednisone, but the exact regimen depends on the specific diagnosis. Therapy for each disorder is discussed in detail in the article on nephrotic syndrome (p. 357).

Other

Proteinuria may be the first and only identifiable urinary abnormality of *interstitial nephritis, diabetic nephropathy,* or congenital renal anomalies that produce *vesicoureteral reflux* or *obstructive uropathy.* Laboratory evaluation should always include BUN, serum creatinine, albumin, total protein, cholesterol and glucose determinations, and a renal ultrasound examination should be done. Appropriate therapy for diabetic nephropathy and congenital renal anomalies are discussed in other articles in this section. Interstitial nephritis, either idiopathic or associated with systemic diseases such as streptococcal infection or sarcoidosis, or secondary to hypersensitivity to drugs, is usually accompanied by a decrease in renal function. Renal ultrasonographic examination reveals only normal to slightly enlarged kidneys. Eosinophils in the urine are characteristic of drug-induced acute interstitial nephritis and can be documented by a Hansel's stain of a spot urine.

With the exception of stopping the offending drug, therapy for interstitial nephritis is nonspecific. If renal failure is severe or persists and if acute inflammation is suspected, a short course of daily prednisone (1 mg/kg/day) may lead to improvement. Therapy should be discontinued in 3 to 4 weeks if improvement in renal function does not occur.

HEMATURIA AND PROTEINURIA

The child with both hematuria and proteinuria almost always has a renal parenchymal lesion (Table 1) and requires a renal biopsy. Before a biopsy is performed, the patient's coagulation status should be checked by a complete blood count with platelet count, prothrombin time, partial thromboplastin time, and bleeding time. Aspirin or nonsteroidal anti-inflammatory drugs should be discontinued, if possible, several days to 2 weeks prior to biopsy. The presence of two kidneys of reasonable size should be confirmed by renal ultrasonography before a percutaneous needle biopsy. Otherwise, an open renal biopsy will be needed.

Once a specific glomerulonephritis is diagnosed, appropriate therapy is possible (see article on glomerulonephritis, p. 357). Occasionally, renal vein thrombosis is the cause of hematuria and proteinuria. It is usually diagnosed by ultrasound examination. Appropriate therapy is outlined in the article on renal vein thrombosis (p. 357).

RENAL TUBULAR DISORDERS

JUAN RODRÍGUEZ-SORIANO, M.D.

CYSTINURIA

Cystinuria is an autosomal recessive disease characterized by the excessive urinary excretion of cystine and dibasic amino acids (lysine, ornithine, and arginine). The basic abnormality is a transport defect present both in renal tubular epithelium and in intestinal mucosa. The increased cystine excretion leads to precipitation in the form of cystine stones. Treatment is indicated only in homozygous subjects and is directed toward the prevention of stone formation and the dissolution of stones that have already been formed.

Because crystallization of cystine depends mainly on its concentration in the urine (crystallization occurs when cystine concentration exceeds 300 mg/L at a urine pH between 4.5 and 7.0, which increases to about 500 mg/L at a urine pH of 7.5 or above), the most important therapeutic measure is the combined administration of large amounts of fluid and alkaline salts. Morning urine should be checked for pH, aiming to obtain values above 7.5. Unfortunately, this regimen has had limited success because, for many patients, especially children, it is often difficult to follow.

An alternative therapy is to decrease urinary excretion of cystine to levels that are below the crystallization range. The safest way to obtain these levels is to restrict salt intake. In adults, the reduction of sodium intake to about 50 mmol/day, along with a high fluid intake, contributes to maintaining a safe range of cystine excretion. Similar data are not yet available for children, but there is no reason to expect a different therapeutic effect.

If stone formation cannot be prevented by decreasing cystine excretion to below the crystallization range, the best option is to initiate treatment with D-penicillamine (Cuprimine). D-Penicillamine (in a divided dose of 30 mg/kg/day), is a dimethylcysteine that reduces cystine excretion by reacting with cystine to form a more soluble mixed disulfide. Its success depends in great part on a careful monitoring of urinary cystine excretion, which should be kept below 200 to 300 mg/day/1.73 m^2. The main disadvantage of this therapy derives from the undesirable side effects of D-penicillamine administration, including fever and rash, leukopenia, proteinuria and nephrotic syndrome, systemic lupus erythematosus, collagen abnormalities, and loss of taste. D-Penicillamine is a powerful vitamin B_6 antagonist, and patients on long-term therapy should always receive a supplementary dose (100 mg/day) of pyridoxine.

Other therapies are of little value in children. A low-methionine diet also reduces cystine excretion, but its value is questioned because of poor patient compliance. Captopril, an angiotensin II–converting enzyme inhibitor, reduces cystine excretion by forming a more soluble compound, but its use in children has not been successful.

FANCONI SYNDROME

Renal Fanconi syndrome represents a clinical entity characterized by a multiple dysfunction of the proximal tubule, which leads to glycosuria, generalized aminoaciduria, hyperphosphaturia, and proximal renal tubular acidosis. Other abnormalities of renal tubular function (tubular proteinuria, hyperuricosuria, hypercalciuria, renal loss of sodium and potassium, diminished concentrating capacity) also may be present. Glomerular filtration rate is not affected initially but may decline secondarily. The main consequences of the tubular dysfunction are growth retardation, polyuria, hypophosphatemic rickets, hypokalemia, and metabolic acidosis. Fanconi syndrome may be either idiopathic or secondary to a variety of causes. Nephropathic cystinosis represents the most important cause of infantile Fanconi syndrome.

The clinical course and prognosis of the syndrome depend on the specific cause. In general, secondary forms may improve or disappear when the cause is avoided or some therapy is possible. In the primary forms, only supportive care may be offered, which aims to treat or prevent rickets, correct the acidosis and hypokalemia, and maintain a normal fluid balance. However, little effect on growth is to be expected.

Supportive Care

Bone lesions of *rickets* and *osteoporosis* are resistant to regular vitamin D therapy and are best treated with oral phosphate supplements and active metabolites of vitamin D. Hypophosphatemia can be partly compensated by oral administration of neutral phosphate (1 to 3 g/day in a divided dose to avoid vomiting, diarrhea, or abdominal discomfort). Various solutions are available. Joulie's solution contains 145 g $Na_2HPO_4 \cdot 7H_2O$ and 18.2 g $NaH_2PO_4 \cdot H_2O$ dissolved in 1 L of water with syrup base and provides 30.4 mg of elemental phosphorus per ml. A marketed product is K-Phos-Neutral, which yields 250 mg of elemental phosphorus per tablet. Calcitriol or 1,25-$(OH)_2D_3$ (Rocaltrol) is given at the initial dose of 15 to 20 ng/kg/day and is increased over several months to a maintenance dose of 30 to 60 ng/kg/day. High doses of vitamin D (up to 2000 to 4000 units/kg/day) or dihydrotachysterol (up to 10 to 25 μg/kg/day) may also be used successfully. As often as monthly check-ups of serum calcium and urinary calcium-to-creatinine ratio are recommended. Repeat renal ultrasonographic studies may provide early detection of nephrocalcinosis. It should be remembered that hypocalcemic tetany can be initiated by acute alkalinization, especially if citrate or bicarbonate is administered at the same time as phosphate.

Patients with Fanconi syndrome waste bicarbonate and thus have *proximal renal tubular acidosis* (RTA). Chronic acidosis interferes with normal growth and contributes to the development of bone lesions. In proximal RTA, treatment must compensate for the urinary losses of bicarbonate and for the endogenous production of acid. Because patients with this disorder often excrete more than 10 per cent of the filtered amount of bicarbonate when the serum level is brought within the normal range, the minimal starting dose of alkali is between 6 and 10 mmol/kg/day; however, larger doses are frequently needed. Alkali administration enhances the urinary loss of potassium, and the preparations used should include both sodium and potassium salts.

Because citrate excretion is not decreased, there is no special need to give the anion in the form of citrate; a mixture of sodium and potassium bicarbonate (1:1) can be given with excellent results. However, bicarbonate ingestion may cause bloating and flatulence; citrate salts are often more palatable. A solution containing 2 g citric acid, 3 g sodium citrate, and 3.3 g potassium citrate/30 ml nonalcoholic syrup base (Polycitra) provides 1 mmol of sodium and 1 mmol of potassium/1 ml. It is better tolerated when diluted in juice, water, or formula. The aim of treatment is to maintain as normal a serum bicarbonate level as possible day and night; thus, doses should be frequent, with the last one as late at night as possible.

In very severe forms of proximal RTA, alkali alone may be ineffective because of the gastrointestinal intolerance to the enormous doses needed or because of rapid loss of the base into the urine. Also, progressive increases in the amount of sodium and potassium salts administered may expand the extracellular fluid volume and be paradoxically followed by a worsening of metabolic acidosis and hypokalemia. In these circumstances, hydrochlorothiazide may be useful because it improves renal bicarbonate reabsorption and allows the dose of alkali to be reduced. The initial dose of hydrochlorothiazide is about 1.5 to 2 mg/kg/day divided into two doses; however, after correction of the acidosis, a smaller dose may be sufficient. An additional benefit of hydrochlorothiazide in patients with Fanconi syndrome is the diminution of urinary calcium and phosphate excretion with subsequent improvement of rickets. However, hydrochlorothiazide administration enhances urinary potassium losses and increases the risk of developing hypokalemia.

Hypokalemia is a frequent finding in Fanconi syndrome and always requires correction. The aim of therapy is to keep serum potassium levels as normal as possible and always above 3.0 mmol/L, if possible. Although potassium is generally given (mixed with sodium citrate) to correct the acidosis, an additive amount may be necessary. A solution of 2 g citric acid and 6.6 g potassium citrate/30 ml nonalcoholic syrup base (Polycitra K) contains 2 mmol of potassium/1 ml. If acidosis is not present, potassium may be given as the gluconate, phosphate, or chloride salt.

When *polyuria* is present, fluid intake must be increased in order to avoid dehydration. A good practice, especially in infants, is to dissolve the required salts in the minimal amount of fluid required for the whole day. Additional water is also given, if necessary. It must be remembered that an excessive fluid intake may lead to overexpansion of extracellular fluid volume and aggravation of proximal tubular dysfunction. Acute management of fluid and electrolyte disturbances may be extraordinarily difficult in infants with Fanconi syndrome secondary to nephropathic cystinosis. In selected cases, it may be useful to administer indomethacin (Indocin, 2 to 5 mg/kg/day). Indomethacin induces a marked improvement in proximal tubular function and reduces the abnormal urinary losses.

Carnitine deficiency may develop in patients with Fanconi syndrome and requires oral L-carnitine supplementation. L-Carnitine (100 mg/kg/day in divided doses every 6 hours) quickly normalizes serum free carnitine levels. Whether muscle carnitine deficiency is also corrected can be assured only by muscle biopsy.

Specific Therapy

Nephropathic cystinosis is an autosomal recessive disorder characterized by the accumulation of cystine within body tissues due to a defect in cystine transport across lysosomal membranes. The increased content of cystine has a deleterious effect on many enzymatic systems and leads to cell death. Many organs are involved, including kidney, thyroid, eye, liver, pancreas, brain, and muscle. The child presents at a young age with Fanconi syndrome; however, a progressive and unremitting glomerular failure develops, and "renal death" takes place before the patient is 10 years of age.

Although supportive care is also of paramount importance, there is strong evidence that *cysteamine* therapy, when started early, may slow down the progression to terminal renal failure. Cysteamine is a free thiol that depletes cystine stores from cells by reacting with cystine to form a cystine-cysteamine mixed disulfide that is able to egress from the cytosolic lysosomes by means of an intact lysine carrier system. Cysteamine is given every 6 hours as an oral cysteamine hydrochloride solution containing 50 mg/ml. The starting dose of 10 mg/kg/day must be increased every 2 weeks to reach a dose of 50 mg/kg/day. Thereafter, the dose must be titrated to maintain leukocyte cystine levels below 1 nmol ½cystine/mg of protein. The dose should not exceed 90 mg/kg/day. This therapy should ideally be given shortly after birth, which is possible when cystinosis is diagnosed early because a sibling was affected. With early treatment, glomerular function is significantly preserved and linear growth is clearly improved. When therapy is started later, especially when glomerular damage has already occurred, the benefit to the kidney is less apparent; however, the therapy may contribute to preserve the function of other organs (eye, thyroid, pancreas, brain, and muscle).

The taste and smell of cysteamine are very repulsive and may result in a high noncompliance rate. Therefore, the use of *phosphocysteamine* is a possible alternative. This drug has cystine-depleting effects similar to those of cysteamine but does not have its offensive odor because cysteamine is formed by intestinal hydrolysis and is quickly absorbed. Corneal crystal deposition may also be improved by the use of cysteamine eye drops, although results are still preliminary.

Unfortunately, although early cysteamine therapy offers some hope for cystinotic patients, many still progress to end-stage renal failure at the end of their first decade. Renal transplantation has represented an important advance because transplanted kidneys do not accumulate cystine and do not suffer a progressive functional deterioration as a consequence of cystine deposits. In fact, the rate of rejection in patients with cystinosis appears to be significantly lower than in children with other chronic renal diseases. The success of renal transplantation has permitted children with cystinosis to live to adulthood, thus allowing the damage of many organs besides the kidney to become evident. The appearance of these complications (hypothyroidism, progressive blindness, diabetes mellitus, pancreatic exocrine dysfunction, myopathy, cerebral atrophy) mandates consideration of the use of cysteamine even after renal transplantation and, probably, for the lifetime of the patient.

RENAL TUBULAR ACIDOSIS

The term renal tubular acidosis is applied to a group of transport defects in the reabsorption of filtered bicarbonate or in the excretion of hydrogen ion or both. The RTA syndromes are characterized by a relatively normal glomerular filtration rate and a metabolic acidosis accompanied by hypokalemia and a normal plasma anion gap. On clinical and pathophysiologic grounds, RTA can be classified as *proximal RTA* (type 2), which is caused by a primary defect in proximal tubular bicarbonate reabsorption; *distal RTA* (type 1), which is caused by an impaired distal hydrogen ion secretion; and *hyperkalemic RTA* (type 4), which is due to impaired ammoniagenesis and is associated with aldosterone deficiency.

Proximal RTA

Proximal RTA may occur in children as a primary and isolated entity or may be accompanied by other proximal tubular defects (Fanconi syndrome). Therapy of proximal RTA as observed in the Fanconi syndrome was discussed previously. When proximal RTA presents as an isolated entity, the correction does not specifically require potassium. Alkali can be given in the form of sodium bicarbonate or sodium citrate (a useful preparation is Shohl's solution, which contains 140 g citric acid and 98 g sodium citrate dissolved in water to a total volume of a liter; 1 ml provides 1 mmol sodium). Primary proximal RTA manifests clinically with growth failure and persistent vomiting in early infancy. Alkali therapy induces a rapid increase in growth rate and can be discontinued after several years without reappearance of symptoms. The self-limited course of infantile proximal RTA contrasts with that of distal RTA, which appears to be persistent even when clinical onset is in infancy.

Distal RTA

Treatment of distal RTA consists of giving enough alkali to maintain correction of the acidosis and normalization of urinary excretion of calcium and citrate. Potassium is also needed, regardless of the serum potassium value, and, in cases of severe hypokalemia, it should be given before correcting the acidosis. Although the effects of sodium bicarbonate on acid-base homeostasis are indistinguishable from those of sodium citrate, the latter should be preferred because it is more effective in increasing urinary excretion of citrate. The amount of sodium and potassium bicarbonate needed to correct the acidosis is often not enough to raise the low citrate excretion. Therefore, treatment is best accomplished with Polycitra. The total dose of citrate is mainly determined by the concomitant excretion of bicarbonate and is equal to the urinary bicarbonate excretion plus about 2 mmol/kg/day to compensate for endogenous acid production. Therapeutic requirements may be as high as 10 to 15 mmol/kg/day during the first years of life, decreasing to about 3 mmol/kg/day in older children.

The aim of treatment is not only to correct the acidosis but also to normalize calcium excretion and thus prevent further development of nephrocalcinosis and nephrolithiasis. Unfortunately, parenchymal calcification already present is not reversible. The efficacy of treatment, when started early in infancy, is demonstrated by normal growth and complete arrest of further nephrocalcinosis. If excessive doses of alkali are used, the overexpansion of extracellular fluid volume leads to a paradoxical increase in urinary calcium excretion, which is rapidly corrected when doses are reduced.

Other therapeutic measures are of little or doubtful value. Vitamin D is generally not needed. Hydrochlorothiazide is not only of limited benefit but is also potentially dangerous because it may aggravate the hypokalemia. Patients treated for distal RTA are at risk of pseudoephedrine intoxication when this drug is used because its renal excretion is minimal in alkalinized urine.

Hyperkalemic RTA

The cause of hyperkalemic RTA should be found in order to manage this disorder adequately. Potassium-retaining drugs should be discontinued at once. If there is extracellular fluid volume contraction, it should be corrected; this is critical in patients with salt-losing aldosterone deficiency. In patients with chronic renal disease and hyporeninemic hypoaldosteronism, treatment decisions should be made from the symptoms and the severity of the hyperkalemia. Acidosis and hyperkalemia may be corrected by high doses of fludrocortisone. Prolonged treatment, however, may be complicated by excessive salt retention, with increased risk of cardiovascular compromise or arterial hypertension. Reduction of potassium intake and potassium-binding resins or, preferably, periodic administration of furosemide will allow the dose of fludrocortisone to be reduced, thus preventing such complications. In many cases, sodium bicarbonate or citrate (~ 2 mmol/kg/day) is also necessary.

Patients with primary or secondary pseudohypoaldosteronism do not respond to exogenous mineralocorticoids and must be treated with salt supplements. Sustained correction of volume contraction is followed, in most cases, by correction of hyperkalemia and metabolic acidosis, without need of additional alkali. In primary pseudohypoaldosteronism, salt supplements (3 to 6 g/day) may be generally discontinued at about 2 years of age without reappearance of symptoms. In exceptional cases, the salt supplement is needed throughout childhood.

Mineralocorticoids are also ineffective in the so-called "chloride-shunt" syndrome or Gordon syndrome. This disease, also called Spitzer syndrome when arterial hypertension is absent, represents an inherited tendency to hyperreabsorb the filtered sodium chloride, which leads to short stature, metabolic acidosis, hyperkalemia, and hyporeninemic hypoaldosteronism. Hypertension is an important feature in adolescents and young adults but not in children. Symptoms are rapidly improved by dietary salt restriction or administration of diuretics. Furosemide has been recommended, but it aggravates the hypercalciuria that is frequently present in this syndrome. The ideal treatment is the administration of hydrochlorothiazide, which is as effective as furosemide in the reversal of hyperkalemia and metabolic acidosis but also corrects the hypercalciuria.

BARTTER SYNDROME

Bartter syndrome, as observed in infants and children, is an autosomal recessive disorder characterized by hypokalemia, metabolic alkalosis, and normal blood pressure despite hyperplasia of the juxtaglomerular apparatus, hyper-reninemia, and hyperaldosteronism. The syndrome starts in infancy with failure to thrive, anorexia, vomiting, polyuria, polydipsia, tendency to dehydration, salt craving, and muscle wasting. Tetany is rare in children and is observed more frequently in adults. Short stature is common in children presenting with the symptoms early in life. More rarely, these children present with rickets, nephrocalcinosis, gout, or oligophrenia. An extremely severe neonatal form is characterized by hydramnios, prematurity, hypercalciuria, and nephrocalcinosis. Bartter syndrome is associated with a chloride reabsorption defect in the distal nephron, which results in potassium wasting, hypokalemia, and increased secretion of prostaglandins. Concomitant elevations of plasma renin activity and angiotensin II stimulate aldosterone secretion but do not cause arterial hypertension because the vasoconstrictive effect of angiotensin II is opposed by the vasodilatory effect of prostacyclin.

Treatment

Treatment of Bartter syndrome must include an attempt to correct the hypokalemia. Potassium chloride supplements (1 to 3 mmol/kg/day, up to 500 mmol/day) are always necessary. The amount needed will change according to the patient, and the supplement must balance the amount of potassium wasted by the kidney. Unfortunately, potassium supplements alone are almost completely ineffective in most cases because the administered potassium is quickly lost into the urine. Addition of spironolactone (Aldactone, 10 to 15 mg/kg/day) or triamterene (Dyazide, 10 mg/kg/day) may be initially effective in the control of the hypokalemia, but this effect is often very transient. The administration of a β-adrenergic inhibitor such as propranolol (1 mg/kg/day) does not offer any additive advantage.

Therapy of Bartter syndrome is today best accomplished by the use of prostaglandin synthesis inhibitors: indomethacin (Indocin, 2 to 5 mg/kg/day); acetylsalicylic acid (aspirin, 100 mg/kg/day); ibuprofen (30 mg/kg/day); or ketoprofen (Orudis, 20 mg/kg/day). Indomethacin is the drug most frequently used and is remarkably well tolerated by these patients, although attention should be paid to signs of intolerance or toxicity such as nausea, vomiting, abdominal pain, peptic ulcer, hematopoietic toxicity, or liver damage. The possibility of developing pseudotumor cerebri should also be considered because it has been reported to occur after both indomethacin and ketoprofen therapy. The early effect of prostaglandin inhibition is spectacular, with improved well-being, strength, and activity, diminution of polyuria and polydipsia, and instauration of normal or even catch-up growth. There is an immediate increase in serum potassium values; these, however, rarely rise above 3.5 mmol/L. Plasma renin activity and aldosterone concentration decrease to a normal range, and the vascular response to angiotensin II or noradrenaline also normalizes. The only renal tubular defect that remains unmodified after indomethacin therapy is the tubular impairment in sodium chloride reabsorption, which is therefore believed to constitute the primary metabolic event.

Addition of magnesium salts should always be considered when hypomagnesemia is present because magnesium deficiency may aggravate potassium wasting. Although many magnesium salts have been used in the treatment of hypomagnesemic states, we consider the use of magnesium chloride ($MgCl_2$), which also compensates for ongoing urinary chloride losses, to be preferable. Each milliliter of a 5 per cent solution contains approximately 0.5 mEq (6 mg) of Mg^{2+}. The total dose should be individualized for each patient and given at intervals of 6 to 8 hours.

The efficacy of long-term use of prostaglandin synthesis inhibitors has been clearly established. With time there is some recurrence of hypokalemia and hyper-reninemia, but clinical improvement is generally maintained. If the symptoms reappear, the dose of indomethacin should be readjusted or a combined therapy of indomethacin and spironolactone should be initiated. In adults, angiotensin II–converting enzyme inhibitors (captopril, enalapril) have been also tried, with conflicting results. There are no data on angiotensin II–converting enzyme inhibitor use in children.

NEPHROGENIC DIABETES INSIPIDUS

Nephrogenic diabetes insipidus (NDI) is an X-linked recessive disorder characterized by a resistance to the antidiuretic action of both endogenous and exogenous vasopressin. The basic defect is unknown, but linkage analysis of affected families has permitted mapping of the NDI gene to the distal long arm of the X chromosome. This gene induces a defect in the functioning of the renal receptors (V_2) for vasopressin, but the vascular receptors (V_1) retain a normal response to the hormone.

Treatment

Therapy consists of lifetime administration of water in amount and frequency necessary to compensate for the obligatory urinary loss, thus avoiding chronic dehydration, hyperelectrolytemia, and secondary neurologic damage. This goal is easily attained in older children and adults, but great difficulties may be encountered in infants, especially when thirst is absent. Administration of solute-poor milk reduces urinary water requirements and helps to maintain an adequate water balance. Occasionally, it is necessary to give water around-the-clock through a gastric tube to allow the infant prolonged periods of rest. This procedure is extremely important to prevent subclinical nocturnal dehydration.

The discovery that hydrochlorothiazide decreases urinary output has enormously facilitated the management of NDI patients, especially during infancy. The decrease in urinary volume observed following administration of the diuretic is accompanied by an increased concentration of urinary solutes and decreased clearance of free water. It has been shown that the effect is mediated through sodium depletion, with increased proximal tubular reaborption of sodium and decreased delivery of fluid to the distal nephron. Hydrochlorothiazide also increases the inner medullary osmolality and thus favors passive water reabsorption from the collecting duct. The recommended dose is 1.5 to 2 mg/kg/day, accompanied by a moderate restriction of salt intake (~ 1.2 mmol/kg/day). Giving sodium chloride in excess interferes with the antidiuretic effect. However, prolonged thiazide therapy increases kaliuresis and may induce the development of profound hypokalemia. The simultaneous administration of potassium supplements is necessary in most cases.

As a result of the limited benefit and possible complications of thiazide administration, other drugs have also been used, generally in association with thiazide therapy. Prostaglandin synthesis inhibitors, such as indomethacin (2 to 5 mg/kg/day), acetylsalicylic acid (100 mg/kg/day), ibuprofen (30 mg/kg/day), or ketoprofen (20 mg/kg/day), have also shown a beneficial effect on urinary output, additive to the antidiuretic effect of hydrochlorothiazide. Hydrochlorothiazide administration reduces urinary output by about 20 to 50 per cent, and indomethacin reduces urinary output by another 20 to 30 per cent. This combined therapy is especially useful in infants and young children. The mechanism by which prostaglandin inhibitors reduce urinary output in patients with NDI is not known but is probably related to a reduction in glomerular filtration rate with a proportional increase in proximal tubular reabsorption of water and sodium. As mentioned in the discussion of Bartter syndrome, prolonged use of prostaglandin synthesis inhibitors may cause renal, gastrointestinal, hematopoietic, and central nervous system complications, and such therapy should be carefully followed.

The safest therapy that can be offered today to infants and children with NDI is the combined administration of hydrochlorothiazide (1.5 to 2 mg/kg/day) and amiloride (0.2 to 0.3 mg/kg/day). This drug combination is marketed in tablets containing 50 mg of hydrochlorothiazide and 5 mg of amiloride hydrochloride. With this therapy, along with moderate dietary salt restriction, urinary volume does not differ significantly from that obtained with combined hydrochlorothiazide-indomethacin therapy, but lesser side effects occur. Amiloride also has an additive antidiuretic effect, probably by further increasing sodium excretion, reducing extracellular fluid volume, and enhancing water and sodium reabsorption in the proximal tubule. Amiloride has antikaliuretic properties, and, when given in association with hydrochlorothiazide, there is no need for potassium supplementation.

ACUTE RENAL FAILURE

KAREN M. GAUDIO, M.D.

Acute renal failure is a frequent clinical problem for the pediatrician, neonatologist, and surgeon. The disorder is characterized by a rapid decline in renal function with progressive azotemia, which is usually, although not always, accompanied by oliguria. It commonly occurs in the postoperative setting of complicated cardiac surgery; following trauma, sepsis, drug toxicity, or severe dehydration; or secondary to hemolytic uremic syndrome or glomerulonephritis.

The aim of the clinician is, first, to reverse any life-threatening abnormality of electrolytes or fluid balance and to maintain homeostasis and euvolemia, and, second, to eliminate or treat any underlying problems that may complicate or prolong renal failure. Thus, the clinician must focus on

1. Maintaining renal perfusion with fluid or other supportive measures.
2. Administering appropriate antibiotics if acute renal failure is associated with sepsis.
3. Investigating the possibility of urinary tract obstruction. Only patients with bilateral obstruction, obstruction of a solitary kidney, or obstruction of the urethral outlet will develop acute renal failure. This may be caused by tumor, stones, or, in the case of neonates, posterior urethral valves.
4. Minimizing the use of nephrotoxins (including radiocontrast dyes, amino glycosides, amphotericin B, antineoplastic agents, and cyclosporin).
5. Supporting the patient nutritionally to prevent catabolism.

Most problems encountered in acute renal failure are treated with standard supportive therapy, although, at times, renal replacement therapy may be necessary.

SHOCK AND DEHYDRATION

In an emergent situation, the child with fluid depletion, regardless of an anuric state, needs replacement with isotonic fluids such as normal saline or Ringer's lactate. The solution should be infused at the rate of 20 ml/kg body weight over 30 to 60 minutes. If bleeding accounts for circulatory insufficiency, blood should be used. If the only cause of anuria is fluid depletion, volume repletion should restore urine flow within 6 hours or less. If fluid resuscitation has not occurred by that time, central venous monitoring may be required to assess volume status.

SUPPORTIVE FLUID THERAPY

Fluid management in children with acute renal failure warrants careful monitoring of blood pressure, weight, fluid intake, and urine output. The estimation of fluid status depends largely on the physical examination as well as on laboratory tests. Fluid intake must be restricted to insensible losses (pulmonary and cutaneous), which are estimated to be one third of daily maintenance fluid requirements in an afebrile child.

It is important to assess each child and the situation carefully. For example, maintenance fluid requirements increase by 12 per cent per degree Celsius above 37°C in a child with fever. Also, in neonates, especially preterm, great care is required to achieve adequate fluid and salt balance because their glomerular filtration rate is low. The renal tubules are immature and unable to handle either salt deprivation or excesses, in part because of immaturity in both the renin-angiotensin-aldosterone system and the distal tubule response to aldosterone. In addition, neonates experience increased insensible losses as a result of greater body surface–to–volume ratios and less cutaneous keratinization. Because the use of phototherapy, warming lights, and humidified oxygen affects fluid losses in premature infants, these therapies must be considered in approximating daily fluid balance and replacement.

Children in the diuretic phase during recovery from acute renal failure or postobstructive diuresis also need special attention to volume and electrolyte losses. Quantitative replacement, especially in the younger child, is preferable. For example, a solution containing the appropriate electrolytes is given in equal amounts of urine excreted. Replacement fluids can be progressively decreased as the renal function returns to normal.

If an appropriate volume of fluids is given, serum sodium

levels will remain stable and the body weight will decrease by 0.5 to 1 per cent per day. If serum sodium levels fall and body weight increases, excess fluids are being given. If serum sodium rises and weight falls, insufficient fluids are being administered.

HYPERKALEMIA

A serum potassium level that is greater than or equal to 7.0 mmol/L is an emergency and necessitates immediate treatment. An electrocardiogram (EKG) is particularly helpful in assessing the pathophysiologic impact of an elevated serum potassium level. Specific changes in EKG tracings are associated with varying degrees of hyperkalemia: (1) widening of the QRS complex, (2) S-T wave depression, and (3) peaked T waves. These EKG changes are not found in every patient with hyperkalemia, and the serum potassium level at which they occur may also vary.

Immediate therapy for hyperkalemia involves intravenous infusion of calcium gluconate, sodium bicarbonate, or glucose and insulin. Ten per cent calcium gluconate (0.5 ml/kg IV over 2 to 4 minutes) is reserved primarily for patients with EKG changes and acts more quickly than alternative therapies. Because of the action of calcium on the myocardium, EKG monitoring should be used when calcium is infused. Despite its brief duration, sodium bicarbonate (2 to 3 mEq/kg over 30 to 60 minutes) is an appropriate agent in patients whose acute renal failure is complicated by acidosis, which may exaggerate the hyperkalemia. However, sodium bicarbonate must be given with caution because it will contribute to volume overload and hypertension and will also favor a decrease in calcium concentrations through the effect of pH on protein charge and increased calcium binding. Glucose (0.5 g/kg) is given with insulin (0.1 units/kg over 30 minutes). These therapies simply shift the potassium from the extracellular to the intracellular space, and the patient usually requires definitive correction of potassium overload, which can be accomplished with either ion exchange resins or dialysis.

Patients with a serum potassium level lower than 7 mEq/L and without concomitant EKG changes can be treated with polystyrene sulfonate ion exchange resins (Kayexalate, 1 g/kg body weight suspended in sorbitol, either orally or rectally). Dosing schedules depend on the individual case but may be every 4 to 6 hours. Children are less successful in retaining the resin rectally than adults, and inflating the balloon of a urinary catheter inserted into the rectum may aid in retention. The volume status of the child must be followed closely because the resin, which exchanges sodium for potassium, will contribute to a volume load. Hyperkalemia of less striking proportions can often be treated with dietary restrictions. In the severely hyperglycemic diabetic patient, correction of the blood glucose may also correct hyperkalemia. Finally, the physician must be alert to the causes of acute renal failure associated with ongoing release of potassium from intracellular stores (e.g., rhabdomyolysis, sepsis, postoperative states, trauma, and tumor-lysis syndrome).

HYPONATREMIA

Manifestations of hyponatremia are related to the central nervous system and include change of mental status, loss of consciousness, or seizures. These symptoms occur when the serum sodium level falls precipitously and are usually not found unless the value is below 120 mEq/L. In such cases, hypertonic saline (3 per cent NaCl), which is approximately 0.5 mEq/ml, can be given cautiously at a rate of 12 ml/kg to increase the serum sodium level by approximately 10 mEq/L. Patients with adequate urine output can be treated with normal saline supplemented by a diuretic. The serum sodium level should not be corrected quickly in order to avoid the dangers of central pontine myelinosis and the risk of permanent central nervous system damage. However, hyponatremia is usually mild, results from continued intake of dilute fluid without adequate amounts of sodium, and can be treated successfully with fluid restriction.

HYPOCALCEMIA AND HYPERPHOSPHATEMIA

In acute renal failure, hypocalcemia is generally the result of hyperphosphatemia and can be treated with oral phosphate binders. However, if hypocalcemia is associated with convulsions, tetany, or cardiac arrhythmias, calcium should be given as a constant intravenous infusion. In children, 10 per cent calcium gluconate solutions are diluted to 2 per cent solutions and given 0.1 mmol calcium/kg/hour. Values of ionized calcium should be monitored every 4 to 6 hours. When acidosis is being corrected concomitantly, hypocalcemia may be corrected more slowly or may actually worsen because alkalinization of serum pH will promote binding of calcium to proteins.

METABOLIC ACIDOSIS

Arterial blood gases should be determined in all patients presenting with acute renal failure; patients with a blood pH less than 7.25 and a bicarbonate level less than 12 mEq/L should receive bicarbonate therapy. Sodium bicarbonate should be given only when there is maximal respiratory compensation (i.e., $P_{CO_2} < 25$ torr) and the acidosis is contributing to other abnormalities (e.g., hyperkalemia). The bicarbonate deficit can be calculated as

$$\text{mEq} = (24 - \text{observed bicarbonate}) \times 0.5 \times \text{body weight}$$

When indicated, half of this amount should be given intravenously over 2 to 4 hours, followed by a repeated check of the acid-base status. The infusion continues at the same rate until blood pH is greater than 7.25 and bicarbonate level is greater than 12 mEq/L.

HYPERTENSION

Hypertension in patients with acute renal failure is frequently due to volume overload and can be managed by attaining euvolemia. However, antihypertensive agents are necessary in symptomatic patients or patients with persistently elevated diastolic pressure above the 95th percentile. Two drugs that are efficacious and safe are hydralazine (0.2 to 0.5 mg/kg per dose IV or IM every 4 to 8 hours, not exceeding 15 mg) and nifedipine (0.3 mg/kg sublingually). In extreme cases, one can use nitroprusside (0.5 μg/kg/minute) or diazoxide (2 to 3 mg/kg IV push). For patients with residual renal function, diuresis can be attempted. In most cases, however, the control of blood pressure is directly linked to the volume status and salt intake, and dialysis may be required for fluid removal.

CONVULSIONS

Many of the previously described problems in acute renal failure may produce seizures, including hyponatremia, hypocalcemia, and hypertension. Correction of these potential causes is important in the treatment of the seizures, which often do not remit unless the underlying disturbance is corrected. Intravenous diazepam (0.2 mg/kg) can be given slowly and repeated at 15-minute intervals. Alternative agents are phenytoin and phenobarbital. Because protein binding of these agents is often diminished in uremia, children may suffer adverse side effects at lower doses than expected unless drug levels, including free concentrations of these agents, are followed.

MEDICATIONS

Aminoglycosides, nonsteroidal anti-inflammatory agents, and radiocontrast media should be avoided in children with acute renal failure because these medications may enhance renal damage. In addition the dose or dosing intervals of many medications need to be adjusted because the kidney is the primary route of excretion from the body. Trompeter has provided a comprehensive review of drug prescribing in children with renal insufficiency (see References). In order to use the tables in that review, one must estimate the glomerular filtration rate. It is important to remember that the serum creatinine increases by 0.5 to 1.5 mg/dl/day with the onset of the acute renal failure. Therefore, during the first several days after onset, the serum creatinine may be numerically elevated to 2 or 3 mg/dl but the overall filtration rate will be very low (<10 ml/minute).

NUTRITION

Infants and children with acute renal failure are at great risk for malnutrition because their metabolic rate per unit body weight is high and their body store of nutrients is low. Therefore, nutritional supplementation is implemented early in children with acute renal failure even if it hastens or increases the requirements for dialysis. A variety of protein supplements of high biologic value and essential amino acid solutions are available in concentrated volumes. Oral or enteral feedings are preferable whenever possible because they are less invasive and more physiologic. Gastric feedings may be used intermittently or continuously and should be given in small amounts of diluted solutions that are gradually increased to meet the estimated needs of the child. Because most of the solutions are hyperosmolar, one may be limited by the development of cramps, abdominal distention, or diarrhea in the patient. If enteral feeding is inadequate for the delivery of the required calories and vitamins needed by each individual child, it can be combined with parenteral methods. Often, many of the more seriously ill and hypercatabolic patients will require nutrition through a central line in conjunction with dialysis in order to receive adequate calories. There are no recipes, however, that eliminate the necessity for assessment of each individual child, including frequent monitoring of weight, blood pressure, and chemistries and adequate quantitation of fluid input and output.

Many metabolic pertubations occur in patients with acute renal failure and contribute to complications observed during nutritional supplementation. For example, glucose intolerance and hyperglycemia may require insulin therapy. Metabolic acidosis and hyperammonemia often occur in small premature infants. Another problem often encountered in the small infant secondary to the use of lipid solutions (necessary to maintain the level of essential fatty acids) is displacement of albumin-bound bilirubin. This phenomenon may cause congestion of small vessels in the lung, thereby complicating the course of hyperbilirubinemia and respiratory distress syndrome. Also, caution should be used in providing lipids to any patient with sepsis, as these compounds are taken up by the reticuloendothelial system and can compromise the activity of this system. Hypermagnesemia, changes in serum calcium and phosphate, and deficits in copper and zinc can generally be controlled by adjustment of the infusate composition. Investigations in the future will need to be directed toward optimal composition of nutritional solutions, the role of nonessential and branched chain amino acids, and other sources of calories.

TABLE 1. Relative Advantages and Disadvantages of Hemofiltration (HF), Peritoneal Dialysis (PD), and Hemodialysis (HD)

Relative Advantages
Simple technique: HF, PD
Continuous: HF, PD
Gentle fluid shifts: HF, PD
No heparin required: PD, ± HF
Easy access: PD
Efficiency: HD (greatest)
Relative Disadvantages
Vascular access required: HF, HD
Hemorrhage possible: HF, HD
Inadequate solute removal: HF
Respiratory compromise: PD
Hyperglycemia: PD
Protein loss: PD
Peritonitis: PD
Requires special staff and equipment: HD, ± HF
Disequilibration: HD
Heparinzation: HD, ± HF
Profound hemodynamic changes: HD, ± HF

RENAL REPLACEMENT THERAPY

Replacement therapy is indicated in the presence of intractable congestive heart failure or pulmonary edema; when electrolyte abnormalities (hyperkalemia, metabolic acidosis, hyponatremia or hypernatremia) do not improve with medical management; and if adequate nutritional supplementation is hindered by fluid restriction. Once the decision to initiate replacement therapy is made, the specific type of procedure (hemofiltration, peritoneal dialysis, or hemodialysis) that would be most beneficial to the clinical situation needs to be addressed. The relative advantages and disadvantages of each type of replacement therapy are listed in Table 1. The choice of procedure depends on the size of the child, the stability of the cardiovascular system, any adjunctive therapy (i.e., the feasibility of using heparin), and the local expertise.

REFERENCES

Feld LG, Cachero S, Springate JE: Fluid needs in acute renal failure. Pediatr Clin North Am 37:337–350, 1990.
Gaudio KM, Siegel NJ: Pathogenesis and treatment of acute renal failure. Pediatr Clin North Am 34:771–787, 1987.
Sweet M, Kher KK, Makker SP: Acute renal failure in children: Etiology, diagnosis, and management. NY State J Med 89:336–342, 1989.
Trompeter RS: A review of drug prescribing in children with end-stage renal failure. Pediatr Nephrol 1:183–194, 1987.

13

Bones and Joints

CRANIOFACIAL MALFORMATIONS

LEONARD B. KABAN, D.M.D., M.D.

The first operation to correct a skeletal jaw deformity was carried out by Simon Hullihen in 1849. This was a mandibular osteotomy to correct a bony deformation secondary to a burn scar contracture of the neck. In the first two decades of the twentieth century, multiple new operations were devised to correct maxillary and mandibular deformities. Techniques were improved, and the biology of these procedures became better understood. By the mid-1970s, correction of maxillary and mandibular deformities with excellent and dependable long-term results was commonplace.

Attempts in the late 1940s to correct major craniofacial anomalies, such as Crouzon syndrome, failed because of inadequate understanding of the anatomy and inadequate surgical exposure techniques. Definitive correction of major skeletal and soft tissue defects of the craniofacial region was first described by the French surgical pioneer Paul Tessier, M.D., in Paris. In the mid-1960s, Tessier developed, refined, and taught operative techniques for correction of these deformities. More importantly, he was a careful observer and described the pathologic anatomy of craniofacial anomalies in great detail. In the 1970s, multidisciplinary craniofacial teams were established in the United States and other countries, and surgeons gained considerable experience (often with Tessier's help) in correcting end-stage craniofacial anomalies with acceptable to excellent results. Both operative time and complication rates were reduced considerably.

In the 1980s, craniofacial surgeons began to correct certain anomalies during infancy and early childhood in an effort to improve growth potential, minimize secondary distortion, and aid in body image development. In addition, principles of craniofacial surgery were applied to the treatment of acute craniofacial trauma, acquired post-traumatic deformities, and reconstruction after craniofacial tumor resection. Advanced imaging techniques, particularly computed tomography (CT) with three-dimensional reconstruction, led to improvements in diagnosis and treatment planning.

In the decade of the 1990s, investigators will be challenged to improve our understanding of the developmental biology of normal and abnormal facial morphology, to further elucidate the genetics of craniofacial anomalies, and to develop new therapeutic methods that will enhance growth of the abnormal craniofacial region. Finally, with advances in molecular biology and genetics, it may be possible to prevent certain craniofacial anomalies.

Craniofacial malformations may be classified as *congenital* and *acquired*. The overwhelming majority of pediatric patients present with congenital malformations, and therefore only these are discussed in this article. Congenital craniofacial malformations include the following categories:

1. Craniosynostosis (craniosynostosis alone; craniosynostosis with mid-face hypoplasia–Crouzon syndrome; craniosynostosis with mid-face hypoplasia and extremity deformity–Apert and Pfeiffer syndromes).
2. Abnormalities of interorbital distance (hypertelorbitism, hypotelorbitism).
3. First and second branchial arch deformities (Treacher Collins syndrome and hemifacial microsomia).
4. Anomalies secondary to cleft lip and palate.

CRANIOSYNOSTOSIS

The estimated incidence of craniosynostosis is 1 in 1000 live births. The facial skeleton is affected in approximately 10 per cent of cases. In patients with craniosynostosis, premature fusion of cranial sutures prevents the normal expansion of the skull, which occurs in response to rapid brain growth during the first year of life. The resultant skull deformity depends on the suture or sutures involved. For example, with premature fusion of the mid-sagittal suture (the skull cannot expand in width), *scaphocephaly,* or a long narrow skull, develops. *Trigonocephaly* is the result of metopic synostosis. With premature fusion of the coronal sutures, acrocephaly or *turricephaly* (a tall or "tower" skull) develops. Unilateral coronal synostosis results in *plagiocephaly* (an asymmetric skull). In patients with plagiocephaly, the affected side of the skull has a flat, posteriorly positioned frontal bone with posterior displacement of the supraorbital rim. To compensate, the contralateral side becomes prominent. Radiographically, the greater wing of the sphenoid bone is distorted in a superior lateral direction. *Hydrocephalus is commonly seen in patients with plagiocephaly, trigonocephaly, and multiple suture synostosis.* It is less commonly seen in patients with Crouzon and Apert syndromes.

The major distinguishing characteristic between Apert and Crouzon syndromes is the complex syndactyly of the hands (and/or feet) with interphalangeal synostosis, symphalangism, and other extremity anomalies present in Apert syndrome. These have been referred to as the "mitten hand" deformity.

Patients with Crouzon, Apert, or Pfeiffer syndrome exhibit

mid-face hypoplasia with shallow bony orbits and resultant exorbitism. They may have divergent strabismus. There is diminished orbital volume resulting from hypoplasia of the greater wing of the sphenoid, ballooning of the ethmoid sinus, and hypoplasia of the maxilla and frontal bone. In severe cases, exposure keratitis and corneal damage may result from the exorbitism. In a small number of patients, progressive visual loss may develop during the first 3 years of life as a result of constriction of the bony optic canals. Inferior positioning of the cribriform plates and widening of the ethmoid sinuses may produce orbital hypertelorism. Zygomatic hypoplasia produces an anti-mongoloid slant to the eyes.

The maxilla or upper jaw is hypoplastic in three dimensions, producing relative prognathism with a normal mandible. The narrow maxillary dental arch results in a cross-bite, and the palate may have a high vault. The nose has been described as "parrot's beak" in appearance.

The mid-face hypoplasia of Apert and Crouzon syndromes is similar. However, Apert patients may be distinguished by the following characteristics: asymmetric exorbitism, more severe lateral canthal dystopia, increased incidence of cleft palate (30 per cent), anterior open bite, seborrheic dermatitis, and a transverse forehead skin furrow. Crouzon syndrome is more common than Apert, but both are inherited with an autosomal dominant pattern. Apert syndrome is characterized by a lower penetrance rate and a higher spontaneous mutation rate than Crouzon syndrome.

Treatment

Infancy

Early treatment of craniofacial synostosis was popularized by Marchac and Renier. *Because of the rapid brain growth that occurs during the first year of life, treatment of craniosynostosis during this time would be expected to alleviate some of the distortion of the skull and mid-face.* The affected portion of the skull is removed and divided into segments, and the pieces are replaced to give the skull a more normal shape. These autografts are loosely positioned and sutured to reconstruct the skull. The abnormal supraorbital rim and nasofrontal region are removed en bloc, advanced anteriorly and inferiorly, and then sutured to the nasal bone, thereby producing a nasofrontal angle. The result is a more normally shaped forehead, supraorbital rim, and nasofrontal angle, all of which are free to grow in response to the expanding brain. This technique is known as the "free-floating forehead" procedure. A high percentage of patients with isolated craniosynostosis exhibit a marked improvement of skull shape after early correction with the free-floating forehead procedure. In contrast, patients with Crouzon and Apert syndromes may show improvement in forehead shape; in the majority of cases, however, mid-face hypoplasia is not improved and needs to be corrected later.

Childhood and Adolescence

Mid-face hypoplasia resulting from craniosynostosis is treated by a LeFort III osteotomy, also known as "mid-face advancement." Via a coronal incision and craniofacial dissection, the mid-face is separated from the base of the skull at the nasofrontal, zygomatic-frontal, zygomatic-temporal, zygomatic-sphenoidal, sphenomaxillary, and nasomaxillary junctions. The mid-face is advanced, and the gaps are bone grafted for stability. Currently, the segments are immobilized and fixed with rigid fixation (i.e., bone plates and screws). When the forehead is retruded, it can be moved forward at the same time as the mid-face (i.e., a frontofacial advancement). Alternatively, the forehead can be advanced as a separate stage followed by a mid-face advancement.

ABNORMALITIES OF INTERORBITAL DISTANCE

Orbital hypertelorism (hypertelorbitism) is a term that describes a physical finding (i.e., increased distance between the bony orbits). It is not a diagnosis and may be associated with a variety of anomalies, including median facial dysraphia, encephalocele, and craniosynostosis. Orbital hypotelorism is less common and is often associated with major intracranial central nervous system anomalies. These patients have a high incidence of mental retardation, blindness and neurologic abnormalities, and a poor long-term prognosis.

Orbital hypertelorism results when the normal progressive narrowing of the orbital axis fails to occur. This is a process that begins during the first 3 months of fetal life and progresses at birth with postnatal development. It has been suggested that median facial malformations resulting in hypertelorbitism develop because of failure of neural crest cell migration into the developing frontonasal mesoderm. The average adult interorbital distance (IOD) is 25 mm in females (achieved by age 13) and 28 mm in males (achieved by 21 years of age). Tessier classified adult patients with orbital hypertelorism on the basis of degree of interorbital widening: *first-degree,* IOD 30 to 34 mm but with almost normal orbital shape and orientation; *second-degree,* IOD 34 to 40 mm; *third-degree,* IOD more than 40 mm, orbits lateralized and cribriform plate prolapsed. Despite the variable anterior orbital divergence, the distance between the interoptic foramina is normal. This anatomic finding makes surgical medial translocation of the bony orbits possible without compromising the optic nerves.

Treatment

Surgical correction of orbital hypertelorism involves a coronal incision, craniofacial dissection, and 360-degree osteotomies around the orbital cavity. The central portion of the nasofrontal complex is excised to permit medial translocation. In the past, this included excision of the nasal septum. Currently, the septum is left intact in an attempt to minimize secondary mid-face growth deficiency.

Most craniofacial teams recommend that hypertelorbitism be corrected after growth is completed. *There is evidence that the operation in growing children is associated with development of secondary mid-face hypoplasia, which requires mid-face advancement during the teenage years.* Despite this problem, the procedure may be recommended in growing children with severe deformities who are having major psychosocial adjustment problems.

FIRST AND SECOND BRANCHIAL ARCH DEFECTS

Classification

First and second branchial arch defects may be classified as (1) symmetric (Treacher Collins syndrome) and (2) asymmetric (hemifacial or craniofacial microsomia).

Treacher Collins Syndrome

Treacher Collins syndrome is an easily recognizable deformity that occurs as an autosomal dominant trait with incomplete penetrance and variable expressivity. The incidence is 1 in 10,000 live births, and about 50 per cent of the patients lack a significant family history of the deformity.

The clinical appearance is variable, and there is a wide spectrum of clinical features. However, it is characteristic of Treacher Collins syndrome that the deformity is bilateral and symmetric. Because the inheritance pattern is quite different from that of hemifacial microsomia, which may also be bilateral (but always asymmetric), it is crucial to make the correct diagnosis.

In Treacher Collins syndrome, there is an anti-mongoloid slant of the palpebral fissures and the external ears are low set and hypoplastic. There is usually a conductive hearing loss and anatomic abnormalities of the middle ear. The inner ear, however, develops normally, as it is not a first or second branchial arch derivative. The nose is large, and the zygomatic bones and arches are hypoplastic. As a result, the orbits are "teardrop" in shape. The mandibular rami are short, and the muscles of mastication are hypoplastic. The chin is retruded. The fundamental deformity in the maxillomandibular portion of the skeleton is a short posterior face height with a short posterior maxilla and mandibular ramus. In addition, the patients often have choanal atresia or varying degrees of nasal airway obstruction. They are therefore mouth breathers. This results in excessive vertical (downward) growth of the anterior maxilla because of lack of contact between the maxillary and mandibular anterior dentition.

The soft tissue defects in Treacher Collins are also quite significant. The patients have coloboma of the lower eyelids and, at the very least, lack of hair on the medial third of the lower eyelid. There is also soft tissue bulk deficiency over the cheeks. It is important to note that patients with Treacher Collins syndrome usually do not have facial nerve involvement, whereas this is a common finding in hemifacial microsomia (HFM).

Hemifacial Microsomia

Hemifacial microsomia is a progressive deformity involving structures of the first and second branchial arches. Unlike Treacher Collins syndrome, hemifacial microsomia is predominantly a unilateral deformity, although 20 to 30 per cent of patients have a subtle contralateral anomaly. Hemifacial microsomia is not usually an inherited disorder but is usually a spontaneous and isolated occurrence (approximately 1 in 5000 live births). It is the second most common craniofacial anomaly after cleft lip and palate.

The physical findings of HFM are the result of progressive asymmetric growth of the affected and normal sides of the face. There is underdevelopment of any or all of the structures of the first and second branchial arches. These include the zygoma, maxilla, mandible, muscles of mastication, trigeminal nerve, upper part of the external ear, and parotid gland. The temporal bone, lower portion of the external ear and middle ear, facial nerve, and muscles of facial expression are second branchial arch derivatives. Mandibular hypoplasia is the earliest skeletal deformity to be clinically evident. Fifteen per cent of patients with hemifacial microsomia have cleft palate, and approximately 40 per cent have cranial nerve deficits, usually the seventh nerve and rarely the fifth nerve. The external ear deformity ranges from mild cupping to absence of the auricle. The asymmetry, high incidence of facial nerve deficits, and inheritance pattern distinguish HFM from Treacher Collins syndrome.

Treatment

Patients with Treacher Collins and HFM syndrome present with a wide spectrum of deformation, and individualized correction is required.

There are two basic approaches to the correction of mid-face hypoplasia in patients with Treacher Collins syndrome. Some surgeons use alloplastic implants over the hypoplastic malar eminences, augmenting them with progressively larger implants as the patients grow. In some cases, the implants are eventually replaced with bone. The approach of most craniofacial surgeons is to use autogenous bone for correction of the skeletal deficiencies. Via a coronal incision and craniofacial dissection, the shape of the orbit is corrected by contour burring of the lateral superior orbital rim. The hypoplastic lateral inferior aspect of the orbit is augmented with bone. Cranial bone grafts are also used to improve zygomatic (cheek) contour. In the past, eyelid defects in patients with Treacher Collins syndrome were repaired at an early age. Today, however, it is recommended that eyelid procedures be deferred until the hypoplastic cheeks are augmented.

When the maxillary and mandibular deformities produce malocclusion, this functional problem is corrected with maxillary and mandibular osteotomies in coordination with orthodontic treatment. Timing of correction is usually in the early teens. The basic approach is to lengthen the posterior height of the maxilla. The operation was described by Tessier. A LeFort II osteotomy is carried out, and the maxilla is rotated in a counterclockwise direction with the nasofrontal suture as the center of rotation. Occasionally, posterior maxillary lengthening is done at the LeFort I level, with the center of rotation at the anterior nasal spine. Bilateral osteotomies of the mandibular rami are performed, and the lower jaw is also rotated. This corrects the occlusion and lengthens the posterior face height. A genioplasty corrects the microgenia (underdevelopment of the mental symphysis of the mandible, resulting in a very small chin).

Hemifacial microsomia is one of the most complex and variable deformities in craniofacial surgery. The basic concept of treatment in the growing child is to elongate the abnormal mandible or to construct a mandible when it is missing. This elongation or construction creates an open bite on the affected side. The space between upper and lower teeth is slowly closed over a period of several years with an orthodontic appliance. This appliance regulates eruption of the maxillary teeth and thereby stimulates maxillary and mid-face growth. The ultimate goal of this treatment is to prevent secondary distortion of the mid-face and thereby achieve facial symmetry. This will minimize the inevitable end-stage deformity of the mandible and mid-face.

In the older child and adult with end-stage deformity, maxillary and mandibular osteotomies and bone grafts are required to elongate the affected mid-face and mandible and to create a horizontal occlusal plane.

Follow-up studies of patients treated in childhood document that early surgical treatment with careful postoperative orthodontic follow-up may indeed stimulate growth on the affected side and minimize secondary distortion in the adjacent structures. Major challenges in the future will be to correct the neuromuscular defects in HFM and to improve techniques of soft tissue and ear reconstruction.

MID-FACE DEFORMITY SECONDARY TO CLEFT LIP AND PALATE

Cleft lip and palate (CL/P) are the most common congenital craniofacial anomalies. Childhood management of CL/P is beyond the scope of this article. (Ralph Millard's three-volume text *Cleft Craft* is a very readable and definitive source for this information.) Mid-face hypoplasia secondary to CL/P is discussed here. This skeletal deformity is commonly treated in the context of a craniofacial anomalies center.

As a result of several or more surgical procedures required to repair CL/P and associated soft tissue anomalies, secondary mid-face hypoplasia develops in 25 to 35 per cent of patients. This is manifested by retrusion of the mid-face (maxilla) with hypoplastic malar eminences. The mandible is usually normal, but there is relative prognathism (or protrusion) of the lower jaw because of the small size of the upper jaw. There may be an oronasal fistula and bony alveolar cleft. There is a resultant malocclusion with the lower teeth anterior to the uppers (Class III malocclusion). The upper jaw may be narrow with a resultant cross-bite (the posterior mandibular teeth occluding lateral to the uppers). The nasal tip is depressed, and the alar bases are flat and widened.

Treatment

The oronasal fistula is usually closed, and the alveolar cleft bone is grafted as a separate stage between ages 8 and 11 years. This corresponds developmentally to the time when the maxillary canine teeth have one-half to two-thirds root development. Mid-face deformity and malocclusion necessitate coordinated surgical and orthodontic treatment. The teeth are aligned so they will fit properly when the upper jaw is moved to the correct position. *Mid-face advancement is carried out during the teenage years, after completion of facial growth. Most commonly, it is a LeFort I level osteotomy but it may be at the LeFort II or III level when necessary.* The contour of the cheeks is augmented with calvarial bone. After correction of the craniofacial skeletal deformity, prosthetic dental rehabilitation may be necessary to replace missing teeth and final revisions of the nose and lip are then performed.

REFERENCES

Marchac D, Renier D: Craniofacial Surgery for Craniosynostosis. Boston, Little, Brown & Company, 1982.

Millard DR Jr: Cleft Craft, Vol III. Boston, Little, Brown & Co, 1980.

Murray JE, Mulliken JB, Kaban LB, Belfer, M: Twenty year experience with maxillo-craniofacial surgery. Ann Surg 190:320, 1979.

DISORDERS OF THE SPINE AND SHOULDER GIRDLE

MICHAEL D. SUSSMAN, M.D.

Disorders of shoulder girdle and spine can be classified as those problems that are congenital, infectious or inflammatory, traumatic, and acquired or developmental. In the pediatric agegroup, one does not see degenerative changes; however, some of these disorders may predispose to degenerative problems in later life. Disorders of the spine may affect neurologic function by applying pathologic mechanical stresses on the spinal cord, and this may have greater impact on function than the primary deformity.

SHOULDER GIRDLE

Congenital Problems

Congenital Pseudarthrosis of the Clavicle. In this entity, there is a discontinuity, which is present at birth, in the midportion of the clavicle. The congenital pseudarthrosis can be easily distinguished from a birth fracture, in that it is painless. The abnormality is usually found on the right side and is probably related to impairment of the development of the clavicle as a result of the juxtaposition of the subclavian artery to the underside of the midportion of the developing clavicle. Congenital pseudarthrosis of the clavicle may also occur in a bilateral form in association with cleidocranial dysostosis.

No treatment is required in infancy, and elective surgical repair of the pseudarthrosis to correct the cosmetic deformity is almost always successful (in contrast to congenital pseudarthrosis of the tibia, which is quite resistant to treatment); repair can be accomplished when the child is old enough so that the structures are large enough for the fixation devices used at the time of surgery. A recent report suggests that early repair without rigid internal fixation is successful if it is performed within the first few years of life. No specific treatment or handling of the child is required prior to repair.

Sprengel's Deformity. The scapula lies adjacent to the cervical region during early fetal development and subsequently descends to its normal position on the posterior thorax. Failure of complete descent of the scapula results in a Sprengel's deformity. In this deformity, the scapula is in an elevated position and is small, malformed, and rotated so that the glenoid faces downward; it also has a superomedial portion that hooks over the upper portion of the thorax. This results in a cosmetic deformity as well as limitation of the mobility of the shoulder because of the fixation and downward inclination of the glenoid. The deformity may be unilateral or bilateral. There is a female preponderance in most series, but this may be due to an ascertainment bias because of the cosmetic nature of this problem. Twenty to 30 per cent of patients may have a supernumerary bone known as the *omovertebral bone,* which connects the elevated, malformed scapula to the axial skeleton.

All patients with Sprengel's deformity should be carefully assessed for anomalies of the spine by radiography and for anomalies of the kidney by ultrasonography. One third of these patients have a mild grade I deformity in which the shoulder joints are almost level, and the deformity cannot be seen with the patient dressed. Those patients with mild deformities should be followed up throughout growth, as there may be progression in the severity of the deformity. One third of the patients have a grade II deformity, in which the asymmetry is mild to moderate but can be appreciated with the patient dressed owing to the asymmetry at the base of the neck. Another third of patients have more severe deformities, which are easily visible and can cause functional impairment.

Patients with grade II or III deformities may undergo surgery prior to age 5 or 6 years to correct the cosmetic appearance. In moderate cases, excision of the superomedial portion of the scapula in an extraperiosteal fashion, leaving the levator scapulae detached, and excision of the omovertebral bone, if present, may suffice. For more severe deformities, the Woodward procedure is recommended. With this technique, the origin of the trapezius is detached and moved caudally in addition to excision of the superomedial angle of the scapula and omovertebral bone. If one waits to perform surgery until the child is older than 7 years, the risk of brachial plexus palsy from compression of the plexus between the scapula and the first rib is increased, so that surgery at a younger age is preferred.

The major goal of surgery is to reduce the cosmetic deformity; however, increased range of motion can also be expected. Scoliosis is common in such patients and may be due to congenital anomalies, or it may develop during the adolescent growth spurt in a pattern similar to that of idiopathic scoliosis. Other associated findings include Klippel-Feil syndrome, rib anomalies, and urogenital system abnormalities.

Snapping Scapula. In this syndrome there is a palpable, audible, and sometimes painful click with elevation and declination of the scapula. This can be due to one or more osteochondromata on the costal surface of the scapula or may be a forme fruste of Sprengel's deformity with a prominent and curved superomedial portion of the scapula. These lesions can be excised surgically when identified.

Acquired Problems

Birth-Related Brachial Plexus Palsy. The most common type of brachial plexus palsy affects the upper, or C5–C6, nerve distribution. This is usually found in large infants and is due to traction on the brachial plexus during delivery. These infants have limited active abduction, external rotation, and elbow flexion; therefore, the arm is held in an adducted, internally rotated, and extended posture.

In the acute phase, no treatment is indicated but the arm should be handled with care to avoid further traction on the injured nerves. At 2 to 3 weeks of age, gentle range of motion can be begun, with concentration on external rotation and abduction. Range of motion should not be forced, and long-term passive splintage should not be used. If elbow flexion is absent when sitting age is reached, an elbow splint should be used to maintain the elbow at 90 degrees to allow for development of active hand use. If the lower plexus is involved, a hand and wrist splint may also be used. Because there are areas that are insensate, close observation should be made to avoid injury to these insensate areas. Improvement is often seen until the age of 2; subsequent to this, however, further improvement is unlikely. The percentage of children who achieve full recovery varies from 10 to 75 per cent, depending on the series. If deficits persist, muscle releases and/or transfers may be done to improve range of motion.

In some cases, a rotational osteotomy of the upper humerus may be performed to improve function. Patients with severe defects persisting past 6 months of age may benefit from surgical exploration of the plexus and grafting to replace destroyed nerves.

Shoulder Dislocation. Congenital dislocation of the shoulder has been reported, but is exceedingly rare. Traumatic shoulder dislocations, likewise, are rare in the pediatric age group but may occur in older teenagers. More frequently, proximal humeral fractures occur with traumatic episodes.

Voluntary dislocation of the shoulder, however, may be seen in this age group, and the dislocation may be multidirectional (i.e., posterior as well as anterior). In general, surgery should be avoided in these patients and physical therapy should be used to strengthen muscles that maintain shoulder alignment. In addition, patients should be counseled not to dislocate their shoulders voluntarily.

Fractures

Fractured Clavicle. This is the most common fracture seen in the pediatric age group. Neonatal clavicular fractures occur with birth trauma, and usually no treatment is required other than gentle handling of the affected extremity. These fractures heal exceedingly rapidly, and infants are usually asymptomatic within a week to 10 days.

In children other than neonates clavicle fractures can be treated with a figure-of-eight dressing to reduce the symptoms. Healing is almost universal, and no reduction is usually necessary because bone remodeling is usually complete. A large amount of fracture callus may occur at the healing site, which may be cosmetically apparent, since the clavicle is directly subcutaneous. However, parents can be counseled that this will resolve in 6 to 12 months.

Fractured Scapula. Fractures of the scapula are very rare in pediatric patients and are usually associated with major trauma. In most cases, scapular fractures can be treated by immobilization of the extremity in a sling until healing occurs.

Fractures of the Upper Humerus. Fractures of the upper humerus usually occur in the proximal metaphysis, 1 to 2 cm distal to the growth plate and not through the growth plate. Although these fractures may be completely displaced, no reduction of the fracture fragments is necessary and manipulation is indicated only if the skin is in jeopardy. Treatment with a collar and a cuff and swathe for 3 to 4 weeks is sufficient. Even in severely displaced fractures, healing and subsequent remodeling can be anticipated and full recovery of function is likely.

SPINE

Congenital Anomalies

Congenital anomalies can occur anywhere in the spine; they may include only a single level or multiple levels or may affect the entire spine. These deformities may affect the growth plate and, therefore, result in progressively increasing deformity.

Most spine anomalies can be classified as failure of segmentation of vertebrae, failure of formation of portions of vertebrae, or combinations of both. Failures of segmentation result in fusion of all or part of one vertebral body to an adjacent vertebral body. If this fusion is partial, the growth plate is absent in the area of fusion but may be present in the unfused area, leading to the development of a progressive deformity. Similarly, if a partially formed vertebra extends over only a portion of adjacent vertebral bodies, the deformity may increase with growth. This asymmetric growth will cause increasing deformity, resulting in progressive scoliosis, kyphosis, or both. Lordosis may occur in those rare cases in which there are multiple congenital fusions of the posterior elements with intact bodies anteriorly.

As with other congenital anomalies, when congenital scoliosis is discovered, the patient should be examined carefully to detect the presence of other anomalies. These may include hypothyroidism or hearing impairment with upper spinal anomalies, and cardiovascular, gastrointestinal, or urogenital anomalies associated with anomalies lower in the spine. Spinal anomalies may also be associated with diastematomyelia or tight filum terminale, which may tether the spinal cord and result in progressive spinal cord dysfunction with growth. For patients with vertebral anomalies who show evidence of neurologic dysfunction or back pain, magnetic resonance imaging (MRI) should be utilized to demonstrate spinal cord anomalies, if present.

In most cases of congenital spine deformity, serial (usually yearly) radiographic follow-up is indicated until growth is finished. If significant progression occurs, posterior spinal fusion, usually without instrumentation, should be performed to prevent further progression of the deformity. Bracing may be indicated to control flexible curves adjacent to anomalous areas, but it is not efficacious in most cases of congenital scoliosis. If posterior fusion alone is insufficient to prevent progression of the deformity, anterior fusion may also be required.

Congenital anomalies in the cervical and upper thoracic spine tend to be less aggressive in terms of producing deformity than those in the lower thoracic and lumbar spine.

Klippel-Feil Syndrome. Any congenital fusion in the cervical spine is known as the Klippel-Feil syndrome. In most cases, this is a total failure of segmentation and, therefore, does not produce scoliosis or kyphosis but limits the linear growth of the cervical vertebrae, resulting in a short neck, low hairline, and limitation of motion of the cervical spine. A high percentage of such patients have hearing problems.

No treatment is necessary for most cases. In exceedingly severe cases in which the cosmetic appearance is unacceptable, resection of the upper two or three ribs, with skin grafting to alter the contours in the shoulder area, may improve the cosmetic appearance.

Occipitocervical Instability. This form of instability, which may present with headache or pain with neck motion, is exceedingly rare and may be seen in combination with fusions in the cervical spine. When detected and documented radiologically, the instability should be treated by fusion of the occiput to the upper cervical spine.

Atlantoaxial Hypermobility. Excessive motion between C1 and C2 may occur in otherwise normal children with an os odontoideum (a hypoplastic odontoid with an ossicle superior to it), in children with skeletal dysplasia due to a hypoplastic odontoid (particularly Morquio's syndrome and spondyloepiphyseal dysplasia congenita), or in children with Down syndrome (owing to alteration and laxity of the restraining ligaments). Diagnosis is made by interpretation of *voluntary* flexion-extension radiographs of the cervical spine with measurement of the distance between the posterior border of the anterior arch of C1 and the anterior border of the odontoid (atlanto-dens interval). It is important not to obtain these radiographs by passively forcing flexion of the neck, since this maneuver could result in injury or even death of patients with hypermobility. An absolute distance of greater than 4 mm of the atlanto-dens interval is abnormal. In the absence of neurologic findings, patients with instability of less than 6 to 7 mm should be observed closely and those with instability of greater amounts should undergo atlantoaxial fusion to prevent progressive myelopathy and/or acute spinal cord damage. If long tract signs, such as clonus, hyperreflexia, Babinski reflex, weakness, or incontinence, are present, MRI scan with flexion should be done to demonstrate cord compression and C1-C2 fusion may be indicated.

Atlantoaxial instability is prevalent in patients with Down syndrome. Even if pathologic laxity is not documented in these patients, they should avoid activities that may place undue stress on the neck, such as tumbling and trampoline exercises. Patients may participate in most recreational sports, with the pediatrician recognizing that their risk of cervical injury is slightly increased. Patients with Down syndrome should undergo radiography initially at age 3 or 4; if the findings are within normal limits, radiography should be repeated every 2 to 4 years, or sooner, if evidence of spinal cord compression is detected.

Pseudosubluxation of C2 to C4 in Children. After experiencing spinal trauma, many children exhibit what appears to be a subluxation of C2 on C3 and/or C3 on C4 on the lateral flexion radiograph of the cervical spine. If this reduces fully in extension, is not greater than 5 mm, and is not associated with other evidence of fracture, such as an increase in the prevertebral soft tissue space, this can be considered normal. Patients should not be overtreated when they exhibit this normal pseudosubluxation.

Developmental Disorders

Idiopathic Scoliosis. Idiopathic scoliosis may present in infancy, although this occurs rarely in the United States and infrequently in the juvenile years. The most frequent onset of idiopathic scoliosis is during the pubertal growth spurt. Small spinal curvatures may occur in 5 to 10 per cent of the preadolescent population, but only 1 in 20 of these requires treatment.

Curves of small magnitude in immature individuals have the potential to progress to severe deformities, so that patients with clinical evidence of spinal asymmetry should be evaluated and treated if progression occurs. Serial radiographs of all patients with spinal asymmetry document the degree of deformity and identify progressive curves, but this approach is costly and results in unnecessary radiation to adolescent children. Therefore, radiography should be reserved for those patients with significant deformities whereas those with milder deformities can be observed clinically.

The degree of deformity may be assessed by measurement of the rib hump or lumbar hump in the forward bend position by using the "scoliometer," as described by Bunnell. This device, adapted from a nautical pitch gauge, is placed in the posterior midline at the point of maximum deformity with the patient in the forward bend position; the angle with which the trunk deviates from the horizontal is then read directly on the scoliometer. This angle of deformity is referred to as the "angle of trunk rotation" (ATR).

Patients with curves of greater than 20 degrees had an ATR of greater than 5 degrees in 99 per cent of the cases examined by Bunnell, giving a very low false-negative rate. There is, however, a significant false-positive rate; thus, some patients with mild curves have an ATR of 5 degrees or more. Therefore, patients with 5 degrees or less ATR do not require radiography. However, if these patients have growth remaining, they should be observed at 6- to 12-month intervals with clinical examination using the scoliometer in order to detect progression. If significant progression is detected (greater than 2 degrees ATR) or if the initial ATR is greater than 5 degrees, a single standing anteroposterior radiograph in boys or a posteroanterior radiograph in girls should be taken using high-speed screens. Girls are seven times more likely to experience progression than boys, and the more immature the patient at the time of initial curve detection, the more likely the curvature is to progress. In addition, there is a strong familial predisposition to scoliosis and patients with a positive family history should be followed up closely.

For curvatures having a Cobb angle of less than 25 to 30 degrees on radiograph, no treatment is necessary; however, follow-up until relative skeletal maturity, which occurs 2 years after menarche in girls and voice change in boys, is indicated to ensure lack of progression. Curves that progress to the range of 25 to 45 degrees in skeletally immature individuals should be treated with an orthosis, usually of the underarm type, until skeletal maturity is achieved. The goal of bracing is to prevent progression of the curvature. In general, most physicians treating scoliosis prescribe 23 hours a day of brace wear; however, there is some evidence that part-time brace wearing (16 hours per day) may be as effective as the 23-hour-a-day program that has been traditional.

Electrical stimulation has been advocated by several groups to prevent progression of scoliosis. This is done at night only by use of transcutaneous electrodes attached to a stimulating device. However, several studies have found this approach ineffective and at present this approach is not recommended.

The Charleston Bending Brace is a scoliosis body brace that overcorrects the curves and is used only 8 hours at nighttime. Preliminary studies of this orthosis indicate it may be quite effective.

Curvatures greater than 45 degrees, in most cases, continue to progress following adolescence and require surgical treatment. Surgery consists of insertion of stainless steel rods onto the posterior (or in some cases, other devices onto the anterior) spine, which partially correct the deformity and hold the curvature in the corrected position, while the spine that has been prepared for fusion by removal of facet joints, decortication, and addition of bone graft heals solidly. The Cotrel-Dubousset system and similar systems that allow multiple sites for hook placement as well as provide correction of sagittal contours have largely replaced the Harrington rod in treatment of idiopathic scoliosis. These systems allow patients to be mobilized rapidly following surgery without the need for a brace; the patients are able to be discharged from the hospital within a week of surgery and are back in school within 2 weeks.

Neuromuscular Scoliosis. Scoliosis is found in a high incidence in quadriparetic cerebral palsy patients as well as in patients with degenerative neuromuscular diseases, such as Duchenne muscular dystrophy and spinal muscular atrophy. Bracing may be indicated in younger patients with cerebral palsy and spinal muscular atrophy and may retard curve progression, but many of such children ultimately require surgery with sublaminar wiring by the Luque technique, which produces excellent curve correction and exceedingly stable fixation, allowing rapid mobilization following surgery.

Bracing is not effective in scoliosis associated with Duchenne muscular dystrophy and may only delay surgery in these boys, thereby subjecting them to surgery at a time when their pulmonary function has deteriorated. Therefore, spinal bracing is contraindicated in boys with Duchenne muscular dystrophy, and these patients should undergo early surgical stabilization as soon as it is apparent that a curvature is developing.

Postural Roundback. Postural roundback is an increase in the normal thoracic kyphosis found in children and adolescents. As long as the kyphosis is flexible, no orthotic treatment is necessary. These patients may respond to physical therapy in the form of thoracic hyperextension and pelvic tilt exercises. Occasionally, if the deformity is severe and progressive, an orthosis may be indicated. Patients should be followed up radiologically for progression or development of structural changes.

Scheuermann's Disease. Scheuermann's disease is characterized by an increased thoracic or thoracolumbar kyphosis associated with changes in the vertebral body consisting of anterior wedging of greater than 5 degrees of at least three vertebra, end-plate irregularity, and Schmorl's nodes. This usually presents in mid to late adolescence and may be associated with back pain and hamstring tightness. Boys are affected more frequently than girls. If the thoracic kyphosis is greater than 45 degrees and there is significant growth remaining, the patient should be treated with an orthosis and physical therapy. Unlike the goal of prevention of progression in patients with scoliosis, actual correction can be achieved and maintained in patients with Scheuermann's disease. Surgical correction may be indicated for patients with severe kyphosis.

Spondylolisthesis. Spondylolisthesis is forward slippage of a vertebral body relative to the adjacent distal vertebral body. This usually occurs when L5 slips forward on S1, and in children this is usually due to a defect in the pars interarticularis, which appears in a predisposed individual during the first decade. Spondylolisthesis may also occur because of congenital deformity and elongation of the pars.

Patients with spondylolisthesis may present with back pain, posterior thigh pain, and evidence of tight hamstrings, or they may be asymptomatic but show evidence of deformity. Clinical examination demonstrates flattening of the buttocks, decreased range of flexion of the spine, and hamstring tightness. Oblique radiographs document the presence of the pars defect, and the severity of the forward slippage should be measured on a standing lateral film.

In order to measure the slippage, the upper border of the sacrum is divided into four quadrants. Grading ranges from grade I for slippage less than 25 per cent to grade V for complete slippage of L5 on S1 (spondyloptosis). Patients with grade I and II spondylolisthesis without significant symptoms should be observed throughout growth for possible progression of the slippage by lateral standing radiographs of the lumbosacral spine on a yearly basis or more frequently if symptoms indicate. Recent studies, however, have indicated that progression is unusual following initial presentation. If there is no evidence of increased slippage, no treatment other than avoidance of high-risk activities, such as football and gymnastics, is required. If the patient is symptomatic, immobilization in a lumbosacral orthosis or cast may decrease symptoms and the patient may be weaned from the orthosis when asymptomatic.

For patients with persistent symptoms or progressive slips of grade III or greater, spinal posterolateral fusion using a massive amount of autogenous graft, usually between L4, L5, and the sacrum, is performed. Only in very severe cases is decompression of the anterior sacrum, anterior fusion, or reduction indicated. Removal of the L5 lamina (Gill procedure) is not indicated and may actually aggravate the instability. When solid fusion is achieved, the symptoms, including the hamstring spasm, will resolve.

Traumatic Injury

Traumatic injuries to the spine may occur at any time during childhood and may be associated with injury to the underlying spinal cord. Injuries that occur at birth may be confused with anterior horn cell disease, since both of these conditions give signs of lower motor neuron damage. However, the spinal cord injury is nonprogressive. In infancy and childhood, spinal cord injury may occur following major trauma without radiographic evidence of bony injury.

The most common cause of vertebral and spinal cord trauma in children is motor vehicle accidents, and appropriate seat restraints are effective in prevention of these disastrous injuries. In the case of complete loss of spinal cord function, no recovery can be expected; with incomplete injuries, recovery may occur. Immediate post-injury treatment of patients with high doses of systemic steroids may reduce the magnitude of neurologic deficit. In either case, the bony injury and instability, if present, should be treated and a rehabilitation program at a center accomplished in treatment of these patients should be instituted. Surgical decompression of the spinal cord is not of any benefit to patients with complete injuries, but in selected patients with incomplete injuries surgery may enhance the resolution of the neurologic deficit by removal of pressure on the spinal cord. Surgery may be necessary to stabilize the associated bony injury. In preadolescents with spinal cord injuries of the upper thoracic and cervical spine, the incidence of scoliosis is exceedingly high and treatment of progressive spinal deformity below the level of injury with an orthosis should be done prophylactically. If progressive scoliosis exceeds 40 degrees, spinal fusion with segmental instrumentation should be done.

Fractures of the Ring Apophysis. With hyperflexion or hyperextension injury of the spine, fragments of the ring apophysis may be separated from the main body of the vertebra and may impinge on the spinal cord, cauda equina, or nerve roots. These fragments can be seen on computed tomography (CT) or MRI studies. When this occurs, the fragments must be surgically removed.

Causes of Back Pain in Children

A variety of entities may cause back pain in children, and it is important to distinguish these from one another by careful history, physical examination, and follow-up of the clinical course. The major causes of back pain are described next.

Spondylolisthesis. Patients with spondylolisthesis usually present with pain that may begin in the back and radiate into the posterior thighs, rarely prior to the age of 10.

Spinal Cord Tumor. The most common presentation of spinal cord tumor is back pain. However, careful physical examination may demonstrate the presence of neurologic dysfunction, and anteroposterior spinal radiographs may show evidence of increased interpedicular distance. Diagnosis is made by MRI or myelography. Treatment consists of neurosurgical excision of the tumor.

Disc Disease. Disc disease may occur in young adolescents and is frequently due to a bulging annulus rather than a herniation of the nucleus. A trial of conservative therapy is indicated in most cases, but a high percentage of patients ultimately require surgical decompression. Because the bulging disc may be central rather than peripheral, patients may present with diffuse, nonradicular pain. Diagnosis can be made by MRI or myelography.

Osteoid Osteoma. Osteoid osteoma is an unusual condition that is thought to be neoplastic. Although the lesions of osteoid osteoma generally appear in the second or third decade, they can occur in young children. They present with nonradiating back pain, which is frequently more apparent at night and classically is relieved by salicylates. Diagnosis can be made by plain radiography, tomography, and technetium-99 scan and confirmed and precisely localized by CT. Treatment of these lesions is by surgical resection, which may be facilitated by injection of the patient with radionuclide and intraoperative use of a radiation-sensitive probe.

Discitis. Discitis may present as back pain with or without leg pain or as pseudoparalysis of the lower extremities. Radiographs may demonstrate a decreased disc space height and end-plate irregularity. Although bacterial cultures of the disc are usually negative, many, if not all, of these cases may be secondary to focal osteomyelitis of the vertebral end-plate. The usual organism is *Staphylococcus,* but occasionally other organisms, including gram-negatives, may be responsible. In the past, many children with discitis were treated successfully with cast immobilization alone. However, 3 to 6 weeks of antibiotic coverage along with cast or brace immobilization of the spine is probably indicated in most cases. An effort should be made to obtain a bacteriologic diagnosis by serial blood cultures and, on occasion, needle biopsy of the vertebral body prior to the institution of antibiotic therapy.

Cord Tether. Tethered cord may present with back pain, although it frequently presents with painless neurologic dysfunction in the lower extremities or secondary incontinence. Patients with a tethered cord secondary to a tight filum terminale also frequently have skin abnormalities, such as café au lait spot, hairy patch, or a dimple at the base of the spine. This entity may be diagnosed by MRI and is treated by surgical release of the tether.

Low Back Strain. Low back strain may be seen in teenagers with acute onset of low back pain without neurologic symptoms or radiographic evidence of bony abnormalities. This is not associated with radicular pain or neurologic changes. Usual treatment is with salicylates or nonsteroidal anti-inflammatory drugs plus an active stretching program.

REFERENCES

Bunnell WP. Spinal deformity. Pediatr Clin North Am 33:1475, 1986.

Bunnell WP. An objective criterion for scoliosis screening. J Bone Joint Surg 66A:1381, 1984.

CONGENITAL DEFORMITIES OF THE ANTERIOR CHEST WALL

ROBERT C. SHAMBERGER, M.D.

STERNAL DEFECTS

Midline sternal defects can be considered in three categories. First, and most severe, are the *defects of the sternum and overlying soft tissues of the chest,* in which the heart is entirely exposed and protruding from the thoracic cavity (ectopia cordis). Affected infants usually have intracardiac defects as well, and despite extensive surgical efforts, they rarely survive.

Second, and less severe, are the *thoracoabdominal defects,* in which the inferior portion of the sternum is cleft but the heart resides within the thoracic cavity and is covered by either a thin layer of skin or omphalocele. Such infants often have a constellation of anomalies termed the *pentalogy of Cantrell,* which consists of defects in the abdominal wall, diaphragm, pericardium, heart, and inferior sternum. Efforts should be made initially to achieve a dermal closure of the defect to prevent sepsis. The cardiac anomaly should then be repaired, prior to soft tissue coverage of the defect, with muscle flaps to minimize the risks of cardiac trauma. Many of these infants can be saved with recent advances in pediatric cardiac surgery, and prognosis is related primarily to the cardiac defect.

Third, and least severe, is the *bifid or cleft sternum,* in which a V-shaped defect of the upper sternum or complete separation of two sternal bars is present but covered with normal skin and subcutaneous tissues. Echocardiography should be performed to exclude the rare associated cardiac anomaly. Closure of the defect is best achieved in infancy, when the chest wall is pliable. This provides protection from trauma to the underlying heart.

PECTUS EXCAVATUM AND CARINATUM

Pectus excavatum—posterior depression of the sternum and costal cartilages—is identified at birth or within the first year of life in 86 per cent of infants who will have the defect. It is present more frequently in males (79 per cent) than females (21 per cent), and a family history of chest wall deformities is often present (37 per cent). Its etiology is unknown. Patients should be evaluated for scoliosis, which is seen in 15 per cent. Although the severity of the depression may change with growth, it rarely resolves entirely. Individuals with particularly severe defects or young males with associated scoliosis should be evaluated for Marfan syndrome. Several series have evaluated cardiopulmonary function in these patients, particularly by means of exercise stress tests. They have demonstrated some impairment from this defect, but the role of conditioning is difficult to assess in these studies. A readily performed and reproducible test to evaluate the impact of the pectus excavatum deformity on cardiopulmonary function has not been defined. Decisions regarding repair must be based on patient and family desires and on the severity of the defect.

Pectus carinatum—anterior protrusion of the costal cartilages and sternum—is identified at birth in only a third of infants who will have the defect. In fact, in almost half the children the defect is not identified until after the 11th birthday, when it appears with the pubertal growth spurt. There is also a male predominance (78 per cent), and a family history of chest wall defects is often present (26 per cent). Etiology is unknown. Indication for repair is primarily the severity of the local protrusion, which generally progresses until full stature is achieved.

POLAND SYNDROME

Poland syndrome is a constellation of anomalies that frequently occur in association; each component of the syndrome can occur with varying severity. Absence of the sternal portion of the pectoralis major muscle, the pectoralis minor muscle, and subcutaneous tissue are found in most patients. Associated thoracic defects may include hypoplasia of the ipsilateral chest wall, and, less frequently, depression of the chest wall or aplasia of the ribs. The latter may require rib grafts for reconstruction. Brachysyndactyly of the ipsilateral middle fingers is seen with variable severity in two thirds of patients with this syndrome. Hypoplasia or absence of the ipsilateral breast (amastia) will necessitate reconstruction in females at puberty with a latissimus dorsi muscle flap and breast augmentation.

ASPHYXIATING THORACIC DYSTROPHY

Infants with asphyxiating thoracic dystrophy (Jeune's disease) are born with a hypoplastic, rigid, bell-shaped chest. Little respiratory motion is present because of the horizontal direction of the ribs. Infants frequently succumb in the perinatal period from pulmonary hypoplasia, but a spectrum of severity is seen in this anomaly. Surgical efforts have been made to enlarge the chest by dividing the sternum and interposing bone grafts or prosthetic material, but no clear improvement in the underlying pulmonary hypoplasia has been demonstrated. Because asphyxiating thoracic dystrophy is inherited in an autosomal recessive pattern, genetic counseling is critical.

REFERENCES

Shamberger RC, Welch KJ: Surgical correction of pectus carinatum. J Pediatr Surg 22:48, 1987.
Shamberger RC, Welch KJ: Surgical repair of pectus excavatum. J Pediatr Surg 23:615, 1988.
Shamberger RC, Welch KJ: Sternal defects. Pediatr Surg Int 5:156, 1990.

ORTHOPEDIC DISORDERS OF THE EXTREMITIES

GEORGE THABIT III, M.D.
and LYLE J. MICHELI, M.D.

Orthopedic disorders of the extremities may be classified broadly into congenital, developmental, and acquired disorders. Congenital problems arise from a failure of formation or differentiation of anatomic structures. Deviation of limb development from the accepted physiologic norm characterizes developmental abnormalities. The majority of acquired disorders of the extremities are the result of mechanical injuries. Sprains, contusions, dislocations, and fractures resulting from acute trauma are responsible for considerable pediatric morbidity. In addition, the cumulative effect of repetitive microtrauma that occurs with organized activities may result in overuse injury: bursitis, tendinitis, apophysitis, and stress fracture, which in the past were encountered primarily in adults.

THE UPPER EXTREMITY

The upper extremity can be divided anatomically into the shoulder mechanism, the upper arm and elbow joint, the lower arm and wrist, and the hand.

The shoulder mechanism consists of four joints: the scapulothoracic, glenohumeral, acromioclavicular, and sternoclavicular. These joints share anatomic and functional associations. In addition, disorders of one joint may result in disorders or dysfunctional compensations at the other sites. Thus, a derangement of the glenohumeral joint, the most complex of the group, may result in dysfunction and pain at any or all of the other joints.

Our examination of the upper extremity focuses on acquired disorders that result primarily from repetitive overuse injury in the child and adolescent. Acute traumatic congenital and developmental causes of upper extremity disability are discussed elsewhere in this section.

Triceps Tendinitis

Posterior elbow pain is a rarely encountered form of overuse injury that occurs with throwing activities. A tender olecranon process is palpable. Radiographs are normal in the acute case but may show bony degenerative changes in the chronic case. Rest is usually curative. Arthroscopic débridement may be considered when osteophyte production causes bony impingement, pain, and loss of elbow motion.

Wrist

DeQuervain's Tendinitis

Focal wrist pain may occur in a variety of athletic settings. DeQuervain's tendinitis is an overuse syndrome presenting as dorsiradial wrist pain over the radial styloid process. Palpable tenderness is present over the abductor pollices longus and flexor pollices brevis tendons as they pass over the distal radius in their respective sheaths. A positive Finkelstein test manifested by provoked pain with first metacarpal flexion and ulnar wrist deviation is usually present. Plain x-ray findings are normal.

Treatment consists of rest, splints, and nonsteroidal medication. Peritendinous cortisone injection may also be useful. Surgical release of the tendon sheaths is recommended in recalcitrant cases.

Stress Fracture of the Wrist

Wrist pain in the gymnast may represent a stress fracture of the distal radius. Point tenderness directly over the dorsum of the distal radius as well as soft tissue swelling helps to identify this entity. Radiographs either appear normal or reveal a sourcil sign, representative of stress concentration in the subchondral bone. Bone scan reveals a marked increase in uptake consistent with the diagnosis of stress fracture.

Treatment consists of cessation of the instigating activity for 4 to 6 weeks. Occasionally, the limb must be immobilized for comfort. When the wrist is nontender, a gradual strengthening program is initiated prior to the resumption of impact sports.

THE LOWER EXTREMITY

Congenital, developmental, and acquired disorders of the lower extremity often result in significant functional disability. Conditions of the hip joint as well as disorders of acute traumatic etiology may be particularly disabling and thus are examined in detail elsewhere in this text.

Congenital Disorders

Lower Limb Deficiency

Congenital deficiency of the femur, tibia, fibula, or foot usually necessitates orthopedic management. Problems that must be addressed to optimize function include limb length discrepancy (LLD), unstable joints, and foot deformity. Complete medical evaluation is necessary to rule out commonly associated musculoskeletal, genitourinary, or cardiac abnormality.

Femoral Deficiency

The spectrum of femoral deformity ranges from a hypoplastic femur requiring limb equalization procedures to an unstable hip joint and abnormal lower limbs. A unilateral deformity associated with a significant length discrepancy and an abnormal foot is best treated by knee fusion, Syme amputation, and early prosthetic restoration. Bilaterality is an indication for prosthetic management.

Tibial Deficiency

Abnormality of the tibia ranges from hypoplasia to complete absence and an unstable knee. A severe club foot may be present because of an abnormal ankle joint. Knee disarticulation with prosthetic management is the usual treatment.

Fibular Deficiency

The presence of limb length inequality and foot deformities determines orthopedic treatment. When projected limb inequality is greater than 12 to 15 cm or when foot deformities are present, amputation and prosthetic restoration are indicated. When the foot is normal and LLD not excessive, limb equalization procedures should be considered.

Congenital Knee and Patellar Dislocation and Subluxation

These unusual conditions are presumed to result from congenital and environmental causes related to in utero fetal positioning and quadriceps muscle fibrosis. At birth, the dislocated knee is found to be hyperextended with the tibia anteriorly displaced on the distal femur. The lateral radiograph not only confirms the diagnosis but also differentiates between the subluxated and dislocated knee, as the two entities appear similar on clinical grounds. On examination, the subluxated knee has better motion with up to 40 degrees of knee flexion. The subluxated knee is usually reducible during the manual exam. The dislocated patella tends to be poorly developed and palpable lateral to the knee joint. Clinical presentation reveals a clicking sensation with knee motion and a flexion deformity. Radiographs demonstrate a laterally displaced patella if ossification has begun.

Treatment of the congenital patellar dislocation consists of surgical release and realignment of structural soft tissue contractures. The subluxated knee usually can be managed with stretching exercises until 90 degrees of knee flexion is achieved. This is followed by resting, splints, and exercises for 4 to 6 weeks. For successful management of knee dislocations, skeletal traction and frequently surgical reduction are required.

Congenital Tibial Bowing

Posteromedial and anterolateral bowing require differentiation, since prognoses are vastly different. Posteromedial bowing usually corrects spontaneously without the need for orthopedic bracing. However, parents must be counseled about the possibility of limb length inequality during childhood development. Contrary to the posteromedial bow, the anterolateral bow is pathologic and often associated with congenital tibial pseudarthrosis. When pseudarthrosis of the tibia occurs, treatment is long and often frustrating. Failure to achieve successful bony union by combinations of non-union excision, bone grafting, internal fixation, and electric stimulation leads to a guarded prognosis. Amputation is recommended after the various surgical reconstruction options have failed to achieve a successful outcome.

Congenital Foot Deformities

Clubfoot. A rigid hindfoot equinovarus in combination with a forefoot adduction and supination deformity is present in 1 in 1000 births. Although a variety of syndromes and neurologic conditions have been associated with the clubfoot deformity, the etiology of the idiopathic clubfoot remains unknown. Vascular, cartilaginous, neurologic, and myopathic growth disturbances all are hypothesized etiologic factors in the orthopedic literature. Plain radiographs reveal the aberrant bony anatomic relationships and provide a means to evaluate treatment modalities.

Initial serial manipulation and cast treatment begin in the newborn nursery. Cast correction is achieved in two stages. Initially, the forefoot deformity is manipulated by applying a medially based forefoot stress and lateral midfoot counterpressure. Concomitantly, the hindfoot varus is subjected to a valgus stress. After correction of these deformities is achieved, the equinus deformity is corrected by applying an ankle dorsiflexion stress during casting. Treatment results are monitored clinically and radiographically such that surgical release is considered for residual deformity at 3 to 6 months of age. A circumferential soft tissue release is performed followed by cast and orthotic management for up to 1 year in order to prevent recurrence.

Pes Planus or Flatfoot. The flexible flatfoot is a common finding in the pediatric foot. Development occurs throughout childhood and proceeds independently of orthotic or shoe management. Treatment is instituted for the symptomatic foot and typically responds to arch supports and shoe modifications to prevent hindfoot valgus and hyperpronation of the forefoot.

Metatarsus Adductus. Forefoot adduction is commonly identified in the neonatal nursery and resolves spontaneously in approximately 90 per cent of cases. Gentle stretching exercises are taught to the adult caregiver to be performed with each diaper change. Should exercises prove inadequate, serial casting on a weekly basis can be performed until correction is achieved. Straight- or reverse-last shoes are prescribed after the desired correction has been obtained. Should the deformity be resistant to manipulation treatment, metatarsal osteotomies performed during early childhood are associated with a high success rate. The previous association between metatarsus adduction and congenital hip dislocation in 10 per cent of cases has recently been challenged, but until further data are presented, repetitive hip examinations should be performed to screen for hip pathology.

Cavus Foot. When a unilateral cavus deformity presents itself, a careful search for the etiology must be performed because idiopathic cavus is usually bilateral and otherwise quite rare. Charcot-Marie-Tooth disease and a variety of other neurologic disorders present with cavus feet. The cavus foot has a high arch, tight plantar fascia, and a tendency to a rigid hindfoot varus. Claw toes and painful plantar calluses complete the clinical description.

Evaluation includes a complete motor and sensory examination, a Coleman block test to evaluate hindfoot rigidity, and, occasionally, electromyelography. Magnetic resonance imaging (MRI) is usually indicated to evaluate the unilateral cavus foot to rule out occult spinal cord deformity such as tethered cord. The block test is performed by placing a block under the lateral border of the foot and observing the effect upon the first metatarsal. The result of this test helps to determine the need for bony hindfoot surgery in addition to forefoot surgery. Lateral radiographs reveal the high arch and plantar flexed forefoot.

Surgical treatment usually consists of soft tissue releases, tendon transfers, and arthrodesis and must be tailored to the severity of the deformity and the age of the child.

Calcaneovalgus. The dramatic appearance of the calcaneovalgus foot often is very alarming to the child's parents. The dorsum of the foot commonly lies adjacent to the anterior aspect of the tibia. In utero positioning is responsible for the foot's appearance and spontaneously resolves with observation. Gentle stretching exercises are often given to the parents to help speed the process. No functional deformity should be anticipated.

Tarsal Coalition. Congenital fusion of the tarsal bone predisposes the adolescent to foot pain, peroneal spasm, and a rigid flatfoot. A stress fracture through the coalition is thought to be responsible for symptoms and often responds to a period of cast immobilization of approximately 6 weeks. Calcaneonavicular and talocalcaneal fusions constitute the most common coalitions requiring treatment. An autosomal mode of inheritance has been determined for calcaneonavicular coalitions and is best identified on oblique radiographs of the foot. Talocalcaneal bars are best defined by computed tomography (CT), which accurately defines the subtalar joint.

Patients with asymptomatic feet require no treatment, and surgery is reserved for the symptomatic coalition that fails to respond to cast immobilization. Surgical resection of the coalition with interposition of local fat or muscle to prevent bar recurrence is the treatment of choice in the absence of tarsal degenerative changes. Triple arthrodesis remains the procedure of choice for failed coalition resections and coalitions associated with arthritic tarsal joints at the time of presentation.

Vertical Talus. The presence of a rigid flatfoot or rocker-bottom foot deformity in the neonate should alert clinicians to the possibility of a congenital vertical talus. Radiographs reveal marked talar plantar flexion and a fixed talonavicular dislocation. The deformity may be isolated or present as part of a syndrome or neurologic disorder.

Initial treatment consists of manipulation and serial casting to stretch the contracted soft tissues. Although conservative treatment alone is variably successful, soft tissues are optimally prepared for the deformative surgical release, which typically is performed at 6 months of age. Beyond 2 years of age, subtalar fusion is recommended in addition to soft tissue release in order to maintain correction.

Toe Deformity. Polydactyly, or "too many toes," is a common abnormality most often affecting the lateral side of the foot. Accessory digits may be simple (all soft tissue) or complex (containing bony elements). Treatment by surgical excision of the most peripheral toes regardless of composition is recommended.

Overlapping Toes. Overlapping of the fifth toe onto the fourth toe usually is asymptomatic, and no treatment is required. However, when symptoms occur secondary to irritation and pressure, conservative measures, such as stretching and splinting, usually fail. When conservative measures fail, partial excision of the proximal phalanx and syndactylization of the fourth and fifth toes provide excellent results.

Developmental Disorders

Physiologic Genu Varum and Genu Valgum

Bowlegged and knock-knee deformities represent opposite ends of the spectrum of normal lower extremity development. Some degree of varus is present in most children prior to 24 months of age. Beyond 2 years of age, continued growth and weight-bearing lead to some degree of valgus deformity, which usually corrects spontaneously by 6 to 8 years of age.

The treatment of angular deformity in the lower extremity should be reserved for situations in which excessive bowing is not expected to resolve spontaneously or cases in which pathologic processes are at work. When excessive bowlegged deformities are encountered and the child is 2 years of age or older, x-rays of the lower extremities are indicated in order to assess bony anatomy and to calculate the metaphyseal-diaphyseal angle. When greater than 11 degrees, this angle predicts the development of pathologic tibia vara *(Blount's disease)*. With angulation less than 11 degrees, spontaneous resolution of the varus deformity is expected. A valgus deformity of 15 to 20 degrees is often associated with foot and knee complaints. Normal valgus measurements range from 5 to 7 degrees in boys and 9 to 11 degrees in girls. Treatment includes medial heel wedges and lower leg braces for the older child and adolescent. Medial physeal stapling may be performed if enough growth remains to correct the deformity, or osteotomy may be utilized if the projected result of stapling proves inadequate to correct the deformity.

Torsional and Angulation Deformities of the Tibia

Tibial Torsion. Intrauterine fetal positioning is responsible for the torsional attitude of the lower limb. Torsion represents a physiologic spectrum of development that typically begins in some degree of internal torsion and with weight-bearing and growth spontaneously derotates to achieve 15 degrees of external torsion by adulthood. Internal tibial torsion, combined with a compensatory external femoral torsion, is more common than external tibial torsion. Clinically, internal torsion, which appears as intoeing and bowleggedness, is noted by most parents or relatives when a child begins to walk. Parental reassurance and observation constitute the standard treatment except in severe cases of internal tibial torsion, when a Dennis-Brown derotation bar may be employed to speed correction.

Tibia Vara (Blount's Disease). By two years of age, physiologic tibia vara usually resolves spontaneously. When varus deformity remains pronounced at 2 years of age, plain radiographs are obtained to help differentiate the severe physiologic varus deformity from pathologic tibia vara. Infantile tibia vara occurs as a result of a disturbance in posteromedial tibial epiphyseal growth and is usually progressive and bilateral. A tibial metaphyseal-diaphyseal angle greater than 11 degrees is predictive of a progressive varus deformity. Early brace treatment occasionally is successful in preventing severe deformity. Failure of conservative treatment should be followed by a proximal tibial osteotomy prior to the development of growth plate damage.

Adolescent tibia vara occurs in the older child, is unilateral, and must be carefully evaluated with tomograms to rule out the presence of a physeal arrest. Surgical treatment calls for tibial osteotomy. If a bony bridge is present at the site of physeal arrest, it must be excised or the rate of deformity recurrence is unacceptably high.

Hallux Valgus and Bunion Deformities. Deformity of the first metatarsal phalangeal joint is a genetically influenced disorder whose expression is greatly affected by environmental factors. The female sex, a hyperpronated foot, a valgus hindfoot, and poorly fitting shoewear may all contribute to the development of the hallux valgus deformity and bunion formation.

Adolescent hallux valgus is often a progressive disorder that does not respond to conservative measures. As the hallux drifts into further valgus, a painful prominence, or bunion, develops over the medial eminence of the first metatarsal phalangeal joint. An anteroposterior weight-bearing foot radiograph allows calculation of the magnitude of metatarsal phalangeal joint angulation.

The choice of surgical procedures is dependent on the degree of deformity. Treatments attempt to diminish symptoms of pain and swelling until skeletal maturity is reached. Shoe orthotics, including a wide toe box, arch supports, and heel wedges, may be prescribed in addition to nonsteroidal anti-inflammatory medications. Disabling pain despite these measures is an indication for surgical correction of the deformity. The surgical results in treating hallux valgus and bunion deformities in adolescents have been poor in contrast to results in adults secondary to the high incidence of deformity recurrence.

Acquired Disorders

Limb Length Inequality

Asymmetric limb growth may result from a number of different orthopedic conditions, including trauma, infection, tumors, and vascular causes. Regardless of the cause, length discrepancies less than 2 cm usually are tolerated well and require no treatment. When associated problems with leg or back pain or apparent scoliosis occur, simple shoe lifts may be added inside or outside the shoe as needed.

Growth patterns are assessed by the Green-Anderson or Moseley methods. Repetitive growth measurements provide an accurate estimate of the projected growth discrepancy at maturity. When the projected discrepancy is 2 to 6 cm, growth plate arrest or epiphysiodesis of the contralateral femur, tibia, or both may be performed at the appropriate time to achieve limb length equalization. When inadequate growth remains to perform epiphysiodesis, leg-shortening procedures of the longer limb may be performed after skeletal maturity is reached. The Ilizarov method of limb lengthening may be considered when a discrepancy is greater than 5 to 6 cm. A gradual distraction of long bone osteotomies obtains the desired length. Although the results of lengthening may be rewarding, the technique is very demanding and fraught with complications.

Cruciate Knee Ligament Injury

The anterior cruciate ligament (ACL) and posterior cruciate ligament (PCL) are the major stabilizers of the knee in the anterior and posterior planes of motion. The history of a twisting injury, a "popping" sensation, and immediate swelling of the knee is diagnostic of an ACL tear more than 80 per cent of the time. Although ACL tears may occur in knee flexion or extension, a PCL injury occurs most commonly from a direct injury to the anterior aspect of the proximal tibia or a hyperextension movement. These injuries may occur as isolated tears or may be associated with meniscal or collateral ligament tears.

Clinical examination of the injured knee reveals increased anterior tibia translation in ACL injuries and posterior translation or "sag" in PCL injuries. Plain radiographs are needed to evaluate the knee for associated bony avulsion injuries. The presence of such fragments mandates early operative repair in order to achieve normal function. MRI and arthroscopy are recommended early in the management of these injuries so that repair or reconstruction of the torn ligament stabilizes and protects the knee from further injury. Quadriceps and hamstring strengthening are essential adjuncts to knee rehabilitation, and the use of a sports brace should be considered.

Collateral Knee Ligaments Injury

The medial collateral ligament (MCL) and lateral collateral ligament (LCL) are commonly injured during contact sports, wherein a varus or valgus stress is imparted to the lateral or medial aspect of the knee. Complete tears of the MCL are often associated with ACL and medial meniscal tears. In the acute setting, the degree of collateral ligament injury is clinically estimated by observing the degree of joint line opening with applied stress under a general anesthetic. Children whose growth plates are still open require a careful assessment, including stress radiographs, to rule out a physeal fracture. After growth plate closure, the incidence of collateral ligament injury increases.

In the absence of associated meniscal or cruciate ligament injuries, the treatment of collateral ligament sprains is nonoperative. Mild *sprains,* defined as tenderness over the ligament and no instability, may be treated with restricted activity and bracing for 3 to 6 weeks. Moderate sprains are partial tears manifested by pain, ecchymosis, swelling, and some degree of instability on examination. The absence of a firm ligament end point distinguishes a partial versus a complete rupture.

Treatment of isolated moderate and severe *tears* of collateral ligaments consists of long leg casting or bracing for approximately 6 weeks. This treatment should be followed by a generalized lower extremity stretching and strengthening program prior to resumption of competitive athletics.

Snapping Hip and Knee Syndrome

Many individuals, especially dancers, gymnasts, and runners, are able to voluntarily produce clicking or snapping sounds around the hip or knee joint. Occasionally, hip and knee pain develops in association with these sounds and is known as the snapping hip and knee syndrome. At the hip, a poorly conditioned and tight iliotibial band or iliopsoas muscle irritates the bursa overlying the greater trochanter or lesser trochanter respectively. X-ray findings of the hips are normal, and treatment consists of rest, a stretching and strengthening program of the respective muscle groups, and an anti-inflammatory medication. These measures are almost always effective, and rarely does surgery have a role in treatment.

When pain occurs along the lateral aspect of the knee and is associated with a popping or snapping sensation, a tight iliotibial band leading to a bursitis is usually responsible. In this syndrome, the knee is free of effusion, which is indicative of intra-articular pathology. Flexion and extension of the knee will clinically demonstrate the tendon pathology. Knee radiographs will be normal.

Treatment consists of iliotibial band stretching exercises and anti-inflammatory medication. Rarely, surgical lengthening or release of the offending tendon is required.

Knee Extensor Mechanism

The knee extensor mechanism consists of the quadriceps and patellar tendons, the patella, and the tibial tubercle. Acute trauma, overuse syndromes, and malalignment induce pain and inflammation, resulting in patellofemoral dysfunction.

In the absence of knee effusion and mechanical signs of internal derangement, activity-related anterior knee pain is the *sine qua non* of patellofemoral dysfunction. Physical findings, including femoral anteversion, genu valgum or recurvature, patella alta, external tibial torsion, and pronated feet, may predispose a child to malalignment and anterior knee pain. Radiographs may be helpful in some cases but, more frequently, are normal. A knowledge of childhood and adolescent knee disorders and a meticulous physical examination are the keys to differentiating the various causes of anterior knee pain.

Patellar and Quadriceps Tendinitis

Also known as "jumper's knee," the patellar tendon and, less frequently, the quadriceps tendon become inflamed and tender secondary to running or jumping activities. Radiographs of the knee typically are normal but may reveal intratendinous calcification.

Treatment consists of quadriceps muscle stretching and strengthening and physiotherapy modalities. Substitution of activities that do not exacerbate the underlying condition permits the athlete to remain in shape until the condition resolves. Steroid injection should be withheld because of the increased risk of tendon rupture following steroid exposure. When conservative treatment fails, surgical débridement of the tendon yields satisfactory results.

Tibial Tubercle Apophysitis (Osgood-Schlatter Disease)

Apophysitis of the tibial tubercle results in pain during running and jumping activities. Symptoms may be exacerbated by climbing stairs or arising from a seated position. The tibial tubercle is tender to palpation and may enlarge to a prominent bump in response to chronic injury. Radiographs usually are normal but may reveal bony fragmentation of the apophysis.

Activity modification, ice, and a quadriceps stretching and strengthening program are the mainstays of therapy. A knee orthosis (infrapatellar strap) dissipates force transmission from the quadriceps to the tibial apophysis and is a valuable adjunctive treatment. Nonoperative treatment is usually successful, and surgery is reserved for cases in which pain and bony fragmentation persist into adulthood despite conservative management. Débridement of inflamed tissue and bone fragments is curative.

Patellar Stress Syndrome and Instability

Peripatellar knee pain commonly occurs during adolescence and results from chronic patellofemoral overloading and/or maltracking. The adolescent, frequently female, complains of persistent, dull, achy anterior knee pain associated with physical activities. Activities that load the knee in moderate to severe flexion produce the highest degree of patellofemoral contact stress. The peripatellar tissues are palpably tender. Retropatellar crepitus may be present with knee motion. The Q-angle (normal males, 10 degrees; females, 15 degrees), formed by a line connecting the anterosuperior iliac spine to the tibial tubercle through the center of the patella, may be excessive and predispose to patellar maltracking and instability. Lateral knee x-rays may reveal the patellar position to be abnormally high (patella alta) or low (patella baja or infera), thus contributing to instability or overloading. The quadriceps muscle may exert an imbalanced force upon the patella such that the vastus lateralis and lateral retinaculum overpower the vastus medialis and predispose to lateral patellar tilting and subluxation. Patellofemoral hypoplasia may also contribute to extensor mechanism instability.

Radiographic evaluation consists of anteroposterior, lateral, and 30-degree axial views. The anteroposterior view provides initial assessment of patellar position; the lateral view best evaluates patellar baja and alta deformities. On the lateral view, the patellar ligament and patellar length should be equal. If the patella is subluxated on a true lateral film, it will appear abnormally dense as a result of the oblique malpositioning. The axial or tangential view best assesses the patellofemoral articulation, including congruency, trochlear hypoplasia, and patellar instability.

Treatment of patellofemoral stress syndrome and malalignment focuses upon quadriceps rehabilitation. Rebalancing the quadriceps mechanism by selective strengthening of the vastus medialis, patellar mobilization, and hamstring stretching forms the foundation of conservative treatment. A variety of braces are available to help center patellar tracking. Occasionally, medial longitudinal arch supports benefit the patient with excessively pronated flat feet by improving lower extremity malalignment. When conservative treatment fails, surgical proximal or distal extensor mechanism realignment procedures may be performed, depending on the nature of the underlying problem.

Osteochondritis Dissecans of the Knee

Localized osteonecrosis of the medial or lateral femoral condyle predisposes the overlying articular cartilage to injury and subsequent detachment with repetitive knee motion. Pain, swelling, and occasionally mechanical symptoms of locking or catching sensations herald the development of osteochondritis dissecans (OCD). Radiographs may reveal the presence of an osteochondral fragment or an irregular femoral condyle, or they may be entirely normal in appearance. MRI provides valuable information and can diagnose the very early case of osteonecrosis prior to cartilage separation. MRI also defines the depth and extent of the lesion, which are usually not apparent on plain radiographs.

Treatment and prognosis are related to the status of the articular cartilage and age of the child. In younger children, there is a better prognosis for any given stage of OCD secondary to the regenerative capacity of immature tissues. Arthroscopic surgical treatment involves some combination of chondral drilling, pinning, and bone grafting or loose body removal, depending on the condition of the cartilage.

Pes Anserine Bursitis

Repetitive trauma to the bursa underlying the sartorius, gracilis, and semitendinosus tendons results in pain and swelling along the anteromedial aspect of the proximal tibia. Pain clearly arises below the medial joint line of the knee, and mechanical knee symptoms are distinctly absent. Runners possessing excessive foot pronation, swimmers, and cyclists are commonly affected.

The mainstays of treatment include ultrasonography, anti-inflammatory medication, and hamstring stretching exercises. Avoidance of inciting activities is necessary during the acute inflammatory phase. Medial longitudinal arch supports are indicated when foot overpronation is present. Rarely, intrabursal steroid injection may be necessary.

Tendinitis

Inflammation of the extrinsic foot tendons commonly occurs secondary to overuse injury and tight muscle-tendon complexes. The Achilles, posterior tibialis, and flexor halluces longus tendons are commonly involved.

Achilles tendinitis presents as tenderness and swelling over the calcaneal insertion of the tendon. Treatment consists of a ⅛-inch heel lift, modification of activities, ice, nonsteroidal anti-inflammatory medication, and a heel cord stretching program.

Pain along the inferomedial aspect of the medial malleolus and at the medial aspect of the navicular characterizes *posterior tibial tendinitis.* Palpable swelling over the course of the tendon is often present. Symptoms are exacerbated by jumping and running activities. Ice, anti-inflammatory medication, and stretching exercises usually are curative. Symptomatic, pronated flat feet may benefit from medial longitudinal arch supports.

Flexor halluces longus tendinitis presents as pain posterior to the medial malleolus and may be confused with posterior tibial tendinitis. Dancers are particularly prone to this tendon injury, in which repetitive tendon microtrauma results in progressive inflammation and stenosis of the flexor halluces longus tendon sheath. Anti-inflammatory medication, ice, and stretching techniques are employed and usually are successful. Surgical release of the tendon sheath is indicated when conservative treatment fails and symptoms become disabling.

Os Trigonum Syndrome

Approximately 10 per cent of the population have an accessory ossicle present on the posterior aspect of the talus. Lateral radiographs of the foot reveal a smooth, rounded ossific density, representing an unfused lateral process of the posterior talus. Most os trigonum ossicles are asymptomatic, and no treatment is necessary. Repetitive or forced foot plantar flexion, as seen in ballet dancers, results in contusions or fractures of the os trigonum. Pain with forced plantar flexion of the foot is diagnostic of the disorder.

Anti-inflammatory medication, ice, and activity modification usually are curative. Should symptoms continue despite conservative treatment, surgical excision of the os trigonum is indicated.

Accessory Navicular Syndrome

Pain at the posterior tibialis tendon insertion in association with an accessory navicular ossicle characterizes this syndrome. Foot radiographs reveal the rounded deformity of the ossicle along the medial border of the navicular. When conservative measures (ice, anti-inflammatory medication, arch supports, intrinsic foot strengthening) fail, surgical excision of the ossicle provides symptomatic relief.

Plantar Fasciitis

The plantar fascia of the foot originates on the plantar medial aspect of the calcaneus and broadly inserts on the midfoot soft tissues and metatarsals. The fascia provides medial longitudinal arch support and is commonly injured by repetitive microtrauma. Periostitis and calcaneal nerve entrapment are postulated causes of heel pain. Weight bearing and morning start-up pain frequently improve after mild activity, only to return later in the day after prolonged activity. Heel cord contracture, which limits ankle dorsiflexion, often accompanies plantar fasciitis. Point tenderness is elicited along the plantar medial aspect of the calcaneus.

Treatment consists of anti-inflammatory modalities and a heel cord stretching program. Weight-relieving arch supports, which stabilize the hindfoot and elevate the heel, are often invaluable. Intrafascial steroid injection may be employed, but fat pad atrophy secondary to steroid use may exacerbate the condition. When all conservative measures have been exhausted, surgical release of the fascia and medial calcaneal nerve decompression may be performed.

THE HIP

PAUL G. DYMENT, M.D.

SEPTIC HIP

Septic arthritis of the hip joint is one of the true emergencies in pediatrics, as prompt surgical drainage of the joint space may prevent destruction of the femoral head and permanent loss of function. Septic hip is associated with an adjacent osteomyelitis, hematogenous seeding, or direct inoculation of bacteria into the joint from trauma. In neonates the most common organisms are *Staphylococcus aureus, Haemophilus influenzae,* group B *Streptococcus,* and gram-negative coliforms; in infants and children from 4 weeks to 4 years, *S. aureus, H. influenzae,* group B *Streptococcus* (especially in those younger than 1 year of age), and group A *Streptococcus;* and in children older than 4 years of age, usually *S. aureus.*

Diagnosis

Diagnosis of septic hip may be difficult in the neonate because the usual symptoms and signs are absent. Instead, the baby presents more like an infant with septicemia, with signs such as lethargy or irritability, refusal to feed, failure to thrive, cyanosis during the feeding, and no fever. Diagnosis in the typical infant or child with a septic hip usually can be readily made because pain and loss of motion are the presenting symptoms. Such children look ill, and the older ones usually have fever, if not chills. The hip joint is kept in flexion, abduction, and slight external rotation, and the proximal thigh may be swollen. Any sort of passive motion of the infected hip will be resisted because it causes pain; the child will not actively move the involved hip. Palpation of the anterior hip joint will reveal tenderness. A distant site of infection, such as paronychia, skin infection, or pneumonia, is frequently present.

In most patients, there is no leukocytosis, and in more than one third, the differential count is normal; thus, the leukocyte count is of limited value. The erythrocyte sedimentation rate (ESR) is a more useful test, with elevation noted in more than 90 per cent of cases, especially after the first 24 to 48 hours of symptoms; however, this value is unreliable in the neonate. Radiographs may show the signs of fluid in the joint space and/or an adjacent osteomyelitis. A radioisotopic bone scan enables an earlier diagnosis to be made than does a radiograph.

The suspicion of a septic hip should lead directly and immediately to an emergent consultation with an orthopedic surgeon for aspiration of the joint. Ultrasonography of the hip is becoming the preferred test to demonstrate fluid in the joint. Following aspiration, it is critical to confirm that the joint has been entered, in case the joint fluid studies are negative. For this reason, the procedure should be performed under fluoroscopic control, or radiopaque dye should be instilled into the joint after aspiration and a radiograph obtained. The joint fluid in septic hip will reveal a high cell count (mainly neutrophilic leukocytes) and decreased glucose; a Gram stain may reveal microorganisms.

Treatment

Antibiotics should be commenced as soon as the diagnosis is made, the initial choice depending on the child's age, the most likely organisms as indicated above, and the results of the Gram stain:

1. *Neonates.* Methicillin IV or IM and cefotaxime IV or IM (doses depend on age and prematurity) for 21 days or longer.
2. *Infants and young children.* Cefuroxime (100 to 150 mg/kg per 24 hours, IV or IM, divided every 8 hours for 21 days or longer.
3. *Children over 4 years.* Nafcillin, 150 mg/kg per 24 hours IV, divided every 6 hours for 21 days or longer, maximum 12 g/day.

The initial antibiotic should be changed to a more appropriate one, if need be, when the synovial fluid culture and sensitivity results are available.

Immediate arthrotomy, within 6 hours after the synovial fluid analysis confirms the diagnosis, should be performed to decompress the joint space to try to prevent destruction of the cartilage (which is permanent and leads to degenerative arthritis).

TRANSIENT SYNOVITIS

Transient synovitis, or "toxic synovitis," is a self-limited syndrome of acute hip pain of unknown etiology. An infectious cause has been postulated because of its frequent association with upper respiratory infection. It has also been thought to be secondary to occult hip trauma, a sort of "contusion of the hip." Its incidence is about 3 in 100, with boys affected twice as often as girls. Most cases occur between ages 3 and 8 years. About 10 per cent of children with symptoms of transient synovitis eventually develop Legg-Calvé-Perthes disease.

About 70 per cent of patients undergo spontaneous resolution of their symptoms within a week, and almost 90 per cent have done so by 4 weeks. There is a 10 per cent chance of recurrence, generally within the first 6 months after the initial episode.

Diagnosis

The cardinal presenting symptom is the acute onset of unilateral hip pain without any history of trauma. There is a limp, and the involved limb is kept preferentially in flexion and external rotation. The patient does not look sick; there is usually no fever, although there may be an upper respiratory infection. The leukocyte count and ESR are either normal or only minimally elevated. Radiographs of the hips should be obtained mainly to help exclude a more serious diagnosis; they will either be normal or reveal some capsular distention. Ultrasound examination can demonstrate the presence of a mild joint effusion, but is generally not necessary. A bone scan is not indicated since either increased or decreased regional activity can be seen.

Treatment

Simple bed rest and insistence on no weight bearing of the involved joint are generally all that is necessary. This therapy should be continued until there is no further pain and until there is a full range of motion. At one time, many youngsters with transient synovitis received skin traction of the joint as part of their initial treatment; however, now this is not believed to be helpful. If symptoms persist, such traction could be instituted but should be done with the hip flexed to 30 to 45 degrees, the position at which hip joint pressure measurements are at a minimum.

It is not known whether the use of a nonsteroidal anti-inflammatory drug will hasten healing, but on theoretical grounds it would be reasonable to prescribe a regular regimen for the anti-inflammatory effect as well as for analgesic action (i.e., ibuprofen, 40 to 50 mg/kg/day, twice or three times daily, for a maximum of 2400 mg/day).

DEVELOPMENTAL DYSPLASIA OF THE HIP

Developmental dysplasia of the hip (DDH), formerly called "congenital hip dislocation" or "congenital hip dysplasia," refers to a condition beginning in infancy in which there is hip instability and dysplasia. The clinical abnormalities range from simple instability, in which the femoral head can be dislocated and reduced out of or into the acetabulum, to a complete dislocation, in which there is loss of contact between the femoral head and acetabulum. The acetabular cavity is frequently both shallower and more vertical than normal, and the ossification of the proximal femoral epiphysis is frequently delayed; thus, the condition consists of not just a simple dislocated hip; there is a dysplastic component.

The incidence is about 1 in 1000 infants. It is more common in baby girls (1 in 300 in contrast to 1 in 2000 for males), and this is consistent with one of the postulated etiologic factors based on experimental data. Neonatal ligamentous laxity may be induced by estrogen followed by progesterone in female guinea pigs but not in male guinea pigs exposed to the same hormones. This laxity, combined with neonatal positioning, appears to be the principal contributing cause. However, there is another group of infants whose diagnosis is not apparent during the newborn screening examination who later are found to have frank acetabular dysplasia. Studies of twins have also revealed a genetic component, with 34 per cent of identical twins but only 3 per cent of fraternal twins affected. The incidence of DDH is increased in certain "high-risk" groups: frank breech position (25 per cent of them have DDH), coexisting torticollis (15 per cent), positive family history (6 per cent), and coexisting metatarsus adductus (1 per cent). It is reasonable to screen high-risk infants with ultrasonography or a single anteroposterior (AP) radiograph at 3 months of age (when the presence of ossification centers makes roentgenographic interpretation more reliable).

Diagnosis

An overemphasis has been placed on the significance of the newborn hip examination. Although it is important to perform hip examination on all newborn babies, since at least 50 per cent of DDH cases will manifest physical abnormalities of the hip during the newborn period, the other cases will be detected several months later, with only the finding of limited hip abduction. Hence, routine screening by physical examination of the hip should continue throughout the first year of life, with negative findings being recorded during each well-child visit.

Newborn

The Barlow modification of the Ortolani test is the standard examination procedure and should be performed as follows. Many examiners prefer the infant to be lying on the mother's lap. The examiner stabilizes the pelvis by holding it between the thumb and fingers of one hand; the other hand grips the leg being examined with the thumb over the femoral triangle, the web between the thumb and index finger over the knee, and the middle finger tip over the greater trochanter. The knee and thigh should be flexed to 90 degrees, and the hip is then abducted to the mid-abduction position. At that point, the middle finger should press forward over the greater trochanter. If there is forward movement of the femoral head, the hip has been dislocated. The examiner then applies an up-and-down force with the thumb several times with the hip in both mid-abduction and adduction position. Hip instability can be detected by a "clunk" as the femoral head slides over the posterior rim of the hip socket. So-called "clicks" can be found in up to 10 per cent of normal infants.

Infancy

The same examination, as just described, should be performed throughout the first year of life; after the first few weeks of life, the signs of hip instability tend to disappear and limited abduction and limb shortening become the most prominent clinical findings. Asymmetric gluteal folds are a good clue to the presence of limb shortening in such infants.

Radiography

By age 3 months, either a single AP radiograph of the pelvis or ultrasonography is the most definitive diagnostic test. Radiography should be performed in all infants with an abnormal Ortolani-Barlow test and in all infants at "high-risk" as listed above, even if the hip examination is normal. The abnormal radiograph will show the acetabular slope to be more oblique than normal, the ossific nucleus either smaller than the normal side or absent, or the metaphysis displaced laterally.

Treatment

Treatment should be prescribed and monitored frequently by an orthopedic surgeon. There is no justification for a primary care physician advising "triple-diapers" in an attempt to force continuous abduction, as was the practice for many years. This only wastes time, when the infant could be successfully managed by conservative means using the Pavlik harness, a simple, effective, inexpensive, and comfortable treatment that has been successful in more than 90 per cent of young infants with DDH. The earlier treatment with the Pavlik harness is started, the more likely it will be successful and the less likely will be the development of avascular necrosis of the femoral head, a complication of splinting. The Pavlik harness works by keeping the hip flexed and abducted and by limiting extension.

If treatment is not begun until infants are older than 6 months of age, they will probably require traction, reduction under anesthesia, and prolonged immobilization using a cast. Children newly diagnosed after age 2 years will probably require open reduction.

LEGG-CALVÉ-PERTHES DISEASE

Legg-Calvé-Perthes disease (LCPD) is an avascular necrosis of the femoral capital epiphysis of unknown etiology. Its incidence is 1 in 20,000; it appears between the ages of 4 and 8. Boys are affected about four times as often as are girls. About 14 per cent of cases are bilateral, and there is a familial predisposition with an incidence of 1 in 35 in family members. There are several associations with this condition: low birth weight, retarded bone age, white race, and previous history of toxic synovitis.

The natural history is for death of all or part of the epiphysis, followed by removal of the dead bone and replacement with new bone, a healing process that takes 2 or 3 years. The healed femoral head may regrow deformed, especially if there has been unrestricted weight bearing or if the lateral part of the head is not contained within the acetabulum (with an indentation of the new bone resulting from pressure from the hard lateral border of the acetabulum). An abnormally shaped femoral head can lead to persistent limitation of motion and premature degenerative arthritis of the hip joint. Modern forms of treatment are designed to allow the femoral head to regrow in a round configuration, thereby preventing later arthritis.

Diagnosis

The insidious appearance of a limp is the most common presenting symptom. There is usually a history of pain in the hip, but sometimes the condition can present with referred knee pain only. This pain is worse with activity and is relieved by rest. Physical examination reveals an antalgic gait, one in which the patient takes a quick step to shorten the time of weight bearing on the affected side. The passive range of motion of the hip reveals limited abduction and internal rotation. There may be atrophy of the thigh or calf muscles and eventually a shortened leg length as the femoral head flattens.

There are four radiographic stages:

In the *initial stage,* the femoral ossific nucleus is smaller than the contralateral one and there is an apparent joint widening as seen in synovitis, probably actually caused by epiphyseal cartilage hypertrophy. The metaphyseal bone appears less mineralized than the epiphysis, and a subchondral radiolucent zone believed to be a stress fracture demarcates the extent of the necrotic fragment. At this stage, a radioisotopic bone scan may show decreased uptake on the affected side.

In the *fragmentation phase,* the epiphysis has areas of radiolucency and radiodensity, the latter presumably representing healing by new bone formation.

In the *reossification stage,* there is increasing homogeneity of the epiphysis and alteration in the shape of the femoral head and neck. During the healing stages, a bone scan can show enhanced uptake.

In the *healed stage,* residual deformities are all that can be seen.

Treatment

Although half of patients with Legg-Calvé-Perthes disease do not need any treatment, the decision whether or not to treat and the close follow-up of all of these patients, whether treated or not, necessitate an orthopedic surgeon with experience in managing this condition. Earlier treatment programs were based on the belief that prevention of weight bearing would prevent the deformities of the head and, therefore, later degenerative arthritis. This required prolonged hospitalization, traction, strict bed rest, and/or a spica cast. However, not only has this resulted in much emotional trauma and financial cost, but prolonged immobilization has not appeared to influence the radiographic course of the disease.

The basic premise of modern-day treatment is *containment,* based on the concept that deformity of the affected epiphysis can best be prevented by containing the femoral head within the depths of the acetabulum, thus allowing the acetabulum to mold the new head. This can be accomplished by either a "broomstick" abduction long leg cast (Petrie cast) or an abduction brace (such as the Scottish Rite orthosis), both of which allow weight bearing and maintenance of hip range of motion. Such an orthosis allows free motion of the knee and ankle, and the child can walk. The cast generally must be worn full time for 6 to 18 months until the radiographic stage of reossification is reached and there is no more risk of further deformity. Patients who do not even require bracing are those in whom the area of avascular necrosis is restricted to only a small portion of the femoral head, such as the anteromedial portion. If the necrosis involves either the lateral portion of the femoral head or the entire head, either a bracing program or surgical intervention is indicated.

Although a bracing program appears to be the treatment of choice, a good deal of compliance is required on the part of the patient and family. Surgical containment procedures, such as a varus osteotomy of the proximal femur (to place the avascular area within the acetabulum), offer the hope of shorter treatment periods; however, there are risks from these procedures and there is no evidence that earlier surgery to contain the hip is preferable to prolonged bracing.

SLIPPED CAPITAL FEMORAL EPIPHYSIS

Slipped capital femoral epiphysis (SCFE), or "adolescent coxa vara," is the condition in which the epiphysis of the proximal femur separates from the metaphysis, causing the femoral metaphysis to move anteriorly and proximally and the epiphysis to slip posteriorly and medially. Although SCFE can result acutely from severe trauma, generally it is due to a more gradual slip originating from chronic abnormal shear forces. It can occur only before the epiphyseal plate closes during late puberty.

The incidence of SCFE is about 2 per 100,000. It occurs twice as often in boys as girls and in blacks more than in whites. About 25 per cent of cases are bilateral, although only 10 per cent are bilateral at the time of initial diagnosis. SCFE is seen between the ages of 9 and 15, in boys later than girls. Almost 90 per cent of affected patients are obese. There is a slight familial tendency, with 5 per cent of these patients having a parent who had also had the condition. If left untreated, limp and limited hip motion will persist, and premature degenerative arthritis can develop by early adulthood.

Diagnosis

If there has been an acute slip, there is a history of trauma and the patient cannot walk. The affected femur is held in external rotation, and passive movements of the hip are painful. In the chronic form, the pain is more varied and frequently is located in the anterior thigh or knee. The latter is a well-known clinical "trap" and is a reason why all children and adolescents with knee pain should have the hip examined. Physical examination will show a limping child with the affected hip kept in external rotation. Internal rotation, abduction, and flexion of the hip are limited.

When the clinical picture is that of SCFE, anteroposterior, lateral, and "frog lateral" radiographs should be obtained. A mild slip is more obvious with the lateral view, on which posterior displacement of the epiphysis is more apparent. Diffuse osteopenia of the metaphysis and widening of the physis are also radiographic characteristics.

Treatment

Once a diagnosis is confirmed radiographically, the patient should be immediately hospitalized; further slipping is prevented by surgical fixation of the epiphysis using threaded pins across the physis or other fixation technique. Manipulation may be attempted to reduce the amount of slippage, but this is associated with a considerable risk of avascular necrosis, a complication of the treatment and not the disease. Thus, if reduction is indicated, it is usually accomplished by an osteotomy of the proximal femur to reposition the femoral head.

BONE AND JOINT INFECTIONS

HUGH G. WATTS, M.D.

Bone and joint infections, if unrecognized, can have devastating consequences for a child. However, if the process is detected early and treated promptly, the expected result is a virtually normal life (with the exception of those who suffered their infections as neonates).

Infections in the bones originate in the blood stream. Additional trauma probably plays a role. The most common bacterial agent is *Staphylococcus aureus*. In children under the age of 4 years, joints are frequently infected by *Haemophilus influenzae, Streptococcus,* and *Streptococcus pneumoniae* with the concomitant threat of spread to the central nervous system (CNS).

In bone infections, the bacteria are carried in the blood stream to the metaphyses adjacent to the growth plates, where the vessels form terminal branches. There the bacteria multiply. If left untreated, the infection spreads peripherally and penetrates through the cortex of the bone and progresses proximally or distally by lifting up the periosteum. The elevation of the periosteum devascularizes the cortex. Subsequently, new bone is formed by the elevated periosteum, leaving the dead cortical bone as a sequestrum. *In bones where the metaphysis is within the capsule of the adjacent joint (classically in the hip, but also in the shoulder, elbow, and laterally in the knee), the infection can penetrate through the cortex into the joint. Thus, it is important to recognize that an infection in a joint may be secondary to an infection that originated within the metaphysis of the bone. This situation necessitates different management than when the infection is localized solely to the joint.*

Children with bone or joint infections usually present with several days of gradually increasing pain in the limb. In infants, the parents may note merely an unwillingness to use a limb. Because children fall very often, a history of trauma is a frequent source of confusion. Other diseases that can mimic an infection are leukemia (5 per cent of leukemias begin as an apparent septic arthritis), neuroblastoma, and, in older children, Ewing's sarcoma. The hip may be the site of transient synovitis ("toxic synovitis") and Legg-Perthes disease. Monarticular arthritis is often only mildly painful and may result in little restriction in the range of motion.

DIAGNOSIS

A precise physical examination of a hurting, frightened child may prove to be a challenge. In infants, pseudoparalysis may be the only physical sign. In small children, the difficulty is localizing the exact focus of the problem. In the assessment of hip joint pain, it is important to compress the wings of the ilium between the examiner's hands so as not to miss an infection of the sacral iliac region.

Laboratory tests are seldom a big help. In neonates, there may be no significant change in the laboratory findings; in older children, the results give only an indication of generalized illness.

Imaging techniques, on the other hand, can be very useful. The loss of fat lines, seen on plain x-ray films of the extremities, should be carefully analyzed. Trauma and cellulitis cause loss of fat lines near the surface, whereas those close to the bone remain intact. With infection, the reverse is found. Changes in the bone itself do not become evident by x-ray for 1 to 2 weeks. Conversely, after the bone infection has been controlled, the plain films show changes for many weeks to months. Severe changes in the bones associated with less severe clinical signs of systemic illness are more likely to be found in Ewing's sarcoma or leukemia. Because the diagnosis is likely to be suspected earlier than in the past (at a time before changes are seen on plain x-rays of the bones), "bone scans," commonly using ^{99m}technetium–labeled diphosphonate, can be useful, particularly in localizing the disease in the bone; results are better yet if lateral as well as anteroposterior views are taken. This makes the needle aspiration more likely to produce a positive culture. The area of the physes (or growth plate) of the bone is always "hot." Because infection begins immediately adjacent to it, the changes seen on scintigraphy may be subtle. Hyperemia due to a joint infection may mask early changes in the metaphysis, which could be the primary site of the infection. If the infection has penetrated the cortex, elevated the periosteum, and devascularized the cortex, the bone scan may show a central "cold" area surrounded by a halo of increased activity. Scans using gallium– and indium–labeled white blood cells have not lived up to their initial promises and usually are not helpful. Ultrasonography of the joints, especially the hip as well as the elbow and ankle, in small infants may be an aid to recognizing fluid in the joints; however, this diagnostic tool is very dependent on the experience of the user. Computed tomography (CT) and magnetic resonance imaging (MRI) are seldom practical tools for the management of osteomyelitis and septic arthritis in children but may be an adjunct if the infection is in the pelvic bones or the spine.

Needle aspiration of the infected focus is a vital part of diagnosis. If a bone scan is anticipated, a prior needle aspiration does not interfere with its interpretation and so may precede the scan. However, obtaining a scan before the aspiration may be a considerable help in localizing the area to be targeted. The place where the aspiration is to be done requires consideration (i.e., treatment room versus operating room or x-ray department). The setting depends on the age of the child and the location of the infection. Because aspirating a hip joint is difficult under the best of circumstances, it is best to prove that the needle is in the joint by using arthrographic dye. Hence, fluoroscopy should be available. In the hip joint, a positive tap mandates opening the joint because it is very difficult to lavage by repeated joint taps with any degree of certainty. Therefore, the original tap is best done in the operating room. The knee, however, is a joint that is readily accessible for repeated taps for lavage, especially in an older child; thus, one may elect to do this in the treatment room. Aspiration of a bone or joint should be done with a stout needle with a trocar that has a bore large enough to allow withdrawal of thick pus (e.g., a No. 18 spinal needle). During bone aspiration, the needle should penetrate the periosteum and then the medullary cavity immediately adjacent to the physis. Since approximately 20 per cent of needle aspirates for osteomyelitis will not produce bacteria, blood specimens for culture should be obtained because they are positive in approximately 50 per cent of the cases. Gram stain of the aspirate can help to identify the organism immediately in half of the cases. In septic arthritis, the yield by Gram stain and culture is lower (50 to 60 per cent). If a swollen joint is to be tapped with the anticipation of lavaging the joint after obtaining a diagnostic specimen, the use of a plastic needle catheter can greatly facilitate the flushing-out process with less likelihood of dislodging the needle during the maneuvering that occurs during switching syringes.

Neonates, especially premature babies, are particularly vulnerable to bone and joint infections, which are often found together and frequently in multiple sites. These patients are often seriously sick with other problems and have few resources to bring to control the infection. Laboratory tests may be normal. In spite of vigilant care, such children can quickly experience total destruction of an infected joint as well as the growth plates of the long bones, leading to lifelong crippling.

TREATMENT (Table 1)

Bone Infections

Acute Hematogenous Osteomyelitis. Three aspects should be considered: (1) treatment of the infection involving the total body, (2) treatment of the bone tissue infection itself, and (3) treatment of the extremity. A child who is generally toxic and vomiting will require intravenous antibiotics. In treatment of bone infection, antibiotics alone are usually sufficient in early cases. If there is evidence of a subperiosteal abscess, the area needs to be drained surgically.

The selection of antibiotics for bone, in contrast to joint infections, is made on the basis that the organism is most likely to be *S. aureus*. Oxacillin is the usual first choice until the culture reports are returned, but cefazolin is used if there is a penicillin allergy; clindamycin is used if there is an allergy to penicillins and cephalosporins. In neonates, who harbor gram-negative organisms and group B streptococci, gentamicin or cefotaxime is added until the sensitivity report is returned.

The route of administration is controversial. Most antibiotics reach adequate tissue levels when given orally. In the past, the intravenous route was used throughout the entire treatment course; current protocols reserve the intravenous route for the first days when the child is toxic and may be unable to swallow the medicine because of vomiting. The added risk of poor absorption from the gut during this period is unwarranted. Intravenous drugs can be given for as little as 2 or 3 days and ordinarily for no more than 1 week. The remainder of the treatment is given orally. The duration of treatment is also controversial. This depends in part on the extent of the disease and the bacteria involved. Although some pediatricians treat for as little as 3 weeks, the common standard is 6 weeks of treatment.

Treating the extremity is best managed by putting it to rest. A light splint to minimize motion is a comforting relief to the child. If the bone involvement is moderate to severe, there is a risk of subsequent pathologic fracture. This is more likely to occur several weeks after the onset of the disease, when the repair process is initiated by osteoclastic reabsorption of bone. Restricted weight bearing may be needed.

Subacute Osteomyelitis. Children with subacute osteomyelitis are more likely to require surgery for the drainage of pus. The antibiotic treatment may be prolonged with oral medication, usually cephalexin, for 2 to 3 months.

Chronic Osteomyelitis. In North America, chronic bone infection in children is most likely to be due to open trauma secondarily involving the bone. When chronic osteomyelitis is observed, one should carefully think of the other diseases (e.g., Ewing's sarcoma and leukemia) as well as the uncommon etiologic agents (tuberculosis or fungi). The increase in the number of children with acquired immunodeficiency syndrome (AIDS) gives a greater likelihood of finding odd organisms.

Sacroiliac Infection. Although commonly designated as a joint infection, usually it is an osteomyelitis in the metaphysis of the ilium adjacent to the sacroiliac joint. The clinical picture is that of vague illness with pain in and around the hip that may be accompanied by limitation of motion of the hip joint. The diagnosis is frequently missed for 1 to 2 months. Characteristically, compression of the pelvis between the palms of the examiner's hands will reproduce the pain. A bone scan is the most likely means of identifying the infection. Because this infection is usually in the ilium adjacent to the joint, aspiration should be directed at the bone rather than the joint.

Punctures of the Foot Through the Shoe. The most common organism causing deep infection resulting from punctures of the sole of the foot (commonly by a nail through a soft "sneaker") is *Pseudomonas*. This infection often becomes evident a week or more after the injury. Treatment commonly involves extensive surgical débridement and appropriate antibiotics, usually gentamicin.

Spine and Discitis. Some authors have questioned whether

TABLE 1. Commonly Used Antibiotics for Infants and Children in Bone and Joint Infection

Antibiotic	Intravenous Dosage	Oral Dosage	Maximum
Ampicillin	100–200 mg/kg/24 hr q 6 hr	—	12 g/day
Amoxicillin	—	25–50 mg/kg/24 hr q 8 hr	
Cefazolin	50–100 mg/kg/24 hr q 8 hr	—	6 g/day
Cefotaxime	100–200 mg/kg/24 hr q 6 hr	—	
Cefuroxime	75–150 mg/kg/24 hr q 8 hr	—	6 g/day
Cephalexin	—	100 mg/kg/24 hr q 6 hr	4 g/day
Chloramphenicol	75 mg/kg/24 hr q 6 hr	50–75 mg/kg/24 hr q 6 hr	
Clindamycin	25–40 mg/kg/24 hr q 8 hr	10–30 mg/kg/24 hr q 8 hr	
Dicloxacillin	—	50–75 mg/kg/24 hr q 6 hr	
Gentamicin	6.0–7.5 mg/kg/24 hr q 8 hr	—	
Oxacillin	150–200 mg/kg/24 hr q 6 hr	—	
Vancomycin	40 mg/kg/24 hr q 6 hr	—	

this is an infection in all cases. However, the consensus is that this is an infection found in older children, immediately adjacent to the metaphysis of the body of the vertebrae, which may penetrate the end plate and lead to a collapse in the disc. The infection may or may not involve the disc itself. Needle aspiration of the disc space is frequently negative and is better directed at the bone adjacent to the end plate. Treatment consists of appropriate antibiotics, and surgery usually is not required. Immobilization in a body jacket relieves the pain. It has been suggested that such immobilization can aid in the treatment of the infection itself.

Sickle Cell Disease. It can be very difficult to differentiate between a sickle crisis and acute osteomyelitis; they may occur together. Usually, bone scans are not helpful in resolving this dilemma, although a bone scan contrasted with a marrow scan may be useful. The organism is commonly *Salmonella* but a wide spectrum of other species, especially *S. aureus,* may be included. It is safest to protect the child with intravenous antibiotics (ampicillin or cefotaxime and cefazolin) until the results of the aspiration cultures become available. In severe involvement, surgical débridement is necessary in spite of the previous concerns for operating on these children.

Brodie's Abscess. This is a low-grade chronic infection in the long bones of the lower extremity found more often in older children. The complaint is pain, and there are rarely any systemic manifestations. Brodie's abscess is seen on the plain x-ray as a very focal lytic area and can be confused with an osteoid osteoma. The treatment is primarily surgical excision. The organism, if one does grow on culture at all, is often *S. aureus* of very low virulence. Although adjuvant antibiotics are used, they probably are not necessary.

Joint Infections

When dealing with an infected joint, one must consider the possibility that the joint infection is secondary to an osteomyelitis of the metaphysis that has penetrated into the joint.

Acute Hematogenous Septic Arthritis. Treatment involves the bacterial infection of the entire body, the treatment of the joint tissues, and care of the extremity.

In children under 4 years of age, the bacteria infecting the joint may include organisms other than *S. aureus* that may spread to the CNS; thus, a different range of antibiotics needs to be used predicated on the age of the child. Neonates are usually treated with gentamicin or cefotaxime in addition to oxacillin to protect against possible gram-negative organisms as well as *Streptococcus* group B. Because *H. influenzae* and *Streptococcus* group A and B are noted in children up to age 4 years, they are usually treated with cefuroxime; children over the age of 4 years are treated with oxacillin or cefazolin. The route of antibiotic administration is as described above for bone (i.e., intravenous for a few days while the child is toxic or vomiting and then conversion to oral antibiotics). Generally, 3 weeks is considered adequate.

When considering the joint itself, one must remember that bacteria alone do not destroy cartilage. The synovium and white blood cells produce lytic enzymes in response to the infection, and these enzymes, in turn, destroy the cartilage cells. Treatment of the joint, therefore, involves not only getting rid of the bacteria but also flushing out the enzymes, which are damaging the cartilage cells. It is extremely difficult to be certain that the needle is in the hip joint. As a consequence, that joint is best managed with an open operation. Other joints may be managed by a second aspiration and flushing of the joint. One needs to balance the morbidity of achieving this by a formal operation in the operating room versus the trauma to the psyche of the patient (and the physician) in doing multiple aspirations with local anesthesia in a small child. In the knee joint, some surgeons prefer the use of an arthroscope. This can be effective unless the treatment has been delayed, at which point adhesions may result in pockets of pus (particularly in the suprapatellar pouch), which readily go unrecognized through the arthroscope and thus are not drained.

Treatment of the extremity itself is controversial. Although motion is important for the nutrition of cartilage tissues, the joint is painful and splinting is the usual first treatment. There is a growing interest in the use of constant passive motion machines (CPMs), but this has not yet proved effective.

Subacute and Chronic Infections of the Joints. Such infections are very uncommon and are usually related to open trauma. They are more likely to necessitate open surgical drainage and, on occasion, synovectomy. With the increase in the incidence of AIDS in children, unusual bacterial involvement in the joint, such as *Mycobacterium, Brucella,* and *Serratia,* must be considered.

TREATMENT OF BONE TUMORS AND LIMB SALVAGE

NORRIS C. CARROLL, M.D.

The annual incidence of primary malignant bone tumors in white children is 5.6 per million, and in black children it is 4.8 per million. Each year in the United States, 320 children under the age of 15 years present with a bone tumor, 60 per cent of which are osteosarcomas. Osteosarcoma is twice as common as Ewing's sarcoma in white children. Ewing's sarcoma is quite rare in black children. Chrondrosarcomas, malignant fibrous histiocytoma, and fibrosarcomas occur very infrequently. In my own practice, chondrosarcoma has been the most common of these three rare tumors.

Modern medicine, with its increased diagnostic awareness, improvements in imaging, new chemotherapeutic regimens, and radiotherapy techniques, has led to dramatic improvements in survival rates for primary malignant bone tumors. With improved surgical techniques, fewer and fewer limbs are being amputated and limb salvage has become accepted as a treatment of choice.

OSTEOSARCOMA

Osteosarcoma can arise in any bone but is most common in the metaphyses of the distal femur, proximal tibia, and proximal humerus. There is an increased incidence of osteosarcoma in children with bilateral retinoblastoma, and there is an increased incidence following irradiation. The most common presenting symptom is pain at the tumor site. The patient and family often assume that the pain is due to an injury. On the plain x-ray, there is mixed destruction and ossification at the tumor site with a wide zone of transition and subperiosteal new bone formation is common.

Staging

All patients must be staged prior to biopsy. Staging leads to better clinical, radiographic, and pathologic correlations because imaging specificity decreases after biopsy. In staging, our team looks at the degree of involvement of the bone, physis, epiphysis, joint, neurovascular bundle, and muscle compartments. We look for lymph node involvement and lung metastases. Magnetic resonance imaging (MRI) is used to determine the tumor margins in the limb. A technetium bone scan is used to look for other sites, and computed tomography (CT) is performed on the lungs to look for pulmonary metastases.

If it is obvious from the staging studies that the child has a malignant bone tumor, the biopsy should be performed by the surgeon who will undertake the definitive surgery. If the child is a candidate for limb salvage, the incision must be excised en bloc with the tumor. This means that a longitudinal, rather than a transverse, incision should be used. The biopsy site should avoid the neurovascular structures and traverse the least number of compartments. The specimen should be taken from the periphery of the tumor, and it is usually not necessary to obtain a biopsy specimen of the bone if there is soft tissue extension. A frozen section should be done to make sure that there is adequate tissue for a definitive diagnosis.

Treatment

The treatment for osteosarcoma is surgery and chemotherapy. There have been trials of intra-arterial chemotherapy with and without preoperative radiation prior to surgery, but my personal preference is for neoadjuvant systemic chemotherapy. The main chemotherapeutic drug has been high-dose methotrexate. Other drugs used in combination include bleomycin, cyclophosphamide (Cytoxan), actinomycin D, doxorubicin (Adriamycin), and cisplatin. Preoperative chemotherapy reduces edema, which facilitates the surgical dissection. It also allows one to assess the efficacy of the drugs being used. One also hopes that it will destroy occult microextensions of the tumor and occult metastases. Following surgery the children receive chemotherapy for 12 to 18 months.

The first priority of surgery is total removal of the tumor with clean margins. The second priority is to preserve function by limb salvage. The criticisms of limb salvage are the risk of local recurrence, the disfiguring aspects of the procedures, and the possible presence of skip lesions. It has been found, however, that limb salvage does not adversely affect survival. Limb salvage options include excision of an expendable bone, replacement with a nonvascularized or vascularized autograft, replacement with an allograft, and replacement with an internal prosthesis.

Some of the problems with these salvage procedures are that children want to lead a vigorous lifestyle, have a growing skeleton, and may present with a large lesion with extensive soft tissue involvement. To solve these problems, we have used the *rotationplasty* for tumors of the distal femur, proximal tibia, and proximal femur. When the *proximal femur* is resected, the knee joint becomes the hip joint, the ankle joint becomes the knee joint, and the calf serves as the quadriceps. When the *distal femur* is resected, the calf becomes the quadriceps and the ankle joint becomes the knee joint. When the *proximal tibia* is resected, the ankle joint becomes the knee joint but the quadriceps maintains its original function as the knee extensor.

Following a rotationplasty, children wear a modified below-knee prosthesis. All of our patients have been good prosthetic users with "active knee" flexion and extension. Because they have a "motorized knee" with swing phase control, their gait is more efficient than that of children with an above-knee amputation.

In the upper extremity, it is possible to resect the clavicle or the scapula and still preserve good function. The proximal two thirds of the humerus can be replaced by a vascularized fibula, as can the distal radius and distal ulna. With neoadjuvant and adjuvant chemotherapy combined with limb salvage, the 5-year, disease-free survival for osteosarcoma has increased to between 50 and 74 per cent.

Approximately one in six children who present with osteosarcoma already have pulmonary metastases. These children usually require an amputation. Even in these children, disease-free survival is possible with aggressive surgery and chemotherapy.

PAROSTEAL OSTEOSARCOMA

Parosteal osteosarcoma is a slow-growing, low-grade malignancy. Again, this tumor occurs in the metaphyses of the major long bones, with the distal femur and the proximal tibia being the most common sites. These lesions usually are not painful. One of my patients who had a large lesion in the posterior aspect of the distal femoral metaphysis presented not because of pain but because she could not flex her knee beyond 80 degrees.

These lesions do not respond to chemotherapy and radiation. The treatment is wide marginal excision.

EWING'S SARCOMA

Ewing's sarcoma is the second most common primary malignant bone tumor in children. It arises from the nonmesenchymal elements of the bone marrow. The most common sites are the femur, pelvis, humerus, clavicle, and fibula.

Clinical Features

The children usually present with a painful mass. They often have a low-grade fever, leukocytosis with a left shift, and an increased erythrocyte sedimentation rate (ESR). Plain x-rays demonstrate a permeative destructive lesion with a wide transition zone. Subperiosteal new bone formation can be seen at the edges of the lesion. It may be difficult to differentiate the tumor from osteomyelitis.

Treatment

When the only treatment option was surgery, the 5-year survival rate was less than 10 per cent. Surgery then took a back seat to radiation therapy. Radiation controlled the tumor initially, but there was a problem with local recurrence and metastatic disease, so that there was a very poor 5-year survival. Survival was even worse in patients with involvement of the pelvis, shoulder girdle, spine, or ribs.

Systemic chemotherapy protocols employing a combination of actinomycin D, cyclophosphamide, Adriamycin, ifosfamide, vincristine, and VP16 have resulted in increased survival in multicenter studies. The best reported results at present are in patients who have undergone resection of the lesion with chemotherapy and radiation. My personal preference is for neoadjuvant chemotherapy, resection of the lesion followed by chemotherapy, and avoidance of radiation because of the risk of inducing an osteosarcoma. The survival rate in children who present with metastases is very poor, the usual treatment includes chemotherapy and radiation alone.

CHONDROSARCOMA

Chrondrosarcomas are very rare neoplasms in childhood. They are slow-growing tumors that do not metastasize early. The primary treatment is surgical. The four children that I have seen with chondrosarcoma were all candidates for limb salvage and were managed by resection of an expendable bone, a replacement autograft, a replacement vascularized autograft, and a rotationplasty.

FIBROSARCOMA

Most fibrosarcomas in children arise in the soft tissues but some can be primarily in bone. The surgical treatment indicated depends on the histologic grade of the lesion, with high-grade lesions warranting a radical excision.

MALIGNANT FIBROUS HISTIOCYTOMA

This tumor is very uncommon in the pediatric population. Whenever possible, the tumor should be treated by a wide surgical excision. The children are given adjuvant chemotherapy. In my experience the prognosis is poor.

ADAMANTINOMA

Another rare tumor is the adamantinoma. I have a lot of respect for this tumor. It is a tumor of uncertain origin that I have seen only in the anterior cortex of the tibia. On plain x-ray it has a characteristic "soap bubble" appearance. Curettage and marginal extracapsular excision invariably lead to a recurrence, whereas with a wide surgical margin one's patient will be cured. There is no indication for chemotherapy.

CONGENITAL HAND AND ARM DEFORMITIES

A. LEE OSTERMAN, M.D.
and GARY DONATH, M.D.

One in every 626 neonates exhibits a congenital anomaly of the upper extremity. Although most of these deformities are minor, one in ten results in significant functional and/or cosmetic derangement.

Many of these anomalies are found in association with abnormalities affecting other organ systems, and some are syndromic. Management of these patients, therefore, requires a coordinated, multidisciplinary approach, including a pediatrician, geneticist, hand surgeon, and hand therapist.

Several classification schemes have been offered to organize upper extremity congenital anomalies. We prefer the classification system presented in Table 1.

TABLE 1. Classification of Congenital Abnormalities

- I. **Failure of Formation**
  - A. Transverse
    1. Amputations
    2. Phocomelia
  - B. Longitudinal
    1. Radial clubhand
    2. Cleft hand
    3. Ulnar clubhand
- II. **Failure of Differentiation**
  1. Simple syndactyly
  2. Complex syndactyly
  3. Radioulnar synostosis
- III. **Duplication**
  1. Polydactyly
- IV. **Overgrowth**
  1. Macrodactyly
- V. **Undergrowth**
  1. Short metacarpals
- VI. **Constriction Bands**
- VII. **Intrinsic Finger Abnormalities**
  1. Camptodactyly
  2. Clinodactyly
  3. Delta phalanx
  4. Kirner's deformity
  5. Symphalangism
- VIII. **Thumb Abnormalities**
  1. Deficient components
     - a. Hypoplasia
     - b. Pouce flottant
     - c. Absent thumb
  2. Extra components
     - a. Triphalangeal thumb
     - b. Duplicated thumb
  3. Disturbance of functional components
     - a. Absent muscle tendon units
     - b. Trigger thumb

The upper limb develops in a proximal to distal direction, with the arm bud appearing on day 26, the hand paddle appearing on day 36, the finger rays appearing on day 41, and finger separation occurring between days 47 and 8 weeks of gestational age. As these developmental changes occur in the upper limb bud, other systems are developing concurrently. Therefore, the association of radial and thumb deficiencies with cardiovascular, gastrointestinal, and hematopoietic disorders is common. Syndactyly, which results from incomplete separation of fingers rays, occurs later in arm bud development and is thus more commonly associated with craniofacial and cutaneous syndromes.

The surgical goals are simply the preservation or improvement of function, particularly power grip and prehension. In children with more proximal upper extremity anomalies, one attempts to improve the ability of the child to place and maneuver the hand in space and to improve the aesthetic appearance.

The timing of surgery for congenital anomalies of the upper extremity is dependent on a number of conditions. In a deformity that threatens the viability of limb or digit as in some cases of constriction band syndrome, correction is required in the first few days of life. If a deformity increases with time and exerts a tethering effect that alters growth, such as *thumb-index syndactyly,* it should be addressed within the first year. Occasionally, staged surgical procedures are required (e.g., radial club hand) and surgical reconstruction should begin early. If developmental patterns of use are influenced by the operation (e.g., index pollicization), it is generally better to perform the surgery when the child is between 1 and 3 years of age. If rehabilitation and therapy are necessary for success (e.g., certain tendon transfers), surgical intervention is often delayed until the child is 4 or 5 years of age. In general, when possible, the majority of any surgical reconstruction should be completed before the child enters kindergarten or first grade.

FAILURE OF FORMATION

Transverse Problems

Amputations

Transverse failure of formation or transverse deficiency (congenital amputation) is classified by the level of amputation. The most common varieties are *adactyly* (absence of the digits), *hemimelia* (absence of the forearm and hand), and *amelia,* (absence of the arm). The incidence of hemimelia is one in 20,000 live births, and the incidence of amelia is one in 270,000 live births. The terminal portion of these congenital amputation stumps may exhibit a variety of configurations, and some may include digital remnants (Fig. 1).

The occasion for surgery in this category is rare, and the hallmark for treatment is prosthetic fitting. The timing of application of prostheses is best summarized by the aphorism "fit to sit." The initial prosthesis is a passive one, and an active prosthesis is usually introduced when coordination is adequate, at 18 to 24 months. Bioelectric systems and other more

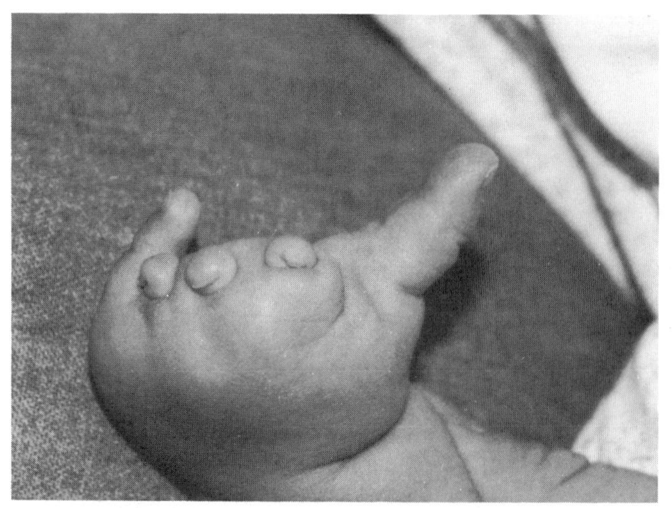

Figure 1. An example of adactyly. In more proximal amputations, such as the short below-elbow amputation, early prosthetic fitting is indicated. In a case such as is seen here, a better solution would be to add digital length to the metacarpal nubbins to provide opposition digits to the relatively normal thumb.

complex prostheses are reserved for later childhood and young adulthood.

Phocomelia

Phocomelia (seal-like arm) is a rare congenital abnormality that was seen in Europe in the late 1950s and related to maternal thalidomide ingestion. Its current incidence is approximately 0.8 per cent of all upper limb anomalies. It is classified into several anatomic types on the basis of the amount of intermediate segment between shoulder and hand. In *type I,* the hand directly attaches to the trunk. In *type II* deformities, a short forearm segment is present between the hand and trunk. In *type III,* the hand articulates with the humerus.

Limb training and prostheses offer the greatest benefit to these patients, and in some cases bone grafting may provide stability and tendon transfers may improve joint motion. A new technique developed in the former Soviet Union, the Ilizarov, uses staged distraction through wires to augment the length of bone and soft tissue. Although its main applications are currently in lower extremity problems, the Ilizarov does appear to have new applications in the treatment of upper extremity failure of formation.

Longitudinal Problems

Radial Clubhand

Radial clubhand is a deformity that includes involvement of the bone, joints, muscle, tendon, and nerves in the forearm (Fig. 2*A*). The severity of the deficiency ranges from hypoplasia of the radius to partial or total absence of the radius. As stated above, radial clubhand is not simply a skeletal deficiency. The thumb is absent or abnormal in 90 per cent of the patients, and the ulna is universally shortened, reaching on average 60 per cent of its normal length, and is often bowed. The radial side of the carpus is frequently deficient; the extensor carpi radialis brevis and longus are absent, and the flexor carpi radialis absent in two thirds of the patients. Larger joints are commonly stiff, particularly in the index and long fingers. Five per cent of patients display significant elbow abnormalities characterized by stiffness in extension, whereas another 5 per cent have shoulder involvement. Associated abnormalities are common, with a particularly high incidence of cardiovascular and blood dyscrasias. Fanconi's syndrome should be ruled out in all patients with radial deficiencies (Table 2).

The treatment of radial clubhand begins in the nursery with static and stretching splints that serve to pull the hand in proper alignment over the forearm. In severe cases, when soft tissue balance cannot be achieved in this manner, early release of tight fascial structures may be necessary.

The goals of surgical treatment are to maximize forearm length, improve digital motion and dexterity, and achieve a more powerful grasp. Although several methods for surgical correction are available, we favor alignment of the carpus over the ulna. The so-called centralization procedure is optimally performed during the child's first year after serial casting has stretched the soft tissue structures (Fig. 2*B, C*). Tendon transfers are a valuable adjunct to the alignment procedure and often obviate the need for wrist arthroscopy, which is performed at the time of skeletal maturity. In children with deficient thumbs, pollicization is generally performed between the first and third years. Power pinch and grip as well as manipulation skills are superior in surgically treated patients. One caveat is a stiff elbow that cannot be mobilized; this may be a contraindication to the centralization procedure.

Cleft Hand Deformity

Cleft hand deformity is characterized by suppression of central growth and a resultant deformity ranging in severity from simple ray separation with normal skeletal structures to the so-called "lobster claw hand" (Fig. 3). This deformity is usually present bilaterally and inherited in a typical dominant pattern. A number of procedures are available that serve to close the skeletal and soft tissue cleft. An important consideration is that the chosen procedure provides an adequate thumb web to allow for opposition. Interestingly, a majority of associated abnormalities include clefts of the feet and cleft lip and cleft palate.

Ulnar Clubhand

Ulnar clubhand is the least common of the longitudinal deficiencies. Its occurrence is sporadic and usually unilateral.

TABLE 2. Syndromes with Radial Defects

Syndrome	Congenital Defect	Inheritance
Holt-Oram	Atrial septal defects	Autosomal dominant
TAR	*T*hrombocytopenia, *A*bsent *R*adius	Autosomal recessive?
Fanconi	Aplastic anemia; skin pigmentation or vitiligo; craniofacial defects, renal defects	
VATER	*V*ertebral *A*bnormalities, *T*racheo-*E*sophageal fistula, *R*adius abnormalities, imperforate anus	Unknown

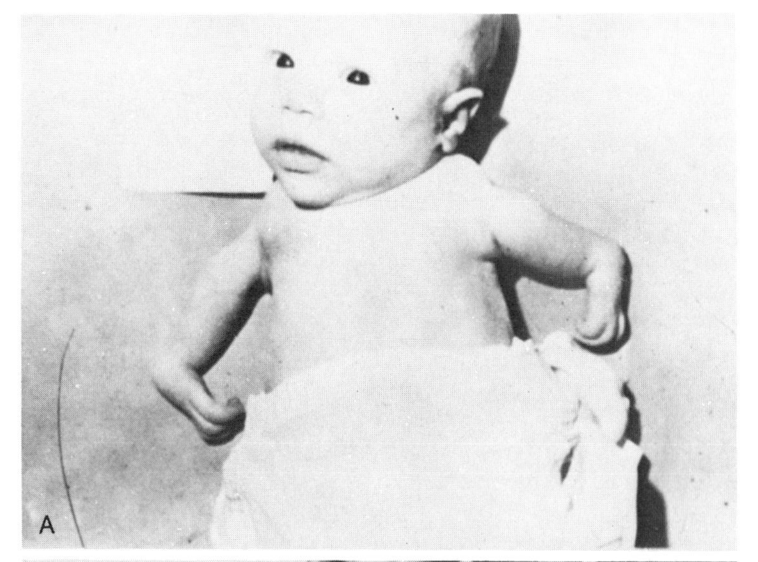

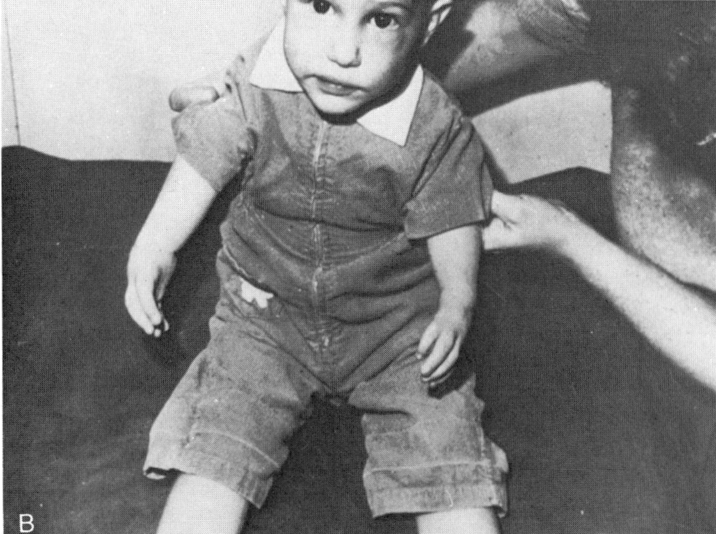

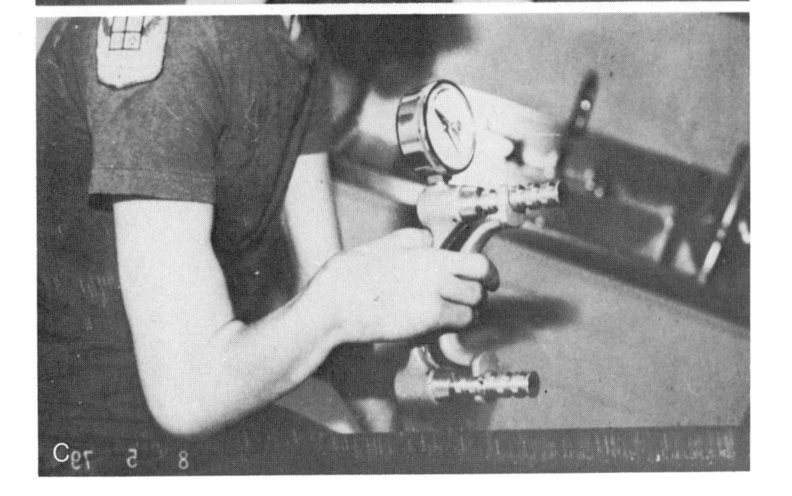

Figure 2. Radial clubhand. *A,* When this is seen in the newborn nursery, initial care includes immediate splinting and stretching exercises. *B,* Child, age 2½ years, after bilateral centralization procedures. *C,* Skeletal maturity following centralization and pollicization in a teenager. Note the persistent relative shortness of the forearm.

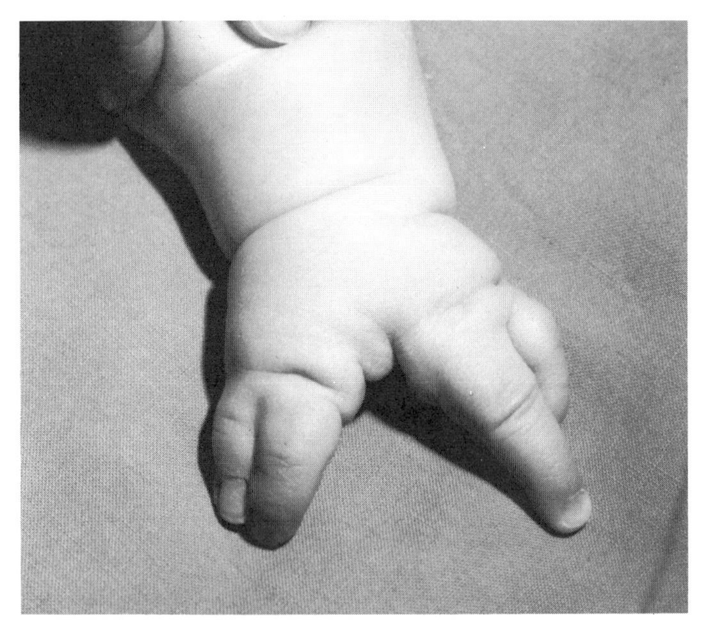

Figure 3. Left hand deformity. Note the relative syndactyly between the ulnar fourth and fifth digits. Treatment would be closure of the defect between the index and ulnar digits with creation of a thumb web space for opposition.

Ulnar clubhand is characterized by ulnar shortening, radial bowing, and digital abnormalities in more than 50 per cent of patients.

Ulnar deficiencies differ from radial deficiencies in several ways: (1) they are one-tenth as common, (2) the hand is generally stable at the wrist and unstable at the elbow, and (3) systemic cardiac, hematologic, and gastrointestinal anomalies are uncommon, whereas other musculoskeletal problems may occur.

Absence of fingers is more common in ulnar clubhand than in radial clubhand. Radial clubhand tends to affect only the thumb and radial digits. In ulnar clubhand, an anlage or fibrous remnant frequently remains. This can cause progressive ulnar deviation of the hand and wrist with growth. When this anlage is present, it should be resected at an early age to prevent this deviation. In older patients with elbow flexion contractures, radial head dislocation, and instability of the forearm, creation of a one-bone forearm provides stability and allows for improved positioning of the hand in space.

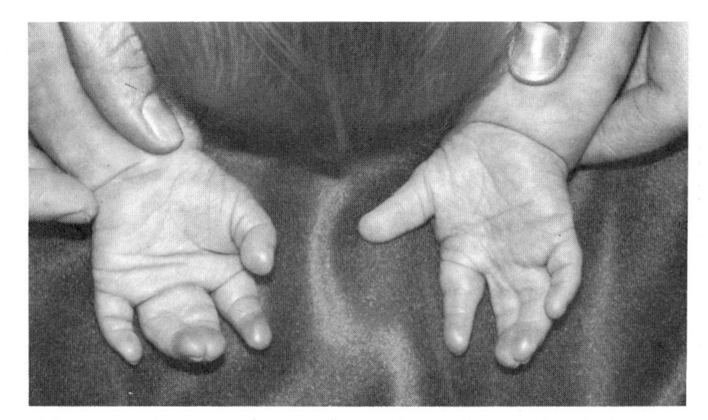

Figure 4. The most common form of complete syndactyly between the middle and ring fingers.

FAILURE OF DIFFERENTIATION

Syndactyly

Syndactyly, or failure of differentiation of tissues between the fingers, can be classified as *simple* (involving skin elements only) (Fig. 4) or *complex* (involving both soft tissue, nail, and skeletal elements) (Fig. 5). Simple syndactyly is further classified as either *complete* or *incomplete* on the basis of the extent of interdigital webbing involved (Fig. 6). It occurs in one of every 2000 to 2500 births and is a sporadic or occasionally genetically determined trait. Boys are more commonly affected than girls, and bilateral symmetric involvement is common. Syndactyly is also a common component of many congenital anomalies, including such syndromes as trisomy 13, 18, and 21; craniofacial syndromes; and cutaneous dermal dysplastic syndromes. These syndromes in which syndactyly is a consistent component are listed in Table 3. The site of syndactyly is most commonly the long and ring fingers followed by the small and ring fingers. The thumb index web is rarely involved (under 5 per cent).

Webbed fingers are an obvious physical defect, and surgical separation is usually beneficial both cosmetically and function-

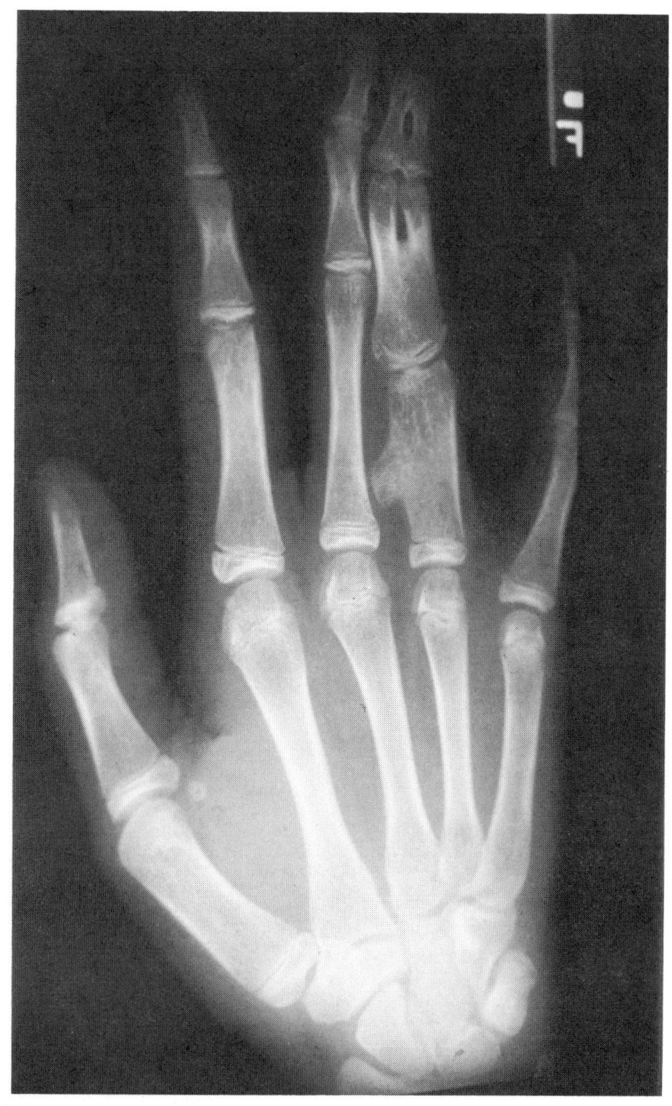

Figure 5. Complex syndactyly with multiple tissues involves bone, tendon, and nerve.

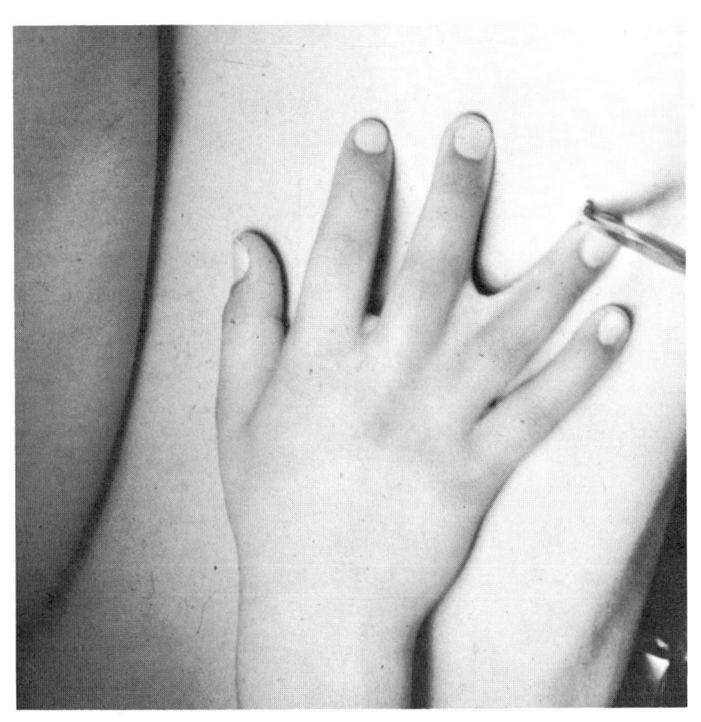

Figure 6. Simple incomplete syndactyly.

ally. The timing of surgical intervention depends on the fingers that are involved. In *simple syndactyly,* separation of fingers of unequal length (border digits) is necessary to prevent a flexion or rotational deformity. *Thumb-index syndactyly* should be corrected by 3 months, and ring and small finger syndactyly should be corrected prior to 2 years. In *triple-digit syndactyly,* staged release is required for vascular security. Only one border of the central digit should be released during a single surgical procedure. Separation of fingers of equal length (long and ring) can be delayed until ages 3 to 4. Some authors believe that such delay allows for better flap definition, as the baby fat is gone, and may decrease the incidence of web creep, which can require late revision in up to 30 per cent of patients. *Complex syndactyly* may require multiple surgical procedures that should be completed by 1 year of age to avoid a progressive deformity and to allow an adequate result to be obtained prior to school age.

Methods for the correction of syndactyly depend on the extent of the web. If only web space deepening is required, local flaps may suffice. With simple complete syndactyly, skin grafting is always required. We prefer to use full-thickness skin grafts from the groin (a near and visible donor site in most patients) and a dorsal rhomboid flap to create the critical padding in the commissure. Zigzag skin incisions are always used. In complex syndactyly, such as *Apert's acrosyndactyly,* our goal is generally to create a three-fingered hand with thumb and digital opposition.

Synostosis

Synostosis (melding in of the bones) can occur anywhere in the arm when two bones are adjacent to each other either in longitudinal or transverse relationships. *Longitudinal synostosis* between the phalanges has a special name *(symphalangism)* and is covered under intrinsic finger abnormalities. Coalition between metacarpal bones is common, with the lunate and triquetrum being the most common carpal coalition, particularly in blacks. Most such carpal coalitions are found in association with the more functionally disabling metacarpal synostosis.

The most common functional synostosis is the *proximal synostosis* between the radius and ulna. The patient presents with a fixed forearm position, with the arm usually positioned in pronation. If this pronation deformity is unilateral and less than 30 degrees, no treatment is indicated. If, however, more than 30 degrees of pronation is present, a derotational osteotomy at the synostosis site is helpful. In bilateral cases, the dominant arm is generally placed in 20 degrees of pronation and the subdominant arm is individualized with a "clapping hands" position most commonly chosen. Corrective surgery, when required, can be done at any age. The circulatory complications are less likely if the patient is under 10 years of age. Attempts at restoring rotational instability to date have failed.

DUPLICATION (POLYDACTYLY)

Polydactyly is a common hand anomaly that is more frequent in blacks than whites. The incidence is 1 in 300 births. Polydactyly can be categorized in three groups on the basis of location of the extra digit:

- Preaxial (radial)
- Central
- Postaxial (ulnar) (Fig. 7)

The extent of the duplication can vary from an extra soft tissue mass, such as a skin tag without any supporting skeletal elements, to a normally appearing extra digit articulating with a bifid phalanx or metacarpal to a fully developed polydactyly when duplication extends through the metacarpal.

Preaxial polydactyly generally involves the thumb. This is discussed under thumb anomalies.

Central polydactyly is often associated with a complex form of syndactyly and is usually bilateral. The ring finger is the most commonly duplicated digit. The most common associated abnormality is syndactyly of the toes.

Postaxial polydactyly of the fifth finger is quite common and

TABLE 3. Syndromes Universally Associated with Syndactyly

Syndrome	Defect	Inheritance
Poland	Pectoral muscle deficient Nipple absent Symbrachydactyly	Sporadic
Apert	Craniosynostosis, hypertelorism Mild mental retardation Complex syndactyly–"mitten hand"	Autosomal dominant
Orofaciodigital (two types)	Cleft tongue and/or palate Hypoplastic facial bones Simple syndactyly	X-Linked dominant Lethal to males Autosomal recessive

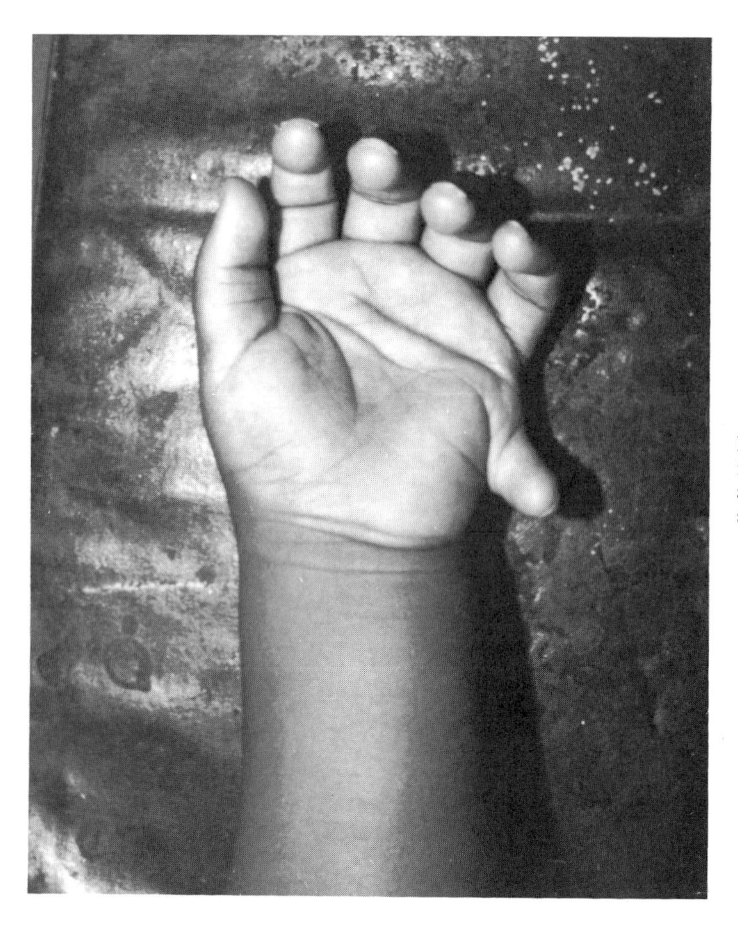

Figure 7. Example of most common postaxial polydactyly. This form is complex in that it is associated with bone and tendon abnormality. Many of the postaxial defects are nothing more than skin tags.

certainly the most common congenital upper extremity anomaly in black infants. It is often paired as an autosomal dominant trait without any associated abnormality in these children. When seen in a white infant, however, it may indicate more serious and systemic abnormalities. More than 40 abnormalities and syndromes have been described as associated with postaxial polydactyly. These include other chromosomal abnormalities, such as trisomy 13, trisomy 18, trisomy B-1, Ellis-van Creveld syndrome, Laurence-Moon-Biedl syndrome, and Meckel syndrome.

Most cases of polydactyly are manifested by soft tissue without skeletal elements involved. The duplicated part is frequently ligated soon after birth and allowed to necrose and fall off. Nevertheless, it is optimal to excise this duplicated part and to close the wound to allow for a cosmetically superior scar and no skin tag remnant. If skeletal elements are present, formal surgical excision is absolutely necessary. A wide variation in anatomic structure exists, and care must be exercised to preserve or replace collateral ligaments (particularly in border digits) as well as neurovascular and tendinous structures.

OVERGROWTH (MACRODACTYLY)

Macrodactyly (gigantism) is the distorted enlargement of a digit that accounts for fewer than 1 per cent of congenital hand anomalies (Fig. 8). Gigantism is characterized by enlargement of all digital components, including bone, neurovascular structures, and cutaneous structures. Macrodactyly most frequently involves the index finger but often follows neural patterns, thus affecting median innervated digits or ulnar innervated digits. The etiology is unclear, but evidence points to such nerve abnormalities as playing a significant role. Fatty infiltration of the digital nerve and neurofibromas have been identified. Other causes of digital enlargements that should be distinguished from gigantism are hemangiomas, lymphangiomas, arteriovenous malformations, and polyfibrous dysplasia.

The involved fingers are unattractive, stiff, and often angulated; indeed, they may compromise the function of the remaining normal digits. The surgical goal in treating macrodactyly is control of the size and growth of the digit. Debulking of skin, soft tissue, and bone are frequently required, and epiphysiodesis is recommended to arrest growth when the finger reaches the adult dimensions. In some cases, amputation of the distorted digit can improve hand function. When median nerve enlargement is present, children may present with nocturnal pain secondary to median nerve compression at the carpal tunnel. In these select patients, carpal tunnel release is indicated. In some situations, neurolysis has been effective in arresting some elements of the progressive digital growth.

UNDERGROWTH (SHORT METACARPALS)

Undergrowth (hypoplasia) is common to all upper extremity abnormalities. Brachymetacarpia (short metacarpals) occurs in many syndromes and should be seen as a sign of a larger disorder. Some of the syndromes and diseases that cause short metacarpals are listed in Table 4. Surgical treatment is rarely indicated, only when the child has a significant cosmetic and functional deformity. When there are multiple, short metacarpals, we prefer the method of *distraction lengthening*. In this technique, the affected metacarpals are osteotomized and distraction devices are positioned. Over the ensuing weeks, gradual lengthening of the bones is performed. Secondary

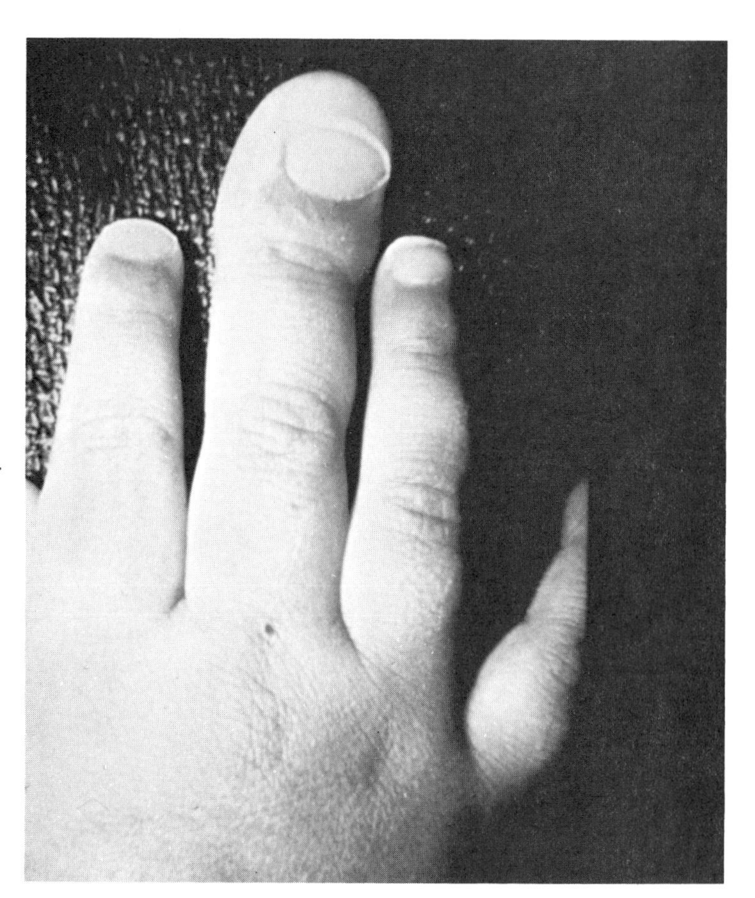

Figure 8. Macrodactyly, long finger.

procedures to remove the device and augment the obtained length with bone grafting are usually required. Such a lengthening procedure is technically demanding and should be done after age 4.

CONSTRICTION BANDS

Congenital constriction bands *(Streeter's bands)* occur in one in 15,000 births (Fig. 9). The circumferential extent and depth of the bands vary, as does the amount of lymphedema distal to the constriction. The band is usually at right angles to the long axis of the affected part, which may be normal up to the constriction. Both orthopedic and oral cavity anomalies are common, with only rare systemic manifestations. The etiology remains controversial; the favored theory is that of amniotic band constriction.

Classification systems relate to the amount of involvement, ranging from:

- 1, Simple constriction rings
- 2, Constriction rings accompanied by deformity of the distal part with or without lymphedema and vascular compromise
- 3, Constriction rings accompanied by fusion of the distal parts with acrosyndactyly
- 4, Intrauterine amputations

Simple constriction rings are shallow and unassociated with distal abnormalities; no treatment is required. When there is distal lymphedema, release of bands is best accomplished by a staged release procedure to avoid vascular compromise of the digit. The band is excised and closed with multiple Z- or W-plasties. For more complex constrictions, both excision of the band and complex local flaps for soft tissue reconstruction are required.

TABLE 4. Syndromes and Diseases Associated with Short Metacarpals

Syndromes
Turner (XO)
Pseudohypoparathyroidism
Pseudo-pseudohypoparathyroidism
Basal cell nevus
Biedmond
Cri du chat
Trichorhinophalangeal
Sybert
Taybi-Linder
Brachydactyly E, A-1, C
Gorman
Tuomaala
Larsen
Diseases
Cretinism
Epiphyseal infection or trauma
Juvenile rheumatoid arthritis
Congenital glaucoma and other eye problems
Sickle cell disease
Multiple epiphyseal dysplasia
Pyruvate kinase deficiency

INTRINSIC FINGER ABNORMALITIES

Camptodactyly

Camptodactyly (bent finger) is a nontraumatic, painless flexion deformity of the proximal interphalangeal joint characterized by a gradual onset and progression. The small finger is the most frequently involved digit, although other fingers may be affected. The flexion contracture ranges from mild

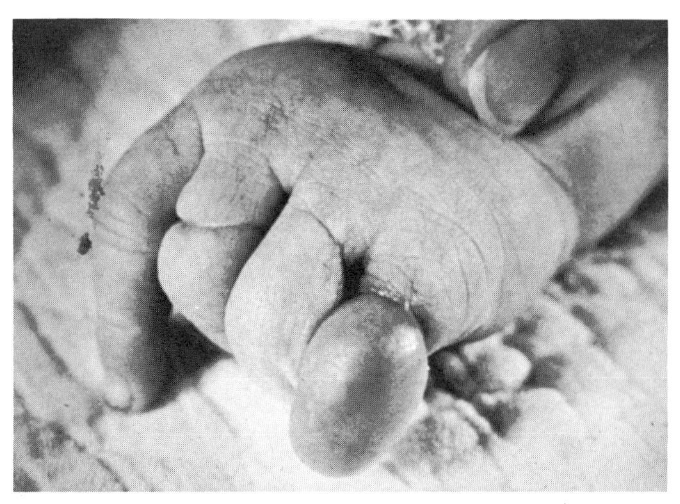

Figure 9. Streeter's bands, multiple fingers. The band on the small finger is causing significant vascular compromise and needs early release. The band on the long finger is not causing compromise but should be released. This is a stage procedure, with only one half of the band being released at one time.

(10 degrees) to severe (90 degrees) and undergoes the greatest change during a growth spurt. When the contracture is greater than 45 degrees, the deformity interferes with glove use, putting the hands in the pockets, and tends to hook onto objects. It is inherited as an autosomal dominant trait with variable penetrance and appears sporadically. Camptodactyly affects girls more frequently than boys. Several etiologic theories have been offered, and a number of anatomic problems have been identified, including abnormal insertion of the flexor tendons and abnormalities of the intrinsic musculature, such as the lumbricales and interossei. Virtually every structure in and about the finger has been blamed.

When the contracture is less than 45 degrees, nonoperative treatment is indicated. Many children may improve with stretching exercises and static and dynamic splinting. When the contracture is greater than 45 degrees, correction of tendon, ligament, and soft tissue contractures are required often with skin grafting. Following surgery, the arc of motion is usually improved but not the range of motion. For example, a 60- to 90-degree arc preoperatively may be converted to a 20- to 60-degree arc postoperatively. With normal metacarpophalangeal joint and distal interphalangeal joint motion, the latter arc is clearly functional. In patients with a radiographic deformity of the proximal phalanx, a wedge osteotomy through the phalangeal neck or fusion of the proximal interphalangeal joint may be required to improve the contracted position.

Clinodactyly

Clinodactyly (radial or ulnar angulation of a digit) is most common in the small finger but may occur in any finger. When present at birth, it is usually not associated with any syndrome; however, in children with Down syndrome, the incidence of clinodactyly ranges from 35 to 80 per cent. In normal children, the incidence varies between 1 and 20 per cent. A functional problem is rarely present, yet many patients request correction for cosmetic reasons.

In general, however, surgical correction is justified only if significant angular deformity interferes with fist making. In these cases, wedge osteotomy and pin fixation have proved helpful.

Delta Phalanx

Delta phalanx is a term applied to an abnormal trapezoid-shaped phalanx that causes clinodactyly with deviation of the digit toward the shoulder side of the bone. The growth plate is longitudinally positioned and C-shaped. This abnormally shaped growth plate accounts for progressive angulation with growth. This abnormality is frequently associated with other abnormalities, including polydactyly, triphalangeal thumb, and cleft hand.

Treatment is surgical and aimed at correcting the angulation. The method most commonly used is wedge osteotomy with and without bone grafting.

Kirner's Deformity

Kirner's deformity is characterized by thickness and curvature of the distal phalanx of the small finger. It is usually bilateral and does not appear until age 8 to 12. Radiographs demonstrate palmar curvature of the phalanx with widening of the growth plate. Treatment necessarily involves multiple wedge osteotomies through the phalanx and K-wire fixation.

Symphalangism

Symphalangism is an autosomal dominant trait characterized by stiffness and poor range of motion of the distal interphalangeal joint. Flatt characterizes three types:

1. *True symphalangism,* with stiff or fused joints but nearly normal phalangeal length.
2. *Symbrachydactyly,* or short stiff digits.
3. *Symphalangism,* with associated abnormalities. Most associated abnormalities involve the hands and feet and are sufficiently common to indicate a skeletal survey. Audiometric evaluation should also be performed.

Treatment is directed to either improving joint motion with hand therapy or arthrodesis to provide a more functional position for the finger. Generally, such a fusion is delayed until the teenage years to avoid growth arrest and thus preserve finger length and appearance.

THUMB ABNORMALITIES

Deficient Components

Thumb deficiencies include hypoplasia, Pouce Flottant, and absent thumb. The independent function of the thumb comprises 50 per cent of the hand function; therefore, with any thumb deficiency, reconstructive efforts are indicated.

Hypoplasia

Three types of small or hypoplastic thumb have been described. *First-degree hypoplasia* is manifested by a slim thumb that is small but contains functioning intrinsic musculature. Impairment is usually minor, and no treatment is indicated.

Second-degree hypoplasia is characterized by poor thenar musculature, a tight thumb web, laxity of the metacarpophalangeal joint, and poor thumb function. Treatment is targeted at the specific deficiency. If the intrinsic muscles are weak or absent, tendon transfers are helpful. If the metacarpophalangeal joint is lax, a capsular stabilizing procedure is indicated. Web space contractures are treated with release and local flap closure or Z- or W-plasty or skin grafting.

When the thumb metacarpal is short and slender, it may be part of a syndrome, such as Holt or Fanconi's syndromes, as mentioned under syndromes associated with radial clubhand. Short or broad metacarpal syndromes, such as Corneoia de Lange syndrome or diastrophic dwarfism, should also be considered.

In *third-degree hypoplasia,* the thumb is not only short but also usually unstable with absent proficient skeletal elements.

This so-called Pouce Flottant (floating thumb) usually contains a rudimentary or absent metacarpal. The thenar compartment is devoid of any intrinsic and extrinsic musculature. Excision and index pollicization offer the best treatment alternative.

Absent Thumb

Total absence of the thumb is commonly seen in radial clubhand. This severe functional and cosmetic deformity should be corrected in a three- or four-fingered hand by pollicization. In more deficient hands, toe-to-thumb microsurgical transfer is indicated. The timing of pollicization relates to the presence of associated conditions, either systemic or in the upper extremity, which precludes early thumb reconstruction. A child first begins to individualize thumb use between 1 and 2 years of age. For that reason, we prefer pollicization in the first 6 to 18 months. In general, the technique involves a transfer of the finger on the neurovascular pedicle, with shortening of the metacarpal to achieve normal thumb and finger length relationships. Positioning of the thumb in opposition and reconstruction of functioning intrinsic musculature is essential. Loss of the transferred finger does occur but is rare. Pollicization is thus one of the most functional and cosmetically rewarding procedures in congenital upper extremity surgery (Fig. 10).

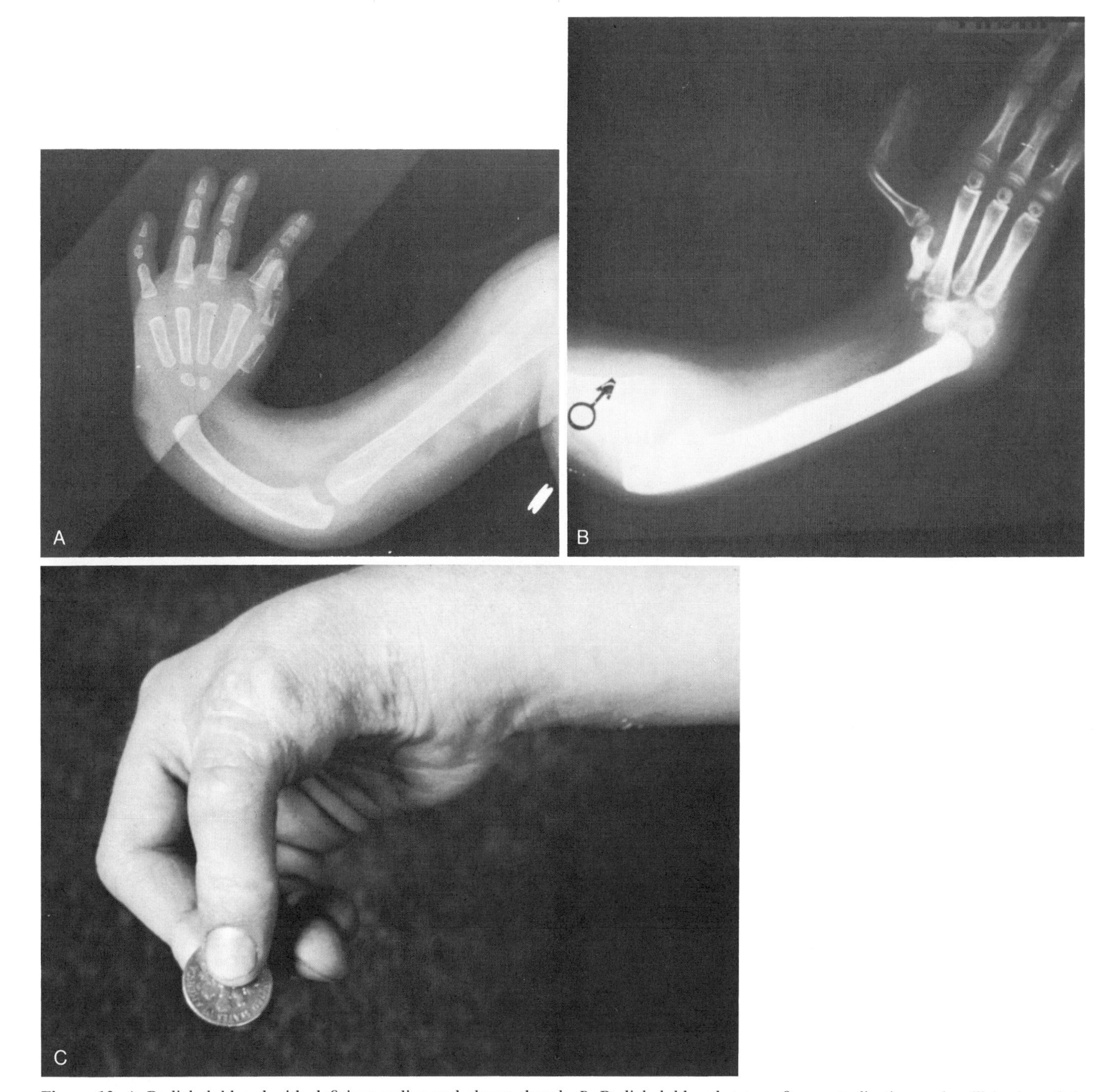

Figure 10. *A,* Radial clubhand with deficient radius and absent thumb. *B,* Radial clubhand status after centralization and pollicization of the index finger. *C,* Pollicized index finger works extremely well and allows fine manipulation of all objects.

Extra Components

Disorders characterized by additional thumb components include triphalangeal thumb and thumb polydactyly.

Triphalangeal Thumb

The triphalangeal thumb contains an extra phalanx between the proximal and distal phalanges. A *type I* deformity characterized by a delta-shaped middle phalanx results in angulation, usually toward the index finger. The *type II* deformity contains a trapezoid-shaped middle phalanx with angulation in the ulnar direction. *Type III* triphalangeal thumb is manifested by a rectangular middle phalanx without angulation. These patterns are often inherited as an autosomal dominant trait and are frequently seen bilaterally.

Treatment is dependent on the shape of the extra phalanx and the presence of angulation. Excessive length and progressive angulation result in weak and awkward pinch and grip and are best treated by osteotomy and pin fixation. If the middle phalanx is small and abnormally shaped, it can be excised.

Duplicated Thumb

Thumb polydactyly occurs in eight of 100,000 births and has been characterized by Wassel on the basis of skeletal pattern. Wassel *types I* and *II* involve duplication at the distal phalangeal level. *Types III* and *IV* are characterized by duplication at the proximal interphalangeal level (Fig. 11), *types V* and *VI* at the carpometacarpal joint level. Wassel *type IV* is the most common thumb polydactyly and involves complete duplication of both proximal and distal phalanges. These thumbs are functionally impaired because they are in poor position for opposition and are often unstable and frequently angulated.

The surgical treatment of Wassel types I and II generally warrant the so-called *Bilhaut-Clouquet procedure.* In this procedure, the central portions of the duplicated phalanges are resected and the remaining portions reapproximated at the midline. Great care is taken to anatomically align the growth plates and the articular surface of the interphalangeal joints and nail beds as well as to preserve the collateral ligaments of each side for stability.

The treatment for the common type IV abnormality depends on the relative size of the two thumb components. Usually, the radial component is deficient and can be excised. Care should be taken to reconstruct the radial collateral ligament. Persistent growth problems may often require further surgery for web space contractures, thumb angulation, or instability or thumb flexion deformity. The treatment for a more complex thumb polydactyly is individualized according to the particular deformity.

Disturbance of Functional Components

Absent Muscle Tendon Units

Congenital muscle and tendon abnormalities of the thumb result from either failure of development or insufficient innervation. The extensor tendon defects of the thumb are most commonly found in the congenitally clasped thumb if the infant holds the thumb in a flexed and adducted position beyond 3 months of age. The deformity usually relates to hypoplasia, as opposed to true absence, of the extensor tendons.

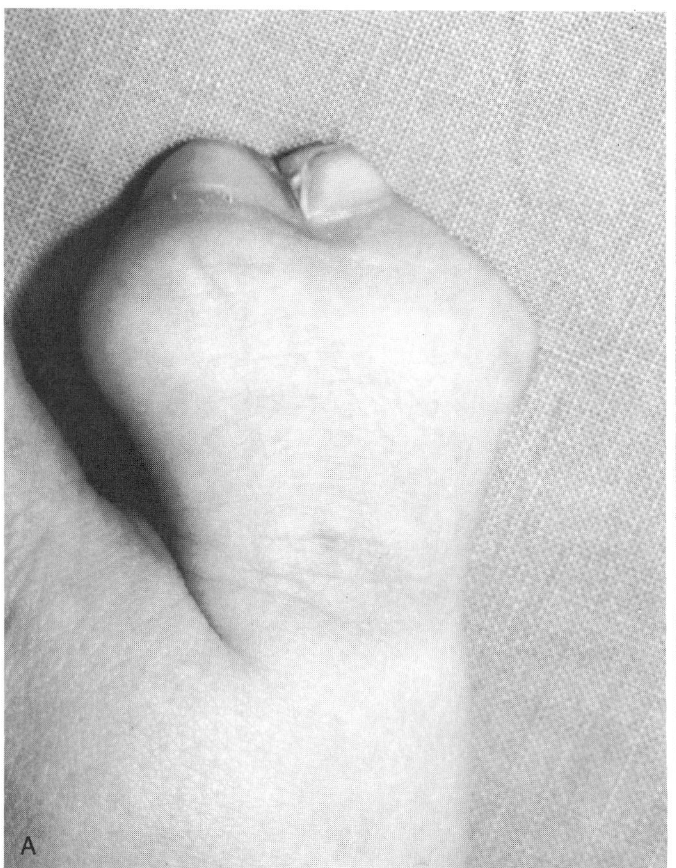

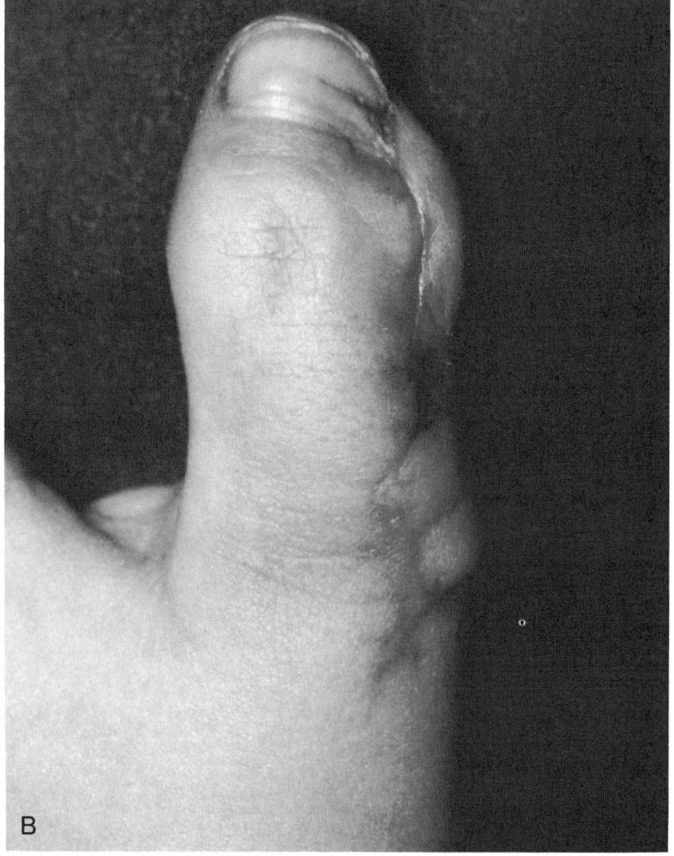

Figure 11. *A,* Classic Wassel's type IV duplicate thumb. *B,* Status after reconstruction, with a merging of the two thumbs and an excellent functional result.

Optimal treatment involves serial extension splinting or casting for a period of 3 to 6 months. If after 3 months some active extension is noted, intermittent and active exercises are encouraged. Most patients respond to this modality, with only a few ultimately requiring surgery. When no extensor function is noted, it can be restored by tendon transfer. Absence of the flexor pollicis longus occasionally occurs, and one can identify this by the lack of an interphalangeal joint crease. In these cases, tendon transfer is generally not helpful. When the terminal joint is unstable, soft tissue stabilization (if the child is skeletally immature) or late fusion is recommended. A flattened thenar eminence and abducted thumb characterizes median innervated intrinsic thenar muscle absence. In this instance, tendon transfers do provide opposition and web space contracture release by four-flap Z-plasty or local flaps are employed.

Congenital Trigger Thumb

Congenital trigger thumb presents as a thumb held in flexion at the interphalangeal joint, as opposed to the metacarpophalangeal joint, in congenital clasp thumb. In trigger thumb, the interphalangeal joint is usually held in 20-degree flexion and attempted passive extension may produce pain or a click. A nodule can frequently be palpated over the flexor pollicis longus at the base of the metacarpal. The initiating pathology—whether a large flexor pollicis longus or a narrow flexor tendon sheath—is still the subject of much debate. Whatever the mechanism, the result is a mechanical obstruction of movement of the flexor pollicis longus tendon. In adults, one can generally identify a click. In children, however, demonstration of the click is unusual. One third of patients spontaneously experience resolution within 6 months with passive stretching or short-term immobilization of the thumb in extension. If the nodule is large and the thumb motion does not improve, surgical release is generally curative.

REFERENCES

Bora FW: The Pediatric Upper Extremity. Philadelphia, WB Saunders Co, 1986.

Dobyns JH, Wood VE, Bayne LG: Congenital Hand Deformities. *In* Green DP (ed): Operative Hand Surgery. New York, Churchill Livingstone, 1988, pp 255–537.

ORTHOPEDIC TRAUMA

JOHN R. GREGG, M.D.
and TAHSIN M. ERGIN, M.D.

GENERAL PRINCIPLES

Children and adolescents, as natural athletes with a keen interest in many and varied physical activities, have always found and will always find ways to hurt themselves. Because of the peculiarities of the developing skeleton, young people suffer from many injuries that are not found in adults. As a consequence, special attention must be given the injured child to ensure that an injury that would be trivial in an adult does not develop into a major problem once the child's growth has been completed.

Children's bones have a much greater number of haversian canals per unit area of cortical bone; as a result, the bones are more porous. Whereas an adult bone fails only in tension in the diaphysis and metaphysis, children's bones may fail in tension (greenstick fracture), compression (torus or buckle fracture), or a combination of the two (plastic deformation or bending fracture).

Biomechanical testing of the elements in the growing bone reveal that the strongest link is the thick periosteal sleeve, which—despite great trauma and displacement of the bone it serves—most commonly remains intact. This accounts for the rarity of open fractures from bone puncture to the outside and the ease with which reduction may be obtained by traction and simple manipulation. The joint capsule and ligaments around the joint are extensions of the periosteal sleeve and, as a result, are equally tough. They serve to transfer stress around a weak link—the epiphysis—to the physis and metaphysis. The epiphysis, although weak, is protected by joint congruity and a compressible shock absorber, the articular cartilage. The weakest link in the chain is the growth plate or physis; this is especially true during the adolescent growth period as the perichondrial ring at the periphery of the physis narrows.

From this information, it can be concluded that children do not sprain ligaments or dislocate joints but, rather, fracture through the physis and/or epiphysis. *This situation makes roentgenographic study of the injured extremity a necessary rather than a precautionary measure.* Complete radiologic evaluation of the site of injury includes at least two views of the fracture at right angles to each other along with the joints proximal and distal to the fracture, as a good general rule. Additional oblique or special views are taken as needed, and additional studies such as computed tomography (CT), bone scan, magnetic resonance imaging (MRI), arteriogram, or arthrogram may still be required. Diagnosis combines this information with the clinical findings of local swelling, deformity (if present), and point tenderness over the fracture site on the bone.

Salter and Harris presented a clinically useful system of five categories in which to classify injuries about the growth plate. A sixth category was later added by Rang (Fig. 1). In general, they are numbered in descending order of frequency and in ascending order of risk of physeal closure.

Type I and II fractures carry a fairly low risk of growth arrest and are fairly easily reduced when recognized and treated acutely.

Type III and IV fractures involve the joint surface in addition to the growth plate and almost always require open reduction and fixation to realign both the joint surface and the growth cartilage accurately. These carry a higher risk of growth arrest, especially when the patient is brought to treatment at a later stage. Failure to achieve accurate reduction also portends poorly for health of the joint cartilage in the future.

Type V and VI injuries are quite sinister in nature and involve the physis. A pure type V injury does not involve disruption of the epiphysis or metaphysis, and therefore it is nearly impossible to arrive at a diagnosis at the time of injury.

These injuries and all crush injuries to the physis are usually recognized at the time that growth arrest becomes clinically apparent; therefore, all injuries that potentially involve the growth plate and possible growth arrest need to be followed carefully, with radiographic follow-up, to ensure that even growth occurs without plate closure, bridge formation, or progressive deformity. Physeal arrest needs to be addressed promptly.

With an intact growth cartilage and periosteal sleeve, growing bones have a tremendous potential to remodel following injury. Large degrees of angulation can be accommodated as the bone and cartilage respond to the application of stress. In general, remodeling can best be expected in fractures near the ends of long bone, with displacement of the fracture in the direction of the plane of movement of the joint, and in children with 2 years or more of skeletal growth remaining. Rotational malalignment, however, does not remodel and cannot be accepted in the reduction of a fracture.

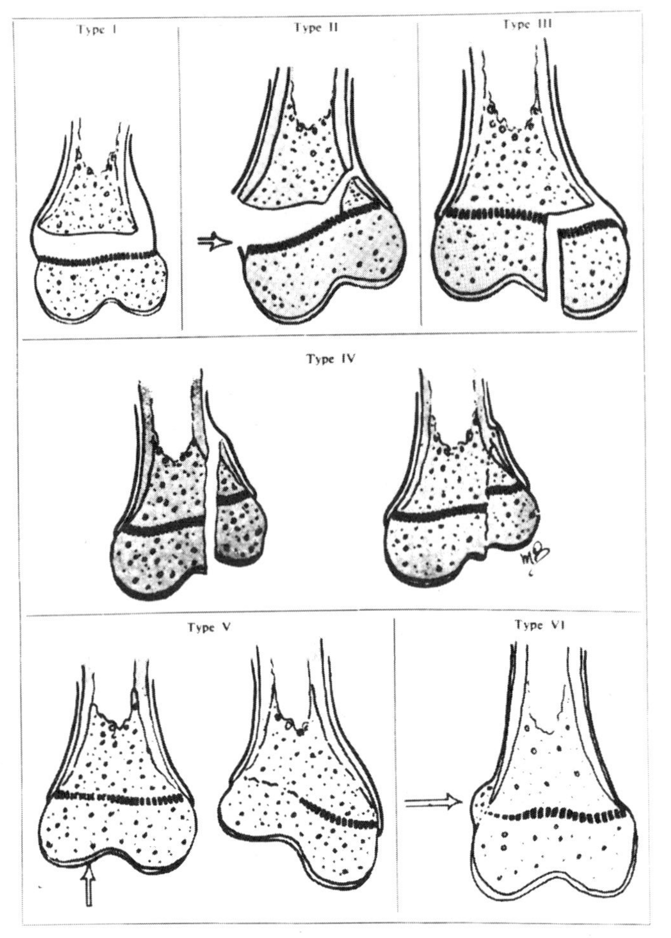

Figure 1. The Salter-Harris classification of physeal fractures, as modified by Rang with the addition of a type VI. See text for a complete discussion of the fracture types. (Rang M: The Growth Plate and Its Disorders. Edinburgh: Churchill Livingstone, 1969.)

Fractures occurring with mechanisms of injury that do not generally produce a fracture are suspicious and need to be thoroughly investigated. Pathologic lesions within the bone, such as unicameral bone cyst, nonossifying fibroma, and enchondroma, are frequently found in children's skeletons and can result in fracture with even minimal trauma. In general, these are best approached by treating and healing the fracture, then treating the underlying lesion as needed. Other conditions have been noted to predispose to injury, including fibrous dysplasia, osteogenesis imperfecta, Ehlers-Danlos syndromes, rickets, renal disease, cerebral palsy, and muscular dystrophy.

CHILD ABUSE

Physicians must have a high index of suspicion regarding injuries to children under the age of 2 because a regular percentage of fractures in this age group will be associated with abuse. Suspicion should be raised when any part of the history of the child's injury is questionable or does not mesh with the physical examination, including the behavior of the child. Dispassionate parents, a delay in seeking treatment, insufficient trauma to have caused the injury seen, and multiple sites of injury or serial injuries are cause for concern. All such patients should be admitted to the hospital and should undergo thorough testing, including a skeletal survey, and the appropriate social work network should be immediately contacted.

Injuries characteristic of child abuse include posterior rib fractures, any fractures of the humerus or femur in a child under 2 years of age, corner epiphyseal fractures, and the presence of subperiosteal new bone. Other manifestations may be observed, including skull and spine fractures, bruises, bites, and burns caused by a cigarette tip or hot water. The penalty for missing a case of child abuse is a 10 per cent chance the child will be dead within 1 year.

MULTIPLE TRAUMA

More and more frequently, children are the victims of major or multiple trauma; they may be hurt when hit by a car as a pedestrian or cyclist, while riding in a car, and in recreational activities in falls from heights, all-terrain vehicles, and dirt bikes. Care for these patients begins in the field and continues on arrival at the hospital. An adequate airway, effective ventilation, and circulating blood volume must be established, monitored and maintained, or supplemented. The cervical spine is stabilized, and the patient is transported with the use of a backboard. Long bone fractures are immobilized temporarily and wounds dressed. Evaluation in the hospital continues with assessment of head, thoracic, abdominal, and pelvic injuries in addition to the spine and extremities. Orthopedic evaluation includes complete documentation of neurologic function; palpation and assessment of all portions of the spine, pelvis and chest, and appendicular skeleton; examination of open wounds; and formulation of a plan of management of all injuries in conjunction with the other members of the trauma team. Portions of the evaluation may best be accomplished at times following induction of anesthesia in order to evaluate the injury more completely and to avoid unnecessary pain to the child. Regional trauma centers are more prevalent in the management of severely injured patients and are best equipped to handle the myriad of problems in these children, although good care can be applied anywhere.

Open fractures require prompt and effective management. Measures to be undertaken in the emergency ward include administration of tetanus toxoid (if more than 5 years has elapsed since the last booster) and/or hyperimmune globulin, intravenous cephalosporin, culture of the wound, and application of a sterile dressing. After the patient is moved to the operating room—which should be no longer than 6 hours from the time of injury—the wound is copiously irrigated using pulsatile lavage; volume is also key. Devitalized tissues along with crushed or necrotic skin margins are débrided. The wound is thoroughly explored, and the bone ends are exposed and cleaned. The wound may be dressed open, with very loose approximation of the margins to reduce retraction and the subsequent need for skin grafts. Delayed primary closure and/or redébridement are performed in 2 to 5 days. Skeletal stabilization may take many forms, depending on the type and location of injury and the presence and severity of other injuries. Simple cast or splint immobilization may be sufficient for some injuries; others may require skeletal traction or smooth pin, external, intramedullary, or plate fixation.

SOFT TISSUE INJURIES

Contusions

Contusions involve direct impact to soft tissues with crushing of the tissues and associated bleeding. Because of increased vasculature, muscles are most susceptible to severe contusion, hematoma formation, and inflammatory response.

Sprains

Sprains occur when a ligament or joint capsule becomes stretched or torn. These tissues are viscoelastic, and the amount of damage done to them is dependent not only on the amount of force applied but also on the rate of application of that force. Sprains may be graded by the amount of damage done to the injured structure.

Grade I sprains involve some tearing of the fibers; however, the ligament integrity is essentially intact with no reduction in range of motion and no increase in joint laxity.

Grade II sprains involve damage to a substantial portion of the ligament with a concomitant increase in joint laxity and loss of motion, but some resistance is met when the joint is stressed.

Grade III sprains show clear-cut joint instability to stress.

Strains

Strains are injuries to a muscle-tendon contractile unit. These injuries may be graded similarly to sprains on the basis of amount of muscle and tendon injured, with complete rupture of a muscle considered a grade III strain.

Management of Soft Tissue Injury

RICE

Rest, ice, compression, and elevation (RICE) should be the mainstay of management in soft tissue injuries.

*R*est allows for pain relief in addition to preventing further damage to tissues and, when accomplished by immobilization, encourages reduction in use of the injured part. This plan should be adhered to over the initial 2 to 3 days following the injury.

*I*ce (cryotherapy) results in vasoconstriction, with a decrease in bleeding and inflammation, reduced edema, and relief of pain when applied. Heat, which results in vasodilation and hyperemia, increased swelling and inflammation, and, frequently, increased pain, should be avoided. Ice chips or ice-water mixtures are sufficiently effective and economical, and they should be applied immediately after the injury when possible and for 20 minutes two to four times daily for 2 to 3 days thereafter.

*C*ompression aids in the control of edema by limiting the volume of the injured compartment and by increasing the interstitial pressure, reducing fluid transudation from the capillary bed. Compression using an elastic bandage should be firm and even but should not result in constriction of arterial supply to or venous return from the injured part. This is particularly true about the elbow and knee.

*E*levation also plays a role in control of edema by improving venous and lymphatic return from the site of injury. This is best accomplished by raising the body part, preferably above the level of the heart, although some elevation is better than none at all.

As the soft tissue injury begins to respond to treatment of the initial acute phase, attention may be turned to the rehabilitative phase. Use of RICE is continued judiciously in this phase, and restoration of function is developed in stages. Recovery of range of motion, followed by strength, endurance, and agility in use of the injured part, is, in turn, encouraged and practiced.

Heterotopic Bone

A special case of soft tissue injury involves the muscle contusion that results in heterotopic bone formation, or myositis ossificans. A contained hematoma may be present within the muscle as a discrete mass. Clinical findings include swelling, pain exacerbated by contraction or passive motion of the muscle, and warmth, often remarkable. Range of motion of the proximal and distal joints is reduced.

Initial treatment consists again of RICE; range-of-motion exercises and massage should be avoided. Once active muscle control is obtained, active range-of-motion exercises are performed. Gradually, muscle strengthening through progressive resistance exercises is introduced and work continues on active range of motion. Passive motion can cause further injury and bone formation. If masses of bone remain in the muscle and cause loss of function, they may be excised, but only after the mass has matured completely—in 12 to 18 months.

COMPARTMENT SYNDROME

Fractures and crush injuries to the extremities may result in large amounts of muscle damage and bleeding. Muscles in the extremities are enveloped by fascia, and as the bleeding and muscle edema develop, the pressure in the muscle compartment increases as the contents of the compartment swell against the fairly inelastic fascial walls. Blood flow to the muscles and nerves in the compartment is gradually compromised and is cut off when pressure in the compartment exceeds the capillary perfusion pressure. Suspicion should be raised by pain out of proportion to the type of injury. Other findings include pain with passive stretch, paresthesias, and reduction of two-point discrimination in sensory distributions. Suspicion should result in immediately splitting encircling dressings and measurement of compartment pressures if the symptoms are unresolved. Various recommendations have been made for the threshold pressure at which fasciotomy is indicated, with many authors recommending that pressures above 30 mm Hg be carefully monitored and fasciotomy performed at pressures above 40 mm Hg. Heppenstall has recommended fasciotomy at compartment pressures within 40 mm Hg of mean arterial pressure. The key is rapid action, since irreversible changes in muscle and nerve can occur after 6 hours of ischemia. The most common sites of compartment syndrome are the volar forearm and the compartments of the lower leg, although the syndrome may also be found in the hand, foot, thigh, and upper arm.

SPECIAL WOUNDS

Bite Injury

Occasionally, lacerations of the skin with or without bony involvement require special attention. The most notable example of this is the human bite wound, which most frequently occurs when hand meets tooth in the delivering of a punch. Skin puncture usually is found on the dorsum of the fourth or fifth metacarpophalangeal joint and may penetrate skin, extensor tendon, joint capsule, and even bone. Any puncture wounds on the hands should be considered possible human bite wounds unless the history is immaculate.

Management consists of irrigation and splinting; intravenous antibiotics, including coverage of both gram-positive (cefazolin), and anaerobic (penicillin G) organisms. Incision and débridement are necessary when a patient presents late with abscess formation.

Nail Puncture Injury

Nail puncture wounds to the foot can cause problems attributable to development of deep bone or joint infection from *Pseudomonas aeruginosa.* The presence of deep infection requires débridement, irrigation, and treatment with intravenous antibiotics for 2 to 6 weeks, bone involvement dictating the latter. Vigilance following nail puncture should be carefully maintained, and antibiotic coverage should be given in the initial period.

SPLINTING

A wide variety of splinting techniques may be used for temporary immobilization and sometimes treatment of extremity injuries. Frequently, initial care of an injury necessitates immobilization for pain relief, protection from further damage, and reduction of swelling—not just letting the bones heal. A simple splint may be fashioned with three to four layers of cast padding, ten to 12 layers of plaster bandage, and a stretch gauze roll or elastic bandage; however, care should be taken not to apply the latter too tightly. Various prepared splint materials are also readily available in both fiberglass and plaster and are simple to apply. Children's skin is sensitive and burns easily. Because plaster splints set with an exothermic reaction, cold water should be used and care should be taken to avoid contact with the skin. When a splint is applied, the position of the splint and extremity must be maintained until the material has set completely.

Upper Extremity Splints

In the upper extremity, useful emergency splints include the volar forearm splint for wrist and hand injuries, the posterior elbow splint for elbow and forearm injuries, radial and ulnar gutter splints for injuries of the thumb or small finger sides of the hand, coaptation splints, and forearm and upper arm sugartong splints for humeral and forearm fractures. In most cases, the arm may be positioned with the elbow flexed 90 degrees, the forearm in neutral rotation, the wrist in slight dorsiflexion, and the hand positioned with the thumb slightly opposed and the metacarpophalangeal and interphalangeal joints slightly flexed, as if the child were holding a can of soda. *If the position of immobilization compromises neurovascular status, it must be immediately changed.* At the time of definitive treatment, the position of the extremity may be changed, depending on the type of injury.

Lower Extremity Splints

In the lower extremity, useful emergency splints include the long posterior or long U-splint placed medially and laterally on the leg for femoral and tibial fractures, medial and lateral coaptation or Jones splints for injuries about the knee, and the short leg posterior and short U-splint for ankle and foot injuries. The leg may be positioned with the knee extended and the ankle in neutral dorsiflexion.

STRESS FRACTURES AND OVERUSE INJURIES

Like high-performance athletes, children perform activities repetitively and occasionally to the exclusion of other activities. As a result, they sometimes become the victims of stress or overuse injuries. These injuries in general respond to rest, ice, and possibly mild anti-inflammatory medication to reduce the initial pain, followed by alteration of the activity that precipitated the injury and stretching and strengthening the muscles in the involved area. To prevent recurrence, a graduated program involving the causative activity is followed in return to participation. Common sites of stress fracture, in addition to those addressed below, are the metatarsals, distal fibula, calcaneus, proximal medial tibial metaphysis in runners, and the pars interarticularis in the vertebral bodies of gymnasts, divers, and football linemen.

Osgood-Schlatter's Disease

Not truly a "disease," this overuse injury is seen in 10 per cent of adolescent athletes. The injury occurs at the infrapatellar tendon insertion into the tibial tubercle apophysis. Repetitive, high-stress activity results in microfractures of the apophysis at the tendon insertion. The highest stresses are obtained in landing from a jump and in decelerating while running; thus, Osgood-Schlatter's disease is found frequently in the left leg of right-handed basketball players and right-footed soccer players.

The patient experiences pain with direct pressure over the apophysis and with activity such as running, jumping, and going up or down stairs. Radiographs are needed in unilateral disease to rule out other pathology. The films may reveal fragmentation and enlargement of the tibial tuberosity or heterotopic bone within the substance of the infrapatellar tendon.

Treatment consists of restriction of painful activity and ice to the tender area when the knee is painful. Use of a neoprene knee support for activities is encouraged, primarily to protect the knee from incident trauma and to let the coach know that an injury is present. Additionally, one may advise stretching out tight hamstring and quadriceps musculature and straight leg resistance exercises (isometric quadriceps contracture), progressing to 10 per cent of the patient's weight for resistance. Patients can participate in sports if they are not limping; however, any limp indicates a need for further rest. There is absolutely no indication for steroid injection or a cast. A cast results in more disability and loss of function than the disease. The problem will ultimately be resolved completely at the time of epiphyseal closure; if the problem remains following closure, radiographs usually reveal an ossicle within the tendon, with symptoms resolving following excision of the ossicle.

Sinding-Larson-Johanson Syndrome

The counterpart to Osgood-Schlatter's disease, this entity is an overstress injury of the infrapatellar tendon insertion to the inferior pole of the patella. Small avulsion ossicles may occasionally be seen at the inferior pole. Treatment of the problem is similar to that for Osgood-Schlatter's disease.

(Sever's) Calcaneal Apophysitis

Because the tendo Achillis is attached to the calcaneal apophysis through numerous Sharpey's fibers, the vertically oriented apophysis is subjected to high shear stress in the performance of running and jumping activity. As with Osgood-Schlatter's disease, the repetitive trauma causes microfractures around the tendon insertion. Symptoms are seen in 1 per cent of adolescent athletes and include pain with running and jumping and tenderness with local pressure over the insertion of the tendo Achillis. The patient frequently has tight heel cords, with ankle dorsiflexion limited to neutral with the knee extended, not the normal 15 degrees. Rest during painful episodes and heel cord and plantar stretching exercises usually resolve the problem, although occasionally a nighttime dorsiflexion splint is needed in young athletes. Radiographs reveal fragmentation and sclerosis of the calcaneal apophysis, which is normal; however, films are necessary to rule out other pathology.

Little League Elbow

A number of entities are found under the classification of Little League elbow. The most widely recognized condition involves overstress of the medial elbow stabilizing structures or repetitive compression injury of the lateral radiocapitellar articulation. On the medial side, overstress or even complete separation of the medial epicondylar apophysis can occur. Point tenderness at the medial epicondyle with loss of complete extension may be found. Radiographs reveal widening of the physis and occasionally fragmentation. On the lateral side, irregular fragmentation of the ossific nucleus of the capitellum or even osteochondral fracture of the capitellum may occur. Pain is lateral, and there is an attendant loss of motion. Loose bodies from fragmentation of the capitellum may cause locking of the elbow joint.

Treatment of these conditions in their milder forms involves rest, provided that the medial epicondyle is not displaced and the capitellar articular surface remains intact. Once the injury heals, which may take 3 to 4 weeks, a progressive rehabilitation program is instituted, with a graduated throwing program following stretching and strengthening of the muscles of the arm. Surgical treatment is needed for fixation of the medial epicondyle if it is displaced or if the elbow is unstable to valgus stress. Excision of loose fragments may be required. The best treatment is prevention, however, and young pitchers should be monitored carefully in the amount of hard throwing they do. Pitchers should pitch no more than six innings per week, with 3 days of rest between outings. Managers should monitor their pitchers closely for throwing mechanics and fatigue.

Little League Shoulder

Overstress that results in a fatigue fracture of the proximal humeral physis has been referred to as Little League shoulder. Previously, many of these injuries remained undiagnosed. The symptoms are nonspecific. Pain with throwing or aching in the shoulder is usual. The proximal humeral physis may be widened radiographically or may show periosteal new bone formation. Rest, followed by a progressive strengthening and then a throwing program, along with teaching of proper throwing mechanics, should treat the problem adequately.

Swimmer's Shoulder

High levels of training are necessary in competitive swimming, even in young age groups; as a result, shoulder pain in childhood and teen swimmers is quite common. After fatigue reduces the athlete's ability to control shoulder motion and position, the humeral head's constant motion causes friction against the rotator cuff and subacromial bursa in the subacromial space. This is exacerbated by the fact that swimmers have increased laxity in the shoulder ligaments and capsule. Hundreds of cycles of shoulder circumduction result in inflammation. Findings include tenderness over the supraspinatus tendon and subacromial bursa, with extent occasionally to the biceps tendon. Pain is produced by forward flexion of the shoulder with adduction and internal rotation. Radiographs, however, are normal.

Treatment consists of rest, followed by a strengthening program for the rotator cuff muscles, with gradual return to swimming. Practice should end for the swimmer when muscle fatigue sets in and when the athlete begins to lose stroke mechanics.

Femoral Neck Stress Fracture

Although not found as frequently as other overstress injuries, stress fracture of the femoral neck has great clinical importance if it progresses to complete fracture, which is a serious complication. The clinical presentation may be nonspecific, with a generalized ache around the groin in the early stages and limping later. Loss of hip motion may be found. Radiographs may show the stress fracture; if findings are negative, a bone scan is diagnostic. The stress fracture may occur on the inferior part of the neck (compression side) or superior part of the neck (tension side).

Treatment of inferior neck stress fractures present on bone scan consists of partial weight-bearing crutch ambulation for 4 to 6 weeks, but the patient may perform nonimpact aerobic exercise if it is not painful. Tension side fractures and all fractures radiographically present should be internally fixed in situ to prevent completion of the fracture.

UPPER EXTREMITY TRAUMA

The upper extremity is very susceptible to injury in children, as there are thousands of ways in which children of all ages can fall onto their outstretched arm. Indeed, when the patient presents to the emergency ward, the history taken frequently reads "fell from the monkey bars landing on . . .".

Clavicle

Medial Clavicular Injury

Injuries to the medial end of the clavicle are rare and are difficult to visualize on routine radiographs. Occasionally, they are seen with cephalic tilt views of the clavicle, although CT scan may be required if the diagnosis remains obscure. Because the medial clavicular epiphysis remains open until age 22, these injuries are commonly epiphyseal fractures, not dislocations. They therefore heal and remodel well, and intervention should be considered only for posterior irreducible displacement with compromise of the great vessels. Management consists of a sling for comfort, with gradual return to activities after 3 to 6 weeks.

Shaft Clavicular Injury

Clavicle shaft fractures in childhood may be difficult to see on radiographs; however, they can easily be found by looking for the clinical signs of fracture in examination of the patient. Swelling, local tenderness, and deformity are usually present. Sling immobilization for comfort is frequently sufficient, but a figure-of-eight clavicle brace is used to maintain length of the clavicle in displaced fractures with overlap. Protection is maintained for 3 to 5 weeks, and remodeling (depending on the age of the patient) and complete rehabilitation are the rule.

Birth Injuries

Birth fractures of the clavicle do occur, more frequently in large infants and in breech presentation. These are usually noted incidentally or as a result of lack of movement of the arm by the infant. They are treated for comfort and heal fully; however, these must be differentiated from proximal humeral epiphyseal separation, osteomyelitis of the shoulder, and brachial plexus traction injuries.

Acromioclavicular Joint Injury

Injuries to the acromioclavicular (AC) joint in skeletally immature patients, as with the medial end of the clavicle, are most commonly epiphyseal fractures rather than ligamentous disruptions. Despite wide displacement of the lateral end of the clavicle, these injuries heal and remodel readily owing to the presence of an intact periosteal tube and intact coracoclavicular ligaments.

Treatment is by clavicle brace or sling for comfort. True subluxations or dislocations of the AC joint are very rare, if they occur at all, but may be seen in late adolescence. They are treated as in adult AC separations, with operative reduction and repair considered only in the case of complete or wide displacement of the clavicle. Generally, return to activities may be pursued in 4 to 6 weeks.

Scapula

Fractures of the scapula are rare; however, the scapula may occasionally appear to be fractured radiographically because of the appearance of secondary centers of ossification from ages 10 to 22. For that reason careful assessment of radiographs, with comparison views, is essential.

Scapular fractures are treated conservatively with rest and gradual mobilization when the patient is comfortable unless displacement of a large glenoid fragment is noted. In that case, operative intervention should be considered to avoid problems of late arthritis or shoulder instability.

Shoulder Dislocation

Atraumatic Injury

True traumatic dislocation of the shoulder is rare in children but may occur more readily in adolescents. In the younger age group, physeal injuries to the proximal humerus are much more common. The nature of this dislocation must be elucidated, as atraumatic *involuntary* dislocation may occur in patients with congenital joint laxity or structural problems and atraumatic *voluntary* dislocations occur in those with psychiatric or emotional problems.

Atraumatic involuntary dislocation is best treated with a rehabilitation program, with emphasis on strengthening all shoulder girdle muscles, especially the internal rotators. Surgery is considered following failure of conservative management. With a voluntary dislocation, attention must be paid to the underlying disorder, although a rehabilitation program may also be beneficial.

Anterior Dislocations

Traumatic anterior dislocation causes disruption of the labral attachment with the glenoid and disruption of the integrity of the middle and inferior glenohumeral ligaments. Treatment is by reduction and immobilization for 3 weeks in adduction and internal rotation. Rehabilitation of atrophied muscles should take place prior to resumption of competitive sports, especially for rotator cuff and subscapularis muscle strengthening.

Despite sufficient treatment as outlined above, recurrence of the dislocation takes place 50 to 90 per cent of the time, with young athletes showing an 82 per cent redislocation rate. These patients frequently require later reconstruction to prevent recurrent dislocations. Numerous repair methods have been described and used effectively, with current recent attention to arthroscopic techniques of capsular plication and Bankart repair (repair of the detached labrum to the glenoid) which, though promising, remain unproven.

Posterior Dislocations

Posterior dislocation is rare, with traumatic posterior dislocations being rarer still. Initial management of traumatic posterior dislocation is conservative with reduction and immobilization. Reconstruction should be considered for those with recurrent problems of posterior instability.

Proximal Humerus

Injuries to the proximal humerus are mostly Salter-Harris type II fractures, with type I injuries occurring in children younger than 5 years old. Because 80 per cent of the longitudinal growth of the humerus results from this physis, these fractures remodel readily. Manipulative reduction with immobilization of the arm at the side or in a spica cast is usually required only with complete displacement of the humeral shaft in older patients. Healing occurs in 3 to 6 weeks, depending on the age of the patient and the degree of displacement, with a gradual progression toward full activities.

Humeral Shaft

With all trauma to the extremities, a complete neurologic assessment of the affected extremity is mandatory. This is especially true with humeral shaft fractures, in which the radial nerve, for a good portion of the length of the bone, lies in close proximity and may be damaged or trapped at the time of fracture or reduction. The nerve is most vulnerable at the junction of the middle and distal thirds of the humerus. Neurologic assessment is performed both before and after reduction with direct attention to the function of the radial nerve. After loss of function, an intact radial nerve usually heals with signs of recovery evident in 8 to 12 weeks. Exploration of the nerve should be performed if recovery does not take place.

Humeral shaft fractures are well managed closed, with closed reduction rarely required, and immobilization in coaptation or sugartong splints and sling is usually sufficient. A hanging cast may also be used. Open reduction and internal fixation are rarely required. Remodeling of the fracture is best if the fracture site is close to the proximal physis.

Elbow

The elbow remains a very frequent site of childhood injuries, and elbow injury is one of the more difficult to manage. The distal humerus itself has four separate ossification centers: the medial epicondyle, the lateral epicondyle, the capitellum and lateral trochlear ridge, and the medial trochlea. The appearance and development of these centers may give the normal distal humeral epiphysis a fragmented or even fractured appearance.

Fractures of the distal humerus may be difficult to evaluate radiographically because true anteroposterior and lateral views are often difficult to obtain in a child in pain. With nondisplaced and minimally displaced fractures, a fracture line may be difficult to find and can be even more challenging in a child, in whom the physis is mostly cartilaginous. A comparison view of the opposite elbow can be most helpful in diagnosis, and an arthrogram of the injured elbow may occasionally be required to evaluate the patient fully.

A number of radiographic keys can be of assistance. On the anteroposterior view, the width of the proximal and distal fragments at the fracture should be equal. On the lateral view, a line along the anterior humeral cortex should pass through the middle of the lateral condylar epiphysis, which in turn should form an angle of about 30 degrees with the humeral shaft. Finally, a posterior olecranon fossa fat pad visible with the elbow flexed is, with few exceptions, indicative of the presence of a joint effusion.

With displaced fractures, the brachial artery and radial, median, and ulnar nerves may become damaged by traction, laceration, or entrapment within the fracture site or joint. Care must be taken to ensure that each of these structures is functioning properly both before and after reduction and/or fixation. Arteriography may be performed if interposition of vessels is suspected.

Supracondylar Fractures

Supracondylar fractures are usually caused by a fall on an outstretched arm, usually with the elbow extended. The peak incidence is in the 5- to 8-year age range, with a gradual decrease in incidence until about age 15. The extension fracture is far more common than the flexion type and may be nondisplaced, greenstick with an intact posterior cortex, or completely displaced.

Treatment for the first two types consists of simple cast or splint immobilization, with a minimal reduction occasionally necessary by flexing the elbow. As with all supracondylar fractures, care must still be taken to ensure that the neurovascular status remains intact. With displaced supracondylar fractures, hospital admission is required to monitor for neurovascular injury and development of compartment syndrome. If there is any question whether the fracture is displaced, the child should be seen immediately by an orthopedist who regularly takes care of this injury. These fractures are best managed with closed reduction and immobilization, if treated early, and with percutaneous Kirschner wire (K-wire) smooth pin fixation, either with two parallel lateral pins or one medial and one lateral pin used in unstable fractures or in those fractures in which reduction may be maintained only in marked flexion. Open reduction is performed for irreducible fractures, open fractures, and neurovascular compromise uncorrected by reduction.

Advantages of pin fixation include improved stability of the reduction, ability to flex and extend the elbow to improve evaluation of the reduction, and increased extension for immobilization to lessen vascular problems. Disadvantages include difficulty in accurately placing the pins with a proper reduction, pin-related problems, and ulnar nerve impingement if a medial pin is used. The pins are removed at 3 weeks, and the cast replaced for an additional week.

Other methods of treatment are lateral or overhead skeletal traction, which requires prolonged hospitalization to monitor reduction but may be used in grossly swollen elbows. Late complications are cubitus varus or gunstock deformity, stiffness, and nerve embarrassment; most neuropraxias recover with observation, and corrective osteotomy may be used to treat malunion.

Lateral Condylar and Epicondylar Fractures

Fractures of the lateral condyle and epicondyle, which are fairly common injuries, are usually found to be Salter-Harris type IV fractures. As such, these fractures, if displaced, necessitate accurate open reduction and internal fixation with K-wires to realign the growth plate and articular surface. Undisplaced fractures may be immobilized, but follow-up is necessary to check for loss of reduction at a time early enough so that something may be done about it. Attendant with these fractures is a risk of late arthritis and growth arrest. True fractures of the lateral epicondyle occur only rarely, but frequently an elbow radiograph appears to suggest this injury. The lateral epicondylar ossification center unites first with the capitellum, then closes laterally. The physician should correlate the radiographic appearance with the clinical examination, using comparison views in assessment.

Physeal Separations of the Distal Humerus

Distal humeral physeal separations occur in children younger than 6 or 7 years of age and masquerade on initial presentation as dislocation of the elbow. These are essentially Salter-Harris type I or II injuries to the entire distal humeral physis. The patient should be admitted to the hospital to closely monitor the neurovascular status of the extremity.

The treatment of choice is closed reduction with casting in extension for 3 weeks; open reduction can lead to cubitus varus and loss of function. For slippery fractures, percutaneous pin fixation with smooth K-wires is occasionally required to maintain reduction.

Medial Epicondylar Fractures

Medial epicondylar fractures are avulsion injuries occurring under valgus stress to the elbow or in association with elbow dislocations. A medial epicondylar injury is significant in that the epicondylar fragment may be displaced completely from the distal humerus and at times may become lodged within the joint. Because the median nerve may also be trapped in the joint, a thorough neurologic assessment is essential. Prior to age 5, comparison views of the uninjured elbow are invaluable and occasionally arthrography is needed to describe the injury fully.

Treatment in a long arm cast is possible unless the epicondyle is displaced, the elbow remains unstable, or the epicondyle or nerve is trapped in the elbow. If any displacement is present, the epicondyle rotates away from the humerus because of the pull of the flexor muscle mass. In such instances, open reduction with K-wire fixation and immobilization with the elbow flexed and the forearm pronated are required. This position relaxes tension on the epicondyle from the common flexor origin.

Medial Condylar Fractures

Fractures of the entire medial condyle occur with a fall on the flexed elbow. Diagnosis is somewhat elusive because the ossific nucleus of the trochlea does not appear until ages 9 to 11. Good clinical examination and comparison views of the opposite elbow are of great help to the physician. Undisplaced fractures can be casted for 3 weeks. Displaced or displaced and rotated fractures require operative reduction, K-wire fixation, and a cast. Stiffness of the elbow and occasionally growth disturbance may result regardless of treatment.

Elbow Dislocations

Elbow dislocations do happen to children, although as stated previously, most commonly occur in association with a fracture, so a complete search for the fracture is necessary. Reduction is performed with the patient under general anesthesia; if joint congruency with fluid motion is not obtained, soft tissue or bone is interposed in the joint and operative reduction is required. An MRI or arthrogram may tell the story best if there is doubt. The elbow stability following reduction must also be checked carefully. Immobilization following reduction is for 1 week in a long arm cast, followed by a cast brace or extension-block splint allowing elbow motion from 15 degrees to full flexion. Full extension of the elbow would allow the reduction to slip.

Proximal Radial Physeal Fractures

Fractures of the proximal radial physis are common; however, damage to the articular surface of the radial head in children is rare, in contrast to the damage in adult injuries. A fall on the outstretched arm is the usual cause, with the elbow in slight valgus and the radiocapitellar articulation accepting the force. The usual patient is 10 or 11 years old. The fracture is through the physis (type I), occasionally with a fragment of the radial metaphysis (type II). True anteroposterior and lateral views of the proximal radius are needed, as treatment choices are based on the degree of angulation and displacement of the radial head. Less than 30 degrees of angulation can be accepted and treated with a cast for 3 weeks. Full return of motion after remodeling is expected. For more than 30 degrees of angulation, closed reduction of the radial head and casting are performed. Open reduction is sometimes needed for unreducible displacement or severe angulation. Even with closed treatment, synostosis of the proximal radius and ulna may ensue. Avascular necrosis of the radial head is rare, but possible.

Olecranon Fractures

Olecranon fractures may usually be treated with cast immobilization, although large amounts of displacement may need to be treated with AO tension band wire fixation. It is important to be sure this is the only injury, and the rest of the arm should be examined carefully.

Pulled Elbow

Pulled or "nursemaid's" elbow may be the most common elbow injury in children. This is because parents and caretakers will often use a forceful pull on the arm to direct a recalcitrant child. The elbow joint is distracted, and the annular ligament slips over the top of the radial head and becomes lodged between it and the capitellum. The child will not use the arm until the subluxed annular ligament is reduced, which many times occurs as the radiology technician supinates the forearm to obtain the anteroposterior radiograph. With traction into extension, supination of the forearm, and flexion, a click is sometimes palpable as reduction occurs. If full flexion is not possible, the radial head is not reduced. A short time later, the child is once again using the arm, usually within 1 to 2 hours. The parents should be cautioned regarding the cause of the problem. For recurrent subluxations, consider casting the child with the elbow flexed 90 degrees and the forearm supinated.

Forearm Fractures

Monteggia Fractures

Monteggia fractures are fractures of the ulnar shaft along with dislocation of the radial head. There are equivalent injuries to this: (1) plastic bending of the ulna with radial head dislocation, and (2) ulna fracture with separation of the proximal radial epiphysis. When the patient presents for treatment, the ulnar fracture is readily noted; however, care must be taken not to miss the radial head dislocation. *For this reason, plain radiographs need to include both the joint above (elbow) and joint below (wrist) the fracture—a good rule to follow in evaluation of all fractures.* Close follow-up of the fracture is needed to ensure that alignment of the ulna and reduction of the radial head are maintained.

Treatment is usually possible with closed manipulation to realign the ulna and to reduce the radial head with traction on the arm in extension, followed by supination, flexion to 90 degrees, and immobilization in a cast. Occasionally, maintenance of radial head reduction requires intramedullary fixation of the ulna to maintain length and alignment. If the radial head is dislocated posteriorly, reduction may be best held in extension.

Greenstick Fractures

Greenstick fractures of both bones of the forearm may be treated by closed reduction; however, the fracture should be completed, by cracking the intact cortex, to reduce risk of recurrence of deformity in the cast and refracture following healing. Angulation of less than 10 degrees must be maintained, or loss of forearm rotation will occur; these fractures are usually diaphyseal, and remodeling is less helpful. Healing with immobilization occurs in 4 to 6 weeks.

Displaced fractures of the ulna and radius should undergo closed reduction, with the physician striving to get the rotation and angulation correct. It should be remembered that one side of the fractured bone will have an intact periosteal sleeve that can be used as a hinge to aid reduction. Cortex-to-cortex apposition is adequate, provided that the alignment and rotation are correct. The arm is immobilized in such a position that the fracture is stable, with the cast carefully formed to provide three-point fixation. Open reduction and internal fixation can be performed if closed treatment fails or in older children. This is a better option than acceptance of an unacceptable position.

Buckle Fractures

Buckle fractures of the distal radius may be found in injury due to the same mechanism. The swelling and tenderness are usually slightly proximal to the distal radial physis, and radiographs may show only a subtle ripple along one cortex or soft tissue swelling. An ulnar styloid fracture may be present. Short arm cast protection for 3 weeks suffices.

Distal Radial and Ulnar Fractures

Fractures of the distal radius and ulna occur primarily in the 6- to 12-year age group and are usually Salter-Harris type I or II. Type I injuries occur in younger children and are frequently nondisplaced. Radiographs are either normal or show subtle widening of the physis. Clinical examination is thus the key, with point tenderness and swelling noted. Reduction is performed only for large amounts of displacement, as remodeling is the rule; the child should be casted for 3 weeks for protection.

Type II injuries are more common in the older patients. These fractures are usually treated closed with reduction and cast immobilization. Again, remodeling is good. Growth disturbance is rare; as with all injuries, however, it can occur. The patient should be checked with radiographs for 6 to 12 months to make sure this does not happen.

Hand Fractures

Several principles are important in the care of hand fractures in children. Fractures of the shafts of the metacarpals and phalanges must be aligned properly, with special attention paid to the rotation of the digits. A good way to check rotation is to flex the finger metacarpophalangeal joints 90 degrees and check the fingernails, which should be aligned evenly. One finger should never be immobilized in order to hold a finger fracture in place; rather, the hand is splinted down to the forearm and two fingers are included in the splint. For almost all injuries, the period of immobilization should be for 3 weeks. This will be sufficient for clinical, but not radiographic, union of the fracture in the hand of most children.

Base of Thumb Fractures

Fractures of the base of the thumb metacarpal occur with hyperextension or abduction of the thumb. These may be metaphyseal fractures or physeal fractures of the basal thumb. Less than 30 degrees of angulation is acceptable because of the mobility of the basal thumb joint, and only thumb spica cast immobilization is required. Salter-Harris type II fractures, if widely displaced, may necessitate open reduction; type III injury, a Bennett fracture equivalent, may necessitate open reduction and K-wire fixation to hold the reduction.

A frequent skiing injury is the so-called "gamekeeper's thumb." Valgus stress is applied to the thumb across the MP joint and results in tearing of the ulnar collateral ligament of the joint in adults and a type III physeal injury in children. A displaced fracture or more than 45 degrees of angulation at the joint, as demonstrated by a stress view, is best treated with repair.

Metacarpophalangeal Joint Dislocation

Metacarpophalangeal joint dislocation may occur with hyperextension of the joint. It may be simple (reducible) or complex (irreducible). For complex dislocations, an operative approach for reduction is required, with removal of interposed volar plate from the joint and extraction of the metacarpal head from a Chinese finger trap of palmar fascia and flexor tendons. Radiographically, the metacarpal is usually found parallel to the proximal phalanx on the lateral view.

Finger and Nail Injuries

Injuries to the tip of the finger and nail bed are very common in children of all ages. With *crush injuries* to the distal phalanx, thorough irrigation is necessary, with repair directed at preservation of the nail bed and proximal nail fold. *Mallet finger* deformity in young children usually is a type I physeal separation and also an open injury. Thorough irrigation of the wound, with antibiotic prophylaxis and reduction of the nail back underneath the proximal nail fold, is required in addition to reduction of the fracture. In older children, the injury is a type III injury of the distal phalanx epiphysis through avulsion by the pull of the extensor tendon. Repair and K-wire fixation are required if the fragment is displaced.

LOWER EXTREMITY TRAUMA

Hip

Hip Dislocations

In children dislocations of the hip occur more often than hip fractures and with less force than that required in adults. Observed primarily in the 12- to 15-year-old age group, posterior dislocation is far more common than anterior dislocation.

Dislocations are usually reduced closed, with the patient treated in Buck's skin traction for 1 to 2 weeks, followed by crutch ambulation to avoid the positions of flexion and adduction for approximately 3 weeks. After reduction, however, it is vital to ensure that a concentric reduction of the hip is obtained. Lack of a concentric reduction implies bone fragments or infolded limbus present within the joint. A careful search for fractures of the femoral head and acetabulum must be conducted, and CT scans are frequently needed for complete assessment. If closed reduction cannot be attained, open reduction is performed—through an anterior approach for anterior dislocations and a posterior approach for posterior dislocations. Bone fragments within the joint may be removed through a posterior approach. Recurrent dislocation is a problem only in patients with excessive ligamentous laxity in conditions such as the Ehlers-Danlos syndrome. The risk of avascular necrosis (AVN) following this injury is approximately 8 to 10 per cent, lower than the rate for adults.

Femoral Neck Fractures

Femoral neck fractures are the result of quite a bit of trauma in children; fortunately, they are fairly infrequent because the risk of complications is high. Avascular necrosis occurs in 30 to 50 per cent and is more of a risk in patients older than 8 years of age. Coxa vara due to malunion is found in 20 to 30 per cent of patients and may warrant corrective osteotomy later. Premature epiphyseal closure depends on the type of injury and can occur in up to 60 per cent.

Traumatic slips of the capital femoral epiphysis may be gently reduced at the time of positioning the hip for fixation and pinned in place with cannulated screws under image intensifier control. The pins should not penetrate the subchondral bone because chondrolysis of the articular cartilage will result. Care must be taken to avoid vigorous reduction with further damage to the epiphyseal vascular supply and increased risk of AVN. There is a 100% risk of AVN if the epiphysis is dislocated.

Transcervical femoral neck fractures are treated with closed reduction and cannulated screw fixation and spica cast immobilization for protection for 4 to 6 weeks. Open reduction may be required for some fractures. There is a 50% risk of AVN with displaced fractures.

Basicervical fractures, with better blood supply to the femoral neck and head, may be treated with spica cast immobilization if they are nondisplaced and by closed reduction and screw or screw and sideplate fixation with spica cast if they are displaced.

Femur

Femoral Shaft Fractures

With fractures of the femoral shaft, it is important to check for the presence of other injuries, to the ipsilateral hip and knee in the trauma victim and to other bones in the possible victim of child abuse. The hip and the knee should be included routinely in the radiographic studies. Careful neurovascular assessment is also required, although findings are frequently negative.

The fracture heals without difficulty as long as the proximal and distal ends of the fracture remain in the same thigh. Overlap or bayonet apposition of the fragments is sufficient in most cases because overgrowth of the femur can make up for up to 2 cm of shortening. The deformity from bayonet position is well hidden by the bulk of the thigh muscle.

In patients ranging from infants to 2 year olds, treatment is by immediate spica cast immobilization, usually with the hip flexed 90 degrees and abducted 45 degrees. Four to 6 weeks is all that is required, and upon removal of the cast the fracture callus will be easily palpable in the thigh.

In patients aged 3 to 10, previous treatment had been with 90/90 skeletal traction using a distal femoral traction pin for 2 weeks until the fracture becomes sticky, followed by spica cast immobilization. This certainly still works. Recent efforts to provide earlier mobilization and reduced hospitalization of the patient have led to immediate spica cast immobilization, a technique used most often in these patients today. Ischial weight-bearing cast braces and external fixation have also been used by some with good results. In association with head injury, external or internal fixation protects patients from themselves.

Adolescent patients, if close to the end of growth, may be treated as adults with intramedullary rod fixation and early mobilization.

Supracondylar and Distal Femoral Fractures

Supracondylar fractures and fractures of the distal femur may be very difficult to properly align because of the pull of the gastrocnemius muscle flexing the distal fragment. If adequate reduction cannot be maintained, internal fixation is required.

Knee

Distal Femoral Epiphyseal Injury

Injuries to the distal femoral epiphysis are seen in the adolescent football player subjected to a clip. Rather than sustaining a tear of the medial collateral ligament, the player sustains a type I or II epiphyseal separation. Valgus stress radiographs of the knee reveal the injury if the diagnosis is in doubt. Because the popliteal artery is closely applied to the distal femur and posterior knee joint, *careful assessment of the vascular supply of the limb is needed and an arteriogram may be required.* Closed reduction and cast immobilization are usually adequate treatment, but open reduction may be required if the injury is irreducible as a result of interposed soft tissue. Admission to the hospital and monitoring for development of compartment syndrome or vascular embarrassment are mandatory. Knee stiffness may result, and the incidence of growth arrest is 50 per cent.

Patellar Fractures

Fractures of the patella are rare but occasionally are found after a direct blow to the patella. They can be treated with immobilization in extension if there is minimal displacement and with a functioning extensor mechanism. Displaced fractures and inability to actively extend the knee indicate a need for operative reduction and fixation using a tension band wire technique. A variant of patella fracture is the sleeve fracture, in which the infrapatellar tendon avulses a fragment of bone from the inferior pole of the patella along with articular cartilage. Internal fixation is necessary if there is displacement.

Lateral Dislocation of the Patella

Lateral patellar dislocation is a common problem in childhood and adolescence. It is observed in patients with valgus angulation, persistent femoral neck anteversion, external rotation of the tibial tubercle, excess tightness of the lateral retinaculum of the knee, or a combination of the above. This is a problem of malalignment. As the patella dislocates and then relocates, damage to the articular surfaces of the patella and trochlea or osteochondral fractures can occur. Hemarthrosis is routinely present.

Initial treatment involves aspiration of the knee, immobilization, and rehabilitation, although repair of a large rent in the medial retinaculum, if present, is advised. Recurrent dislocation dictates consideration of realignment procedures. If osteochondral fragments are present within the knee, they are removed if small or are reduced and fixed with absorbable pins if large.

Intercondylar Eminence Fractures

Intercondylar eminence fractures of the tibia are the equivalent of the torn anterior cruciate ligament in the adult; in the child, however, the bone yields to the stress applied before the ligament. These fractures occur with valgus rotational stress on the knee, or hyperflexion occasionally, and result in a hemarthrosis that is impressive. The tibial eminence fracture may be nondisplaced, hinged, or displaced. The knee is aspirated for comfort, and the leg casted with the knee in full extension for nondisplaced and reducible hinged fractures. Displaced and irreducible fractures require internal fixation, which may be done open or arthroscopically, to reduce the risk of symptomatic instability. Despite this treatment, increased laxity of the anterior cruciate ligament may be seen following healing.

Proximal Tibial Epiphyseal Fractures

As noted previously with distal femoral epiphyseal injuries, vascular problems can occur with fractures of the proximal tibial epiphysis. Careful assessment is required; the presence of pulses does not preclude the presence of injury with an intimal tear. The popliteal artery is tethered to the epiphysis by the geniculate vessels and is easily injured. Admission to the hospital and an arteriogram are needed, most notably with displaced fractures, and the patient needs to be monitored for compartment syndrome. The injury is usually a type I or II and can be treated with reduction and cast immobilization. If a vascular repair or reconstruction is needed or if the fracture is type III or IV, open reduction with internal fixation is necessary.

Avulsion of Tibial Tubercle

Avulsion of the tibial tubercle at the attachment of the infrapatellar tendon is found primarily in patients aged 14 to 16 years. Open reduction and internal fixation are needed if the fractures are displaced or if they occur at the level of the tibial physis. Nondisplaced or minimally displaced fractures may be treated with a cast in extension.

Meniscal Tears

Meniscal tears occur in children and can be treated with arthroscopic-assisted resection or repair as appropriate. Magnetic resonance imaging of the meniscus is very helpful in delineating the pathology. Repairable lesions are vertical tears through the meniscosynovial junction or in the most peripheral 25 per cent of the meniscus. The remainder of the meniscus is not sufficiently vascular to heal following repair. Discoid lateral meniscus is the cause of "snapping knee" and, when torn, can be a cause of locking and knee pain in children. Loose fragments of meniscus causing symptoms necessitate removal along with meniscoplasty performed along the remaining meniscal substance to form a more normal-appearing meniscal rim.

Tibia and Fibula

Tibial Shaft Fractures

Fractures of the tibial shaft for the most part can be treated with cast immobilization. They heal readily in young patients in 6 to 8 weeks. One must be careful to avoid varus or valgus angulation of more than 5 to 10 degrees. Slight varus is preferable to slight valgus, as the deformity is more noticeable in valgus because the tibia is immediately subcutaneous medially. Wedging the cast can correct alignment problems. One must also be careful to avoid rotational malalignment of the foot because excessive internal or external rotation of the foot will most certainly be noticed by the patient and parents. A cast with a foot-thigh angle equal to the opposite leg or 0 (zero) degrees is used if one is in doubt. Operative treatment is rarely required, but it may be an option with intramedullary fixation in those nearing skeletal maturity.

Occasionally, pins incorporated into the cast may be needed to maintain length and alignment. The fibula may remain intact with fracture of the tibial shaft and may undergo plastic bowing. The cast must be molded carefully to prevent the fracture from migrating into varus or valgus.

Other Tibial and Fibular Fractures

The limping child younger than 2 years old may be found to have a *toddler fracture,* a spiral nondisplaced fracture of the tibia. This fracture heals readily and without displacement, but a cast should be used for protection for 3 weeks. Problem fractures include *displaced proximal metaphyseal fractures,* as damage to the vascular trifurcation can occur, and *greenstick fractures of the proximal metaphysis.* These latter fractures, unless reduced well and held, can result in overgrowth medially with progressive valgus of the tibia. These fractures should be casted in extension with varus molding.

Ankle

Type I Injury

Type I epiphyseal separations of the distal fibular physis is the pediatric equivalent of the ankle sprain. Cast immobilization for 3 weeks is indicated, and displacement is rare.

Type II Injury

A *type II separation of the distal tibial physis* can occur with greenstick fracture of the fibula. This injury can be treated closed. Despite angulation of up to 20 degrees, results are good because of remodeling, with growth disturbance a rare complication.

Type III Injury

The *Tillaux fracture* is a type III epiphyseal injury to the lateral aspect of the distal tibial physis. Most likely, it occurs as an avulsion injury at the site of attachment of the anterior tibiofibular ligaments under external rotation stress. Closed reduction and cast immobilization can be performed. However, open reduction and internal fixation are required if displacement is 2 mm or more. This is an intra-articular fracture, and care must be taken to avoid incongruity of the ankle joint.

Combined Type II and III Injury

The *triplane fracture* of the ankle combines a type II injury with a type III injury (Tillaux). Radiographs can be difficult to interpret, and a CT scan can be invaluable to fully evaluate the reduction of the fracture. If there is any question at all as to whether the closed reduction is adequate, open reduction and internal fixation should be performed. This injury involves possible epiphyseal arrest and joint incongruity and must be treated aggressively. The CT scan may also be helpful with Tillaux fracture evaluation.

Type III or IV Injury

Medial malleolar fractures are type III or IV physeal injuries and should be treated as such, with accurate reduction to realign the physis and articular surface and internal fixation to maintain it. There is a high incidence of bridge formation with these fractures, especially those treated nonoperatively.

Foot

Several fractures are worth mentioning in the foot; however, most of those not mentioned respond well to cast immobilization for 3 to 6 weeks until healed.

Phalangeal Fractures

Fractures of the phalanx require little more than buddy taping, as all of them will heal readily. Fractures of the bones of the great toe, however, may require more aggressive care if they are displaced or intra-articular to prevent early degenerative changes along this mobile weight-bearing ray.

Metatarsal Stress Fractures

Stress fracture of the fifth metatarsal base can occur in residual clubfoot deformity due to increased weight bearing on the lateral border of the foot. The base of the fifth metatarsal can also be the site of avulsion injury with inversion injury owing to the pull of the peroneus brevis. Displacement is rare. This stress fracture may be treated with weight-bearing casts. In the residual clubfoot situation, however, the deformity ultimately may need to be addressed.

Talar Fractures

Fractures of the talus are rare and may be divided into neck and body fractures. Talar neck fractures are usually nondisplaced and heal with cast immobilization; reduction and internal fixation may be needed in displaced fractures.

Talar body fractures are frequently displaced, requiring open reduction and internal fixation. They are associated with an increased incidence of AVN.

Calcaneal fractures are rare in children, and most commonly can be managed closed with non weight-bearing cast immobilization. Hospital admission may be needed to monitor swelling and to provide elevation.

Osteochondral fractures of the dome of the talus occur following 1 per cent of ankle injuries. They are frequently diagnosed late because acute stage and even delayed radiographs may not be diagnostic. The common sites of occurrence are the anterolateral and posteromedial dome of the talus. Persistent ankle pain or fluid within the ankle following an ankle injury should alert one to the possibility, and MRI is usually diagnostic. The lesions may be staged, with compression injury without delineation of an osteochondral fragment amenable to conservative cast treatment; however, they must be watched carefully for progression. For partial or complete delineation of an osteochondral fragment, with or without separation, arthroscopic débridement of the fragment and curettage to bleeding bone are necessary.

REFERENCES

Gregg JR, Das M: Foot and ankle problems in the adolescent and preadolescent athlete. Clin Sports Med 1:131–147, 1982.

Landry GL, Gomez JE: Management of soft tissue injuries. *In* Dyment PG (ed): Adolescent Medicine: State of the Art Reviews. Philadelphia, Hanley & Belfus, Inc, 1991.

Oliver JH: Stress fracture of the lower extremity. *In* Torg JS, Welsh RP, Shephard RJ (eds): Current Therapy in Sports Medicine, 2nd ed. Philadelphia, Decker Inc, 1990.

Salter RB, Harris WR: Injuries involving the epiphyseal plate. J Bone Joint Surg 45A:587–622, 1963.

14

Muscles

TORTICOLLIS

RICHARD J. MIER, M.D.

Torticollis means "twisted neck" and describes a condition in which the head is persistently laterally flexed and rotated on the neck. The most common cause of *congenital* torticollis is fibrous shortening of the sternocleidomastoid (SCM) muscle. Possible etiologic factors include intrauterine positioning, hemorrhage, or birth trauma. The muscular foreshortening draws the head into lateral flexion and produces rotation to the contralateral side, with the chin pointing away from the lesion. Other positional deformities may be present, including hip dysplasia; facial asymmetry may develop if the restriction is persistent. An olive-shaped fibrous mass often appears during the early postnatal period and usually regresses by the end of the first year of life. Intrauterine torticollis may be maternal (due to fibroids) or fetal (due to a congenital myopathic process). Most often, no specific cause is apparent.

Malformations of the cervical spine such as vertebral fusion (the Klippel-Feil sequence) may be associated with torticollis presenting at birth. On examination, affected children have low hairlines and short necks. Odontoid aplasia may also be associated with torticollis. *Failure to diagnose the cause of the torticollis accurately may result in neurologic catastrophe if physical therapy is attempted.* Computed tomography (CT) may be necessary to exclude these vertebral anomalies because the immature spine may not demonstrate the abnormality on radiograph.

Spinal malformations predispose to injury, and torticollis at birth may also be due to fracture or dislocation even if the delivery is not traumatic in the usual sense of the word. Gastroesophageal reflux may be associated with abnormal torticollis-like head and neck positioning as the infant reacts to the discomfort of reflux esophagitis (Sandifer syndrome). This may be present early enough to appear to be a congenital lesion.

Acquired torticollis is frequently due to such benign causes as minor soft tissue trauma or viral myositis. Any inflammatory condition affecting tissues of the neck, including adenitis, pharyngitis, retropharyngeal abscess, cellulitis, or sinusitis, may cause torticollis. It is sometimes difficult to distinguish these conditions from rotatory atlantoaxial subluxation, which is not rare in children and may itself be related to upper respiratory infections, minor trauma, or such chronic inflammation of the atlantoaxial joint as occurs with juvenile rheumatoid arthritis (JRA).

Other less common causes of acquired torticollis include medications (particularly the phenothiazines), myositis ossificans progressiva, ocular strabismus, and tumors of the posterior fossa, brain stem, or cervical spine. One case due to pseudotumor cerebri has been reported.

Spasmodic torticollis may be the manifestation of a segmental or focal dystonia. Such dystonic reactions are a result of a variety of uncommon *heredodegenerative diseases.* A small number of children have also been described with paroxysmal torticollis, sometimes associated with headache, vomiting, or ataxia. Subsequently, these children sometimes experience more typical symptoms of migraine. There frequently is a family history of either paroxysmal torticollis or classic migraine.

Congenital muscular torticollis generally responds well to physical therapy, assuming that vertebral anomalies have been excluded. Therapy can be performed at home by gentle but persistent lateral flexion of the head to stretch the contralaterally tightened SCM muscle. Rotation of the head toward the side with the tightness can be done simultaneously. Ten to 20 repetitions, holding the head momentarily at maximal range, will usually suffice if done three or four times daily. Referral to a physical therapist is recommended so that progress and compliance may be monitored. Children presenting late (after 1 year of age), particularly if they exhibit significant facial asymmetry, may not respond to physical therapy and will frequently require surgery, usually SCM release, followed by postoperative physical therapy and splinting.

A complete evaluation, including CT (for suspected bony lesions) and/or magnetic resonance imaging (for soft tissue or cord lesions), is useful in the older child with acquired torticollis if symptoms are severe or persistent or if the cause is not apparent. Rotatory atlantoaxial subluxation often responds to traction, although open reduction and fusion are sometimes necessary in children with long-standing refractory symptoms. Surgical consultation is appropriate under these circumstances, particularly if neurologic signs or symptoms are present.

REFERENCES

Canale ST, Griffin DW, Hubbard CN: Congenital muscular torticollis: A long-term follow-up. J Bone Joint Surg 64:810, 1982.

CONGENITAL MUSCULAR DEFECTS

RICHARD J. MIER, M.D.

The category of congenital muscular defects comprises a large number of disparate conditions. These disorders may be subgrouped into those representing either embryologic absence of a specific muscle or group of muscles (e.g., Poland anomaly) or those representing intrinsic abnormalities of muscle itself (e.g., central core myopathy).

PRIMARY DEFECTS

Disability due to these abnormalities varies widely, depending on the site and degree of the defect, and may be of no importance, of only cosmetic importance, or of serious functional significance. Therapy, when available, is primarily surgical and is oriented toward reparative or transfer procedures.

An archetypal example of isolated congenital lack of muscle development is Poland anomaly, consisting of unilateral absence of the costal and sternal portions of the pectoralis major muscle, often with synbrachydactyly of the ipsilateral hand and other mesodermal defects of the upper ipsilateral chest (skin hypoplasia, nipple absence, or hypoplasia). Poland anomaly is thought to be a local defect of mesodermal development and is generally not hereditary; there is no specific therapy.

Similar congenital hypoplasia syndromes have been described involving the depressor anguli oris muscle, resulting in the asymmetric crying facies syndrome—important because of its association with congenital heart disease, genitourinary malformations, and other anomalies. Electrophysiologic studies may be required to distinguish muscular absence in this syndrome from true facial nerve palsy. Duane syndrome represents replacement of the ocular abducens muscle by a fibrous band and causes failure of abduction of the affected side and retraction of the globe when adduction is attempted. Congenital absence of the trapezius, quadratus femoris, and serratus major muscles has also been described.

SECONDARY MUSCULAR DISRUPTION SYNDROMES

Secondary muscular disruption syndromes are not uncommon at birth and manifest themselves as a result of other, more primary processes. They occur, for example, as a result of congenital limb deficiency syndromes (such as radial hypoplasia) or as a result of massive fetal urinary tract dilatation, associated with deficiency of the muscles of the anterior abdominal wall (prune-belly syndrome).

INTRINSIC MUSCLE DISEASES

Intrinsic muscle disease may also be manifested at birth. Included are such "benign" causes for early proximal hypotonicity as nemaline myopathy, central core disease, and myotubular myopathy. Elevations of muscle enzymes are often modest, if present at all; electrophysiologic studies are often normal. Structural or ultrastructural changes on microscopy permit categorization and prognostication, which is often, but not invariably, good.

Several of the muscular dystrophies may also be present at birth. The most prominent is congenital muscular dystrophy, inherited as an autosomal recessive disease and having a slow, somewhat unpredictably progressive course. One variant is associated with mental retardation (Fukuyama), and one with striking congenital joint contractures (Ullrich disease). Diagnosis depends on the results of muscle biopsy.

Additionally, several of the dystrophic myotonic disorders may present at birth, including the congenital form of myotonic dystrophy. Usually hypotonic at birth, these infants have a weak cry and suck, often exhibit arthrogryposis, and are frequently mentally retarded. Therapy is supportive, and orthopedic procedures may be necessary to improve function.

INFANTILE HYPOTONIA

HERBERT E. GILMORE, M.D.

Normal muscle tone is maintained by the activity of the gamma motoneuron system. Central control of tone is mediated through the basal ganglia, cerebellum, and brain stem (mainly vestibular) nuclei. From these centers, rubrospinal, reticulospinal, and other extrapyramidal pathways carry impulses to gamma motoneurons in the intermediate and anterior horns of the spinal cord. From there, impulses are relayed through the nerve roots, peripheral nerves, and myoneural junction to the muscle spindle and somatic muscle cells. When the activity of any of these areas is disrupted, hypotonia can develop. These pathways are different from those used for central control of strength (mainly corticospinal tract); thus, hypotonia is often present without weakness.

Infantile hypotonia is caused by disorders that affect the nervous system at various levels. Table 1 lists the major diseases affecting each site. Evaluation of the hypotonic infant includes clinical and laboratory analyses appropriate to each anatomic site. A careful history and thorough physical, neurologic, and developmental examinations are crucial to determine the direction of further investigations. Often during the general physical examination, specific "visual diagnoses" can be made. Table 2 lists these disorders and the major clinical criteria for diagnosis. During the neurologic examination, specific attention must be paid to the muscle bulk, form, and strength. Infants with hypotonia of central origin do not exhibit early weakness and atrophy. Those with anterior horn cell, peripheral nerve, or muscle disease exhibit early weakness and atrophy, sometimes resulting in chest wall and extremity deformities (pectus carinatum, pes valgus, claw-hand). In peripheral nerve disease, weakness and atrophy are proportional to hypotonia; in muscle disease, they are greater than hypotonia. The deep tendon reflexes are normal or slightly depressed early on in patients with muscle disease; in those with anterior horn cell or peripheral nerve disease, they are markedly hypoactive or absent; and in those with central disease, they are normal early and accentuated later. The presence of persistent ankle clonus and Babinski sign beyond 18 months of age suggests central or spinal cord disease.

Sometimes the anatomic localization of or specific diagnosis for hypotonia can be determined clinically, making laboratory investigations necessary. Such investigations may include magnetic resonance imaging, cerebrospinal fluid analysis, chromosome analysis, serum amino acid and urine organic acid determinations, creatine phosphokinase levels, electromyographic and nerve conduction velocities, as well as other metabolic testing (lactate, pyruvate, ammonia), depending on the clinical findings. The main goal of such investigations is to identify treatable (amino and organic acidopathies) or inherited disorders (Duchenne muscular dystrophy). After a specific diagnosis is established, the appropriate therapy can be instituted.

CLINICAL COURSE AND PROGNOSIS

The clinical course and prognosis of infants with hypotonia depend on its cause, anatomic distribution, and severity. In general, patients with spinal muscular atrophy, progressive metabolic disorders, and some myopathies, especially Du-

TABLE 1. Causes of Infantile Hypotonia

Central Nervous System Diseases
Perinatal hypoxia-ischemia
Congenital infections (TORCH syndrome, HIV)
Encephalitis, meningitis
Head trauma
Hydrocephalus
Syringobulbia
Brain tumors: medulloblastoma, pontine glioma
Chromosomal disorders: trisomy 13, 21
Prader-Willi syndrome
Birth defect syndromes
Cerebral dysgenesis
Tuberous sclerosis
Neurofibromatosis
Peroxisomal disorders (Zellweger syndrome, neonatal adrenoleukodystrophy)
Amino and organic acidopathies (hyperglycinemia, glutaric aciduria)
Ornithine transcarbamylase deficiency
Lysosomal storage diseases (GM_1 gangliosidosis, Krabbe's disease, metachromatic leukodystrophy)
Other progressive leukoencephalopathies (Pelizaeus-Merzbacher, Canavan's, Alexander's disease)
Spinal Cord Diseases
Infantile spinal muscular atrophy (Werdnig-Hoffmann syndrome)
In utero viral arthrogryposis
Poliomyelitis
Trauma: C-1–C-2 subluxation, C-5–C-6 distraction
Severe perinatal hypoxia-ischemia
Nerve Root and Peripheral Nerve Diseases
Postinfectious polyradiculoneuropathy (Guillain-Barré syndrome)
Infantile polyneuropathies
Myoneural Diseases
Myasthenia gravis: transient, persistent
Infantile botulism
Muscle Diseases
Congenital myopathies (myotubular, mitochondrial, nemaline rod, etc.)
Congenital muscular dystrophy
Duchenne type and Becker muscular dystrophy (older infants)
Infantile myotonic dystrophy
Polymyositis
Carnitine deficiency
Acid maltase deficiency (Pompe's disease)
Combined Central and Peripheral Diseases
Mitochondrial encephalomyopathies
Fukuyama type muscular dystrophy
Neuroaxonal dystrophy
Metachromatic leukodystrophy
Familial dysautonomia (Riley-Day syndrome)
Non-Neurologic Diseases
Ehlers-Danlos syndrome
Sepsis
Dehydration
Malnutrition
Hypothyroidism
Hypothermia

Abbreviations: HIV, human immunodeficiency virus.

chenne type muscular dystrophy, have a poor prognosis. These patients usually experience significant progressive weakness with associated hypotonia. Patients with mild hypotonia having no specific cause will often exhibit significant spontaneous improvement. Those with generalized hypotonia usually have a more protracted clinical course than those with focal (mainly lower extremity) hypotonia.

Patients with hypotonia having a central nervous system cause (see Table 1) have a broad spectrum of prognoses, from

TABLE 2. Disorders Associated with Hypotonia for Which a Clinical Diagnosis Can Be Made

Disorder	Clinical Criteria
Perinatal hypoxia-ischemia	Cerebral palsy, strabismus, developmental delay
Encephalitis/meningitis	Stiff neck, fever
Head trauma	Battle sign, raccoon eyes, skull fracture, other signs of trauma
Hydrocephalus	Progressive macrocephaly, setting-sun sign, suture separation
Brain tumor	Papilledema, ophthalmoplegia, titubation, dysmetria, focal weakness
Down syndrome	Characteristic facial features, Brushfield's spots (iris), simian crease
Prader-Willi syndrome	Undescended testicles, almond-shaped eyes, small hands and feet, failure to thrive
Birth defect syndromes	Multiple malformations in three or more organ systems
Cerebral dysgenesis	Microcephaly, dysmorphic features
Tuberous sclerosis	Ash-leaf spots (Wood's lamp examination of skin)
Neurofibromatosis (type 1)	>6 café au lait spots by 1 year of age, axillary freckling, Lisch nodules, cutaneous neurofibromas
Zellweger syndrome	High forehead, facial anomalies, organomegaly
Pelizaeus-Merzbacher disease	X-linked, pendular nystagmus, head-nodding
Alexander's, Canavan's disease	Macrocephaly without hydrocephalus, leukodystrophy on CT/MRI
Lysosomal storage disorders	Organomegaly, cherry-red spot (ocular fundi)
Ornithine transcarbamylase deficiency	Episodic ataxia, drowsiness, coma
Glutaric aciduria, type I	Macrocephaly, choreoathetosis
Hyperglycinemia	Microcephaly, cerebral dysgenesis on MRI
Werdnig-Hoffman disease	Tongue fasciculations, areflexia, occasional arthrogryposis
In utero viral arthrogryposis	Multiple, fixed joint contractures at birth
Myasthenia gravis/infantile botulism	Diurnal fluctuating hypotonia and weakness, eyelid droop, ophthalmoplegia
Myotonic dystrophy	"Tenting" of upper lip, "fish mouth," facial diplegia, percussion myotonia; myotonic response in mother
Duchenne type and Becker's muscular dystrophy	Calf hypertrophy, accentuated lumbar lordosis, Gowers' sign
Acid maltase deficiency (Pompe's disease)	Large tongue, heart murmur; radiographic cardiomegaly
Riley-Day syndrome	Temperature instability, underdeveloped or absent fungiform papillae of the tongue, gastrointestinal disturbances, labile blood pressure, lack of tears, swallowing incoordination
Ehlers-Danlos syndrome	Ligamentous laxity, "loose skin," double-jointedness, family history of similar signs

Abbreviations: CT, computed tomography; MRI, magnetic resonance imaging.

a benign course in some infants with perinatal hypoxia-ischemia, encephalitis, meningitis, and trauma to a progressive course in patients with leukoencephalopathies, lysosomal storage diseases, and other progressive metabolic disorders. An intermediate degree of hypotonia is seen in patients with chromosomal disorders, such as Down syndrome. Patients with Prader-Willi syndrome have severe hypotonia at onset, with rapid improvement to normal tone by 1 year of age. Infants with central nervous system hypotonia usually exhibit other characteristics (cognitive delay, visual and hearing impairment) that determine poor prognosis; hypotonia is usually not the major concern in such infants.

Patients with spinal cord disease, on the other hand, often suffer severe hypotonia and weakness, which pose major problems for them. Infants with type 1 spinal muscular atrophy (SMA) (Werdnig-Hoffmann disease) experience early onset of severe, progressive hypotonia and weakness, resulting in death by 1 year of age. Those with type 2 SMA exhibit onset of disease from 2 to 12 months of age and are often able to sit and stand but can never walk; most of them die in the first decade. Patients with type 3 SMA display symptoms at 1 to 2 years of age and can sometimes walk but are most often confined to a wheelchair.

Congenital SMA can cause fixed joint contractures, which are difficult to differentiate from arthrogryposis resulting from in utero viral infection of the anterior horn cell. Differentiation of the two disorders is important, however, because infants with arthrogryposis do not experience progressive deterioration as do infants with SMA. Thus, it should not be assumed that all infants with congenital arthrogryposis have SMA with a poor prognosis.

Most infants with Guillain-Barré syndrome do well and have full recovery of function; a few require prolonged ventilatory assistance.

Neonatal myasthenia gravis (MG) is either transient or persistent. Transient MG is due to passive transfer of antiacetylcholine receptor antibodies from the affected mother to the infant. Symptoms of weak suck, dysphagia, ptosis, and lack of spontaneous movements occur hours or days after birth and last for several weeks. In persistent MG, onset is usually after many days and prolonged treatment is required (see later).

Infantile botulism is a transient disorder that lasts 2 to 8 weeks regardless of treatment. As in Guillain-Barré syndrome, some patients require ventilatory assistance; apnea and sudden death have been reported.

Most congenital myopathies are benign and transient, but congenital muscular dystrophy and myotubular, mitochondrial, reducing-body, and carnitine deficiency myopathy are progressive. Older infants with Duchenne type muscular dystrophy experience a slowly progressive course and are usually wheelchair-bound by age 10 to 12 years; those with the milder Becker form are often ambulatory well into their teenaged years or twenties. Patients with acid maltase deficiency (Pompe's disease) experience severe hypotonia and weakness, and most die of cardiac failure.

Patients with both central and peripheral nervous system involvement experience a variable course that is dependent on the cause. Patients with neuraxonal dystrophy and metachromatic leukodystrophy (MLD) usually exhibit progressive deterioration and have a poor prognosis. Those with mitochondrial encephalomyopathies experience a variable course that is dependent on the specific subtype and response to therapy (see later). In general, patients with cytochrome *c* oxidase deficiency exhibit progressive deterioration and have a poor prognosis (except for those with rare benign type); patients with Leigh disease experience a variable course that is dependent on the specific enzyme abnormality.

THERAPY

General Treatment

Regardless of the cause of hypotonia, many affected infants require physical and occupational therapy; those with developmental delay should be enrolled in early intervention programs. Orthopedic interventions (splints, braces, surgery) are required for infants with joint instability or contractures. Infants with significant swallowing difficulties often require feeding via nasogastric tube or gastrostomy, and those with severe respiratory distress often require ventilatory support.

The following is a summary of specific therapies for disorders that cause infantile hypotonia.

Transient non-neurologic disorders, such as sepsis, dehydration, malnutrition, hypothermia, and hypothyroidism, should be promptly identified and corrected. Experimental trials are ongoing regarding the efficacy of prenatally administered indomethacin to reduce the effects of hypoxia-ischemia on the neonatal brain. Additionally, improvements in neonatal care should reduce postnatally acquired hypoxic-ischemic hypotonia. Congenital infections (TORCH syndrome, human immunodeficiency virus) should be promptly identified, and treatment with antiviral medication should be considered, if appropriate. Bacterial meningitis should be promptly identified and treated. Hydrocephalus should be treated, if deemed clinically appropriate, either medically (serial lumbar puncture, acetazolamide and furosemide) or surgically (external drainage, ventriculoperitoneal shunt). Management of brain tumors requires a combined medical, neurosurgical, and oncologic approach.

Patients with chromosome disorders, Prader-Willi syndrome, and identifiable but untreatable progressive central nervous system disorders (e.g., neuraxonal dystrophy, MLD) should be referred to appropriate subspecialty clinics because management of their problems requires a multidisciplinary approach.

Specific Treatment

Several treatments are available for Guillain-Barré syndrome. These include prednisone (3 mg/kg/day, tapered over 10 days to 2 mg/kg/day and continued until improvement is noted); plasmapheresis, effective mainly within the first week of illness, especially for patients requiring mechanical ventilation (reduces time on ventilator and in intensive care unit); and, more recently, intravenous immunoglobulin (IVIg).

Initial treatment of infants with MG is with pyridostigmine syrup (Mestinon, 4 to 10 mg orally every 4 hours); dosage adjustments are made according to clinical response. Alternatively, neostigmine (0.5 mg/kg orally every 4 hours) may be used. If pyridostigmine is administered parenterally, only 1/30 of the oral dose should be given. Significant cholinergic side effects (diarrhea, bradycardia) can occur in patients after initial treatment with pyridostigmine. Patients with transient MG usually do not require treatment longer than 4 to 6 weeks. Those with persistent MG require treatment indefinitely. Prednisone (2 mg/kg/day), intermittent plasmapheresis, and/or thymectomy may be required in certain cases. Although antibiotics and botulinum antitoxin have been used in the treatment of infantile botulism, there does not appear to be any difference in outcome using these measures compared with supportive treatment (parenteral or nasogastric feedings, ventilatory support).

The number of identifiable and treatable inborn errors of metabolism that can cause infantile hypotonia increases yearly. A partial listing of these disorders and their specific treatments is given in Table 3. Unfortunately, in many of these disorders,

TABLE 3. Treatable Inborn Errors of Metabolism Causing Infantile Hypotonia

Disorder	Treatment
Aminoacidopathies and organic acidurias	Elimination diets Vitamins (e.g., B_{12}, 1–3 mg/day IM; Biotin, 5–20 mg/day)
Nonketotic hyperglycinemia	Sodium benzoate, 125–250 mg/kg/day Diazepam, 1–3 mg/kg/day Choline, 1–4 g/day Folic acid, 2 mg/day
Glutaric aciduria, type I	Sodium benzoate, 125–250 mg/kg/day Lysine restriction diet Riboflavin, 200–300 mg/day Baclofen, 2 mg/kg/day
Hyperammonemia due to ornithine transcarbamylase deficiency	Sodium benzoate, 125–250 mg/kg/day
Carnitine deficiency	L-Carnitine, 100 mg/kg/day
Pyruvate carboxylase/ pyruvate dehydrogenase deficiency	Thiamine, 100–1000 mg/day
Mitochondrial myopathies (e.g., cytochrome *c* oxidase deficiency)	Riboflavin, 100 mg/day Coenzyme Q_{10}, 120 mg/day
Lactic acidosis due to mitochondrial disorders	Dichloroacetate, 100 mg/kg/day (limited availability) Sodium citrate, 2–3 mEq/kg/day
Neonatal adrenoleukodystrophy	?Oleic acid ?Plasma exchange ?Bone marrow transplant

the treatments are palliative and do not alter ultimate poor prognosis.

The parents or guardians of infants with progressive infantile spinal muscular atrophy, muscular dystrophy, and other progressive neuromuscular disorders (i.e., progressive cytochrome *c* oxidase deficiency, leukoencephalopathies) should be informed that these infants will invariably develop life-threatening respiratory and swallowing difficulties, necessitating gastrostomy tube placement and ventilatory support. Given the irreversible nature of these disorders, the appropriateness of such measures is often questioned by families and their treating pediatricians. Often, hospital ethics committees, lawyers, and the courts are called upon to assist in the decision to withhold these therapies. Psychologic support should be offered early to the families of such infants.

MUSCULAR DYSTROPHY AND RELATED MYOPATHIES

IRWIN M. SIEGEL, M.D.

Muscular dystrophy is the general term for a group of chronic diseases that have in common abiotrophy—that is, progressive degeneration of skeletal musculature—leading to atrophy and weakness, often contracture and deformity, and motor disability.

Recent investigation has identified the gene for Duchenne type muscular dystrophy (DMD) as well as Becker's muscular dystrophy at the XP21 locus of the short arm of the X chromosome. Its protein product (dystrophin) has been characterized. As of this writing, a variety of experimental techniques, including myoblast transfer and genetic engineering of cloned genes, are in progress. Chromosome localization of other myopathic genes, including those for Emery-Dreifus myopathy, myotonic dystrophy, facioscapulohumeral muscular dystrophy, and central core disease, has been achieved. It is hoped that specific therapies for these hereditary muscular dystrophies will be forthcoming. Meanwhile, we must establish an early diagnosis and initiate an energetic treatment program to obtain optimal function in children afflicted with muscular dystrophy, delaying disability until a cure is available.

GENERAL THERAPY

Management of the patient with a muscle disease should be aggressive and multidisciplinary. Treatment is best administered by a team that includes pediatric, neurologic, genetic, physiatric, and orthopedic consultants. Additionally, occupational therapists, physical therapists, and medical social workers or psychologists can assist the patient and the family. Speech and dietary therapy, as well as subspecialty consultation (for instance, gastrointestinal and cardiopulmonary care), provide a thorough approach to the problems of comprehensive management.

Medications

There is no effective drug treatment for muscular dystrophy, except in those myopathies that are due to the absence of a specific metabolite, for which replacement therapy will sometimes help (e.g., muscle carnitine deficiency), or in muscle disease secondary to endocrinopathy (e.g., hypothyroidism), in which appropriate therapy of the primary condition can alleviate the secondary myopathy.

Although the myotonia of dystrophia myotonica can be relieved by a variety of agents, the dystrophia (weakness) remains. Agents used are phenytoin (Dilantin, 100 mg two or three times a day) or quinine* (200 mg three times a day). Both procainamide and prednisolone, although mentioned in the literature, have undesirable side effects and are not suggested. Corticosteroids have resulted in at least temporary increase of strength in DMD. It has also been noted that a growth hormone inhibitor (mazindol) restrains weakness and contracture in this disease. Studies with these drugs are ongoing.

Cardiac

Cardiomyopathy is believed to be present in more than 80 per cent of patients with DMD; however, the child may not show clinical evidence of heart disease because his or her restricted activity serves to maintain a precarious status quo. In muscular dystrophy, four clinical pictures may reflect the presence of cardiomyopathy in both primary and secondary disease: (1) dilatation of the cardiac chambers, (2) cardiac conduction anomalies, (3) hypertrophy of the ventricular walls, and (4) minor clinical signs, including nonspecific anomalies as well as electrocardiographic and echocardiographic findings.

Treatment is along conventional lines, with the administration of cardiac glycosides, diuretics, calcium channel blockers or beta-blockers, or antiarrhythmic medications, as indicated.

Respiratory

Pneumonitis, secondary to decreased pulmonary function and poor respiratory toilet with aspiration, is frequently encountered in those in advanced stages of the muscular dystrophies; therefore, periodic evaluation to monitor restrictive pulmonary disease is an integral part of any treatment regimen.

*This use is not listed by manufacturer.

Reduction in chest compliance, secondary to progressive weakness of respiratory musculature, requires an ongoing program of pulmonary rehabilitation. This may include diaphragmatic breathing exercises, postural drainage, chest percussion, proper humidification, and training in the use of various respiratory aids. Vigorous treatment of upper respiratory infections requires pharyngeal suction and intermittent positive pressure breathing, as well as appropriate antibiotic therapy. Decreased respiratory function in DMD can result in cor pulmonale with cardiomyopathy and right heart failure. Diminished vital capacity secondary to a weakened chest bellows leads to a restrictive ventilatory defect.

Clinical findings include inability to cough, reduction in chest compliance, and weakness of the respiratory musculature. Chronic alveolar hypoventilation, sometimes seen as the pickwickian syndrome in obese, wheelchair-confined patients, has been reported. Sleep hypoxemia (REM-related) is not uncommon in advanced DMD.

Low-flow oxygen augmented by protriptyline (5 mg two or three times a day) has been effective in treating this condition. Mechanical ventilation of patients in the terminal stages of DMD can often be managed at home without a tracheostomy, utilizing apparatus such as the rocking bed, plastic-wrap ventilator, chest-abdomen cuirass respirator, and pneumobelt.

Dietary

Because obesity accelerates functional disability, nutrition should be carefully monitored throughout the course of muscular dystrophy but particularly after wheelchair confinement. A well-balanced, vitamin-supplemented diet of at least 2400 calories for an active child and 1200 calories for one who is confined to a wheelchair is suggested. Patients are encouraged to choose fruits and vegetables as alternatives to high-calorie snacks and high-fiber foods and fruit juices to aid in maintaining normal elimination. Only small amounts of dairy products are included because of their mucus-producing tendency.

Smooth muscle can be involved in DMD, leading to (1) pharyngeal weakness with aspiration; (2) gastric atony with distention and altered peristalsis; (3) decreased or uncoordinated esophageal movement with dilatation and delay at the esophagogastric junction; (4) colonic dilatation, pseudo-obstruction, or volvulus; (5) small-bowel obstruction, malabsorption, or ileus; and (6) hypocontractility of the gallbladder with an increased incidence of cholelithiasis. All of these conditions are treated in the conventional manner.

Wheelchair-bound patients tend to reduce their fluid intake and are often reluctant to ask for toileting assistance, retaining urine as long as possible. Such urinary stasis predisposes to infection. In addition to ensuring adequate fluid intake, one should recommend foods such as cereals, meat, poultry, and fish, as well as cranberry juice, which all lower urine pH because of their acid residues. If undernutrition is a problem, hyperalimentation utilizing a dietary additive containing low potassium and middle-chain triglycerides can supplement daily food intake.

Constipation can be due to inactivity, problems with gastrointestinal transit time or other dysfunction, decreased fiber and fluid intake (overuse of highly refined, low-fiber foods), poor toileting habits, hypokalemia, or bad meal patterning. Dietary measures rather than medications are preferred in the treatment of constipation.

When deglutition is difficult because of posterior pharyngeal and upper esophageal weakness, swallowing can be facilitated by instruction in proper positioning while eating, eating slowly, and sitting upright for a time after meals; one should also introduce soft foods into the patient's diet. Myotonic patients should avoid cold foods or fluids, which may cause pharyngeal myotonia.

Psychosocial

In addition to coping with the psychologic problems imposed by a progressively disabling disease, children with muscular dystrophy face the same problems of peer interaction, body image, family adjustment, and sexuality that all normal youngsters must resolve in the process of maturing. Supportive psychiatric intervention made available at times of psychosocial crises can avert critical emotional damage, and empathic counseling of both the patient and the family throughout the course of the illness is an important part of total management.

A higher incidence of mental retardation and decreased intellectual function has been noted in patients with DMD than in normal or other control groups. Verbal ability is affected more often than performance intelligence quotient. Lower intelligence does not protect against the development of psychiatric disorder in these patients. The psychosocial management of children with DMD (as well as their families) requires diagnostic procedures that quickly and accurately reflect primary disturbances. The Kinetic Family Drawing Test* is one such projective evaluation that has been used to assess the attitudes of DMD children and their normal siblings.

Whenever possible, it is desirable to keep children with muscular dystrophy in the mainstream in their regular neighborhood school. In the treatment of muscular dystrophy, the family is also the patient; group therapy has proved valuable in assisting parents and normal siblings by helping them to develop insight and to increase communication by sharing experiences.

The treating physician must offer intelligent and empathic advice, correlating definite therapy with an ongoing program of patient and parent counseling during the early diagnostic phase of treatment. Preventive psychiatry is useful, particularly during puberty. Attention paid to the psychosocial aspects of muscular dystrophy can add productive life to the years available to these patients.

MOTOR DISABILITY

Physical and Occupational Therapy

Because muscular activity enhances protein synthesis (the danger of rapid loss of strength because of inactivity in DMD is well documented), it is imperative that the patient with muscular dystrophy be kept as mobile as possible for as long as feasible. The physical therapist systematically assesses weakness, imbalance, and contracture and provides submaximal exercise, gait training, and contracture stretching. As the child grows, surface area increases by the square of each linear increment, and volume by its cube. This "scale effect" explains why a child with a condition limiting the ultimate muscle mass may eventually lose the ability to ambulate, even though the disease is arrested or only slowly progressive. Gradient measurement of strength and functional ability by the physical therapist aids in indicating appropriate times for contracture release and bracing.

The occupational therapist determines the patient's ability to attend to the tasks of daily living, assisting him or her through a variety of techniques and devices, such as lift and transfer equipment, clothing adaptations, and special mattresses. The occupational therapist also evaluates the patient's home environment, mobility status, problems with lifting, transfer, and toileting, nighttime management, and communication status. A sensitive, intelligent program of occupa-

*See J Am Phys Therap Assoc 60:293–298, 1980.

tional therapy anticipates when changes of function may occur, altering patient and parent expectations and programming accordingly.

Wheelchair Care

Wheelchair confinement is a critical incident, both physiologically and psychologically, in the life of a patient with muscular dystrophy. Special wheelchair adaptations—for example, balanced forearm orthoses facilitating the use of the hands for feeding, writing, and other utilitarian tasks—can be prescribed to increase both comfort and function. Electric wheelchairs are available for those patients with insufficient strength to manage the standard model. Use of the wheelchair can often enable the homebound, nonambulatory patient to again travel within the community.

ORTHOPEDIC MANAGEMENT

Orthopedic complications are found in most of the muscular dystrophies. Central core disease (one of the congenital myopathies) can present at birth with congenital dislocation of the hips. Neonatal dystrophia myotonica is frequently complicated by severe clubfeet. In addition to weakness and contracture, particularly of the heel cords, in children with dermatomyositis, subcutaneous or intramuscular calcification or both often develop. In DMD, lower extremity contracture progresses until talipes equinovarus and weakened pelvic balance, produced by hip flexion contracture, prohibit ambulation. Patients develop a stance and gait typified by hip flexion and abduction, increasing lumbar lordosis, and equinocavovarus. Eventually, patients can no longer maintain a line projected from their center of gravity behind the center of rotation of their hips, in front of the center of rotation of their knees, and within their base of support. Ambulation stops at this point.

Properly timed surgery and bracing have helped selected patients to continue standing and walking anywhere from 2 to 5 years, thus significantly delaying confinement to a wheelchair with its inevitable downhill course.

Surgical management should permit early postoperative mobilization, as even brief restraint can lead to rapid loss of strength. *Anesthesia must be closely monitored, with particular attention paid to preventing gastric dilatation or potassium overload, to ensuring adequate ventilation, and to avoiding the singular danger of malignant hyperthermia in this class of disease.*

For the patient experiencing increased difficulty with walking because of lower extremity contracture, percutaneous hip flexor, bipolar tensor fascia lata, and heel cord tenotomies, followed by extremity bracing, have proved effective in maintaining ambulation. Percutaneous tarsal medullostomy or osteoclasis with soft tissue release has been successful in treating late equinocavovarus with rigid bony deformity. Isolated forefoot adduction is corrected by percutaneous metatarsal osteotomy. Increased intracompartmental pressure in the calves, which accelerates muscle degradation, can be relieved by percutaneous fasciotomy. Postsurgical orthotic management employs molded plastic appliances that are considerably lighter than steel or aluminum braces, yet equally sturdy. In cases of facioscapulohumeral dystrophy in which shoulder weakness significantly interferes with upper extremity function, scapular stabilization has been performed.

Scoliosis

Because paraspinal weakness is symmetric, spinal curvature is unusual in the walking Duchenne dystrophic patient or in the child with limb-girdle dystrophy. Asymmetric muscle weakness, leading to scoliosis in the ambulatory patient, can occur in Becker's muscular dystrophy, sometimes in childhood dystrophia myotonica, and often in childhood facioscapulohumeral muscular dystrophy. These spinal curves, when severe and progressive, can be surgically stabilized.

In most patients with DMD, paralytic scoliosis develops as a complication of wheelchair confinement. A variety of external spinal containment systems, such as thoracic jackets or special wheelchair seating designed to keep the pelvis level and to shape and hold the spine in the upright extended position, can retard such deformity.

Spinal fusion has been successfully used to correct and stabilize scoliosis in heritable neurologic conditions such as spinal muscular atrophy, familial dysautonomia, Charcot-Marie-Tooth disease, and Friedreich's ataxia. Such surgery is also increasingly performed in properly selected wheelchair-confined Duchenne dystrophic patients with rapidly decompensating scoliosis.

Spine arthrodesis is usually indicated in a wheelchair-bound DMD patient with an unstable curvature of 35 to 40 degrees if his or her vital capacity falls within 35 to 40 per cent of predicted normal. With early surgery, these curves can often be corrected to near neutral. A variety of techniques are available, including compression-distraction instrumentation, L-rod segmental spinal stabilization, and anterior fusion. The preferred method depends on the nature of the individual case. Spinal stabilization eliminates discomfort, improves body image, frees the upper extremities from their supportive role for more functional use, enhances cardiorespiratory function, and facilitates transfer. With a progressive curve unresponsive to external containment, if respiratory parameters are adequate to survive surgery, spinal fusion can prove an excellent method of handling this otherwise serious complication of wheelchair constraint.

Fractures

Fractures in muscular dystrophy are most frequently seen in the long bones and are more common in patients who have fallen from wheelchairs than in braced patients still ambulating. Such fractures are usually only slightly displaced, and there is not much pain because there is little muscle spasm. They heal without complication in the expected time and should be treated with minimal splintage (mold and sling for humeral fractures, light walking casts for fractures of the femur), with the pediatrician encouraging continued independent function as long as possible.

SUMMARY

Treatment in muscular dystrophy should be prospective and aimed at maintaining maximal function so that patients can remain independent for as long as possible. Early diagnosis is important not only to enable genetic counseling concerning future pregnancy and screening of female siblings but also to stage physical therapy to delay muscle contracture. Surgery, when indicated, must anticipate realistic functional goals (transfer, standing, walking) and enable immediate postoperative mobilization. Bracing should be suitably provided and orthoses appropriately constructed to ensure maximal support with minimal weight. Spinal deformity must be prevented when feasible and appropriately treated when present. Maximal function in wheelchair-confined patients can be enhanced through the use of appliances that encourage proper sitting posture and utilize residual strength. Complications must be anticipated and vigorously treated. Attention must be paid to the psychic as well as the somatic aspects of these diseases.

Optimal treatment of the patient with muscular dystrophy should be multidisciplinary, aggressive, and conducted in an atmosphere of intelligent concern. This approach minimizes the frustrating aspects of these diseases while maximizing the benefits obtained through available care. In this manner, the quality of life for the patient with muscular dystrophy can be significantly enhanced and life expectancy extended.

MYASTHENIA GRAVIS

DAVID M. DAWSON, M.D.
and DAVID LACOMIS, M.D.

Myasthenia gravis (MG) begins before the age of 17 years in about 11 per cent of all cases; it is rare before age 10 years. The illness may be *acquired* (autoimmune) or *genetic* in origin.

ACQUIRED MYASTHENIA GRAVIS

Acquired MG includes *transient neonatal* MG and *juvenile* MG. Antibodies (Abs) to acetylcholine receptors (AChR) in muscle are believed to be present in both types; however, they are not always measurable. Abs to AChR cause a postsynaptic impairment in neuromuscular transmission, resulting in fatigue and weakness.

Transient Neonatal Myasthenia Gravis

In transient neonatal MG, the Abs originate in the affected mother and cross the placenta. Symptoms last days to weeks and occur in only 10 to 15 per cent of the infants of myasthenic mothers. The severity of the illness in the mother may not be correlated with the child's symptoms; therefore, mothers with only mild or moderate MG may have a severely affected child.

Treatment

Supportive Care. In transient neonatal and all other types of MG, supportive care is crucial. Airway protection and oxygenation must be maintained, and nutritional status must be maximized. Intubation, mechanical ventilation, and enteral feeding may be required. Good general nursing care, aimed especially toward preventing infection, is equally important.

Anticholinesterase Drugs (ACEDs). These agents are the mainstay of therapy, and they may be required for days to weeks. ACEDs should be started if bulbar or respiratory symptoms occur, as they do in about 80 per cent of cases. Neostigmine was introduced first and has been used successfully for diagnosis and treatment of MG in neonates. However, most clinicians now prefer pyridostigmine (Mestinon) for all forms of MG, partly because it has fewer muscarinic side effects. Intubated neonates can be given pyridostigmine either intramuscularly or slowly intravenously (Table 1). When symptoms are severe but oral feeding is possible, intramuscular pyridostigmine can be given 30 minutes prior to feedings. If oral medication can be tolerated, the syrup form of pyridostigmine is most convenient. It is best to start with lower doses and to increase the dose or frequency of dosing gradually while monitoring for muscarinic and nicotinic types of cholinergic toxicity. Muscarinic toxicity manifests itself by diarrhea, salivation, vomiting, lacrimation, and bradycardia. Atropine generally reverses these effects. Nicotinic side effects may occur later; they include weakness, fasiculations, and cramps.

Because of the transient nature of the disorder and the exogenous source of Abs, steroids and immunosuppresive agents are not indicated. However, exchange transfusions have been shown to be effective in several cases.

Juvenile Myasthenia Gravis

Juvenile MG generally begins after 1 year of age, with a mean age of onset of 8 years. The clinical characteristics are similar to those of the adult form.

Treatment

Anticholinesterase Drugs. ACEDS, usually oral pyridostigmine, are the first line of treatment (Table 1). They often result in good, although not total, control of symptoms. Generally, this is the only form of treatment for purely ocular weakness. The dose is titrated upward in order to control symptoms without causing significant toxicity. Few patients require more than 500 mg/day; many manage well on 180 mg/day. If there is bulbar weakness, a dose should be given just before meals. Dose effects generally last 3 to 4 hours. The timed-release preparation is often useful when given at bedtime. If patients cannot take oral medications (e.g., perioperatively) or if only swallowing function is impaired, parenteral pyridostigmine can be administered (slowly if given intravenously).

Edrophonium (Tensilon) is short-acting and is used primarily for the diagnosis of MG (Table 1). One fifth of the total dose is administered intravenously while heart rate and blood pressure are monitored. If there is no significant bradycardia or increase in respiratory secretions, the remainder of the dose is given either incrementally (in young children) or in one or two doses (in older children). Several clinical signs and symptoms, such as vital capacity and muscle strength and fatigability in several muscle groups, must be checked before and after edrophonium is given. The increase in strength occurs within 2 to 5 minutes and lasts about 30 minutes.

Steroid Therapy. If symptoms are disabling despite optimal pyridostigmine, prednisone is usually begun, preferably with alternate-day therapy (60 mg/m^2 or 2 mg/kg every other day given in the morning). Because their condition may worsen during the first week or so of treatment, patients starting steroid therapy should be hospitalized. Many patients will require potassium supplements and antacids or H_2 receptor blockers. If symptoms stabilize, prednisone may be slowly tapered over months but a maintenance dose may be required.

Thymectomy. The indications for thymectomy are somewhat controversial. Clearly, the procedure is indicated for all patients with a thymoma; but this is a very rare problem in childhood. Older studies recommended thymectomy only for severe MG that did not respond to optimal medical management. The current trend is toward earlier thymectomy,[1] either after treatment with ACEDs alone or after stabilization with other treatment modalities. Prospective, randomized trials have not been done, but retrospective data indicate that 60 to 70 per cent of adult myasthenics improve after thymectomy.

Thymectomy is best performed in centers that have demonstrated low morbidity from the procedure. In this setting, the morbidity from a successful, potentially curative thymectomy is lower than the morbidity from long-term steroid use. Optimally, all thymus and mediastinal fat are removed. Either a transsternal or a transcervical approach may be used. In order to control symptoms throughout the perioperative period, *plasmapheresis* is usually performed prior to surgery.

Myasthenic Crisis. This refers to severe weakness with bulbar and respiratory compromise occurring during the course of the disease. Myasthenic crisis is often difficult to separate from *cholinergic crisis* resulting from ACED toxicity. The presence of muscarinic side effects usually indicates toxicity, and an edrophonium test (Table 1) can also be

TABLE 1. Anticholinesterase Drugs Used for Diagnosis and Treatment of Myasthenia Gravis

Drug	Route	Availability	Dose in Infants	Dose in Children	Comment
Pyridostigmine (Mestinon)	IV, IM	5 mg/ml in 2-ml ampules	0.05–0.15 mg/kg up to q 3–4 hr	1.0–1.5 mg per dose q 3–4 hr	IV/IM dose is equivalent to 1/30 of p.o. dose
Pyridostigmine (Mestinon)	p.o.	12 mg/ml syrup; 60-mg tablet 180 mg sustained-release tablet	4–10 mg up to q 3–4 hr	30–45 mg q 3–8 hr	Each dose is typically effective for 3–4 hr Sustained-release tablets may be most useful at bedtime in adolescent patients
Neostigmine bromide (Prostigmin)	p.o.	15-mg tablet	1–2 mg up to q 2–4 hr	7.5–15 mg up to q 2–4 hr	IV/IM dose is 1/30 of p.o. dose
Edrophonium (Tensilon)	IV	10 mg/ml in 1-mg ampules	0.15–0.2 mg/kg total	0.2 mg/kg total; maximum, 10 mg	For diagnosis only. Give 1/5 total dose as test dose; if tolerated, give remainder incrementally. Monitor BP and heart rate. Atropine (0.01 mg/kg up to 0.4 mg) can block or reverse muscarinic effects.

Abbreviations: IV, intravenously; IM, intramuscularly; q, every; p.o., by mouth; BP, blood pressure.

helpful. The test dose (0.04 mg/kg) is given while monitoring muscarinic effects, strength in multiple muscle groups, and respiratory function. If there is improvement in all measures, the patient may be in myasthenic crisis and should benefit from higher doses of ACEDs. If there is worsening in any measure, overdose nicotinic effects may be present at some receptors (cholinergic crisis). However, in crisis situations, there is often a combination of myasthenic and cholinergic-induced weakness. Thus, the best solution is to discontinue ACEDs, institute supportive care, and begin plasmapheresis. Three to five exchanges are performed during the course of a week. Improvement occurs within a few days in most patients. Once the patient improves, other forms of medical treatment (including ACEDs and steroids) can be restarted; thymectomy can be considered.

Problems Associated with Treatment. *Pitfalls in the treatment of all forms of MG include administration of drugs that can exacerbate weakness. These include aminoglycosides, procainamide, quinidine, curare, succinylcholine, and possibly calcium channel blockers and beta-blockers.* Sedatives and narcotics may be dangerous if respiratory or bulbar symptoms are present. Infections should be managed aggressively. Other associated autoimmune disorders, such as hyperthyroidism and diabetes mellitus, should be sought and treated appropriately.

Finally, *immunosuppressive agents* such as azathioprine have not been well studied in children and are not recommended, although they are effective in long-term care of adults.

GENETIC MYASTHENIA GRAVIS

Genetic forms of MG are very rare and generally present at birth or during infancy as the clinical entity of *familial infantile (congenital) MG*. An affected relative is usually identified. Abs to AChR are absent, and the diagnosis is made by neurophysiologic or sophisticated ultrastructural techniques.[2] Numerous defects involving pre- and postsynaptic transmission of AChR are being identified. Some presynaptic defects involve abnormal AChR resynthesis or transport, or abnormal uptake of choline by the nerve terminal. These disorders are usually responsive to modest doses of ACEDs. Congenital end-plate acetylcholinesterase deficiency, however, is a postsynaptic defect that is refractory to ACEDs. Similarly, there is no known effective treatment for another postsynaptic disorder, the so-called slow channel syndrome. Corticosteroids or other immunomodulators are not helpful in treating genetic forms of MG.

REFERENCES

1. Adams C, Theodorescu D, Murphy EG, Shandling B: Thymectomy in juvenile myasthenia gravis. J Child Neurol 5:215–218, 1990.
2. Engel AG: Congenital myasthenic syndromes. J Child Neurol 3:233–246, 1988.

PERIODIC PARALYSIS

RICHARD T. MOXLEY III, M.D.
and ROBERT C. GRIGGS, M.D.

Recognition and accurate diagnosis are often the major challenges in the treatment of periodic paralysis. Most patients present before their 20th birthday—those in early childhood for paramyotonia and potassium-sensitive (hyperkalemic) periodic paralysis, and those in adolescence for hypokalemic periodic paralysis. When diagnosis is first considered, exclusion of other disorders associated with weakness and abnormal serum potassium (K^+) is necessary. Initial attacks require careful documentation before treatment is initiated. Provocative testing is needed in most patients both to establish the diagnosis and to assist in predicting responses to treatment. The recent definition of a gene defect in a family with potassium-sensitive periodic paralysis in the alpha subunit of the sodium channel (on chromosome 17) heralds an era of more specific diagnosis.

HYPOKALEMIC PERIODIC PARALYSIS

Acute Attacks

During paralytic episodes, potassium is invariably low. Unless the patient is unable to swallow or is vomiting, potassium should be administered orally. A preparation of potassium chloride (KCl) is usually indicated (typically 0.35 mEq/kg per dose as 25 per cent KCl) and may have to be repeated. Because oral KCl has an unpleasant taste, it is helpful to have the solution chilled and to have the patient drink chilled water both before and after dosing. This helps avoid inducing nausea and decreases the bitter taste of the preparation. During severe attacks, serum electrolytes and electrocardiogram (EKG) should be monitored at half-hour intervals until the attack resolves. The exact total dosage of potassium depends on the severity and duration of the attack and on the response to the initial dose.

If patients are unable to take oral potassium, intravenous KCl may be necessary. The diluent for such treatment is of concern because both 5 per cent glucose and physiologic saline cause a transient lowering of serum potassium. A concentration of at least 60 mEq/L of KCl must be used if either of these diluents is employed. *Because intravenous glucose increases insulin release and can acutely enhance insulin-mediated potassium uptake by body tissues, saline is usually the diluent of choice.* Intravenous treatment is reserved for severely affected patients and requires careful monitoring of electrolytes, EKG, respiratory function, strength, and urinary output. Intravenous KCl-containing solutions should be administered slowly.

Prevention of Attacks

The prophylactic administration of potassium salts is seldom successful in preventing attacks, even when given in large doses on a daily basis. Patients subject to frequent attacks should undergo a trial with agents to prevent attacks. Most patients respond to the carbonic anhydrase inhibitor acetazolamide with complete cessation of attacks. Treatment is usually effective within 24 to 48 hours, and attacks recur promptly after treatment is discontinued. The effective daily dosage is quite variable (2 to 20 mg/kg in divided doses) but is usually that which produces a metabolic acidosis, as indicated by an elevation of serum chloride and a depression of bicarbonate. In severe cases, it may be necessary to give acetazolamide at 6-hour intervals.

In some patients, acetazolamide may worsen the disorder. Potassium-sparing agents such as triamterene may be effective in these patients. Dietary management, including the avoidance of carbohydrate and sodium loads, may be effective. Occasionally, diet is the sole treatment; more often, however, it is useful as an adjunctive treatment.

Chronic acetazolamide treatment presents certain hazards, most notably the formation of renal calculi. Patients on acetazolamide should undergo periodic abdominal ultrasound studies and should maintain good hydration to ensure a high urine output. *Sulfonamides should not be prescribed concurrently because a sulfonamide nephropathy may be produced.* Frequent but less troublesome side effects include dysgeusia for carbonated beverages, paresthesias, mild anorexia, and osteomalacia.

Treatment and Prevention of Progressive Weakness

Patients with frequent attacks of all types of periodic paralysis may experience persistent interattack weakness. Acetazolamide prevents and improves such weakness in many patients. Those unresponsive to acetazolamide may respond to the chloruretic carbonic anhydrase inhibitor dichlorphenamide. The dose has to be individualized, and typically ranges from 25 to 50 mg two to three times daily in adults. Doses for children have not been established.

Thyrotoxic hypokalemic periodic paralysis rarely occurs in childhood, and its treatment is markedly different from that of other forms of hypokalemic periodic paralysis. Potassium administration is indicated for acute attacks, but acetazolamide markedly worsens patients. Treatment consists of management of underlying thyrotoxicosis. Propranolol is strikingly effective in preventing attacks, even while patients remain thyrotoxic and have hypokalemia.

POTASSIUM-SENSITIVE (HYPERKALEMIC) PERIODIC PARALYSIS

Acute Attacks

Hyperkalemic periodic paralysis is often a misnomer because the serum potassium may remain within the normal range during attacks. The disorder, therefore, is defined by the development of weakness with potassium loading. Acute attacks are often so mild that treatment is unnecessary. Oral carbohydrate administration in the form of sugar solutions is preferable to potassium-containing fruit juices and soft drinks. Attacks are seldom severe enough to require intravenous therapy. If a severe attack does occur, it will respond to standard measures used to treat hyperkalemia, that is, intravenous glucose, insulin, or sodium bicarbonate.

Prevention of Attacks

Many patients, particularly those with slight, infrequent attacks, do not require chronic treatment. Acetazolamide in a dose sufficient to produce a mild kaliopenia (usually 3 mg/kg two or three times a day) will prevent attacks and has the added benefit of ameliorating myotonia, which may be present in some patients manifesting primarily as stiffness. Side effects (particularly paresthesias) often limit patient acceptability. For this reason, thiazide diuretics are the agents of choice. Chlorothiazide (10 mg/kg in two divided doses daily) prevents attacks. Hypokalemia and weakness can develop in these patients, as in normal people, when they take thiazides. Thiazide dosage should be kept low enough to prevent this occurrence. The use of inhaled β-adrenergic agents such as albuterol (one or two puffs) has been found useful in alleviating attacks. Occasionally, patients with potassium-sensitive periodic paralysis have associated ventricular ectopy. β-adrenergic agents should not be used in such patients, and their care should be coordinated with a cardiologist. Interattack weakness can also develop in potassium-sensitive periodic paralysis. Because repeated attacks of weakness may contribute to persistent weakness, patients should be encouraged to take prophylactic medication.

NORMOKALEMIC PERIODIC PARALYSIS

There are only rare, well-documented cases of patients with so-called normokalemic periodic paralysis who have not been found to have features identical to those of hyperkalemic periodic paralysis. Treatment is similar in these cases.

PARAMYOTONIA CONGENITA

Myotonia, manifesting primarily as stiffness, is a more disabling feature of this disorder than the paralysis that is caused by cold exposure plus exercise. The myotonic stiffness is sometimes severe after sudden movements or a sudden fright. Occasionally, patients with paramyotonia congenita have periodic attacks of weakness associated with hyperkalemia. This periodic weakness occurs primarily in the morning and is usually mild to moderate in severity. The myotonic stiffness and the paralysis caused by cold exposure plus exercise can be abolished by treatment with mexilitene, a drug similar in structure to lidocaine, which is frequently used to control cardiac arrhythmias. Usually, mexilitene (150 to 200 mg two to three times daily) controls these symptoms. Gastrointestinal complaints and light-headedness are the most common side effects, and they decrease or vanish when the medication dose is lowered. Simple maneuvers such as avoiding exposure to cold are often sufficient treatment for mild cases of paramyotonia congenita.

Those cases involving paramyotonia congenita with hyperkalemic periodic paralysis usually require a combination of the therapeutic agents to control both disorders. Mexilitene controls the stiffness and cold-induced weakness. Thiazide diuretics are necessary to control the attacks of hyperkalemic periodic weakness. Acetazolamide is not recommended for treatment in this circumstance. Some patients have experienced attacks of quadriplegia after acetazolamide therapy.

INFLAMMATORY MYOPATHIES

OWEN B. EVANS, M.D.

The inflammatory myopathies are the most frequent cause of acquired muscle disease and can be classified into three groups: dermatomyositis, polymyositis, and inclusion-body myositis. *Eighty per cent of children with dermatomyositis respond to therapy. Similar therapies are used in the treatment of polymyositis, although the response is less predictable. There is no effective therapy for inclusion-body myositis.*

STEROID THERAPY

It is generally agreed that steroids are effective in ameliorating the signs and symptoms of dermatomyositis. The starting dose is 2 to 3 mg/kg/day of prednisone in two divided doses. Within days the fever usually remits, and within a week the serum enzyme concentrations are reduced. After about 2 weeks, there is improved strength. At this point, the steroid dose can be changed to alternate-day therapy to reduce adrenal suppression by tapering the alternate daily dose over 1 week. Some recommend continued daily therapy to achieve maximal effectiveness. The total daily dose can be reduced by 10 mg/week until 50 mg/day is reached and then can be reduced by 5 mg/week until a maintenance dose of 10 to 20 mg/day is achieved.

During the initial period, the child should be observed frequently to monitor strength and the serum enzymes. If there is clinical deterioration or a rise in serum enzymes, the dose of prednisone should be increased to 2 mg/kg/day and tapered more slowly. The typical treatment period is 2 years for those who respond to steroids. If the drug is discontinued too soon, there may be relapses and the long-term prognosis may be worse.

Complications of steroid therapy are potentially serious but are usually well tolerated. Cushingoid appearance and temporary growth delay are common. Hypertension, hyperglycemia, cataracts, and increased susceptibility to infections are uncommon in my experience. Because severe, potentially fatal varicella may occur in a susceptible child on steroids, varicella exposure should be avoided in a child who has not had this disease; zoster immune globulin should be administered if exposure occurs. Osteoporosis is occasionally encountered, and vertebral compression fractures can occur. One pitfall of high-dose steroid therapy is a superimposed steroid myopathy that may obscure the clinical signs of the underlying disease.

CYTOTOXIC DRUGS

Problems arise in the child who does not respond to steroids or who requires such large doses of steroids that intolerable side effects emerge. The use of cytotoxic drugs has been found to be beneficial in some patients as an adjunct to steroids. Methotrexate (1 to 2 mg/kg/week either orally or IM; maximum, 25 mg) can be given with regular monitoring of liver functions and complete blood counts. The prednisone can be tapered by 5 mg/week until a maintenance dose is achieved with minimal side effects. Azathioprine (Imuran, 2 mg/kg/day) can also be used in a similar fashion. Patients who are clearly deteriorating despite maximal doses of steroids and cytotoxic therapy pose special problems. Plasmapheresis, total body irradiation, and intravenous immunoglobulins have been efficacious in a few selected patients.

The typical rash does not improve as rapidly as the muscle weakness. Normally, no specific therapy is needed, and steroid application is of no benefit. Patients should use sunscreens generously because the rash is photosensitive. Calcinosis is a severe complication and can practically encrust the patient when extensive. Systemic steroids may reduce the subcutaneous deposits; however, neither steroids nor chelation has been effective in my experience. A serious complication is secondary bacterial infections of ulcerative vasculitic lesions or areas where calcium deposits have protruded through the skin. Vigorous antibiotic therapy and wound care may be necessary to prevent local or systemic spread of such infection.

Physical therapy must be instituted early in the course of the illness to help prevent contractures and to maintain mobility. Patients who have a chronic, unremitting course are in need of rehabilitation services to provide occupational therapy and orthopedic appliances to maintain mobility and independent function.

15

Skin

SKIN DISORDERS OF THE NEONATE

JOAN E. HODGMAN, M.D.

CARE OF THE NORMAL SKIN

The normal skin of the neonate needs no special care. Cleansing should be gentle, with warm water alone or with mild nonmedicated soap followed by thorough rinsing. The newborn skin is hyperkeratotic, presumably because the immersion of the fetus in amniotic fluid has prevented shedding of the outermost layers. Peeling of this thick keratotic layer is a normal phenomenon that starts within the first day or two after birth in the term infant.

In the postmature infant, the process is accentuated and peeling may be present at birth. Creams or other emollients designed to treat this "dry" skin are contraindicated, as they contribute to maceration and enhance bacterial growth. Note that the skin's protective function is primarily limited to the outermost layer, the stratum corneum. Injury or maceration of the stratum corneum destroys this barrier and provides a portal of entry for pathogenic organisms and toxic chemicals. Many common practices in the nursery encourage maceration, such as exposure to warm, humid environments in incubators, occlusive dressings, and prolonged contact with a plastic mattress. Adhesive tape effectively peels the stratum corneum and should be used sparingly. The common practice of covering puncture wounds with adhesive tape strips has no justification except for hemostasis.

Initial Bath

The function of the initial bath is primarily aesthetic—that is, to remove blood and secretions acquired during birth. The initial bath must be postponed until the infant's temperature is stable, and care must be taken to avoid cooling the infant during the bathing. *Vernix should not be vigorously removed, as it probably provides a protective covering and disappears naturally over time.*

Chlorhexidine gluconate in 4 per cent solution is used for the initial bath after the infant's temperature is stable in many centers, including our own, to decrease colonization by staphylococcal bacteria. The active agent is bactericidal on contact and binds with skin protein, leaving an active residue. Daily baths with this compound are not necessary but may be instituted temporarily during outbreaks of staphylococcal infection. We recommend bathing infants in the neonatal intensive care unit with chlorhexidine weekly. The primary source for colonization by pathogenic bacteria is the hands of nursery personnel. Meticulous hand washing using soaps or detergents containing antibacterial preparations needs to be rigorously enforced for all individuals in contact with infants.

Umbilical Cord

The umbilical cord should be carefully cleaned, as it becomes colonized early. The application of triple dye has been effective in our nursery, but alcohol and antibacterial ointments have also been recommended.

Pre-term Skin

Care of the skin in a premature infant does not differ essentially from that in a term infant. The skin of the premature infant is more fragile and more permeable than that of the mature infant; consequently, greater care is necessary to prevent injury and absorption of chemicals.

TRAUMA

Ecchymoses and Petechiae

Ecchymoses and petechiae, which are regularly found over the infant's presenting part, resolve spontaneously and should not cause concern. In difficult deliveries, hemorrhage and erosions may be present as well. No special therapy is needed for erosions or hemorrhage, but the lesions should be kept clean and dry.

Caput Succedaneum

Caput succedaneum is an edematous swelling resulting from pressure changes over the infant's presenting part. It usually occurs on the vertex but may involve the genitalia in breech deliveries. Even when edema may be alarming, it decreases markedly in the first 24 hours following birth and treatment is unnecessary. The use of vacuum extraction for delivery may accentuate the findings. *An exaggerated caput that has not regressed in 24 hours is reported as a precursor to neonatal herpes infection.*

Cephalohematoma

Cephalohematoma is a swelling beneath the scalp resulting from subperiosteal hemorrhage over one of the bones of the skull, most commonly the parietal. The swelling is limited by the suture lines, and it increases in size during the first few days as a result of absorption of fluid. The condition is benign, and aspiration is contraindicated because of the risk of introducing infection. The breakdown and reabsorption of hemoglobin increases the likelihood of jaundice in the first days of life.

Hemorrhage

Hemorrhage below the galea but outside the skull has been erroneously referred to as a giant cephalohematoma; however, it carries a more serious prognosis. Without the constraint of the periosteum, hemorrhage in this area may be large enough to induce cardiac failure from hypovolemia and to require urgent replacement transfusion or exchange transfusion.

Pressure Necrosis

Pressure necrosis is seen following prolonged labor and delivery, especially in large infants. The most common sites are the parietal bosses of the skull and the zygoma. With improved control of the pregnant diabetic and with the practice of cesarean section for large infants, the incidence of pressure necrosis has markedly decreased. The lesions are sterile until rupture of the skin occurs. Exudate should be obtained for stain and culture to determine pathogenic organisms. The presence of normal skin flora is not an indication for antibiotic treatment. The lesions are indolent and heal slowly. Saline compresses may be useful early to aid in débridement, but then the lesions should be kept clean and dry. Infants may be safely discharged from the nursery during the healing process. Scarring is minimal, even with facial lesions.

Iatrogenic Injury

Iatrogenic injury to the skin is common during perinatal care. Invasive intrauterine diagnostic procedures, such as amniocentesis, may result in injury to the fetus. Small lacerations or scars from puncture sites are the usual findings, although more serious injury may infrequently be found. With internal fetal monitoring, pressure necrosis of the scalp at the site of monitor placement is a common finding. The resulting sterile abscess must be differentiated from infection and treated expectantly. Wet compresses for débridement and drainage may be useful, but antibiotics are not indicated.

Lacerations may occur during incision of the uterus for cesarean section. These usually involve the scalp but may occur over any body part that underlies the incision site. Fortunately, the lesions heal rapidly with minimal scarring.

Intensive care of the newborn infant involves extensive monitoring of vital signs. Most of the monitors require fixation to the skin, with consequent disruption of the stratum corneum. Heated sensors for determination of transcutaneous gases may leave small first- or second-degree burns. Scarring and depigmentation may result. The problem may be particularly troubling in immature black infants, who make up a disproportionate number of infants needing intensive care. Heel sticks used to obtain blood specimens may introduce infection unless careful attention is paid to aseptic technique.

Necrotic Lesions

Necrotic lesions of no clear etiology are occasionally present at birth. These occur most often on the lower extremity and involve the skin and the underlying tissues. They are asymmetric and display various stages of healing. The degree of scarring depends on the extent of the lesion. Necrotic lesions appear to be the result of local vascular accidents in utero.

SKIN DISORDERS

Cutis Aplasia

Cutis aplasia is an uncommon congenital defect that consists of localized absence of the dermis and epidermis. Inheritance is uncertain, but familial cases suggest an autosomal mode. Differentiation from injury at birth is important. Lesions, which may be single or multiple, are most common on the vertex of the scalp. Defects in the skull, which heal spontaneously within the first 6 months of life, are frequently present beneath the scalp defects. When lesions appear on the trunk or legs, they are bilateral and symmetric. Lesions heal by developing a smooth atrophic scar devoid of appendageal structures. Cosmetic surgery to improve the appearance of the scar is rarely necessary.

Transient Skin Lesions

Milia

Milia occur in term infants as superficial white epidermal inclusions of 1 to 2 mm, usually limited to the face. They exfoliate upon normal peeling, and no treatment is required.

Mongolian Spots

Mongolian spots are flat, poorly circumscribed, brown to slate-blue, large macular lesions present at birth. They are most commonly found over the lower sacrum and buttocks but may have a more general distribution over the back and extensor surfaces of the extremities. Mongolian spots occur most frequently in infants of dark-skinned races. They tend to disappear with age, and no treatment is needed.

Sebaceous Hypertrophy

Sebaceous hypertrophy occurs primarily in the glands over the nose, which enlarge in response to hormonal changes at birth. The sebum is usually white but becomes yellow-stained if the infant becomes jaundiced. They are benign and regress spontaneously. A rare exaggeration of this process has been called "acne of the newborn."

Miliaria Crystallina

Miliaria crystallina (sudamina) is the sweat rash seen in mature newborn infants. The lesions are small, superficial vesicles containing a clear fluid. They are the result of increased sweat production under humid conditions in which hygroscopic swelling of the stratum corneum obstructs the follicular outlets. The condition is best treated by decreasing the temperature and humidity of the infant's environment.

Sucking Blisters

Sucking blisters may be noted at birth over the dorsum of the hand and on the fingers. The lesions occur in large, active infants and occasionally are hemorrhagic. They are harmless but must be differentiated from congenital blistering disorders, such as epidermolysis bullosa.

Toxic Erythema

Toxic erythema of the newborn is a benign, self-limited condition of healthy infants during the first week of life. It is related to maturity, being uncommon in the preterm infant but occurring in 50 per cent of term infants. The lesions usually appear during the first 48 hours but, rarely, may be present at birth. Sites of predilection are the chest, buttocks, shoulders, and proximal extremities. The central area of the face, the scalp, and the palms and soles are spared. The initial lesion is a blotchy erythematous macule with a central small papulovesicle. Well-developed lesions may appear pustular. The vesicles contain eosinophils that can be demonstrated by smear. The cause of toxic erythema of the newborn is unknown; there is no indication of allergy, and treatment is unnecessary. The lesions, which are superficial, dry and peel upon normal exfoliation of the newborn skin.

Transient Neonatal Pustular Melanosis

Transient neonatal pustular melanosis is invariably present at birth and is limited to healthy dark-skinned infants. The condition appears in infants of Mexican extraction as well as in black newborns. Three characteristic types of lesion are present simultaneously: (1) small pustules on a narrow erythematous or nonerythematous base; (2) dried pustules identifiable by their collar of scale; and (3) pigmented macules. Smears indicate polymorphonuclear leukocytes and debris, and cultures are negative. As with toxic erythema, the etiology is unknown.

No treatment is necessary, and isolation of the infant is not required. The pigmented macules may persist for several months but eventually fade.

Nevi

Vascular Nevi

Vascular nevi are among the most common lesions seen in the newborn. The nevus simplex, or salmon patch, occurs on the nape in at least 40 per cent of infants and has been called the "stork bite" because of its ubiquity. The same flat capillary nevi may be seen on the face above the eyebrows, on the upper eyelids, around the alae nasi, and on the upper lip. The facial lesions always regress spontaneously. Approximately 10 per cent of lesions on the nape of the neck are reported to persist into adulthood.

Nevus Flammeus

The nevus flammeus (port-wine stain) is also a flat capillary nevus but the prognosis is more ominous. These lesions do not regress and are frequently associated with hemangiomas in the underlying structures. The association of nevus flammeus in the region of the first branch of the trigeminal nerve with cortical lesions in the brain is known as the *Sturge-Weber syndrome.* Diagnostic ultrasonographic examination should be performed before discharge from the nursery. Ocular involvement may result in childhood glaucoma. The skin lesions can be obliterated with pulse-dye laser therapy. Treatment, which may necessitate several stages, should be started in early infancy so that it may be completed before school entrance.

Capillary Nevus

The raised capillary nevus, or *strawberry mark,* is never seen at birth; rather, it appears during the neonatal period. The earliest manifestation is the appearance of a small depigmented area centered by dilated capillaries that enlarge rapidly to form the characteristic tumor. These lesions ultimately regress, and benign neglect is the most satisfactory therapeutic plan for most established tumors. When the location of the hemangioma presents a problem, destruction by argon laser is recommended. If the lesion is detected in its earliest stage, it can be completely ablated by laser with excellent cosmetic results.

Cavernous Hemangioma

Eighty per cent of cavernous hemangiomas also regress during the first few years and should be watched expectantly. Steroids have accelerated the regression of these tumors but should be tried early when the tumor is large or in a hazardous location. Oral prednisone (2 to 3 mg/kg per 24 hours) should be given for a 4-week period, followed by a tapered dosage during the next 2 weeks. If rebound occurs following initial involution, a second or third course of steroids may be instituted.

A small number of cavernous hemangiomas are associated with significant complications that may be life-threatening. These vary from sepsis in the infant with large venous lakes to heart failure in the infant with arteriovenous anastomoses. Hypertrophy of the underlying structures may occur, especially when the tumor involves an extremity *(Klippel-Trénaunay syndrome).* Hemorrhage from trapping of platelets within the hemangioma may appear early in infancy *(Kasabach-Merritt syndrome).* In lesions that do not respond to steroids, a combined approach using laser and other ablative techniques under the direction of a plastic surgeon is recommended.

Nevus Sebaceus

Nevus sebaceus consists of skin-colored, hairless plaques with a surface texture like that of an orange peel. They occur most commonly at the hairline and are also seen on the face and ear. They can safely be watched during childhood but may develop basal cell carcinomas after adolescence.

Pigmented Nevi

Pigmented nevi in the newborn are considered to pose an increased risk for malignant change, but the actual risk for small lesions is not well defined. Careful notation of the size and location of the lesions is essential so that changes can be detected during follow-up. A pictorial record is recommended. Large pigmented nevi, which may cover major portions of the trunk and buttocks and are accompanied by satellite lesions in other locations, pose a serious health risk for the affected infant. Development of melanoma within these nevi is a common complication.

Treatment is directed toward removal of the extensive lesions. With new techniques of tissue expansion and tissue culture, staged excision of these extensive lesions is achievable.

Infections (Table 1)

Listerial Infection

Listeria monocytogenes is the only bacterial infection that may result in pustules present at the time of birth. Transmission of infection is transplacental following bacteremia in the mother. The lesions appear over the trunk and extremities as discrete, dull-red macules with central pustulation. Diagnosis is made by smear and culture of the lesions and by culture of the mother's and infant's blood. Parenteral antibiotics are

TABLE 1. Treatment for Skin Infections in the Neonate

Drug	Indication	Route	Dose
Acyclovir	Neonatal herpes	IV	30 mg/kg/24 hr in 3 divided doses × 10–14 days
Penicillin			
Aqueous	Congenital syphilis	IM or IV	50,000 units/kg/24 hr in 2 divided doses × 10 days
Procaine	Congenital syphilis	IM	50,000 units/kg/24 hr daily × 10 days
Ampicillin	Neonatal listerial infection	IM or IV	50–75 mg/kg/24 hr in 2–3 divided doses
Methicillin	Neonatal staphylococcal infection	IM or IV	50–100 mg/kg/24 hr in 2–3 divided doses
Vancomycin	Neonatal staphylococcal infection	p.o. or IV	30–45 mg/kg/24 hr in 2 or 3 divided doses
Prednisone	Cavernous hemangioma	p.o.	2–3 mg/kg per 24 hr once daily × 4 weeks

indicated, and ampicillin (50 to 75 mg/kg every 12 hours) is the antibiotic of choice.

Congenital Syphilis

Congenital syphilis manifests itself at birth as a bullous dermatitis involving the palms and soles. Diagnosis is made by demonstrating spirochetes in the bullous fluid or by serologic tests of mother and infant. The lesions are infectious until treatment is started. The drug of choice is penicillin (50,000 units/kg either aqueous in divided doses every 12 hours IM or IV, or procaine IM daily for 10 days).

Herpes

Herpes simplex virus infection may present with vesicles at birth or during the first days of life. The skin lesions may be associated with encephalitis or disseminated infection. The vesicles consist of groups of tense, roughly circular "pox" lesions that are most frequently seen on the face and scalp but that may occur over any part of the body. In the term infant, the lesions may be limited to two or three vesicles; in the preterm infant, extensive vesicles may coalesce into bullae. Occasionally, the lesions follow a zosteriform distribution. Diagnosis is confirmed by examination of scrapings from the base of a vesicle and by culture of vesicular fluid.

Parenteral antiviral therapy is indicated no matter how benign the local lesions appear because of the danger of systemic involvement. Although both adenine arabinoside and acyclovir are effective, acyclovir (30 mg/kg/day IV divided into three doses for at least 10 to 14 days) is the treatment of choice because it requires less intravenous fluid for administration and is less toxic. Recurrent crops of skin lesions can be expected to appear during the first several months.

Pyogenic Skin Infection

Pyogenic skin infections are most frequently caused by staphylococci but may also be due to the beta-streptococcus. The most common manifestation is small, grouped, superficial pustules surrounded by narrow erythematous zones, although occasionally the lesions appear as superficial bullae. The most common sites are periumbilical and genital. Involvement of deeper structures results in subcutaneous abcesses and paronychia.

Even though the infant rarely shows systemic symptoms, systemic antibiotics should be given. The newborn localizes infection poorly, and superficial infection may progress to sepsis and osteomyelitis. The initial choice of drug depends on the antibiotic sensitivity pattern of recent nursery infections. Until sensitivities are available, it is prudent to assume that staphylococci will be penicillin-resistant. Methicillin (50 to 100 mg/kg per 24 hours in two or three divided doses) or vancomycin (30 to 45 mg/kg per 24 hours in two or three divided doses) may be given, depending on the maturity and postnatal age of the infant.

"Scalded Skin" Syndrome

A toxin produced by a particular strain of *Staphylococcus* may be responsible for a more generalized bullous eruption, the *scalded skin syndrome.* In addition to parenteral antibiotics, infants with this latter condition require careful attention to fluid and protein intake because of potential large losses due to exudation from the lesions.

DIAPER DERMATITIS

SHARON S. RAIMER, M.D.
and BEN G. RAIMER, M.D.

Countless phone calls and office visits to physicians are made each year seeking guidance in the treatment of diaper dermatitis. This problem is undoubtedly best addressed in a preventive manner by providing instructions to new parents during the neonatal period regarding proper perineal hygiene for their infant—a task easily handled by a health care extender. Hands-on demonstrations for bathing, cord care, and diapering are encouraged. Also, the American Academy of Pediatrics provides a publication for distribution to parents on perineal care and diaper rash.

A suitable protocol for the prevention of diaper dermatitis should include the following:

1. Gently cleanse the skin of the perineal area, particularly after a bowel movement, using a mild soap such as Dove. Stool, especially diarrhea stool, is irritating to infant skin.
2. Choose diapers (cloth or disposable—parent's choice) that are absorbent, fit snugly, and *permit no plastic to touch the infant's skin.*
3. Change diapers frequently (soon after soiled); check frequently.
4. Use "overnight" diapers, add extra-absorbent pads, or awaken and change infant every 4 to 6 hours at night (after usual feedings is probably most sensible).
5. Use "diaper wipes" sparingly; after they are used, alternate with plain soap and water washes.
6. Keep the infant's room from becoming too warm; avoid excessive humidity.
7. Soak and wash cloth diapers thoroughly; avoid fabric softeners and/or harsh detergents.
8. Avoid use of dusting powders.

General instructions for parents when diaper dermatitis does appear should state:

1. Wash the area with mild soap (e.g., Dove) and water.
2. Pat the area dry with a soft towel, or blow dry using hair dryer on low heat.
3. Leave area uncovered when possible (no diaper); for example, when the infant is napping, place diaper under the infant.

SPECIFIC CONDITIONS

Chafing and Irritant Dermatitis

Mild chafing and irritation frequently resolve with an application of an ointment such as white petrolatum (Vaseline) or zinc oxide. Chafing may be prominent at the edge of the diapers, which results from the rubbing of the diapers on damp skin, but should respond to emollients.

Candidal Dermatitis

Candida in the diaper area generally responds to topical agents such as the imidazoles (e.g., clotrimazole [Lotrimin, Mycelex] or miconazole [Micatin], which are now over-the-counter agents) and nystatin cream (applied lightly two to three times a day).

More rapid response can be obtained by applying an anti-inflammatory agent, preferably 1 per cent hydrocortisone cream, directly over the anticandidal cream or by mixing them in equal proportions before application. Mycolog is not an ideal preparation for diaper dermatitis because it contains triamcinolone, a mid-strength topical steroid. Triamcinolone may cause local atrophy of skin and, more important, adrenal suppression, as it is readily absorbed through inflamed skin and absorption is enhanced by the occlusive effects of a diaper. If Mycolog is used, parents should be advised to limit the period of application to less than 2 weeks. Mycolog II, which contains no neomycin, a potent topical sensitizer, is preferable to Mycolog. Lotrisone contains the potent topical steroid betamethasone diproprionate (Diprosone) and should be avoided altogether in the diaper area.

If the eruption fails to respond to topical agents or if thrush is present, oral nystatin should be prescribed. Also, the breasts of nursing mothers should be treated with topical agents when *Candida* is present in the infant. Recalcitrant candidal infections suggest possible immunosuppression.

Seborrheic and Atopic Dermatitis

Seborrheic dermatitis is very common in infants 3 months of age and younger. It frequently presents as cradle cap (scaling behind the ears) and an eruption in intertriginous areas, particularly the groin. Atopic dermatitis is more common in infants 3 months of age and older and less consistently involves the diaper area.

Both types of dermatitis generally respond to 1 per cent hydrocortisone cream. Dermatitis in the diaper area is frequently secondarily infected with *Candida,* in which case the application of an anticandidal cream, as suggested previously, promotes resolution of the dermatitis.

Psoriasis

Psoriasis in infants may present as a well-demarcated plaque or plaques in the groin that are recalcitrant to treatment. Although dramatic in appearance, the eruptions appear to be relatively asymptomatic unless secondarily infected with *Candida* or bacteria.

Treatment with potent topical steroids should not be used in the diaper area, as they are readily absorbed. Application of 1 per cent hydrocortisone cream or ointment when the disease is flaring usually results in moderate improvement. Treatment for secondary infection with *Candida* or bacteria should be given when appropriate. Protecting the eruption from the irritation of stools by applying an ointment such as zinc oxide may be helpful. Moderate sunlight exposure, taking care not to allow sunburn of the infant, is frequently beneficial. The eruption generally clears when the infant is out of diapers and dry for a majority of the day.

Bacterial Infections

Bullous impetigo is not rare in the diaper area. Because the bullae rupture readily in this area, the impetigo clinically presents as annular scaling plaques that are slightly oozy near the margin. Limited involvement will generally respond to the topical antibiotic mupirocin (Bactroban). Extensive infections and infections in very young infants are more appropriately treated with systemic antibiotics.

Persistent erythema and tenderness in the perianal area suggest a *streptococcal infection.* The diagnosis can generally be confirmed by obtaining a specimen from the moist skin in the area for culture. Treatment is with an appropriate systemic antibiotic.

Congenital syphilis, currently on the rise, may present with condylomata lata or annular scaling lesions in the groin area. Treatment is with aqueous crystalline penicillin G or procaine penicillin G (50,000 units/kg daily for 10 days).

Dermatophyte Infections

Tinea is uncommon in the diaper area of infants but should be considered in a groin eruption that has a well-demarcated border. Dermatophyte infections generally respond to most available topical antifungal agents. Naftifine (Naftin) is currently the only topical antifungal agent that is fungicidal rather than fungistatic.

Viral Infections

Condyloma acuminatum and *molluscum contagiosum* infections occasionally occur in the diaper area of infants. Infections most frequently appear to be acquired from routine care and handling of the infant or from maternal exposure at birth, but the possibility of child abuse should be considered. Sexual abuse should strongly be considered if herpes simplex virus infection occurs in the groin of an infant. Treatment of these infections is discussed in the articles on the specific disease entities.

Cytomegalovirus may present as an eroded diaper dermatitis in an immunosupressed infant. Treatment with ganciclovir may possibly be of benefit.

Granuloma Gluteale Infantum

Granuloma gluteale infantum starts as an inflammation in the diaper area that is treated with potent topical steroids. A variable number of reddish-brown nodules develop on the inner thigh and perineal area. The topical steroids should be discontinued, and the lesions will resolve spontaneously over a period of a few months.

Recalcitrant Diaper Dermatitis

Recalcitrant dermatitis from a number of noninfectious causes frequently respond to a mixture of hydrocortisone powder (to a concentration of 1 per cent) and nystatin (15 g) in 60 g of zinc oxide ointment. Other diagnoses not discussed, such as Letterer-Siwe disease and acrodermatitis enteropathica, also should be considered when the diaper dermatitis is recalcitrant.

ALLERGIC CONTACT DERMATITIS

SUSAN BAYLISS MALLORY, M.D.

Allergic contact dermatitis (ACD) is a form of eczematous dermatitis in which a chemical agent, such as a plant, medicine, cosmetic, fabric, or metal, is the local inciting factor. The configuration of skin lesions, as well as the site involved, may give clues to the causal agent. Patch testing may confirm the diagnosis but is usually not necessary in the more common causes of ACD, such as poison ivy.

TREATMENT

Treatment can be divided into two major categories: prevention and management.

Prevention

Avoidance of the provocative allergen is necessary in curing contact dermatitis. Cross-reacting allergens should also be avoided. A detailed history may be needed to find the offending agent. Patients should understand that they may become allergic to a substance or chemical at any time after initial exposure and that it actually takes time to become sensitized to a certain agent.

Hyposensitization to poison ivy is not practical routinely and is not recommended. Side effects, such as vesicular or urticarial eruptions and pruritus ani, occur in the majority of patients, and complete desensitization is not accomplished.

Barrier creams, such as polyamine salts of a linoleic acid dimer, can be used as topical prophylaxis if applied prior to exposure. This type of agent is available as Stokogard-Gard Outdoor Cream* and must be washed off within 8 hours.

Management

The pruritus and oozing of acute ACD may be treated with compresses for débridement and a cooling effect. Simple baths or wet wraps with tap water are satisfactory. Burow's solution (aluminum sulfate and calcium acetate; Domeboro) can be added for a drying effect. Towels or bandages should be moist but not dripping; they should be left in place for 15 minutes to 1 hour but not allowed to dry. This procedure can be repeated as many times as needed. Plain calamine lotion also has a drying effect.

When the acute weeping eruption subsides or if the dermatitis is mild, potent topical steroid creams, lotions, or ointments can help reduce inflammation. Weaker topical steroids, in classes 6 and 7, have little effect on significant ACD. Potent topical steroids are more effective (i.e., Diprolene, Lidex, Temovate) and are recommended except on the face, groin, and axillae. In these areas, hydrocortisone 1 per cent is adequate. Caution should be given to the adult-sized patient if he or she is using more than 45 g/week of a potent steroid because suppression of the pituitary-adrenal axis may occur.

Systemic administration of corticosteroids may be indicated in severe or very extensive dermatitis (oral prednisone, beginning at 1 mg/kg/day and tapering slowly over 2 to 3 weeks). Intramuscular triamcinolone has a prolonged effect and is erratically absorbed and is therefore not recommended. Oral dose packs of steroids (e.g., Medrol Dosepak) usually last 6 days; however, in ACD, lesions can continue to form up to 2 to 3 weeks after a single exposure. Therefore, oral steroids should be given for a 2- to 3-week period.

The administration of an oral antihistamine, such as hydroxyzine or diphenhydramine, may decrease pruritus mainly because of its soporific effect and may therefore be most useful at bedtime. Topical anti-itching preparations, such as benzocaine or diphenhydramine (Benadryl), are of only temporary benefit and may be potential sensitizers. Therefore, these preparations are not recommended.

The most common contact allergens in childhood differ from country to country. In the United States, poison ivy, neomycin, nickel, rubber chemicals, formaldehyde, balsam of Peru, and benzocaine are the most common contact allergens. Neomycin is found in otic preparations, topical antibiotic creams, and some prescription combination topical medications. Nickel can be found in earrings, jewelry, and snaps on clothing, including infant clothing. With pierced ears becoming more common in boys, nickel dermatitis of the ear lobes is likely to increase in this population. Shoes can contain rubber chemicals. Clothing, particularly that made with permanent-press material, can contain formaldehyde and may need to be washed several times before it is worn. Cosmetics and hand lotions can contain formaldehyde releasers and balsam of Peru or other fragrances. Benzocaine is found in topical anti-itching creams, particularly those for sunburn or poison ivy.

Educating a sensitive patient to avoid these substances can greatly reduce episodes of ACD. Recognizing local plants that cause contact dermatitis also is beneficial. Occasionally, an extensive history may be needed to find the source of ACD. For instance, a dog may run in the woods and pick up and carry poison ivy oleoresin (plant sap) to its owner by means of its fur. Only by diligently searching for these sources of ACD will a physician find them.

If a child has recurrent or persistent ACD, patch testing for specific allergen identification may be useful. Patch testing involves placing the suspected substance on the skin for 48 hours, removing the patch, and reading it at 72 hours, looking for the typical eczematous dermatitis. Because false-positive and false-negative results are common, patch tests should be performed by a physician skilled at reading them. When a contact allergen is confirmed by this method, avoidance of the substance is necessary for the dermatitis to clear. Lists of products that contain these chemicals are usually available in a physician's office where patch testing is routine.

*Manufactured by Stockhausen and available through Dermatologic Lab & Supply, Inc., 201 Ridge, Council Bluffs, IA 51503, or 1-800-831-6273.

ATOPIC DERMATITIS

ELLIOT F. ELLIS, M.D.

Atopic dermatitis is an inflammatory skin disease that characteristically occurs in individuals with a genetic predisposition to form immunoglobulin E (IgE) antibodies. Typically a disease of infancy and childhood, atopic dermatitis is a harbinger of the subsequent development of other atopic diseases. The disease has a characteristic morphology and distribution: facial and extensor involvement in infants and flexural involvement in older children. Characteristic of atopic dermatitis is lichenification, a peculiar thickening of the skin and accentuation of the normal skin markings (secondary to chronic scratching and rubbing) and intense pruritus (which must be controlled to treat the disease successfully). During infancy, the skin eruption is typically exudative and secondary infection with *Staphylococcus aureus* is common. Studies of the natural history of atopic dermatitis, which most often has its onset at 2 to 3 months of age, have shown that by 5 years of age, in the great majority of cases, the skin disease has undergone remission.

TREATMENT

Therapy is directed toward identifying and eliminating factors that exacerbate the skin lesions, treating infection, and controlling the pruritis and scratching.

Nonspecific Measures

Like the nasal mucous membranes in allergic rhinitis and the airways in asthma, the skin in atopic dermatitis is hyperresponsive to environmental irritants. One should therefore avoid wearing wool garments (loose-fitting cotton clothing is best) and occlusive fibers such as nylon; extremes of heat, leading to sweating, or cold, leading to chilling; overbathing, especially taking hot baths and scrubbing the skin vigorously with soap; and, in infancy, crawling around on rugs. During laundering, clothing should be rinsed thoroughly to remove residual soap and/or detergents that may be irritating to the skin. Although often overlooked, the fingernails must be trimmed as short as possible to prevent injury due to scratching. During an episode of itching, an infant or young child can abrade and injure his or her skin greatly over the course of minutes by vigorous scratching if the nails are not cut short.

Specific Measures

Therapy for Infection

Infection of the skin, most often with *S. aureus,* is very common in exacerbations of atopic dermatitis, particularly in infancy, when the wet, weepy skin provides an ideal culture medium for bacterial growth. Topical antibiotics are a waste of time, and systemic treatment is mandatory. Dicloxacillin (12 to 25 mg/kg/day every 6 hours) and cephalexin (Keflex) (25 to 50 mg/kg/day every 6 hours), which are both available as generics and therefore relatively inexpensive, are effective in most instances.

Herpes simplex virus infection of the skin is an uncommon complication that rarely becomes disseminated and that can be successfully treated with povidone-iodine (Betadine) compresses. Very rarely, particularly in childhood, the skin may become infected with a dermatophyte. This complication responds to systemic administration of griseofulvin (10/mg/kg/day up to a maximum of 500 mg a day for 4 weeks).

Bathing

There are two schools of thought regarding the bathing of patients affected with atopic dermatitis. The proponents of the Scholtz type regimen forbid bathing and instead recommend cleansing with Cetaphil, a nonlipid lotion, followed by application of a corticosteroid solution. Most parents do not favor this regimen because they dislike not being able to bathe their infant or child.

The other belief is that regular bathing may be very helpful in the management of atopic dermatitis if performed correctly. The idea of the soaking bath is to hydrate the skin. Over the course of 20 minutes, water is absorbed into the stratum corneum. The use of soap is minimized, and, immediately following the bath the skin is patted dry (*not* rubbed) with a soft, absorbent towel. Within 3 minutes, corticosteroid ointment is applied to the affected areas, and a lubricant is applied (e.g., Nutriderm cream or lotion or Lac-Hydra 12 per cent lotion). The purpose of the lubricant is to seal the water into the skin and to prevent evaporation. Bath oils, if used, should be added at the end of the bath, not at the beginning (if added at the beginning, they coat the skin and prevent hydration). Bathing, done appropriately, can be very useful in reducing the itching associated with dry skin, which is a characteristic of patients with atopic dermatitis, even in areas uninvolved by the dermatitis.

Corticosteroids

The topical application of corticosteroids to areas of active dermatitis is the cornerstone of therapy. Hydrocortisone 1 per cent cream is very safe for regular therapy but is often not potent enough for the more severe forms of dermatitis. A mid-strength topical corticosteroid (e.g., triamcinolone 0.1 per cent in an ointment base) is a good product and has the substantial advantage of being available as a generic with great savings in cost. Other, more potent fluorinated steroids may be necessary on areas of thick skin, such as the hands and feet, but should be avoided on areas of thin skin, particularly the face. Thinning of the skin and the development of telangiectasias and striae are distressing complications of the unrestricted application of potent fluorinated corticosteroids. An ointment is preferred to a cream, particularly if it is applied immediately after hydrating the skin, because it is better at sealing water into the skin. Topical corticosteroid ointments are particularly well absorbed when applied to hydrated skin.

Generally, the use of systemic steroids is avoided because, as effective as they are, discontinuation of the drug is frequently associated with an exacerbation of the skin disease. However, systemic corticosteroids are occasionally necessary to bring the skin disease under control. In patients with the most severe forms of atopic dermatitis, the maintenance use of an alternate-day prednisone regimen may be necessary to provide the patient with satisfactory control of the dermatitis.

Antipruritics

There are no drugs that are uniformly successful in controlling itching. However, antihistamines with potent central nervous system sedative effects appear to be the best. Hydroxyzine (Atarax, Vistaril), (2.0 mg/kg per 24 hours in two divided doses) and diphenhydramine (Benadryl), (5 mg/kg per 24 hours in two divided doses) are both widely used in the treatment of atopic dermatitis in infants and children. Doxepin, a tricyclic agent (starting dose 25 to 50 mg/day), is effective in many instances and has the advantage of once-a-day dosing. The nonsedating antihistamines, such as terfenadine, are less effective in the control of pruritus of atopic dermatitis than the conventional sedating antihistamines. This finding supports the central effect of the antihistamines, rather than a peripheral effect, as the mechanism of antipruritic action.

Aspirin, in some cases, is very useful in relieving itching. Generally, higher doses of aspirin than are ordinarily prescribed are required; in young infants, one must be alert to the possibility of producing salicylism.

Coal-tar preparations are rarely used today; exposure to ultraviolet light, as effective as it is in some cases of atopic dermatitis, is not widely used because of the fear of subsequent development of skin cancer.

In some infants and young children with severe atopic dermatitis flares, a method of immobilizing the extremities to prevent scratching, proposed originally by Louis Webb Hill, a pioneer pediatric allergist, is very useful. After the child is bathed and the skin hydrated, a topical corticosteroid ointment is applied to the extremities. This is followed by application of gauze (alternatively, an old sheet can be cut up and used) to wrap the entire extremity beginning distally. An Ace bandage is then applied and secured. The pressure of the dressing seems to relieve the itching and to prevent scratching of the skin, particularly at night, when much of the damage is done. The dressing is removed the following morning. There is often a remarkable improvement in the condition of the skin as a result of the child's not being able to scratch during the night. This treatment is also very effective in breaking the scratch-itch-scratch cycle that is responsible for the perpetuation of the disease. During the daytime, elbow restraints (the kind used for infants who have had cleft lip repair) are useful in preventing scratching. These restraints, known as No-No Pediatric Arm Restraints,* are available in four sizes and cost from $12 to $17 per pair.

Diet

The role of food allergy in the pathogenesis of atopic dermatitis, particularly during infancy and childhood, has been debated for many years. Recent studies have clearly demonstrated a significant association between ingestion of certain dietary items and flare of the skin in children with atopic dermatitis. The foods most often involved are eggs, milk, peanuts, soy, and wheat. Therefore, an empiric trial of elimination of these dietary items is indicated.

Control of Inhalant Allergens

The role of inhalant allergens, such as the house dust mite, in atopic dermatitis is controversial. Anecdotally, in some children, the elimination of exposure to house dust mites has an ameliorating effect on skin disease. Whether house dust mites act as an inhalant or as a contact allergen is not known.

---

*H & H Research, 286 West Brown, Birmingham, MI 48009.

Neurogenic and Psychologic Factors

Neurogenic and psychologic factors have long been known to play a role in atopic dermatitis. When the infant with atopic dermatitis is upset—for example, during the course of the physical examination—he or she will begin to cry and at the same time scratch vigorously. Parents need a lot of support to deal with the affected infant or child. They need to understand that atopic dermatitis is a chronic disease for which the fundamental cause is unknown. Although there is no cure, the dermatitis can be treated; and, with the passage of time, the prognosis is good.

Hospitalization

Hospitalization should certainly be considered for patients with severe, infected atopic dermatitis. Relocating the infant or child from the home environment to a controlled setting in the hospital, where the infected dermatitis can be treated is often very useful. To get the skin disease under control, initial therapy involves compresses of cool water or Burow's solution (1:40), antibiotics, and corticosteroids; the extremities can be wrapped to prevent scratching, and elimination diet therapy can be started.

URTICARIA

STANLEY M. FINEMAN, M.D.

Urticaria is commonly encountered in clinical practice and may affect up to 20 per cent of the population at some time. The disorder, also known as hives, is readily recognized by its characteristic pruritic, erythematous, raised lesions that blanch with pressure. The lesions may be small and well circumscribed or coalescent and generalized.

Acute urticaria is most common in children and young adults and is frequently self-limited, lasting less than 6 weeks. Chronic urticaria persists for at least 6 weeks and is more common in adults, particularly females.

The lesions of urticaria are caused by edema of the upper dermis of the skin, with dilatation and increased permeability of the capillaries. Angioedema can accompany urticaria and may be caused by similar pathologic changes occurring in the dermis and subcutaneous tissues. The lesions of angioedema differ in that they are usually not pruritic and they consist of deeper dermal and subcutaneous swellings.

The approach to a patient with urticaria or angioedema must begin with a sound understanding of the various causes and the classification of these conditions (Table 1).

TABLE 1. Classification of Urticaria and Angioedema

Immunologic
Anaphylactic (type I Gell-Coombs)
Cytotoxic (type II Gell-Coombs)
Immune complex (type III Gell-Coombs)
Papular urticaria
Anaphylactoid
Hereditary angioedema (HAE)
Histamine-releasing agents
Aspirin
Physical Factors
Dermographism
Pressure urticaria
Cold urticaria
Cholinergic urticaria
Solar urticaria
Vibratory angioedema
Systemic Conditions
Cutaneous mastocytosis
Systemic mastocytosis
Infectious
Collagen vascular disease
Neoplasms
Hormone imbalance
Psychogenic factors
Episodic angioedema and eosinophilia
Idiopathic

ETIOLOGY AND CLASSIFICATION

Immunologic Origin

Urticaria and angioedema may be considered to be of immunologic origin when specific antigens, antibodies, or sensitized cells are identified.

Anaphylactic hypersensitivity may be the most common immunologic mechanism producing acute urticaria. The most common antigens causing urticaria through this mechanism include foods (particularly fish, shellfish, eggs, and nuts); medications (particularly penicillin and sulfonamides); insect stings, and animal dander and saliva (contact urticaria).

Cytotoxic antibodies are responsible for urticaria that accompanies transfusion reactions.

Antigen antibody complexes may also trigger the complement pathway and cause mediator release. Serum sickness is a classic example of a type III hypersensitivity reaction and may be manifested as urticaria, arthralgias, and fever.

Papular urticaria involves small pruritic papules and wheals that usually present on the lower extremities of children. These lesions are triggered by the bites of certain insects such as mosquitoes and fleas. The lesions may be persistent; they have been attributed to a biphasic reaction to the saliva and mouth parts of the insect, which are left on the skin after the bite. The immediate wheal may be secondary to a type I allergic reaction, and the delayed component may be a type IV or lymphocyte-mediated reaction.

Anaphylactoid Origin

Anaphylactoid reactions may involve certain immunologic pathways but do not require the presence of a known specific antibody.

Hereditary angioedema (HAE) is an autosomal dominant condition that is characterized by recurrent attacks of nonpruritic, painful angioedema involving the skin and mucosa of the upper respiratory and gastrointestinal tracts. The most significant manifestation is life-threatening upper respiratory obstruction, which may occur in as many as 25 per cent of affected persons. Various factors that initiate an attack include minor trauma, emotional stress, change in environmental temperature, or infections.

Patients with HAE are deficient in C1 esterase inhibitor (C1INH), which is a protein that inhibits the function of activated C1 in the complement pathway. The lack of this globulin leads to unwanted activation of the complement cascade. Through analysis of serum from patients with HAE, a deficiency of C1INH and a low level of C4 can be detected. In 15 per cent of patients, the C1 esterase protein may be of normal quantity but dysfunctional.

Histamine-releasing agents include certain medications, foods, and chemicals that have been shown to cause urticaria by direct degranulation of mast cells with subsequent histamine release. These substances include opiates (codeine and morphine), muscle relaxants (curare, *d*-tubocurarine), dextran, bile salts, polymyxin, thiamine, radiographic contrast material, and certain foods such as strawberries, tomatoes, citrus fruits, and lobster.

Aspirin may directly cause urticaria. However, this effect may be mediated by aspirin's ability to block the cyclooxygenase pathway of arachidonic acid metabolism. This may result in the enhanced formation of leukotrienes and other chemical mediators. Other preparations that inhibit cyclooxygenase and may also aggravate urticaria include indomethacin, phenylbutazone, and other nonsteroidal anti-inflammatory agents. Various artificial coloring agents, such as tartrazine yellow number 5, and benzoic acid derivatives may also cause difficulty in aspirin-sensitive patients with urticaria. Aspirin and these agents have been shown to exacerbate symptoms in 40 per cent of patients with chronic urticaria or angioedema from other causes.

Physical Factors

Dermatographism (dermographia) is the most common form of physical urticaria. It has been reported to occur in up to 5 per cent of the general population. Dermatographism has also been reported in as many as 20 per cent of patients with chronic urticaria. It is easily elicited by stroking the volar forearm, which should be done in all patients presenting with urticaria and angioedema.

Pressure urticaria is triggered by the direct application of pressure to the skin in sensitive patients. Deep and painful swellings may occur 4 to 6 hours after the application of pressure. The palms, soles, and buttocks are the most commonly involved sites.

Cold urticaria can be either acquired or hereditarily transmitted. The most common form of cold urticaria is the acquired idiopathic type. In these patients, the lesions develop upon exposure of skin surfaces to changes in temperature.

Cholinergic urticaria is probably the second most common form of physical urticaria. It is manifested by pruritic wheals, which are 2 to 3 mm in size, with surrounding erythematous flares. These lesions usually develop after vigorous exercise with sweating, with exposure to warm temperatures, or with emotional stress. Exercise-induced anaphylaxis, on the other hand, is triggered by exercise and not by direct heat.

Solar urticaria is relatively uncommon and is characterized by the appearance of pruritic erythematous wheals within minutes following exposure to sunlight.

Vibratory angioedema is a rare condition that is associated with swellings following prolonged exposure to vibration. It may be associated with intense pruritus as well. An inherited form has been described.

Systemic Conditions

Urticaria or angioedema can be the presenting sign of an underlying systemic illness. *Mastocytosis* is characterized by an increased accumulation of mast cells in the skin (cutaneous form) and in other organs (systemic form). *Urticaria pigmentosa* is a mild form of mastocytosis in which the mast cells accumulate in the skin. Mild stroking of the skin *(Darier's sign)* elicits urtication in these lesions, which may have increased pigmentation.

Urticaria can be associated with infectious agents. Viral infections may be the most common triggers of urticaria in children. Urticaria is frequently present in the preicteric phase of hepatitis B and early in the course of infectious mononucleosis. Subclinical bacterial infections have also been attributed to causing urticaria. Urticaria may also occur in patients with systemic lupus erythematosus, rheumatoid arthritis, and Sjögren syndrome.

Urticaria has been associated with neoplasms, particularly lymphomas. Carcinoma of the colon, rectum, and lungs has been reported to be associated with urticaria.

Hormone imbalances, such as occur in hyperthyroidism and pregnancy, have been identified as causing urticaria.

Psychogenic factors, such as anxiety and emotional stress, frequently play a major role in chronic urticaria. It is quite common for patients to have exacerbations during periods of stress.

Idiopathic Factors

The cause of urticaria and angioedema may remain elusive in as many of 70 to 80 per cent of patients with chronic symptoms. The diagnosis of idiopathic urticaria and angioedema remains one of exclusion.

DIAGNOSTIC APPROACH AND DIFFERENTIAL DIAGNOSIS

The evaluation of a patient presenting with urticaria and angioedema begins with a thorough history and careful physical examination. Not infrequently, the cause of the urticaria may be elicited from the history or may be suspected on physical examination (particularly with contact urticaria or papular urticaria). Asking the patient what he or she thinks is causing the hives may yield the etiologic factor responsible for the urticarial episode. One should always make specific inquiry regarding allergenic factors such as foods or inhalant allergens, medications or food additives, artificially colored preparations, and aspirin. Specific inquiry regarding temperature changes and other systemic symptomatology, such as arthritis or fevers with infections, should also be made.

In most patients with acute urticaria, laboratory procedures are not helpful. In patients with chronic urticaria, a general screening panel to eliminate the possibility of an underlying condition may be helpful. It is usually recommended that one obtain a complete blood count, erythrocyte sedimentation rate, and urinalysis.

Further specific diagnostic tests should be conducted only when certain predisposing conditions are suspected. It has been estimated that allergens trigger hives in less than 3 per cent of all patients with chronic urticaria. It is generally not helpful to obtain a serum immunoglobulin E or specific allergy skin test in patients with chronic urticaria unless the history suggests allergy as a cause.

TREATMENT

The optimal treatment for urticaria and angioedema is the identification and removal of the triggering factors. This is particularly helpful for urticaria secondary to allergies or physical factors. Avoidance of aspirin, benzoates, and tartrazine and other azodyes may be beneficial. In many cases, urticaria is a self-limited condition that requires little treatment other than the relief of the associated pruritis.

Antihistamines are the drugs of first choice. Hydroxyzine, diphenhydramine, and cyproheptadine have been the cornerstone of therapy for urticaria. These classic H_1 antagonists are effective, but the problem of sedation may limit their usefulness in certain patients. The recommended initial dose of hydroxyzine is 2 mg/kg/day in divided doses. Gradual increases in the dose may be necessary to control symptoms. It has also been suggested that combining two H_1 antagonist agents may provide added benefit to certain patients. The recommended starting dose for diphenhydramine is 5 mg/kg/day. The initial dose of cyproheptadine is 0.2 mg/kg/day.

The newer, nonsedating H_1 antagonists include terfenadine, loratadine, astemizole, and cetirizine. At this time, only terfenadine and astemizole are approved for use in the United States. Neither are approved for use in children less than 12 years of age.

Doxepin is a tricyclic antidepressant with H_1 and H_2 antagonist properties. It is shown to be effective in selective patients with chronic urticaria. Calcium channel blockers, such as ketotifen and nifedipine, have been shown to be useful in physical urticarias, particularly when used in combination with H_1 antagonists. Other studies have shown the benefit of combining H_1 antagonists with H_2 blocking antihistamines, such as cimetidine, for effective control of urticaria symptomatology. Cimetidine is available in tablet form (200, 300, 400, and 800 mg) and oral liquid form (300 mg/5 ml). The use of cimetidine is not approved by the Food and Drug Administration for children less than 16 years of age, but it has been used in doses of 20 to 40 mg/kg/day in certain cases.

Adrenergic agents may be useful in severe acute urticaria and angioedema. For life-threatening symptoms such as laryngealedema, epinephrine should be administered subcutaneously (1:1000 aqueous epinephrine, 0.01 ml/kg up to 0.3 ml). This can be repeated every 20 minutes for recurrent symptoms. Oral adrenergic agents, such as ephedrine or terbutaline, have been used in combination with H_1 antagonists but have been found to be of limited usefulness in patients with urticaria and angioedema.

Corticosteroids should be reserved for severe disease when other agents have been unsuccessful in controlling the symptomatology. Topical corticosteroids are not efficacious in urticaria. Systemic treatment with corticosteroids is usually begun with 2 mg/kg/day of prednisone. The prednisone dose can gradually be tapered and then discontinued. The use of long-term corticosteroid therapy should be limited to patients that have not responded to other treatment modalities. The lowest possible daily or alternate-day dose of prednisone should be used.

Patients with HAE require special attention. Acute attacks should be treated with adrenalin, corticosteroids, and antihistamines, but the response may be suboptimal. Anabolic steroids, such as danazol, have been useful in the long-term management of patients with HAE.

Patients with mastocytosis may benefit from oral cromolyn, which is now available in the form of capsules (Gastrocrom). The starting dose is 20 mg/kg/day in divided doses.

ERYTHEMA NODOSUM

ALDO VINCENT LONDINO, JR., M.D.

Erythema nodosum (EN) is one of a variety of disorders that lead to inflammatory lesions of adipose tissue known as panniculitis. Normal adipose tissue is organized around a vascular plexus. The adipocytes are grouped in lobules that have a central artery and peripheral vein in the fibrous septa, which separates the lobules. Panniculitis is therefore classified as either lobular or septal. EN, a septal panniculitis, is believed to be a type 3 hypersensitivity reaction to a multitude of agents and processes. The pathologic lesion is relatively nonspecific. Early, there is an acute inflammatory reaction in the lower dermis and in the interlobular septa involving the veins. As the lesions mature, a granulomatous infiltrate develops at the junction of the dermis and the subcutaneous fat.

CLINICAL FEATURES

EN is most often seen in winter and spring. It is three times more common in females than males. Although EN can occur at any age, it occurs more frequently in the young than in the old. The lesions, consisting of crops of painful subcutaneous erythematous nodules that appear bruise-like while developing or fading, may be accompanied by fever and malaise. The nodules are bilateral, multiple, and in different stages of development. The lesions are most frequent and obtain their greatest size in the lower extremities; however, more generalized lesions, including facial EN, have been described.

TABLE 1. Associations of Erythema Nodosum

Streptococcal infection
Inflammatory bowel disease
Yersiniosis
Campylobacter jejuni dysentery
Tuberculosis
Coccidioidomycosis
Histoplasmosis
North American blastomycosis
Cat-scratch fever
Trichophyton infection
Behçet syndrome
Sulfonamides
Bromides
Oral contraceptives
Sarcoidosis
Idiopathic

Joint symptoms occur in about 75 per cent of patients, ranging from arthralgias, monarthritis, pauciarthritis, and a migratory polyarthritis. An acute periarthritis of the ankles with bilateral hilar adenopathy and EN is an acute form of sarcoidosis known as *Löfgren syndrome* and generally implies a favorable prognosis. Articular symptoms may antedate the skin lesions. The remainder of the clinical syndrome depends on the underlying cause.

DIAGNOSIS

The differential diagnosis of nodules on the legs includes nodular liquifying panniculitis, lupus profundus, vasculitis, and other forms of panniculitis (i.e., panniculitis with pancreatic cancer). Rarely, EN can follow a chronic or protracted course in which the lesions may ulcerate and leave hyperpigmented changes. This situation must be differentiated from erythema induratum. Multiple diseases and drugs can be associated with EN (Table 1). The evaluation of EN involves a complete blood count, urinalysis, chest radiograph, anergy panel, including purified protein derivative, trichophytin test, antistreptolysin-O titer, and other studies based on history or physical examination. Biopsy is not always necessary.

THERAPY

Erythema nodosum can usually be treated with elevation of the legs, rest, and anti-inflammatory medication. Oral potassium iodide has also been used effectively. Although corticosteroids may hasten recovery, they are rarely, if ever, indicated. The physician must also provide reassurance to the patient while excluding more serious associated diseases that may require specific therapy.

DRUG REACTIONS AND THE SKIN

PAUL J. HONIG, M.D.

Drug reactions occur at a rate of 3 per 1000 courses of therapy in the general population. Hospitalized patients are more likely to experience a reaction to a drug than outpatients because of their frequency of exposure. The rate of adverse events depends on the particular medication used (e.g., 59 adverse events per 1000 drug courses of trimethoprim-sulfamethoxazole compared with 0.2 reactions per 1000 courses of chloral hydrate). Children are less likely to experience undesirable side effects than adults as a result of their decreased exposure to drugs and a reluctance of physicians to use systemic therapy in the pediatric population.

Drug reactions occur on an immune or nonimmune basis. Any of the four types of immunologic mechanisms (immunoglobulin E–mediated, immune complex, cytotoxic, or cell-mediated) can be involved. Adverse reactions also occur on the basis of overdosage, specific toxicity, common side effects of a particular drug, or unusual drug interactions. Many times, the exact pathophysiology is not identified.

The appearance of drug reactions is nonspecific and may mimic almost any known dermatosis. Therefore, one cannot make a diagnosis of a drug reaction on the basis of the appearance of the rash alone. However, certain patterns should make one suspicious of the presence of an adverse reaction:

1. Urticaria constitutes the most common expression of drug sensitivity.
2. Maculopapular eruptions similar to a viral exanthem are the second most common skin change seen. This pattern poses a difficult problem because children are frequently infected by viruses.
3. Erythema multiforme is often secondary to drugs. However, recent observations suggest that the majority of cases of erythema multiforme may be due to herpes simplex virus or other infectious agents.
4. Vasculitis may occur.
5. Erythema nodosum may occur.
6. Photosensitive cutaneous eruptions may occur.
7. Toxic epidermal necrolysis may occur.
8. Fixed drug eruptions (i.e., recurrent, circumscribed, erythematous to brown plaques that recur at the same site with each exposure to the offending medication) may occur.

THERAPY

Essential to the management of any drug reaction is the identification and elimination of the offending medication. Historical information frequently overlooked includes

1. Drugs ingested by mother during pregnancy (newborn with skin changes).
2. Medications given to nursing mothers (the amount of drug excreted in mother's milk varies from drug to drug).
3. Topically applied preparations (enhanced absorption through children's skin due to greater surface area-to-body weight ratio—e.g., steroids or salicylic acid).
4. Medications for other family members ingested accidentally.
5. Over-the-counter preparations not considered to be "medications" by patients.

Treatment must be individualized. Minor reactions frequently disappear once the offending agent is discontinued. Persistent pruritus can be controlled with oral antihistamines. More severe, persistent reactions may respond to oral antihistamines (e.g., diphenhydramine, hydroxyzine) and/or oral steroids. If blistering occurs, attention to fluid and electrolyte balance and secondary infection is important. With mucous membrane involvement, an ophthalmologist must be consulted to rule out the presence of corneal changes. Hospitalization should be considered in toxic patients with severe skin involvement that may include extensive exfoliation.

Stevens-Johnson syndrome and drug-induced toxic epidermal necrolysis (conditions at the most severe end of the drug reaction spectrum) demand special consideration. The literature suggests that steroid therapy of these conditions are of no value, will prolong hospital stays, and may in fact be harmful. However, many clinicians think that steroid preparations are helpful. Steroid therapy (i.e., an equivalent of prednisone, 1 to 2 mg/kg/day) should be reserved for the toxic patient whose condition is rapidly worsening. Steroids must be started within the first 2 to 3 days of the eruption to be effective. Thereafter, existing damage probably cannot be reversed. If the patient continues to progress after 5 days of steroid therapy, the medication should be discontinued.

Patients receiving steroids must be carefully monitored for infection (i.e., complete blood cell count, periodic wound culture, periodic blood culture). When skin denudation involves greater than 20 per cent of the child's body surface area, steroid therapy should not be used at all. Open lesions respond to compressing with solutions such as Burow's solution and topical silver sulfadiazine. Broad-spectrum antibiotic coverage is started if patients have unusual temperature fluctuations or changes in level of consciousness. Urethral involvement may produce urinary retention and secondary infection. Therefore, urinary output must be monitored. If denudation progresses to greater than 25 per cent of body surface area, the patient should be transferred to a burn unit. Plasmapheresis has been used when all else has failed.

REFERENCES

Arndt KA, Jick H: Rates of cutaneous reactions to drugs: A report from the Boston Collaborative Drug Surveillance Program. JAMA 235:918–923, 1976.
Orton PW, Huff JC, Tonnesen JG, et al: Detection of a herpes simplex viral antigen in skin lesions of erythema multiforme. Ann Intern Med 101:48–50, 1984.

ERYTHEMA MULTIFORME

JAMES E. RASMUSSEN, M.D.

Patients with erythema multiforme (EM) can have a spectrum of illness ranging from trivial to life-threatening. Mild EM manifests itself as ringed erythematous lesions on the palms and soles (target or iris lesions). The next grade of severity involves more widespread papular lesions and perhaps a few blisters. When the blisters become severe, the patient is defined as having erythema multiforme major. Other major forms of EM are Stevens-Johnson syndrome (SJS), which features blisters on mucous membranes such as the lips, mouth, eyes, rectum, penis, and vagina; and toxic epidermal necrolysis (TEN), the most severe and widespread form of EM.

Patients with minor varieties of EM usually need no specific therapy and have a self-limited disease that resolves without any sequelae. Minor varieties are frequently associated with outbreaks of herpes simplex virus and can often be controlled through the prophylactic use of acyclovir. More severe varieties of EM are usually due to allergies to drugs, which should be discontinued immediately when the diagnosis is suspected. Unfortunately, even though the offending drug is withdrawn, the disease usually proceeds through its natural course, which is 10 to 21 days to recovery.

GENERAL CARE

Patients with minor degrees of EM need no specific therapy but may respond to prophylactic therapy with acyclovir. Patients with more widespread forms of EM usually require hospitalization and frequently need admission to a burn unit for surgical management.

The first major problem in the care of these patients is adequate fluid and electrolyte intake because most find it difficult if not impossible to eat or drink. Consequently, considerable care must be given to intake and output, calories, proteins, electrolytes, and urine output. Second, considerable attention must be paid to the patient's damaged skin. Topical antibiotics, antiseptics, artificial skin, and other new types of membranes have all been advocated. There is probably no reason to use one of these over another because the epithelium regenerates naturally. It is not necessary to resort to skin grafting.

Third, prompt attention should be given to the eyes by a competent ophthalmologist, who may wish to insert an irrigating shield in the form of a contact lens to help diminish problems with adhesions.

SPECIFIC THERAPY

Patients with severe varieties of EM should be carefully screened for drug allergies. These are responsible for probably 80 to 90 per cent of cases of SJS and TEN. Suspected drugs should be discontinued immediately, and drugs in the same family should not be readministered.

Corticosteroids are of no proven value in the treatment of EM. Seven studies have evaluated patients treated with and without corticosteroids, and all have come to the same conclusion: The use of corticosteroids does not improve the rate of healing and may actually be associated with a higher morbidity and mortality.

COMPLICATIONS

Twenty to 30 per cent of patients with inflammation of ocular conjunctiva suffer corneal scarring, lid adhesions, and dry eyes. Consequently, their care should be carefully coordinated with that of a competent ophthalmologist.

Severe varieties can produce permanent loss of hair and nails, and scarring may occur if secondary cutaneous infection has been prominent. Dark-skinned patients will also notice considerable irregularity in their pigmentation for months to years following recovery, but this is usually not a permanent problem. Hair and nails usually regrow but in some instances not completely.

Sepsis, gastrointestinal bleeding, and kidney and liver failure are the most common causes of death. The prognosis is the worst in older patients with more than 50 per cent of their skin involved, a low white blood cell count, and associated organ failure.

PAPULOSQUAMOUS DISORDERS

SIDNEY HURWITZ, M.D.

SEBORRHEIC DERMATITIS

Seborrheic dermatitis (SD) is a term used to describe an erythematous, scaly, or crusting eruption that appears primarily in the seborrheic areas (those with the highest concentration of sebaceous glands)—namely, the scalp, face, and postauricular, presternal, and intertriginous areas.

Seborrheic dermatitis of the scalp is best managed by the use of an antiseborrheic shampoo; those containing sulfur or salicylic acid, or both, are generally satisfactory. Individuals with more stubborn involvement, however, may use shampoos containing pyrithione, tars, or selenium sulfide. If the scale is extremely thick and adherent, P & S liquid (a specifically formulated liquid that helps facilitate the removal of scales) and a topical corticosteroid lotion (alone or in combination with 3 to 5 per cent sulfur precipitate or salicylic acid, or both) may be used.

Lesions of SD on other areas of the body respond rapidly to topical corticosteroids. Because it is advisable to avoid high-potency fluorinated steroids on the face, medium-potency topical preparations, such as Aclovate, DesOwen, Tridesilon, or Westcort, or low-potency hydrocortisone formulations may be used.

Blepharitis may be managed with warm water compresses followed by a gentle, nonirritating baby shampoo; mechanical removal of scales when necessary; and, at times, topical sulfacetamide (Sulamyd) ointment or sulfacetamide with 0.5 per cent prednisolone (Metimyd). However, corticosteroids must be used with caution on the eyelids.

PSORIASIS

Psoriasis is a common inherited disorder characterized by erythematous, scaly papules or plaques with a predisposition for the elbows, knees, extensor surfaces of the limbs, genitalia, scalp, and lumbosacral area. Psoriatic involvement of the nails is also seen in 25 to 50 per cent of patients. Pitting, probably the best known and most characteristic nail change, is generally seen as small, irregular pits or depressions. Other nail changes include discoloration, subungual hyperkeratosis, crumbling and grooving of the nail plate, and onycholysis (separation of the nail plate from the nail bed).

Although studies suggest that childhood psoriasis usually portends a severe course in adult life, spontaneous remissions occur at times and most patients generally respond well to currently available therapeutic measures. Accordingly, most patients, with a little effort, can do much to control the cutaneous aspects of the disorder. Topical corticosteroids, alone or in combination with tar formulations, are often the mainstay of therapy. Although high-potency topical corticosteroids are invaluable in short-term management of severe recalcitrant lesions, most patients respond quite well to medium- or low-potency steroid formulations. Topical corticosteroids have replaced tars to a great extent in the treatment of many forms of dermatitis. Nevertheless, tars still remain a highly effective therapeutic modality for the management of patients with psoriasis and other chronic dermatoses.

Most psoriatic patients also benefit from ultraviolet light therapy and sunlight exposure and are thus frequently better during the summer months. Advantage should be taken of this in planning the summer activities of the psoriatic child. For those who can arrange to be exposed to sunlight on a regular basis, it can be an important aspect of therapy. Caution is recommended, however, to reduce sunburning, sun damage, and photosensitization. Thus, a sunscreen formulation with a sun protective factor (SPF) of 15 or greater should be used on uninvolved areas, and one with a SPF of 6 or 8 may be used on affected cutaneous areas.

Psoriasis of the scalp frequently responds to tar shampoos (DHS Tar, Ionil T Plus, Polytar, Pentrax, T-Gel, T-Sal, or Sebutone). Topical corticosteroid lotions (Elocon, Lidex, Synalar, or Valisone) once or twice a day in conjunction with tar shampoos are also beneficial. When scaling and crusting are particularly thick and resistant to therapy, incorporation of 3 to 5 per cent salicylic acid to the steroid lotion and P & S liquid, as in the treatment of SD, will soften the scales and help facilitate their removal.

LICHEN PLANUS

Lichen planus is a dermatosis of unknown cause characterized by small, shiny, flat-topped, polygonal, reddish or violaceous, intensely pruritic papules with a predilection for the flexural surfaces of the wrists, legs, genitalia, and mucous membranes.

There is no specific treatment for lichen planus. Symptomatic relief, however, can be obtained by systemic antihistamines, ataractics such as hydroxyzine (Atarax or Vistaril), topical corticosteroid preparations, topical antipruritics, intralesional corticosteroids, and, on rare occasions, a short course of systemic corticosteroids. Mucous membrane lesions usually require no treatment. When these lesions are symptomatic, eroded, or ulcerated, however, topical anesthetics such as Benadryl elixir, Xylocaine viscous, topical corticosteroids (Kenalog in Orabase), or intralesional corticosteroids can be beneficial.

PITYRIASIS ROSEA

Pityriasis rosea is an acute, benign, self-limiting disorder of undetermined origin that follows a distinctive pattern, usually reaches its height within a period of a few days to a week, and generally resolves spontaneously within a period of 6 to 12 weeks.

Most patients require no treatment beyond reassurance as to the nature and prognosis of the disorder. Pruritus, if present, usually responds to topical antipruritic lotions combining menthol and camphor (Sarna), pramoxine-containing formulations (such as PrameGel, Pramosone, or Prax), calamine lotion, and mild topical corticosteroid formulations. Exposure to ultraviolet light or sunlight generally tends to hasten resolution of lesions, and, in the summertime, it is not uncommon to see pityriasis rosea on sun-protected areas of the body and little or no evidence of the eruption on sun-exposed areas in affected patients.

PITYRIASIS RUBRA PILARIS

Pityriasis rubra pilaris is a chronic skin disorder characterized by small follicular papules, disseminated yellowish-pink scaly plaques surrounding islands of normal skin, and hyperkeratosis of the palms and soles.

Treatment depends on suppression of hyperkeratinization. Mild forms may require topical corticosteroids, emollients, and keratolytic agents; in severe cases, oral vitamin A (50,000 units twice a day for children, and 150,000 to 600,000 units once a day for adolescents) has been used, but patients must be observed for signs of vitamin A toxicity. After several months of continuous therapy, oral vitamin A may be discontinued for periods of 2 or 3 months or more in an effort to avoid signs of toxicity. Although oral vitamin A may at times be supplanted by the use of synthetic retinoids (Accutane or Tegison), complications associated with use of these agents limit their usefulness in children.

PITYRIASIS LICHENOIDES (Mucha-Habermann Disease)

Pityriasis lichenoides is a self-limiting disorder characterized by crops of macules, papules, or papulovesicles that tend to develop central necrosis and crusts soon after they arise. The disorder occurs in two forms: an acute form (*p*ityriasis *l*ichenoides *e*t *v*arioliformis *a*cuta, also known as PLEVA or Mucha-Habermann disease), seen primarily in children; and a chronic form, more commonly noted in adolescents and young adults.

Antipruritics and lubricants, although not curative, may be helpful in ameliorating the symptoms. Topical corticosteroids, tar preparations, and exposure to ultraviolet light or sunlight have been employed with varying degrees of success in the treatment of persistent or chronic forms of the disorder. In addition, tetracycline (for older children and adults) and eythromycin (30 to 50 mg/kg/day, with a maximum of 1 or 2 g a day for older children and adults) for a period of 1 or 2 months can also be helpful.

CHRONIC NONHEREDITARY VESICULOBULLOUS DISORDERS OF CHILDHOOD

WALTER W. TUNNESSEN, JR., M.D.

The chronic nonhereditary vesiculobullous disorders of childhood constitute a confusing group and require the expertise of an experienced dermatologist using established dermatoimmunology and dermatopathology laboratories to assist in arriving at the correct diagnosis. The disorders are quite rare in children, but it is important to be aware of their existence to separate them from some of the more common disorders they mimic, such as bullous impetigo and bullous papular urticaria. Most of the chronic bullous disorders require treatment with drugs that have significant side effects and toxicities, for which treated children must be monitored.

DERMATITIS HERPETIFORMIS

Dermatitis herpetiformis (DH) is a rare disorder in children, occurring much less commonly than in adults, for whom the incidence rate is estimated to be 1 to 2 in 100,000. The rash of DH is characterized by the appearance of small pink to red papules that frequently become vesicular and, less frequently, reach a bullous state. The lesions are often preceded by a burning sensation or pruritus. Persistent pruritus results in severe excoriation, potentially hiding the vesiculobullous component of DH. Another characteristic of the disorder is the symmetric distribution of the lesions. The lesions occur most commonly on the extensor surfaces of the limbs, but they also occur on the shoulders, trunk, sacral area, perineum, neck, scalp, face, and palms.

One of the most interesting aspects of DH is its association with gluten enteropathy. Unlike celiac disease, patients affected with DH usually do not have diarrhea and wasting. Less than 15 per cent of children with DH have evidence of clinical enteropathy. Nonetheless, biopsy of the small intestine will reveal evidence of villous atrophy in 85 to 95 per cent of patients with DH irrespective of their symptoms. Elimination of gluten from the diet will ameliorate the villous atrophy in all those affected and will result in clearing of the cutaneous eruption in about 80 per cent. It may take months before the dietary restrictions result in clinical response. Although a gluten-free diet seems to be the therapy of choice, this diet is extremely difficult to follow because of its restrictions. The protein fractions of wheat, barley, rye, and oats must be avoided; however, these vegetable proteins are fairly pervasive in our diet. The diet is also expensive, and the patient will require the help of a skilled pediatric nutritionist.

Drug therapy with either sulfapyridine or sulfone derivatives (dapsone) is usually effective, but it is fraught with dangers of toxicity. In most cases, affected children will require a combination of dietary and drug therapy. The drugs are tapered as rapidly as possible once the cutaneous manifestations are under control, but they are rarely able to be discontinued unless adherence to the gluten-free diet is strict. Sulfapyridine is used in a dose of 60 to 200 mg/kg/day in four divided doses, with a maximum dose of 2 to 4 g. The side effects from sulfapyridine include nausea, vomiting, headache, and fever; however, of much greater concern are the serious complications: serum sickness, agranulocytosis, hemolytic and aplastic anemias, exfoliative dermatitis, and hepatorenal toxicity. Dapsone is given in a dose of 2 mg/kg/day, with a maximum daily dose of 400 mg/day. Its toxicities mostly affect the hematopoietic system and include hemolysis, methemoglobinemia, leukopenia, and agranulocytosis. A glucose-6-phosphate dehydrogenase (G-6-PD) level must be obtained before beginning dapsone and sulfapyridine because of the risk of inducing severe hemolysis. During treatment, blood counts must be closely monitored with both drugs, and liver function tests must be obtained intermittently with dapsone. Even with a normal G-6-PD, dapsone must frequently be tapered because of a decrease in hemoglobin.

Topical therapy with emollients and antipruritics may be of some help in reducing the inflammation and pruritus. Unfortunately, the disorder persists into adulthood in most affected children.

CHRONIC BULLOUS DERMATOSIS OF CHILDHOOD

Chronic bullous dermatosis of childhood (CBDC), also known as linear immunoglobulin A (IgA) dermatosis of childhood, is quite rare but probably more common than DH in children. Debate has centered over whether CBDC is a distinct entity or simply a form of DH or childhood bullous pemphigoid. The characteristic immunofluorescent and immunoelectron microscopic findings support the belief that it is a separate category. Linear IgA deposits are found at the dermoepidermal junction on immunofluorescent studies.

Most cases of CBDC present in the first decade, usually before age 5 years. The associated vesicles and bullae tend to be large and tense. They occur most frequently on the lower trunk, perineum, and lower extremities. A characteristic finding is the clustering of the bullae in pear-shaped ellipses in an arrangement resembling a "string of jewels." Pruritus is variable, as is mucous membrane involvement. The course is one of remissions and exacerbations. Although in most children the disease was thought to remit in a few months to years, extension to adulthood is not uncommon.

The treatment of CBDC is similar to that of DH, using sulfapyridine or dapsone. Systemic steroids may be needed as adjunct therapy in resistant cases. Local therapy is helpful for pruritus, irritation, and infection.

CHILDHOOD PEMPHIGUS

Pemphigus vulgaris occurs even more rarely in children. In contrast to DH and CBDC, oral lesions are the rule. Erosive stomatitis may be the presenting complaint, preceding the appearance of the cutaneous vesiculobullous eruption. The lesions are accompanied by severe pain, as well as pruritus, and they tend to enlarge from the borders with a positive Nikolsky sign. On direct immunofluorescent staining, IgG antibodies to epidermal intercellular cement substance are present. Remissions rarely occur. Aggressive therapy is usually required with high doses of systemic corticosteroids (prednisone, 2 to 6 mg/k/day for 6 to 8 weeks) before tapering is successful.

Pemphigus foliaceus is considered a form of pemphigus vulgaris but is less severe. It is characterized by a pruritic, painful dermatitis that usually begins on the scalp, suggesting seborrheic dermatitis or impetigo. As the lesions progress, they acquire an eczematous appearance. Laboratory findings are similar to those of pemphigus vulgaris. Fortunately, high-potency topical corticosteroids may control the disorder; however, systemic steroids and, less commonly, sulfapyridine or sulfones may be necessary.

JUVENILE BULLOUS PEMPHIGOID

Juvenile bullous pemphigoid is a rare disorder characterized by large, tense bullae of the skin as well as oral erosive lesions. The lesions occur most frequently on the lower abdomen, anogenital region, and thighs. Direct immunofluorescence demonstrates linear IgG deposition along the basement membrane. The disorder is often, but not always, self-limiting. Systemic steroids (prednisone, 1 to 2 mg/k/day) are often necessary to control the disease, although topical steroids may be helpful.

DISCOID LUPUS ERYTHEMATOSUS

BERNARD COHEN, M.D.

Discoid lupus erythematosus (DLE) defines a pattern of clinical disease characterized by "disc" or coin-shaped cutaneous lesions found most commonly on sun-exposed sites. Although findings in DLE are usually confined to the skin, nearly 15 per cent of individuals with systemic lupus erythematosus (SLE) will develop discoid lesions and many patients with DLE experience at least mild systemic symptoms.

CLINICAL FINDINGS

DLE is a chronic persistent disease that may last for years. The eruption develops most commonly on the face, followed by the scalp and ears. Occasionally, lesions spread to the extremities and trunk. Localized lesions are only rarely associated with SLE. However, widespread involvement both above and below the neck may impart a higher risk for systemic disease.

The cutaneous eruption begins with slightly infiltrated, erythematous, violaceous papules and plaques with adherent scale and prominent follicular hyperkeratosis. When the scale is peeled away, the undersurface reveals a characteristic "carpet tack" appearance from the retained follicular keratin plugs. Expanding plaques develop peripheral hyperpigmentation and central atrophy and hypopigmentation. Lesions may become confluent on the face and scalp, producing extensive, disfiguring scarring and pigmentary changes. Thick, warty scale (hypertrophic DLE) may develop in old burned-out plaques, particularly at their periphery. Malar plaques on the face may demonstrate a butterfly pattern. Follicular destruction on the scalp leads to widespread, permanent, cicatricial alopecia. Involution of the eruption without scarring may also occur. The lips and mucous membranes, particularly the buccal mucosa and gingiva, may develop silvery-white scaling and ulceration. Patients with chronic scarring in these sites require close observation because of the risk of development of squamous cell carcinoma.

LABORATORY FINDINGS

Diagnostic changes of DLE on cutaneous biopsy of involved sites include hyperkeratosis with follicular plugging, thinning, and flattening of the outer layers of the epidermis, lymphocytic perivascular and periappendageal infiltration of the dermis, edema, vasodilatation, and mild hemorrhage in the upper dermis. However, histologic findings may be subtle and may vary with the evolution of clinical lesions.

Some individuals with DLE demonstrate a biologic false-positive result for syphilis, positive rheumatoid factor, low-titer antinuclear antibody, slight increase in gamma globulin, minimal decrease in complement, and mild hematologic abnormalities. However, progressive laboratory changes should suggest the possibility of SLE.

TREATMENT

Although fewer than 5 per cent of patients with DLE will develop SLE, all patients with active cutaneous lesions should be evaluated at least twice yearly with a thorough interval history, physical examination, and selective laboratory studies (complete blood count, erythrocyte sedimentation rate, platelet count, antinuclear antibody, urinalysis, and complement).

Individuals who give a history of exacerbation of disease after sun exposure should be counseled regarding sun avoidance and the use of sunscreens and sunblocks. Protective clothing with tightly woven materials, hats, long sleeves, and long pants are particularly useful during the summer months. Beach vacations and mid-day exposure should be discouraged. Sunscreens with a sun protective factor of 15 or higher should be applied to all exposed surfaces at least 15 minutes before going outdoors from April until October. Opaque make-up provides an excellent sun shield, and many enhancement cosmetics contain sunscreens. Patients living in the Sun Belt states may require year-round sunscreen protection. Extra precautions should also be taken at high elevations, in arid climates, in windy conditions, and while skiing because of increased exposure to ultraviolet light.

In all patients, medical cover-up cosmetics may be a useful adjunct to therapy. Excellent cosmesis is achieved with products such as Covermark (Lydia O'Leary) and Dermablend (Florey Roberts). These agents are hypoallergenic, relatively water-resistant, and blend well with normal pigment. They are, however, occlusive and consequently comedogenic.

Limited discoid plaques may respond within several weeks to medium-potency topical steroids (e.g., Aristocort 0.1%, Valisone 0.1%). Thicker plaques may require high-potency topical agents (e.g., Diprolene, Psorcon, Temovate) and may also be used for several weeks with close clinical monitoring. Overzealous application of topical agents may result in atrophy and hypopigmentation. Resistant localized plaques may be treated with small quantities (0.1 to 0.2 ml/papule) of intralesional steroids (e.g., Kenalog, 10 mg/ml diluted with 2 per cent xylocaine to 2.5 to 5 mg/ml) before proceeding to systemic therapy.

In patients with widespread or resistant cutaneous disease antimalarials, chloroquine (250 mg/day) or hydroxychloroquine (200 to 400 mg/day), are the most effective treatment. Ophthalmologic examinations should be obtained before starting therapy and then every 6 months during treatment because of the risk of antimalarial retinopathy. If possible, therapy should be discontinued during winter remissions. Lesions resistant to individual agents may respond to a combination of chloroquine, hydroxychloroquine, and quinacrine.

Individuals with rapidly progressive, disfiguring DLE, particularly on the face, improve quickly with oral prednisone (0.5 to 1.0 mg/kg/day in two divided doses) in combination with a single dose of an antimalarial. The systemic corticosteroid can usually be tapered over 4 to 6 weeks while the antimalarial begins to take effect.

FUNGAL INFECTIONS OF THE SKIN

RICHARD E. FITZPATRICK, M.D.

DERMATOPHYTE INFECTIONS

Dermatophytes are fungi with an enzymatic system that allows invasion and colonization of keratinized tissue. This factor limits infection to the skin, hair, and nails. Clinical infections are classified according to body location. Some dermatophyte species are so highly specialized that they exclusively infect humans and tend to cause very chronic infection (*Trichophyton rubrum*), whereas other species are predominantly animal parasites and, when involved in human infection, may produce an intense acute inflammatory reaction (*Microsporum canis*).

Dermatophyte infections are extremely common worldwide, to the extent that 90 per cent of adult men are infected at least transiently at some time during their life, and 20 per cent of the population has an ongoing chronic infection. Though tinea infections are considered rare or unusual in infants and young children, an appropriate index of suspicion is necessary to make the diagnosis, as these infections are often overlooked or misdiagnosed. Tinea capitis, tinea faciale, and tinea corporis are common in children aged 5 to 12, whereas tinea cruris and tinea pedis are common in adolescents (Table 1).

Most of the dermatophyte infections, but especially tinea capitis, behave as a familial disease. The presence of a dermatophyte in one family member acts as a source of infection for others. The spread of infection is either through direct contact with infected lesions or contact with flakes of skin, nail fragments, or hair infected with dermatophytes. Such contact is often indirect, through sharing of contaminated combs, brushes, clothing, shoes, socks, towels, blankets, sheets, and headgear, or even through house dust and flooring surfaces. Repeated contact over a prolonged period is generally necessary to spread the infection from one person to another, but this may occur in as many as 75 per cent of family members.

Moisture, skin hydration, and heat are critical factors in the establishment of clinical infection. The incidence of infection as well as the severity of symptoms and extent of lesions are all directly proportional to environmental heat and humidity. When these two conditions are not present, infections may be subclinical and asymptomatic, and infectivity and spread are low.

A secondary skin eruption representing an allergic reaction to the dermatophyte, termed an "id" reaction, occurs in some patients. In children, this occurs most commonly with tinea capitis and is predominantly truncal and may be scarlatiniform, seborrhea-like, eczematous, or similar to pityriasis rosea or erythema multiforme. In adolescents, it occurs with inflammatory tinea pedis and presents as papular and vesicular lesions on the sides of the fingers, palms, and wrists.

Diagnostic Procedures

Because the clinical presentations so closely simulate a variety of other dermatologic diseases, confirmation of the presence of dermatophyte hyphae by microscopic examination or culture is essential. The active margin of the lesion should be scraped with a No. 15 Bard-Parker blade to obtain relatively large pieces of keratinous material. Suppurative or macerated areas should be avoided. Scrapings for culture can be placed in a dermatophyte test medium or on a glass slide with 20 per cent potassium hydroxide (KOH) preparation and a coverslip in place for direct examination. These laboratory procedures have an 80 to 90 per cent accuracy rate if performed correctly.

Hyphae are visible as highly refractile, long-branching threads that course through cells; chains of spores are often visible as well (Fig. 1). The major artifact to be differentiated is the very visible interlacing periphery of keratinized epidermal cells. This artifact diminishes if the scraping is given adequate time (10 to 15 minutes) to soak in the KOH preparation.

TABLE 1. Relative Incidence of Dermatophytoses

Years	Tinea Capitis	Tinea Corporis	Tinea Faciale	Tinea Pedis	Tinea Cruris	Tinea Unguium
0–4	+	+	+	–	–	–
5–12	+ + + +	+ + +	+ + +	+/–	+/–	–
13–18	+	+ +	+	+ +	+	+/–

Tinea Capitis

Tinea capitis is primarily a disease of black children younger than 11 years of age. It occurs most commonly in urban, overcrowded areas. The racial prevalence is poorly understood. The essential feature is invasion of hair by the dermatophyte, resulting in broken-off hairs. Two types are seen (Table 2).

In the United States today, "black-dot" tinea capitis, caused by *T. tonsurans*, is the most common clinical presentation. A chronic noninflammatory course follows. Black dots appear from hair breaking at the skin surface, resulting in patches of baldness studded with black dots. Lesions are small (often only 2 to 3 hairs per lesion) and result in polygonal indistinct lesions with normal hairs intermixed. If extensive, a diffuse alopecia results. Scaling of the scalp mimics seborrheic dermatitis. Infected family members, often asymptomatic, represent the main source of infection. Because adult scalps can be infected, the mother may act as a continuing source of infection for other children.

"Gray-patch" ringworm is the more classic disease pattern, caused primarily by *M. canis* and *M. audouini*. This pattern involves hairs breaking off a few millimeters above the scalp, usually affecting about 95 per cent of the hairs in an area, and a dense scale on the scalp surface. This results in a clinical picture of several distinctive annular patches of hair loss and scale. It is uncommon for more than 50 per cent of the scalp to be involved.

The differential diagnosis of these conditions includes seborrheic dermatitis, psoriasis, alopecia areata, trichotillomania, traction alopecia, impetigo, pyoderma, secondary syphilis, and cicatricial alopecia.

Tinea Corporis

Tinea corporis refers to lesions on the glabrous skin of the trunk or limbs. In children, these lesions most commonly occur from contact with lesions of an infected animal (usually a kitten or puppy) or as secondary spread from lesions of tinea capitis. In adolescents, lesions result from the spread from other primary sites of infection: tinea pedis, tinea cruris, or tinea unguium.

Characteristically, the lesion is a red scaly annular patch with central clearing and an active advancing margin—classic "ringworm." Some lesions may persist for years, but the majority will resolve spontaneously after a few months. The more inflammatory the lesion, the shorter the duration.

The differential diagnosis includes psoriasis, nummular eczema, contact dermatitis, granuloma annulare, impetigo, and pityriasis rosea. One source of confusion in diagnosis is alteration of the appearance of lesions by the application of topical steroid creams after misdiagnosis. Bizarre clinical pictures may result, including hypopigmented lesions, acneiform papules, folliculitis, inflammatory papules, striae, and atrophy.

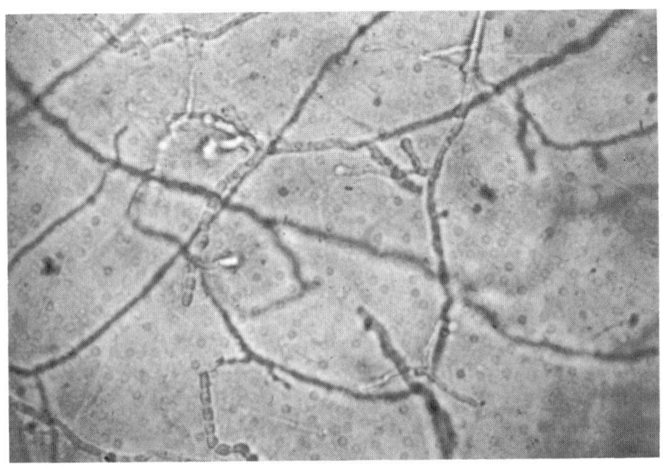

Figure 1. Potassium hydroxide preparation of epidermal scraping. Highly refractile, branching hyphae can be seen coursing through these epidermal cells.

Tinea Faciale

This is simply tinea corporis located on the face. Some lesions may be light-sensitive and may simulate systemic lupus erythematosus or polymorphous light eruption. It occurs most commonly from contact with infected pets.

Tinea Cruris

Tinea cruris refers to lesions of the groin, perineum, and perianal region. It is rare in infants and children but more common in adolescents.

The upper, inner aspect of the thighs is usually involved in a bilaterally symmetric fashion. Lesions are normally absent from the scrotum but may extend to the intergluteal fold and even out onto the buttocks. The lesion is characterized by a sharply marginated, scaling border at the periphery and may be quite inflammatory.

The differential diagnosis includes flexural psoriasis, seborrheic dermatitis intertrigo, erythrasma, neurodermatitis, and atopic dermatitis. In the infant, *Candida albicans* may produce similar lesions.

Tinea Pedis

Tinea pedis, or "athlete's foot," is by far the most common dermatophyte infection in humans. It is primarily an infection of the interdigital spaces and plantar surface of the feet related to the heat and maceration that result from wearing shoes. Prior to 7 years of age, the incidence is negligible and thereafter rises, 1 per cent being infected at age 7 to 8, 6 to 9 per cent by age 12, and 20 per cent by age 20.

Peeling, maceration, and fissuring of the skin between the toes is typical. The lesions are very persistent but may be subclinical except during periods of high temperature and humidity. With successive exacerbations, the eruption spreads to the plantar surface, sides, and dorsum of the foot. *T. rubrum* tends to cause chronic infection with dry, scaling, hyperkeratotic patches of the soles. Nails are often involved as well. *T. mentagrophytes* tends to cause vesicular lesions, single or grouped, often on the instep. These lesions are very pruritic and rupture, leaving a jagged collarette scale.

The differential diagnosis includes erythrasma, intertrigo, psoriasis, ichthyosis, eczema, and contact dermatitis.

TABLE 2. Tinea Capitis

Causative Dermatophyte	Fluorescence with Wood's Light	Potassium Hydroxide Examination	Clinical Pattern	Inflammatory Response	Spontaneous Resolution	Infection of Adults
Microsporum canis *Microsporum audouini*	Brilliant green	Hyphae inside hair Spores outside hair	Circular patches of hair loss	+ + Kerion formation "id" reaction	Months to years	No
Trichophyton tonsurans	None	Hyphae inside hair Spores inside hair (endothrix)	Irregular, ill-defined polygonal patterns of hair loss	+/− Asymptomatic carrier state described	Decades to lifetime	Yes

Tinea Unguium

Tinea unguium (or infection of the nails) usually occurs in association with tinea pedis. Infection begins in the lateral nail folds and extends under the lateral nail to the nail bed. The nail bed epithelium becomes irritated and produces soft keratin. This accumulation of subungual hyperkeratosis is the most characteristic feature of tinea unguium. Involvement is usually asymmetric and often includes only one or two nails. Early infection is characterized by subungual hyperkeratosis, brownish discoloration of the nail, and separation of the nail from the nail bed along the lateral borders, causing a yellow-white discoloration. Later in the course, the nail becomes thicker and the distal edge crumbles and becomes irregular.

The differential diagnosis for dystrophic nails includes psoriasis, eczema, lichen planus, warts, contact dermatitis, and pyogenic granuloma.

Treatment of Dermatophyte Infections

Topical Therapy

With the exception of tinea capitis, tinea unguium, and chronic tinea pedis, most lesions caused by dermatophyte infections respond to treatment with topical antifungal creams. Occasionally, these lesions require systemic therapy.

Treatment with topical agents should generally be continued for at least 1 week beyond clinical resolution because these medications are fungistatic and require elimination of fungal elements through turnover of the epidermis. For this reason, treatment should generally be continued for a minimum of 4 weeks.

Modern agents include the imidazoles: clotrimazole (Lotrimin, Mycelex), miconazole (Micatin), econazole (Spectazole), and tioconazole. Miconazole and tioconazole have been released as over-the-counter agents, as has the non-imidazole haloprogin (Halotex). All of these agents are safe and effective broad-spectrum topical antifungal agents.

Aclopirox (Loprox) is another non-imidazole antifungal agent that has proven to be equally efficacious. Naftifine (Naftin), an allylamine, is at least as effective as the imidazoles and has been shown to have an earlier onset of action. In addition, it has fungicidal-type activity and, because of its ability to concentrate in the epidermis, allows once-daily dosing without compromising effectiveness.

Systemic Therapy

The drug of choice for treatment of tinea capitis and tinea unguium is griseofulvin. Like the topical agents, griseofulvin is fungistatic, and therefore reliance is placed on noninfected griseofulvin-impregnated tissue replacing infected tissue through normal growth processes.

Griseofulvin is generally well tolerated, but side effects include headache, gastrointestinal disturbances, urticaria, pruritus, photosensitivity and transient leukopenia. Laboratory monitoring with periodic complete blood count and SMA 20 panels is recommended.

The ultramicroscopic form (Gris-peg, Fulvicin P/G) is absorbed better and is recommended. Dosages are listed in Table 3. For tinea capitis, one single oral dose of 3 g has been shown to be effective and is useful when treating an unreliable patient. In addition, the use of selenium sulfide shampoo (2½ per cent twice a week) is helpful in removing spores and fungal elements in the treatment of tinea capitis.

Ketoconazole is a newer broad-spectrum antifungal agent that has proven effective against dermatophytes. However, because of hepatotoxicity that occurs in a symptomatic form in 1 in 12,000 patients and has resulted in hepatic necrosis and death in two patients, it is generally considered a drug to be used in patients who are intolerant of griseofulvin or whose infection has been unresponsive to griseofulvin. Monitoring of hepatic function with periodic blood tests is essential.

CANDIDIASIS

Candidiasis or moniliasis is an acute or chronic fungus infection involving the skin or mucous membranes. *C. albicans* exists most commonly as a nonpathogenic colonist on pre-existing cutaneous lesions or in the gastrointestinal tract or vagina. Infection occurs by transmission from one individual to another. It is harbored in the vagina in up to 35 per cent of normal women, and this is often the source of infection in newborns.

Clinical disorders caused by *Candida* can be classified as (1) infection of mucous membranes, (2) infection of the skin, and (3) chronic mucocutaneous candidiasis.

Diagnostic Procedures

Because *Candida* can be found in large numbers as a saprophyte, it is sometimes difficult to interpret the nature of its presence. The demonstration of true segmented mycelia (budding cells and filaments) in a KOH preparation (see discussion under dermatophye infections) suggests a pathogenic state, as these are formed only after invasion of tissue. The demonstration of *C. albicans* by culture on Sabouraud's

TABLE 3. Griseofulvin Dosage and Therapy

Dosage (7.3 mg/kg/24 hr)		Therapy	
Weight (lb)	*Daily Dosage Range (mg)*	*Site*	*Duration of Therapy*
35–60*	125–187.5	Scalp	4–8 wk
60–100	187–375	Skin	3–4 wk
100–125	317–453	Palms and soles	8–12 wk
		Fingernails	4–9 mo
		Toenails†	6–18 mo

*Dosage has not been established for children 2 years of age or younger.
†Requires an increase in dosage by a factor of 50 to 100 per cent.

media is of no significance by itself. The direct examination via KOH preparation is of much more significance because of the ability to document budding spores and mycelia. This laboratory data must be considered in relationship to the anatomic location of the lesion and the clinical presentation in order to arrive at a correct diagnosis.

Infection of Mucous Membranes

Thrush. Oral candidiasis is the most common manifestation of thrush. The tongue and/or other oral surfaces are covered with discrete patches of a creamy white pseudomembrane, which are almost pure colonies of the fungus. The lesions may extend to the corners of the mouth, forming cracks and fissures covered with the creamy material, a condition known as perleche.

Oral thrush in the newborn is usually a complication of vulvovaginal-vaginal candidiasis present at the time of delivery. This can be prevented by administering a suspension of 100,000 units of nystatin in 1 ml of water into the infant's mouth on the 2nd, 3rd, and 5th days of life.

The presence of oral thrush in an infant other than a newborn requires investigation into the general health status of the patient, as it occurs much more readily in the presence of diabetes and other endocrine disturbances, immune disorders, vitamin deficiencies, malnutrition, or neoplasia.

Vaginitis. Newborn infants acquire candidal vaginitis in the same manner that they acquire thrush: from maternal infection during birth. A white or yellow curdy discharge is the most characteristic sign. Labial swelling and erythema with thrush-like patches may be present as well. As with thrush, when it appears in an older infant or child, underlying systemic disorders need to be excluded.

Infection of the Skin

Candidal Intertrigo. The most characteristic lesion of candidal intertrigo is a well-defined weeping erosion with scalloped edges and an intense red base. Satellite flaccid vesiculopustular lesions outside the main plaque are common and make the clinical picture more diagnostic. The areas of involvement are the groin, axilla, prepuce and glans penis, intergluteal cleft, and interdigital spaces. Intertrigo, seborrheic dermatitis, psoriasis, contact dermatitis, tinea, and impetigo are in the differential diagnosis, but they may also be pre-existing conditions that predispose to infection. Diabetes, obesity, and the use of systemic antibiotics also are predisposing factors.

Candidal Paronychia. Edema and erythema of the paronychial tissue and occasional purulent drainage from the nail fold are characteristic of candidal paronychia. Paronychial involvement always precedes nail changes in candidiasis. The absence of subungual hyperkeratosis and of thickening or crumbling of the nail plate differentiates this nail dystrophy from tinea. Candidal paronychia generally occurs in conjunction with mucous membrane involvement or as a secondary manifestation of the systemic disorders previously mentioned.

Diaper Dermatitis. This occurs most commonly during the 2nd to 4th months of life. When *C. albicans* is a causative agent, the intertriginous areas are usually affected and the lesions are typical of those described as candidal intertrigo. The eruption generally starts in the perianal area and spreads to involve the perineum and upper thighs. Predisposing factors include dampness and maceration, irritation from urine and feces, and contact or irritant dermatitis from rubber or plastic pants or laundry detergents and fabric softeners. Diaper dermatitis may also be a secondary infection in infants with oral or vaginal candidiasis.

In addition to treatment with appropriate antifungal creams, treatment includes keeping the area as dry as possible by changing diapers frequently, discontinuing occlusive plastic or rubber pants, and using powder frequently.

Chronic Mucocutaneous Candidiasis

Chronic mucocutaneous candidiasis is a progressive infection associated with underlying lymphocytic disorders, especially congenital thymic disorders. Symptoms generally begin during infancy with thrush or intertrigo, which are very resistant to therapy and spread to the scalp and glabrous skin. Large polycyclic plaques, resembling ringworm or psoriasis but with thick hyperkeratotic crusts, are typical. *C. albicans* proliferates in the crusts.

Defective cell-mediated immunity is a constant feature of this syndrome, but systemic candidiasis rarely occurs. When cell-mediated immunity is restored to normal, the cutaneous lesions resolve.

Treatment of Candidiasis

The first principle in treatment of candidiasis is to look for an underlying condition and to correct it. Once this has been accomplished, treatment of candidiasis will be successful using the following measures.

The treatment of all cutaneous infections requires avoidance of excessive moisture and maceration; application of antifungal creams will then effectively eliminate *C. albicans.*

In thrush, nystatin (100,000 units four times per day for 10 days) is administered by oral suspension and may be placed directly on lesions. Nystatin may be administered as a vaginal tablet containing 100,000 units and should be inserted twice daily for 7 to 14 days for vulvovaginal candidiasis.

The newer antifungal creams, the imidazoles, have a broad spectrum and are effective against *C. albicans.* This group includes miconazole (Micatin, Monistat) and econazole (Spectazole). In addition, the newer non-imidazoles are equally effective and include cicloprox (Loprox) and naftifine (Naftin). These creams and lotions should be used on areas of infection involving the skin for a period of 7 to 14 days.

TINEA VERSICOLOR

Tinea versicolor is a noninflammatory, asymptomatic, superficial fungal infection of the stratum corneum. It causes whitish to brown macular patches of superficial scale, often becoming confluent and covering large areas of the torso and proximal extremities. Direct examination of the scale reveals the causative fungus, *Malassezia furfur.* Its characteristic appearance on KOH examination is that of "spaghetti and meatballs": short filaments and grape-like clusters of budding cells. This fungus has been shown to be identical to the fungus *Pityrosporum orbiculare,* a normal inhabitant of the skin. This suggests that the condition is actually an overgrowth during conditions of heat and moisture of an organism that is part of the normal skin flora. In some typical areas, as many as 50 per cent of the population may be affected.

Tinea versicolor is common in adults and adolescents but has been considered rare in children by most authors. However, a recent survey of a mycology clinic in Italy found the condition not infrequent in patients aged 5 months to 13 years. One significant difference in pediatric patients was facial involvement—found to be present in 50 per cent of the pediatric cases but unusual among adults.

Treatment

All of the topical broad-spectrum antifungal creams are effective against tinea versicolor, including the imidazoles: miconazole (Micatin, Monistat), clotrimazole (Lotrimin, Mycelex), econazole (Spectazole), ciclopro (Loprox), and naftifine (Naftin). These should be applied once or twice daily for 2 to 3 weeks until clear. Selenium sulfide suspension is effective as well. Recurrences are common, as the source of infection appears to be from the normal skin flora.

REFERENCES

Fitzpatrick RE, Newcomer VD: Dermatophytosis and candidiasis. *In* Feigin RD, Cherry JD (eds): Textbook of Pediatric Infectious Diseases 2nd ed. Philadelphia, WB Saunders Co, 1984, pp 818–855.

Terragni L, Lasagni A, Oriani A, Gelmetti C: Pityriasis versicolor in the pediatric age. Pediatr Dermatol 8:9–12, 1991.

WARTS AND MOLLUSCUM CONTAGIOSUM

JOSEPH W. LANDAU, M.D.

WARTS

Warts are skin tumors produced by the human papillomavirus (HPV). More than 60 different types of HPV have been identified on the basis of their DNA sequences. These types have been associated with a variety of different clinical entities, including common, flat, plantar, and anogenital warts. The vast majority of these warts are benign. Certain HPV types, such as 16, 18, and 31 found in some anogenital warts, have been associated with genital dysplasias and carcinomas. Malignant transformation is also more likely to occur in warts in patients with the rare genetic disorder epidermodysplasia verruciformis and with various other types of immunosuppression.

Treatment

Common, flat, and plantar warts, particularly in children, will usually resolve spontaneously in several years. Treatment is often desired, however, to remove painful or cosmetically disfiguring warts and to prevent spread. No currently available treatment is specific, completely safe, and totally effective. The selection of any treatment must consider the age and pain tolerance of the child and the location of the wart. Treatment should produce negligible scarring and minimal disability. Warts in immunosuppressed patients occur more frequently, are widespread, and are difficult to treat.

Common and Plantar Warts

Initial treatment of common and plantar warts with salicylic acid and/or lactic acid in liquid vehicles, in plaster dressings, or in a karaya gum patch is relatively safe for home use. As part of this treatment, paring of the warts and application of 25 per cent trichloroacetic acid every few weeks in the physician's office is helpful. Common warts on the extremities can be treated with liquid nitrogen applications. This treatment is very effective if the patient can tolerate the pain. Several applications at 2- to 3-week intervals may be required. The application of cantharidin in collodion is another in-office method that is sometimes effective. Electrodesiccation is an excellent method of removing one or two common warts. Local anesthesia is necessary with this method, and scarring may occur.

Aggressive therapy is not recommended for plantar warts because any scarring on the sole may be very painful. Caution is always advised in patients with compromised peripheral circulation.

Flat Warts

Flat warts can be treated with mild peeling agents containing benzoyl peroxide, salicylic acid and lactic acid preparations, and tretinoin. Slight peeling and erythema are desirable. Several months of treatment are often required. Liquid nitrogen and electrodesiccation must be used with extreme caution on the face.

Recalcitrant Warts

Additional methods of treating recalcitrant warts are currently being studied. The superiority of these methods over conventional modalities and their safety in children have not been established. These methods include CO_2 laser vaporization, topical 5-fluorouracil, intralesional bleomycin, sensitization to dinitrochlorobenzene or squaric acid dibutyl ester, interferons, and systemic retinoids.

Anogenital Warts

Management of anogenital warts is more complex. The usual transmission is sexual, and additional studies are indicated to exclude other possibly coexistent sexually transmitted diseases. Women should have a pelvic examination and a Papanicolaou smear. Most cervical HPV infections and some lesions in men may be entirely invisible without the application of 3 to 5 per cent acetic acid and magnification. In children, the presence of anogenital warts is suggestive but not conclusively indicative of sexual abuse. Perianal warts in the absence of other genital warts is suggestive of anal intercourse and, in men, of homosexuality.

Office treatment of external anogenital warts includes local application of cryotherapy, 50 per cent trichloroacetic acid, podophyllin, and electrosurgery. Other methods include 5-fluorouracil, interferon, and laser ablation. A topical solution of podifilox, a purified derivative of the active ingredient in podophyllin, has recently been approved for self-treatment of genital warts by patients older than children. Patients with cervical, vaginal, intraurethal, and rectal warts should be managed by appropriate specialists.

MOLLUSCUM CONTAGIOSUM

Molluscum contagiosum is a common skin disease produced by a member of the poxvirus group. It is characterized by single or multiple asymptomatic, translucent, pearly papules from 2 to 15 mm in diameter with central umbilication. Some papules may become inflamed prior to their disappearance. The usual sites of involvement are the trunk, face, and extremities in children, and the anogenital region in sexually active adolescents. In young children, the presence of the papules predominantly in the anogenital region may denote sexual abuse. The disease is benign and generally clears spontaneously within several years.

Treatment

Treatment is not absolutely essential but may be desired in order to prevent spread and improve appearance. Neither systemic nor specific antiviral therapy is available. Daily topical application for 4 to 6 weeks of weak peeling agents, such as benzoyl peroxide gels, salicylic acid and lactic acid preparations, and tretinoin, is sometimes successful. Some mild degree of irritation is expected and is desirable. The in-office application of cantharidin in collodion at 2- to 3-week intervals is effective and reasonably well tolerated. Other procedures include the removal of each papule with a sharp curet and the superficial incision of each papule followed by expression of the contents with a comedo extractor. These minor surgical procedures can be performed rapidly, often without local anesthesia. Light electrodesiccation and application of liquid nitrogen are other methods of destroying the lesions. Treatment must often be repeated several times at monthly intervals as new lesions appear.

SCABIES AND PEDICULOSIS

STEPHEN E. GELLIS, M.D.

SCABIES

The diagnosis of scabies may be difficult. It combines good history taking and close inspection for burrows and typical nodules. Alterations caused by secondary infection or prior treatment with topical steroids may mask the usual findings.

Treatment

When therapy is recommended, all close contacts should be simultaneously treated to prevent later reinfection. In most circumstances, the treatment of choice is 5 per cent permethrin cream (Elimite). The medication should be applied to the entire body surface, including the head and face of infants. In older children and adults, treatment of the face and scalp can be omitted. Care should be taken to apply medication carefully underneath the fingernails and to the skin folds. The medication is left on overnight or from 8 to 12 hours. It is then removed by a bath or shower.

After treatment, clothing and bed sheets should be changed. All apparel worn in the previous several days can be set aside in a sealed plastic bag for 1 week or laundered or dry cleaned. In a heavily infested patient, a second treatment 1 week later may be recommended. It is important to inform patients that the lesions and pruritus may persist for up to 1 month after treatment.

Alternative treatments for adults and for children older than 1 year of age include 1 per cent gamma benzene hexachloride (lindane or Kwell). It can be applied in a similar manner to permethrin. Because of possible neurotoxicity when used excessively in small infants, gamma benzene hexachloride is best avoided in infants, in pregnant women, and in nursing mothers. For these three populations, 6 per cent precipitated sulfur compounded in petrolatum is an alternative. This is applied on 3 consecutive days.

PEDICULOSIS

Head Lice

Pediculosis capitis is a common infestation seen in young school-aged children. Spread occurs from close contact with infected children and from shared hats, combs, and brushes. Patients have pruritus and may show secondary infection with adenopathy.

Treatment

Permethrin 1 per cent (Nix creme rinse) is an effective and safe preparation that is applied after the scalp has been washed with regular shampoo. It is left on the scalp for 10 minutes. Removal of the dead egg cases (nits) for cosmetic reasons can be accomplished with a fine-toothed comb. If removal is difficult, the eggs can be loosened by rinsing the hair with a formic acid formulation (Step 2 creme rinse) or a 1:1 mixture of white vinegar and water. All symptomatic family members should be treated simultaneously. If live insects are seen beyond 1 week, a second application can be used.

Alternative therapy includes (1) gamma benzene hexachloride (Kwell, Scabene) in shampoo form (not recommended for infants, pregnant women, and nursing mothers because of the potential neurotoxicity); and (2) pyrethrins (A-200, RID), which are available over the counter and are applied as shampoos.

Pediculosis Pubis

Phthirus pubis is a species of lice that mainly inhabits the pubic area but occasionally spreads to eyelashes, axillae, beards, and scalps. The lice are spread by sexual contact or exposure to clothing, bedding, or towels. The treatment is the same as for head lice. Sexual partners should be treated simultaneously. All clothing, bedding, and towels should be washed and dried to destroy remaining ova.

Pediculosis Palpebrarum

Pediculosis of the eyelashes can be treated with twice-daily application of petrolatum for 1 week.

DISORDERS OF PIGMENTATION

SERGE A. COOPMAN, M.D.
and KENNETH A. ARNDT, M.D.

The color of human skin is the cumulative result of the absorption and scattering of specific wavelengths of light by both intrinsic pigments (e.g., melanin, hemoglobin) and extrinsic pigments (e.g., carotene). A clinical picture of hyperpigmentation or hypopigmentation can originate from a variety of underlying pigment anomalies. This overview is limited to pigment disorders related to the melanin-producing system. These conditions, some of which are very common, can be a cause of profound cosmetic concern in young patients and their parents, and, on occasion, they may be a presenting sign of a serious systemic disorder.

HYPERPIGMENTATION

Diagnosis

Common congenital hyperpigmented lesions include nevi, lentigines, café au lait spots, and dermal melanosis. Nevi and nevoid disorders are discussed on p. 504.

Lentigines

Lentigines are well-circumscribed brown macules, usually less than 0.5 cm in size, that may be congenital or acquired. Histologically, they show an increased number of melanocytes along the basal layer of the epidermis as well as elongated epidermal rete ridges. Lentigines are usually a sporadic finding of no consequence, but they can occur in the context of several syndromes.

Centrofacial lentiginosis is an autosomal dominant condition characterized by the occurrence of lentigines in a butterfly distribution over the nose and cheeks. In this condition, there are often associated neurologic and orthopedic abnormalities.

Peutz-Jeghers syndrome is an autosomal dominant disorder in which perioral lentiginosis is characteristically associated with intestinal polyposis and, occasionally, anomalies of the skeletal, cardiovascular, and genitourinary system.

LEOPARD syndrome is an acronym for a rare autosomal dominant disease consisting of *l*entigines, *e*lectrocardiographic abnormalities, *o*cular hypertelorism, *p*ulmonary stenosis, *a*bnormalities of the genitals, *r*etardation of growth, and *d*eafness.

Moynahan syndrome consists of lentigines, dwarfism, mental retardation, mitral stenosis, and genital hypoplasia.

LAMB and *NAME* are acronyms denoting cardiocutaneous syndromes that consist of *l*entigines, *a*trial *m*yxomas, mucocutaneous myxomas, and *b*lue nevi; and *n*evi, *a*trial *m*yxomas, myxoid neurofibromas, and *e*phelides, respectively.

Lentigines are to be distinguished from *freckles* (ephelides), which are small light-brown macules occurring exclusively on sun-exposed areas that usually become darker and more conspicuous in response to ultraviolet light. Freckles are not present at birth but develop during early childhood and tend to fade in adult life. Histologically, there is increased melanization but no increase in the number of melanocytes. In rare cases, however, excessive freckling during infancy may be a sign of a photosensitivity disorder such as xeroderma pigmentosum.

Café au Lait Spots

Café au lait spots are uniformly colored, well-defined light-brown macules that are relatively common as an isolated finding in the newborn. Histologically, these lesions show increased melanin in melanocytes and keratinocytes. Café au lait spots can also be seen in several syndromes, of which type I *neurofibromatosis* (von Recklinghausen's disease) is the most prevalent. Neurofibromatosis, an autosomal dominant disorder with a high incidence of spontaneous new mutations, is characterized by the presence of six or more café au lait spots having a diameter larger than 5 mm in prepubertal children, and larger than 15 mm in adults; axillary "freckling" (Crowe's sign); neurofibromas; Lisch nodules (hamartomas of the iris); as well as a variety of neurologic, skeletal, endocrine, and cardiovascular abnormalities. The café au lait spots may be present at birth, with their number usually increasing during childhood; the axillary "freckles," actually small café au lait spots, generally develop at a later age. Large café au lait spots in a unilateral or segmental distribution are suggestive of *Albright syndrome,* a sporadically occurring disease characterized by precocious puberty and fibrous dysplasia of the bones.

Dermal Melanosis

Dermal melanosis is a term denoting the deposition of melanin in the dermis. The pigment can be present in dermal melanocytes, in melanophages, or in the form of extracellular deposits. Because of Tyndall scattering of the short-wavelength components of light, the lesions display a bluish or slate-gray color. Dermal melanosis is responsible for the hyperpigmentation of the *Mongolian spot,* a bluish-gray macule commonly seen in the lumbosacral area of newborns principally of Asian and dark-skinned races. The intensity of the hyperpigmentation decreases gradually after birth, and most mongolian spots disappear before the age of 10 years.

A similar clinical and histologic picture is seen in *nevus of Ota* and *nevus of Ito.* These grayish-brown lesions, often intermingled with small darker maculae, are permanent and occur in skin areas supplied by the first and second division of the trigeminal nerve (nevus of Ota) or in the shoulder and neck region (nevus of Ito). In nevus of Ota, pigmented macules are often present on adjacent mucosae as well. In the majority of cases, the lesions are present at birth, but they may occasionally develop during childhood or even later in life.

Dermal melanosis is also a characteristic of *incontinentia pigmenti* (Bloch-Sulzberger syndrome), an X-linked dominant condition featuring three sequential clinical stages: (1) an acral vesicular eruption occurring in utero or in the first weeks of life; (2) the development of acral verrucous papules, usually between 2 and 6 weeks of age; and (3) the appearance of a characteristic whirled or "marble-cake" hyperpigmentation, usually developing on the trunk along the so-called lines of Blaschko between 2 weeks and 6 months of age. The third stage is characterized by pigment incontinence and the presence of dermal melanophages. The hyperpigmentation usually fades gradually over the years. There are often associated dental, ocular, and central nervous system abnormalities. The disease is lethal to the male fetus in utero.

Miscellaneous Lesions

In addition to these primary lesions of hyperpigmentation and their clinical presentation, a number of other conditions must be noted. Several types of *pigmentary demarcation lines* are frequent in dark-skinned individuals. This phenomenon is caused by natural variations in melanin distribution and is therefore without pathologic significance. Common pigmentary demarcation lines include Futcher's type A lines, which are dorsoventral lines on the upper anterior aspects of the arms, and Futcher's type B lines, which are located on the posteromedial aspect of the lower extremities.

Postinflammatory hyperpigmentation is a very frequent finding that can occur after almost any inflammatory skin condition, especially in dark-skinned individuals. The history usually provides the clue to the diagnosis. The hyperpigmentation may last for many months or even persist indefinitely because of melanin retention in dermal melanophages.

Acromelanosis is a patchy hyperpigmentation of the dorsal digits in infancy that usually fades in childhood. Histologically, there is increased basal melanization. In another, probably hereditary variant of acromelanosis, however, there is progressive involvement of other body parts (acromelanosis progressiva).

Poikiloderma congenitale of Rothmund-Thomson, an X-linked recessive disorder, is characterized by hyperpigmented patches following an erythematous skin rash, as well as by cataracts, microdentia, microcephaly, and mental retardation.

Dyskeratosis congenita, usually inherited as an X-linked recessive trait, consists of reticular hyper- and hypopigmented atrophic macules, nail dystrophy, keratoderma palmare et plantare, alopecia, dental dystrophy, mental retardation, and anemia.

In *Fanconi syndrome,* hyperpigmented macules are seen in conjunction with pancytopenia, microcephaly, and a high incidence of malignancy.

Therapy

As a first step in the clinical approach to a disorder of hyperpigmentation, sporadic lesions have to be distinguished from those that occur in syndromes in which other anomalies may exist. An appropriate investigation should be undertaken in patients with the latter type. Qualified medical advice in disorders of cosmetic significance is no superfluous luxury, however, because these conditions can in some cases interfere adversely with the normal psychosocial development of the child.

Therapy of hyperpigmentation is generally directed at diminishing the contrast between dark and light areas of skin.

Freckles

The best management of freckles, if any is desired, consists of the application of sunscreen agents with a high sun protection factor (SPF; at least 15). This also protects the child with a fair complexion from acute and chronic hazards of sunlight exposure such as sunburn and subsequent photodamage and skin cancer.

Lentigines

Treatment of lentigines is not advised; however, when treatment is sought for cosmetic purposes, it can be attempted with hydroquinone bleaches (as discussed later), liquid nitrogen cryosurgery, shave excision, or lasers (Q-switched ruby or YAG laser, the CO_2 laser at low-power density, or the pulsed-dye laser at 504 nm).

Café au Lait Spots

Treatment of café au lait spots is not indicated.

Postinflammatory Hyperpigmentation

Treatment of postinflammatory hyperpigmentation represents a common clinical problem. If the hyperpigmentation is caused by a chronic or recurrent inflammatory skin condition, prompt institution of adequate topical anti-inflammatory therapy is essential to minimize the occurrence of new lesions. As a rule, the therapies available for postinflammatory hyperpigmentation are particularly ineffective if the pigment is situated in the dermis. The persistence of melanin in pigment-laden macrophages can therefore result in permanent cosmetic disfigurement.

A Wood's lamp examination (long-wavelength ultraviolet light) of the lesion should be performed prior to the institution of therapy to determine whether the excess melanin is located in the epidermis (enhanced contrast with Wood's lamp) or dermis (decreased contrast with Wood's lamp). A Wood's lamp examination is generally not useful in dark-skinned individuals. If necessary, a skin biopsy with specific melanin staining (e.g., silver Fontana-Masson stain) can confirm the localization of the pigment.

The standard bleaching agent in clinical use is hydroquinone in a 2 to 4 per cent topical vehicle (Melanex, Eldoquin), applied twice daily over at least several months. Concomitant use of sunscreens is essential to avoid further ultraviolet light–induced darkening of the affected areas. Some authors have advocated use of a combination formula containing various concentrations of hydroquinone, retinoic acid, and hydrocortisone. Side effects of topical hydroquinone include contact sensitization, occurrence of a paradoxical hyperpigmentation referred to as pseudo-ochronosis (especially in blacks after chronic use), and pigmented colloid milium. The topical 20 per cent monobenzyl ether of hydroquinone (Benoquin) causes a complete and often irreversible depigmentation and is not indicated for the treatment of hyperpigmentation.

Dermal Melanosis

Cosmetic cover-ups (e.g., Dermablend, Covermark) are usually the only realistic therapeutic option for dermal melanosis and for many of the hereditary syndromes in which hyperpigmentation occurs.

HYPOPIGMENTATION

Diagnosis

Disorders of hypopigmentation can be subdivided into melanocytopenic disorders, in which melanocytes are absent or reduced (e.g., vitiligo, piebaldism), and melanopenic disorders, in which melanocytes are present but melanin content is subnormal (e.g., tuberous sclerosis, albinism). The distinction between complete absence and decreased content of pigment is often facilitated by use of the Wood's lamp. This is especially true in fair-skinned individuals and in most infants because of their light skin color.

Melanocytopenic Disorders

Vitiligo

Vitiligo is a common acquired disorder characterized by a symmetric pattern of well-circumscribed depigmented macules resulting from a loss of melanocytes. Sites of predilection are the periorificial areas, the skin overlying bony prominences, the groin, the axillae, and the oral mucosa. In some cases, vitiligo manifests itself in a segmental, dermatomal distribution. Hairs within the areas of depigmentation are often depigmented as well. The amelanotic areas and their extent are more apparent with Wood's lamp illumination. Vitiligo has been associated with an atopic constitution and several autoimmune diseases, including thyroid disease (both hyper- and hypothyroidism), Addison's disease, pernicious anemia, insulin-dependent diabetes mellitus, alopecia areata, and uveitis. There is a positive family history in approximately one third of cases. Vitiligo can occur within the context of the rare *Vogt-Koyanagi-Harada syndrome,* in conjunction with uveitis, signs of meningeal irritation, hearing loss, alopecia, and poliosis.

Piebaldism and Waardenburg Syndrome

Piebaldism is an autosomal dominant, stable disorder characterized by a white forelock of the scalp and circumscribed areas of hypomelanosis, especially on the anterior trunk and the extremities. Hyperpigmented macules are characteristically seen in these patches of leukoderma. The lesions are present at birth. Piebaldism is also a feature of the Waardenburg syndrome, a rare autosomal dominant condition characterized by depigmented areas of hair or skin or both, as well as by congenital sensorineural deafness, iris heterochromia, a broad nasal root, and dystopia canthorum. Both piebaldism and the Waardenburg syndrome have been reported in association with Hirschsprung's disease.

Melanopenic Disorders

Tuberous sclerosis (Pringle-Bourneville disease) is an autosomal dominant condition with a relatively high rate of spontaneous new mutations, characterized by ash-leaf–shaped hypopigmented macules, facial angiofibromas, periungual fibromas (tumor of Koenen), and shagreen patches (collagen hamartomata presenting as skin-colored, rough plaques, often in the lumbosacral region). Mental retardation, seizures, and intracranial calcifications are commonly seen in these patients. Ash-leaf spots, which are areas with reduced pigmentation resulting from an arrest in the maturation of melanosomes, occur most frequently on the trunk or lower extremities. These lesions can be found in at least 80 per cent of affected individuals upon careful examination using the Wood's lamp, and they may represent the earliest sign of the disease.

Hypomelanosis of Ito (incontinentia pigmentia achromicans) is a sporadic condition characterized by whirled, hypopigmented macules that tend to follow Blaschko's lines. The lesions are often but not always present at birth. The underlying defect is a decreased number of melanosomes in melanocytes and keratinocytes. A variety of associated abnormalities have been described, with mental retardation being the most common.

Disorders of pigment dilution are caused by widespread or generalized defects of melanin synthesis or transport.

Oculocutaneous albinism is a group of inherited disorders of the pigment system, most of which are transmitted in an autosomal recessive pattern, characterized by an absence or decreased content of melanin in the skin, hair, and eyes. Photophobia is usually present. A funduscopic examination and quantification of hair bulb tyrosinase activity may be helpful in identifying the subtype of albinism.

Hermansky-Pudlak syndrome is a rare multisystem disorder characterized by albinism, a bleeding diathesis, pulmonary fibrosis, ocular abnormalities, and ceroid deposits in various organs.

Chédiak-Higashi syndrome is a rare autosomal recessive syndrome featuring hypopigmented patches, recurrent pyogenic infections, peripheral neuropathy, and ocular anomalies.

In *phenylketonuria,* an autosomal recessive disease, a generalized pigment dilution is often seen in addition to mental retardation and seizures.

Pityriasis alba is a common disorder in children of school age, characterized by slightly scaly hypopigmented macules with indistinct borders that usually occur on the face and neck. The condition is frequent in atopic children. The lesions usually fade spontaneously over time.

Pityriasis (tinea) versicolor is a common skin disease in older children and young adults characterized by slightly scaly, hypo- or hyperpigmented macules that typically occur on the upper trunk or neck. The condition is caused by the lipophilic yeast *Pityrosporum orbiculare,* and a microscopic examination of scales demonstrates short hyphae and spores.

Postinflammatory hypopigmentation may occur after a wide variety of skin disorders, and is particularly common in association with burns, pityriasis lichenoides chronica, tuberculoid leprosy, and treponematoses such as pinta, yaws, or secondary syphilis. Spontaneous recovery is expected but may require a long time. Hypopigmentation can also occur in areas of atrophic scarring in disorders such as chronic discoid lupus erythematosus, morphea, and lichen sclerosus et atrophicus. Pigment anomalies in these conditions are often permanent.

Therapy

As with disorders of hyperpigmentation, an investigation for associated systemic anomalies should be conducted when indicated. Skin protection from the harmful effects of ultraviolet radiation is essential in all individuals with cutaneous hypopigmentation and can be accomplished with sunscreens having a SPF of at least 15. The use of sunscreens also minimizes the difference in tanning response upon ultraviolet light exposure of hypopigmented and normal skin and, hence, minimizes the color contrast. In many congenital disorders of hypopigmentation, the only useful therapy consists of the use of camouflage agents (Dermablend, Covermark).

Vitiligo

In vitiligo, partial spontaneous repigmentation can occur, but complete normalization of the skin is rare. Repigmentation is mainly the result of a migration of melanocytes from hair follicles and is therefore first seen in the perifollicular areas. Localized vitiligo patches can be treated with moderate to potent topical steroids. Patients with extensive forms of vitiligo can benefit from PUVA therapy, in which oral or topical 8-methoxypsoralen or oral trimethylpsoralen is combined with long-wavelength ultraviolet light irradiation or, occasionally, regular sun exposure (PUVA-SOL). This therapy will lead to repigmentation in many patients, but at least 100 to 200 treatment sessions are usually required to achieve a substantial response. The treatment is therefore time-consuming and expensive, and the response of cosmetically important areas, such as the hands, is usually very limited. Camouflage agents are often still needed for these parts of the body. PUVA therapy is generally not recommended for children younger than 10 years of age because of potential toxicity.

A more radical treatment for patients with extensive vitiligo may be indicated in dark-skinned individuals because of the disfiguring contrast between depigmented and normal skin. This therapy consists of a permanent total skin depigmentation with the topical 20 per cent monobenzyl ether of hydroquinone.

Pityriasis Alba

Effective therapies for pityriasis alba include moisturizers and mild hydrocortisone or tar preparations.

Pityriasis Versicolor

Pityriasis versicolor can be treated with shampoos containing selenium disulfide, zinc pyrithione, or ketoconazole; antifungal creams containing imidazole derivatives (ketoconazole or clotrimazole); and a short course of oral ketoconazole. The condition tends to recur, even after apparently successful treatment.

PHOTODERMATOSES

MOISE L. LEVY, M.D.

Dermatoses due to exposure to sunlight are generally easy to appreciate from the distribution of the cutaneous findings in affected individuals. The challenge to physicians is dealing with the wide variety of causes for photosensitivity reactions seen in patients. Such problems can be purely environmental in origin, based in genetic or metabolic diseases, the result of systemic illnesses, drug-related, or idiopathic.

DRUG-INDUCED PHOTOSENSITIVITY

Photodistributed skin eruptions should raise concern for drug-induced photosensitivity. Frequent offenders include tetracycline derivatives, sulfonamides, phenothiazines, and thiazides. Additional medications, such as amiodarone, and certain nonsteroidal anti-inflammatory agents, e.g., naproxen (and other phenyl propionic acid derivatives), have been implicated in drug-induced photosensitivity as well. Obviously, discontinuation of the suspected drugs should be attempted if at all possible. Diligent application of sunscreens should also be employed.

COLLAGEN VASCULAR DISEASES

Lupus erythematosus (LE) is a well-known systemic illness that can be marked by acute or chronic photosensitivity. The diagnosis can, at times, be difficult to confirm. An "acquired" form of LE, neonatal lupus erythematosus (NLE), is essential to recognize. This condition is often marked by a primary photodistributed dermatitis and, in some infants, by congenital heart block. The skin lesions in NLE may be annular and either papulosquamous, plaque-like, or atrophic, as well as morbilliform in appearance. Dermatomyositis, like LE, will frequently show varying degrees of photosensitivity, often marked by erythematous plaques.

Treatment consists of sunscreen use, occasional applications of topical corticosteroids, or antimalarials such as hydroxychloroquine.

GENETIC AND METABOLIC DISEASES

A number of genetic and metabolic diseases should be included in this discussion and can usually be distinguished on the basis of clinical or laboratory data. Examples include Rothmund-Thomson syndrome, ataxia-telangiectasia, Bloom and Cockayne syndromes, xeroderma pigmentosum, and the group of porphyrias.

Of the porphyrias, erythropoietic protoporphyria (EPP) is dominantly inherited and is seen in children aged 2 to 5 years. This condition is marked by itching or burning, which is followed by vesiculation and ultimately scarring over exposed surfaces after exposure to long-wavelength ultraviolet light (UVA). Other porphyrias may be seen in children but are much less common.

Again, management involves sun protection. Beta-carotene has proved quite useful in some cases of EPP. Many of the other disorders carry an increased risk of development of cutaneous or internal malignancies, necessitating cautious, long-term evaluation of affected patients.

ENVIRONMENTAL PHOTODERMATITIS

Photodermatitis can result from a variety of agents found in deodorant soaps, perfumes, and plants such as limes and figs. Many of these photoreactions are due to furocoumarins, which, when exposed to light, result in skin disease marked by erythema, vesiculation, and oozing. The often bizarre-shaped hyperpigmentation that results is sometimes confused with bruising from physical abuse.

Management, of course, involves avoidance of sun exposure and treatment of the acute reaction with mild topical corticosteroids. The postinflammatory hyperpigmentation generally resolves spontaneously over weeks to months.

POLYMORPHOUS LIGHT ERUPTION

The diagnosis of polymorphous light eruption describes a group of diseases characterized by a photodistributed eruption marked by eczematous patches, erythematous papules or plaques, or, at times, vesicles, which may resolve with superficial scarring. This group of diseases is believed to result primarily from short-wavelength ultraviolet light (UVB), although some cases are demonstrated to result from UVA exposure. It must be emphasized that the diagnosis is one of exclusion.

Treatment is necessarily based on protection from excessive sun exposure. The routine use of sunscreens is essential. In selected individuals, the use of antimalarial agents, such as hydroxychloroquine, or beta-carotene has proved useful in controlling these eruptions.

NEVI AND NEVOID TUMORS

ARTHUR R. RHODES, M.D., M.P.H.

The term *nevus,* derived from Sanskrit and Latin, refers to any abnormality that is related to conception, gestation, or postnatal development and stems from a hereditable or embryogenic fault. Nevus is commonly used to describe congenital and acquired lesions that may be neoplasms or hamartomas. A hamartoma is an abnormal mixture of tissue elements or an abnormal proportion of a single element normally present at the site that grows and develops at virtually the same rate as normal components and is not likely to result in compression of adjacent tissues (in contrast to neoplastic proliferations). The term nevus is also used histopathologically to describe a kind of cell (i.e., the nevomelanocyte) in nevomelanocytic nevus; the term may be used to describe nevomelanocytic, melanocytic, vascular, and epidermal lesions.

NEVOMELANOCYTIC AND MELANOCYTIC NEVI

Congenital Nevomelanocytic Nevus

Congenital nevomelanocytic nevi (CNN) are pigmented, benign neoplasms that are present at birth and are composed of nevomelanocytes in the epidermis and/or dermis. CNN occur in about 1 per cent of newborns, regardless of race. There appears to be no sex predilection. The prevalence in blacks and Asians appears to be twice that in whites.

CNN are defined as "small" if lesions can be excised and the wound defect closed primarily without flaps or grafts (i.e., usually <3 cm in diameter). "Large" CNN do not meet the definition of small, and "giant" CNN constitute a subset of the large, occupying a major portion of a major anatomic site. The prevalence of CNN that are greater than 99 mm in diameter is about 1 in 20,000 newborns, and that of giant CNN is about 1 in 500,000 newborns.

Small CNN are responsible for 3 to 15 per cent of cutaneous melanomas. "Giant" CNN are responsible for fewer than 0.1 per cent of melanomas. The estimated lifetime melanoma risk for people with giant CNN is about 10 per cent, whereas that for individuals with small CNN is 1 to 5 per cent. Of those melanomas associated with giant CNN, approximately half are diagnosed within the first 3 to 5 years of life. Of the melanomas associated with small CNN, the malignant potential is rare in patients younger than 12 years of age. Melanoma developing in small and large CNN occurs in whites and nonwhites.

All children with CNN, regardless of nevus size, should be evaluated to determine if a given lesion is suspected of being histologically typical, atypical, or malignant. Atypical varieties of nevomelanocytic nevi (regardless of age of patient at onset or size of nevus) should be considered for immediate excision, even if general anesthesia is required. Large varieties of CNN should be considered for surgical excision even in the first year of life, particularly darkly pigmented lesions or lesions that have an irregular surface. The first sign of malignant change in large CNN may be a palpable nodule. An alternative approach for benign-appearing large (but not giant) CNN is photographic follow-up and examination at 3- to 5-month intervals until excision can be performed safely, usually within the first several years of life. Risks of surgery and multiple general anesthetics as well as an infant's general health are all considered in the decision-making process. Large CNN should be observed using visual inspection (for color or surface change) and palpation (for a deep nodule). CNN affecting the head or neck area may be associated with leptomeningeal melanocytosis, which may be asymptomatic (and undetectable with current imaging techniques) or associated with obstructive hydrocephalus, seizures, or even melanoma.

Management of children with small CNN is still somewhat controversial because the precise lifetime melanoma risk is not clear. However, small CNN (by definition) are readily amenable to surgical excision and rarely show malignant change before puberty. Therefore, lesions that have a benign appearance can be followed up photographically until the end of the first decade of life, when they can be excised using local anesthesia and while parents still exert control over a child's health care. Excision at the end of the first decade is usually preferable to lifetime follow-up unless a lesion involves a vital structure and excision would compromise function. Parents should be counseled about the malignant potential of congenital nevi and the signs and symptoms during monthly home examinations that indicate the need for immediate evaluation.

Acquired Nevomelanocytic Nevus

Typical acquired nevomelanocytic nevi usually appear after the first 3 to 6 months of life, enlarge with body growth, and regress in later life. Approximately 75 to 85 per cent of adults have one or more acquired nevi, regardless of race. Approximately 16 to 40 per cent of children have one or more acquired nevi by age 3 years. The vast majority of acquired nevi may be left alone.

Guidelines for Excision

In regard to the indications for excision of nevi, each case must be individualized. The following guidelines may be useful:

1. *Cosmetic removal.* Desire on the part of a mature adolescent to have a nevus removed is sufficient indication for excision. Often, patients find darkly pigmented nevi cosmetically "displeasing." Pathologists will frequently detect histologic dysplasia and even melanoma in lesions removed solely for "cosmetic" purposes (by unsuspecting clinicians).
2. *Continual irritation.* Nevi exposed to continual physical irritation and that demonstrate periodic enlargement and/or discoloration are best excised to avoid confusion with neoplasia.
3. *Hidden sites.* There is a finite risk (albeit small) of melanoma arising in any nevomelanocytic nevus. Therefore, it may be reasonable to advise all affected individuals to practice periodic self-examination of nevi for symptomatic or asymptomatic change. Nevi that are difficult or impossible to follow up because of hidden location (i.e., hairy scalp or perineum) ought to be considered for excision, particularly lesions that are darkly pigmented and/or occurring in individuals with a family and/or personal history of melanoma and/or atypical (dysplastic) nevi.

There can be no rules about wholesale removal of nevi based on anatomic site alone. Lesion location (i.e., palms, soles, or genitalia, or beneath a belt, brassiere strap, or collar) is not sufficient grounds for excision of asymptomatic and benign lesions. It cannot be emphasized too strongly, however, that very darkly pigmented nevi on palms, soles, and mucosal surfaces should be viewed with suspicion and evaluated accordingly, regardless of the patient's race. On the basis of a very low prevalence in whites, pigmented nevi of nail beds and conjunctivae in this population should be evaluated for biopsy or follow-up. However, because of their high prevalence in darkly pigmented races, pigmented nevi of nail beds should be assessed on an individual basis in this population. Rapidly growing pigmented nail nevi, particularly those with pigmentation involving the nail fold, should be evaluated for histopathologic examination.

4. *Atypical appearance.* Atypical appearance of a nevus is reason enough to recommend excision. In a white individual, the most important gross features in a given lesion that may suggest an increased likelihood of atypical histology include relatively large diameter (≥ 5 mm), very dark pigmentation, haphazard and/or asymmetric distribution of pigmentation, or "fried egg" appearance. Other "atypical" features include irregular borders and/or poor demarcation from surrounding skin and heterogeneous or asymmetric topography. It has been said that presence of hair in a nevus excludes malignancy. In fact, congenital "hairy" nevi may develop melanoma. (Usually, the nodule of melanoma lacks hair.) Pigment pattern assessed using high magnification of the mineral oil–coated surface may be useful in differentiating benign from malignant melanocytic tumors.
5. *Atypical evolution.* Nevi usually grow in proportion to overall body growth for a given anatomic location. During the toddler years and puberty, growth of nevi may be striking. During growth spurts, all nevi in a given individual should be changing together. Any nevus undergoing independent growth requires expert evaluation. In general, a sudden and rapid change in color, size, or topography should be regarded as suspicious for neoplastic evolution. Although there are nonmalignant causes of atypical change (i.e., trauma, infection, and irritation), biopsy may be required to be certain about the pathology of a given lesion.
6. *Lesions posing a potential risk.* Several well-defined and clinically recognizable nevi appear to have a high risk for developing melanoma. Such lesions warrant either prophylactic excision or careful photographic follow-up indefinitely. These lesions include lentigo maligna (old age group, on sun-damaged skin), CNN, dysplastic melanocytic nevus, dysplastic and/or congenital nevus spilus, cellular blue nevus, and varieties of darkly or irregularly pigmented melanocytic proliferations on acral or mucosal surfaces. Also associated with an increased melanoma risk are a large number of prominent moles, a family or personal history of melanoma, age older than 12 years, sun-induced freckles, and excessive sun exposure and sun sensitivity.

Methods of Excision

Complete removal of benign-appearing nevi may be accomplished by elliptic excision or deep saucerization. Leaving a partially excised nevus, regardless of initial pathology, is fraught with potentially alarming repigmentation and/or regrowth simulating neoplasia (pseudomelanoma); this is not always the case, however, and individual judgment should be exercised. Lesions with an atypical histologic pattern should be excised completely or observed closely for malignant change if complete excision is not feasible without compromising function or causing mutilation.

Incisional biopsy, even for melanoma, is necessary at times, particularly for lesions that cannot be excised easily and that require histopathologic diagnosis before further therapy can be recommended. Although excisional biopsy is desirable, incisional biopsy of melanoma is not associated with an adverse prognosis. Destructive modes of therapy (electrodesiccation, cryotherapy, dermabrasion) should not be considered in the usual treatment of nevi. Although dermabrasion has been used to eliminate pigmentation of nevi, residual nevus cells in the dermis are to be expected, cosmetic outcome is often unpredictable, and recurrence with worrisome clinical and histopathologic features may complicate management.

Dysplastic Melanocytic Nevus

A subset of acquired nevi consists of dysplastic melanocytic nevi (DMN). DMN should be suspected in relatively large (≥ 5 mm diameter), irregularly formed nevomelanocytic nevi and also in any child who has one or more nevi at least 5 mm in diameter. (The presence of five nevi at least 5 mm in diameter in white adults increases the melanoma risk tenfold.)

DMN is manifested by a disordered proliferation of variably atypical intraepidermal melanocytes. This histopathologic picture is intermediate between typical nevi and melanoma. DMN occur in 2 to 5 per cent of white adults, but onset occurs during the first decade of life. If DMN are not present by age 20 years, they are unlikely to occur. DMN may occur in the presence or absence of a personal or family history of cutaneous melanoma. In the absence of a personal or family history of melanoma, the estimated melanoma risk associated with the presence of one or more DMN is increased sevenfold to more than 20-fold. In the presence of a family history of melanoma, the melanoma risk may be increased more than 100-fold and metastatic melanoma has been reported at age 10 years for lesions hidden in the hairy scalp. DMN are potential precursors of melanoma as well as markers of increased risk.

Management of children with one or more DMN is an area of ongoing discussion. The goal of management is to remove lesions that raise clinical suspicion of melanoma before metastasis occurs. The following guidelines must be individualized:

1. It is advisable to confirm the diagnosis of DMN by excising one or two of the most atypical lesions to provide a more solid basis for making additional management recommendations. Pathologic diagnosis is not mandatory. Even without histology, periodic follow-up can be recommended for children who have slightly irregular DMN, a prominent number of nevi, and/or one or more large nevi, in which the histology in any single nevus is not likely to be sufficiently atypical to firmly establish the diagnosis of DMN.

2. For children who have only one or two lesions suspicious for being DMN, excision is reasonable but periodic examination is required for a lifetime. Affected children may be expected to have new DMN over time. Prophylactic removal of numerous DMN is impractical, mutilating, and will not obviate the need for periodic examination. Lesions that are difficult to monitor (i.e., hairy scalp, perianal area) should be considered for prophylactic excision. Other lesions to be considered for prophylactic excision include those that are extremely atypical in gross appearance, those that are documented to be new or changing, those in patients for whom medical follow-up is deemed likely to be inadequate, and those in immunosuppressed patients.

3. For children who have numerous DMN, clinical photographs are invaluable for detecting changing lesions or "new" lesions over time.

4. Self-examination should be practiced every 4 to 6 weeks using full-length mirrors and hand-held mirrors for difficult-to-examine sites. Family members should be enlisted to assist in these examinations and should be made aware of signs and symptoms in a nevus that indicate the need for immediate evaluation. Patients with DMN should be examined every 3 to 6 months by a physician who is expert in the evaluation of nevi, depending on the "activity" and gross abnormalities of nevi and the demonstrated risk of melanoma in the individual or kindred.

5. Patients who have undergone excision of DMN (and/or melanoma) in the past and who have no pigmented lesions remaining should still be followed up yearly for evidence of new lesions. The relationship between hormonal factors and the progression of DMN to melanoma is unknown. Patients with DMN (or melanoma) who are pregnant or taking reproductive hormones should be observed closely.

6. All bloodline relatives in melanoma-prone families should be examined at least once for DMN and/or melanoma, and, if unaffected, at least yearly until age 20 years. For people with DMN or melanoma, with or without a family history of melanoma or DMN, it is prudent to recommend examination of first-degree bloodline relatives for DMN and melanoma. These examinations should be started at about age 5 or 6 years.

7. Ultraviolet radiation (UVR) exposure, to either artificial or natural sources, may promote cellular alterations in genetically "initiated" melanocytes in DMN (or even in normal skin in such individuals) that may permit the formation of new DMN or *de novo* melanoma, cause progression of pre-existing DMN to melanoma, or adversely affect immune surveillance of neoplastic progression. People who have DMN should avoid sunbathing, getting red in the sun, or being exposed during the peak intensity hours of 10 A.M. to 3 P.M. during spring and summer. Wearing a cover-up made of tightly woven fabric and applying a sunscreen with a maximum sun protection factor (SPF) to body sites that cannot be covered easily are recommended to protect exposed sites during sun exposure.

8. Eye care given to patients with DMN is controversial. Although there are case reports of ocular melanoma associated with DMN and/or cutaneous melanoma, such cases are likely to be coincidental. Ophthalmologic examinations conducted in patients with DMN in the familial melanoma setting failed to reveal intraocular melanoma or atypical choroidal nevi, and 6 years of observation of 14 melanoma-prone families with DMN failed to reveal ocular melanoma. Uveal melanoma and cutaneous melanoma do not appear to be etiologically linked through the presence of DMN. Until there is more conclusive information, individuals with DMN, whether or not there is a personal or family history of melanoma, should receive the same level of eye care as recommended for the general population.

9. Complete surgical excision is the current method of removing suspicious DMN, either to establish the diagnosis or to prevent melanoma progression in suspicious lesions. For patients with hundreds of DMN, excision of each and every lesion is impractical. Destructive modes of therapy are to be avoided. All excised nevi should be subjected to histopathologic examination. The use of topical 5 per cent 5-fluorouracil and topical tretinoin to remove DMN is currently experimental (and not very reliable, in fact).

Halo Nevus

Nevomelanocytic nevi that are surrounded by a rim of depigmentation are called halo nevi. The halo phenomenon may occur in one or more acquired nevi as well as in other varieties of skin lesions. CNN, both large and small, may occasionally develop the halo phenomenon. The depigmented halo is usually devoid of melanocytes. The cause of the depigmentation is unknown. Approximately 0.9 per cent of adults and 0.1 per cent of 3 year olds have one or more halo nevi.

In benign halo nevi, the nevus is centered symmetrically in the area of depigmentation. The central nevus may remain pigmented or may become depigmented and even regress over time. Melanoma of the skin may occasionally present with a depigmented halo; however, unlike benign halo nevi, the depigmented halo associated with melanoma is asymmetric and the central nevus usually has an atypical appearance.

The appearance of halo nevi should trigger a careful examination of the skin for associated features, including atypical nevi, melanoma, and vitiligo. A Wood's lamp examination may be required to visualize halo nevi (and vitiligo) in lightly pigmented individuals. Vitiligo occurs in 18 to 26 per cent of patients who have halo nevi, and 20 per cent (range 0.5 to 50 per cent) of vitiligo patients have halo nevi. Halo nevi may be associated with poliosis, Vogt-Koyanagi-Harada syndrome, pernicious anemia, a personal or family history of cutaneous melanoma and/or dysplastic nevi, and, very rarely, ocular melanoma. The number of halo nevi per person may be one or many, the frequency of multiple lesions being 25 to 50 per cent of cases. Usually, only one or a few pigmented lesions in a given individual are affected; in rare instances, however, dozens of lesions may occur. Any nevus in any anatomic site may be involved, but the posterior torso is most commonly affected.

Lesions are usually asymptomatic. Ultraviolet radiation may cause redness and even blistering in the perinevic halo. If no abnormalities are detected, treatment should consist of periodic examination for associated diseases and protection of the depigmented areas of the skin with clothing or high-SPF sunscreens to prevent sun damage and epidermal skin cancer.

Nevus Spilus

Nevus spilus (derived from Greek *spilos,* "spot"; thus, a genetic anomaly that is spotty) is defined as circumscribed tan pigmentation consisting of lentigo simplex (brown macular pigmentation composed of epidermal melanocytic hyperplasia), in which more darkly pigmented raised or flat speckled melanocytic and/or nevomelanocytic hyperplasias are present. Most lesions are relatively small, but giant varieties occur. There are no associated abnormalities or conditions in the vast majority of cases. Lesions are usually acquired but occasionally appear at birth. Nevus spilus occurs in 2 per cent of children aged 8 to 16 years. There does not appear to be a sexual predilection.

Although there are nine well-documented cases of melanoma developing in contiguity with nevus spilus, there can be no absolute rules about managing affected patients. Small lesions usually have a minor cosmetic deficit. Very large lesions may be more disturbing, especially those occupying a large anatomic area. Complete excision is often difficult. Clinical appearance, history of stability or instability of pigmented elements, congenital or noncongenital onset, and perceived risk of developing melanoma may help to determine treatment. The speckled melanocytic and/or nevomelanocytic elements of *congenital nevus spilus* should be evaluated for prophylactic excision or followed photographically for suspicious change. Atypical-appearing, new, and/or unstable elements in nevus spilus should be evaluated for histopathologic examination to exclude melanoma.

Epithelioid Cell and/or Spindle Cell Nevomelanocytic Nevi

Epithelioid cell and/or spindle cell nevomelanocytic nevi (EC-SC nevi) are unique, usually acquired, usually benign melanocytic tumors differing grossly and histopathologically from typical acquired nevi but are so alarming in their clinical presentation and sufficiently bizarre histologically that they cause diagnostic confusion with melanoma. Other terms for EC-SC nevi include Spitz's juvenile melanoma, benign juvenile melanoma, Spitz's tumor, prepubertal melanoma, and compound melanocytoma.

EC-SC nevi are not restricted to children. About two thirds of cases occur in persons older than 14 years of age. There appears to be no sexual predilection. Published cases have been described primarily in whites; a small number of cases have been reported in darkly pigmented races. Familial aggregation does not usually occur. The incidence of EC-SC nevi is about 1/15 as common as cutaneous melanoma.

The most common variety of the EC-SC nevus is the solitary, asymptomatic, pink or red, hairless, firm, dome-shaped, verrucous or smooth-surfaced telangiectatic papule or nodule. Very darkly pigmented lesions constitute a minority of EC-SC nevi, that is, up to 7 per cent of cases. The diameter of a EC-SC nevus ranges from several millimeters to several centimeters, but in more than 90 per cent of cases the tumor is less than 10 mm in diameter. The duration of solitary EC-SC nevi before presentation is usually less than 9 months. In a minority of cases, lesions have been present for many years; a congenital history has been documented for some lesions. Indeed, of the 13 original cases reported by Sophie Spitz in 1948, six cases were described as having been present since birth. Lesions usually show an increase in radial size over time, some gradual and others rapid. Lesions may occur anywhere, but the dominant location is the head or neck (42 per cent), followed by the upper extremities (21 per cent), torso (21 per cent), and lower extremities (16 per cent). EC-SC nevi tend to spare palms, soles, and mucous membranes.

Although the bizarre histology and frequent occurrence of dermal inflammation may cause diagnostic confusion, EC-SC nevi can usually be differentiated from melanoma. Nonetheless, tumors believed to have a histologic pattern identical to that of EC-SC nevi may occasionally metastasize.

Nonpigmented varieties of EC-SC nevi may resemble juvenile xanthogranuloma, hemangioma, pyogenic granuloma, molluscum contagiosum, primary dermal nevomelanocytic nevus, solitary mastocytoma, granuloma (i.e., sarcoid, foreign body reaction), insect bite reaction, and dermatofibroma. Pigmented varieties of EC-SC nevi may appear similar to nodular melanoma, dysplastic nevus, fibrous histiocytoma, sclerosing hemangioma, appendage tumor, keloid, and unusual varieties of acquired junctional and compound nevomelanocytic nevus. Warty variants of EC-SC nevi may be confused with verruca vulgaris, seborrheic keratosis, and epidermal nevus. Histologic examination is required to establish the diagnosis of EC-SC nevi.

Conservative total excision with 5- to 10-mm lateral margins, depending on location, is the author's treatment of choice for the EC-SC nevus. Incompletely excised lesions may recur, and recurrent lesions may lead to diagnostic confusion. Recurrences related to incomplete excision may occur because of inapparent junctional activity extending beyond the elevated portion of the tumor and/or deep dermal involvement extending laterally from the main body of the tumor. Treatment of the rare presentation of numerous EC-SC nevi requires individual judgment and periodic examination using clinical photographs to aid in the assessment of new or changing lesions.

The natural history of EC-SC nevi is unknown because the lesions are usually singular and histologic confirmation is required to establish the diagnosis. The concern is that some varieties of a EC-SC nevus may progress to melanoma or represent melanoma from the outset.

DERMAL MELANOCYTOSIS AND MELANOCYTOMA

Congenital Dermal Melanocytosis (Mongolian Spot)

Congenital dermal melanocytosis, also known as mongolian spot, refers to a "rest" of melanoblast-derived, melanin-producing cells that normally migrate through the dermis on their way to epidermal destinations, presenting as blue-gray macules at birth. Most lesions of dermal melanocytosis occur on the sacrogluteal region or shoulders. Lesions may be single or multiple and may vary in size from a few millimeters in diameter to involvement of large areas. Rarely, dermal melanocytosis may be generalized.

There is no malignant potential associated with ordinary varieties of congenital dermal melanocytosis. No treatment is necessary. Disappearance within the first 5 years of life occurs in the vast majority of cases. About 4 per cent of lesions persist to adulthood.

Nevus of Ota and Nevus of Ito

Nevus of Ota, also called nevus fuscoceruleus ophthalmomaxillaris, is a unilateral slate-gray and blue-brown, speckled macular pigmentation usually occurring in the distribution of the first and second divisions of the trigeminal nerve and involving the periorbital, temporal, malar, and/or frontal areas of the facial skin. Skin pigmentation may be black, black-purple, blue-black, deep blue, slate-blue, purple-brown, or faint brown, and intensity of pigmentation may vary from day to day, particularly in females. Pigmentation also may be noted in the ipsilateral scleral connective tissue. Lips, oral palate, and nasal mucosa also may be involved. Occasional lesions are bilateral.

Approximately 50 per cent of cases are congenital or appear very early in childhood, with the remainder developing by the second decade of life. Lesions occur mostly in Asians and blacks, rarely in whites. The prevalence has been reported to be 0.2 to 0.8 per cent of Japanese outpatients. Familial aggregation has been reported. There appears to be a female predominance. Rare cases are associated with sensorineural deafness. Nevus of Ito, or nevus fuscoceruleus acromiodeltoideus, has the same clinical features as nevus of Ota except that lesions are located on the scapula and deltoid area.

The pathology of nevus of Ota and nevus of Ito is similar, with melanin-producing melanocytes and melanin-laden macrophages usually in the superficial reticular dermis. The more superficial location of melanin in these lesions (compared with congenital dermal melanocytosis) is responsible for their brownish cast.

Nevus of Ota has been associated with leptomeningeal melanocytosis and leptomeningeal melanoma as well as with melanoma developing from the iris, choroid, orbit, and uveal tract. Melanoma developing in the skin of nevus of Ito also has been reported. Patients with nevus of Ota and nevus of Ito should be observed periodically for signs and symptoms of early melanoma. Excision, dermabrasion, or laser surgery should be considered on an individual basis. Repeated cryotherapy has been reported to help fade pigmentation temporarily. Cosmetic cover-up may be helpful. Pigmentation may fade with time.

Blue Nevus

Types of Blue Nevi

The cutaneous blue nevus (dermal melanocytoma) consists of an acquired or congenital blue, blue-gray, or blue-black papular, nodular, or plaque-like aggregate of aberrant dermal melanocytes actively producing melanin. Three types of cutaneous blue nevi are recognized: (1) common blue nevus, (2) cellular blue nevus, and (3) combined blue nevus–nevomelanocytic nevus.

The *cellular blue nevus* differs from the *common blue nevus* in that it is usually larger, more elevated, more aggressive locally, usually congenital, and occasionally associated with development of melanoma. Common blue nevi are usually not noted until after the first decade of life. About 3 per cent of Japanese males aged 18 to 26 years have one (or occasionally more) common blue nevi. About 0.5 per cent of white adults have a common blue nevus. Common blue nevi are usually singular. Multiple blue nevi have been reported in association with a syndrome consisting of periorificial lentigines, atrial or ventricular cardiac myxoma, and mucocutaneous myxomas (LAMB syndrome).

Common blue nevi are usually acquired, solitary, asymptomatic blue, blue-gray, or blue-black papules, usually smaller than 10 mm in diameter. Lesions occur anywhere, but about half the cases occur on the dorsa of hands and feet. Cellular blue nevi are blue-gray or blue-brown nodules or plaques, 1 to 3 cm in diameter and occasionally larger. About half of cellular blue nevi are located on the buttock or sacrum. Very large congenital blue nevi have been reported.

Combined blue nevus–nevomelanocytic nevus and a compound variant of blue nevus are usually excised as atypical nevi or suspected melanomas that have a blue-brown and/or blue-black color, variable size, and smooth or slightly irregular surface.

In the common blue nevus, dermal melanocytes appear as melanin-containing fibroblast-like cells grouped in irregular bundles admixed with melanin-containing macrophages, intimately associated with excessive production of fibrous tissue in the mid or upper reticular dermis. In the cellular blue nevus, there are usually components of common blue nevus associated with fascicles of spindle-shaped cells with ovoid nuclei and abundant pale cytoplasm with little or no melanin and often epithelioid cells, present in the dermis and often subcutaneous fat, in nests, bundles, and neuroid forms, with little or no intervening stroma. In the combined blue nevus–nevomelanocytic nevus, there is a typical nevomelanocytic nevus or spindle cell and/or epithelioid cell nevus in the epidermis and/or dermis.

Diagnosis and Treatment

Blue nevi may be confused clinically with sclerosing hemangioma, dermatofibroma, histiocytoma, glomus tumor, primary or metastatic melanoma, pyogenic granuloma, pigmented spindle cell nevus, and traumatic tattoo. For definitive diagnosis, biopsy is necessary. Mongolian spots, nevus of Ota, and nevus of Ito also are accumulations of melanin-producing melanocytes in the dermis, but, unlike typical blue nevi, these forms of dermal melanocytosis are congenital, usually broad in extent, and macular.

Common blue nevi that are stable for many years in an adult usually demand no therapy. Sudden appearance of a blue nodule, expansion of a pre-existing blue nodule, a congenital blue nodule, or a relatively large blue nodule or plaque ($\geq$10 mm in diameter) demands evaluation for histopathologic examination. Excision should include subcutaneous fat to ensure complete removal of deep dermal melanocytes, which are frequently present in the subcutaneous tissue of cellular blue nevi.

At least a dozen cases of melanoma developing in association with cellular blue nevus have been described. Cellular blue nevi should be evaluated for excision because of their malignant potential.

VASCULAR LESIONS

Vascular lesions may be separated into ectasia, malformation, and tumorous proliferation. Capillary ectatic lesions may be transient (salmon patch) or relatively permanent and even progressive (nevus flammeus). Vascular malformations may be superficial and/or deep and are permanent. Tumorous capillary endothelial proliferative lesions may be benign and reversible (capillary hemangioma) or malignant (angiosarcoma).

Transient capillary ectatic lesions are apparent at birth and usually regress by 2 years of age. Varieties of permanent capillary ectatic lesions (nevus flammeus) also are usually apparent at birth and are often progressive in cosmetic and/or functional deformity. Vascular malformations involve larger blood vessels, are usually apparent within the first few years of life and often at birth, and are usually slowly progressive in their cosmetic and functional deformity. Benign tumorous endothelial proliferative lesions (i.e., strawberry hemangioma) are usually apparent within the first year of life, have a rapidly progressive course within the first few months of life, and regress in more than 90 per cent of cases by the end of the first decade of life.

It is important to be able to distinguish the various types of vascular lesions in order to offer timely and appropriate therapy or to withhold therapy if appropriate.

Capillary Ectatic Lesions

Transient Capillary Ectasia

One of the most common skin lesions in the newborn is the salmon patch, also called angel's kiss, nevus simplex, and macular hemangioma. Lesions occur as single or multiple blanchable pink macules over the eyelids, forehead, and glabella in 40 per cent of normal newborns. Compared with nevus flammeus, salmon patches are smaller in diameter, less intense in color, and transient in nature. Salmon patches become more intensely red with crying or fever. The pathology of this lesion is presumed to be focal dilatation of capillaries. The cause is not known. The vast majority of eyelid salmon patches fade within 1 year, whereas glabellar lesions are more persistent.

Capillary ectasia occurs on the neck in 50 per cent of newborns and is called erythema nuchae (stork bite, Unna's nevus). Capillary ectasia on the neck tends to be more persistent than facial lesions. Nuchal lesions are still visible in 50 per cent of cases at 1 year of age and in 25 per cent of cases in adults.

Treatment is usually not necessary for salmon patches or erythema nuchae. Fading is the rule for the former, and hair usually camouflages the latter.

Nevus Flammeus

Nevus flammeus, also called port-wine stain or telangiectatic nevus, is apparent at birth in 0.3 per cent of infants and consists of progressive capillary ectasia (but no endothelial proliferation) and increased numbers of vessels in the superficial dermis (and later involving deep dermis).

There is a sharply demarcated area of macular pink, deep red, or purple (or jet black in darkly pigmented skin). The surface is usually flat in early childhood, but a thickened surface frequently occurs over time. Small polypoid papules occur later in life and consist of proliferations of thick- and thin-walled vessels and surrounding stroma. Very pale lesions may become less visible over time, but even pale lesions become apparent with vasodilatation from crying, heat, or flushing.

Lesions may occur anywhere on the skin but are found most commonly on the face. Mucous membranes may be involved. Lesions may be a few millimeters in size or occupy a significant portion of body surface. Extensive lesions on extremities may be associated with soft tissue and/or bony hypertrophy (see discussion of Klippel-Trénaunay-Weber syndrome later). Involvement of the face in the ophthalmic division of the fifth cranial nerve (V1) may be associated with central nervous system (CNS) disease (see discussion of Sturge-Weber syndrome next). Glaucoma is possible if the eyelid is involved. Eye and/or CNS complications are most frequently seen when the nevus flammeus simultaneously involves V1, V2, and V3 trigeminal sensory areas, but involvement of V2 alone and V2 and V3 alone also may be associated with eye and/or CNS complications. In 91 per cent of patients with eye and/or CNS complications, the nevus flammeus involved both the upper and the lower eyelids; only 9 per cent had involvement of the lower eyelid alone. Glaucoma is rare if only the upper eyelid is involved with nevus flammeus. Total involvement of V1 is much more likely to be associated with CNS disease than is partial involvement of V1. Bilateral nevus flammeus is a risk factor for CNS disease.

Sturge-Weber Syndrome. Also called encephalofacial or trigeminal angiomatosis, the syndrome consists of nevus flammeus involving the first branch of the trigeminal nerve and at least one of the following manifestations: ipsilateral vascular malformation or calcification of the meninges and cerebral cortex, focal motor seizures, and hemiparesis contralateral to facial lesions. Familial aggregation is the exception. Nevus flammeus is usually unilateral but may be bilateral. Similar lesions may occur at any site, and intraoral involvement may present as vascular hyperplasia of the lips, maxillary gingiva, tongue, and/or buccal mucosa. Cerebral calcification is progressive but is evident only after the second year of life in 90 per cent of cases. Seizures occur in up to 80 per cent of patients, manifesting before age 1 year in 50 per cent of cases. Behavior disturbance and mental deficiency may occur.

Computed tomography (CT) scan and nuclear magnetic resonance imaging (MRI) of the brain will usually visualize the vascular malformation. Ocular manifestations occur in up to half the cases in the form of angiomatosis of the conjunctiva, iris, or choroid, manifested as congenital or late-onset glaucoma, enlargement of the eyeball, angioma of the choroid, hemianoptic defects, and optic atrophy. Prognosis of Sturge-Weber syndrome depends on the extent of cerebral involvement and progression. Anticonvulsant therapy and neurosurgical intervention are often helpful. Excessive vascular change of the gingiva may require surgical excision, sclerosing solutions, and x-irradiation.

Treatment. Treatment of cutaneous nevus flammeus may not be necessary if lesions are pale and inconspicuous. Conspicuous lesions may require camouflage make-up. Argon laser therapy is useful for darker lesions in older children. The flashlamp-pulsed tunable dye laser may be useful for very young children, with little or no scarring resulting, but local discomfort of treatment usually requires restraint, heavy sedation, or general anesthesia. Any eyelid involvement, upper or lower, warrants ophthalmologic investigation.

Vascular Malformation

Vascular malformations, also known (probably incorrectly) as cavernous hemangiomas, appear at birth in 90 per cent of cases as soft and compressible, bluish-red subcutaneous tumors. Unlike strawberry hemangiomas, vascular malformations grow in proportion to body growth and continue to progress after age 12 months. There may be more rapid growth during puberty. Lesions are composed of vascular channels lined by flat and mature endothelium, without evidence of endothelial proliferation or an increased labeling index. Lymphatic elements may be present and may predominate in some cases. Vascular malformations are hemodynamically low flow, compared with arterial malformations, which are high flow. Vascular malformations may be associated with underlying skeletal distortion, hypertrophy, erosion, hypoplasia, and demineralization.

Evaluation by a plastic surgeon is indicated when the lesion's true nature is suspected. Functional and cosmetic deformity tend to persist and worsen.

Capillary Hemangioma

Capillary or strawberry hemangioma is a vascular abnormality occurring in 1 to 3 per cent of normal newborns and 9 per cent of infants between the ages of 1 and 12 months. The frequency is higher in preterm infants. About 90 per cent of lesions occur within the first month of life. Lesions are singular in 80 per cent of cases. Rarely, there may be hundreds of lesions.

Superficial lesions begin as a red macule that develops into a strawberry mass with well-circumscribed borders. Deep lesions appear as a spongy blue mass. Lesions grow rapidly for 6 to 8 months and then stabilize for a time before beginning to regress, usually not growing after age 12 months. Eighty per cent of cases exhibit maximal growth and are less than double their original size during the first 2 years of observation. Fewer than 5 per cent of cases triple in size, and 2 per cent quadruple in size. Superficial hemangiomas disappear by age 5 years in 50 per cent of cases, by age 7 years in 70 per cent, and by age 9 years in 90 per cent, leaving an area of pale and/or redundant skin. Fewer than 5 per cent of cases result in cosmetic deformity. Deeper hemangiomas usually regress as well, whereas vascular malformations continue to progress. Histologically, the proliferative phase is characterized by endothelial hyperplasia, with and without lumen formation, and a high labeling index. The involuting phase shows fibrous and fatty infiltration, diminished cellularity, and a labeling index that approaches zero.

Treatment

Generally, no therapy is needed. However, if a lesion encroaches on vital structures, intervention may be necessary. Lesions may respond to injected and systemic corticosteroid therapy during the rapidly proliferative phase of growth. Cryotherapy and laser may be useful in some cases. Ionizing radiation is not advisable in the usual case. Lesions may erode and become infected during spontaneous resolution. Orbital involvement requires ophthalmologic evaluation. Prolonged mechanical closure of eyes or encroachment of the globe (or compression of the optic nerve) during infancy may result in amblyopia or failure to achieve stereoscopic vision.

Syndromes Associated with Vascular Nevi

Multiple Diffuse Cutaneous Hemangiomas (Diffuse Neonatal Hemangiomatosis). These hemangiomas may be present at birth or develop during the first few weeks of life and also involve the liver, gastrointestinal tract, CNS, and/or lungs. Complications include arteriovenous shunts, high-output cardiac failure, hepatic dysfunction, gastrointestinal hemorrhage, respiratory tract obstruction, thrombocytopenia, and CNS compromise. Systemic corticosterioid therapy should be considered for compromise of vital organ function by space-occupying lesions, bleeding, or hematologic complications.

Sacral Hemangiomas. These hemangiomas may be associated with imperforate anus, renal anomalies, bony deformities of the sacrum, lipomeningomyelocele, and skin tags in the genital and sacral areas.

Lumbar cutaneous hemangioma has been associated with tethered spinal cord in asymptomatic infants. Neurologic deficits develop if the tethering is not released. Tethering can be detected using MRI. Because spinal laminae are poorly calcified in infants, plain lumbosacral spine radiographs in infants will not show tethered cords and may not register occult spina bifida. Other common stigmata of occult spinal dysraphism include subcutaneous lipoma, a hairy tuft, a prominent dimple, or a midline sinus tract or skin defect.

Blue Rubber Bleb Nevus Syndrome. This syndrome involves the association of one or more painful, compressible, cutaneous vascular malformations of the venous type with similar lesions in the gastrointestinal tract (mostly small intestine or colon) and is present at birth or very early childhood. Adult onset has been described. Major complications include anemia, bleeding (rectal, stomach, nasal), and orthopedic problems. Most cases are sporadic, but familial aggregation may occur. This syndrome requires early recognition and aggressive intervention using sclerosing techniques or laser surgery for gastrointestinal lesions. Treatment of cutaneous and skeletal involvement is dependent on cosmetic and functional deformity.

Maffucci Syndrome. This disease is characterized by vascular overgrowths or malformations (hemangiomas, phlebectasias, and lymphangiomas) and dyschondroplasia, usually appearing at the end of the first decade of life as hard nodules on the fingers or toes and elsewhere followed by pathologic fractures and skeletal deformities. Maffucci syndrome occurs more frequently in males and has a 30 per cent chance of malignancy (chondrosarcoma or angiosarcoma). Management consists of surgical excision of bothersome nodules or lesions suggestive of malignancy.

Cobb Syndrome. This syndrome consists of a nevus flammeus or angiokeratoma in a dermatomal distribution on the trunk or extremity associated with intraspinal arteriovenous malformation, involving a sharp sensory level, spastic paralysis, and decreased sensation to all stimuli at the same level as the cutaneous lesion.

Klippel-Trénaunay-Weber Syndrome. This disease consists of vascular malformation (i.e., port-wine stain, capillary hemangioma, cavernous hemangioma, phlebectasia, arteriovenous fistula, and/or lymphangioma) associated with hypertrophy of soft tissue and bone (length and breadth) on an extremity. Cutaneous lesions may simulate Kaposi sarcoma. Complications include infection and functional deformity. Treatment is palliative.

Kasabach-Merritt Syndrome. This syndrome consists of thrombocytopenia, microangiopathic hemolytic anemia, and consumptive coagulopathy associated with a rapidly enlarging capillary hemangioma, vascular malformation, or hemangioendothelioma. Skin lesions may be as small as 5 to 6 cm in diameter. Mortality ranges from 20 to 30 per cent. A 2- to 4-week course of systemic corticosteroid therapy may be helpful in preventing further growth of the lesion and perhaps restoring normal clotting.

Gorham Syndrome. This disease consists of cutaneous hemangiomas in association with osteolysis and fibrosis of bone ("disappearing bones"). The cause of bone resorption is not known. Gorham syndrome does not appear to aggregate in families. The disease first manifests in early childhood, involving one or more bones. There is no associated malignancy.

ORGANOID NEVI

Epithelial Nevi

Epithelial nevi are circumscribed developmental defects of epidermal structures consisting of epidermal hyperplasia. Lesions appear as single or multiple, well-demarcated, hairless, linear, flesh-colored to hyperpigmented verrucous plaques usually involving a small area of body surface. These nevi may appear at birth, but more often they appear during early infancy or childhood and occasionally even during early adulthood. Small lesions are usually not associated with any other abnormalities. Very extensive lesions may be unilateral or bilateral and may be associated with skeletal defects, vascular anomalies, and serious CNS disease. Underlying anomalies include kyphoscoliosis, vertebral defects, short limbs, phocomelia, osseous hypertrophy, abnormalities of eyes and teeth, angiomas of skin and CNS, mental retardation, and seizures. Associated abnormalities are usually present within the first several years of life. Epithelial neoplasia (basal cell carcinoma and squamous cell carcinoma) may occur rarely.

Therapy should be withheld until the lesion is fully evolved, which may take several years. Therapy for relatively small lesions should be individualized and includes surgical excision, cryotherapy, electrodesiccation and curettage, and dermabrasion of the lesion plus underlying reticular dermis. Large lesions may be difficult or impossible to remove without extensive grafting. Removal of excessive and often foul-smelling hyperkeratosis in very large lesions may be accomplished using judicious use of topical keratolytics.

Nevus Sebaceus

Nevus sebaceus is a congenital hamartoma of malformed sebaceous glands and other epidermal appendageal elements. Lesions occur in 0.3 per cent of newborns as a single, circumscribed, slightly elevated, hairless, yellow to orange or red, linear or oval plaque. The most common locations are the face and scalp. Rarely, extensive lesions involve half the face or scalp, associated with ocular dermoids, ocular colobomata, cerebral cysts, mental retardation, seizures, and skeletal abnormalities. No race is spared, and there is no sex predilection. Lesions usually remain stable throughout life. Risk of malignant degeneration is estimated to be 5 to 10 per cent; mostly epithelial carcinoma is found, but other epithelial tumors may occur. Treatment consists of careful periodic observation for neoplasia during infancy and early childhood, followed by surgical excision (if easily accomplished) around the time of puberty.

Becker's Nevus

Becker's nevus (pigmented hairy epidermal nevus, Becker's melanosis, nevus pigmentosus et tardus, nevoid melanosis) is a variety of organoid hamartoma involving epidermal, melanocytic, and dermal elements. Lesions consist of solitary, concurrent, light-brown, macular, blotchy pigmentation associated with a normal or slightly increased number of melanocytes producing abnormally increased amounts of melanin, plus hypertrichosis. Lesions are most common on the anterior and/or posterior torso in a unilateral distribution. Most lesions first appear as macular pigmentation during the first decade, followed by hypertrichosis in the second decade. Sixty per cent of lesions develop in patients by age 15 years. (Similar lesions have been reported to be congenital.) Lesions occur in 0.5 per cent of males and are about one fifth as common in females.

Treatment is usually not necessary. There is no malignant potential. Hair may be shaved or epilated. Pigmentation may temporarily respond to nonscarring cryotherapy or laser. Another lesion in the same spectrum of abnormality is the arrector pili hamartoma (smooth muscle hamartoma), which usually appears at birth and consists of hypertrichosis, slight pigmentation, and slight induration. This hamartoma has no malignant potential and may be confused with congenital nevomelanocytic nevus.

OTHER SKIN TUMORS

MARY K. SPRAKER, M.D.

Most skin tumors are uncommon in children, but when a lesion does occur it is important that it be diagnosed accurately, because some of these tumors indicate underlying systemic disease, some require surgical intervention, and an occasional lesion is malignant.

FACIAL LESIONS

The following lesions are most frequently found on the face and therefore may be confused with acne if they are not carefully examined.

Angiofibromas, inaccurately called *adenoma sebaceum* in the older literature, are the small (1 to 4 mm) pink or flesh-colored papules seen in association with tuberous sclerosis. They generally begin during early childhood but occasionally are not present until puberty. As the patient ages, the lesions become somewhat larger. They can be effectively treated with cryosurgery, electrodesiccation and curettage, or dermabrasion if removal is necessary for cosmetic reasons. Occasionally, a lesion may be solitary; in that case, it is not associated with tuberous sclerosis.

Although *trichoepitheliomas* may occur as solitary lesions in early adult life, the other form of the disorder, which is dominantly inherited, begins during childhood or at puberty and is associated with multiple lesions. Small (2 to 5 mm) flesh-colored papules and nodules are seen on the central area of the face. Solitary lesions should be excised; however, with multiple lesions, excision is unnecessary. Instead, they are treated with electrodesiccation, cryotherapy, or dermabrasion. Although most trichoepitheliomas are benign, there is disagreement in the literature about whether some of these lesions eventually evolve into basal cell carcinomas.

Trichofolliculomas also occur on the face. These flesh-colored papules or dome-shaped nodules classically have a central pore with a protruding tuft of fine hair. The lesion is best treated by surgical excision.

Syringomas frequently first appear during adolescence. Small (1 to 3 mm) yellowish papules are seen. They occur on the lower eyelids in more than half of affected patients. Other common locations include the sides of the neck, trunk, extremities, and genital area. It is estimated that one fifth to one third of children with Down syndrome have syringomas. Treatment is necessary only for cosmetic reasons and consists of destruction by electrodesiccation, cryotherapy, or surgical excision.

Basal cell carcinomas are slow-growing, locally invasive but rarely metastasizing malignant skin tumors that are all too common in older adults but are also seen occasionally in children. They occur most commonly in individuals with fair skin who have been exposed to the sun. Over the past decade, we have been seeing more adolescents with basal cell carcinomas on the face, which are frequently mistaken for acne. The lesions begin as small (2 mm) erythematous papules that have a clear or translucent quality and often contain telangiectasias. They enlarge slowly and may undergo some central necrosis and crusting. Occasionally, basal cell carcinomas are pigmented and resemble nevi, or they may be sclerosing and resemble scars.

In the *basal cell nevus syndrome,* multiple basal cell carcinomas are associated with other abnormalities, including temporal bossing, dental cysts, bifid ribs, intracranial calcifications, ovarian fibromas, and, rarely, medulloblastoma. The disorder is inherited in an autosomal dominant fashion. Skin lesions usually first appear at puberty, although they may occur much earlier.

It is important that basal cell carcinomas be completely removed because the carcinoma may recur locally if the excision is not complete. The lesions can be surgically excised or removed by curettage and electrodesiccation.

RED-BROWN LESIONS

Pyogenic Granulomas. These solitary, red-to-brown, vascular pedunculated nodules, 5 mm to 1 cm in diameter, may develop rapidly on any cutaneous surface. The lesions are round and well circumscribed and clinically may resemble small capillary hemangiomas. The cause is unclear, but it is thought that trauma to the skin in the presence of pyogenic bacteria results in a reactive proliferative vascular process. These lesions are usually easy to treat. They can be shaved or snipped off parallel to the skin, and the base electrodesiccated. The specimen is usually sent for a pathologic examination to confirm the diagnosis and to differentiate this benign lesion from other conditions, including a Spitz nevus or amelanotic melanoma.

Urticaria Pigmentosa. It is not uncommon for the pediatric dermatologist to see children with one or two localized lesions of urticaria pigmentosa known as *mastocytomas.* These red-brown or yellow-brown papules or nodules urticate when rubbed (Darier's sign). They are composed of collections of mast cells in the dermis that release histamine when the skin is traumatized, resulting in the characteristic urtication. Children with just a few of these lesions rarely have systemic symptoms.

Other children, however, have myriads of smaller yellow to red-brown macules or papules that are also composed of mast cells and therefore urticate with stroking. When the disease is this extensive, it is known as *urticaria pigmentosa.* Many children have only cutaneous symptoms of the disease, consisting of itching and, sometimes, blister formation. Approximately 10 per cent of patients, however, have systemic involvement, since mast cells can also accumulate in almost any body organ or tissue, including the bones, liver, spleen, and lymph nodes. Patients with systemic symptoms may have flushing attacks, hypotension, headaches, tachycardia, pruritus, diarrhea, and, rarely, blood clotting abnormalities. These symptoms can be severe and life-threatening.

Patients with cutaneous disease alone generally require no therapy unless the lesions are symptomatic; then antihistamines usually help to control pruritus or blistering. The prognosis in most patients is excellent, since the lesions resolve spontaneously in time. Children with numerous lesions should avoid aspirin, codeine, morphine, procaine, and polymyxin B because these nonspecific releasers of histamine may cause systemic symptoms. Patients with systemic symptoms may be treated with oral cromolyn, cimetidine combined with an H_1 antihistamine, or ultraviolet A phototherapy with psoralen (PUVA). Children with many cutaneous lesions should have a complete blood count periodically to check for the presence of mast cell leukemia, which has been reported in a small number of patients.

Juvenile Xanthogranulomas. These yellow to red-brown papules and nodules can be solitary or multiple. They may occur anywhere on the body but are common on the head and neck. They resolve spontaneously after several years. In most patients, this is a benign and self-limited problem; however, the disease can also occur in other body organs, including the lung, pericardium, meninges, liver, spleen, and testes. Systemic involvement usually is asymptomatic and requires no treatment or evaluation. However, if lesions are present in the eye, glaucoma or hemorrhage may occur in the absence of treatment. Therefore, any child with this disease should be examined by an ophthalmologist.

Eccrine Poromas. This benign cutaneous tumor, which arises from the sweat duct unit, usually occurs in older adults but has been reported in adolescents. Firm, reddish nodules, 2 to 12 mm in diameter, are usually seen on the dorsal surface of the foot. The treatment of choice is surgical excision.

FLESH-COLORED LESIONS

Follicular Cysts. This lesion, which is also known as an *epidermal* or *sebaceous cyst,* is a discrete, slowly growing, elevated, firm nodule that may occur anywhere on the body but is commonly seen on the face, scalp, and back. The cyst contains a cheesy white material that has a sour odor. The treatment is surgical excision. The entire cyst, with its epidermal lining, must be removed to prevent recurrence.

Pilomatrixomas. These uncommon, solitary, deep nodules occur only in children and adolescents. A 0.5- to 2-cm flesh-colored or reddish-blue nodule is seen on the face, neck, or upper extremities. Treatment is surgical excision.

Neurofibromas. These soft polypoid lesions, which "buttonhole" or invaginate into the underlying dermis when pressure is applied to their surface, may first appear in childhood. Solitary lesions may occur in otherwise normal individuals. However, when multiple lesions are present, they are a cutaneous marker for the dominantly inherited disease *neurofibromatosis.*

Connective Tissue Nevi. These single or multiple, slightly raised, skin-colored oval lesions may occur anywhere on the body and may be a sign of an inherited condition. Biopsy shows them to be composed of collagen or elastic fibers. The *shagreen patch* seen in tuberous sclerosis is actually a large connective tissue nevus. In the *Buschke-Ollendorff syndrome,* multiple widespread connective tissue nevi are present in association with osteopoikilosis.

Lipomas. These benign nodules, which are soft and rubbery in consistency, may occur on any part of the body. They are composed of mature fat cells. Treatment is not required unless the lesions are large enough to cause a cosmetic problem.

Recurring Digital Fibromas of Childhood. These smooth, shiny, erythematous nodules occur on the distal phalanges of infants and young children. The management of these lesions is controversial. There are several case reports of spontaneous involution. Of lesions surgically excised, 70 per cent recur. Dissection down to the periosteum is necessary.

Dermatofibromas. Dermatofibromas are small (1 mm to 3 cm) dermal nodules that are fixed to the skin but move freely over the subcutaneous fat. They may occur anywhere on the body. They range from flesh-colored to brown. Treatment is unnecessary unless there is a cosmetic problem. Treatment options include cryotherapy and surgical excision.

SCARS AND KELOIDS

Damaged dermis heals with a *scar* that is initially pink. The color gradually fades to a permanent white, and the scar appears shiny. New scars may be elevated or *hypertrophic* before they finally flatten and contract, within 6 months to 1 year after the original injury. Scars must be differentiated from *keloids,* which are an exaggerated connective tissue response to skin injury. Keloids appear long after the original injury and slowly increase in size beyond the area of the original wound.

Although hypertrophic scars usually necessitate no therapy, as they will flatten in time, keloids do not resolve spontaneously and may continue to enlarge slowly. They can be treated with intralesional injections of corticosteroids; if this fails, surgery can be attempted if it is needed for cosmetic reasons. Surgical excision must be done with care, and intralesional steroids are usually injected both at the time of excision and periodically during the postoperative period to prevent recurrence of the keloid.

THE GENODERMATOSES

AMY S. PALLER, M.D.

The genodermatoses are inherited cutaneous disorders; many are associated with abnormalities of other organs as well. Most genodermatoses may be classified within the following categories: keratinizing disorders, ectodermal dysplasias, disorders of collagen and elastic tissue, neurocutaneous disorders, blistering diseases, photosensitivity disorders, pigmentary abnormalities, disorders of metabolism, and tumor syndromes.

Appropriate management requires an understanding of the clinical features of these genodermatoses, the genetic risks for patients and their families, and the possibility of prenatal diagnosis. For many of the genodermatoses, little therapy is available other than supportive care and avoidance of exacerbating agents. In all of these disorders, however, genetic counseling is an important means of therapy. Prenatal diagnosis is possible for many of the genodermatoses by fetal skin biopsy or evaluation of fetal DNA, often by restriction fragment length polymorphisms if other family members are affected and linkage to the abnormal gene can be established.

KERATINIZING DISORDERS

The keratinizing disorders are a group of genodermatoses that includes the ichthyoses and palmoplantar keratodermas.

Ichthyoses

Because all of the ichthyoses are characterized by dryness and excessive scaling, therapy is directed toward preventing loss of water, rehydration of the stratum corneum, and elimination of the scaling. *Ichthyosis vulgaris,* the most common form of ichthyosis, is an autosomal dominant condition, whereas *recessive X-linked ichthyosis* (RXLI), due to a deficiency of a sulfatase, manifests only in male patients.

Prenatal diagnosis of the ichthyoses is available by fetal skin biopsy, performed between the 16th and 18th weeks of gestation. The Foundation for Ichthyosis and Related Skin Types (FIRST) is an excellent source of information and support for patients and families with ichthyosis (FIRST, P.O. Box 20921, Raleigh, NC 27619-0921).

Treatment

Both ichthyosis vulgaris and RXLI are disorders of excessive retention of stratum corneum rather than hyperproliferation, and patients with these disorders respond well both to keratolytic agents to remove scales and to the application of good lubricants, particularly immediately after bathing. Alpha-hydroxy acids, such as lactic acid and glycolic acid, are commercially available as Lac-Hydrin lotion (12 per cent lactic acid), Epilyt lotion (<5 per cent lactic acid in propylene glycol), and LactiCare (5 per cent lactic acid). Glycolic acid may be purchased as Aquaglycolic lotion (5 per cent) and is also available as a shampoo for patients with affected scalps.

Urea preparations may also be helpful in softening skin and increasing hydration and are found commercially in creams, lotions, or ointments in concentrations up to 25 per cent (Ultramide lotion). Propylene glycol (40 to 60 per cent) may be compounded in hydrophilic ointment and applied under occlusion with good results. Salicylic acid is also an effective keratolytic agent in concentrations of 3 to 10 per cent, but frequent applications to large areas of the body surface may lead to significant absorption and the risk of salicylate toxicity (Keralyt is a preparation of 6 per cent salicylic acid in propylene glycol). Topical retinoic acid (Retin-A) may be beneficial as a keratolytic agent but may be irritating. Retin-A should always be introduced gradually—for example, every other day, beginning with the lowest concentration (0.025 per cent cream), until the limits of tolerance are established.

The more severe forms of ichthyosis include *classic lamellar ichthyosis* and *congenital ichthyosiform erythroderma,* both usually autosomal recessive, and *epidermolytic hyperkeratosis* (bullous ichthyosiform erythroderma), an autosomal dominant disorder that often results from spontaneous mutation. Although some improvement often occurs with the use of lubricants and keratolytic agents, patients with these hyperproliferative disorders do not respond as well to topical agents as do patients with ichthyosis vulgaris and RXLI.

Patients with epidermolytic hyperkeratosis frequently have a foul smell as a result of macerated scale with extensive bacterial colonization, and secondary cutaneous infections develop. Antibacterial scrubs, such as chlorhexidine, may be added to bath water, and systemic antibiotics may be required to control secondary infections.

The systemic retinoids isotretinoin (Accutane) and etretinate (Tegison) have caused significant improvement, particularly in patients with classic lamellar and congenital ichthyosiform erythroderma, but are associated with a number of potential side effects when used chronically. Of greatest significance is the effect of retinoids on bone growth in children, including premature closure of the epiphyses. In addition, the retinoids are potent teratogens and should be avoided in fertile female patients. Because relatively high doses and long-term use of systemic retinoids are necessary for patients with keratinizing disorders, the many possible complications preclude their use for most patients.

Palmoplantar Keratodermas

Patients with palmoplantar keratodermas show diffuse or punctate thickening of the stratum corneum of the palms and/or soles. Most forms of palmoplantar keratoderma are inherited as autosomal dominant disorders.

Treatment

The thickened stratum corneum may be mechanically removed by soaking the hands or feet for 20 minutes, rubbing with a pumice stone to remove desquamating stratum corneum, and applying an effective keratolytic agent, such as 6 to 16 per cent salicylic acid, under occlusion. For patients with severe, disabling forms of palmoplantar keratoderma, systemic retinoids may be used temporarily for intermittent relief. Skin grafts to the palms or soles have also been applied when patients have functional impairment.

PACHYONYCHIA CONGENITA

Pachyonychia congenita is an autosomal dominant disorder that is characterized by marked thickening and yellowing of all fingernails and toenails, a process that tends to begin in infancy. Palmoplantar keratoderma, hyperhidrosis, oral leukokeratosis, follicular keratosis, and, in some families, steatocystoma multiplex may be associated.

Treatment

The keratoderma may be treated with keratolytic agents, such as 60 per cent propylene glycol or 6 per cent salicylic acid in propylene glycol, under occlusion, as mentioned previously. The nails are kept under control by frequent filing and, in some cases, by surgical avulsion with scraping of the matrix to prevent regrowth.

FAMILIAL BENIGN PEMPHIGUS

Familial benign pemphigus (Hailey-Hailey disease) is an autosomal dominant disorder that usually becomes manifest in adolescence or young adulthood. Recurrent crops of vesicles, bullae, and crusted erosions develop, particularly in the axillae, groin, and perineal areas and on the neck.

Treatment

Because heat, humidity, and friction are precipitating factors, air-conditioning, avoidance of tight and excessive clothing, and weight loss, if appropriate, may be helpful. The intermittent use of systemic antibiotics (particularly tetracycline) is often useful, and topical corticosteroid preparations may decrease the associated discomfort for some patients. In severe cases, the involved areas have been excised and replaced with grafts.

ECTODERMAL DYSPLASIAS

Hidrotic ectodermal dysplasia is an autosomal dominant disorder characterized by sparse hair, nail dystrophy, and hyperkeratotic palms and soles.

Hypohidrotic ectodermal dysplasia, an X-linked recessive disorder, is the most common form of ectodermal dysplasia. Affected patients show partial absence of eccrine glands, sparse hair, dental abnormalities, and insufficient mucous and lacrimal gland secretion. Patients have very similar facial features and often have associated atopic dermatitis. Most severely affected patients are male, but female heterozygotes may also show extensive manifestations. Many patients present in infancy with unexplained fevers owing to the inability to sweat and remove heat.

Treatment

Air conditioning, dousing frequently with water, increasing fluid intake, wearing cool clothing, and avoiding excessive physical exertion are useful means to reduce the need for sweating.

Because of the frequent absence of teeth and ineffectual conical incisors, early dental examination and fitting for a dental prosthesis by 2 years of age improves mastication, cosmetic appearance, and facial development. Permanent dental implants are now available for teenagers and adults.

Saline nasal sprays and application of intranasal petrolatum or a topical antibiotic can help patients with dry nasal mucosa. Artificial tears can be used for patients with defective lacrimation. Topical corticosteroid preparation and good lubrication diminish the cutaneous dryness and pruritus of patients with associated atopic dermatitis. Plastic surgery and psychiatric intervention may be necessary for patients who are severely limited in their lifestyle or have difficulty with their appearance.

The National Foundation for Ectodermal Dysplasias (NFED) is a support group for patients with ectodermal dysplasia and their families (NFED, 219 East Main, P.O. Box 114, Mascoutah, IL 62258).

ACRODERMATITIS ENTEROPATHICA

Acrodermatitis enteropathica is an autosomal recessive disorder that occurs in early infancy as periorificial and acral vesiculobullous, pustular, and eczematous lesions. Irritability, alopecia, nail dystrophy, diarrhea, stomatitis, and secondary bacterial and candidal infections are often associated.

Patients respond to zinc supplementation within days with decreased irritability, diarrhea, and skin lesions. Zinc levels should be monitored once to twice yearly to determine proper maintenance zinc supplementation.

NEUROCUTANEOUS DISORDERS

Neurofibromatosis is an autosomal dominant disorder with a 50 per cent rate of spontaneous mutation. Affected patients may have disfiguring tumors, skeletal abnormalities, speech and learning disabilities, and an increased risk of malignant neoplasms. The major clinical criteria for diagnosis are multiple café au lait macules, Lisch nodules (iris hamartomas), and neurofibromas.

If cosmetically objectionable, the superficial neurofibromas may be removed completely by surgical excision (leaving a scar) or transiently by dermabrasion. The new lasers that remove cutaneous pigmentation may prove useful for patients with many café au lait spots.

Tuberous sclerosis also is inherited in an autosomal dominant manner, with a 75 per cent rate of spontaneous mutation. Most patients with tuberous sclerosis have seizures, and 60 per cent of patients have mental retardation. Cardiac rhabdomyomas, renal angiomyolipomas and cysts, and retinal gliomas also frequently occur. The cutaneous abnormalities of this multisystemic disorder include facial angiofibromas (adenoma sebaceum), periungual and subungual fibromas, and collagenomas (shagreen patches).

The elevation and discoloration of facial angiofibromas may be reduced by dermabrasion and/or laser therapy. Surgical removal of periungual fibromas may also be attempted, but lesions tend to regrow.

TUMOR SYNDROMES

The autosomal dominant disorder *basal cell nevus syndrome* is characterized by the early development of multiple basal cell carcinomas associated with frontal bossing, palmoplantar pits, epidermal and jaw cysts, intracranial calcifications, and bifid ribs. Patients also have an increased risk of developing other neoplasms, particularly ovarian fibromas and medulloblastomas.

Basal cell carcinomas should be removed entirely by electrodesiccation and curettage or by surgical excision. Sun protection and avoidance should be instituted early. The long-term administration of low-dose isotretinoin (Accutane) decreases the development of carcinomas, but its use is not appropriate in children.

EPIDERMOLYSIS BULLOSA

Epidermolysis bullosa (EB) is a heterogeneous group of inherited blistering disorders.

Prenatal diagnosis of EB is possible by fetal skin biopsy. The Dystrophic Epidermolysis Bullosa Research Association (DEBRA) provides information and support for patients and families with EB (DEBRA of America, Inc., 141 Fifth Avenue, Suite 7S, New York, NY 10010).

Treatment

Patients with the autosomal dominant epidermolytic forms (EB simplex, Weber-Cockayne syndrome) tend to worsen in summer months, and efforts to decrease hyperhidrosis and humidity and to treat open bullae with topical antibiotics usually suffice.

In contrast, patients with the more severe dystrophic and nondystrophic forms, such as EB letalis and recessive dystrophic EB (both autosomal recessive), require extensive attention by parents and nursing personnel. Mechanical trauma may be reduced by use of a mattress with a soft fleece covering, gentle handling, use of nonadherent dressings, and avoidance of tape in contact with the skin. Semiocclusive dressings have helped to reduce the incidence of blister formation in some affected patients. Sterile aspiration of blister fluid may prevent blister extension and alleviate discomfort. The application of topical antibiotics, particularly mupirocin (Bactroban), should be used to prevent secondary infection and promote healing. Patients with large areas of denuded skin should be kept in isolation to decrease the risk of sepsis and treated similarly to burn patients. Fluid and electrolyte balance should be maintained through intravenous administration of fluids, and systemic antibiotics are necessary if infection ensues.

Patients with severe EB need nutritious caloric supplementation to grow appropriately, and consultation with a dietitian is often helpful. A soft diet and, if ineffective, bougienage and/or surgery may be needed in patients with esophageal involvement and dysphagia.

Individuals with the recessive dystrophic form of EB have extensive residual scarring at sites of blistering, particularly on the hands and feet. Physiotherapy and extensive surgical intervention ("degloving") with subsequent splinting may ameliorate the fusion deformities ("mitten deformity") that result from scarring and may restore hand function. Although phenytoin (Dilantin) has been reported anecdotally to reduce blister formation in patients with recessive dystrophic EB, a recent multicenter double-blind trial failed to find any usefulness of phenytoin therapy.

REFERENCES

Alper JC (ed): Genetic Disorders of the Skin. St. Louis, Mosby Year Book, 1991.

Fine J-D, Bauer EA, Briggaman RA, et al: Revised clinical and laboratory

criteria for subtypes of inherited epidermolysis bullosa. J Am Acad Dermatol 24:119–135, 1991.
Provost TT, Farmer ER (eds): Current Therapy in Dermatology. Philadelphia, BC Decker, 1985.
Williams ML: The ichthyoses—pathogenesis and prenatal diagnosis. Pediatr Dermatol 1:1–24, 1983.
Worobec-Victor SM, Shanker DB, Bené-Bain MA, Solomon LM: Genodermatoses. *In* Schachner LA, Hansen RC (eds): Pediatric Dermatology. New York, Churchill Livingstone, 1988, pp 311–443.

DISORDERS OF THE HAIR AND SCALP

JAMES E. RASMUSSEN, M.D.

GENERAL APPROACH TO DIAGNOSIS

Patients with diseases of the hair and scalp should be approached in a systematic fashion in order to make an accurate diagnosis. One logical approach is to consider whether the disease is congenital or acquired, and then whether the process is localized or diffuse. Only the more common disorders are considered here. (See Table 1.)

Congenital Localized

Aplasia Cutis Congenita

Aplasia cutis congenita presents as a round hairless scar that is usually well healed at the time of birth. Occasionally, erosions may be present. The disease is inherited in a dominant fashion.

Nevus Sebaceus of Jadassohn

Nevus sebaceus is a "birthmark" with differentiation toward sebaceous glands. It always presents at birth with a hairless, oval to linear, yellow-orange, slightly raised plaque that further thickens around the time of puberty. In 5 to 10 per cent of these lesions, low-grade malignancies develop in the third through fifth decades. Consequently, prophylactic excision is usually suggested when feasible. Large lesions may be associated with seizures, mental retardation, vascular, and skeletal disorders.

Congenital—Diffuse

There are a wide variety of uncommon to rare congenital disorders of the hair shaft. They feature twisting and thinning of the shaft with increased hair breakage, mostly at points of trauma (such as the sides of the scalp and the back of the neck). The specific hair shaft defect can usually be determined by viewing plucked hairs mounted on a glass slide under light or polarizing microscope. (A detailed discussion of the morphology of these defects is beyond the scope of this article.) In addition, several of these syndromes feature major widespread metabolic disease, such as trichothiodystrophy and Menkes syndrome. Currently, there is no specific treatment for any of these disorders.

TABLE 1. Disorders of Hair and Scalp

	Congenital	Acquired
Localized	Aplasia cutis Nevus sebaceous	Alopecia areata Tinea capitis Trichotillomania Psoriasis
Diffuse	Hair shaft disorders Monilithrix Menkes syndrome Trichothiodystrophy	Telogen effluvium Seborrheic dermatitis Folliculitis Psoriasis

Acquired—Localized

Alopecia Areata

Alopecia areata is one of the more common causes of hair loss in children and young adults. It usually begins as a noninflammatory circular area with complete hair loss. The proximal ends of shed hairs have small dystrophic bulbs. Tugging at hairs in the margin of expanding lesions usually removes multiple loose hairs (a positive "pull test"). The margins of the lesions also contain short, broken hairs called "exclamation points." Alopecia areata may involve from 1- to 2-cm lesions to diffuse hair loss. Hair in other areas, such as the eyebrows, eyelashes, beard, and axillary and pubic areas, may also be lost. The cause is unknown but probably represents an autoimmune phenomenon. All patients should be evaluated for the presence of underlying endocrine and other autoimmune processes, but these are often not present.

There is no generally effective therapy for alopecia areata, but topical steroids are useful for localized areas. Ultraviolet light and the antipsoriatic drug anthralin may also be useful, but these modalities take long periods of time to be effective. Therapy using chronic contact allergens (dinitrochlorobenzene, squaric acid) has also produced good results, but requires a physician experienced in their use. Topical minoxidil has a low rate of efficacy. Systemic steroids and cyclosporine are effective but are not safe for long-term use.

The prognosis is uncertain, with smaller patches usually resolving spontaneously. Patients with generalized hair loss often do not experience permanent regrowth.

Tinea Capitis

Tinea capitis due to *Trichophyton tonsurans* is a common cause of hair loss in prepubertal patients. This organism has a predilection for black patients for reasons that are not fully known. In the past, individual cases or large epidemics were due to *Microsporum canis* and *Microsporum audouini,* but these are uncommon to rare causes today. *T. tonsurans* does not fluoresce under a Wood's lamp, and, consequently, this method of evaluation is of little use in making the diagnosis. Only culture and potassium hydroxide preparation of scraped hairs are successful in identifying the causative organisms today.

The treatment of tinea capitis is griseofulvin (10 to 15 mg/kg, either microsized or ultramicrosized, in two to three divided doses or as a single dose, depending on the reliability of parents, given with fatty food for a period of 6 to 16 weeks). Ketoconazole is less effective and should not be routinely used. Topical antifungals offer very little because they do not penetrate into the hair follicle. Shampooing with selenium sulfide (Selsun and others) decreases the period of infectiousness but does not hasten recovery.

Trichotillomania

Trichotillomania is a common cause of hair loss most often seen in adolescent females. The patient typically presents with a history of a bizarrely patterned area of incomplete hair loss that is usually noninflammatory. Hairs are of varying lengths, and the pull test is negative. Many hairs are broken flush with the scalp, giving the appearance of ragged stubble. The patient usually does not notice loose hairs in the brush or after shampooing. Most patients are not significantly concerned about the problem and are usually brought in at the request of parents. The diagnosis is based on the irregular margination, lack of inflammation, and hairs of varying lengths.

There is no uniformly successful therapy. Topical steroids and lubricants can be given for their placebo effect as well as to make the hairs greasy and difficult to pluck. For small, localized patches, the prognosis is usually good, with spontaneous resolution in a period of months. Larger areas of hair loss are usually indicative of an underlying psychologic disorder, and these patients should be carefully considered for psychiatric referral. The oral drug clomipramine has clearly been shown to be effective in a double-blind cross-over study, but it is associated a number of significant side effects.

Acquired—Diffuse

Telogen Effluvium

Telogen effluvium is an uncommon cause of hair loss in children and young adults. It occurs after a major systemic illness, such as a seizure or a severe infection. It can also occur following major accidents, general anesthesia, and childbirth. Two to 8 weeks after the metabolic insult, the patient's growing hairs, which have been put into a resting phase, are shed when new hairs begin to emerge from the resting follicles. This produces a diffuse pattern of hair loss that is usually not severe, but the number of loose hairs will alarm the patient. The diagnosis depends on the history of the antecedent metabolic insult, coupled with the history of rapid hair loss—the period in which the hairs come out, revealing small resting roots (telogen phase). No therapy is necessary, and the process is usually self-limited to 4 to 8 weeks.

Seborrheic Dermatitis

Seborrheic dermatitis is a common problem in the first 2 to 6 months of life and is usually called "cradle cap." Other varieties of seborrheic dermatitis in older patients merge with atopic eczema, yielding scaly patches at the scalp margin and behind the ears. It is important to rule out the possibility of tinea capitis in young children who present with a clinical picture of seborrheic dermatitis.

The treatment of cradle cap is usually mild shampoos (baby shampoo) and emollients, such as mineral oil or olive oil. Shampoos indicated for treatment of adult seborrheic dermatitis (Sebulex) are usually not indicated in the first year of life. Mild topical steroid lotions (Synalar .01%) are useful for short periods of time.

Folliculitis

Scalp folliculitis can be produced by bacteria, trauma, or chemicals. There is no easy way to distinguish these three sources, and therapy must frequently be directed at all of them if present. Folliculitis is most commonly seen in patients who use hair pomades and tight braids. This combination of mechanical traction and occlusion frequently produces bacterial, traumatic, or chemical inflammation. Hair loss is usually not severe unless traction is a major component.

The treatment of folliculitis is directed at relieving the traction and reducing the chemical occlusion of the follicular mouth; topical or systemic antibiotics are used. The topical antibiotics useful in the treatment of acne (Cleocin T) are easily applied to the scalp because they are in vehicles that evaporate and do not leave a gummy mess. Systemic antibiotics, such as erythromycin, are also excellent choices.

Psoriasis

Psoriasis is a common problem but is usually not limited to the scalp. In children with this disease, often there are guttate lesions widely spread over the body, including the face and scalp. Occasionally, large plaques may be limited to the scalp. The clinical presentation of psoriasis in the scalp is quite characteristic. Sharply marginated areas of bright erythema are covered with a thick, heavy, yellow to white adherent scale. Hair loss is usually not significant unless the patient has been mechanically removing the scales. A family history of psoriasis is found in approximately 30 to 60 per cent of individuals. Also common is a preceding history of a streptococcal sore throat or upper respiratory infection, particularly when the lesions are in the guttate form.

Therapy is directed toward treating the antecedent infection if present. In addition, mild topical steroids (Synalar .01%) and tar shampoos on a daily basis are somewhat effective. Psoriasis of the scalp is fairly resistant to treatment, however. Recent evidence has suggested that *Pityrosporum ovale* may be involved in the pathogenesis of psoriasis of the scalp. Ketoconazole topical cream or shampoo may be effective, but at least 1 to 2 months of therapy would be required.

DISORDERS OF THE SEBACEOUS GLANDS AND SWEAT GLANDS

STEPHEN E. GELLIS, M.D.

DISORDERS OF THE SEBACEOUS GLANDS

Acne, a common skin problem that is seen to some extent in almost all patients, may begin in children as young as 8 years. Whereas some teenagers may be overly concerned about what appears to be mild acne, others may deny the presence of a severe problem. Often, it is the parent who expresses the most concern and whose involvement may be viewed negatively by the adolescent.

It is important to obtain a history that includes the date of onset of the problem; family history; presence of other medical problems, including endocrine disorders; current medications; prior therapies; and external factors, such as activities that may exacerbate acne (e.g., athletic endeavors requiring helmets or shoulder padding or involvement in food preparation with exposure to grease-filled kitchens).

Next, an assessment of the type and degree of skin involvement is made. *Mild acne* is characterized by open and closed comedones (plugged sebaceous follicles) with little erythema. *Moderate acne* cases show pustules, papules, and erythema with early scar formation. *Severe acne* cases involve multiple inflamed nodules with significant scarring.

The treatment should be individualized. A patient who has a tendency to produce postinflammatory hyperpigmentation following minor comedonal acne may require aggressive systemic treatment.

Mild Acne

Mild acne can be successfully managed with topical preparations. These include benzoyl peroxide, retinoic acid, and topical antibiotics. It is important to explain to the patient that topical preparations are applied not only to the lesions but also to the areas in which the lesions tend to form.

Benzoyl Peroxide

The easiest and least expensive treatment for mild acne is benzoyl peroxide, which reduces bacteria, produces desquamation, and lowers sebum production. It is available over the counter and by prescription in soaps, washes, creams, gels, and scrubs. The concentration ranges from 2.5 to 10 per cent.

Benzoyl peroxide is usually applied to the skin twice a day. The main side effect is excessive drying, which can be avoided by selecting the lower-strength products or those that are compounded with emollient bases and by decreasing the frequency of application.

Retinoic Acid (Retin-A)

For extensive numbers of comedones not responding to benzoyl peroxide, retinoic acid can be added. Retinoic acid produces desquamation and reduces comedones. It is available in various strengths. The cream forms are less irritating than the gels and the liquid preparation. The available forms are, in increasing strength and irritancy: 0.025 per cent cream, 0.05 per cent cream, 0.1 per cent cream, 0.01 per cent gel, 0.025 per cent gel, and 0.05 per cent liquid. The medication is usually applied at night, confining the application of benzoyl peroxide to another time of day. Simultaneous application of both agents may produce inactivation. Retinoic acid should be applied to dry skin to minimize irritation. Some redness and peeling are desired. If irritancy occurs, the frequency of application should be reduced. Patients should be told to expect some possible worsening of the condition in the first 1 to 2 months of use. Use in fair-skinned individuals during the summer may have to be curtailed because of increased sensitivity to the sun.

Topical Antibiotics

If a small number of inflammatory lesions are present, a topical antibiotic can be used along with benzoyl peroxide and retinoic acid. The most commonly prescribed topical antibiotics include erythromycin and clindamycin. They are available in gels, creams, and solutions and are applied twice a day.

Moderate Acne

Moderate acne characterized by extensive inflammatory lesions often necessitates initial treatment with systemic antibiotics to avoid the development of scarring. This is undertaken in combination with the previously discussed topical preparations.

Oral Antibiotics

The most commonly used oral antibiotics include tetracycline, erythromycin, minocycline, and doxycycline. The initial choice may be determined by cost and convenience.

Tetracycline is best absorbed on an empty stomach. Because an empty stomach is an unusual occurrence in most male teenagers, erythromycin may be a better choice in this patient population. The starting dose for both tetracycline and erythromycin is usually 1 g/day divided into two, three, or four doses. School schedules and other activities make twice-a-day administration the most practical. The dose can be increased to 1.5 g.

Tetracycline may cause an increased tendency for vaginal yeast infections to develop. It can also cause a photosensitivity in some patients. Another potential complication of both tetracycline and erythromycin is interference with the effectiveness of birth control medication. This may be due to alterations in the metabolism of the oral contraceptive. Patients should be warned to take additional contraceptive precautions if breakthrough bleeding occurs. Once improvement occurs, the antibiotic dose may be lowered.

For minocycline and doxycycline, an initial dose of 50 to 100 mg is prescribed. This can be increased up to a total of 200 mg/day. Minocycline can produce dizziness and hyperpigmentation, which is first noticeable along the hard palate or over the anterior tibias. If such side effects occur, the drug should be discontinued.

Severe Acne

13-*cis Retinoic Acid*

For severe acne consisting of inflammatory nodules and scarring that fails to respond to conventional treatments, 13-*cis* retinoic acid (Accutane) may be considered. It should be prescribed only by those familiar with the potential complications. Accutane must not be used in patients who are pregnant or who may become pregnant while undergoing treatment.

Major fetal abnormalities related to Accutane have been reported. Women of childbearing age should be counseled on the risk to a fetus if the drug is taken while pregnant. A negative pregnancy test should be obtained 2 weeks prior to initiating treatment. Treatment can begin on day 2 or 3 of the next menstrual cycle. An effective form of contraception should be used beginning 1 month before treatment and continuing until 1 month after its cessation. The usual course of treatment is 20 weeks.

Other side effects include dry skin causing epistaxis, cheilitis and conjunctivitis, pseudotumor cerebri (particularly when Accutane is given with tetracycline), depression, fatigue, muscle ache, and skeletal hyperostosis. Abnormal laboratory findings seen in some patients include hypertriglyceride and elevated sedimentation rates. The usual dose is 1 mg/kg.

Steroids

Intralesional steroid injections offer another useful therapy for inflammatory nodules. Triamcinolone acetonide at a concentration of 2.5 to 5.0 mg/ml can be injected intralesionally into a nodule. Resolution usually results within 24 hours.

Before commencing any form of acne treatment, it is important to be sure that the patient and parent have a clear understanding of the pathophysiology of acne. The most commonly held misconceptions relate to the role of greasy food and poor hygiene.

DISORDERS OF THE SWEAT GLANDS

Foot

Hyperhidrosis of the feet is usually exacerbated by occlusive sneakers, boots, or shoes. From a repetitive cycle of wetting and drying, fissuring may develop. In the acute stage, treatment consists of application of emollients or, in some instances, topical steroids. Prevention of hyperhidrosis can be accomplished with the use of absorbent powders (Zeasorb), avoidance of occlusive footwear, frequent changes of shoes and socks, and application of emollients to prevent drying.

Axilla and Palm

Hyperhidrosis of the axillae and palms can be a socially upsetting condition. Aluminum hexahydrate (Drysol), applied nightly for up to 1 week, will reduce sweating, which can then be maintained by less frequent application. When no response is seen, Drysol can be applied and occluded by plastic wrap overnight for several consecutive nights until the sweating is reduced. In unresponsive patients, an alternative is iontophoresis, which produces physical blockage of sweat ducts. Iontophoresis can be accomplished with a battery-powered home unit (Drionic).

SUN PROTECTION IN THE PEDIATRIC POPULATION

LAWRENCE A. SCHACHNER, M.D.

In 1989, the National Institutes of Health convened a consensus development conference on sunlight, ultraviolet radiation, and the skin. Key issues relevant to pediatric health care providers were reviewed, including (1) whether there are specific factors that influence children's susceptibility to solar ultraviolet radiation that make them particularly vulnerable to its adverse effects and (2) whether adverse ultraviolet-induced changes can be prevented.

SKIN CANCER INCIDENCE

It is estimated that nearly two thirds of an individual's lifetime ultraviolet radiation dose is received by 18 years of age. Recent statistical analysis has revealed that people born in the 1930s have a 1 in 1500 lifetime risk for melanoma, as opposed to those born in 1990, whose risk is more on the order of 1 in 100. Indeed, melanoma is the most rapidly increasing cancer in incidence over the past two decades. More than one fourth of melanomas develop in patients younger than 40 years of age, and melanoma is the most frequent cancer of women aged 25 to 29 and the second most frequent in women aged 30 to 35.

This increase in melanoma and in other non-melanoma skin cancers may be related to three main factors: (1) the major shift of the United States population as a whole southward, closer to the equator; (2) the popularity of suntans in recent decades; and (3) the worsening depletion in the protective ozone layer of the earth's atmosphere. In short, for environmental and societal reasons, young people are receiving, on average, more ambient ultraviolet radiation, resulting in an increase in melanoma and non-melanoma skin cancer.

SUSCEPTIBILITY

Predictable intrinsic factors influence children's susceptibility to ultraviolet radiation. These include skin that easily burns and does not tan, light eyes and hair color, the presence of multiple nevi, and a tendency toward freckling. Myriad intrinsic inherited and acquired disorders can also heighten susceptibility. In addition, for the average well child, evidence exists to suggest that there are age-related structural and immunologic differences that make sunburns and other acute and chronic sun exposures more dangerous to humans in the first two decades of life.

REDUCING CANCER RISK

How can we diminish the effect of ultraviolet radiation on pediatric skin? There are reasonable and appropriate measures that, if utilized, will probably reduce this generation's risk of skin cancer by more than 80 per cent. These measures include the following.

Clothing

Cotton clothing offers increased protection to sun exposure and, because of its light weight, will be better tolerated both in long-sleeved shirts and long pants. Caps or hats with visors protect more than 70 per cent of the face and offer photoprotection of the skin and eyes alike.

Chemical Sunscreens

Sunscreens should be used during appropriate times of the year on a daily basis. A combined UVB/UVA protective sunscreen with a sun protection factor (SPF) of at least 15 that is both sweatproof and waterproof should be applied 30 minutes before exposure and reapplied if exposure is prolonged during the course of the day.

Policies of Sun Exposure

Regional policies that reduce or stop the forced sun exposure of children during the peak sun hours in day care centers, schools, camps, etc., should be encouraged. On a sunny May or June day, more than 60 per cent of solar UVB radiation reaches the surface of the earth between 10:00 A.M. and 3:00 P.M. *Scheduling physical education classes, marching bands, and other outdoor activities before 10:00* A.M. *and after 3:00* P.M. *can greatly diminish a child's daily ultraviolet radiation dose.*

Avoidance of Artificial Tanning Devices

There are no safe, healthy tans and no safe, healthy tanning devices. The pediatrician should lead the campaign to educate the public that the more than 1 million daily exposures to artificial tanning devices are a hazard to young people's health.

SUMMARY

If one can establish appropriate guidelines for clothing and sunscreens and modify time of sun exposure, the current mortality rate of one American dying each hour from skin cancer can be dramatically decreased.

TREATMENT OF MALIGNANT MELANOMA IN CHILDREN

BERNETT L. JOHNSON, JR., M.D.

Malignant melanoma, when compared with other cutaneous malignancies, is an uncommon tumor. There does appear to be some increase in the incidence of this tumor type owing to today's behavior of continued and persistent sun exposure. In children, the greatest source for the development of malignant melanoma is the congenital nevus. The predicted incidence for the development of melanoma in those with congenital nevi is almost two and a half times that for those who do not have similar lesions. Melanomas in children also arise from acral sites, including the nail bed, palms, and soles. There is a reported increased incidence of melanoma in patients with dysplastic nevus syndrome. True dysplastic nevus syndrome is relatively uncommon, although there are many reports of sporadic dysplastic nevi. Whether the presence of sporadic dysplastic nevi indicates an increased risk for melanoma is debatable.

TREATMENT

The treatment of malignant melanoma in children is the same as for adults. The critical issue in the treatment of melanoma is its early recognition and diagnosis. In large congenital nevi, early recognition of small lesions is often difficult, if not impossible, because of the milieu in which the melanoma has developed. Those areas in congenital nevi that become nodular, grow suddenly, or change their characteristics, including becoming inflamed and itchy, should be attended to with haste and a biopsy of the lesion performed. Because congenital nevi of the large garment type often occupy large body areas, excisional surgery for the entire nevus containing the melanomas is not feasible. Melanomas that arise in dysplastic nevi or on acral surfaces should be removed *in toto.*

The histologic assessment provides an aid for further therapy. Malignant melanomas that are in the radial growth phase and occupy only the superficial layer of the papillary dermis (level II thin melanoma) are considered zero-risk melanomas, and complete excision is the treatment of choice. Malignant melanomas that are considerably thicker (> 1 mm) should also be totally excised, and the patient followed. Whether one should perform an incontinuity or a later node dissection is still open to question. There are some clinicians who believe that if nodes are palpable at the time of the primary excision, an incontinuity node dissection should be done along with the excision of the melanoma.

Therefore, the treatment of melanoma depends on the histologic assessment of thickness and depth, the presence or absence of lymph nodes, and the presence or absence of other signs of dissemination. For those patients who develop lymph nodes subsequent to the excision of the primary lesion, therapy, in many instances, is only excision of the affected nodes and continued careful follow-up. Melanomas that are disseminated, involving multiple organ systems as well as diffuse cutaneous metastases, can be treated with a host of cancer chemotherapeutic agents, including imidazole, carboximide, or a regimen of clophosphamide, vincristine, and dactinomycin, their number and type depending on the oncology service of the institution at which the child will be treated. There are no specific chemotherapeutic agents that are equally effective in the eradication of disseminated malignant melanoma, and chemotherapy in children has been as ineffective as in adults.

New therapies are on the horizon for melanoma that include the use of interferons, interleukins, new vaccines, and new cancer therapeutic drugs. The National Cancer Institute continues to lead in the development of new and innovative therapies in melanoma.

The therapy of melanoma should not be viewed with pessimism, especially when lesions are diagnosed early and the histologic assessment is that of a thin melanoma. Perhaps the most disconcerting to treat are those children who have large congenital nevi, whose potential risk for the development of melanoma is always in the fore. The best means of treating melanoma is for a physician to engage in judicious, prudent, and prompt follow-up and to have an eye for change and detail.

16

The Eye

THE EYE

LEONARD APT, M.D.

GENERAL CONSIDERATIONS OF EYE DISORDERS

Eye disorders that may be recognized and treated by the pediatric practitioner are stressed in this article. For the most part, these disorders are the simple inflammations of the eye and its adnexa. Children with most other ocular diseases should be referred to an ophthalmologist. It is our recommendation that instrumentation other than that required to remove a superficial foreign body be avoided by the nonophthalmologic physician.

As in other areas of medicine, the key to successful therapy of eye disorders is precise diagnosis. An accurate diagnosis is derived from a careful history, a systematic inspection of the visible eye structures, ophthalmoscopy, and appropriate laboratory studies. The history should include details about the symptoms and their duration, preceding illnesses or trauma, and contact with others with similar symptoms. Thorough inspection of the eye with good illumination is imperative. One must gain the child's confidence and cooperation to accomplish this. Forceful closure of the eyelids by the patient causes the eyeball to roll up and thus conceal the cornea. Forceful separation of the eyelids by the physician with the placement of inadvertent pressure on the globe may rupture a thin or perforated cornea or globe in patients having a history of trauma. In some instances, a sedative or general anesthetic may be necessary to satisfactorily relax a child for an ocular examination.

Since a child's primary care physician is often consulted first when an eye problem arises, it is necessary that he or she be aware of the manifestations of a serious eye disease. Knowledge of certain danger signs is of particular importance in dealing with "red eye," a common presenting complaint that varies in significance from a benign conjunctivitis to a blinding or life-threatening intraocular disease. A serious or potentially serious eye disease should be considered if any of the following signs or symptoms is present:

1. *Visual disturbance*—reduced acuity, diplopia, "spots" before the eyes, reduction in part of the field of vision.
2. Severe *pain* or *photophobia* suggests corneal, intraocular, or orbital disease. A corneal abrasion or foreign body may be the cause.
3. *Opacities* in the cornea, lens, or vitreous. A corneal opacity may be overlooked if a bright focal light aimed obliquely is not used. Opacities in the lens or vitreous can be seen as dark areas outlined in the red ophthalmoscopic reflex.
4. *Pupils*—irregularities in size or shape are seen after trauma or with intraocular inflammation.
5. Persistent *discharge* or *red eye* after several days of supposedly adequate treatment.

General Remarks About Local Therapy

In young children, medication in ointment form has certain advantages over liquid preparations; contact time on the eye is longer, and there is less tendency for the ointment preparation to undergo dilution from crying, with subsequent loss of the medication. As a consequence, instillations of ointments are required less frequently. On the other hand, drops may be easier to instill, are less messy, and do not temporarily blur the vision. In some children, it is often more convenient to use drops during the day and ointment at bedtime.

The pediatric practitioner should not prescribe local eye anesthetics for a painful eye for use at home. Local anesthetics tend to retard corneal healing. Furthermore, injury to an anesthetized eye by the parent or child may occur unintentionally.

A plea is made for the nonophthalmologic physician to avoid the indiscriminate use of local corticosteroids or combination drug products that include corticosteroids for the treatment of nonspecific inflamed or irritated eyes. Corticosteroids are effective antiallergic and anti-inflammatory agents, but they may retard healing, allow the progression of serious viral (e.g., herpes simplex) and/or fungal infections of the eye, or lead to glaucoma and cataract with prolonged use. The pediatric practitioner should make it a general rule that when an antibiotic or corticosteroid eye preparation is given in the absence of a definitive diagnosis, the patient is to be referred to an ophthalmologist if no distinct improvement occurs in 1 or 2 days.

Useful Local Eye Preparations

Diagnostic Stain. Stains are used to delineate abrasions, ulcerations, and foreign bodies of the cornea and conjunctiva.

FLUORESCEIN STRIPS. Strips of filter paper impregnated with fluorescein are commercially available in sterile packages. Fluorescein strips are desirable because the sterility of a fluorescein solution is difficult to maintain, particularly against contamination with *Pseudomonas* organisms. The dry or slightly moistened strip is merely touched to the conjunctival fornix. No flushing of the eye is needed.

Rose Bengal Solution. This dye stains devitalized epithelium. It is useful in demonstrating changes in the conjunctiva and cornea in Sjögren's syndrome and in exhibiting the dendrites in herpes epithelial keratitis.

Local Anesthetics. Local anesthetics are used to alleviate pain in order to examine the eye with convenience or to anesthetize the cornea and conjunctiva prior to the removal of a foreign body (Table 1).

The most widely used local anesthetics are tetracaine and proparacaine. Tetracaine aqueous solution has the advantages of high anesthetic potency, great stability, resistance to bacterial and fungal contamination, and low cost. The disadvantages are the moderate burning sensation with initial instillation of the drug and the mild congestion of the conjunctival vessels that it evokes. Proparacaine causes little or no discomfort on instillation, is not toxic, and has a rapid onset, but it has a much shorter duration of action than tetracaine. The minimal stinging and burning of proparacaine constitute a practical advantage of its use in infants and children.

Mydriatics and Cycloplegics. Weak mydriatics merely dilate the pupil. Strong mydriatics, in addition to dilating the pupil, temporarily relax or paralyze accommodation (the act of focusing at near objects) by acting on the ciliary muscle. For ophthalmoscopy alone, a weak mydriatic is all that is needed, since relaxation of accommodation often is unnecessary. Mydriasis lasts only a few hours. Cycloplegic drugs are used principally to measure refractive errors, to immobilize the ciliary muscle in inflammatory conditions of the uveal tract, and to dilate the pupil to avoid posterior synechiae formation in cases of iridocyclitis.

The useful drugs for this purpose are as follows:

Mydriatics (minimal or virtually no cycloplegic effect)
- Tropicamide (Mydriacyl) 0.5%
- Cyclopentolate 0.2% with phenylephrine 1% (Cyclomydril)
- Phenylephrine (Neo-Synephrine) 2.5, 10%

Cycloplegics
- Atropine 0.5, 1, 2, 3%
- Scopolamine 0.25%
- Homatropine 2, 5%
- Cyclopentolate (Cyclogyl) 0.5, 1, 2%
- Tropicamide (Mydriacyl) 1%

Atropine is the most potent cycloplegic drug and is the longest acting: 7 to 14 days. Mydriasis begins within 30 to 40 minutes after instillation of the drug, and maximum cycloplegia occurs in about 32 hours. The lower concentrations of the drug should be used in infants and young children because toxic amounts of the drug may be absorbed systemically. It is important to realize that toxic quantities of atropine can be absorbed. For example, a 1 per cent solution provides 0.5 mg of atropine with each drop or 1 mg when a drop is instilled into each eye. Assuming that only 50 per cent of the administered drug is absorbed systemically, a 5-kg infant receives ten times the usual systemic therapeutic dose (0.05 mg) and a 20-kg child receives 2.5 times the usual therapeutic dose (0.2 mg). Similar comparisons can be made for other topically applied drugs. Pressure over the lacrimal sac when the solution is instilled helps to prevent absorption of the drug through the nasopharyngeal mucosa. Use of atropine in ointment form allows less chance of absorption of the drug through the lacrimal drainage system.

Scopolamine is also a potent cycloplegic. It produces the same toxic symptoms as atropine. Mydriasis begins within 40 minutes; cycloplegia is maximal in 60 to 90 minutes and gradually subsides in 3 to 6 days.

Homatropine is a less potent cycloplegic drug than atropine or scopolamine. The higher concentrations produce full mydriasis within 30 minutes, and maximum cycloplegia is reached in 1 to 2 hours. Recovery from cycloplegia occurs in 36 to 48 hours. Toxicity from homatropine eye drops is infrequent. Instillation causes a burning sensation.

Cyclopentolate (Cyclogyl) produces rapid mydriasis and cycloplegia. Mydriasis appears in 15 minutes, and maximum cycloplegia is reached in 30 to 75 minutes after instillation of the drug. Recovery of accommodation takes place in 6 to 24 hours; mydriasis can persist beyond 24 hours. The cycloplegia, when maximal, is as profound as that obtained with atropine. Systemic toxicity is similar to that produced by atropine except that visual and tactile hallucinations are a more striking feature. The 2 per cent concentration should be avoided in infants.

Tropicamide (Mydriacyl) in the 1 per cent concentration is an ultra-short-acting cycloplegic. The 0.5 per cent preparation is principally a mydriatic. Mydriasis and cycloplegia occur simultaneously in 15 to 30 minutes. The duration of maximal cycloplegia is only 10 to 20 minutes. Recovery from cycloplegia likewise is rapid: 30 minutes to 4 hours. Tropicamide is used primarily as a mydriatic in pediatric patients because of its transient effect on accommodation. Local or systemic toxic effects are rare.

TABLE 1. Local Anesthetics for Ocular Use

Generic Name	Trade Name	Concentration
Tetracaine solution	Pontocaine	0.5%
Tetracaine ointment	Pontocaine	0.5%
Proparacaine solution	AK-Taine	0.5%
	Alcaine	0.5%
	I-Paracaine	0.5%
	Kainair	0.5%
	Ophthaine	0.5%
	Ophthetic	0.5%

EYELID DISORDERS

Blepharitis ("Granulated Eyelids")

Blepharitis is a common, chronic, recurrent inflammation of the lid margins characterized by redness, crusting, burning, irritation, itching, loss of eyelashes, and conjunctival irritation.

Two types are recognized by inspection. Clinical differentiation is of practical importance because knowledge of the cause aids in determining the specific treatment.

Staphylococcal Blepharitis. The most common cause of inflammation, crusting, and irritation along the lid margins in children is staphylococcal blepharitis. Although the findings of accumulated secretions with inflammation of the eyelid margins are quite characteristic, smears, specimens for culture, and sensitivity tests can readily be obtained to confirm the diagnosis. The scales at the base of the lashes often are hard and tenacious. In more severe cases, ulcers and pustules may appear on the eyelid margins. Toxic products of the bacteria may cause an accompanying conjunctivitis. A hypersensitivity reaction to staphylococcal antigens may produce an inflammatory keratitis.

Treatment. Lid hygiene, whereby scales are removed from the eyelid margins, is the mainstay of treatment of staphylococcal blepharitis. Moist compresses for 5 to 10 minutes may be needed to first loosen the scales before they are removed by mechanical scrubbing with a clean washcloth or cotton-tipped applicator moistened with diluted baby shampoo or commercial products intended for eyelid cleansing, such as Eyescrub (CooperVision Pharmaceuticals, Inc.) and OcuSoft Lid Scrub (Cynacon/OcuSoft, Inc.). The topical antistaphylococcal preparations most useful for treatment are erythromycin, bacitracin, and sulfacetamide ophthalmic ointments or drops (Table 2). After removal of the scales, the medication is placed between the eyelid and globe at bedtime. In severe cases a combined antimicrobial-steroid agent (Table 3) is sometimes helpful to reduce the inflammation in the eye and on the eyelid caused by the Staphylococcus itself or by the hypersensitivity reaction that may accompany the infection. The use of drops during the day and ointment at bedtime often is more convenient. Prolonged use of neomycin should be avoided because of the risk of an allergic reaction. Tonometry is indicated if corticosteroid therapy is long term. General measures, such as the daily use of antibacterial soap to control skin staphylococci, also are worthwhile.

Seborrheic Blepharitis. In seborrheic blepharitis, greasy scales and flakes are found along the eyelashes; seborrhea of the scalp usually coexists. A helpful sign in differentiating staphylococcal from seborrheic blepharitis is that conjunctivitis or keratitis usually is absent in the latter.

TREATMENT. Lid hygiene, as described above, is similarly effective in the treatment of seborrheic blepharitis. Sulfacetamide has antiseborrheic activity, but the commonly used antibiotics do not. For the successful therapy of seborrheic blepharitis, it is imperative to treat the seborrhea that usually exists in other areas, e.g., scalp, eyebrows, or ears. Diluted baby shampoo, Eyescrub, or OcuSoft Lid Scrub may similarly be used to facilitate hygiene of the lid margins and lashes.

TABLE 2. Topical Antibiotic and Sulfonamide Eye Preparations

Generic Name	Trade Name	Concentration
Drops		
Chloramphenicol solution	Chloromycetin	0.16–0.5%
	AK-Chlor	0.5%
	Chloroptic	0.5%
	Ophthochlor	0.5%
Ciprofloxacin	Ciloxan	0.35%
Gentamicin solution	Garamycin	0.3%
	Genoptic	0.3%
	Gentacidin	0.3%
	Gentrasul	0.3%
	Gent-AK	0.3%
Norfloxacin	Chibroxin	0.3%
Polymixin-B solution		10,000–25,000 U/ml
Sulfacetamide solution	AK-Sulf	10% & 15%
	AK-Sulf Forte	30%
	Bleph-10	10%
	Isopto Cetamide	15%
	Ophthacet	10%
	Sodium Sulamyd	10% & 30%
	Sulf-10	10%
	Sulfair-15	15%
	Sulten-10	10%
Sulfisoxazole solution	Gantrisin	4%
Tetracycline suspension	Achromycin	1%
Tobramycin solution	Tobrex	0.3%
Ointments		
Bacitracin	AK-Tracin	500 U/g
Chloramphenicol	AK-Chlor	10 mg/g
	Chloromycetin	10 mg/g
	Chloroptic S.O.P.	10 mg/g
Chlortetracycline	Aureomycin	10 mg/g
Erythromycin	AK-Mycin	5 mg/g
	Ilotycin	5 mg/g
Gentamicin	Garamycin	3 mg/g
	Genoptic S.O.P.	3 mg/g
	Gentacidin	3 mg/g
	Gentrasul	3 mg/g
	Gent-AK	3 mg/g
Sulfacetamide	AK-Sulf	10%
	Bleph-10 S.O.P.	10%
	Cetamide	10%
	Sodium Sulamyd	10%
Sulfisoxazole	Gantrisin	4%
Tetracycline	Achromycin	10 mg/g
Tobramycin	Tobrex	3 mg/g

TABLE 3. Topical Antimicrobial-Corticosteroid Eye Preparations

Generic Name	Trade Name
Drops	
Chloramphenicol + hydrocortisone (suspension)	Chloromycetin-hydrocortisone
Gentamicin + prednisolone (suspension)	Pred-G
Neomycin + hydrocortisone (suspension)	AK-Neo-Cort
	Cor-Oticin
	Neo-Cortef
	Ortho Drops
Neomycin + dexamethasone (solution)	Neo-Decadron
Neomycin + polymyxin B + hydrocortisone (suspension)	Cortisporin
	Triple-Gen
Neomycin + polymyxin B + prednisolone (suspension)	Poly-Pred
Neomycin + polymyxin B + dexamethasone (suspension)	AK-Trol
	Dexacidin
	Infectrol
	Maxitrol
Sulfacetamide + fluorometholone (suspension)	FML-S
Sulfacetamide + prednisolone (suspension)	AK-Cide
	Blephamide
	Isopto Cetapred
	Metimyd
	Ophtha P/S
	Or-Toptic M
	Predamide
	Predsulfair
	Sulfamide
	Sulphrin
Sulfacetamide + prednisolone (solution)	Optimyd
	Vasocidin
Tobramycin + dexamethasone (suspension)	TobraDex
Ointments	
Chloramphenicol + polymyxin B + hydrocortisone	Ophthocort
Neomycin + dexamethasone	Neo-Decadron
Neomycin + polymyxin B + bacitracin + hydrocortisone	Coracin
	Cortisporin
Sulfacetamide + prednisolone	AK-Cide
	Blephamide S.O.P.
	Cetapred
	Metimyd
	Predsulfair
	Vasocidin

Hordeolum (Stye)

External Hordeolum. This is an acute localized pyogenic infection (usually staphylococcal) of the sebaceous glands (Zeis or Moll) along the lid margin. The localized area of redness, swelling, and tenderness appears on the lid margin at the base of the eyelash. A small yellow area of suppuration appears in a day or so. With rupture of the abscess, pain diminishes. Recurrences are common.

TREATMENT. In the early stages warm, moist compresses applied for 20 minutes three or four times daily hasten localization of the infection. Pressure should not be applied to speed up this process. When the hordeolum is entirely localized, pointing through the epidermis, it is then incised to allow the pus to drain. An antistaphylococcal ointment (bacitracin, erythromycin, or sulfacetamide) applied locally four to six times daily is helpful in aborting the suppuration and preventing spread of the infection. Treatment should be continued for about 1 week after the stye has healed to prevent further infection in other hair follicles.

Internal Hordeolum. This acute purulent infection involves one of the meibomian glands (meibomian stye). The area of localized redness, pain, swelling, or abscess appears on the conjunctival rather than the skin side corresponding to the location of the gland. Spontaneous rupture is less frequent than with the external stye. Recurrences are common.

TREATMENT. Treatment is the same as for external hordeolum.

Chalazion

Chalazion is a common, chronic granulomatous meibomian gland infection of unknown cause. In contrast to the acute purulent infection of this gland (internal hordeolum), there is little or no pain or tenderness unless there is a superimposed secondary pyogenic infection. Symptoms are slight. A slow-growing, hard, round mass localized in the tarsus points more commonly to the conjunctival than to the skin side. If large enough, the mass will distort vision. The tumor may remain the same size, may ulcerate through the surface and leave some remains, or may be absorbed gradually over a few weeks or months.

TREATMENT. If warm moist compresses, eyelid scrubs with diluted baby shampoo or commercial eyelid cleansers, and topical antibiotic-corticosteroid therapy do not appreciably reduce the size of the mass in a few weeks, an intralesional injection of a corticosteroid or incision and evacuation of the chalazion should be performed. For recurrent chalazia, the use of an antibacterial ointment at bedtime and several times a day and weekly massage of the meibomian glands to express secretions may be helpful.

CONJUNCTIVAL DISORDERS

Conjunctivitis

Conjunctivitis ranks with blepharitis as one of the most common external ocular inflammations. Inflammation of the conjunctiva may be microbial, allergic, or traumatic in origin. It may be acute, subacute, or chronic. In the differential diagnosis of the acutely inflamed eye, conjunctivitis can be differentiated from iritis and glaucoma by the presence of a discharge (often bilateral), normal or unaffected vision, normal pupil size and reaction to light, and normal intraocular pressure.

Bacterial Conjunctivitis. Because certain bacteria cause distinct clinical features of bacterial conjunctivitis, the following classification is possible.

ACUTE BACTERIAL (MUCOPURULENT) CONJUNCTIVITIS ("PINK EYE"). The most common causative microorganisms are *Staphylococcus aureus,* pneumococcus, *Haemophilus influenzae,* and beta-hemolytic *Streptococcus.* Intense bulbar but minimal tarsal inflammation is seen. Epithelial keratitis is rare except in the staphylococcal form. Petechial hemorrhages are most common with pneumococcal and *H. influenzae* infections. The disease is highly contagious. It may last several weeks if untreated. The eyelids seal overnight from drying of the products of inflammation.

HYPERACUTE (PURULENT) CONJUNCTIVITIS. Purulent discharge occurs with intense bulbar and tarsal conjunctivitis and chemosis. The gonococcus and, much less commonly, the meningococcus are the main etiologic agents. Meningococcal conjunctivitis may accompany meningitis.

CHRONIC BACTERIAL CONJUNCTIVITIS. *S. aureus* is not only a frequent cause of acute conjunctivitis but also the most common microorganism causing chronic bacterial conjunctivitis. Aerobic, gram-negative bacilli may also cause acute, subacute, and chronic conjunctivitis. *Proteus mirabilis, Klebsiella pneumoniae, Serratia marcescens,* and *Escherichia coli* are common organisms implicated in such cases. Any of the bacteria that cause the more acute forms of conjunctivitis may be found here. Typically, the eye feels worse (itching, irritation, foreign body sensation) at night or in the morning. Blepharitis is common. The palpebral conjunctiva is chronically inflamed, but the bulbar conjunctiva is little affected, if at all. In the staphylococcal type, marginal infiltrates, ulcers, and epithelial erosions of the cornea are frequently seen. Loss of cilia may result. *Moraxella lacunata* characteristically produces redness, most intense near the inner and outer canthi (angular conjunctivitis). *Staphylococcus* can also cause an angular conjunctivitis.

TREATMENT. The best guide for specific therapy is established by showing etiologic bacteria in smears and cultures and then testing the sensitivity to various antimicrobial agents. From a practical standpoint, this seldom is done. Often the conjunctivitis is treated empirically with a topical broad-spectrum antibiotic or sulfacetamide (Tables 2 and 4). The drug prescribed should produce few or no local sensitivities and should be one that is used infrequently in the treatment of systemic disease. Bacitracin, neomycin, polymyxin B, and sulfacetamide are such drugs. If no improvement occurs in several days, specimens for culture are obtained, antibiotic sensitivity studies are done, and the appropriate antibiotic is used.

Corticosteroids have been combined with antimicrobial agents in ophthalmic preparations (Table 4) to reduce the inflammatory and possibly the allergic reactions to the bacterial infection. It is best to avoid corticosteroids because of their adverse effect on latent or potential herpes simplex infections and because of a false impression of control of the inflammatory response by the anti-inflammatory action of corticosteroids. Prolonged corticosteroid use also can cause increased intraocular pressure and cataract.

In severe forms of bacterial conjunctivitis, systemic therapy may be needed. In cases of uncomplicated conjunctivitis, the eyes should not be patched. To avoid infections in other sites or other people, clean and separate cloths should be used for cleansing the eye area.

Viral Conjunctivitis. There is no specific therapy for viral conjunctivitis. The adenovirus is one of the most common agents. Therapy consists in combating secondary bacterial

TABLE 4. Topical Antimicrobial Combination Eye Preparations

Generic Name	Trade Name
Drop	
Polymyxin B + neomycin	Statrol
Polymyxin B + neomycin + gramicidin	AK-Spore Neocidin Neosporin Neotricin
Polymyxin B + trimethoprim	Polytrim
Polymyxin B + trimethoprim	Polytrim
Ointments	
Polymyxin B + bacitracin	AK-Poly-Bac Polysporin
Polymyxin B + neomycin	Statrol
Polymyxin B + bacitracin + neomycin	AK-Spore Neosporin Neotal Mycitracin
Polymyxin B + chloramphenicol	Chloromyxin
Polymyxin B + oxytetracycline	Terramycin

infections by the local use of broad-spectrum antibiotics or a sulfonamide and in relieving symptoms by the use of hot or cold compresses and local astringents or vasoconstrictors (Table 5).

Adenoviral Conjunctivitis. The adenoviruses produce two well-organized infections: pharyngeal-conjunctival fever and epidemic keratoconjunctivitis.

Pharyngeal-Conjunctival Fever. This infection is seen mostly in children and is characterized by fever, malaise, sore throat, preauricular and cervical lymphadenopathy, and a follicular conjunctivitis. The palpebral conjunctiva is red, and there is a copious watery discharge. The disease usually is caused by adenovirus type 3 and less frequently by types 4 and 7 or other serotypes. It is self-limited, lasting about 10 days. Contaminated swimming pools, even chlorinated, are frequent sources of infection.

There is no specific therapy. Isolation precautions should be taken. Symptomatic relief can be given with cold compresses, topical decongestants (Table 5), and sunglasses. Sulfacetamide ophthalmic ointment has been used to prevent secondary bacterial infection.

Epidemic Keratoconjunctivitis. This infection is highly contagious and actually may occur in epidemics. Types 8 and 19 adenovirus are the most frequent causes, but other serotypes may be etiologic. There is a sudden onset of conjunctival congestion, chemosis, profuse tearing, and epithelial keratitis but little secretion. The infection may also be manifested as a pseudomembranous conjunctivitis. Physicians and hospital personnel may spread the disease. The exudate contains predominantly mononuclear cells, sometimes many polymorphonuclear cells if there is a pseudomembranous reaction, but no inclusions. A few days after onset, preauricular lymphadenopathy appears on the affected side. After about 15 days, subepithelial infiltrates may develop in the cornea. The corneal opacities usually clear in several months but on occasion may never clear completely.

Because of its communicability, great care should be exercised in the handling of objects used around the eye. Patients admitted to the hospital should be isolated. Topical broad-spectrum antibiotics have been used to prevent secondary infection. In severe cases, topical corticosteroids in low concentrations may be used to treat the severe conjunctivitis or keratitis if herpes simplex infection is excluded.

TABLE 5. Topical Vasoconstrictor, Astringent, and Antihistaminic Preparations

Generic Name	Trade Name
Vasoconstrictors	
Naphazoline (0.1%)	AK-Con Albalon Muro's Opcon Nafazair Naphcon Forte Opcon Vasocon Regular
Naphazoline (0.03%)	Comfort Eye Drops
Naphazoline (0.025%)	Naphazoline
Naphazoline (0.02%)	VasoClear
Naphazoline (0.012%)	Allerest Clear Eyes Degest 2 Estivin II Naphcon
Phenylephrine (0.12%)	AK-Nefrin Isopto Frin Prefrin
Tetrahydrozoline (0.05%)	Murine Plus Optigene Soothe Visine
Vasoconstrictors with Astringent or Antihistamine	
Naphazoline (0.02%) + zinc sulfate (0.25%)	VasoClear A
Naphazoline (0.05%) + antazoline (0.5%)	Albalon-A Vasocon-A
Naphazoline (0.025%) + pheniramine (0.3%)	AK-Con-A Opcon-A Naphcon-A
Phenylephrine (0.125%) + pheniramine maleate (0.5%)	AK-Vernacon
Phenylephrine (0.12%) + pyrilamine (0.1%)	Prefrin-A
Phenylephrine (0.12%) + zinc sulfate (0.25%)	Phenylzin Zincfrin
Tetrahydrozoline (0.05%) + zinc sulfate (0.25%)	Visine A.C.

Chlamydial (Inclusion) Conjunctivitis. The disease takes different forms in newborns (see Conjunctivitis Neonatorum for treatment details) and in older children and adults (usually referred to as adult inclusion conjunctivitis). The causative organism is *Chlamydia trachomatis* serotypes D, E, F, G, H, I, J, and K.

In newborns a mucopurulent or purulent papillary conjunctivitis appears 5 to 14 days after vaginal delivery. Sequelae usually do not occur, but occasionally a mild superior micropanus and flat conjunctival scarring are seen, especially if treatment is delayed. Diagnosis can be easily made by microscopic examination of a Giemsa-stained conjunctival smear because the typical basophilic granular intracytoplasmic inclusions in epithelial cells are prevalent. (Additional diagnostic tests are given in the discussion of conjunctivitis neonatorum.)

In adolescents and adults, chlamydial conjunctivitis most often results from exposure to infected genital secretions. Occasionally, transmission of inclusion conjunctivitis occurs in poorly chlorinated swimming pools. An acute mucopurulent follicular conjunctivitis appears, usually in one eye and often with preauricular adenopathy. Corneal involvement with superficial epithelial keratitis and marginal subepithelial infiltrates can occur. Because few inclusions are seen in Giemsa-stained conjunctival smears in adult inclusion conjunctivitis, diagnosis usually is made by isolation of the agent in cell culture or by immunofluorescent assay.

Treatment. Treatment consists of full doses of oral tetracycline (in children older than 8 years of age) or erythromycin for 2 or preferably 3 weeks. Sexual consorts should also receive systemic antibiotic therapy. Pregnant women are treated with oral erythromycin. Topical 1 per cent tetracycline or 0.5 per cent erythromycin is not necessary for patients receiving full oral therapeutic doses of antibiotics, but local therapy often is prescribed for additional relief and prevention of bilateral infection. Topical therapy alone is not advisable because the effect is slow or partial and the infection usually is not limited to the eye.

Trachoma. This disease is one of the leading causes of blindness in some parts of the world. Contrary to general belief, it exists also in the United States. Trachoma is endemic among the native American Indians, in a few localities in the South and Southwest, and in immigrant populations from endemic areas. The causative organism is *C. trachomatis* serotypes A, B, and C. The organism is of low infectivity, but the infection occurs under conditions of poor sanitation and hygiene. The clinical picture is that of chronic bilateral conjunctival redness, mild itching, and watery discharge with scant exudate. In the early stages, trachoma is indistinguishable from a mild bacterial conjunctivitis. Cytoplasmic inclusion bodies, morphologically identical to those found in inclusion blennorrhea, although fewer in number, are present in conjunctival scrapings. In untreated cases, inflammation of the conjunctiva continues over a period of months or years, producing papillary and then follicular hypertrophy followed by scarring. With progression of the disease, the cornea becomes opacified, vascularized, and scarred and vision is severely impaired. Some of the ocular complications are due to secondary bacterial infection.

TREATMENT. Trachoma is effectively treated with a 3-week course of oral tetracycline or erythromycin (30 mg/kg/day in four divided doses). Erythromycin is used instead of tetracycline in pregnant women and children under 8 years old. Topical tetracycline or erythromycin therapy alone can cure trachoma, but the response time is longer. Topical antibiotic therapy usually is given along with systemic therapy because it decreases the intensity of the conjunctival inflammation and counteracts secondary bacterial infection—a factor contributing to scar formation. Concurrent topical corticosteroids should be avoided because (1) signs and symptoms of the primary eye disease could be masked, (2) rebound of the disease may occur when the corticosteroid is discontinued, and (3) reactivation of a concomitant herpes virus infection is liable to occur. Eyelid deformities are treated surgically.

Exanthematous Conjunctivitis. The exanthems such as measles, chickenpox, and smallpox may be accompanied by an acute conjunctivitis. No specific treatment is given unless secondary bacterial infection occurs. If the cornea becomes involved, an ophthalmologist should be consulted for further treatment.

Vaccinia Conjunctivitis. Ocular vaccinia is rarely seen now since smallpox vaccination no longer is routinely recommended. Autoinoculation or inoculation from a contact may lead to a conjunctivitis or serious corneal involvement.

TREATMENT. Treatment of the conjunctival lesions with a topical antiviral agent may help prevent development of keratitis. Vidarabine (Vira-A) and trifluridine (Viroptic) are probably more effective than idoxuridine (Stoxil, Herplex). Vidarabine is given as a 3 per cent ointment five times daily. Trifluridine 1 per cent drops are given every 2 hours while the patient is awake (maximum 9 drops/day). Idoxuridine is given as a 0.1 per cent solution every hour during the day and every 2 hours at night or as a 0.5 per cent ointment every 6 hours. Hyperimmune vaccinial gamma globulin (VIG) may be used topically (100 mg/ml) every 2 hours. If there is considerable eyelid and conjunctival involvement but no keratitis, VIG may be given intramuscularly (0.6 ml/kg body weight) and repeated in 48 hours if no improvement occurs. VIG is not given or is used with caution if the cornea is involved because of experimental evidence that antigen-antibody complexes within the cornea from administration of VIG may aggravate the keratitis and cause persistent stromal edema. Topical antibiotics may be used to prevent superinfection.

Conjunctivitis Neonatorum (Ophthalmia Neonatorum). Any inflammation of the conjunctiva of the newborn is considered in this category. The inflammation may be due to the chemical irritant silver nitrate or to an infection acquired from an infected birth canal during parturition. The infection may be (1) bacterial (staphylococcus; streptococcus; pneumococcus; *Neisseria* species, e.g., *N. gonorrhoeae, N. meningitidis; Haemophilus* species; coliform organisms; or other bacteria), (2) chlamydial (see Chlamydial [Inclusion] Conjunctivitis), or (3) viral (herpes simplex).

The incidence of blindness from gonococcal conjunctivitis has been dramatically reduced by prenatal treatment of the mother and by routine topical use of 1 per cent silver nitrate solution or an appropriate antibiotic in each eye of the infant within 1 hour after birth. Erythromycin (and, less commonly, tetracycline) in recent years have replaced silver nitrate as the prophylactic agents of choice in most newborn nurseries. The reason for the change is that these antibiotics are effective against *C. trachomatis*—currently the most common cause of infectious ophthalmia neonatorum—as well as *N. gonorrhoeae*. Also, the antibiotics do not cause a chemical conjunctivitis. Silver nitrate has been thought to be ineffective against *C. trachomatis*. Recently, however, the drug has been shown to have some activity against the organism. Although most strains of *N. gonorrhoeae* at present are sensitive to erythromycin and tetracycline, there is the distinct danger of encountering an increasing number of resistant strains. Resistance to silver nitrate over the years has not been a factor. Since gonococcal ophthalmia neonatorum is a rapidly blinding disease when not treated promptly, whereas chlamydial ophthalmia neonatorum is not, some pediatricians still prefer the use of silver nitrate. They fear that they may encounter an antibiotic-resistant strain of *N. gonorrhoeae*. Infants born to mothers with untreated gonorrhea should be treated prophylactically with a single injection of aqueous crystalline penicillin G (15,000 units intravenously or intramuscularly if full-term and 20,000 units if birth weight is under 2000 g).

The time of onset of conjunctivitis after exposure to the etiologic agent is helpful in the diagnosis. In general, the onset times are 1 to 2 days for silver nitrate, 2 to 4 days for *N. gonorrhoeae*, 4 to 7 days for other bacteria, 2 to 4 days for herpes simplex, and 5 to 14 days for *C. trachomatis*. The definitive diagnosis, however, is made from studies that include (1) examination of Gram- and Giemsa-stained scrapings from the tarsal conjunctiva, (2) bacterial cultures of scrapings and exudates, (3) additional chlamydial identification tests, such as cell culture of conjunctival scrapings, immunoglobulin antibody titers, monoclonal antibody test on conjunctival smears, and enzyme-linked immunoassay, and (4) other herpes simplex identification tests such as viral culture, recognition of specific herpes simplex virus antigen by immunofluorescence in conjunctival scrapings, and detection of herpes simplex virus particles by electron microscopic examination.

TREATMENT. Active treatment of neonatal gonococcal ophthalmia consists of (1) hospitalization with isolation for 24 hours after initiation of treatment, and (2) ceftriaxone sodium (50 mg/kg/day, maximum 125 mg, in a single dose intravenously or intramuscularly for 7 days). Initial therapy with a third-generation cephalosporin (ceftriaxone or cefotaxime) has replaced penicillin as first-line treatment because of the increased prevalence of penicillin-resistant *N. gonorrhoeae*. If the gonococcal isolate, however, is found susceptible to penicillin, aqueous crystalline penicillin G (100,000 U/kg/day) may be given intravenously in two doses or intramuscularly in four doses for 7 days. Topical erythromycin ointment commonly is instilled four to six times daily even though local therapy is not required when systemic therapy is used. Frequent irrigation of the eye with saline to eliminate discharge is helpful. Caregivers should be treated with tetracycline or an appropriate penicillin taken orally.

Other bacteria cause neonatal conjunctivitis but have less propensity for corneal involvement. Microscopic examination of Gram-stained conjunctival scrapings and discharge is useful for selection of initial antibiotic therapy. Bacterial specimens of conjunctival scrapings and discharge should be obtained for culture and sensitivity tests should be performed at the outset to properly guide further therapy. Most gram-positive pathogens respond to 0.5 per cent erythromycin ointment; gram-negative organisms are treated with 0.3 per cent gentamicin or tobramycin drops or ointment. If initially one is uncertain of the etiologic agent, a broad-spectrum antimicrobial drug or drug combination (see Tables 2 and 4) may be given until results of the culture and sensitivity studies are returned. *Pseudomonas* conjunctivitis can be particularly serious, especially in premature infants. Prompt topical therapy with gentamicin or tobramycin for several weeks is indicated. If response is poor, subconjunctival injections are given twice daily until cultures are negative. Systemic gentamicin or tobramycin is given if there are other foci of infection or if the conjunctivitis continues to progress.

Chlamydial conjunctivitis is treated with systemic therapy because many infants also have nasopharyngeal infection and chlamydial pneumonia may develop. Oral erythromycin (50 mg/kg/day) is given in four divided doses for 2 weeks along with topical tetracycline or erythromycin ointment instilled four times daily. All caregivers should be treated with erythromycin (30 mg/kg/day for 3 weeks) to avoid reinfecting the infant.

Herpes simplex conjunctivitis should be treated in association with an ophthalmologist because serious ocular sequelae may occur, namely, keratitis, cataracts, chorioretinitis, and optic neuritis. Infected infants must be isolated. Topical antiviral therapy consists of 1 drop of 1 per cent trifluridine instilled every 2 to 3 hours while the infant is awake, with 0.5 per cent idoxuridine ointment used at bedtime until 3 days after healing appears complete (usually within 2 weeks). If no response occurs within 1 week, therapy with systemic acyclovir (30 mg/kg/day in 3 divided doses, given intravenously for a minimum of 2 weeks) may be considered. Topical and systemic corticosteroids should be avoided because they exacerbate herpes simplex infections.

Mucocutaneous Ocular Diseases. Treatment of the conjunctivitis associated with the mucocutaneous diseases, such as erythema multiforme, Stevens-Johnson syndrome, and Reiter's syndrome, is mostly nonspecific, since the etiologic agent is unknown. Precipitating factors may be drugs, food allergy, or infections. Mild soothing eye drops with or without astringent and vasoconstricting properties (see Table 5) may be used. Steroids used locally (Table 6) or systemically may be helpful in controlling the allergic and inflammatory phases of the disease, but they must be used judiciously. Drugs such as the sulfonamides and antibiotics should be avoided, for they have been known to precipitate erythema multiforme and Stevens-Johnson disease. A local antibiotic should be used only when a secondary bacterial infection occurs. The pediatrician should choose a suitable antibiotic that the patient has not previously used or one that unquestionably was not associated with the present episode. In severe cases, visual function can be seriously impaired because of lack of tears, symblepharon formation, corneal ulcer, perforation, and panophthalmitis in Stevens-Johnson disease and scleritis, interstitial keratitis, and hypopyon uveitis in Reiter's disease. Because of the seriousness of the eye complications, it is advisable for an ophthalmologist to treat the ocular aspects of these diseases.

Allergic Forms of Conjunctivitis

SIMPLE ALLERGIC CONJUNCTIVITIS. The clinical manifestations of these nonspecific conjunctival inflammations are acute edema of the lids and conjunctiva, itching, photophobia, lacrimation, mild injection of the palpebral and bulbar conjunctiva, and a scanty, stringy discharge. Conjunctival papillae and follicles are not present. An occasional eosinophil is present in the smear of the conjunctival scraping. There may or may not be a direct relation to an allergen, such as a pollen (hay fever), cosmetic, or drug.

Treatment. Treatment consists of (1) removal of the offending agent if possible, (2) desensitization to the allergen, and (3) symptomatic relief with the use of local vasoconstrictors with or without antihistamines, astringents, cromolyn sodium 4 per cent solution (Opticrom), and—only during the acute phase of severe cases—corticosteroids (Tables 5 and 6). Steroids should be avoided, if possible, and used only under special circumstances supervised by an ophthalmologist. The disadvantages of the steroids, i.e., activation of herpes simplex keratoconjunctivitis and bacterial and fungal infections, must be kept in mind. Cataracts and glaucoma have been seen in children as well as in adults who have used topical corticosteroids for long periods. If vasoconstrictors with or without antihistamines (local and systemic) or cromolyn sodium drops control the allergic reaction, steroids should not be used.

TABLE 6. Topical Corticosteroid Eye Preparations

Generic Name	Trade Name	Concentration
Drops		
Dexamethasone alcohol (suspension)	Maxidex	0.1%
Dexamethasone sodium phosphate (solution)	AK-Dex	0.1%
	Baldex	0.1%
	Decadron	0.1%
Fluorometholone (suspension)	FML	0.1%
	Fluor-Op	0.1%
	FML Forte	0.25%
Medrysone (suspension)	HMS	1%
Prednisolone acetate (suspension)	Econopred	0.125%
	Econopred Plus	1%
	Pred Mild	0.12%
	Pred Forte	1%
Prednisolone sodium phosphate (solution)	AK-Pred	0.125% & 1%
	Inflamase Mild	0.125%
	Inflamase Forte	1%
	Metreton	0.5%
Ointments		
Dexamethasone sodium phosphate	AK-Dex	0.05%
	Baldex	0.05%
	Decadron	0.05%
	Maxidex	0.05%
Fluorometholone	FML	0.1%

VERNAL CONJUNCTIVITIS. This is a bilateral chronic conjunctivitis accompanied by symptoms that usually become worse in the spring and last throughout the warm months. The cause is thought to be allergic. The onset is between 5 and 15 years. The severity of the symptoms tends to become milder with the passing years. This condition is characterized by intense itching, lacrimation, photophobia, conjunctival injection, a stringy conjunctival discharge, and, at times, a milky pseudomembrane. Giant papillary hypertrophy develops in the tarsal conjunctiva, especially the upper, to give the typical "cobblestone" appearance. The lesions may cause a corneal "shield ulcer" (called such because of the shape of the epithelial defect). Papillary hypertrophy in the limbal region appears as gray elevated lesions. Many eosinophils are seen in the smear of the conjunctival exudate.

Treatment. In mild cases, symptoms may be relieved by topical vasoconstrictors, topical and oral antihistamines, and cold compresses. More serious disease warrants topical cromolyn 4 per cent (Opticrom) eye drops instilled four times daily. Cromolyn inhibits the degranulation of conjunctival mast cells, thereby preventing the release of histamine. The action of cromolyn is prophylactic in that it prevents the release of this mediator of inflammation.

If further control of the disease is required, topical corticosteroids (Table 6) are used. To suppress symptoms in severe disabling disease, it may be necessary to use the corticosteroid every 2 hours, perhaps supplemented by small oral doses. As improvement occurs, corticosteroid therapy is reduced as soon as possible to the minimum therapeutic dosage. Fluorometholone (FML) is the topical corticosteroid often preferred over the more potent preparations, such as dexamethasone and prednisolone, because it is effective locally yet has less tendency to increase intraocular pressure with continued use. The prolonged use of any corticosteroid, however, carries the risk of glaucoma, herpes simplex infection activation, and cataract. Topical cromolyn sodium in many cases has eliminated the need for topical corticosteroids or has reduced its use to once or twice a day.

Beta-radiation, cryoablation, and surgical excision of giant papillae have been used, but the papillae usually recur. Desensitization of the patient to allergens has had little effect on the disease. Symptoms usually subside or disappear with cool or cold weather.

PHLYCTENULAR KERATOCONJUNCTIVITIS. The phlyctenule is a small, hard, red elevated nodule surrounded by hyperemic vessels. It appears most commonly at the limbus to involve both the bulbar conjunctiva and the cornea. The lesion is a subepithelial collection of neutrophils and mononuclear cells, including lymphocytes, macrophages, and plasma cells that ulcerate but usually heal. Recurrences, especially with secondary infection, may result in corneal opacification. The outstanding clinical manifestations are intense photophobia and lacrimation. The disease has been regarded as a hypersensitivity reaction of the conjunctiva and cornea to a product of the tubercle bacillus, other bacteria such as the staphylococcus, or fungi.

Treatment. Since malnutrition is frequently a part of the disease, general measures such as improving the diet and hygiene are important. A topical corticosteroid or antimicrobial-corticosteroid combination (see Tables 3 and 6) is effective in treating the disease and the secondary infection that may be present. For patients who do not respond to corticosteroids or who experience corticosteroid complications, oral erythromycin or tetracycline (for patients older than 8 years) has proved effective. Investigation for a systemic disease, such as tuberculosis, should be made.

Nonspecific Conjunctival Hyperemia. External irritants (smoke, smog, fumes, or swimming pool or ocean water) or factors such as inadequate rest or asthenopia (eyestrain) may produce conjunctival hyperemia. Astringent eye drops with or without a vasoconstrictor (see Table 5) relieve this nonspecific inflammation. A complete eye examination should be performed if the symptoms are associated with eyestrain.

The pediatrician must consider specific diseases, such as ataxia-telangiectasia and familial dysautonomia (Riley-Day syndrome), before settling on a diagnosis of nonspecific conjunctival hyperemia.

CORNEAL DISORDERS

In general, diseases of the cornea mandate early attention by an ophthalmologist. Even so-called minor infections of this portion of the eye can lead to serious ocular complications, including blindness, if they are not promptly and correctly handled by the skilled specialist. A safe rule to follow for the nonophthalmologic physician is that all diseases and injuries of the cornea (including foreign bodies) should be seen promptly by an ophthalmologist. It is important, therefore, for pediatricians to learn the symptoms and signs of corneal disease to enable them to recognize this diagnostic possibility.

Patients with corneal disease may have photophobia, lacrimation, blepharospasm, pain, decreased vision, ocular discharge, hyperemia of the superficial and deep conjunctival vessels (circumlimbal flush), corneal opacity, small pupil if secondary iritis exists, and often a history of trauma. Inspection of the cornea with intense oblique focal illumination is often necessary to see a foreign body or a lesion.

The treatment of corneal diseases is not reviewed in detail because therapy should be carried out by the ophthalmologist.

Corneal Ulcers and Infections

Careful examination of the ocular adnexa is important because inflammation of the cornea may be secondary to other diseases, e.g., blepharitis, trichiasis, trachoma, the "cobblestone" papillae of vernal conjunctivitis, conjunctivitis, scleritis, iritis, or dacryocystitis. Systemic disease and poor general physical condition must be evaluated, for they may contribute to the development of a corneal infection.

Ulcers of the cornea can be easily seen by placing a drop or two of sterile fluorescein solution or a moistened fluorescein paper strip (Fluor-I-Strip) into the conjunctival sac and then washing out the excess with isotonic saline solution. Studies to determine the cause of corneal ulcer include Gram and Giemsa stains of smears and scrapings, cultures (bacterial, viral, and fungal), and antimicrobial sensitivity tests when cultures are positive.

Simple Corneal Ulcer. This lesion may result from direct infection after a break of the epithelial barrier by trauma or by disturbances in the metabolism of the epithelium from causes such as vitamin A deficiency, corneal exposure, and neurotrophic disease.

Central Corneal Ulcer. Central ulcers have an intense purulent reaction in and around the ulcer, with occasional extension into the deeper layers of the cornea or an exudative reaction in the anterior chamber (hypopyon); most are bacterial. The gram-positive cocci most likely to produce central corneal ulcers are *S. aureus, Staphylococcus epidermidis, Streptococcus pneumoniae,* and *Streptococcus pyogenes.* The most common gram-negative causative bacteria are *Pseudomonas aeruginosa, Moraxella lacunata,* and Enterobacteriaceae (*Proteus, Serratia, E. coli,* and *Klebsiella*). The ulcers may develop after trauma or appear in association with a dacryocystitis.

TREATMENT. Corneal ulcers are best managed by the ophthalmologist. Before antimicrobial treatment is started, smears and cultures of the ulcer material should be prepared and sensitivity studies to various antimicrobial agents should be pursued. To accomplish these studies in young children, a general anesthetic may be required. Until these studies indicate the antimicrobial drug of choice, fortified topical antibiotics, such as cefazolin (50 mg/ml) and gentamicin or tobramycin (15 mg/ml), effective against a wide range of gram-positive and gram-negative bacteria, should be used at hourly intervals. Mixtures that contain bacitracin or gramicidin, neomycin, and polymyxin B are available (see Table 4). Gentamicin plus bacitracin may also be used. Local therapy alone may be all that is required in the superficial ulcers. In the more severe corneal ulcers, systemic and subconjunctival antibiotic therapy may be necessary. Cycloplegic medication is usually given because of the accompanying iridocyclitis. Local corticosteroid therapy is avoided because it interferes with tissue reparative processes and immune responses. Ulcers that progress in spite of vigorous medical therapy may benefit from covering the ulcer with a conjunctival flap, closure of the eyelids with adhesions (tarsorrhaphy), or replacement of the ulcer site by a keratoplasty.

Marginal Corneal Ulcer. Marginal ulcers may be sterile and may represent a toxic or hypersensitivity reaction to bacterial infection, usually staphylococcal, of the conjunctiva or eyelid.

TREATMENT. Topical corticosteroids usually cure the sterile

toxic or hypersensitivity type of ulcer in 3 to 4 days. The infectious blepharitis and conjunctivitis can be treated with bacitracin if the primary infection is due to *Staphylococcus, Streptococcus,* or *H. influenzae.* A tetracycline or sulfonamide is also effective against these bacteria as well as *Moraxella lacunata.*

Phlyctenular Keratoconjunctivitis. See page 527.

Herpes Simplex Virus Keratitis (Dendritic Keratitis). This form of keratitis is a common corneal disease in childhood. The widespread and indiscriminate use of local steroids increases the severity of the infection and the ocular complications such as corneal perforation and loss of the eye. Dendritic keratitis is the most important corneal disease leading to loss of vision in the United States. Herpes simplex infections of the cornea tend to be chronic, leaving opaque scars that impair vision. Recurrent infections are frequent.

The patient complains of mild irritation and has photophobia, lacrimation, and blurred vision. A recent history of an infection of the respiratory tract with "cold sores" on the face is often elicited. Fever, trauma, menstruation, and psychic stress may be other precipitating factors. The dendrite-shaped ulcer (seen best with fluorescein or rose bengal staining) and decreased corneal sensitivity characterize this type of keratitis.

TREATMENT. The principal treatment previously had consisted of the removal of the virus-containing epithelium by mechanical débridement. Chemotherapy with the topical antiviral drugs idoxuridine (Herplex, Stoxil), vidarabine (Vira-A), and trifluridine (Viroptic) is known to be effective against herpes simplex keratitis. These drugs interfere with DNA synthesis. The response to topical antiviral therapy is best when the infection is limited to the epithelium. With stromal involvement, these drugs are less effective or ineffective. Of the three antiviral agents, trifluridine has been the most effective, probably because of its greater solubility than either idoxuridine or vidarabine. One drop of the 1 per cent solution is instilled every 2 hours while the patient is awake for a maximal daily dose of 9 drops. Healing of uncomplicated ulcers occurs in 1 to 2 weeks. As the epithelial defect heals, the antiviral therapy can be tapered to 5 drops daily but it should be continued for about 1 week after healing to prevent immediate recurrences.

Although corticosteroids are generally contraindicated in herpes simplex keratitis, in the less acute inflammatory form with stromal involvement known as *disciform herpetic keratitis,* restricted use of a topical corticosteroid, such as prednisolone acetate 1 per cent, can be helpful if used concurrently with trifluridine if the epithelium is healed. Disciform herpetic keratitis is believed to be a hypersensitivity reaction to the viral antigens. If the keratitis is progressive in spite of medical treatment, a conjunctival flap, tarsorrhaphy, or lamellar keratoplasty may be required. A topical cycloplegic agent, such as 1 per cent atropine or 0.25 per cent scopolamine, is helpful in keeping the eye comfortable.

Herpes Zoster Keratitis. The diagnosis is usually made from the characteristic skin lesions and their distribution along the ophthalmic division of the trigeminal nerve. The skin of the tip of the nose and the eye are often simultaneously involved, since the nasociliary nerve innervates both sites (positive Hutchinson's sign). An iridocyclitis usually accompanies the corneal involvement.

TREATMENT. Commercially available topical antiviral agents generally are ineffective. Topical ophthalmic acyclovir has shown benefit but is not available commercially in the United States. A 3 per cent ophthalmic ointment is available through compassionate plea request from the Burroughs Wellcome Company.

Although corticosteroids (without antiviral agents) are contraindicated in herpes simplex keratitis, they frequently relieve the keratitis and iridocyclitis of herpes zoster. Severe involvement of post-herpetic neuralgia may be alleviated by systemic use of corticosteroids. The incidence of neuralgia, however, is not high in young patients. The steroids act primarily as an anti-inflammatory agent. Corticosteroids should be avoided or used with extreme caution in immunosuppressed patients for fear of dissemination of the disease. Correspondingly, fulminating herpes zoster has developed in patients who were receiving systemic corticosteroids for other diseases. Thus, it is wise to delay start of corticosteroid therapy in the otherwise healthy patient for 3 to 5 days after appearance of the eruption to enable the host's immune system to be mobilized. Intravenous or oral acyclovir given within the first 72 hours of the onset of herpes zoster ophthalmicus has been particularly beneficial. Its use, especially in immunosuppressed patients, is indicated for severe corneal or uveal involvement and visually threatening complications such as proptosis, chorioretinitis, or optic neuritis. The oral dose of acyclovir (Zovirax) is 800 mg five times a day for 10 days in immunocompetent adult patients; effective oral dosage has not been established in pediatric patients. In immunosuppressed patients, the acyclovir dosage is 5 to 10 mg/kg or 500 mg/m^2 intravenously every 8 hours for 5 to 7 days.

Cycloplegic eye drops are used along with topical corticosteroids for the iridocyclitis. Antibiotics to control secondary bacterial infection may reduce severe scarring of the cornea.

Vaccinia Keratitis. Topical antiviral drugs are used for vaccinia infection of the cornea (see Vaccinia Conjunctivitis). Trifluridine is the agent of choice because of better corneal permeability. Cycloplegics are used to relieve the iritis. Vaccinia immune globulin (VIG) is not used because experimental studies indicate that delayed immune reactions occur in the cornea from its use and these reactions lead to prolonged stromal edema. Topical antibiotics may be given twice daily to prevent superinfection.

Exanthematous Keratitis. Measles (rubeola) and its complications are less often seen now because of routine immunization of young children with live attenuated measles virus. A keratitis with multiple epithelial erosions causes photophobia. The keratoconjunctivitis usually is mild and self-limited. The available topical antiviral agents are not effective. Microbial superinfection is prevented or treated with topical antibiotics.

Chickenpox (varicella) rarely causes serious ocular disease. In addition to a mild conjunctivitis, varicella may produce a punctate or dendritic keratitis that is similar to but not caused by herpes simplex infection. Although there is no conclusive evidence that topical antiviral drugs are efficacious, claims of their value in the acute phase of epithelial keratitis have been made. Trifluridine 1 per cent (Viroptic), 1 drop five times daily, may be helpful. Cycloplegics are used for the uveitis that may accompany the keratitis. Topical antibiotics are given to prevent or treat microbial superinfection.

Smallpox (variola) has been essentially eliminated by vaccination measures. Direct corneal involvement can occur, but most lesions heal spontaneously and leave minimal scars. Severe infections, however, may lead to corneal ulcers that become secondarily infected with bacteria and result in dense scars. Adequate antiviral therapy is not available. Cycloplegics are used for any accompanying iridocyclitis. Topical antibiotics prevent secondary bacterial infections.

Superficial Punctate Keratitis. Thygeson's superficial punctate keratitis is characterized by scattered, fine, punctate infiltrations in the superficial corneal layers, usually of both eyes. The lesions favor the pupillary area and require magnification to be seen. Vision may be appreciably reduced. The lesions are nonulcerative, but most stain with fluorescein. Healing may take several years in the untreated case, but no scarring or vascularization occurs. The disease is thought to be caused by a virus. Drugs, exposure, and staphylococcal infections, however, may produce the same signs and symptoms. The symptoms are photophobia, lacrimation, pain, conjunctival infection, and decreased vision. Preauricular lymphadenopathy may be present.

TREATMENT. Topical use of a corticosteroid such as FML usually is beneficial. Steroid dosage is tapered rapidly. Since recurrence of keratitis is common, periodic use of the steroid (e.g., 1 drop once or twice weekly) may be sufficient to keep the patient asymptomatic. Antiviral drugs are not recommended because they can cause scarring beneath the lesions. Cycloplegics usually are not needed. Local antibiotics are used if there is a bacterial infection. The use of soft contact lenses to reduce symptoms has also been helpful.

Fungal Corneal Ulcers. The incidence of keratomycosis has increased in recent years. Local antibiotic and steroid therapy seems to be an important factor in this increase. Fungi infect the cornea after a break in the epithelium from trauma or damage by inflammation. Numerous fungi, including those previously regarded as nonpathogenic, have been cultured from these indolent, slowly progressive corneal ulcers. A fungal etiology should be considered if an ulcer does not respond to antibiotic therapy. Identification of the fungus is made by examination of scrapings obtained with Gram, Giemsa, and potassium hydroxide stains and by culture on Sabouraud's agar or blood agar at room temperature.

TREATMENT. Natamycin (Natacyn) is the initial drug of choice for both yeast and filamentary forms; a 5 per cent suspension is given every 1 to 2 hours for 3 to 4 days, then reduced to 1 drop six to eight times daily for 2 to 3 weeks. If no response occurs and filamentous organisms are isolated, miconazole (Monistat) 1 per cent prepared from the injectable solution is given every hour initially. If yeast forms *(Candida)* do not respond to topical natamycin, then nystatin (Mycostatin, Nilstat) is used—1 drop of 25,000 units/ml hourly—or the powder may be dusted onto the lesion. Flucytosine 1 per cent, prepared from oral capsules, has been used hourly for *Candida* infections. Amphotericin B (Fungi-zone) 0.15 per cent solution applied hourly is effective against a group of pathogenic and saprophytic fungi, including *Candida, Coccidioides, Cryptococcus, Histoplasma, Blastomyces,* and *Sporotrichum.* For corneal perforations or intraocular extension of *Candida* and filamentous fungi (except *Fusarium*), miconazole may be given subconjunctivally and intravenously. Oral flucytosine may also be effective. Oral ketaconazole has been reported to be helpful for severe keratomycoses. For nonhealing ulcers, a conjunctival flap may be required. A penetrating keratoplasty may provide a cure if the entire area of infection can be encompassed. Cycloplegics are used for an accompanying iridocyclitis. Broad-spectrum antibiotics are applied to combat bacterial superinfection.

Interstitial Keratitis. Most cases of interstitial keratitis in children occur as complications of congenital syphilis. Tuberculosis and leprosy are rare causes. Symptoms of intense photophobia, lacrimation, pain, and gradual loss of vision, ultimately in both eyes, occur between 5 and 15 years of age. Inflammation and vascularization involve the deep layers of the cornea. The cornea assumes a ground-glass appearance with orange-red areas ("salmon patches") due to vascularization. The reaction normally begins to subside in 1 to 2 months, sooner when topical or systemic corticosteroids are given. Ghost vessels, seen with magnification, remain in the corneal stroma after the inflammation has subsided. An associated uveitis or choroiditis is common. These serious ocular manifestations are less often seen today because of intensive systemic antiluetic and topical corticosteroid therapy. Other signs of congenital syphilis may be seen, such as saddle nose, deafness, and notched teeth. The serologic tests for syphilis give positive results. Interstitial keratitis may represent an allergic response, since *Treponema pallidum* is not found in the cornea during the acute stage.

TREATMENT. There is no specific treatment for syphilitic interstitial keratitis. Systemic acute syphilis should be treated with penicillin, but the treatment does not affect the corneal disease. Topical steroids relieve the symptoms. Systemic steroids are valuable if the local steroids do not adequately control the symptoms. Some physicians believe that steroid therapy may prolong the disease. The accompanying iridocyclitis is helped by the local steroids, but in addition a strong cycloplegic such as atropine 1 per cent should be instilled daily. For severe corneal scarring, a corneal transplant is indicated but only if damage to other parts of the eye does not preclude a good visual outcome. In the rare case when tuberculosis is the cause of the interstitial keratitis (usually unilateral), the systemic infection is treated.

Corneal Drying and Exposure. The following diseases are associated with the complications of corneal drying and exposure: (1) *keratitis sicca,* the result of a lacrimal gland insufficiency; (2) *exposure keratitis,* developing after facial nerve palsies, exophthalmos, and prolonged periods of unconsciousness; (3) *neuroparalytic keratitis,* seen after interruption of function of the trigeminal nerve; (4) *familial dysautonomia* (Riley-Day syndrome), corneal complications occurring from the congenital absence or deficiency of tears and corneal hypesthesia. Corneal infection may lead to intraocular infection and loss of the eye.

TREATMENT. The cornea should be protected with artificial tears used hourly or less often as needed. The many different products available commercially attest to the variability in patient relief. The principal bases in the liquid preparations include (1) methylcellulose, (2) ethylcellulose, (3) polyvinyl alcohol, and (4) polyvinylpyrrolidone polymer. The lubricant ointments contain petrolatum, lanolin, and mineral oil. For patients who need frequent tear replacement, a soluble insert of hydroxypropylcellulose (Lacrisert) is available. Sodium hyaluronate (Healon) 0.1 per cent solution has been helpful in some patients. The use of a soft contact lens in association with frequent artificial tear instillation helps to maintain a satisfactory precorneal tear film. To conserve tears, temporary closure of the lacrimal punta can be accomplished with silicone or polytef (Teflon) plugs or with cyanoacrylate glue; permanent closure is achieved with electrocautery or argon laser. Temporary closure of the puncta may be used to predict whether the patient will have epiphora following permanent closure. In severe cases, a moist chamber can be made by applying an occlusive plastic shield across the eyes or by wearing flush-fitting goggles. Lastly, a temporary or permanent tarsorrhaphy may be required to protect the cornea.

SCLERAL AND EPISCLERAL DISORDERS

Episcleritis

A localized inflammation of the tissue between the conjunctiva and sclera is characteristic of episcleritis. The patient has slight pain, photophobia, and tenderness in the area. The localized patch of hyperemia and the absence of a discharge distinguish episcleritis from conjunctivitis. Episcleritis can occur as an isolated disease or in association with a systemic disorder, most commonly a collagen disease such as rheumatoid arthritis. The condition often is self-limited. About one third of the patients have uveitis as well.

TREATMENT. Local vasoconstrictor drops (see Table 5) are

helpful, but topical steroid medication (see Table 6) may give better relief of symptoms. A cycloplegic such as scopolamine 0.25 per cent, 1 drop two times daily, is instilled into the eye if there is an anterior uveitis. A systemic disorder should be sought and treated. Oral oxyphenbutazone (Tandearil) or indomethacin (Indocin) has been reported to be effective in the treatment of persistent episcleritis. Oxyphenbutazone is not available at present in the United States.

Scleritis

Inflammation of the deeper scleral tissue is more severe and appears more purplish than in episcleritis. It may be localized, diffuse, or nodular. Pain, photophobia, and tenderness may be intense. An associated anterior uveitis is frequently present. Scleritis may be seen with systemic diseases such as the collagen diseases (particularly rheumatoid arthritis), tuberculosis, syphilis, brucellosis, and gout. The severity of the scleritis is often directly related to the severity of the systemic disease.

TREATMENT. In the acute phase, an occasional patient may respond to topical corticosteroid therapy but topical anti-inflammatory agents usually are ineffective. Systemic nonsteroidal anti-inflammatory drugs or a corticosteroid generally is necessary. The nonsteroidal drugs are tried first. If long-term corticosteroid therapy is needed for recurrent or persistent episcleritis or scleritis, periodic examination for increased intraocular pressure and cataract should be performed. In the severe necrotizing form of scleritis, topical steroids may hasten corneal and scleral melting. Systemic steroids may be needed for severe posterior scleritis. Scopolamine 0.25 per cent is instilled into the eye two times daily if an anterior uveitis is present. The systemic disease is actively treated.

It is of interest that scleritis may develop in patients receiving salicylates or systemic corticosteroids for a disease such as rheumatoid arthritis. The addition of topical steroid therapy is rarely of value in such a situation. Subconjunctival corticosteroid injections must be avoided because the sclera often is thin and may perforate after injection of the drug. Cases of severe scleritis may necessitate the use of immunosuppressive drugs. If scleral ectasia and impending perforation of the globe occur, scleral grafting may be necessary.

UVEITIS

Inflammation of the uveal tract is a serious disease because it often leads to severe visual impairment or blindness. Early diagnosis and treatment are important to prevent the ocular complications. The damaging effect of the disease often is subtle in children. There may be few or no subjective complaints or obvious signs of the disease during episodes of recurrent or chronic inflammation.

Uveitis has been popularly classified as nongranulomatous and granulomatous. *Nongranulomatous uveitis* more often involves the anterior uvea, producing the following symptoms and signs: acute onset with pain, redness, photophobia, blurred vision, circumcorneal flush, miotic or irregular pupil, and, on slit-lamp examination, the presence of fibrin and cells in the anterior chamber and fine white keratic precipitates on the posterior surface of the cornea.

Granulomatous uveitis appears more frequently as a posterior uveitis with a slow onset, minimal redness, pain or photophobia, normal or slightly miotic pupil, and vision less than one would expect from the mild external manifestations of the disease. Large, yellow-gray "mutton-fat" keratic precipitates are seen on the posterior surface of the cornea with the slit lamp. Iris nodules are often visible. On ophthalmoscopy single or multiple yellow or white exudative lesions are seen in the choroid with or without vitreous haze.

Uveitis presents a difficult therapeutic problem because, although numerous causes are suspected, in only relatively few cases is a specific etiologic agent detected. Studies indicate that there is a higher incidence of nongranulomatous uveitis in patients with autoimmune disorders, such as juvenile rheumatoid arthritis, sarcoidosis, systemic lupus erythematosus, and the like. Granulomatous uveitis may result from the actual invasion of the uveal tract by an organism, but organisms are rarely isolated or demonstrated. Granulomatous uveitis may be caused by toxoplasmosis (the infection most frequently incriminated), syphilis, tuberculosis, brucellosis, leptospirosis, viruses, fungi, nematodes, and sarcoidosis.

TREATMENT. The management of uveitis consists of (1) thorough medical evaluation of the patient in search for a specific cause (the primary care physician should work closely with the ophthalmologist), (2) specific treatment if the cause is found or if one is highly suspected, and (3) nonspecific ocular treatment to minimize the complications from the inflammatory process (often this is all that is or can be done).

Nonspecific treatment should include the following:

Cycloplegics to dilate the pupil to prevent posterior synechiae and to put the iris and ciliary body at rest. This reduces pain from the ciliary and pupillary spasm and decreases the inflammatory protein response in the aqueous humor. Scopolamine 0.25 per cent or atropine 1 per cent solution or ointment, instilled once or twice daily, is the favored cycloplegic agent.

Mydriatics further help the cycloplegic in obtaining wide pupillary dilatation and thus prevent or break up posterior synechiae. A drug such as phenylephrine 2.5 per cent (Neo-Synephrine) is an effective mydriatic and also decreases hyperemia by its vasoconstricting properties.

Corticosteroids, applied locally or given by subconjunctival injection, may be used to treat anterior uveitis. The subconjunctival route usually is reserved for the more severe forms of anterior uveitis in which a higher and prolonged concentration of the drug is desired. Topical steroid drops or ointment (see Table 6) can be used initially every 1 to 4 hours, depending on the severity of the disease, then less often as improvement occurs.

Steroids should be given systemically in the more severe forms of anterior uveitis if local or subconjunctival medications are not beneficial. Posterior uveitis also usually requires systemic therapy. The daily dosage in children is 1 to 2 mg/kg body weight of prednisone up to a maximum of 80 mg. The equivalent dose of another corticosteroid may be used. One should use the minimum dose necessary to achieve a reasonable effect and for the shortest time needed to control the inflammation. The toxic effects and contraindications to the corticosteroids for short-term and long-term therapy must be kept in mind.

Treatment for active *ocular toxoplasmosis* deserves special mention. It consists in the combined use of pyrimethamine (Daraprim) and sulfadiazine. The concomitant use of systemic corticosteroids is controversial and generally is reserved for acute, progressive lesions in the macular area or optic nerve. Pyrimethamine is given orally twice daily in the total daily dosage of 2 mg/kg up to 150 mg for 1 to 3 days, then 1 mg/kg up to 25 mg daily for 4 weeks. The sulfadiazine* dosage is 120 to 150 mg/kg/day orally in four divided doses up to 4 g/day for 4 weeks. In the acute fulminating cases, clinical improvement is seen in 2 to 3 weeks. Pyrimethamine should be avoided in pregnant patients because it can cause congenital malformations. Clindamycin and (in Europe) spiramycin have been used instead of pyrimethamine.

Weekly urinalysis for sulfadiazine crystaluria or evidence of

*Manufacturer's precaution: Sulfadiazine is not recommended for use in children under 2 months of age.

kidney irritation should be ascertained. Since pyrimethamine is a folic acid antagonist, folinic acid (3 mg intramuscularly or orally twice weekly) should be given to prevent hematologic toxicity (e.g., bone marrow suppression, especially thrombocytopenia).

LACRIMAL APPARATUS DISORDERS

Infantile Dacryostenosis

Normally the nasolacrimal drainage system is patent throughout its length at birth. Failure of the nasolacrimal duct to canalize completely leads to persistent tearing *(epiphora)* of one eye or both eyes in the first weeks of life. Contrary to a common belief, most newborn infants produce tears in the first week of life. Persistent tearing from dacryostenosis without dacryocystitis can be differentiated from conjunctivitis and corneal disease by the lack of conjunctival inflammation. The diagnosis of infantile glaucoma must also be excluded. Usually, significant dacryostenosis is followed promptly by dacryocystitis.

TREATMENT. Most cases of infantile dacryostenosis clear spontaneously with further canalization of the nasolacrimal duct in the first 6 to 8 months of life. Massaging the contents of the lacrimal sac properly down through the nasolacrimal duct four to six times daily may be helpful. Topical antibiotics usually are not prescribed if there is no secondary infection. Persistent obstruction generally leads to dacryocystitis (see Infantile Dacryocystitis).

Infantile Dacryocystitis

Obstruction of the nasolacrimal duct usually leads to infection of the lacrimal sac (dacryocystitis) by the common pyogenic bacteria. Excess tearing is then replaced by mucopurulent discharge and some conjunctival redness. There may be an acute distention of the lacrimal sac with overlying redness, pain, and tenderness. Occasionally, a lacrimal sac abscess ruptures and forms a draining fistula. In the differential diagnosis of infantile dacryocystitis, one must exclude infantile glaucoma as well as conjunctival or corneal disease.

TREATMENT. Since most cases of obstructed nasolacrimal ducts clear spontaneously in the first 6 to 8 months of life, medical treatment consisting of massage and topical antibiotic medication is advisable in this age period. Massaging the nasolacrimal sac area properly empties the sac of purulent material, and the downward pressure tends to increase hydrostatic pressure to rupture the obstructing membrane located usually at the lower end of the duct. The author's preferred treatment program consists of massage of the nasolacrimal sac area four to six times daily followed by the instillation into the inner canthus of a broad-spectrum drop (not ointment) such as gramicidin-neomycin-polymyxin B (see Table 4) for 4 to 7 days. Sulfacetamide drops may be used if the discharge is not predominantly purulent.

If signs of obstruction reappear, a second course of massage and topical antimicrobial therapy is given. If the two separate courses of treatment are not curative, I then irrigate the lacrimal sac and probe the nasolacrimal duct using light general anesthesia. By this time, the infant usually is older than 6 months of age, but age is no contraindication to this procedure if skillful anesthesiologists are available. The success rate of simple irrigation and probing begins to diminish after 12 months of age and even more so after 18 months of age. Severe infections of the lacrimal sac are treated with systemic antibiotics. An abscess of the lacrimal sac calls for a probing of the sac and nasolacrimal duct. If the abscess cannot be decompressed successfully, incision and drainage are required.

To properly guide antimicrobial therapy in cases of chronic, recurrent, or severe infection, it is advisable to obtain smears for Gram-stain examination, cultures, and antibiotic sensitivity studies.

A single probing with irrigation usually eliminates the obstruction and infection. Occasionally, the procedure must be repeated. If the nasolacrimal duct cannot be opened by probing, intubation of the nasolacrimal system with silicone tubing for a short period or an external dacryocystorhinostomy may be required to restore drainage of tears into the nose. The operation usually is not performed before the age of 3 years.

One exception to delaying the probing of obstructed ducts until after 6 to 8 months of age or after several trials of medical treatment is in the management of congenital nasolacrimal duct obstruction associated with congenital mucocele *(dacryocystocele)*. This condition usually is apparent in the newborn nursery and is manifested by a bluish swelling over the lacrimal sac, occasionally mistaken for a hemangioma. Diagnosis is aided by ultrasonography. Treatment consists of immediate probing of the lacrimal system.

CELLULITIS

Preseptal and Orbital (Postseptal) Cellulitis

The term preseptal cellulitis refers to an inflammation located anterior to the orbital septum. Thus, signs of orbital involvement (i.e., proptosis, ophthalmoplegia, decreased vision) are absent. The clinical findings are limited to the eyelids and periorbital tissues and are characterized by erythema and edema of these tissues; conjunctivitis, chemosis, and fever may also be present. Preseptal cellulitis may result from eyelid trauma with subsequent infection, skin infections, spread of infection in the eyelid or periorbital region (e.g., hordeolum, conjunctivitis, dacryocystitis), upper respiratory infection, sinusitis, and bacteremia. Causative organisms include staphylococci, streptococci, *H. influenzae,* and anaerobes. The *H. influenzae* organism is more likely to be encountered in children, especially those younger than 5 years; a magenta discoloration of the skin of the eyelids is distinctive.

Preseptal cellulitis should not be considered a benign disease. Infections caused by virulent organisms may enter the vascular system and progress to orbital and intracranial involvement. Therefore, most patients are hospitalized for treatment.

Bacteriologic studies involving the conjunctiva, nasopharynx, and blood (Gram-stained smears, cultures, antibiotic sensitivity tests) should be initiated. Radiography and computed tomography (CT) of the orbital and sinus areas are ordered if there is any indication of orbital inflammation, sinusitis, fracture, or foreign body. If a fluctuant mass is present, surgical drainage of the mass is performed and smears and cultures of the drained material are assessed. If no area of fluctuation is present, percutaneous aspiration of the swollen area with smear and culture of the aspirated material should be considered for possible detection of the causative organism. If a causative organism cannot be found, broad-spectrum antibiotic therapy is recommended until results of the bacteriologic studies are returned. At present our preference is full parenteral doses of a penicillinase-resistant penicillin such as oxacillin or nafcillin and chloramphenicol. The latter drug is effective against *H. influenzae,* including ampicillin-resistant strains, streptococcal species, and anaerobes, and it has good tissue penetration ability. For patients allergic to penicillin, vancomycin is given. An alternative regimen is the use of cefotaxime, ceftriaxone, or cefuroxime. Antibiotic therapy usually is given for 1 to 2 weeks. Appropriate antibiotics may be given orally when there is clear clinical improvement.

Orbital Cellulitis

Orbital (postseptal) cellulitis designates an inflammation behind the orbital septum. Most often the cause is direct extension of a bacterial infection from the paranasal sinuses. Other causes include extension of infection from facial cellulitis, orbital trauma, dental abscess, and bacteremia. The organisms most frequently responsible are *S. pneumoniae*, group A beta-hemolytic streptococci, *S. aureus*, *H. influenzae* (especially in young children), and non–spore-forming anaerobes. The characteristic clinical findings are erythema and edema of the eyelids and periorbital tissues, proptosis, painful limitation of eye movement (ophthalmoplegia), decreased vision, and often symptoms of toxicity with fever and leukocytosis.

It is imperative that orbital cellulitis be recognized promptly and treated aggressively. Progressive inflammation within the orbit may lead to decreased vision and blindness. Extension of the process may result in meningitis, central nervous system abscess, and death from cavernous sinus thrombosis.

TREATMENT. Treatment is carried out in the hospital. Consultation with an otolaryngologist is advisable. Bacteriologic studies, orbit and sinus radiographs, and orbital CT scans as described for preseptal cellulitis should be obtained. If on admission Gram stain smears of material obtained from the nose and throat, infected sinus, or surgical drainage of an acutely compromised orbit are not informative for selection of appropriate initial antibiotic therapy, then broad-spectrum antibiotic therapy is given as for preseptal cellulitis. Results of culture and antibiotic sensitivity studies may dictate a change in the choice of antibiotics. Treatment usually is given for 2 to 3 weeks or at least 7 to 10 days after the patient is afebrile and decided clinical improvement has been seen.

A subperiosteal or orbital abscess may result from progression of an acute ethmoiditis and could lead to compression of the optic nerve and blindness. Intensive antibiotic therapy early in the formation of the periosteal abscess, that is, when limitation of globe movement is minimal and vision is unaffected, may make surgical intervention unnecessary. The diagnosis of early subperiosteal abscess by CT scan is not always accurate.

GLAUCOMA

Primary Glaucoma

Primary congenital, infantile, or developmental glaucoma occurs in the first few years of life owing to abnormal development of the aqueous drainage structures. Twenty-five per cent of cases are present at birth, over 75 per cent appear by 3 months of age, and 90 per cent are evident within the first year of life. Both eyes are involved in about 75 per cent of the cases. Most instances occur sporadically, but some show a hereditary trait (autosomal recessive). Infantile glaucoma may occur alone or associated with other congenital anomalies, such as aniridia or the syndromes of Axenfeld, Sturge-Weber, or Lowe.

Classic clinical manifestations are tearing, photophobia, cloudy cornea, corneal enlargement, and excess cupping of the optic disc. Corneal enlargement does not occur after 2 to 3 years of age because the coats of the eye become more rigid.

TREATMENT. Without prompt, effective treatment permanent blindness occurs at an early age. Treatment primarily is surgical. Surgery is directed at the trabecular aqueous drainage meshwork in the form of goniotomy, external trabeculotomy, or trabeculectomy. Operations may be repeated several times if necessary. Glaucoma can be controlled by surgical means in 75 per cent of the uncomplicated cases. Recently, valve implants (such as the Molteno) have been used with some success in intractable cases. When these operations fail, filtration surgery or ciliary body destruction with cryotherapy or ultrasound may be attempted.

Medical treatment with topical antiglaucoma drugs, such as the beta-adrenergic blocking agents (timolol, levobunolol, betaxolol), pilocarpine, and epinephrine products, or systemic therapy with a carbonic anhydrase inhibitor such as acetazolamide (Diamox), are rarely of long-term value and are generally ineffective. These drugs may be used (1) preoperatively, as an adjunctive measure; (2) intraoperatively, to help control residual elevation of intraocular pressure; or (3) judiciously, when surgery has been only partially effective.

Acetazolamide is used in infants for a short period only (for example, preoperatively) because the drug can produce serious metabolic acidosis and electrolyte imbalance. The oral dosage for infants and children is 10 to 20 mg/kg/day in three or four divided doses; intravenous dosage is 5 to 10 mg/kg every 6 hours. In neonates, use the lower dosage at 12-hour intervals.

The hyperosmotic agent mannitol is occasionally used immediately preoperatively to lower the intraocular pressure. The drug is given intravenously over a 30- to 40-minute period as a 10 per cent solution. The total dose is 1 to 1.5 g/kg body weight. Maximal ocular hypotensive effect is reached in 1 hour, and the effect may last up to 6 hours. Catheterization is advised if the drug is given during surgery when the patient is receiving a general anesthetic.

Because vision may be reduced in part by a refractive error or anisometropic amblyopia, appropriate spectacle or contact lens wear and intensive amblyopia therapy are important aspects of treatment.

Juvenile Glaucoma

Juvenile open angle glaucoma may appear in the latter half of the first decade or in the second decade of life. The young patient may be asymptomatic until irreversible visual damage has occurred. The classic presenting features of a young, black, myopic patient with a positive family history of early-onset glaucoma (autosomal dominant inheritance trait) calls for an intraocular pressure measurement and examination of the optic discs for cupping even if the youngster is asymptomatic.

TREATMENT. Treatment for juvenile glaucoma is the same as that for adult open angle glaucoma.

Secondary Glaucoma

Secondary glaucoma may have many causes, including lens dislocation, iridocyclitis, hemorrhage into the eye, tumors (for example, retinoblastoma), retinopathy of prematurity, juvenile xanthogranuloma of the iris, metabolic disorders, and topical corticosteroid use.

TREATMENT. Treatment may be complex and is carried out by the ophthalmologist.

RETINOBLASTOMA

Retinoblastoma, although a relatively rare malignant tumor, is the most common primary intraocular malignancy in infants and children. The incidence of retinoblastoma is about one case in every 20,000 live births. The tumor may be present at birth (detected often by routine examination in families known to have retinoblastoma) but most often is discovered before 3 years of age. The average age of detection is about 17 months. Extraocular extension with histologically proved orbital retinoblastoma is associated with an overall 3-year mortality rate of 91 per cent. Mortality from retinoblastoma results from central nervous system involvement by extension along the optic nerve or by hematogenous metastases from the choroid to other organs, most commonly bone, liver, kidney, and adrenal glands. In the United States, advanced disease at presentation is rare. In cases of early diagnosis, in which the tumor remains confined within the eye and early treatment is provided in modern centers, the mortality rate is much decreased. In the past 100 years, the overall mortality rate of retinoblastoma has decreased from 95 per cent to 9 per cent in the United States.

The occurrence of retinoblastoma is largely sporadic (i.e., there is no previous history of the tumor), but a significant proportion of cases are familial. *Nonhereditary retinoblastoma,* comprising 60 per cent of all cases, represents a sporadic somatic mutation and tends to be unilateral and unifocal. It is estimated that 10 to 15 per cent of patients with sporadic, unilateral retinoblastoma transmit the disease to their offspring. In contrast, *hereditary retinoblastoma,* comprising approximately 40 per cent of all patients, can arise after inheritance of a predisposing germ-line mutation from an affected parent (approximately 10 per cent of cases) or through acquisition of a new germinal mutation (approximately 30 per cent of cases). Hereditary retinoblastoma cases exhibit a high degree of penetrance, are usually bilateral and multifocal, and are marked by an earlier age of onset. The hereditary, bilateral cases often do not reflect a previous family history of the tumor. A patient with bilateral retinoblastoma or a family history of retinoblastoma has a 50 per cent probability of transmitting the disease to his or her offspring. The risk estimate of the offspring of healthy siblings or healthy children of a patient with familial retinoblastoma is about 1 in 15. The birth of an affected child to such a person, however, establishes that individual as an unaffected carrier and the risk factor becomes 1 in 2. Patients with hereditary retinoblastoma are also at increased risk for not only "radiation-induced" neoplasms in the field of ocular irradiation but also second cancers different from retinoblastoma. Most are osteogenic sarcomas in and out of the field of radiation.

The risk to children of patients with unilateral sporadic cases of retinoblastoma (usually the nonhereditary type) is about 5 per cent. The risk of disease in siblings of the sporadic cases is about 1 per cent.

Genetic predisposition to the inheritance of retinoblastoma has been demonstrated in those born with a partial deletion of the long arm of chromosome 13. Partial loss of band 14 (region 13q14) has been hypothesized to result in faulty retinal development, which may predispose to the development of retinoblastoma. Patients with small 13q14 deletions usually have no phenotypic abnormalities other than retinoblastoma. Patients with larger deletions often have other congenital abnormalities, including mental retardation. Studies have demonstrated that the locus for autosomal dominant retinoblastoma is closely linked to the locus for the enzyme esterase D. Quantitation of esterase D levels has been shown to be a quick and objective means of identifying 13q14 deletion carriers in cases in which conventional chromosomal analysis has proved inadequate. Other studies have demonstrated the location of the gene responsible for the nondeletion form of hereditary cases to be also in region 13q14. In order to provide accurate counseling to the parents of a child with retinoblastoma, genetic evaluation of all retinoblastoma patients should include chromosome analysis using high-resolution prophase banding, determination of esterase D activity, and family studies.

The gene for retinoblastoma recently has been partially cloned. There is little doubt that the process will be completed. Genetic evaluation in the future with all the new developments at hand will then enable the physician or counselor to specify which patients with retinoblastoma are at risk for second nonocular malignancies and for producing future children with the tumor.

Awareness of a positive family history results in earlier diagnosis of the tumor in both unilateral and bilateral cases. The most common presenting sign of retinoblastoma is leukokoria, or "white pupil." Other presenting signs may include strabismus resulting from impairment of vision, ocular inflammation, anisocoria, heterochromia iridis, red painful eye, glaucoma, hyphema, and hypopyon.

Before treatment is initiated, a number of diagnostic studies may be performed to help establish an accurate diagnosis and the degree of tumor involvement. They include (1) the basic diagnostic evaluation (history, physical, and ocular examination); (2) ocular ultrasonography (A and B scans); (3) computed tomography (also detects an associated pinealoblastoma or "trilateral retinoblastoma"); (4) aqueous enzyme levels of lactic dehydrogenase (LDH) and phosphoglucose isomerase (PGI), including plasma concentrations of these enzymes for ratio comparisons; (5) anterior chamber tap for cytologic studies of possible tumor cells; and (6) bone marrow and cerebrospinal fluid samples for cytologic studies if tumor spread is suspected.

TREATMENT. Of greatest significance in determining the treatment modality for retinoblastoma is the stage of the disease at the time of diagnosis. For this reason, it is imperative that the patient with leukokoria be referred to an ophthalmologist immediately. Extraocular extension of the tumor invariably is associated with a poor prognosis. The classification of eyes with retinoblastoma is based on tumor size, number of tumors, and location. The smaller, the fewer, and the more posteriorly located in the retina the tumors are, the better is the overall prognosis. If the disease is unilateral, examination of the fellow eye reveals no disease, and the search for metastasis is negative, enucleation of the involved eye is usually advised. In rare instances, unilateral cases with a favorable classification may be treated in lieu of enucleation.

Generally, in bilateral cases, one eye has far advanced changes requiring enucleation whereas the remaining eye has a more favorable classification allowing nonsurgical therapy. In rare instances, when there is far advanced bilateral disease that would result in complete blindness despite treatment, bilateral enucleation is indicated to ensure the best chance for survival. It should be noted that some parents may refuse permission to remove both eyes.

In patients requiring enucleation, the surgeon should attempt to remove at least 10 mm of optic nerve to determine whether invasion has occurred. If the tumor has spread to the optic nerve and there is no evidence of extraocular spread, external beam radiation and chemotherapy have been used. The remaining eye must be examined thoroughly at 3- to 6-month intervals for several years.

Supravoltage external beam irradiation may be recommended as a primary mode of therapy if useful vision is salvageable and tumor growth is not advanced enough to require enucleation. The total tumor dose is about 400 rads. Episcleral plaque radiotherapy (cobalt-60, iridium-192, iodine-125) has been used to treat solitary tumors less than 12 mm in diameter and 8 mm thick; a target dose of 3500 to 4000 rads is given to the apex of the tumor.

The indications for chemotherapy in retinoblastoma are controversial. The merit of using chemotherapy as a prophylactic measure following enucleation for unilateral sporadic retinoblastoma and for patients having local treatment of tumors confined to the eye is unsettled. A combination of antitumor drugs such as cyclophosphamide (Cytoxan) and vincristine (Oncovin) has been used when there is metastatic disease or extraocular orbital involvement. Nonetheless, extraorbital spread invariably is fatal.

Photocoagulation and cryotherapy have been used as primary modes of therapy when a tumor is small, solitary, unilateral, and extrafoveal. These modalities have been used most often for recurrent or residual tumors following incomplete destruction by radiation therapy.

The prognosis for survival has been dramatically improved in recent years because of earlier diagnosis, better visualization of the entire retina by the use of indirect ophthalmoscopy, and improved radiotherapeutic and chemotherapeutic techniques. No longer is retinoblastoma a hopeless disease. A survival rate up to 90 per cent has been reported in patients whose prognosis was favorable at the time that treatment was begun.

OCULAR TRAUMA

Prompt and appropriate care after eye injury often saves useful vision; poor management may lead to blindness. Improper initial eye care by the nonophthalmologic physician usually results from unfamiliarity with a few fundamental rules in the correct handling of the patient with ocular trauma.

To determine the ocular structures involved and the extent of the injury, it is imperative to examine closely the external and visible structures of the eyes with good illumination and magnification and to perform ophthalmoscopy. An accurate history is essential. Testing the patient's visual acuity before treatment is important for diagnostic, prognostic, and medicolegal reasons. If an adequate examination cannot be performed by the nonophthalmologic physician, the patient should be referred to an eye physician for further care. The nonophthalmologic physician should not be the one to decide whether or not an eye injury is minor except in obvious situations such as occur with a superficial conjunctival foreign body.

Foreign Bodies

Conjunctival foreign bodies can usually be safely flushed out with a stream of isotonic saline solution or removed with a sterile moistened cotton applicator. If the history suggests that a foreign body is the likely cause of the eye symptoms and none is found on the bulbar or lower palpebral conjunctiva of the cornea, the upper eyelid should be everted for inspection. The use of a local anesthetic, such as 0.5 per cent proparacaine (see Table 1), facilitates the examination.

Corneal foreign bodies may be difficult to see unless adequate local anesthesia, oblique lighting, and magnification (loupe or slit-lamp biomicroscopy) are used. Fluorescein stain helps to delineate the foreign body. One drop of sterile 2 per cent fluorescein solution or a fluorescein strip is placed in the conjunctival sac and the excess washed out with isotonic saline solution. Patients with corneal foreign bodies that are not easily removed by irrigation or with the wipe of a moistened sterile cotton applicator should be referred to an ophthalmologist for further treatment. If the foreign body is dislodged, fluorescein is again added to the eye to determine the extent of the corneal abrasion. Unless the abrasion is minute (less than 1 mm), a broad-spectrum antimicrobial agent, such as sulfacetamide, or a combination of bacitracin or gramicidin, neomycin, and polymyxin B is instilled into the eye and the eye is covered with a patch for 24 hours. If the abrasion is not superficial or is large (more than a few millimeters), an antibiotic is instilled and a patch is applied. The patient should then be seen by an ophthalmologist. The cornea should be re-examined in 24 hours in all cases after the removal of a foreign body for the presence of a secondary infection in the abraded area. Metallic foreign bodies frequently leave a localized rust stain (rust ring). This is best removed by an ophthalmologist using slit-lamp magnification. An untreated corneal infection may lead to corneal ulceration, intraocular infection, and loss of the eye.

Children with *intraocular foreign bodies* (suspected or known) must be referred immediately to an eye physician. If there will be a delay of a few hours before the child is seen by an ophthalmologist, the physician should test the visual acuity, instill a cycloplegic drug and a broad-spectrum antibiotic into the eye, and start systemic antimicrobial therapy. Ampicillin, gentamicin, or chloramphenicol in full dose has been widely used for potential or active intraocular infections because of the broad spectrum of antibacterial activity and the ability to penetrate the ocular tissues. It is important to know that small, missile-like foreign bodies may penetrate the globe and cause transient pain or no pain at all. When a history suggests the possibility of penetration of the eye by a high-velocity foreign body, the patient should be referred to an ophthalmologist for thorough evaluation. Radiographs and computed tomography may help to confirm the suspicion of an intraocular foreign body.

Corneal Abrasions

Corneal abrasions are handled in the same way as described for the abrasion that remains after removal of a corneal foreign body.

Lacerations

Lacerations that involve the eyelid margin or the lacrimal apparatus should be treated by the ophthalmologist. Permanent notching may result from improper lid margin repair. Superficial minor lacerations of the eyelid and brow, however, may be closed with fine sutures by the experienced nonophthalmologic physician after careful evaluation of the levator palpebrae for normal function, determination of good visual acuity, and examination to rule out trauma to the globe. Laceration or perforating injury to the globe is an ocular emergency. Examination by the nonophthalmologist should be limited because lid squeezing may cause expulsion of intraocular tissues. The eye should be covered and the patient sent immediately to an ophthalmologist.

Contusions

Contusion injuries of the globe and the surrounding tissues are usually produced by blunt objects. The effects may be minor or serious, obvious or inapparent, immediate or delayed. Therefore, careful study by an ophthalmologist and sufficient follow-up are necessary. A blunt injury to the eye may result in ecchymosis of the eyelid ("black eye"), subconjunctival hemorrhage, abrasion or rupture of the cornea, anterior chamber hemorrhage (hyphema), laceration of the iris, cataract, dislocated lens, vitreous hemorrhage, retinal edema or hemorrhage, retinal detachment, rupture of the choroid, optic nerve injury, or rupture of the globe. All these complications, except for the eyelid ecchymosis, require expert eye care.

Traumatic hyphema is defined as the presence of blood in the anterior chamber of the eye. It commonly results from a contusion injury to the eye or may stem from a perforating eye injury. Child abuse may be suspected. It may appear as a blood-fluid level in the anterior chamber between the cornea and the iris or as a diffuse hemorrhage in the aqueous humor. It is imperative that a patient with a hyphema be referred for ophthalmologic evaluation promptly, as more extensive injury to the internal and more posterior structures of the eye may be present.

An important goal of treatment is to prevent vision-threatening complications. A particularly serious complication is recurrent or secondary hemorrhage. The occurrence ranges from 3 to 38 per cent. It is difficult to predict which patients will experience rebleeding. Rebleeding may occur within the first 6 days of injury, most often between 3 and 5 days. Secondary hemorrhage predisposes to (1) acute glaucoma with subsequent optic nerve damage and atrophy, (2) corneal blood staining, a particular concern in children younger than 6 years because amblyopia may result from visual deprivation, and (3) peripheral anterior synechiae formation, which may lead to chronic glaucoma. Glaucoma may also ensue from traumatic recession of the iris angle where aqueous fluid normally leaves the eye.

Controversy exists over the ideal treatment plan for hyphema patients. Disagreement prevails regarding the value of absolute bed rest, binocular patching, need for hospitalization, use of various drug regimens, and surgical procedures. Lack of agreement probably is due in part to the types of cases encountered. In general, this author prefers to hospitalize infants and children to permit close observation. In the uncomplicated case wherein most hyphemas clear in 5 to 6 days, ordinarily the management plan consists of bed rest with bathroom privileges and monocular eye patch for 5 days, cautious ambulation on the 6th day, and discharge from the hospital on the 7th day. Aspirin is avoided because of its possible effect on bleeding time. Miotics and cycloplegics usually are not used. A topical corticosteroid and atropine are prescribed if iritis develops.

To reduce the incidence of secondary hemorrhage, some physicians recommend the prophylactic use of an antifibrinolytic agent such as aminocaproic acid (Amikar) in the dosage of 50 to 100 mg/kg body weight up to 30 g/day orally for 5 days. Another antifibrinolytic drug, tranexamic acid (Cyklokapron), is available in tablet and intravenous injection forms for use in hemophiliacs who are to undergo dental extraction; the drug has been used abroad to prevent rebleeding in traumatic hyphema. These drugs reduce lysis of the initial clot until the primary ruptured blood vessels heal. Systemic corticosteroids (equivalent to an adult dosage of prednisone, 40 mg/day for 5 days) also have been advocated by some ophthalmologists to prevent secondary hemorrhage. Although some ophthalmologists recommend the systemic use of either aminocaproic acid or corticosteroids in all cases of traumatic hyphema (because the rebleeding rate may not depend on the size of the hyphema), the low incidence of rebleeding, especially in the less severe hyphemas, coupled with the high cost (principally aminocaproic acid) and possible side effects of these drugs, has deterred their routine use. The fibrinolytic agent tissue plasminogen activator (tPA) may prove of clinical value in the future when used at the proper time. It has been reported to be effective in accelerating the clearance of hyphema in the experimental animal.

If glaucoma occurs, a topical beta-blocker such as timolol maleate, is given. If it is ineffective, ocular hypotensives such as oral acetazolamide (Diamox) or intravenous mannitol may be needed. If medical therapy fails to control elevated intraocular pressure, surgical removal of the aqueous humor or clot material may be necessary.

Sickle cell hyphema merits special attention. Patients with either the trait or the disease are at increased risk for complications of hyphema because their circulating erythrocytes tend to sickle in the acidic, hypoxic environment of the aqueous humor. Sickle cells have difficulty passing through the outflow drainage system of the eye and thus can lead to an acute secondary glaucoma with blindness from retinal or optic nerve infarction. Initial laboratory screening for sickle cell trait or disease therefore is important for patients who are black, Hispanic, or of Mediterranean origin. These patients must be observed closely for a rise in intraocular pressure so that medical or surgical treatment can be initiated promptly.

Burns

Thermal burns of the eyelids are treated as burns of the skin elsewhere. Burns of the cornea are treated by irrigation with water or saline solution and an antibiotic ointment before the patient is sent to an ophthalmologist.

Chemical burns of the conjunctiva and cornea are treated immediately by irrigation with water or isotonic saline solution. Time should not be lost in trying to neutralize the chemical. Serious damage may occur in a matter of minutes. Moreover, the heat generated by such a reaction may lead to further damage. Alkali burns of the cornea are more serious than those caused by acids because alkalis are not precipitated by the tissue proteins as are the acids.

Immediate irrigation should be carried out for at least 30 minutes in the case of alkalis. The eye can be held under the water faucet stream. Local anesthetics may be used to relieve the pain. A local antibiotic ointment can be inserted into the conjunctival sac, and the patient is sent as soon as possible to an ophthalmologist for further care.

STRABISMUS

Strabismus is a misalignment of the eyes that occurs in about 3 per cent of children. Depending on the nature of the eye misalignment, strabismus is categorized as *esotropia* (eyes turned in), *exotropia* (turned out), *hypertropia* (up), or *hypotropia* (down). Strabismus can occur in the newborn (most commonly congenital esotropia), but it is most likely to occur in infancy or early childhood (most commonly accommodative esotropia). Many young infants appear to have strabismus but actually have normal ocular alignment. This "false strabismus," or *pseudostrabismus,* is usually caused by a wide nasal bridge and prominent epicanthal folds, which obscure the medial conjunctiva and give the appearance of esotropia *(pseudoesotropia).* The apparent resolution of a pseudostrabismus as the child grows older is the basis for the mistaken notion that some infants outgrow their strabismus. This can lead to a false sense of security, which delays referral of an infant or child to an ophthalmologist for evaluation and treatment of a true strabismus.

Monocular strabismus is a common cause of *amblyopia,* that is, decreased vision or "lazy eye." At least 3 per cent of children have amblyopia. Approximately half of the cases are secondary to strabismus, and most of the others are due to an uncorrected refractive error in one eye. The unfortunate aspect of the problem is that in most instances this form of visual impairment could have been prevented if the patient had been seen early in childhood by an ophthalmologist.

When strabismus is present in an infant or child, the brain actively suppresses the image from the strabismic eye to avoid double vision and confusion. As a consequence, vision fails to develop properly in the deviating eye, and it becomes amblyopic ("lazy"). Normal vision and binocular function are not present at birth. These functions mature rapidly during the first years of life and become relatively fixed by the age of about 6 years. To reach the goal of 20/20 vision with normal binocular fusion, clear images must be presented to both foveae simultaneously throughout the early years of life. With proper ocular alignment, similar images from each eye are relayed along the visual pathway in the brain, where the two images are ultimately perceived as one. This binocular visual fusion permits the appreciation of depth perception, or *stereopsis.* In the presence of monocular strabismus, vision does not develop fully. If normal binocular vision does not develop by about age 4 years because of amblyopia and strabismus, correction of the strabismus after this age is unlikely to provide fully normal fusion. If amblyopia is not treated by appropriate occlusion of the normal eye or by other means before the age of about 6 years, it is unlikely that one can effect substantial improvement of vision in the amblyopic eye thereafter.

It is important for the pediatrician to keep in mind that diseases such as retinoblastoma, intraocular infection, congenital cataract, or other eye abnormalities may be manifested early in life as a transient or constant strabismus. The pediatrician should not take the responsibility of delaying the referral of the patient unless he or she can absolutely rule out serious ocular disease or the presence of a true strabismus rather than pseudostrabismus.

TREATMENT. The earlier strabismus therapy is initiated, the better is the prognosis for a functional as well as a cosmetic cure. No infant or child is too young to have an eye examination and to have treatment initiated. Although fusion is not necessary for good vision, its presence is a powerful force for maintaining ocular alignment after treatment of strabismus.

The first goal in the treatment of strabismus is obtaining good vision in each eye. The best way to stimulate vision in an amblyopic eye is to correct an underlying refractive error (if present) and to patch the good eye. Occlusion therapy generally is given full time if vision is poor and is tapered to part time as the vision improves. Occlusion therapy is continued until the best visual acuity is reached.

The second goal is correction of the strabismus. This commonly is accomplished by one or more of the following measures:

- Corrective lenses or spectacles
- Miotic therapy (drugs)
- Orthoptics (eye exercises)
- Surgery

Spectacles or Contact Lenses. Corrective lenses generally are effective for the accommodative forms of esotropia. In children with moderate or high degrees of hyperopia, greater accommodation is required to see clearly. Because of the synkinetic reflex of accommodation and convergence, the eyes may overconverge and become esotropic. Proper correction of the refractive error with lenses or spectacles decreases the need for accommodation and thus lessens convergence.

Another type of accommodative strabismus is seen in children who are not highly hyperopic but who have an exaggerated accommodative-convergence ratio at near fixation. These patients usually respond to bifocals to reduce the need for increased accommodation with near targets.

Miotic Therapy. Also effective in selected patients with exaggerated accommodative-convergence ratio are the cholinesterase inhibitor miotics isoflurophate (Floropryl, DFP) and echothiophate iodide (Phospholine iodide). These drugs induce "peripheral" rather than "central" accommodation by their action on the ciliary body and thus lessen convergence. Potential toxic effects (usually from excessive dosage or use) must be kept in mind. They include headache, conjunctival hyperemia, rhinorrhea, abdominal pain, nausea, vomiting, diarrhea, excess salivation, hypotension, and potential ocular (iris cysts) and systemic side effects (such as prolonged apnea if a general anesthesia preceded by succinylcholine should need to be administered).

Orthoptics. Orthoptics (eye exercises) conducted by a trained technician (orthoptist) or doctor in certain circumstances may help to treat amblyopia and suppression, increase fusion ability, and stereopsis. Orthoptics are more commonly effective in cases of intermittent strabismus and may be useful before or after surgery or during both periods.

Surgery. When nonsurgical methods of treatment do not or cannot satisfactorily correct the strabismus, surgery is performed on the extraocular muscles. Although surgery at times may be performed for "cosmetic reasons," it is often performed with the goal of promoting binocular fusion by aligning the eyes in those patients in whom there is a reasonable expectation of obtaining some fusion. Fusion is more likely to be achieved if the strabismus is corrected early in life. The most common strabismus procedures performed are recession and/or resection operations. In a *recession* procedure, a rectus muscle is cut from its insertion onto the sclera and recessed, or moved back, from its insertion to weaken the pull of the muscle. In a *resection* operation, a segment of the rectus muscle is removed and the shortened muscle is then reattached to its site of original insertion in order to strengthen the action of the muscle. Surgery may be performed on one or both eyes in spite of the appearance of a monocular strabismus. More than one operation may be needed to correct the strabismus. In older children and adults, an "adjustable suture" technique may be used to "fine tune" the eye position later on the day of surgery or on the first postoperative day.

Botulinum Toxin. An alternative to surgery in special circumstances is the injection of botulinum toxin (Oculinum) into an overacting rectus muscle to temporarily weaken its action. This drug is also used for the treatment of blepharospasm associated with dystonia, including benign essential blepharospasm. It has been found successful, for example, in patients with transient sixth nerve palsies to prevent contracture of the opposing overactive medial rectus muscle. The younger patient may require a general anesthetic for the procedure. Treatment with Oculinum in patients younger than 12 years remains investigational.

17

The Ear

FOREIGN BODIES IN THE EXTERNAL EAR

ELLEN M. FRIEDMAN, M.D.

Young children frequently put foreign objects in the external auditory canal. Commonly retrieved objects are beads, earrings, pieces of food, wads of paper, and toy parts. These objects may not cause any symptoms, or, depending on their position, they may inflict pain, vertigo, or hearing loss.

Anatomically, the size, shape, and curvature of the external auditory canal is highly variable. The ear is innervated by cranial nerves V, VII, and X, and its substantial vascular supply is covered by rather thin skin. These anatomic factors, as well as patient mobility, can make the removal of a foreign body from the external auditory canal a challenging procedure.

TREATMENT

One's first attempt to remove a foreign object from the external auditory canal is the best chance to be successful because subsequent attempts may be compounded by pain, bleeding, external canal swelling, poor visibility, and decreased patient cooperation. Therefore, the initial attempt at foreign body removal is enhanced by adequate sedation, adequate restraints, proper illumination, and appropriate-sized instruments.

Chloral hydrate is a suggested sedative and has been used with great success. Whereas general anesthesia is rarely necessary when adequate sedation is achieved during the early stages of management, multiple attempts with additional trauma may mandate that the procedure be performed in the operating room.

If adequate restraints are not enforced, the result may be a laceration of the external auditory canal skin, perforation of the tympanic membrane, or ossicular dislocation. The papoose may be used to further limit patient mobility.

The office microscope is very useful for foreign body removal; however, an otoscope with an operating head may also yield adequate illumination. Microsized instruments, such as the alligator or Tobey forceps are necessary.

Alternatively, irrigation may also successfully flush out a foreign body; however, this technique should be avoided when the object is hydrophilic and might swell with irrigation. Live insects, which are commonly retrieved foreign bodies, may be removed by placing several drops of mineral oil in the external auditory canal and then flushing out the insect. Forceps removal of live insects should be avoided because a portion of their barbs may remain embedded in the skin of the external auditory canal.

OTITIS MEDIA

JOHN S. O'SHEA, M.D.

By their third birthday, about two thirds of all children will have had at least one episode of acute middle ear infection (i.e., otitis media). Half of these children will experience no more than one additional episode, whereas the other half will continue having recurrences, usually dissipating, however, before elementary school age. The condition rarely occurs among adolescents and is even rarer in adults, only 1 to 2 per cent of whom ever get otitis media. It remains unknown, however, how many adult otitis media patients were themselves affected as children.

The mainstay of treatment for most patients with otitis media is antimicrobial therapy. Although some cases resolve spontaneously without such therapy, it has generally been found that patients treated are much more likely to experience a prompt resolution both of symptoms and of other frequent, often subtler complications such as hearing loss. Moreover, populations in which there is frequent antimicrobial treatment of middle ear disease have been reported to have fewer children with chronic hearing loss, mastoiditis, or intracerebral infections.

The development of otitis media usually requires the presence of both an infectious agent and some functional or anatomic abnormality of the eustachian tube. Inhaled irritants, allergens, bottle feeding, and attendance at day care centers may also have roles. Tube abnormality is found more frequently in young children than in older children or adults, in certain families and ethnic groups, and in patients with facial maldevelopment or generalized neurologic difficulty.

In approximately one third of children with otitis media, *Streptococcus pneumoniae* is present in middle ear fluid; in one fourth, *Haemophilus influenzae* (generally nontypable) is present. For the past decade, there has been an increase in the reported frequency of *Branhamella catarrhalis* in the fluid. Streptococci (of assorted variety besides pneumococci), staphylococci, gram-negative bacilli, and anaerobic bacteria continue to be found occasionally. Recognized bacterial pathogens, however, are not found in the middle ear fluid of one quarter of patients with otitis media. Beta-lactamase activity has been noted during the past decade in variably increasing frequency in both *H. influenzae* and *B. catarrhalis* isolates from middle ear fluid. Furthermore, recent emphasis has been placed on the frequently simultaneous occurrence of respiratory sinus disease in patients with otitis media.

TREATMENT

Acute Otitis Media

Acute otitis media is most often treated initially with either amoxicillin or trimethoprim-sulfamethoxazole (TMP-SMZ). As noted in Table 1, the former is given in three divided daily doses and the latter in two. Amoxicillin, other penicillins, or cephalosporin should be avoided in children who appear likely to have had a severe prior reaction to any of those drugs. Although the reactions may not truly be dangerous, such past reactions can discourage the parent from adhering to the antimicrobial regimen prescribed, as can cost or other barriers to acquiring the medicine.

Within 2 days of beginning therapy, the child should be improved, with any fever, pain, or anorexia diminished. Tympanic membrane rupture (with drainage of middle ear fluid into the external auditory canal) and other acute complications (such as mastoiditis, meningitis, labyrinthitis, and facial paralysis) become less likely as other symptoms abate. Pain is often relieved abruptly upon rupture of the tympanic membrane.

If there is no convincing improvement in 2 days after therapy has been initiated, beta-lactamase–producing bacteria resistant to the initial antimicrobial will often be found when tympanocentesis is performed. Correspondingly, if one changes the therapy to an antimicrobial resistant to beta-lactamase without performing tympanocentesis, improvement often ensues. Amoxicillin with clavulanic acid, cefaclor, or cefixime is usually chosen in the absence of previous reactions. Alternatively, erythromycin or TMP-SMZ (if not used initially) can be used. Continued lack of improvement after this change in therapy warrants either tympanocentesis or consideration that the child may have persistent otitis media (as discussed later).

In any event, once accompanied by improvement, antimicrobial therapy should be continued for a total of 10 to 14 days. If the patient improves clinically, follow-up evaluation, including audiometry when feasible, should be deferred until 1 or 2 weeks after the completion of antimicrobial therapy. This practice appears adequate and lessens the likelihood of undue concern and expense often associated with the finding of mild tympanic membrane malfunction or hearing loss, each of which usually abates in 3 or 4 weeks after onset.

Although frequently employed, antihistamines and decongestants, given separately or in combination, have little effect on the course of acute otitis media. Analgesics, however, tend to be underutilized. Acetaminophen, sometimes administered with codeine, should be considered for periodic administration during the initial treatment of children with obvious or suspected pain in whom a more serious condition (especially meningitis or mastoiditis) is unlikely to be masked. Topical analgesics are of variable help when placed in the external auditory canal.

TABLE 1. Antimicrobials for Otitis Media

Drug	Dosage (kg/day)
Amoxicillin	40–50 mg in 3 doses
Amoxicillin w/ clavulanic acid	40–50 mg in 3 doses
Cefaclor	40–50 mg in 3 doses
Cefixime	8 mg in 1 dose
Erythromycin	40–50 mg in 4 doses
Trimethoprim-sulfamethoxazole (TMP-SMZ)*	TMP 8 mg-SMZ 40 mg in 2 doses

*According to manufacturer, not recommended for infants younger than 2 months of age.

Recurring Otitis Media

Recurrences of otitis media are usually associated with the same organisms in the middle ear fluid as initial cases. Therapy is thus similar for both types.

Frequent recurrences can sometimes be averted successfully with continuous antimicrobial "prophylaxis." Recent studies indicate that the daily administration of one dose of amoxicillin (20 mg/kg) or sulfisoxazole (50 mg/kg) is often effective. The latter is not recommended by the manufacturer for infants under 2 months of age. Although results are still not proven, it may be beneficial to administer purified polysaccharide pneumococcal antigens to children older than 2 years of age with frequent recurrences. Recent evidence indicates that purified polysaccharide *H. influenzae* vaccine, conjugated with diphtheria toxoid, can protect toddlers and older children from invasive disease due to type B organisms. *This vaccine is not effective, however, for "prophylaxis" of recurrent otitis media, because the nontypable* Haemophilus *organisms, which are much more commonly found than those of type B, are usually not covered.*

Persistent Otitis Media

Persistent otitis media is often accompanied by long-lasting hearing impairment and learning difficulties. Several studies have shown that both of these difficulties, if of fairly brief duration, can be reversed quite promptly after successful treatment of the underlying middle ear disease. How long these problems persist without treatment is not fully known, but some appear to remain indefinitely.

Generally, children with persistent otitis media should be treated with antimicrobials, as in acute otitis media, until there is resolution or until the problem has lasted for 2 to 3 months. In the latter situation, studies indicate that myringotomy can be effective in restoring hearing and learning abilities to predisease status, at least temporarily. Not yet determined is whether tympanostomy tubes should be inserted at the time of myringotomy or whether improvement remains after the incision in the tympanic membrane has begun to heal. There is evidence that adenoidectomy, not necessarily with tonsillectomy, might also be helpful, at least temporarily, for persistent cases, particularly when they are accompanied by an obvious effusion in the middle ear. Antihistamines and decongestants have repeatedly been found ineffective in published studies.

LABYRINTHITIS

MARGARET A. KENNA, M.D.

The term labyrinthitis refers to inflammation of the labyrinth, or inner ear structures. It does not specify whether the perilymph, endolymph, or bony labyrinth is the site of involvement. However, symptoms do not occur unless the membranous labyrinth is involved in the inflammatory process. The initial location of the cause of the labyrinthitis may also determine the presenting symptoms.

Most labyrinthitis in children occurs secondary to acute or chronic bacterial or viral infections. These types of labyrinthitis can be divided into several categories.

SUPPURATIVE (PURULENT) LABYRINTHITIS

Suppurative labyrinthitis occurs when bacteria invade the inner ear from the middle ear, other areas of the temporal bone, meninges, or cerebrospinal fluid (CSF) or by hematogenous spread. Symptoms include severe vertigo, often accompanied by nausea and vomiting, and sensorineural hearing loss. Common causes of acute suppurative labyrinthitis include acute otitis media (AOM), lateral semicircular canal fistula secondary to cholesteatoma, and meningitis.

To treat suppurative labyrinthitis, an unusual and severe condition, one needs to identify the bacterial organism involved. If AOM is the cause of the condition, tympanocentesis or wide myringotomy (sometimes with the placement of a ventilating tube) to drain the middle ear and obtain material for culture should be performed and appropriate systemic antimicrobials should be given. If the patient does not improve after these measures, *mastoidectomy* may be indicated (especially if other complications of AOM are impending, such as meningitis). When a lateral canal fistula associated with chronic suppurative otitis media with or without cholesteatoma is identified, mastoidectomy, culture of mastoid contents, and systemic antimicrobials are recommended. If bacterial meningitis is considered to be the cause of suppurative labyrinthitis, the condition usually resolves when the meningitis is treated with the appropriate systemic antimicrobial. If the meningitis was thought to result from suppurative otitis media, material may need to be obtained from the middle ear for culture, and the middle ear drained. If incapacitating vertigo persists despite these measures, labyrinthectomy may rarely need to be considered.

Suppurative labyrinthitis is nearly always associated with some degree of sensorineural hearing loss, frequently severe. All children need to undergo complete audiometric evaluation when the acute disease process has improved. Evaluation of hearing in both ears separately is necessary, as there may be profound hearing loss in one ear but usable hearing in the other. If the child cannot cooperate for behavioral testing, auditory brain stem evoked response testing should be performed. If hearing loss is identified, immediate counseling is necessary for habilitative and rehabilitative purposes. If a conductive hearing loss associated with persistent middle ear fluid is identified, ventilating tubes may need to be inserted. If the child has persistent dysequilibrium, vestibular evaluation should be undertaken; the patient may need physical therapy.

If the suppurative labyrinthitis resulted from acute or chronic middle ear and mastoid disease, the child may need further middle ear and mastoid surgery, such as tympanoplasty or ossicular reconstruction, after the acute labyrinthitis has been treated.

SEROUS LABYRINTHITIS

Serous labyrinthitis is a sterile inflammatory process that usually occurs secondary to a contiguous infection, such as otitis media or mastoiditis (acute or chronic). It is currently thought that bacterial toxins cross the round window membrane (or enter through a congenital or acquired defect) but that actual bacterial invasion does not occur. The symptoms may include dysequilibrium and hearing impairment, although not usually as severe as in suppurative labyrinthitis.

The management of serous labyrinthitis consists of treating the underlying disorder with systemic antimicrobials and, in the case of otitis media, wide myringotomy. Hearing should be evaluated as soon as the child is well enough; although it is uncommon for total deafness to develop from serous labyrinthitis, permanent sensorineural hearing loss can occur.

VIRAL LABYRINTHITIS

Viral labyrinthitis occurs as a result of invasion of the inner ear by a virus. The viruses best known to cause labyrinthitis include mumps, measles, influenza, varicella, and herpes. Congenital rubella is also associated with severe malformations and hearing impairment. Infants with congenital cytomegalovirus can also have severe sensorineural hearing loss. It is suspected that other viruses, especially in utero, may be responsible for some of the hearing losses noted at or shortly after birth. Identifying these agents has been difficult because the in utero event happens remotely from the time of diagnosis.

If a child has measles or mumps, a hearing evaluation should be conducted. As with all other types of labyrinthitis, the hearing loss associated with viral labyrinthitis should be evaluated as early as possible so that amplification and educational intervention can be initiated. If the child experiences acute symptoms of dysequilibrium, bed rest, fluids, and medications such as meclizine (Antivert), diazepam, or droperidol may be effective. When there are chronic symptoms of dysequilibrium, complete vestibular evaluation is required.

SYPHILITIC LABYRINTHITIS

Syphilitic labyrinthitis is a very specific type that can often be identified and treated, with improvement in the hearing and vertiginous symptoms. The histopathology is twofold. First, syphilis may cause a meningo-neuro-labyrinthitis in early congenital syphilis and in the acute meningitides in secondary and tertiary syphilis. Second, osteitis of the temporal bone may be the predominant form, with secondary involvement of the membranous labyrinth.

Diagnosis is made by serum fluorescent treponemal antibody absorption test and positive CSF serologic studies. The symptoms include sudden, fluctuating, or progressive hearing loss with or without vestibular symptoms.

Treatment includes high-dose penicillin and high-dose, long-term steroids. Symptoms of hearing loss and vertigo may stabilize or improve on this regimen but relapse (especially the hearing loss) may occur if steroids are discontinued.

PERILYMPHATIC FISTULA

A perilymphatic fistula (PLF) is a connection between the middle and the inner ears and can act as a conduit to the inner ear for viruses, bacteria, or toxins, resulting in labyrinthitis and/or meningitis. PLFs can be congenital or acquired (usually traumatic) in nature and may be silent. Symptoms include fluctuating or progressive sensorineural hearing loss and vertigo. A PLF may not be suspected until multiple bouts of meningitis have occurred, and even then can be very difficult to identify.

Treatment consists of middle ear exploration and closure of the PLF, as well as the management of any associated infectious complications.

INJURIES TO THE MIDDLE EAR

ELLEN M. FRIEDMAN, M.D.

The ear, because of its location, is fairly vulnerable to trauma. Trauma to the middle ear may be seen with or without an injury to the pinna, external auditory canal, or inner ear. As with all trauma cases, one must begin with a thorough history and physical examination. Although middle ear injuries are not life-threatening, they may account for significant functional morbidity.

Patients with middle ear trauma may present with a variety of symptoms, including otorrhea, aural bleeding, severe pain, hearing loss, vertigo, nausea, or tinnitus. The presence of any symptoms other than subjective hearing loss may indicate extensive middle ear or inner ear damage. Specifically, if the injury is limited to a tympanic membrane perforation, then vertigo, nausea, or tinnitus is usually not present. Therefore, when such symptoms are exhibited, suspicion concerning further injury should be raised.

CLASSIFICATION

Middle ear trauma is routinely divided into several categories, including head trauma, direct trauma, indirect trauma, or barotrauma.

Head trauma resulting in middle ear injury is usually the result of a motor vehicle accident. Patients with these injuries frequently suffer severe hearing loss, which is usually irreversible and sensorineural in nature.

Direct trauma refers to cases in which there is a direct injury to the tympanic membrane or middle ear. These injuries are most commonly caused by the patient placing foreign bodies such as bobby pins or cotton-tipped applicators in the external auditory canal either intentionally or iatrogenously during cerumen or foreign body removal. Uncommonly, thermal injuries may occur when molten material explodes in the air and may cause direct middle ear damage. Most cases of direct trauma result in tympanic membrane perforation alone; however, ossicular dislocation may also occur.

Barotrauma occurs in conjunction with changes in atmospheric pressure and is most commonly seen in deep-sea scuba divers or with air flight descent.

Indirect trauma occurs following a slap injury to the pinna and usually results in a tympanic membrane perforation.

PHYSICAL EXAMINATION

Middle ear trauma may result in a variety of problems. Although the most common injury is an isolated tympanic membrane perforation, perilymph fistula or ossicular dislocation or subluxation may also occur. The initial examination of a traumatized ear is performed once any existing blood is removed from the external auditory canal. This evaluation is best performed under the microscope with suction in order to avoid further insult to a tympanic membrane that is possibly not intact. It is of utmost importance to determine whether a patient with a traumatic tympanic membrane perforation has other concomitant ear injuries, in which case the management will differ. Indicators of a perilymph fistula or other inner ear injuries are the presence of vertigo, nausea, or tinnitus.

DIAGNOSIS

To help delineate the extent of the injury, several tests are useful. Tuning fork tests are used to assess the possibility of a sensorineural hearing loss. A vibrating 512-frequency tuning fork should be placed in the center of the patient's forehead (Weber's test). If the sound lateralizes to the uninjured ear, there is a high likelihood of a sensorineural hearing loss in the traumatized ear (i.e., perilymph fistula). Unfortunately, young children may have difficulty repetitively cooperating during this test. Another test used to investigate the possibility of a perilymph fistula is the fistula test, which is performed at the bedside. The fistula test is carried out in the following manner: Using a pneumatic otoscope and the appropriate speculum, one applies positive pressure for approximately 15 seconds. The patient is then questioned concerning vertigo and examined for the presence of nystagmus. When the fistula sign is positive—that is, the patient has vertigo or nystagmus—there is a high likelihood of a perilymphatic fistula.

An audiogram should be obtained when the patient is stable in order to evaluate the presence and nature (conductive or sensorineural) of the hearing loss. Computed tomography of the temporal bones is helpful in ruling out the possibility of a temporal bone fracture and can frequently show in exquisite detail the area of the ossicular mass, thereby revealing ossicular dislocation.

TREATMENT

Once the diagnosis and extent of the injury are established, treatment is somewhat controversial. Traumatic tympanic membrane perforations may be handled either by a conservative method of observation with water precautions or by early surgical intervention (i.e., tympanoplasty). The literature supports a watchful waiting approach if the injury is limited to an isolated tympanic membrane perforation. There is a very high rate of spontaneous healing associated with these isolated injuries, which would avert the need for surgical intervention. However, ossicular dislocation associated with trauma is associated with an improved outcome when the diagnosis is established early and surgical intervention is initiated as early as possible. With early surgery, the ossicles may be realigned without adhering to and scarring the floor of the middle ear space.

Although malleus fractures and incus fractures have been reported, it is most common for the incus, which is the least tethered of the ossicles, to be involved with trauma. If the stapes is unaffected by the trauma, the resulting hearing loss will most likely be mainly conductive in nature. When there is subluxation of the stapes, the ear usually sustains a mixed hearing loss with a significant sensorineural component. The sensorineural component most likely will be irreversible. When an oval window or round window fistula is suspected, early surgical intervention is imperative. During surgery, these areas are examined under the microscope and plugged with fat or muscle fascia. By sealing these areas, the surgeon may be able to prevent further sensorineural hearing loss, to stabilize the hearing, and to create a barrier to extension of middle ear infections to the intracranial cavity.

REFERENCES

Kristensen S, Juul A, Gammelgaard NP, et al: Traumatic tympanic membrane perforations: Complications and management. Ear Nose Throat J 68:503–516, 1989.

Turbiak T: Ear trauma. Emerg Med Clin North Am 5:243–251, 1987.

HEARING LOSS

GERALD B. HEALY, M.D.

The failure to identify and diagnose hearing loss in children may have a devastating effect on intellectual and emotional development. The actual incidence of hearing loss in children is unknown, but it is certain that almost all children will suffer a temporary conductive hearing loss associated with otitis media at least once before the age of 8 years. In either congenital or acquired deafness, there is usually a time lag in detection and treatment. It is imperative that both the primary care physician and the specialist keep this time to the barest minimum if the devastating effects of hearing loss are to be avoided.

CLASSIFICATION

Acquired Conductive Type

Acute Otitis Media with Effusion

Acute otitis media with effusion (AOME) (see also article on otitis media, p. 537) is one of the most common diseases of early childhood. It is defined as the presence of a middle ear effusion with signs of systemic toxicity. The patient presents with marked distortion of the tympanic membrane, including erythema, thickening, and, occasionally, bulging. If prompt therapeutic intervention is not carried out, the tympanic membrane may rupture, thereby producing a purulent otorrhea.

Medical management continues to be the main modality of therapy. Amoxicillin (40 to 50 mg/kg/day for patients weighing under 20 kg; or 750 mg/day for those weighing over 20 kg); Augmentin (40 to 50 mg/kg/day); and cephaclor (40 to 50 mg/kg/day) are the most common antibiotics used in the treatment of this disorder. In patients with penicillin sensitivity, erythromycin (30 to 50 mg/kg/day) and sulfisoxazole (120 mg/kg/day) may be used.

If rupture of the tympanic membrane has occurred, topical antimicrobial therapy should be added to systemic treatment in the form of an antimicrobial-cortisone otic preparation. This ensures that a secondary external otitis will not develop from the infected material coming from the middle ear space. Topical therapy is also helpful in sterilizing the middle ear, as it gains access through the spontaneous perforation. Spontaneous perforations secondary to acute otitis media with effusion usually resolve without surgical intervention.

Occasionally, it may be necessary to obtain an aspirate of the middle ear space when initial antimicrobial therapy is not proving effective. Middle ear fluid should also be obtained in patients younger than 30 days old when acute otitis media with effusion develops. *Tympanocentesis* (aspiration of the middle ear) is performed by inserting a 18- to 22-gauge spinal needle attached to a tuberculin syringe through the inferior-posterior portion of the tympanic membrane. Before aspiration is performed, material from the external canal must be obtained for culture, and then the external canal cleansed with an appropriate topical agent such as iodine or alcohol. The culture is helpful in determining whether the organisms obtained from the middle ear are contaminants from the canal or actual pathogens from the middle ear space.

Recurrent Otitis Media with Effusion

Recurrent otitis media with effusion may occur with almost every respiratory tract infection in some children. Prophylactic antimicrobials have been advocated for prevention. This modality of therapy appears useful in children who do maintain a middle ear effusion between acute suppurative episodes. Amoxicillin appears to be the agent most useful for this purpose. Recently, sulfisoxazole has not proved as effective as previously thought for prophylaxis.

Patients with recurrent acute suppurative episodes who maintain an effusion between bouts should be considered for surgical intervention. Antimicrobial prophylaxis usually does little to resolve the effusion with the resultant conductive hearing loss. Myringotomy and the insertion of a ventilation tube have proved effective for many of these patients. This type of intervention should also be considered in patients who show significant antibiotic sensitivity.

Chronic Otitis Media with Effusion

Chronic otitis media with effusion (COME) is the most common cause of hearing loss in children under 10 years of age. It is defined as the presence of a middle ear effusion without clinical evidence of systemic toxicity. The diagnosis is confirmed by pneumo-otoscopy and impedance audiometry. Therapy is usually directed toward restoring eustachian tube function to normal.

Medical therapy for this process has been somewhat controversial. Widespread use of antihistamines or antihistamine-decongestant preparations has been fairly unrewarding. Clinical trials have also proved that this type of therapy has little effectiveness.

More recently, antibiotic therapy has been used with a moderate degree of success. Patients are usually treated with the agents used for AOME, but therapy is continued for a minimum of 21 days.

Steroid therapy has been advocated for COME and may play some role in the resolution of this process. A few controlled clinical trials have been undertaken and seem encouraging, but more data are necessary before large numbers of children are committed to this form of therapy.

Autoinflation techniques may yield reasonable results in resolving middle ear effusion. These techniques may be taught to older children; they include Valsalva-type maneuvers, such as occluding the nose, closing the mouth, and asking the child to attempt to blow the nose. Other techniques, such as having the child blow up a balloon with the nose occluded, can accomplish the same thing. In some patients, normal middle ear pressures will be re-established with this simple form of therapy.

Surgical intervention should be reserved for patients who demonstrate prolonged abnormality of the middle ear space. Patients with effusions persisting for more than 12 weeks, causing a conductive hearing loss of greater than 15 decibels, should be considered for this form of therapy. In addition, patients who demonstrate severe atelectasis of the middle ear space with marked retraction of the tympanic membrane are also surgical candidates. These patients are at a high risk for the development of cholesteatoma, and the severe negative pressure will not clear with medical management in most cases.

Myringotomy with the removal of middle ear effusion, coupled with the insertion of a ventilating tube, represents the mainstay of surgical therapy. The tube usually extrudes spontaneously anywhere from 6 to 12 months after insertion. A general anesthetic is needed in young children, but the procedure may be done on an ambulatory basis if there are no other significant underlying medical conditions.

Adenoidectomy has proved effective in reducing the recurrence of middle ear effusion in patients who have required more than one set of ventilation tubes. Controlled clinical trials have been conducted to prove the efficacy of adenoidectomy in this disease process.

External Otitis

Other, less frequent causes of acquired conductive hearing loss include pathology of the external ear canal. Most commonly, this is in the form of external otitis. This process usually presents with pain secondary to intense inflammation of the external canal, with the accumulation of a significant amount of desquamated epithelium.

Treatment involves mechanical irrigation of the debris from the ear canal followed by topical antibiotic therapy in the form of antimicrobial-cortisone otic drops.

Trauma

Trauma to the ear may result in perforation of the tympanic membrane and/or ossicular chain disruption. This may or may not be associated with an actual fracture of the temporal bone. Most traumatic perforations heal spontaneously if the ear is kept free from infection. Care must be taken in the immediate post-injury period to keep the ear dry; water precautions should be explained to the patient.

If ossicular disruption has occurred, exploration of the middle ear space is indicated. Repositioning of the traumatized ossicle or ossicles may be feasible. The use of autograft bone or cartilage or prosthetic material may be required to re-establish ossicular continuity. All patients should undergo a thorough audiologic evaluation before surgery is undertaken.

Tumors

Tumors, both benign and malignant, can occur in the external auditory canal as well as in the middle ear space. The first presenting symptom may be a conductive hearing loss due to the mass effect.

Treatment depends on the underlying cause.

Chronic Otitis Media

Chronic otitis media refers to an infection of the middle ear space associated with a persistent perforation of the tympanic membrane and otorrhea. This chronic inflammatory process may or may not be associated with cholesteatoma. Characteristically, gram-negative organisms are responsible for this process. Chronic otitis media is almost always associated with hearing loss and may be due to perforation of the tympanic membrane or from actual destruction of parts or all of the ossicular chain due to chronic infection.

If cholesteatoma can be absolutely ruled out, parenteral medical therapy may be attempted to control recurrent otorrhea. This therapy should be used in conjunction with a topical antimicrobial-cortisone otic preparation. No adverse effect on inner ear function has ever been demonstrated from the use of such topical therapy in humans.

Surgical intervention is always indicated in patients in whom cholesteatoma is present, the objective being to excise all irreversibly diseased tissue and to reconstruct defective hearing wherever possible by the use of bone or cartilage or by the insertion of a prosthetic implant. When persistent tympanic membrane perforation is present, reconstruction is often accomplished by grafting with fascia from the temporalis muscle. Occasionally, these procedures must be combined with a mastoidectomy if disease has spread from the middle ear space into the mastoid complex.

Congenital Conductive Type

Defects associated with congenital conductive hearing loss may affect the external ear, the middle ear, or both.

Congenital conductive hearing loss has been reported in association with defects involving almost all other organ systems. Thorough investigation, including audiologic studies, radiographic evaluation of the temporal bones, and a complete search for other systemic defects, must be undertaken before any treatment plan can be determined.

Aural atresia is more commonly unilateral than bilateral. If audiologic evaluation confirms the presence of normal hearing in the unaffected ear, therapy in the affected ear may be delayed. In the past, therapy was generally geared to restoration of a cosmetically acceptable auricle on the affected side. However, modern imaging techniques and methods of microsurgery have provided alternative options for surgical intervention in these cases. In addition, implantable hearing aids have provided an alternative to reconstructive surgery. Their usefulness in young children has yet to be demonstrated, however.

Isolated middle ear ossicular deformities have been reported on a congenital basis. Deformities may affect any of the three ossicles, either singly or in conjunction with deformities of an adjacent ossicle. Treatment options include either amplification or surgical exploration in an attempt to remodel the deformed ossicle(s) by microsurgical approaches.

Acquired Sensorineural Type

The etiology of acquired sensorineural hearing loss may be infectious, traumatic, or neoplastic.

Infection

Labyrinthine Infection. Labyrinthine infection may be either viral or bacterial in origin. The associated hearing loss may or may not be associated with vertigo. Multiple viruses and bacteria have been implicated.

No specific therapy has proved effective in altering the course of well-established disease. Immunizations in early childhood are vitally important as a prophylaxis against viral attack on the labyrinth. Both measles and mumps have been implicated in the development of sensorineural hearing loss in the pediatric population.

Meningitis. Meningitis, whether of viral or bacterial cause; may produce a profound sensorineural hearing loss. It is the most common cause of this type of hearing loss in children. Recent studies, however, have indicated that treatment of the acute infection with high-dose corticosteroid therapy may significantly alter the development of hearing loss in this infectious process. Corticosteroids may be particularly effective in those cases caused by bacterial infection.

Trauma

Concussion. Concussive injuries to the temporal bone, with or without associated fractures, may produce sensorineural hearing loss. Unfortunately, no specific treatment has been defined to reverse the loss sometimes seen. Occasionally, patients who have sustained concussive-type injuries to the head develop symptoms of unilateral hearing loss associated with vertigo or unsteadiness. Fistulas of the round or oval windows have been demonstrated in some of these patients.

Surgical exploration of the middle ear and closure of the fistula with a soft tissue graft have restored hearing in some patients.

Acoustic Trauma. Acoustic trauma may produce sudden or progressive sensorineural hearing loss. Occasionally, there is some spontaneous improvement in hearing, but there is no known effective treatment to restore damaged hair cells. Guidance about using ear protection in noisy atmospheres and warnings against the use of high-intensity recording devices must be provided to patients and families.

Neoplastic

Acoustic tumors involving the eighth cranial nerve may cause sensorineural hearing loss. Such tumors are exceedingly rare in children, however.

Drugs

Many drugs have been implicated in the etiology of acquired sensorineural hearing loss. Aminoglycoside antibiotics such as kanamycin and gentamicin are known to be toxic to the auditory and vestibular systems. Diuretics such as furosemide are also harmful to the inner ear and should be used with appropriate monitoring in children. This is especially true in patients with impaired renal function. The hearing loss associated with these various agents is usually irreversible, and there is no known treatment.

Hyperbilirubinemia

Hyperbilirubinemia is a recognized cause of sensorineural hearing loss. This once significant contributor is now almost extinct as a cause of pathology to the inner ear.

Congenital Sensorineural Type

Classification

Congenital sensorineural hearing loss may be either *genetic* or *nongenetic* in origin. The most common type of genetic deafness is recessive in origin, but dominant types as well as sex-linked neural deafness can also occur. These various abnormalities may be associated with other systemic defects.

Nongenetic deafness has its origin most commonly in perinatal hypoxia and occasionally in prenatal infection. Prenatal rubella was a primary cause of this problem, but today the incidence has been dramatically reduced. Other causes include cytomegalic inclusion disease, congenital toxoplasmosis infection, and congenital syphilis, as well as maternal herpes and measles. Ototoxic drug administration during the prenatal period is also a recognized cause. Prevention is paramount because treatment is unknown.

Treatment

Habilitation of hearing-impaired children assumes great importance when dealing with those with acquired and congenital sensorineural deafness. The parents and child must be professionally counseled and guided during the traumatic period when the diagnosis is first made. The pediatrician, otolaryngologist, audiologist, and a teacher of hearing-impaired children must be intimately involved as a team to habilitate these patients.

The use of a hearing aid is of prime importance in patients with acquired and congenital sensorineural deafness. Whether the child is a candidate for an aid becomes an extremely important question. The answer lies in whether the patient is better able to communicate with those around him or her with the hearing aid or without it. Any child with a moderate to profound hearing loss is a potential candidate for a hearing aid. It is vitally important that it be fitted early so that the natural development of speech and language is not impaired.

A variety of educational programs are available for hearing-impaired children, and parents must be guided to take advantage of these opportunities so that the natural intellectual development of the child is not jeopardized.

More recently, the introduction of the cochlear implant has offered some potential for those patients in whom no peripheral hearing is demonstrable. Its effectiveness in postlingually deaf children is rapidly becoming established. Continued evaluation of this device must be undertaken, as it offers significant potential for these patients.

The primary physician must also be mindful that hearing-impaired children are afflicted from time to time with the ordinary otologic problems of childhood such as otitis media. Problems of the middle ear space must be dealt with appropriately and urgently. Middle ear effusion may significantly impair these children such that an already moderate sensorineural hearing loss may be immediately converted to a profound one. This will render a hearing aid useless. Vigilance must be maintained in the care of these patients so that they can lead productive and meaningful lives.

18

Infectious Diseases

NEONATAL SEPTICEMIA, MENINGITIS, AND PNEUMONIA

XAVIER SAEZ-LLORENS, M.D.
and JANE D. SIEGEL, M.D.

Neonatal septicemia is a clinical state in which there is invasion of the blood stream by a bacterial pathogen accompanied by systemic signs of infection during the first month of life. In approximately 20 to 25 per cent of these bacteremic infants, meningitis will develop and in some of them bacterial invasion of other organs will occur as well.

The incidence of neonatal sepsis has been reported to be as low as 0.3 to as high as 10 per 1000 live births. This incidence depends on many factors, such as geographic area, rate of premature deliveries, obstetric risk factors, technical sophistication of the nursery, and liberal use of antibiotics during labor. Regardless of the incidence, systemic bacterial infections are still associated with high case fatality rates and substantial morbidity in the surviving infants. As a result of an immature immunologic system, exposure to invasive procedures, and prolonged nursery stay, the largest incidence of neonatal systemic infections is observed among premature infants. *For example, the rate of neonatal group B streptococcal early-onset disease has been reported to vary from 1.1 per 1000 among infants with birth weights greater than 2500 g to 26.2 per 1000 among infants with birth weights between 501 to 1000 g.*

The majority of neonatal bacterial infections occur during the first 5 days of life and are classified as early-onset septicemias. Ninety-five per cent of early-onset group B streptococcal infections occur within the first 3 days of life. These early systemic infections occur most commonly as a result of direct contact by the infant with microorganisms colonizing the maternal genital tract or the contaminated amniotic fluid and less often by the transplacental route. Currently, the usual pathogens responsible for early-onset disease include group B streptococci *(Streptococcus agalactiae), Escherichia coli* and other gram-negative bacilli, *Listeria monocytogenes,* and enterococci.

Late-onset infections may occur as early as 5 days of age but are more commonly recognized after the first week of life. These can be caused by some of the organisms associated with early-onset disease, such as group B streptococci and *L. monocytogenes,* in which case meningitis is the usual clinical manifestation. Nosocomially acquired bacteria account for the larger number of these late-onset infections. Thus, *Staphylococcus aureus,* coagulase-negative staphylococci, *Pseudomonas aeruginosa,* and other gram-negative bacilli, such as *E. coli, Klebsiella pneumoniae, Enterobacter cloacae,* and *Salmonella* species, are the usual offending agents. In addition, those infants requiring invasive procedures and broad-spectrum antimicrobial agents will be more susceptible to severe fungal infections, with *Candida albicans* isolated most frequently. Once the infants are discharged from the nursery and exposed to the household environment, older newborns can also be affected by pathogens commonly seen beyond the neonatal period, such as *Haemophilus influenzae* type b and *Streptococcus pneumoniae.*

Tables 1 and 2 show the etiologic agents in bacterial sepsis and meningitis and associated case fatality rates for 20 years (1969–1989) at Parkland Memorial Hospital of Dallas. This distribution of neonatal pathogens is similar to that reported from many nurseries in the United States and other developed countries. Of note, the microorganisms most frequently isolated from infants with nosocomial infection has shifted from a gram-negative rod predominance in the early 1970s to a

TABLE 1. Etiologic Agents in Neonatal Bacterial Sepsis, Parkland Memorial Hospital, 1969–1989*

Organism	No. (%)	Death (%)
Group B *Streptococcus*	277 (37)	47 (17)
Escherichia coli	127 (17)	43 (34)
Other gram-negative enteric (GNE) rods	76 (10)	28 (37)
Staphylococcus aureus†	94 (13)	20 (21)
Enterococcus	79 (10)	6 (13)
Staphylococcus coagulase-negative	56 (7)	3 (5)
Pseudomonas aeruginosa	17 (2)	13 (76)
Listeria monocytogenes	5 (1)	1 (20)
Streptococcus pneumoniae	4 (1)	0
Haemophilus influenzae type b	3 (1)	1 (33)
Nontypable *H. influenzae*	5 (1)	1 (20)
Neisseria meningitidis	1 (0)	0
Miscellaneous	5	2 (40)
Polymicrobial‡	50	15 (30)
TOTALS	799	180 (23)

*Based on all cases of bacterial sepsis (early- and late-onset) managed at Parkland Memorial Hospital at Dallas. There were 204,505 deliveries. (Sepsis rate per 1000 live births was 3.9.)

†51 Methicillin-resistant *S. aureus* strains (54 per cent) isolated in the last five years.

‡Mostly caused by GNE rods and anaerobes.

TABLE 2. Etiologic Agents of Neonatal Bacterial Meningitis (Parkland Memorial Hospital, 1969–1989*)

Organism	No. (%)	Death (%)
Group B *Streptococcus*	136 (53%)	23 (17%)
Escherichia coli	48 (19%)	11 (23%)
Other gram-negative enteric rods	32 (12%)	8 (25%)
Listeria monocytogenes	17 (7%)	0
Enterococcus	6 (2%)	1 (17%)
Staphylococcus aureus	5 (2%)	2 (40%)
Streptococcus pneumoniae	3 (1%)	0
Pseudomonas aeruginosa	2 (2%)	1 (50%)
Haemophilus influenzae type b	2 (1%)	0
Neisseria meningitidis	2 (1%)	0
Miscellaneous	4	1 (25%)
TOTALS	257	47 (18%)

*Based on all cases of bacterial meningitis managed at Parkland Memorial Hospital at Dallas. There were 204,505 deliveries. (Meningitis rate per 1000 live births was 1.3.)

clear predominance of coagulase-negative staphylococci and other gram-positive cocci in the 1980s and early 1990s.

SEPTICEMIA

Diagnosis

The primary objective of the clinician who cares for infants at risk for neonatal infection is to identify and treat promptly all infected patients on the basis of the likelihood that obstetric risk factors, clinical signs, and/or selected laboratory tests will identify infected infants and that the asymptomatic neonate with bacteremia is at high risk for development of rapidly progressive disease. We believe that a second objective should be to avoid excessive diagnostic investigations and unnecessary use of antimicrobial agents for a prolonged period of time. For these purposes, we have designed guidelines (Figs. 1 and 2) to help clinicians in their diagnostic and therapeutic decisions for asymptomatic or symptomatic premature and term infants at risk for infection. Nevertheless, these guidelines should supplement, rather than replace, the clinical judgment of an experienced pediatrician.

The inclusion of lumbar puncture in the admission sepsis work-up of the asymptomatic infant with obstetric risk factors or of the premature infant with respiratory distress has been the subject of several studies published recently. *We conclude from these studies that examination of cerebrospinal fluid (CSF) is not indicated in the initial diagnostic evaluation of asymptomatic infants whose mothers have obstetric risk factors for neonatal infection.* However, greater caution is advised with the premature infant with respiratory distress because a rare case of meningitis will not be diagnosed without CSF evaluation. Lumbar puncture is always performed in any infant with a positive blood culture.

Treatment

Drug Therapy

Infants with suspected sepsis during the first 5 days of life are treated with a combination of a penicillin (usually ampicillin) and an aminoglycoside. Ampicillin is preferred over penicillin for its better in vitro activity against *L. monocytogenes,* enterococci, and some gram-negative bacilli, including nontypable *H. influenzae.* The choice of the aminoglycoside (gentamicin, tobramycin, netilmicin, or amikacin) is guided by the prevalence of resistant strains within an individual nursery. Use of third-generation cephalosporins (cefotaxime or ceftazidime), instead of aminoglycosides, should not be recommended routinely for empiric therapy of suspected sepsis because of the rapid emergence of resistance associated with the excessive use of these agents in a closed unit.

For infants older than 5 days of age, antimicrobial agents active against staphylococci (methicillin, vancomycin) are included. Vancomycin has the advantage over methicillin of good activity against coagulase-negative staphylococci, enterococci, *Listeria,* and the methicillin-resistant strains of *S. aureus* (MRSA). Vancomycin is not a first-line drug for treatment of infections caused by *Listeria* because clinical failures have been reported.

Once the etiologic agent has been identified, antibiotic therapy is tailored according to the results of in vitro susceptibility testing (see Table 3). *L. monocytogenes* and enterococci warrant treatment with ampicillin, whereas group B streptococci respond to either penicillin or ampicillin. Although ampicillin alone is sufficient to treat *L. monocytogenes* infections, an aminoglycoside is added for its synergistic activity against group B streptococci and enterococci in serious infections or infections with delayed clinical or bacteriologic response. The rarely occurring tolerant strains (showing a 32-fold difference between the in vitro minimal inhibitory and the minimal bactericidal concentrations) of group B streptococci require addition of an aminoglycoside for complete killing. In such cases, cefotaxime alone can be used alternatively. For patients with serious infections with gram-negative enteric pathogens (e.g., abscesses, meningitis) or with suboptimal clinical response to initial treatment, third-generation cephalosporins, with or without an aminoglycoside, are the preferred antimicrobial agents. For systemic infections with *P. aeruginosa,* a regimen of ceftazidime or ticarcillin combined with an aminoglycoside is generally used. Metronidazole, clindamycin, or ticarcillin offers adequate coverage for anaerobic bacteria sometimes isolated with other organisms in the blood of neonates with necrotizing enterocolitis and/or gastrointestinal perforation. Chloramphenicol is no longer recommended for treatment of neonatal infections because of its bacteriostatic mechanism of action against most gram-negative pathogens, its potential antagonism with bactericidal drugs against group B streptococci and gram-negative enteric bacilli, and the necessity of monitoring its serum drug concentrations to avoid either toxic or subtherapeutic levels.

Blood cultures are repeated 24 to 48 hours following institution of antibiotic therapy to document sterilization. If bacteremia persists, further diagnostic evaluation is necessary to rule out errors in antimicrobial dosages, subtherapeutic levels of antibiotics, infection with a tolerant or resistant strain, an occult focus of infection (e.g., abscess), or the presence of infected foreign bodies (e.g., indwelling catheters) that need to be removed. Persistence of signs of infection despite negative cultures should prompt the clinician to consider a fungal or viral etiology and to perform more extensive diagnostic studies. The antigen detection of group B streptococcus by latex particle agglutination kits has more than 95 per cent sensitivity and specificity when applied to CSF or fresh concentrated urine samples. Occasionally, however, perineal contamination may cause false-positive results in heavily colonized neonates in the absence of invasive disease when the urine is obtained by bag collection.

The usual duration of treatment of most uncomplicated episodes of sepsis is 7 to 10 days. Longer courses of therapy are indicated for the treatment of infections disseminated to the meninges or osteoarticular sites. The intravenous route of drug administration is preferred, but the intramuscular route can be used temporarily for most antimicrobial agents if there is an adequate muscle mass and appropriate peripheral perfusion and cardiovascular function.

Infants treated with vancomycin or aminoglycosides require

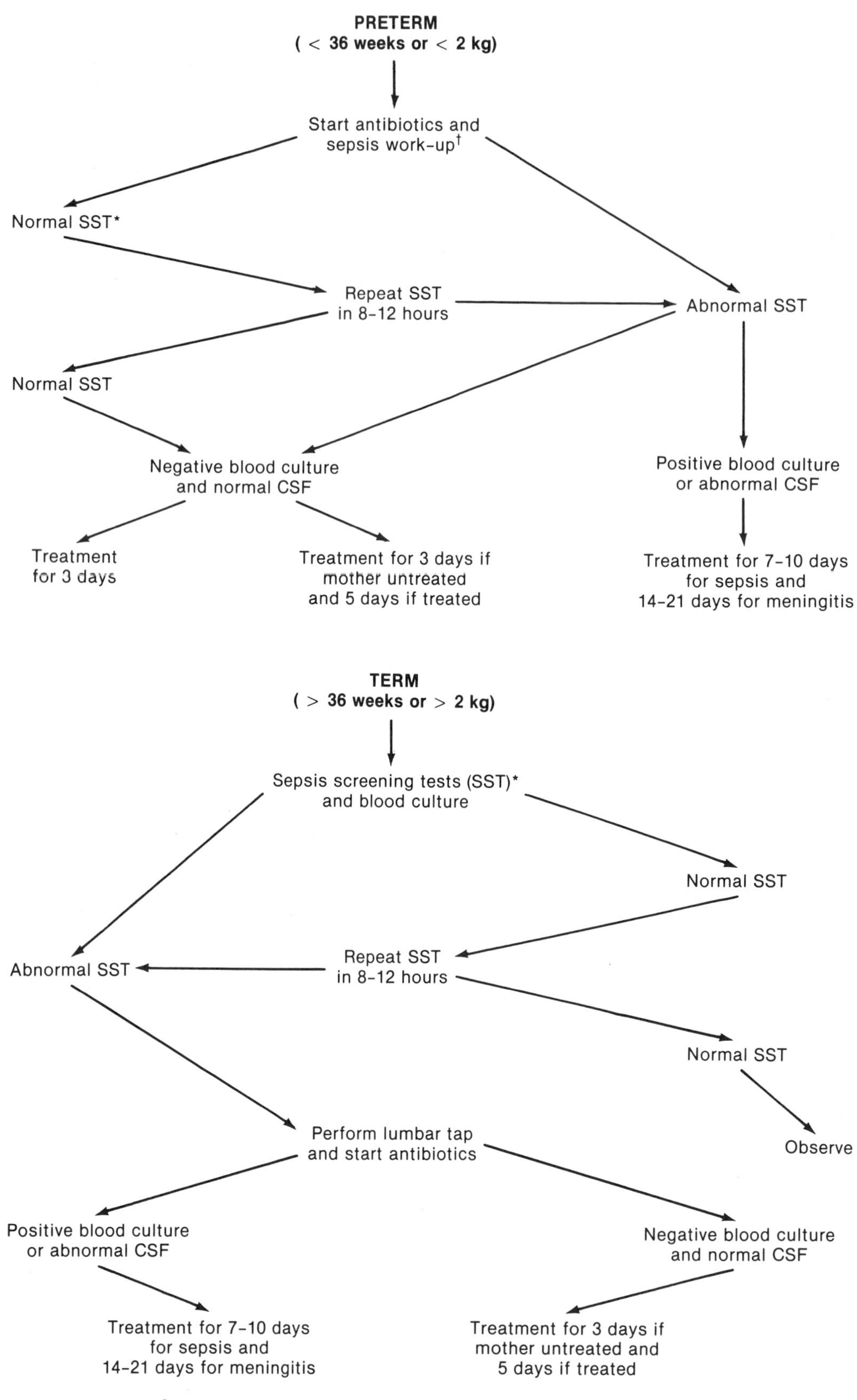

Figure 1. Recommended diagnostic and therapeutic approaches for asymptomatic preterm and term newborns with obstetric risk factors. Risk factors include prolonged rupture of membranes (PROM) for at least 18 hours; maternal fever; uterine tenderness; cloudy amniotic fluid; foul-smelling amniotic fluid, placenta, or infant; or persistent fetal tachycardia. I/T, immature/total neutrophils; CSF, cerebrospinal fluid; SST, sepsis screening test(s); WBC, white blood cell count.

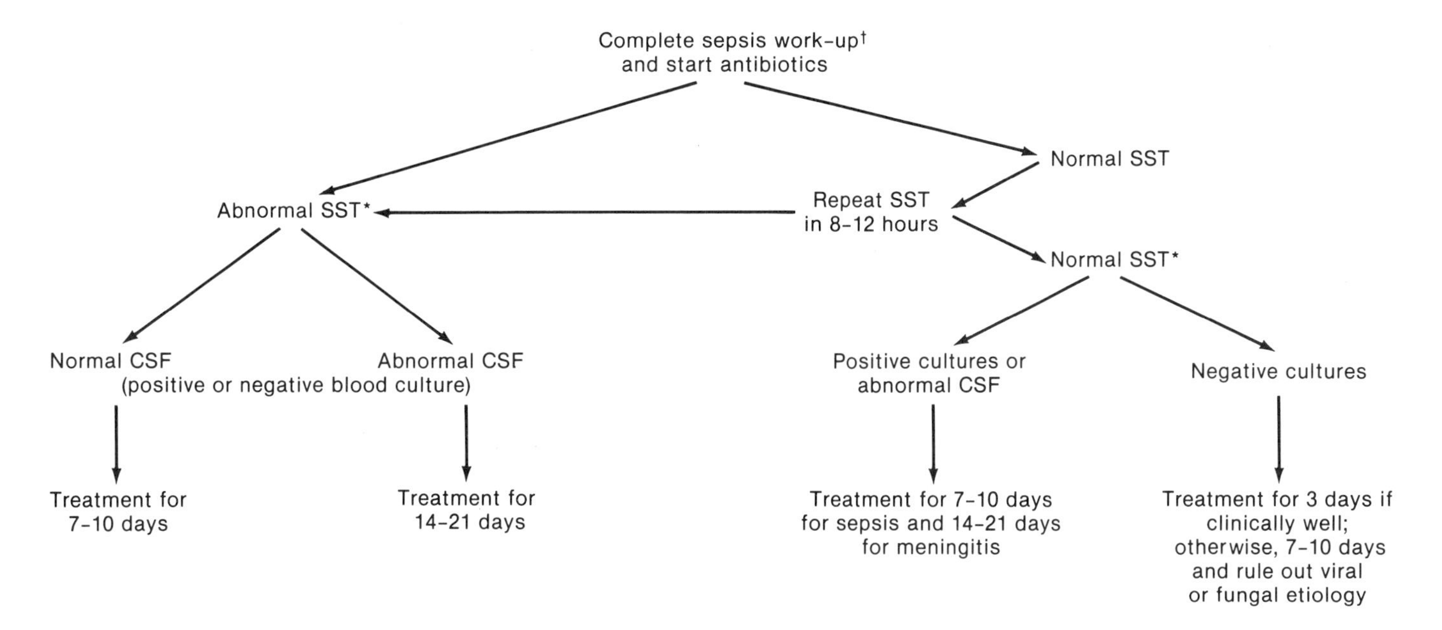

*WBC < 5000/mm^3 or I/T ratio > 0.2 or C-reactive protein > 1.0 mg/dl

†SST plus urine, blood, and CSF cultures; urine and CSF analysis; and chest X-ray

Figure 2. Recommended diagnostic and therapeutic approaches for the symptomatic term or preterm newborn. I/T, immature/total neutrophils; CSF, cerebrospinal fluid; SST, sepsis screening test(s); WBC, white blood cell count.

monitoring of the drug peak and trough serum concentrations to avoid either toxic or subtherapeutic levels. Recommended peak concentrations are 5 to 8 μg/ml for gentamicin, tobramycin, and netilmicin and 20 to 30 μg/ml for amikacin and vancomycin. Trough levels should be less than 2 μg/ml for gentamicin, tobramycin, and netilmicin and less than 10 μg/ml for amikacin and vancomycin.

Supportive Care

In addition to appropriate antimicrobial therapy, general supportive care is vital to optimize recovery from septicemia. The need for ventilatory support, volume expansion with fresh frozen plasma, replacement of blood or platelets, correction of electrolytes and other metabolic abnormalities, and early initiation of parenteral nutritional fluids must be determined. The role of adjunctive therapeutic modalities, such as granulocyte transfusions, intravenous gammaglobulin, and exchange transfusions, is currently of limited or inconclusive value. Efficacy of intravenous gammaglobulin for prevention of sepsis in infants weighing less than 1500 g has not yet been proven despite the completion of several trials, two of which were well-designed, large, multicenter, placebo-controlled studies. Promising adjunctive therapeutic possibilities for the future include use of specific monoclonal antibodies against bacterial cell wall components (e.g., endotoxin) or of the agents directed against inflammatory mediators (e.g., cytokines).

MENINGITIS

Treatment

Drug Therapy

Bacteremia usually precedes the development of meningitis. Meningitis may complicate as many as 25 per cent of bacteremias in neonates. Thus, the empiric antimicrobial therapy is the same as for neonatal septicemia. After appropriate specimens for CSF and blood culture are obtained, ampicillin and an aminoglycoside are recommended. Therapy is then adjusted, depending on results of cultures and susceptibility testing. For group B streptococci, penicillin or ampicillin alone is generally adequate, although the addition of an aminoglycoside to the regimen is preferred by many investigators for a synergistic effect. For potential synergistic activity, ampicillin, with or without a short course of an aminoglycoside, is the preferred choice for meningitis caused by *L. monocytogenes.*

For gram-negative bacillary meningitis, the traditional combination therapy of ampicillin and an aminoglycoside has been used extensively. Because the concentration of aminoglycosides in the subarachnoid and ventricular fluid may be suboptimal, sterilization of CSF is often delayed and this probably contributes to the high incidence of adverse neurologic outcome seen in this age group. Third-generation cephalosporins, such as cefotaxime and ceftazidime, possess extraordinary in vitro activity against gram-negative enteric bacilli and *Pseudomonas,* respectively; achieve high serum and CSF concentrations; and are well tolerated by newborns. Such favorable properties make these antibiotics our choice once the pathogen causing meningitis has been properly identified as a gram-negative rod. We usually combine an aminoglycoside with cefotaxime for at least the first 10 days of treatment of meningitis caused by *Enterobacter, Serratia,* or *Citrobacter* species and with ceftazidime for *P. aeruginosa,* to avoid development of resistance and for possible synergistic activity. Ceftriaxone is not recommended for use in neonates because of its potential to displace bilirubin from albumin-binding sites and its marked suppression of the normal intestinal flora.

Because of the high propensity for development of brain abscess in meningitis caused by Citrobacter *diversus (75 per cent versus <10 per cent for other gram-negative rods), appropriate imaging studies—computed tomography (CT) or magnetic resonance imaging (MRI)—and neurosurgical consultation for needle aspiration and/or excision are recommended early in the course.*

When staphylococci are believed to be responsible for men-

TABLE 3. Recommended Dosage Schedule* in Treatment of Neonatal Sepsis and Meningitis

		Dosages (mg/kg) and Intervals of Administration				
		< 1200 g	*1200–2000 g*		*> 2000 g*	
Antibiotic	**Route**	*0–4 wk*	*0–7 Days*	*> 7 Days*	*0–7 Days*	*> 7 Days*
Amikacin	IV, IM	7.5 q18–24h	7.5 q12–18h	7.5 q8–12h	10 q12h	10 q8h
Ampicillin	IV, IM					
Meningitis		50 q12h	50 q12h	50 q8h	50 q8h	50 q6h
Other diseases		25 q12h	25 q12h	25 q8h	25 q8h	25 q6h
Aztreonam	IV, IM	30 q12h	30 q12h	30 q8h	30 q8h	30 q6h
Cefazolin	IV, IM	20 q12h	20 q12h	20 q12h	20 q12h	20 q8h
Cefotaxime	IV, IM	50 q12h	50 q12h	50 q8h	50 q12h	50 q8h
Ceftazidime	IV, IM	50 q12h	50 q12h	50 q8h	50 q12h	50 q8h
Ceftriaxone	IV, IM	50 q24h	50 q24h	50 q24h	50 q24h	75 q24h
Cephalothin	IV	20 q12h	20 q12h	20 q8h	20 q8h	20 q6h
Chloramphenicol	IV, PO	25 q24h	25 q24h	25 q24h	25 q24h	25 q12h
Clindamycin	IV, IM, PO	5 q12h	5 q12h	5 q8h	5 q8h	5 q6h
Erythromycin	PO	10 q12h	10 q12h	10 q8h	10 q12h	10 q8h
Gentamicin	IV, IM	2.5 q18–24h	2.5 q12–18h	2.5 q8–12h	2.5 q12h	2.5 q8h
Imipenem	IV, IM	20 q18–24h	20 q12h	20 q12h	20 q12h	20 q8h
Kanamycin	IV, IM	7.5 q18–24h	7.5 q12–18h	7.5 q8–12h	10 q12h	10 q8h
Methicillin	IV, IM					
Meningitis		50 q12h	50 q12h	50 q8h	50 q8h	50 q6h
Other diseases		25 q12h	25 q12h	25 q8h	25 q8h	25 q6h
Metronidazole	IV, PO	7.5 q48h	7.5 q24h	7.5 q12h	7.5 q12h	15 q12h
Mezlocillin	IV, IM	75 q12h	75 q12h	75 q8h	75 q12h	75 q8h
Oxacillin	IV, IM	25 q12h	25 q12h	25 q8h	25 q8h	25 q6h
Nafcillin	IV	25 q12h	25 q12h	25 q8h	25 q8h	25 q6h
Netilmicin	IV, IM	2.5 q18–24h	2.5 q12–18h	2.5 q8–12h	2.5 q12h	2.5 q8h
Penicillin G	IV					
Meningitis		50,000 U q12h	50,000 U q12h	75,000 U q8h	50,000 U q8h	50,000 U q6h
Other diseases		25,000 U q12h	25,000 U q12h	25,000 U q8h	25,000 U q8h	25,000 U q6h
Penicillin G Benzathine	IM		50,000 U (one dose)	50,000 U (one dose)	50,000 U (one dose)	50,000 U (one dose)
Procaine			50,000 U q24h	50,000 U q24h	50,000 U q24h	50,000 U q24h
Ticarcillin	IV, IM	75 q12h	75 q12h	75 q8h	75 q8h	75 q6h
Tobramycin	IV, IM	2.5 q18–24h	2.5 q12–18h	2.5 q8–12h	2.5 q12h	2.5 q8h
Vancomycin	IV	15 q24h	15 q12–18h	15 q8–12h	15 q12h	15 q8h

Adapted from Nelson JD: Antibiotic therapy for newborns. *In* Pocketbook of Pediatric Antimicrobial Therapy, 10th ed. Baltimore, Williams & Wilkins, 1991–1993.
*For infants weighing less than 1.2 kg, smaller doses and longer intervals between doses may be advisable (see Prober et al. Pediatr Infect Dis J 9:111, 1990).

ingitis (e.g., in infants with ventriculoperitoneal shunts), vancomycin is combined with an aminoglycoside.

To ensure sterility of the CSF, another specimen is obtained for culture after 24 to 48 hours of therapy. If the second culture results are positive after 48 hours for group B streptococci and *Listeria* and 72 hours for gram-negative bacillary organisms, the susceptibilities of the pathogen must be reviewed carefully and the antibiotic concentrations and/or their bactericidal activities in blood and CSF measured. Consideration is then given to the need for modifying the antimicrobial regimen and performing cranial imaging studies to identify a localized collection of infected fluid, cerebritis, or brain abscess.

The duration of therapy for uncomplicated meningitis caused by group B streptococci and *Listeria* is 14 days. For enterococcal and gram-negative bacillary meningitis, a minimum of 21 days (or 14 days after the first negative CSF culture if sterilization is delayed beyond 7 days) is recommended.

Supportive Care

Supportive care of the newborn with meningitis is similar to that of the infant with sepsis. Neurologic examination with measurement of the head circumference is performed daily. Seizures are managed with phenobarbital and/or phenytoin. Fluid requirements are adjusted to avoid hypotensive states and to maintain adequate systemic blood pressure and cerebral perfusion. Fluids are restricted if there is evidence of volume retention secondary to inappropriate antidiuretic hormone (ADH) secretion or increased if there is evidence of dehydration. Frequent determination of weight, urinary output, and serum and urine electrolytes is helpful in guiding fluid management during the first 48 hours. Placement of a ventriculoperitoneal shunt is usually necessary if hydrocephalus develops. At the conclusion of therapy, we recommend a head CT study and evaluation of hearing status using brain stem auditory evoked responses. *Efficacy of steroids as adjunctive therapy to improve outcome from bacterial meningitis in newborns has not been determined. However, markedly elevated levels of interleukin (IL-I) have been detected in the CSF of neonates with gram-negative meningitis and correlated with an increased incidence of neurologic sequelae and fatality. Therefore, it is likely that steroids will be beneficial as in older infants with* H. influenzae *type B meningitis.*

PNEUMONIA

Etiology

Pneumonia in the neonatal period is most commonly acquired during birth, when the newborn infant is exposed to microorganisms colonizing the maternal birth canal, or in utero, as a result of direct inhalation and/or aspiration of contaminated amniotic fluid. In these instances, pneumonia is usually seen as a part of the early-onset sepsis and can be difficult to differentiate from uncomplicated hyaline membrane disease. Although group B streptococci are the most common agents implicated, gram-negative coliforms can also be the responsible pathogens. *Chlamydia trachomatis* is acquired by the same route, but the resulting pneumonia does not become manifest until the end of the first month of life.

A newborn can also acquire pneumonia through the transplacental route—in which case it is part of a generalized congenital disease. Rubella virus, cytomegalovirus, herpes simplex virus, *Toxoplasma gondii, Treponema pallidum, Mycobacterium tuberculosis,* and *L. monocytogenes* are examples of pathogens that infect infants via this route of transmission. *L. monocytogenes,* cytomegalovirus, and herpes simplex virus are more likely to be acquired at the time of delivery and *M. tuberculosis* after delivery.

Pneumonia can also develop in the infant, usually a premature neonate, after contact with contaminated nursery equipment and other intensive care technical devices, in which case the likely etiologic agents are *S. aureus* and a variety of gram-negative rods. Additionally, when the infant is discharged from the hospital and exposed to the household environment, viruses become the predominant organisms causing pneumonia, the most frequent being respiratory syncytial virus (RSV), parainfluenza, and adenovirus.

Other rare and still not well-defined etiologic factors in pneumonia in newborns are *Ureaplasma urealyticum* and *Pneumocystis carinii,* the former implicated in cases of bronchopulmonary dysplasia and the latter seen in severely malnourished or immunodeficient infants.

Treatment

Drug Therapy

Initial empiric antimicrobial therapy for pneumonia in the newborn is the same as that for early-onset septicemia or meningitis and consists of ampicillin and an aminoglycoside. For late-onset infections or suspected nosocomially acquired pneumonias, an antistaphylococcal agent (methicillin, vancomycin) combined with an aminoglycoside should be used. If infection with *P. aeruginosa* is likely, addition of ceftazidime or ticarcillin to the aminoglycoside is recommended.

Infants with *Chlamydia* pneumonia generally present with mild to moderate respiratory distress, a dry and repetitive cough, absence of fever, bilateral, diffuse interstitial infiltrates on chest roentgenograms, and a peripheral eosinophilia. The diagnosis is confirmed by antigen detection in nasopharyngeal secretions or in conjunctival scrapings in the presence of conjunctivitis. Erythromycin is the drug of choice, and the mother and her sexual partner(s) are treated with tetracycline.

Antiviral therapy is limited. Ribavirin aerosol is recommended for treatment of progressive severe RSV pneumonitis in the healthy neonate or less severe disease in any infant with congenital heart disease or immunodeficiency or in the premature infant with bronchopulmonary dysplasia.

Intravenous acyclovir is indicated for treatment of herpes simplex pneumonitis. Although there is limited experience in neonates, amantadine initiated within the first 48 hours is beneficial for severe influenza A pneumonia. Efficacy of ganciclovir for treatment of congenital cytomegalovirus infection is currently under investigation, but the preliminary results do not look encouraging.

The duration of antibiotic therapy is usually 3 weeks for pneumonias caused by *S. aureus, Pseudomonas,* or gram-negative enteric organisms and 10 to 14 days for those caused by group B streptococci, *Listeria,* or *Chlamydia* or other agents.

Supportive Care

Supportive therapy frequently includes supplemental oxygen, mechanical ventilation, chest physiotherapy, and nutritional support. Thoracentesis for diagnostic and therapeutic purposes is usually indicated, and placement of a closed chest tube is recommended when an empyema is present. Pleural fluid must be examined carefully to exclude chylothorax. Chyle in the pleural space is milky or yellow in an infant who has been fed, but it is clear in the infant who has not been fed recently. Chyle is characterized by a high white blood cell count, predominantly lymphocytes, and an elevated lipid and protein content.

REFERENCES

Klein JO, Marcy SM: Bacterial sepsis and meningitis. *In* Remington JS, Klein JO (eds): Infectious Diseases of the Fetus and Newborn Infant, 3rd ed. Philadelphia, WB Saunders Co, 1990, pp 601–644.

Mustafa MM, McCracken GH: Perinatal bacterial diseases. *In* Feigin RD, Cherry JD (eds): Textbook of Pediatric Infectious Diseases, 3rd ed. Philadelphia, WB Saunders Co, 1992, pp 891–924.

Nelson JD: Antibiotic therapy for newborns. *In* 1991–1992 Pocketbook of Pediatric Antimicrobial Therapy, 7th ed. Baltimore, Williams & Wilkins, 1987, pp 16–17.

Siegel JD: Sepsis neonatorum. *In* Oski FA, De Angelis C, Feigin RD, Warshaw JB (eds): Principles and Practice of Pediatrics. Philadelphia, JB Lippincott, 1990, pp 471–479.

BACTERIAL MENINGITIS AND SEPTICEMIA BEYOND THE NEONATAL PERIOD

SHELDON L. KAPLAN, M.D.

BACTERIAL MENINGITIS

Once the diagnosis of bacterial meningitis is suspected or established in a child, antibiotics are the most important components of therapy. Although the *Haemophilus influenzae* type b protein-conjugate vaccines undoubtedly will change the distribution of organisms causing bacterial meningitis in pediatrics, the three most common organisms for infants and children 3 months to 10 years old remain *H. influenzae* type b, *Streptococcus pneumoniae,* and *Neisseria meningitidis.* In the United States, approximately 30 per cent of systemic *H. influenzae* type b isolates are ampicillin-resistant. Chloramphenicol-resistant and ampicillin-resistant isolates are unusual but do occur. The incidence of *S. pneumoniae* isolates that are fully or relatively resistant to penicillin is unknown but may be increasing. Such organisms have diminished susceptibility to penicillin as a result of alterations in penicillin-binding proteins. Therefore, all systemic isolates of *S. pneumoniae* should be screened routinely for susceptibility to penicillin. Cefotaxime and ceftriaxone are highly active against all three of these common pediatric pathogens.

In children with underlying deficiencies in host defense, meningitis may develop as a result of the standard highly encapsulated organisms or an unusual pathogen may be the etiologic agent. *Listeria monocytogenes, Salmonella* sp., nontypable *H. influenzae, Moraxella catarrhalis,* and gram-negative enterics are examples of such organisms. *Staphylococcus aureus* and gram-negative organisms may cause meningitis following neurosurgical procedures or complicated head trauma. These same bacteria, in addition to anaerobes, when isolated from cerebrospinal fluid (CSF), should raise the suspicion of dermal or enteric sinuses leading to the subarachnoid space. The antimicrobial therapy for these unusual forms of bacterial meningitis must be determined on an individual basis, depending on the results of in vitro susceptibility testing.

For otherwise normal children, 3 months to 10 years of age with presumed bacterial meningitis, regardless of Gram stain findings or the results of rapid antigen tests, initial empiric therapy with either cefotaxime (200 mg/kg/day in four divided doses every 6 hours) or ceftriaxone (100 mg/kg/day in two divided doses every 12 hours) intravenously is generally recommended. The combination of ampicillin (300 to 400 mg/kg/day in four or six divided doses) plus chloramphenicol (75 to 100 mg/kg/day in four divided doses) is also acceptable. However, because the use of chloramphenicol requires monitoring of serum concentrations of chloramphenicol (ideal peak levels are between 15 and 25 μg/ml), and several other drugs (phenobarbital, phenytoin) may alter the pharmacokinetics of chloramphenicol, it is far simpler to avoid chloramphenicol administration unless there is a specific reason not to do so. In areas where ampicillin and chloramphenicol-resistant *H. influenzae* type b have been encountered, this combination is probably not optimal for initial empiric therapy. For children with a history of anaphylaxis to penicillin, chloramphenicol is an agent of first choice.

Once an organism is isolated and the antimicrobial susceptibility is determined, antimicrobial therapy can be modified (Table 1). For ampicillin-susceptible *H. influenzae* type b, ampicillin remains the agent with the least adverse side effects. Cefotaxime or ceftriaxone is continued for ampicillin-resistant isolates. Diarrhea is the most common complication of these agents. *Gallbladder "sludge" may be detected by ultrasonography in children receiving ceftriaxone, but this finding rarely leads to clinical symptoms.* Aq penicillin G remains the agent of choice for completing treatment of meningitis due to penicillin-susceptible strains of *S. pneumoniae* or *N. meningitidis.* Although the optimal therapy for pneumococcal meningitis (when strains fully or relatively resistant to penicillin are isolated) has not been established, published experience indicates that either chloramphenicol or cefotaxime is effective for susceptible isolates. *Cefuroxime should not be considered an adequate agent for the treatment of bacterial meningitis because delayed sterilization of CSF and a greater incidence of hearing loss are associated with this agent compared with other antibiotics.*

The antimicrobial management of meningitis due to other bacteria is determined by in vitro susceptibility testing of the isolate (Table 2). A penicillinase-resistant penicillin is the agent of choice for treating meningitis due to methicillin-susceptible *S. aureus.* Vancomycin is recommended for treating meningitis due to *S. aureus* when the isolate is methicillin-resistant or when the child is allergic to penicillin. Vancomycin (60 mg/kg/day in four divided doses every 6 hours) is administered over 60 minutes, which appears to decrease adverse effects. For treatment of meningitis, peak serum concentrations of vancomycin between 35 and 40 μg/ml and trough levels less than 10 to 15 μg/ml are desirable. If the patient has renal dysfunction, the dose of vancomycin is modified.

The third-generation cephalosporins, especially cefotaxime, are the most commonly administered agents for treating meningitis due to gram-negative bacilli. Although the addition of an aminoglycoside may provide for synergistic activity, there is no proof that this is necessary or optimal. In selected patients who have persistently positive lumbar CSF or ventricular fluid cultures, intraventricular administration of an aminoglycoside may be beneficial. *Ceftazidime appears useful for treating* Pseudomonas *meningitis.* The optimal antibiotic therapy for *Salmonella* meningitis is not known. Relapses have been reported with both ampicillin and chloramphenicol despite in vitro susceptibility and prolonged administration. Cefotaxime has been found to be successful treatment for several patients with *Salmonella* meningitis. Trimethoprim-sulfamethoxazole should be considered in patients who are not responding to therapy as expected.

TABLE 1. Suggested Antibiotics for Treatment of Bacterial Meningitis in Infants Beyond 3 Months of Age

Organism	Antibiotic	Dose (mg/kg/day)	Interval (Hours)
Haemophilus influenzae type b	Ampicillin*	300–400	4–6
	Cefotaxime	200	6
	Ceftriaxone	100	12
	Chloramphenicol	75–100	6
Streptococcus pneumoniae			
Penicillin-susceptible	Aqueous penicillin G	300,000 U	4–6
Relatively or fully penicillin-resistant	Cefotaxime or Chloramphenicol	As above	
	or Vancomycin	60	6
Neisseria meningitidis	Aqueous penicillin G	As above	

*Ampicillin-susceptible strains.

TABLE 2. Antimicrobial Therapy for Bacterial Meningitis Caused by Unusual Pathogens

Organism	Antibiotic	Dose (mg/kg/day)	Interval (Hours)
Staphylococcus aureus			
Methicillin-susceptible	Nafcillin, oxacillin	200	6
Methicillin-resistant	Vancomycin	60	6
Gram-negative enteric	Cefotaxime ± Aminoglycoside*	200	6
Listeria monocytogenes	Ampicillin ± Aminoglycoside*	300	4–6
Salmonella sp.	Ampicillin	300–400	4–6
	Chloramphenicol	75–100	6
	Cefotaxime	200	6
Pseudomonas sp.	Ceftazidime	150–200	6–8

*Aminoglycoside can be discontinued after 7 days.

Duration of Therapy

For otherwise uncomplicated courses of bacterial meningitis, 10 days (some authorities favor 7 days) of antibiotic therapy is adequate for *H. influenzae* type b and *S. pneumoniae* meningitis. Meningococcal meningitis is treated satisfactorily after 7 days. Gram-negative enteric meningitis generally is treated for a minimum of 21 days and at least 2 weeks after the CSF is sterile, whichever is longer. In some cases, sterilization may take several days or even weeks. Two weeks of therapy is usually adequate for *S. aureus* meningitis.

If some complication occurs or if the child remains febrile despite adequate therapy, a longer treatment course is generally indicated. I usually continue to treat children who remain febrile for more than 8 days without any specific evidence of a suppurative complication for a 2-week course after an evaluation for possible causes of prolonged fever has been unrevealing (Table 3). In my experience, prolonged fever in a child being treated appropriately for bacterial meningitis frequently is not associated with any documented

TABLE 3. Potential Sources of Prolonged or Secondary Fever in Children with Bacterial Meningitis

Nosocomial infections
- Diarrhea
- Pneumonia
- Viral upper respiratory tract infection
- Urinary tract infection
- Phlebitis

Suppurative complications
- Septic arthritis
- Pericarditis
- Pleural or subdural empyema
- Brain abscess (very rare)

Immune complex arthritis

Inadequately treated meningitis

Drug fever

cause. It is debatable whether the presence of a subdural effusion is an adequate explanation for persistent fever. However, a subdural tap may be indicated in such a child who has a rapidly growing head circumference, vomiting, bulging fontanelle, or other symptoms and signs of increased intracranial pressure (ICP).

A second lumbar puncture is not necessary for the management of older infants and children with meningitis caused by the three most common pathogens when the patient is responding to therapy as expected. However, if meningitis is caused by an unusual organism or if there is any concern about the patient's response to treatment, a second analysis of the CSF can be helpful.

Supportive Care

For children who are not in shock, poorly perfused, or markedly dehydrated, some degree of fluid restriction initially appears useful to prevent exacerbation of cerebral edema. Children are not allowed to drink or eat anything until they are clearly alert enough not to aspirate what they ingest. Generally, a multielectrolyte-containing solution (one-fourth to one-half normal saline plus potassium at 20 to 40 mEq/L in 5 per cent dextrose) is infused intravenously at approximately two thirds of normal maintenance requirements or at 1000 to 1200 ml/m^2 per 24 hours. Once the serum sodium level reaches or remains at 135 mEq/L or above, the volume of fluid infused can be gradually increased; by 24 to 48 hours, most patients are receiving maintenance rates (1500 to 1700 ml/m^2/day). Serum electrolytes (osmolalities are optimal), urine-specific gravity, and urine output are monitored frequently during the first several days after admission to help guide fluid management.

If perfusion is poor or if the child is hypotensive, measures are required to reverse these processes. In most instances, additional fluid volumes of 10 to 20 ml/kg of normal saline are all that is necessary to normalize perfusion. For children more critically ill, the placement of central venous lines and a urinary catheter is required for accurate measurements of central venous pressure (CVP) and urine output, respectively, which are important guides for fluid management. Dopamine or dobutamine may be indicated if perfusion remains inadequate despite appropriate fluid administration and if CVP indicates that there is a risk for pulmonary edema. Wide swings in blood pressure should be avoided, since cerebral blood flow may be adversely affected.

Normally, no special measures other than elevating the head of the bed 30 degrees and careful fluid management are indicated for combating the increased ICP associated with bacterial meningitis. However, progressive lethargy, increasing muscle tone, and further bulging of the fontanelle may indicate advancing increased ICP. Unequal or dilated pupils, impaired ocular mobility, bradycardia, apnea, or decorticate or decerebrate posturing are signs of cerebral herniation and indicate that more aggressive measures are needed to decrease ICP. Intubation and hyperventilation to a P_{CO_2} of approximately 25 to 30 torr should rapidly decrease ICP (but may also decrease cerebral blood flow). Mannitol (0.5 to 2.0 g/kg) is infused over 30 minutes and may help to reduce cerebral edema and thus ICP.

The routine administration of dexamethasone is recommended by some authorities, although I believe that its efficacy requires further clarification. The safety and efficacy of dexamethasone in children with pneumococcal meningitis due to strains relatively or fully resistant to penicillin are unknown. Nevertheless, on the basis of available information, if dexamethasone is to be used, it should be administered as soon as the first dose of antibiotic is administered. The regimen of dexamethasone suggested is 0.15 mg/kg per dose every 6 hours intravenously for the first 4 days (16 doses). One must be certain to discontinue therapy at this time or as soon as bacterial meningitis is no longer a consideration. It is common for fever to recur once dexamethasone therapy is discontinued. Gastrointestinal bleeding may also occur more frequently in patients receiving dexamethasone. Thus, H_2 blockers should be administered if dexamethasone is employed.

Seizure Management

Approximately 20 to 30 per cent of children with bacterial meningitis will have seizures sometime during the acute illness, with most of the seizures occurring prior to or within 48 hours of admission. For brief, generalized seizures that occur early in the illness, phenytoin (5 to 10 mg/kg loading dose) or phenobarbital (5 to 20 mg/kg loading dose), administered intravenously once or twice followed by maintenance doses, is generally adequate to control seizure activity. Usually, anticonvulsants can be discontinued by the time of discharge or shortly thereafter in these instances. However, for seizures that are prolonged, focal, or difficult to control or that develop later in the hospital course, prolonged anticonvulsant therapy may be necessary. The subsequent onset of epilepsy usually is associated with damage to the brain parenchyma (such as might occur secondary to infarction related to vasculitis), as demonstrated by computed tomography of the brain.

Prevention

For children with *H. influenzae* type b meningitis, rifampin (20 mg/kg per dose, maximum dose 600 mg) is recommended for 4 consecutive days to eradicate nasopharyngeal colonization, which is not reliably accomplished with therapy for the meningitis. This can be administered at the end of or after completing antibiotic therapy. Following *H. influenzae* type b meningitis, unimmunized children under 2 years of age should receive an *H. influenzae* type b polysaccharide-conjugate vaccine (one licensed for administration at 2 months of age) according to the age-appropriate schedule. Children who have acquired meningitis or other invasive infection due to *H. influenzae* type b despite receiving *H. influenzae* conjugate vaccines appropriately should be evaluated for immunoglobulin and immunoglobulin subclass deficiencies. For meningococcal meningitis, rifampin can be administered as above or in a dosage of 10 mg/kg every 12 hours for four doses.

Follow-up Evaluation

Because sensorineural hearing loss is one of the more common neurologic sequelae of bacterial meningitis, it is routine to test hearing just prior to or within a month of patient discharge from the hospital. If a hearing loss is detected that is expected to interfere with developing vocabulary and learning, careful follow-up and intervention are obviously mandatory. Any concern regarding intellectual development should prompt a formal developmental assessment.

SEPTICEMIA AND BACTEREMIA

Etiology

As with meningitis, a relatively small group of bacteria is responsible for the vast majority of bacteremias in normal children. *S. pneumoniae*, *H. influenzae* type b, and *N. meningitidis* are, again, among the most common isolates, and each may be associated with "outpatient" or "unsuspected" bacteremia. *S. aureus*, *Salmonella* sp., and most recently group A streptococcus are also important pathogens frequently isolated from blood cultures.

S. aureus sepsis should always be considered in the critically

TABLE 4. Empiric Antibiotic Therapy for Septicemia and Bacteremia in Normal Children

Age	Likely Organisms	Antibiotics	Dose (mg/kg/day)
Child up to 5 years	*Haemophilus influenzae* type b	Cefotaxime	150
		or	
	Streptococcus pneumoniae	Ceftriaxone	50–100
		or	
	Neisseria meningitidis	Cefuroxime (meningitis excluded)	150–200
Suspected source			
Skin or wound infection	*Staphylococcus aureus*	Add nafcillin/ oxacillin to above	150
	Group A streptococci		
Abdominal source	Gram-negative enterics	Clindamycin	30–40
		+	
	Anaerobes	Ampicillin	200
	Pseudomonas aeruginosa	+	
		Aminoglycoside	—
Urinary tract infection	Gram-negative enterics	Cefotaxime	150
		or	
		Ceftriaxone	50–100
		or	
		Aminoglycoside	7.5
Older child or Adolescent	*S. aureus*	Nafcillin	150
	N. meningiditis	+	
	S. pneumoniae	Cefotaxime	150

ill child, especially adolescents. A preceding skin infection or lesion may heighten the suspicion of *S. aureus* or group A streptococcal bacteremia. In otherwise normal children, gram-negative enterics may cause bacteremia in association with pyelonephritis or diarrhea. Children with defects in host immunity may develop bacteremia with the same "community-acquired pathogens" observed in normal children, but they also are at increased risk for infections due to a wide variety of bacteria, especially during hospitalization.

Functional or anatomic asplenia can be associated with overwhelming bacteremia caused by highly encapsulated microorganisms, particularly *S. pneumoniae.* The presence of foreign material, such as a catheter or central line, enhances the risk of bacteremia due to both gram-positive (*S. epidermidis,* other coagulase-negative staphylococci, *S. aureus, Streptococcus*) and gram-negative bacteria. Colonization of the respiratory or urinary tracts with gram-negative enterics and *P. aeruginosa* as a result of endotracheal intubation, or placement of a urinary catheter, respectively, certainly can lead to entry of gram-negative organisms into the blood stream and subsequent sepsis. The empiric administration of antibiotics to children with suspected septicemia takes into account these factors as well as the likely antimicrobial susceptibility pattern of the probable pathogen(s).

Diagnosis and Treatment

The history and physical examination of a child with suspected septicemia are performed carefully but in a timely manner. Blood specimens (preferably two) as well as specimens of urine, other fluids (CSF, joint fluid, pleural fluid), and other sites as deemed appropriate are obtained for culture, and empiric antibiotic therapy is initiated as soon as possible. For critically ill patients, antibiotics are infused intravenously immediately after a specimen is drawn for culture. If septicemia is suspected but blood specimens cannot be drawn for some reason, antibiotics are still administered and specimens can be obtained as soon as possible thereafter.

Guidelines for initial empiric therapy are outlined in Tables 4 and 5. Once a pathogen is identified, the antibiotic regimen is modified on the basis of antimicrobial susceptibility pattern as well as the safety profile of the agent.

Normal children sick with bacteremia without meningitis or other foci of infection due to *H. influenzae* type b, *S. pneumoniae,* or *N. meningitidis* generally should receive parenteral antibiotics until they are afebrile for 48 to 72 hours, after which a 10-day course of therapy can be completed with an appropriate oral agent. *One must be certain of patient compliance for completing the outpatient therapy.* Route and duration of therapy in children with foci of infection are determined by the specific site of the infection (as in osteomyelitis and pneumonia). Deficiencies of terminal complement components are associated with meningococcal infections. Therefore, a screening test, such as total serum complement activity (CH_{50}), should be performed in children with nonepidemic and certainly recurrent meningococcal infection.

Bacteremia in febrile young children without a focus of infection but who otherwise do not appear severely ill is frequently referred to as "occult," "unsuspected," or "outpatient." These previously healthy children usually are between 3 and 36 months of age, have a fever greater than 39°C, and a peripheral white blood cell count $\geq$ 15,000/mm^3. Approximately 5 to 10 per cent of such children will have a bacteremia due to *S. pneumoniae* (80 per cent), *H. influenzae* type b (10 per cent), or other organism (*Salmonella* sp., *N. meningitidis*). Various approaches have been advocated in detecting and managing this entity. Other than a blood culture, no laboratory test—including total peripheral white blood cell count, erythrocyte sedimentation rate, or C-reactive protein—has acceptable sensitivity or specificity for predicting the presence of bacteremia.

Furthermore, the results of two randomized studies comparing placebo to empiric antibiotic therapy in these patients are conflicting. Therefore, the approach to the febrile child with possible occult bacteremia must be handled on an individual basis, with several management strategies being reasonable. The reliability of the parents and the ability to contact

TABLE 5. Empiric Antibiotic Therapy for Septicemia and Bacteremia in Immunocompromised Children

	Likely Organism	Antibiotics	Dose (mg/kg/day)
Community-acquired	*Haemophilus influenzae* type b	Nafcillin/oxacillin	150
		+	
		Cefotaxime	150
	Streptococcus pneumoniae	or	
		Nafcillin/oxacillin	
	Gram-negative enterics	+	150
		Aminoglycoside	
	Staphylococcus aureus	+	—
		Extended-spectrum penicillin*	
Central line present	*S. aureus* *Staphylococcus epidermidis*	Consider vancomycin rather than nafcillin/oxacillin	40
Hospital-acquired	Gram-negative enteric, *Pseudomonas* sp., methicillin-resistant staphylococci	Dependent on antimicrobial susceptibility of hospital pathogens	—

*Especially for neutropenic child. Ceftazidime (150 mg/kg/day) can be substituted for the aminoglycoside plus an extended spectrum penicillin (ticarcillin, piperacillin).

and communicate with the family are important factors to consider when outpatient management is to be undertaken.

Under the proper circumstances, one approach is to obtain a blood specimen for culture, if bacteremia is suspected, and to initiate oral therapy with amoxicillin with or without an initial parenteral dose of an antibiotic. Although the efficacy and safety of ceftriaxone therapy in the empiric treatment of occult bacteremia are currently unknown, the rationale is to administer a single intramuscular dose (50 mg/kg) followed by oral therapy with amoxicillin. If the blood culture is negative at 48 to 72 hours, antibiotics can be discontinued. Modification of therapy may be necessary if the condition of the child changes prior to receipt of the blood culture results. Management of children with a positive blood culture is dependent on their clinical condition when the physician is notified that the blood culture is positive. For such children who are afebrile, with normal behavior, and normal physical findings at follow-up, a second blood specimen is obtained and therapy is continued on an outpatient basis. A careful reassessment is required for children who remain febrile, have persistent or newly developed symptoms, or who now have abnormal physical findings. A focal infection, such as meningitis, septic arthritis, or pneumonia, among others, may have developed in these patients, who then should be hospitalized for appropriate re-evaluation and antibiotic therapy.

Other physicians may choose not to initiate empiric antibiotic therapy for these children, since bacteremia will not be present in 90 per cent or more. Whatever decision regarding antibiotic administration is made, careful follow-up and communication with the family regarding the child's condition and progress are the key factors in allowing different approaches to this clinical problem.

REFERENCES

Jaffe DM, Tanz RR, Davis AT, Henretig F, Fleisher G: Antibiotic administration to treat possible occult bacteremia in febrile children. N Engl J Med 317:1175–1180, 1987.

Kaplan SL: Recent advances in bacterial meningitis. Adv Pediatr Infect Dis 4:83–110, 1989.

Klein JO, Feigin RD, McCracken GH Jr: Report of the task force on diagnosis and management of meningitis. Pediatrics 78 (Suppl):959–982, 1986.

STAPHYLOCOCCAL INFECTIONS

JAMES K. TODD, M.D.

Staphylococci cause a wide variety of infections ranging from furunculosis to toxic shock syndrome. Successful therapy depends on the proper choice of antibiotics as well as secondary treatments appropriate to the varying modes of pathogenesis.

ANTIBIOTIC FACTORS

Table 1 lists the antibiotics frequently used or recommended for treatment of staphylococcal infections. It is generally accepted that the tetracyclines, chloramphenicol, and the sulfonamides—as well as the penicillinase-susceptible penicillins (e.g., penicillin, ampicillin, amoxicillin)—usually are not satisfactory for the treatment of beta-lactamase–producing staphylococci. In general, the penicillinase-resistant penicillins (e.g., nafcillin, oxacillin, dicloxacillin) or first- or second-generation cephalosporins (e.g., cefazolin, cephalexin, cephradine) are considered drugs of choice. The third-generation cepalosporins (e.g., cefotaxime, ceftriaxone) are not recommended for treatment of severe *Staphylococcus aureus* infections. Some strains of *S. aureus* (the so-called MRSA [methicillin-resistant *S. aureus*]) and many strains of coagulase-negative *Staphylococcus* (e.g., *S. epidermidis*) are resistant to the penicillinase-resistant penicillins and cephalosporins. Most remain susceptible to vancomycin. Many *S. aureus* strains may be effectively treated with clindamycin or erythromycin, and many coagulase-negative staphylococci are susceptible to rifampin, which should be used only in combination with a second drug. *For some superficial infections, topical therapy with mupirocin may be effective but this should never be used alone in patients with deep infections or those with systemic manifestations.* Selection of appropriate therapy depends on the in vitro susceptibility of the organism as well as considerations of the severity of illness, route of administration, potential side effects, tolerance of the patient, and the relative costs.

Current evidence suggests that, in proper dosage, the penicillinase-resistant penicillins are equivalent in therapeutic efficacy in spite of quite divergent levels of protein binding. The cephalosporins are less likely than the true penicillins to cause acute, severe hypersensitivity reactions (e.g., anaphylaxis) in penicillin-allergic patients. Primary cephalosporin hypersensitivity also is known to occur. Although methicillin has been implicated most commonly in causing a drug-related reversible nephritis, many other penicillins and cephalosporins have been reported to do likewise.

In extremely serious infections caused by *S. aureus*, additional therapeutic considerations may be indicated. Meningitis secondary to *Staphylococcus* is rare in absence of an indwelling foreign body but may be refractory to therapy. The penetration of the cephalosporins into the cerebrospinal fluid (CSF) is limited. In general, the penicillinase-resistant penicillins are preferred for treating staphylococcal infections of the central nervous system (CNS) if the organisms are demonstrated to be susceptible in vitro.

Patients with *S. aureus* sepsis and a refractory focus may remain bacteremic in spite of antibiotics. Drainage or removal of sequestered foci may be instrumental in curing such infections. The use of a penicillinase-resistant penicillin plus an aminoglycoside (and/or rifampin) may demonstrate a synergistic or additive combination antibiotic effect in vitro and may be useful in selected patients.

In summary, the choice of a primary agent to treat staphylococcal infections depends very much on personal preference and experience. As always, careful monitoring for therapeutic efficacy and side effects is imperative.

TREATMENT

Route and Duration of Therapy

Route of Administration

Oral antistaphylococcal agents can be selected for primary therapy of minor infections unlikely to be associated with bacteremia. Children with infections potentially accompanied by positive blood cultures should be treated by the parenteral route initially until all signs and symptoms have abated (afebrile, normalized leukocyte count, decreased erythrocyte sedimentation rate, resolved local signs). *One of the most exciting improvements in the therapy for serious staphylococcal infections relates to the accumulation of evidence that parenteral therapy may be replaced by oral therapy after documented clinical improvement of the patient, assuming that proper attention is paid to the details of transition.* Critical to the substitution of oral therapy is (1) a knowledge of the in vitro susceptibility of the causative organism, (2) the availability of an appropriate oral agent that can give blood levels comparable to those being achieved parenterally, (3) assurance of compliance with the drug administration schedule, and (4) ultimate documentation that the oral levels actually being achieved (as measured by the serum

TABLE 1. Antibiotics Used for Staphylococcal Infections

Antibiotic	Indications: Severity of Infection (Major)	Indications: Severity of Infection (Minor)	Route of Administration	Dosage (mg/kg/day): Age (<1 Month)‡	Dosage (mg/kg/day): Age (>1 Month)	Adult Daily Maximum (g)	Relative Toxicity
Oxacillin	+	+	IV, p.o.	50–150	50–200	12	+
Nafcillin	+	−	IV	50–150	50–200	12	+
Dicloxacillin	(+)*	+	p.o.	NR	25–100	6	+
Cefazolin	+	−	IV	NR	50–150	6	+
Cephradine	(+)*	+	IV, p.o.	NR	50–150	8	+
Cephalexin	(+)*	+	p.o.	NR	25–100	6	+
Vancomycin	+	−	IV	20–30	40	2	+ + +
Erythromycin	−	+	p.o.	20–30	30–50	4	+
Clindamycin	+	+	IV, p.o.	10–20	20–40	4.8	+ +
Gentamicin (tobramycin)	(+)†	−	IV, IM	4–7.5	3–7.5	300 mg	+ +
Rifampin	(+)†	−	p.o.	NR	10–20	600 mg	+ +

*After initial control with parenteral antibiotic.
†Always use in combination with another antistaphylococcal antibiotic.
‡May require modification of dose or frequency in premature infants and newborns younger than 7 days of age.
Abbreviations: NR, not recommended; p.o., by mouth; IV, intravenous; IM, intramuscular.

bactericidal assay) are comparable with those achieved parenterally against the patient's own organism (see Monitoring Therapy). It should be remembered that higher-than-usual doses of oral antibiotics will sometimes be required to achieve levels similar to those being produced parenterally. Oral dosages approaching 50 to 100 mg/kg/day of oral cephalosporin or penicillinase-resistant penicillin should be used initially and the frequency of administration be maintained on a 6-hour schedule. At present, there is little evidence to support the use of oral therapy in treating CNS or heart infections.

Duration of Therapy

Duration of treatment of staphylococcal infections is a matter of opinion rather than fact. Superficial infections may be treated for 7 to 10 days, whereas more severe involvement seems to require longer therapy. A practical rule is to treat serious infections at least 2 weeks beyond all clinical signs of infection (fever, local signs, positive blood culture) and at least 3 weeks overall.

Chronic infections (especially chronic osteomyelitis) may necessitate months of appropriate treatment, since the healing process and penetration of antibiotics to the site of infection may not be as efficient as in acute infection.

Occasionally, staphylococcal infections have been noted to continue to persist (or drain) in spite of long-term penicillin or cephalosporin treatment. Empiric therapy with clindamycin (which has a different method of action) has been successful in some of these refractory infections, which presumably are related to cell wall–deficient bacterial variants acting as "persisters."

Surgical Therapy

Because of the great propensity of *S. aureus* to form abscesses, it is recommended that these be surgically drained, whenever possible, to hasten recovery. A patient with documented bacteremia or a deep focus of infection may have other subclinical foci that cannot always be cured by antibiotics alone. Patients with proven *S. aureus* bacteremia who do not become afebrile within 48 to 72 hours of appropriate antimicrobial therapy, or who remain bacteremic, should be investigated thoroughly for other foci. The gallium scan has proved to be a very effective means of identifying occult foci that may benefit from drainage procedures. Prospective surgical drainage may result in shorter hospitalization as symptoms (fever, toxicity) are alleviated.

Perhaps the most dramatic recoveries will be seen in infections caused by staphylococci related to indwelling vascular lines. Any patient with a documented staphylococcal bacteremia should be examined thoroughly for the presence of such foreign bodies. Although high-dose antimicrobial therapy might control the infection, it rarely cures it without removing the focus of infection. *Central venous lines are especially dangerous because of the additional risk of development of a right-sided endocarditis.*

Similarly, staphylococcal infections involving prostheses, such as ventriculoperitoneal or ventriculoatrial shunts, are best treated by removal of the offending foreign body. Intensive antibiotic therapy may cure 5 to 30 per cent of these infections, whereas early removal results in total cure and allows for early replacement of a sterile shunt. If prosthetic devices of critical physiologic importance or major surgical complexity are involved (e.g., prosthetic heart valves, orthopedic devices), intensive antibiotic therapy may be attempted; duration of therapy, however, must be prolonged, and the persistence of symptoms ultimately may necessitate replacement of the foreign body in the case of heart valves or prolonged drainage in the case of orthopedic devices. In these cases, the addition of clindamycin for 10 days at the end of therapy may be helpful.

Monitoring Therapy

The final proof of therapeutic success is the continued absence of signs and symptoms in the absence of antibiotic therapy. In vitro susceptibility does not invariably guarantee therapeutic success, especially if a foreign body, abscess, or host deficiency state exists. Minimum inhibitory concentrations and minimum bactericidal concentrations should be ascertained in refractory cases.

The serum bactericidal assay (serum killing power) can be used to assess the adequacy of blood levels being achieved against the patient's own organism. Adequate antibiotic therapy appears to be present when the nadir (low point) level is at least 1 to 8 (or the blood antibiotic level is eight times the minimum inhibitory concentration of the patient's organism). If oral therapy is chosen after a period of parenteral antibiotic administration, the serum bactericidal assay after an oral dose is compared with an assay after a parenteral dose. If levels are equivalent in a patient already documented to be improving, continued improvement may be expected, assuming good compliance with the prescribed oral regimen and close clinical follow-up.

Clinical Infections (Table 2)

General Culture Procedures

S. aureus and *S. epidermidis* are components of the normal flora of the nasopharynx, throat, skin, and genital tract. Cultures of these permissive sites, when positive, reflect colonization but not necessarily infection. In general, cultures of ordinary sterile body sites—blood, CSF, middle ear, sinus, lymph node, lung tissue, or abscess aspirate—should take precedence.

Central Nervous System

Meningitis and Brain Abscess. *S. aureus* meningitis or brain abscess is a rare occurrence except after penetrating head injury. Penicillinase-resistant penicillins are preferred in treatment.

Ventriculitis. Shunt or vascular device infections with coagulase-negative staphylococci are optimally treated with vancomycin and rifampin, followed by removal of the shunt and parenteral treatment with high doses of appropriate antibiotics, depending on the in vitro susceptibility results. The shunt usually can be replaced safely whenever evidence of increased intracranial pressure becomes manifest. It is not advisable to try to "sterilize" an infected device in situ with intraventricular and parenteral antibiotics, as the foreign body seems to protect the organism from complete killing and the majority of patients will still require eventual shunt replacement.

Upper Respiratory Tract Infections

Mastoiditis. Acute mastoiditis should be treated like osteomyelitis (see below).

Otitis Media. Acute or chronic staphylococcal otitis media usually is accompanied by a perforated tympanic membrane. Oral antistaphylococcal agents and facilitated drainage of the ear (cotton wick externally) are recommended.

Sinusitis. Chronic sinusitis may be caused by *S. aureus* and can be treated with oral antistaphylococcal agents. Surgical drainage may be necessary when topically applied decongestant cannot promote drainage of the affected sinus.

Peritonsillar Abscess. Peritonsillar abscesses are often caused by *S. aureus*. Parenteral therapy is indicated, and drainage is a priority if the area is palpably fluctuant.

Cervical Lymphadenitis. Cervical lymphadenitis caused by *S. aureus* is usually unilateral, occurs in younger children, and is less frequent than that caused by group A streptococcus. Initially, in cases of unilateral lymphadenitis, specimens from the throat, and possibly the nose, are obtained for culture to incriminate the group A streptococcus; penicillin or erythromycin is given. If patients fail to respond, a needle aspirate of the node can be performed for culture and oral antistaphylococcal therapy is begun. Even if a staphylococcal etiology is documented and focal inflammation is controlled, fever may continue until several days to weeks later, when the node becomes fluctuant and requires drainage. There is very little evidence that acute pharyngitis is caused by *S. aureus*. Isolation of this organism from the throats of symptomatic children *is not* an indication for therapy.

Pulmonary Infections

Staphylococcal pneumonia and empyema seem to occur less frequently than in the past but are still causes of morbidity in newborns and malnourished children. Diagnosis can be made only by a lung, direct tracheal, or pleural aspirate or positive blood culture; nasopharyngeal, throat, or "sputum" cultures are not reliable in diagnosis. High-dose parenteral antibiotic therapy is indicated in staphylococcal pneumonia. Chest tubes are certainly indicated if the patient deteriorates rapidly secondary to a pyopneumothorax, which can be life-threatening. A diagnostic thoracocentesis is always indicated before therapy, and as much fluid as possible should be removed. Chest tube drainage is indicated if the fluid reaccumulates or causes significant distortion of the lung and interferes with

TABLE 2. Treatment of Clinical Staphylococcal Infections

Infection	Etiologic Agent	Initial Antibiotic Route	Additional Therapy
Meningitis	*Staphylococcus aureus*	IV	
Brain abscess	*Staphylococcus aureus*	IV	Surgical drainage
Ventriculitis (shunt)	Coagulase-negative staphylococcus	IV	Shunt removal
Mastoiditis	*Staphylococcus aureus*	IV → p.o.	Drainage if no improvement in 72 hours
Otitis media	*Staphylococcus aureus*	p.o.	Promotion of drainage
Sinusitis	*Staphylococcus aureus*	p.o.	Medical/surgical drainage
Peritonsillar abscess (cellulitis)	*Staphylococcus aureus*	IV → p.o.	Drainage if infection fluctuant
Cervical lymphadenitis	*Staphylococcus aureus*	p.o.	Drainage if infection fluctuant
Pneumonia-empyema	*Staphylococcus aureus*	IV	Chest tubes as needed
Endocarditis	*Staphylococcus aureus*	IV	Valve removal if poor patient response
	Staphylococcus aureus	None	Fluids
Urinary tract infection	Coagulase-negative staphylococcus	p.o.	
Osteomyelitis	*Staphylococcus aureus*	IV → p.o.	Drainage if infection not improved in 72 hours
Arthritis	*Staphylococcus aureus*	IV → p.o.	Surgical drainage
Furunculosis	*Staphylococcus aureus*	p.o.	
Abscess	*Staphylococcus aureus*	IV → p.o.	Surgical drainage
Cellulitis	*Staphylococcus aureus*	p.o.	
Scalded skin syndrome	*Staphylococcus aureus*	p.o.	
Toxic shock syndrome	*Staphylococcus aureus*	IV	Intensive support; drainage of focus
Bacteremia	*Staphylococcus aureus*	IV	
Septicemia	*Staphylococcus aureus*	IV	Gallium scan and appropriate drainage
Phlebitis	Coagulase-negative staphylococcus	IV	Line(s) removal

ventilation. It usually is not possible to remove all of the pleural fluid. With adequate antibiotics and time, however, the chest generally heals and returns to a normal radiologic appearance and pulmonary functioning, even though convalescence may be prolonged.

Cardiac Infections

Staphylococcal endocarditis occurs in patients abusing intravenous drugs, those with prosthetic heart valves, and occasionally in children with congenital heart disease. High-dose, long-term parenteral antibiotics are indicated; sometimes the potentially additive combination of a penicillinase-resistant penicillin and aminoglycoside may be useful. Removal of infected tissue (valve prosthesis) may be indicated for severe embolic episodes, refractory congestive heart failure, or persistent bacteremia.

Urinary Tract Infections

Urinary tract infections caused by coagulase-negative staphylococci are increasingly more common. Oral therapy is effective, but a thorough urinary tract evaluation should be completed in boys to discover urologic abnormalities that might require surgery.

Bone and Joint Infections

Osteomyelitis. Children with acute osteomyelitis should undergo a diagnostic needle aspirate of the bone on admission. If purulent material is present or the cortex is destroyed or if the patient fails to respond in 48 to 72 hours, surgical drainage is indicated. There is little evidence that antibiotic irrigants are necessary or effective after appropriate drainage procedures. After control of the symptoms and inflammation with parenteral staphylococcal therapy, oral therapy has proved quite successful in completing at least 3 weeks of total treatment as long as comparable serum levels are achieved. In the case of chronic osteomyelitis, more extensive surgery and a much longer period of oral antibiotic therapy may be required.

Arthritis. Septic arthritis may accompany osteomyelitis or occur separately. Surgical drainage of critical joints (hip) is recommended and may hasten recovery of others also. Again, oral therapy can be considered once all symptoms and signs of inflammation are controlled.

Skin Infections

Furunculosis. Recurrent furunculosis is a common problem caused by *S. aureus,* and although oral therapy and local drainage result in rapid healing of the lesions, new lesions may appear after the discontinuation of antibiotic therapy. Most patients with recurrent furunculosis do not have any glaring host defense deficiencies and do not seem to have trouble with systemic infection or other organisms. Often, recurrences are related to continued colonization with a particularly virulent strain of *Staphylococcus.* This colonization may be controlled by using hexachlorophene soaps and by early treatment of new lesions. Some patients will demonstrate an increased gamma E immunoglobulin (IgE) and abnormalities of chemotaxis.

Subcutaneous Abscess. Deep soft tissue abscesses (carbuncles) usually require surgical drainage as well as oral therapy.

Cellulitis. Cellulitis may be caused by *S. aureus* and is often indistinguishable from that caused by group A streptococcus. Usually, an entry wound is apparent, although it may appear to be minor. Human bite wounds may be a source of local staphylococcal infections. Needle aspiration should be performed and specimens from the wound should be obtained for culture if purulent material is present. Oral antibiotic therapy is usually sufficient, although toxic-appearing patients should be treated with parenteral therapy until blood cultures are negative.

Scalded Skin Syndrome. The scalded skin syndrome (*toxic epidermal necrolysis*) is a spectrum of exanthematous manifestations of a toxin produced by phage group II staphylococci. These organisms may not actually be invading the host; more often, they are colonizing the nasopharynx and allowing systemic absorption of the toxin, which causes injury to the granular cell layer of the skin. This results in a painful erythema that may go no further than a scarlet fever–like illness but also may progress to the formation of bullous lesions. Ritter syndrome, bullous varicella, bullous impetigo, Lyell syndrome, and toxic epidermal necrolysis all fall into this latter category. The toxic effect is self-limited and rarely serious, although there may be extensive skin involvement. Disseminated staphylococcal disease, which may develop in newborns with Ritter syndrome, should be treated with parenteral antistaphylococcal therapy. Older children seem to suffer only from the toxemia, and there is no conclusive evidence that antistaphylococcal agents alter the course of the illness once the rash is fully developed. Nonetheless, it is recommended that oral therapy be used to prevent the spread of these toxigenic strains. Local skin therapy is often overdone. Most of these children are at little risk for secondary infection, as the basal layers of the skin are still intact. Adequate fluid support and oral antibiotics are usually all that are indicated, although patients should be reassured that the acute appearance of the exanthem does not necessarily imply significant scarring as long as secondary infection does not occur.

Toxic Shock Syndrome. This infection has recently been described and is related to a newly recognized toxin produced by certain *S. aureus* strains. It is seen primarily in older children who present with pharyngitis, fever, watery diarrhea, myalgia, hyperemic conjunctiva, and a diffuse scarlatiniform erythroderma. The condition may progress rapidly to include a high-output shock with capillary leakage of fluid, renal failure, disseminated intravascular coagulation, liver function abnormalities, and shock lung. Blood cultures are often negative, and this severe illness has been attributed to the release of a toxin from a colonized or locally infected site. Intensive supportive therapy is indicated, with major efforts at maintaining blood pressure. Parenteral antistaphylococcal antibiotics are used along with drainage of the infected focus. In severe cases, parenteral corticosteroids and/or intravenous immunoglobulin may be effective. Recovery is accompanied by a marked desquamation of the palms and soles.

Systemic Infections

Bacteremia. Many of the focal infections already described may be accompanied by bacteremia.

Disseminated Staphylococcal Septicemia. This infection has recently increased in frequency, especially in older children, and is characterized by a high-level staphylococcal bacteremia associated with multiple foci of sequestered infections, including the lung, heart, bone and joints, skin, CNS, and kidney. Any child with documented staphylococcal bacteremia and an obvious focus of infection who does not become afebrile within 48 to 72 hours on appropriate antistaphylococcal therapy should be thoroughly investigated for other foci. A chest film is indicated to look for evidence of pulmonary emboli or infection, and a gallium scan has been very useful in identifying other soft tissue or sequestered foci. These children may be critically ill, and thorough drainage of all foci may be required before the septicemia can be controlled.

Phlebitis. Vascular infections associated with bacteremia may be caused by either coagulase-negative staphylococcus or *S. aureus* and usually are related to an indwelling vascular catheter. Once infection is documented, most vascular lines should be removed and systemic antibiotic therapy should be instituted until all signs of infection are abated. It sometimes may be possible to sterilize such an infection, leaving the foreign body in place; however, this should not be attempted in patients with signs of systemic illness. Routine culture of catheter tips is not useful.

Neonatal Staphylococcal Infections

With the decrease in routine usage of hexachlorophene in newborn nurseries, there has been an associated resurgence of staphylococcal nosocomial infections. Newborns in intensive care nurseries are at highest risk owing to poor nutrition, indwelling vascular lines, and abnormalities of lung and skin. Nonetheless, colonization may occur in normal newborns in the nursery and focal or systemic staphylococcal infection may develop any time after hospital discharge. It is critical that all neonatal units specify an infection control coordinator and that all physicians taking care of children initially hospitalized in that unit notify the coordinator if a staphylococcal or other infection is documented within the first month of life. Routine screening cultures of newborns being discharged from such units usually are not productive unless evidence of an increased incidence of actual staphylococcal infection is reported. Some staphylococci are relatively benign, and a high level of colonization will not be accompanied by an increased frequency of actual infection. On the other hand, virulent strains of *Staphylococcus* may become established in a nursery unit and can cause frequent staphylococcal infections in spite of a low rate of colonization. Routine screening of hospital personnel is not recommended unless there is evidence of a definite outbreak caused by a single strain. Because colonies of staphylococci are often similar in appearance, even though they may be of differing phage types, it is important to save organisms thought to be associated with an outbreak of staphylococcal infection so that microbial typing can be pursued to confirm a common etiology.

Once a true outbreak of infection rather than colonization is confirmed, the nursery should be placed on a strict cohort system, with strong emphasis on gowning and strict hand washing before the handling of any infant. Bathing with hexachlorophene may be instituted as long as care is taken to rinse infants well after bathing. Premature infants may be at greater risk for hexachlorophene toxicity if they are bathed frequently. The application of triple dye or an iodophor in alcoholic solution or other topical antistaphylococcal agent to the cord area may be effective in reducing colonization and subsequent infection. The use of topical antibiotic gels to the cord area tends to promote a moist medium for secondary colonization and infection and, therefore, should not be a primary method for controlling an outbreak. All newborns with proven infection should be isolated separately, gown and glove precautions should be taken, and personnel with proven active infection (as distinguished from colonization) should be excluded from contact with the patients.

REFERENCES

Christensen GD: The confusing and tenacious coagulase-negative staphylococci. Adv Intern Med 32:177, 1987.

Craven DE, Reed C, Kollisch N, et al: A large outbreak of infections caused by a strain of *Staphylococcus aureus* resistant to oxacillin and aminoglycosides. Am J Med 71:53, 1981.

Flynn PM, Shenep JL, Stokes DC, Barrett FF: In situ management of confirmed central venous catheter–related bacteremia. Pediatr Infect Dis 6:729, 1987.

Haley RW, Hightower AW, Khabbaz RF, et al: The emergence of methicillin-resistant *Staphylococcus aureus* infections in United States hospitals. Ann Intern Med 97:297, 1982.

Righter J: Treatment of coagulase-negative staphylococcal infections: Dilemmas for laboratory and clinician. J Antimicrobial Chemother 20:459, 1987.

Sabath LD: Mechanisms of resistance to beta-lactam antibiotics in strains of *Staphylococcus aureus*. Ann Intern Med 97:339, 1982.

Sheagren JN: *Staphylococcus aureus:* The persistent pathogen. N Engl J Med 310:1368, 1984.

Todd JK: Toxic shock syndrome. Clin Microbiol Rev 1:432, 1988.

GROUP A STREPTOCOCCAL INFECTIONS

MICHAEL RADETSKY, M.D., C.M.

Group A beta-hemolytic streptococcus *(Streptococcus pyogenes)* is the most frequent cause of acute bacterial pharyngitis, the antecedent event to acute rheumatic fever. It also causes a spectrum of cutaneous infections, may spread to the lungs and other deep organs, and may lead to acute poststreptococcal glomerulonephritis. *Severe invasive streptococcal syndrome,* a newly described systemic illness of high mortality, is the most recent manifestation of this highly pathogenic organism.

MICROBIOLOGIC PROPERTIES

Group A streptococci are Gram-stain–positive cocci that grow as pairs or short to moderate chains on 5 per cent sheep blood agar plates. Organism recovery is enhanced when the medium contains trimethoprim-sulfamethoxazole to suppress the growth of normal oral flora. Colonies are 1 to 2 mm in diameter and are surrounded by comparatively large zones of complete (beta) hemolysis. Strains that produce abundant hyaluronic acid capsules appear mucoid. Organism virulence depends on the presence of the antiphagocytic M-protein cell wall antigen, which also forms the basis for classification into more than 80 different serotypes.

Numerous extracellular products are produced by group A streptococci. Streptolysins O (oxygen-labile) and S (oxygen-stable) damage cell membranes and are hemolytic. Enzymes that degrade DNA (DNases A, B, C, D), hyaluronidase, streptokinase, and various proteases are spreading factors that facilitate the rapid propagation of organisms through tissue planes. Antibody to streptolysin O (ASO), DNase B (ADB), and multiple antigenic determinants (Streptozyme) are the marker serologies for recent (but not acute) streptococcal infection. Pyogenic exotoxins A, B, C, formerly called "scarlet fever erythrogenic toxins," not only produce rashes but also are pyogenic, cytotoxic, mitogenic, and immunosuppressive. Pyogenic exotoxins have been implicated in the severe invasive streptococcal syndrome.

STREPTOCOCCAL PHARYNGITIS

Epidemiology

Streptococcal pharyngitis is a common infection of children and young adults. Serogroup A causes virtually all these episodes. Serogroup C, and perhaps G, may cause episodic pharyngitis in college-aged adolescents, but only rarely, if ever, in younger children. Pharyngitis, with or without uvular or palatal involvement, occurs in children at any age, including those younger than 3 years. The infection is spread by direct contact via either saliva or droplets, but food or water-borne outbreaks are well described. Acutely infected individuals readily transmit virulent M-protein positive organisms. Even without therapy, the numbers of streptococci, the M-protein content, and the risk of transmissibility decline with time. An asymptomatic carrier state exists, which at times may represent 5 to 15 per cent of school-aged children.

Clinical Manifestations

The prototype case of streptococcal pharyngitis begins 2 to 4 days after exposure with a sore throat, an abrupt fever, headache, and malaise. Vomiting and abdominal pain also occur. Physical findings include erythema and edema of the pharynx, exudative tonsillitis, characteristic (though infrequent) palatal petechiae, and tender, enlarged, symmetric anterior cervical lymph nodes. In the absence of fever and pharyngitis, group A streptococci are rarely found.

This "classic" presentation occurs only in the minority of cases, since the clinical spectrum of streptococcal pharyngitis is wide. Mini-symptomatic or asymptomatic infections occur and may induce subsequent seroconversion. In fact, one third to two thirds of cases of acute rheumatic fever victims have no clear-cut memory of a preceding sore throat. The manifestations of streptococcal infection are more mild in infants and in individuals with prior tonsillectomies.

Complications

Peritonsillar cellulitis, peritonsillar abscess, and retropharyngeal abscesses all may contain group A streptococci but usually contain mixed oral flora as well. Pharyngeal streptococci may occasionally participate in infections of adjacent structures, such as the sinuses, the preseptal orbital tissues, and the middle ear.

Acute rheumatic fever (ARF) and acute poststreptococcal glomerulonephritis (AGN) are the nonsuppurative complications of streptococcal pharyngitis. Appropriate antimicrobial therapy within 7 to 9 days of the onset of illness will reduce the subsequent risk of ARF by 90 per cent. The risk of AGN, however, is not altered by the use of antimicrobials.

Diagnosis

A diagnostic strategy for streptococcal pharyngitis relies on certain established principles:

1. The basic purpose of diagnostic streptococcal testing is to prevent ARF.
2. The major risk factor for ARF is a personal or family history of prior ARF.
3. The general incidence of ARF in the United States is low, but rheumatogenic M-protein serotypes cause local epidemic disease.
4. Prompt treatment of streptococcal pharyngitis with antimicrobials is most likely to meaningfully accelerate patient recovery in severe clinical disease.
5. The contagious spread of streptococci is ablated with 24 hours of antimicrobial therapy.
6. The carrier rate of streptococci may be high, especially among school-aged children.
7. The clinical assessment of acute pharyngitis can predict the absence of group A streptococci with accuracy (negative predictive value of 97 per cent) but cannot reliably predict its presence (positive predictive value of 36 per cent at a prevalence of 15 per cent).
8. The throat culture remains the gold standard for streptococcal detection.
9. Rapid streptococcal test kits are accurate when positive but may be falsely negative up to 40 per cent of the time.

Therapy

Penicillin is the drug of choice for confirmed streptococcal pharyngitis. Intramuscular benzathine penicillin G may be given in a single dose of 600,000 units for patients weighing less than 60 pounds and 1,200,000 units for patients greater than 60 pounds. Alternatively, oral penicillin V may be used in a dose of 250 mg three times daily for 10 days. Less frequent dosing intervals or a shorter duration of therapy has not been validated for the prevention of ARF.

For penicillin-allergic patients, erythromycin estolate (20 to 40 mg/kg/day) or erythromycin ethyl succinate (40 mg/kg/day) divided into three to four doses should be given for 10 days with a maximum total daily dose of 1 g. Trimethoprim-sulfamethoxazole, sulfonamides, and tetracyclines do not cure streptococcal pharyngitis. Symptomatic relief can be provided with acetaminophen (10 to 15 mg/kg per dose every 3 to 4 hours), salt-water gargles, hard candy, popsicles, and fluids.

Follow-up

If the acute illness resolves, a second culture of the throat is not recommended. Five to 30 per cent of patients will have pharyngeal group A streptococci cultured after proper therapy, but the risk of ARF in these patients and the protective efficacy of re-treatment are not known and are thought to be small in normal individuals. Only if the patient has a history of ARF, if an outbreak of ARF is occurring, or if symptoms persist or recur should there be a second throat culture. If streptococci are found, a single re-treatment course with penicillin should be given without a subsequent second culture. In exposed families, the only members who require throat cultures are those who are symptomatic and those with a history of ARF.

Prevention of Recurrent Acute Rheumatic Fever

Individuals who have already experienced one episode of ARF are at high risk for recurrent attacks. Recurrences may occur after asymptomatic infection. Prevention of further attacks depends on a policy of continuous antimicrobial prophylaxis ("secondary prevention"). The standard choice for this purpose is benzathine penicillin (1,200,000 units intramuscularly at 4-week intervals). However, because of the declining serum drug levels toward the end of the dosing interval, experts now recommend that this schedule be shortened to dosing every 3 weeks in areas where the risk for ARF is high. Oral penicillin V (250 mg twice daily) or sulfadiazine (0.5 g once daily for patients under 60 pounds and 1.0 g once daily for patients over 60 pounds), is the recommended oral drug for this purpose.

STREPTOCOCCAL PYODERMA

Inadvertent intradermal inoculation of colonizing group A streptococci and direct finger inoculation of sores, bites, or abrasions are the antecedents for streptococcal pyoderma. Depending on the depth of the skin involvement, the infection may produce clinical impetigo, ecthyma, erysipelas, cellulitis, fasciitis, or a mixture of clinical types. For unexplained reasons, ARF does not occur after streptococcal pyoderma. However, skin infections with nephritogenic strains do cause acute glomerulonephritis regardless of antimicrobial therapy. *S. aureus* may coinfect streptococcal pyoderma or may be the primary infecting organism. In one recent culture survey, 60 per cent of acute impetigo cases were due solely to *S. aureus*.

Therapy

Antimicrobial therapy for culture-proven group A streptococcal pyoderma is penicillin. However, if a site culture is not definitive, then antimicrobials suitable for both *S. aureus* and group A streptococcus must be chosen. Since cephalexin has recently become a generic drug, it has emerged as the oral antimicrobial of choice for the ambulatory therapy of pyoderma because of its pleasing taste, its gastric tolerance, its price, and its suitable spectrum. For impetigo, topical mupirocin has also proved effective.

SEVERE INVASIVE STREPTOCOCCAL SYNDROME

This recently described syndrome has now been seen both sporadically and in clusters throughout the United States. Reported mortality has been as high as 30 per cent. The causative agent is a pyrogenic exotoxin–producing group A streptococcus. Generally, the afflicted individual has no predisposing factor, and either a focal, suppurative streptococcal infection of the soft tissues or lung (65 per cent) or streptococcal bacteremia without a focus (35 per cent) develops. Secondarily infected varicella is one common setting for this sequence. The disease evolves rapidly with fever, systemic toxicity, shock, and multiple organ failure.

Therapy

Successful therapy consists of early recognition, intravenous penicillin (300,000 units/kg/day divided every 4 hours) and full critical care support commensurate with the degree of illness. Surgical débridement of suppurative soft tissue foci is recommended when possible.

GROUP B STREPTOCOCCAL INFECTIONS

CAROL J. BAKER, M.D.
and MORVEN S. EDWARDS, M.D.

Therapy for group B streptococcal (GBS) infections is based on the tenet that bacteremia is the initial event in the pathogenesis either of early-onset or late-onset infection. With early-onset disease, the risk for penetration of mucous membrane barriers and subsequent bacteremia correlates with the magnitude of the maternal genital inoculum. Unless specifically excluded by lumbar puncture results, spread to the meninges must be assumed when antimicrobial therapy is initiated. Documented meningeal involvement occurs in 30 per cent of early-onset and 60 per cent of late-onset infections and influences the dose and duration of therapy as well as other aspects of supportive management.

TREATMENT

Empiric Therapy

In the usual setting, antimicrobial therapy for infection due to GBS must be initiated while culture results are pending. Initial therapy generally consists of intravenous ampicillin and an aminoglycoside for the treatment of this as well as other neonatal pathogens (Table 1). Irrespective of birth weight, infants with suspected or proven meningitis and those in whom the clinical condition will not permit lumbar puncture should receive ampicillin (300 mg/kg/day) in combination with an aminoglycoside, usually gentamicin. This combination is more effective than ampicillin or penicillin G alone in the in vitro and in vivo killing of most GBS strains.

Specific Therapy

Penicillin G remains the drug of choice for the treatment of infections caused by GBS, since susceptibility to this agent is uniform. Once GBS has been identified and its penicillin susceptibility verified, penicillin G or ampicillin alone is sufficient for the treatment of these infections. The optimal dose and duration of therapy are dictated by the focus and severity of infection, since most reported relapses of infection can be attributed to inadequate dosage or length of therapy. Other facts important when considering appropriate dose are the following:

TABLE 1. Antibiotic Therapy for Neonatal Group B Streptococcal Infections

Type of Infection	Antibiotic (Dose)	Duration
Suspected meningitis (initial empiric therapy)	Ampicillin (300 mg/kg/day) *plus* Gentamicin (5–7 mg/kg/day)*	Until cerebrospinal fluid sterility *and* penicillin susceptibility documented
Suspected sepsis† (initial empiric therapy)	Ampicillin (150 mg/kg/day) *plus* Gentamicin (5–7 mg/kg/day)*	Until blood stream sterility documented
Bacteremia	Ampicillin (150 mg/kg/day) *or* Penicillin G (200,000 units/kg/day)	10 days
Meningitis	Penicillin G (400,000–500,000 units/kg/day)	14 days minimum
Arthritis	Penicillin G (200,000–300,000 units/kg/day)	2 to 3 weeks
Osteomyelitis	Penicillin G (200,000–300,000 units/kg/day)	3 to 4 weeks
Endocarditis	Penicillin G (200,000–300,000 units/kg/day)	4 weeks

*Monitor serum concentration to maintain a peak level of 5 to 10 μg/ml and a trough of less than 2 μg/ml.

†Assumes lumbar puncture to exclude meningitis has been performed and that cerebrospinal fluid has no detectable abnormalities.

1. The minimal inhibitory concentration (MIC) of GBS to penicillin G is approximately tenfold greater than that of group A streptococci.
2. The amount of penicillin G achievable in the cerebrospinal fluid (CSF) is at best 10 to 20 per cent of serum levels.
3. The inoculum of GBS in the CSF of infants with meningitis is often high (10^7 to 10^8).
4. High doses of penicillin G and ampicillin are safe in the newborn. Therefore, to ensure rapid bacterial killing, especially in patients with meningitis, relatively high doses of penicillin G or ampicillin are recommended for both early-onset and late-onset infections.

Once CSF sterility is documented in infants with meningitis (usually within 36 hours of therapy) *and* susceptibility to penicillin G is verified, penicillin G alone (400,000 to 500,000 units/kg/day) is given (Table 1). Intravenous therapy should be continued for a minimum of 14 days, longer if the course is particularly severe, if the infant has concomitant ventriculitis, or if there is delayed sterilization of the CSF. In the last circumstance, the presence of an unsuspected suppurative focus (subdural empyema, brain abscess, obstructive ventriculitis, or septic thrombophlebitis) should be suspected and excluded by appropriate studies. At the completion of therapy, a second lumbar puncture should be done to determine whether the CSF findings are consistent with adequate therapy or suggest the need for additional treatment. Examples of the latter include polymorphonuclear cells in excess of 20 per cent of the total cells or a protein level in excess of 150 to 200 mg/dl. These findings may occur in infants with severe cerebritis, extensive parenchymal destruction with focal suppuration, severe vasculitis, or a combination of these.

Infants with bacteremia *without* meningitis should receive intravenous ampicillin or penicillin G for 10 days (Table 1). A shorter duration of therapy has no documented efficacy, and relapses, although rare, have been reported under these circumstances. Patients with septic arthritis, osteomyelitis, or endocarditis should be treated with intravenous penicillin G for 2 to 3 weeks (arthritis), 3 to 4 weeks (osteomyelitis), and 4 weeks (endocarditis) (Table 1). Oral therapy has no place in the management of infants with GBS infections. Alternative agents, such as the cephalosporins and vancomycin, are active against GBS in vitro, but their efficacy is unknown and they are not recommended in the usual clinical situation.

When suppurative foci occur, they should be drained. For septic arthritis, involvement of the hip, and often the shoulder, dictates open surgical drainage. For other joints, needle aspiration on one or two occasions usually achieves adequate drainage. For osteomyelitis, open curettage of necrotic metaphyseal bone is required in most patients, and in all cases diagnostic needle aspiration of the involved metaphyseal area should be performed to determine the etiologic agent *before* or within 24 hours of the initiation of antibiotic therapy. In the infant younger than 2 months of age who presents with an indolent course, pseudoparalysis of an arm, and a metaphyseal lytic lesion, the propensity of GBS for the humerus, especially the proximal end, is an important clue that this agent is involved.

Supportive Therapy

The importance of prompt, vigorous, and careful supportive therapy in the successful treatment of serious GBS infections in infants cannot be overstated. In infants with early-onset infection accompanied by pneumonia, the need for ventilatory assistance should be anticipated before the onset of apnea or respiratory failure. The prompt treatment of shock in its early phases is critical. Persistent metabolic acidosis and delayed capillary refill are characteristic of this phase. All patients with signs of circulatory or respiratory failure or meningitis should be cared for in a neonatal or pediatric intensive care unit or transferred to one as promptly as possible. When present, hypoxemia or severe anemia should be corrected, seizures should be controlled with anticonvulsants, and acidosis should be treated. In addition, fluid and electrolyte status should be monitored meticulously.

Adjunctive therapies for life-threatening GBS infections that are aimed at correction of "deficient" host defense mechanisms are under investigation. These include use of intravenous human immune globulins and leukocyte transfusions in neutropenic patients. Neither therapy has proven efficacy, and although these methods might be employed for individual patients, they should be considered investigational.

Recurrent Infections

In infants with recurrent infection, suppurative foci should be excluded or treated if present, as should humoral immune deficiency. Quantitative immunoglobulins should be determined to exclude the latter. Tube dilution susceptibility testing of the GBS isolate should be done to ensure in vitro susceptibility to penicillin G. If the reason for the recurrence remains unknown, it is likely that mucous membrane infection with GBS, which is not predictably eradicated by even parenteral therapy with penicillins, is the source. *Although controlled studies supporting the use of oral rifampin (20 mg/kg/day once daily for 4 days) at the conclusion of parenteral therapy have not been performed for such patients, such use of this agent may eradicate the source of infection.*

Preventive Therapy

The continuing magnitude and severity of GBS infections in infants has led to many investigations aimed at their prevention. Administration of penicillin G at birth is not effective in the prevention of early-onset infection because most GBS infections have their onset in utero. However, *selective intrapartum prophylaxis* for women known to have genital or anorectal GBS infection during pregnancy is effective in the prevention of early-onset GBS infections in infants. Maternal prophylaxis consists of intravenous ampicillin (an initial dose of 2 g followed by 1 g every 4 hours) until delivery. Selection criteria are based on the known increased risk of systemic infections in infants when predisposing conditions exist in maternal GBS carriers, including premature rupture of membranes, preterm delivery, prolonged rupture of membranes, chorioamnionitis, and/or intrapartum maternal fever. Therapy in infants born to women given prophylaxis should be individualized. Term, healthy infants may require none, symptomatic infants obviously should be treated with broad-spectrum antibiotics pending laboratory results, and preterm infants may be given empiric therapy until laboratory results and clinical course clarify their need.

The second mode of prevention—*immunoprophylaxis*—remains investigational. This method is based on the observation that immunity to GBS depends on antibody to the capsular polysaccharides of these organisms. These antibodies, in combination with complement and polymorphonuclear leukocytes, allow for opsonization, phagocytosis, and bacterial killing of GBS. Since most pregnant women are "deficient" in these type-specific GBS antibodies, active immunization of women with polysaccharide or polysaccharide-protein vaccines has been advocated as a method for prevention. Similarly, use of human immune globulins has been suggested as a method to correct antibody "deficiencies." However, existing intravenous preparations contain low concentrations of antibodies specific for GBS, therefore suggesting that the volume required would be prohibitive. Further, if globulins were administered to the infant, these would be suitable only for prevention of late-onset infections. Before these methods of prophylaxis can be recommended, additional studies must be done.

LISTERIA MONOCYTOGENES INFECTION

R. BORTOLUSSI, M.D.
and J. R. EVANS, M.D.

Listeria monocytogenes is a small, aerobic, motile, gram-positive rod widely distributed in animal species and in the environment. Human infections occur both sporadically and in epidemics through consumption of contaminated food, often dairy products. Nosocomial outbreaks through fomites have also been reported. Since *Listeria* tolerates a wide range of temperatures, storage by refrigeration may not suppress growth of the organism and improper pasteurization may not kill all organisms.

CLINICAL PICTURE

Listeria is a pathogen that affects hosts that are moderately to severely immunocompromised. Perinatal infection may be unrecognized in the mother but causes abortion, preterm labor, or serious, often fatal, infection in the fetus or newborn. Maternal infection during pregnancy is transmitted transplacentally to the fetus, but transmission may be interrupted if infection is recognized and treated prenatally.

Neonatal listeriosis, by far the most common pediatric form of infection, has been classified into "early-onset" or "late-onset" forms on the basis of distinct clinical characteristics (Table 1). Non-neonatal cases are rare in the pediatric age group, but *Listeria* may cause infection in immunocompromised children, particularly after renal transplantation. Because of the severity of *Listeria* disease, rapid institution of therapy is important to prevent death or severe sequelae; antimicrobials effective against *Listeria* should be administered after appropriate specimens are taken for culture but before reports are available.

TREATMENT

The results of antibiotic susceptibility testing of clinical isolates of *L. monocytogenes* have often been contradictory, and most antibiotics are not bactericidal for *Listeria.* Ampicillin with gentamicin has proved to be the most reliably synergistic combination of antibiotics and remains the treatment of choice for systemic *Listeria* infections. Penicillin and gentamicin are also highly effective. Although resistance to the penicillins is rare, when used alone, ampicillin or penicillin is bacteriostatic only. Therefore, a combination of an aminoglycoside and a beta-lactam antibiotic is recommended, particularly in neonates or other immunocompromised patients.

During the first week of life, therapy should be with ampicillin (100 mg/kg/day) given intravenously in two divided doses; from the second to fourth week of life, 200 mg/kg/day in three divided doses is given. Thereafter, the recommended dosage is 200 to 400 mg/kg/day in four to six divided doses, depending on the severity of the infection. The dosage of gentamicin in the first week of life is 5 mg/kg/day IV or IM, divided into two doses. Serum drug levels should be monitored to avoid toxicity and to ensure continued appropriate dosage levels. After 1 week of life in the term infant, 7.5 mg/kg/day of gentamicin in three divided doses is recommended, again with monitoring of serum drug levels. Although maintenance of therapy for 2 weeks is usually sufficient, 3 weeks of antibiotics or longer may be necessary in cases of *Listeria* meningitis, particularly in the immunocompromised host, as there have been reports of relapse after 10 to 17 days of therapy. Usually after 2 weeks of combined therapy and negative cultures, gentamicin may be discontinued.

In vitro studies have usually shown susceptibility of *L. monocytogenes* to tetracycline, erythromycin, sulfonamides, chloramphenicol, trimethoprim-sulfamethoxazole, and rifampin. *Listeria* is resistant to cephalosporin antibiotics. Trimethoprim-sulfamethoxazole is the recommended treatment in non-perinatal listeriosis in patients with penicillin allergy, but it is not recommended for use in perinatal infections because of the concern of sulfonamide's displacement of bilirubin from albumin and increased risk for kernicteris.

TABLE 1. Features of Early-Onset and Late-Onset *Listeria* Infection

	Early-Onset	Late-Onset
Age	0–7 Days	7–45 Days
Risk factors	Prematurity	None
	Maternal fever	
Clinical features	Meconium stained at birth	Insidious onset
	Sepsis	Fever
	Nodular rash with erythematous base	
	Pneumonia	Meningitis
Mortality	Up to 50%	5–15%

Trimethoprim-sulfamethoxazole also appears to be very effective in *Listeria* meningitis, and some authors suggest this may become the treatment of choice for *Listeria* meningitis. Vancomycin with an aminoglycoside has also shown in vitro bactericidal activity against *Listeria,* and this combination has been used successfully in several reported cases.

MANAGEMENT OF PREGNANCY

Women with listeriosis in pregnancy should be promptly treated with ampicillin. For pregnant women who present with flu-like symptoms, blood cultures are necessary and, in time of high *Listeria* prevalence rates, strong consideration should be given to presumptive treatment with ampicillin. Although it has not been proven that early antenatal *Listeria* treatment can prevent abortion, preterm labor, or an affected newborn, a number of reports in the literature strongly suggest an improved outcome; this approach may decrease the continued high mortality in perinatal disease. Supportive measures are also important, particularly in the premature infant in whom infection with *Listeria* is an additional, often fatal, complication.

REFERENCES

Gunther G, Philipson A: Oral trimethoprim as follow-up treatment of meningitis caused by *L. monocytogenes.* Rev Infect Dis 10:53–55, 1981.

Spitzer PG, Hammer SM, Karchmer AW: Treatment of *L. monocytogenes* infection with trimethoprim-sulfamethoxazole: Case report and review of the literature. Rev Infect Dis 8:427–430, 1986.

DIPHTHERIA

BARBARA W. STECHENBERG, M.D.

Diphtheria is an acute infection caused by *Corynebacterium diphtheriae.* Both generalized and localized symptoms follow production and elaboration of toxin by toxigenic strains. The diagnosis of diphtheria should be made on clinical grounds because delay in therapy may pose a serious risk from continued toxin production and dissemination.

TREATMENT

Antitoxin Therapy

Treatment of diphtheria is predicated upon neutralization of free toxin and eradication of the organism with antibiotics. The only specific treatment is antitoxin of equine origin, which should be administered on the basis of site of infection, degree of toxicity, and duration of illness.

The antitoxin must be given as early as possible by the intravenous route in a single dose sufficient to neutralize all free toxin. One dose is given to avoid the risk of sensitization from repeated doses. A history of prior sensitization to horse serum should be obtained, and testing for sensitivity to horse serum should be performed prior to administration of the therapeutic dose. This can be accomplished with a drop of a 1:10 dilution of the antitoxin for conjunctival testing; a positive reaction is demonstrated by tearing or conjunctivitis within 10 to 30 minutes. More commonly, 0.1 ml of a 1:100 dilution is used for intracutaneous testing with a positive reaction, demonstrated by the development of a wheal and/or erythema up to or greater than 10 mm within 20 minutes. If the patient is sensitive to the antitoxin, desensitization is necessary. Several regimens that utilize slowly increasing doses at 20-minute intervals are available. This procedure should be accomplished by trained personnel familiar with the treatment of anaphylaxis.

Intravenous administration of antitoxin results in more rapid excretion of antitoxin into saliva, preventing further absorption of free toxin from the oropharynx. The dosage of antitoxin is empiric and is dependent on the site of the diphtheritic membrane, the degree of toxicity and swelling, and the duration of illness. The dosage does not depend on age or size of the patient. Mild nasal or pharyngeal diphtheria can be treated with 40,000 units of antitoxin; moderately severe pharyngeal diphtheria, with 80,000 units. Severe pharyngeal or laryngeal disease should be treated with 100,000 to 120,000 units; this dose should be given to patients with mixed clinical symptoms, brawny edema, or disease of greater than 48 hours' duration. The antitoxin is available from the Centers for Disease Control (CDC), Atlanta.

An immediate allergic reaction to the infusion of antitoxin may be seen in approximately 16 per cent of patients. Serum sickness may develop in 10 to 30 per cent of recipients of antitoxin, usually 5 to 14 days after infusion. This is acceptable in light of the marked reduction in morbidity and mortality with its use.

Antibiotic Therapy

Antibiotics are not a substitute for antitoxin but are important for eradication of the organism. Either erythromycin or penicillin constitutes effective therapy. Erythromycin (40 mg/kg/day) may be given orally or intravenously for 14 days. The intravenous form is associated with a significant incidence of thrombophlebitis. Penicillin may be given as aqueous procaine penicillin G intramuscularly at 300,000 units for those weighing less than 10 kg or as 600,000 units for those weighing greater than 10 kg once daily for 14 days. Elimination of the organism should be documented by three consecutive negative cultures 24 hours apart after cessation of therapy. Either of these regimens would also be effective in eradicating group A streptococci, which may complicate up to 30 per cent of cases.

In patients with cutaneous diphtheria, lesions should be cleansed vigorously with soap and water. Antibiotic therapy, either oral erythromycin or penicillin, should be given for 10 days. Antitoxic therapy probably is of no value in this form, but some authorities give 20,000 units of antitoxin if there is no sensitivity to it.

Carriers of *C. diphtheriae* should be identified and treated with antibiotics. Oral erythromycin in the dosage noted above is appropriate for a 7-day course. Alternatives include oral penicillin or benzathine penicillin at a dosage of 600,000 units for children weighing less than 30 kg and 1,200,000 units for those weighing more than 30 kg. Two consecutive cultures at least 24 hours apart should be assessed after treatment. If the result is positive, re-treatment may be necessary.

Supportive Therapy

Patients with diphtheria, other than cutaneous, should be hospitalized. Bed rest is important and may be necessary for 2 to 3 weeks. Serial electrocardiograms should be obtained two or three times a week for 4 to 6 weeks to detect myocarditis as early as possible. If myocarditis is present, absolute bed rest and cardiac monitoring should be enforced. The patient may be digitalized carefully if heart failure develops. In severe cases of myocarditis, prednisone (1 to 1.5 mg/kg/day for 2 weeks) may be helpful.

Patients with respiratory tract diphtheria should be in strict isolation until follow-up cultures are negative. Patients with cutaneous diphtheria should be on contact isolation until follow-up cultures after therapy are negative.

Maintenance of hydration and nutrition is important. Parenteral nutritional support may be necessary. Close observation for airway obstruction is required. Secretions should be suctioned. Regular checks of the quality of the voice and the gag reflex may offer clues to obstruction. Patients with laryngeal disease may require bronchoscopy and/or intubation for relief of obstruction. Careful observation for signs of other organ involvement is necessary. Neurologic complications, such as palatal paralysis, may complicate respiratory and nutritional support.

Immunization with diphtheria toxoid is required following recovery because, in at least half of the patients who recover from diphtheria, adequate immunity does not develop.

Care of Contacts

Care of exposed persons depends on immunization status and likelihood of compliance with prophylaxis. Carriers should be identified as noted above. If a contact has clinical evidence of disease, specimens are obtained for culture and treatment with antitoxin and antibiotics is begun at once.

Asymptomatic, previously immunized close contacts should receive a booster dose of an appropriate immunizing agent (DTP, DT, or dT) if they have not received a booster in the last 5 years.

In underimmunized, asymptomatic close contacts or those in whom the immunization status is unknown, specimens for culture are obtained and erythromycin or benzathine penicillin is initiated, as for carriers. Active immunization with DTP, DT, or dT, depending on age, should be instituted. The prophylactic use of antitoxin is not warranted.

PROGNOSIS

Prior to the use of antitoxin and the availability of antibiotics, the mortality was 30 to 50 per cent, mainly in children younger than 4 years of age. At present the mortality is less than 5 per cent. The elimination of diphtheria as a threat depends on the universal use of active immunization.

PERTUSSIS

MELVIN I. MARKS, M.D.

Pertussis continues to be a major problem in developing countries and in other poorly immunized populations. *In the United States, for example, there were 10,468 cases reported from 1986 to 1988 with a case fatality rate of 0.3 per cent.* The term "pertussis" is reserved for respiratory infection due to the bacterium *Bordetella pertussis;* however, pertussis-like syndromes are occasionally noted in association with infection due to *Bordetella parapertussis, Bordetella bronchiseptica, Chlamydia trachomatis,* adenovirus, and combinations of these microorganisms. Age of the patient, immunization status, virulence of the bacteria, and stage of the disease are major determinants of the clinical expression.

TREATMENT

Supportive Care

The younger the patient, the more important the supportive care in cases of pertussis due to *B. pertussis.* In fact, respiratory compromise due to obstructive secretions, aspiration of secretions and/or vomitus, and central nervous system complications (apnea, seizures) are the major causes of severe morbidity and death in this infectious disease. These are most prevalent in infants in the first year of life, particularly those under 6 months of age. Hence, these patients with pertussis need to be assessed very carefully for two features: One is the severity of the clinical disease, and the other is the ability of the family to provide appropriate supportive care. There should be no hesitation about admitting such patients to the hospital. This should probably be done with all infants under 6 months of age and with many under 1 year of age. For example, a brief period of in-hospital training may be necessary to help parents learn how to observe the child and how to manage the secretions, vomiting, and paroxysmal episodes.

Infants most commonly come to medical attention during the early paroxysmal stage, when a variety of stimuli will precipitate a paroxysm; this is often followed by vomiting and occasionally by apnea, cyanosis, and severe distress. It is important, therefore, to provide the most comforting quiet environment. Pollutant-free air and a solicitous, caring observer are most important. Infants are often most calm in the arms of their mother or other caretakers. Invasive procedures, such as blood taking, suctioning, and measurement of vital signs, should be kept to a minimum and are probably best done immediately after a paroxysm, when there is some refractoriness to further coughing. Suctioning should be gentle, and it should be used in addition to the head-down position for handling excessive secretions and vomitus. Adequate hydration and nutrition are important because excessive secretions and vomiting can disturb fluid and electrolyte balance and the nutritional status of the host in a dramatic fashion. Humidified oxygen should be administered to patients with cyanosis and apnea and when blood gas levels indicate true hypoxemia. The risks and benefits of masks, tents, and other methods for administering oxygen need to be weighed carefully in such cases. Humidified air in a mist tent is contraindicated.

Respiratory isolation is important because pertussis is so highly contagious. Nonetheless, immune individuals (e.g., the child's mother) who are providing constant care for the patient should avoid wearing masks if possible. Similarly, isolation should be carefully enforced but should not be a deterrent to observation. Infants with paroxysmal pertussis under 6 months of age and those with apnea should never be left alone because apnea, convulsions, and aspiration are frequent and life-threatening complications.

Antibiotic Therapy

Erythromycin estolate is the most active drug against *B. pertussis* in vitro and in vivo and should be administered in all cases. This is done primarily to reduce contagiousness, although administration of the drug may reduce the severity of the disease if given during the catarrhal phase. The appropriate dosage of erythromycin estolate is 50 mg/kg/day, given orally in divided doses every 6 hours for 14 days. Respiratory isolation can be relaxed after approximately 5 days of erythromycin therapy, since the bacteria will be eliminated from the nasopharynx during this period of time in almost all patients. Fourteen days of therapy are recommended because bacteriologic relapses have been reported with shorter durations.

Although chloramphenicol, trimethoprim-sulfamethoxazole, ampicillin, fluoroquinolones, and some cephalosporins (cefoperazone and cefotaxime) are active in vitro against *B. pertussis*, there is limited clinical experience with these agents for the prevention and treatment of pertussis.

Occasionally Useful Therapy

Adrenal corticosteroids have been used in infants with particularly severe paroxysmal disease in an effort to reduce the host's inflammatory response, which is thought to be mediated by toxins elaborated by these bacteria. Although preliminary studies indicate this and some bronchodilators (such as albuterol* and salbutamol*) reduce the severity of paroxysms and other complications of the disease, there are insufficient controlled studies to justify their use on a routine basis. Currently, prescription of these pharmacologic agents should be limited to hospitalized infants with severe paroxysmal disease under careful observation for the known toxicities of these agents. Corticosteroids (beta-methasone, in oral doses of 0.075 mg/kg/day, or hydrocortisone, in intramuscular doses of 30 mg/kg/day) can be given for 2 days and then in gradually tapered dosages for 1 week. Albuterol (0.5 mg/kg/day) can be given during the severe paroxysmal stage. Intubation and ventilation may be useful in selected cases.

Knowledge of the complications of pertussis is important in order to diagnose and manage bronchopneumonia, otitis media, apnea, and convulsions. Other manifestations of the disease, such as rectal prolapse and petechiae, may be referable to the extreme pressures developed during the paroxysmal stage and may occasionally be attributed to therapies as well.

Prevention

Avoidance of exposure and appropriate immunization with pertussis vaccine are most effective. *Remember that subclinical infection is common in immunized family contacts.* Exposed susceptible individuals under 7 years of age should receive a booster dose of vaccine if their primary series of immunizations (three doses, each separated by at least 4 weeks, plus booster doses at 18 months and 4 to 6 years) is incomplete or if more than 2 years have elapsed since immunization. Immunization can be initiated shortly after birth in epidemic situations and in highly endemic regions. Erythromycin can also be administered at the time of exposure or at the earliest onset of catarrhal symptoms in exposed susceptible individuals at any age.

To avoid outbreaks in closed populations, erythromycin and strict respiratory isolation may be necessary for all subjects regardless of age or immunization status. The recommended dose is 40 to 50 mg/kg/day (maximum 1 g/day) in three to four divided doses for 10 days. Hospital staff should wear masks, and patients should be isolated in single rooms with negative pressure ventilation.

Household or similarly close contacts should be excluded from day care (or cohorted with other contacts) for 14 days or until they have been taking erythromycin for at least 5 days. Patients may be considered noninfectious after at least 5 days of erythromycin and after cough is gone (or 3 weeks after the onset of the paroxysmal cough—whichever is first). Immune globulin has no proven value in the prevention or treatment of pertussis.

*The safety and efficacy of these agents in children younger than 12 years of age have not been established.

PNEUMONIA

GEORGES PETER, M.D.

The diagnosis of pneumonia in infants and children can be readily established by the patient's history, physical examination, and chest roentgenogram, but the microbial etiology of the pneumonia is much more difficult to determine. Clinical findings, the white blood cell count and differential, and roentgenogram do not always readily distinguish viral from bacterial pneumonia. Microbiologic tests also are often unrevealing. In the United States, fewer than 5 per cent of children with pneumonia have positive blood cultures. Although bacterial antigen can be detected in sera, urine, or pleural fluid in as many as 25 per cent of such patients, its presence is not always specific for the bacterial etiology of pneumonia. In many cases of pneumonia in children, no etiology is established.

TREATMENT

Antimicrobial Therapy

The decision to give antimicrobial therapy is most often based on the physician's assessment of the probability of bacterial infection. Factors in this decision and the choice of antimicrobial therapy include clinical findings, particularly respiratory distress and severity ("toxicity") of the illness; the most likely viral and bacterial pathogens for the patient's age; immunologic competence of the host; and epidemiologic factors. These include the current predominant cause of respiratory illness in the community (for example, influenza or *Mycoplasma pneumoniae*), exposure of the patients to other children (e.g., at home or in day care) with respiratory tract infection, season, and possible nosocomial acquisition of infection. In young children, the majority of cases are caused by respiratory viruses; in school-aged children, *M. pneumoniae* is a major cause. Some children with bacterial pneumonia also appear to have a viral component to their illness resulting from a preceding upper respiratory tract viral infection.

In mildly ill patients with presumed viral pneumonia, withholding antimicrobial therapy is appropriate if follow-up can be ensured. In cases of viral pneumonia, antimicrobial therapy does not affect the clinical course or risk of secondary bacterial infection. In cases in which a bacterial pathogen is isolated, the antimicrobial choice is determined by its antimicrobial susceptibilities. In hospitalized patients, antimicrobials are initially administered parenterally, usually intravenously. Once the patient improves and in children managed as outpatients, oral therapy is given.

Antimicrobial Selection (Tables 1 and 2)

Neonates (Younger Than 1 Month)

Therapy is indicated in all neonates with pneumonia. The causes of perinatally acquired pneumonia are those that cause neonatal sepsis and most commonly are group B streptococci and gram-negative enteric bacteria, especially *Escherichia coli.* Nontypable *Haemophilus influenzae* also has been common in some centers. Thus, empiric administration of ampicillin and an aminoglycoside, such as gentamicin or tobramycin, is appropriate. Because *Pseudomonas* sp. are unlikely pathogens for early-onset pneumonia (less than 7 days after birth), cefotaxime can be substituted for the aminoglycoside in initial therapy. Severe pneumonia that develops after the first few days of life can be due to herpes simplex virus (HSV). Acyclovir is indicated for neonates with suspected or proven HSV pneumonia. In late-onset pneumonia, *Staphylococcus aureus* is a potential cause. In recent decades, however, staphylococcal pneumonia has become uncommon. In low-birth-weight infants with coagulase-negative staphylococcal bacteremia, respiratory symptoms can occur; however, this organism is not an established cause of pneumonia.

Infants 1 to 3 Months

Viruses and *Chlamydia trachomatis* are the predominant causes. *C. trachomatis* typically causes an afebrile pneumonitis in young infants. Other causes include the major bacterial pathogens for older infants and children (*Streptococcus pneumoniae* and *H. influenzae* type b). *S. aureus* is an important consideration for the infant who was in a special care nursery experiencing nosocomial staphylococcal infections.

Cefotaxime is effective against most of the common bacterial pathogens for this age group and is an appropriate choice for the febrile, ill-appearing infant with pneumonia. For infants who are not severely ill and in whom *S. aureus* is not a likely cause, ceftriaxone is a reasonable alternative. If *S. aureus* is a major consideration or is proven to be the cause, the infant should be treated with a penicillinase-resistant penicillin, such as nafcillin or oxacillin. In the unusual circumstance of methicillin-resistant staphylococcal pneumonia, vancomycin is indicated. If *S. aureus* etiology is proven, a sweat test should be performed because the initial presentation of cystic fibrosis can be staphylococcal pneumonia.

When *C. trachomatis* pneumonia is suspected, oral erythromycin or sulfisoxazole is the drug of choice. This infection can be rapidly diagnosed by direct immunofluorescence or enzyme immunoassay of nasopharyngeal secretions.

Respiratory syncytial virus (RSV), an important cause of pneumonia in this age group, also can be rapidly detected in nasopharyngeal secretions by enzyme immunoassays. In infants with underlying immune, cardiac, or pulmonary disease and those with severe RSV infection (as indicated by increasing hypoxia and increasing hypercapnia), ribavirin is recommended. Ribavirin, which is expensive, should not be prescribed for infants who are mildly ill with RSV pneumonitis.

Children 3 Months to 4 Years

The most common causes in this age group are respiratory viruses, including RSV. Ribavirin is indicated for high-risk infants or those with severe disease, as described for infants 1 to 3 months of age. The most important bacterial causes currently are *S. pneumoniae* and *H. influenzae* type b, but the incidence of *H. influenzae* disease is expected to decrease with the advent of recommended *Haemophilus* immunization at 2 months of age. For children who require hospitalization because of either age or degree of illness, intravenous cefuroxime is an appropriate choice in view of its excellent *in vitro* activity against the likely bacterial pathogens, including ampicillin-resistant *H. influenzae* type b and *S. aureus*. Cefuroxime is also active against strains of *S. pneumoniae* relatively resistant to penicillin, which may account currently for approximately 10 per cent of clinically significant pneumococcal isolates in the United States. Ceftriaxone (intravenously or intramuscularly) is an alternative for children with suspected pneumonia due to *S. pneumoniae* or *H. influenzae* type b. If no organism is isolated or implicated by rapid antigen testing of nasopharyngeal secretions for RSV or *C. trachomatis* or of serum or urine for pyogenic bacterial antigen (e.g., pneumococcal polysaccharide antigen), cefuroxime (or ceftriaxone) should be continued. In patients from whom *S. pneumoniae* or *H. influenzae* type b susceptible to ampicillin is isolated, aqueous penicillin G or ampicillin, respectively, should be substituted for cefuroxime.

Once the patient is afebrile, has improved symptomatically, and is able to take medications by mouth, an oral antimicrobial can be substituted for the parenteral agent. In children with proven bacterial etiology, the choice of oral drug is determined by the in vitro susceptibilities of the bacterium. However, since often a bacterial cause has not been proven, the selection is empiric. Amoxicillin, ampicillin, amoxicillin-clavulanic acid, trimethoprim-sulfamethoxazole, erythromycin-sulfisoxazole, cefaclor, or cefuroxime axetil is each a reasonable choice (unless ampicillin-resistant *H. influenzae* type b is highly suspected, in which case amoxicillin is not an appropriate drug). The specific choice is based on price, adverse effects, patient acceptance, and personal preferences. If group

TABLE 1. Parenteral Antimicrobials for Children with Pneumonia

Agent	Spectrum of Activity	Dose—mg/kg/day	Comments
Acyclovir	Herpes simplex, varicella-zoster	30 in 3 doses (q 8 hr)	Dose adjustment required in renal failure
Aminoglycosides Gentamicin Tobramycin Amikacin	Gram-negative enteric bacilli (*Escherichia coli, Klebsiella pneumoniae, Proteus* sp.), *Pseudomonas aeruginosa*	Gentamicin: 3.7–7.5 in 3 doses (q 8 hr) Tobramycin: 3–7.5 in 3 doses (q 8 hr) Amikacin, 15–30 in 3 doses (q 8 hr)	Aminoglycoside selection depends upon bacterial susceptibilities in the hospital; serum concentrations should be monitored and the dose reduced in renal dysfunction
Amphotericin B	*Candida* sp., other fungi	0.5–1.0 once daily (q 24 hr)	Renal function and serum potassium concentrations should be monitored
Ampicillin	*Streptococcus pneumoniae,* other streptococci (groups A and B, enterococci), *Haemophilus influenzae* type b (ampicillin-susceptible)	200 in 4 doses (q 6 hr)	
Cefazolin	*Staphylococcus aureus, S. pneumoniae,* other streptococci	50–100 in 3 doses (q 8 hr)	For use in penicillin-allergic patients
Cefotaxime	*H. influenzae* type b, gram-negative enteric bacilli, streptococci, *S. aureus, Moraxella catarrhalis**	100–150 in 3–4 doses (q 6–8 hr)	—
Ceftazidime	Gram-negative enteric bacilli, *P. aeruginosa*	125–150 in 3 doses (q 8 hr)	—
Ceftriaxone	*H. influenzae* type b, gram-negative enteric bacilli, streptococci, *M. catarrhalis**	50–80 in 1–2 doses (q 12–24 hr)	Moderate activity against *S. aureus*
Cefuroxime	*S. pneumoniae, H. influenzae* type b, *S. aureus* streptococci, *M. catarrhalis**	100–150 in 3 doses (q 8 hr)	
Chloramphenicol	*H. influenzae, M. catarrhalis,** streptococci, *S. pneumoniae,* anaerobes	50–75 in 4 doses (q 6 hr)	Serum concentrations should be monitored
Erythromycin	*Mycoplasma, pneumoniae, Chlamydia trachomatis, Legionella pneumophila*	20–50 in 4 doses (q 6 hr)	Thrombophlebitis may occur
Extended-spectrum penicillins Ticarcillin Piperacillin Mezlocillin	Gram-negative enteric bacilli, *P. aeruginosa,* streptococci	200–300 in 4 doses (q 6 hr)	Used in combination with an aminoglycoside
Ganciclovir	*Cytomegalovirus*	10 in 2 doses (q 12 hr)	Consultation with a specialist indicated
Nafcillin, oxacillin	*S. aureus, S. pneumoniae*	150–200 in 4–6 doses (q 4–6 hr)	
Penicillin G	*S. pneumoniae*	50,000–250,000 units in 4–6 doses (q 4–6 h)	In severe disease or infections caused by relatively resistant *S. pneumoniae,* higher dosage given q 4 hr is indicated
Ribavirin	Respiratory syncytial virus (RSV)	Aerosol for 3 to 7 days	Expensive
Trimethoprim-sulfamethoxazole	*Pneumocystis carinii,* gram-negative enteric bacilli, (except *Pseudomonas* sp.)	20 of trimethoprim/100 of the sulfamethoxazole in 4 doses (q 6 hr)	
Vancomycin	Methicillin-resistant staphylococci	40 in 4 doses (q 12 hr)	Serum concentrations should be monitored; dose reduction in renal dysfunction

*Formerly termed *Branhamella catarrhalis.*

TABLE 2. Oral Antimicrobials for Children with Pneumonia

Agent	Daily Dose—mg/kg/day (Adult Dose/day)
Amantadine*	8.8 in 2 doses for children 1–9 yr (maximum dose, 150 mg/day); 200 mg (total daily) in 2 doses for children >9 yr
Amoxicillin	25–50 in 3 doses (0.75–1.5 g)
Amoxicillin-clavulanic acid	20–40 of amoxicillin component in 3 doses (0.75–1.5 g)
Ampicillin	50–100 in 4 doses (2–4 g)
Cefaclor	20–40 in 2 or 3 doses (0.75–1.5 g)
Cefixime	8 in 1 or 2 doses (400 mg)
Cefuroxime axetil	250–500† in 2 doses (0.25–1.0 g)
Cephalexin	25–50 in 4 doses (1–4 g)
Cephradine	25–50 in 2–4 doses (1–4 g)
Cloxacillin	50–100 in 4 doses (2–4 g)
Dicloxacillin	12.5 25 in 4 doses (1–2 g)
Erythromycin (available in base, sterate, ethyl succinate, and estolate preparations)	20–50† in 2–4 doses (1–2 g)
Erythromycin-sulfisoxazole	40 of erythromycin/120 of sulfisoxazole in 3–4 doses
Penicillin V	25,000–50,000 U in 3 or 4 doses
Sulfisoxazole	100–150 in 4 doses
Trimethoprim-sulfamethoxazole	8 of trimethoprim/40 of sulfamethoxazole in 2 doses (320 mg of trimethoprim/1.6 g of sulfamethoxazole)

*Dosage regimens vary for different preparations.
†For influenza A.

A streptococcus is the cause, trimethoprim-sulfamethoxazole is not appropriate.

These oral antimicrobials also are appropriate for initial therapy of nonhospitalized patients with presumed bacterial pneumonia. In the United States, amoxicillin is most commonly recommended. However, if the child has received amoxicillin, ampicillin, or penicillin for another infection, such as otitis media, in the preceding month, the likelihood of ampicillin-resistant *H. influenzae* is increased and a drug active against ampicillin-resistant *H. influenzae* type b should be considered. Appropriate drugs include amoxicillin-clavulanic acid, erythromycin-sulfisoxazole, and cefuroxime axetil. If the patient does not improve or clinically worsens while receiving amoxicillin, one of these drugs or parenteral therapy with cefuroxime or ceftriaxone should be given in place of amoxicillin. Hospitalization may be indicated.

During influenza A outbreaks, if the child has other clinical features consistent with influenza and is seriously ill, amantadine therapy should be considered. In addition, secondary bacterial infection due to *S. pneumoniae, H. influenzae,* or *S. aureus* is a possibility.

In developing countries, the World Health Organization recommends daily intramuscular procaine penicillin, oral trimethoprim-sulfamethoxazole, or oral ampicillin (or amoxicillin) for 5 days for treatment of pneumonia in nonhospitalized infants and children.

Children 5 Years and Older

M. pneumoniae is the leading cause of pneumonia in children over 5 years. Erythromycin therapy is appropriate and also is effective treatment of pneumococcal pneumonia. If *M. pneumoniae* is considered clinically unlikely, penicillin is adequate therapy, as *S. pneumoniae* is the major pyogenic bacterial pathogen in this age group. If the child is 9 years of age or older, tetracycline is equally effective for established *M. pneumoniae* infections but is not recommended for pneumococcal pneumonia.

For the otherwise normal child 5 years of age or older who is hospitalized with pneumonia, intravenous aqueous penicillin G or cefuroxime is appropriate initial therapy. If pneumonia complicates a preceding viral infection that has been caused by influenza or varicella, *S. aureus* is also a possibility and cefuroxime is the indicated drug. If staphylococcal disease is proven or highly likely, nafcillin or oxacillin is recommended.

Duration of Therapy

A total of 7 to 10 days of antimicrobial therapy, irrespective of the route of administration, is generally adequate treatment of bacterial pneumonia in an otherwise normal child. However, patients with complications of pneumonia, pleural effusion, or empyema require 2 to 4 weeks of therapy; duration in patients with staphylococcal empyema is 3 to 4 weeks. Initial therapy is given parenterally followed by oral therapy once the patient is afebrile and clinically improved.

For *Chlamydia* pneumonia, 14 days of therapy is recommended. *M. pneumoniae* infection is treated for 10 days. Ribavirin for RSV infection is given for 3 to 7 days, depending on the patient's response.

Nosocomial Pneumonia

Nosocomial viral respiratory infections are common, especially in the winter, and are caused by RSV or influenza, depending on the currently prevalent virus in the community. Hospital-acquired bacterial pneumonias occur primarily in children who are intubated and receiving mechanical ventilation. Fever, a change in the character of the sputum, and new pulmonary infiltrates on chest roentgenogram suggest possible pneumonia in such patients. The bacterial etiologic agents usually are organisms that colonize the orotracheal airway. Initially, antibiotic therapy is directed against the organisms colonizing the host and the known nosocomial pathogens (in accordance with their antimicrobial susceptibilities) within the intensive care unit. In general, an aminoglycoside is included in the initial antibiotic regimen, since gram-negative bacterial colonization is common in this setting. However, the bacterial etiology of nosocomial pneumonia in children is infrequently proven. If methicillin-resistant *Staphylococcus* is endemic within a unit, vancomycin should also be considered in the initial therapy.

Pneumonia in the Immunocompromised Host

Deciding which antimicrobial agent(s) to administer to children with pneumonia who are immunocompromised, such as from human immunodeficiency virus (HIV) infection or chemotherapy for leukemia, is difficult. The likely pathogens differ with the nature of the underlying host immunologic abnormality. Children with neutropenia secondary to chemotherapy are susceptible to gram-negative bacterial infections. Usually, an aminoglycoside and an extended-spectrum beta-lactam, such as mezlocillin, piperacillin, or ceftazidime, is an appropriate regimen. The addition of an antistaphylococcal penicillin or vancomycin is appropriate if the child has an indwelling central line and, thus, is prone to gram-positive bacteremia.

Infection due to *Pneumocystis carinii* should always be considered when patients with HIV infection or leukemia or those who are receiving chemotherapy present with fever, coughing, hypoxia, and diffuse alveolar infiltrates. Parenteral trimethoprim-sulfamethoxazole should be administered promptly in such cases. Other opportunistic organisms, such as *Candida* sp., *Aspergillus* sp., and cytomegalovirus, should also be considered in immunocompromised patients with pneumonia. Amphotericin B is indicated for children with suspected or proven fungal pneumonia. Cytomegalovirus pneumonia is common in allogenic bone marrow transplant recipients and is treated with ganciclovir and intravenous immune globulin. Consultation with an infectious disease or other specialist is usually warranted in the management of an immunocompromised patient with pneumonia and possible opportunistic infection.

S. pneumoniae and *H. influenzae* type b are the predominant pathogens in children with acquired immunodeficiency syndrome (AIDS) and those with congenital hypogammaglobulinemia. Hence, cefuroxime is an appropriate choice for initial therapy for pneumonia in these patients. Ceftriaxone is an alternative if the child is not seriously ill and if *S. aureus* is not a major concern.

Causes of pneumonia in children with sickle cell anemia include *S. pneumoniae, H. influenzae* type b, *M. pneumoniae,* and *Chlamydia pneumoniae.* Infections due to *Mycoplasma* or *Chlamydia* can be more severe than in the normal host and are treated with erythromycin (or tetracycline in children 9 years of age or older).

Hospitalization

Children with pneumonia often can be managed as outpatients. For close observation, however, hospitalization is usually indicated for young infants; children with underlying disease predisposing to pulmonary infections; immunocompromised patients; acutely ill children with respiratory distress, including tachypnea, accessory respiratory muscle use, or hypoxemia; and those with significant pleural effusion. Pulse oximetry is an excellent means for assessing arterial oxygen saturation and the resulting need for hospitalization. The ability of the child to take oral medications as well as the compliance of the family or caretaker in giving prescribed antimicrobial therapy is another consideration. Hospitalization is also indicated for children treated initially as outpatients with oral therapy whose clinical course deteriorates with appropriate therapy.

Other Considerations

Pleural Fluid

A diagnostic thoracentesis is indicated initially for cultures and other microbiologic tests, cell count, and chemical tests (protein, glucose, and pH). In addition, therapeutic drainage is required when empyema is suspected, when the accumulation of fluid is large enough to impair respiration, or when fever persists. In cases of small effusions, one thoracentesis may be sufficient. If empyema or large volumes of fluid are present, drainage by a closed system with a chest tube under negative pressure may be required until drainage is complete.

Supportive Care

Maintenance of adequate oxygenation, hydration, and acid-base balance is indicated. Respiratory failure necessitates intubation and mechanical ventilation. Symptomatic therapy with antipyretics and, in some cases, with antitussives may be helpful.

Tuberculin Test

The possibility of pulmonary tuberculosis should always be considered in a child with pneumonia. An intermediate-strength Mantoux (5 tuberculin units) skin test is indicated if the child does not respond to therapy as expected, has a history of possible exposure to a person with tuberculosis, or is from a high-risk population, such as foreign-born persons from high prevalence areas (for example, in Asia, Africa, or Latin America) or low-income groups.

Follow-up

A critical aspect of the management of the child with pneumonia is follow-up care. The child should be evaluated 24 to 48 hours after the diagnosis has been made, either by re-examination or, if the family is reliable, by telephone contact. The child should be subsequently re-examined approximately 10 to 14 days later.

Second Chest Roentgenogram

If a normal child with pneumonia responds promptly to antibiotic therapy, is clinically well, and has normal physical findings at follow-up, another chest roentgenogram at 6 weeks is optional. However, a chest roentgenogram is indicated if the child has continuing symptoms and signs of pneumonia or if foreign body aspiration or congenital malformation is suspected.

MENINGOCOCCAL DISEASE

MARTHA L. LEPOW, M.D.

The patient with meningococcal disease is frequently an infant or young child who most commonly presents with an acute illness characterized by fever, toxicity, and a petechial, maculopapular, or purpuric rash. The cerebrospinal fluid (CSF) may or may not be abnormal. Shock and disseminated intravascular coagulation are frequent. Invasive meningococcal infections can be complicated by arthritis, myocarditis, pericarditis, or pneumonia. Serogroups B, C, Y, and W-135 are prevalent in the United States.

Disease occurs most frequently in children younger than 5 years, with the peak attack rate in the 6- to 12-month age group. A second period of increased incidence occurs in 18- to 20-year-olds when they are in college or in the armed forces.

Diagnosis is by Gram's stain and culture of infected fluids, including buffy coat of blood. Antigen detection by latex agglutination of CSF or urine with group-specific meningococcal antisera may allow rapid diagnosis, although specificity may be lacking for group B.

TREATMENT

Treatment should be initiated immediately after specimens for blood culture are obtained and before laboratory studies are complete. Cerebrospinal fluid examination may be deferred if the patient's condition is unstable. In the young child, initial treatment should include antimicrobial coverage appropriate for the other major causes of sepsis and meningitis, including *Haemophilus influenzae* type b, many of which are resistant to ampicillin; *Streptococcus pneumoniae;* and occasionally gram-negative bacteria and *Listeria.*

Several options are available in antibiotic treatment. If the diagnosis is confirmed, penicillin G (400,000 U/kg/day in four to six divided doses) may be given. Ceftriaxone (100 to 150 mg/kg/day in two divided doses) can be used intravenously (IV) for meningitis for the first 48 hours and then once daily IV or intramuscularly (IM) at 75 mg/kg for the duration of therapy. Other alternatives include cefotaxime (200 mg/kg/day in four divided doses). When the etiology is confirmed (after 24 to 48 hours), the treatment can be changed to IV penicillin; if ceftriaxone is used initially it can be continued.

Chloramphenicol sodium succinate (100 mg/kg/day in four divided doses) used to be the most commonly used antimicrobial drug for initial treatment of bacterial meningitis in children along with ampicillin. The necessity for monitoring levels to avoid acute bone marrow suppression and the remote possibility of idiosyncratic aplastic anemia have made the newer effective cephalosporins the first-line drugs of choice in acute pyogenic meningitis in infants and children. If the etiology of the meningitis is not known and the infant is younger than 8 weeks of age, ampicillin should be added if third-generation cephalosporins are used until listerial infection is ruled out. In the case of penicillin allergy, either a third-generation cephalosporin or chloramphenicol can be used. One advantage of chloramphenicol is that oral absorption is excellent; once the patient is stable, this route may be used for completion of the treatment course but the dosage may need to be lowered. Whenever chloramphenicol is used beyond 3 days, the serum concentration should be measured and the dose modified to maintain a peak level below 25 μg/ml and a trough of 5 to 10 μg/ml. The accepted duration of treatment for meningococcemia and meningitis is 7 days.

Dexamethasone (0.15 mg/kg every 6 hours for 4 days) has been shown to be effective in lowering the incidence of the hearing loss in *H. influenzae* type b meningitis in a study of pyogenic meningitis; the number of evaluable patients with meningococcal meningitis was too small for significance. Nonetheless, there were no significant adverse effects noted. For the optimal effect, dexamethasone should be given before or concurrent with the first dose of antibiotic therapy in children. There are no data on the use of dexamethasone in meningitic infants younger than 2 months of age. In rare instances, upper gastrointestinal bleeding has been noted with this treatment and examination of stools for melena and measurements of hemoglobin are indicated during this therapy.

Children who present with fulminant meningococcal disease with multiple organ involvement, disseminated intravascular coagulation, hypotension, and coma require careful monitoring and appropriate therapy to preserve organ function. These patients are best treated in an intensive care setting, where monitoring as well as pharmacologic intervention is available. Administration of IV hydrocortisone (10 mg/kg), repeated at variable frequencies along with blood products and fluids has been used for treatment of septic shock. (See discussion of septic shock, p. 636.) Correlates of poor prognosis are meningococcemia without meningitis, hypotension with a systolic blood pressure of less than 70 mm Hg in children up to 14 years of age, presence of petechiae for less than 12 hours prior to admission, hyperpyrexia (rectal temperature of greater than 40°C), peripheral leukocytosis of less than 15,000/mm^3, or thrombocytopenia (<100,000 platelets/mm^3). Patients who have two or more of these signs are severely ill and require constant vigilance and intensive care. Mortality rate is about 10 per cent for all forms of meningococcal disease.

On presentation, respiratory isolation should be established. Traditionally, isolation for 24 hours has been recommended in a private room. At times the patient's condition requires that care be delivered in a multibed room. If strict respiratory isolation cannot be maintained for 24 hours, rifampin (20 mg/kg/day in two divided doses for 2 days) should be given to assist with abbreviating the potential period of infectiousness.

Household contacts, hospital personnel who have been in intimate contact with the patient's bodily fluids, and day care contacts should receive rifampin prophylaxis, 600 mg every 12 hours for four doses in adults and 20 mg/kg/day in two divided doses for 2 days, with a maximum individual dose of 600 mg for children aged 1 to 12 years (rifampin is contraindicated in pregnancy). For infants younger than 1 month, 10 mg/kg/day in two divided doses for 2 days should be given. The incubation period is from 1 to 10 days but most often is less than 4 days. Observation for illness in exposed individuals—even after prophylaxis—is prudent.

Ceftriaxone (in a single intramuscular dose of 125 mg for children younger than 12 years and 250 mg for adults) is effective in eradicating the group A carrier state, and data may be forthcoming for use with other strains. This drug would have the advantages of easier administration, availability, and safety in pregnancy.

A serogroup-specific quadrivalent polysaccharide meningococcal vaccine against groups A, C, Y, and W-135 *Neisseria meningitidis* is available in the United States. Although the group A component is immunogenic in young infants (with a two-dose schedule), response to the other components is poor in infants under 2 years of age. The vaccine should be administered routinely to children 2 years and older in high-risk groups, including those with functional or anatomic asplenia and those with terminal complement component deficiencies. It could be used as an adjunct to chemoprophylaxis to control outbreaks of disease caused by serogroups represented in the vaccine and may be of benefit to travelers to countries where hyperendemic or epidemic disease is recognized.

INFECTIONS DUE TO ANAEROBIC COCCI AND GRAM-NEGATIVE BACILLI

LISA M. DUNKLE, M.D.

INCIDENCE

Anaerobic infections occur less frequently in infants and children than in adults, probably because the compromise of tissue health and integrity due to trauma or disease (which predisposes to invasion by anaerobic organisms) is less common in children. When anaerobic infections do occur, they generally involve flora endogenous to the child's skin or gastrointestinal tract and are frequently polymicrobial. Aerobic organisms commonly coexist in such infections and may contribute to the pathogenicity of the anaerobes by further reducing the oxygen tension of devitalized tissues.

TREATMENT

Prompt and thorough surgical débridement as well as adequate antimicrobial therapy is required for these pathophysiologically complicated infections. Hyperbaric oxygen therapy has been advocated for some deep-seated infections; however, there is little experience with this modality in children and, under no circumstances, can it replace appropriate surgical and medical intervention. Although surgical débridement may be the only therapy required in some localized abscesses or decubitus ulcers without signs of systemic involvement, antibiotics are indicated whenever systemic manifestations of infection are present or when suppuration has either extended into or threatened to spread into surrounding tissue.

Selection of Antimicrobials

Selection of antimicrobial agents for anaerobic or mixed infections is simplified when culture results of reliable specimens are available. This is rarely the case, however, because of the difficulty encountered in obtaining appropriate specimens and the relatively slow growth of anaerobes in the laboratory. Therefore, most patients must be treated empirically on the basis of suspected, rather than established, pathogens. Fortunately, the types of organisms involved in many anaerobic infections and their antimicrobial susceptibility patterns tend to be predictable. Gram-stained smears of infected material, together with the observation of foul odor, may be invaluable in the rapid identification of anaerobic infection.

Other factors to be considered in the choice of antimicrobial agents include the pharmacologic characteristics of various drugs, their potential toxicities, their effect on normal flora, and their bactericidal activity. The antimicrobial agents chosen should provide for adequate coverage of most expected pathogens at the site of the infection. Some commonly used broad-spectrum agents possess these qualities, but for most anaerobic infections, agents should be chosen specifically for their activity in these circumstances.

Specific Antimicrobial Drugs

Table 1 lists the antimicrobial agents most useful for the infections that commonly involve anaerobic organisms and the appropriate dosages and route(s) of administration. Choices of other agents should be relied on only when specific results of culture and susceptibility testing are available.

Penicillins

Penicillin G is the drug of choice for infecting strains that are susceptible to this drug. These organisms include virtually all gram-positive and most gram-negative anaerobic strains other than *Bacteroides fragilis.* Some strains of *Bacteroides,* such as the *B. melaninogenicus* group and *B. oralis,* as well as strains of *Clostridium, Fusobacterium* species, and microaerophilic streptococci occasionally demonstrate resistance to penicillin, usually resulting from beta-lactamase production. Some of these strains are inhibited by concentrations of 8 to 32 units/ml of penicillin G. In these instances, administration of very high dosages of penicillin G may eradicate the infection. Although ampicillin, amoxicillin, and penicillin generally are equally active, methicillin, nafcillin, and the isoxazolyl penicillins have unpredictable activity and frequently are inferior to penicillin G. Carbenicillin and ticarcillin are active against *B. fragilis* because of the high serum level that can be achieved; however, penicillin G is also active against *B. fragilis* in this concentration. Resistance to these agents is present in up to 30 per cent of *B. fragilis* strains.

Clavulanic acid and sulbactam are beta-lactamase inhibitors that resemble the nucleus of penicillin but differ in several ways. They irreversibly inhibit beta-lactamase enzymes produced by some Enterobacteriaceae, staphylococci, and beta-lactamase–producing *Bacteroides* species (*B. fragilis* group and some strains of *B. melaninogenicus* and *B. oralis*). When used in conjunction with a beta-lactam antibiotic, they render the antibiotic effective in treating infections caused by beta-lactamase–producing bacteria. Combination of amoxicillin or ticarcillin with clavulanate or sulbactam results in agents to which over 98 per cent of the *B. fragilis* group are susceptible; however, resistance to penicillins due to other mechanisms is present in a small number of aerobic and facultative bacteria. Nonetheless, the amoxicillin-clavulanic acid combination probably represents the most useful agent available in the treatment of simple animal and human bite wounds that commonly involve a multiplicity of organisms, including aerobic and anaerobic and gram-positive and gram-negative strains.

Chloramphenicol

Although it is a bacteriostatic drug, chloramphenicol is one of the antimicrobial agents most active against anaerobes. Resistance is rare. Failures to eradicate infections, including bacteremia, with chloramphenicol have been reported; however, this drug has been used for more than 25 years as first-line therapy for anaerobic infections. It is regarded as a good choice for treatment of serious anaerobic infections when the nature and susceptibility of the infecting organisms are unknown, especially infections involving the central nervous system (CNS). The potential toxicity of chloramphenicol must be borne in mind, including the low risk of aplastic anemia, dose-dependent leukopenia, and "gray syndrome" in newborns and patients with impaired hepatic glucuronidation.

Cephalosporins

First-Generation. The first-generation cephalosporins are less active than penicillin G, and most strains of *B. fragilis* and many of *B. melaninogenicus* are resistant on the basis of cephalosporinase production.

Second-Generation. Cefoxitin, a second-generation cephalosporin, is relatively resistant to cephalosporinase and is

TABLE 1. Antimicrobial Agents for Anaerobic and Mixed Infections

Site	Drug	Dose	Route of Administration
Pulmonary	Clindamycin	20–40 mg/kg/day	IV, p.o.
Parapharyngeal	Penicillin G	10–12 million units/m^2	IV
Abdominal	Clindamycin (with aminoglycoside)	20–40 mg/kg/day	IV, p.o.
Pelvic	Cefoxitin	100–150 mg/kg/day	IV
Skeletal	Clindamycin	20–40 mg/kg/day	IV, p.o.
Soft Tissue	Cefoxitin	100–150 mg/kg/day	IV
Central nervous system	Chloramphenicol	50–100 mg/kg/day	IV, p.o.
	Metronidazole (with penicillin)	30 mg/kg/day	IV, p.o.
Minor soft tissue (bites)	Amoxicillin/clavulanate/(Augmentin)	20–40 mg/kg/day	p.o.
Others	Imipenem	No pediatric dose available	IV
	Tetracyclines	40 mg/kg/day	p.o.
	Ciprofloxacin	250–750 mg twice daily	p.o.

therefore effective against most *B. fragilis* strains. Cefoxitin is active in vitro against at least 95 per cent of strains of *B. fragilis* at a level of 32 μg/ml but is relatively inactive against most species of *Clostridium* (including *C. difficile*) other than *Clostridium perfringens.* Clinical experience with cefoxitin has shown it to be effective in eradication of most anaerobic infections. It is used successfully for surgical prophylaxis because of its complementary activity against aerobic enteric gram-negative rods. Cefoxitin does not cross the blood-brain barrier and should not be used for CNS infections.

Third-Generation. Cefotetan exhibits a similar spectrum but is less active against some members of the *B. fragilis* group, which may constitute as many as 30 to 50 per cent of the *Bacteroides* isolates from patients. Third-generation cephalosporins exhibit unpredictable activity against anaerobes and may be effective against as few as 50 per cent of *B. fragilis.*

Clindamycin

Clindamycin exhibits a broad range of activity against both gram-positive and gram-negative anaerobic organisms and has proved its efficacy in clinical trials. Approximately 95 per cent of the anaerobic bacteria isolated in clinical practice are susceptible to easily achievable levels below 3 μg/ml. There are reports of resistant strains associated with clinical infections, although these are uncommon. Because clindamycin cannot be demonstrated to cross the blood-brain barrier efficiently, it should not be administered in cases of CNS infections. It is frequently used in combination with aminoglycosides for infections of the abdominal cavity and pelvis and represents first-line therapy for these infections. It is particularly useful in deep-seated purulent infection, such as osteomyelitis, because of its ease of entry into leukocytes. Because of the increasing frequency of penicillin resistance among oral anaerobes, clindamycin represents an excellent choice for the treatment of necrotic pulmonary infection, such as lung abscess due to aspiration. Although the primary toxicity recognized with clindamycin is colitis, it should be kept in mind that colitis is associated, probably more frequently, with a number of other antimicrobial agents, such as ampicillin and all the cephalosporins, and may occur in seriously ill patients in the absence of previous antimicrobial therapy. The occurrence of colitis in pediatric patients is very rare.

Metronidazole

Metronidazole shows excellent bactericidal activity against most obligate anaerobic bacteria, such as *B. fragilis,* other species of *Bacteroides, Fusobacterium,* and *Clostridium.* More than 90 per cent of gram-negative obligate anaerobes are susceptible to less than 2 μg/ml of metronidazole. However, most strains of gram-positive anaerobes, including gram-positive cocci, nonsporulating bacilli, microaerophilic streptococci, *Propionibacterium acnes,* and *Actinomyces* species, are almost uniformly resistant. Aerobic and facultative anaerobes, such as coliforms, are usually highly resistant. As such, metronidazole should not be used alone as therapy for clinical anaerobic infections that are usually mixed.

Clinical experience in adults and limited experience in children indicate the efficacy of metronidazole in the treatment of infections caused by gram-negative anaerobes, including intra-abdominal sepsis, infections of the female genital tract, and especially infections of the CNS. However, it is not effective in therapy of gram-positive anaerobic pulmonary infections. Thus, when gram-positive or mixed infection is suspected, additional agents effective against these organisms, such as penicillin G, should be administered. Metronidazole may be particularly advantageous in CNS infections because of its excellent penetration into the CNS. Penicillin must be administered concurrently in these cases.

Other Drugs

Imipenem-Cilastatin (Thienamycin). This drug is active against a wide variety of aerobic and anaerobic gram-positive and gram-negative organisms. It possesses excellent activity against beta-lactamase–producing *Bacteroides* species and is effective as a single agent for the treatment of mixed aerobic-anaerobic infections. However, at present, data in children are limited, and this drug is not yet approved for use in this age group.

Tetracyclines. Because of the development of resistance by virtually all types of anaerobes, tetracyclines no longer represent useful therapeutic alternatives for anaerobic infections. The new tetracycline analogues, doxycycline and minocycline, are more active than the parent compound, but the use of any of these agents is not recommended in children under 8 years of age because of adverse effects on teeth and bone.

Erythromycin. Like tetracyline, erythromycin should no longer be relied on for empiric therapy because resistance has developed in a large proportion of strains.

Vancomycin. Vancomycin is effective against all gram-positive anaerobes but is inactive against gram-negative species. Little clinical experience has been gained in the treatment of anaerobic bacteria using this agent.

Quinolones. The quinolones (ciprofloxacin, norfloxacin) are active against most gram-positive anaerobic species, but are generally not active against gram-negative species. Even in adolescents for whom quinolones may be used appropriately, they do not generally represent a satisfactory choice for the treatment of mixed anaerobic infections.

INFECTIONS CAUSED BY *HAEMOPHILUS INFLUENZAE* TYPE B

EUGENE D. SHAPIRO, M.D.

In the United States, *Haemophilus influenzae* type b (Hib) has been the most common cause of bacterial meningitis and of other serious bacterial infections in children beyond the neonatal period. With the introduction of conjugate vaccines that are effective even in infants, the incidence of serious Hib infections should diminish substantially. Nevertheless, Hib will continue to be a major cause of invasive infections in children. Appropriate treatment depends on the specific type of infection.

TREATMENT

General Principles

Antimicrobial treatment of Hib is directed at rapid sterilization of the site of the infection. For many years, ampicillin was the drug of choice. However, in the late 1970s, strains of Hib that produce beta-lactamase began to increase in prevalence. Chloramphenicol was used to treat organisms that were resistant to ampicillin. More recently, second- and third-generation cephalosporins have been licensed and many appear to be highly efficacious against Hib. In some instances, these cephalosporins offer advantages over older agents because of differences in their pharmacokinetics or in their toxicities.

Other bacteria (specifically *Streptococcus pneumoniae* and *Neisseria meningitidis)* may produce clinical illnesses in children similar to those caused by Hib. There is usually a delay of at least 48 hours until the causative organism is isolated from cultures and its antimicrobial susceptibility is determined. Consequently, empirical antimicrobial therapy usually is begun before the causative organism is identified. Such empirical therapy should include agents (such as ampicillin and chloramphenicol) or a single agent (such as cefotaxime, ceftriaxone, or cefuroxime) that is effective against ampicillin-resistant as well as ampicillin-susceptible strains of Hib. Once the organism is isolated and its antimicrobial susceptibility is ascertained, therapy should be directed against the specific strain that is responsible for the infection.

The prevalence of ampicillin resistance among strains of Hib ranges from 10 per cent to as high as 50 per cent in different areas of the United States. Although most ampicillin-resistant strains of Hib produce beta-lactamase, some strains are resistant to ampicillin by other mechanisms. Consequently, organisms that do not produce beta-lactamase are not necessarily susceptible to ampicillin. Treatment of serious Hib infections should include antimicrobials that are effective against ampicillin-resistant strains until antimicrobial susceptibility tests have been completed. Chloramphenicol-resistant strains have remained rare in the United States, although they are found commonly in some foreign countries. The susceptibility of strains of Hib to chloramphenicol and to the newer cephalosporins should also be determined for all invasive infections.

Finally, there have been rare reports of the isolation, in an individual patient, of organisms from the blood and from the cerebrospinal fluid (CSF) that differ in their antimicrobial susceptibility. Consequently, antimicrobial susceptibility tests should be performed on all isolates that are recovered from normally sterile sites.

Specific Antimicrobials (Table 1)

Ampicillin

Ampicillin has been used for many years as a first-line drug for the treatment of infections caused by Hib. It remains highly effective for infections that are caused by susceptible organisms.

Chloramphenicol

Chloramphenicol is also highly effective against strains of Hib that produce beta-lactamase as well as against most beta-lactamase–negative strains. However, there are strains of Hib that are resistant to chloramphenicol. Chloramphenicol penetrates the blood-brain barrier very well. In addition, because it is usually well absorbed from the gastrointestinal tract, in instances in which parenteral therapy is difficult or impossible to administer, adequate concentrations of this drug may be achieved in the serum and in the cerebrospinal fluid after orally administered doses.

Unfortunately, because of its toxicity, treatment with chloramphenicol must be carefully monitored. Chloramphenicol causes a predictable, dose-dependent suppression of the bone marrow. In addition, especially in very young infants, very high serum concentrations of chloramphenicol (usually higher than 50 μg/ml) may lead to cardiovascular collapse and the "gray baby syndrome." Furthermore, metabolism of chloramphenicol may vary from person to person and may be affected by the concurrent administration of a number of other drugs such as anticonvulsants or rifampin. Consequently, when chloramphenicol is used for more than 2 days, serum concentrations should be monitored. Peak concentrations (obtained 30 minutes after completion of an intravenous dose or 90 minutes after an oral dose) should be in the range of 15 to 25 μg/ml.

TABLE 1. Guidelines for Antimicrobial Treatment of Invasive *Haemophilus Influenzae* type B Infections*

Type of Infection	Antimicrobial	Dosage
Meningitis	Ampicillin	200–400 mg/kg/day divided q 6 hr (maximum 12 g/day)
	or	
	Cefotaxime	150–200 mg/kg/day divided q 6–8 hr (maximum 10 g/day)
	or	
	Ceftriaxone	75–100 mg/kg/day divided q 12 hr (maximum 2 g/day)
	or	
	Chloramphenicol†	75–100 mg/kg/day divided q 6 hr (maximum 4 g/day)
Focal invasive infections without meningitis (i.e., pneumonia, cellulitis, epiglottitis, arthritis) or bacteremia alone	Ampicillin	100–200 mg/kg/day divided q 6 hr (maximum 12 g/day)
	or	
	Cefotaxime	100–150 mg/kg/day divided q 6–8 hr (maximum 10 g/day)
	or	
	Ceftriaxone	50–75 mg/kg/day divided q 12–24 hr (maximum 2 g/day)
	or	
	Cefuroxime	100–150 mg/kg/day divided q 8 hr (maximum 6 g/day)
	or	
	Chloramphenicol†	75–100 mg/kg/day divided q 6 hr (maximum 4 g/day)

*It is assumed that the antimicrobial susceptibility of the responsible strain is known.
†Serum concentrations should be monitored.

Finally, because of the rare but potentially fatal aplastic anemia that is an idiopathic reaction caused by exposure to chloramphenicol, many physicians now prefer to use second- or third-generation cephalosporins, which have a much wider therapeutic index.

Cephalosporins

First-generation cephalosporins have poor antimicrobial activity against Hib. Cefuroxime (a second-generation cephalosporin) and cefotaxime and ceftriaxone (both third-generation cephalosporins) are extremely potent against virtually all strains of Hib. Because there have been several reports of delayed sterilization of the CSF in patients with Hib meningitis who were treated with cefuroxime, many experts will not use cefuroxime if Hib meningitis is suspected or confirmed. Because of its long half-life, ceftriaxone, administered twice or even just once a day, can be used to treat serious Hib infections. Consequently, ceftriaxone is an attractive agent for treatment of Hib—especially for home therapy of stable patients. Because these drugs (especially the third-generation cephalosporins) are expensive and have a very broad spectrum of antimicrobial activity, if the strain of Hib that is isolated is susceptible to ampicillin and the patient is being treated in the hospital, in general it is advisable to switch from the cephalosporin to ampicillin.

Duration and Mode of Treatment

As with many other infections, the recommended duration of treatment for Hib more often is based on custom than on scientific data. Recommendations should be viewed as general guidelines, with room for modifications for the individual patient whose clinical illness is more or less severe than usual or whose clinical course is complicated by unusual factors. Nevertheless, it is clear that different types of infections caused by Hib should be treated for different durations.

Meningitis

It has been traditional to treat Hib meningitis for 10 to 14 days. More recently, some studies have shown that 7 to 10 days of treatment is adequate for many patients. In general, treatment should be administered parenterally (intravenously) for the entire duration. It is necessary to attain high concentrations of the antimicrobials in the blood because the concentration of an antimicrobial in the CSF generally is only a small proportion (5 to 15 per cent) of that attained in the blood. Furthermore, this proportion may decrease as the patient's clinical condition improves and the inflammation of the meninges resolves. Chloramphenicol differs from the other recommended agents because it is well absorbed when it is administered orally and high concentrations are attained in the CSF (~50% of the concentration in serum) independent of meningeal inflammation. Consequently, if compliance can be ensured, it is acceptable to treat meningitis with chloramphenicol administered orally. In general, however, this approach should be reserved for when the patient is not vomiting, when there is a compelling reason why antimicrobials cannot be administered parenterally, and when serum concentrations of chloramphenicol can be monitored.

Patients with meningitis may require special supportive therapy. In addition, because a substantial proportion of patients with meningitis have the syndrome of inappropriate secretion of anti-diuretic hormone (SIADH), the input and output of fluids and electrolytes should be carefully monitored initially and the amount of fluids administered modified as necessary.

Some recent studies have indicated that the potent anti-inflammatory drug dexamethasone (0.6 mg/kg/day every 6 hours for 4 days), when given shortly before or concurrent with the initiation of antimicrobial treatment, may reduce the hearing loss and perhaps other neurologic sequelae associated with Hib meningitis. Additional studies are under way to try to confirm these findings. Until then, physicians should, after weighing the benefits and risks, consider the use of dexamethasone for patients with Hib meningitis on a case-by-case basis.

Epiglottitis

Because of the risk of complete obstruction of the trachea, epiglottitis is a medical emergency. Initial therapy should be directed at securing the airway through nasotracheal or orotracheal intubation (best accomplished by a trained expert under controlled conditions in the operating room). Tracheostomy is an alternative when intubation is impossible. Initial antimicrobial treatment should be administered intravenously after the airway is secure; orally administered treatment may be started when the patient can take fluids by mouth and is customarily continued for 7 days. The endotracheal tube may be removed when the inflammation has subsided (usually within 2 to 3 days).

Arthritis and Osteomyelitis

Except for Hib arthritis of the hip joint (which should promptly be drained surgically), appropriate antimicrobial treatment alone usually is adequate to treat Hib arthritis of other joints without surgical drainage. Parenteral treatment with an appropriate antimicrobial should be administered for at least 5 to 7 days. If the clinical response is good (as evidenced by the absence of fever, decreased signs of inflammation, and a reduction in the erythrocyte sedimentation rate), a patient may receive the remainder of a 2- to 3-week course of antimicrobial treatment as an outpatient. This may be given either as a single daily dose of ceftriaxone (50 mg/kg/day with a maximum of 2 g/day) or, if compliance can be ensured, as a course of orally administered antimicrobials (amoxicillin, 100 mg/kg/day three times a day or cefuroxime axetil, 75 to 100 mg/kg/day twice daily or cefaclor, 100 to 150 mg/kg/day three times a day).

For osteomyelitis, a similar approach to treatment may be used. In general, patients with osteomyelitis should receive a more prolonged course of antimicrobial treatment (at least 3 to 4 weeks; some experts treat for a total of 6 weeks) than patients with Hib arthritis. As with arthritis, antimicrobials should be administered orally only if compliance can be ensured. It may be worthwhile to check the adequacy of serum concentrations of the antimicrobial by measuring the peak concentration in the serum (obtained 2 hours after an orally administered dose). Doses of antimicrobials to treat osteomyelitis are similar to those used to treat arthritis.

Cellulitis

Although children with Hib cellulitis may be clinically ill, this manifestation of Hib infection usually responds well to antimicrobial treatment. Fever usually resolves promptly, but the local inflammation may not begin to decrease until 24 to 48 hours after treatment is initiated. Prolonged fever may be a sign of concomitant infection (such as meningitis or arthritis) at another site. After the child has become afebrile and the signs of inflammation begin to decrease (usually within 2 to 4 days), a switch may be made to an orally administered antimicrobial to complete a 7- to 10-day course.

Pneumonia

As with cellulitis and arthritis, initial treatment should be with a parenterally administered antimicrobial; however, in children who are not severely ill, orally administered antimicrobials alone may be adequate to cure the infection. If the child responds well to parenteral treatment (with prompt defervescence and decreased respiratory distress), parenteral treatment may be discontinued after 3 to 5 days. Therapy then should be continued with an orally administered agent for a total of 10 days of combined parenteral-oral therapy.

Occult Bacteremia

Because of the common practice of obtaining specimens of blood for culture in febrile outpatients with no apparent focus of infection, physicians will sometimes be informed that a child was bacteremic with Hib 24 to 48 hours earlier. There has been controversy about how such children should be managed, since the outcome of such children ranges from spontaneous recovery to the subsequent development of Hib meningitis. Because of the substantial risk that children with occult bacteremia with Hib will have a focal infection, all such children promptly should be re-evaluated and a careful search for a focus should be made. If no focus is found but the child is febrile, another blood culture is recommended and the patient should be hospitalized and treated with parenterally administered empiric antimicrobials pending the results of antimicrobial susceptibility tests. If no focus of infection subsequently becomes apparent and defervescence occurs, after 2 to 5 days parenteral treatment may be changed so the patient may complete a 7- to 10-day course of therapy with orally administered drugs.

If the child with occult Hib bacteremia is afebrile and appears well on re-evaluation, specimens of blood for culture should be obtained again. Such a patient may be managed as an outpatient with a single daily dose of ceftriaxone (50 mg/kg/day) until the second blood culture is known to be sterile and it is apparent that the child is well and has no focus of infection. Whether more prolonged, subsequent oral treatment for such children is indicated is unknown.

Other Infections

Treatment of other, less common manifestations of Hib infection should be tailored to the type of infection. Thus, children with *empyema* may need a chest tube to drain the pleural exudate in addition to 10 to 14 days of antimicrobial treatment. Children with *pericarditis* may need to have a partial or complete pericardiectomy in addition to more prolonged antimicrobial treatment. Children with Hib *endocarditis* should be treated for 6 weeks. Children with *purpura fulminans* caused by Hib will need to have extensive supportive therapy in an intensive care unit in addition to antimicrobial treatment.

Chemoprophylaxis

Close contacts, younger than 4 years of age, of patients with invasive Hib infections are at increased risk for invasive Hib infection. The degree of increased risk is inversely related to age (for children older than 3 months). In close contacts of children with Hib infections (such as household and day care workers), very high rates of colonization with Hib have been demonstrated. Because of the high prevalence of colonization and the frequent and relatively intimate contact among members of households and among children who attend day care centers, there is an increased likelihood that noncolonized members of the group will encounter and eventually become colonized with Hib. In susceptible individuals, invasive disease may follow colonization.

Ideally, children should be protected by prior immunization with one of the licensed conjugate vaccines against Hib. However, not all children will have been immunized and, in any case, the vaccines are not 100 per cent effective. Consequently, chemoprophylaxis to prevent Hib infection may be indicated. The goal of chemoprophylaxis is to protect the susceptible child from acquiring Hib from contacts by eliminating colonization with Hib in all members of the group of close contacts (the household or day care group). Adults and older children in such groups may transmit Hib to susceptible children even though they are at little risk for invasive infection themselves. Consequently, if there are susceptible children younger than 4 years of age in a household in which a case of Hib disease occurs, rifampin should be administered to all members of the group.

Rifampin

Although recommendations for chemoprophylaxis to prevent secondary Hib infections in households have been widely accepted, there has been disagreement about the use of rifampin for children enrolled in day care centers. First, because the data on the risk of secondary Hib infection among children who attend group day care are conflicting, some believe that the risk is too low to justify the effort of getting all of the children in a day care classroom to take rifampin. Furthermore, because there usually are many different physicians involved, it often is difficult to institute a uniform policy. In addition, in the day care setting, children who are treated may soon become re-colonized with Hib from untreated siblings.

Rifampin (20 mg/kg per dose, maximum 600 mg per dose, once a day for 4 days) is given. It should not be administered to pregnant women. Rifampin turns urine, saliva, and tears a reddish-orange color and may permanently stain soft contact lenses.

INFANT BOTULISM

SARAH S. LONG, M.D.

In most cases, infant botulism occurs through unavoidable circumstances, when an infant under 12 months ingests *Clostridium botulinum* spores. There is no tissue invasion or inflammation. The organism colonizes the intestine and elaborates a potent neurotoxin that is absorbed and binds irreversibly to terminal axons, preventing release of acetylcholine. Symmetric descending paralysis follows, with impairment of muscles controlled by cranial nerves and then those of trunk, extremities, and diaphragm. Autonomic impairment leads to atonic gut and bladder as well as fluctuating blood pressure, heart rate, skin tone, and diminished lacrimation and salivation. More than 1000 cases of infant botulism have been reported since the recognition of this entity in 1976. Cases have occurred in all states, with disproportionately high numbers in Hawaii, California, Utah, and Pennsylvania—probably reflecting soil concentration of spores. The pathophysiology of infant botulism (intoxication following in vivo proliferation) is distinct from food-borne botulism (intoxication) and wound botulism.

TREATMENT

The challenge of management is to recognize the diagnosis early, to prevent sudden catastrophic hypoxemia, and to sustain vigilance over weeks of intensive care in anticipation of regeneration of nerve endings and return of muscle function. The success of treatment depends entirely on meticulous attention to protect the airway, provide adequate ventilation and nutrition, and prevent complications of hospitalization.

Respiratory Management

Respiratory arrest is the primary cause of morbidity and mortality. Respiratory failure is more frequently due to loss of strength of intercostal and diaphragmatic muscle than to bulbar dysfunction. It may occur following days of progressive paresis or occasionally may take place so rapidly as to simulate the idiopathic sudden infant death syndrome.

The patient must be observed in an intensive care unit with continuous monitoring for at least 48 hours to determine the progression of disease. Most patients require intubation and ventilation. Impairment of the ability to cough, gag, and swallow and to move against gravity indicates a loss of reserve muscle strength. Intubation should be performed to protect the airway at this time. Waiting for fatigue, apnea, tachypnea, hypercarbia, or hypoxemia is inappropriate because sudden respiratory arrest and hypoxic encephalopathy or death can occur. Optimal positioning, frequent suctioning, and nasogastric feeding may help to avoid endotracheal intubation in more mildly affected patients. Tracheostomy is rarely necessary and should not be performed "prophylactically" in these immobile patients, who have little traumatic injury to the subglottic airway if care is taken in choosing the tube and in performing suctioning. Atelectasis and pneumonia are frequent complications that are somewhat avoidable. Accidental extubation during manipulation for suctioning, physiotherapy, and positioning must be carefully avoided. Plugging of the endotracheal tube is a serious and not infrequent event that necessitates immediate and experienced reaction. Most patients require intubation for two to three weeks. Criteria for extubation are the return of gag, cough, and sustained motion against gravity.

Nutrition

Decreased gut motility, impaired gag and swallowing function, increased work of breathing during feeding, and fatigue preclude oral feedings in almost all patients. Within a few days of hospitalization, however, continuous nasogastric feeding should be attempted and is almost always successful. Intravenous alimentation is infrequently required over any length of time. The caloric requirement of the immobile infant on a ventilator is approximately two thirds of that normally predicted. Saline enema is judiciously used to obtain a stool specimen for diagnosis or to relieve impaction if necessary. Therapeutic benefit in removal of toxin is not proven. Cathartics are contraindicated because they do not affect bowel motility. Significant fluid or electrolyte imbalance is infrequent except as part of initial dehydration, iatrogenic complication, or inappropriate secretion of antidiuretic hormone, which occurs in up to 20 per cent of patients (usually in association with ventilation). Oral feedings should not be resumed until the swallow and gag reflexes are normal and the infant has sustained strength against gravity and has tolerated bolus nasogastric feedings. Many patients receive nasogastric feedings at home after discharge.

Antimicrobial Therapy

Neither antibiotics effective against *C. botulinum* nor specific antitoxin appears to shorten the course of illness. Aminoglycosidic antibiotics should be avoided because they contribute to blockade at the neuromuscular junction. Fever and an abnormal white blood cell count suggest a complicating infection. Penicillin or ampicillin is usually sufficient therapy for secondary bacterial pneumonia but should not be used prophylactically. Middle ear and sinus infection can occur, especially in conjunction with nasogastric tube presence. Urinary tract infection is not infrequent and is probably related to atony of the bladder. The number of laboratory tests, days of intravenous access, and use of antibiotics should be aggressively limited to obtain the best outcome with the fewest complications.

Infection Control

There is no reported case of person-to-person transmission in the home or hospital. *C. botulinum* is present ubiquitously in nature and is present in the patient's stool. Isolation is not necessary. Good hand washing should be practiced, with the bigger risk being the patient's falling victim to hospital-acquired viral or bacterial infection.

PSYCHOSOCIAL ISSUES

Families require continuous support and counseling. In the usual case, there are days of diminishing strength (frequently to complete paralysis), days to weeks of no change, and then very slow return of function. Although return of function is constant over weeks, it is not constant over hours or a day, because there may be multiple "setbacks." Intensive care providers require continuous encouragement to sustain minute-to-minute vigilance over weeks. Families know that an excellent outcome is dependent on avoidance of mistakes, and they may assume a policing role. This adversely affects the patient's care and can usually be avoided if a team concept is established early.

SHIGELLOSIS

MYRON M. LEVINE, M.D., D.T.P.H.
and KAREN KOTLOFF, M.D.

Shigellosis is an acute infection of the intestinal tract mainly involving the terminal ileum, colon, and rectum caused by bacteria of the genus *Shigella*. The spectrum of illness is broad, extending from subclinical infections to mild, watery diarrhea to fulminating dysentery manifested by high fever, chills, toxemia, tenesmus, and the passage of multiple scanty stools of blood and mucus. Four species or groups of *Shigella* are recognized *S. sonnei* (the most frequent type isolated in industrialized countries and a problem among children attending day care centers), *S. flexneri*, *S. boydii*, and *S. dysenteriae*. One serotype, *S. dysenteriae* 1, the so-called Shiga's bacillus, causes particularly severe disease in less developed countries.

TREATMENT

The therapy for shigellosis can be divided into four phases: (1) emergency treatment of life-endangering complications, (2) specific antimicrobial drugs, (3) supportive measures, and (4) health education.

Potentially Life-Endangering Emergencies

The early stage of clinical illness due to *Shigella* is often characterized by watery diarrhea that, particularly when accompanied by fever, can lead to dehydration in infants. Severe dehydration must be vigorously treated with intravenous infusions (30 to 40 ml/kg) of Ringer's lactate, isotonic saline, or similar solutions to restore the intravascular volume and to correct shock and acidosis. This should be followed by continued oral rehydration with glucose-electrolyte solution.

Convulsions are a well-recognized complication of shigellosis in young children. Airway obstruction due to aspiration of stomach contents and head trauma can occur during loss of consciousness, as with convulsions of any cause. Convulsions should be treated with intravenous diazepam (0.2 to 0.5 mg/kg up to 10 mg) or phenobarbital (10 mg/kg). The high fever usually associated with *Shigella* convulsions in young children may be lowered with oral acetaminophen and by sponging the child in a tepid water bath.

Specific Antimicrobial Therapy

Results of multiple placebo-controlled clinical trials have shown that certain antimicrobials significantly decrease the duration of fever, diarrheal illness, and excretion of *Shigella* in infections due to sensitive strains. This cumulative experience, bolstered by the fact that humans are the natural reservoir and host of this infection, constitutes a compelling rationale for treating all persons suffering from *Shigella* dysentery with antimicrobials. However, this must be tempered by the realization that only a few antimicrobials have proven clinical efficacy (even though many more show considerable anti-*Shigella* activity in vitro) and that increasing use of these effective antibiotics eventually results in the emergence of resistant *Shigella* strains. The increasing prevalence of resistance has been a recurring theme in the treatment of shigellosis. For example, sulfonamides, the drug of choice in the 1940s, were of little practical value by the mid-1950s. Oral ampicillin (100 mg/kg daily in four divided doses for 5 days) became the treatment of choice for pediatric shigellosis in the 1960s. Oral trimethoprim-sulfamethoxazole (10 mg/kg trimethoprim and 50 mg/kg sulfamethoxazole daily in two divided doses for 5 days) replaced ampicillin as the first line of specific therapy in the early 1970s, when resistance to ampicillin became widespread. Recently, nalidixic acid (55 mg/kg daily in four divided doses for 5 days) has become important as strains resistant to trimethoprim-sulfamethoxazole have become increasingly prevalent.

The usual clinical indication for treatment with antibiotics is the child who presents with fever and overt dysentery (blood and mucus in stools). Trimethoprim-sulfamethoxazole and nalidixic acid are presently considered the antimicrobials of choice in the treatment of *Shigella* dysentery. If a particular epidemic strain (or local endemic strains in general) are known to be sensitive to ampicillin, that drug may also be used. In the relatively unusual situation in which a hospitalized child has severe illness with a *Shigella* strain that proves to be resistant to all the first-line antimicrobials mentioned above, limited recent experience suggests that parenteral ceftriaxone (50 mg/kg given once daily intravenously or intramuscularly for 5 days) constitutes effective therapy. The newer quinolone antibiotics, such as ciprofloxacin and norfloxacin, are quite useful in treating shigellosis in adults but, regrettably, are not recommended for pediatric use because they cause arthropathies in young animals given extended courses of therapy. It should be noted, however, that nalidixic acid causes similar arthropathies in young animals, yet is used in pediatrics without recognized adverse reactions of this type. It is possible that in the future short courses (2 to 3 days) of therapy with these antibiotics will be shown to be safe and effective in treating *Shigella* dysentery in children.

Supportive Measures

Agents such as diphenoxylate, loperamide, and tincture of opium, which suppress intestinal motility, should not be given to the child with dysentery, as some animal model and clinical data suggest that these agents may exacerbate the infection. There is no convincing evidence that common antidiarrheal preparations, such as kaolin-pectin formulas, lactobacilli, or bismuth-salicylate, have a significantly beneficial effect on the clinical or bacteriologic course of shigellosis; nor is there evidence that these agents are deleterious or contraindicated.

Health Education

Shigella infections are readily transmitted from person to person by direct contact with minute numbers of bacteria (as few as ten *Shigella* organisms can initiate clinical infection). Consequently, it is imperative to impress upon patients and their family contacts the importance of hand washing with soap after defecation.

UNUSUAL COMPLICATIONS

Several severe complications are recognized to be associated with shigellosis; however, they are rare. The hemolytic-uremic syndrome, leukemoid reactions, and hypoproteinemia are well recognized as complications of Shiga (i.e., *S. dysenteriae* 1) dysentery, which occurs in many less developed countries. Reiter's syndrome of reactive arthritis, conjunctivitis, and urethritis rarely occurs in patients with *S. flexneri* or *S. dysenteriae* infections who have histocompatibility antigen HLA-B27. Rectal prolapse can occur in infants with severe dysentery. It must be emphasized that these severe complications are uncommon, and their treatment is not considered in this article.

TYPHOID FEVER

MYRON M. LEVINE, M.D., D.T.P.H.
and PABLO VIAL, M.D.

Typhoid fever is an acute, generalized infection of the reticuloendothelial system, intestinal lymphoid tissues, and gallbladder caused by *Salmonella typhi*. The peak incidence of typhoid fever usually occurs in school-aged children. A virtually identical form of enteric fever—paratyphoid fever—is caused by *Salmonella paratyphi* A and B. Uncommonly, other serotypes, such as *Salmonella typhimurium*, can cause enteric fever in young infants or immunocompromised children. Infection is acquired by ingesting contaminated food or water. Following an incubation of 8 to 14 days, clinical illness begins with malaise, fever (which increases in step-wise fashion), headache, and abdominal discomfort. Intestinal hemorrhage and perforation are among the most common serious complications of acute typhoid fever, each occurring in approximately 0.5 per cent of cases. With varying frequency in different areas of the world, typhoid fever can sometimes be manifest in an unusually severe form characterized by extreme toxemia, delirium, and obtundation.

THERAPY

The management of children with acute typhoid fever (mild or severe) should include specific antibiotic therapy, general supportive measures, and the treatment of more common severe complications.

Antimicrobial Therapy

Since the late 1940s, oral chloramphenicol has been the drug of first choice for treatment of typhoid fever in less developed countries because of its high efficacy, practicality, and low cost. Indeed, the advent of chloramphenicol has modified typhoid fever from a 3- to 5-week illness with a 10 to 20 per cent case fatality rate to an illness of approximately 1 week with a case fatality below 1 per cent. The recommended dosage of chloramphenicol for children is 50 mg/kg/day in four divided doses (maximum 750 mg every six hours) for a total of 14 days; fever usually subsides within 3 to 7 days but up to 15 per cent of children experience relapses. Chloramphenicol can be given intravenously until the preferred oral route can be tolerated, but intramuscular administration should be avoided because absorption is poor.

Several considerations and events have conspired to tarnish the previously pre-eminent role that chloramphenicol played in the treatment of typhoid fever: (1) A relapse rate of approximately 8 to 15 per cent, (2) the possible occurrence of irreversible aplastic anemia in approximately 1 in 40,000 to 1 in 100,000 patients in certain populations, (3) on occasion, a Herxheimer-like "toxic crisis," and (4) large epidemics due to chloramphenicol-resistant strains in Mexico (1972), Vietnam (1973), Peru (1980), India, and Bahrain (1990).

The occurrence of several large epidemics due to chloramphenicol-resistant *S. typhi* has led to the use of alternative antibiotics, including amoxicillin, trimethoprim-sulfamethoxazole (TMP-SMZ), and ciprofloxacin (in adults). Amoxicillin is well absorbed from the intestine. Children are given 100 mg/kg/day in four divided doses for 14 days. Children who are allergic to penicillin can be treated with oral TMP-SMZ in a dose of 8 mg/kg/day of TMP and 40 mg/kg/day of SMZ in two divided doses for 14 days. Considerable experience with TMP-SMZ has demonstrated that it is comparable in efficacy to chloramphenicol in approximately 90 per cent of cases; in 10 per cent of cases, the clinical response is somewhat delayed. No matter which appropriate antimicrobial is employed in a sensitive infection, the clinical response in typhoid fever is slow. In general, two days of therapy are required before the fever begins to abate and a normal temperature is not reached for 5 to 7 days.

During the past few years, *S. typhi* strains have been isolated from patients in the Indian subcontinent and in the Persian Gulf region that show resistance to amoxicillin-ampicillin and TMP-SMZ as well as to chloramphenicol. In adults, such infections can be readily treated with ciprofloxacin (500 mg every 12 hours) or norfloxacin (400 mg every 12 hours) for 14 days. However, because there remains concern about the possible occurrence of arthropathy and damage to growth cartilage if these quinolone derivatives are given to children (based on animal studies), their pediatric use is not presently recommended. Consequently, at present, in order to treat such unusual multiply resistant infections in children, one must turn to yet other alternatives for which clinical experience is still quite limited. These include several third-generation cephalosporins (cefotaxime, ceftriaxone, cefoperazone) and furazolidone. Although ceftriaxone must be administered intravenously or intramuscularly, it can be given just once daily (80 mg/kg) for 7 to 10 days, and in small series it has proved to be 85 to 90 per cent effective in treating acute typhoid fever in children. It must be reiterated that the use of these expensive, parenteral cephalosporin antibiotics should be limited to infections with *S. typhi* when resistance to the first-line antibiotics is known or strongly suspected. In developing countries, treatment of such multiply resistant infections can be pursued with oral furazolidone (10 mg/kg/day in four divided doses) for 14 days.

General Supportive Measures

Water and electrolyte losses from the high fever and the occasional diarrhea associated with typhoid fever in children must be amply replaced; daily maintenance fluid requirements should be increased by 10 per cent for each degree of fever above 99°F. Salicylates and acetaminophen should not be routinely used because they sometimes result in abrupt changes in temperature, hypotension, and even shock. Body temperature should be lowered by sponging with tepid water. Older children often experience constipation. In general, one should exercise caution and not administer laxatives or enemas to avoid precipitating intestinal hemorrhage. If constipation is problematic, oral lactulose can be administered. This nonabsorbable disaccharide is a gentle physiologic softener of stool.

Treatment of Complications

Approximately 5 to 15 per cent of children with typhoid fever experience relapses that are clinically milder than the primary illness and are readily treated with a second course of antibiotic. The initial treatment of intestinal hemorrhage is conservative and involves blood transfusions. In contrast, should intestinal perforation occur, surgical intervention is now regarded as the treatment of choice.

In areas of the world such as Jakarta, Indonesia, where a virulent clinical form of typhoid fever is not uncommon and is characterized by severe toxemia, delirium, and obtundation, intravenous dexamethasone therapy (3 mg/kg initially, followed by 1 mg/kg every 6 hours for 48 hours) is indicated to reduce the case fatality rate. Steroids should be reserved for this particular clinical presentation only and are not for routine use in the treatment of typhoid fever.

Osteomyelitis is an uncommon complication of typhoid fever that requires more prolonged antimicrobial therapy (at least 4 weeks), preferably with intravenous ampicillin followed by oral amoxicillin.

Depending on their age and sex, a few patients with acute typhoid fever become chronic gallbladder carriers of *S. typhi.* Young children rarely become carriers. The carrier state most readily follows typhoid fever in older women who have some form of prior gallbladder disease. In such adults, ciprofloxacin (750 mg twice a day for 28 days) or norfloxacin (400 mg twice a day for 28 days) can cure up to 90 per cent of chronic carriers without cholecystectomy.

Immunoprophylaxis

Since December 1989, a new live oral typhoid vaccine, strain Ty21a (Vivotif Berna), has been licensed for use in children 6 years of age and older. Four doses are taken at a schedule of one enteric-coated capsule each on days 1, 3, 5, and 7. This vaccine, which causes no significant adverse reactions and provides a moderate level of protection, should be given to children traveling to typhoid-endemic areas and to pediatric contacts of chronic carriers.

NONTYPHOIDAL SALMONELLOSIS

KAREN L. KOTLOFF, M.D.

Nontyphoidal salmonellosis (NTS) continues to be an important public health problem in the United States. During the past 30 years, there has been a steady increase in the incidence of reported NTS, a trend that has been attributed to widespread contamination of foods from animal sources, particularly eggs, poultry, beef, and milk. Furthermore, successful treatment is complicated by a growing percentage of human infections caused by multi-antibiotic resistant strains traced to livestock that have been fed subtherapeutic doses of antibiotics for growth promotion.

More than 2000 serotypes of *Salmonella* have been described; however, the majority of clinical illness seen in the United States in recent years is due to *S. typhimurium, S. enteritidis, S. newport, S. infantis,* and *S. heidelberg.* The clinical manifestations of infection may vary according to the infecting strain. For example, *S. cholera–suis* usually produces severe illness with bacteremia. Antibiotic resistant strains, in contrast to sensitive strains, have been associated with high case-fatality rates. Host factors also influence the clinical spectrum of disease, which is more severe at the extremes of age and in the presence of certain underlying conditions, such as malignancy and other causes of immunodeficiency, sickle cell disease and other hemolytic anemias, ulcerative colitis, and cardiovascular malformations. Patients with human immunodeficiency virus (HIV) infection are particularly susceptible to a syndrome of severe salmonellosis characterized by prolonged diarrhea, weight loss, persistent or recurrent bacteremia, and widely disseminated infection.

Acute, self-limited enterocolitis sometimes accompanied by bacteremia is the most common clinical manifestation of NTS infection. The diarrhea is usually watery, but it may contain blood, mucus, and fecal leukocytes. Associated headache, abdominal pain, fever, and vomiting may occur. The reported incidence of *Salmonella* bacteremia is highest during the first year of life, with a peak during the first 3 months, when it is seen in 5 to 45 per cent of infants with *Salmonella* enterocolitis. In a small proportion of patients, most of whom are young infants, severe extraintestinal infection may develop, manifesting as life-threatening sepsis or focal infections in the meninges, bones, lungs, or elsewhere.

THERAPY

In an effort to prevent systemic complications of NTS, many experts advocate treating *Salmonella* enterocolitis during the first 3 months of life; however, this recommendation has been the subject of much controversy. It is not known whether empiric therapy can effectively confine *Salmonella* to the intestine, and this approach is not without risks. Antibiotics can convert asymptomatic intestinal carriage to systemic illness, prolong *Salmonella* excretion, increase the risk of symptomatic and bacteriologic relapse, and promote the development of antimicrobial resistance. Furthermore, in several randomized placebo-controlled trials, antibiotics were of no proven efficacy in the treatment of uncomplicated NTS enterocolitis.

Thus, antimicrobial therapy should not be used in the normal host to treat asymptomatic carriage or uncomplicated enterocolitis. Antibiotic therapy should be considered in the management of intestinal infection for infants younger than 3 months and those with underlying conditions that may predispose them to disseminated infection, particularly if spontaneous improvement has not occurred. All patients with suspected or proven NTS who appear "ill" or "toxic", who have documented bacteremia, or who have an extraintestinal focus of infection should receive antibiotics.

Ampicillin (200 to 300 mg/kg per 24 hours IV divided every 4 to 6 hours), chloramphenicol (50 to 100 mg/kg per 24 hours IV or orally divided every 6 hours), or trimethoprim-sulfamethoxazole (trimethoprim, 10 mg/kg per 24 hours, plus sulfamethoxazole, 50 mg/kg per 24 hours orally divided every 8 to 12 hours) can be used to treat susceptible strains. The third-generation cephalosporins appear to be highly effective in curing systemic infection, including meningitis, which was previously associated with a high mortality rate. Furthermore, they can be used to treat infections with strains resistant to standard antibiotics. Cefotaxime (150 to 200 mg/kg per 24 hours IV divided every 6 hours) has been most widely used, but ceftriaxone (100 mg/kg per 24 hours IV divided every 12 hours) also shows promise. Quinolone antibiotics, such as ciprofloxacin, have been reported to be effective as treatment of systemic salmonellosis in both immunocompetent and immunodeficient patients and as chronic suppressive therapy in HIV infection; however, these agents are not approved for use in children younger than 18 years because they induce permanent cartilaginous damage in young animals. Although many other antibiotics are active in vitro, antibiotic susceptibility correlates poorly with clinical response.

Duration of therapy is influenced by the site of infection and characteristics of the host. Patients with bacteremia should be treated for 14 days, whereas those with localized infections, such as osteomyelitis and meningitis, and those with HIV infection should receive 4 to 6 weeks of therapy. To prevent relapse after treatment of *Salmonella* bacteremia in HIV-infected patients, some authorities advocate the use of long-term suppressive therapy with oral agents (ampicillin or amoxicillin).

CAMPYLOBACTER INFECTIONS

MARIAN G. MICHAELS, M.D., M.P.H.

Campylobacter species are recognized as major causes of acute bacterial enterocolitis and, less commonly, of systemic disease. These organisms enjoy a worldwide distribution and in many geographic areas are the most prevalent bacterial enteropathogens. The incidence of *Campylobacter* infection in developed nations is highest during infancy, with a second peak in early adulthood.

TRANSMISSION

The chief reservoir for *Campylobacter* species is the animal kingdom, especially birds. They are the principal source of infection for livestock such as poultry, which in turn are the main source of transmission to humans. Additional sources of *Campylobacter* infection include unpasteurized milk, untreated water contaminated by wild birds, and household pets with diarrhea. Person-to-person transmission, though less common than that seen for other enteric pathogens, has been documented, particularly involving young children.

CLINICAL MANIFESTATIONS

Enterocolitis, the most common clinical manifestation of *Campylobacter* infection, is primarily caused by *C. jejuni* and, to a lesser extent, by *C. coli* and *C. upsalensias.* Clinically, the disease is difficult to distinguish from other bacterial causes. However, it often has a nonspecific prodrome of fever, headache, and myalgia and is typically accompanied by crampy abdominal pain. Half of the patients have blood in the stool. Usually, the illness is benign and self-limited; in such cases, treatment is aimed at symptomatic relief and restoration or maintenance of hydration.

A wide variety of extraintestinal complications of *Campylobacter* infection have been reported. Reactive arthritis, Guillain-Barré syndrome, and hemolytic uremic syndrome follow gastrointestinal illnesses; however, bacteremia, endocarditis, and meningitis may appear without preceding gastrointestinal complaints. *C. fetus* has been more commonly associated with systemic illness, especially in immunocompromised hosts or those at the extremes of age.

Neonatal infections can range from benign bloody diarrhea to fulminant meningitis and death. Both *C. jejuni* and *C. fetus* can cause severe neonatal disease. It is believed that transmission generally occurs at delivery, but there is evidence for intrauterine infection as well.

TREATMENT

Prospective trials in both adults and children have demonstrated that erythromycin terminates gastrointestinal shedding of *Campylobacter* within 24 to 72 hours; however, bacteriologic cure is not consistently accompanied by relief of symptoms. This lack of observed efficacy may have been due to delayed initiation of antibiotics. On the other hand, treatment does not appear to lead to a prolonged carrier state. Treatment with antibiotics is advisable in day care or preschool settings to diminish shedding and prevent potential spread. A trial of antimicrobial therapy is also warranted for patients with severe or persistent symptoms.

Erythromycin is the drug of choice. The dose is 30 to 50 mg/kg/day divided in four doses for 5 to 7 days. In adults, tetracycline and ciprofloxacin represent reasonable alternatives. Women in the third trimester of pregnancy who have suspected or proven *Campylobacter* infection should be considered for erythromycin treatment.

Aminoglycosides are first-line treatment for systemic illness.

The dose of gentamicin is 7.5 mg/kg/day intravenously divided every 8 hours. Duration is dependent on the underlying immune status of the host, the response to antimicrobial therapy, and the site of infection. Generally, treatment is given for 2 to 4 weeks. Chloramphenicol or cefotaxime is the preferred agent for meningitis caused by susceptible strains.

Prevention, through use of good hand-washing practices, milk pasteurization, water treatment, thorough cooking of meat, and proper disposal of soiled diapers in hospital settings, remains an important method of control.

Helicobacter pylori Infection

H. pylori (formerly *C. pylori*), has been associated with primary gastritis both in adults and children. In vitro testing indicates that the organism is usually sensitive to ampicillin and cephalothin as well as to other antimicrobial agents to which *Campylobacter* species are susceptible. Antibiotics that are active at a low pH, such as amoxicillin, appear to be more effective than erythromycin. Still, a relatively high relapse or reinfection rate has been documented after discontinuation of amoxicillin. Amoxicillin dosage is 25 to 50 mg/kg/day, divided into three doses; ampicillin dosage is 50 mg/kg/day (maximum, 1 g/day), divided into four doses.

Bismuth salts appear to enhance the efficacy of amoxicillin and ampicillin. Bismuth subsalicylate is administered as a 1.75 per cent liquid suspension, four times a day. The dosage is 30 ml per dose in adolescents and adults, 15 ml per dose for 9- to 12-year-olds, 10 ml per dose for 6- to 9-year-olds, and 5 ml per dose in 3- to 6-year-olds. The recommended duration of therapy is 3 to 6 weeks.

REFERENCES

Drumm B, Sherman P, Chiasson D, Karmali M, Cutz E: Treatment of *Campylobacter pylori*–associated antral gastritis with bismuth subsalicylate and ampicillin. J Pediatr 113:908–912, 1988.

Skirrow MB: *Campylobacter*. Lancet 336:921–923, 1990.

Tauxe RV, Hargrett-Bean N, Patton CM, Wachsmuth IK: *Campylobacter* isolates in the United States, 1982–1986. MMWR 37:1–14, 1988.

YERSINIA ENTEROCOLITICA INFECTIONS

MARGARET B. RENNELS, M.D.

Yersinia enterocolitica is an enteropathogen that invades the intestinal mucosa; it may be taken up by the mesenteric lymphatics and from there reach the blood stream. Yersinial infections are more common in Canada and northern European countries than in the United States. The organism may be acquired by the fecal-oral route from infected humans or animals or from contaminated animal products or water. There are also reports of transmission through blood transfusions; presumably, the donors had transient, asymptomatic bacteremia.

CLINICAL FEATURES

Clinical manifestations of infection depend on the age and immune status of the individual and the virulence of the infecting strain. The most common presentation in young children is enterocolitis, typically consisting of fever, malaise, anorexia, abdominal pain, vomiting, and diarrhea (which may contain blood and leukocytes). Enterocolitis is usually self-limited, with resolution of symptoms within 2 weeks of onset. Older children and young adults may present with right lower-quadrant abdominal pain from involvement of the terminal ileum and mesenteric lymph nodes. This so-called "pseudoappendicitis syndrome" is difficult to distinguish from true appendicitis and has resulted in "outbreaks" of appendectomies. Sepsis and metastatic seeding may occur in immunocompromised individuals. Postinfectious manifestations occasionally seen are polyarthritis, Reiter syndrome, and erythema nodosum; the pathogenesis of these entities is unclear.

TREATMENT (Table 1)

In Vitro Sensitivities

Because *Y. enterocolitica* is capable of producing beta-lactamase, typically it is resistant to most penicillins (penicillin, ampicillin, methacillin, oxacillin) and first-generation cephalosporins. Most isolates are sensitive to aminoglycosides, chloramphenicol, tetracycline, trimethoprim-sulfamethoxazole (TMP-SMX), quinolones (pefloxacin, ofloxacin, ciprofloxacin), third-generation cephalosporins, and piperacillin.

It is important to be aware that in vitro sensitivity does not necessarily mean that the antibiotic will be effective in vivo. Yersiniosis is largely an intracellular infection; thus, only antibiotics that penetrate cells in active forms may be suitable. Optimal antibiotic choice, dose, and length of therapy have not been determined through prospective clinical trials; one has to rely on anecdotal experience and retrospective series for guidance.

Recommendations

There is general agreement that uncomplicated gastroenteritis and mesenteric adenitis in normal children do not necessitate antibiotic therapy. It may be prudent, however, to treat high-risk individuals, such as persons with hemoglobinopathy, iron overload, immunodeficiency, and neonates. Antibiotics that appear to be useful are TMP-SMX (5 to 10 mg/kg/day of TMP orally, divided in three doses), or in children over 8 years of age, doxycycline (2 to 4 mg/kg/day orally, divided into two doses). The quinolones may prove to be very useful in adults but, unfortunately, should not be used in children because of the potential for damage to articular cartilage.

Bacteremic disease and extraintestinal infection have been treated successfully either with gentamicin (3 to 7.5 mg/kg/day IV, every 8 hours), TMP-SMX (10 mg/kg/day TMP IV, divided into three doses) or chloramphenicol (50 to 100 mg/kg/day orally or IV, four times daily). It is recommended that at least one of these drugs be used to treat serious infection. Although most isolates are sensitive in vivo to third-generation cephalosporins, failures have been reported with these drugs. Until more experience is gathered, a third-generation cephalosporin should not be used alone for treatment of serious *Y. enterocolitica* infections. Length of therapy is extrapolated from experience with other gram-negative enteric infections; for example, meningitis should be treated for a minimum of

TABLE 1. Therapy for *Yersinia enterocolitica* Infections

Recommended Drugs
Chloramphenicol
Doxycycline
Gentamicin
Trimethoprim-sulfamethoxazole
Drugs Not Recommended
Penicillin
Ampicillin
Methacillin
Oxacillin
Cephalosporins, first-generation
Quinolones

3 weeks after documentation of negative cerebrospinal fluid cultures, and sepsis is treated for 2 weeks.

Postinfectious syndromes have not been thought to benefit from antimicrobial therapy. Prospective, randomized trials have not been carried out, however, and the recent demonstration of yersinial antigens in synovial fluid cells suggests that a trial of antibiotic therapy may be warranted.

BRUCELLOSIS

EDWARD J. YOUNG, M.D.

Brucellosis is a communicable disease of domestic and wild animals caused by a small gram-negative coccobacillus belonging to the genus *Brucella.* Natural hosts include cattle *(B. abortus),* goats *(B. melitensis),* swine *(B. suis),* and dogs *(B. canis),* and the incidence of human brucellosis relates to the prevalence of the disease in animals. Humans are always accidental hosts, contracting the disease by direct or indirect contact with infected animals or their carcasses or secretions. The bacteria are shed in large numbers in the milk of infected animals, and unpasteurized dairy products are a common source of human disease. Although brucellosis was once believed to be rare in children, it is now recognized that persons of all ages are susceptible to infection with *Brucella,* especially in areas hyperendemic for the disease.

CLINICAL FEATURES

Brucellosis in humans is characterized by a multitude of nonspecific somatic complaints, with a paucity of abnormal physical findings. Fever, lymphadenopathy, and occasionally hepatosplenomegaly are notable findings. The brucellae are facultative intracellular pathogens that localize in organs rich in elements of the reticuloendothelial system, such as lymph nodes, liver, spleen, and bone marrow. Like typhoid fever, brucellosis can be an enteric infection in which systemic manifestations overshadow gastrointestinal findings. Serious complications include meningitis, infective endocarditis, and osteoarticular and genitourinary infections.

DIAGNOSIS

A definitive diagnosis is made by recovery of brucellae from blood, bone marrow, or other tissues. In the absence of bacteriologic confirmation, the diagnosis rests with demonstrating high or rising titers of specific antibodies in the serum. A variety of serologic methods have been applied to brucellosis, but agglutination tests continue to be the most widely used technique.

TREATMENT

A variety of antimicrobial agents have in vitro activity against *Brucella* species, but tetracyclines continue to be the most commonly used drugs. Doxycycline (100 mg twice daily by mouth) continued for 4 to 6 weeks is effective therapy for uncomplicated brucellosis. Some authors report a high rate of relapse with tetracycline monotherapy of brucellosis; therefore, other agents have been used in combination therapy. Commonly, streptomycin (20 to 40 mg/kg/day), in divided intramuscular injections to a maximum of 1 g/day, has been given with tetracycline for the first week or two of therapy.

Other aminoglycosides are as effective as streptomycin in reducing the rate of relapse. Rifampin (20 mg/kg/day) by mouth has also been used in combination with tetracycline (doxycycline), but this combination appears to be less effective than the combination of doxycycline plus aminoglycoside. For children younger than 8 years of age, for whom tetracycline therapy is contraindicated, combination drugs, such as trimethoprim-sulfamethoxazole (TMP-SMZ), have been used with success. The usual compounded dose of (80 mg trimethoprim and 400 mg sulfamethoxazole) is generally given as four tablets per day; alternatively, two double-strength tablets per day can be used.

Although most quinolones have in vitro activity against *Brucella,* there is limited experience with these compounds and their role in human brucellosis remains unclear. Because of reports of high relapse rates when quinolones have been used as monotherapy, it is likely that, as with rifampin, they will be most useful in combination with other drugs, such as doxycycline.

The preferred treatment for complications, such as *Brucella* meningitis and endocarditis, for which bactericidal concentrations of antimicrobial agents are required, is less well defined. Third-generation cephalosporins penetrate well into cerebrospinal fluid (CSF), but there is limited experience with these drugs in neurobrucellosis. TMP-SMZ also achieves acceptable CSF levels and has been used successfully for *Brucella* meningitis with prolonged (4 to 12 months) administration. Combinations of doxycycline and rifampin, with and without TMP-SMZ, have also been used for *Brucella* meningitis. The role of steroids, in conjunction with antibiotics, for neurobrucellosis remains unclear. *Brucella* endocarditis, like neurobrucellosis, has generally been treated with combination drug therapy; however, cures are infrequent without adjunctive valve replacement surgery.

REFERENCES

Ariza J, Gudiol F, Pallares R, et al: Comparative trial of rifampin-doxycycline versus tetracycline-streptomycin in the therapy of human brucellosis. Antimicrob Agents Chemother 28:548–551, 1985.

Hall WH: Modern chemotherapy for brucellosis in humans. Rev Infect Dis 12:1060–1099, 1990.

Lubani MM, Dudin KI, Sharda DC, et al: A multicenter therapeutic study of 1100 children with brucellosis. Pediatr Infect Dis J 8:75–78, 1989.

TULAREMIA

WALTER T. HUGHES, M.D.

Francisella tularensis is one of the most virulent bacteria causing human disease, but it is remarkably susceptible to antibiotics introduced during the acute stage of the infection. Type A strains are found only in North America, are associated with rabbits and tick vectors, and account for 70 to 90 per cent of all cases of tularemia. Without treatment 5 to 7 per cent of infected patients die. Type B strains are less virulent, rarely cause fatal disease, and are associated primarily with rodents and aquatic animals.

TREATMENT

Streptomycin, gentamicin, tetracycline, and chloramphenicol have been used successfully for the treatment of tularemia.

Most commonly used in the past, streptomycin is given in the dosage of 20 to 30 mg/kg/day in two equally divided doses intramuscularly for 7 to 10 days. The total daily dose should not exceed 2.0 g. Ototoxicity, which is primarily vestibular, is the most serious adverse effect; nephrotoxicity is rarely a problem with the usual doses. Recent studies with streptomycin are lacking, and the drug may not be readily available in some areas.

Gentamicin is an alternative to streptomycin and may be

equally effective, although comparative studies in children have not been done. The dose of gentamicin is 5.0 mg/kg/day in two or three equally divided doses intramuscularly or intravenously. Vestibular and auditory ototoxicity and nephrotoxicity are adverse side effects encountered in a few patients. Both streptomycin and gentamicin are bactericidal for *F. tularensis,* and relapses rarely occur after a course of treatment. Other aminoglycosides have not been adequately tested to judge their effectiveness in tularemia.

Tetracycline and chloramphenicol are also effective in the treatment of this infection; however, they are bacteriostatic, and relapses occasionally occur with courses of treatment given for less than 2 weeks. Tetracycline may be given orally in the dose of 30 mg/kg/day in four equally divided doses (not to exceed a total dose of 2.0 g). The intravenous tetracycline preparation is given in the dose of 20 mg/kg/day in four equal doses (not to exceed a total dose of 2.0 g). Tetracycline should be avoided in infants and children younger than 9 years of age because of the staining effect on developing teeth. Chloramphenicol is given in the dosage of 50 to 100 mg/kg/day in four equally divided doses (not to exceed a total daily dose of 2.0 g), orally or intravenously. Aplastic anemia is a rare complication of chloramphenicol therapy. The course of treatment with either tetracycline or chloramphenicol is usually about 2 weeks.

Despite the high virulence of *F. tularensis,* person-to-person transmission rarely occurs. The Centers for Disease Control in Atlanta recommends drainage-secretion precautions for open lesions. No isolation is required for pulmonary or other systemic forms of the disease. Laboratory personnel should be forewarned of specimens sent for culture because once the organism replicates in culture, it is hazardous.

Defervescence occurs in about 48 hours with most cases treated early in the course of the infection. In nonfatal cases in which treatment is started late in the infection (e.g., with chronic draining lesions), little impact of antibiotic therapy may be evident and slow recovery can be expected. Relapses are more likely in patients treated early in the course with bacteriostatic drugs for less than 2 weeks. Lifelong immunity follows the primary infection. The overall mortality rate in treated cases of tularemia is less than 1.0 per cent.

PREVENTION

Documented cases should be reported to the local health department so that high-risk areas may be identified for the institution of control measures.

Impervious gloves should be used in handling rabbits and other wild animals killed by hunters or found dead of unknown causes. Meat to be consumed should be thoroughly cooked. *F. tularensis* survives freezing. One should avoid drinking raw water from creeks, rivers, or lakes.

Children in tick-infested areas should be disrobed and inspected at least daily for adherent ticks. Hairy portions of the body are prime sites. The tick should be removed with forceps or a gloved hand. An attempt should be made not to burst the tick, since infected tissues and fluids may be expelled, sometimes reaching the eyes. Domestic pets should be regularly inspected and deticked. Tick repellents, such as diethyltoluamide or dimethylphthalate, may be used for the prevention of tick adherence.

The use of antibiotics prophylactically for tick bites or contact with suspect animals is not warranted and, when used, may only serve to prolong the incubation time.

REFERENCES

Evans ME, Gregory DW, Schaffner W, McGee ZA: Tularemia: A 30-year experience with 88 cases. Medicine 64:251–269, 1985.

Mason WL, Eigelsbach HT, Little SF, Bates JH: Treatment of tularemia, including pulmonary tularemia with gentamicin. Am Rev Respir Dis 121:39–45, 1980.

Uhari M, Syrjälä H, Salminen A: Tularemia in children caused by *Francisella tularensis* biovar *palaearctica.* Pediatr Infect Dis J 9:80–83, 1990.

PLAGUE

MARIA D. GOLDSTEIN, M.D.

ETIOLOGY

Plague is caused by *Yersinia pestis,* a small, pleomorphic, gram-negative bacillus. In the United States today, *Y. pestis* is endemic in the rodent populations of 15 western states. Plague in this country is predominantly rural and is transmitted to humans by the fleas of infected wild rodents.

People living in the rural areas of the American Southwest may acquire plague by one of the following mechanisms: (1) the bite of the flea of an infected wild rodent or, less commonly, an infected domestic animal; (2) the inhalation of infected droplets from a case of pneumonic plague; and (3) direct blood stream infection via a break in the skin during the skinning and eviscerating of an infected animal. Most cases of plague in the United States occur between April and September. There is no gender difference in attack rate; 60 per cent of the cases occur in people under the age of 20, and 35% of cases occur in Native Americans.

CLINICAL MANIFESTATIONS

The bubonic form of plague is by far the most common presentation, the infection being localized in the regional lymph nodes and resulting in a bubo, an extremely tender often visible swelling of the lymph nodes. The septicemic form of plague may or may not be associated with buboes. The onset of the illness is usually abrupt, with fever, malaise, weakness, headache and, occasionally, gastrointestinal symptoms. Meningitis may sometimes occur late in the course of the illness in spite of antibiotic treatment.

Pneumonic plague is very rare, especially as a presenting symptom, but is usually fulminant and very infectious. Therefore, all plague patients should be isolated until pneumonia has been ruled out or the patient has been treated with antibiotics for 48 hours. Health care workers tending plague victims in whom pulmonary disease has not been ruled out should wear face masks that include eye protection.

TREATMENT

Successful treatment of plague rests in its prompt diagnosis. Classic bubonic plague presentation in an endemic area is easy to diagnose. The nonspecific presentation of septicemic plague makes its early diagnosis more difficult, and therefore a high degree of suspicion is necessary. In endemic areas or in patients with a history of recent travel to endemic areas, treatment of community acquired sepsis should include an aminoglycoside because of the possibility of plague.

Antibiotic Therapy

The antibiotics with the greatest proven efficacy in the treatment of plague are streptomycin and tetracycline.

Streptomycin, Tetracycline, Chloramphenicol

Streptomycin is the drug of choice for severe plague, including septicemic and pneumonic plague. It is given in a dosage of 20 to 30 mg/kg/day intramuscularly, initially in four divided doses, in an effort to avoid sudden release of massive doses of endotoxin, and later in two divided doses, for a total of 10 days or for 2 to 4 days after fever lysis.

Tetracycline (30 to 40 mg/kg/day in four divided doses) may be used in uncomplicated cases of bubonic plague in adults and children over 8 years of age.

Plague meningitis is best treated with chloramphenicol (50 to 100 mg/kg/day intravenously in four to six divided doses). Chloramphenicol may also be used as an adjunct to the other antibiotics.

Aminoglycosides and Sulfonamides

Aminoglycosides, such as kanamycin (15 mg/kg/day in three divided doses, up to 1.5 g/day) and gentamicin (7.5 mg/kg/day in children and 3 to 5 mg/kg/day in adults) are also probably effective against plague, but experience with them is limited.

Sulfonamides, including sulfadiazine and the trisulfapyridines at a loading dose of 25 mg/kg and then 75 mg/kg/day orally in four divided doses, may also be effective. Trimethoprim-sulfamethoxazole has been used successfully in a few instances.

Penicillins and Cephalosporins

Penicillins, semisynthetic penicillins, and cephalosporins, although effective in vitro, are considered to be only partially effective in vivo.

Intravenous Fluids and Glucocorticoids

Besides the prompt institution of appropriate specific antibiotics for treating the infection, in cases of shock the usual supportive therapy with intravenous fluids and glucocorticoids should be considered.

PREVENTION AND CONTROL

Hospitalized patients with plague must be isolated with respiratory precautions to prevent secondary spread due to pneumonic plague until the patient has been receiving appropriate antibiotics for 48 hours. Contacts should receive chemoprophylaxis with tetracycline (0.5 g four times a day for 7 days) if older than 8 years or a sulfonamide (150 mg/kg/day in four divided doses) if younger than 8 years. A plague vaccine is available and recommended for laboratory and field personnel who are exposed to *Y. pestis* on a regular basis.

In areas of high endemicity, surveillance for epizootics and periodic community education must be high priorities. Other measures should include extensive use of insecticides in fields and housing areas, domestic animal flea control, and avoidance of wild rodents.

REFERENCES

Hull HF, Montes J, Mann JM: Septicemic plague in New Mexico. J Infect Dis 155:113–118, 1987.

Kaufman AF, Boyce JM, Martone WJ: Trends in human plague in the United States. J Infect Dis 141:522–524, 1980.

TUBERCULOSIS

LAURA S. INSELMAN, M.D.

INCIDENCE

The overall case rate of tuberculosis in the United States declined until 1984. Subsequently, this trend reversed, leading to a high rate of 10.4 cases/100,000 population in 1991. This apparent resurgence is due, in part, to the large influx of the foreign-born population into the United States in the late 1970s, but it is also recognized in the native-born population. In addition, the spread of human immunodeficiency virus (HIV) infection, homelessness, crowded living conditions, lack of access to medical care, and the increasing incidence of drug-resistant tuberculosis have contributed to the rise in the number of cases of tuberculosis. The resurgence in tuberculosis has occurred in both children and adults and appears to continue on its upward trend at present. An increasing proportion of extrapulmonary tuberculosis has been identified in all age groups. Many of these cases have manifestations that differ from earlier classic descriptions of the disease—miliary tuberculosis in a completely asymptomatic child, clinically advanced tuberculous meningitis with repeatedly normal cerebrospinal fluid examinations, and growth of tubercle bacilli in a pleural effusion.

CHEMOTHERAPY PRINCIPLES

Chemotherapy for tuberculosis is directed toward the eradication of the tubercle bacilli in both extracellular and intracellular sites harboring large and small numbers of organisms, the prevention of the emergence of drug-resistant strains of *Mycobacterium tuberculosis*, and the prevention of the complications of tuberculosis. To accomplish this, in the longer therapeutic regimen previously used, two drugs, at least one of which was bactericidal, were utilized to treat most types of pulmonary and localized extrapulmonary tuberculosis. Three drugs were employed for more intensive initial therapy for widespread pulmonary involvement, as, for example, endobronchial tuberculosis, and for systemic disease. These guidelines were based on the number of bacilli anticipated in a lesion, with more drugs required for larger numbers of organisms.

Short-Course Chemotherapy. Until recently, daily treatment for 1 to 2 years was the recommended therapeutic regimen for pulmonary tuberculosis. Short-course chemotherapy using two bactericidal drugs, isoniazid and rifampin, and supplemented by pyrazinamide either as a daily or an intermittent regimen for 6 to 9 months appears to be as effective as longer treatment for uncomplicated pulmonary tuberculosis. This regimen results in sputum conversion in more than 90 per cent of patients by the third treatment month, has a reported relapse rate of only 1 to 2 per cent after completion, improves patient compliance, and is less costly.

Short-course chemotherapy should not be used when sterilization of the sputum or clinical response in the early phase of treatment fails to occur; when either isoniazid or rifampin cannot be utilized because of drug toxicity or intolerance; when drug-resistant bacilli are present; or when "complicated" pulmonary disease, such as tuberculous empyema or bronchopleural fistula, tuberculous meningitis, congenital tuberculosis, and other medical conditions, such as diabetes mellitus, silicosis, malignant disease, HIV infection, and immunosuppression, occur.

There are two possible short-course regimens. In the 9-month regimen, isoniazid and rifampin are prescribed daily for 2 months and then either daily or twice weekly for the next 7 months. In the 6-month regimen, isoniazid, rifampin, and pyrazinamide are prescribed daily for 2 months, with isoniazid and rifampin prescribed either daily or twice weekly for the next 4 months. Dosage guidelines are listed in Table 1.

Intermittent therapy (twice weekly) is administered only if patient compliance can be ascertained. The drugs are prescribed for a minimum of 6 months after the sputum culture no longer grows *M. tuberculosis*. Therapeutic efficacy is not augmented by use of pyrazinamide for more than 2 months and is reduced by substituting ethambutol or streptomycin

TABLE 1. Short-Course Chemotherapy for Tuberculosis

Drug	Daily Regimen	Intermittent Regimen
Isoniazid*	10–20 mg/kg/day†	20–40 mg/kg/dose‡
Rifampin*	15–20 mg/kg/day§	10–20 mg/kg/dose‖
Pyrazinamide	15–30 mg/kg/day††	50–70 mg/kg/dose
Ethambutol**	15–25 mg/kg/day§§	50 mg/kg/dose
Streptomycin	20–40 mg/kg/day△	25–30 mg/kg/dose
Prednisone	1–2 mg/kg/day△△	—

*The hepatic toxicity of isoniazid and/or rifampin may be increased and may cause one or both to be discontinued when administered concomitantly. The Centers for Disease Control recommend that the isoniazid dose not exceed 10 mg/kg/day and that the rifampin dose not exceed 15 mg/kg/day when these drugs are used concurrently.
**Manufacturer's warning: Ethambutol is not recommended for children under 13 years of age.
†Maximum, 300 mg/day.
‡Maximum, 900 mg/dose.
§Maximum, 600 mg/day.
‖Maximum, 600 mg/dose.
††Maximum, 2 g/day.
§§Maximum, 1500 mg/day.
△Maximum, 1 g/day.
△△Maximum, 60 mg/day.

for pyrazinamide. Although pyrazinamide has not had widespread utilization in children in the United States, it is becoming an important drug with increasing use of the 6-month regimen.

Ethambutol is included initially if isoniazid resistance is suspected. If isoniazid resistance does occur, two new drugs that demonstrate in vitro inhibition of *M. tuberculosis* are added or substituted for at least 1 year. One or both of these drugs should be bactericidal.

The following recommendations for chemotherapy of children with tuberculosis are based on the use of the short-course treatment regimens. These guidelines may be individualized when appropriate, and, in certain situations, such as treatment of adolescents with chronic pulmonary tuberculosis or children with HIV infection, the longer treatment regimen may be advisable (Table 2).

TYPES OF TUBERCULOSIS

Purified Protein Derivative (PPD) Conversion

The presence of a positive reaction to an intermediate-strength Mantoux test and the absence of radiographic changes and physical signs or symptoms suggestive of tuberculosis indicate that exposure to tuberculosis (i.e., infection without disease) has occurred. Pulmonary tuberculous lesions are presumably present but are too small to be radiographically identified and cause clinical manifestations.

A positive tuberculin skin test in a child indicates recent exposure to tuberculosis. Any child with a positive tuberculin skin test reaction who never received previous therapy for tuberculous infection or disease or previous immunization with the bacillus Calmette-Guérin (BCG) antigen is considered a recent PPD converter and should receive appropriate evaluation and treatment.

TABLE 2. Long-Course Chemotherapy for Tuberculosis

Drug	Daily Regimen	Maximum Dose
Isoniazid*	10–20 mg/kg/day	300 mg/day
Rifampin*	15–20 mg/kg/day	600 mg/day
Pyrazinamide	15–30 mg/kg/day	2 g/day
Ethambutol†	15–25 mg/kg/day	1500 mg/day
Streptomycin	20–40 mg/kg/day	1 g/day
Prednisone	1–2 mg/kg/day	60 mg/day

*The hepatic toxicity of isoniazid and/or rifampin may be increased and may cause one or both to be discontinued when administered concomitantly. The Centers for Disease Control recommend that the isoniazid dose not exceed 10 mg/kg/day and that the rifampin dose not exceed 15 mg/kg/day when these drugs are used concurrently.
†Manufacturer's warning: Ethambutol is not recommended for children under 13 years of age.

Therapy consists of isoniazid, 10 to 15 mg/kg/day (maximum 300 mg), given daily for 9 months in the short-course regimen or 12 months in the longer treatment course. Isoniazid is prescribed prophylactically to prevent the development of widespread extrapulmonary tuberculosis, which could originate from the radiographically unidentifiable pulmonary lesions and spread hematogenously. Such systemic disease, particularly meningitis and miliary tuberculosis, is more likely to occur in children. In addition, prophylactic isoniazid may prevent the further development of pulmonary lesions. Prophylactic treatment extended beyond 1 year does not provide greater protection.

Pulmonary Tuberculosis

Mediastinal Lymphadenopathy. Enlarged tuberculous hilar lymph nodes are present radiographically as part of the primary tuberculous complex, which also consists of the primary tuberculous lesion in the lung parenchyma and its associated lymphatic vessels. If calcification occurs in the primary lesion, the Ghon complex is formed. Mediastinal lymphadenopathy without the radiographically identifiable primary parenchymal lesion is the most frequent type of pulmonary tuberculosis in children.

Treatment consists of isoniazid and rifampin as a daily or intermittent short-course regimen (see Table 1). If intermittent or 6-month treatment is utilized or if there is widespread disease or naturally impaired host immunity, pyrazinamide is added for two months (see Table 1). If the longer regimen is used, isoniazid and either rifampin or ethambutol are prescribed for 12 months (see Table 2).

Pneumonia. A radiographic tuberculous pneumonic process indicates local and/or bronchogenic extension of the primary tuberculous complex. The treatment regimen includes isoniazid, rifampin, and pyrazinamide as a daily or intermittent short-course regimen (see Table 1). If the longer regimen is used, isoniazid and either rifampin or ethambutol are prescribed for 12 months (see Table 2).

Pleural Effusion. A tuberculous pleural effusion can result from extension of a subpleural site of infection but may also represent a hypersensitivity reaction to tuberculin. The effusion usually has small numbers of tubercle bacilli, and therefore cultures may not always indicate the presence of the organisms.

Treatment consists of a combination of isoniazid, rifampin, and pyrazinamide as a daily or intermittent short-course regimen (see Table 1). In the longer treatment regimen, isoniazid and either rifampin or ethambutol are prescribed for 12 to 18 months (see Table 2). Occasionally, in order to enhance resorption of the fluid, prednisone is given until the effusion has diminished (see Tables 1 and 2).

Endobronchial. Endobronchial tuberculosis results from erosion of tuberculous caseous lymph nodes into a bronchus, causing partial or complete airway obstruction. A sinus tract may form, allowing passage of caseous material into the bronchus.

Isoniazid, rifampin, and pyrazinamide are prescribed as a daily or intermittent short-course regimen (see Table 1). In order to reduce the size of the enlarged caseous lymph nodes and thereby decrease the airway inflammation, prednisone may be added for 6 to 12 weeks or until wheezing and dyspnea subside (see Table 1). In the longer treatment regimen, isoniazid and rifampin are prescribed for 12 months, with the optional addition of prednisone (see Table 2).

Miliary. Lymphohematogenous dissemination of *M. tuberculosis* from a tuberculous pulmonary site can result in diffuse, nodular, millet-sized lesions throughout both lungs and other organs. Treatment consists of isoniazid, rifampin, and pyrazinamide in a daily 9-month regimen (see Table 1). Streptomycin may be added for 1 to 3 months (see Table 1). In the longer treatment course, isoniazid and rifampin are prescribed for 12 to 18 months, with the addition of pyrazinamide for 2 months, streptomycin for 3 months, or ethambutol for 3 to 6 months (see Table 2). If acute respiratory distress occurs, prednisone is added in either regimen until dyspnea or cyanosis resolves (see Tables 1 and 2).

Chronic. Chronic pulmonary tuberculosis usually occurs in adolescents and adults but may be manifested in the younger age group. It occurs in individuals who have been previously infected with *M. tuberculosis* and may result from either reactivation of the latent infection (i.e., endogenously acquired) or from acquisition of a new infection (i.e., exogenously acquired). Isoniazid and either rifampin or ethambutol are prescribed for 12 to 18 months (see Table 2). Use of isoniazid, rifampin, and pyrazinamide in a daily short-course treatment schedule for these unstable pulmonary lesions may be indicated only if compliance can be assured (see Table 1). Otherwise, the longer treatment regimen is preferred.

Extrapulmonary Tuberculosis

Meningitis. Tuberculous meningitis results from hematogenous spread of tubercle bacilli. Like miliary tuberculosis, meningitis is associated with a 100 per cent mortality rate if it is untreated and is particularly likely to occur in children under 4 years of age.

Treatment includes isoniazid and rifampin daily for 12 months in the shorter regimen (see Table 1) and 12 to 18 months in the longer treatment regimen (see Table 2), with the addition of pyrazinamide for 2 months and/or streptomycin for 1 to 3 months in either therapeutic protocol. Prednisone is utilized for 6 to 12 weeks in order to decrease the intracranial pressure.

Skeletal, Superficial Lymph Nodes, Gastrointestinal, Renal, Pericardial, Dermatologic, Endocrinologic, Genital, Ophthalmologic, and Upper Respiratory Tract. Chemotherapy of each of these forms of extrapulmonary tuberculosis is similar and consists of isoniazid, rifampin, and pyrazinamide in a 9-month short-course regimen (see Table 1). Alternatively, isoniazid and either rifampin or ethambutol may be prescribed in the longer treatment regimen (see Table 2) for 18 to 24 months for skeletal tuberculosis, 24 months for renal tuberculosis, and 12 to 18 months for the other forms of extrapulmonary disease.

In addition, therapy is directed at the specific organ system involved. For example, in skeletal tuberculosis, accessible abscesses are surgically drained, and weight-bearing structures, such as the hip and vertebrae, are immobilized. The presence of a paravertebral abscess, spinal cord compression, or progression of the disease process despite chemotherapy is an additional indication for surgery. In tuberculosis of the superficial lymph nodes, surgical excision of the nodes is combined with antituberculous chemotherapy if the size of the nodes is increasing or, in order to prevent spread of tubercle bacilli, if spontaneous drainage will occur. Pericardial surgery may be necessary in tuberculous pericarditis if tamponade or constriction develops. In renal tuberculosis, intravenous pyelography, ureteral calibration, urinalyses, urine cultures, and renal function tests are performed periodically during and for approximately 10 years following chemotherapy to evaluate the development of complications. Follow-up after completion of chemotherapy for the other organ systems is also indicated to detect complications and permanent changes resulting from tuberculosis.

SPECIAL SITUATIONS

Congenital Tuberculosis. Chemotherapy for a newborn with congenital pulmonary tuberculosis includes isoniazid, 10 mg/kg/day, and rifampin, 15 mg/kg/day, for 12 months. Treatment for congenital systemic and extrapulmonary tuberculosis is directed along the previously mentioned longer treatment guidelines for these conditions, with streptomycin often used as a third antituberculous chemotherapeutic agent, if indicated. Short-course chemotherapy has not been evaluated for congenital tuberculosis and is not currently recommended in this age group. As with any serious infectious disease in the newborn, the presence of central nervous system involvement, even if asymptomatic, must be determined.

Newborn Infant of Tuberculous Mother. The neonate and mother are separated after delivery until the neonate is adequately protected, either with isoniazid prophylaxis or with BCG immunization, and until the mother's treatment renders her noninfectious. These measures are employed to prevent the newborn from acquiring tuberculosis.

If the infant's initial tuberculin skin test reaction and chest radiograph are negative, then either isoniazid prophylaxis or BCG immunization is administered. If isoniazid is used, it is prescribed for 1 year at a dose of 10 mg/kg/day. Conversion of the tuberculin skin test reaction is evaluated every 3 months by Mantoux testing; if a positive reaction occurs, further investigation is warranted for the possible development of tuberculous disease despite isoniazid prophylaxis. If the skin test reaction remains negative, isoniazid is frequently continued for 1 year even if the mother is theoretically noninfectious without bacilli in her sputum. This protection is employed because the mother may still shed bacilli with subsequent respiratory tract infections.

If the initial tuberculin skin test reaction and chest radiograph are negative and BCG immunization is used, the infant and mother are separated until the infant's tuberculin skin test reaction becomes positive. If either the initial tuberculin skin test reaction or chest radiograph is positive, then the infant is evaluated and treated for congenital tuberculosis.

Antituberculous drugs are secreted in breast milk, although in small amounts. Thus, recommendations regarding breast-feeding for a noninfectious mother taking antituberculous chemotherapy should be individualized, with evaluation of the advantages of breast-feeding and the possible risks of drug toxicity to the infant.

Pregnancy. Although guidelines for chemotherapy of tuberculosis during pregnancy are not well established, two drugs are used for treatment of intrapartum active pulmonary disease. Isoniazid and rifampin are usually prescribed, and, if isoniazid resistance is suspected, ethambutol is added. Either the 9-month short course or the longer treatment regimen may be used. Isoniazid, rifampin, streptomycin, and ethambutol cross the placenta. However, only streptomycin has a definite adverse effect—ototoxicity—on the fetus. The possibility of teratogenicity of pyrazinamide is unknown at present, and this drug should be avoided during pregnancy.

Therapy for other manifestations of tuberculosis during pregnancy varies according to individual circumstances. Isoniazid prophylaxis for a recent tuberculin skin test conversion or antituberculous chemotherapy for untreated, inactive pulmonary disease may be given either during or after pregnancy. The risk for development of tuberculosis is greatest during the first year after infection and may, therefore, necessitate the use of isoniazid prophylaxis during pregnancy in some instances. Isoniazid prophylaxis is often begun after the first trimester. Therapy is not necessary in pregnant women with long-standing tuberculin skin test conversions or with previously treated, inactive pulmonary disease.

The presence of tuberculosis during pregnancy is not an indication for a therapeutic abortion. When the disease is properly treated during pregnancy, the prognosis is excellent for the mother and fetus. After delivery, the mother and newborn are separated and the infant is evaluated and treated as previously described.

Human Immunodeficiency Virus Infection. The relatively longer chemotherapeutic regimens are recommended for treatment of tuberculosis with HIV infection because of the presence of profound and extended immunodeficiency. Antituberculous drugs are prescribed for at least 6 months following three negative culture specimens, and total therapy is administered for a minimum of 9 months. However, more prolonged regimens may be used, including the administration of isoniazid indefinitely. If resistance or toxicity is present with isoniazid or rifampin, antituberculous therapy is prescribed for a minimum of 12 months following culture conversion and total therapy is prescribed for a minimum of 18 months. Isoniazid prophylaxis should be administered for at least 1 year.

Exposure in the Home. Any child who has been in contact with an adult in the home with active tuberculosis should be evaluated for exposure or disease due to tuberculosis. If the Mantoux intermediate tuberculin skin test reaction and chest radiograph are negative, isoniazid prophylaxis, 10 to 15 mg/kg/day (maximum 300 mg), is prescribed for at least 3 months. Tuberculin skin test conversion may not have occurred yet, and isoniazid is employed to prevent the development of infection. If the skin test reaction remains negative and if exposure to active tuberculosis is no longer present, isoniazid can be discontinued. If the skin test reaction becomes significant, which, in this setting, is interpreted as having at least 5 mm of induration, then additional evaluation and therapy are necessary.

Exposure Outside the Home. Mantoux tuberculin skin testing is sufficient evaluation of a child exposed to active tuberculosis in a school, camp, or day care center. If the tuberculin skin test reaction is negative, no treatment is necessary, provided that the contact with active tuberculosis is broken. If the tuberculin skin test reaction is positive and the chest radiograph is negative, isoniazid prophylaxis is prescribed for 9 to 12 months. Usually an adult, rather than another child, with active tuberculosis is the source of exposure in these settings.

Drug Resistance. Both primary and secondary antituberculous drug resistance has become increasingly important in the United States, particularly with the recently arrived foreign-born from Southeast Asia and the Caribbean. Drug resistance is prevented by the simultaneous use of at least two antituberculous agents, usually isoniazid and rifampin. If resistance to either one occurs, two new drugs to which the tubercle bacillus is sensitive are either substituted or added and treatment is prescribed for at least 12 to 18 months. One or both of these drugs should be bactericidal. A drug that demonstrates in vitro resistance may still be included because its in vivo activity may differ. If therapy is started prior to the availability of sensitivity data, in a geographic area in which multiply drug-resistant tuberculosis is prevalent, two antituberculosis drugs such as capreomycin and kanamycin, in addition to isoniazid and rifampin, should be initiated.

If prophylaxis is prescribed for exposure to an isoniazid-resistant strain of *M. tuberculosis,* rifampin, 15 to 20 mg/kg/day (maximum 600 mg), may be used alone or in combination with isoniazid, 10 to 15 mg/kg/day (maximum 300 mg), for 1 year. However, these regimens have not been evaluated for efficacy in prevention of tuberculous disease.

CHARACTERISTICS OF ANTITUBERCULOUS DRUGS

Isoniazid. Since its introduction in 1952, isoniazid has become the primary drug in the treatment of tuberculosis in children. It is a hydrazide of isonicotinic acid, is bactericidal, and affects both intracellular and extracellular organisms. It exerts its action in cavities, caseous tissue, and pulmonary alveolar macrophages by possible inhibition of the biosynthesis of mycolic acids in the mycobacterial cell wall and inhibition of enzymes within the bacilli. Peak plasma concentrations of 3 to 5 μg/ml are attained by 2 hours after ingestion, with therapeutic levels persisting until 6 to 8 hours. The drug easily penetrates almost all tissues and fluid collections, including cerebrospinal fluid. It is metabolized by the liver and excreted by the kidney.

Isoniazid is administered orally or, for widespread disease, intramuscularly or intrathecally, as one daily dose, usually in the morning. Dosages of isoniazid for the daily and intermittent short-course regimens differ, with higher doses in the intermittent regimen following the initial 2-month daily treatment whereas the dose remains unchanged in the daily regimen (see Table 1).

Adverse effects of isoniazid include neurotoxicity and hepatotoxicity. Peripheral neuritis associated with isoniazid administration is due to increased pyridoxine excretion and is prevented by the daily ingestion of 10 mg of pyridoxine (maximum 50 mg) for every 100 mg of isoniazid administered. Pyridoxine supplementation is prescribed in adolescents and adults, including pregnant women, but is usually unnecessary in young children with adequate nutrition and without predisposition to peripheral neuropathy. Isoniazid-induced neurotoxicity may also cause convulsions, optic neuritis, tremors, ataxia, toxic encephalopathy, and memory disturbances.

The incidence of hepatotoxicity resulting from isoniazid alone or in combination with rifampin is much lower in children than adults, even when both drugs are used. The hepatic injury usually occurs within the first 3 months of therapy and is transient, with the elevated liver enzyme levels frequently returning to normal despite continuation of the drug. In general, isoniazid is administered if the serum aspartate aminotransferase (glutamic oxaloacetic transaminase) level is below three times normal and clinical manifestations of liver disease are absent. The risk of isoniazid-associated hepatitis is increased with alcohol ingestion.

Other side effects of isoniazid include hematologic reactions, with anemia, agranulocytosis, and thrombocytopenia; vasculitis, including a lupus erythematosus–like syndrome; hypersensitivity, with skin rashes, fever, and eosinophilia; gastrointestinal disturbances; and arthritic symptoms of arthralgias and joint pains. Isoniazid potentiates the actions of carbamazepine, phenytoin, barbiturates, acetaminophen, and vitamin D, resulting in toxicity of the central nervous system (somnolence, confusion, ataxia) and liver. Dosages of these drugs are often decreased during their administration with isoniazid. Metabolic acidosis, hyperglycemia, seizures, and coma can result from isoniazid overdose. Pyridoxine administered in an amount equal to that of ingested isoniazid can reverse the manifestations of overdose.

Rifampin. The combination of isoniazid and rifampin has become the most effective treatment of tuberculosis in children. Rifampin is produced by *Streptomyces mediterranei* and was introduced as an antituberculous agent in the 1960s. It is bactericidal to intracellular and extracellular organisms, causing suppression of mycobacterial RNA chain formation by inhibiting the DNA-dependent RNA polymerase. It penetrates easily into most tissues, macrophages, and fluid collections but only across an inflamed blood-brain barrier. Peak serum levels of 7 μg/ml are attained by 3 hours following ingestion. The drug is metabolized by the liver and excreted by the kidney and gallbladder.

Rifampin is administered orally or intravenously, in one daily dose, usually in the morning. Its absorption may be delayed by para-aminosalicylic acid, and administration of both drugs should be separated by 8 to 12 hours.

The primary adverse effect of rifampin is hepatotoxicity, as with isoniazid. Rifampin causes secretions, including urine, stool, saliva, sweat, tears, and sputum, to become a benign red-orange color and may discolor contact lenses. It can also cause gastrointestinal disturbances; hematologic reactions, with anemia, thrombocytopenia and leukopenia; hypersensitivity, with dermatitis, fever, eosinophilia, stomatitis, hemolysis, and renal insufficiency; neurotoxicity, consisting of drowsiness, ataxia, confusion, and headache; and cell-mediated immunosuppression. Therapy administered less frequently than twice weekly or in doses greater than 1200 mg/day may result in the hepatorenal syndrome, thrombocytopenia, or autoimmune anemia.

Rifampin enhances the hepatic metabolism of coumadin, quinidine, digoxin, oral contraceptives, corticosteroids, oral hypoglycemic agents, verapamil, beta-blockers, theophylline, chloramphenicol, ketoconazole, cyclosporine, anticonvulsants, narcotics, and methadone, resulting in a decrease in their serum levels and subsequent effects. Increased serum rifampin concentrations caused by diminished hepatic uptake of rifampin occur with halothane and probenecid, while decreased concentrations occur with ketoconazole. Rifampin overdose can result in a red-orange discoloration of skin and secretions but not sclera; gastrointestinal irritation; angioedema; somnolence; diffuse pruritus; and elevated liver enzymes.

Pyrazinamide. Pyrazinamide is utilized as a third drug in short-course chemotherapy of tuberculosis. It is synthesized from nicotinamide, is probably bactericidal to intracellular organisms in an acid environment, and penetrates well into tissue and fluid, including cerebrospinal fluid. Peak serum levels of 45 μg/ml occur within 2 hours after ingestion, and the drug is excreted by the kidney.

Pyrazinamide is administered orally in three to four divided doses per day. Pharmacokinetic data are presently unavailable for its use in children.

Side effects include hepatotoxicity, which is rare even when the drug is given with isoniazid and rifampin, hyperuricemia, gastrointestinal irritation, dermatitis, and arthralgia. There are no known drug interactions.

Ethambutol. Ethambutol* is sometimes used as an alternative to rifampin in the longer treatment regimen, as an additional antituberculous agent in multidrug regimens, and with rifampin or isoniazid for an 18-month regimen if one of these two drugs cannot be employed because of intolerance or resistance. Ethambutol is a synthetic alcohol that is bacteriostatic to intracellular and extracellular organisms, causing inhibition of RNA synthesis. It attains peak serum levels of 5 μg/ml within 4 hours after ingestion; concentrates within erythrocytes, which may act as its storage for entry into the plasma; and is excreted by the kidney.

Ethambutol is administered orally in one daily dose, usually in the morning. It is prescribed in high doses (25 mg/kg/day) for the first 6 to 8 weeks and in low doses (15 mg/kg/day) subsequently. A higher dose (50 mg/kg/dose) is used in the intermittent regimen.

Adverse effects of ethambutol include ocular toxicity, which may result in unilateral or bilateral optic neuritis, diminished visual acuity, central scotoma, absence of red/green color perception, and a defect in the peripheral visual field. The incidence and intensity of the ocular toxicity are related to the dose and duration of therapy, usually not occurring with the lower dosage and subsiding upon discontinuation of the drug. Visual acuity and red/green color perception, even in young children, should be tested before, during, and after administration of ethambutol.

Other side effects of ethambutol include hyperuricemia, which frequently occurs by the third week of treatment and results from diminished renal clearance of urate; gastrointestinal irritation; hypersensitivity, with fever, dermatitis, and joint pain; and central nervous system alterations, with headache and mental confusion. Ethambutol is not associated with any known drug interactions.

Streptomycin. Streptomycin is often used in multidrug regimens for treatment of severe systemic tuberculosis, such as miliary or meningeal disease. As an aminoglycoside and a product of *Streptomyces griseus,* it inhibits ribosomal protein synthesis. It is bactericidal to extracellular organisms in cavities and, to a lesser degree, to intracellular organisms, where its action is primarily bacteriostatic. It does not easily penetrate fluid collections and crosses the blood-brain barrier only if the barrier is inflamed. Cell membrane transport of streptomycin is oxygen-dependent, and the drug's antimicrobial activity is markedly diminished in the anerobic milieu of a tuberculous abscess. Peak serum levels of 25 to 50 μg/ml are attained within 2 hours after administration, and the drug is excreted by the kidney.

Streptomycin is administered intramuscularly either once daily or, in severe disease, as a 12-hour regimen initially for a few days and then once a day. Adverse effects of streptomycin include ototoxicity and nephrotoxicity, which are more likely to occur with increased dose and duration of therapy. Ototoxicity may be manifested as vestibular, with vomiting, vertigo, tinnitus, headaches, and nystagmus, and as auditory, with hearing loss, which may be irreversible. Audiograms and tests of vestibular function should be performed before, during, and after therapy with streptomycin.

Although nephrotoxicity is less likely with streptomycin than with other aminoglycosides, albuminuria, cylindruria, and oliguria can occur. Additional side effects of the drug include hypersensitivity, with fever, dermatitis, eosinophilia, and stomatitis; hematologic reactions, with agranulocytosis, anemia, and thrombocytopenia; and peripheral neuritis. Streptomycin may potentiate the effects of neuromuscular blocking agents, ethacrynic acid, aminoglycosides, polymyxin B, and cephalosporins. Elevated serum levels of streptomycin occur with probenecid and result in enhancement of its effects. Overdose in infants causes respiratory depression, hypotonia, and coma.

Adrenocorticosteroids. Corticosteroids are used in combination with antituberculous drugs to treat tuberculosis in children in certain situations. They are often employed to diminish intracranial pressure in tuberculous meningitis, decrease the alveolar-capillary block causing cyanosis in miliary disease, promote fluid absorption in symptomatic pleural and pericardial tuberculous effusions, and enhance shrinkage of tuberculous lymph nodes in endobronchial disease.

The drugs are administered intravenously or intramuscularly in divided doses initially if the patient is seriously ill or orally as one daily dose for less symptomatic disease. Prednisone is frequently used as the oral preparation.

Adverse effects of corticosteroids include pituitary-adrenal

*Manufacturer's warning: Ethambutol is not recommended for children under 13 years of age.

suppression, growth inhibition, osteoporosis, behavioral disturbances, cataracts, myopathy, electrolyte imbalance, and peptic ulcer. Corticosteroids enhance the action of neuromuscular blocking agents and decrease the effect of calcium salts. Rifampin, barbiturates, and phenytoin cause suppression of the effects of corticosteroids.

Other Drugs. Para-aminosalicylic acid, capreomycin, kanamycin, cycloserine, and ethionamide are second-line antituberculous drugs used to treat tuberculosis when toxicity or resistance to isoniazid and rifampin occurs. They are not utilized in short-course chemotherapy. Except for para-aminosalicylic acid, their use in children is limited.

Para-aminosalicylic acid is bacteriostatic to extracellular organisms and diffuses readily into tissues but not cerebrospinal fluid or macrophages. It is administered orally in a dose of 200 mg/kg/day (maximum 12 g) in three divided doses after meals to decrease gastrointestinal irritation. Side effects include hepatotoxicity, pancytopenia, eosinophilia, thyroid imbalance, and hypokalemia.

Capreomycin and kanamycin are bactericidal to extracellular organisms, are prescribed intramuscularly in doses of 15 to 30 mg/kg/day (maximum 1 g), and can cause nephrotoxicity and vestibular and auditory ototoxicity.

Cycloserine and ethionamide are bacteriostatic to intracellular and extracellular organisms. They are prescribed orally in doses of 15 to 20 mg/kg/day (maximum 1 g). Cycloserine can cause seizures, psychosis, and skin rashes, while gastrointestinal irritation, hepatotoxicity, and hypersensitivity can occur with ethionamide.

SUPPORTIVE THERAPY

General supportive measures, including adequate nutrition and avoidance of unnecessary exposure to other infections, which may further compromise the body's defense mechanisms, are important in the care of a child with tuberculosis. Unless the child is acutely ill, bed rest is not required.

The need for hospitalization varies according to the type and extent of disease. Ideally, all children with recent PPD conversions or with tuberculous disease should be hospitalized to obtain appropriate culture material, ascertain tolerance and compliance with medications, investigate household contacts for exposure to tuberculosis, identify and initiate treatment of the index case, and remove all sources of active tuberculosis from the environment before returning the child home. In addition, hospitalization provides an opportunity for family education concerning the importance of the medications and follow-up care. However, this may not be practical, and the decision to hospitalize children with recent PPD conversions or asymptomatic pulmonary tuberculosis may have to be individualized. All children with symptomatic pulmonary, extrapulmonary, or systemic tuberculosis should be hospitalized until the previously mentioned goals have been accomplished and the disease is under control.

If acid-fast bacilli are present on sputum smears, isolation is required until further smears are negative, which usually occurs by 2 weeks after antituberculous therapy has begun. Isolation is unnecessary for children without sputum or without an open wound growing tubercle bacilli.

PREVENTION

The best prevention of tuberculosis is the minimization of exposure by identification and treatment of the index case and chemoprophylaxis of infected individuals. All cases of tuberculosis should be reported to the local health department.

BCG Vaccine. The protection afforded by the BCG vaccine, a derivative of *Mycobacterium bovis*, is controversial. The vaccine varies in potency, efficacy, and immunogenicity and has resulted in serious reactions, including BCG osteomyelitis, dissemination of BCG infection, anaphylaxis, and death. In addition, conversion of the Mantoux tuberculin skin test reaction caused by the immunization results in loss of negativity of the skin test as an index of subsequent exposure to active tuberculosis.

In the United States, the vaccine is employed when compliance with isoniazid prophylaxis cannot be assured in an individual with a negative Mantoux tuberculin skin test and negative chest radiograph who has been subject to repeated exposure to active tuberculosis. The vaccine is also used for asymptomatic children with HIV infection who are at increased risk for tuberculosis. It is administered intradermally at doses of 0.05 ml for neonates and 0.10 ml for older children and adolescents. If the Mantoux tuberculin skin test reaction does not become significant 6 to 8 weeks later, BCG is readministered and the tuberculin skin test is repeated 6 to 8 weeks after that time. The size of the induration of the skin test reaction resulting from a BCG immunization usually measures 5 to 9 mm in diameter. The vaccine is not used for patients with burns, skin infections, corticosteroid therapy, immunosuppression, or children with HIV infection who are symptomatic or unlikely to develop tuberculosis. The vaccine is also not administered during pregnancy.

LEPROSY

(Hansen's Disease)

ROBERT H. GELBER, M.D.

Leprosy (Hansen's disease) is a chronic infectious disease caused by *Mycobacterium leprae*. It is only rarely fatal but, owing to the predilection of the causative agent for peripheral nerves, may cause insensitivity (particulary temperature, pain, and fine touch), myopathy, and resultant deformity. The World Health Organization (WHO) estimates that there are 12 to 15 million cases worldwide.

The successful treatment of leprosy requires long-term compliance with an appropriate antimicrobial regimen, recognition of and considered intervention for a variety of immunologically determined reactional states, the patients' cooperation in protecting insensitive parts from further damage, and skilled reconstructive and cosmetic surgery for established disabilities and deformities. Compliance in any disease requiring prolonged therapy is often inadequate. This may be an especial problem in leprosy because of the lack of troublesome symptoms both initially and particularly after some months or years of treatment and, also, because of reactional symptoms often perceived by the patient to be the result of therapy itself. Because of social stigma, patients and their parents are often fearful of institutionalization and rejection by other family members and friends, do not seek medical attention for a diagnosis that they suspect, or reject the diagnosis and therapy when offered by a professional.

Sociocultural fears and expectations decidedly affect patients' lives. Many patients believe their disease is a result of some wrongdoing. Upon diagnosis patients frequently remove themselves from the life of their families. They may begin to use separate dishes and toilet facilities and to sleep alone. Because of the belief in certain cultures that the disease is in the blood and because in some countries it had been the practice to separate children at birth from affected parents, patients frequently believe that they should not parent children. Children with established deformities become stigmatized and often are ridiculed by their peers. Both functional and cosmetic repairs are integral to the success of medical therapy and allow patients to live normally in society. Education and counseling are necessary initially and on a continuing basis to help patients comply with therapy and not allow certain cultural and psychosocial aspects of the diagnosis themselves to contribute to debilitation.

Leprosy is a disease with a distinct clinicopathologic spectrum. The great majority of pediatric patients, fortunately, have the generally milder tuberculoid (paucibacillary) form of the disease. Patients with tuberculoid leprosy have one or a few hypopigmented, anesthetic macules often with erythematous borders and/or evidence of asymmetric peripheral neuropathy, most commonly of the ulnar nerve. Tuberculoid patients have dermal granulomata; few, if any, acid-fast bacilli; and demonstrable cellular immunity to *M. leprae.* On the other pole of the spectrum, lepromatous (multibacillary) patients have nodular and infiltrated skin lesions, later but more symmetric peripheral neuropathy, and frequently *chronic nasal congestion.* On skin biopsy, lepromatous patients have numerous acid-fast bacilli in the dermis and highly vacuolated or "foamy" macrophages. There is an absence of protective cellular immune responses to the causative mycobacterium. Patients in the middle of the spectrum, borderline leprosy, have features of both polar forms.

TREATMENT

Chemotherapy

The mean age of onset of leprosy is in the twenties, and in many patients the first signs of the disease develop in the first decade or two of life. Pediatric disease is generally mild and without substantial peripheral neuropathy. Because initiation of therapy largely arrests subsequent neuropathy and deformity, early disease detection and initiation of treatment are critical to prevention of serious neuromuscular sequelae. Unfortunately, the very places where the disease is most prevalent are poor and lacking in medical infrastructure, hence the unavailability of the long-term therapy and care required for a salutary outcome. As a consequence, fewer than half of the patients worldwide receive any therapy whatsoever.

Dapsone

Because of the enormous numbers of *M. leprae* and the lack of cell-mediated immunity to *M. leprae,* the lepromatous form of leprosy presents the greater therapeutic difficulty. Dapsone (4,4′-diaminodiphenylsulfone, or DDS) is still the agent of choice for treating all forms of leprosy (Table 1). It is the only agent approved for general use as treatment of leprosy in the United States and has the virtues of being relatively safe, effective, and inexpensive. Dapsone is available in 25-mg and 100-mg tablets. In lepromatous leprosy, administration of dapsone should be initiated and maintained as a single adult daily dose of 100 mg. Suggested pediatric doses are the following: for ages 2 to 5 years, 25 mg three times weekly; for ages 6 to 12 years, 25 mg daily; and for ages 13 to 18 years, 50 mg daily. Although previously leprologists had built up to the maintenance dose slowly and discontinued dapsone during reactions, particularly erythema nodosum leprosum (ENL), these measures no longer appear reasonable. Dapsone is cross-allergenic with sulfonamides and should not be initiated in patients with a history of sulfa allergy. It may cause a hemolytic anemia, particularly in patients deficient in glucose-6-phosphate dehydrogenase (G-6-PD), and may result in dose-related methemoglobinemia and sulfhemoglobinemia in certain patients. Early in therapy, the "sulfone syndrome" (associated with an initially morbilliform rash followed by an exfoliative dermatitis, and at times a mononucleosis-type blood picture, fever, lymphadenopathy, hemolytic anemia, and hepatic dysfunction) uncommonly occurs and corticosteroids in addition to discontinuation of dapsone may be necessary.

TABLE 1. Pediatric Dosage of the Most Important Antimicrobials for Leprosy

Drug	Dosage		
	2–5 Years of Age	*6–12 Years of Age*	*13–18 Years of Age*
Dapsone	25 mg three times weekly	25 mg/day	50 mg/day
Rifampin*	150 mg/day	300 mg/day	600 mg/day

*Dosage is 10 to 20 mg/kg, not to exceed 600 mg/day.

Dapsone monotherapy of lepromatous leprosy may result in the development of dapsone-resistant relapse. This becomes clinically apparent with the development of new lesions despite continued dapsone administration and occurs at a minimum of 5 years after the initiation of dapsone therapy. The risks for dapsone-resistant relapse vary between 2.5 and 40 per cent in different series. Regular full-dose dapsone monotherapy results in the lower percentage of dapsone-resistant relapse, whereas lower-dosage regimens and intermittent adherence to therapy predispose to the higher percentage of resistant relapse. Because of the potential of resistant relapse, borderline and lepromatous leprosy ideally should be treated with at least two effective agents. Furthermore, even after 10 or more years of dapsone therapy, lepromatous leprosy patients harbor viable, dapsone-sensitive *M. leprae* "persisters." *It remains unclear what risk these persisters pose for clinical relapse if therapy is discontinued, and hence the safety of ever discontinuing treatment for lepromatous leprosy is uncertain.*

In certain remote regions, where patients do not have access to medical facilities and cannot be expected to take medication regularly, the repository sulfone DADDS* (225 mg intramuscularly every 77 days in adults and proportionally less according to weight in children) might be substituted for dapsone in all forms of leprosy. However, resulting plasma levels of DDS are low and the potential for developing dapsone resistance is of sufficient magnitude that treatment of the lepromatous form of the disease with this agent alone should be avoided if at all possible.

Rifampin

In both animal and human studies, rifampin has proved to be significantly more potent than dapsone against *M. leprae.* It is available in 150-mg and 300-mg capsules. A single daily adult dose of 600 mg is recommended, and proportionately less is used for children, generally 150 mg daily for ages 2 to 5 years; 300 mg daily for ages 6 to 12 years; and 600 mg daily for ages 13 to 18 years, depending on body weight (10 to 20 mg/kg, not to exceed 600 mg/day). Rifampin turns the urine orange-red. Because it may be hepatotoxic, rifampin should be avoided in all patients with established liver dysfunction. *Discontinuation of rifampin followed by reinstitution has been associated with severe and even fatal episodes of thrombocytopenia and renal failure.* There is no available information on what duration of rifampin together with dapsone will prevent drug-resistant relapse and whether such combination chemotherapy for any duration will allow discontinuation of therapy without subsequent relapse from "persisters." Furthermore, the cost of daily rifampin, about $300 per adult patient-year, is prohibitively expensive in most developing nations where leprosy

*DADDS (4-4′ diacetyl-diaminodiphenylsulfone) is not available in the United States.

is a problem; hence the WHO recommends monthly rifampin for the therapy of leprosy.

Second-Line Drugs

Particularly because of allergy to sulfones and in the therapy of sulfone resistance, other second-line antimicrobial agents may be necessary to treat leprosy.

Clofazimine* (Lamprene) appears as potent as dapsone against *M. leprae.* In adults, 50 to 100 mg orally daily or two to three times weekly is an effective alternative to dapsone administration. Its administration, unfortunately, is associated with a red-black discoloration of the skin, which may be unnoticeable in blacks and other dark-skinned persons but is cosmetically unacceptable to many people with lighter complexions. Clofazimine-induced gastrointestinal side effects of a mild-to-moderate degree affect some patients.

Ethionamide† is even more active than dapsone against *M. leprae* and, when utilized, should be given in a once-daily adult dosage of 250 to 375 mg and proportionally less in children. Unfortunately, gastrointestinal intolerance to ethionamide is common, as is liver dysfunction, particularly when it is used together with rifampin. Indeed, if such a combination is utilized, liver function tests should be carefully monitored.

Streptomycin (1 g three times weekly intramuscularly in adults and proportionally less in children) is as potent as dapsone against *M. leprae.* However, because of its potential for nephrotoxicity and eighth nerve damage, no more than 1 year's therapy can be recommended. Hence, streptomycin should be used only with another agent that can be administered on a longer-term basis.

New Agents

Minocycline, some of the newer macrolide antibiotics, particularly clarithromycin, and a number of fluoroquinolones have been found to be bactericidal against *M. leprae* in mice. Minocycline and two of the fluoroquinolones, pefloxacin and ofloxacin, have been more rapidly effective than either dapsone or clofazimine in clinical trial. Thus, there are prospects that new antimicrobials may emerge to further improve the therapy of leprosy.

Response to Therapy

On therapy, tuberculoid macules may resolve somewhat, disappear entirely, or remain unchanged. Their anesthesia or hypoesthesia properties may also respond variably to therapy. Lepromatous infiltration does not begin to improve noticeably for a few months. Effective antimicrobials, however, do prevent new lesions and the progressive neuropathy of untreated disease from appearing. It is important that both clinician and patient understand these expectations.

Regimens to Treat Leprosy

Because of growing concerns with the emergence of secondary and even primary dapsone resistance, the WHO in 1981 developed some novel treatment recommendations. Triple-drug therapy was suggested for adults with multibacillary leprosy: rifampin (600 mg once monthly, supervised; dapsone (100 mg daily); clofazimine (300 mg once monthly, supervised, plus 50 mg daily). The WHO recommends that this therapy be maintained for at least 2 years, preferably until skin smears are bacteriologically negative (negativity generally occurs in 5 years) and that all therapy then be discontinued. For adult patients with paucibacillary disease, dapsone (100 mg daily) and rifampin (600 mg monthly, supervised) are recommended for a total of 6 months. My own experience suggests that primary dapsone resistance is most uncommon, the few resistant strains being only partially resistant and sensitive to levels achieved by generally recommended dapsone doses. Furthermore, patients harboring partially dapsone-resistant strains respond clinically to dapsone. In the United States, the author recommends dapsone sensitivity studies in newly diagnosed patients; if high-level dapsone resistance is found, multibacillary patients should receive rifampin daily and clofazimine three times weekly and paucibacillary patients should receive rifampin daily alone.

Monthly rifampin and the reduced duration of therapy recommended by the WHO for both tuberculoid and lepromatous leprosy are largely a result of important economic considerations in developing countries. Because such economic considerations are not particularly relevant in the United States and Western Europe and because there is limited clinical experience with these reduced durations, the author has not adopted monthly rifampin or these reduced courses of therapy. For multibacillary leprosy, the author and authorities at the G. W. Long Hansen's Disease Center advise rifampin daily for 3 years and dapsone daily lifelong. The author treats paucibacillary leprosy with dapsone daily for 5 years. Authorities at the G. W. Long Hansen's Disease Center treat adult paucibacillary leprosy with dapsone (100 mg daily for 3 to 5 years) and with rifampin (600 mg daily for the first 6 months).

Reactions and Their Management

In about 50 per cent of patients with lepromatous leprosy, the syndrome of erythema nodosum leprosum (ENL, lepra type 2 reaction) may develop, generally within the first few years of antimicrobial therapy. This syndrome may consist of one or a number of the following manifestations: crops of erythematous, painful skin papules that remain a few days and may pustulate and ulcerate, being most commonly found on the extensor surface of the extremities; fever that may be as high as 105°F (40.5°C); painful neuritis that may result in further nerve damage; lymphadenitis; uveitis; orchitis; and occasionally large-joint arthritis and glomerulonephritis. Histopathologically, this syndrome is secondary to a vasculitis and is probably the result of immune complexes. The clinical manifestations may be mild and evanescent or severe, recurrent, and occasionally fatal.

Patients with borderline leprosy may show signs of inflammation, usually within previous skin lesions, and painful neuritis, which may cause further nerve damage and occasionally fever (lepra type 1 reactions). If these occur prior to therapy, they are termed "down-grading reactions"; if these occur during therapy, usually within a few weeks or months of the start of treatment, they are termed "reversal reactions." Therapy is required in the presence of neuritis, with skin inflammation of a sufficient extent that ulceration appears likely, or for cosmetic reasons, especially if lesions involve the face.

Because the majority of cases of childhood leprosy are tuberculoid and because the described reactional states occur in borderline and lepromatous leprosy, reactions are not really as much a problem in affected children as they are in adults.

Corticosteroids are effective in ENL, and generally even the most severe cases can be controlled with adult doses of prednisone (60 mg). In this respect, I have not found alternate-day steroids useful. Individual ENL papules resolve in a matter of days, and control can be best judged by the assessment of the prevention of new manifestations. When episodes are controlled, steroid doses can be tapered and then discon-

*Clofazimine is available from the G. W. Long Hansen's Disease Center, Carville, LA 70721.

†This use of ethionamide is not listed by the manufacturer.

tinued, generally in 1 to 4 weeks. If ENL appears to be recurrent, thalidomide is the drug of choice for its control and prevention. The dosage must be individualized, and the minimal amount necessary to control ENL manifestation is advised; in adults, generally 100 to 400 mg in a single evening dose is sufficient. In the United States and Canada, thalidomide is available to licensed physicians participating as co-investigators on the investigational license sponsored by Dr. Robert Hastings, G. W. Long Hansen's Disease Center. In the United States, there are a number of National Ambulatory Hansen's Disease Clinics and private physicians licensed to prescribe thalidomide. (For information, call 800–642–2477.) An occasional patient, despite thalidomide therapy, may still require corticosteroids to prevent recurrent ENL.

Because of thalidomide's potential for causing severe birth defects, including phocomelia, it should not be administered to women in the childbearing years. Side effects include tranquilization (to which tolerance generally develops rapidly), leukopenia, and constipation.

Clofazimine, although slow in onset of action and only moderately effective in adult doses of 300 mg/day, may enable one to reduce the steroid requirement for therapy of ENL.

Thalidomide is of no value for lepra type 1 reactions. Corticosteroids are usually effective in controlling these reactions in adult doses of prednisone (40 to 60 mg/day), but generally they must be maintained at a lowered dose for a few months to prevent recurrence. Clofazimine may be of some value in decreasing the steroid requirement in these reactions in the same dose as in the treatment of ENL, but it is not as effective in lepra type 1 reactions.

Rehabilitation

Follow-up visits should always include examination of the feet, and plantar ulcers must be vigorously treated with specific antibiotics, débridement, and either bed rest or a total-contact walking cast until healed. Judicious use of extra-depth shoes with molded inserts or specially molded shoes is crucial to prevent recurrence. Tendon transfers to permit substitutions of innervated for denervated muscles may provide patients with more functional use of hands, correct foot drop, and enable them to close their eyes so that corneal trauma and its sequelae will not lead to blindness. If maximal results are to be expected, reconstructive surgery should not be initiated until patients have received at least 6 months of therapy directed against *M. leprae* and at least 6 months have passed since signs of reaction have abated. When possible, mechanical devices may help the severely deformed, and special job training may be necessary to prevent trauma and further disability.

Prophylaxis

The close, prolonged, intimate contact of household members of lepromatous patients poses some risk for the development of subsequent disease (about 10 per cent in endemic countries and 1 per cent in nonendemic locales). Although tuberculoid leprosy is not contagious, family members of tuberculoid patients may be incubating disease obtained from the same source. The author recommends that household contacts of patients be examined annually for 5 to 7 years, preferably by a physician experienced in leprosy. Health workers and casual contacts appear to be at no significant risk. Therefore, when patients are hospitalized, no isolation requirements are necessary.

Trials of chemoprophylaxis with sulfones have at most been marginally effective. Thus, they are not generally recommended. Bacille Calmette-Guérin (BCG) vaccination has been successful in some locales and not in others. It is not generally recommended. In the future, however, vaccines utilizing heat-killed *M. leprae* alone and combined with BCG or *M. leprae* products may prove more efficacious in inducing the necessary protective cellular immunity. Specific and sensitive serodiagnosis of leprosy has recently become possible owing to the presence of circulating antibodies, particularly of the IgM class, directed at an *M. leprae*–specific phenolic glycolipid in nearly all lepromatous patients and about two thirds of tuberculoid patients. It is hoped that early serodiagnosis during the long incubation period may soon prove feasible and useful in leprosy control.

THE ATYPICAL MYCOBACTERIA

ANN M. APALSCH, M.D.
and KENNETH E. SCHUIT, M.D., Ph.D.

The nontuberculous, or atypical, mycobacteria are ubiquitous microbes of relatively low virulence found in soil and water. In this article, for purposes of simplicity, we refer to these bacteria as MOTT (mycobacteria other than tuberculosis). The species that most frequently cause disease in children are *M. avium–intracellulare* (MAC for *M. avium–intracellulare* complex), *M. scrofulaceum,* and *M. kansasii.* Infections are also caused by *M. chelonei, M. fortuitum, M. marinum,* and *M. xenopi.*

PRESENTATION AND NATURAL HISTORY

Children with infections caused by MOTT classically present with chronic cervical lymphadenitis. Typically, patients are between 1 and 5 years and healthy, living in an urban area and with no history of exposure to tuberculosis. The nodes are usually unilateral and nontender; they involve the cervical or preauricular chains close to the mandible and can become matted and confluent. The lesions are often violaceous in color and minimally tender. With time, the skin may thin, and occasionally a sinus tract or ulcer develops. Fever and other constitutional findings are uncommon. Patients generally seek medical evaluation some weeks after appearance of the mass. The responsible species is usually MAC (in 70 to 80 per cent of cases) or *M. scrofulaceum* (20 to 30 per cent) but varies with region.

Localized skin lesions associated with trauma can result in abscess formation or draining lesions and are usually due to *M. fortuitum* or *M. chelonei.* Painless papules associated with lesions sustained in swimming pools or fish tanks are caused by *M. marinum.*

Unusual presentations of MOTT infections in children include disseminated disease and nonpulmonary focal infections in presumably normal hosts, pulmonary disease in patients with cystic fibrosis, and opportunistic infections in patients with acquired immunodeficiency syndrome (AIDS).

DIAGNOSIS

The diagnosis of MOTT adenitis should be suspected clinically in any patient with persistent, nontender cervical nodes. Other important diagnostic considerations are pyogenic and tuberculous adenitis. Pyogenic adenitis is usually more tender, erythematous, and warm to touch. Tuberculous adenitis is more often bilateral and more likely to occur in noncervical nodes than is MOTT adenitis.

In areas where tuberculosis is common, the differentiation between tuberculous adenitis and adenitis caused by MOTT may be difficult. Three important diagnostic clues should be sought as important issues in favor of the diagnosis of tuberculous adenitis: (1) the history of exposure to an individual with active tuberculosis, (2) an abnormal chest x-ray suggestive of primary tuberculosis, and (3) positive tuberculin skin tests in the patient and family members. Other diagnoses to be entertained in a patient with chronic lymphadenitis include cat-scratch disease, viral infections, toxoplasmosis, tumors, and congenital anomalies.

In the past, antigens prepared from a number of the more common MOTT species were available for purposes of skin testing (PPD-B, PPD-G). These antigens are not currently available. The mycobacterial skin tests that are available (PPD-T and the Tine) are not consistently reliable in the diagnosis of MOTT. These tests help to diagnose mycobacterial infection but do not differentiate in a reliable fashion between MOTT and tuberculous disease.

Today, the diagnosis of MOTT cervical adenitis is made on the basis of clinical evaluation and, if necessary, on excisional biopsy. The "gold standard" for the diagnosis of MOTT adenitis is excisional biopsy with histologic evidence of caseating granuloma, demonstration of acid-fast bacilli, and positive culture. Culture and speciation of the mycobacteria can take several weeks, and up to 50 per cent of cultures may remain sterile.

Diagnosis of other infections, including cutaneous and pulmonary disease, rests on having a high index of suspicion and on careful culture procedures. Skin lesions should be drained. In patients with chronic pulmonary disease (including cystic fibrosis), microscopic examination should be undertaken and specimens of sputum or bronchoscopic washings should be obtained for culture. In patients with suspected disseminated disease, special blood culturing techniques should be employed because routine blood culture media will not support growth of MOTT.

TREATMENT

In general, MOTT infections are not life-threatening and will resolve without specific therapy. Complete resolution may take months, causing considerable cosmetic concern but little functional compromise. MOTT species should be considered resistant to the commonly used antituberculous drugs. In vitro sensitivity testing is necessary to determine which, if any, antituberculous drugs may be helpful against any given strain.

Lymphadenitis

Diseased lymph nodes that are small and do not drain or affect the overlying skin do not warrant treatment. The recommended treatment for lymphadenitis of significance is excisional biopsy, a procedure that can be of diagnostic value as well. Simple needle aspiration or incision and drainage is not recommended because of the possibility that a fistula or chronically draining lesion will result.

Treatment with antituberculous compounds is not recommended unless there is a possibility that the patient has tuberculosis. If, for example, the patient has a documented tuberculous contact, an abnormal chest x-ray, or a strongly reactive PPD-T (>15 mm), presumptive treatment for extrapulmonary tuberculosis is recommended until definitive results are available. If relapse occurs, the advisability of a second excision versus excision plus chemotherapy is controversial. Antituberculous therapy should be considered when complete excision is not an option.

Disseminated Disease

Pulmonary or disseminated disease caused by MOTT is unusual in children; thus, no randomized, controlled treatment trials have been undertaken. However, most authorities recommend prolonged treatment with at least three antituberculous agents, the choice of which should be based on in vitro sensitivity testing. Agents that should be tested routinely include rifampin, isoniazid, pyrazinamide, streptomycin, and ethionamide. In some cases, newer drugs such as clarithromycin, ansamycin, clofazimine, and a quinolone may be considered. (Because of its effect on connective tissue development, the use of the quinolones in children should be avoided if possible). Treatment of MOTT infections in children with AIDS is complicated by profound immune suppression in these patients.

Cutaneous lesions, caused by the rapidly growing mycobacteria or by *M. marinum*, should be removed surgically if possible. Minocycline or doxycycline has been used to treat skin lesions caused by *M. marinum* in children older than 8 years of age.

Patients with MOTT infections do not need to be isolated, as person-to-person spread does not occur. The only exception to this rule is in the child with cavitary or draining lesions in whom the diagnosis of tuberculosis has not been ruled out.

SYPHILIS

PABLO J. SANCHEZ, M.D.

Since 1986, there has been a steady increase in the incidence of primary and secondary syphilis in the United States. This increase has been greatest among blacks and Hispanics in such large urban areas as New York City, Miami, Los Angeles, and Detroit, and is largely due to the exchange of drugs, particularly crack cocaine, for sex with multiple partners of unknown identities. Such practice makes partner notification, a traditional syphilis control measure, virtually impossible. Most disturbing has been the overrepresentation of cases among women that has resulted in a dramatic rise in the incidence of congenital syphilis. In 1990, more than 2800 cases of congenital syphilis were reported to the Centers for Disease Control (CDC) in Atlanta. Moreover, the role of *Treponema pallidum* as a cofactor for transmission of the human immunodeficiency virus (HIV) has made syphilis a major public health problem for the 1990s.

TREATMENT

Penicillin remains the drug of choice for treatment of both acquired and congenital syphilis. A serum concentration of 0.018 μg/ml is required to ensure adequate killing of the organism and must be maintained for 7 days in early cases and up to 3 weeks in late disease. No penicillin-resistant isolate has yet been recovered.

All patients with reactive serologic findings for syphilis should be counseled concerning the risks of HIV infection and tested for HIV antibody.

Persons Exposed to Syphilis

A person exposed sexually to a patient with early syphilis may be infected yet seronegative if the exposure occurred within the previous 90 days. In such a case, the person should be treated presumptively with benzathine penicillin G (50,000 U/kg intramuscularly [IM], with a maximum dose of 2.4 million units). The efficacy of either tetracycline or ceftriaxone is less. Combination therapy with ceftriaxone and doxycycline, recommended for treatment of gonorrhea, is probably effective against incubating syphilis.

Early Syphilis (Primary, Secondary, and Early Latent Syphilis of Less Than One Year's Duration)

The recommended treatment is a single intramuscular injection of benzathine penicillin G (50,000 U/kg IM, not to exceed 2.4 million units). Alternative regimens for nonpregnant, penicillin-allergic adult patients include doxycycline (100 mg orally two times a day for 2 weeks) or tetracycline (500 mg orally four times a day for 2 weeks). Both are equivalent therapies; compliance, however, is improved with doxycycline because fewer doses are required, it can be taken with meals, and it is associated with less gastrointestinal irritation. Tetracycline and doxycycline are not recommended for children younger than 9 years of age because of the risk of dental staining. The use of erythromycin has resulted in higher rates of failure as well as poor compliance secondary to gastrointestinal side effects. Ceftriaxone (250 mg intramuscularly once a day for 10 days) also appears to be effective therapy, although clinical experience is limited.

Nontreponemal antibody titers should decline fourfold by 3 months following treatment with primary or secondary syphilis or by 6 months with early latent infection. Failure of serologic titers to decrease appropriately is reason for cerebrospinal fluid (CSF) examination and re-treatment unless reinfection can be established as the cause.

Late Latent Syphilis of More Than One Year's Duration

Benzathine penicillin G (50,000 U/kg IM, maximum 2.4 million units), administered 1 week apart for 3 consecutive weeks, is the treatment of choice. For nonpregnant penicillin-allergic patients, doxycycline (100 mg orally twice a day for 4 weeks) or tetracycline (500 mg orally four times a day for 4 weeks) may be given but only after CSF examination has excluded neurosyphilis. Other indications for lumbar puncture in these patients include neurologic signs or symptoms, treatment failure, serum nontreponemal antibody titer greater than 1:32, other evidence of active syphilis, such as aortitis, gumma, or iritis, and a positive HIV antibody test. If results of the CSF examination are consistent with neurosyphilis, a regimen appropriate for neurosyphilis is indicated. Tetracycline or doxycycline should not be given to children younger than 9 years because of the risk of dental staining.

Quantitative nontreponemal serologic testing should be performed 6 and 12 months after treatment. If serologic titers increase fourfold or if there is recurrence or persistence of clinical signs, re-evaluation for possible neurosyphilis and re-treatment is recommended.

Neurosyphilis

The recommended treatment of neurosyphilis is intravenous (IV) aqueous crystalline penicillin G (200,000 to 300,000 U/kg/day, or 50,000 U/kg every 4 to 6 hours) for 10 to 14 days. The maximum adult dose is 12 to 24 million units/day (2 to 4 million units IV every 4 hours) administered intravenously for 10 to 14 days. If outpatient compliance can be ensured, an alternative regimen consists of daily aqueous procaine penicillin G (2.4 million units IM) plus probenicid (500 mg orally four times a day), both for 10 to 14 days. Some authorities follow both of these treatment regimens with benzathine penicillin G (50,000 U/kg IM, maximum adult dose 2.4 million units), for 3 successive weeks. Patients with a history of penicillin allergy should be skin-tested and desensitized if necessary. Amoxicillin (6 g combined with 2 g of probenicid daily), doxycycline (200 mg twice daily), and ceftriaxone (1 g daily for 14 days) have been used as alternative regimens. However, insufficient clinical data and follow-up are available for any of these regimens to be recommended.

A follow-up CSF examination should be performed every 6 months until findings are normal. CSF pleocytosis that has not improved significantly by 6 months or failure of CSF results to become normal by 2 years after therapy are indications for re-treatment.

Syphilis in Pregnancy

Pregnant women should be treated with the penicillin regimen appropriate for the stage of syphilis. Benzathine penicillin G remains the drug of choice for treatment of maternal infection and prevention of congenital syphilis. The efficacy in early syphilis is approximately 98 per cent. Tetracycline and doxycycline are contraindicated during pregnancy because both can result in staining of decidual teeth. Tetracycline also has been associated with temporary impairment of long bone growth and with hepatic toxicity in pregnant patients who have impaired renal function. Erythromycin should not be used because of unpredictable maternal serum levels and transplacental transfer, leading to a high risk of failure to cure infection in the fetus. Pregnant women with a history of penicillin allergy should be skin tested and, if necessary, desensitized according to the protocol established by Wendel et al. (see References).

Follow-up consists of monthly quantitative serologic testing until delivery. Criteria for re-treatment are similar as for nonpregnant individuals.

Syphilis in HIV-Infected Patients

Patients coinfected with syphilis and HIV can be treated for syphilis with a regimen similar to that for patients who lack HIV antibody. Penicillin therapy, however, should be used whenever possible in these patients. Moreover, careful and frequent clinical and serologic follow-up at 1, 2, 3, 6, 9, and 12 months after treatment is indicated. If nontreponemal antibody titers have not declined fourfold by 3 months with primary or secondary syphilis or by 6 months in early latent syphilis, or if the titer has increased fourfold at any time, then a CSF examination should be performed and the patient re-treated with a neurosyphilis regimen unless reinfection can be established as the cause of the increased titer.

Congenital Syphilis

The decision to treat an infant for congenital syphilis is based on the clinical presentation, previous serologic test results and treatment of the mother, and results of serologic testing of the infant and mother at the time of delivery. Treatment at birth is required for the following situations:

1. The infant is symptomatic.
2. There is no documented maternal treatment before delivery.
3. Maternal treatment has been inadequate or unknown.
4. The mother has been treated with drugs other than penicillin.
5. The mother has been appropriately treated previously for syphilis, but there is evidence of reinfection during the pregnancy, either by physical examination or a fourfold increase in serologic test result.
6. The mother has been treated within 4 weeks of delivery.
7. Adequate follow-up of the infant is uncertain.

Infants who are 4 weeks of age or younger and who have proven or highly probable disease (i.e., symptomatic infants or asymptomatic infants with an abnormal CSF examination, abnormal bone radiographs, or laboratory evaluation) should be treated for 10 to 14 days with either: (1) aqueous crystalline penicillin G (50,000 U/kg [IV] every 12 hours for the first 7 days of life and every 8 hours beyond 1 week of age); or (2) aqueous procaine penicillin G (50,000 U/kg IM once daily).

Similar infants who are older than 4 weeks of age should receive aqueous penicillin G (50,000 U/kg IV every 6 hours for 10 to 14 days).

The treatment of the asymptomatic infant with a normal CSF, laboratory, and radiographic findings is dependent on maternal treatment history and HIV status. If maternal treatment was nonexistent, inadequate, unknown, or with erythromycin, a 10-day course of either aqueous penicillin G or procaine penicillin G is preferred by such authorities as the CDC. Alternatively, a single intramuscular injection of benzathine penicillin G (50,000 U/kg) can be administered with follow-up serologic testing of the infant (see later). Failure of a single injection of benzathine penicillin G administered to three asymptomatic infants has been reported. These infants were delivered of mothers with early syphilis and were not fully evaluated for evidence of congenital syphilis at delivery. These treatment failures have been attributed to the inability of penicillin to adequately penetrate and achieve treponemicidal concentration in certain sites such as the aqueous humor and central nervous system. Infants born to women coinfected with syphilis and HIV may be at higher risk for infection with *T. pallidum.* It is not known whether coinfected infants respond to treatment for congenital syphilis differently from infants uninfected with HIV. For these reasons, asymptomatic infants born to coinfected mothers should receive a 10-day course of IV aqueous penicillin G or IM procaine penicillin G rather than a single IM dose of benzathine penicillin.

Asymptomatic infants born to mothers treated for syphilis within 4 weeks of delivery can be treated with a single IM dose of benzathine penicillin G (50,000 U/kg) unless the mother is coinfected with HIV, in which case a 10-day course of penicillin may be preferred. If the mother received adequate therapy more than 4 weeks before delivery, the infant does not require any treatment if adequate follow-up can be ensured. Benzathine penicillin G is adequate therapy for these infants if the evaluation is normal, if adequate follow-up cannot be ensured, or if the mother is HIV-antibody positive. These infants are at low risk for congenital infection.

Infants with reactive serologic tests for syphilis require frequent clinical evaluation and serologic follow-up with RPR/VDRL titers and MHA-TP/FTA-ABS tests.* This can be incorporated into routine pediatric care at 2, 4, 6, 12, and 15 months. The nontreponemal serologic tests of most uninfected infants will become nonreactive within 6 months. Persistent stable titer beyond 1 year is an indication for re-evaluation and re-treatment with aqueous penicillin G (50,000 U/kg IV every 6 hours for 10 to 14 days). A reactive treponemal test beyond 15 months of age, seen in approximately 70 per cent of symptomatic infants, confirms the diagnosis of congenital syphilis. For infants whose initial CSF findings are abnormal, a second lumbar puncture is performed 6 months after therapy. An abnormal result at this time also is an indication for re-treatment with aqueous penicillin G (50,000 U/kg IV every 6 hours for 10 to 14 days).

JARISCH-HERXHEIMER REACTION

The Jarisch-Herxheimer reaction occurs in both adults and infants within 2 to 12 hours after the initial treatment of syphilis with antibiotics, especially penicillin. This acute systemic reaction is characterized by fever, myalgias, headache, vasodilation with flushing, hypotension, and tachycardia. In pregnant women, uterine contractions, fetal tachycardia and decelerations, and decreased fetal movements may occur. Symptoms may last for up to 24 hours and are usually associated with treatment of early syphilis. The exact etiology is unclear; it may be due to the release of endotoxin by the spirochetes. There is no proven preventive treatment, although aspirin may ameliorate the symptoms.

*RPR, rapid plasma reagin (test); VDRL, Venereal Disease Research Laboratory; MHA-TP, microhemagglutination assay for *T. pallidum* antibody; FTA-ABS, fluorescent treponemal antibody–absorbed.

REFERENCES

Wendel GD, Stark BJ, Jamison RB, et al: Penicillin allergy and desensitization in serious maternal/fetal infections. N Engl J Med 312:1229–1239, 1985.

LEPTOSPIROSIS

WILLIAM T. SPECK, M.D.

ETIOLOGY

Leptospirosis is a generalized infection of humans and animals caused by spirochetes of the genus *Leptospira.* The pathogenic leptospira belongs to the species *L. interrogans,* which contains more than 200 pathogenic serovars in 23 serogroups.

Animal infection varies from inapparent to fatal; once infected, animals can excrete large numbers of organisms in the urine for extended periods of time. Humans become infected following contact with the urine or tissues of infected animals. *Leptospira* enters humans through moist, and preferably abraded, skin and/or through the mucous membranes of the eye or nasopharynx.

TREATMENT

Despite the in vitro sensitivity of *Leptospira* to penicillin and tetracycline and the efficacy of these agents in experimental infection, their effectiveness in human leptospirosis remains controversial, as many people recover without treatment. Controlled trials suggest that administration of antibiotics within the first 4 days of illness shortens the clinical course and decreases the severity of infection. Accordingly, when the diagnosis of leptospirosis is considered possible or probable and the patient has been ill for less than 1 week, treatment with penicillin or tetracycline (in children older than 12 years) should be initiated. Parenteral penicillin G (6 to 8 million units/m^2 per 24 hours in six divided doses for 7 days) is recommended.

In patients allergic to penicillin, tetracycline (10 to 20 mg/kg/day) should be administered orally or intravenously in four divided doses for 7 days. A Jarisch-Herxheimer reaction has been observed in patients treated with penicillin; however, the reaction has not proved to be of sufficient severity to prevent penicillin use. Leptospirosis has been prevented in American service personnel stationed in the tropics by administering doxycycline (200 mg once a week) as prophylaxis.

General supportive care is mandatory in the management of critically ill infants and children. Complications, which may include hemorrhage, disseminated intravascular coagulation, thrombocytopenia, hepatitis, myocarditis, meningitis, and renal failure, must be dealt with accordingly. There is no evidence to suggest a role for corticosteroids in the treatment of leptospirosis.

RAT-BITE FEVER

BARRY DASHEFSKY, M.D.

Rat-bite fever is a term applied to two similar but distinct clinical syndromes currently occurring rarely in the United States. Both are characterized by the abrupt onset of high, often intermittent fever, rash, musculoskeletal complaints, and constitutional symptoms that are caused by microorganisms usually transmitted by biting rodents. The more common entity in the United States—streptobacillary fever—is caused by *Streptobacillus moniliformis*. It typically presents within 3 (up to 5) days after a rat bite that heals promptly without producing significant regional lymphadenopathy and features a pink maculopapular or petechial rash on the extremities (in 75 per cent of cases) and nonsuppurative migratory polyarthritis or arthralgia (in 50 per cent of cases). Streptobacillary fever may also be acquired by ingestion of contaminated food or milk (Haverhill fever) and may be manifested additionally by pharyngitis. Untreated, the illness usually subsides within 3 weeks, although it may be complicated by a chronic, relapsing course of arthritis; the development of subcutaneous abscesses or other focal disease, most significantly endocarditis; and a mortality rate of 10 per cent.

Less common in the United States, "classic" rat-bite fever (or *sodoku*) is caused by *Spirillum minus*. Typically, after an incubation period of 14 to 18 days (range 7 to 21 days), it presents with ulceration of an initially healed rat bite in association with prominent regional lymphadenopathy and a rash consisting of large purple to reddish-brown macules and occasional indurated plaques; joint involvement is rare. Untreated, infection with *S. minus* usually resolves within 3 to 8 weeks; however, multiple relapses of fever and rash may occur over months or years; suppurative complications and death are very rare.

TREATMENT

Both varieties of rat-bite fever are treated similarly and respond promptly and readily to antimicrobials. Recommended treatment is procaine penicillin G (20,000 to 50,000 U/kg/day, up to 1.2 million units, IM in one to two doses), or penicillin G (50,000 U/kg/day, up to 2.4 million units, IV in four to six doses) for 7 to 10 days. Oral penicillin V (1 to 2 g daily in four divided doses for the same duration) is considered to be a satisfactory alternative.

For penicillin-allergic patients, options include tetracycline (30 to 50 mg/kg/day, maximum daily dose 2 g, orally or IV in four doses) for patients 9 years of age or older; streptomycin (20 to 30 mg/kg/day, maximum daily dose 4 g, orally or IV in four doses); or chloramphenicol (50 to 75 mg/kg/day, maximum daily dose 4 g, orally or IV in four doses). For treating endocarditis, penicillin G (150,000 to 250,000 U/kg/day, maximum daily dose 20 million units, IV in four to six divided doses for at least 4 weeks) is recommended; streptomycin, or presumably another aminoglycoside, may be a helpful adjunct.

Additional treatment issues include care of local bite wounds, drainage of abscesses as necessary, and implementation of standard guidelines for tetanus prophylaxis. Gloves should be used for touching any infective material until 24 hours of effective antimicrobial therapy has been completed. The major preventive measure is rodent control.

REFERENCES

Holroyd KJ, Reiner AP, Dick JD: *Streptobacillus moniliformis* polyarthritis mimicking rheumatoid arthritis: An urban case of rat bite fever. Am J Med 85:711–714, 1988.

Roughgarden JW: Antimicrobial therapy of rat bite fever. Arch Intern Med 116:39–54, 1965.

Shackelford PF: Rat bite fever. *In* Feigin RD, Cherry JD (eds): Textbook of Pediatric Infectious Diseases, 2nd ed. Philadelphia, WB Saunders Co, 1987, pp 1257–1260.

PNEUMOCYSTIS CARINII PNEUMONITIS

WALTER T. HUGHES, M.D.

Pneumonitis caused by *Pneumocystis carinii* is usually fatal if untreated. With specific antimicrobial therapy, about 75 per cent of patients can be expected to recover if treatment is begun early. Because the infection usually occurs in immunocompromised patients and a definitive diagnosis requires an invasive procedure, such as bronchoalveolar lavage or open lung biopsy, management consists of close attention to complications from the underlying primary disease and the diagnostic procedures. Thus, associated or secondary viral, bacterial, or fungal infections may occur and pneumothorax or pneumomediastinum may complicate the diagnostic procedure. Hypoxia with low arterial oxygen tension (PaO_2) is regularly present, whereas carbon dioxide retention is unusual and the arterial pH is frequently increased. Unlike other infections in the immunosuppressed host, *P. carinii* infection remains localized entirely to the lungs, with rare exception.

When *P. carinii* pneumonitis is recognized as the first illness of an infant or child, a careful search should be made for an underlying disease.

TREATMENT

Specific Therapy. Trimethoprim-sulfamethoxazole (TMP-SMZ)* and pentamidine isethionate are equally effective in the treatment of *P. carinii* pneumonitis, but TMP-SMZ is the drug of first choice because of its low toxicity and easy availability.

TMP-SMZ may be given orally or intravenously. The oral dose is 20 mg trimethoprim and 100 mg sulfamethoxazole/kg/day, divided into four parts at 6-hour intervals. It is advisable to give half of the calculated daily dose initially as a loading dose when the oral route is used. TMP-SMZ is available in tablet form ("regular size" with 80 mg trimethoprim, 400 mg sulfamethoxazole and as a "double-strength" tablet with twice these amounts). An oral suspension contains 40 mg trimethoprim and 200 mg sulfamethoxazole per 5 ml. The intravenous preparation is available in 5.0-ml ampules containing 80 mg trimethoprim and 400 mg sulfamethoxazole. Each 5.0-ml ampule must be added to 125 ml of 5 per cent dextrose in water. The dosage for intravenous use is 15.0 mg trimethoprim and 75.0 mg sulfamethoxazole/kg/day divided in three to four equal doses. Each dose is infused over a 60-minute period. From available data, peak serum levels of 3 to 5 μg/ml of trimethoprim and 100 to 150 μg/ml of sulfamethoxazole seem to be the optimal ranges.

The adverse and toxic side effects are essentially those of sulfonamides, and although they are uncommon, they include transient maculopapular rash, nausea, vomiting, diarrhea, neutropenia, agranulocytosis, aplastic anemia, megaloblastic anemia, hemolytic anemia, methemoglobinemia, Stevens-Johnson syndrome, allergic reactions, toxic nephrosis, and drug fever. Folic acid deficiency has occurred rarely. It is reversible by folinic acid (10 to 25 mg daily). Folinic acid does not interfere with the therapeutic effects of the drug. Patients with acquired immunodeficiency syndrome (AIDS) have a higher rate of adverse reactions than other patients.

Pentamidine is the drug of second choice because of its high frequency of adverse effects. Pentamidine is administered as a single daily dose of 4 mg/kg intravenously infused over a period of 1 hour for 10 to 14 days. If improvement is apparent after 5 days of treatment, this may be reduced to 3

*Manufacturer's precaution: Not recommended for infants younger than 2 months of age.

mg/kg/day. The total dosage should not exceed 56 mg/kg. The drug may also be given by intramuscular injection if use of the intravenous route is not possible. Intramuscular injections should be given deeply into the anterolateral aspect of the thigh.

Adverse effects include induration, abscess formation, and necrosis at injection sites; nephrotoxicity; hypoglycemia or, rarely, hyperglycemia; hypotension; alteration in liver function; tachycardia; hypocalcemia; nausea and vomiting; skin rash; anemia; hyperkalemia; and thrombocytopenia.

Isolation. Animal studies indicate that *P. carinii* is transmitted by the airborne route. It is advisable to use respiratory isolation procedures to distinguish active cases of *P. carinii* pneumonitis from other compromised individuals at high risk for this infection.

Supportive Measures. Oxygen should be administered by mask as needed to maintain the PaO_2 above 70 mm Hg. The fraction of inspired oxygen (FIO_2) should be kept below 50 volumes per cent, if possible, to avoid oxygen toxicity, since oxygen therapy usually is required for relatively long periods.

Assisted or controlled ventilation is indicated in patients with arterial oxygen tension less than 60 mmHg at FIO_2 of 50 per cent or greater. Those with acutely elevated $Paco_2$, without pH changes and with or without hypoxemia, should be considered candidates for ventilatory therapy.

Studies of adults with AIDS suggest that a corticosteroid, such as prednisone, given early in the course of patients with moderately severe *P. carinii* pneumonitis (arterial-alveolar oxygen gradient of 35 mmHg or greater) results in an improved survival rate. No detailed studies have been reported in children and non-AIDS patients. The dose recommended in patients older than 13 years of age with AIDS by an expert committee is prednisone (40 mg twice daily for 5 days and then 20 mg twice daily for 5 days, followed by 20 mg daily) until the antimicrobial treatment is completed.

Fluid and electrolyte quantities are calculated by the patient's needs, but the solution should contain 5 or 10 per cent glucose to help prevent hypoglycemia during pentamidine therapy. Metabolic acidosis must be corrected.

Bacterial pneumonia or sepsis may occur in association with *P. carinii* pneumonitis. In the seriously ill patient with marked neutropenia (absolute neutrophil count less than 500 mm^3) or evidence of bacterial infection, antibiotics should be given. Oxacillin (200 mg/kg/day) and gentamicin (5 to 7 mg/kg/day) are administered intravenously until the results of cultures are known.

Efforts should be made to improve the nutritional status of the patient by dietary means even during the acute stage of the disease. Multivitamins should be given empirically. The value of intravenous alimentation has not been determined.

A blood transfusion is given if the hemoglobin level is lower than normal. The hemoglobin content must be sufficient to result in an arterial oxygen content of 15 to 20 ml/dl of blood at an arterial oxygen tension of 100 mmHg.

Pneumothorax may be a complication of the diagnostic procedures. If it is mild with no adverse effect on respiration, close observation is adequate. If it is more extensive, insertion of a thoracotomy tube with a water seal drainage system is necessary.

Parameters to Monitor

1. Assess serum immunoglobulin. At the onset of the illness, administer immune serum globulin (0.66 ml/kg [165 mg/ml]) the immunoglobulin G level is below 300 mg/dl.

2. Perform roentgenograms of the chest daily until there is clinical evidence of improvement. If needle aspiration of the lung, lung biopsy, or endotracheal brush catheter technique has been used as a diagnostic procedure, chest roentgenograms should be made at 30 minutes, 4 hours, and 12 hours after the procedure to detect pneumothorax.

3. Determine hemoglobin, white blood cell count and differential, and platelets daily.

4. Measure body weight, intake, and output daily.

5. Measure arterial blood gases: pH, $Paco_2$, PaO_2, and base excess or deficit initially and as often as necessary, according to severity of clinical course.

6. Measure serum electrolytes: sodium, chloride, potassium, and carbon dioxide content every 3 days, or more frequently if indicated.

7. Monitor total serum proteins, albumin, and globulin every 3 days. Hypoalbuminemia may occur.

8. Monitor blood pressure, pulse, and respiratory rate every 4 hours or more often if the condition is critical.

9. For patients receiving pentamidine, check blood urea nitrogen (BUN), creatinine, and urine every 3 days. If the BUN exceeds 30 mg/dl or serum creatinine is greater than 1.5 mg/dl, withhold pentamidine for 1 or 2 days. Monitor blood glucose 4 to 6 hours after each injection of pentamidine. Administer glucose if blood glucose value is less than 40 mg/dl. Monitor serum glutamic-oxaloacetic transaminase (SGOT) every 3 days; withhold pentamidine for 1 to 2 days if evidence of hepatic toxicity exists; and monitor serum calcium and phosphorus every 3 days. If the serum inorganic phosphate level becomes increased and the calcium level becomes decreased from normal values on the basis of renal insufficiency, give calcium lactate (15 to 20 g/day) or calcium carbonate (5 to 8 g/day orally). The diet should be low in phosphate, and 25,000 to 50,000 units of vitamin D are given orally. For patients with renal impairment and receiving trimethoprim-sulfamethoxazole, the dosage should be regulated on the basis of serum drug levels. Measurement of serum levels of the sulfonamide is adequate. The level of free sulfonamide should be maintained with peak values between 100 and 150 μg/ml measured 2 hours after the oral dosage.

Experimental studies suggest that diaminodiphenylsulfone (dapsone), trimetrexate with leucovorin, sulfadoxine-pyrimethamine (Fansidar), primaquine-clindamycin, and a new hydroxynaphthoquinone (566C80) may be effective in *P. carinii* pneumonitis.

EXPECTED COURSE

Fever, tachypnea, and pulmonary infiltrates usually persist with little change for 4 to 6 days. If no improvement is apparent after a week of therapy, concomitant or secondary infection most likely exists. These infections have included bacterial pneumonia or sepsis, systemic candidiasis, aspergillosis, cryptococcosis, histoplasmosis, and cytomegalovirus inclusion disease as well as other viral infections. *P. carinii* pneumonitis may recur several months after apparent recovery in 10 to 15 per cent of cases.

PREVENTION

P. carinii pneumonitis can be prevented by chemoprophylaxis with TMP-SMZ.* Dosage is one-fourth the therapeutic dose, 5 mg/kg of trimethoprim and 25 mg/kg of sulfamethoxazole per day in two divided doses. The protection is afforded only while the patient is receiving the drug. Aerosolized pentamidine has been found to be effective in preventing *P. carinii* pneumonitis in adults with AIDS. However, similar studies in children are lacking.

Recommendations from a panel of experts have been published (MMWR, Vol 40, March 15, 1991) for the preven-

*This use is not listed by the manufacturer.

tion of *P. carinii* pneumonitis in infants and children with AIDS. Trimethoprim-sulfamethoxazole prophylaxis is recommended for all who have had a prior episode of the pneumonitis; for HIV-seropositive patients 1 to 12 months of age, with CD4 lymphocyte counts of below 1500 cells per mm^3; for those 12 to 24 months of age, with counts less than 750 cells per mm^3; for those 24 months to 6 years of age, with counts less than 500 cells per mm^3; and for those over 6 years of age, with counts less than 200 cells per mm^3. More details are provided in the journal report.

MEASLES

EDWARD A. MORTIMER, JR., M.D.

Measles is an acute, systemic viral infection that in the past affected nearly all children in the United States and therefore was classified as one of the usual childhood diseases. A severe disease, it is manifested by a course of approximately 7 days with high fever; moderately severe respiratory symptoms, including coryza, conjunctivitis, and cough; the classic enanthem (Koplik's spots); and a characteristic rash. Besides the severity of the acute illness, the importance of the disease in the United States has been measured by its complications, particularly otitis media, pneumonia, measles encephalitis, and, rarely, subacute sclerosing panencephalitis (SSPE). In the past, mortality in the United States was largely a result of pneumonia; perhaps because of better nutrition, antibiotics, and other factors, deaths from the disease declined remarkably even before widespread use of the vaccine.

Even today, however, the situation in the remainder of the world is very different. The World Health Organization (WHO) estimates for 1990 indicated that of the 120 million babies born in the Third World annually, 800,000 (0.7 per cent) succumbed to measles before their fifth birthday. Undoubtedly, complicating factors, such as low birth weight, malnutrition, recurrent diarrhea, and other infections, contribute to this high mortality. Thus, measles remains a severe disease.

CONTROL OF MEASLES

Control of measles and its associated morbidity and mortality depends on timely active immunization of all eligible children. Treatment of the illness is only symptomatic; its bacterial complications are susceptible to therapy, but the more serious neurologic and other sequelae are not. Passive immunization of susceptible children with immune serum globulin is useful only in occasional instances when exposure is recognized early.

Live, Attenuated Measles Vaccine

Isolation and propagation of the measles virus in 1954 led to the development and licensure of inactivated and live, attenuated vaccines in 1963. Since 1967, only the live vaccine has been used. A single dose of properly administered measles vaccine induces seroconversion and clinical immunity in more than 95 per cent of recipients. Available preparations include monovalent measles vaccine; measles vaccine combined with live, attenuated rubella vaccine (MR); and the familiar formula that comprises live, attenuated measles, mumps, and rubella vaccines (MMR)—the preparation of choice for routine immunization since 1971. There is no biologic advantage to administering measles, mumps, or rubella vaccine in monovalent form.

In the United States, it was originally recommended that children receive measles vaccine at 9 months of age, but the preferred age was raised first to 12 months and in 1976 to 15 months because of interference with the immune response by small amounts of persisting transplacental maternal antibody. From 1976 until 1989, a single dose of MMR at 15 months of age was recommended as a routine policy; in 1989 this policy was changed to include a second dose of MMR.

Rationale for Two-Dose Measles Vaccine Policy

The widespread use of measles vaccine in the United States has resulted in a remarkable decline in disease incidence and a shift in the age distribution of cases. Indeed, in 1983 only 1497 cases and four deaths were reported. Since then, however, there has been a considerable increase, with an estimate of nearly 30,000 cases and 89 deaths in 1990. Most of these cases occurred in localized rather than sporadic outbreaks. Rates have increased primarily in preschool children and young adults; school-aged children have been less affected because of school entry requirements. Prior to the use of measles vaccine, 90 per cent of all measles cases occurred in children younger than 10 years and only about 3 per cent in persons 15 years and older. With widespread immunization, the incidence has decreased markedly in all age groups, particularly in elementary school–aged children. Indeed, in 1990 48 per cent of all cases occurred in children younger than 5 years and 47 per cent in persons 10 years and older. Of the nearly 30,000 individuals with measles in 1990, 18 per cent represent vaccine failures, 44 per cent should have been vaccinated but were not, and in the remaining 38 percent the vaccine was not indicated under current guidelines (most were younger than 16 months of age). Thus, a major reason for this recrudescence of measles appears to be failure to achieve high rates of measles immunization in preschool children who are unaffected by school entry laws; vaccine failures, either primary (failure of the vaccine to "take") or secondary (waning immunity) in a few instances, are also important.

Vaccine Failures

Vaccine failures, as evidenced by clinical measles in a previously immunized child (or failure of seroconversion in studies of efficacy), have been reported in 5 to 10 per cent of children. Many, if not most, of these can be attributed to any of three factors: improper handling of the vaccine, administration at too young an age, or simultaneous use of immune serum globulin. The vaccine is susceptible to inactivation by light or by warmth during transport or storage (breaks in the "cold chain"); it should always be transported and stored until use at or below 45°F (8°C), although the current preparation is more thermostable than that prior to 1979. The vaccine also should not be exposed to bright light unnecessarily.

As noted, administration of properly stored and handled vaccine may nonetheless be associated with failure to immunize because of persistent maternal antibody; the younger the infant, the higher the proportion of failures. Many of the cases of measles occurring during outbreaks in previously immunized persons are so explained. Accordingly, for some years, it was a recommended (and frequently mandatory) policy to reimmunize all children who received measles vaccine prior to their first birthdays and it was considered acceptable to reimmunize those who were vaccinated between 12 and 15 months.

Some vaccine failures are attributable to the simultaneous administration of immune globulin to many children who received measles vaccine prepared from the less attenuated Edmonton B strain of virus between 1963, when it was first licensed, and 1975, when it was replaced by the further attenuated vaccine. Immune globulin was given to ameliorate the excessive reactions from Edmonton B vaccine, and some physicians did continue to use it in conjunction with the further attenuated vaccine. Unfortunately, although the immune serum globulin reduced reaction rates, it also prevented the acquisition of active immunity in some children, particularly those who received the further attenuated vaccine.

There is evidence of vaccine-induced immunity waning to the point of clinical susceptibility to measles in rare individuals. Such a phenomenon might occur because measles vaccine produces lower antibody titers than does natural disease and, more importantly, because the near disappearance of the disease has resulted in lack of a booster effect from casual exposure to the disease (the "street car" booster).

Recommendations for Vaccine Use

For routine childhood preventive care, the first dose of measles vaccine, given as MMR, is administered when the child is 15 months old. Simultaneous administration of other vaccines, including diphtheria and tetanus toxoids and pertussis vaccine adsorbed (DTP), and live attenuated or inactivated poliovirus vaccine (OPV or IPV) does not interfere with immune responses or enhance reactivity. Although precise data are not yet available, it is likely that *Haemophilus influenzae* b conjugated vaccine (HbCV) may be given with MMR, OPV, and DTP. Therefore, when there is concern about whether a child will be brought back for subsequent care, it is acceptable to give all four vaccines (MMR, DTP, OPV or IPV, and HbCV) simultaneously at different sites at age 15 months. Otherwise, some physicians may prefer to give MMR at 15 months and defer the other three until the child is 18 months of age.

In 1989, both the U.S. Public Health Service and the American Academy of Pediatrics recommended adding a second dose of measles vaccine, given as MMR, as part of the routine childhood immunization schedule. The American Academy of Pediatrics recommends the second dose at about 12 years; the U.S. Public Health Service advises the second dose simultaneously with DTP and OPV (or IPV) at the time of kindergarten entry (4 to 6 years). Either approach is acceptable. Some communities affected by high rates of measles have recommended the first dose as early as 9 months and the second at 18 months. Under any schedule, at least 1 month should elapse between the two doses. It is likely that more general agreement as to the optimum ages for the two doses will occur as experience is gained. Currently, several enhanced potency measles vaccines for infants are under study, particularly for use in the developing world.

There are certain circumstances, including outbreaks and foreign travel, in which special considerations are necessary. For full review of these considerations and all aspects of the changed vaccine policy and its rationale, the reader should consult the recommendations of the U.S. Public Health Service Immunization Practices Advisory Committee (ACIP) (MMWR 38:S1–S18, December 29, 1989).

Reactions to Measles Vaccine

Because measles vaccine produces a "mild" measles infection, side effects may be anticipated in some recipients. The most frequent of these is fever, usually appearing 6 days after inoculation. Although fever is usually slight and lasts only a few days, in approximately 10 per cent of children it may reach 103°F (39.4°C) or more. Less commonly, transient, nondescript rashes occur. Measles vaccine does not appear to cause the neurologic sequelae (acute encephalitis and SSPE) that occur following the disease. Although there have been isolated anecdotal reports of acute encephalitis following the vaccine, their rarity suggests that they probably represent coincidence and not causation. Similarly, if measles vaccine causes SSPE, the rate must be only a minute fraction of that from natural measles since the incidence of SSPE in the United States has declined remarkably following widespread use of the vaccine.

Children with a past or family history of convulsions are at slightly increased risk of a febrile convulsion secondary to vaccine-induced fever. Because short febrile convulsions are considered harmless (though distressing), such a history is not considered a contraindication to measles vaccine on the basis that the disease risk is far greater. Because fever is most apt to occur 5 to 12 days following immunization, some physicians may wish to advise antipyretic prophylaxis with acetaminophen during those days. Unless the child is already receiving anticonvulsant medications, these drugs are probably of little value because of the weeks required to attain satisfactory levels. As with any vaccine or other medication given to children, the benefits and risks should be explained to the parents.

A unique problem is presented by those individuals, now young adults, who received killed measles vaccine during the years it was licensed (1963 to 1967). Up to 1 million children received the killed vaccine. The vaccine was abandoned when it became apparent that protection was transient and that children exposed to measles 2 or more years later experienced a severe type of measles with high fever, unusual rash, edema, pneumonitis, and other findings (atypical measles). Such persons also exhibit greater reactivity to subsequent live measles vaccine; a few have quite severe reactions resembling atypical measles. However, because atypical natural measles is far more severe than the vast majority of reactions to the live vaccine in these persons, most authorities advise administering the live vaccine with adequate warning to the patient. Reimmunization of those who received killed vaccine or vaccine of unknown type is particularly important for those who travel to other countries where measles is common.

CONTRAINDICATIONS TO MEASLES VACCINE

Prior Immunization

Prior immunity to measles, mumps, or rubella, whether acquired from disease or by immunization, is *not* associated with untoward reactions to MMR and is therefore of no concern.

Egg Sensitivity

Live measles vaccine is propagated in chick embryo cell culture. In recent years, rare potentially serious immediate allergic reactions to the vaccine have been unquestionably related to egg sensitivity. Therefore, children with a clear history of an immediate anaphylactic response to egg ingestion (hives, oropharyngeal swelling, hypotension) should not receive measles vaccine.

Immunocompromised States

Except for children with human immunodeficiency virus (HIV) infection, children with congenital immune deficiencies and those whose immune systems are compromised by immunosuppressive therapy should not receive measles vaccine because of the risk of enhanced infection with the vaccine virus. For most children receiving intense immunosuppressive therapy, the vaccine may be delayed until treatment is discontinued. Low-dose therapy is not a contraindication. Because recipients of the vaccine do not transmit the virus, immunodeficient persons are not jeopardized by the immunization of others, including siblings.

MMR is safe for asymptomatic HIV-infected children and should be given. Because incomplete data suggest that symptomatic HIV-infected children, including those with AIDS, do not incur serious untoward effects, MMR should be considered, although immune responses may be blunted.

Neomycin Allergy

Measles vaccine contains small amounts of neomycin but no other antibiotic. The rare individual who has experienced an anaphylactic response to topical or systemic neomycin should not receive the vaccine. Contact dermatitis from neomycin is not a contraindication, although a small, transient nodule may develop at the injection site.

Pregnancy

Although there is no empiric evidence that measles vaccine (or any live vaccine, including that for rubella) is deleterious to the fetus, pregnant women should not receive measles vaccine on theoretical grounds and to avoid confusion about causation of any adverse outcome of the pregnancy. Immunization of children of pregnant women with MMR poses no risk to such women because none of the three vaccine components has been shown to be transmissible to susceptible contacts.

Prior Receipt of Immune Serum Globulin

Human immune serum globulin contains substantial amounts of measles antibody, which may interfere with a measles vaccine "take." Therefore, administration of the vaccine to any child who has received immune serum globulin should be deferred for at least 3 months after receipt of the globulin.

Acute Illness

Because children repetitively display evidence of mild, transient respiratory infections with little or no fever and because there is no confirmed evidence of deleterious interaction between these minor illnesses and the receipt of measles vaccine or of interference with acquisition of immunity, the decision to administer measles vaccine in the presence of such symptoms should be determined by individual circumstances, including the likelihood that the child will return for a subsequent visit.

PASSIVE IMMUNIZATION

Immune serum globulin (ISG) prevents or modifies measles in exposed susceptible individuals, depending on the dose administered and when given as soon as possible after exposure (no later than 6 days). Preventive doses of ISG (0.25 ml/kg intramuscularly, maximum dose 15 ml) should be given to all infants between 6 and 24 months of age and to all nonimmune immunodeficient persons exposed to measles, because of the high incidence of complications in such children. Infants younger than 6 months of age may be presumed to be immune. An alternative approach for certain susceptible, immunocompetent individuals older than 1 year exposed within the previous 72 hours is to administer measles vaccine because vaccine-induced immunity appears promptly, often prior to the development of the clinical disease.

For nonimmunized children older than 2 years who are exposed to measles, a modifying dose of ISG may be given (0.04 ml/kg as a single injection). This dose may be expected to ameliorate the severity of the disease if given within 6 days and nonetheless permit the development of active immunity. Unless modified (mild) measles develops, these children should receive measles vaccine 3 months after receipt of ISG.

ISG should not be used to control measles outbreaks in schools or communities. Instead, all persons at risk of exposure born since 1957 should receive measles vaccine unless they have proof of physician-diagnosed measles or immunization with two doses of live vaccine beginning at 12 months or older. In such situations, ISG should be given only to individuals for whom the vaccine is contraindicated and to infants 6 to 24 months of age with documented exposure to the disease.

MANAGEMENT

The treatment of measles is symptomatic only. ISG does not modify the course or prevent complications once symptoms have begun. Prophylactic antibiotics do not prevent secondary infection. Acetaminophen (15 mg/kg) may be given as often as every 4 hours for symptomatic relief. Symptoms of the disease are such that bed rest during the febrile stages is not difficult to enforce. Mild cough suppressants may be given but usually have little effect.

A frequent problem that has arisen since the advent of the vaccine is that of misdiagnosis because an increasing number of physicians have never seen measles. If there is doubt, a practical approach to diagnosis is to have the patient seen by an older physician who has past experience with the disease.

Important in the management of measles is recognition and treatment of complications. Most common is bacterial otitis media, which requires appropriate antimicrobial therapy. In the past, mastoiditis frequently ensued. Pulmonary complications include bronchiolitis, especially in infants, and pneumonia, which may be lobar or bronchopneumonic in distribution. Suspicion of pneumonia usually arises when symptoms worsen late in the course of the disease or fever fails to subside with full appearance of the rash. A chest radiograph may be required for diagnosis. Pneumonia may be bacterial in origin, especially if lobar, and should be treated with antimicrobial drugs. Rarely, pneumothorax or pneumomediastinum occurs. Occasionally, inflammation of the upper airway progresses to obstructive laryngotracheitis and may require tracheostomy.

Other rare complications include appendicitis, presumably secondary to lymphoid hyperplasia; abdominal pain and vomiting in the course of measles or early in convalescence suggest this possibility. Acute measles encephalitis, estimated to occur in about 1 per 1000 cases, usually appears near the end of the course of the disease or early in convalescence. Persistent or recurring fever, somnolence, irrational behavior, vomiting, and convulsions are frequent manifestations. Treatment is symptomatic; neurologic consultation is advisable.

RUBELLA AND CONGENITAL RUBELLA

PHILIP R. ZIRING, M.D.

The decline in the incidence of rubella and congenital rubella since licensure of live attenuated rubella virus vaccines in 1969 has been one of the most notable achievements of modern medicine. The last major epidemic of rubella in the United States in 1964 was accompanied by rubella infection in one in every 100 pregnancies and the birth of approximately 20,000 infants with rubella-associated defects. More than 100 million doses of rubella vaccine have been administered in the United States since 1969, which brought the predictable 7-year cycles of rubella epidemics to a conclusion. So dramatic has this change been that by 1989 there was only one case of congenital rubella nationwide reported to the Centers for Disease Control (CDC) in Atlanta.

Rubella and congenital rubella are considered in this article because, despite their low incidence, they remain matters of concern for pediatricians. Sporadic cases of rubella still occur, especially in clusters among older adolescents and young adults who have not had the disease or been immunized and in susceptible persons immigrating to the United States. There is a great need to maintain a high level of awareness about the importance of immunization and the safety and efficacy of rubella vaccine. Furthermore, there is an ongoing concern for the thousands of patients with congenital rubella, many of whom were victims of the 1964 epidemic who are now entering the third decade of life and who are at risk for development of new clinical manifestations of this disorder.

Since 1988, when an all-time low of 225 cases of rubella were reported to the CDC, there has been a distressing increase in cases throughout the United States, with more than 1000 cases reported in 1990. In California, which reported half of all the cases in the nation, 81 per cent occurred in young adults, the vast majority of whom had no history of rubella immunization. Eleven confirmed cases of congenital rubella syndrome were reported in 1990; nine of the patients were multihandicapped infants born in southern California.

RUBELLA

In general, rubella (German measles, 3-day measles) can be considered among the mildest viral illnesses. In fact, a significant percentage of adults and even larger numbers of children may undergo infection that is completely asymptomatic. Although often pruritic, the rash generally responds to simple antihistamine treatment. There may be an associated sore throat, tender lymphadenopathy, and low-grade fever, which are responsive to analgesics. It is most important to recall that the patient is highly contagious for a period of time beginning a few days prior to the onset of rash until 1 to 2 weeks after the rash clears. During this time, it is important to avoid exposure of the patient to a woman who may be in early pregnancy and whose rubella susceptibility status is unknown.

The most important common complication of rubella is postinfectious arthralgia or arthritis, principally involving the small joints of the hands and feet. Although these joint symptoms sometimes are quite painful and may recur periodically for an extended period of time, they always clear completely without residua. Thrombocytopenia of mild degree is not uncommon and usually resolves without treatment. Thrombocytopenic purpura is a rare complication, which should prompt thorough hematologic investigation to ensure that there is no other underlying cause. Postinfectious encephalitis is seen in rubella far less often than in measles and usually responds to simple supportive measures.

CONGENITAL RUBELLA

It is most useful to consider the clinical manifestations of congenital rubella in three stages: those that are present and identifiable at birth, those that are developmental and appear only as the infant grows older, and those late manifestations that may not be clinically apparent until the second decade of life or beyond.

Disorders Apparent in the Neonatal Period

The rubella-associated birth defects that are apparent at birth are a result of rubella virus interference with cell growth and cell division in the fetus. They include defects of the eye (cataract, glaucoma, and retinopathy), of the heart (stenosis of the main pulmonary artery and/or its branches, patent ductus arteriosus, and other less common heart defects less commonly seen), central nervous system (sensory neural hearing loss and other evidence of brain injury), bone marrow (anemia, thrombocytopenia, and defects of the immune system), and general intrauterine growth retardation. The management of these disorders differs little from that used when such defects result from other diverse etiologies.

A few clinical issues are especially worth remembering. For example, surgery for congenital glaucoma must be performed promptly after diagnosis in the neonatal period to guard against permanent visual loss from high intraocular pressure. Surgery for congenital cataracts, on the other hand, can often be deferred until as late as 1 year of age, when optimum surgical results are often obtained. Surgery for a uniocular rubella cataract has rarely been rewarded by useful vision in the operated eye. Sensorineural hearing loss is the most common clinically significant consequence of rubella infection during the first 4 months of pregnancy and must be ruled out in every infant suspected of having congenital rubella. The hearing impairment may be unilateral or bilateral and ranges in severity from mild to profound and may be manifest at all frequencies. Early diagnosis through testing of infants by skilled audiologists followed by early amplification with hearing aids and enrollment in auditory training programs can often spell the difference between an individual capable of speech and one unable to communicate orally.

Developmental Disorders

As the infant passes beyond the neonatal period, other disorders of a developmental character may appear. Mental retardation is more likely and more severe the earlier in pregnancy the infection takes place and is often complicated by the presence of impairment of vision and/or hearing. The enrollment of these infants in preschool enrichment programs often helps them to make maximum use of their residual abilities and assists the family with needed training and support.

Symptoms of spastic cerebral palsy are usually not apparent until the first year of life. In such cases, close follow-up by neurologists, orthopedists, physiatrists, and physical, occupational, and speech therapists skilled in the management of physically handicapped children can often be helpful in management related to ambulation, sitting, feeding, and other skills of daily living.

Behavioral disorders occur commonly and are often complicated by the presence of sensory defects or mental retardation. Extreme restlessness and hyperactivity or symptoms of autism often prove difficult to manage. The results of the use of stimulant medication, tranquilizers, or barbiturates have generally been disappointing. More success has followed the use of mild sedatives such as diphenhydramine (Benadryl) or psychotropic agents such as thioridazine (Mellaril). Consultation with child psychiatrists and behavioral psychologists may also be helpful.

Late Manifestations

Clinical disturbances of endocrine function in children and young adults with congenital rubella are now well recognized. Patients with hypothyroidism or hyperthyroidism have been described, with identification of rubella virus antigen in the thyroid gland of at least one child with Hashimoto's thyroiditis. The most common endocrine disturbance seems to be insulin-dependent diabetes mellitus, with up to 20 per cent or more of patients having some evidence of this disorder by the second decade of life. Interest has been focused on the association of insulin-dependent diabetes mellitus in children with congenital rubella, predominantly with certain human leukocyte antigen (HLA) phenotypes, especially DR3 and B8. In such cases, the rubella infection of the islet cells in utero seems to have acted as a "trigger" in the expression of insulin-dependent diabetes mellitus in children who are so genetically predisposed. Early diagnosis of these disorders through measurement of antibodies directed against thyroid and islet cells is now becoming more commonplace. The interpretation of such tests and their therapeutic implications may often best be carried out in consultation with a pediatric endocrinologist.

Several patients with congenital rubella have been reported with progressive rubella panencephalitis, a degenerative disorder of the central nervous system apparently caused by an exacerbation of rubella infection within the brain. Although few patients have been so identified thus far, it is important to be alert to the existence of this entity in patients with congenital rubella who undergo deterioration in behavior, intellectual performance, or motor function or develop seizures.

PREVENTION

As noted, immunization of most children at approximately 15 months of age and selected adults who are shown to be rubella seronegative has resulted in a dramatic decline in the incidence of rubella and congenital rubella. The RA 27/3 strain of virus grown in human diploid cell culture may be given alone or in combination with other live attenuated virus vaccines (measles, mumps). A single inoculation of this vaccine produces durable immunity, although the antibody levels achieved may be lower than that following natural rubella infection.

The American Academy of Pediatrics has responded to the recent resurgence of rubella and congenital rubella syndrome in the United States by recommending that children be given a second dose of measles, mumps, and rubella (MMR) vaccine upon entry to middle (or junior high) school at 11 to 12 years of age. It is also urgent to redouble our efforts to see that *all* infants are immunized at 15 months of age and that women of childbearing age who have no serologic evidence of ever having received rubella vaccine or having had rubella are immunized.

Ongoing surveillance conducted by the CDC in regard to the risk to the fetus of inadvertent rubella immunization of a susceptible woman in early pregnancy has taken place since the introduction of the vaccine. It has been well established that vaccine virus so inoculated can be recovered from the fetus, but evidence is still lacking that this vaccine virus is teratogenic. Numerous such pregnancies have gone to term with no evidence of congenital rubella birth defects present in the offspring. Pregnant women so exposed should be counseled regarding the *theoretical* risks posed by such vaccination, but they may be reassured at this time regarding the lack of known association with congenital rubella birth defects. Side effects of vaccination are similar (although generally milder) than those seen in natural rubella, with transient arthralgias and arthritis being the most common clinical conditions observed.

VARICELLA-ZOSTER VIRUS INFECTION

ANNE A. GERSHON, M.D.

Varicella-zoster virus (VZV) causes two diseases, varicella and zoster. Varicella is the primary infection, and zoster is the secondary infection, resulting from reactivation of latent VZV. Zoster develops in about 15 per cent of individuals, but by far most cases occur in the elderly rather than in the young. Zoster most often occurs in immunocompromised patients. Both diseases are characterized by a vesicular skin eruption: generalized in varicella, but localized and unilateral in zoster. Varicella is usually a mild, uncomplicated illness in children, but it can be severe or fatal in the immunoincompetent.

TREATMENT OF VARICELLA

For most varicella infections in children, no specific therapy is required. Itching can be alleviated with calamine lotion or appropriate doses of antihistamines. Aspirin should not be administered for fever in order to prevent the complication of Reye syndrome. Bathing is essential to prevent bacterial skin superinfection. Oatmeal baths may also provide relief from itching. Superinfections of skin or lung (usually caused by staphylococci or streptococci) that follow varicella should be treated with an antistaphylococcal penicillin until the offending organism is identified.

Antiviral therapy for treatment of chickenpox is available in the form of the DNA inhibitor acyclovir (ACV). Whether to treat otherwise healthy children with ACV administered orally, nevertheless, is problematic. ACV shortens the clinical illness, but only by about 1 day. It has no effect on the incidence of complications, nor does it hasten the return to school. ACV may be more useful for treatment of adults, whose illness tends to be more severe, than of children whose illness is most often mild and self-limited. It may be useful, however, to treat selected children, such as older adolescents, and secondary household cases.

Acyclovir given orally must be administered within 24 hours after onset of rash to have an effect. The dosage is 80 mg/kg/day, divided into four doses, given for 5 days. ACV is available as a suspension (200 mg per 5 ml) and as 200-mg capsules.

Adverse effects are minimal, consisting of maculopapular rash and abdominal discomfort. Long-term effects of ACV, although predicted to be inconsequential, are not yet fully known. Latent infection with VZV is not prevented or cured with any currently available antiviral drug. The cost of a course of oral ACV for a child is about $35.

ACV is mainly indicated for treatment of immunocompromised patients who are at great risk for severe varicella infection. In this case, it should be given intravenously, in a dosage of 500 mg/m^2 per dose, three times a day (1500 mg/m^2/day) in patients with normal renal function. The dosage of acyclovir for patients with abnormal renal function (creatinine clearance less than 50 ml/minute/1.73m^2) should be smaller (usually one half to one third) than that routinely employed in order to prevent toxic concentrations of the drug from developing.

Immunocompromised patients with varicella who have not been passively immunized or received varicella vaccine previously (see later) should be admitted to the hospital and treated with ACV as soon as the diagnosis of varicella is made, even if there are only a few skin lesions. Successful antiviral therapy has been associated with administration of intravenous ACV within the first 3 days after onset of illness. Children at high risk for severe varicella include those with underlying malignancy (especially leukemia and lymphoma) for which they are receiving therapy, children with congenital or acquired immunodeficiency, and those receiving large dosages of steroids for any reason (1 mg/kg/day or more of prednisone or its equivalent).

In children with an underlying malignancy, consideration would be given to temporary postponement of chemotherapy. Baseline chest radiographs plus evaluation of blood gases and serum transaminase levels should be performed. Mechanically assisted ventilation should be used when it is necessary. The dosage of steroids should be decreased to physiologic levels, if possible, but stress doses may be given to severely ill children. Steroids should not be stopped abruptly.

Intravenous acyclovir therapy is usually given for 5 to 10 days, although in some instances a shorter or longer interval may be used. Discontinuing ACV in patients who cease experiencing new lesions for a period of several days, who have become afebrile, and who are clearly recovering is reasonable. It is not uncommon, however, for patients in the early stages of severe varicella to appear to be stable for 1 or 2 days and then to have new lesions, presumably secondary to another bout of viremia. Therefore, care should be taken not to stop acyclovir therapy too soon in immunocompromised patients.

Relatively common adverse effects of ACV include phlebitis due to the high pH of the intravenous solution (in about 15 per cent), reversible elevation of serum creatinine (in about 5 per cent), hive-like rash (in about 5 per cent), and nausea and vomiting (in about 1 per cent). Elevation of serum creatinine is a result of precipitation of the drug in the renal tubules when it is administered at a high concentration. This can be prevented by allowing at least 1 hour for infusion of each dose and maintaining good hydration. Rare toxicity includes encephalopathic manifestations, such as tremors, confusion, and agitation.

Because zoster is a secondary infection, the prognosis is generally better than for varicella, even in the immunocompromised. Otherwise healthy children in whom zoster develops rarely need specific antiviral therapy. Although it is usually not a life-saving measure, it is prudent to treat immunocompromised children if zoster develops in order to hasten healing and prevent dissemination. Whether to treat with the oral or intravenous formulation of ACV depends on the condition of the patient. Those with early and mild infections may be started on oral therapy and observed closely, but those with extensive rashes and/or toxicity (such as fever) should be given intravenous medication, at least to begin therapy. Doses of ACV for zoster are the same as for varicella.

VZV is not as susceptible to acyclovir in vitro, as is herpes simplex virus (HSV), and there is also considerable variability of susceptibilities of different strains of VZV to the drug. An intravenous dose of 500 mg/m^2 results in blood concentrations that are significantly above levels inhibitory to VZV, but oral administration of acyclovir at the usual adult dosage for HSV (200 mg, five times a day) probably will not. Therefore, the dose of oral ACV for a large adolescent (or adult) is 4 g/day, in five divided doses (four capsules five times a day). Only about 20 per cent of orally administered acyclovir is absorbed.

It is difficult to make recommendations concerning antiviral therapy for patients with central nervous system (CNS) involvement with VZV because the underlying pathogenesis of this complication is unknown and no controlled studies of the efficacy of antiviral therapy have been performed. Some clinicians elect to treat only immunocompromised patients with CNS involvement. This rationale is based on the likelihood that at least part of the problem in immunocompromised patients is a result of viral multiplication; this would be unlikely in immunologically normal patients. Children with cerebellar ataxia as a complication of chickenpox invariably recover without specific treatment.

Vidarabine is now the second-line drug for treatment of VZV infections, mainly since it is more toxic than ACV. If for some reason ACV cannot be given, vidarabine can be used for high-risk patients. The dosage is 10 mg/kg/day intravenously, administered once a day over a period of 12 hours, usually for 5 days. There are no data concerning the simultaneous use of both drugs for VZV infections; because of potential toxicity, this is not recommended.

PREVENTION OF VARICELLA

Varicella-Zoster Immune Globulin (VZIG)

VZIG was licensed by the Food and Drug Administration (FDA) in 1981. It is distributed in Massachusetts by the Massachusetts Public Health Biological Laboratory and elsewhere by the American Red Cross through local blood centers. Although VZIG is effective when administered up to 3 to 5 days after exposure, it should be given as soon as possible. The dose is 125 U/10 kg, with a maximum dosage of 625 U intramuscularly. The cost of one vial containing 125 U of VZIG is $75. VZIG should be readministered to high-risk children who are closely re-exposed to VZV 3 weeks following a first exposure for which VZIG was given.

Since varicella is a self-limited illness in otherwise healthy children, passive immunization should not be administered to them. The amount of VZV antibody in VZIG is about ten times higher than that in immune serum globulin (ISG). ISG, therefore, is of little use for prevention of varicella since the amount that must be given is unacceptably high. The efficacy of intravenous immunoglobulin (IVIG) for passive immunization against varicella has not been determined.

VZIG today is mainly used to prevent severe varicella in exposed susceptible children who are at high risk for development of severe or fatal varicella; this group includes immunocompromised children and newborn infants whose mothers have active varicella at the time of delivery. Candidates for whom VZIG is recommended by the Centers for Disease Control (CDC) in Atlanta, Georgia, are listed in Table 1.

High-risk infants and children should receive VZIG if they have had a close exposure to varicella or zoster (Table 2). They should be considered to be susceptible to varicella if there is no prior history of chickenpox (or uncertainty). The decision to administer VZIG to an immunocompromised child should not be based on an antibody titer because of the possibility of a false-positive antibody test. In contrast, however, VZIG is not indicated for healthy adults unless they are proven to be susceptible by laboratory testing because most adults are immune. It is therefore advised that the blood be tested for VZV antibodies in adults with no past history of varicella who are likely to be closely exposed to VZV. Then, should a close exposure occur, VZIG could be given.

Children with human immunodeficiency virus (HIV) infection are also at high risk for severe varicella infection. Management should be similar to that for immunocompromised children and adults. Even those children who have been receiving IVIG for treatment of AIDS should receive VZIG

TABLE 1. Candidates for Whom Varicella-Zoster Immune Globulin Is Indicated

1. No previous history of clinical varicella

   and

2. Underlying condition:
   a. Leukemia, lymphoma
   b. Congenital or acquired immunodeficiency
   c. Immunosuppressive therapy (including prednisone)
   d. Newborn infant of mother with onset of varicella within 5 days before delivery and 2 days after delivery
   e. Premature infant born after more than 28 weeks' gestation whose mother has no prior history of varicella
   f. Premature infant born before 28 weeks' gestation

   and

3. Significant exposure (see Table 2)

Modified from Centers for Disease Control: MMWR 33:84–100, 1984.

TABLE 2. Indications for Use of Varicella-Zoster Immune Globulin

1. Continuous household contact,

or

2. Playmate contact, greater than 1 hour indoors,
3. Hospital contact: in same two- or four-bed room or in adjacent beds in large ward; face-to-face contact with an infectious employee or patient;

or

4. Newborn contact with (a) infected mother *and* within 3 days of contact (preferably given sooner; in some cases may give up to 5 days after exposure) *and* (b) high risk for severe varicella (see Table 1)

Modified from Centers for Disease Control: MMWR 33:84–100, 1984.

if there is no past history of varicella and a close exposure has occurred.

Infants whose mothers have active varicella at delivery should receive VZIG. This includes infants whose mothers have the onset of chickenpox 5 days or less prior to delivery or within 48 hours after delivery. The dose of VZIG for infants is 125 units intramuscularly (Table 3). Usually varicella is mild after VZIG, although occasionally severe varicella may develop in an infant. Passively immunized infants should be observed carefully, but usually this can be done on an outpatient basis. Should an infant develop an extensive skin rash (more than 100 vesicles) or evidence of pneumonia, intravenous ACV should be administered.

VZIG can electively be given to infants under 1 week of age if their siblings at home have active varicella, especially if the mother has no history of chickenpox. It might also be given to infants younger than 1 week of age whose mothers have varicella. Infants exposed to mothers with zoster are not expected to develop severe varicella because they have high antibody titers and therefore do not require prophylactic VZIG.

Nosocomial spread of varicella in neonatal nurseries is a rare phenomenon. Low-birth-weight infants, however, may have undetectable titers of antibodies to VZV. Therefore, it is recommended that newborn infants exposed to VZV weighing less than 1000 g or of less than 28 weeks' gestation be passively immunized (see Table 1). Varicella has been observed in infants with pre-existing maternal transplacental antibodies when exposed to VZV, but it is usually a modified illness. This may be one reason that varicella in infants between 1 and 6 months of age is characteristically mild.

TABLE 3. Summary of Recommended Doses of Drugs for Varicella Infections

Acyclovir (ACV)

Oral: For healthy children with chickenpox (or zoster in selected patients): 80 mg/kg/day, divided into four doses, given for 5 days; maximum single dose, 800 mg (4 capsules). For large adolescent (or adult): 4 g/day, divided into five doses (4 capsules 5 times a day).

Intravenous: For immunocompromised patients with normal renal function: 1500 mg/m^2/day, divided into 3 doses (500 mg/m^2 per dose). For patients with abnormal renal function (creatinine clearance less than 50 ml/minute/1.73 m^2) dosage should be smaller (usually one half to one third).

Vidarabine (Ara-A)

Intravenous: 10 mg/kg/day once a day over a period of 12 hours, usually for 5 days

Varicella-Zoster Immune Globulin (VZIG)

Intramuscular: 125 U for each 10 kg of body weight, with a maximum dosage of 625 U; for infants, 125 U.

Zoster occurs despite serum antibody to VZV, and patients with zoster manifest brisk increases in VZV antibody titer. VZIG, therefore, is of no use in treating or preventing zoster.

Varicella Vaccine

A live attenuated varicella vaccine was developed in Japan about 20 years ago. This vaccine is licensed in some European countries and in Japan and Korea, but it is not yet licensed in the United States. The vaccine is highly protective in immunocompromised children and healthy adults, and there is great interest in vaccinating healthy children on a routine basis. Not all vaccinees are completely protected, however. Some experience a mild breakthrough illness following an exposure. However, varicella vaccine has been 100 per cent effective in preventing severe varicella. It is rare to need to use antiviral therapy in vaccinated leukemic children with a breakthrough illness.

Leukemic children can be given varicella vaccine if they have been in remission for at least 1 year. Two doses of vaccine 3 months apart are administered. Chemotherapy must be stopped 1 week before and after the first vaccination. In those who are immunized, there is a 50 per cent chance of a vaccine-associated rash developing 1 month later; about half require antiviral therapy for this rash, which may be given either orally or intravenously, depending on the extent of the rash and other symptoms such as fever. Vaccinees with a rash may also transmit the vaccine-type virus to about 15 per cent of other varicella susceptibles with whom they have close contact.

VARICELLA IN PREGNANCY

Varicella can be severe in pregnant women, and careful follow-up is indicated; treatment with acyclovir should be used in severe cases, such as those complicated by pneumonia. An unusual fetal syndrome (low birth weight, skin scarring, hypoplastic limb, mental retardation) occurs in about 2 per cent of infants born to women with varicella in the first or second trimester of pregnancy. Ultrasonography may be used to assess the condition of the fetus in some instances. Usually, termination of pregnancy is not recommended, although each case must be individualized.

REFERENCES

Balfour HH, Kelly JM, Suarez CS, et al: Acyclovir treatment of varicella in otherwise healthy children. J Pediatr 116:633–639, 1990.

Centers for Disease Control. Varicella-zoster immune globulin for the prevention of chickenpox. MMWR 33:84–100, 1984.

Gershon AA, LaRussa P, Steinberg S: Live attenuated varicella vaccine: Current status and future uses. Semin Pediatr Infect Dis 2:171–178, 1991.

HERPES SIMPLEX VIRUS INFECTIONS

STEVE KOHL, M.D.

Herpes simplex virus (HSV) infection is a common illness in children. In both normal and immunocompromised children, it may cause a wide variety of syndromes. Because it is easily treated when diagnosed early, the clinical index of suspicion must be high, especially in several settings, such as the neonate with vesicular lesions, unexplained seizures, spinal fluid pleocytosis, or even a sepsis-like syndrome. In the older child, focal encephalitis is the hallmark of HSV encephalitis. Unfortunately, because many other conditions can mimic this illness, a brain biopsy may still be necessary to diagnose HSV encephalitis and especially to exclude other treatable causes. In the immunocompromised child, mucositis, atypical erosive, necrotic, or papular skin lesions, or more invasive disease (pneumonitis, hepatitis, or a severe sepsis-like syndrome) may result from HSV infection.

TREATMENT

Neonatal Herpes Infection

A neonate with any manifestation of HSV from the most trivial vesicular lesion to the worst syndrome of disseminated disease must be treated with anti-HSV therapy immediately to prevent disease progression. Two drugs have been demonstrated to be equally effective in the therapy of neonatal HSV infection (Table 1). These include acyclovir (30 mg/kg/day in three divided doses, each infused over a 1-hour period, intravenously) and vidarabine (30 mg/kg/day in one dose infused over 12 hours).

Because of the lower fluid load required for administration, most clinicians prefer acyclovir. The typical duration of therapy is 14 to 21 days, regardless of the apparent trivial nature of some cases (e.g., local skin or eye infection) Five to 10 per cent of these infants will experience a serious recurrence of infection in the first month of life, whereas a much larger number (up to 50 per cent) will have recurrent skin infection. It has become our practice to treat any first recurrent infection in the first month with intravenous therapy for 14 days, beginning with vidarabine, pending viral drug sensitivity, to treat for the possibility of a yet to be reported acyclovir-resistant variant in the neonate.

TABLE 1. Summary of Drugs Used to Treat Herpes Infection*

Neonatal	Acyclovir: IV, 30–45 mg/kg/day in 3 divided doses for 14–21 days Vidarabine: IV, 30 mg/kg/day in single dose
Gingivostomatitis	Acyclovir: IV, 15 mg/kg/day in 3 divided doses Acyclovir: oral, 200 mg 5 × day (not to exceed 80 mg/kg/day) for 7–10 days
Ocular	Trifluorothymidine: 1% ophthalmic solution, 1 drop each 2 hr, maximum 9 drops, then 1 drop each 4 hr (5 drops per day) not to exceed 21 days
Encephalitis	Acyclovir: IV, 30 mg/kg/day in 3 divided doses for 14–21 days
Genital	
Primary disease	Acyclovir: oral, 200 mg 5 × day for 10 days, (not to exceed 80 mg/kg/day) Acyclovir: IV, 15 mg/kg/day in 3 divided doses for 5–7 days
Recurrence	Acyclovir: oral, 200 mg 5 × day for 5 days (not to exceed 80 mg/kg/day)
Chemosuppression	Acyclovir: oral, 200 mg 3–5 × day (not to exceed 80 mg/kg/day) for up to 12 months
Immunocompromised host	As for gingivostomatitis, duration as warranted clinically; in severe cases, may use doses of acyclovir: IV, 30 mg/kg/day in 3 divided doses Vidarabine: IV, 15 mg/kg/day in 1 dose over 12 hr Foscarnet†: IV, 120 mg/kg/day in 3 divided doses

*Oral acyclovir is not approved for use in children; informed consent is recommended. One capsule is 200 mg; 1 teaspoon of suspension is 200 mg.
†Foscarnet is not licensed to treat HSV infection.

A large number of surviving neonates will continue to have recurrent skin lesions in the first year of life. These lesions are usually not treated with antiviral chemotherapy. Those patients with localized skin disease originally, with three or more skin lesion recurrences in the first 6 months of life, are at increased risk of eventual long-term neurologic sequelae. A study utilizing chronic oral acyclovir therapy to prevent these recurrences and possibly improve outcome is ongoing. Interestingly, it is among these chronically treated patients that an acyclovir-resistant isolate has been observed.

Ancillary therapy for the neonate generally includes intensive care often necessitating ventilation, control of seizures, therapy for disseminated intravascular coagulopathy, and careful monitoring of areas with extensive skin lesions for secondary bacterial infection. If the eyes are involved, the use of a topical antiviral (trifluorothymidine in particular, one drop per eye each 2 hours) in conjunction with ophthalmologic consultation is advised. The neonate must be maintained in a private room with contact isolation. Respiratory isolation is also necessary in the neonate with HSV pneumonitis.

Therapy for the neonate exposed, but not yet infected (as in the case of a child born to a mother with genital lesions or a known positive culture for HSV at delivery) remains problematic. Because the attack rate in this setting to a child born to a mother with primary HSV infection is high (30 to 50 per cent), most would initiate anticipatory antiviral therapy, after appropriate culture, even in the well-appearing child. In the child born of a mother with recurrent illness, the lower attack rate (1 to 3 per cent) has generally allowed for a strategy of culture of the child at 24 to 48 hours of age and then only treating the child if its cultures for HSV are positive, or if symptoms of neonatal HSV infection are manifested.

As a result of the high rate of HSV infection concordance in multiple births, if one of twins or triplets has HSV infection, the entire group should be treated for HSV infection pending culture and careful child observation.

Gingivostomatitis

As a primary infection, typically in young children, gingivostomatitis is a bothersome, and at times very painful, illness lasting 7 to 10 days. The local oral and pharyngeal lesions can lead to poor fluid intake, resulting in dehydration. Conservative therapy includes bland fluids (apple juice, liquid gelatin, lukewarm broth) and ice popsicles. At times, intravenous rehydration is necessary. Acetaminophen is useful for fever and pain relief. Most pediatricians have shied away from the use of local anesthetics, such as viscous lidocaine, because of the short duration of pain relief and the risk that the child will further traumatize temporarily anesthetized and friable tissue.

In the moderately or severely ill child or in the child hospitalized for intravenous hydration, acyclovir (15 mg/kg/day in three divided doses intravenously) will probably shorten the duration of illness and viral shedding (Table 1). There are no sizable controlled studies utilizing either intravenous or oral acyclovir in this setting, but extrapolating from other similar manifestations of HSV (as genital disease) suggests that even in mild to moderate forms of illness, oral acyclovir (200 mg per dose four to five times per day, not to exceed a total dose of 80 mg/kg/day) will shorten the duration of illness. This is not an approved use of acyclovir.

Recurrent oral herpes (fever blisters) is generally of such mild severity and short duration that antiviral therapy is unwarranted. In patients with unusually severe recurrences, oral therapy should be considered (dosage as in primary infection). In patients with particularly frequent and severe recurrences, chronic suppressive acyclovir therapy may be contemplated (200 mg per dose, two to three times per day, not to exceed 80 mg/kg/day). This is especially useful in the patient who has erythema multiforme or aseptic meningitis syndrome associated with herpetic recurrences. These recommendations are not approved for children, and this must be carefully explained to the parents with consent.

Local Cutaneous Herpetic Infection

In some instances, HSV infection may develop on the skin, usually involving a digit (the herpetic whitlow), or the face (often associated with trauma), or trunk (as in a wrestler or rugby player). These infections should be treated as noted above for oral infection, again with the knowledge that to date there are no controlled trials proving the efficacy of acyclovir in these particular settings.

Ocular Infection

Herpes may cause blepharitis, conjunctivitis, keratitis, and, less commonly, retinitis. The practitioner is urged to care for such a patient in conjunction with a knowledgeable ophthalmologist.

Several licensed topical drugs increase the healing rate of herpetic eye infection (Table 1). These include trifluorothymidine (1 per cent, one drop every 2 hours, maximum nine drops, then one drop every 4 hours, maximum of 21 days), vidarabine (3 per cent ophthalmic ointment, five times daily; a different agent is substituted if there is no healing in 7 to 9 days) and idoxuridine (0.1 per cent ophthalmic ointment or solution). Trifluorothymidine appears to be the drug of choice and the least irritating to the eye itself. Orally administered acyclovir has been used to treat herpetic keratoconjunctivitis. Ophthalmologists may also utilize steroid therapy and ophthalmoplegics concomitant with the use of antivirals. The primary care physician is cautioned against the use of steroids in cases of conjunctivitis, because without antiviral therapy their use worsens herpetic eye infection. Although topical interferon-alpha and topical acyclovir are effective in therapy of HSV ocular disease, they are not licensed or available in ophthalmic preparations in the United States.

Encephalitis

HSV is the most common cause of sporadic fatal encephalitis in the United States. The fatality rate of untreated HSV encephalitis is 75 to 80 per cent. It typically presents as a focal encephalitis, but only about one half of cases presenting in this fashion are due to HSV. Brain biopsy is currently the only definite way to diagnose HSV encephalitis and to exclude conditions that mimic it unless reliable HSV polymerase chain reaction tests of the cerebrospinal fluid (CSF) are available. The constellation of localized findings on a computed tomogram, electroencephalogram, or brain scan, age over 30 years and CSF pleocytosis is highly associated with HSV encephalitis. Unfortunately, similar diagnostic criteria do not specifically exist for the pediatric patient.

Nonspecific therapy for the patient with HSV encephalitis includes intensive care management of a variety of neurologic complications, including increased intracranial pressure, often necessitating invasive intracranial monitoring procedures; maximum efforts to control the all too common severe and prolonged seizures; meticulous fluid management; and, at times, ventilatory support. Care is best administered in a tertiary level pediatric intensive care unit by a team consisting of intensivists, neurologists, neurosurgeons, and infectious disease experts.

Specific antiviral therapy is acyclovir (30 mg/kg/day in three divided doses, intravenously for 14 to 21 days) (Table 1). The outcome of HSV encephalitis is very dependent on the neurologic status of the patient at the time of administration of acyclovir. Thus, early institution of therapy—usually prior to definitive diagnosis and, it is hoped, prior to progression to semicoma or coma—is indicated. Therapy generally does not obscure the diagnosis if brain biopsy is performed within 24 hours. The role of corticosteroids is unstudied and controversial.

Apparent recurrences of encephalitis after cessation of therapy may be due to noninfectious, autoimmune-like phenomenon or recrudescence of HSV infection. Brain biopsy may be necessary to determine the need for therapy with anti-inflammatory agents or acyclovir, respectively.

The mortality rate of HSV encephalitis in the pediatric population is 5 to 10 per cent. Patients surviving HSV encephalitis usually need rehabilitation care of various types, depending on the neurologic damage sustained.

Genital Infection

Primary genital or *rectal herpes* is a painful, debilitating condition. Local care includes keeping lesions dry and clean. Some relief from periurethral pain may be achieved by urinating into a water-filled bathtub.

As in oral disease, in patients sick enough to be hospitalized, IV acyclovir (15 mg/kg/day in three divided doses) reduces symptoms, promotes healing, and decreases viral shedding (Table 1). In less severe cases, oral acyclovir (200 mg five times per day for 10 days) has similar, but slightly less dramatic, effects. Therapy of primary infection does not prevent subsequent recurrences.

Topical acyclovir has statistically significant effects but is much less useful than the systemically administered drug.

Recurrent herpes, if severe enough to warrant treatment, responds to oral acyclovir (one capsule [200 mg] five times a day for 5 days). In the patient with frequent or severe recurrences, the use of suppressive acyclovir (one capsule three to five times per day for up to a year) will have dramatic results, with an 80 to 90 per cent reduction of recurrence rate. The use of acyclovir in this setting must be carefully individualized. It is not a licensed use in children. Often the first recurrence after stopping acyclovir chemosuppression is perceived as one of the patient's most severe recurrences. Breakthrough recurrences are usually not due to viral resistance, although that may occur. In that situation, the next recurrence usually reverts to an acyclovir-susceptible virus strain.

Immunocompromised Host

Any manifestation of HSV infection in the immunocompromised host, as in the neonate, mandates therapy. Although topical therapy with acyclovir ointment is moderately effective, the mainstay of therapy is oral or intravenous acyclovir or vidarabine (Table 1). In anything but the most trivial HSV infection, one generally commences therapy with an intravenous preparation, usually acyclovir (15 mg/kg/day in three divided doses) because of the relative ease of administration in contrast to vidarabine. As the patient improves, therapy may be finalized with the oral preparation (dosage as for oral HSV infection). In patients with central nervous system (CNS) or disseminated disease, the intravenous acyclovir dose should

TABLE 2. Dosage Adjustment of Intravenous Acyclovir in Patients with Renal Insufficiency

Creatinine Clearance (ml/minute/1.73 m²)	Intravenous*		Oral†	
	Dose (mg)	*Dose Interval (hr)*	*Dose (mg)*	*Dose Interval (hr)*
Over 50	5	8	200	4 (5 × day)
25–50	5	12	200	4 (5 × day)
10–25	5	24	200	4 (5 × day)
0–10	2.5	24	200	12 (2 × day)

*Dosage for those conditions in which 15 mg/kg/day is typical dosage. Higher doses (30 mg/kg/day) with appropriate adjustment utilized in patients with encephalitis, in neonates, and in the severely ill immunosuppressed patient.
†Oral use not licensed in the pediatric population. Total daily dose not to exceed 80 mg/kg.

be 30 mg/kg/day in three divided doses. Duration of therapy is a clinical decision depending on state of healing of lesions.

In the HSV-seropositive patient about to be subjected to immunosuppression, as for induction therapy of cancer or transplantation, the risk of severe HSV recurrence is considerable and prophylactic oral or intravenous acyclovir has been shown to be beneficial. Similarly, in the chronically immunocompromised patient, as in those with acquired immunodeficiency syndrome (AIDS), primary immunodeficiency disease, or chronic immunosuppression, who is subjected to frequent or severe recurrent HSV infection, prophylactic oral acyclovir (200 mg three to five times per day, not to exceed 80 mg/kg/day) is effective in suppressing HSV recurrence. Cessation of prophylactic therapy usually results in prompt HSV recurrence.

It is particularly in the immunocompromised patient who is treated intermittently or chronically with acyclovir that acyclovir-resistant viruses have arisen. These are manifested by an absence of response or a poor response to therapy with acyclovir. In this setting, vidarabine is indicated pending viral susceptibility tests. A new relatively toxic drug—foscarnet—has shown promise in patients with HSV not responding to either acyclovir or vidarabine and may be the drug of choice for acyclovir-resistant HSV infection.

DRUG THERAPY

Acyclovir

Acyclovir is the mainstay of therapy for HSV infection. An oral preparation exists (one capsule contains 200 mg, one teaspoon of 5 ml contains 200 mg), but there are no licensed anti-HSV pediatric indications or dosages. Thus, when the oral preparation is used, this must be explained and written consent may be advisable.

Acyclovir is converted to the active antiviral by a series of phosphorylation steps in vivo, the first being mediated by an HSV enzyme, thymidine kinase (TK). Thus, TK-deficient viruses are resistant to acyclovir. The concentration of acyclovir inhibiting most acyclovir-susceptible HSV-1 isolates is 0.2 μg/ml, and 0.5 μg/ml for HSV-2 isolates. The major side effects of oral acyclovir are gastrointestinal (nausea, vomiting—3 per cent), and headache, or rash. The major side effects of intravenous acyclovir are phlebitis (15 per cent), increased serum creatinine levels (5 per cent), and rash. Less commonly, neurologic problems (lethargy, confusion, tremor, seizures, coma) and nephrotoxicity are reported. These are associated with elevated drug levels and reversed upon cessation of therapy. Nephrotoxicity can usually be avoided by maintaining hydration.

Acyclovir has been shown to blunt both the humoral and cellular immune response to HSV. Therapy of primary HSV infection with acyclovir has been associated with a more severe first recurrence in adults with genital infection. There are no analogous clinical data in the pediatric setting. Acyclovir has no effect on latent virus or on subsequent recurrence rates after cessation of acute or chronic therapy.

The dosage adjustment for patients with renal insufficiency is outlined in Table 2.

Vidarabine

As noted, vidarabine is essentially a back-up drug for acyclovir, generally reserved to treat acyclovir-resistant isolates. The drug is a nucleoside derivative and inhibits HSV by interfering with DNA polymerase. It is quite insoluble (1 mg per 2.2 ml of infusion fluid), necessitating large infusion volumes. This often makes its administration impractical in the neonate and encephalitic patient. The major side effects are gastrointestinal problems (anorexia, nausea, vomiting, diarrhea, increased liver function tests), suppression of the hematopoietic system, and neurologic problems (tremor, dizziness, hallucinations, ataxia, seizures). The neurologic symptoms have been seen especially in leukemic patients who have previously received antineoplastic treatment intrathecally.

REFERENCES

Kohl S: Postnatal herpes simplex virus infection. *In* Feigin RD, Cherry JD (eds): Textbook of Pediatric Infectious Diseases, 3rd ed. Philadelphia, WB Saunders Co, 1992.

Whitley R, Arvin A, Prober C, et al: A controlled trial comparing vidarabine with acyclovir in neonatal herpes simplex virus infection. N Engl J Med 324:444–449, 1991.

MUMPS

GREGORY F. HAYDEN, M.D.

No specific therapy is currently available for this self-limited illness. The selection of treatment, if any, depends solely upon the presence and severity of particular signs and symptoms. The spectrum of clinical illness is broad. Many infections are subclinical and require no therapy. Many children with mild clinical cases also benefit from therapeutic restraint. Occasional antipyretic-analgesic therapy with acetaminophen or aspirin may be used for symptomatic fever and general discomfort. Those relatively few children with severe or complicated cases may require more intensive supportive measures, sometimes including hospitalization.

MANAGEMENT OF SPECIFIC FEATURES

Appropriate management varies according to the manifestations of mumps that are encountered.

Parotitis. A regular diet is often well tolerated, but if chewing is painful, a soft diet with generous fluids will be appreciated. If acidic, sour, or highly seasoned foods induce pain, a bland diet is advisable. Analgesic therapy with acetaminophen often relieves parotid discomfort; aspirin can also be helpful but may make matters worse if it is allowed to dissolve in the mouth. Warm or cold compresses may provide local relief. Anecdotal reports suggest that a short course of corticosteroids may reduce intense parotid swelling and pain, but such therapy has not prevented the development of contralateral parotid involvement. This mode of treatment remains experimental and cannot be recommended.

Meningitis and Encephalitis. The spectrum of central nervous system (CNS) involvement is broad, ranging from asymptomatic lymphocytic pleocytosis in the cerebrospinal fluid (common) to severe encephalitis (rare). Acetaminophen or aspirin may relieve associated headache. Lumbar puncture sometimes relieves the headache associated with mumps but is indicated only for diagnostic purposes. Children with severe CNS involvement may require hospitalization for bed rest, analgesic-antipyretic therapy, and carefully monitored parenteral fluid therapy. Hospitalization is not required for mild, typical CNS involvement as long as the etiology has been established as mumps with reasonable certainty. Limited experience in the former Soviet Union suggests that interferon therapy can shorten the course of CNS involvement associated with mumps, but these preliminary findings need to be confirmed in a double-blind clinical trial.

Pancreatitis. Mild elevation of pancreatic enzymes in the absence of symptoms is frequent. Clinically apparent pancreatitis is unusual, but parenteral fluid therapy may be necessary for those children with abdominal pain and severe vomiting associated with pancreatitis. Acetaminophen therapy may sometimes relieve pain adequately. Narcotic agents can be used for severe pain but can potentially induce biliary spasm, with transient elevations of plasma amylase and lipase levels. Antiemetic therapy is not recommended.

Orchitis. About 20 to 30 per cent of postpubertal male patients with mumps are affected by orchitis, usually unilateral. Analgesia with acetaminophen or aspirin may relieve associated discomfort, but narcotic agents may be required. Bed rest, intermittent application of ice packs, and gentle support of the affected testis may also be helpful. Anesthetic block of the spermatic cord has been reported to relieve pain but should be reserved for severe cases refractory to less extreme measures. Treatment with systemic corticosteroids has been reported to decrease fever associated with orchitis but has not been documented to accelerate the resolution of orchitis or to reduce the incidence of subsequent atrophy. Diethylstilbestrol therapy and surgical incision of the tunica albuginea are likewise of largely unproven benefit and should be used infrequently, if at all.

There is no evidence that bed rest reduces the risk of orchitis. When given after the onset of illness, standard immunoglobulin (Ig) does not prevent orchitis or otherwise modify the clinical course. In previous years, a human hyperimmune globulin (mumps immune globulin, or MIG) was sometimes given to young men with early mumps in the hope of preventing the subsequent development of orchitis. The efficacy of such therapy was controversial, however, and this expensive preparation is no longer commercially available.

Patients and their parents may benefit from reassurance about normal reproductive function following mumps orchitis. Only about 25 per cent of cases of orchitis are bilateral, and in only a fraction of young men with such cases does progressive testicular atrophy develop. Subnormal sperm counts have occasionally been observed among such patients, but this impairment of fertility is generally partial and may be temporary. Contrary to popular belief, mumps orchitis does not cause impotence and rarely, if ever, results in frank sterility.

Very limited experience in Germany suggests that interferon therapy may help to prevent the late complications of mumps orchitis; however, these preliminary observations need to be confirmed in larger, controlled studies.

Arthritis. Salicylate therapy is often ineffective in treating the arthritis occasionally associated with mumps. A short course of corticosteroids or nonsteroidal anti-inflammatory agents is more likely to be helpful.

Other Manifestations. Other rare manifestations of mumps may include myocarditis, thyroiditis, nephritis, hepatitis, mastitis, epididymitis, oophoritis, and thrombocytopenia. These manifestations may be treated with a combination of careful monitoring, general supportive care, and symptomatic therapy.

Isolation. Hospitalized patients should remain in respiratory isolation until the parotid swelling has subsided or other manifestations have cleared. Attempts to isolate patients at home and in the community are less useful because patients are often contagious before the onset of parotid swelling and because persons with inapparent infection can nevertheless be contagious.

Treatment of Contacts. The comprehensive treatment of a child with mumps includes counseling family members and other close contacts about their risk for development of mumps and informing them what preventive measures are available. When one is planning a suitable course of action, the first step is to determine whether the exposed persons are likely to be susceptible to mumps. Laboratory testing is, unfortunately, of only limited value. The presence of mumps-neutralizing antibodies reliably indicates immunity, but this assay is time consuming, expensive, and not generally available. The mumps skin test and the commonly available serologic tests for mumps are not adequately sensitive to be clinically useful.

In most instances, estimation of susceptibility must therefore depend on simple historical information. A definite history of previous mumps illness or immunization strongly suggests immunity and provides grounds for reassurance. In contrast, a negative history of mumps illness is poorly predictive of mumps susceptibility; approximately 90 per cent of adults with such histories are immune on the basis of previous, unrecognized infection.

If susceptibility to mumps is nevertheless suspected, what can be done? Standard Ig is not effective in preventing mumps infection. The efficacy of even the higher potency MIG in this setting was questionable. It is uncertain whether the administration of live mumps vaccine after exposure can prevent or modify illness. In deciding whether to recommend vaccine, several considerations apply. On the positive side, adverse reactions to mumps vaccine are uncommon, and there is no increased risk of adverse reactions following the vaccination of an immune person. Vaccination after exposure is not known to increase the severity of incubating mumps. If the recognized exposure has not resulted in incubating infection, live mumps vaccination should provide protection against subsequent exposures. On the negative side, vaccination after exposure has never been demonstrated to be effective, and the vaccination (and vaccinator) may wrongly be blamed for the manifestations of mumps illness that develop after the vaccination. *Contraindications to live mumps vaccination include immunodeficiency, anaphylactic allergy to neomycin, severe febrile illness, pregnancy, and receipt of Ig or blood products within 3 months.* Persons with anaphylactic allergy to ingested egg should receive mumps vaccine only with caution according to published protocols for skin testing and rapid desensitization. If vaccination is considered, these limitations and uncertainties should be described in sufficient detail that the involved persons understand what benefits can reasonably be expected.

INFLUENZA

TERRENCE L. STULL, M.D.

Influenza pandemics occur almost yearly during the winter months in the United States. Even between these pandemics, approximately 10 to 40 per cent of children are infected with influenza each year. Influenza infections commonly result in school absenteeism, emergency room visits, and hospitalization of children. Although certain symptoms are characteristic of influenza, laboratory confirmation is needed for a specific diagnosis; rapid tests for the diagnosis of influenza infections are becoming available.

Annual prophylactic immunization against influenza is recommended for children who are at increased risk for acquiring the infection and for experiencing severe disease or complications. Amantadine is effective for prophylaxis and for specific therapy of early infections.

CLINICAL MANIFESTATIONS

Most influenza infections in children result in coryza, cough, and fever; these infections cannot be distinguished clinically from respiratory tract infections caused by other agents. More specific signs include headache, malaise, myalgia, and chills. Infants may present with signs compatible with sepsis. Less commonly, influenza infections may present with abdominal pain, vomiting, renal failure, or dysfunction of the central nervous system.

DIAGNOSIS

The specific diagnosis of influenza infection necessitates isolation of the virus from tissue culture; this can usually be accomplished in 2 to 3 days. Recently, methods for the rapid detection of influenza antigens in nasopharyngeal specimens or sputum by immunofluorescence and immunoassay have become available. If these rapid methods prove to be accurate, they should markedly improve the accuracy of therapeutic decisions and provide increased confidence in the decisions concerning therapy.

TREATMENT

Nonspecific supportive therapy, including bed rest, cough suppressants for nonproductive cough, and hydration therapy, is useful for symptomatic relief from influenza. To control fever in young children at risk of convulsions, acetaminophen is recommended because aspirin usage has been associated with Reye syndrome.

Both amantadine hydrochloride (Symmetrel, DuPont) and its structural analogue, rimantadine hydrochloride, are useful in the prevention of influenza A infections in unimmunized individuals (Table 1). These compounds are also effective for treatment of influenza A infections if therapy is initiated within 48 hours of the onset of symptoms, but are not useful against influenza B infections.

The recommended dose for children older than 1 year and younger than 9 years of age is 4.4 mg/kg/day given orally as two doses; the maximum recommended dose in this age group is 150 mg/day. Amantadine is available in both syrup (50 mg per 5 ml) and capsule (100 mg) forms. The dose recommended for older children is 200 mg/day given as two divided doses. Rimantadine is not yet commercially available; however, it may become the preferred drug because it has comparable efficacy and reduced toxicity.

TABLE 1. The Use of Amantadine in Influenza

Age (Years)	Dosage	Interval	Maximum Dose
1–8	2.2 mg/kg	12 hours	150 mg/day
≥9	100 mg	12 hours	

Chemotherapy should be considered for children with severe disease or who are at risk for severe disease or complications. Therapy with amantadine should continue 2 to 5 days, depending on the clinical course of the illness. For high-risk patients receiving prophylaxis, therapy should be considered until the risk of exposure has been eliminated or until 2 weeks after immunization is completed.

The role of aerosolized ribavirin, which has in vitro activity against both influenza A and B, is being investigated.

COMPLICATIONS

The most common complications of influenza infections, such as croup and pneumonia, result from localized viral infection of the respiratory tract. In patients with persistent fever, secondary bacterial infections (e.g., otitis media, sinusitis, pneumonia) should be suspected. Although most of these infections are due to *Haemophilus influenzae* and *Streptococcus pneumoniae*, *Staphylococcus aureus* may cause severe pneumonia.

Central nervous system involvement, such as convulsions, warrants investigations to rule out bacterial meningitis, encephalitis, and Reye syndrome.

IMMUNIZATIONS

Annual immunization against influenza is recommended for high-risk children, including (1) children with chronic cardiovascular or pulmonary conditions, including asthma; (2) children with other chronic conditions such as diabetes mellitus, renal dysfunction, hemoglobinopathies, or immunosuppression, requiring regular medical attention; (3) children at risk for Reye syndrome because of long-term aspirin therapy; and (4) children who live with high-risk individuals.

Two doses of inactivated, trivalent vaccine are given 1 month apart for the primary immunization of children 12 years of age or younger. Subsequent immunizations for these children, depending on the antigenic drift of the viruses, may be given in one dose. All immunizations for older children may be given in one dose. Subvirion (split) virus vaccine should be used in children 6 months to 12 years of age; whole-virus or split virus vaccine may be used on older children. The dosage varies, and the package insert should be read to determine the recommendations each year.

Limited information is available for infants under 6 months of age, and immunization is not recommended. Children with anaphylactic hypersensitivity to chicken or eggs should undergo skin testing; if results confirm the hypersensitivity, influenza immunization should not be given. The improvements in techniques to achieve purified vaccine components have reduced the risk of vaccine-related side effects.

RABIES

MARK S. PASTERNACK, M.D.

Rabies is a viral zoonosis endemic among a variety of terrestrial mammals. It is transmitted to humans either through direct contact with infected wild animals or through infection of domestic animals and pets with subsequent human infection. Disease in humans is manifested by progressive encephalitis, which is virtually always fatal. Consequently, the management of rabies focuses on the prevention of disease in exposed individuals through passive and active immunization (post-exposure prophylaxis), the pre-exposure immunization of individuals who are at increased risk of contracting rabies as a result of professional or recreational activities, including travel, and the immunization of pets (to reduce the possibility of rabies in a household vector). Although currently less than one human case is diagnosed each year in the United States, thousands of cases of animal rabies are reported to the Centers for Disease Control annually, while more than 10,000 individuals are treated for possible exposure, and tens of thousands of cases of human rabies occur each year in underdeveloped countries.

HUMAN RABIES

As noted above, within the United States rabies in man is extraordinarily rare. Because of the potentially long incubation period, past rabies exposures (i.e., attacks by animals abroad, exploration of caves) may not be recalled and rabies may not be considered in the initial differential diagnosis. The incubation period of rabies is highly variable, depending on the inoculum and site of infection. Although the incubation period commonly ranges between 20 and 90 days, clinical rabies has been reported months or even years after presumed exposure.

Clinical Features

Illness begins with an initial febrile prodrome, with malaise, headache, and nonlocalizing symptoms; in some cases, there may be paresthesias at the site of infection. The prodromal phase lasts from 2 to 10 days, when acute neurologic disease supervenes. Early encephalitic symptoms include intermittent agitation, hyperactivity, and disorientation and may include neck stiffness and seizures. Laryngospasm and spasms of the pharyngeal musculature after attempted ingestion of liquids are responsible for classic hydrophobia. In an acutely ill and febrile patient, the presence of prominent brain stem findings with relatively clear sensorium (without an alternative explanation) strongly supports the diagnosis of rabies.

A variety of additional neurologic findings may be present, including hyperactive or absent deep tendon reflexes and flaccid symmetric or asymmetric paralysis ("dumb rabies"). A mild mononuclear pleocytosis is present in the cerebrospinal fluid (CSF) in the majority of patients, with variable CSF protein and fluid pressure. After several days, the encephalitic phase progresses to coma and subsequent death by respiratory arrest in untreated patients. Intensive care unit support has prolonged the lives of patients with rabies for weeks, usually until a fatal complication supervenes.

Diagnosis

The diagnosis of rabies is best confirmed by neck skin biopsy and immunofluorescence testing. The patient should be isolated, and staff should use barrier (gown and glove) and respiratory precautions. Caregivers who have wound or mucous membrane contamination by the patient's secretions or tissues, or who are bitten, must undergo post-exposure prophylaxis.

POST-EXPOSURE MANAGEMENT

Rabies virus is present in the saliva of rabid animals, and transmission usually occurs following bite wound injuries; however, virus may be present on animal claws and transmitted by scratch, by contamination of a pre-existent wound or abrasion by animal saliva, or, rarely, by aerosol exposures in areas such as caves containing aerosolized virus from rabid bat secretions or in laboratories engaged in the study or production of rabies virus.

Rabies transmission is typically initiated by an unprovoked attack by a rabid animal. All injuries inflicted by wild carnivorous animals should be evaluated for rabies prophylaxis. Bites sustained during the feeding or handling of an apparently healthy domestic animal are considered "provoked." Documenting an unprovoked attack, especially with young children, may be problematic, and infected animals may shed rabies virus in saliva for several days prior to the onset of symptoms. Hence, in addition to the type of exposure, epidemiologic considerations are crucial in the management of possible rabies exposures.

Criteria for Prophylaxis

The decision to initiate post-exposure prophylaxis is made on the basis of (1) the animal species responsible for the initial attack, (2) the prevalence of rabies in this species in the local area, (3) the nature of the animal contact, (4) the animal's rabies immunization status, and (5) the availability of the attacking animal for monitoring or direct tissue examination.

Generally, bites by carnivorous wild animals, particularly skunks, raccoons, bats, or foxes and other predators, mandate post-exposure prophylaxis. Conversely, attacks by small rodents, such as squirrels, rats, and mice, do not warrant prophylaxis, although larger species (e.g., woodchucks) can harbor rabies. Petting a rabid animal or coming into contact with its excreta does not demand prophylaxis. When rabies is present in wild animals in the local area, attacks by unimmunized dogs or cats also require prophylaxis unless the domesticated animal can be captured for 10-day quarantine (in the case of pets) or examination (in the case of strays). Fully vaccinated dogs or cats have been reported to develop rabies only rarely.

Quarantined domestic animals should be monitored by a veterinarian or animal control officer and killed for examination if signs of disease develop. Captured wild animals should be killed and the head submitted for rabies testing. In addition to performing brain immunofluorescence examinations to confirm animal rabies, local and state health authorities offer expert consultative advice regarding the prevalence of rabies in a given area among different animal species and the need for post-exposure prophylaxis in individual cases.

Wound Care

Prompt and thorough local wound care is the foundation of post-exposure management. Wounds must be copiously irrigated with soap and water, and puncture wounds should be irrigated by catheter. Tetanus immunization status should be reviewed and prophylaxis administered if indicated, and antibiotics should be administered as clinically indicated.

Specific immunoprophylaxis should begin as promptly as possible, preferably within 24 hours of attack. Passive immunization with human rabies immune globulin (HRIG) confers protection to the victim before rabies vaccine can elicit protective antibody. HRIG is administered at a dose of 20 IU of HRIG/kg, with half of the dose infiltrated into the soft tissues around the wound and the remainder administered intramuscularly in the gluteal area. If HRIG is not immediately available, it should be administered as soon as possible, but it probably offers little benefit if given beyond 7 to 8 days after active immunization with rabies vaccine is begun. HRIG is not required if complete pre-exposure prophylaxis or earlier post-exposure prophylaxis has been administered.

Vaccines

In the United States, two inactivated, tissue culture–derived rabies vaccines are available for human use: a human diploid cell vaccine (HDCV) and an aluminum phosphate-adsorbed vaccine (RVA) derived from fetal rhesus lung diploid cell culture. In both instances, 1 ml of vaccine is given intramuscularly initially and on days 3, 7, 14, and 28 thereafter in the deltoid (or anterolateral aspect of the thigh in children). The vaccine should not be given in the same limb as the HRIG. If the captured domestic animal is observed for 10 days and remains well, or if it is killed and findings are negative for rabies by immunofluorescence testing, the immunization series initiated at the time of animal attack may be discontinued. Although both vaccines reliably evoke protective neutralizing antibodies in normal hosts, immunocompromised individuals receiving rabies immunizations should be tested for the development of neutralizing antibodies.

Localized side effects, such as pain, swelling, and induration, as well as mild to moderate systemic toxicity, including fever, headache, and myalgias, are common but should not interrupt the immunization series. Instead, symptomatic treatment with analgesics or anti-inflammatory, antipyretic agents (e.g., aspirin) as well as antihistamines should be employed.

A variety of post-exposure immunization schedules are employed outside the United States, including the use of equine antirabies antiserum, intradermally administered tissue culture–derived rabies vaccines, and vaccines derived from nerve tissue. If post-exposure prophylaxis has been initiated abroad, additional therapy may be necessary when the patient returns to the United States; the state or local health department should be consulted for specific advice.

PRE-EXPOSURE PROPHYLAXIS

Individuals at increased risk for rabies exposure include veterinarians, animal handlers, laboratory workers engaged in rabies research and virus production, spelunkers, and travelers residing for extended intervals in areas where there is endemic canine rabies. Primary pre-exposure vaccination with human diploid cell rabies vaccine (HDCV) can be administered in three 1-ml intramuscular doses on days 0, 7, and 21 or 28, or as three 0.1-ml intradermal doses according to the same schedule. Immunocompromised recipients should undergo intramuscular vaccine immunization and be tested for the development of neutralizing antibodies. Individuals receiving chloroquine prophylaxis for malaria also require the intramuscular vaccine immunization regimen because chloroquine interferes with the antibody response to HDCV.

Individuals with the highest ongoing risk of rabies exposure should undergo serologic monitoring of immune status at 6-month intervals and should receive boosters as needed to maintain adequate neutralizing titers. Individuals at moderate risk should undergo serologic monitoring at 2-year intervals or should simply receive booster immunizations at this interval. Serologic monitoring and booster doses are not required for those with low risks of exposure once the primary vaccination series is completed. If previously vaccinated persons are exposed to rabies, they should receive two additional doses of vaccine (1 ml, given intramuscularly) on days 0 and 3 days thereafter. Such individuals do not require the administration of HRIG and do not require the complete five-dose post-exposure vaccine regimen.

An immune complex–like reaction is seen in some individuals receiving booster doses of HDCV but is not common in primary immunization recipients. This reaction has been attributed to nonvirion constituents in HDCV; if it occurs, subsequent boosters should be administered with an alternate inactivated diploid cell rabies vaccine. Rabies Vaccine Inactivated (Diploid Cell Origin)-Dried,* a purified human diploid cell vaccine, has not been associated with this reaction.

*Connaught Laboratories, Stillwater, Pa. Phone: 1–800–VACCINE.

INFECTIOUS MONONUCLEOSIS AND EPSTEIN-BARR VIRUS RELATED SYNDROMES

CIRO V. SUMAYA, M.D.

Epstein-Barr virus (EBV), a member of the herpesvirus group, is a common infectious agent worldwide. EBV infections have an important interrelationship with age, socioeconomic status, and disease. In developing countries and poverty pockets of developed countries, infections by this virus develop very early in childhood and are predominantly asymptomatic. With onset of the EBV infection in older children and young adults, as seen more in the higher socioeconomic strata of developed countries, there is a much greater likelihood for the consequence to be infectious mononucleosis (IM). This EBV-induced disease consists of a triad of typical clinical (fever, tonsillopharyngitis, cervical adenitis, and hepatosplenomegaly), hematologic (lymphocytosis with atypical formation), and serologic (heterophil antibody, specific EBV antibody) findings. It is clear, though, that typical IM may occur at the earlier end of the age spectrum, including young infants.

EBV regularly establishes a lifelong latent infection of B lymphocytes and endothelial cells of the oropharynx and possibly the uterine cervix. In selected patients, usually with an underlying immunocompromised state, reactivation of the previously quiescent (latent) infection may lead to deleterious effects, such as lymphoproliferative and lymphomatous complications. On rare occasions, primary EBV infections have also produced severe and prolonged disease with eventual death.

LABORATORY DIAGNOSIS

The clinical suspicion of EBV IM is confirmed by the laboratory detection of a lymphocyte count of at least 50 per cent accompanied by an atypical lymphocyte count of at least 10 per cent of peripheral white blood cells and a positive heterophil antibody test. The most widely used method to determine these heterophil antibodies is the rapid slide agglutination test. The slide test employing sensitized horse erythrocytes and a guinea pig kidney adsorption step (some kits include a beef cell antigen absorption step also) has a false-positive rate of less than 10 per cent and detects heterophil antibody in at least 80 to 90 per cent of adult and adolescent cases of IM. Interpretation of agglutination by the reader is the variable most likely to account for false-positive and possibly false-negative results. A heterophil antibody response is often not detected in very young children. Heterophil antibody responses also may not be detectable early in the course of EBV IM and in some cases (10 per cent) are absent during the entire disease course. A smaller proportion of heterophil-negative episodes of IM are produced by cytomegalovirus, *Toxoplasma gondii,* human immunodeficiency virus (HIV), adenovirus, possibly rubella, or other as yet unknown agent(s).

Specific EBV serologic testing is not indicated in typical episodes of IM but may be needed in cases lacking a heterophil antibody response or in heterophil antibody-positive cases that are unusually severe or atypical. The serologic response associated with an acute EBV infection is characterized by the following pattern: IgM antibodies to EB viral capsid antigen (VCA), raised IgG antibodies to VCA and early antigen (EA) complex, and an absent or low level of antibodies to EB nuclear antigen (EBNA). In acute EBV IM, the antibody response to EA complex classically is directed to diffuse (D) component; the anti-EA response in other forms of EBV infection is more likely directed to restricted (R) component.

TREATMENT

A specific diagnosis of IM should reassure both patient and parents, as the illness usually follows a self-limited (albeit at times severe) course taking 2 to 3 weeks. Symptomatic measures can include the use of acetaminophen for the acute febrile illness, saline gargles for relief of pharyngitis, and intake of sufficient fluid. Penicillin therapy is probably prudent for those patients who have a positive throat culture or antigen test for group A beta-hemolytic streptococci. Ampicillin or amoxicillin should not be given because these medications may elicit a generalized rash in many patients with IM. Bed rest or reduction of activity can be decided on the basis of individual tolerance and severity of clinical manifestations. Patients with splenomegaly should avoid strenuous activities and, in particular, contact sports because of the risk of splenic rupture. Another uncommon, potentially life-threatening complication is the development of respiratory obstruction due to the acutely inflamed tonsillar and pharyngeal tissue. The latter patients may need to be hospitalized for close supervision and begun on a short (4- to 5-day) course of steroids equivalent to 40 mg/m^2/day of prednisone based on anecdotal evidence that this may reduce pharyngeal inflammation and preclude the need for invasive procedures. Trials of intravenous or oral acyclovir in patients with IM have resulted in a transient reduction of viral shedding, but only minimal or no amelioration in duration or severity of symptoms. Other antiviral agents do not appear to produce any beneficial results.

CLINICAL COURSE

Routine Course

The acute symptoms and fever usually last a few days to 2 weeks. It is not uncommon, however, for splenomegaly to last 2 or 3 months. Up to 6 or so months may elapse before the patient fully recovers; the course of recovery may be interrupted by temporary setbacks or periods of no improvement.

Complications

Fortunately, most of the complications, including severe ones, are transient and lead to no sequelae. Nonetheless, the presence of significant complications such as pneumonia, bone marrow dysfunction, hepatitis, renal abnormalities, and neurologic problems may require consultation with a specialist. In some cases, the use of steroids may be warranted, although the evidence for their beneficial effect is unclear.

In selected individuals who are unable to muster an adequate T cell immune response to the infection, an overwhelming lymphoproliferative disease, characterized by EBV-infected B cell dissemination that may involve multiple organs, may develop. This is well illustrated by the rare genetic condition, X-linked lymphoproliferative syndrome, described in young male kindred in whom the primary EBV infection usually produces a fatal illness. Conversely, an overly intense T cell immune response has been considered a cause of hypogammaglobulinemia and other immunodepressive-type events following IM. Children with a variety of congenital immunodeficiencies and acquired immunocompromised states, in particular organ transplant recipients and those with an underlying HIV infection, may at times also experience severe EBV disease with ultimate lymphoproliferation or lymphomatous sequelae. Acyclovir administration has been reported to reduce or resolve EBV-associated lymphoproliferative lesions in organ transplant recipients; variable results have been noted in the use of acyclovir plus interferon and possibly gamma globulin in patients with severe multisystem EBV disease. It is speculated that an intense, chronic EBV infection is largely responsible for the development of Burkitt's lymphoma in young African children.

Chronic Fatigue Syndrome

In this debilitating condition there is a pattern of complaints of long-standing fatigue, low-grade intermittent fever, neuropsychologic problems, and sore throat, among others. However, chronic fatigue syndrome is commonly unaccompanied by objective physical signs. The original controversial association with a persistent EBV infection generated by a somewhat abnormal EBV serologic response in affected individuals is now viewed as an epiphenomenon probably reflecting a generalized mild and variable dysfunction of the immune system. The cause, pathogenesis, and specific treatment of this poorly defined, debilitating condition remain unclear. It should be kept in mind that significant chronic infectious, collagen vascular, or oncologic diseases may produce similar manifestations early in their course, with specific treatment possibly available.

CAT-SCRATCH DISEASE

ANDREW M. MARGILETH, M.D.

Cat-scratch disease (CSD) usually presents as a chronic (at least 3 weeks) lymphadenitis in the cervical or axillary region and is commonly benign and self-limiting. The cause is a gram-negative pleomorphic bacillus that has been obtained from skin, blood, pleural fluid, lymph node, and liver cultures. The adenopathy (at least 10 mm) is usually regional and tender initially in 80 per cent of patients. However, in one third of patients, multifocal adenitis may occur. Following cat contact (95 per cent) and/or scratches (66 per cent) prior to the onset of adenopathy, the patient or parent often notes a primary inoculation skin papule or eye lesion. About 80 per cent of patients are under 21 years of age. Adenopathy persists for several weeks to months and gradually resolves spontaneously. However, 10 to 15 per cent of CSD patients have atypical clinical manifestations, which include the oculoglandular syndrome of Parinaud, systemic disease with or without hepatosplenomegaly, thrombocytopenic purpura, osteomyelitis, and breast tumor.

Systemic disease (severe malaise, weight loss, prolonged fevers, fatigue, encephalopathy) occurs in 1 to 2 per cent of patients. Morbidity appears to be more severe in adolescents and adults. Recently, severe disseminated systemic disease, characterized by hepatic and/or splenic abscesses, neuroretinitis, pleuritis, and generalized lymphadenitis with epithelioid angiomatosis and bone marrow involvement, has been noted in immunocompromised patients. Paradoxically, CSD in patients with acquired immunodeficiency syndrome (AIDS) have responded dramatically to commonly used antibiotics.

Cat-scratch skin test antigens, which have been used since 1947, constitute a safe, reliable, and specific (90 to 98 per cent) means of diagnosis. More than 6000 doses of the skin test antigen have been used with no reports of disease transmission or serious reactions. Positive tests in persons without active disease are reported in family members of CSD patients, animal workers, cat lovers, healthy adults, and patients who previously had the disease.

THERAPY

General Treatment

In most patients, no therapy is required. Conservative management of CSD consists of careful observation over several (usually 2 to 6) months, during which time spontaneous involution of the lymphadenopathy should occur. Bed rest is usually not required; however, extreme fatigue may be lessened by frequent bed rest. The patient should avoid trauma to the involved enlarged node. The local application of heat may provide relief and decrease swelling over several days. We have noted less pain, more rapid involution, and occasionally spontaneous drainage, particularly from fluctuant lesions with application of warm, moist compresses applied to areas of adenopathy and also to primary inoculation sites for 30 to 60 minutes, four to six times daily.

Fever occurs in one third of patients with CSD. Antipyretics and analgesics, such as aspirin (65 mg/kg/day in six doses) or acetaminophen (60 mg/kg/day in six doses), are advised for the tender adenitis.

If suppuration occurs (10 to 15 per cent of patients), incision and drainage are not recommended because a chronic sinus tract discharge may occur and persist for several or more months. Needle aspiration relieves painful adenopathy and provides material for culture. After one or two aspirates, the patient usually becomes symptom-free within 24 to 48 hours.

The following technique is used for needle aspiration. After the skin is washed with povidone-iodine (Betadine) cleanser, an 18- or 19-gauge needle is inserted through 1 to 2 cm of normal unanesthetized skin at the base of the mass to avoid a chronic sinus tract in the event that a tuberculous lesion is present. Surgical incision of the nodes is usually not indicated unless one suspects a noninfectious etiology, such as a neoplasm.

Specific Treatment

Systemic Antibiotics

A relatively healthy child or adolescent with typical CSD probably does not need antibiotic therapy. In the few CSD patients with prolonged fever, systemic symptoms and/or severe lymphadenitis, each of four drugs was effective at least 50 per cent of the time:

1. Oral trimethoprim-sulfamethoxazole (6 to 8 mg/kg/day, [trimethoprim component] in two divided doses for 7 days) may bring about prompt improvement.
2. Rifampin (10 to 20 mg/kg/day in two to three doses for 7 to 14 days) may be effective. Maximum dose daily is 600 mg.
3. For children over 12 years of age, ciprofloxacin (20 to 30 mg/kg/day in two divided doses for 7 to 14 days) may be very effective.
4. In the rare, severely ill patient, gentamicin sulfate (5 mg/kg/day in three divided doses intramuscularly) has been quite effective within 72 hours.

Other Antibiotics and Medications

Commonly used antibiotics are not effective in patients with typical CSD. However, patients with AIDS and CSD may respond to erythromycin, doxycycline, or antimycobacterial antibiotics.

Anticonvulsants for several weeks or months may be helpful for the patient with CSD encephalitis.

The use of oral corticosteroids cannot be recommended at this time. Anecdotally, we know of several patients severely ill with systemic disease who responded to prednisone (2 mg/kg for 24 hours for 5 to 7 days or longer).

PROGNOSIS

The prognosis is excellent: Lymphadenopathy usually regresses spontaneously in 2 to 6 months. One attack of CSD appears to confer lifelong immunity in children. However, three adults experienced a recurrence of lymphadenopathy 6 to 13 months after the initial diagnosis of CSD. Fatal complications and irreversible sequelae have not been documented. Those patients with encephalitis have recovered completely.

PREVENTION

The patient with CSD does not require isolation or quarantine. The disease cannot be spread directly from one person to another. Because the animals involved are invariably healthy, disposing of the cat or dog is not recommended. CSD develops in about 5 per cent of family members, usually within a 2- to 3-week period of each other. The declawing of pet cats can reduce CSD incidence. Because there are a large number of households with cats worldwide (approximately 50 million households in the United States), CSD will be difficult to prevent and will continue to be seen in general practice. The most common pitfall in diagnosis of CSD is failure to inquire about animal contact and/or scratches, especially by a cat or dog. The pediatrician should always ask the child about contact with a neighbor's or relative's animal. Intimate cat contact, usually with a kitten, is common.

REFERENCES

Carithers HA, Margileth AM: Cat scratch disease: Acute encephalopathy and other neurologic manifestations. Am J Dis Child 145:98–101, 1991.

Margileth AM: Antibiotic therapy for cat scratch disease: Clinical study of therapeutic outcome in 268 patients and a review of the literature. Pediatr Infect Dis J 11:474–478, 1992.

Relman DA, Loutit JS, Schmidt TM, et al: The agent of bacillary angiomatosis. N Engl J Med 323:1573–1580, 1990.

LYME DISEASE

EUGENE D. SHAPIRO, M.D.

Lyme disease, caused by the spirochete *Borrelia burgdorferi,* is transmitted by ticks of the *Ixodes* species (*Ixodes dammini,* the deer tick, in the eastern United States and *Ixodes pacificus* on the West Coast). Infection with *Borrelia burgdorferi* results in a wide spectrum of clinical manifestations, from asymptomatic seroconversion to encephalomyelitis. Because the disease has been recognized only recently, there are limited data about optimal treatment regimens and about long-term outcomes after treatment, especially in children. It is likely that as more information becomes available and as new antimicrobials are licensed, some of the following recommendations will change. In addition, because in many instances there are no data from clinical trials of treatment of children, the recommendations are extrapolated from studies conducted with adults.

DIAGNOSIS

Although this article is not intended to address the issue of diagnosis, because of extraordinary publicity about Lyme disease in the lay press, an exception must be made for this disease, since misdiagnosis is so common. Indeed, the most common reason for failure of treatment of Lyme disease is misdiagnosis.

The problem is that methods of confirming that the organism is present in a patient (e.g., culture, antigen detection, or histopathology) have poor sensitivity and, in any case, appropriate specimens often are unavailable. Consequently, much reliance has been placed on serologic tests, such as enzyme-linked immunosorbent assays, that document antibody response to the organism. *Unfortunately, many of these tests, except in laboratories with exceptionally rigid standards of quality control, are unreliable, with unacceptably high rates of false-positive and false-negative results. In addition, because patients often do not produce measurable antibodies until 4 to 6 weeks after the onset of the infection, most patients with early Lyme disease will not have antibodies to* B. burgdorferi *that are detectable by conventional means.*

Clinical manifestations are the most important factor in making the diagnosis. Physicians must evaluate the results of antibody tests critically. Patients with atypical symptoms are unlikely to have Lyme disease even if the antibody test is positive. In questionable cases such as these, the tests should be repeated in a reference laboratory before treatment is initiated. It is hoped that within the next few years serologic tests that are more specific and better standardized will become available.

TREATMENT

Appropriate treatment depends on stage of disease and clinical manifestations. Stages are generally divided into early and late disease.

Early Disease

Erythema Migrans

The first clinical manifestation of Lyme disease is erythema migrans, a characteristic expanding, erythematous, annular rash that occurs at the site of the tick bite. The lesion may (or may not) demonstrate clearing in the center. The center may also become vesicular or, rarely, necrotic in appearance. The single erythema migrans lesion may or may not be accompanied by systemic symptoms such as fever and myalgias. Often, dissemination occurs, with the development of multiple erythema migrans lesions accompanied by systemic symptoms. Occasionally, early Lyme disease manifests as a flu-like illness without erythema migrans (because the rash either is absent or is unrecognized). Because specific antibodies usually are not yet detectable in this stage of the illness, without the rash the diagnosis rarely can be made.

The recommended treatment regimens for early Lyme disease are shown in Table 1. Doxycycline and amoxicillin are considered to be equivalent in their therapeutic efficacy. There have been a slightly larger proportion of clinical treatment failures when erythromycin was used to treat early Lyme disease. Consequently, erythromycin should be used only when there are contraindications to the use of both amoxicillin and doxycycline. In the future, erythromycin as an alternative agent may be replaced by azithromycin (a macrolide antimicrobial that is not yet licensed in the United States), cefuroxime, or other antimicrobials if clinical trials confirm preliminary data about their efficacy. Amoxicillin and doxycycline, respectively, have largely replaced penicillin and tetracycline as standard agents for treatment because they are better absorbed, are equally potent or more potent in vitro against *B. burgdorferi*, and may be administered less frequently. Doxycycline should *not* be administered to children younger than 9 years of age because it may discolor the teeth. Although 21 days of treatment usually is recommended for early Lyme disease, a shorter course of treatment (10 days) may be effective but should be reserved for children with a single erythema migrans lesion and no systemic symptoms.

Occasionally, a Jarisch-Herxheimer reaction, characterized by fevers and myalgias, occurs shortly after antimicrobial treatment is begun. This reaction is generally short-lived and should be treated with nonsteroidal anti-inflammatory agents. Antimicrobial therapy should not be altered.

TABLE 1. Antimicrobial Treatment of Lyme Borreliosis

A. Early Lyme Disease

1. *Erythema migrans and disseminated early disease without focal findings.*
   Doxycycline, 100 mg b.i.d. for 21 days (do not use in children <9 years of age)
   or
   Amoxicillin, 50 mg/kg/day divided t.i.d. (maximum 500 mg per dose) for 21 days

   An alternative agent for those who cannot take either amoxicillin or doxycycline is erythromycin, 30–50 mg/kg/day divided q.i.d. (maximum 250 mg per dose) for 21 days.
2. *Bell's palsy*
   Treat as for erythema migrans for 21–30 days (do not use corticosteroids).
3. *Carditis*
   Treat as for late neurologic disease.
4. *Meningitis*
   Treat as for late neurologic disease.

B. Late Lyme Disease

1. *Arthritis*
   Initial treatment is the same as for erythema migrans except treat for 30 days. If symptoms fail to resolve after 2 months or there is a recurrence, treat as for late neurologic disease.
2. *Neurologic disease**
   Ceftriaxone, 50–80 mg/kg/day in a single dose (maximum 2 g) for 14–21 days IV or IM
   or
   Penicillin G, 200,000–400,000 units/kg/day (maximum 20 million units/day) divided q 4 hr IV for 14–21 days.

*For isolated palsy of the facial nerve, see A.2 above.

Bell's Palsy

Paralysis of the facial nerve, which also is usually a manifestation of early disseminated Lyme disease, often occurs while erythema migrans is still present and before antibodies to *B. burgdorferi* are detectable. The outcome of Bell's palsy due to Lyme disease generally is excellent (with or without antimicrobial therapy); resolution usually occurs within 4 to 6 weeks. The purpose of antimicrobial treatment is to prevent late manifestations of Lyme disease. If Bell's palsy is the only neurologic manifestation of Lyme disease, the outcome with orally administered antimicrobials is as good as the outcome with parenteral treatment (which, consequently, is not necessary). The oral regimens should be administered for 21 to 30 days (Table 1).

Corticosteroids are unnecessary and may be contraindicated. Although pleocytosis sometimes may be present in the cerebrospinal fluid, there is no evidence, without other neurologic symptoms (such as meningitis or radiculitis), that parenteral therapy is necessary for such patients. Nevertheless, some physicians prefer to treat patients with pleocytosis with parenteral antimicrobial therapy.

Carditis

Lyme carditis, which usually presents with abnormalities of the conduction system (especially different degrees of atrioventricular block), is very rare in children. If it does occur, it usually is a manifestation of relatively early disseminated disease and should be treated as noted in Table 1.

Meningitis

Aseptic meningitis is a rare manifestation of disseminated Lyme disease. It may be accompanied by other focal neurologic signs and symptoms. Treatment with parenterally administered ceftriaxone or penicillin is indicated.

Late Disease

Arthritis

Monarticular or oligoarticular arthritis of large joints (typically the knee) is the classic manifestation of late Lyme disease. A number of different treatment regimens have been used for Lyme arthritis, the superiority of any one of which has not been convincingly demonstrated. Persistence of symptoms after treatment ("treatment failure") occurs in a relatively small proportion of patients with either orally administered or parenterally administered antimicrobials. Presumably, in most instances persistent synovitis is due not to the failure to kill *B. burgdorferi* but, rather, is caused by either autoimmunity or reactive inflammation.

If there are no concomitant neurologic symptoms, Lyme arthritis initially should be treated with orally administered amoxicillin or doxycycline. If symptoms persist several months after treatment, a single course of parenterally administered penicillin or ceftriaxone should be administered.

Neurologic Symptoms

Encephalitis, encephalopathy, and radiculoneuritis are rare manifestations of Lyme disease in children. It is important to document either serum antibodies against *B. burgdorferi* and pleocytosis in the cerebrospinal fluid or concentration of antibodies against *B. burgdorferi* in the cerebrospinal fluid of patients suspected of having Lyme disease of the central nervous system. Chronic fatigue alone and other nonspecific symptoms, in the absence of objective abnormalities that are demonstrable by physical examination, nerve conduction tests, or psychometric tests, have not been shown to be associated with Lyme disease. The above-mentioned neurologic syndromes should be treated with parenterally administered antimicrobials—either ceftriaxone or penicillin. As with arthritis, it may take some time after treatment for the symptoms to resolve.

Tick Bites

There have been no studies that demonstrate that prophylactic antimicrobials are indicated for people in endemic areas who are bitten by ixodid ticks. Data indicate that the risk of Lyme disease developing after a recognized bite is very low. Such patients should be treated only if symptoms or signs of Lyme disease develop.

CYTOMEGALOVIRUS INFECTION

SERGIO STAGNO, M.D.

CONGENITAL INFECTION

Cytomegalovirus (CMV) is the most common viral agent to cause congenital infection in humans, affecting from 0.2 to 2.2 per cent of all live births. It may result from either primary infection acquired during gestation or a recurrent maternal infection (reactivation or reinfection) in seropositive women. Approximately 5 per cent of the estimated 35,000 infants born annually in the United States with congenital CMV infection have overt signs and symptoms at birth, with generalized disease commonly referred to as "cytomegalic inclusion disease" (CID). Another 5 per cent have milder or atypical involvement, and 90 per cent are born with subclinical infection. Most, but not all, symptomatic congenital CMV infections result from primary infection.

TREATMENT

A small number of systemically administered antiviral agents have been used in therapeutic trials of CMV infection, mostly in immunosuppressed patients, normal adults with mononucleosis syndrome, and infants with symptomatic congenital infections. Most trials with idoxuridine, 5-fluoro-2′-deoxyuridine, cytosine arabinoside, adenine arabinoside, acyclovir, leukocyte interferon, interferon stimulators, transfer factor, or combinations of these agents have proved very disappointing in the treatment of symptomatic congenital infections. During therapy, these compounds cause reductions in the amount of virus excreted but the effect is short-lived. With the exception of vidarabine and acyclovir, drug-related toxicity is a significant problem.

Similarly, the use of leukocyte interferon and transfer factor has yielded mixed results. Toxicity and variability of interferon preparations, combined with the highly variable effect on viral excretion and the lack of controls, have rendered these small studies difficult to interpret. The toxic effects of interferon included poor weight gain, transient elevation of serum glutamic-oxaloacetic transaminase (SGOT), and fever.

Thus far, it has been impossible to verify clinical efficacy in any of these studies. Besides the fact that suppression of viral replication has been only transient, other confounding factors are the wide spectrum of disease resulting from congenital infection, the unpredictable natural course of the illness, and the fact that many patients had incurred irreversible damage before birth.

The most recent addition to the armamentarium is ganciclovir, 9-[1,3-dihydroxypropoxymethyl] guanine, which in preliminary studies has proved partially effective in the treatment of CMV retinochoroiditis and pneumonitis in immunosuppressed transplant patients. No controlled studies of treatment of congenital CMV infection are yet available.

One report describes the result of a phase I–II protocol in which 37 infants with severe symptomatic congenital CMV infection were treated with either 8 mg/kg/day or 12 mg/kg/day (individual doses administered at 12-hour intervals) for a total of 6 weeks. The study included serial clinical, pharmacokinetic, virologic, audiometric, and ophthalmologic evaluations. One infant died on day 9 of therapy, and 23 of the 27 completed the course of therapy. Ganciclovir administration was discontinued in five patients because of neutropenia (two), necrotizing enterocolitis (one), worsening of liver function tests (one), and bacterial infection (one). Retinal hemorrhages developed in four infants during ganciclovir therapy or shortly after discontinuation of treatment. Of equal importance was the suggestion of improved hearing in treated patients with evidence of hearing impairment at the onset of treatment. Given these observations, the National Institutes of Allergy and Infectious Diseases (NIAID)–sponsored collaborative antiviral study group is undertaking a randomized controlled study to determine the efficacy of ganciclovir for symptomatic congenital CMV infection (12 mg/kg/day as above).

Asymptomatic Infection

Infants with asymptomatic infection or with mild disease do not require antiviral therapy. Passive immunization has not been tried, but it is doubtful that it will ever work for treatment of congenital infections because the cases are identified weeks and months after the infection occurred in utero. Vaccines have not received extensive study as a means of preventing acquisition of CMV infection during pregnancy, and their efficacy is unknown.

Postnatal Infection

CMV infections are quite common during the first years of life. Transmission results from direct or indirect person-to-person contact through exposure to breast milk, genital secretions, saliva, and urine or from transfusion of blood and blood products. With the exception of immunocompromised patients and premature infants, clinically apparent disease is very uncommon. Infection may result in mononucleosis-like syndrome, pneumonitis, polyneuritis, and retinitis. In immunocompromised patients, a temporary reduction or suppression of chemotherapy may result in clinical improvement. Ganciclovir has been used to treat life-threatening CMV infections in immunocompromised hosts (bone marrow and cardiac transplant recipients and patients with acquired immunodeficiency syndrome [AIDS]). CMV infections of various sorts in adult patients have responded to ganciclovir given at a dose of 10 mg/kg/day (individual doses administered at 12-hour intervals) for 2 or 3 weeks, followed by once-a-day maintenance of 5 mg/kg administered until regression of clinical manifestations.

CMV retinitis and gastrointestinal disease appear to be clinically responsive to therapy but, like viral excretion, recur upon cessation of therapy. Early experience with CMV pneumonitis was very discouraging with no reduction in mortality or morbidity. Drug toxicity with ganciclovir is extensive and includes neutropenia, thrombocytopenia with bleeding, liver dysfunction, reduction in spermatogenesis, and gastrointestinal and renal abnormalities.

The experience with ganciclovir in pediatric patients has been extremely limited. Passive immune prophylaxis in combination with ganciclovir has been used in bone marrow recipients with CMV pneumonia on the assumption that this complication has an immunopathologic as well as a viral element. The use of hyperimmune plasma or globulin in recipients of bone marrow and kidney transplants has resulted in significant reduction of symptomatic CMV disease but not in prevention of infection. The prophylactic efficacy of immunoglobulin is more striking in situations in which primary CMV infections carry a high risk of morbidity, such as in bone marrow transplantation. One recommended regimen is 1.0 g/kg of immunoglobulin given as a single intravenous dose beginning within 72 hours of transplantation and once weekly thereafter until day 120 after transplantation.

The use of a live attenuated vaccine (Towne strain) has resulted in a modest reduction in morbidity caused by primary CMV infection. This marginal benefit does not justify the use of this vaccine at this time. Other types of vaccines, such as subunit and recombinant vaccines, remain to be developed.

PREVENTION

CMV is not very contagious, and horizontal transmission requires close direct contact with secretions that contain the virus and less likely fomites. The risk of transmission by blood or blood products can be eliminated by selecting CMV-negative blood donors or using deglycerolized, frozen red blood cells or cotton-wool filters to render the transfusates CMV-"free." For the time being, the use of blood products from seronegative donors remains the only proven and safe method to prevent post-transfusion infection after transfusion of leukocytes and platelets. Another proven method to reduce CMV infections is to select CMV-negative donors for organ transplants. This is particularly important in CMV-negative allograft recipients.

MYCOPLASMA INFECTIONS

JULIA A. McMILLAN, M.D.

Mycoplasmas are bacteria without cell walls that are ubiquitous agents of infection among plants and animals, including humans. The mycoplasmal species known to be responsible for human infection include *Mycoplasma pneumoniae, Mycoplasma hominis,* and *Ureaplasma urealyticum.*

INFECTIONS CAUSED BY *MYCOPLASMA PNEUMONIAE*

Respiratory tract infection due to *M. pneumoniae* affects all age groups and all levels of the respiratory tract. That *M. pneumoniae* infection occurs in children under 5 years of age has been determined by retrospective serologic studies, but the absence of a history of significant lower respiratory infection among the seropositive preschool children in these studies indicates that *M. pneumoniae* infection in this age group is usually responsible only for upper respiratory tract symptoms. Laryngotracheobronchitis (croup) in young children has also been attributed to *M. pneumoniae* in a minority of cases. Among school-aged children, approximately 20 per cent of pneumonia episodes can be attributed to *M. pneumoniae,* and that proportion increases to as high as 50 per cent among college students and military recruits.

Clinical Presentation

In adolescents and young adults infected with *M. pneumoniae,* coryza and other signs and symptoms of upper respiratory tract infection, including pharyngitis, may develop. The majority of adolescents and young adults who seek medical attention for *M. pneumoniae* infection, however, have lower respiratory tract involvement. Pneumonia due to *M. pneumoniae* is typically characterized by the gradual onset of malaise, generalized aching, sore throat, headache, and fever. Symptoms may progress to include a nonproductive cough, chills, and chest pain; in some patients nausea, vomiting, and diarrhea develop. The pneumonia due to *M. pneumoniae* is often referred to as "atypical," largely because of its gradual onset, nonproductive cough, and paucity of auscultatory findings relative to the complaints of the patient. The chest x-ray may be positive in the presence of minimal evidence of pneumonia on physical examination and may reveal either an interstitial or alveolar pattern. When infiltrates are seen, they are usually unilateral, and pleural fluid is apparent on chest x-ray in approximately 20 per cent of patients. M. pneumoniae *infection has also been shown to be important in precipitating exacerbations of reactive airway disease.*

Diagnosis

The diagnosis of pneumonia due to *M. pneumoniae* is best made on clinical grounds and on awareness of the organism's presence in the community. Culture of *M. pneumoniae* is a cumbersome and time-consuming procedure not undertaken by most clinical laboratories, and the serologic tests available are not specific enough to be clinically helpful. Cold agglutinin antibodies are said to be positive in 50 to 90 per cent of patients with *M. pneumoniae* pneumonia but are less likely to be present in younger children or in patients with modest lower respiratory tract involvement. Cold agglutinin antibodies may also be present in patients with viral pneumonia.

Nonrespiratory Complications

A wide range of nonrespiratory illnesses have been attributed to *M. pneumoniae* infection. Hemolytic anemia due to cold agglutinin antibodies occurs but is rarely clinically significant. Rash, including erythema multiforme, central nervous system complications, and monoarticular arthritis, are unusual, but the association has been clearly documented in anecdotal reports. Life-threatening, and sometimes lethal, respiratory disease occasionally associated with severe hemolysis has been described.

Treatment

Since mycoplasmas have no cell wall, they are not susceptible to the antibiotic effects of penicillins or cephalosporins. Both erythromycin and tetracycline are effective in treating lower respiratory tract infection due to *M. pneumoniae*, although tetracycline should not be prescribed for children younger than 8 years of age. A 7-day course of oral therapy is usually sufficient; however, relapses do occur and a course of 10 to 14 days may avoid this problem. In vitro studies suggest that two new oral antibiotics, azithromycin and clarithromycin, may be effective in the treatment of *M. pneumoniae* infection. Clinical studies are as yet inadequate. There is no evidence that antibiotic therapy is helpful in treating the nonrespiratory complications of *M. pneumoniae* infection.

GENITAL MYCOPLASMAS

U. urealyticum and *M. hominis* are the organisms usually referred to as the genital mycoplasmas. The presence of *U. urealyticum* in the adult genital tract has been associated with infertility, chorioamnionitis, urethritis, prostatitis, and urinary calculi, whereas *M. hominis* has been implicated as a cause of postpartum septicemia and pyelonephritis. The difficulty in determining the importance of these two mycoplasmas as causes of human disease lies in the frequency with which they are found in the genitourinary tract of asymptomatic individuals. *U. urealyticum* can be recovered from the vagina of up to 80 per cent of adult women, and *M. hominis* infects or colonizes as many as 50 per cent. These organisms are less frequently found in asymptomatic adult men, but *U. urealyticum* has been recovered from as many as 50 per cent of sexually active men without genitourinary complaints.

Isolation of either *U. urealyticum* or *M. hominis* from a site which is normally sterile provides better evidence of their importance in disease. Both organisms have been found in the joint fluid of hypogammaglobulinemic patients with arthritis, and *M. hominis* has been recovered from blood, cerebrospinal fluid (CSF), and pleural fluid of patients with clinical evidence of septicemia, meningitis, and pneumonia or empyema.

Anecdotal reports of significant disease related to the genital mycoplasmas among newborn infants during the 1980s led to investigation of the importance of these organisms as causes of neonatal lung disease, disseminated infection, and meningitis. *Ureaplasma* has been recovered from autopsy specimens of multiple organs and the placentas of infants who died because of pneumonia and disseminated infection. Serologic studies and microbiologic investigation have suggested a link between *U. urealyticum* and premature delivery, in utero growth retardation, and chronic lung disease in premature infants.

Both *M. hominis* and *U. urealyticum* have been found in the CSF of term and preterm infants being evaluated for meningitis, and *U. urealyticum* has been isolated from the CNS of patients with intracranial hemorrhage and hydrocephalus. The importance of these findings is uncertain, since the majority of infants with CSF cultures positive for *M. hominis* recover without therapy or improve while being treated with antibiotics not likely to be effective against *M. hominis*. The relationship between the genital mycoplasmas and disease in neonates is provocative, however, and a search for virulence markers or specific antibodies that can be correlated with disease rather than colonization will undoubtedly uncover a role for these organisms in the diseases of newborn infants.

Diagnosis

Recovery of the genital mycoplasmas from clinical specimens is now possible using commercially available prepared media. A determination of the need for therapy must be made on the basis of clinical findings, the site from which the organism is recovered, and the status of the patient's immune system. *Antibiotic therapy for all patients, whether neonate or adult, from whom genital mycoplasms are isolated cannot be recommended at this time.*

Treatment

Erythromycin (40 mg/kg/day) and tetracyclines are generally effective in treating infections caused by *U. urealyticum*, although erythromycin resistance has been reported. Sulfonamides and clindamycin are not effective in treating infection caused by *U. urealyticum*. Tetracycline resistance on the part of *U. urealyticum* (as much as 20 per cent) and *M. hominis* (as much as 40 per cent) has also been detected in some series. *M. hominis* is always resistant to erythromycin and sulfonamides, and thus far always sensitive to clindamycin. Tetracycline (25 to 50 mg/kg/day) or doxycycline (4 mg/kg/day) is recommended for the treatment of either *U. urealyticum* or *M. hominis* in most patients older than 8 years of age. A 10-day course of oral therapy is generally appropriate for patients with genitourinary tract infection. Prolonged intravenous therapy may be required to treat arthritis, pneumonia, or neonatal infection. In critical situations when *M. hominis* has been demonstrated or is suspected to be a pathogen, intravenous clindamycin may be indicated. Genital mycoplasma isolates from patients not responding to therapy or who have central nervous system or disseminated disease should be tested for antibiotic resistance.

VIRAL PNEUMONIAS

FREDERICK W. HENDERSON, M.D.

INCIDENCE

The incidence of viral pneumonia is highest in preschool children, with a broad peak in disease incidence between 2 and 5 years of age. Respiratory syncytial virus (RSV) is the single most important cause of viral bronchopneumonia in childhood; infections with the parainfluenza viruses, influenza viruses, and adenoviruses account for most other cases of viral pneumonia in the previously healthy young child. Measles virus (rubeola) is an occasional cause of pneumonia in unimmunized children. Children with inborn or acquired conditions that compromise immunologic defenses are at risk for pneumonias due to varicella zoster virus, herpes simplex virus, and cytomegalovirus, agents that rarely cause pneumonia in the healthy child. These children are also at increased risk for more severe and prolonged pneumonias due to common respiratory viruses, including RSV, parainfluenza virus type 3, and influenza A viruses. In children with human immunodeficiency virus (HIV) infections, diffuse lymphoid interstitial pneumonia may develop. Neonates are at risk for herpes simplex and cytomegalovirus pneumonias.

DIAGNOSIS

In most children with viral pneumonia, there is a 1- to 3-day prodrome of symptoms of upper respiratory infection with gradual progression of the clinical illness to involve the lower respiratory tract. The clinical diagnosis is made when fine crackles, either localized or generalized, are heard on auscultation. The outpatient assessment of illness severity has been facilitated with use of pulse oximetry to identify children with unsuspected hypoxemia. Apnea can be a complication of viral pneumonia in young infants, particularly those who have been born prematurely.

Bacterial secondary infection is not an important element in most cases of community-acquired viral pneumonias in children. This has been particularly well studied for RSV infections but is probably also true of parainfluenza virus and adenovirus pneumonias. Rapidly progressive pneumonias can occur in children with influenza virus infections; most represent complicating bacterial pneumonias, but fulminant primary influenza viral pneumonia occurs rarely. Nosocomial bacterial pneumonias can complicate the intensive care required for children with severe viral lower respiratory infections.

Using knowledge of the epidemicity of viral respiratory infections, one can make a presumptive etiologic diagnosis for many children with viral pneumonia. Recently, rapid laboratory diagnosis of respiratory infections by viral antigen detection techniques has become more widely available. This is particularly true for RSV infections, and rapid laboratory confirmation of other viral infections is likely to become more commonplace in the near future. Nasopharyngeal secretions obtained within the first 3 to 5 days of illness contain the highest concentrations of viral antigens and represent appropriate specimens for rapid diagnosis.

TREATMENT

Most healthy children with viral pneumonia have relatively mild illnesses and do not require hospital care; these illnesses resolve without specific therapy. When wheezing is present, bronchodilators may provide symptomatic relief. Differentiating more severely ill children with uncomplicated viral pneumonias from those with bacterial infections can be difficult for the clinician. When there is concern about an etiologic role for bacteria in preschool children with pneumonia, antibiotic treatment appropriate for infection with *Streptococcus pneumoniae, Haemophilus influenzae,* and *Staphylococcus aureus* can be employed. Although bronchopneumonia due to *Mycoplasma pneumoniae* occurs most commonly in school-aged children, this organism can also cause disease in preschool children. In hospitalized children, supplemental oxygen is indicated to alleviate hypoxemia and chest percussion may facilitate resolution of atelectasis. Antiviral therapy is available for more severe respiratory syncytial virus, influenza A virus, varicella-zoster virus, herpes simplex virus, and cytomegalovirus pneumonias.

Ribavirin

Ribavirin is approved for treatment of RSV pneumonia and bronchiolitis. Most children with RSV pneumonia experience uncomplicated clinical illnesses of mild to moderate severity; these children do not require antiviral treatment. Ribavirin therapy should be considered for children with severe illness or at risk for development of severe disease, including those with cystic fibrosis, asthma, bronchopulmonary dysplasia, congenital heart disease, neuromuscular disorders, a history of premature birth, and immunocompromising conditions.

The drug is administered by the aerosol route, and a small-particle aerosol generator is provided by the manufacturer. A 20 mg/ml solution of ribavirin in water is nebulized into an oxygen hood or tent for 12 to 18 hours a day for 3 to 7 days. Administration of the drug to children requiring mechanical ventilation is complicated, necessitates special expertise, and has not been approved by the Food and Drug Administration (FDA). However, a recent report indicated that previously healthy children who required mechanical ventilation for respiratory failure due to RSV pneumonia improved significantly more rapidly when treated with ribavirin. Ribavirin administration by mechanical ventilator should be considered experimental and limited to centers with approved protocols for utilizing this technique. Contamination of room air with ribavirin occurs when the drug is administered by oxygen hood or tent. Because ribavirin is teratogenic in laboratory animals, pregnant women should be protected from environmental exposure.

Amantadine

Amantadine is approved for treatment and prophylaxis of influenza A virus infections. The oral dose for children 1 to 9 years of age (and those weighing less than 45 kg) is 4.4 mg/kg/day divided in two doses, not to exceed 150 mg/day. For older children, the dose is 200 mg/day divided in two doses. The duration of treatment is 2 to 7 days. Dosage adjustment is required for patients with impaired renal function. The clinical benefits of treatment are most apparent when therapy is initiated within 24 to 48 hours of onset of the influenza syndrome.

Acyclovir

Acyclovir is effective therapy for herpes simplex virus and varicella-zoster virus infections. Patients with pneumonia caused by these agents should receive intravenous treatment. The dose for herpes simplex infections in children older than 1 year of age is 750 mg/m^2/day divided every 8 hours; for children 1 month to 1 year old without associated encephalitis, 15 to 20 mg/kg/day; for full-term neonates, 30 mg/kg/day; and for premature neonates, 20 mg/kg/day. Therapy for varicella pneumonia is 1500 mg/m^2/day divided every 8 hours in children older than 1 year of age, and 30 mg/kg/day for children under 1 year old. Dosage adjustment is required for patients with impaired renal function.

Ganciclovir

Ganciclovir can be administered together with cytomegalovirus immune globulin to patients with established cytomegalovirus pneumonia; the dose is 10 mg/kg/day intravenously divided every 12 hours. Recent data indicate that symptomatic CMV pneumonia can be prevented with ganciclovir therapy (10 mg/kg/day divided every 12 hours for 2 weeks, then 5 mg/kg/day for 5 days a week for 10 weeks) in bone marrow transplant recipients with asymptomatic pulmonary CMV infections detected by shell-vial culture of bronchoalveolar lavage specimens obtained on the 35th post-transplant day.

Zidovudine

Zidovudine (AZT) (720 mg/m^2/day orally in four divided doses) is approved therapy for children with HIV infection. Whether this treatment has any impact on the course of the lymphoid interstitial pneumonia that occurs in approximately 30 per cent of infants and toddlers with HIV infection remains undefined.

VIRAL HEPATITIS

RICHARD D. AACH, M.D.

Viral hepatitis is the term applied to infection primarily or exclusively involving the liver and is due to at least five distinct viral agents: hepatitis A, hepatitis B, hepatitis C, hepatitis D (or delta hepatitis), and hepatitis E.

HEPATITIS A

Hepatitis A is the most common type viral hepatitis and produces the mildest illness. Formerly called "infectious" or "epidemic" hepatitis, it is primarily transmitted from person to person by the fecal-oral route. Exposure typically occurs among children in the household, particularly in conditions of poor sanitation. Outbreaks of hepatitis A from ingestion of fecally contaminated drinking water or food are well documented but uncommon. Only rare instances of transfusion-associated hepatitis A have been reported.

Hepatitis A is caused by the hepatitis A virus (HAV), now known to be a 27-nm enterovirus, which has been given the designation of type 72. It is excreted in the stool 1 to 2 weeks before any clinical manifestations of hepatitis are evident, usually before the serum enzymes begin to rise, and remains detectable for up to several weeks after infection is first evident.

The incubation period is approximately 30 days, with a range of 15 to 45 days. Most HAV infections in children are asymptomatic and only rarely accompanied by jaundice. Deaths due to hepatitis A are very unusual. Infection is self-limited, usually lasting less than 2 weeks, and does not result in chronic infection or a hepatitis A carrier state.

The diagnosis of acute hepatitis A is made by detecting gamma M immunoglobulin (IgM) class antibody to HAV (IgM-anti-HAV) in the serum. IgM-anti-HAV appears early, during the acute stages of infection, and lasts about 6 months. Thereafter, anti-HAV resides in the IgG fraction, which, if found, is indicative of prior infection and immunity to hepatitis A but not to the other types of viral hepatitis. Approximately 25 to 50 per cent of adults living in metropolitan areas in the United States have serologic evidence of prior HAV infection.

Prevention

General Measures

Good personal hygiene cannot be overemphasized. Scrupulous hand washing and thorough cleaning of food utensils have been effective in controlling the spread of hepatitis A. HAV is destroyed by heat sterilization at 100°C for 10 minutes or autoclaving properly for 15 minutes. Chlorination of water has not been shown to be viricidal for HAV.

Passive Immunization

Standard immune globulin (IG) is highly effective in preventing hepatitis A or in lessening its clinical manifestations if given before or early enough after exposure.

Post-exposure Prophylaxis

Post-exposure prophylaxis is recommended if direct personal exposure to hepatitis A has occurred. This will usually be for household contacts. IG is not routinely recommended in other settings, such as schools, offices, or factories, where spread of infection is unlikely unless there is clear-cut evidence of an outbreak of infection. For maximum protection, IG should be given as soon as possible after exposure is recognized, within 1 week of contact. The recommended dose of IG is 0.02 ml/kg of body weight given intramuscularly (IM).

Pre-exposure Prophylaxis

IG is also recommended for susceptible individuals traveling to or working in areas where hepatitis A is highly endemic. It is advisable to first determine the immune status of the individual by testing for anti-HAV in the IgG fraction (IgG-anti-HAV). If the test is negative, indicating that the person is not immune, IG should be given in a dose of 0.02 ml/kg of body weight IM, with repeated doses every 4 to 5 months if exposure is ongoing.

Active Immunization

A licensed HAV vaccine is not available. Live attenuated and inactivated vaccines are currently under evaluation.

Treatment

Treatment of acute hepatitis A, as for all other types of viral hepatitis, is supportive. No medications have been effective in terminating infection or lessening its duration. Management consists of limiting activity to that which is tolerated, a well-balanced nutritious diet, and multivitamins. Hospitalization is indicated when there is inanition and dehydration due to inadequate oral intake or when there is evidence of hepatic failure (e.g., hepatic encephalopathy, clotting disturbance). Intravenous fluids and hyperalimentation may be required. In instances of fulminant hepatic failure, admission to the intensive care unit is indicated to monitor the patient's cardiopulmonary status, maintain fluid and electrolyte balance, and correct clotting deficiencies if bleeding occurs.

HEPATITIS B

Hepatitis B was recognized as a distinct type of viral hepatitis following the discovery of the Australia antigen, now designated as the "hepatitis B surface antigen," or HBsAg. Hepatitis B, along with non-A, non-B hepatitis, was formerly called "serum hepatitis" or "homologous serum jaundice" because it is spread percutaneously, primarily by contaminated blood and blood components. Transmission also occurs following sexual exposure as well as perinatally from infected mother to her newborn at the time of childbirth or during the first few months of life. It is estimated that there are 250,000 new cases of hepatitis B annually in the United States, mainly among intravenous drug abusers and their contacts.

Hepatitis B is caused by the hepatitis B virus (HBV), a member of the hepadnavirus family, which also infects the woodchuck, ground squirrel, and Peking duck. HBV is 45 nm in diameter. It has a surface coat of antigen (HBsAg) that surrounds an inner core on which is "core" antigen (HBcAg) within which is double-stranded DNA, DNA polymerase, and a third antigen, HBeAg. Free HBsAg is usually produced in large amounts during the process of HBV replication. HBsAg (and HBV) can be detected in the serum of most patients for up to a month before the onset of clinically evident hepatitis.

The mean incubation period is 90 days, with a range of 60 to 180 days. Most infections are anicteric and self-limited. The mortality rate from fulminant hepatitis B is approximately 1 per cent. Hepatitis B can result in chronic hepatitis and a chronic carrier state. The risk is related to the age and the immune status of the infected individual. *Infection is followed by chronicity in 90 per cent of newborns but in only 3 to 10 per cent among adults.* Chronic hepatitis B also follows acute infection more frequently when it occurs in immunocompromised individuals, as a result of either another illness or immunosuppressive agents. Cirrhosis of the liver and hepatocellular carcinoma are recognized as possible late complications of hepatitis B.

The diagnosis of hepatitis B is made by detecting HBsAg in the serum. A few infected individuals do not have levels of HBsAg high enough to detect when tested. However, hepatitis B can be strongly suspected in these patients by finding antibodies to HBcAg (anti-HBc) in the IgM fraction in association with abnormal liver tests indicative of acute viral hepatitis. Chronic hepatitis B is diagnosed by finding HBsAg in the serum for at least 6 months. The finding of anti-HBs and/or IgG-anti-HBc is indicative of full recovery from and immunity to hepatitis B.

Prevention

General Measures

Because contaminated blood is the most common source of HBV, strategies for prevention have been directed toward minimizing the risk of transmission by identifying the infected carrier. All donors in the United States are routinely screened for HBsAg and anti-HBc before transfusion. The use of disposable needles, syringes, and tubing as well as careful sterilization of all nonreusable equipment is a vital part of the strategy of prevention. Minimizing the amount of blood to that which is necessary, autologous transfusions, single-unit products for clotting factors, and Cohn fractionation of blood proteins are other effective measures of prevention.

Immunoprophylaxis

The strategy for prevention of hepatitis B infection recommended by the U.S. Public Health Services Immunization Practices Advisory Committee is to vaccinate all individuals who are at high risk for infection. *Universal HBsAg screening of pregnant women is recommended so that newborns at risk for perinatally acquired infection can be protected by immunoprophylaxis.*

Two basic products are available: hyperimmune B immune globulin (HBIG) and hepatitis B vaccines. HBIG is immune globulin derived from the plasma of donors that has been preselected to contain a high titer of anti-HBs. The anti-HBs titer is greater than 100,000 by radioimmunoassay and is used when temporary passive protection is indicated following exposure to HBV. HBIG is drawn only from HIV-negative donors and is carefully treated to be HIV-free as well.

Two types of vaccines are available, one consisting of highly purified alum-absorbed inactivated HBsAg particles obtained from hepatitis B carriers, and the other is a recombinant vaccine produced in yeast. The plasma-derived vaccine, first licensed in 1981, is no longer being manufactured; it is used only for immunocompromised patients, including patients on chronic hemodialysis, and individuals sensitive to yeast. Both vaccines are safe and more than 85 per cent effective in preventing hepatitis B if given according to the recommended regimen. Efficacy among immunocompromised persons is much less. Pregnancy is not a contraindication for vaccination if otherwise indicated. No adverse effects following vaccination have been observed among patients who have chronic hepatitis B or are HBV carriers. Furthermore, no interference with other vaccines has been demonstrated.

Pre-exposure Prophylaxis

The hepatitis B vaccines are used to provide long-lasting protection against hepatitis B among susceptible individuals. Universal vaccination is now recommended for all newborns. The vaccine is also recommended for the following groups of individuals: health care professionals; clients and staff of institutions for the developmentally disabled; hemodialysis patients and staff; sexually active gay males; illicit intravenous drug users; recipients of frequent blood transfusions, including patients with clotting disorders likely to receive clotting-factor concentrates; household and sexual contacts of HBV carriers; adoptees from countries with high HBV endemicity; heterosexually active persons with multiple partners; inmates of long-term correctional facilities; and international travelers who will be residing in an area with a high HBV carrier rate.

The duration of protection of the HBV vaccines is unknown. Approximately 30 to 50 per cent of persons with an adequate vaccine response lose demonstrable anti-HBs, but protection appears to persist. As a result, a booster dose and anti-HBs screening are not routinely recommended within 7 years of vaccination for adults or within 5 years for infants who received vaccine at the time of delivery. However, some experts recommend a booster dose in situations when there is clear-cut exposure to HBV and the previously vaccinated patient is found to be anti-HBs negative.

The primary vaccination series consists of three intramuscular doses given at 0, 1, and 6 months in the deltoid muscle. The dose for each vaccine currently available is found in the printed material that accompanies each product.

Pre-vaccination screening to determine whether the patient is susceptible to hepatitis B is recommended only when there is a high probability of immunity due to prior exposure. The patient's serum should be tested for the presence of anti-HBs or anti-HBc. Post-vaccination anti-HBs screening is recommended only in individuals who are likely to obtain a suboptimal response, e.g., chronic hemodialysis patients.

Post-exposure Prophylaxis

Susceptible persons should be vaccinated after exposure to hepatitis B in the following situations: percutaneous or permucosal exposure to HBsAg positive body secretions, such as might occur due to an accidental needle stick or sexual exposure; perinatal exposure of an infant born to an HBsAg-positive mother; and exposure of an infant under 12 months old to a caregiver who has acute hepatitis B infection.

A regimen of two doses of HBIG in doses of 0.06 ml/kg of body weight IM is recommended after percutaneous or permucosal exposure. The first dose should be given as soon as possible after exposure, preferably within 48 hours, and the second dose 1 month later. This regimen is about 75 per cent effective in preventing hepatitis B. For sexual exposure, a single dose of HBIG is 75 per cent effective if given within 2 weeks of exposure. If exposure to HBV is likely to be ongoing, either in an occupational or a household setting, concurrent hepatitis B vaccination is also recommended. *The full vaccine course should be administered, in which case the second dose of HBIG is not necessary if exposure followed an accidental stick.* This regimen has the advantages that it is less costly than giving HBIG twice and it provides long-term immunity. *It is important to give HBIG and the vaccine at different sites.*

Prevention of Neonatal Hepatitis B

For newborns of mothers who are HBsAg-positive, both HBIG and hepatitis B vaccine should be administered. HBIG (0.5 ml) should be given IM within the first few hours of life after the infant has become physiologically stable. Vaccine in the appropriate infant dose can be given at the same time or before the infant is discharged at a site different from that for IG. The same vaccine dose should be repeated 1 and 6 months later. This regimen is 85 to 95 per cent effective in preventing the development of hepatitis B. The infant should be tested for HBsAg and anti-HBs at 12 to 15 months of age to determine whether therapy has been successful. The presence of anti-HBs is indicative of immunity, whereas the finding of HBsAg is indicative of hepatitis B infection—which is almost certainly chronic.

Treatment

Treatment of acute hepatitis B is supportive, as described for hepatitis A. No therapeutic agent has been shown to be effective in shortening the period of infection or in decreasing the likelihood of chronic infection. Corticosteroids have no role in the treatment of acute hepatitis B, for they increase viral replication and are associated with a higher risk of chronic HBV infection and hepatitis.

Administration of high-dose anti-HBs and transfer factor has been used to terminate the chronic carrier state without effect. Anti-HBs does not benefit patients with fulminant hepatitis B.

Studies conducted in adults have demonstrated that a 3- to 6-month course of interferon-α therapy in doses ranging from 5 to 10 million units given daily or three times a week subcutaneously will induce a clinical remission in approximately 40 per cent of patients and eradicate infection in about 10 per cent. These figures may underestimate the long-term beneficial effects because additional patients who clinically respond initially to interferon are more likely over time to lose all evidence of HBV infection than chronic hepatitis B patients who do not receive interferon. Predictors of a clinical response include a high initial serum aminotransferase level and a low level of circulating HBV-DNA. Pretreatment for 6 weeks with corticosteroids just prior to interferon may increase the rate of response of patients with low aminotransferase levels. Interferon may precipitate hepatic failure in patients with advanced liver disease and is contraindicated in this setting.

Indications for interferon therapy of children with chronic hepatitis B have not been established, and the agent has not yet been approved for treatment of this condition. Only a few studies on the effect of interferon on children with chronic hepatitis B have been conducted. A 6-month course of interferon-α_{2b} three times a week resulted in a serologic, biologic, and histologic remission in approximately 50 per cent of 36 Spanish children with chronic hepatitis B. Remission was sustained in the majority of children who responded. The higher dose was well tolerated and resulted in a slightly higher response rate in this study, but other experience indicates that not all children tolerate doses in this range. Asian children (and adults) do not respond as well as whites to interferon therapy, and this is also true of patients who are co-infected with HIV.

HEPATITIS D

Hepatitis D, or delta hepatitis, is the most virulent type of viral hepatitis. First discovered in the late 1970s, it always accompanies hepatitis B infection and therefore is spread in the same manner as HBV. It is endemic in the Mediterranean Basin and is found primarily among intravenous drug abusers in Western Europe and the United States.

Delta hepatitis is due to a unique defective viral agent, HDV, which has a surface coat of HBsAg that surrounds an inner core with its unique antigen (HDAg) and a genome consisting of RNA. HDV requires the helper function of HBV to replicate and survive. It can be acquired simultaneously as a co-infection with HBV or can superinfect a person who has chronic hepatitis B.

HDV infection is typically clinically evident and may be severe. Fulminant hepatitis has been observed in 10 to 40 per cent of chronic hepatitis B patients who become superinfected with HDV. Those who survive superinfection are prone to a more severe course of chronic hepatitis B and D, with the early development of cirrhosis and hepatic compromise. The diagnosis of hepatitis D is made by finding anti-HD (IgG or IgM) in the serum. Hepatitis D should be suspected in any patient who experiences a severe episode of acute viral hepatitis or a very aggressive course of chronic hepatitis.

Prevention

Because HDV cannot survive in the absence of HBV, the strategy of prevention of delta hepatitis is the prevention of hepatitis B infection, as discussed earlier.

Treatment

Experience with interferon therapy of delta hepatitis is limited. Improvement has been observed in about 50 per cent of those treated, but relapse occurs when therapy is stopped.

HEPATITIS C (AND NON-A, NON-B HEPATITIS)

Parenterally transmitted non-A, non-B hepatitis is the major cause of post-transfusion hepatitis. Like hepatitis B, it was formerly called serum hepatitis and homologous serum jaundice. The diagnosis of non-A, non-B hepatitis was made strictly on the basis of excluding hepatitis A and B until 1988, when a causative viral agent, the hepatitis C virus, or HCV, was identified. HCV is a 35- to 50-nm RNA-enveloped virus that bears homology to the flaviviruses and pestiviruses. It is not known whether this is the only non-A, non-B agent, but current evidence indicates that HCV is the principal cause of post-transfusion hepatitis and probably the sole cause of chronic non-A, non-B hepatitis following hemotherapy.

Hepatitis C has a mean incubation period of approximately 50 days with a range of 14 to 180 days. Infection is usually mild, and only about 20 to 25 per cent of patients have symptoms or icteric illness. Chronic hepatitis and a prolonged HCV carrier state occur in 50 per cent of infected individuals. Chronic hepatitis C is usually indolent but over many years can lead slowly to the development of cirrhosis in about 20 to 25 per cent of persons. Hepatocellular carcinoma has recently been associated with long-term HCV infection as well.

The diagnosis of hepatitis C is made by ruling out hepatitis A and B and by the finding of antibodies to HCV (anti-HCV) in the patient's serum. *Not all individuals with hepatitis C undergo seroconversion. With the tests currently available, anti-HCV does not appear until 12 to 16 weeks after onset, and its appearance may be delayed for as long as a year. Furthermore, falsely positive anti-HCV test results may be seen in other forms of chronic liver disease and illnesses associated with hypergammaglobulinemia.* Confirmatory assays are under development that should improve the specificity of serologic tests for hepatitis C.

Prevention

Clinical trials that evaluated the efficacy of IG in preventing non-A, non-B hepatitis, and presumably that due to HCV, have given conflicting results. As a result, there are no official recommendations for prophylaxis of hepatitis C. However, when there is clear-cut parenteral exposure to HCV, it seems reasonable to administer IG in a dose of 0.06 ml/kg of body weight IM as soon as possible.

The risk of perinatal transmission of hepatitis C is presently unknown. Some studies have shown very little or no evidence of transmission from infected mothers to their newborns, whereas infection acquired in this fashion has been observed in other investigations, particularly when the mother is HIV-positive or has high serum aminotransferase levels. No data are available about the possible role of IG in the prevention of perinatal transmission of non-A, non-B hepatitis and hepatitis C.

A hepatitis C vaccine is not available. The ability to clone HCV and characterize its genome makes it possible to develop candidate vaccines for its prevention.

Treatment

Several trials of interferon-α_{2b} have been conducted in adults with chronic hepatitis C. Interferon (3 million units three times a week for 6 months) resulted in a clinical remission in about 50 per cent of those treated that was sustained in 50 per cent of those who responded. Relapses usually occurred within the first 6 months after therapy was discontinued. Re-treatment with interferon usually resulted in a second clinical remission among those persons who experienced relapse.

Interferon has been approved by the U.S. Food and Drug Administration (FDA) for use in adults. Additional studies are in progress to identify a more optimal regimen for control and cure of chronic HCV infection. Information is not yet available on the effect of interferon in children with chronic non-A, non-B and hepatitis C.

HEPATITIS E

Hepatitis E, formerly called "epidemic" or "enterically transmitted (ET) non-A, non-B" hepatitis, is the most recently characterized type of viral hepatitis. To date, about 20 epidemics of hepatitis E have been described, all due to ingestion of contaminated water. Hepatitis E has been observed primarily in the Far East, particularly India, Pakistan, and Burma, but outbreaks also have been documented in Russia, Africa, and Mexico.

Hepatitis E is due to a 30- to 35-nm RNA virus with features of a calcivirus, an agent transmitted enterically and known to give rise to diarrhea in children. The mean incubation period is 45 days. *Complications are infrequent except for pregnant women, in whom the risk of fulminant hepatitis and death can be as high as 5 to 10 per cent.* Infection is self-limited and does not give rise to chronic hepatitis. The diagnosis is made epidemiologically and by excluding the other types of hepatitis. There is a serologic assay, but it is used only in the experimental laboratory at present.

Prevention

Whether IG is effective in preventing hepatitis E is unknown. Because the incidence in the United States is very low, it is highly likely that IG prepared in this country will not be very protective.

Treatment

Like the other types of viral hepatitis, acute hepatitis E should be treated supportively.

ENTEROVIRUSES

LAURENCE B. GIVNER, M.D.

The *Picornavirus* family is made up of small (from Greek, *pico*), single-stranded RNA viruses, approximately 20 to 30 nm in size. Among these is included the genus *Enterovirus,* so named because it inhabits the gastrointestinal tract. The virus is acid-stable (necessary for survival during transit through the stomach), and stable at room temperature for several days. The enteroviruses currently include polioviruses 1, 2, and 3; coxsackieviruses A1-A24 and B1-B6; the echoviruses (32 serotypes); enteroviruses 68-71; and hepatitis A virus, also called enterovirus 72 (see article on viral hepatitis, p. 616).

PREVENTION

Paralytic poliomyelitis has been eradicated in the United States through the use of active immunization in childhood. The rare cases (a few annually) now reported are associated with the use of the oral, attenuated live virus vaccine itself. This has prompted re-evaluation of the continued use of this vaccine versus return to use of the parenteral, inactivated virus vaccine, especially with the recent development of new, enhanced potency inactivated vaccines. In this country, the vaccine now recommended for general use in children is the live, oral vaccine. The inactivated vaccine is recommended for immunodeficient hosts and their close contacts.

Prevention of most other enteroviral infections is best accomplished through the use of good, consistent hand-washing techniques, as these viruses are spread primarily by the fecal-oral route. Health care workers must be especially mindful of these precautions.

TREATMENT

Treatment of enteroviral infections is generally supportive. Physicians caring for these patients must be aware that enteroviral disease may affect multiple organ systems, although the patient may complain of symptoms referable only to the predominant system involved.

Specific antiviral therapy of enteroviral infections is limited to the use of human immune globulins in patients with chronic enteroviral (usually echovirus) meningoencephalitis in association with agammaglobulinemia. Such patients may benefit from periodic infusions of pooled human IgG intravenously; intraventricular administration also may be necessary for some of these patients.

Although the human IgG preparations for intravenous use contain antibodies against the common enteroviruses, their use in the treatment (or prevention) of other enteroviral infections, such as overwhelming enteroviral sepsis in the young infant, cannot be recommended because of the lack of controlled studies. Enteroviral infection should be considered, however, in the young infant with overwhelming sepsis when properly obtained culture specimens reveal no bacteria. Antibacterial therapy should be given, however, until a bacterial etiology has been ruled out. Supportive care continues unchanged in either case.

Myopericarditis

The enteroviruses (especially the coxsackie B viruses) may be responsible for up to 50 per cent of cases of acute myocarditis; pericarditis also may be present in these patients. Consequently, the enteroviruses account for a large percentage of cases of dilated cardiomyopathy. At the time of presentation, the degree of illness varies from the asymptomatic or mildly ill adolescent to the newborn with immediately life-threatening cardiac decompensation.

In the treatment of acute myocarditis, many have considered the use of steroids to decrease the inflammatory response, thereby perhaps limiting the resultant damage to the myocardium. *Such therapy cannot be recommended,* however, in view of (1) the deleterious effect of steroids noted in murine models of myocarditis, (2) concern regarding the use of agents to blunt the immune response during an active infection, and (3) the lack of well-controlled clinical trials.

Supportive care is the mainstay of therapy for myocarditis. A cardiologist should be involved in the care of most, if not all, of these patients. After careful evaluation, the asymptomatic or mildly ill patient may require only limitation of activities and attention to fluid status with continued close follow-up as an outpatient. The more severely affected patient will require inpatient care with intensive cardiac monitoring, especially for the occurrence of dysrhythmias; should they occur, prompt antiarrhythmic therapy may be necessary. The development of congestive heart failure may require the use of diuretics, inotropic drugs, or angiotensin-converting enzyme (ACE) inhibitors for afterload reduction. Anticoagulant therapy may be necessary if chronic dilated cardiomyopathy develops in order to prevent embolic phenomena.

Aseptic Meningitis

The enteroviruses circulate primarily in the summer and early fall months, and during these seasons cause most cases of aseptic (routine bacterial culture-negative) meningitis. In older patients, an antipyretic or analgesic usually is all that is necessary. Occasionally, older patients with more severe illness or those unable to tolerate oral fluids may require hospitalization. Often, the initial lumbar puncture confers relief to those suffering the effects of increased intracranial pressure (headache, vomiting) due to aseptic meningitis; this alleviation of symptoms may be useful in the differentiation of aseptic from bacterial meningitis. The young infant, however, should be routinely hospitalized and given broad-spectrum parenteral antibacterial therapy (e.g., ampicillin and cefotaxime) because rapid differentiation from bacterial meningitis (especially due to *Listeria monocytogenes*) is difficult. If appropriate cultures subsequently reveal no bacteria, antibacterial therapy then may be discontinued. Differentiation from herpes simplex infection (for which antiviral therapy is indicated) also may be difficult in the newborn. Fluid restriction may be of benefit to those hospitalized with aseptic meningitis in order to decrease intracranial pressure and to avoid the inappropriate secretion of antidiuretic hormone. Fluid and electrolyte status should be closely monitored in such patients, with special attention to serum sodium concentration. Following aseptic meningitis in the first year of life, some studies have demonstrated long-term neurologic sequelae, especially in language development. However, these findings have not been consistent in all studies. The outlook for the vast majority of children is excellent.

Herpangina and Hand-Foot-and-Mouth Disease

The coxsackieviruses cause most cases of herpangina, and coxsackievirus A16 is the major causative agent of hand-foot-and-mouth disease. These relatively "benign" illnesses may require symptomatic therapy—antipyretics for relief of fever or analgesics for relief of the pain and discomfort due to oral lesions. The oral discomfort may be alleviated by chilled fluids, such as popsicles, or by systemic analgesics. Some recommend use of topical analgesics; however, concern for overuse makes them less desirable. Occasionally, parenteral fluids are necessary to avoid dehydration due to decreased oral intake.

Acute Hemorrhagic Conjunctivitis

Recently, outbreaks of acute hemorrhagic conjunctivitis have been described, usually as a result of enterovirus 70. This illness generally is self-limited. However, secondary bacterial infection may be heralded by increased purulence of the ocular discharge. In such cases, topical antibacterial therapy is indicated. Attention to good hand washing is especially important in attempts to limit the spread of this highly contagious illness.

ASEPTIC MENINGITIS

LEONARD B. WEINER, M.D.

Aseptic meningitis is a general term applied to acute meningeal inflammatory processes that are not the result of infection with pyogenic bacteria. Usually recognized causes include viruses, parasites, unusual bacteria, pharmacologic agents, and toxins. The most common etiology is viral, with enteroviruses, respiratory viruses, and herpes group viruses most frequently encountered. Seasonal influence is an important feature of certain causes of viral meningitis; not only does enteroviral etiology predominate in the summer and early fall; it may also be responsible for greater than a 70 to 80 per cent incidence of infection overall in infants with viral meningitis. *When enteroviral meningitis occurs in neonates, it may be only one component of a multisystem infection that includes myocarditis, hepatitis, pneumonia, and encephalitis.* Many of the agents known to cause viral meningitis, regardless of the age of the patient, can also produce encephalitis. Tuberculous and fungal meningitis, meningitis due to *Mycoplasma* species, syphilis, and Lyme disease are examples of nonviral processes that may produce an aseptic meningitis syndrome.

DIAGNOSIS

The diagnosis of aseptic meningitis is usually made by the exclusion of pyogenic bacteria from the cerebrospinal fluid (CSF) utilizing appropriate cultures. A compatible history should include failure of routine blood and/or CSF bacterial cultures to grow, coupled with an acute clinical picture of headache, meningeal irritation, and fever in a patient who has not received antibiotic pretreatment. Culture results may not be available for at least 48 hours and infants younger than 12 months of age with viral meningitis often are as ill-appearing as those with bacterial meningitis. *Such infants should receive intravenous antibiotics for presumptive bacterial meningitis until the culture results are known.* Older children with viral meningitis are generally not as ill-appearing as their counterparts with bacterial meningitis and can be treated expectantly.

CSF findings are variable and may range from those clearly indicative of a viral etiology to those mimicking bacterial meningitis, especially when determined early in the course of illness. CSF cell counts of less than 300 white blood cells (WBCs) per cubic millimeter (mm^3) with a mononuclear cell predominance, a normal CSF protein level, and normal CSF–to–blood glucose ratio are characteristic of viral meningitis; however, many studies of enteroviral meningitis in infants have demonstrated that the initial CSF may have greater than 300 WBCs per mm^3 with a 60 per cent or greater polymorphonuclear predominance. CSF hypoglycorrhachia, in the range of 25 to 55 mg/dl, has been well documented in enteroviral, herpes simplex virus (HSV), mumps, and arboviral meningitis. Impressively low CSF glucose levels (0 to 10 mg/dl) are characteristic of tuberculous and fungal meningitis and are associated with concomitant elevations of CSF protein (>200 mg/dl).

Because most of the pathogens responsible for aseptic meningitis cannot be readily defined by simple culture techniques, the diagnosis relies on enhanced organism recognition by specialized culture and/or antigen detection methods. The latter, often in a rapid test format, may eventually prove useful in CSF but at present are limited to research laboratories. Examples of these include direct detection of HSV, enteroviral and other viral antigens by enzyme immunoassay, polymerase chain reaction (PCR), and DNA/RNA probes. In the future, fungal and tuberculous meningitis may also be defined by PCR or probe technology. "Shell-vial" cultures for virus significantly shorten the identification time for HSV, CMV, and certain other viruses, but culture yields are generally low in viral meningitis except in neonates and the immunocompromised.

TREATMENT

Therapy for fungal and tuberculous meningitis is discussed elsewhere. Treatment of HSV and varicella-zoster virus with acyclovir, treatment of CMV with ganciclovir, the use of IVIG for enteroviral meningitis in the immunocompromised, and the use of IVIG and/or convalescent maternal plasma in neonatal enteroviral disease have demonstrable therapeutic effectiveness.

Increased antidiuretic hormone secretion has been detected in children with viral meningitis, although specific intravenous fluid adjustment is rarely required. Dexamethasone therapy is now recommended in the early management of presumed bacterial meningitis, and this has resulted in the administration of steroids to a number of children whose ultimate diagnosis was viral meningitis. Information to date indicates that no measurable adverse effects have occurred in these circumstances. Because most children hospitalized with viral meningitis are infants and are likely to be infected with enteroviruses, enteric isolation precautions are indicated.

Long-term central nervous system sequelae following enteroviral meningitis have not been documented in a recent study of infants who had mild acute illnesses. However, infants with severe neurologic disabilities during the acute episode, such as coma, seizures, or focal neurologic deficits, may be at greater risk for long-term problems.

PSITTACOSIS

CAROL F. PHILLIPS, M.D.

Psittacosis (ornithosis) is a zoonotic disease usually acquired by inhaling infected particles from bird secretions or droppings or by handling carcasses of infected birds. Occasionally, there is intrafamilial spread. The disease can be transmitted by healthy birds, is rare in children, and has no seasonality. The incubation period is usually 7 to 14 days.

CLINICAL FEATURES

The clinical picture consists of an abrupt onset of high fever, chills, sweating, severe headache, myalgia, vomiting, or diarrhea. A dry cough usually appears several days into the illness, and pneumonia is common. Rarely, hepatitis, arthritis, endocarditis, severe anemia, pulmonary embolism, erythema nodosum, Guillain-Barré syndrome, transverse myelitis, or disseminated intravascular coagulation occurs. Untreated, severe illness persists for 2 to 3 weeks.

DIAGNOSIS

Isolation of the organism should be attempted only by experienced laboratory personnel. The diagnosis is usually made by demonstrating a significant rise in the complement fixation (CF) titer of blood specimens between the time of acute illness and convalescence or a single CF titer of at least 32. This test measures a common chlamydial group lipopolysaccharide antigen. Findings are positive in patients infected with *Chlamydia pneumoniae* (TWAR agent). Patients with *C. pneumoniae* usually have a milder disease and no history of contact with birds. There is not prolonged immunity, and reinfections occur. The chest radiograph usually shows atypical pneumonia, but lobar consolidation can occur. The erythrocyte sedimentation rate is usually elevated.

TREATMENT

Tetracycline (30 to 40 mg/kg/day) is the treatment of choice for patients older than 8 years. Erythromycin (40 mg/kg/day) can be used in younger children. Most patients are afebrile after 48 hours. Therapy should be continued for 2 weeks.

Bed rest, oxygen, adequate fluids, and antipyretics are supplemental therapy. Hospitalized patients should be placed in respiratory isolation.

RICKETTSIAL DISEASES

JON S. ABRAMSON, M.D.

Rickettsial diseases include Rocky Mountain spotted fever (RMSF), ehrlichiosis, Q fever, Mediterranean spotted fever, typhus, and scrub typhus. The organisms causing these infections are transmitted through the bites of blood-sucking arthropods. Mediterranean spotted fever, typhus, and scrub typhus infections are uncommon in the United States today and are not further discussed in this article.

ROCKY MOUNTAIN SPOTTED FEVER

Treatment

Empiric antibiotic treatment for RMSF is necessary in many patients because (1) a definitive diagnosis usually cannot be made before the 2nd week of illness with currently available laboratory tests and (2) delaying treatment until a diagnosis is confirmed can lead to mortality approaching 25 per cent. Tetracycline (and related derivatives such as doxycycline) and chloramphenicol are the only two antibiotics with proven clinical efficacy in treating RMSF. Older patients usually receive tetracycline for suspected RMSF, but both the American Academy of Pediatrics and the Centers for Disease Control in Atlanta recommend using only chloramphenicol for children younger than 9 years of age because of the potential for tetracycline to stain teeth. However, a strong case in favor of using tetracycline in young children can be made:

1. Staining of teeth by tetracycline appears to be dose-related, and it is extremely unlikely to occur in a child given one or two short courses (usually 5 to 7 days are adequate) of tetracycline for RMSF.
2. Chloramphenicol therapy causes, on rare occasions (~1 in 30,000 courses), idiosyncratic, non–dose-related, often fatal aplastic anemia. (Many patients are treated annually for presumptive RMSF, making it likely that aplastic anemia will occur if chloramphenicol is used to treat each suspected case of RMSF.
3. Chloramphenicol has a narrow therapeutic-toxic ratio, and serum levels of the drug are difficult to predict. (Therefore, even during short-course therapy, it is prudent to measure levels, which makes treatment more problematic.)
4. Human ehrlichiosis, a potentially fatal disease, can be difficult to differentiate clinically from RMSF. (Currently, tetracycline is the only antibiotic with proven efficacy against this disease [see below]).

For these reasons, many physicians choose to treat children of all ages with tetracycline (or its analogues) instead of chloramphenicol for presumed RMSF.

In some patients who are seriously ill on presentation, the

differential diagnosis may involve other pathogens (e.g., *Neisseria meningitidis* and *Haemophilus influenzae*) in addition to *Rickettsia rickettsii.* Chloramphenicol is preferred in these patients because of its better coverage for these other pathogens. Both tetracycline and chloramphenicol are "rickettsialstatic" rather than "rickettsialcidal." Once major vascular damage has occurred, these drugs will inhibit the growth of the organism but may not substantially change the course of the disease. Other therapeutic measures often required in these patients include hospitalization, ventilatory support, and intravenous fluid resuscitation for hypovolemia resulting from capillary leakage.

Prevention

Useful measures for preventing RMSF include:

- Wearing long clothing and using insect repellent in wooded areas
- Inspecting frequently for ticks (usually it takes several hours for a tick to engorge with the host's blood and cause infection)
- Removing ticks using an instrument (e.g., tweezers)
- Pulling the tick from as close to the skin surface as possible with a steady, even force

Finally, ticks should not be touched with bare hands or split open.

Only a small percentage (<10 per cent) of ticks are infected with *R. rickettsii.* Therefore, prophylactic antibiotics should not be given to everyone with a history of tick bite. Instead, treatment should be reserved if symptoms and signs compatible with RMSF develop.

EHRLICHIOSIS

Human ehrlichiosis is an acute febrile illness caused by *Ehrlichia canis* or a closely related rickettsial species. In some geographic areas, the incidence of human ehrlichiosis may exceed that of RMSF. Many of the symptoms and signs are similar to that seen with RMSF. Human ehrlichiosis was thought to be a benign, self-limited illness. However, the disease appears to be associated with substantial morbidity and mortality resulting from pulmonary, renal, and central nervous system manifestations, thus making early treatment prudent.

Treatment

Both tetracycline and chloramphenicol have been used in the treatment of ehrlichiosis. In canine ehrlichiosis, only tetracycline has been efficacious. Controlled studies to examine the efficacy of these antibiotics for treatment of human ehrlichiosis have not been reported. Therefore, tetracycline is currently the treatment of choice for ehrlichiosis in children and adults.

Although the exact duration of treatment is unknown, it appears that a short course of therapy, like that used for RMSF, is adequate. The preventive measures noted above for RMSF are also important in preventing human ehrlichiosis.

Q FEVER

Q fever is caused by the rickettsial organism *Coxiella burnetti* and domestic animals (e.g., goats, sheep, and cattle) are the primary reservoir. The rickettsia is shed periodically from animals, and as little as one organism can cause disease in children and adults. The patient usually presents with retrobulbar headache, high fever with shaking chills, myalgia, chest pain, and sometimes pneumonia, hepatitis, endocarditis, and encephalitis.

Treatment

Q fever often resolves without specific therapy, but chronic infection can occur, making treatment prudent. Tetracycline (or one of its analogues) for 2 weeks is the treatment of choice for acute Q fever. Other antibiotics have not been effective. Therefore, although the treatment period is longer than that for RMSF or ehrlichiosis, it is reasonable to use tetracycline in children younger than 9 years of age (even 2 weeks of tetracycline therapy is unlikely to lead to cosmetically important staining of teeth). Some authorities recommend combining tetracycline with trimethoprim-sulfamethoxazole or rifampin for the treatment of chronic forms of Q fever (e.g., endocarditis). Researchers using Q fever vaccines in high-risk individuals (e.g., abattoir workers) suggest that they may be adequate in preventing disease, but these vaccines are not currently licensed for use in the United States.

CHLAMYDIA INFECTION

MARGARET R. HAMMERSCHLAG, M.D.

The genus *Chlamydia* includes a group of obligate intracellular parasites with a unique developmental cycle with morphologically distinct infectious and reproductive forms. All members of the genus have a gram-negative envelope without peptidoglycan, share a genus-specific lipopolysaccharide antigen, and utilize host adenosine triphosphate (ATP) for the synthesis of chlamydial protein. The genus now contains three species, *C. trachomatis, C. psittaci,* and the recently described *C. pneumoniae* (TWAR strain).

DIAGNOSIS

Diagnosis can be made by isolation of the organisms in tissue culture. Several non-culture methods are available for the diagnosis of *C. trachomatis* infection, including enzyme immunoassay (EIA), direct fluorescence antibody tests (DFA), and DNA probes. All three categories of tests are approved for detection of *C. trachomatis* in cervical and urethral specimens from adolescents and adults. The EIAs and DFAs have additional indications for use in conjunctival and nasopharyngeal specimens from infants with suspected chlamydial conjunctivitis and pneumonia. Antigen-detection tests and DNA probes are not approved and should not be used on genital (vaginal or urethral) and rectal specimens from prepubertal children or for any forensic purposes. The tests are not accurate at these sites.

Since infection with *C. pneumoniae* has been described only recently, culture and serologic analysis is available only at a limited number of research laboratories in the United States. The complement fixation (CF) test can be of use for the serologic diagnosis of psittacosis and lymphogranuloma venereum (LGV).

INFECTION DUE TO *C. TRACHOMATIS*

Eye Infection

Neonatal inclusion conjunctivitis usually presents 5 to 14 days after birth. Clinical presentation is variable, ranging from minimal injection and discharge, to severe injection with chemosis, pseudomembrane formation, and copious, mucopurulent discharge. The conjunctivae may be quite friable and bleed when stroked with a swab.

The treatment of choice is oral erythromycin suspension (50 mg/kg/day in four divided doses for 10 to 14 days). Topical therapy is not indicated and is generally ineffective.

Pneumonia

Infantile chlamydial pneumonia usually presents between 1 and 3 months of age. Infants are usually afebrile and tachypneic. Rales are usually heard on auscultation. Wheezing is rare. The chest radiograph shows hyperinflation with variable infiltrates. Peripheral eosinophilia (>400 cells per mm^3) is also present.

Infants with *C. trachomatis* pneumonia should be treated with erythromycin. The dosage schedule is the same as for chlamydial conjunctivitis.

Uncomplicated Urethral, Cervical, and Rectal Infections

C. trachomatis is the major identifiable infectious cause of nongonococcal urethritis, responsible for 30 to 50 per cent of cases. In women the organism can cause mucopurulent cervicitis and salpingitis. Salpingitis may eventually lead to tubal obstruction, infertility, and an increased risk of ectopic pregnancy. However, the great majority of chlamydial genital infections are asymptomatic.

The treatment of choice in adolescents is doxycycline (100 mg twice a day for 7 days). Alternative therapy is erythromycin (2 g/day for 7 days). Sexual partners should also be treated.

Lymphogranuloma Venereum

LGV is a sexually transmitted disease caused by the L_1, L_2, and L_3 serotypes of *C. trachomatis.* The infection is characterized by an initial transient genital papule or ulcer followed by the development of inguinal adenopathy, which may break down and form fistulas. This presentation is more common in men. Because the lymphatic drainage of the vulva is to the retroperitoneal nodes, women are more likely to present in the tertiary stage of the disease with rectovaginal fistulas and strictures.

Tetracycline (500 mg four times a day) or doxycycline (100 mg twice a day) should be given for 3 to 6 weeks.

INFECTION DUE TO *C. PNEUMONIAE* (TWAR)

C. pneumoniae appears to be a primary human respiratory pathogen. Clinical presentations include asymptomatic respiratory infection, a flu-like illness with pharyngitis, sinusitis with headache, bronchitis, and atypical pneumonia. The organism has been isolated from pleural fluid of a patient with pneumonia. Spread appears to be person to person via aerosol droplets. Multiple members of households may be infected.

Therapy is not well defined. In children, oral erythromycin suspension 50 mg/kg/day in four divided doses for 2 to 3 weeks is recommended. In adolescents, it appears that up to 21 days of either doxycycline (100 mg twice a day) or erythromycin (500 mg four times a day) may be necessary.

INFECTION DUE TO *C. PSITTACI*

C. psittaci is a ubiquitous animal pathogen. Infection in humans is usually due to exposure to animals, most commonly birds, and is usually respiratory. Onset is abrupt, accompanied by high fever. Headache is frequent. Rales are usually heard on auscultation, and the chest radiograph reveals variable infiltrates and frequently pleural effusions.

Recommended treatment is tetracycline (500 mg every 6 hours orally for 7 to 10 days). Erythromycin (2 g/day for 7 to 10 days) can also be used.

HISTOPLASMOSIS

BERNHARD L. WIEDERMANN, M.D.

Most cases of histoplasmosis in children and in adults are mild, self-limited, and often asymptomatic infections. Therefore, most infected children require no specific therapy. However, a few special instances merit antifungal therapy and are addressed here.

DISSEMINATED HISTOPLASMOSIS

The disseminated form of the disease is most often seen in young infants. Mortality is high if the patient remains untreated. Amphotericin B is the drug of choice and is given in dosages similar to those used for treating other fungal infections (Table 1).

Typically, a test dose of 0.1 mg/kg (maximum 1 mg) is given intravenously over 1 hour. If there are no adverse effects, such as arrhythmia, anuria, hypotension, or hypersensitivity reaction, further drug is given the same day, to total 0.25 mg/kg for the first day's treatment. An infusion time of 2 hours is probably sufficient. The following day, the dosage is increased to 0.5 mg/kg, and further daily increases to 1.0 mg/kg can be scheduled over the subsequent 2 days. Maintenance therapy (1.0 mg/kg/day or 1.5 mg/kg two or three times weekly), infused over 4 hours, is continued until a total dosage of 30 mg/kg has been administered. Although there are anecdotal reports of survival with lower total doses of amphotericin, published experience with these shortened regimens has been minimal.

At the onset of amphotericin B therapy, renal function and serum potassium and magnesium concentrations should be monitored approximately every other day for evidence of renal insufficiency, hypokalemia, and hypomagnesemia. Later in the course, weekly monitoring is sufficient if the patient is stable. Hypokalemia is particularly common and may be managed with oral supplements in most cases. Renal insufficiency may necessitate lowering the dose of amphotericin B administered in order to lessen nephrotoxicity, but excretion of amphotericin is not altered in oliguric states.

Acute reactions, such as fever, chills, and nausea, are usually easily managed. Pretreatment with diphenhydramine hydrochloride (1.25 mg/kg) or acetaminophen (10 to 15 mg/kg) is helpful; hydrocortisone (0.5 mg/kg) may be given as an intravenous bolus. Ibuprofen may also be helpful but carries the theoretic risk of worsening nephrotoxicity and is not

TABLE 1. Summary of Drug Treatment for Histoplasmosis

Amphotericin B: 0.25–1.0 mg/kg/day IV over 2–6 hr, or 1.0–1.5 mg/kg per dose every other day or q 3 days, usually to total dose of 30 mg/kg; usual maximum* 2–2.5 g total dose
Ketoconazole: 6 mg/kg/day q 12 hr; maximum 400 mg/day for histoplasmosis
Diphenhydramine hydrochloride: 1.25 mg/kg per dose IV or IM prior to amphotericin B infusion; maximum 50 mg
Meperidine: 1.0–1.5 mg/kg/dose IV or IM prior to amphotericin B infusion; maximum 50 mg
Acetaminophen: 10–15 mg/kg/dose p.o. prior to or following amphotericin B infusion; maximum 650 mg
Hydrocortisone: 0.5 mg/kg IV prior to amphotericin B infusion; maximum 50 mg

*Maximum doses listed here are specifically for the indications in this article and may differ from maximum dosages used for other purposes.

recommended. Patients with more severe reactions may respond to meperidine (1.0 to 1.5 mg/kg) IV. Heparin (1 unit/ml) may be added to the infusate to minimize thrombophlebitis. If pretreatment for acute reactions is necessary, it should be noted that the reactions tend to diminish later in the course of therapy; withdrawal of the pretreatment medications should be attempted after 2 or 3 weeks of amphotericin treatment.

Ketoconazole has been used successfully for treatment of disseminated histoplasmosis in selected adults but has not been well studied in children. The drug might be considered, however, for "step-down" therapy in some children who show improvement after several days of amphotericin therapy rather than switching to intermittent amphotericin administration. The usual pediatric dosage is 6 mg/kg/day orally twice daily, with a maximum dose of 400 mg daily.

Gastric upset with nausea and vomiting is the most common side effect, although hepatitis (1 in 10,000 to 15,000 patients) has been noted. Also, because ketoconazole can lessen adrenal testosterone synthesis with long-term use and may blunt adrenal response to adrenocorticotropic hormone (ACTH), it should be used with caution in patients with adrenal histoplasmosis. Ketoconazole interferes with metabolism of many drugs, including isoniazid, rifampin, phenytoin, and cyclosporin; thus, levels of these drugs must be monitored if concomitant ketoconazole use is necessary.

ACUTE PULMONARY HISTOPLASMOSIS

Most patients with acute pulmonary symptoms due to histoplasmosis do not require therapy. However, some individuals may experience more severe, acutely life-threatening illness and should receive amphotericin B therapy in dosages as suggested above. A more rapid increase in dosage every 12 hours initially may be used. This form of disease probably does not require a full 30 mg/kg regimen of amphotericin; 10 to 15 mg/kg may be sufficient if there has been a good clinical response.

The role of steroid therapy for these patients is unclear. Ketoconazole is not recommended as initial therapy for this situation because of the delay in achieving therapeutic response.

CHRONIC CAVITARY HISTOPLASMOSIS

The chronic cavitary form of disease is extremely uncommon in children, and recommendations for treatment are based primarily on adult studies. Amphotericin B administration may be required in individuals with progression of symptoms, persistence of cavitation beyond 6 to 8 weeks, or capsule thickness greater than 2 mm; however, these guidelines are somewhat arbitrary and should be tailored to the individual. Ketoconazole may be a suitable alternative for immunocompetent patients, but the optimal duration of therapy is unclear.

SYMPTOMATIC LOCALIZED HISTOPLASMOSIS

Occasionally, therapy is indicated for localized histoplasmosis when symptoms related to the site of the disease occur. Pulmonary disease causing spinal nerve root irritation, enlarging mediastinal granuloma causing airway compromise, and fistulas are some examples.

Ketoconazole, given for a period of 3 to 6 months, is probably the treatment of choice when symptoms persist beyond a few weeks and a delay in clinical response of several days is not critical. Surgical management is sometimes necessary, particularly to repair fistulas, but there is a risk of spillage of contents of caseous nodes or other infected material and caution should be used. If spillage occurs, treatment with amphotericin B or ketoconazole is indicated.

HISTOPLASMOSIS IN IMMUNOCOMPROMISED HOSTS

Histoplasmosis may cause illness in immunocompromised hosts either by primary infection or by reactivation. The risk for dissemination is higher than in immunocompetent individuals. For the reasons cited above, amphotericin B is preferred over ketoconazole for initial therapy in these patients. Ketoconazole is likely to be useful for continuing suppressive therapy after a course of amphotericin B and has been given in adults with acquired immunodeficiency syndrome (AIDS). Although relapse has occurred in such patients receiving ketoconazole, overall results have been fairly positive. For AIDS patients with histoplasmosis, ketoconazole suppression should probably be continued indefinitely.

OTHER THERAPY

Promising Treatments

Many newer antifungal agents are in various stages of clinical trials for treatment of histoplasmosis. Itraconazole, an oral triazole, has high in vitro activity against *Histoplasma capsulatum* and has been used successfully as sole therapy in both normal and immunocompromised patients. Fluconazole also has good activity against *H. capsulatum*, but preliminary studies in human diseases are not encouraging. Liposome-encapsulated amphotericin B and the methyl ester form of amphotericin B both allow for use of higher amphotericin B doses with less toxicity and appear promising for treatment of histoplasmosis. It is possible that some of these newer agents will be effective for treatment of some forms of histoplasmosis in the near future.

Indications for Surgery

The primary need for therapeutic surgical intervention in histoplasmosis is in patients with obstruction of thoracic structures (vascular airway, esophagus) caused by large mediastinal masses or for fistulous tracts. However, fibrosing mediastinitis and calcifications are probably not amenable to surgical intervention. Prophylactic excision of asymptomatic large mediastinal nodes (enlarging "histoplasmomas") has not been shown to be of benefit.

SUMMARY

Most patients with histoplasmosis, including those with mild symptoms, do not require any specific therapy. The self-limited nature of this infection complicates evaluation of therapeutic efficacy of newer agents, and the paucity of symptomatic disease in children has necessitated reliance on results of treatment of adult disease for development of treatment guidelines for children.

COCCIDIOIDOMYCOSIS

JANET R. GILSDORF, M.D.

Coccidioidomycosis, a localized or disseminated infection caused by the dimorphic fungus *Coccidioides immitis*, is endemic to the southwestern United States, including the central valley of California (from which Valley Fever derives its name), southern Arizona, New Mexico, and southwestern Texas. Coccidioidomycosis is relatively uncommon outside of these endemic areas, but because of increased travel and prolonged survival of immunocompromised patients, it may be seen in children from other regions.

THERAPEUTIC OPTIONS

Prior to the advent of antifungal agents, disseminated coccidioidomycosis was associated with a very high mortality rate. Fortunately, since amphotericin B has become available, many patients have been successfully treated. However, amphotericin B is associated with many undesirable side effects, including fever, chills and rigors, diminished renal glomerular filtration, and electrolyte abnormalities that may compromise adequate therapy.

More recently, the imidazole agents, including ketoconazole and miconazole, have become available and have proved to be effective in some patients infected with *C. immitis.* Ketoconazole is available in 200-mg tablets that must be divided or compounded into powders for administration to young children. Although ketoconazole is considerably safer than amphotericin B to administer, it has resulted in a decrease in testosterone levels in a few male patients, particularly at high doses. The effect of this endocrinologic toxicity on pubertal adolescent boys is not clear. Miconazole is available only in a parenteral form.

Recently, the triazole fluconazole has become available. Fluconazole does not show the testosterone-inhibiting effect of ketoconazole and is available in 50-, 100-, and 200-mg tablets, thus making it somewhat easier to achieve accurate dosing in children. Only limited studies of the use of fluconazole are available in children and dosing guidelines based on a clear understanding of its pharmacokinetics in children are not available.

Itraconazole is a new oral triazole that has undergone study in adults with a variety of fungal infections, including coccidioidomycosis, with promising results. Further studies are needed to understand the role of itraconazole in the treatment of pediatric fungal infections of all types, including coccidioidomycosis.

Imidazole antifungal drugs may interact with other drugs; ketoconazole levels are depressed with concurrent administration of rifampin. Both ketoconazole and fluconazole increase serum levels of cyclosporine. Fluconazole may also increase phenytoin levels. The choice of antifungal agents for the treatment of infections with *C. immitis* depends on the clinical presentation and the site of infection, and the duration of therapy ranges from no therapy to lifelong therapy.

PRIMARY DISEASE

In children, as in adults, primary acquisition of coccidioidomycosis is through the pulmonary route by inhalation of arthroconidia, which are the infectious phase of *C. immitis.* Asymptomatic infection develops in approximately two thirds of normal individuals who acquire *C. immitis* by this route. Those with symptomatic disease usually present with a syndrome characterized by anorexia, fever, cough, and chest pain. In addition, an erythematous rash may be seen early in the course of infection or a delayed hypersensitivity type rash of erythema nodosum may occur in the course of the infection. In the vast majority of normal individuals, this form of infection is benign and treatment is not warranted. Antifungal agents have not been investigated for their role in reducing the symptoms of these benign infections.

A unique method of acquisition of disease occasionally seen in children is primary cutaneous inoculation. Although usually described in laboratory workers, some children have acquired the disease through trauma with inoculation of the arthroconidia from contaminated environmental sources. This type of infection may result in a local nodule or ulcer that then disappears over several weeks and requires no therapy. However, local spread of direct-inoculation–acquired disease to regional lymph nodes with ulceration and drainage has been described, which responds well to therapy (see below).

DISSEMINATED DISEASE

Slowly Evolving Infection

Although the majority of healthy individuals experience a benign, self-limited disease when infected with *C. immitis,* about 1 per cent of normal children as well as adults have evidence of disseminated disease. The risk of disseminated spread is considerably higher among certain ethnic groups, including Filipinos, Asians, American Indians, and blacks. Disseminated disease limited to subcutaneous soft tissues, skin, or regional lymph nodes can be successfully treated with oral ketoconazole at a dose of 5 to 10 mg/kg/day twice daily or once a day. Although efficacy studies have not been conducted in children, success in slowly evolving disseminated disease in adults with fluconazole has been very encouraging; a suggested dose in children would be 3 to 5 mg/kg/day orally once daily. Some investigators prefer to initiate treatment with amphotericin B for several weeks until evidence of clinical improvement is seen and then continue the antifungal therapy with oral ketoconazole or fluconazole. Optimal duration of therapy for these infections is variable and depends on the response to therapy and the state of immunocompetency. Improved outcome may also be achieved by local surgical excision of infected nodes or cutaneous nodules.

Rapidly Progressing or Bone and Joint Infection

Rapidly progressive coccidioidomycosis, miliary disease, multiorgan system disease, or infections of poorly perfused spaces such as bones or joints require more intensive and aggressive antifungal therapy. The standard therapy for these infections is intravenous amphotericin B. After a test dose of 0.5 to 1 mg (depending on the age of the child), therapy is

TABLE 1. Drugs Used in Treatment of Coccidioidomycosis

Drug	Indication	Route	Dose
Amphotericin B	Fungal infections	IV	0.75 to 1.0 mg/kg/day, initial dose 0.25 mg/kg; increase daily dose by 0.25 mg/kg increments to final dose
Miconazole	Coccidioidomycosis meningitis	intraventricular	3–5 mg every day
Ketoconazole	Fungal infections	p.o.	5–10 mg/kg/day q.d. or b.i.d.
	Coccidioidomycosis meningitis	p.o.	15–20 mg/kg/day q.d.
Fluconazole	Fungal infections	p.o.	3–5 mg/kg/day q.d.
	Fungal meningitis	p.o.	Dose not established in children; 400 mg every day in adults

initiated at 0.25 mg/kg/day and increased daily by 0.25 mg/kg to a daily dose of 0.75 or 1.0 mg/kg/day. These relatively high doses are tolerated much better in children than in adults but may result in toxicity from the drug that cannot be tolerated by the patient. In this situation, oral fluconazole (3 to 5 mg/kg/day once a day in children) has been shown in some adults to provide effective therapy when amphotericin B cannot be tolerated or in amphotericin B treatment failure. Again, duration of therapy for rapidly progressive and serious disseminated coccidioidomycosis is unclear and depends on the rapidity of clinical improvement and on the immunocompetency of the patient.

MENINGITIS

C. immitis meningitis has been a notoriously difficult infection to treat. In the past, intrathecal or intracisternal instillation of amphotericin B offered the best outcome but still mortality was about 50 per cent. Recent evidence suggests that *C. immitis* meningitis in children can be successfully treated with a combination of oral ketoconazole (15 to 20 mg/kg/day) once a day with daily intraventricular instillation of 3 to 5 mg of miconazole via an indwelling Ommaya reservoir. Children seem to show greater improvement on this type of therapy than adults, possibly because coccidioidomycosis meningitis in children is more likely to be manifested as ventriculitis with early development of hydrocephalus; in adults, basilar inflammation is more prominent. A few patients initially begun on ketoconazole and intraventricular miconazole have been successfully maintained with prolonged oral ketoconazole alone.

Although fluconazole has not been used extensively for *C. immitis* meningitis in children, clinical trials in adults are very promising. Fluconazole penetrates well into the cerebrospinal fluid and does not exhibit the suppression of gonadal and adrenal steroidogenesis seen with ketoconazole. No dosing guidelines for fluconazole in *C. immitis* meningitis are available for children; the adult dose is 400 mg/day. Although the duration of treatment for *C. immitis* meningitis is also unclear, most patients require lifelong therapy.

NEONATAL INFECTION

Several reports have suggested intrauterine transmission of coccidioidomycosis from mother to fetus. In addition, several other infants with neonatally acquired disease have been reported. The infection appears to be particularly virulent in these young infants, and the majority have died, with the diagnosis made at autopsy. Successful treatment, however, with amphotericin B has been described.

INFECTION IN IMMUNOSUPPRESSED INDIVIDUALS

Because transplant recipients, patients with hematologic or lymphoproliferative malignancies, and patients with acquired immunodeficiency syndrome are at greatly increased risk for disseminated disease, aggressive antifungal therapy needs to be instituted immediately and continued for the duration of their immunosuppressed state. The onset of immunosuppression from any of these causes may reactivate previously latent and well-contained coccidioidomycosis.

INFECTION DURING PREGNANCY

Possibly because of the increased level of estrogenic hormones, pregnant women are at an extremely high risk for development of disseminated disease, particularly in the third trimester. Again, aggressive antifungal therapy needs to be initiated and their infants monitored carefully for evidence of intrauterine-acquired infection.

MONITORING EFFICACY OF THERAPY

In addition to clinical parameters of response to antifungal therapy, changing levels of antibodies against *C. immitis* may indicate progression of disease or response to therapy. Decreasing levels of complement-fixing antibodies in the serum or in the cerebrospinal fluid, when measured at 1- to 2-month intervals, along with an improving or stable clinical course suggests efficacy of treatment. Anti–*C. immitis* antibodies, as measured by quantitative immunodiffusion, also correlate with disease activity and may be particularly helpful in patients whose sera are anti-complementary because of immune complex formation.

CYSTICERCOSIS

LOUIS M. WEISS, M.D., M.P.H.
and MURRAY WITTNER, M.D., Ph.D.

The pork tapeworm, *Taenia solium,* is one of the most common tapeworms of humans. Infection with its larval form, or *Cysticercus,* is a common cause of central nervous system (CNS) disease in endemic areas. When humans (or hogs) ingest mature eggs, the embryos hatch (stimulated by gastric juice, intestinal enzymes, and bile), enter the circulation, and are transported throughout the body. They then enter and encyst in striated muscle and other tissues, where, in 10 to 11 weeks, they become infective larvae termed *Cysticercus cellulosae.* Cysticerci are bladder-like cysts in which protoscolex has developed. Symptomatic disease can result when these larvae become encysted in the CNS, eye, or heart. Often, symptoms occur when the cysts die and are believed to be due in part to the host's inflammatory response.

Human infection with cysticerci is found wherever adult *T. solium* infection is common. Thus, human cysticercosis is often encountered in Mexico, South and Central America, Africa, India, and parts of China. In Mexico, autopsy studies have demonstrated this parasite in 3.5 per cent of the population. Although the usual onset of symptoms is within 7 years of acquiring the infection, the onset of symptomatic disease has occurred in patients who left endemic areas 30 years before. In some cases, disease has occurred within 6 months of exposure. Recently, an "outbreak" of neurocysticercosis was reported in an orthodox Jewish community apparently acquired from recently emigrated domestic employees from Latin America.

CLINICAL FEATURES

The clinical manifestations depend on the number, anatomic localization, swelling, and expansion of the cysts, as well as the inflammatory response of the host. Cysticerci have been found in almost every tissue and organ of the body. Except in eye lesions, the cyst often provokes the development of a fibrotic capsule. CNS lesions often provoke seizures and in endemic areas may be the leading cause of seizure disorders. A cyst located in the ventricles may cause noncommunicating hydrocephalus; rarely, a ball-valve mechanism can occur, causing sudden blockage and syncope. In the basilar cisterns, cysts may cause communicating hydrocephalus and cranial nerve palsy. A proliferating or racemose form may develop in this location, and the prognosis is poor. Heavy cyst burdens may be associated with dementia and personality changes. Ocular cysticercosis can manifest as disturbances of vision, scotoma, free-floating parasites in the vitreous, or retinal detachment. *In some cases, the retinal lesion has been misdiagnosed as retinoblastoma, and the eye has been enucleated.* Rarely, myositis may also develop, although skeletal muscle involvement is usually asymptomatic.

DIAGNOSIS

In any person with CNS manifestations who is from an endemic area, the diagnosis of CNS cysticercosis should be considered. Computed tomographic scanning should help demonstrate active cysts with edema, old calcified cysts, or hydrocephalus in 70 to 80 per cent of cases. Magnetic resonance imaging (MRI) may be more sensitive to active lesions with edema but is less sensitive to old calcified lesions. At present, no comparative studies are available that assess which is the more useful imaging modality. Calcified cysticerci can often be seen by roentgenographic examination; thus, multiple comma-shaped or arc-like calcifications in the brain or soft tissues are suggestive of cysticerci. Careful physical examination may reveal subcutaneous cysticerci, which can be obtained for biopsy. In selected patients—that is, those with hydrocephalus or aseptic meningitis—myelography to demonstrate extraventricular cysts may be useful.

Serologic studies are useful in diagnosis. Specimens of cerebrospinal fluid (CSF) and serum should be examined in suspected cases, although CSF is often more sensitive than serum in establishing the diagnosis. In addition, the presence of an active meningitic profile in the CSF is an indication to treat the infection. CSF eosinophilia is present in a small number of cases. Recently, a western blot technique has replaced the indirect hemagglutination (IHA) test as the diagnostic test at the Centers for Disease Control (CDC). This procedure has essentially precluded previous problems of cross-reactivity with *Echinococcus.* The reported sensitivity and specificity of the western blot are 98 per cent and 99 per cent or more, respectively in patients with multiple cysts. In patients with a solitary cyst, the sensitivity is lower (about 70 per cent). Recent studies have shown that the immunoblot (western blot) and double diffusion tests for hydatid disease may cross-react with sera from patients with cysticercosis. These tests are available from the CDC.

Even though the yield is low, patients with cysticercosis should have stool examinations for *T. solium.* Family members should also be screened. Heavy CNS infections in children may possibly be due to autoinfection in children harboring adult *T. solium.*

TREATMENT

With the advent of praziquantel, the treatment of CNS cysticercosis has changed dramatically. Praziquantel, at 50 mg/kg/day in three divided doses for 14 days, in controlled studies has been shown to be successful in reducing the number of cysts and the CNS symptoms. However, severe reactions, including death, with this therapy, probably resulting from the death of the cysticerci and subsequent host inflammatory response, have been reported. For this reason, treatment is indicated only in patients with symptomatic neurologic disease, active meningitis, or hydrocephalus. Ocular cysticercosis is a contraindication to therapy. Steroids should be administered to reduce inflammation—prednisone, 1 to 3 mg/kg/day, starting 2 to 3 days before therapy. Praziquantel is of no benefit when all of the cysticerci are calcified. As the natural history of an isolated, asymptomatic cyst is usually benign, there is debate about the use of praziquantel in this setting. We do not routinely treat patients with parenchymal cysts whose symptoms can be controlled with appropriate medication, such as antiseizure drugs or medication for headaches. Other investigators recommend treatment in all cases to decrease the incidence of seizures.

Alternative drugs with reported success in CNS cysticercosis are albendazole (15 mg/kg for 30 days), metrifonate (7.5 mg/kg for 5 days), and flubendazole. Metrifonate has also been reported to be effective for ocular disease. In many parts of the world, albendazole has replaced praziquantel as the drug of choice for cystercosis. However, albendazole is not available in the United States except as an investigational agent. Steroids are also used with albendazole (same dose as with praziquantel). Steroids are reported to cause higher serum levels of albendazole. Anecdotally, racemose disease appears to respond to albendazole treatment.

Patients with hydrocephalus often require shunts. If intraventricular cysts are present, shunt obstruction may occur. This obstruction can be treated by simple ventriculostomy with cyst removal. Resection of parenchymal cysts should be reserved for intractable seizures unresponsive to medical therapy, so that an epileptic focus may be removed. Basilar cistern adhesions may require lysis if involvement of the optic chiasm has resulted in compromised vision.

PREVENTION

Prevention of cysticercosis is the same as that for any parasitic infection transmitted by the fecal-oral route. Given the recent "outbreak" of neurocysticercosis related to domestic employees recently emigrated from endemic regions, it is reasonable to do stool examinations on such employees for *T. solium.*

MUCORMYCOSIS

(ZYGOMYCOSIS)

W. THOMAS CORDER, M.D.
and STEPHEN ARONOFF, M.D.

Mucormycosis, also known as zygomycosis, is an infection caused by fungi commonly found on bread, fruit, and soil. Mucormycosis is rare and is seen most often as an opportunistic infection in patients with diabetic ketoacidosis, debilitation, agranulocytopenia, or immunosuppression. Nearby construction activity may present an independent risk factor for susceptible individuals. In particular, the infection has reportedly been transmitted to a neonate by contaminated parenteral feeding solution. Infections are usually acute and rapidly fatal.

The most common forms of mucormycosis are rhinocerebral, pulmonary, intestinal, and cutaneous.

CLASSIFICATION

Rhinocerebral. The fungus is suspected to invade through the mucous membranes of the nasal passages or sinuses or through the soft palate. Symptoms can include unilateral headache, eye irritation, periorbital edema, epistaxis, nasal discharge, and pain over the affected sinus (maxillary or frontal). Areas of black necrosis can be seen in the nose, medial maxillary wall, and turbinates or on the palate. Ecchymoses and periorbital cellulitis can occur. A discharge of "black pus" is pathognomonic. Direct extension to the central nervous system, lethargy, and coma can occur.

Pulmonary. The course is similar to that of pulmonary aspergillosis and is characterized by fever and pulmonary infiltrates. Pulmonary vascular thrombosis and infarction are late sequelae. Extension to the central nervous system is not uncommon and is usually fatal.

Intestinal. Intestinal disease follows ingestion of fungi by susceptible persons. Symptoms, which may vary according to site and extent, include abdominal pain, diarrhea, hematemesis, and hematochezia. Ulcers can be found throughout the intestinal tract and may result in thromboses and gangrene.

Cutaneous. Cutaneous mucormycosis is a particular danger to burn patients. Skin infection has also been reported with the use of Elastoplast bandages over wounds and adhesive tape over an intravenous site.

DIAGNOSIS

Definitive diagnosis requires histologic examination of biopsy or affected material because blood cultures and direct cultures from affected tissue are often sterile. Negative cultures cannot exclude the diagnosis. Multiple biopsies may be needed to make the diagnosis. Histologically, broad, coenocytic hyphae are found invading tissue. The organisms are known to invade arterial walls to produce an arteritis and thrombosis that results in infarction of the distally perfused area.

TREATMENT

Therapy consists of correction of underlying problems (such as diabetic ketoacidosis), surgical débridement, and drainage. Hyperbaric oxygen has been used experimentally in the rhinocerebral form. Amphotericin B is the antifungal agent of choice. Side effects from amphotericin B include bone marrow suppression, nephrotoxicity, hypokalemia, fever, chills, headache, nausea, anorexia, phlebitis, and hypomagnesemia. Hypercalciuria, renal tubular acidosis, and acute hepatic failure can also occur. Baseline renal function, liver function, hematologic values, and electrolytes should be obtained before administration and should be followed throughout the course of therapy.

To minimize side effects, the patient can be premedicated with acetaminophen (10 to 15 mg/kg per dose), and diphenhydramine (1.25 mg/kg per dose) 30 minutes before and 4 hours after infusion. If toxic symptoms still occur, the patient may also be premedicated with hydrocortisone (1 mg/kg per dose up to 25 mg) or this can be added to the intravenous solution. The drug is mixed with D_5W to a concentration of 0.1 mg/ml and pH > 4.2. A test dose of 0.1 mg/kg (up to maximum of 1.0 mg) is infused over 20 to 30 minutes. The patient's temperature and vital functions are followed for the next 4 hours. If the test dose is tolerated well, the remainder of a 0.25 mg/kg dose may be given over the next 4 to 6 hours. The dose is increased in daily increments of 0.25 mg/kg per dose until a daily dose of 0.4 to 0.6 mg/kg is reached. This dose is given daily until the patient's condition stabilizes or improves, and then it can be given every other day until the total dose is administered. In adults the total dose is usually in the range of 2 to 4 g. The total dose for children is unknown; according to extrapolation of the adult range, the total dosage for a child would be 15 to 30 mg/kg.

SUMMARY

Mucormycosis is a rapidly progressive fulminant disease that is usually associated with a fatal outcome. A high degree of clinical suspicion and a prompt histologic examination of material submitted for biopsy are needed to make an early diagnosis. Rapid diagnosis and early institution of therapy provide the best chance for improved outcome.

TOXOCARA CANIS INFECTIONS

J. JEFFREY MALATACK, M.D.

Toxocara canis is a species of roundworm that parasitizes dogs. However, when it infects humans, it can cause a clinical pathologic entity that typically presents with abdominal pain, hepatosplenomegaly, cough, wheeze, pulmonary infiltrates, and urticaria or papular skin eruptions. This infection, known as visceral larva migrans (VLM), is contracted when infective *T. canis* ova are ingested by a human.

MECHANISMS OF INFECTION

The dog infected by *T. canis* provides a host in which the parasite can mature into the adult form in the intestinal tract. The mature *T. canis* female can lay as many as 200,000 ova a day. These ova are excreted by the dog via the stool into the soil. Infection in dogs is worldwide and, consequently, so is human infection, although most cases are reported from the temperate areas. The frequent use of city parks and green areas by pets has caused heavy contamination of the soil and sandboxes in these areas. One study of the parks in a large United States city revealed one of three soil samples to contain *T. canis* ova.

Children are most frequently infected. The mechanism of infection appears to be due to ingestion of soil by the 1- to 4-year-old child. A second mechanism has also been appreciated, in which petting infected dogs can transmit ova to the petter's hand; subsequently, hand-to-mouth activity can lead to an infection. Adults may become infected from soiled hands or from eating food or drinking water contaminated with the ova.

Once an ovum gains access into the human intestinal tract, it becomes a larva and begins to "migrate" first by burrowing into the intestinal wall, then using venous channels to enter the liver, triggering eosinophilic abscesses and granuloma formation, which may calcify in time. The larva also migrates to the lungs but fails to penetrate the alveoli—a necessary step for the larva to return to the intestinal tract to mature. Respiratory symptoms of wheezing and cough ensue. The larva in heavy infections may migrate and reach the heart (where it can lead to heart failure), kidneys, spleen, brain, eyes, and other tissues. The infected patient's symptoms depend on the organ involved, the quantity of infecting larvae, the migrating larva's mechanical effect on the organ's function, and immune response. The acute symptoms last 3 to 4 weeks, but complete resolution may take as long as 18 months. Rarely, in heavy infection, death due to cardiac involvement or blindness due to eye involvement may occur.

In infected individuals, in addition to clinical features, invariably the eosinophil count is significantly elevated. Typically, the total leukocyte count increases to greater than 30,000 with 20 to 80 percent eosinophils. Hypergammaglobulinemia and elevated isoagglutinins (anti-A and anti-B titers greater than 1:1024) are usually present. Chest x-ray may show infiltrates, and calcified granuloma may be noted. When the brain is a site of migrating larvae, cerebrospinal fluid (CSF) may have an eosinophilic pleocytosis and a seizure disorder with electroencephalographic localized ictal activity may develop. When the eyes are involved, usually the patient's clinical complaint is unilateral visual impairment or strabismus is noted by the parent. The lesion itself is also unilateral and painless.

Most infestations with *T. canis* are asymptomatic, and only when the load of infesting larvae is substantial does VLM develop. It is also worth noting that although *T. canis* is the most frequent cause of cases of VLM, it is not the only cause of VLM. *Toxocara cati,* which normally infects cats, *Boylisascaris peocyonis,* which normally infects raccoons, and probably other ascarids that have a complete host/parasite relationship with other mammals can cause VLM in humans.

MANAGEMENT

Preventive Measures

Management begins with an understanding of the life cycle of *T. canis* in the dog. It is known that puppies and lactating bitches are responsible for most *T. canis* excreted into the environment. Adult nonparous dogs are infrequent carriers of *Toxocara* infection. This is because larvae in the intestinal tract burrow out of the intestine, lodging in the somatic tissues where they become dormant. Reactivation of larval migration occurs during pregnancy, both infecting the fetal pup in utero or newborn pups via lactation and reaching the intestinal tract and maturing to an ova-excreting postpartum adult. Uninfected adult dogs can become infected by ingesting eggs from dog feces or eating small rodents that harbor the larvae in their tissues or by ingesting infected soil. Consequently, controlling *T. canis* infection can be enhanced by:

1. Eliminating ownerless dogs who are not purged of ascarids at appropriate times.
2. Enforcing of leash laws and "pooper scooper" ordinances.
3. Protecting playground play areas from possible contaminated dog feces (i.e., cover sandboxes, fence in playground areas to exclude dogs).
4. Good hand washing after playing in soil.
5. Supervising children's play to avoid soil and sand eating.

Additionally, deworming of the parous dog or cat during the last 2 weeks of gestation and lactation can diminish the infection in pups. If preventive deworming is not accomplished, newborn kittens and pups and lactating dog and cat mothers should be treated for intestinal *Toxocara* infections at 2-week intervals for 12 weeks after parturition. Infants and young children are not to play with pups and kittens that have not been dewormed until they are inculcated with good hand-washing behavior after petting an animal. Additionally, for the child who ingests soil and sand, pets should be disallowed until the ingesting behavior has ceased. Adult dogs and cats should be treated prophylactically twice a year. If, however, the dog has had positive stool findings, treatment should be guided by subsequent stool examination. Deworming is best done under direction of a veterinarian who can suggest the appropriate drug and drug dosage.

Definitive Diagnosis

Perhaps because prevention efforts are only sporadically adhered to, the child occasionally may be both symptomatic and have positive classic laboratory support of the diagnosis of VLM. Specific diagnosis can be further confirmed by the use of an enzyme-linked immunoabsorbent assay (ELISA), which uses embryonic *Toxocara* eggs as antigens. This ELISA is 92 per cent specific and 78 per cent sensitive. For a definitive diagnosis, liver biopsy, which may give direct histologic evidence of larval infestation, is necessary. However, liver biopsy is rarely necessary if the clinicopathologic picture is clear prior to it.

TREATMENT

Treatment of the infected child should be based on the severity of the child's symptoms. In the absence of significant symptoms, the child need not be treated, aside from elimination of the source of further infestation. Treatment, when necessary, is primarily supportive, with routine antibronchospastic therapy for the child with bronchospasm. Corticosteroids can be very helpful in controlling the inflammatory response, including the bronchospasm.

Specific anthelmintic therapy is only somewhat effective. Thiabendazole (25 mg/kg twice a day for 5 to 7 days) has been tried to hasten larval destruction. Since thiabendazole prolongs the half-life of theophylline, it is best to discontinue theophylline at least 48 hours before starting thiabendazole. Some authors report that the use of thiabendazole may be associated with increased atopic symptoms (perhaps due to increased antigen release) and believe anthelmintics should always be used in conjunction with corticosteroids. Thiabendazole is frequently associated with adverse reactions, including nausea, vomiting, and epigastric pain. Rarely leukopenia, intrahepatic cholestasis, and Steven-Johnson syndrome have been reported. Two alternative drugs have been used as treatment. Diethylcarbamazine (6 mg/kg/day in three divided doses for 2 to 3 weeks) and mebendazole (1 g three times a day for 21 days) have each given equivocal results.

Ocular Larva Migrans

Treatment of ocular larva migrans (OLM) is even less satisfying than treatment of VLM. Systemic anthelmintic drugs have shown equivocal results. Topical and intraocular steroids may decrease the inflammatory changes. Visible larvae close to the macula may successfully undergo laser photocoagulation. Vitrectomy has been used for vitreous traction. Usually, as with VLM, OLM is self-limited; however, partial or total visual impairment infrequently results from nematode-induced endophthalmitis and retinal granuloma formation. Disease, and hence visual impairment, when it does occur is most often unilateral. Close ophthalmologic management and follow-up are required.

REFERENCES

Goldsmith R, Heyneman D: Tropical Medicine and Parasitology. Norwalk, Conn, Appleton and Lange, 1989.
Noble ER, Noble GA, Schad GA, et al: Parasitology: The Biology of Animal Parasites. Philadelphia, Lea and Febiger, 1989.

MALARIA

COY D. FITCH, M.D.

Malaria is an ancient and well-understood disease, for which there has been adequate treatment for several centuries. Cinchona bark, a source of quinine, was introduced by American Indians to the Jesuits, who then introduced it in Europe more than three centuries ago. Nevertheless, the disease continues to be a major threat to 1.6 billion people who live in tropical and subtropical areas. *Each year in tropical Africa alone, there are probably 90 million clinical cases of malaria, with as many as a million children dying from the disease.* Efforts have been made to eradicate the disease by controlling mosquitoes, but those efforts have been unsuccessful.

MECHANISM OF INFECTION

Of the more than 100 species of malaria parasites, only four naturally infect human beings: *Plasmodium malariae, Plasmodium vivax, Plasmodium ovale,* and *Plasmodium falciparum.* These protozoan parasites have two hosts, human beings and female anophelene mosquitoes of several species. The parasites undergo sexual reproduction in the mosquito, and the progeny (sporozoites) are infectious for the human host when injected by the bite of the mosquito. In human beings, the parasite reproduces asexually, first in the liver and then in erythrocytes. As part of the erythrocytic stage, female and male gametocytes are produced and are available for ingestion by mosquitoes, thus allowing the life cycle to be repeated.

The periodic chills and fever of malaria coincide with the asexual, erythrocytic reproduction of parasites and probably result from the release of toxic substances when erythrocytes more or less synchronously rupture to release their broods of new parasites (merozoites). *P. vivax, P. ovale,* and *P. falciparum* produce a typical periodicity of chills and fever of 48 hours (tertian). For *P. malariae,* the typical interval is longer, 72 hours (quartan). *P. vivax, P. ovale,* and *P. malariae* usually cause self-limited disease if the patient remains untreated, although relapses or recrudescences may occur after long periods of time. In fact, patients infected with *P. malariae* may harbor parasites for decades and transmit them when they donate blood for transfusion. In the case of *P. vivax,* it is well established that the liver stage of the parasite persists asymptomatically and gives rise to multiple recrudescences many weeks or months after the initial attack. *P. falciparum* does not persist in the liver stage, but it is the parasite that causes severe disease, including death.

Early in the course of malaria, the characteristic periodicity of chills and fever may not be present, and the disease may easily be mistaken for influenza or another febrile illness. Indeed, *P. falciparum* infections often fail to produce tertian chills and fever before the parasitemia is so great that there is extensive morbidity with central nervous system symptoms (cerebral malaria) or acute respiratory distress. Therefore, a travel history may be the key to early diagnosis of malaria in non-endemic areas. Once suspected, malaria can usually be diagnosed by examining Giemsa-stained thick and thin blood films. An experienced examiner can identify the species of malarial parasite from the blood film. Other diagnostic tests, such as DNA probes, are under development but are not in general clinical use.

Not only is *P. falciparum* the most virulent malaria parasite for human beings, it has a propensity to develop resistance to antimalarial drugs, including chloroquine, quinine, and pyrimethamine. Chloroquine resistance has been reported from most countries endemic for *P. falciparum,* although in West Africa it still has a focal distribution. In Southeast Asia and South America, the phenomenon is more widespread. Fortunately, the parasites usually are not totally resistant and parasitemia can be suppressed by chloroquine, quinine, or mefloquine. The other three species of malaria parasites show relatively little tendency to develop drug resistance.

TREATMENT

The best antimalarial drugs fall into three classes: (1) quinoline derivatives and related drugs (which include quinine, chloroquine, and mefloquine), (2) dihydrofolate reductase inhibitors, and (3) sulfonamides. The latter two classes show synergism against malaria when combined, as in Fansidar, which includes 25 mg of pyrimethamine and 500 mg of sulfadoxine in each tablet. Certain other antimicrobials, including tetracycline, erythromycin, lincomycin derivatives, and fluoroquinolines, have antimalarial activity, but they are relatively slow to act and otherwise are not superior to the other drugs in our armamentarium. Because of the threat of drug-resistant *P. falciparum,* several potential new antimalarials are under development.

Chloroquine is still the drug of choice for large areas of the world, including West Africa. It is given orally in four doses over a 3-day period to achieve a total dose of 20 to 25 mg of the base per kg of body weight. Approximately 300 mg of chloroquine base are contained in a 500-mg chloroquine phosphate tablet. For older children and adults, the maximum recommended dose of chloroquine base is 600 mg in the first dose, 300 mg 6 hours after the first dose, and 300 mg on each of the next two days. For young children, the dose should be kept on the low side because these patients are especially susceptible to chloroquine toxicity. Other drugs closely related to chloroquine (quinacrine, amodiaquine, hydroxychloroquine) may be used if chloroquine is not available.

When chloroquine-resistant *P. falciparum* is suspected, quinine sulfate or mefloquine hydrochloride (Lariam) is the drug of choice, despite the fact that the parasite may have a low level of cross-resistance to either drug. The dose of quinine is 20 mg/kg of the salt daily for 10 to 14 days. This dose is divided into three parts and taken orally after meals. The maximum dose of quinine for older children and adults is 650 mg of the salt three times daily for 10 to 14 days.

The therapeutic dose of mefloquine is 15 to 25 mg of the base per kg as a single oral dose. The maximum recommended dose of mefloquine is 1250 mg.

In addition to quinine or mefloquine, Fansidar should be added to the treatment regimen. For adults, the dose of Fansidar is two to three tablets as a single dose; for children 9 to 14 years of age, two tablets; for children 4 to 8 years of age, one tablet; and for children under 4 years of age, one-half tablet. If Fansidar cannot be used because of hypersensitivity, one of the antimicrobials mentioned earlier may be added.

When the patient is gravely ill, as with cerebral malaria or acute respiratory distress syndrome from *P. falciparum,* and cannot take oral medication, quinine or quinidine intravenously is the drug of choice. Each drug is a stereoisomer of the other and is approximately equally potent as an antimalarial agent. Each carries significant risk when used intravenously, and its use by this route can be justified only in emergencies.

The intravenous dose of quinine is 20 mg of the base per kg per day. One third of this dose, not to exceed 600 mg of the base, is diluted in 200 ml or more of normal saline and infused slowly over a period of 4 hours. These infusions may be repeated at 8-hour intervals only for as long as the patient is unable to take oral medication. During the use of intravenous quinine or quinidine, the patient should be monitored for hypoglycemia, hypotension, cardiac arrhythmias, and neurologic toxicity.

If the patient has a prior history of intravascular hemolysis associated with the use of quinine, parenteral chloroquine may be used instead of quinine. An initial dose of 3.5 mg of the base per kg is administered intramuscularly. This dose may be repeated at 6- to 12-hour intervals, but the total daily dose of chloroquine base intramuscularly should not exceed 10 mg/kg. Alternatively, a continuous intravenous infusion of 0.83 mg of chloroquine base per kg per hour may be used for up to 30 hours. Overdosage with chloroquine may produce respiratory depression, cardiovascular collapse, shock, convulsions, and death, especially in infants and children. As soon as possible, therefore, oral treatment should be started, through a stomach tube, if necessary, and supplemental therapy with Fansidar or alternative antimicrobial should be instituted.

Because the sporozoites of *P. vivax, P. ovale,* and possibly *P. malariae* may persist in the liver for long periods of time, it is necessary to eradicate them to achieve a complete cure (radical cure). For this purpose, the therapeutic armamentarium is limited to one drug, primaquine. Chloroquine, quinine, and the other drugs used to treat the erythrocytic stage are ineffective against the liver stage. To achieve a radical cure, in addition to the standard treatment with chloroquine, primaquine phosphate is given in a daily dose of 0.3 mg of the base (approximately 0.5 mg of the salt) per kg for 14 days. The maximum dose for older children and adults is 15 mg of the base (26.5 mg of the salt) daily for 14 days. It is not necessary to use primaquine to treat infections with *P. falciparum* because this parasite does not persist in the liver.

Side Effects from Antimalarials

In addition to the toxicities that have already been mentioned, each of the antimalarial drugs has side effects. For example, chloroquine may cause pruritus in blacks, and in very large amounts (prolonged use with a cumulative dose exceeding 100 g) it may cause retinal damage.

Quinine and quinidine may cause cinchonism (tinnitus, headache, visual disturbances, nausea, and sometimes severe gastrointestinal, neurologic, and cardiovascular symptoms). Primaquine may cause oxidative hemolysis of glucose-6-phosphate dehydrogenase (G-6-PD)–deficient erythrocytes. Pyrimethamine may cause megaloblastic anemia. Mefloquine may cause psychoses and convulsions.

Finally, sulfonamides may cause the Stevens-Johnson syndrome or a serum sickness–like syndrome. These toxicities are relatively unusual, however, except for the oxidative hemolysis provoked by primaquine in susceptible individuals.

PREVENTION OF MALARIA

International travelers to areas endemic for malaria should receive advice on how to avoid mosquito bites and on chemoprophylaxis of malaria. Because anopheline mosquitoes primarily feed at night, travelers are advised to wear clothing covering most of the body, stay indoors, or use mosquito nets at night. A mosquito repellent, such as *N,N*-dimethylmetatoluamide (DEET), may also be helpful.

Recommendations for chemoprophylaxis of malaria are difficult and change frequently because consideration must be given to the increasing geographic distribution of chloroquine-resistant *P. falciparum* and the toxicities of the available chemoprophylactic agents. Chloroquine is still the safest and most effective drug for malaria prophylaxis, although its use does not guarantee protection from chloroquine-resistant *P. falciparum.* When used prophylactically, chloroquine is taken in a single weekly dose of 5 mg of the base per kg, not to exceed 300 mg, beginning 1 week before travel and continuing for 4 weeks after leaving the malarious area. It is also prudent for the traveler to carry a single therapeutic dose of Fansidar to be taken if chills and fever occur and if medical help is not immediately available.

After travel to an area endemic for *P. vivax, P. ovale,* or *P. malariae,* it is prudent to recommend a course of treatment with primaquine, as previously discussed, to eliminate the possibility of persistence of the parasites in the liver. The use of primaquine in this way should be limited to people who exhibit normal G-6-PD activity in the erythrocytes.

For travelers to areas where chloroquine-resistant *P. falciparum* is prevalent, the Centers for Disease Control (CDC) in Atlanta recommends mefloquine alone as the drug of choice. It is taken as a single weekly dose of 250 mg beginning 1 week before the travel and continuing for four weeks after leaving the malarious area. Mefloquine is not recommended for travelers with known hypersensitivity to the drug, for children under 30 pounds in weight, for pregnant women, for anyone involved in tasks requiring fine coordination and spatial discrimination, or for anyone with a history of epilepsy or psychiatric disorders.

Because the recommendations for malarial chemoprophylaxis change frequently, the physician giving advice to international travelers should keep abreast of the most current information. A country-by-country listing of the risk of malaria is published periodically in the *Weekly Epidemiological Record* by the World Health Organization, and recommendations from the CDC may be found in the *Morbidity and Mortality Weekly Report.* The CDC encourages consultation by maintaining a Malaria Hotline: phone number, (404) 639–1610.

BABESIOSIS

PETER J. KRAUSE, M.D.

Babesiosis is a hemolytic disease caused by intraerythrocytic protozoa and transmitted by ticks. Many of the clinical features are similar to those of malaria. Although babesiosis has been recognized since biblical times as an important disease in livestock and is known to affect a wide variety of wild and domestic animals, the first human case was not described until 1957. Since that time, it has been recognized with increasing frequency in humans in different areas of Europe and the United States, including California, Minnesota, Washington State, Wisconsin, and endemic areas in southern New England and New York.

Babesiosis has been considered to be a disease primarily affecting adults, but recent studies indicate that children are infected at least as frequently. Children, with the possible exception of newborn infants, are thought to have milder illness than adults.

Two *Babesia* species have been found to cause disease in humans, *B. microti* in North America and *B. divergens* in Europe. The primary reservoir for *B. microti* in eastern North America is the white-footed mouse (*Peromyscus leucopus*). The primary vector is *Ixodes dammini,* which is the same tick that transmits *Borrelia burgdorferi,* the etiologic agent of Lyme disease. The white-tailed deer *(Odocoileus virginianus)* is an important host for the tick but is not a reservoir for *B. microti.* Domestic animals such as the dog may carry the adult *I. dammini* but do not appear to be important hosts for the ticks and are not infected with *B. microti.* Babesiosis has also been reported to be transmitted by blood transfusion. Most human cases of babesiosis occur in the summertime.

CLINICAL FEATURES

The clinical manifestations of babesiosis range from subclinical illness to fulminating disease resulting in death. Immunocompromised patients are more susceptible to severe babesial infection, especially patients who are asplenic or who have acquired immunodeficiency syndrome (AIDS). Overt signs and symptoms begin after an incubation period of 1 to 4 weeks from the beginning of tick feeding. In most cases, there is a gradual onset of malaise, anorexia, and fatigue, followed by intermittent temperature to as high as 40°C (104°F) and one or more of the following: chills, diaphoresis, myalgia, arthralgia, nausea, and vomiting. Less commonly noted are emotional lability and depression, hyperesthesia, headache, sore throat, abdominal pain, conjunctival injection, photophobia, weight loss, and nonproductive cough.

The findings on physical examination are generally minimal, often consisting only of fever, mild splenomegaly, hepatomegaly, or both. Pharyngeal erythema, jaundice, and retinopathy with splinter hemorrhages and retinal infarcts are noted occasionally.

Laboratory tests may show mild to moderately severe hemolytic anemia and elevations in the reticulocyte count, liver function tests, blood urea nitrogen, creatinine, and erythrocyte sedimentation rate. The leukocyte count is normal to slightly decreased with a "left shift."

The illness usually lasts for a few weeks to several months with prolonged recovery. Parasitemia may continue for as long as 10 months.

DIAGNOSIS

Specific diagnosis of babesiosis is made by microscopic identification of the organism by Giemsa stain of blood smears and by detection of babesial antibodies by one of several serologic tests. Multiple thick and thin blood smears should be examined because only a few erythrocytes are infected in the early stage of illness, when most people seek medical attention. Of the commonly used serologic tests, the indirect immunofluorescent antibody (IFA) assay is the most reliable. When babesiosis is suspected but not demonstrated by blood smears or antibody studies, blood from the patient can be injected into hamsters with subsequent demonstration of *B. microti* in the blood of the inoculated animal within 2 to 4 weeks. Serologic tests for Lyme disease should be performed in all suspected cases of babesiosis since co-infection with Lyme disease can occur and may result in severe illness.

TREATMENT

No drug developed for therapy of babesiosis has been completely effective. Because many patients experience a mild clinical course and recover without specific antibabesial chemotherapy, it is recommended that therapy be reserved for moderately to severely ill patients.

The combination of clindamycin (20 mg/kg/day every 6 hours intramuscularly [IM] or intravenously [IV], maximum 2400 mg/day) and quinine (25 mg/kg/day every 8 hours orally, maximum 1950 mg/day) is the therapy of choice for babesiosis. There have been six reported cases of babesiosis in children or adults treated with clindamycin and quinine who experienced prompt clearing of parasitemia and diminution of clinical signs and symptoms. There has also been a report of failure of this combination.

Pentamidine (240 mg/day IV) and trimethoprim-sulfamethoxazole (3 g/day orally) have recently been used successfully to treat a case of *B. divergens* in France. Exchange blood transfusions have been used successfully in splenectomized patients with life-threatening babesial infection. Exchange transfusion can decrease the degree of parasitemia rapidly and remove toxic byproducts of babesial infection, but it should be used only in the most severe infections.

Effective *B. bovis* and *B. bigemina* vaccines have been developed for use in cattle, but there is no *B. microti* vaccine.

TOXOPLASMOSIS

GREGORY A. FILICE, M.D.

Toxoplasma gondii is an ubiquitous protozoan parasite that infects about half of all humans during their lifetimes. Postnatal infections in healthy children are usually mild or asymptomatic. In contrast, congenital infection may lead to severe problems in infected infants. Women who become infected during pregnancy and who choose not to interrupt the pregnancy should be treated to prevent congenital infection or lessen its severity. Primary infection or reactivation of latent infection can be devastating to profoundly immunosuppressed children, and they should be treated to arrest the process.

There have been few studies of therapy for pregnant women or congenitally infected infants. Systematic studies of therapy for immunosuppressed patients are just now being conducted in those with the acquired immunodeficiency syndrome (AIDS). Recommendations are based largely on clinical experience, and clinicians should be prepared to modify their approach in particular clinical circumstances on the basis of a knowledge of the pathogenesis of *T. gondii* infection.

CLINICAL ILLNESS

Acute Acquired Infection in Immunocompetent Children

Most immunocompetent children who become infected with *T. gondii* are asymptomatic. One person in ten has a mild, self-limited illness 1 to 3 weeks after infection, usually characterized by fever and lymphadenopathy. Rare manifestations of acute acquired toxoplasmosis include encephalitis, myocarditis, hepatitis, pneumonitis, polymyositis, or persistent fevers. The syndrome is not specific, and the diagnosis is usually made by serology or lymph node histology.

Retinochoroiditis

Isolated retinochoroiditis is usually a late manifestation of congenital toxoplasmosis and then is usually bilateral. In contrast, retinochoroiditis occurs in fewer than 1 per cent of cases acquired by people with intact host defenses postnatally, and then it is usually unilateral. Retinochoroiditis also occurs in severely immunocompromised people with systemic toxoplasmosis.

Toxoplasmosis in Immunosuppressed Children

Children with profoundly deficient cell-mediated immunity are at risk for severe toxoplasmosis, usually from reactivation of latent infection. Common associated conditions include lymphoid malignancies, organ transplantation, and AIDS. The risk of toxoplasmosis in solid organ transplant recipients is greatest when a seronegative recipient receives an organ from a seropositive donor. In this case, the parasite is transmitted with the organ. The risk in bone marrow transplant recipients is greatest when a seropositive recipient receives marrow from a seronegative donor. In this case, immune cells transplanted with the marrow would not recognize latent *T. gondii* in the recipient.

The most commonly recognized manifestation is encephalitis, which often progresses to necrosis. Other common manifestations include pneumonitis, myocarditis, and fever without focal findings. Diagnosis and management are complicated by the fact that severely immunosuppressed people often have other opportunistic infections.

Toxoplasmosis in Pregnancy

Like other healthy adults, pregnant women with acute toxoplasmosis are symptomatic only 10 per cent of the time. In areas of high incidence (e.g., more than one case of congenital toxoplasmosis per 1000 live births), screening for antibodies to *T. gondii* should be done for all seronegative women before pregnancy and at monthly intervals during pregnancy to detect asymptomatic or mild infections. In areas of lower risk, which include many regions of the United States, the risk does not warrant monthly screening unless an individual woman's activities place her at high risk. The risks of transmission to babies born to mothers with primary infection during the first, second, or third trimester are 15, 20, and 60 per cent, respectively. Congenital transmission from healthy mothers infected before conception is exceedingly rare. The risk is increased for mothers with severely deficient cellular immunity, especially those with AIDS.

For screening, IgG antibodies to *T. gondii* should be measured first. Women seropositive before pregnancy need not be tested again. If the first test is done after conception, a positive IgG test should be followed by a test for IgM or IgA antibodies. The interpretation of positive serologic results when the first titer has been obtained during pregnancy can be difficult. In the first 6 to 8 weeks after infection, gamma G immunoglobulin (IgG) titers are usually unstable; a stable IgG titer in the first 2 months of pregnancy usually signifies infection acquired before pregnancy. After this time, if the IgG titer is greater than 2000 or if there is IgM antibody, there is a substantial likelihood that infection was acquired during pregnancy.

Diagnosis of Fetal Infection

If infection is suspected in a woman during pregnancy, attempts at fetal diagnosis should be made. Between 18 and 28 weeks of gestation, fetal blood should be obtained and tested for the titer of IgM antibodies against *T. gondii* and concentrations of total IgM antibodies, gamma glutamyl transpeptidase (GGT), lactate dehydrogenase, white blood cells, platelets, and eosinophils. A portion of the blood clot should be inoculated into mice for culture. Amniotic fluid obtained at the same time should be concentrated by centrifugation and inoculated into mice. Every 2 weeks, fetal ultrasound examinations should be performed to determine the size of cerebral ventricles and the thickness of the placenta and to seek evidence for fetal ascites, hepatomegaly, or intracranial calcification.

Congenital Infection

Infection acquired in utero can result in abortion, prematurity, stillbirth, or congenital infection. Only a minority of children with congenital infection are symptomatic at birth. As a rule, the earlier the mother was infected during pregnancy, the worse the disease. If asymptomatic babies are not treated, the majority will develop ocular and perhaps neurologic or other abnormalities later in life. Because treatment appears to reduce the risk of sequelae, all congenitally infected children should be treated.

In cases of suspected congenital toxoplasmosis, samples of the placenta, including one near the insertion of the cord, (total ~100 g) should be homogenized, trypsinized, and inoculated into mice. IgG and IgM titers should be determined at birth and periodically afterward on infant sera. IgA antibody titers may be determined in place of or in addition to IgM titers.

Presence of IgM or IgA antibody to *T. gondii* is strongly suggestive of the diagnosis. Each can be of maternal origin if there has been a leak in the placental barrier, but both antibodies have short half-lives and should disappear rapidly. If IgM or IgA antibody persists or increases in titer, congenital infection is confirmed. One fourth of congenitally infected infants will have IgM detectable by the IgM immunofluorescence antibody test (IgM-IFA) and three fourths will have IgM detectable by the double-sandwich IgM enzyme-linked immunosorbent assay (DS-IgM-ELISA). IgG crosses the placenta, and the half-life in the infant is approximately 30 days, which makes early diagnosis by IgG difficult. Titers should be followed monthly. If titers do not fall or if they begin to increase, the diagnosis is confirmed.

THERAPEUTIC APPROACH

Drugs

The combination of pyrimethamine and sulfadiazine is the standard therapy for toxoplasmosis. The combination has been used extensively in humans and is synergistic against experimental infections in mice. Other agents demonstrate activity in vitro or in experimental animals, but they have generally been less active than the combination of pyrimethamine and sulfadiazine. Several new agents are under active investigation, and these recommendations may be superseded over the next few years.

Pyrimethamine

Pyrimethamine (Daraprim, Chloridin, Malocide), a substituted phenylpyrimidine, inhibits folic acid production in *T. gondii* by interfering with dihydrofolate reductase. It is orally absorbed and has a half-life of 4.5 days in adults. I usually use 1 to 2 mg/kg/day, up to a maximum of 50 mg, for the first 2 days and 1 mg/kg/day, up to a maximum of 25 mg, thereafter. Daily doses of 50 mg for prolonged periods have been required in some adults with AIDS. After 4 to 6 weeks of therapy, I give pyrimethamine three times a week because of its long half-life. For newborns with congenital infection, I give 2 mg/kg/day for the first 2 days, 1 mg/kg/day for the balance of 2 months (~58 days), and then 1 mg/kg/day three times a week.

The major toxicity of pyrimethamine is reversible, dose-related bone marrow depression. Platelets are most commonly depressed, although leukopenia and anemia also occur. Pyrimethamine can also cause headache, gastrointestinal discomfort, and a bad taste. Complete blood counts should be performed once or twice a week while the patient is taking pyrimethamine. Folinic acid can be absorbed by mammalian cells, but not by *T. gondii,* and it has been suggested that hematologic toxicity may be prevented or treated with folinic acid (citrovorum factor, leucovorin), 5 to 15 mg/day.

Large doses of pyrimethamine are teratogenic in animals. Teratogenicity in humans has not been documented, but the drug should be avoided in the first 16 weeks of pregnancy. I recommend it for documented fetal infection after 20 weeks of gestation (see below) because I believe that the potential benefits outweigh the potential risks in the latter half of pregnancy.

Sulfonamides

Sulfonamides inhibit *T. gondii* by preventing normal use of para-aminobenzoic acid in folate metabolism. Sulfadiazine and trisulfapyrimidines (sulfapyrazine, sulfadimidine, and sulfamerazine) are most active; all other sulfonamides are much less active. The half-life of sulfadiazine is 11 hours. I give a loading dose of 75 mg/kg (maximum 4 g) followed by 100 to 150 mg/kg/day in two divided doses (maximum 6 to 8 g/day). For newborns with congenital infection, I use 100 mg of sulfadiazine or triple sulfonamides per kg per day in two divided doses.

A wide variety of toxicities have been associated with sulfonamides, including hemolytic anemia, aplastic anemia, agranulocytosis, thrombocytopenia, crystalluria, hepatitis, nephritis, neuritis, anorexia, nausea, vomiting, and reactions due to sensitization. Manifestations of sensitization include rash, arteritis, erythema multiforme, photosensitivity, serum sickness, and drug fever.

Spiramycin

Spiramycin, a macrolide antibiotic, is active against *T. gondii* in experimental animals, and there is clinical, uncontrolled evidence that it is effective in pregnant women. The usual dose is 100 mg/kg/day in two to four divided doses.

Spiramycin has minimal toxicity, limited almost entirely to nausea, vomiting, diarrhea, and allergic skin rashes. Spiramycin is approved for use in Canada, Mexico, and Europe, but not in the United States. It can be obtained on an investigational basis for treatment of toxoplasmosis in pregnant women.*

Clindamycin

Clindamycin has activity against *T. gondii* in experimental animals, but its efficacy in humans is unproven. It is concentrated in the choroid, iris, and retina and has been used to treat retinochoroiditis. The usual dose for adults is 15 to 40 mg/kg/day in four divided doses, although up to 4800 mg/day has been used. Neonates should be treated with 15 to 20 mg/kg/day; children over the age of 1 month should be treated with 20 to 40 mg/kg/day, depending on severity of the infection.

The most important toxicity of clindamycin is diarrhea, especially from *Clostridium difficile* colitis. Other untoward effects include rashes, transaminase elevations, granulocytopenia, thrombopenia, and anaphylaxis. Clindamycin has been administered locally through subconjunctival injection, but the toxicity of local therapy appears to outweigh the potential benefits.

Corticosteroids

Corticosteroids have been used to reduce inflammation in toxoplasmosis, especially for sight-threatening ocular disease or encephalitis. There is anecdotal evidence that it is effective in ocular disease, but it should always be used in conjunction with antiprotozoal therapy. I use prednisone (1 to 2 mg/kg/day, up to 75 mg/day maximum) or the equivalent for sight-threatening or progressive ocular disease. There is no good evidence that corticosteroids are effective for inflammation elsewhere in the body, including the central nervous system.

Therapy in Specific Clinical Circumstances

Acute Acquired Infection in Immunocompetent Children

Most immunocompetent children with acute toxoplasmosis do not require treatment. Fevers may necessitate antipyretic therapy. If symptoms are unusually severe or prolonged, I use pyrimethamine and sulfadiazine. Where spiramycin is available, it may be used as a less toxic, though probably less effective, alternative. In the unusual cases when organs other than lymph nodes are clinically involved, I use antimicrobial therapy to prevent significant organ dysfunction.

Retinochoroiditis

Peripheral lesions that do not noticeably affect vision can be observed without chemotherapy. If lesions progress, affect vision, or threaten important structures (i.e., macula, maculopapillary bundle, or optic nerve), pyrimethamine and sulfadiazine should be given. By 10 days, the borders of retinal lesions should sharpen and vitreous haze should disappear. Treatment should be continued for 3 to 4 weeks after lesions cease to appear active. Steroids should be used in cases involving the macula, maculopapillary bundle, or optic nerve, always in conjunction with antiparasitic chemotherapy. Clindamycin appears to be an alternative for patients who cannot be treated with pyrimethamine and sulfadiazine.

Disease in Immunosuppressed Patients

Symptomatic toxoplasmosis in patients with severe T cell dysfunction should be treated with pyrimethamine and sulfonamides. The response is often slow and incomplete, and prolonged courses with high doses are often necessary. Toxoplasmosis is common and particularly difficult to control in persons with AIDS, and experiences with these patients are redefining our approach to treatment. Persons with AIDS frequently become sensitized to sulfonamides and require nonstandard approaches. A few have been treated successfully with clindamycin and pyrimethamine. Others have been treated with 50 to 75 mg of pyrimethamine per day alone.

Toxoplasmosis recurs in at least 50 per cent of persons with AIDS after therapy has been discontinued. To prevent relapse, I maintain patients with AIDS who have had one episode of clinical reactivation on therapy with pyrimethamine and sulfadiazine for life. The dose must often be tailored to avoid toxicity and still maintain effective blood levels. Other drugs, alone or in combination, have been used to prevent relapse, but none has emerged as an effective substitute for continual therapy with pyrimethamine and sulfadiazine.

Infection During Pregnancy

If toxoplasmosis is acquired during pregnancy, the parents and physician must decide between termination of the pregnancy and chemotherapy. If the pregnancy is continued, the mother should take 1 g spiramycin three times daily to decrease the incidence of fetal infection. Attempts to diagnose fetal infection should be made as described above. If fetal infection is documented, the option of terminating the pregnancy arises again. If the decision is to continue with the pregnancy, I prescribe 3-week courses of pyrimethamine, sulfadiazine, and folinic acid, alternating with 3-week courses of spiramycin for the duration of the pregnancy.

Congenital Infection

Newborns with documented toxoplasmosis should be treated for 1 year. I give 2-month cycles, each consisting of a course of pyrimethamine, sulfadiazine, and folinic acid for 21 days, alternating with spiramycin for the balance of the cycle. If a newborn appears healthy and testing has not yet confirmed or excluded the possibility of congenital toxoplasmosis, I prescribe one of these cycles while diagnostic efforts are continued.

*Division of Antiviral Drug Products, Food and Drug Administration, Washington, DC. Telephone number: (301) 443–9550.

REFERENCES

Daffos F, Forestier F, Capella-Pavlovsky M, Thulliez P, Aufrant C, Valeni D, Cox WL: Prenatal management of 746 pregnancies at risk for congenital toxoplasmosis. N Engl J Med 318:271–275, 1988.

CHOLERA

GERALD T. KEUSCH, M.D.
and JEFFREY K. GRIFFITHS, M.D.

The term cholera not only applies to the infection caused by *Vibrio cholerae* but also historically has been applied to any rapidly progressive, profound, watery diarrhea that leads to severe dehydration and shock. In the past decade, it has become evident that an endemic focus exists in the United States along the Gulf Coast. The cholera vibrio is a marine organism; with its natural habitat in brackish water, it readily contaminates shellfish that are eaten raw or partially cooked (crabs or oysters), and it is by this means that the infection is transmitted in the United States.

EPIDEMIOLOGY

Cholera has long been endemic in the Indian subcontinent, with periodic global pandemics occurring at least since 1817, when the first such worldwide spread of the disease was recorded. Cholera gained its reputation as a killer disease by the high mortality associated with untreated infection during epidemic spread, which often exceeded 50 per cent. In 1961, the present pandemic and the world's seventh began when the El Tor variant of *V. cholerae* spread from the Celebes Islands, reaching Africa in the 1970s, and Latin America at the beginning of 1991. The latter outbreak has been explosive since the first cases were identified in Peru in January 1991. Within 9 months, approximately 300,000 cases had been recorded. By the rapid implementation of good case management, the mortality was kept to under 1 per cent, primarily in individuals failing to reach medical care until dehydration and shock were irreversible.

The cholera vibrio is a noninvasive organism that induces profound alterations in electrolyte and water transport across the small-bowel mucosa. In endemic regions, cholera is primarily a pediatric disease, although adults are affected to a lesser extent. Cholera is generally spread through unchlorinated drinking water, but food can become contaminated within the household or in the markets and can be the vehicle for infection. The organism is rather acid-sensitive; susceptibility is markedly enhanced in people with reduced gastric acidity for any reason, whether due to gastritis, postduodenal ulcer surgery, or use of H_2 blockers. The disease varies in severity from one person to another; in its most severely purging form, profuse diarrhea may develop and progress to shock and death within a matter of a few hours. This process is due to fecal losses of electrolytes, base, and fluid; there are no direct systemic effects of the organism.

PATHOPHYSIOLOGY

Cholera is the best understood of the infectious diarrheas. The clinical disease can be reproduced in experimental animals and humans by oral administration of a protein, cholera toxin, produced by the *Vibrio* locally in the small bowel. This toxin is an enzyme that covalently transfers the adenosine diphosphate (ADP)–ribose moiety from nicotine adenine dinucleotide (NAD) to its target, the G regulatory protein of the adenylate cyclase complex. With this modification of the enzyme, the catalytic unit is maintained in the "on" position and cyclic adenosine monophosphate (*c*AMP) is continuously made for the life of that cell. *c*AMP is used as a biologic messenger within cells; in the small-bowel epithelium, it signals a reduction in the active absorption of sodium and an increase in the active secretion of chloride. NaCl thus accumulates in the intestinal lumen along with water, which follows passively to maintain isosmolarity. Diarrhea results when the volume exceeds the reabsorptive capacity of the remainder of the bowel.

The cholera stool is rich in sodium, potassium, and bicarbonate (Table 1), losses rapidly leading to dehydration and metabolic acidosis and sometimes to hypokalemic renal failure. With the high volume, which is passed without pain, the typical cholera stool quickly loses its fecal characteristics, appearing as a pale, opaque, yellow-white fluid with flecks of mucus and a nonfecal slightly "sweet" odor. This is often called "rice-water stool" because it looks like the water in which rice is washed. Vomiting is prominent early and may continue as metabolic acidosis becomes established. Muscle and abdominal cramps can occur secondary to hypokalemia, and hypoglycemia is often present as a result of diminished food intake and exhaustion of carbohydrate stores, especially in children with limited gluconeogenic response, as is found associated with underlying malnutrition. Cholera patients are often obtunded, and hypoglycemic seizures occur in some.

TABLE 1. Electrolyte Composition of Cholera Stool

	Sodium (Na) (mEq/L)	Potassium (K) (mEq/L)	Chloride (Cl) (mEq/L)	Bicarbonate (HCO_3) (mEq/L)
Children	135	15	90	30
Adults	100	25	90	30

The good news in the pathophysiology is that because the altered gut function is specifically due to natural *c*AMP-dependent mechanisms, there is no structural damage to epithelial cells. Thus, other transport systems remain intact, including sodium-coupled substrate uptake, such as that mediated by glucose. In this way, each actively absorbed glucose molecule is accompanied by one cotransported sodium. Because this process requires chloride and water absorption to maintain electroneutrality and isosmolarity, the presence of glucose and sodium in the lumen leads to net absorption of isotonic fluid. With oral ingestion of glucose-salt solutions, it is possible to rehydrate mild to moderate dehydration in this manner and to maintain fluid balance in severe dehydration after initial correction with parenteral fluids.

TREATMENT

Oral Replacement Therapy

On the basis of the pathophysiology of cholera, the urgent, and often the only, therapeutic requirement is replacement of fluids and salts and the restoration of acid-base balance. The discovery of the sodium co-transport mechanism has permitted the development of oral rehydration therapy (ORT); its early administration can prevent severe dehydration, whereas later treatment necessitates replacement of existing as well as continuing fluid losses.

Several formulas for oral solutions have been produced (Table 2). These may take the form of premixed salts, sugar and base packaged in foil, or home-mixed salt and sugar preparations. The original World Health Organization (WHO) ORT formula has a high sodium content of 90 mEq/L to cover the large losses of sodium in cholera stool. It is effective in other diarrheas as well, but patients with other types of diarrhea do not need as much sodium. WHO has continued to foster this single solution for simplicity and ease of use in the Third World, where cholera is highly endemic. Commercial formulas are marketed with lower sodium, especially in the developed world, and although they are less ideal for treating cholera, they are effective.

Recently, cereal-based ORT has become popular because the complex carbohydrates in the cereals impose less osmotic burden, lead to a reduction in stool volume losses, and provide more nutrients than glucose-based ORT. Rice-based ORT has been the most studied of these solutions, and a commercial rice-ORT is now available in the United States.

Intravenous Fluids

When dehydration is severe, the purging rate is high (>100 ml/kg/day), or the patient is already in shock, oral replacement is not rapid enough and intravenous fluids must be given very quickly. In the severely dehydrated person (loss of ≥ 10 per cent of body weight), 100 ml/kg of Ringer's lactate solution, or an equivalent fluid, should be given in the first 4 hours, with half delivered over the first 30 to 60 minutes. Initial maintenance fluids are then administered at 10 ml/kg/hour. A dose of 60 to 80 ml/kg is given initially for patients with moderate dehydration (losses of 5 to 10 per cent of normal body weight) and with inability to take ORT because of vomiting, ileus, or state of consciousness. *Hesitation in vigorous rehydration is a cardinal mistake.* Although serum potassium levels may appear normal at first, this is a spurious finding because of effects of acidosis; when bicarbonate-containing

TABLE 2. Comparison of Commonly Available and World Health Organization (WHO) Oral Rehydration Formulas

Rehydration Solution	Sodium (mEq/L)	Potassium (mEq/L)	Chloride (mEq/L)	Bicarbonate (mEq/L)	Glucose
WHO formula (ORS)	90	20	80	30	20 g/L
Rehydralyte (Ross)	75	20	65	30	25 g/L
Resol (Wyeth)	50	20	50	34	20 g/L
Ricelyte (Mead Johnson)	50	25	45	34	Rice*
Infalyte (Fisons)	50	20	40	30	20 g/L
Pedialyte (Ross)	45	20	35	30	25 g/L

*Rice solids, 30 g/L.

fluids are administered, potassium concentration rapidly falls. Therefore, potassium is added to the intravenous solution even though the patient may be anuric at that time; urinary output usually returns within 4 hours of initiating rehydration.

Glucose Replacement

Once the patient is rehydrated, maintenance is almost always possible by the oral route by matching output. Therefore, it is important to monitor stool volumes; this can be done simply by placing the patient on a so-called cholera cot, which has an opening with a chute leading to a container with a graduated dip stick. Cholera cots can be made anywhere in the world and are extremely useful. Hypoglycemia should be assumed in any patient with altered consciousness or with seizure activity. If blood sugar cannot be assessed, a bolus of 1 to 2 ml of 25 per cent glucose can be given for every 10 kg of body weight and glucose added to the intravenous fluid to provide 100 mg/kg/hour.

Antibiotics

The course of the illness can be shortened by administration of antibiotics to which the organism is sensitive, although drug resistance is a growing problem. Tetracycline (30 mg/kg in four divided doses for 3 days) is the antimicrobial of choice in the developing world owing to its availability, cost, and the minimal risk of dental staining or bone deposition because of the small amount of tetracycline given. Ampicillin (50 mg/kg/day) and trimethoprim-sulfamethoxazole (8 mg/kg/day of trimethoprim and 40 mg/kg/day of sulfamethoxazole) are useful alternatives, as are erythromycin and chloramphenicol. The new 4-fluoroquinolones are highly effective; however, restrictions by the Food and Drug Administration in the United States limit their use to individuals under the age of 17 because of the still unproven risk of cartilage damage. In adults, a single oral dose of 2 g of tetracycline or 300 mg of doxycycline provides good clinical response. Unfortunately, multiple drug resistance has already emerged in the current Latin American epidemic, no doubt fostered by uncontrolled use of antimicrobials. At this writing, strains resistant to tetracycline, trimethoprim-sulfamethoxazole, and chloramphenicol but sensitive to ampicillin, erythromycin, furazolidone, and ciprofloxacin are being commonly isolated.

PREVENTION AND CONTROL

Environmental sanitation and safe water are the essentials for cholera control. This is why epidemic cholera no longer exists in the developed world and why the developing countries remain so affected. Where epidemics are occurring, chlorine levels need to be higher than usual in municipal water systems, especially when these are only intermittently pressurized. Where water tank trucks are used, addition of 1 mg/L of free chlorine is necessary. The general public should be told to boil all water for consumption, to avoid seafood or cook it well, and to avoid street food and beverages. Cooked food should be eaten while it is hot; raw vegetables should be avoided; pots and dishes should be washed in soap and rinsed in clean, disinfected water; and hand washing with soap and water before handling, preparing, or eating foods and after defecation should be encouraged.

Although major efforts are under way to develop a cholera vaccine no useful licensed product yet exists. The old parenteral vaccine does not provide effective protection.

SEPTIC SHOCK

FIONA H. LEVY, M.D.
and ROBERT K. CRONE, M.D.

Septic shock occurs in 5 to 30 per cent of patients with bacterial sepsis and is associated with a fatality rate of 45 to 98 per cent. Although septic shock is frequently associated with gram-negative bacteremia, other organisms have been identified as causative agents. Within the pediatric population, these pathogens vary with age, underlying medical condition, and clinical setting (Table 1).

DIAGNOSIS

An early diagnosis of septic shock requires recognition of those patients predisposed to its development. The risk factors for development of septic shock can be host-related or treatment-related. Host-related factors include extremes of age, malnutrition, immunodeficiency, chronic health problems, and trauma. Treatment-related factors include surgical or invasive procedures, antibiotic use, immunosuppression, and hospital environment.

CLINICAL PRESENTATION

Shock is defined as inadequate perfusion relative to tissue metabolic requirement. It is the host's response to the multiplying microorganisms that results in the clinical spectrum of septic shock. Typically, septic shock is represented as a clinical continuum from "warm" to "cold." In this description, the hallmark of "warm" shock is a decrease in peripheral vascular resistance and a resultant hyperdynamic circulation. The clinical correlates of this include tachycardia; tachypnea; wide pulse pressure with normal mean arterial pressure; bounding pulses; warm, dry skin; and irritability and restlessness. Secondary to relative hypovolemia and direct myocardial depression, "warm" shock progresses to "cold" shock with its associated increase in peripheral vascular resistance and hypodynamic circulatory state. In this phase, the clinical presentation is one of tachycardia, hypotension, narrow pulse pressure, shallow rapid respiration, thready pulses, cold clammy skin, oliguria, cyanosis, metabolic acidosis, and hypoxia. Blood pressure is not always a good indicator of the adequacy of perfusion in children because their ability to peripherally vasoconstrict is so efficient that central blood

TABLE 1. Pathogens of Septic Shock in Children

Neonates
Group B beta-hemolytic streptococci
Enterobacteriaceae
Listeria monocytogenes
Infants and Young Children
Haemophilus influenzae type b
Streptococcus pneumoniae
Staphylococcus aureus
Neisseria meningitidis
Older Children
Streptococcus pneumoniae
Neisseria meningitidis
Staphylococcus aureus
Immunocompromised Children
Enterobacteriaceae
Staphylococcus aureus
Pseudomonas sp.
Candida albicans

pressure may be normal despite impending circulatory collapse.

TREATMENT

The management of septic shock can be divided into three areas: (1) respiratory stabilization, (2) hemodynamic stabilization, and (3) antimicrobial therapy. Effective management requires simultaneous and continual evaluation with concurrent treatment of the patient. At any time during this process, the severity of the child's illness may also warrant transfer to a regional pediatric center.

Respiratory Stabilization

When a child presents with suspected septic shock, the resuscitation begins with the ABC's (airway, breathing, and circulation). First, through a cursory physical examination it is important to determine whether the child's airway is patent. At this time, the more seriously ill patient with an altered level of consciousness and/or cardiovascular instability may require intubation and mechanical ventilation to achieve airway protection and control. If the airway is secure, the issue becomes whether oxygen exchange and ventilation are adequate. Assessment of this process can be made with the aid of continuous oximetry and frequent determination of arterial blood gases. Even the stable child should be placed on supplemental humidified oxygen via nasal cannula or face mask. If the arterial blood gases reflect hypercarbia or hypoxemia or the child is requiring increasing levels of supplemental oxygen to maintain adequate oxygen saturation and PaO_2, intubation and mechanical ventilatory support are again recommended.

Hemodynamic Stabilization and Assessment

An assessment of the child's circulation encompasses two areas: intravascular volume status and myocardial performance. These are interrelated, as cardiac output is equal to the product of heart rate and stroke volume, and stroke volume is determined by preload, afterload, and myocardial contractility.

Intravascular Volume Status

Evaluation of intravascular volume status involves physical examination and often invasive monitoring. Clinical evidence of intravascular hypovolemia includes diminished peripheral pulses, cool mottled extremities, and increased capillary refill time. It is important at this point to distinguish between intravascular volume status and total body fluids. In septic shock, capillary endothelial leak develops. Although a child may require large volumes of resuscitative fluids and may become grossly edematous, intravascular volume is often still depleted. Other methods of assessing volume status include determination of metabolic acidosis, measurement of urine output, determination of central venous pressure (CVP) directly or indirectly by echocardiography. The presence of a metabolic acidosis is determined through the evaluation of arterial blood gases. The arterial blood pH is the single best laboratory indicator of the adequacy of perfusion. Placement of a Foley catheter allows accurate measurement of urine output, which ideally should be greater than 1 ml/kg/hour. CVP is measured through placement of a central venous catheter within the thorax. The CVP acts as a measure of preload or cardiac filling. No ideal CVP exists, but a low value (< 5 cm H_2O) is suggestive of hypovolemia, and a high CVP (>10 cm H_2O) of myocardial dysfunction.

When interpreting an absolute CVP measurement, one must remember that external influences, such as positive pressure ventilation and structural anomalies, may cause the numerical value to be artificially elevated or depressed. Alternatively, echocardiography allows a rapid and noninvasive assessment of intravascular volume status and myocardial function. In addition, it allows the physician to rule out any structural cardiac anomalies that might complicate the resuscitative effort. The drawback, however, is that sophisticated equipment and skilled technicians are required for the performance and interpretation of pediatric cardiac echocardiograms.

Assuming that the patient is hypovolemic, the treatment is volume expansion. This necessitates the establishment of venous access, which is often extremely difficult to accomplish in a child in septic shock. Peripheral access may be attempted; however, this is often unsuccessful in a child with poor peripheral perfusion. For this reason, long periods of time should not be spent attempting the insertion of peripheral lines; one should move rapidly to alternative methods, including intraosseous infusion, saphenous vein cutdown, or central vein cannulation. In children under the age of 5, intraosseous access can be established with the placement of a short-beveled trocar needle into the anteromedial surface of the tibia. Once secured, this catheter allows access to the central circulation and infusion of all types of fluids and medications. Saphenous vein cutdown is a reliable form of venous access because the position of the saphenous vein is very consistent. Central venous cannulation can be achieved through accessing the femoral, internal jugular, external jugular, and subclavian veins. However, placement of lines in these vessels is associated with severe complications and should be attempted only by skilled individuals.

Volume expansion will increase the heart's preload and, therefore, overall cardiac output. This can be accomplished with three types of fluid: (1) crystalloid (normal saline or Ringer's lactate), (2) colloid (albumin, hetastarch, or dextran), and (3) blood products. Under most clinical conditions, volume expansion can be adequately achieved using crystalloid solutions, with colloids and blood products as the fluid of choice if a known deficit (i.e., hypoalbuminemia or coagulopathy or anemia) is present. A coagulopathy may be the result of either decreased production of clotting factors or an increased consumption; in either case, it can be ameliorated with the slow infusion of fresh frozen plasma given in 10 ml/kg aliquots. In the case of any stressed state such as septic shock, an effort should be made to maintain a hemoglobin in the range of 12 to 15 mg/dl; this increases the patient's oxygen-carrying capacity and may improve oxygen delivery to the tissue. This can be accomplished through the transfusion of packed red blood cells in volumes of 10 to 15 ml/kg.

When fluids are initially administered, a bolus of 10 to 20 ml/kg of a crystalloid solution should be given rapidly, followed by an additional 10 ml/kg if no improvement is noted. If the patient continues to show evidence of poor cardiac output, one needs to decide whether this is the result of poor myocardial function or of continued hypovolemia. At this point, either an echocardiogram or a CVP will help in the assessment. A low CVP is consistent with persistent hypovolemia, and an elevated CVP suggests impaired cardiac contractility. The physical examination is also very helpful. Enlarging liver span, rales, and jugular venous distention also point toward myocardial dysfunction. If this is the case, early intervention with inotropes and afterload reduction may be necessary. It is not unusual, however, to find that the child in septic shock requires numerous fluid boluses; these should be given repeatedly and rapidly in 10 ml/kg aliquots. After every bolus, it is important to reassess hemodynamic status, as hypovolemia may become complicated by myocardial dysfunction. During this rapid volume expansion, respiratory status may decline requiring the initiation of positive pressure ventilation. If the patient continues to be hypotensive and poorly perfused despite fluid therapy, it may be necessary to augment an already normally functioning or hyperdynamic myocardium in order to preserve myocardial, renal, and cerebral perfusion.

Myocardial Performance

Effective cardiac contractility is dependent on (1) adequate heart rate, (2) presence of a sinus rhythm, and (3) adequate contractile strength.

Heart Rate. In children, adequate heart rate is determined by age and clinical situation, with young infants and critically ill children requiring faster heart rates. Normal ranges of heart rate are as follows: neonates, 120 to 160; infants, 80 to 120; and children, 60 to 80. These "normal" values may need to increase to provide adequate cardiac output in times of stress such as septic shock. The most efficient way for a neonate to increase cardiac output is through an increase in heart rate, as stroke volume is relatively fixed. With this in mind, the treatment of septic shock includes ensuring that the child's heart rate and rhythm are sufficient to produce an adequate cardiac output. Heart rate can be maximized with β-adrenergic agents, such as dopamine, dobutamine, epinephrine, and isoproterenol, or with vagolytic agents, such as atropine.

Rhythm. Treatment of abnormal cardiac rhythm should be guided by the nature of the aberrant rhythm.

Contractility. Improving myocardial contractility can be achieved by eliminating any ongoing negative inotropic influences and by providing agents that improve the strength of myocardial contraction (positive inotropic agents).

NEGATIVE INFLUENCES. Negative inotropic influences include hypoxemia, hypoglycemia, hypocalcemia, and severe acidosis with a pH below 7.25. These metabolic aberrations should be treated immediately. Hypoxemia should be eliminated through the use of supplemental oxygen and/or mechanical ventilation. Hypoglycemia can be avoided with the continual monitoring of serum glucose and by providing an ongoing source of dextrose with a maintenance intravenous infusion. This dextrose-containing solution should not be used as the fluid for volume expansion boluses. If hypoglycemia develops (glucose < 80), it can be treated with the administration of 1 to 2 ml/kg of $D_{50}W$ in the neonate or infant and 1 to 2 ml/kg of $D_{50}W$ in the older child. Hypocalcemia can be treated using intravenous infusions of calcium gluconate given as 100 mg/kg. Care should be taken when infusing calcium, which is an extremely caustic substance. Metabolic acidosis is the result of systemic hypoperfusion and impaired oxygen utilization, with an uncoupling of oxygen delivery and extraction at the cellular level. To treat this, it is important to treat the underlying cause; however, in the meantime, one can also use sodium bicarbonate given in doses of 1 to 2 mEq/kg by slow intravenous push. The use of sodium bicarbonate should never replace attempts to improve perfusion through the use of fluid resuscitation and inotropes.

POSITIVE INOTROPIC AGENTS. These agents increase the strength of myocardial contraction. They can be divided into multiple categories, including sympathomimetic amines, xanthines, and cardiac glycosides.

Sympathomimetic amines work through the stimulation of adrenergic receptors and include dopamine, dobutamine, and epinephrine. The achieved effect is dose-dependent and correlates with the type of adrenergic receptor, which is preferentially stimulated. There are four types of receptors to be concerned with at this point: alpha-one (α_1), beta-one (β_1), beta-two (β_2), and delta (Δ). α_1-Receptors are located in the peripheral and coronary circulations as well as the lungs; stimulation of these receptors results in vasoconstriction and bronchoconstriction. β_1-Receptors are cardiac and reside in the SA node, the AV node, and both atria and ventricles. Stimulation of these receptors leads to an increase in heart rate (*chronotropy*) and an increase in contractile strength (*inotropy*). β_2-Receptors control peripheral vasodilation and bronchodilation. Finally, Δ (dopaminergic)-receptors mediate renal and splanchnic vasodilation.

Dopamine is usually the first drug of choice in the setting of septic shock. At low doses of 3 to 5 μg/kg/minute, it stimulates dopaminergic receptors leading to renal vasodilation and, it is hoped, to increased urine output. From 5 to 20 μg/kg/minute, dopamine is primarily a β-adrenergic agent, with the resultant increase in heart rate, myocardial contraction, and peripheral vasodilation. These higher infusion rates up to 20 μg/kg/minute do not usually cause peripheral vasoconstriction as they do in adults; however, greater than 20 μg/kg/minute may stimulate α_1-receptors, causing an increase in systemic vascular resistance.

Another initial agent of choice is dobutamine, which is a purely beta agent and can be used in doses of 5 to 20 μg/kg/minute depending on the desired amount of chronotropy, inotropy, and peripheral vasodilation.

Epinephrine is usually considered the pressor of last resort; however, in the moribund child, it should be the agent of choice. Low-dose epinephrine (0.1 μg/kg/minute) is primarily a β-agonist; at higher doses (0.5 μg/kg/minute) it becomes an α-agonist with only minimal beta effect. In the moribund child, this increase in alpha (peripheral) tone increases the diastolic blood pressure and hence increases coronary perfusion pressure and maintains coronary blood flow and oxygen delivery in the face of intractable hypotension.

Xanthines include theophylline and amrinone, both phosphodiesterase inhibitors. Although theophylline is rarely used clinically, amrinone is being used with increasing frequency because it exhibits both positive inotropic and afterload reducing properties. It works through a different mechanism than do the sympathomimetic amines and, therefore, can be used as adjunctive therapy. It is given with a divided loading dose of 1.5 to 6 mg/kg and then in drip form at 10 to 20 μg/kg/minute. Extreme caution should be exercised because the loading dose can result in profound hypotension and because the drug's ongoing use is associated with a decrease in platelet production.

TABLE 2. Antibiotic Treatment of Septic Shock in Children

Patient	Drug	Dosage
Neonate (0–4 weeks)	Ampicillin	50 mg/kg per dose q 8 hr < 7 days and q 6 hr > 7 days
	and Gentamicin	2.5 mg/kg per dose q 12 hr < 7 days and q 8 hr > 7 days
Infant (1–3 mo)	Ampicillin	50 mg/kg per dose q 6 hr
	and Cefotaxime	50 mg/kg per dose q 6 hr
Young child (3 mo–5 yr)	Cefotaxime	50 mg/kg per dose q 6 hr
Older child (>5 yr)	Nafcillin	150 mg/kg/day divided q 6 hr
	and Cefotaxime	50 mg/kg per dose q 6 hr
Immunocompromised child	Vancomycin	10 mg/kg per dose q 6 hr
	and Ceftazidime	50 mg/kg per dose q 8 hr

Finally, the cardiac glycosides are relatively weak inotropic agents and have little place in the initial management of septic shock; the risk of toxicity is high in the metabolically unstable patient.

Afterload Reduction. Although positive inotropic agents work to increase myocardial contractile force, another way to improve cardiac output is by decreasing left ventricular afterload. Although used less frequently in septic shock, it may be necessary to decrease an inappropriately elevated systemic vascular resistance or to decrease the work of a failing heart by decreasing a relatively normal systemic vascular resistance. This can be achieved through the use of β_2-agonists, such as dobutamine and isoproterenol; α_1-antagonists, such as phentolamine and tolazoline; or direct vasodilators, such as sodium nitroprusside and nitroglycerine. These agents must be used with caution, and often the patient will require additional fluid therapy to fill the newly expanding vascular space. Any patient undergoing treatment with afterload reduction should have an intra-arterial, and probably a pulmonary artery, catheter to allow for the continuous monitoring of blood pressure, cardiac output, and systemic vascular resistance.

Antibiotics

The final phase in the management of septic shock is the determination and institution of appropriate antimicrobial therapy. Initial antimicrobial therapy is usually broad spectrum, with the choice dependent on the patient's age and clinical condition. Laboratory tests that can help in the choice of appropriate agents include blood, urine, and cerebral spinal fluid cultures; Gram stains; and latex agglutination tests for bacterial antigens. Clearly, the importance of any of the tests is far outweighed by the priority of stabilizing the patient. Although the choice of agents varies in different institutions, some recommendations can be found in Table 2.

IMMUNIZATION PRACTICE

JANET R. GILSDORF, M.D.

ROUTINE CHILDHOOD IMMUNIZATION

As newer, more effective, and safer vaccines become available, and as our understanding of the strengths and weaknesses of current vaccines improves, recommendations for routine childhood immunizations change. Table 1 incorporates some of the recent changes.

The *Haemophilus influenzae* b (Hib) conjugate vaccines containing the polysaccharide capsule conjugated to CRM 197 protein (HbOC; Hib TITER, Lederle) and to *Neisseria meningitidis* group B outer membrane protein (PRP-OMP Pedvax HIB, Merck) have been licensed for use in children as young as 2 months of age. Curiously, these vaccines are given on differing schedules; HbOC is given at 2, 4, and 6 months with a booster dose at 12 to 15 months, whereas PRP-OMP is given at 2 and 4 months, with a booster dose at 12 months. Although any conjugate Hib vaccine may be given at 15 months of age or greater irrespective of the type of vaccine used for the initial series, the doses given in the primary series must be the same vaccine, either PRP-OMP or HbOC.

Recent outbreaks of measles among previously vaccinated high school and college-aged young adults suggest waning immunity following childhood immunization with measles vaccine. Thus, complete measles immunization includes a primary dose at age 15 months and a booster dose either at school entry (age 4 to 6 years) or at middle or junior high school entry (age 12 to 13 years). Outbreaks of measles in inner city preschool children suggest that these children are inadequately immunized. Fewer than half of inner city preschool children in many areas are thought to be appropriately immunized against measles.

Prompted by concerns of toxicity of whole cell pertussis vaccines, several acellular pertussis vaccines have been in clinical trial in the United States. One vaccine, ACEL-IMUNE, composed of the pertussis components filamentous hemagglutinin (FHA), pertussis toxoid (PT), pertactin (Pn), and type 2 fimbriae as well as diphtheria toxoid and tetanus toxoid, has been licensed for the fourth and fifth doses of the DPT series. Ongoing clinical trials may result in licensure of this product, or other acellular vaccines, for use in younger children.

OTHER IMMUNIZATIONS

Pneumovax

Use of Pneumovax may prevent bacteremic infections caused by *Streptococcus pneumoniae* in susceptible children. The vaccine contains polysaccharide antigens of 23 of the most common invasive serotypes and is recommended for use in children older than age 2 years with sickle cell disease, functional or anatomic asplenia, nephrotic syndrome, human immunodeficiency virus (HIV) infection, or Hodgkin's lymphoma. Although the duration of Pneumovax-induced immunity is unclear and local reactions to the vaccine may be increased on a second vaccination, some centers are recommending reimmunization with Pneumovax 3 to 5 years after primary immunization for children at especially high risk of overwhelming pneumococcal infections. Data on the efficacy of Pneumovax to prevent otitis media are incomplete.

Hepatitis B

Numerous studies have documented the efficacy of hepatitis B vaccine in preventing this disease among newborn infants of hepatitis B carrier mothers and other susceptible individuals. The vaccines now in use (Recombivax HB and Engerix

TABLE 1. Recommendations for Immunization‡

Age	Diphtheria-Pertussis-Tetanus Vaccine	Polio Vaccine	Measles-Mumps-Rubella Vaccine	*Haemophilus influenzae* Type b Vaccine: *HbOC*	*or* *PRP-OMP*
2 months	DPT	OPV		HbOC	PRP-OMP
4 months	DPT	OPV		HbOC	PRP-OMP
6 months	DPT			HbOC	
12 months					PRP-OMP
15 months			MMR	HbOC†	
18 months	DPT	OPV			
4–6 years	DPT	OPV	Measles or MMR		
12–13 years			Measles* or MMR*		
14–16 years	Td				

*If not given at 4 to 6 years (school entry).
†May use any conjugate Hib vaccine for this dose.
‡Hepatitis B vaccine is recommended at birth, 1 to 2 months, and 6 to 18 months *or* at 1 to 2 months, 4 months, and 6 to 18 months.

B) consist of purified hepatitis B surface antigen (HBsAg) obtained from cultures of yeast that contain a plasmid encoding for HBsAg. The vaccine is recommended for children at risk of exposure to hepatitis B (such as newborns of hepatitis B carrier mothers, children undergoing renal dialysis, children living in a household with a hepatitis B carrier, or children with a needlestick exposure. In addition, some advisory bodies have recommended hepatitis vaccine for all American infants.

IMMUNIZATION OF IMMUNOCOMPROMISED CHILDREN

Children treated with immunosuppressive drugs or those with a primary immunodeficiency disease should not receive vaccines that contain live microbial agents, such as bacille Calmette-Guérin (BCG), poliovirus (TOPV), measles, mumps, rubella (MMR), and yellow fever vaccines. Normal children receiving short-term doses of steroids or low to moderate doses of steroids over the long term may receive live virus vaccines. Household contacts of immunocompromised children may be given MMR, as these vaccine viruses are not shed by vaccines, but they should not receive OPV (they may get IPV instead). Data on efficacy of many non-live virus vaccines in immunocompromised children are not complete, but influenza vaccine, *H. influenzae* b vaccines, and pneumococcal vaccines should be used in susceptible immunocompromised children as they may benefit from their use.

SIMULTANEOUS ADMINISTRATION OF VACCINES

Hib conjugate vaccines, DPT, OPV (or IPV), hepatitis B, and MMR may be given in any combination in different syringes at different sites on the same day without a reduction in immune response to any of the vaccines.

FEDERAL VACCINE INJURY COMPENSATION

In 1988, the National Childhood Vaccine Injury Act was enacted to compensate the families of children suffering certain documented adverse effects from receipt of vaccines. Standardized risk-benefits statements must be used in obtaining informed consent for use of vaccines. The medical record and the patient-retained immunization record should contain the following data: month, day, and year of administration; name, manufacturer, lot number, and date of expiration of the vaccine; site and route of administration; and name of person administering the vaccine. Certain adverse events occurring following vaccination must be reported to the Centers for Disease Control in Atlanta or to the U.S. Food and Drug Administration.

FUTURE VACCINES

Efficacy and immunogenicity trials of acellular pertussis, varicella, cytomegalovirus, and human immunodeficiency virus vaccines are being conducted in the United States. Recommendation for appropriate uses of these vaccines await the completion of these studies.

REFERENCES

Centers for Disease Control: General recommendations on immunizations. MMWR 38:205–227, 1989.
Report of the Committee on Infectious Disease ("Red Book"), 22nd ed. Elk Grove Village, Ill, American Academy of Pediatrics, 1991.

CLOSTRIDIUM DIFFICILE

NANCY E. VINTON, M.D.

Clostridium difficile is a gram-positive, rod-shaped bacterium that reproduces via spore formation. It may be either a normal inhabitant or an opportunistic pathogen among the microbial flora of the human colon. The spectrum of colonization by *C. difficile* in humans ranges from asymptomatic colonization as a "silent reservoir" to the pathognomonic "pseudomembranous" colitis (PMC), a watery, mucus-laden diarrhea with occasional frank blood. PMC can be diagnosed endoscopically by the presence of yellowish-white plaques (containing neutrophils, fibrin, cell debris, and mucin), interspersed with normal-appearing colonic mucosa, often with rectal sparing. However, *C. difficile* may also present as "benign," guaiac-negative, loose stools or as a "nonspecific" enterocolitis with guaiac-positive or frankly bloody diarrhea. The spectrum of disease is primarily dependent on toxin-mediated events, not bacterial invasion.

Of the various presentations, only PMC is clinically diagnostic of *C. difficile* infection, which otherwise remains a diagnosis of exclusion. The confusion about the etiologic role of *C. difficile* in less severe forms of diarrhea is due to our current lack of understanding and diagnostic abilities, as is discussed below. The role of *C. difficile* as a potential pathogen, however, cannot be taken lightly. In its most severe form, toxin-mediated sequelae may include protein-losing enteropathy with secondary hypoalbuminemia and hypogammaglobulinemia, toxic megacolon, and perforation but, more commonly, fever, hypovolemia, hypotension, and shock. The mortality from overwhelming *C. difficile* enterocolitis remains high, at 10 to 20 per cent, in spite of the most advanced pediatric intensive care measures now available.

Alterations of the native colonic microflora disrupt what is termed the "colonization resistance" of that intestinal microenvironment. Hence, many studies have shown a strong relationship of antibiotic therapy, either oral or intravenous, and *C. difficile* infection. The loss of the competitive and inhibitory nature of the anaerobic flora during antibiotic therapy may allow for the colonization or overgrowth and subsequent infection with *C. difficile.* Nearly every antibiotic has been implicated.

Penicillins (beta-lactamase–sensitive or –resistant), cephalosporins, and clindamycin are most often causative; sulfamethoxazole-trimethoprim and metronidazole least often—the main difference between these drugs being their ability to disturb the anaerobic flora of the intestine. The more severe the form of infection, the higher the incidence of *C. difficile* toxin; i.e., only 10 to 25 per cent of cases with benign diarrhea will be positive whereas PMC will be 100 per cent positive. In many benign cases, simply discontinuing antibiotics results in the disappearance of the *C. difficile* and related symptoms. More severe forms of enterocolitis, however, require specific treatment of the *C. difficile* organism, as described below, to resolve the infection and toxin-associated symptoms.

The pathologic effects of *C. difficile* result from its ability to elaborate an enteropathogenic (toxin A) and a cytopathogenic (toxin B) toxin. Both toxins are produced simultaneously, act synergistically, and are neurotoxins, as are those of other *Clostridium* species, such as *C. perfringens* and *C. botulinum.* Toxin A is known to bind to a brush border membrane glycoprotein receptor and to cause toxicity by several mechanisms. Toxin A stimulates fluid secretion, increases permeability at cellular tight junctions, induces actin depolymerization and intracellular calcium release, and, probably most importantly, mediates a chemotactic neutrophilic infiltration leading to necrosis of enterocytes and subsequent enterocolitis.

Toxin B is a glycosylated protein with subunits whose action is not receptor-mediated and that causes actin depolymerization. Toxin B is less virulent and apparently cannot produce a disease state in the absence of toxin A. Antitoxin A and B antibodies are produced after exposure to *C. difficile.* By 3 years of age, the sera of 60 to 70 per cent of children contain antitoxin antibodies, with *C. difficile* cultures being negative. There is no evidence to suggest that such antibodies, although detectable throughout life, convey any protection to future exposure.

When *C. difficile* specimens are obtained for culture from the stool of either an asymptomatic or symptomatic patient, only 30 to 50 per cent of positive cultures show detectable toxin production. Conversely, a stool may test positive for toxin but will not grow the organism on culture. This finding is indicative of the limitations in current diagnostic abilities and understanding of the disease process. On a technical level, it can be a tedious task to grow this organism. Thus, assays to detect toxin as evidence of *C. difficile* infection have been developed. However, most of these toxin assays identify the presence of toxin B, which is detectable at very low concentration either by the ease of an enzyme-linked immunosorbent assay (ELISA) or the immediacy of cytopathic effects in tissue culture. One commercially available assay does not test for either toxin A or B but rather for a nontoxic protein component also found in other species of *Clostridium* besides *C. difficile.* Assays for toxin A, the putative agent of greatest virulence and major determinant of disease severity, are available but also limited in predictive value.

TABLE 1. Therapy for *Clostridium Difficile* Enterocolitis

Medication	Route	Interval	Single Dose	Duration
Antibiotics*				
Vancomycin				
Initial/relapse	p.o./p.r./IV	t.i.d./q.i.d.	10 mg/kg	2–? weeks
Maximum†			125–500 mg	
Metronidazole				
Initial/relapse	p.o./IV	t.i.d./q.i.d.	5 mg/kg	2–? weeks
Maximum			250–500 mg	
Bacitracin				
Relapse	p.o.	q.i.d.	500 units/kg	2–? weeks
Maximum			25,000 units	
Rifampin				
Relapse	p.o.	b.i.d.	5 mg/kg	2–? weeks
Maximum			600 mg	
Toxin-Binding Agents				
Cholestyramine				
Relapse	p.o.	t.i.d./q.i.d.	750 mg = ½ tsp/kg	2–? weeks
Maximum			4 g = 1 scoop = 1 tbs	
Psyllium seed fiber				
Relapse	p.o.	b.i.d./t.i.d.	750 mg = ½ tsp/kg	2–? weeks
Maximum			3.4 g = 1 tbs	
Recolonization Agents				
Lactobacillus (Lactinex, *acidophilus*)				
Relapse	p.o.	q.i.d.	10 mg/kg	3 weeks
Maximum			1 g = 1 pkt	
Saccharomyces boulardii‡				
Adult	p.o.	b.i.d.	500 mg = 2 caps	2 months
Normal feces	p.r.		?	

*Approximate pediatric doses.
†Usual adult dose.
‡Laboratories Biocodex, France.
Abbreviations: p.o., orally; p.r., per rectum; q.i.d., four times a day; b.i.d., twice a day; t.i.d., three times a day; IV, intravenous.

TREATMENT (Table 1)

Treatment options for *C. difficile* infections in the adult or pediatric population are limited as a result of antibiotic sensitivities of the organism. Vancomycin (monitoring serum levels for renal toxicity) and metronidazole are the only two intravenous antibiotics appropriate for the systemically ill child with *C. difficile*–associated enterocolitis (nonspecific colitis or PMC). Because the latter is much less expensive, it has become more commonly used as the drug of first choice. Additional antibiotic coverage for gram-negative and anaerobic organisms is appropriate in the presence of sepsis or shock from an enteric source. For the infant or child who presents with enterocolitis at the time of diagnosis of Hirschsprung's disease, rectal decompression and gentle irrigation with vancomycin (250 to 500 mg/30 to 60 ml normal saline every 6 to 8 hours), using a soft red Robinson rubber tube No. 30 to 32 French, approximately 4 to 6 cm into the rectum, may help to stabilize the patient prior to decompression via colostomy.

Initial interventions may need to be primarily resuscitative to overcome the acute effects of hypovolemia and shock. An intravenous normal saline bolus of 20 ml/kg or more may be necessary, followed by pressor support. Additionally, 25 per cent (salt-poor) albumin at 1 g/kg may be given intravenously to treat intravascular volume depletion and hypoalbuminemia subsequent to protein-losing enteropathy. These patients usually present with peripheral edema. More recent evidence indicates that replacement therapy with intravenous immune gammaglobulin may be helpful in recovery, even in those patients with normal serum levels of immunoglobulin. Parenteral nutrition, peripheral or central, should be started in any patient with an expected loss of intestinal use or function of greater than 1 week in duration or with hypoalbuminemia upon initial presentation.

Once stable, as with those patients suffering from more benign forms of *C. difficile* infection, the patient should receive the chosen antibiotic orally to decontaminate the gastrointestinal tract more thoroughly. A short term of therapy, 7 to 14 days, may be all that is required to control an initial episode. It is unclear whether treatment completely eradicates *C. difficile* from the intestinal tract or reduces it to undetectable levels long enough to prevent overgrowth until "colonization resistance" of the intestinal microflora is restored. Relapses, however, are common, occurring in approximately 10 to 30 per cent of cases, even though follow-up cultures and/or toxin assays may be negative prior to discontinuation of antibiotics. Studies vary, but overall recurrence rates do not seem to differ between vancomycin or metronidazole therapy. Prolonged pulsatile or tapering antibiotic regimens (up to 4 to 6 weeks) theoretically allow for treatment of the recurrent infection and for subsequent germination of any remaining spores, which only then will become sensitive to antibiotic effects. Alternative oral antibiotics that have been used for chronic relapse include bacitracin (minimal toxicity due to limited intestinal absorption) and rifampin (only in infants older than 3 months of age).

Toxin-binding agents, such as cholestyramine and psyllium seed fiber, may be useful adjunctive therapy in treatment of chronic relapse. Recolonization agents have also been employed in an attempt to recreate an approriate milieu among the colonic microflora and, thus, to enhance the re-establishment of colonization resistance. *Lactobacillus acidophilus, Saccharomyces boulardii* (approved only as an investigational new drug in the United States), and even normal feces (per rectal infusion) have been successful in a few cases recalcitrant to pulsatile or tapering antibiotic therapy.

GONOCOCCAL INFECTIONS

BARRY DASHEFSKY, M.D.

Infection with *Neisseria gonorrhoeae* is the most common reportable infectious disease in the United States; an estimated three quarters of a million reported and 1 to 2 million unreported cases occurred in 1989. Although most prevalent among young adults, more than 25 per cent of reported cases involve pediatric-aged patients, especially teenaged girls between the ages of 15 and 19 years. Although, as with sexually transmitted diseases (STDs) in general, most cases of childhood gonococcal infection are attributable to voluntary (albeit frequently unacknowledged) sexual activity, practitioners must also be highly alert and responsive to the less frequent cases associated with perinatal transmission and sexual abuse.

The most significant recent change in the management of gonococcal infections reflects a decade-long increase in the number of isolates that are resistant to traditionally used antimicrobial regimens. Plasmid-mediated, penicillinase-producing *N. gonorrhoeae* (PPNG), which is resistant to penicillins; chromosomally mediated resistant *N. gonorrhoeae* (CMRNG), which is resistant to a wide array of antibiotics; and plasmid mediated tetracycline resistant *N. gonorrhoeae* (TRNG) accounted for 13 per cent of nationally surveyed isolates in 1989. *As a consequence, as of 1989, ceftriaxone has supplanted penicillin (or ampicillin or amoxicillin) as the empiric antimicrobial of choice for treating most proven or presumed gonococcal infections.* Certainly, penicillin or other candidate agents remain appropriate therapeutic alternatives when specific susceptibility data so signify.

GENERAL MANAGEMENT CONSIDERATIONS

Because multiple STDs often coexist, the suspicion or diagnosis of gonococcal infection should generally result in testing for the presence of other STDs, including *Chlamydia trachomatis;* syphilis; and, depending on local prevalence, human immunodeficiency virus (HIV). With a similar rationale, sexually active patients diagnosed as having an STD should be vaccinated against hepatitis B virus.

Because *C. trachomatis* frequently co-infects patients with gonococcal infection (in up to 25 per cent of men and 45 per cent of women with acute urogenital gonorrhea), in the absence of accurate test data that definitively exclude this possibility in a specific case, patients who are treated for suspected or documented gonococcal infection should also be routinely treated concomitantly with a second agent effective against *C. trachomatis*. In nonpregnant patients 9 years of age or older, such additional treatment of uncomplicated infections should be accomplished with doxycycline (100 mg orally twice daily) or tetracycline (500 mg orally four times daily) for 7 days. In pregnant patients or patients younger than 9 years, either erythromycin (10 to 12.5 mg/kg [maximum dose 500 mg] orally four times daily) or, in patients older than 1 month of age, sulfisoxazole (37.5 mg/kg [maximum dose 2 g] orally four times daily) for 7 days may be used.

A serologic test for syphilis (STS) should be performed in all patients with documented or suspected gonococcal infection. Although all regimens recommended for treatment of *N. gonorrhoeae* utilizing penicillins or cephalosporins are adequate to treat incubating syphilis, the same cannot be said for therapies using spectinomycin, tetracyclines, erythromycin, or quinolones. Therefore, if any of the latter agents are used, an STS should be repeated 4 to 6 weeks after treatment.

Hospitalization and parenteral therapy are generally indicated for at least initial treatment of all forms of gonococcal infection in neonates as well as for systemic infection in older patients. In addition, because of substantial risks of poor compliance with prescribed treatment and long-term morbidity among adolescent patients with complicated genital infection, such as pelvic inflammatory disease (PID), a low threshold for hospitalization of this population is advised. Admission is warranted whenever the diagnosis of PID is uncertain, abscess is suggested, compliance with or tolerance of oral medications is suspect, the patient is pregnant, or a previous attempt at outpatient management has failed. Any patient with PID who is managed as an outpatient should be reassessed within 2 to 3 days.

Newborns and prepubertal children who are hospitalized with gonococcal infection require contact isolation precautions until 24 hours of effective therapy has been completed.

Because involuntary sexual contact after the neonatal period is the most likely mode of acquisition of gonococcal infection in prepubertal children younger than 9 years of age and because it must also be suspected in adolescents who are not sexually active, documentation of gonococcal infection in these populations mandates a careful and thorough evaluation for sexual abuse. Genital, rectal, and pharyngeal specimens should be obtained for culture. Diagnosis of gonococcal infection in cases of suspected abuse should be established by positive cultures confirmed by at least two different biochemical, enzymatic, or serologic tests. Because sexually abused children are considered to have a low but uncertain risk of acquiring STDs, in the absence of demonstrated infection they need not be treated presumptively unless the perpetrator is known to be infected, the parents prefer treatment, or follow-up cannot be ensured.

SPECIFIC TREATMENT REGIMENS

Both the clinical manifestations and the appropriate specific therapies for childhood gonococcal infections vary with age. For the most part, treatment regimens have not been evaluated in pediatric populations; recommendations are based on controlled observations in adult patients. Adult dosage routines are used for children weighing more than 45 kg. Selected recommendations deriving from a large number of options for management of specific clinical problems due to gonococcal infection follow. For detailed guidance, the reader is referred to the most recent recommendations of the U.S. Centers for Disease Control.

Neonatal Infections

Gonococcal infections of neonates include ophthalmia, scalp abscesses, and disseminated disease, such as sepsis, meningitis, arthritis, and endocarditis. Gonococcal disease at any site should prompt a careful evaluation for systemic infection. With the presumption that infection was acquired from the mother, both the mother and her sexual contacts should be evaluated and treated for the implicated STDs.

In general, both local and non-meningitic systemic neonatal gonococcal infection should be treated with either ceftriaxone (25 to 50 mg/kg/day IV or IM in a single dose) or cefotaxime (25 to 75 mg/kg/day IV or IM in two to three doses) for 7 days. Some advocate the use of a single dose of ceftriaxone (50 mg/kg up to 125 mg) for treating uncomplicated ophthalmia. Penicillin G (100,000 U/kg/day IV in two to four divided doses for 7 days) is an acceptable alternative for treating infection associated with susceptible isolates. Gonococcal ophthalmia should also be managed with eye irrigation using buffered saline at least hourly until the discharge has resolved. Topical antibiotics are inadequate alone and unnecessary adjuncts to parenteral therapy.

For gonococcal meningitis, ceftriaxone (50 mg/kg/day IV or IM in one or two doses) or cefotaxime (50 to 75 mg/kg/day IV or IM in two or three doses) for 10 to 14 days is recommended. For susceptible isolates, penicillin G (100,000 to 150,000 U/kg/day IV in two to four doses for 10 to 14 days) is an alternative.

Ceftriaxone must be used cautiously in neonates with hyperbilirubinemia. The pain associated with intramuscular injection of ceftriaxone may be ameliorated by the use of a lidocaine diluent.

Infections in Prepubertal Children and Adolescents

After the neonatal period, gonococcal infection most frequently affects the genital tract. In prepubertal girls, this is most commonly manifest as vaginitis and, in boys, as urethritis. Following puberty, endocervicitis, urethritis, and PID are the most common expressions in female adolescents; urethritis and epididymitis in adolescent males. Pharyngeal, rectal, and conjunctival infection as well as systemic disease, including pyogenic arthritis and tenosynovitis, arthritis-dermatitis syndrome with sepsis (also referred to as disseminated gonococcal infection, or DGI), and, less commonly, osteomyelitis, pneumonia, meningitis, and endocarditis also occur in children and adults of all ages.

For uncomplicated urogenital, rectal, or pharyngeal gonococcal infection, outpatient management consisting of a single IM dose of ceftriaxone (125 mg for patients weighing less than 45 kg and 250 mg for those weighing 45 kg or more) is recommended. For older children and adults, alternative regimens (except for pharyngeal infection, for which ceftriaxone alone affords reliable treatment) include cefixime (400 or 800 mg orally in one dose); cefuroxime axetil (1 g orally taken once with 1 g of probenecid); cefotaxime (1 g IM once); or ceftizoxime (500 mg IM once). Patients who are allergic to penicillins and cephalosporins should be treated with spectinomycin (40 mg/kg [maximum dose 2 g] IM once). For nonpregnant patients older than 16 years, ciprofloxacin (500 mg orally once) or norfloxacin (800 mg orally once) is an alternative (which apparently also is effective in eradicating pharyngeal infection). For penicillin-susceptible isolates, either procaine penicillin G (100,000 U/kg [maximum dose 4.8 million units] IM once) or amoxicillin (50 mg/kg [maximum dose, 3 g] orally once), administered with probenecid (25 mg/kg [maximum dose 1 g]) is a well-established treatment option.

PID is usually caused by infection with *N. gonorrhoeae, C. trachomatis,* gram-negative enteric bacilli, or anaerobes, either alone or in combination. Because of the difficulty of determining the specific cause in a given case, empiric therapy should consist of a broad-spectrum antimicrobial regimen that is sufficient to treat most, if not all, candidate pathogens such as cefoxitin or ceftriaxone, combined with doxycycline. (See discussion on pelvic inflammatory disease, p. 840.)

Similarly, epididymitis is usually attributable to *N. gonorrhoeae, C. trachomatis,* or gram-negative enteric bacilli. Recommended treatment is ceftriaxone (250 mg IM once), followed by 10 days of either doxycycline (200 mg/day orally in two divided doses) or tetracycline (2 g/day orally in four divided doses) for children 9 years of age or older. For children younger than 9 years, 10 days of erythromycin (50 mg/kg/day [maximum daily dose 2 g] orally in four doses) is appropriate.

Non-septicemic gonococcal ophthalmia usually can be successfully treated with a single dose of ceftriaxone (50 mg/kg [maximum dose 1 g] IM) and saline irrigation. Patients with severe cases may require hospitalization and ceftriaxone at the same dosage schedule for 5 to 7 days.

Systemic gonococcal infection other than meningitis and endocarditis should be treated with ceftriaxone (50 mg/kg/day [maximum dose 1 g] IV or IM once daily) or cefotaxime

(50 mg/kg/day [maximum daily dose 3 g] IV or IM in three doses) for 7 to 10 days. For penicillin-allergic and cephalosporin-allergic patients, spectinomycin (40 mg/kg/day [maximum daily dose 4 g] IM in two divided doses for 7 to 10 days) is recommended. Penicillin G (150,000 U/kg/day [maximum daily dose 10 million units] IV in four to six divided doses) or equivalent penicillin agents may be substituted when the susceptibility of the isolate permits. In older, reliable patients, following symptomatic resolution the balance of therapy may be completed on an outpatient basis using cefuroxime axetil (500 mg orally twice daily); amoxicillin with clavulanic acid (500 mg orally three times daily); or, subject to age and pregnancy restrictions, ciprofloxacin (500 mg orally twice daily).

Management of gonococcal arthritis may require additional therapeutic modalities appropriate for any case of pyogenic arthritis (see discussion on pyogenic [or septic] arthritis, p. 442); however, antimocrobial treatment alone typically suffices to effect an excellent outcome.

Patients with disseminated gonococcal infection should be evaluated carefully for evidence of meningitis or endocarditis. Meningitis should be treated with ceftriaxone (100 mg/kg/day [maximum daily dose 2 to 4 g] IV or IM in one or two doses) or cefotaxime (200 mg/kg/day [maximum daily dose 8 to 10 g] IV in three or four doses) for 10 to 14 days. Alternative agents for susceptible strains include penicillin G (250,000 U/kg/day [maximum daily dose 10 to 20 million units] IV in four to six doses for 10 to 14 days); or, for penicillin-allergic and cephalosporin-allergic patients, chloramphenicol (100 mg/kg/day [maximum daily dose 2 to 6 g] IV in four doses for 10 to 14 days), with careful monitoring of blood levels. Treatment for endocarditis, using the same agents and dosage schedules, should be extended to at least 4 weeks. The occurrence of gonococcal meningitis or endocarditis or recurrence of DGI should prompt an evaluation for possible complement deficiency.

CONTROL AND PREVENTIVE MEASURES

Early detection of gonococcal infection affords the best chance for a satisfactory therapeutic outcome. Accordingly, routine screening of sexually active adolescents as well as all pregnant women (at the time of the first prenatal visit and again late in pregnancy) is recommended. Infected pregnant women may be treated with standard regimens, except that doxycycline and tetracycline should be avoided.

Universal ophthalmic prophylaxis is indicated in order to prevent gonococcal ophthalmia neonatorum. Either 1 per cent aqueous silver nitrate solution, 1 per cent tetracycline ointment, or 0.5 per cent erythromycin ointment should be instilled once in the eyes as soon as possible but no later than 1 hour after birth; the eyes should not be subsequently irrigated. These regimens do not dependably prevent chlamydial infection.

Despite the high degree of efficacy of ophthalmic prophylaxis, newborns delivered to women with untreated gonorrhea should receive a single dose of ceftriaxone (25 to 50 mg/kg [maximum dose 125 mg] IM or IV).

All cases of gonococcal infection should be reported to public health authorities in order to facilitate surveillance and contact tracing.

Sex partners of infected patients should be identified, evaluated, and usually presumptively treated for the implicated STDs.

Although currently recommended regimens are reliably effective in curing gonococcal infection, in order to permit timely recognition of the emergence of additionally resistant strains, at least a representative sample of gonococcal isolates should be subjected to antibiotic susceptibility testing. Likewise, all isolates associated with treatment failure should be evaluated to guide retreatment.

Because therapeutic failure following treatment with the combination of ceftriaxone and doxycycline is very rare, "test of cure" cultures are not routinely required for gonococcal infections treated with this regimen. However, a second specimen should be obtained for culture approximately 4 to 7 days after completion of any other therapeutic regimen. In addition, the selective use of "rescreening" cultures obtained 1 to 2 months after treatment is recommended irrespective of treatment regimen in order to permit the early detection of reinfection.

Education regarding issues of sexuality and transmission of STDs is the most important and potentially most beneficial element of strategies for controlling and preventing infection. Infected patients need to be instructed to defer additional sexual activity until after successful completion of a course of treatment. Harder still is teaching adolescents the lesson that, barring sexual abstinence, the (proper) use of barrier contraceptives, such as condoms, affords the only available means of minimizing (not eliminating) the risk of acquiring STDs.

REFERENCES

Centers for Disease Control: 1989 Sexually transmitted diseases treatment guidelines. MMWR 38 (No. S-8):21–27, 1989.

Committee on Infectious Diseases, American Academy of Pediatrics: Gonococcal Infections. *In* Report of the Committee on Infectious Diseases, 22nd ed. Elk Grove Village, Ill, American Academy of Pediatrics, 1991, pp 211–219.

Moran JS, Zenilman JM: Therapy for gonococcal infections: Options in 1989. Rev Infect Dis 12(S6):S633–S644, 1990.

CANDIDIASIS

KWANG SIK KIM, M.D.

Candida albicans is probably the most important variety of *Candida* that is pathogenic to humans. Other clinically significant *Candida* organisms include *C. tropicalis, C. glabrata, C. lusitaniae, C. pseudotropicalis, C. stellatoidea, C. krusei, C. parapsilosis,* and *C. quilliermondii. Candida* causes a wide spectrum of diseases, as described in this article.

TYPES OF CANDIDAL INFECTIONS

Cutaneous and Oropharyngeal Candidiasis

This form of candidal infection is common and in nonimmunocompromised patients usually responds to topical antifungal agents. For diaper dermatitis, topical nystatin, clotrimazole, or miconazole applied four times a day is the recommended therapy. Thrush responds to 100,000 units/ml of oral nystatin suppression. In infants, 1 ml should be applied to each side of the mouth four times a day until the lesions resolve. In older children, up to 4 ml four times a day can be given. Perlèche and paronychia can be treated with one of the topical antifungal agents. When the nail is involved (onychia), oral antifungal therapy will be needed (e.g., ketoconazole).

Chronic Oral *Candida* Infection Associated with Chronic Mucocutaneous Candidiasis and Immunosuppression

In more persistent and extensive oral candidiasis in patients with underlying immunosuppression, treatment may be undertaken with ketoconazole, intravenous miconazole, fluconazole, or a short course of parenteral amphotericin B, particularly for patients with severe neutropenia or severe mucositis.

Urinary Candidiasis

Candiduria may represent bladder infection, renal parenchymal infection, or a manifestation of disseminated diseases. In most instances, however, the finding of yeast in urine reflects improper collection and processing of urine samples. For candidal infection confined to the bladder without an indwelling catheter, oral flucytosine therapy may be adequate. For patients requiring indwelling bladder catheterization, continuous irrigation with amphotericin B in a concentration of 1 mg/dl (10 μg/ml) for 5 to 7 days is usually successful. If urine cultures continue to yield *Candida,* systemic antifungal therapy with flucytosine or amphotericin B plus flucytosine is indicated. The combination of amphotericin B plus flucytosine is indicated for renal parenchymal infection and infections associated with fungus ball formation.

Peritoneal Candidiasis

There is no well-established therapy for peritoneal candidal infection. Intraperitoneal lavage with amphotericin B along with removal of catheter has been successfully used for patients requiring peritoneal dialysis, but systemic amphotericin B should be employed, particularly when disseminated candidiasis cannot be excluded.

Catheter-Related Candidemia

Removal of the catheter and initiation of parenteral amphotericin B therapy (a total dose of 5 to 10 mg/kg) should be sufficient for most cases in which there is no evidence of deep-seated or disseminated candidiasis.

Deep-Seated or Disseminated Candidiasis with or without Candidemia

This form of candidiasis continues to provide a major diagnostic and therapeutic challenge to clinicians, and includes sepsis, pneumonia, arthritis, osteomyelitis, endocarditis, endophthalmitis, and hepatosplenic candidiasis. Disseminated candidiasis is most frequently encountered in the immunocompromised host and premature infants with the following predisposing factors: broad-spectrum antibiotic therapy, malignant hematologic diseases, cytotoxic or steroid therapy, intravascular catheters, central parenteral alimentation, gastrointestinal surgery, or pathology. Amphotericin B (a total dose of 30 to 40 mg/kg) with or without flucytosine is recommended.

TREATMENT

Antifungal Agents

Amphotericin B

Amphotericin B, despite its considerable toxicity, remains the principal antifungal agent for deep-seated or disseminated candidiasis. The basic mechanism of antifungal activity of amphotericin B has been ascribed to its binding to sterols in the fungus cell membrane, with a resultant increase in the membrane permeability. Most of the *Candida* species are inhibited by amphotericin B in vitro. The drug is fungistatic, but it can be fungicidal at high concentrations. Resistance to amphotericin B is rare, but there have been several reports of amphotericin B–resistant yeasts that include *C. albicans, C. tropicalis, C. lusitaniae, C. krusei, C. parapsilosis,* and *C. quilliermondii.*

Administration. Amphotericin B should be administered intravenously to patients for whom adequate medical supervision and nursing care are available. The drug is very irritating, and care must be taken so that no perivascular or subcutaneous leakage occurs. The drug should be prepared in a concentration of 0.1 mg/ml or less in 5 per cent dextrose in water (not in saline because the drug will precipitate). Infusion times can vary from 2 to 6 hours, based on the patient's tolerance, but no less than 1 to 2 hours per infusion. Light shielding of the infusion bottle is unnecessary during drug administration.

Amphotericin B is usually started at a testing dose of 0.1 mg/kg (maximum 1 mg). Subsequent doses of amphotericin can be increased in daily increments of 0.1 to 0.25 mg/kg/day or as rapidly as possible to a maximal dose of 1 mg/kg/day for severely ill patients. For a patient who requires aggressive therapy, if a test dose is well tolerated, the remainder of an initial dose of amphotericin B (e.g., 0.25 mg/kg) can be completed on day 1 of therapy. The speed of incremental increase depends on the patient's tolerance of the drug and toxicity. The tolerance to amphotericin B varies substantially from patient to patient. The pharmacology of intravenously administered amphotericin B remains incompletely understood, but the drug has a long half-life. Thus, after the clinical response and tolerance to doses are established, it is possible to give the drug on an alternate-day schedule or two to three times per week for consolidation therapy.

Side Effects. Amphotericin B induces abnormalities of renal function and inhibits erythropoiesis. Hypokalemia, increases in blood urea nitrogen and creatinine, and anemia are common but are not an indication for discontinuance. Dosage adjustments are not necessary with pre-existing renal impairment. Sodium supplementation may decrease the nephrotoxic potential of amphotericin B. If decreased renal function occurs, the daily dose can be decreased by 50 per cent, or the dose can be given every other day. Interruption of amphotericin B therapy may be needed if rapid decline in renal function occurs. Careful monitoring of patients' renal and electrolyte status is required (at least biweekly). Concurrent administration of carbenicillin or ticarcillin may exacerbate the hypokalemia.

Fever, chills, headache, nausea, and vomiting may develop during the infusion of amphotericin B. Depending on the patient's tolerance, an antiemetic (e.g., diphenhydramine), antipyretics (e.g., acetaminophen), meperidine (for chills), or ibuprofen (for chills and fever), may be required 30 minutes before the infusion. In some patients, hydrocortisone may be added to the infusion to minimize severe reactions.

Flucytosine

Flucytosine (5-FC) is well absorbed orally, is excreted via the kidney, and has been used for urinary candidiasis as a single agent. More commonly, however, 5-FC is used in combination with amphotericin B in the treatment of disseminated candidiasis or prolonged candidemia. Many clinical isolates of *Candida* are susceptible to 5-FC concentrations of less than 5 μg/ml, but as many as 25 per cent of isolates have been reported to be resistant to 5-FC. Resistance to 5-FC frequently develops when the drug is used alone. Thus, determination of susceptibility of *Candida* to 5-FC should be made in all instances. If the organism is susceptible to 5-FC, this drug should be used to treat deep-seated or disseminated candidiasis, although no prospective data are available comparing the efficacy of combined amphotericin B plus flucytosine versus amphotericin B alone.

5-FC is usually given in a dosage of 50 to 150 mg/kg in four divided doses. The major toxicity is bone marrow suppression (e.g., leukopenia), which seems to be related to serum concentrations greater than 100 μg/ml. Thus, serum drug levels should be measured to be certain to keep the level below 100 μg/ml. For patients with renal impairment, the dosage interval needs to be increased (e.g., every 12 hours for 50 per cent decrease in renal function). When 5-FC is used with amphotericin B (a nephrotoxic drug), serum levels of 5-FC should be determined periodically.

Imidazoles

Clotrimazole

Topical preparation of clotrimazole is available for cutaneous and vaginal candidiasis.

Miconazole

Topical preparation of miconazole is useful for cutaneous and vaginal candidiasis. Intravenous preparation (20 to 40 mg/kg/day in three divided doses) has been used for selected cases of mucocutaneous candidiasis with limited success but is associated with a rather high incidence of adverse reactions.

Ketoconazole

Ketoconazole has been used for chronic mucocutaneous candidiasis (5 to 10 mg/kg/day orally in two or three divided doses for 5 to 6 weeks), but its efficacy for candidal esophagitis is not established. The common side effects are gastrointestinal reactions. Rarely, hepatitis develops, an indication for discontinuance.

Fluconazole

Fluconazole is well absorbed orally and can be given either parentally or orally. The dose is the same for both routes (3 to 6 mg/kg/day). The drug has a long half-life and is given once daily. The drug is excreted into the urine in high concentrations; thus, dosage modification is required in patients with renal impairment. Fluconazole is approved for the treatment of oropharyngal and esophageal candidiasis, but its efficacy in children is not established.

ASPERGILLOSIS

MICHAEL GREEN, M.D., M.P.H.

Invasive aspergillosis is the second most frequent mycotic infection in children with altered defense mechanisms. The lung is the major site of infection in such patients. Hematogenous dissemination occurs in 20 to 50 per cent of infected patients and most commonly affects the central nervous system and the gastrointestinal tract. Less frequently, the paranasal sinuses serve as the primary site of infection, which can lead to contiguous spread into the central nervous system. In disseminated disease, *Aspergillus* can also be recovered from the skin and most other organs.

PROGNOSIS

The outcome of immunocompromised children with invasive aspergillosis is disappointing. Survival is uncommon in patients with ongoing impairment of host defenses. Efforts to improve the immune status of infected patients have not been effective. Granulocyte transfusions have been used without apparent benefit in a small number of infected patients with either persistent neutropenia or chronic granulomatous disease. The use of granulocyte transfusions should be further discouraged because this treatment is associated with severe pulmonary reactions in some patients. The use of the recently licensed recombinant granulocyte colony-stimulating factor offers some promise, but no data are available to assess its efficacy in the treatment of aspergillosis. Withdrawal of immunosuppressive therapy in organ transplant recipients is indicated, but—with the exception of pulmonary disease—outcome is exceedingly poor in these patients even when immunosuppressive medications are discontinued.

TREATMENT

Amphotericin B

Amphotericin B remains the drug of choice for children with invasive aspergillosis. The drug must be suspended in an electrolyte-free solution (water or D_5W) at a concentration not to exceed 0.1 mg/ml. It is not necessary to shield the drug from light because usual infusion times of 1 to 6 hours do not lead to light inactivation of conventional doses. An intravenous test dose of the drug (0.1 mg/kg, maximum 1.0 mg) infused over 1 to 2 hours is given to the patient who has not been recently treated with amphotericin. The child should be monitored carefully for the development of acute toxicity, including bronchospasm or seizures. If the test dose is tolerated, a second dose of 0.5 mg/kg is given approximately 6 to 12 hours later. This and all subsequent doses are given over 4 to 6 hours. The child then receives the full daily maintenance dose of 1.0 mg/kg the following day. The optimal duration of therapy for children with invasive aspergillosis is unknown. Retrospective review of surviving patients suggests that a minimum of 6 to 8 weeks may be required.

Acute Effects

Acute toxicity, manifested as chills, fever, rigors, nausea, and vomiting, occurs commonly during the infusion of amphotericin B. These reactions seem to occur less frequently in children than in adults and may be minimized by increasing the infusion time or by using premedications. Acetaminophen (10 to 15 mg/kg orally) and diphenhydramine hydrochloride (1.25 mg/kg orally or intravenously), given 30 minutes before infusing amphotericin B, are helpful in decreasing or preventing these reactions. We use this combination routinely in all children being treated with amphotericin B. A second dose with acetaminophen is recommended if the infusion is incomplete after 4 hours. Intravenously administered meperidine hydrochloride (1.0 to 1.5 mg/kg) is given acutely to patients who develop rigors during the infusion and, subsequently, is given just prior to the dose of amphotericin B throughout the remainder of the child's treatment course. Patients whose reactions are refractory to other measures may benefit from the addition of hydrocortisone (0.5 to 0.7 mg/kg) to the infusion.

Chronic Effects

Chronic effects of amphotericin B therapy include electrolyte disturbances, renal insufficiency, and, uncommonly, anemia. For these reasons, serum electrolytes, blood urea nitrogen, creatinine, and a complete blood count should be obtained prior to the institution of therapy. These laboratory values are then followed two to three times per week on therapy. Patients experiencing hypokalemia should receive potassium supplementation. In patients who experience marked renal insufficiency, switching to alternate-day therapy at the same dose of 1.0 mg/kg usually results in a notable improvement of renal function.

Combination Therapy

Combination antifungal chemotherapy has been recommended by some investigators in the treatment of invasive aspergillosis. These recommendations are based on in vitro and animal model data suggesting synergistic inhibition or killing and improved outcome when amphotericin B is used in combination with either 5-flucytosine or rifampin. Although no data from controlled clinical trials are available, the poor outcome seen with this disease has led us to recommend combination chemotherapy in the majority of patients with invasive aspergillosis. We recommend 5-flucytosine given orally (75 to 150 mg/kg/day in four divided doses). Because of associated toxicity, drug levels should be monitored (therapeutic range: 50 to 100 μg/ml). Rifampin (20 mg/kg/day) has been used less commonly, usually in patients with severe hematologic abnormalities who were not considered to be candidates for 5-flucytosine.

Alternative Antifungal Agents

The poor outcome of invasive aspergillosis and concerns over the toxicity of amphotericin B have led to the search for alternative antifungal agents. The encapsulation of amphotericin B into liposomes appears to allow for the use of increasing dosages of the drug within the liposome with little acute toxicity. Although the initial experience appears promising, only limited, uncontrolled results are currently available in the treatment of invasive aspergillosis with liposomal amphotericin B, and we cannot recommend its use at this time.

Itraconazole

Itraconazole, an *N*-substituted triazole, is active in vitro and in vivo, utilizing a murine model of aspergillosis. However, it has been less effective than amphotericin B in the treatment of experimental aspergillosis in a rabbit model. Initial, limited uncontrolled experience in adults has been promising, and this drug probably represents a significant advance in the therapy of invasive aspergillosis. To date, however, there are no published studies in pediatric patients, and the exact role of itraconazole in the treatment of aspergillosis remains to be determined.

Fluconazole, another new and recently licensed triazole agent, does not appear to be useful in the treatment of this disease.

Surgery

Many authors recommend surgical débridement of infected tissue for patients with invasive aspergillosis. It is clear that some sites of infection may require surgery while in others the role of surgery is less clear. In patients with uncorrectable immunodeficiencies, it is likely that resection of a localized area of aspergillosis may be life-saving.

Allergic Bronchopulmonary Aspergillosis

Allergic bronchopulmonary aspergillosis is a hypersensitivity response to inhalation of the spores of *Aspergillus fumigatus*. This noninvasive disease is typically seen in patients with illnesses associated with poor pulmonary clearance (such as cystic fibrosis or asthma). Patients inhale spores that grow in the bronchial lumen, shedding antigen into the tissue and provoking an inflammatory response. The disease can be chronic and can lead to severe lung destruction in some patients. Corticosteroids and chest physiotherapy are the mainstays of treatment. Steroids are given initially at a dose of 0.5 mg/kg/day for 2 weeks, followed by the same dose on alternate days for the next 3 months. The patient may then be weaned from the steroids. Patients who experience relapse may require chronic steroid therapy.

REFERENCES

Denning DW, Stevens DA: Antifungal and surgical treatment of invasive aspergillosis: Review of 2,121 published cases. Rev Infect Dis 12:1147–1201, 1990.

Mendelson EB, Fisher MR, Mintzer RA, et al: Roentgenographic and clinical staging of allergic bronchopulmonary aspergillosis. Chest 87:334–339:1985.

Patterson R, Greenberger PA, Halwig M, et al: Allergic bronchopulmonary aspergillosis. Arch Intern Med 146:916–918, 1986.

ENTAMOEBA HISTOLYTICA INFECTION

WILLIAM J. KLISH, M.D.

Human infection with *Entamoeba histolytica* is common throughout the world and has been estimated to cause approximately 100,000 deaths per year. It is the third most common cause of death from parasitic infection.

EPIDEMIOLOGY

Up to 500 million people are infected throughout the world at any one time, and approximately one fifth are symptomatic. The prevalence of infection varies widely, depending on local conditions and is less than 1 per cent in Canada and Alaska, approximately 5 per cent in the contiguous United States, and as high as 40 per cent in tropical areas. Age influences the prevalence of infection, with children under 5 years affected less than other age groups. Prevalence is higher in people confined to institutions. Symptoms such as diarrhea or dysentery are seen in 2 to 8 per cent of infected individuals. Although amebic hepatic abscess appears less commonly in children than adults, it is found as a complication in 1 to 9 per cent of patients with intestinal disease. *E. histolytica* infection is not a common cause of traveler's diarrhea, but it has been reported in as many as 6 per cent of cases in some studies.

The human being is the natural host and reservoir for *E. histolytica;* however, dogs, pigs, and monkeys also have been implicated. Filth, flies, and cockroaches have been shown to be important mechanical vectors of the cysts. Fecal-oral transmission can occur through contaminated water or foods such as vegetables. Infected food handlers play a major role in transmission of infection. Major outbreaks have occurred in the United States, but person-to-person spread is the predominant form of transmission. *E. histolytica* is a common commensal organism in the homosexual population.

CLINICAL FEATURES

Amebiasis is the term used to define an infection with *E. histolytica.* However, infection can result in a wide range of clinical syndromes, including asymptomatic infection, amebic colitis, or extraintestinal amebiasis, which is usually a hepatic abscess. Eighty to 90 per cent of infected individuals are asymptomatic carriers. The incubation period for illness varies but is usually 2 to 4 weeks. A patient can present with very mild symptoms to severe fulminating disease. Most patients present with a gradual onset of cramping abdominal pain, malaise, and frequent stools. Tenesmus can occur with rectal involvement. Stools are mucoid and usually blood-stained. Diarrhea may persist for weeks but can fluctuate with alternating periods of constipation. The disease may occasionally present as acute dysentery, with fever, profuse bloody diarrhea, and dehydration. Physical examination usually reveals tenderness throughout the lower abdomen. Complications of acute dysentery include hemorrhage, stricture, or intestinal perforation with peritonitis or ameba formation.

Hepatic amebiasis and abscess can occur within days, months, or years after the onset of bowel infection. In up to 50 per cent of cases, no clear history of amebic colitis is obtained. Symptoms include fever, right-sided abdominal pain, chest pain, respiratory distress, and hepatomegaly. Pain is usually in the right upper quadrant of the abdomen, with

TABLE 1. Treatment of Amebiasis

Drug	Dosage
Asymptomatic Carrier	
Iodoquinol (formerly diiodohydroxyquin)	40 mg/kg/day in 3 doses × 20 days Adult dose: 650 mg t.i.d. × 20 days
or	
Diloxanide furoate (furamide)	20 mg/kg/day in 3 doses × 10 days Adult dose: 500 mg t.i.d. × 10 days
or	
Parmomycin	25–30 mg/kg/day in 3 doses × 7 days
Mild to Moderate Intestinal Disease	
Metronidazole	35–50 mg/kg/day in 3 doses × 10 days Adult dose: 750 mg t.i.d. × 10 days
plus	
Iodoquinol	35 mg/kg/day in 3 doses × 10 days Adult dose: 750 mg t.i.d. × 10 days
or	
Parmomycin	25–30 mg/kg/day in 3 doses × 7 days
Severe Intestinal Disease	
Metronidazole	35–50 mg/kg/day in 3 doses × 10 days Adult dose: 650 mg t.i.d. × 10 days
plus	
Iodoquinol	35 mg/kg/day in 3 doses × 10 days Adult dose: 650 mg t.i.d. × 10 days
or	
Dihydroemetine	1–1.5 mg/kg/day IM in 2 doses for up to 5 days (max: 90 mg/day)
plus	
Iodoquinol	35 mg/kg/day in 3 doses × 10 days Adult dose: 650 mg t.i.d. × 10 days
Hepatic Abscess	
Metronidazole	35–50 mg/kg/day in 3 doses × 10 days Adult dose: 700 mg t.i.d. × 10 days
plus	
Iodoquinol	35 mg/kg/day in 3 doses × 10 days Adult dose: 650 mg t.i.d. × 10 days
or	
Dehydroemetine	1–1.5 mg/kg/day IM in 2 doses for up to 5 days (max: 90 mg/day)
followed by	
Chloroquine phosphate	10 mg base/kg/day × 2–3 weeks (maximum 300 mg base) Adult dose: 600 mg base (1 g)/day × 2 days
plus	
Iodoquinol	35 mg/kg/day in 3 doses × 10 days Adult dose: 650 mg t.i.d. × 10 days

radiation to the right shoulder and lateral chest wall caused by inflammation of the diaphragm and pleura.

Physical examination commonly reveals a large tender liver. Chest examination may reveal rales, decreased breath sounds, and a friction rub. Jaundice is an ominous sign. Hepatic abscesses develop in fewer than 1 per cent of patients with intestinal amebiasis.

DIAGNOSIS

Demonstrations of *E. histolytica* trophozoites and cysts in feces remains the definitive diagnostic test. If stool examination is done correctly, results will be positive in more than 90% of infected patients. Stool samples should be examined with a saline wet mount immediately while they are still warm. Motile trophozoites containing ingested red blood cells will be seen. Nonpathogenic strains of intestinal amebas are not erythrophagic. Stool samples can be preserved in a fixative such as polyvinyl alcohol or formalin ethylacetate for later examination. This allows concentration of the specimen and increased sensitivity of the test. The examination of rectal mucosal scrapings collected during proctoscopy increases the positive yield. Trophozoites can be seen in colonic biopsy tissue in approximately 50 per cent of cases.

Serologic tests for amebiasis are also available. Indirect hemagglutination (IHA) is strongly positive (titer greater than 1:256) in 85 to 90 per cent of cases of either invasive colonic disease or liver abscess. Because patients with liver abscess usually do not have concurrent diarrhea, stool findings are frequently not positive. Serology, liver scanning, ultrasound examination, and needle aspiration are sometimes needed to establish a diagnosis.

TREATMENT

Recommended drug therapy for amebiasis is listed in Table 1. The site of involvement and severity of disease determine the combination of drugs used. Iodoquinol has been reported to cause optic atrophy in rare cases. Diloxanide furoate can be used alternatively. Metronidazole is not a very effective luminal amebicide and thus should be used with another drug. Dehydroemetine should be used with caution because it may cause severe side effects; these include cardiotoxicity, which can lead to a fatal myocardiopathy; arrhythmias with T-wave changes; and renal complications.

Uncomplicated, deep, unruptured liver abscess may be managed medically. For refractory cases or impending rupture of the abscess, percutaneous needle aspiration or open surgical drainage is necessary.

Prophylaxis for travelers to endemic areas is not recommended. Exercising caution in unsanitary conditions is the best prophylaxis.

GIARDIASIS

JUAN N. WALTERSPIEL, M.D.

Giardia lamblia is the most common intestinal parasite in humans worldwide. Infection and colonization are more frequent in children than in adults. Oral transmission by cysts excreted in stool occurs from person to person and through fecally contaminated food and water supplies. The spectrum of infection ranges from asymptomatic to failure to thrive and malabsorption.

TREATMENT

Treatment usually results in prompt improvement, although in some patients symptoms persist for weeks in spite of appropriate therapy. In these instances, stools should be retested for *Giardia* antigens. Poor compliance or an underlying immunodeficiency should be considered before medications are changed. Susceptibility testing is not available. Immunocompromised patients might require several courses of treatment. Treatment of asymptomatic carriers is not recommended because the benefits and risks have not been established. Drugs available for treatment of patients with giardiasis are furazolidone, quinacrine hydrochloride, metronidazole and its derivatives (Table 1).

Furazolidone

The drug of choice for children under 5 years of age is furazolidone (Furoxone). It is available in 100-mg tablets and as an oral suspension with the unusual formulation of 50 mg/15 ml, which in more common terms equals 16.6 mg per 5 ml or per teaspoon. Cure rates range from 70 to 80 per cent. Side effects are rare and include mild gastrointestinal disturbances, reversible hypersensitivity reactions, brown discoloration of urine, and occasional hemolysis in patients with glucose-6-phosphate dehydrogenase deficiency. Disulfiram-like reactions can occur (vasodilatation, vomiting, hypotension) with alcohol consumption during and within 4 days of furazolidone treatment. Children can unknowingly be exposed to alcohol as an ingredient of several pediatric elixirs. Nasal decongestants and methylphenidate (Ritalin) should not be given concomitantly.

Quinacrine

Quinacrine hydrochloride (Atabrine) is available in 100-mg tablets. Although this is the most effective drug for the treatment of giardiasis, its unpleasant taste makes it an unacceptable first choice for children. Cure rates in those who are compliant range from 90 to 100 per cent. About one third of children under 5 years of age will experience nausea and vomiting, and more than two thirds will have yellow discoloration of the skin. Psoriatic lesions can be exacerbated with this drug. Behavioral changes caused by quinacrine have been described in adults. Quinacrine also causes mild disulfiram-like reactions. No mutagenic or carcinogenic effects have been demonstrated, and it is the least expensive agent available.

TABLE 1. Antimicrobial Therapy of Giardiasis

Antimicrobial Agent	Dose
First Choice	
Furazolidone (Furoxone)	8 mg/kg/day, divided q 6 hr × 10 days orally, not to exceed 400 mg/day
Alternatives	
Metronidazole (Flagyl)	15 mg/kg/day, divided q 8 hr × 7 days orally, not to exceed 750 mg/day
or	
Ornidazole (not available in United States)	40 mg/kg once orally, not to exceed 1.5 g
or	
Tinidazole (not available in United States)	50 mg/kg once orally, not to exceed 2 g
or	
Quinacrine (Atabrine)	6 mg/kg/day, divided q 8 hr × 10 days orally, not to exceed 300 mg/day

Metronidazole

Metronidazole (Flagyl) is available in 250-mg tablets. These can be crushed and made into a suspension that leaves a metallic aftertaste. A tasteless benzoyl-metronidazole preparation is available as oral suspension (Flagyl-S) in some countries but not in the United States. Its efficacy varies from 50 per cent for single-dose regimens to 97 per cent for 7- to 10-day regimens. Side effects in children are minimal. Uncommon reactions are dizziness, vertigo, ataxia, paresthesia, dysuria, and dark urine. Disulfiram-like reactions can occur during and within 4 days of therapy. The drug is not approved by the U.S. Food and Drug Administration for treatment of giardiasis in children because of its mutagenic potential in bacteria. In animals, therapeutic concentrations given over a prolonged period of time increased the incidence of mammary tumors. Conversely, in humans no evidence of cancer associated with the use of metronidazole has ever been demonstrated.

Tinidazole and Ornidazole

Tinidazole and ornidazole are chemically related to metronidazole. They are currently not available in the United States. Cure rates and side effects are comparable to metronidazole. The advantage is the one time dose. Ornidazole (with three brand names) is given at 40 mg/kg, not to exceed 1.5 g once. Tinidazole (with nine brand names) is given at 50 mg/kg/day, not to exceed 2 g as single-dose therapy.

PINWORMS

ANDREW H. URBACH

Pinworm infestation is caused by the helminth *Enterobius vermicularis*. It is the most common and ubiquitous parasitic worm worldwide. Estimates suggest that 20 per cent of children in the United States harbor this endemic parasite. Humans are the only natural host, with a particular predilection for children in cosmopolitan, temperate settings. The organism crosses socioeconomic barriers but is more common in crowded institutional environments. This spindle-shaped parasite is transmitted by the fecal-oral route, but food, drink, fomites and possibly inhaled dust have been implicated. Following ingestion of pinworm eggs, the larvae hatch and migrate to the distal ileum, cecum, and ascending colon, where the adult male and female worms live and mate. The gravid female, which is 8 to 13 mm long, subsequently travels to the anus, where she lays an average of 11,000 eggs and dies. These very adhesive, colorless eggs proceed to reinitiate the *E. vermicularis* life cycle.

CLINICAL SYMPTOMS

The deposition of pinworm eggs and the distal migration of the adult in the perianal area cause the pruritus ani that is the hallmark of this infection. The intense itching that ensues facilitates continued infestation by the manual transmission of eggs to other body sites. Many clinical symptoms have been attributed to pinworms, including pruritus vulvae, vaginal discharge, dysuria, restlessness, irritability, and insomnia. As a result of intense itching, eczematous dermatitis, hemorrhage, and secondary bacterial infection occur. The manual transfer of eggs from site to site on the body and the mobility of the adult worm itself account for the reports of ectopic locations for pinworm infestation. Included are vaginitis, salpingitis, peritonitis, tubovarian abscess, urethral involve-

TABLE 1. Treatment of Pinworms

Drug	Dosage	Forms	Possible Side Effects
Mebendazole* (Vermox)	100 mg in a single dose (adults and children); repeat in 2 weeks	Chewable tablets (100 mg each)	Rarely, transient abdominal pain and diarrhea
Pyrantel pamoate (Antiminth)	11 mg/kg in a single dose (maximum: 1 g/dose); repeat in 2 weeks	Suspension (50 mg/ml)	Anorexia, nausea, vomiting, cramps, diarrhea, transient elevation of aspartate aminotransferase
Piperazine citrate (Vermizine)	65 mg/kg/day for 7 days (maximum: 2.5 g/dose)	Tablets (250 mg each) Suspension (100 mg/ml)	Nausea, vomiting, diarrhea; may exacerbate seizure disorders

Adapted from Jones JE. Pinworms. Am Fam Physician 38:159–164, 1988.
*Not for children under 2 years old or pregnant women.
Note: Three negative perianal preparations 1 week apart indicate eradication of the parasite.

ment, hepatic granuloma, pulmonary "coin" lesions, conjunctivitis, ear infestation, and even invasion of the human embryo.

Clinical symptoms often suggest the diagnosis, which is confirmed by the "Scotch tape" test. The test is optimally performed on three to five successive mornings before the child arises, bathes, or defecates. Adhesive tape is pressed against the perianal area and is then applied to a microscopic slide to allow detection of eggs. The direct use of stool for egg detection is effective only 5 per cent of the time and, therefore, is not recommended.

TREATMENT

Treatment is best accomplished with pyrantel pamoate (11 mg/kg orally for one dose) or mebendazole (100 mg orally [same for all body weights] for one dose); this regimen is repeated in 2 weeks (Table 1). Many authors recommend treating all family contacts of the index case. Patients and families can be reassured that although pinworms are disturbing, they rarely cause serious disease.

PREVENTION AND PROGNOSIS

Prevention necessitates attention to personal hygiene, specifically careful hand washing before meals and after toilet use, fingernail care, and avoidance of thumb sucking and scratching of affected areas. Washing and drying clothes and linens, washing toilet seats, and careful vacuuming of bedrooms of affected individuals may be helpful. Shaking infested linens may perpetuate the disease process. The initial housecleaning process need not be repeated. Reassurance that pinworm infestation is not a result of uncleanliness may assuage the parental guilt often associated with the infestation.

Prognosis is excellent, although a high carrier rate results in frequent reinfection.

REFERENCES

Chaudhry AZ, Longworth DL. Cutaneous manifestations of intestinal helminthic infections. Dermatol Clin 7:275–290, 1989.

Jones JE. Pinworms. Am Fam Physician 38:159–164, 1988.

ASCARIASIS

MICHAEL KATZ, M.D.

Ascaris lumbricoides, a large nematode, is found mainly throughout the tropical and subtropical world. *It is estimated that world prevalence of ascariasis exceeds one billion.* The importance of this infection in the United States relates primarily to the recent arrivals of immigrants from Southeast Asia and from other parts of the Third World. However, occasional children in some rural parts of the United States are also infected.

ETIOLOGY

The most serious clinical manifestation of *Ascaris* infection relates to its early migratory phase. When eggs that have incubated in soil for about 2 weeks and have embryonated are ingested with food, larvae hatch in the small intestine, penetrate the mucosa and enter the venous circulation. When they reach capillaries of the lungs, they break out into the alveoli and begin ascending through the respiratory tree. After reaching the pharynx, they are swallowed and in the small intestine mature into adult worms. During the migratory phase—depending on their number—the larvae can cause an inflammatory reaction, characterized by eosinophilic infiltration. In severe cases, the patient may be overwhelmed by this type of pneumonitis; however, in an average case, this phase remains unnoticed.

After the worms in the small intestine mature into adults, they begin to lay eggs or produce sperm; the fertilized eggs are deposited in the soil with feces. This happens if there are no sanitary facilities, and often the process is enhanced by the use of human feces as fertilizer. Adult worms occasionally migrate aberrantly and can cause obstruction of the bile duct and even can perforate the intestine and cause peritonitis. Such an aberrant migration can be a consequence of fever. Worms can also be regurgitated and vomited and can be passed intact with feces. Very heavy infections—when a hundred or more worms get matted in the intestine—can result in a mechanical obstruction.

Malnutrition has been attributed to the presence of *Ascaris,* but the data supporting this contention are imprecise. It is likely, however, that in states of marginal nutrition *Ascaris* does play a negative role.

DIAGNOSIS AND TREATMENT

Diagnosis depends on the identification of the characteristic eggs in the stool by microscopic examination. Treatment should be carried out at the time the diagnosis is made. Pyrantel pamoate, given orally at 11 mg/kg once is curative. An alternative drug, mebendazole, is equally effective by the oral route at 100 mg twice a day (regardless of weight) for 3 days. The advantage of a single-dose administration of the first drug is obvious. The patient or the family should be warned that successful treatment will make the worms immobile and that they will be eliminated with feces a day or so after the drug has been administered. Treatment of the pulmonary phase of this infection—very rarely recognized as such and manifested only in an endemic area—is entirely symptomatic, but in severe cases corticosteroids may be required.

PREVENTION

Ascaris infection is wholly avoided by eating only boiled produce. Primary prevention is based on sanitary disposal of feces.

TRICHINOSIS

JOSE IGNACIO SANTOS, M.D.
and JOSE LUIS ROMERO, M.D.

Trichinosis is a systemic disease caused by the presence of the larvae of the tissue nematode, *Trichinella spiralis,* in skeletal muscle, heart, brain, and gastrointestinal tract of the susceptible host. Humans acquire trichinosis by the ingestion of undercooked meat, generally pork, containing viable, encysted *Trichinella* larvae. After ingestion, these larvae hatch in the intestine and mature into adults, which in turn produce and release larvae that invade the intestinal wall and enter the blood stream, ultimately encysting in skeletal muscle cells.

Although trichinosis was common in the United States up until a few decades ago, autopsy studies reveal a marked decrease in parasitism from 16 per cent to less than 1 per cent in recent years. The same is true in Mexico, where trichinosis is reported only sporadically and is generally associated with outbreaks related to improperly cooked pork sausage.

The clinical manifestations of trichinosis correlate with the load of larvae in tissues and the degree of the host's allergic response to them, which may range from asymptomatic to fatal. The incubation period from the time of the ingestion of the infected meat also correlates with the number of viable larvae ingested; this may be as short as 2 days but generally ranges from 5 to 15 days.

STAGES OF DISEASE

There are three stages of disease:

- Intestinal
- Muscle
- Convalescent

The intestinal stage is associated with diarrhea, pain, nausea, and vomiting, but may be asymptomatic.

Muscle invasion is the second stage, in which edema of the eyelids and face is the most consistent finding. Other features include fever, myalgias, weakness, and eosinophilia. Myocarditis is the most frequent and serious complication, and patients with 100 to 5000 larvae per gram of tissue may die from involvement of the heart, between 4 to 8 weeks after infection. Abnormal electrocardiographic findings have been reported in up to 20 per cent of cases of acute trichinosis.

The convalescent stage which begins after the 2nd month, is marked by continued myalgias and muscle weakness in untreated individuals.

DIAGNOSIS

From a laboratory standpoint, eosinophilia is the most common finding. Muscle enzymes, such as aldolase and creatine phosphokinase, are commonly elevated. Because antibody titer rises do not occur until 3 weeks into the illness, serologic studies with indirect immunoflourescence, enzyme-linked immunosorbent assay (ELISA), or the bentonite flocculation test may help to confirm the diagnosis but are not useful in the management of severely ill patients. Similarly, although there is a commercially available skin test antigen, the skin test becomes positive after the 3rd week. Biopsy of a tender muscle often reveals *Trichinella* larvae under low-power microscopic magnification.

TABLE 1. Therapy for *Trichinella spiralis* Infection

Drug	Pediatric Dosage
Prednisone (for severe symptoms)	1–2 mg/kg/day
Thiabendazole	25 mg/kg twice a day for 5 days
Mebendazole	5 mg/kg/day for 5 days

TREATMENT (Table 1)

Although various drugs are active against the adult parasites in the intestinal tract, no drug has been shown to be effective in controlled clinical trials against circulating and encysting larvae. The drug of choice for treating the intestinal parasite and thus for helping to reduce the number of larvae reaching the circulation is thiabendazole (Mintezol). Thiabendazole also has some activity against the larvae in muscle, and its anti-inflammatory activity may produce symptomatic relief by reducing the fever and the inflammatory response. Thiabendazole doses have not been standardized for adults or children, and the dosage regimen approved by the U.S. Food and Drug Administration makes no adjustment for weight or age. The dose commonly recommended for children is 25 mg/kg twice daily for five days.

Mebendazole (Vermox) also has activity against circulating and encysting larvae, making it a useful alternative; it may become the future drug of choice. The dose recommended by the World Health Organization for children is 5 mg/kg/day for 5 days. Simultaneous administration of prednisone (1 to 2 mg/kg/day) may prevent the paradoxical worsening of symptoms (Herxheimer reaction) associated with the initial phases of therapy in acute trichinosis.

Corticosteroids at pharmacologic doses may also be used in patients with severe central nervous system or myocardial involvement but should never be used alone because that may intensify the disease.

SCHISTOSOMIASIS

MARK W. KLINE, M.D.

EPIDEMIOLOGY

Schistosomiasis is a disease of diverse clinical manifestations caused by several related species of trematodes. *Schistosoma mansoni* is widespread in Africa and is the only human schistosome endemic to the Western hemisphere, with foci in South America and the Caribbean. *Schistosoma haematobium* is endemic throughout Africa and in parts of Southwest Asia and the Middle East. *Schistosoma japonicum* and *Schistosoma mekongi* are endemic only to the Far East.

It is estimated that between 200 and 300 million individuals worldwide are infected with one of these organisms. World travel has spread the disease well beyond its historical geographic distribution to North America and Europe. In the United States alone, more than 400,000 individuals may be infected with one of the human schistosomes. Transmission

TABLE 1. Treatment of *Schistosoma* Infections

Drug	Dose	Indication
Praziquantel	20 mg/kg p.o. × 3 in 1 day	Schistosomiasis
Oxamniquine	15 mg/kg p.o. × 1*	*S. mansoni* infection
Metrifonate	10 mg/kg p.o. every 2 weeks × 3	*S. haematobium* infection

*African strains of *S. mansoni* require a dose of 60 mg/kg, given in four divided doses over two days.

of infection is not possible in the United States because of absence of obligate snail intermediate hosts; however, recognition of the clinical features of the disease in travelers from endemic areas is important for early institution of therapy and prevention of complications.

STAGES OF DISEASE

Schistosomiasis can be differentiated into three distinct clinical phases:

1. Schistosome dermatitis, or swimmer's itch, which occurs with initial infection.
2. Katayama fever, a serum sickness–like immunologic reaction that occurs when deposition of eggs commences days or weeks after initial infection.
3. Chronic schistosomiasis, which may evolve over a period of months or years with granuloma formation and fibrosis of liver, ureters and bladder, or distant organs.

Definitive diagnosis of schistosomiasis is based on the demonstration of viable eggs in stool, urine, or tissues.

TREATMENT (Table 1)

Praziquantel is the drug of choice for treatment of all types and clinical phases of schistosomiasis. The recommended dose is 60 mg/kg, given in three divided doses in one day. Praziquantel therapy generally is well tolerated, with only occasional mild adverse effects, such as abdominal discomfort, headache, or rash.

Oxamniquine, given in a single oral dose of 15 mg/kg, is an alternative to praziquantel for treatment of *S. mansoni* infection. For infection caused by African strains of *S. mansoni,* a larger dose of oxamniquine is needed: 60 mg/kg, given in four divided doses over 2 days. Potential adverse effects of oxamniquine include drowsiness, dizziness, and headache. Convulsions may occur in individuals with pre-existing seizure disorders.

S. haematobium infection can be treated with metrifonate (10 mg/kg, administered on three occasions at 2-week intervals). Potential adverse effects of metrifonate include abdominal discomfort and bronchospasm.

PROGNOSIS

The prognosis of schistosomiasis is excellent when treatment is initiated early. Rare complications of schistosomiasis include schistosomal cor pulmonale, transverse myelitis, and intracranial mass lesions. Late effects of chronic schistosomiasis, including cirrhosis of the liver and portal hypertension in addition to ulcerative or fibrotic changes of the ureters and bladder, are not entirely reversible with therapy.

ROTAVIRUS

PAUL A. OFFIT, M.D.

Infectious diarrhea is an important cause of disease and death worldwide. Each year an estimated 3 to 5 billion cases of diarrhea account for 5 to 10 million deaths. Since their identification as a human pathogen in the early 1970s, rotaviruses have been found to be the most important cause of acute infectious gastroenteritis in infants and young children both in developed and developing countries. In the United States, rotavirus infection accounts for approximately 65,000 to 70,000 hospitalizations and 200 deaths per year.

TREATMENT

At present there is no specific antiviral therapy for ameliorating acute infection. Therefore, efforts to manage acute rotavirus-induced gastroenteritis and dehydration center around oral rehydration and maintenance therapies. However, the most efficient and cost-effective means of dealing with rotavirus infection will be disease prevention via the development of a safe, inexpensive vaccine.

For most children throughout the world with dehydration secondary to acute rotavirus-induced gastroenteritis, fluid management consists of an oral rehydration regimen currently recommended by the World Health Organization (WHO) and the United Nations Children's Fund (UNICEF). The WHO-UNICEF solution contains glucose (111 mmol/L), sodium (90 mmol/L), potassium (20 mmol/L), chloride (80 mmol/L), and base (as either citrate or bicarbonate at 10 mmol/L). The carbohydrate-to-sodium ratio of approximately 1.2:1 takes best advantage of the co-transport of sodium and glucose across the intestinal mucosal surface and offers an efficient means of both providing calories and replacing electrolyte losses.

Unfortunately, the current approach to oral rehydration and maintenance fluid therapy for many children in the United States with viral-induced gastroenteritis is often inappropriate. Therapy often consists of "clear liquids," such as fruit juices, tea, carbonated beverages, or homemade glucose-electrolyte solutions. In addition, feeding of solid foods is often delayed until diarrhea is resolved. There are several problems with this approach:

1. Clear fluids often contain less than 5 mmol/L of sodium, potassium, chloride, and base and are unlikely to replace electrolytes lost during viral enteritis.
2. Homemade solutions containing salt and sugar lack the needed potassium and base.
3. Intestinal absorption of food occurs even in severe diarrhea. Some foods, including rice, wheat, and potatoes, actually increase absorption of sodium and water from the intestine and provide more calories than either rehydration solutions or clear fluids.

A sensible approach to outpatient fluid management has been recommended by The American Academy of Pediatrics Committee on Nutrition:

1. Oral rehydration solutions may be used to treat mild, moderate, or severe dehydration.
2. Rehydration fluid therapy should consist of glucose-electrolyte solutions containing 75 to 90 mmol/L of sodium.
3. Maintenance fluid therapy should consist of glucose-electrolyte solutions containing 40–60 mmol/L of sodium. Rehydration fluids may be used to provide maintenance therapy when given with water, breast milk, or low-carbohydrate juices.

4. Carbohydrate-to-sodium ratios should not exceed 2:1 for either rehydration or maintenance therapy.
5. Feeding should be reintroduced within 24 hours of the onset of diarrhea and may include breast milk, diluted formula, or diluted milk for infants and rice cereal, potatoes, or bananas for older infants and young children.

Although frequent spoon feedings of small amounts of fluid demand an enormous amount of time and patience, oral rehydration therapy may be administered instead of intravenous fluid therapy to children with even severe vomiting and diarrhea. The obvious benefits of avoiding the cost, trauma, and potential nosocomial infections associated with hospitalization clearly outweigh the time it takes to teach parents how to administer fluids slowly. Unfortunately, because intravenous fluid therapy has long been used successfully in this country, there is a reluctance among both physicians and parents to adopt an oral rehydration regimen.

Antisecretory drugs (e.g., bismuth subsalicylate), antimotility drugs (e.g., diphenoxylate, atropine, loperamide), absorbents (e.g., kaolin), antiemetics (e.g., phenothizines), and antibiotics do *not* play a role in either amelioration of acute infection, prevention of reinfection, or management or prevention of fluid losses.

PREVENTION

Since the late 1970s, investigators in the United States and Finland have examined the efficacy of candidate rotavirus vaccines. Because animal rotaviruses are better adapted to growth in tissue culture than most human strains, candidate vaccine strains are currently of either simian or bovine origin. In addition, animal rotavirus strains are less well adapted to growth in the human intestinal tract than human strains and are, therefore, less likely to cause undesirable side effects.

Unfortunately, to date rotavirus vaccines administered to infants and young children have been inconsistent in inducing protection against moderate or severe disease. However, because protection against rotavirus disease is regularly induced after natural infection, development of a successful vaccine should be within reach. Given the devastating impact of this infection both in the United States and developing countries, the benefits of developing a successful vaccine would be substantial.

REFERENCES

Avery ME, Snyder JD: Oral therapy for acute diarrhea: The underused simple solution. N Engl J Med 323:891–894, 1990.

ACQUIRED IMMUNODEFICIENCY SYNDROME

ROBERT N. HUSSON, M.D.

The current therapy of pediatric human immunodeficiency virus type I (HIV-1) infection has been limited to date; however, new treatment options can be expected to evolve rapidly throughout the rest of the decade. The development and approval of new antiretroviral and adjunctive agents, new and expanded indications for treatment, better-defined dosing based on pharmacokinetic principles, and new approaches to prophylaxis and treatment of secondary infections should all contribute to improved therapy of HIV infection and its consequences. National Institutes of Health (NIH)–sponsored clinical trials, in which a large number of HIV-infected children are enrolled, will continue to play a major role in this development and will continue to be a source of new treatment options beyond those that are approved for routine use in HIV-infected children.*

This article describes current practice and anticipated developments in the antiretroviral therapy of HIV infection, certain aspects of adjunctive therapy, and the prophylaxis and therapy of secondary infections in HIV-infected children. It must be emphasized, however, that HIV infection causes chronic multisystem disease and that this infection occurs disproportionately among socially and economically disadvantaged populations. Comprehensive care in a multidisciplinary setting, with access to social service systems as well as to pediatric medical subspecialties, is thus necessary to provide optimal care for these children.

ANTIRETROVIRAL THERAPY

The precise detail in which the molecular mechanisms of the replicative cycle of HIV-1 are known has led to several approaches to interrupt this process in vitro that may lead to useful antiviral agents in vivo. The goal of antiretroviral therapy is to arrest the replication of HIV-1, which causes the immune destruction and neurologic dysfunction that are the hallmarks of HIV disease in infants and children. Early treatment with combinations of active drugs may someday allow HIV-infected children to anticipate a normal life span without major complications of HIV infection. Ultimately, it is hoped that therapies directed at eliminating HIV from the body, resulting in a cure, may be developed.

The first agents found to have anti–HIV-1 activity were the 2′,3′-dideoxynucleosides, which act through inhibition of the virus-specific reverse transcriptase. To date, this is the only class of drugs that has been developed as efficacious antiretroviral therapy. Agents that interfere with several of the other steps in virus replication, including receptor-binding and virus-specific protease activity, among others, are currently in various stages of preclinical and clinical testing.

Nucleoside Analogues

3′-azido-2′,3′-dideoxythymidine (zidovudine, azidothymidine, ZDV, AZT) is the prototype of the dideoxynucleoside analogues and was the first drug approved for the treatment of HIV infection in children. These agents are thought to act by selective inhibition of the virus-encoded reverse transcriptase through competitive substrate inhibition and chain termination. As such, they are active against an early step in the viral replication pathway and theoretically can prevent infection of susceptible cells in an HIV-infected individual. They are not active against the virus once it has completed the reverse transcription process and has become integrated into the cell's genome.

The approved pediatric indication for zidovudine therapy is for symptomatic HIV-1–infected children (Class P-2 by the Centers for Disease Control classification system outlined in Table 1) as well as asymptomatic children with laboratory evidence of HIV-related immune impairment. An abnormally low CD4 cell number is accepted as the major laboratory marker of HIV-mediated immunosuppression; however, normal CD4 counts for young children have only recently been determined and these counts change markedly over the first few years of life. At present there is no consensus on the CD4 count at which therapy should be introduced for asymptomatic infants. Young infants with low CD4 counts are often symptomatic, however, so that treatment is frequently initiated

*Information regarding clinical trials that are available for children may be obtained by calling phone number 1–800–TRIALS–A.

TABLE 1. Classification of Human Immunodeficiency Virus (HIV) Infection in Children

Class	Subclass	Description
Class P-0:	**Indeterminate infection in children under 15 months of age**	
Class P-1:	**Asymptomatic infection**	
	Subclass A:	Normal immune function
	Subclass B:	Abnormal Immune function: hypergammaglobulinemia, decreased T4 lymphocyte count or T4:T8 ratio, or decreased total lymphocyte count
	Subclass C:	Immune function not tested
Class P-2:	**Symptomatic Infection**	
	Subclass A:	Nonspecific findings (causes other than HIV excluded, two or more findings persisting for more than 2 months): fever, failure-to-thrive, weight loss $>10\%$ of baseline, hepatomegaly, splenomegaly, generalized lymphadenopathy, parotid enlargement, or persistent (≥ 3 loose stools per day) or recurrent (≥ 2 episodes with dehydration within a 2-month period) diarrhea
	Subclass B:	Progressive neurologic disease
	Subclass C:	Lymphoid interstitial pneumonitis
	Subclass D:	Secondary infectious disease
		D-1: Those listed in the CDC definition of AIDS:
		Bacterial: mycobacterial (disseminated or noncutaneous extrapulmonary), nocardiosis
		Fungal: esophageal, bronchial or pulmonary candidiasis; extrapulmonary cryptococcosis; disseminated histoplasmosis; coccidiomycosis
		Parasitic: Pneumocystis carinii pneumonia, disseminated toxoplasmosis (onset ≥ 1 month of age), chronic cryptosporidiosis or isosporiasis, extraintestinal strongyloidiasis
		Viral: cytomegalovirus disease (onset ≥ 1 month of age), chronic mucocutaneous or disseminated herpes simplex disease (onset ≥ 1 month of age), progressive multifocal leukoencephalopathy
		D-2: Recurrent serious bacterial infections (two or more within a two year period) including sepsis, meningitis, pneumonia, abscess of an internal organ, and bone or joint infection.
		D-3: Other specified infections:
		Oral candidiasis (persisting 2 months)
		Two or more episodes of herpes stomatitis within 1 year
		Multidermatomal or disseminated herpes zoster
	Subclass E:	Secondary cancers
		E-1: Those listed in the CDC definition of AIDS:
		Kaposi's sarcoma, B-cell non-Hodgkin's lymphoma, primary central nervous system lymphoma
		E-2: Other possibly HIV-related malignancies
	Subclass F:	Other possibly HIV-related disorders:
		Hepatitis, cardiopathy, nephropathy, dermatitis, hematologic disease

Adapted from Centers for Disease Control: Classification system for human immunodeficiency virus (HIV) infection in children under 13 years of age. MMWR 36:225–235, 1987.

on the basis of symptoms. The CD4 count used as an indication for treatment of asymptomatic adults, less than 500/mm^3, is an appropriate CD4 cell count for beginning zidovudine therapy in older children (older than 6 years of age).

The recommended dose of zidovudine, based on pediatric clinical trials is 180 mg/m^2 per dose given every 6 hours around the clock. This dose has been found to be active in HIV-infected children, with many patients showing improvement in clinical well-being, growth, immunologic parameters, virologic parameters, and neurologic function. Many children, however, experience toxicity at this dose, primarily bone marrow suppression manifested as clinically significant anemia and granulocytopenia.

In adults, comparatively much lower doses have been found to be as effective as higher doses in all respects, with the possible exception of improved neurologic function in patients with encephalopathy. A recently completed NIH-sponsored trial in children comparing the 180 mg/m^2, every-6-hour zidovudine regimen with a 90 mg/m^2 every-6-hour regimen should provide important information on the efficacy of low-dose zidovudine in children. On the basis of the marked improvements in cognitive function observed in an early pediatric study and because of the potential for achieving greater central nervous system activity by maintaining constant plasma levels of zidovudine, an ongoing study in the Pediatric Branch of the National Cancer Institute (NCI) is evaluating the role of zidovudine given by continuous intravenous infusion in children with documented HIV encephalopathy.

Our approach is to initiate oral zidovudine at the recommended dose of 180 mg/m^2 every 6 hours, with clinical and laboratory monitoring for evidence of toxicity on a monthly or bimonthly basis. Patients with more advanced HIV disease may require more frequent follow-up. Included in the laboratory monitoring are complete blood count with differential, liver function tests, creatine phosphokinase (CPK) as well as immunologic (CD4 counts) and virologic (p24 antigen) monitoring on a less frequent basis. Periodic neurologic and neuropsychometric evaluations are also extremely valuable as measures of treatment response or disease progression.

Neutropenia (polymorphonuclear cell plus band form count less than 500 to 750/mm^3) is an indication for temporary discontinuation of zidovudine followed by dose reduction. Significant anemia (hemoglobin below 7.5 to 8.0 g/dl) can be managed by transfusion on an intermittent basis; however, a persistent transfusion requirement (one transfusion per month for 2 or more months, or two transfusions in less than 2 months) is an indication for dose reduction. Other causes of anemia (e.g., iron deficiency, lead poisoning, hemoglobinopathy) should be investigated thoroughly, with the awareness that the macrocytosis caused by zidovudine will obscure the usual changes in red blood cell indices that would indicate other causes of anemia.

Dose reduction to 120 mg/m^2 every 6 hours often allows continuation of zidovudine therapy in patients who experienced toxicity at the higher dose. Recurrence of hematologic toxicity at this reduced dose level can be problematic. Further dose reduction, alternative antiretroviral therapy, or adjunctive therapy may be necessary to maintain red blood cell or white blood cell parameters. Unfortunately, no data exist on the efficacy of low-dose zidovudine in children, access to other antiretroviral therapies is limited, and adjunctive therapies (such as granulocyte colony-stimulating factor and erythropoietin), although commercially available, have not been approved for this indication in children and are very expensive.

Additional less common toxicities of zidovudine include a mitochondrial myopathy, headache, nausea, and insomnia. The myopathy is suggested by weakness and muscle tenderness in association with elevation of CPK. Characteristic histopathology on muscle biopsy confirms this diagnosis and is an indication for discontinuation of zidovudine. The other adverse effects noted can usually be managed symptomatically; however, they rarely may be severe enough to require dose reduction or even discontinuation.

Viral resistance to zidovudine has been demonstrated to occur in a significant proportion of patients receiving the drug, especially those with more advanced HIV disease and presumably a higher viral load. The clinical significance of viral drug resistance remains to be determined; however, this issue may prove to be of critical importance in the long-term therapy of HIV infection.

Other Dideoxynucleosides

2',3',-Dideoxyinosine (Didanosine, ddl)

The Food and Drug Administration (FDA) approved ddl in October 1991 for adults and children who were unable to take zidovudine because of toxicity or disease progression. Prior to its approval, this agent was evaluated extensively in adults and, to a lesser extent, in children through clinical trials and through a novel expanded-access program. The simultaneous approval of ddl for adults and children, along with its approval primarily on the basis of data from uncontrolled trials, are both landmarks in the process of approval of therapies for AIDS and other life-threatening diseases.

A phase I/II study conducted in the Pediatric Branch of the NCI provides much of the available information on the use of ddl in children. As was the case with zidovudine, many children receiving ddl showed improvement in clinical status, weight gain, immunologic parameters, virologic parameters, and neurologic function. Importantly, hematologic toxicity, the major toxic result from zidovudine, was not a significant problem in this study. Pancreatitis, however, occurred in a small proportion of children in this study, especially at higher doses—a finding similar to the experience that has accumulated in adult ddl recipients. The apparent dose dependence of this toxicity and the relatively lower doses of ddl recommended for clinical use in children should make this an uncommon complication of ddl therapy. Painful peripheral neuropathy, seen at high doses in early adult studies, is rare in children at the doses currently being evaluated. An important finding from this study is the low oral bioavailability and the marked interpatient variability in absorption of ddl.

The pediatric dose of ddl recommended by the manufacturer is 200 mg/m^2/day divided in two daily doses, although investigators have used doses of 270 mg/m^2/day with little serious toxicity. The optimal dose of this agent in HIV-infected children remains to be defined. ddl is acid-labile and must be taken with an antacid in order to prevent degradation of the drug by stomach acid. ddl has therefore been formulated as a chewable, dispersible, buffered tablet; as a buffered powder for oral solution in single-dose packages; and as a powder for oral solution that is reconstituted with water and liquid antacid, thus providing several options for pediatric administration. The bioavailability of these formulations may differ, and extensive pediatric pharmacokinetic data exist only for the oral solution administered with liquid antacid.

Careful monitoring of children receiving ddl is essential. Monthly or bimonthly clinical and laboratory evaluation for drug tolerance and disease status should be performed as described for zidovudine recipients. In addition to the laboratory tests previously noted, measurement of serum amylase and/or lipase may be useful. Asymptomatic hyperamylasemia does not appear to be a specific indicator of impending pancreatitis, however, and we do not use it as an indication to discontinue ddl therapy. Measurement of serum lipase or fractionation of serum amylase into salivary and pancreatic forms may prove more specific in screening for subclinical pancreatic inflammation. Elevation of amylase or lipase in association with signs or symptoms of pancreatitis (nausea, vomiting, abdominal pain) is an absolute indication for discontinuation of ddl pending further patient evaluation. Patients should be monitored for symptoms of peripheral neuropathy, which presents as pain, numbness, or tingling of the hands or feet. The occurrence of these symptoms warrants discontinuation of ddl pending evaluation. A retinal examination with dilatation should be performed at least every 6 months, based on the occurrence of peripheral retinal atrophy with depigmentation in four children receiving ddl in the NCI study.

Although ddl is approved for use in patients intolerant of zidovudine or who experience clinical or immunologic deterioration while receiving zidovudine, neither of these concepts is precisely defined. Decisions to change antiretroviral therapy, therefore, require careful consideration, and subspecialist consultation may be appropriate. As ddl comes into widespread clinical use, significant improvement in our understanding of pediatric dosing, pharmacokinetics, toxicities, and antiviral activity can be anticipated.

2',3',-Dideoxycytosine (Zalcitabine, ddC) and Other Nucleosides

The most potent anti-HIV nucleoside evaluated thus far, ddC has been less widely evaluated than zidovudine or ddl. It appears to be active in vivo, but its use has been limited by toxicities, including painful peripheral neuropathy, rash, and oral ulcerations. ddC has been evaluated as part of an alternating regimen with zidovudine and is well tolerated in this setting, although the benefit of an alternating regimen over zidovudine alone is not known. Lower doses of ddC, as a single agent and as a component of combination therapies, are being evaluated in adults and children for evidence of activity with reduced toxicity. The Food and Drug Administration recently approved ddC for use in adults in combination with zidovudine.

Numerous other nucleoside analogues are in various stages of development, with the goals of increased antiviral potency, decreased toxicity, prolonged half-life, and better central nervous system penetration. It is expected that this class of drug, led by zidovudine and ddl, will be the mainstays of antiretroviral therapy for the immediate future.

Other Antiretroviral Agents

The complexity of the life cycle of HIV-1 that makes it such a formidable pathogen also provides several potential targets for antiretroviral therapy. Agents directed at many of these targets are being developed and hold the promise for much improved therapy of HIV infection.

A number of non-nucleosides with in vitro anti-HIV activity that act by inhibition of reverse transcriptase have been developed. The rapid emergence of resistance to these drugs, however, may limit their clinical utility.

The interaction between HIV-1 and its specific receptor, the CD4 molecule found on the surface of some T lymphocytes, has been a target for antiretroviral therapies. A truncated form of this CD4 molecule was found to have in vitro activity in blocking infection by HIV-1. Clinical trials to date have demonstrated the safety of this agent, but there is little evidence of antiviral activity in vivo. Variants of CD4 as well as other receptor-blocking agents, such as small peptides, are being developed and may ultimately prove more useful as therapeutic agents.

HIV-1 encodes a specific protease that is required for expression of several viral genes. A number of specific inhibitors of this protease have been developed and have been found to exhibit anti-HIV activity in vitro. Although clinical testing of these agents has just begun, protease inhibitors hold great promise as potent, specific anti-HIV drugs.

Other agents that are still in the preclinical or very early stages of clinical development include, among others, antisense oligonucleotides, high-titer anti-HIV immune globulin, and interferons.

ADJUNCTIVE THERAPY

Included in the category of adjunctive therapy are agents without specific antiviral activity that act to ameliorate the deleterious effects of HIV infection or of drug therapy for HIV infection.

Erythropoietin

Anemia secondary to zidovudine is improved by erythropoietin in HIV-infected adults with low endogenous levels of erythropoietin. The use of erythropoietin in children is not established; however, it is expected that a comparable subgroup of HIV-infected children might benefit. Starting doses in adults range from 50 to 100 units given three times per week, with adjustments based on response. A recent study in the Pediatric Branch, NCI, evaluated the use of erythropoietin in HIV-infected children with zidovudine-induced anemia and found it to be well tolerated but with limited beneficial effects.

Granulocyte Colony-Stimulating Factor

Granulocyte colony-stimulating factor is also useful in maintaining adequate granulocyte counts in HIV-infected adults and is associated with minimal side effects. Doses ranging from less than 1 to 20 μg/kg/day, administered by subcutaneous injection, appeared to be beneficial in children with a history of zidovudine-related neutropenia in a recent study in the Pediatric Branch, NCI.

Intravenous Immunoglobulin

Intravenous immunoglobulin (IVIG) has been used extensively in children with HIV infection in an attempt to prevent the recurrent bacterial infections to which these children are prone. The value of this approach has not been clearly defined, although one study has indicated efficacy at a dose of 400 mg/kg given every 4 weeks in preventing bacterial infection among the subgroup of symptomatic HIV-infected children with CD4 cell counts greater than 200/mm^3. An ongoing NIH–sponsored study is evaluating the role of IVIG in preventing bacterial infection in HIV-infected children receiving zidovudine. There is no consensus on the use of IVIG in this patient population, with approaches ranging from treatment of all symptomatic children, to treatment only of children with a prior history of recurrent bacterial infections, to minimal use of this treatment modality.

THERAPY OF SECONDARY PROCESSES

Information regarding the therapy of many secondary processes is presented in other articles in this volume. Information of particular relevance to the treatment of HIV-infected children is presented here.

Lymphocytic Interstitial Pneumonitis

Lymphocyte interstitial pneumonitis (LIP) occurs in a significant proportion of HIV-infected children, generally in those who survive infancy with relatively high CD4 cell counts. Generally a slowly progressive lymphoproliferative process, LIP is often asymptomatic and may be diagnosed on chest radiograph in the absence of symptoms. In some children, this process becomes symptomatic, with shortness of breath and desaturation at rest or with exercise. In symptomatic children, a short course of corticosteroids may be beneficial, but it is essential to rule out an intercurrent infectious process as the cause of respiratory symptoms prior to initiating steroids. Prednisone (2 mg/kg/day in divided doses) is given for 2 to 4 weeks, followed by a taper to 1 mg/kg as a single dose on alternate days. Pulmonary function testing with measurement of blood oxygen saturation at baseline, following daily steroid therapy, and during follow-up is useful to determine the individual patient's response to steroid therapy as well as the persistence of this response.

Pneumocystis carinii Pneumonia

P. carinii infection is the most common presentation of AIDS in children and is a major cause of mortality in HIV-infected children. First-line treatment remains trimethoprim-sulfamethoxazole (TMP-SMX) at a dose of 20 mg/kg/day of trimethoprim in four divided doses. The daily dose should not exceed 960 mg of TMP. Monitoring of serum TMP or SMX levels may be useful in this setting. Intravenous pentamidine isethionate as a single daily infusion of 4 mg/kg is an alternative agent with similar efficacy but increased side effects.

Lack of response to initial therapy for the first few days is typical of patients with this illness and does not indicate drug failure. Lack of response after 4 to 5 days may be an indication to change (or add) therapy; however, the crucial issue of when to adjust anti-pneumocystis therapy remains unresolved. Alternatives to TMP-SMX and pentamidine include agents such as trimetrexate, dapsone-trimethoprim, clindamycin, and others, but the efficacy of these agents relative to TMP-SMX remains to be determined. Short-course corticosteroids are of benefit in adults with moderate to severe *P. carinii* infection, when used early after presentation. Given the poor outcome of *P. carinii* infection in children, use of steroids with similar indications seems warranted.

Important new information regarding the ranges of CD4 cell counts in normal infants and children has led to a recent major revision of guidelines for prophylaxis of *P. carinii* infection in HIV-infected children.* These guidelines are presented in Table 2, with prophylaxis recommendations based on age and CD4 cell count for children born to HIV-positive mothers, for children who are definitively HIV-infected, and for children who are HIV-seropositive whose infection status is not yet determined. The recommended regimen is TMP-SMX, with 150 mg/m^2/day of TMP divided in two doses given on 3 consecutive days per week. Alternatives for children who cannot take TMP-SMX include aerosolized pentamidine for older children (300 mg on a monthly basis), or oral dapsone (1 mg/kg/day). Intravenous pentamidine (4 mg/kg every 2 to 4 weeks) has been used as well, but its efficacy is unknown.

---

*More detailed discussion of these guidelines is presented in a publication from the National AIDS Information Clearinghouse, P.O. Box 6003, Rockville, MD 20850.

TABLE 2. Indications* for *Pneumocystis carinii* Pneumonia Prophylaxis Based on Age and CD4 Cell Count†

Age	CD4 Count to Initiate *P. carinii* Prophylaxis	CD4 Count Requiring Monthly Monitoring
1–11 months	<1500	1500–2000
12–23 months	<750	750–1000
24–71 months	<500	500–750
6 years or older	<200	200–300

Data from Centers for Disease Control: MMWR 40 (No. RR-2), 1991. Copies are available from the National AIDS Information Clearinghouse, P.O. Box 6003, Rockville, MD 20850.

*These prophylaxis indications are for children known to be HIV-infected, children who are HIV-seropositive but of undetermined infection status, and children of unknown infection and sero-status who are younger than 12 months of age and who were born to an HIV-infected mother. Children in these categories whose CD4 cell count is not known should begin prophylaxis pending the results of T cell subset analysis. Children whose CD4 cell percentage is less than 20% should have prophylaxis initiated regardless of the absolute CD4 cell count.

†CD4 counts are CD4-positive lymphocytes per cubic millimeter.

Cytomegalovirus

Cytomegalovirus (CMV) causes retinitis and colitis in HIV-infected children. Treatment of CMV disease is limited at present. Ganciclovir is the agent of choice for children. Therapy for CMV retinitis is initiated at 10 mg/kg/day in two divided doses for 2 to 3 weeks until visible remission occurs, after which maintenance therapy (5 mg/kg/day in a single dose) can be administered. Relapse after weeks to months is common, and patients may respond to a second course at 10 mg/kg/day. Treatment of CMV colitis generally does not require maintenance therapy, although relapse may occur. A major toxicity of ganciclovir is bone marrow suppression, making the concomitant use of high-dose zidovudine and ganciclovir difficult.

Phosphonoformate (foscarnet) is also approved for the treatment of CMV retinitis in adults and may be associated with improved survival. As is the case with ganciclovir, breakthrough disease progression appears to be a common outcome in patients with CMV retinitis receiving long-term foscarnet. There are few data on the use of foscarnet in children; accordingly, its use should be limited to pediatric patients with progressive retinitis despite therapy with ganciclovir.

Herpes Simplex Virus and Varicella-Zoster Virus

Herpes simplex virus (HSV) may cause a particularly severe gingivostomatitis as a primary or recurrent infection in HIV-infected children. Treatment with oral or intravenous acyclovir is warranted in severe cases, as described elsewhere in this book. Varicella-zoster virus (VZV) infection has been a major problem in HIV-infected children. Susceptible children who are exposed to chickenpox should receive Zoster Immune Globulin as soon as possible within 96 hours of exposure.

Treatment with intravenous acyclovir at a dose of 1500 mg/m^2/day in three divided doses, with vigorous hydration, is warranted for acute chickenpox in the HIV-infected child. Recurrent dermatomal zoster as well as persistent diffuse cutaneous varicella lesions is a major problem for some HIV-infected children. These manifestations usually respond to intravenous acyclovir; however, recurrences may occur once acyclovir is discontinued. The role of suppressive oral acyclovir in this setting is not known but is likely to be limited because of its poor oral bioavailability.

Mucosal Candidiasis

Candidal infection is present in nearly all symptomatic HIV-infected children. Oral candidiasis can often be controlled with oral nystatin suspension (2 to 6 ml four times per day) or clotrimazole lozenges (five times per day). Although the nystatin suspension is convenient for infants, clotrimazole lozenges are generally more effective in children who are old enough to use them. Ketoconazole (5 mg/kg/day in one or two divided doses) or fluconazole (3 to 6 mg/kg/day as a single dose) is useful for treating refractory oral candidiasis and as therapy for esophageal candidiasis. Fluconazole appears to be more effective than ketoconazole for the treatment of esophageal candidiasis in HIV-infected adults. Intravenous amphotericin B remains the treatment of choice for patients with candidiasis that is not responsive to these oral agents.

Mycobacterium avium Complex Infection

M. avium infection occurs as a systemic process in severely immunocompromised HIV-infected adults and children, causing syndromes of recurrent fever, bone marrow suppression, abdominal pain, and diarrhea. No consistently effective treatment has been demonstrated, although combinations of three or more drugs, including amikacin, ethambutol, rifampin or rifabutin, clofazamine, ciprofloxacin, or others, may be beneficial in some patients. Several new agents, including new macrolides with increased in vitro activity against *M. avium,* are being evaluated for the treatment of this infection. A phase I pediatric trial of clarithromycin, among the most active of the new macrolides, is being conducted in the Pediatric Branch of NCI. Rifabutin appears to be effective prophylaxis against *M. avium* in adults with low CD4 counts and is being studied for this indication in children.

Recurrent Bacterial Infections

Treatment of recurrent bacterial infections makes use of standard antimicrobial agents specific for the pathogen involved, as discussed elsewhere. Presumptive therapy pending culture results should have a broad spectrum of antibacterial activity because of the wide diversity of gram-negative and gram-positive organisms to which HIV-infected children are susceptible.

Other Infections

HIV-infected children are susceptible to a wide variety of other opportunistic and nonopportunistic infections, such as toxoplasmosis and intestinal parasitic disease caused by organisms including *Cryptosporidium, Giardia lamblia, Isospora belli,* and *Microsporidium.* Treatments for these infections are discussed elsewhere in this book.

VAGINITIS AND URETHRITIS

LOUIS FRIEDLANDER, M.D.

Vulvovaginal complaints in adolescent females are exceedingly common. Sole reliance on symptoms, including dysuria, pruritus, and vaginal discharge to distinguish between upper tract disease and additional lower tract problems (e.g., cervicitis, cystitis), is often misleading.

A detailed sexual and general medical history as well as the physical examination will help to distinguish leukorrhea from pathologic entities. Appropriate use of simple laboratory tests may clarify the presumptive diagnosis of vaginitis, cystitis, urethritis, or cervicitis. Identification of the specific etiologic agent will determine pharmacologic therapy and preventive measures.

LEUKORRHEA

Physiologic leukorrhea refers to a normal (physiologic) increase in vaginal discharge (leukorrhea) due to estrogen stimulation. Mucoid endocervical secretions combine with sloughed vaginal epithelial cells and normal bacteria to form a physiologic vaginal discharge.

This condition is often noted during the first few days or weeks in newborns and often in girls around menarche. At birth, the secretion is sterile and has a pH of 5.0 to 6.0. As maternal estrogens fall the infant's vulvovaginal tissue becomes thin and alkaline (pH 7.0 to 8.0). At puberty, the genital tract becomes estrogenized. The prepubertal vagina becomes colonized with flora rich in anaerobic bacteria (in particular *Bacteroides* species), *Staphylococcus epidermidis*, and yeasts. *Ureaplasma* and *Gardnerella vaginalis* occur in 20 to 25 per cent of females who have not commenced sexual activity. Acidic pH 5.0 to 5.5 results from the action of lactobacilli on epithelial cell glycogen to produce lactic acid.

Physiologic leukorrhea is variable in quantity and is usually a clear white or gray mucoid discharge that is not associated with itching, irritation, or odor. There is usually no sign of inflammation of the vagina or vulva. The labia may be sodden from excessive secretions.

It is important to reassure the patient that the condition is physiologic and does not represent sexually transmitted disease (STD) or genital injury. Frequent changes of cotton undergarments to help to absorb the leukorrhea, and frequent bathing is all that is required.

VULVOVAGINITIS IN PREPUBERTAL FEMALES

Vulvovaginitis in prepubertal females, common in preschool and school-aged children, may be due to nonspecific factors, meaning that no specific microbe is found. Causes include improper perianal hygiene; foreign bodies, such as toilet paper; and fecal contamination. Chemical irritation can result from laundry detergents, bubble-baths, perfumed toilet paper, soaps, use of sprays, and pinworms. Vulvovaginitis may be induced by gastroenteritis *(Shigella, Salmonella)* and respiratory tract infection *(Haemophilus influenzae, Neisseria meningitidis)*.

Skin microbes such as beta-hemolytic streptococcus and *Staphylococcus aureus* can lead to vaginal discharge. Isolation of sexually transmitted pathogens or evidence of genital trauma should raise the question of sexual abuse.

Complaints of itching, burning, dysuria, and malodorous discharge result from irritation, rubbing, and scratching of the genital area.

Treatment of Nonspecific Vulvovaginitis

Treatment depends on recognition and elimination of underlying local causes. Attention should be given to proper toilet procedures, avoidance of exposure to local irritants, and removal of foreign bodies, such as paper and fecal material.

Pinworms *(Enterobius vermicularis)* are treated with Mebendazole (Vermox, 100 mg orally in a single dose) or pyrantel pamoate (11 mg/kg up to 1 g in a single dose).

Treatment of respiratory, gastrointestinal, and skin infection is discussed elsewhere.

VAGINITIS IN THE ADOLESCENT

There is often a specific etiology for the symptomatic adolescent who complains of vaginal discharge. Information should be obtained regarding the quality, quantity, and odor of the discharge; associated pruritus; dysuria; sexual activity; and contraceptive practices. Careful evaluation should include measurement of vaginal fluid pH, wet mount, potassium hydroxide (KOH) examination of the vaginal fluid for detection of yeast infections, endocervical culture for *Neisseria gonorrhoeae*, and antigen detection tests for *Chlamydia trachomatis*. A Gram-stained smear of endocervical secretions and a Papanicolaou smear are obtained.

Patients with urinary tract symptoms should undergo urine culture in addition to the evaluation for sexually transmitted pathogens.

BACTERIAL VAGINOSIS*

Bacterial vaginosis, formerly called *Haemophilus* or *Gardnerella vaginalis* vaginitis or nonspecific vaginitis, is the most common cause of malodorous vaginal discharge in sexually active individuals. *G. vaginalis* is a gram-negative, facultative, surface anaerobe that rarely causes gross vulvovaginal inflammatory changes or pruritus. Several other anaerobic bacteria, including motile, curved, gram-negative anaerobic rods (classified Mobiluncus) are involved in this complex syndrome, which is poorly understood.

Diagnosis is based on a thin, grayish-white, homogeneous, frequently frothy vaginal discharge that has a foul-smelling "fishy" odor, a vaginal fluid pH greater than 4.5, a positive whiff test (amine odor when KOH is added to the vaginal fluid) and clue cells (epithelial cells studded with numerous gram-negative bacilli on its surface) on examination of a wet preparation of vaginal secretions. The vagina shows no inflammatory changes. Vulvar pruritus is not common.

Treatment

Treatment is directed towards the eradication of the high level of anaerobic bacteria in the vagina.

Oral metronidazole (Flagyl, Metryl, Protostat), 2 g taken initially and again in 48 hours, or 500 mg orally twice daily for 7 days, is usually effective. Problems with use include metallic taste, reversible neutropenia, and lowered seizure threshold. Metronidazole favors overgrowth of *Monilia* infection. Patients should be warned not to drink alcohol because nausea and vomiting may occur (Antabuse-type reaction). The use of metronidazole is contraindicated during the first 20 weeks of pregnancy.

Oral clindamycin (Cleocin HCl, 300 mg three times daily for 7 days) may be effective.

During pregnancy, Augmentin (amoxicillin and potassium clavulanate, 500 mg three times a day for 7 to 10 days) is used, but it is not effective in all cases.

Because sexual partners often harbor the organism in the urethra, their treatment is recommended if there is a recurrence. Use of condoms is recommended.

TRICHOMONAS VAGINALIS VAGINITIS

Trichomonas vaginalis vaginitis is characterized by a malodorous vaginal discharge that is homogeneous yellow-green or frothy with a vaginal pH greater than 4.5. The vagina and cervix may be erythematous, and occasionally punctate hemorrhages or strawberry spots are seen on the cervix. Severe cases may involve excoriation of the vulva or inner thighs. Ten per cent of cases are asymptomatic and, when observed, should be treated because of increased pathogenicity in the upper genital tract. Examination of wet preparations reveals numerous unicellular, pear-shaped, flagellated organisms (protozoa) usually twice the size of normal leukocytes.

Treatment

The only effective treatment for *T. vaginalis* vaginitis is metronidazole. A single 2-g dose appears to be as effective as

*Formerly called *Haemophilus* or *Gardnerella vaginalis* vaginitis or nonspecific vaginitis.

the 7-day treatment regimen and is the preferred regimen for most adolescents. Treatment of sexual partners is recommended to prevent treatment failure. When a single dose is not tolerated, metronidazole (250 mg three times a day for 7 days) may be given in divided doses.

Adjunctive therapies for symptomatic relief include acidification with vinegar or Aci-Jel douches.

During the first half of pregnancy, when metronidazole is contraindicated, clotrimazole (Mycelex, Gyne-Lotrimin, 100 mg tablets intravaginally at night for 7 days) is prescribed. This preparation is thought to act by lowering the pH of secretions, thereby preventing reproduction of trichomonads.

CANDIDA VAGINITIS

The predominant organism is *Candida albicans (Monilia albicans)* in 90 per cent and *Torulopsis glabrata* in 10 per cent of patients. Characteristic findings include vaginal and vulvar erythema, vulvar edema, pruritus (often intense), and the presence of a thick, white, odorless discharge that resembles cottage cheese. Diagnosis is confirmed by microscopic findings of yeast forms on a KOH preparation or by culturing the organism on Nickersen's medium.

Predisposing factors to yeast infection include:

1. Eradication of bacterial normal flora through use of broad-spectrum antibiotics or metronidazole.
2. Increase in glycogen content in vaginal epithelial cells with lowering of pH as in pregnancy, diabetes, and birth control medications.
3. Debilitating illness, iron-deficiency anemia, and corticosteroids.
4. Constant reinfection exposure from intestinal reservoir, contaminated soaps, infected male partners, practice of orogenital sex from transmission in saliva.
5. Increase in heat or moisture—obesity; tight, or nylon undergarments; or allergy.

Candidiasis may also be chronically recurrent in otherwise healthy subjects.

Treatment

Several regimens have been recommended:

- Clotrimazole (500 mg vaginal tablet in a single dose)
- Miconazole nitrate (Monistat 3), 200 mg as a vaginal suppository inserted one time daily for 3 days
- Butaconazole nitrate 2 per cent cream (Femstat), one applicatorful intravaginally one time daily for 3 days

Each is as effective as longer courses of therapy even in cases of recurrent infection.

Terconazole (0.4 per cent vaginal cream, Terazole 7, an 80-mg suppository, Terazole 3) has been introduced once at night for three nights or vaginal cream for 7 nights.

In resistant cases, painting the vagina, cervix, and vulva with 1 per cent gentian violet (Genepax) daily for 3 or 4 days gives rapid relief despite the fact that this procedure is messy and stains clothing.

Acute vulvitis may be relieved with warm sitz baths with baking soda and hydrocortisone ointment. Pruritus is relieved with white vinegar douches.

For recurrent and persistent candidiasis, use of an oral antifungal medication helps to eliminate candidal organisms from the intestinal tract to reduce reinfection in the vagina. Ketoconazole (Nizoral) 400 mg daily for 2 weeks, followed by 100 mg daily for 6 months, may be given. Liver enzymes should be checked for hepatic toxicity. Nystatin (500 mg three times daily for 2 weeks to 6 months) may be used.

Loose-fitting clothing and cotton underwear should be worn. Avoid tight or nylon undergarments.

In cases of recurrent yeast infections, male partners should be carefully screened and treated for evidence of local disease (e.g. balanitis). The use of condoms is strongly advised.

URETHRITIS

Symptoms of dysuria, discomfort, pain, and itching range from trivial to disabling. Urethral discharge, more frequently recognized in males, may be scanty to mucopurulent and white, yellow, green, or brown. Discharge is expressed by pressure on the urethra. Specimens of material obtained by calcium alginate urethral swabs will reveal polymorphonuclear leukocytes. Gram stain may reveal gram-negative intracellular diplococci. Nongonococcal urethritis (NGU) cannot be ruled out. As a result of the great clinical overlap between gonorrhea and NGU, diagnosis cannot be made solely on clinical grounds. Appropriate tests will identify trichomonads, *Ureaplasma urealyticum,* candidiasis, and *G. vaginalis.*

Urethritis may accompany noninfectious disease (e.g. Stevens-Johnson syndrome) and chemical irritation from vaginal chemicals used by the sexual partner.

Dysuria, the result of primary herpes genital infection, should be confirmed by culture and scrapings of the base of the ulcer stained with Giemsa stain (Tzanck preparation) showing multinucleated giant cells highly suggestive of herpes.

Because ulcerations may be secondarily infected, positive bacterial cultures must be interpreted with caution. Visual examination and urethroscopy may be indicated to exclude noninfectious states. Urethral caruncle (a reddened, tender, polypoid excrescence protruding from the urethral meatus) and urethral prolapse (a circular eversion of the mucosa at the urethral meatus) may be associated with dysuria, frequency, and hematuria. These lesions should be differentiated from urethritis by careful examination. Surgical treatment is usually indicated.

ACUTE URETHRAL SYNDROME

In acute urethral syndrome, dysuria, frequency, urgency, and nocturia occur with no apparent evidence of urinary tract infection. Bacterial pathogens are not isolated. This condition appears to be due to sexually transmitted pathogens (e.g., *Chlamydia* or *Ureaplasma*) and treated accordingly. Asymptomatic urethral infection in males and females is well recognized as a cause of spread of STD. It is therefore mandatory to treat asymptomatic sexual partners at the time of presentation.

BLASTOMYCOSIS

THOMAS G. MITCHELL, Ph.D.

Blastomycosis is a chronic disease characterized by granulomatous and suppurative lesions. The infection is initiated by inhalation of the thermally dimorphic fungus *Blastomyces dermatitidis.* From the lung, dissemination may occur to any organ but occurs preferentially to the skin and bones. Blastomycosis is endemic to eastern parts of the United States, but little is known about its prevalence. *B. dermatitidis* cannot be readily isolated from nature, and a good skin test is not available for population surveys of exposure to *B. dermatitidis.* Unlike histoplasmosis and coccidioidomycosis, blastomycosis does not occur frequently in immunocompromised patients, such as those with acquired immunodeficiency syndrome

(AIDS). There have been almost a dozen reports of outbreaks of blastomycosis attributed to common exposure to *B. dermatitidis,* and many cases have been associated with river banks. Investigations have yielded important information about the natural history of blastomycosis, and several pediatric cases have occurred during outbreaks of blastomycosis.

The primary pulmonary infection may be inapparent to severe. Even if the infection is inapparent, dissemination may ensue to the skin, bones, or other sites. If the pulmonary episode is severe, the generalized systemic disease may develop and may involve multiple organs. In cases associated with outbreaks, the incubation period was 3 to 12 weeks and spontaneous recovery can follow primary blastomycosis. Overall, most cases occur in adult males, but in pediatric blastomycosis, children of both sexes are equally susceptible.

Most cases in children are recognized as acute blastomycosis. Patients with symptomatic, primary pulmonary infection may present with symptoms of mild respiratory infection, including cough, chest pain, and high fever as well as numerous other complaints. The primary pulmonary infection may persist locally, spread to other organ(s), or both. Alternatively, the pulmonary lesion may heal by fibrosis and absorption, leaving no residual evidence of infection. In patients whose pulmonary lesions have resolved, dissemination, generally to the skin, may already have occurred. If the pulmonary focus becomes more severe, an acute to chronic lung infection may develop. Patients with chronic pulmonary blastomycosis usually present with cough, low-grade fever, loss of weight, night sweats, and other problems. The most common forms of pulmonary involvement are infiltration, cavitation, pneumonia, or nodules.

A wide variety of symptoms, pathology, and radiographic appearances may be observed in blastomycosis. After the lung, the most frequently involved organs are the skin, bones, and genitourinary tract, followed by the central nervous system, liver, or spleen. Less often, the lymph nodes, thyroid, heart, adrenal, omentum, gastrointestinal tract, muscles, and pancreas may become infected.

DIAGNOSIS

Blastomycosis is best diagnosed by positive culture or direct examination of sputum, skin lesion, or other specimen. *B. dermatitidis* grows on most routine culture media to produce a mold with variable macroscopic features and conidia. Its identification is confirmed by growth on a rich medium at 37°C and conversion to the characteristic yeast form; alternatively, a *B. dermatitidis*–specific antigen (exoantigen A) may be extracted and identified by an immunodiffusion test using reference antisera and antigen. In a 37°C culture, histopathologic sections or fresh calcofluor white or potassium hydroxide preparations, *B. dermatitidis* forms large (8 to 15 μm) single-budding yeast cells with highly refractory cell walls and a broad attachment between the bud and parent yeast cell. In tissue sections, the yeasts are better seen with periodic acid–Schiff or methenamine silver stains. Because the tests for complement-fixing antibodies and delayed skin reactivity lack specificity and sensitivity, they are not helpful unless the patient is negative to heterologous fungal antigens; even then, positive, monospecific serologic tests to *B. dermatitidis* may not indicate active infection. Serologic tests for antibodies to the specific antigen A, which can be detected by the immunodiffusion test or an enzyme immunoassay, are more suggestive of infection, but negative tests do not exclude blastomycosis.

TREATMENT

As indicated by the outbreak cases, immunocompetent individuals with primary blastomycosis may not require therapy. However, the patient with proven, primary pulmonary infection that is mild and resolves spontaneously without treatment must be closely observed for at least 2 years after primary infection because of the possible occurrence of reactivation blastomycosis. Patients with protracted, severe, or progressive primary infection or chronic pulmonary or disseminated blastomycosis require treatment.

Ketoconazole

Ketoconazole is recommended for less severely infected patients (i.e., blastomycosis that is neither life-threatening nor involving the central nervous system). A dose of 400 mg/day for 6 months is effective in most adult patients, but patients must be closely observed because relapses have occurred with ketoconazole therapy. For difficult cases, treatment with higher doses (800 mg/day) for more than 6 months, if tolerated, may be effective. The adverse effects of ketoconazole include liver toxicity and reversible hormonal imbalances (e.g., gynecomastia) as well as nausea, pruritus, dizziness, or headache. In the future, other azoles, such as itraconazole or fluconazole, may prove effective.

Amphotericin B

B. dermatitidis is quite susceptible to amphotericin B, which is the recommended treatment for patients with severe disease (e.g., involvement of several organs), those with meningitis, or immunocompromised patients with blastomycosis, and patients who do not respond to ketoconazole. In adults, a total dose of at least 2 g is required to eradicate all the organisms. When a dose of 1.5 g or less is administered, the relapse rate is significant.

The protocol for administration of amphotericin B and monitoring renal function is similar to its application for other mycoses. An initial test dose of 1 or 5 mg in adults is administered intravenously in a solution of 5 per cent glucose, deoxycholate, and buffer. The dose is gradually increased by 5 to 10 mg/day to a maximal daily administration of 0.5 to 1.5 mg/kg. Most patients experience toxic side effects, including renal dysfunction, fever, anorexia, phlebitis, hypokalemia, nausea, chills, headache, and anemia. Administration is interrupted when blood levels of urea nitrogen reach 40 to 50 mg/dl or 3.0 to 3.5 mg/dl of creatinine. Blastomycosis in patients with AIDS may require maintenance therapy following the initial course of treatment with amphotericin B, similar to the management of histoplasmosis in patients with AIDS.

For children, the test dose of 0.1 mg/kg (maximum dose 1 mg) should be followed by 0.25 mg/kg at 4 hours later and 0.5 mg/kg after 24 hours. Beyond 48 hours, 1 mg/kg/day is administered. Pediatric as well as adult patients must be closely monitored for adverse reactions.

Blastomycosis has been reported in pregnant women, and the infection may or may not be transmitted to the infant. Pregnant patients have been treated with amphotericin B without congenital or toxic effects in the fetus.

Surgery

Corrective surgery may be necessary as an adjunct to antibiotic treatment. Because of the occurrence of relapse or reactivation blastomycosis, patients should be observed for years after treatment and resolution of disease.

FEVER OF UNKNOWN ORIGIN

J. CARLTON GARTNER, JR.

From early times, fever has been regarded as a cardinal symptom of disease. Unfortunately, many consider fever a disease itself and not a physiologic response to stimuli. In the past few years, the precise mechanism of fever production has been elucidated. Numerous infectious or immunologic agents (exogenous pyrogens) induce monocytes or fixed tissue macrophages to release interleukin-1 (endogenous pyrogen). Among the myriad effects of this polypeptide (or group of peptides) is an increase in synthesis of certain prostaglandins in the anterior hypothalamus—raising the set-point of body temperature.

Accurate measurement and normative data are necessary before pursuit of a body temperature reading as elevated. Rectal temperature is regarded as the best practical method for approximating core body temperature. Oral temperature is influenced by respiratory rate and recent liquid intake. Electronic thermometers have largely replaced standard glass-mercury instruments but should be recalibrated periodically. The next development will be further perfection of instruments that will measure middle ear temperature by infrared emissions. Several studies have demonstrated that temperature in children is less precisely regulated than in adults and tends to be higher, especially in infants and toddlers. More than 50 percent of the 18-month-old-children in a study by Bayley and Stolz had a rectal temperature above 100°F.

Although fever for a few days is part of the course of many minor pediatric illnesses (and is the chief complaint in about one third of office visits), more persistent fever without obvious localizing signs (FWLS) is less common, and perhaps 5 to 10 per cent of children who present for outpatient evaluation will fall into this category. Some will have bacteremia.

True fever of unknown (or undetermined) origin (FUO) is rare. Definitions of the entity vary; however, in adults at least 3 weeks of fever without a diagnosis after 1 week of hospital evaluation is a generally accepted one. Unfortunately, definitions in pediatric studies vary from 5 to 7 days of fever to 3 weeks outpatient or 1 week inpatient evaluation without a diagnosis.

Some general conclusions are as follows:

1. Infectious diseases are most common, with respiratory tract infection predominant, followed by urinary tract, nervous system, and bone infections.
2. Uncommon presentation of common infections is the rule.
3. Younger children tend to have self-limited or more minor illness.
4. Collagen-vascular disease (e.g., juvenile rheumatoid arthritis, systemic lupus, rheumatic fever, Kawasaki disease) is next in frequency, followed by neoplastic disease. Many children recover without a diagnosis.

DIAGNOSIS

Several principles should be followed in the evaluation of children with FUO. Fever must be carefully documented by medical personnel. A detailed and repeated history along with meticulous physical examination is more likely to yield a diagnosis than is the laboratory or an imaging technique. Helpful screening tests that mandate further observation are an elevated sedimentation rate and reversal of the albumin-globulin ratio. Bone marrow examination and/or culture are most helpful when there are progressive abnormalities of the blood count involving several cell lines or in the immunocompromised child. Newer imaging procedures, such as computed tomography, are useful when symptoms and signs are localized, for example, to the abdomen.

TREATMENT

Obviously, once a diagnosis is established, the treatment for the individual disease can be initiated—and the current edition of this text may be extremely helpful. Once again, several principles apply. It is not necessary to treat minor elevations of body temperature as this may be helpful in combating the illness. Although the pattern of fever is not often helpful in arriving at a precise diagnosis, one should avoid overtreatment so that a helpful pattern may be discerned—such as the twice daily elevation, followed by subnormal temperature of rheumatoid arthritis. Characteristic rash may be seen only with the highest temperature rise.

Acetaminophen (10 to 15 mg/kg every 4 to 6 hours) is the drug of choice for routine treatment. Presumptive therapy with antimicrobial agents is indicated only rarely, and specimens for culture must be obtained before therapy is instituted. Indications for this therapy might be an immunocompromised host, presumptive endocarditis or pyelonephritis, or tuberculosis (especially with central nervous system involvement).

Several treatable disorders that may present as FUO have emerged over the past few years.

Sinusitis

Sinusitis of a subacute or chronic nature is frequently underdiagnosed. Presenting symptoms may be cough, fever, nasal discharge, malaise, headache, and fatigue. Often patients have been treated, but for a limited period. At least 3 to 4 weeks of a broad-spectrum semisynthetic penicillin (such as amoxicillin-clavulanic acid) has been successful.

Cat-Scratch Disease

Cat-scratch disease has recently emerged as a systemic disorder that may affect the nervous system or liver and may not be associated with adenopathy. Diagnosis is usually obtained by direct silver stain (Warthin-Starry) of tissue, but may occasionally be confirmed by a positive skin test. Numerous antimicrobial agents have been utilized, of which gentamicin has been perhaps the most promising. Recently, several adult patients showed a dramatic response to ciprofloxacin (500 mg twice daily).

Tuberculosis and Syphilis

Tuberculosis and syphilis have re-emerged as major pathogens in the AIDS and intravenous drug abuse era. Although presentations are similar to those of a previous era, the clinician must be aware of late perinatal syphilis as well as perinatal tuberculosis, which may present as true FUO. Therapy for the latter condition may need to be very aggressive (similar to the immunocompromised host) and may include streptomycin in addition to the usual agents (isoniazid, rifampin, pyrazinamide).

Collagen-Vascular Disease

Rheumatic Fever

Among the collagen-vascular diseases, rheumatic fever has re-emerged as a serious problem. Although the Jones criteria need to be fulfilled, occasional patients may present with prolonged fever only. Careful and repeated physical examinations along with selective laboratory testing should yield the information necessary to make the diagnosis. Aspirin in moderate doses (50 to 75 mg/kg/day) is usually dramatically effective for the joint symptoms and prophylactic penicillin (250 mg bid of penicillin V) is warranted.

Kawasaki Disease

Kawasaki disease is diagnosed clinically with multisystem involvement (fever, rash, adenopathy, conjunctival injection, mucous membrane involvement, extremity changes). Several patients were described who had coronary aneurysms yet did not meet all criteria for the diagnosis. In addition, infants younger than 6 months of age may have an atypical course. As treatment with gamma globulin has dramatically lessened complications, patients who may have the disease should be treated. The standard regimen is now 2 g/kg as a single infusion. Aspirin is given concomitantly (100 mg/kg/day) in four doses until systemic symptoms disappear, at which time the dose maybe decreased to about 5 mg/kg as a single daily dose until follow-up echocardiographic results are normal.

Periodic Fever

Periodic fever sometimes is considered under the heading of FUO. While entities such as familial Mediterranean fever and brucellosis are discussed separately in this book, the clinician should be aware of a newer entity "periodic fever, aphthous stomatitis, pharyngitis" syndrome. Patients with this disorder have almost cyclical symptoms not accompanied by neutropenia. The long-term outlook is excellent, but the symptoms may be quite troublesome. A short course of steroid therapy has been suggested for acute exacerbations.

REFERENCES

Gartner JC: Fever of unknown origin. Adv Pediatr Infect Dis 7:1–24, 1992.

Larson EB, Featherstone HJ, Petersdorf RG: Fever of undetermined origin: Diagnosis and follow-up of 105 cases, 1970–1980. Medicine 61:269–292, 1982.

Lorin MI, Feigin RD: Fever without localizing signs and fever of unknown origin. *In* Feigin RD, Cherry JD (eds): Textbook of Pediatric Infectious Diseases, 3rd ed. Philadelphia, WB Saunders Co, 1992.

PARVOVIRUS INFECTION IN CHILDREN

JOHANNA GOLDFARB, M.D.

Human parvovirus infection is most often an asymptomatic or mild, nonspecific illness. Infection occurs only once, usually in childhood, and is associated with seroconversion. About 60 per cent of adults have antibodies, suggesting the presence of an earlier infection.

Several clinical presentations of parvovirus infection are now being recognized; the most common is erythema infectiosum or "slapped cheek" disease. Also known as "fifth's disease" (the fifth exanthematous disease of childhood), this is a mild, self-limited entity in normal children and no therapy is required. Epidemics occur in winter and spring. Other associated syndromes include acute aplastic crisis in individuals with chronic hemolytic anemia (Table 1), bone marrow suppression in immunocompromised children and adults, arthralgias and arthritis in adults, and hydrops in the fetus infected during the second trimester.

TREATMENT

Erythema Infectiosum

No treatment is necessary. The rash occurs late in the infection and coincides with the development of antibodies. Children are no longer infectious by the time the diagnosis is made.

TABLE 1. Chronic Anemias Associated with Parvovirus Infection–Induced Acute Aplastic Crisis

Sickle cell disease
Hereditary spherocytosis
Pyruvate kinase deficiency
Sickle C hemoglobulin anemia
Autoimmune hemolytic anemia
Thalassemia

Acute Hemolytic Crisis

Treatment is directed at supporting the child through the acute self-limited crisis. A significant drop in hematocrit to levels as low as 5 g/dl occurs over the first days, with reticulocyte counts of zero (0) in some cases. Transfusions are frequently necessary to treat congestive heart failure or to prevent cardiac compromise. Reticulocytosis signals the end of the crisis. Children with acute aplastic crisis are contagious (often for prolonged periods) and should be kept in respiratory isolation while hospitalized because of the nosocomial spread of infection.

Immunocompromised Status

Treatment with immune serum globulin has been successful in a small number of patients with lymphocytic leukemia or acquired immunodeficiency syndrome (AIDS) who had documented chronic parvovirus infection with associated bone marrow suppression. Treatment courses of 400 mg/kg/day of intravenous immunoglobulin (IVIG) given for 5 to 10 days have been used successfully to clear persistent parvovirus infection and to reverse the bone marrow suppression.

Reversal of the immunosuppressed state (i.e., discontinuation of chemotherapy) has also aborted persistent infection and resulted in seroconversion and resolution of the marrow suppression. The immunocompromised patient with acute or chronic infection with parvovirus should be considered contagious and appropriately isolated when in the hospital.

Pregnancy

Infection during pregnancy carries no increased risk for the mother. However, maternal infection, especially during the second trimester, is associated with fetal hydrops. Because routine parvovirus antibody screening is not available commercially, evaluation of a pregnant woman for parvovirus infection usually involves testing at the Division for Viral Diseases of the Centers for Disease Control, arranged through the local State Health Department. The presence of maternal IgM parvovirus antibody suggests acute infection and a risk for fetal infection. Intrauterine blood sampling by cordocentesis for IgM antibody testing has been used to diagnose fetal infection. The fetus must be closely observed for signs of hydrops, which, untreated, carries a mortality rate of up to perhaps 80 to 90 per cent. Intrauterine blood transfusion has been successfully used to treat hydropic fetuses with resolution of the hydrops and continuation of pregnancy to term.

A high index of suspicion of parvovirus is required because infection in the mother will likely be nonspecific or asymptomatic. Pregnant women exposed to children during an erythema infectiosum outbreak should be screened to determine serologic status. Immune women cannot transmit the infection to their unborn children.

PREVENTION OF INFECTION

Prevention of parvovirus in these settings is difficult. By the time infection can be diagnosed, usually with an outbreak of erythema infectiosum, affected children are no longer contagious. Respiratory spread appears to be the likely mode of transmission and occurs in the days prior to the onset of rash. Those at risk for serious disease, including individuals with chronic hemolytic anemia, immunosuppressed hosts, and pregnant women, should be counseled about these risks.

In the hospital, children with acute infection should be kept in respiratory isolation. Nosocomial spread to other parents as well as to health care personnel caring for infected children has been reported.

No data yet suggest that immune globulin is effective in passive protection. Therefore, it is not recommended for contacts of infected children.

19

Allergy

ALLERGIC RHINITIS IN CHILDREN

GAIL G. SHAPIRO, M.D.

Allergic rhinitis is the most common cause of chronic nasal congestion in children. Its features include mucosal membrane edema and mucus hypersecretion secondary to an immunologic reaction between environmental antigens and nasal mucosal mast cells and basophils. Although all people have such mucosal cells, only allergic individuals have cell-bound immunoglobulin E (IgE) that specifically interacts with antigens (allergens) to set off an inflammatory event. The conjugation of cell-bound IgE and allergen molecules results in the release of chemical mediators that are capable of causing vasodilation, increased mucosal permeability, increased mucus production, influx of inflammatory cells, and increased sensitivity to subsequent allergen exposure.

This nasal allergic reaction may result in isolated mast cell mediator release. In this case, mediators such as histamine, prostaglandin D_2, toluene-sulfo-trypsin arginine methyl (TAME) esterase, and kinins produce direct and reflex-mediated changes in nasal vascular permeability and mucus secretion that are relatively short-lived. In other cases, this early-phase reaction is followed hours later by a late-phase reaction. It is thought that chemotactic mediators from the early event stimulate inflammatory cell influx (e.g., eosinophils, neutrophils) into the nasal membranes. These inflammatory cells play a role in the late-phase reaction. In addition, basophils, which are present in the stimulated respiratory epithelium, play a major role by secreting more histamine, TAME esterase, and kinins. Consequently, an allergen exposure creates a disorder that greatly outlives its duration. Even days after a significant exposure, inflammatory changes may still be noticeable in the nasal airway.

DIFFERENTIAL DIAGNOSIS

Although allergic rhinitis is an extremely common cause of chronic rhinitis in children, other problems require consideration.

Infectious rhinitis secondary to unrecognized sinusitis brings nonallergic children to the allergist's office rather frequently.

Nonallergic rhinitis with eosinophilia resembles allergic rhinitis identically on examination; however, allergy testing is negative and the etiology of the nasal disease is unknown. The problem is uncommon before puberty.

Vasomotor rhinitis is nasal membrane edema and mucus hypersecretion of unknown etiology, but it is probably due to autonomic imbalance in the nasal airway. Secretions tend to be thin, watery, and acellular on microscopic examination. This diagnosis is much more common in middle-aged adults than in children.

Nasal polyposis is another inflammatory problem of unknown etiology, but may be associated with allergic rhinitis. Nasal polyps in children recall the diagnosis of cystic fibrosis, which is the most common cause of this problem in childhood.

Rhinitis medicamentosa refers to nasal membrane inflammation secondary to overuse of vasoconstrictive nose sprays. These products should be avoided.

Structural problems, including septal deviations, unilateral choanal atresia, tumors, and foreign bodies, are unusual causes of chronic rhinitis in children.

Adenoidal hypertrophy is a common cause of upper airway congestion that can be confused with allergic rhinitis. A very static congestion free of rhinorrhea, not fluctuating with environmental changes and unresponsive to antihistamines and decongestants suggests an adenoid problem.

DIAGNOSIS

The usual features of allergic rhinitis are nasal congestion, rhinorrhea, sneezing, and nasal itching. Some patients complain of constantly feeling as if they have a cold. Some experience itching of the palate or ear as a result of common fifth cranial nerve innervation of the nose and ear canal. Youngsters may habitually rub their noses or make strange facial gestures to overcome nasal pruritus. A dark periorbital appearance has won the name "allergic shiner." Allergic rhinitis may be an etiologic factor for chronic or recurrent acute sinusitis as well as for eustachian tube dysfunction and middle ear problems, including infections, effusions, and conductive hearing loss.

Allergic rhinitis may be episodic or continual, depending on the spectrum of allergens affecting the patient; this is to some degree age-related. Infants and toddlers may have allergic rhinitis as a manifestation of food allergy, although it is uncommon for this to occur without coexisting dermatitis and gastrointestinal symptoms. After age 3 years, foods are rare causes of rhinitis. In early childhood, perennial allergic rhinitis is most often caused by dust mite and pet antigens. By about 5 years of age, children have experienced enough seasonal pollen exposure to manifest pollen-induced rhinitis. Older children may have year-round "perennial rhinitis" or only seasonal pollenosis (usually in spring and summer, although warmer regions will have pollen year-round). In general, trees pollinate in early spring, followed by grasses and then weeds in summer. Ragweed season, the major problem pollen in the eastern and midwestern United States, extends from mid August until the first frost, usually in mid October.

Individuals with year-round allergic rhinitis typically have sensitivity to dust mite, mold, and/or animal antigens and may also react to pollen. Aggravating allergens must be sought in multiple locations if the child spends time with parents who do not live together or if an out-of-home baby-sitter or a day care setting is used. See Table 1 for environmental considerations in allergic rhinitis.

DIAGNOSTIC TECHNIQUES

Microscopic Evaluation

The microscopic evaluation of nasal secretions provides valuable information in making a diagnosis. The patient blows his or her nose into plastic wrap; alternatively, a swab can be used to obtain the specimen. The secretions are wiped onto a glass slide, which is then heat-fixed and stained with Hansel's stain.

The presence of over 5 to 10 per cent eosinophils per field suggests allergic rhinitis. However, the less common problems, nonallergic rhinitis with eosinophilia and nasal polyposis (with or without concomitant allergic rhinitis), cannot be discounted. A predominance of polymorphonuclear cells suggests infectious rhinitis, most likely related to a viral syndrome if the condition is acute, or, if more long-standing, to bacterial rhinosinusitis. If there are watery secretions that yield few cells, vasomotor rhinitis is quite likely, although it is possible that the patient has allergic rhinitis but is currently asymptomatic.

Skin Testing

Allergy skin testing plays an important role in distinguishing allergic rhinitis from other diagnostic possibilities. Extracts of common aeroallergens are applied to the epidermis in such a way as to reproduce the interaction of environmental allergen and mast cell–bound IgE that occurs in the nose. Initial testing is usually carried out by an epicutaneous method (e.g., prick, puncture, or scratch). A drop of an extract of each allergen in question is applied to the skin, and a needle is used to pierce the skin superficially, enough to bring antigen and mediator-containing cells into contact. Within 15 to 20 minutes, a wheal and flare will appear if significant amounts of histamine are released.

There is a good correlation between positive epicutaneous skin testing to inhaled allergens and clinical symptoms on exposure. Because this testing is not always adequately sensitive, intradermal skin testing may be needed. A small quantity of allergen is directly injected into the epidermis. Again, a wheal-and-flare reaction occurring within 15 to 20 minutes of exposure indicates IgE reaction against the allergen. The correlation between positive intradermal test and actual symptoms from exposure to a particular allergen is less commanding than epicutaneous test reactions.

An alternative approach to diagnosis is in vitro measurement of allergen-specific IgE. The patient's serum is incubated with an inert carrier material coated with allergen. Serum IgE to specific allergen will react with the allergen-carrier complex to form an IgE-allergen-carrier complex that can be radiolabeled and then quantitated. The prototype of this is the radioallergosorbent test (RAST). In general, such in vitro methods are more costly and less sensitive than skin testing and are rarely preferable.

The decision to perform skin tests or to treat allergic rhinitis empirically depends on the chronicity and severity of the problem. For some situations, brief courses of antihistamines or decongestants will provide satisfactory relief so that in-depth evaluation is unnecessary. Sometimes, a determination of total serum IgE may be helpful, giving general information concerning the patient's allergic status. Because total serum IgE is elevated in approximately only one half of allergic rhinitis patients, it is helpful when positive but not when negative.

TREATMENT

Avoidance

The common allergens provoking allergic rhinitis are house dust mites, molds, animal proteins, and pollens. Insect antigens (especially from cockroaches) are important in certain parts of the United States. The most effective therapy is avoidance of the inciting allergens. In the case of animal exposures, this may represent severe sacrifice. One must weigh the patient's emotional attachment to a pet against the degree of disease involvement and relief through other modalities.

House dust mites are ubiquitous microscopic creatures that live off human skin scales. They thrive in climates with high relative humidity, and they avoid ambient daylight. They are thus abundant in stuffed furniture, mattresses, and carpets, where they leave fecal particles that are more antigenic than the mites themselves.

Dust mites do not survive extremes of boiling and freezing and do not proliferate in dry relative humidity. Their effects may be minimized by such measures as decreasing moisture, removing carpets, and encasing mattresses in nonporous plastic covers (Table 2). Hot-water washing of bedding, including pillows and blankets, on a 1- to 2-week basis appears to be helpful. Placing stuffed toys that cannot be washed in a hot dryer or freezer may be helpful, although little firm data exist to validate these measures. Acaricides (dust mite killers) are in their infancy. Benzyl benzoate powder is commercially available for application to carpets on an every-6-month basis. Evaluations of its effectiveness are conflicting. Tannic acid solution (3 per cent) is also available commercially for application to carpets and upholstery every 1 to 3 months. Although it does not kill mites, tannic acid appears to denature mite and pet antigens, rendering them nonimmunogenic.

Mold avoidance also involves measures to decrease household humidity. Heating and cooling systems should be checked to eliminate mold reservoirs. A layer of heavy plastic (Visqueen) in the crawl space of a home will decrease moisture problems and mold. A dehumidifier may be necessary at times. An application of liquid laundry bleach removes mold growth on window frames and bathroom tiles.

Pollen avoidance is extremely difficult because pollens are so widespread at certain times of year. Keeping doors and windows closed and using air conditioning effectively filters most pollen from the home. This is ineffective, however, for individuals with an outdoor-oriented lifestyle. Similarly, it is impractical where air conditioning is unnecessary for temperature control. High-efficiency filters (electrostatic precipitators, *h*igh-*e*fficiency *p*articulate *a*ir filters) remove particulate matter, including pollens, mold spores, and mites. They, too, are most effective if doors and windows are kept closed. The correlation between high-efficiency filter use and control of rhinitis symptoms is unclear.

Although environmental control is the theoretic ideal for managing allergic rhinitis, it is difficult to institute and to sustain. The impressive improvement that is seen in many patients who have accomplished these preventive measures encourages one to continue providing these recommendations. Nevertheless, complicated lifestyles involving such confounding factors as rental homes, dual-parent custody of children, and day care settings are important factors that force the use of other approaches.

TABLE 1. Environmental Considerations in Allergic Rhinitis

Examples of Factors Meriting Consideration	Reasons for Consideration
Home Construction	
Heating system	
Radiator	
Forced air	Possibility for central filtering of forced air systems
Wood	Pollutants from wood stoves
Baseboard	Poor air circulation and mold growth from noncirculating baseboard heat
Humidity	More humid, greater likelihood of dust mite and mold
Cleaning Regimen	
Ownership of vacuum cleaner	
Frequency of dusting and vacuuming	May influence dust mite population in the home
Frequency of cleaning drapery and carpet	
Household Contents	
Age of carpeting and furnishings	The older these items, the more likely they are as sources of dust mites
Quantity of overstuffed articles	
Pets	Source of animal allergies
Bedroom	
Carpeting, window coverings	Dust mite likely in carpets, overstuffed mattresses, and furniture
Mattress	
Bedding materials	Feathers in bedding attract dust mites and are allergens themselves
Stuffed toys	
Ambient Air Quality	
Exposure to tobacco smoke	Pollutants and irritants
Exposure to wood stove	

From Shapiro GG: Allergic rhinitis due to inhalant factors. *In* Rohel RR (ed): Conn's Current Therapy; Philadelphia, WB Saunders Co, p 644, 1988.

Pharmacologic Intervention

Antihistamines

Antihistamines are first-line therapy for allergic rhinitis. They competitively inhibit the allergic mediator histamine at its receptor sites. Although there are both H_1 and H_2 receptors in the tissues of the upper airway, H_1 receptors are most relevant to allergic rhinitis. Antihistamines block both the vasodilation that results from stimulation of the blood vessels by H_1 receptor–histamine interaction and the mucous gland hypersecretion and sneezing that result from reflex initiation consequent to the stimulation of H_1 receptors on sensory nerves by histamine. In terms of symptomatic benefit, antihistamines are most effective for diminishing nasal itch and hypersecretion but do not effectively decrease mucous membrane swelling.

Antihistamines are classified on the basis of chemical structure; some newer agents are considered "miscellaneous" because they do not fall into the established six categories (Table 3). If one becomes familiar with a representative drug from each of several classes, one can alternate between these because tachyphylaxis or adverse side effects often make alternate choices necessary.

Terfenadine and astemizole are the first antihistamines approved by the U.S. Food and Drug Administration (FDA) that do not cross the blood-brain barrier. They do not usually cause drowsiness. Although terfenadine is FDA-approved in the United States for children older than 12 years of age, it is available in a liquid form in other parts of the world and has been used successfully in younger children. The customary dose is 60 mg (one tablet) twice daily. Its potency is similar to that of chlorpheniramine, but it is much more expensive. Astemizole differs from terfenadine in that it has a much slower onset and much longer duration of action. The customary dose is 10 mg (one tablet) daily. The activity of astemizole is so prolonged that it must be discontinued a month or more prior to allergy skin testing to avoid histamine-induced wheal suppression. Most other antihistamines need to be discontinued for only 24 to 48 hours prior to testing.

Decongestants

The oral decongestants phenylpropanolamine, phenylephrine, and pseudoephedrine are α-adrenergic agents capable

TABLE 2. Environmental Control Suggestions

Exposure	Intervention
Airborne irritants	Avoid tobacco smoke, wood stoves, noxious fumes
Dust mites	Remove carpet if possible; use acaricides if not:
	1. Tannic acid solution 3%*: Spray on carpets and stuffed furniture every 6 months (denatures mite and pet antigen but does not kill mites).
	2. Benzyl benzoate: Spread on carpets every 2–3 months (denatures antigen and kills mites with repeated use).†
	Place zippered plastic cover on mattress and box spring cover.
	Wash pillow, blankets, and sheets in hot water weekly.
Mold	Decrease humidity in home to <50% relative humidity.
	Apply bleach-containing cleaners to visible mildew.

*Available from Allergy Control Product, Inc., 96 Danbury Road, Ridgefield, CT 06877.
†Acarosan, Fisons Corporation, P.O. Box 1766, Rochester, NY 14603.

TABLE 3. Classification of Commonly Used Antihistamines

Class	Generic Name	Trade Name	Suggested Dose for Childen (mg/kg/24 hr)	Suggested Dose for Adults
Ethanolamine	Diphenhydramine hydrochloride	Benadryl	5.0	25–50 mg q.i.d.
	Carbinoxamine maleate	Clistin	0.8	4–8 mg q.i.d.
Ethylenediamine	Tripelennamine hydrochloride	PBZ	5.0	25–50 mg q.i.d.
Alkylamine	Chlorpheniramine maleate	Chlor-Trimeton Teldrin	0.35	4 mg q.i.d.
	Brompheniramine maleate	Dimetane	0.35	4 mg q.i.d.
	Triprolidine hydrochloride	Actidil	0.18	2.5 q.i.d.
Phenothiazine	Promethazine hydrochloride	Phenergan	0.5	12.5–25 mg q.i.d.
	Methdilazine	Tacaryl	0.3	16–32 mg q.i.d. (as b.i.d. or q.i.d.)
Piperazine	Hydroxyzine hydrochloride	Atarax, Vistaril, Durrax	2.0	10–20 mg q.i.d.
Piperidine	Cyproheptadine hydrochloride	Periactin	0.25	4–20 mg q.i.d.
Miscellaneous	Terfenadine	Seldane	—	60 mg b.i.d.
	Astemizole	Himanal	—	10 mg q.d.

From Shapiro GG: Allergic rhinitis due to inhalant factors. *In* Rohel RR (ed): Conn's Current Therapy; Philadelphia, WB Saunders Co, p 646, 1988.

of producing nasal mucous membrane vasoconstriction adequate to reduce edema. They work well in conjunction with antihistamines. There are currently a large number of combination products, containing both antihistamine and decongestant. Although fixed-combination preparations are convenient and increase compliance, they prevent individualized dose adjustments. However, because little is currently known about dose-response relationships and kinetics of most of these preparations, they remain practical and popular.

Topical decongestants are poor choices for treating chronic rhinitis. With repeated use, they tend to cause less sustained decongestion, leading both to overuse and to rebound vasodilation with increased congestion. This iatrogenic congestion is known as rhinitis medicamentosa.

Cromolyn

Cromolyn, long used for asthma therapy, is an alternative to antihistamines as primary therapy for treatment of allergic rhinitis. Nasalcrom is a 4 per cent solution of cromolyn that is used as a nasal spray and may act by preventing release of allergic mediators. The usual dose is one spray per nostril three to six times daily; each spray delivers 5.2 mg of cromolyn. Cromolyn is effective only as a prophylactic agent and, for best results, must be used regularly rather than after symptoms occur. Adverse effects are uncommon and benign. These include transient sneezing, nasal stinging, and headache.

Corticosteroids

Nasal administration of corticosteroids is an extremely effective therapy for allergic rhinitis. It is usually used for brief intervals when the previously mentioned agents are inadequate. Corticosteroids appear to diminish histamine release and to alter the pathways that lead to the production of mediators from arachidonic acid.

Until recently, available corticosteroid nasal sprays were systemically absorbed to a significant degree. Intranasal beclomethasone (Beconase, Vancenase) and flunisolide (Nasalide) are highly active topically and are very poorly absorbed from the mucosa. The portion that is swallowed and absorbed from the gastrointestinal tract is rapidly metabolized to an inactive form. These new preparations have greatly improved the safety of long-term topical corticosteroid therapy. They are generally used for several weeks during rhinitis exacerbations, although longer treatment periods may be needed during pollen seasons and for especially severe, chronic, perennial rhinitis. Often, therapy with antihistamines and decongestants is continued. Customary dosage is 2 puffs per nostril two to four times daily. This is usually well tolerated; most complaints relate to nasal stinging and nosebleeds, which remit when use of the drug is discontinued. Perforation of the nasal septum has been reported but is extremely uncommon.

Systemic corticosteroid therapy is rarely needed for allergic rhinitis. In patients who have severe involvement that appears refractory to other therapy, a short course of oral, short-acting steroid (e.g., prednisone) is helpful. Long-term use puts the patient at risk for a long list of steroid-induced adverse effects, which may well be more worrisome than the initial rhinitis complaints. Intramuscular steroid injection has produced unsightly keloid formation and subcutaneous fat atrophy, which have been the basis for malpractice suits. Injection of steroids into the turbinates has been associated with blindness due to intra-arterial embolization of the mixture.

Conclusion

Reasonable certainty about the cause of rhinitis will dramatically help one's success rate with medical management. A patient with vasomotor rhinitis will not benefit from nasal steroids or cromolyn. Decongestants as well as antihistamines (with their atropine-like drying effect) are most useful. For nonallergic rhinitis with eosinophilia, antihistamines and decongestants may be of some benefit but topical nasal steroids offer best results. Patients with nasal polyposis may require a short course of relatively high dose daily steroid therapy (40 to 60 mg each morning for 1 week in an adult or 1 mg/kg in children), followed by chronic use of a topical nasal steroid. Chronic infectious rhinitis, similarly to sinusitis, necessitates appropriate antimicrobial therapy in addition to decongestants. In rhinitis medicamentosa, the initiating agent must be removed. The use of a topical nasal steroid spray aids in weaning the patient from the topical decongestant.

IMMUNOTHERAPY

Immunotherapy, also known as "desensitization" or "hyposensitization," is the injection of allergens into an immunologically sensitive individual for the purpose of building tolerance to those allergens. Many studies attest to its usefulness, provided that appropriate patients are selected and that appropriate allergenic extract and dosing are used. Immunotherapy is usually reserved for those allergic individuals who continue to have recalcitrant disease after optimal avoidance measures and pharmacologic intervention have been investigated. Frequently, these patients suffer from sensitivity to pollens that are present much of the year, thus reducing the impact of environmental control measures. Immunotherapy is ordinarily limited to such patients because it is a costly investment of time and money. Usually, patients receive injections once to twice weekly for several months and eventually reach a monthly regimen, which continues for several years. After this, most patients who have had symptomatic benefit will continue to benefit because of maintained immunologic tolerance to the specific allergens to which they were immunized.

Prior to initiating immunotherapy, one should confirm a patient's sensitivity to allergens by skin testing. Only clinically significant allergens with such skin test verification should be added to the treatment mixture. Therapy is usually confined to house dust mite, pollen, and mold allergies. Evidence of efficacy with mold antigens is limited. Recently, standardized cat antigen for immunotherapy has become commercially available.

Immunotherapy is usually initiated at a concentration of allergenic extract one order of magnitude less than that which produces a 5-mm wheal on prick skin testing. Frequently, this is a 1:100,000 concentration. Patients receive 0.05 ml of this concentration, and, with subsequent injections once or twice weekly, advance to 0.5 mg. They then begin receiving injections with the 1:10,000 concentration and progress as before, eventually reaching the 1:1000 and finally the 1:100 concentration. A maintenance dose (usually 0.2 or 0.3 ml) is then selected and given every 2 to 4 weeks. There are many variations of this schedule, but all follow the principle of gradual progression from a dilute to a concentrated antigen mixture.

Benefits of immunotherapy are often achieved in the first year. Most patients receive it for 3 to 5 years. After this time, many of those who have responded seem to retain symptomatic benefit even when immunotherapy is discontinued. Responsiveness is thought to relate to production of IgE-blocking antibodies, down-regulation of IgE production, and decreased releasability by mediator-containing cells (i.e., mast cells and basophils).

Physicians who administer immunotherapy must be prepared to treat anaphylaxis. Patients are most at risk as they progress to higher antigen doses. Nevertheless, anaphylaxis can occur at any time. Life-threatening anaphylaxis occurs most commonly immediately after the injection. For this reason, patients should remain in the clinic for 30 minutes after the injection so that they can be observed for possible systemic complications. Quite commonly, patients experience local reactions at the injection site. If a large immediate or late-phase local reaction occurs, the dose should be decreased and then advanced slowly if reactions diminish.

ASTHMA

THOMAS F. SMITH, M.D.

The prevalence of asthma and the rate of death from asthma are increasing in the United States as well as in other countries for uncertain reasons. Because asthma is such a widespread disease that has such a significant impact on health and health care expenditures, the Coordinating Committee of the National Asthma Education Program recently convened an expert panel to develop guidelines to improve the detection and treatment of asthma. The panel's report[1] should be required reading for all health care professionals dealing with patients with asthma.

Asthma is a chronic lung disease that has the following three characteristics[1]:

1. Airway obstruction that is reversible (but not completely in some patients).
2. Airway inflammation.
3. Increased responsiveness to a variety of stimuli.

Asthma is an extremely variable disease; patients with asthma present with a variety of signs and symptoms that vary in degree of severity from patient to patient as well as within each patient over time. Thus, treatment regimens must be individualized and must account for changes in degree of airway obstruction and inflammation. Because asthma is a chronic illness in which there usually are acute exacerbations, treatment must include a continuous care plan that will minimize airway inflammation, control symptoms, and prevent or minimize exacerbations.

Management of asthma should have the following goals:

1. Maintenance of normal activities (including exercise).
2. Maintenance of normal (or as close to normal as possible) pulmonary function.
3. Prevention of symptoms, including cough, chest congestion, and shortness of breath.
4. Prevention of recurrent exacerbations of asthma.
5. Avoidance of adverse effects from asthma medications.

Accomplishing these goals requires that asthma therapy have multiple components:

1. Education of the patient and the patient's family.
2. Environmental control measures.
3. Comprehensive pharmacologic therapy with a written plan to increase or decrease the level of therapy according to degree of airway obstruction and inflammation.
4. Immunotherapy, which may benefit certain children with asthma.
5. Objective monitoring measures to guide the patient, the patient's family, and the physician in use of medicines and to permit assessment of the success of the therapy.

It is important to emphasize the role of airway inflammation in asthma. Although it has long been recognized that fatal asthma is associated with marked inflammation in airways, it is now apparent that airway inflammation is present even in patients with mild asthma. Furthermore, there appears to be a direct relationship between degree of airway inflammation and level of both airway hyper-reactivity and clinical symptoms. Thus, therapy of asthma must include strategies to prevent or reduce airway inflammation.

PATIENT EDUCATION

Health education by the clinician is a powerful tool for helping patients acquire the motivation and competence to control their asthma.[1] This education must begin at the time of diagnosis and be an integral part of continuing care. It should be part of each patient encounter, whether in the office, in an urgent care setting, or in the hospital. Patient education should include helping patients and their families understand asthma, helping them learn and practice skills needed to control asthma, and acknowledging their efforts. An important part of this process is the establishment of a partnership between the patient, the patient's family, and the clinician, which, in turn, will improve adherence to the treatment plan and promote improvement in asthma control.

These objectives are not achieved by simply providing information. It is unlikely that any part of the treatment plan will be instituted correctly or completely, if at all, unless this three-way partnership is in place and unless the patient and the patient's family understand the goals of therapy and the treatment plan.

Areas and topics that are important parts of patient education have been discussed in detail elsewhere.[1] They include information about the definition of asthma and its chronic nature, signs and symptoms of asthma, characteristic changes in the airways of asthma patients, asthma triggers and how to avoid them, role of medicines in asthma therapy, and criteria for beginning or increasing medications to prevent onset of symptoms. Each patient encounter should include a review of proper use of medicines (especially metered-dose inhalers and home nebulizing equipment); home use of peak expiratory flow rate monitoring and of symptom and medication diaries; and use of written guidelines to maintain and alter therapy. Education must also address fears and misconceptions about asthma and asthma medicines as well as patient and family feelings about asthma. Finally, education must address family understanding of, support for, and adherence to all parts of the treatment plan.

AVOIDANCE OF ALLERGENS, IRRITANTS, AND RESPIRATORY VIRUSES

Avoidance of factors that increase airway inflammation is preferable to treatment of inflammation with medicines.[2] The two primary factors that increase airway inflammation in childhood asthma are allergy and viral respiratory infections. Furthermore, once the airway is inflamed, it becomes responsive to nonspecific irritants. Therefore, environmental measures that reduce exposure to allergens and irritants, and strategies that address exposures to viral respiratory infections, are an essential part of the management of asthma.

Allergens

The importance of allergy in childhood asthma cannot be overstated. It has been reported that between 75 and 85 per cent of patients with asthma have positive immediate hypersensitivity skin test reactions to common inhalant allergens. Furthermore, it has been shown that both childhood asthma and airway hyperresponsiveness are significantly correlated with allergy, as determined by serum immunoglobulin E (IgE) level. Therefore, it is important to consider allergy as the major cause of airway inflammation in asthmatic children. Allergy to inhalant allergens is common in children 3 years of age and older, although it may be present in younger children. On the other hand, food allergy is a more common cause of asthma in infants than it is in older children.

Indoor Allergens

Avoidance of indoor allergens is accomplished by removing warm-blooded animals from the home and by instituting control measures for house dust mites, cockroaches, and indoor molds. Mite allergy is a major component of asthma in most parts of the United States and deserves special attention. In the Southeast, at least 60 per cent of children with asthma have positive skin test reactions to mites, often as the single positive reaction. High levels of mite allergen are found in mattresses, pillows, bedding, stuffed animals, upholstered furniture, and carpeting. House dust mite precautions are listed in Table 1. (See preceding article on allergy.)

TABLE 1. Patient Guide: House Dust Mite Control Measures

Routine Precautions

1. Wash bedding (including blankets) in hot water every 2 weeks.
2. Enclose mattresses and box springs on all beds in zippered, dust-proof encasings.
3. Wash pillows in hot water every 2 weeks or encase them in zippered, dust-proof encasings.
4. Wash stuffed animals in hot water every 2 weeks or remove them.
5. Use air conditioners spring through fall to reduce humidity. Use a dehumidifier in damp basements.
6. Avoid overhumidification. Avoid ventilating houses in humid climates by opening windows. Avoid humidifiers.

Heroic Precautions

1. Remove all carpeting or treat carpeting with 3% tannic acid to denature mite allergens and treat with benzyl benzoate to kill mites.
2. Remove upholstered furniture, cover it in plastic, or treat it with 3% tannic acid and benzyl benzoate.

Mite content in homes can be decreased considerably by hot-cycle washing of bedding (including blankets and pillows) and stuffed animals and by encasing mattresses (and pillows that are not washed) in zippered plastic covers. Mites require greater than 50 per cent humidity to survive, and mite numbers in homes in humid climates can be reduced by using either air conditioning or heat rather than ventilating the home by opening windows. Mite content is decreased further by removal of carpeting and upholstered furniture. Mite (and animal) allergen in homes can be reduced by 3 per cent tannic acid treatment of carpeting and upholstered furniture; this denatures the mite allergen found in high concentrations in mite fecal particles but does not kill mites. Mite numbers in homes can be reduced by using benzyl benzoate (Acarasan), an acaricide currently marketed in a form to treat carpets.

Cockroach exposure is more difficult to reduce and is usually accomplished only with the assistance of professional exterminators. Indoor mold exposure also is reduced by lowering humidity in homes by using either air conditioning or heat; dehumidifiers may be useful as well. Use of humidifiers in homes should be discouraged. Indoor air-cleaning devices may give some benefit but generally are less useful than simply decreasing the source of the allergen. Cleaning air ducts and vents in the home is a logical adjunctive measure to decrease indoor allergen exposure. Asthma caused by allergy to animals is usually easily treated by avoidance measures. Control of asthma caused by allergy to mite, cockroach, or mold usually requires the addition of pharmacotherapy or immunotherapy.

Outdoor Allergens

Avoidance of outdoor allergens, such as pollens and mold spores, is more difficult than is avoidance of indoor allergens. Exposure to outdoor allergens can be reduced by keeping the windows in the patient's home closed and controlling indoor temperature with either air conditioning or heat. Washing the child's hair before bedtime also has been advocated to reduce exposure to pollen caught in hair during outdoor play. However, airway inflammation because of outdoor allergens usually requires seasonal pharmacotherapy or immunotherapy.

Irritants

Avoidance of indoor irritants is also an important part of the therapy of childhood asthma. Parents should be told that inflamed airways are sensitive to irritants, and decreasing particle and irritant load in a child's environment is an important part of treating respiratory diseases. Families of children with asthma should be cautioned that tobacco smoke releases gases, particles, and odors into the environment that are harmful and unnecessary. People should not be allowed to smoke in the homes of children with asthma or in the vehicles in which they travel; smoking indoors or in the car even when the child is not present should not be permitted. Indoor pets also add to the particulate irritant load of a home, and having warm-blooded pets indoors should be discouraged. Other sources of irritants in homes include wood-burning stoves and strong odors and sprays, and exposure to these should be avoided as well.

It should be noted that simple allergen-avoidance measures are warranted in all children with asthma, even if they are not yet allergic. It is reasonable to request that the family have only outdoor pets and that "routine" house dust mite precautions be taken (see Table 1). Permitting an asthmatic child with a negative skin test to have an indoor warm-blooded pet is kind-hearted but not logical, considering the risk of sensitization from intimate continuous exposure to the allergen.

Respiratory Viruses

Respiratory viruses also commonly cause airway inflammation in children with asthma, and they are the principal trigger of asthma in infants and young children. Respiratory viruses are acquired most easily from other children, and control of asthma in an infant or child who attends a day care center or who has older siblings in school or a day care setting may be particularly difficult. Parents may be a source of respiratory viruses, especially if their occupation or avocation includes exposure to children. Avoidance of day care settings is usually beneficial to young children with asthma; unfortunately, for economic reasons, this is often not possible for families to accomplish. Immunization against influenza is warranted yearly.

Exercise Participation

Of the common triggers of asthma in children, the one *not* to be avoided is exercise. Participation in exercise is an essential part of childhood for both physical health and psychosocial reasons. Although exercise frequently causes symptoms in asthmatic children who have inflamed airways, prophylaxis and therapy of airway inflammation rather than avoidance strategies should be emphasized. Avoidance of physical education classes, in particular, should be discouraged. It should be noted that a child with asthma may experience symptoms during exercise that are not related to asthma. Commonly, these result from decreased physical conditioning or fear of exercise-induced asthma (EIA) because of previous poor control of asthma. These children should be

TABLE 2. Dosages for Therapy in Childhood Asthma

Drug	Mode of Administration	Dosage
β₂-Agonists		
Inhaled	Metered-dose inhaler	2 puffs q 4–6 hours
Examples: albuterol,	Dry powder inhaler	1 capsule q 4–6 hours
metaproterenol, bitolterol,	Nebulizer solution*	Albuterol: 5 mg/ml; 0.1–0.15 mg/kg in 2 ml of saline q 4–6 hours,
terbutaline, pirbuteral		maximum 5.0 mg
		Metaproterenol: 50 mg/ml; 0.25–0.50 mg/kg in 2 ml of saline q 4–6 hours, maximum 15.0 mg
Oral		
Liquids		
Albuterol		0.1–0.15 mg/kg q 4–6 hours
Metaproterenol		0.3–0.5 mg/kg q 4–6 hours
Tablets		
Albuterol		2- or 4-mg tablet q 4–6 hours; 4-mg sustained-release tablet q 12 hours
Metaproterenol		10- or 20-mg tablet q 4–6 hours
Terbutaline		2.5- or 5.0-mg tablet q 4–6 hours
Cromolyn Sodium		
Inhaled	Metered-dose inhaler	1 mg/puff; 2 puffs b.i.d.–q.i.d.
	Dry powder inhaler	20 mg/capsule; 1 capsule b.i.d.–q.i.d.
	Nebulizer solution	20 mg/2-ml ampule; 1 ampule b.i.d.–q.i.d.
Theophylline		
Liquid		Dosage to achieve serum concentration of 5–15 μg/ml
Tablets, capsules		
Sustained-release tablets, capsules		
Corticosteroids		
Inhaled†		
Beclomethasone		42 μg/puff; 2–4 puffs b.i.d.–q.i.d.
Triamcinolone		100 μg/puff; 2–4 puffs b.i.d.–q.i.d.
Flunisolide		250 μg/puff; 2–4 puffs b.i.d.
Oral‡		
Liquids		
Prednisone		5 mg/5 ml
Prednisolone		5 mg/5 ml
		15 mg/5 ml
Tablets		
Prednisone		1, 2.5, 5, 10, 25, 50 mg
Prednisolone		5 mg
Methylprednisolone		2, 4, 8, 16, 24, 32 mg

*Premixed solutions are available. It is suggested that the per-kilogram dosage recommendations be followed.
†Consider use of spacer devices to minimize local adverse effects.
‡For acute exacerbations, doses of 1–2 mg/kg in single or divided doses are used initially and then modified. Reassess in 3 days, as only a short burst may be needed. There is no need to taper a short (3- to 5-day) course of therapy. If therapy extends beyond this period, it may be appropriate to taper the dosage. For chronic dosage, the lowest possible alternate-day morning dosage should be established.

TABLE 3. Dosages for Drugs in Acute Exacerbations of Asthma in Children

Drug	Available Form	Dosage	Comment
Inhaled β_2-Agonist			
Albuterol			
Metered-dose inhaler	90 μg per puff	2 inhalations every 5 minutes for total of 12 puffs, with monitoring of PEFR or FEV_1 to document response	If not improved, switch to nebulizer. If improved, decrease to 4 puffs every hour.
Nebulizer solution	0.5% (5 mg/ml)	0.1–0.15 mg/kg/dose up to 5 mg every 20 minutes for 1–2 hr (minimum dose 1.25 mg/dose) 0.5 mg/kg/hr by continuous nebulization (maximum dose 15 mg/hr)	If improved, decrease to 1–2 hr. If not improved, use by continuous inhalation.
Metaproterenol			
Metered-dose inhaler	650 μg per puff	2 inhalations	Frequent high-dose administration has not been evaluated. Metaproterenol is not interchangeable with β_2-agonists albuterol and terbutaline.
Nebulizer solution	5% (50 mg/ml)	0.1–0.3 cc (5–15 mg). Do not exceed 15 m	
	0.6% unit dose vial of 2.5 ml (15 mg)	As above 5–15 mg. Do not exceed 15 mg	
Terbutaline			
Metered-dose inhaler	200 μg per puff	2 inhalations every 5 minutes for a total of 12 puffs	
Injectable solution used in nebulizer	0.1% (1 mg/l ml) solution in 0.9% NaCl solution for injection Not FDA-approved for inhalation		Not recommended because not available as nebulizer solution. Offers no advantage over albuterol, which is available as nebulizer solution.
Systemic β-Agonist			
Epinephrine Hydrochloride	1:1000 (1 mg/ml)	0.01 mg/kg up to 0.3 mg subcutaneously every 20 minutes for 3 doses	Inhaled β_2-agonist preferred
Terbutaline	(0.1%) 1 mg/ml solution for injection in 0.9% NaCl.	Subcutaneous 0.01 mg/kg up to 0.3 mg every 2–6 hr needed. Intravenous 10 μg/kg over 10 minutes loading dose. Maintenance: 0.4 μg/kg/minute. Increase as necessary by 0.2 μg/kg/minutes and expect to use 3–6 μg/kg/minute	Inhaled β_2-agonist preferred
Methylxanthines			
Theophylline	Aminophylline (80% anhydrous theophylline)	Loading dose*: If theophylline concentration known: every 1 mg/kg aminophylline will give 2 μg/ml increase in concentration Loading dose*: If theophylline concentration unknown: —No previous theophylline: 6 mg/kg aminophylline —Previous theophylline: 3 mg/kg aminophylline Constant infusion rates*: Infusion rates to obtain a mean steady-state concentration of 15 μg/ml: *Age*	
		1–6 months	0.5 mg/kg/hr aminophylline
		6 months–1 year	1.0 mg/kg/hr aminophylline
		1–9 years	1.5 mg/kg/hr aminophylline
		10–16 years	1.2 mg/kg/hr aminophylline

Table continued on following page

TABLE 3. Dosages for Drugs in Acute Exacerbations of Asthma in Children *Continued*

Drug	Available Form	Dosage	Comment
Corticosteroids			
Outpatients	Oral prednisone, prednisolone, or methylprednisolone	1–2 mg/kg/day in single or divided doses	Reassess at 3 days because only a short burst may be needed. No need to taper dose.
Emergency department or hospitalized patients	Methylprednisolone IV or PO	1–2 mg/kg/dose every 6 hr for 24 hr then 1–2 mg/kg/day in divided doses q 8–12 hr	Length depends on response. May only need a few days.

*Check serum concentration at approximately 1, 12, and 24 hours after starting the infusion.
Abbreviation: FDA, U.S. Food and Drug Administration.

treated with understanding, support, and encouragement; avoidance of exercise only prolongs or amplifies the problem.

PHARMACOLOGIC THERAPY (Tables 2 and 3)

Medicines used for treatment of asthma fall into two categories: those that treat airway inflammation and those that treat symptoms of asthma. Anti-inflammatory agents used for asthma include cromolyn sodium (Intal), nedocromil sodium (Tilade), corticosteroids, and other anti-inflammatory compounds. Symptomatic treatment of asthma is accomplished with bronchodilators such as β_2-adrenergic agonists, methylxanthines, and anticholinergics. According to current understanding, if airway inflammation is controlled, symptomatic treatment will be unnecessary. Thus, more than occasional symptoms or need for symptomatic treatment or suboptimal pulmonary functioning suggests that airway inflammation is present, and anti-inflammatory therapy is necessary. *The management of asthma should stress the prevention and control of the disease rather than the treatment of symptoms after they have occurred. Avoidance of triggers of asthma is the most logical first step in therapy, but avoidance strategies are rarely completely successful in managing asthma; almost all children with asthma require some pharmacologic therapy.*

In treating children with asthma, the pediatrician must provide adequate pharmacotherapy to establish control of the disease as quickly as possible. Complete control of asthma implies that the child has no symptoms, has normal activities, can exercise without symptoms, has normal airflow rates, and has little daily variation in peak expiratory flow rate (see later). Complete control is a reasonable goal for most asthmatic children. A child whose asthma is out of control requires therapy both with medicines that treat airway inflammation and with those that treat symptoms. Once control has been established, medicines should be reduced to the lowest level needed to maintain control. In general, routine use of medicines that treat symptoms (i.e., bronchodilators) is stopped before use of anti-inflammatory medicines is stopped to prove that the latter are not needed. If asthma then becomes out of control, therapy should be accelerated rapidly to re-establish control. Pharmacotherapy of asthma is thus a continuing process of decreasing medicines if the child's asthma is under control and increasing them if it is not. Maintenance therapy is needed for some children with asthma, but it is usually needed seasonally (e.g., all spring or all winter); the need for maintenance therapy in a well child should be reassessed at regular intervals.

With all of these therapeutic options, *the optimal way to treat lung disease pharmacologically is by treating the lung directly—that is, inhalation therapy for asthma is superior to oral or parenteral therapy.* Inhalation therapy is superior because it provides maximum dosing of medicines directly to the affected organ while minimizing adverse effects of the medicines on other organs. However, deposition of particles into the lung is limited by airway caliber and airflow characteristics, including airflow velocity and turbulence. Thus, inhalation therapy has decreased efficacy in infants and young children, in tachypneic patients, and in patients with airflow obstruction. Furthermore, deposition of particles into the lung requires transoral inhalation. Nasal inhalation (such as may occur when using a facemask for inhalation of nebulized medications) delivers little if any medicine directly into the lung because of the superb filtering capability of the nose.

The use of metered-dose inhalers (MDIs, or "puffers") deserves special mention. MDIs offer a convenient means of delivering antiasthma medicines to the lung, and they can be effective if used properly. An adult using the device properly can deliver only about 13 per cent of a metered dose into the lung; efficiency is decreased in children, whose airways are smaller and further decreased when there is airflow obstruction. Steps for proper inhalation are listed in Table 4. Patients who are treated with MDIs should be required to demonstrate that they can use these devices at regular intervals. The use of drug delivery systems or holding chambers (such as InspirEase, Inhal-Aid, or AeroChamber) or other "spacers" or extenders (such as a rolled sheet of notebook paper) should be considered for patients receiving steroid inhalers and for young children or other patients who may have difficulty accomplishing the optimum technique for inhalation. Spacers decrease the amount of medicine deposited in the mouth (and therefore usually prevent oropharyngeal candidiasis as a complication of steroid inhalation) and may increase the amount of medicine inhaled into the lung.

Medicines

Anti-inflammatory Medicines

Anti-inflammatory medicines used to treat asthma include cromolyn sodium, nedocromil sodium, corticosteroids, and other anti-inflammatory compounds.

Cromolyn Sodium and Nedocromil Sodium. Cromolyn sodium (Intal) and nedocromil sodium (Tilade) are unrelated, potent, nonsteroidal anti-inflammatory drugs. Both are virtually devoid of side effects, in large part because they are poorly absorbed. Administered early, both cromolyn and nedocromil will inhibit early-phase and late-phase allergen-induced airway narrowing as well as acute airway responses to exercise; chronic use has been shown to decrease airway hyperreactivity (presumably by decreasing airway inflammation). When compared with cromolyn, nedocromil appears to be more potent in inhibiting airway responses to nonallergen challenges (such as sulfur dioxide and adenosine); it may require less frequent daily dosing as maintenance therapy; and it may provide sooner overall response. However, nedocromil currently is not approved in the United States for use in children younger than age 12 years.

Corticosteroids. These anti-inflammatory drugs are the most effective in the treatment of asthma. Like cromolyn and nedocromil, they block late-phase allergen-induced airway narrowing and decrease airway hyperreactivity. Inhaled corticosteroids are useful in the maintenance management of moderate and severe asthma, and they may play a role in the management of mild asthma as well. In moderate dosing, inhaled corticosteroids have minimal, if any, systemic effects. Immediate benefit may not be evident because suppression of symptoms and improvement in lung function may require several weeks or more of treatment. Oral steroids are used for patients whose airflow obstruction prevents deposition of inhaled steroids into the lung or who cannot use inhalation devices reliably. They are also required during times of stress by asthmatic patients with adrenal suppression because of previous steroid therapy.

It is appropriate to prescribe an oral corticosteroid and inhaled anti-inflammatory drugs simultaneously in patients expected to need the inhaled anti-inflammatory drugs after the oral agent is discontinued, in patients who are learning to use inhaled devices, and in patients who need the protective effect of cromolyn or nedocromil for exercise or other challenge. It may be that nedocromil has some steroid-sparing (i.e., reduces amount of corticosteroid) effect, and thus it may be appropriate to use both nedocromil and a corticosteroid simultaneously in the chronic management of an asthmatic patient who is steroid-dependent. Cromolyn has not been shown to have a steroid-sparing effect.

Other Anti-inflammatory Agents. Antihistamines such as clemastine and ketotifen, calcium antagonists, methotrexate, gold salts, and intravenous immunoglobulin are additional anti-inflammatory agents that have been used to treat asthma. The antihistamines studied have been found to have relatively weak anti-inflammatory activity and are not very useful clinically. Calcium antagonists studied in asthma also have relatively weak anti-inflammatory activity. Both methotrexate and oral gold are potent anti-inflammatory agents that have been reported to benefit some patients with severe steroid-dependent asthma; neither have been studied adequately to recommend their use in childhood asthma. There has been a recent report of the use of high-dose intravenous immunoglobulin to treat children with severe asthma, but controlled clinical trials are necessary to determine its role in asthma therapy. Methotrexate, gold salts, and intravenous immunoglobulin should all be regarded as experimental therapies to be considered only after conventional therapeutic strategies have been exhausted.

One other medicine deserves consideration as part of anti-inflammatory therapy. Troleandomycin (TAO) is a macrolide antibiotic that decreases the hepatic elimination of both theophylline and methylprednisolone. Although it has no anti-inflammatory properties of its own, TAO permits reduction in methylprednisolone dosage in steroid-dependent patients with severe asthma.

TABLE 4. Patient Guide: Correct Use of a Metered-Dose Inhaler

General Directions

1. Check that there is medicine in the canister at regular intervals.
   a. Put the canister (not the plastic mouthpiece or cap) into a cup of water.
   b. If it sinks to the bottom, it is full. If it floats upright on the surface, it is half full. If it floats sideways on the surface, it is empty.
2. Administer bronchodilator medicines before anti-inflammatory medicines.
3. Consider the use of drug delivery systems or holding chambers (such as InspirEase, Aerochamber, or Inhal-Aid) or other "spacers" or extenders (such as a rolled sheet of notebook paper) if you are using steroid inhalers or if the patient is a young child or someone who may have difficulty accomplishing the optimum technique for inhalation as described below.

Specific Steps

1. Shake the canister vigorously.
2. Put the mouthpiece on the canister if not using a spacer. If using an AeroChamber, Inhal-Aid, or similar spacer, insert mouthpiece into appropriate opening on the spacer. If using InspirEase, connect mouthpiece to reservoir bag, untwist bag, and insert canister into plastic stem on mouthpiece.
3. Sit up straight or stand up.
4. Take a *big* breath in, then breathe out slowly to the usual place. Do not force air out of your lungs.
5. If not using a spacer, position inhaler with canister above mouthpiece and hold the inhaler with mouthpiece 1 to 2 inches in front of the mouth with mouth wide open. *Do not* put your lips around the mouthpiece.
   If using a spacer, hold mouthpiece of the spacer in your mouth between your teeth with your lips around it.
6. If not using a spacer, begin breathing in *slowly*. Just after you start to breathe in, press down on the canister firmly to release one dose of medicine and keep breathing in.
   If using a spacer, press down on the canister firmly to release one dose of medicine into the spacer and breathe in *slowly*.
7. Finish taking a slow, deep breath. It should take 5 to 10 seconds. Breathe in as deeply as possible.
8. Hold your breath for at least 5 seconds. Try to hold your breath for 10 seconds.
9. If not using a spacer or if using an AeroChamber-type spacer, breathe out slowly through your nose. If using InspirEase, breathe out into the bag and repeat the inhalation cycle as recommended by the manufacturer.
10. If you are experiencing airflow obstruction, subsequent doses of bronchodilator or anti-inflammatory medicines may be more effective if you wait 15 minutes between doses. It is not necessary to wait between doses of anti-inflammatory medicines.
11. If you see the medicine float out of your nose or mouth, it never made it into your lungs! Repeat the dose (but only one more time).
12. Each night, wash mouthpiece (only) and dry thoroughly.

Bronchodilators

The three types of bronchodilating drugs currently used in the United States are β_2-adrenergic agonists (β_2-agonists), methylxanthines, and anticholinergics.

β_2-Adrenergic Agonists. The most widely used bronchodilators are the β_2-agonists. These agents act on β_2-adrenergic receptors on airway smooth muscle to cause muscle relaxation, resulting in bronchodilation; they may also reduce mediator release from mast cells and basophils. β_2-Agonists are available in oral formulations (liquids, plain tablets, and sustained-release tablets) and in metered-dose aerosols, aerosol solutions, and even a dry-powder preparation for inhalation. Inhaled therapy as compared with oral therapy has a faster onset of action, produces more bronchodilation and fewer systemic adverse effects, and achieves desired results at lower doses.

There is little difference between the various β_2-agonists available. The β_2-agonist most commonly prescribed in the United States is albuterol, which in other countries is called salbutamol. By inhalation, albuterol has onset of action within 15 minutes and duration of action of 4 to 6 hours in most patients. Albuterol liquid and tablet formulations taken orally have onset of action within 30 minutes and duration of action similar to that which occurs with inhalation; sustained-release albuterol tablets may produce bronchodilation for as long as

12 hours. Longer-acting β_2-agonists that are inhaled are currently undergoing clinical trials.

The β_2-agonists should be prescribed in the form, amount, and frequency needed to achieve maximum control of symptoms and maximum bronchodilation while causing minimum if any adverse effects. It should be noted that prolonged regular administration of β_2-agonists has been associated with increased airway reactivity and diminished control of asthma, and most recently it has been suggested that prolonged use of high doses of β_2-agonists may increase mortality from asthma. Therefore, the basic goal of therapy should be to minimize airway inflammation so that therapy with β_2-agonists (or any bronchodilator) is not needed. *Certainly, exceeding three-to four-times-a-day administration of an inhaled β_2-agonist on a daily regular basis is not recommended.*

Methylxanthines. These agents also are potent bronchodilators; in addition, they may benefit asthma patients by improving diaphragmatic muscle contractility and decreasing respiratory muscle fatigue, accelerating mucociliary transport, enhancing cardiovascular function, and reducing mediator release from mast cells. Although methylxanthines have been shown to inhibit the late-phase response to allergen challenge, they do not decrease airway reactivity. They are not effective when administered by inhalation and must be given orally or intravenously.

The principal methylxanthines used to treat asthma are theophylline or its salts (aminophylline or oxtriphylline). Short-acting methylxanthines, such as dyphylline, should be avoided. It is recommended that serum levels be maintained between 10 and 15 μg/ml unless complete bronchodilation is achieved at lower levels; higher levels are associated with an increased incidence of adverse effects. Bronchodilation may be seen within 30 minutes after dosing with a liquid form or rapidly absorbed tablet, with peak serum levels achieved 1½ to 2 hours after dosing. Dosing guidelines for theophylline have been detailed elsewhere.[1] Sustained-release oral preparations have a long duration of action and are particularly useful for chronic therapy; they are not suitable for acute administration, however.

Although methylxanthines are potent bronchodilators, they cannot be considered first-line therapy for asthma because of their narrow therapeutic ratio, the variability in their metabolism (both between patients and in response to intervening factors, such as intercurrent viral respiratory infections), and unwanted effects (such as central nervous system stimulation) that may occur with relatively low serum levels. They are useful in childhood asthma because they may produce additional bronchodilation when used in combination with β_2-agonists; they may provide bronchodilation in children who have difficulty using inhalation treatments; and their long duration of action in the sustained-release forms may decrease frequency of medicine administration.

Anticholinergics. When inhaled, anticholinergic drugs produce bronchodilation by reducing intrinsic vagal tone to the airways. Inhaled atropine sulfate and atropine methylnitrate and inhaled ipratropium bromide (Atrovent) block bronchoconstriction caused by inhaled irritants; they have also been shown to be beneficial as adjunctive therapy in acute asthma. In addition, they are likely to be beneficial in asthmatic children with cough (especially cough during and after viral respiratory infection) and with symptoms provoked mechanically or by emotions (e.g., by full, forced respiration, laughing, or crying).

Unlabeled Use of Approved Drugs

Many of the medicines useful in the management of asthma in children are not labeled for use in children below a given age. Lack of approval does not mean disapproval, however. Drugs licensed for use in the United States may be prescribed by licensed physicians based on available information regarding safety and effectiveness. Use of a drug not specifically approved for use in children below a given age must be differentiated from use of a drug that is contraindicated in children because studies have shown it to be unsafe or ineffective. Nonetheless, prudence dictates that unlabeled use of approved drugs be reserved for situations in which alternative drugs labeled for such use are not available or are less effective.

Strategies for Pharmacotherapy

Several different basic strategies are useful in treating children with asthma, depending on their clinical situation. As noted previously, children who present with a history of chronic symptoms, whose asthma is therefore out of control, require therapy both with medicines that treat airway inflammation and with those that treat symptoms. Once control has been established, medicines should be reduced to the lowest level needed to maintain control. On the other hand, children whose asthma has been in control but is now slipping out of control are appropriately treated with an increase in medications. Children with a severe exacerbation of asthma deserve aggressive treatment with a maximum pharmacologic regimen (Table 3). Finally, the following special situations warrant particular consideration.

Therapy for Chronic Symptoms or Airflow Obstruction

As noted previously, it is important to provide adequate pharmacotherapy to establish control of the disease as quickly as possible. Patients who present with a history of chronic symptoms (either intermittent or continuous) can be presumed to have airway inflammation. Those found to have airflow obstruction incompletely responsive or unresponsive to bronchodilator therapy also should be presumed to have airway inflammation. Therapy for these patients must include treatment of inflammation as well as therapy for symptoms. Patients without airflow obstruction or who have only mild airflow obstruction after bronchodilator treatment should receive cromolyn sodium, nedocromil sodium, or corticosteroid by inhalation. Patients who have more than mild airflow obstruction, those who have marked airway reactivity, and those who are unable to inhale medicines into the lung reliably should receive an oral corticosteroid.

It is reasonable to prescribe oral corticosteroids initially for patients who may later benefit from inhaled anti-inflammatory drugs in order to relieve airflow obstruction that might limit deposition of inhaled medicines into the lung and in order to give patients time to master use of a MDI. In these situations, prednisone (1 mg/kg) or an equivalent dose of an alternative preparation may be given morning and night (maximum dose usually no more than 60 to 80 mg/day) for 3 to 5 days. If the patient is well at this time, prednisone may be discontinued; tapering is usually not needed after such a short course of therapy. Patients who still have persistent obstruction or airway reactivity after 5 days of twice-a-day dosing may be given prednisone (1 mg/kg) every other day in the morning until sufficient clinical response is seen; this dose is then decreased in steps at 2-week intervals before being discontinued, assuming that clinical response is maintained.

In addition to anti-inflammatory drugs, patients who have chronic symptoms or airflow obstruction should receive bronchodilator therapy, both to relieve symptoms and to maximize airway caliber. The latter is especially important if inhaled anti-inflammatory medicines are being used. Bronchodilators should be prescribed in the form, amount, frequency, and combination needed to achieve maximum control of symptoms and maximum bronchodilation while causing minimum if any adverse effects.

After a patient's symptoms of asthma have resolved and lung function has normalized, the patient's medicine regimen should be reduced in steps to determine the smallest amount of medicine needed to maintain control of asthma. For example, if a patient has remained well on no oral steroid therapy (or the lowest dose possible) for 2 weeks, regular daily bronchodilator therapy should be discontinued or reduced. Likewise, if a patient requires only occasional treatment with a bronchodilator, any inhaled anti-inflammatory therapy should be discontinued or reduced. Decreases in therapy are usually made in steps (e.g., three-times-a-day dosing is reduced to twice-a-day dosing) every 1 to 2 weeks, although more frequent reductions in dosage are appropriate if symptoms and airflow obstruction both were mild and resolved rapidly. The optimum situation would be to administer only one medicine as infrequently as possible; however, the goals of asthma therapy listed at the beginning of this article may not be achieved by this approach.

Therapy for Increasing Symptoms or Airflow Obstruction

Once the minimum amount of medication needed for control of asthma has been established, there should be a "step-care" pharmacologic plan for increasing medications if increasing symptoms or airflow obstruction should occur. Patients requiring dosing with a β_2-agonist no more than twice a week have asthma that is under control. If symptoms occur more often or if peak flow variability is unacceptable (see later), regular use of an anti-inflammatory drug is recommended. In children, a trial with cromolyn should be instituted before an inhaled corticosteroid is prescribed. Increased need for β_2-agonist therapy or decreased duration of its effect indicates that increased anti-inflammatory therapy is needed. This increased therapy may be accomplished by increasing the frequency of dosing with cromolyn or by the addition of or increasing the dose of an inhaled corticosteroid. A sustained-release theophylline preparation should be added as a third-line drug if additional control of symptoms is necessary. Administration of a steroid orally should be the final step.

The rate at which therapy is accelerated depends on the degree and progression of symptoms or airflow obstruction. Mild symptoms or airflow obstruction might be approached with reasonable trials of a given level of therapy before going up a step; more severe or rapidly progressing symptoms or airflow obstruction necessitate rapid, decisive increases in therapy.

Therapy for Severe Symptoms or Airflow Obstruction

Patients who present with severe symptoms or with severe airflow obstruction should be treated with maximum antiasthma therapy. This includes:

1. Oxygen to maintain oxygen saturation (SaO_2) >93 to 95 per cent.
2. Inhaled β_2-agonist administered repetitively or continuously.
3. Theophylline or aminophylline to achieve a serum level of 10 to 15 μg/ml.
4. Systemic corticosteroid.

Oxygen is the first drug for severe asthma; patients with significant airflow obstruction are hypoxemic, and treatment with a β_2-agonist may increase hypoxemia by increasing perfusion to the lung more than ventilation. Albuterol is specifically recommended as the inhaled β_2-agonist for children with severe symptoms because of its safety when administered in frequent, high doses. Although intravenous theophylline or aminophylline has not been shown to produce additional bronchodilation when combined with β_2-agonist in the emergency department setting, a recent study has suggested that the addition of aminophylline decreases rate of hospitalization. Systemic corticosteroid is warranted for patients who have had prolonged symptoms or who have airflow obstruction that is not rapidly and completely relieved with bronchodilator treatment. Methylprednisolone (1 to 2 mg/kg orally or intravenously followed by 1 mg/kg given every 4 to 6 hours) is recommended for patients with severe symptoms or airflow obstruction in the emergency department or hospital.

Although treatment with anticholinergics, hydration, and chest physical therapy may be beneficial in selected children, they are not part of the routine management of severe asthma. Hydration is more important for infants and young children, who may become dehydrated because of increased fluid loss via the respiratory tract and decreased oral intake. Overhydration should be avoided because it may cause pulmonary edema in patients with severe airflow obstruction. Chest physiotherapy, including chest percussion or vibration and postural drainage, may benefit children who have mucus hypersecretion or atelectasis as part of their asthma. Mucolytics and sedation should not be given to children with severe exacerbations of asthma. Antibiotics should be reserved for children with clear evidence of bacterial infection, such as purulent secretions or lobar consolidation on chest radiograph.

Children with severe airflow obstruction must be monitored closely, both in the emergency department and in the hospital if necessary. Those with impending respiratory failure should be treated in an intensive care unit. A trial of intravenous terbutaline may be considered for children in an intensive care unit who have progressive respiratory compromise in spite of oxygen, continuous inhalation of albuterol, intravenous theophylline or aminophylline, and intravenous methylprednisolone. Children with elevated P_{CO_2} that is rising should be intubated and mechanically ventilated.

After a patient's symptoms of asthma have begun to decrease and lung function has begun to normalize, the patient's medicine regimen should be reduced in steps. As described previously, the rate of reduction should be determined by the level of symptoms and airflow obstruction. However, concerns about adverse effects from prolonged or high dosing should be weighed against the goal of healing the airway as rapidly as possible.

Exercise-Induced Asthma

Exercise usually causes symptoms in asthmatic children who have inflamed airways. However, participation in exercise is an essential part of childhood, for both physical health and psychosocial reasons. Children who experience EIA should receive prophylactic treatment. The majority of children will experience complete ablation of EIA by pretreatment with an inhaled β_2-agonist, usually given within an hour of anticipated exercise. The majority will also gain complete protection by pretreatment with inhaled cromolyn or nedocromil. A few children require the combination of inhaled β_2-agonist and inhaled cromolyn for complete prophylaxis of EIA. Young children who cannot use a MDI or who do not have a home nebulizer may be treated with an oral β_2-agonist given at least 30 minutes before exercise. Such children may also be treated with a rapidly absorbed theophylline given 1 to 2 hours before exercise, but theophylline is less effective than are β_2-agonists in blocking EIA. It should be kept in mind that EIA is a reflection of airway reactivity and airway inflammation. Thus, frequent episodes of EIA warrant institution of anti-inflammatory therapy (see previously).

Virus-Induced Asthma

Viral respiratory infections commonly cause exacerbations of asthma in children, especially in young children. Early institution of therapy with a corticosteroid has been shown to decrease the duration and severity of virus-induced exacerbations of asthma in children, and treatment with corticosteroid at the first sign of illness should be considered in children with an established pattern of severe asthma from viral respiratory infections. Patients and their families should be alert for early signs of an exacerbation of asthma when the patient experiences a viral respiratory illness so that asthma medicine may be started or increased promptly.

Nocturnal Asthma

Children with asthma commonly experience an increase in symptoms at night. This may occur because of changes in lung function and airway regulation with recumbency and sleep, circadian changes in hormones and mediators, and exposure to allergens in the bedroom, among other reasons. Children with nocturnal asthma need attention to their sleeping environment and anti-inflammatory therapy to decrease airway hyperreactivity. While waiting for these measures to take effect, such children may also benefit from dosing with a sustained-release theophylline preparation or a sustained-release β_2-agonist tablet, because inhaled β_2-agonists currently used are unlikely to provide adequate bronchodilation for the duration of sleep.

Severe, Chronic Asthma

Fewer than 5 per cent of children with asthma have severe, chronic symptoms that warrant intensive anti-inflammatory and bronchodilator therapy at all times. All steroid-dependent asthmatic children require thorough investigation for contributing factors, such as allergy, sinusitis, gastroesophageal reflux, and immunodeficiency. Innovative therapeutic alternatives to reduce oral steroid dosage that have been proposed for such children include treatment with high-dose inhaled steroid, TAO, methotrexate, gold, and intravenous immunoglobulin. Experimental therapies such as these should be considered only after conventional therapeutic strategies have been exhausted.

IMMUNOTHERAPY

Avoidance of allergens by allergic children is preferable to treatment with any other mode of therapy. However, allergen immunotherapy should be considered when (1) avoidance is difficult (e.g., house dust mites or cockroaches) or impossible (e.g., outdoor aeroallergens such as pollens), and (2) appropriate medicines fail to control allergic asthma or an untoward level of therapy is needed to maintain control. Allergen immunotherapy (also called allergen hyposensitization) in double-blind studies has been shown to decrease symptoms of asthma and airway reactivity. Allergen immunotherapy is different from desensitization to an allergen, such as might be done for patients who are allergic to penicillin but require therapy with this drug. Desensitization provides benefit only while the allergen is being given; no protective long-term immunity results from this measure.

Allergen immunotherapy should be reserved for patients who have demonstrable allergy (by allergy testing) that correlates with their clinical history. Response to immunotherapy is specific for the allergens included in the vaccine and is dependent on the dose administered; small doses of an allergy extract, even given over time, are not likely to generate protective immunologic responses. Immunotherapy is given in three phases. First, the dose of allergen given is increased in small increments until the patient is able to tolerate injection of the "maintenance" dose. The maintenance dose is calculated to be large enough to generate protective immunologic responses. Second, this maintenance dose is given until a therapeutic response is achieved. Third, the frequency of injections is decreased in steps to maintain the beneficial response.

While building to the maintenance dose, injections are usually given one to four times each week, depending on the time the patient has to receive injections and the urgency to generate a clinical response. Maintenance injections are usually given once or twice a week until a beneficial response is seen; afterward, the interval between injections is increased in steps over 4 to 6 weeks. Immunotherapy injections should always be given in a medical facility where both personnel and equipment are available, because life-threatening reactions may (but rarely do) occur. Immunotherapy is usually continued for 3 to 5 years in patients who experience clinical benefit. If there is no evidence of response within 2 years, it should be stopped. Although there are true treatment failures, a more common reason for lack of success of immunotherapy is use of inadequate amounts of allergen to generate beneficial immunologic responses, either because of poor quality extracts or because of attempts to include too many allergens in a single injection (thereby diluting all of them).

OBJECTIVE MEASUREMENT OF LUNG FUNCTION

Pulmonary function testing is essential to the management of pulmonary diseases, including asthma. It is especially important in children with asthma because the child's reports of symptoms, the parent's assessment of the child's clinical status, and the physician's physical findings on examination often do not correlate with objective measurements of lung function. Many children simply cannot sense mild to moderate levels of airflow obstruction and experience no symptoms; others are reluctant to admit to having symptoms of asthma because such an admission risks restricting their activities and having to take medicines.

Lung function should be assessed objectively at each visit to the physician. It is important to determine each child's best lung function test results because comparison of results to "per cent predicted" (which actually are mean values for a similar population) may be misleading. Testing before and after provocation (such as exercise provocation by free running) is useful to gauge degree of airway hyperreactivity or the protective effects of medicines. Testing before and after bronchodilator use (e.g., before and after the child uses a MDI) also may gauge airway reactivity and airway inflammation: a large change in airway caliber reflects the former, whereas incomplete bronchodilation reflects the latter.

Testing is best accomplished using a spirometer, which measures forced vital capacity (FVC), 1-second forced expiratory volume (FEV_1), and forced expiratory flow between 25 and 75 per cent of vital capacity (FEF_{25-75}). Units that provide expiratory flow-volume curves provide additional useful information. Airflow obstruction in asthma usually occurs primarily in small airways. This is first reflected in decreased flow at lower lung volumes, best seen in FEF_{25-75} or on flow-volume loop. Further obstruction will also compromise FEV_1. Finally, hyperinflation of the lung will restrict FVC.

Measuring peak expiratory flow rate (PEFR, or peak flow) with a peak flow meter has been advocated for the office assessment of lung function in asthma. Unfortunately, peak flow (which occurs at high lung volume) usually decreases only after there is moderate to severe airflow obstruction, and

TABLE 5. Patient Guide: Steps for Measurement of Peak Expiratory Flow Rate

1. Make certain that the peak flow meter reads zero or is at base level.
2. Stand up (or sit up straight).
3. Take in as deep a breath as possible.
4. Put the peak flow meter in your mouth between your teeth and place your lips tightly around it. Keep your tongue away from the mouthpiece.
5. Blow out as hard and as fast as possible.
6. Repeat this process (steps 1 to 5) two more times.
7. Discard values if coughing.
8. In your peak flow diary, record the highest of the three measurements obtained.

a normal peak flow does not guarantee completely normal lung function. Despite this reservation, measuring peak flow at home can be very useful in monitoring and managing asthma. Inexpensive, reliable portable peak flow meters are available for home use. The proper technique for peak flow assessment is described in Table 5.

It has been suggested that a series of peak flow zones be established to guide management at home.[1] A goal of therapy is that all peak flow measurements be at least 80 per cent of the patient's personal best, although peak flows ideally should vary less than 10 per cent. Consistent readings within this "green zone" suggest that the patient's asthma is under control. Readings between 50 and 80 to 90 per cent of the patient's personal best (the "yellow zone") indicate that the patient's asthma is not under control and that an increase in medicine is needed. A reading that is below 50 per cent of the patient's personal best (the "red zone") warrants immediate bronchodilator treatment and physician notification; further intervention is mandatory if the reading does not return to the yellow or green zone. The child's peak flow meter should be marked with green, yellow, and red tape to make these zones obvious, and these zones should be marked on the peak flow diary pages as well.

Patients with asthma are first asked to measure their peak flows in the morning and evening for several weeks to give them practice with the device and to establish their best measurement. Those receiving inhaled or oral β_2-agonist therapy should measure peak flows before and after dosing both morning and evening. The best of three efforts should be recorded on a peak flow diary sheet, which also permits plotting of the results; plotting the results allows the patient and the patient's family to visualize lung function more easily than can be done from the readings alone. Readings consistently in the green zone suggest that the patient's medicines might be reduced. A patient who is well on no medicines or on a maintenance therapy might be asked to make peak flow measurements only in the morning upon arising (since this is when peak flow is most likely to be decreased), either daily or on certain days of the week. Of course, peak flow measurements should be made whenever there is a question about clinical status.

WRITTEN GUIDELINES FOR PATIENTS AND FAMILIES

Written guidelines for patients and their families are important to promote adherence to the treatment plan and to achieve improvement in asthma control (Table 6). Patients and their families should be given written instructions for mite avoidance (see Table 1), use of a MDI (see Table 4), and use of a peak flow meter (see Table 5). Patients should also be given peak flow diary pages.

Most important, all patients with asthma should have written guidelines that include specific instructions about use of medicines and an "action plan" for the management of symptoms or airflow obstruction.[1, 2] The action plan should include:

1. The symptoms and peak flow measurements that warrant an increase in therapy and exactly what this increase should be.
2. What to do if symptoms or low peak flow measurements persist in spite of an increase in therapy.
3. Criteria for beginning or increasing oral steroid dosing.
4. Criteria for contacting the patient's physician.
5. Specific criteria for seeking emergency medical care.

The action plan also should include criteria for determining wellness (e.g., no symptoms for the previous 2 weeks and peak flows >80 per cent of personal best) and instructions for decreasing therapy in steps if the child is well.

SPECIAL CONSIDERATIONS

Control of rhinitis, which often occurs in children with asthma, is likely to benefit overall control of asthma, and therapy of rhinitis should be part of therapy of asthma. Children with rhinitis frequently experience sinusitis, and sinusitis has been shown to contribute to the worsening of asthma.

Gastroesophageal reflux occurs more commonly in patients with asthma than it does in those without asthma, but its role in causing symptoms of asthma is controversial. The relationship between chest symptoms and gastroesophageal reflux in infants is particularly difficult to assess because the majority of infants normally have some reflux.

CHILDREN AT HIGH RISK OF ASTHMA-RELATED DEATH

It should be appreciated that certain children are at high risk of death from asthma. These children require intensive education, close monitoring, and prompt medical care. They include children with a history of:

1. Respiratory failure requiring intubation.

TABLE 6. Items to be Included in Written Guidelines for Patients and Families

1. Instructions for instituting environmental precautions.
2. How to use a nebulizer and metered-dose inhaler, if prescribed.
3. Instructions for home monitoring of peak flow (children ≥5 years of age).
4. Specific instructions about use of medications: dose, frequency of administration, adverse effects to report to the physician.
5. How to monitor signs, symptoms, and peak flow rates to detect increasing airflow obstruction as early as possible.
6. Criteria for initiating or modifying treatment (including signs, symptoms, and peak flow measurements).
7. Guidelines for increasing dose or adding medication.
8. List of other actions to take in managing an acute episode of asthma (e.g., remove precipitating trigger, avoid strenuous physical activity, stay calm).
9. Guidelines for contacting physician (e.g., symptoms persisting longer than 2 days, symptoms requiring bronchodilator more than every 4 hours).
10. Specific criteria for seeking emergency medical care (e.g., peak flow <50% of personal best that is unresponsive to bronchodilator; cyanosis).
11. Guidelines for decreasing medication when well.

Adapted from Guidelines for the Diagnosis and Management of Asthma. National Asthma Education Program Expert Panel Report. National Heart, Lung, and Blood Institute, National Institutes of Health, Publication No. 91-3042, 1991.

2. Admission to an intensive care unit because of asthma.
3. Frequent hospitalizations or emergency room visits in the previous year.
4. Current or recent use of systemic corticosteroids.
5. Past history of syncope or hypoxic seizure from asthma.
6. Serious psychiatric disease and psychosocial problems.
7. Lack of access to medical care.

An additional important risk factor is a child's inability to sense airflow obstruction. It is unfair to ask such a child to judge by subjective criteria how well his or her asthma is controlled, and use of medicines should certainly not be determined by subjective feeling. Although many children benefit from using a peak flow meter to help monitor and manage their asthma, use of peak flow measurements is mandatory in children younger than age 5 years who cannot tell when they are wheezing.

REFERENCES

1. Guidelines for the Diagnosis and Management of Asthma. National Asthma Education Program Expert Panel Report. National Heart, Lung, and Blood Institute, National Institutes of Health, Publication No. 91–3042, 1991.
2. Hargreave FE, Dolovich J, Newhouse MT: The assessment and treatment of asthma: A conference report. J Allergy Clin Immunol 85:1098–1111, 1990.

SERUM SICKNESS

LEONARD BIELORY, M.D.

ETIOLOGY

Serum sickness, as described in 1905 by Emil von Pirquet and Bela Schick in their classic study "Die Serum Krankheit," consisted of a spectrum of clinical findings that included fever, malaise, cutaneous eruptions (primarily urticaria), arthralgia, lymphadenopathy, edema, and albuminuria. Their patients were primarily children in whom one or a combination of these symptoms developed 6 to 10 days after an initial exposure to heterologous antisera used to treat various infectious diseases. The administration of heterologous antisera remained the major cause of serum sickness until the advent of modern drug therapy.

Currently, the most frequently encountered medications producing serum sickness include penicillins, sulfonamides, streptomycin, cephalosporins, thiouracils, and hydantoins. Penicillin is the most common agent implicated in the induction of serum sickness, although it is unusual with dosages under 2 g/day. Sulfonamides have recently been associated with an increase in serum sickness–like reactions in patients infected with the human immunodeficiency virus (HIV). However, the medications producing the highest and most consistent frequency of serum sickness reactions are still the heterologous proteins, which are used for crotalid and arachnid envenomation; for treatment of specific clostridial infections and rabies; and as immunosuppressive agents for the prevention of organ allograft rejection or to precondition patients about to receive allogeneic organs.

TREATMENT

The treatment of serum sickness is either prophylactic or symptomatic. Most patients with serum sickness are probably never seen by the physician because the clinical spectrum of complaints is very similar to that which the public perceives as the "flu", and patients are apt to treat themselves with fluids, aspirin, and bed rest. It is usually only the rare circumstance of a frightening cutaneous eruption or severe arthralgia that brings a person to the attention of a physician for medical treatment.

Prophylaxis

For prophylactic treatment, all physicians should maintain up-to-date vaccinations of their patients, as recommended by the American College of Physicians Committee's Guide for Adult Immunization and by the Red Book of the American Academy of Pediatrics, in order to immunize them against those diseases still treated with heterologous antisera. Heterologous antisera are still in use in several underdeveloped countries for acute diphtheria. All individuals traveling to underdeveloped countries should be vaccinated for endemic infectious agents, as recommended by the Centers for Disease Control in the *Morbidity and Mortality Weekly Report.* Individuals may contact their local or state health departments to locate the closest "certified" immunization center.

Symptomatic Treatment

Symptomatic treatment is based on the severity and extent of the patient's complaints. First, if possible, the offending antigen should be eliminated. It is known from animal models that elimination of antigen will lead to rapid resolution of immunopathologic damage. Symptomatic treatment usually involves the use of combinations of antipyretics, analgesics, glucocorticoids, and antihistamines.

Antipyretic medications such as the salicylates, as noted by von Pirquet and Schick, are of some benefit in ameliorating the febrile response but have relatively little effect on the arthralgia or the various cutaneous eruptions. In addition, the use of salicylates at an antipyretic dose range of 10 to 15 mg/kg must be considered in light of their effect on platelet function, because some serum sickness patients develop thrombocytopenia. Acetaminophen as an antipyretic may be a better choice in thrombocytopenic individuals. Furthermore, the concern of the enhanced risk of Reye syndrome in children with a respiratory disease or chickenpox has resulted in the use of antipyretic medications other than aspirin (e.g., acetaminophen).

Other symptoms, particularly those associated with proteinuria or arthralgia, usually warrant treatment with a "burst" of glucocorticoids. "Burst" glucocorticoid therapy involves the use of prednisone (1 to 2 mg/kg/day in divided doses for 7 to 10 days). This is followed by consolidation to once-a-day doses coinciding with the normal diurnal (A.M.) variation of cortisol levels and then tapering the drug by 10-mg and then by 2.5-mg decrements until the prednisone is discontinued within a period of about 3 to 4 weeks.

Antihistamines have proved to be of value in the treatment of generalized urticaria and pruritus, including such medications as diphenhydramine (Benadryl, 50 mg every 4 hours [1 mg/kg in children]) or, alternatively, hydroxyzine (Atarax, Vistaril, 25 mg every 4 hours [0.3 mg/kg in children]). The prophylactic value of antihistamines in serum sickness has not been proven, but these drugs may be useful. Doses of diphenhydramine or cyproheptadine are started 4 days prior to the expected onset of serum sickness and continued for a period of 1 to 2 weeks. Marked urticarial eruptions or angioedema is usually treated with aqueous epinephrine (1:1000, 0.01 ml/kg subcutaneously with a maximum of 0.3 to 0.5 ml every 15 minutes for three doses). If attacks of angioedema recur after use of the preceding treatment, intramuscular aqueous epinephrine suspension (Sus-Phrine) can be used (1:200, 0.005 ml/kg, with a maximum of 0.2 ml every 6 hours).

If large amounts of heterologous antisera are required over a course of days, the usual precautions as recommended by the manufacturer should be strictly followed. Skin testing with the antigen and appropriate controls should be done prior to administration of the heterologous protein. If there is an immediate hypersensitivity reaction, desensitization may be required to prevent anaphylaxis. However, desensitization does not prevent the occurrence of serum sickness.

Glucocorticoids in the form of prednisone (or intravenous methylprednisolone, 1 mg/kg/day in three or four divided doses) should be started concomitantly with the first dose of heterologous antisera. This dose should be increased to 1.5 mg/kg/day at the first sign of serum sickness, maintained for 3 or 4 days or as long as the heterologous protein must be given, then tapered by 10-mg decrements every 2 or 3 days to 30 mg, then tapered by 5-mg decrements every 2 or 3 days to 10 mg, and then tapered by 2.5-mg decrements over the course of a week. If the antigen persists longer than expected and the patient has a breakthrough of symptoms while steroids are being tapered, the dose at which the symptoms reappeared (usually between 10 and 20 mg of prednisone) should be doubled. The steroids may then be decreased on alternate days rather than daily in 10-mg decrements every two or three cycles until a dose of 30 mg is reached, then tapered by 5-mg decrements every two or three cycles until 20 mg is reached, and then tapered by 2.5-mg decrements every two or three cycles until the alternate-day dose has been discontinued. If exacerbations occur on the off days, one should increase the dose to a previous level that controlled the symptoms and then taper even more slowly. When the alternate-day therapy is achieved, it is maintained for 2 to 4 weeks to permit the hypothalamic-pituitary-adrenal (HPA) axis to recover and is then tapered by 5 mg a week. The alternate-day regimen has been shown to cause far less HPA axis suppression and to result in fewer opportunistic infections.

In cases necessitating the readministration of heterologous antisera, in which the "accelerated" form of serum sickness is expected within 24 to 72 hours after administration, the concomitant use of glucocorticoids, as described previously, is recommended. One should also be extremely careful of the possibility of anaphylaxis because the patient has had a previous exposure to the heterologous protein.

Local reactions at the site of intramuscular injections of heterologous antisera during the course of serum sickness can range from a mild urticarial eruption to a severely indurated granulomatous lesion. Treatment usually involves the use of oral antihistamines for the mild reaction and systemic "burst" of glucocorticoids for the severe reaction.

REFERENCES

Bielory L, Gascon P, Lawley TJ, et al: Human serum sickness: A prospective, clinical, immunological, and immunopathological analysis of 35 patients treated with antithymocyte globulin. Medicine 67:40–57, 1988.

ALLERGIC GASTROINTESTINAL DISORDERS

DOUGLAS H. SANDBERG, M.D.

Although this article is devoted to immunoglobulin E (IgE) antibody–mediated allergic reactions to foods, it should be understood that other immunologic mechanisms may be involved in some patients, including type III (Arthus reaction) and type IV mechanisms. These mechanisms are not well understood; however, treatment methods are similar in all of them.

Gastrointestinal symptoms that may be caused by food hypersensitivity include nausea and/or vomiting, diarrhea, enteritis with malabsorption and/or failure to thrive, abdominal pain and bloating, colitis, intestinal loss of serum proteins and/or blood, and eosinophilic gastroenteritis. In some children, these symptoms may be accompanied by involvement of the skin and the upper and/or lower respiratory tract. Other children may have symptoms or signs confined to the gastrointestinal tract.

The basic principles governing the management of these gastrointestinal disorders have not changed very much in the past several years, although there is continuing debate among physicians as to the best approach to the treatment of allergic problems. Identification of specific allergens and subsequent avoidance of those agents remain the primary methods of clinical management. An equally important aspect of treatment is prevention of development of sensitivities.

DIAGNOSIS

Clinical History

Diagnostic approaches to allergic gastrointestinal disorders include an accurate and detailed clinical history, including:

1. Circumstances surrounding the onset of symptoms and signs.
2. Chronologic progression of symptoms.
3. Any treatments and response to those treatments.
4. Specific foods that appear to be implicated as provoking agents (amounts of the foods needed to trigger a reaction, method of food preparation, and awareness of other foods eaten at approximately the same time prior to a reaction).

This clinical history is more helpful when symptoms are intermittent rather than constant.

A diet diary is frequently helpful, particularly if a separate symptom diary is kept simultaneously over a period in which several episodes occur. It is preferable to record episodes of a single major symptom rather than to note all symptoms occurring within the time period.

Laboratory Tests

Laboratory tests may also be helpful in diagnosis. Positive skin prick tests have been shown to be predictive of IgE-mediated hypersensitivity to specific foods; however, they are not very accurate for identifying reactions mediated by other immunologic mechanisms. In vitro IgE radioallergosorbent test (RAST) (or other tests such as fluorescent allergosorbent test [FAST] and enzyme-linked immunosorbent assay [ELISA], which provide essentially the same information) may also identify specific food allergens but is somewhat less sensitive than skin tests. RAST is useful in specific circumstances in which skin tests would be difficult to perform (i.e., children with diffuse dermatitis). Interpretation of test results is through correlation with the clinical history and with confirmation by open (or preferably blind) food challenges.

Other methods used by some physicians (including various methods for provocation of symptoms or neutralization) are still considered by most allergists to be investigational or, as in the case of cytotoxic food testing and measurement of serum IgG antibodies to specific foods, unreliable.

Elimination Diets

Elimination diets may also be valuable in relating diet to a specific gastrointestinal disorder. A number of caveats apply, however. Symptoms should be severe enough to warrant a severe diet, and markedly restricted diets should be used for short periods (1 to 4 weeks). Careful attention to ensuring nutritional adequacy of such diets is important.

During elimination diets, careful written diet and symptom diaries should be maintained. In certain instances, very restricted diets (e.g., Tolerex*, Nutramigen†) for periods of 1 to 2 weeks are valuable. If improvement is observed, eliminated foods should be returned to the diet one at a time, with close observation for appearance of targeted symptoms. Again, it is preferable that the foods be added in a single or double-blind manner to avoid subjective bias. For small children, the food may be simply disguised in other food; for older children, powdered foods hidden in opaque gelatin capsules are ideal.

Challenges should not be carried out if there is a clinical history of anaphylaxis. For investigation of severe symptoms, such challenges usually require in-hospital administration. Challenges preceded by periods of avoidance of more than 4 days but less than 2 weeks are more likely to produce easily observable reactions. When possible, quantitative data such as number of bowel movements, white and/or red blood cells in stool, and episodes of vomiting should be recorded during elimination periods as well as during food challenges. For patients with complicated problems, these diets and challenges are best supervised by a physician experienced in these techniques.

MANAGEMENT

Avoidance of Allergens

Avoidance of offending allergens is still the preferred method of management of allergic disorders. For infants, the necessary period of avoidance may be quite variable. However, for most infants with milk allergy, milk may be returned to the diet somewhere after 1 year of age without observable adverse effects on the gastrointestinal tract. In general, after a period of avoidance of a food of 6 weeks to 3 months, cautious reintroduction may be attempted, with close observation for return of symptoms. If a reaction does occur, the food should be eliminated for an additional period of 2 to 3 months and the process repeated. If reintroduction is successful, tolerance may sometimes be lost if there is unusually heavy use of the food in the diet. With appropriate education, parents often become adept at monitoring the child's diet. In most children, gastrointestinal symptoms related to food allergy tend to subside by age 3 to 5 years.

Medications

The use of drugs in the treatment of allergic gastrointestinal disorders has generally been disappointing. Antihistamines (both H_1 and H_2 blockers), adrenal corticosteroids, and oral cromolyn sodium have been used with only occasional or partial success. Treatment with nonsedating H_1-type antihistamines, such as astemizole, allows use of somewhat higher doses of the drug and may very occasionally reduce symptoms such as abdominal pain.

Two clinical entities in which corticosteroid therapy has been shown to be effective are allergic gastroenteritis with protein-losing enteropathy and eosinophilic gastroenteritis.

Use of oral cromolyn sodium for prevention of reactions to food is moderately expensive but relatively free of important side effects or toxicity. For infants younger than 6 months of age, the dose is 20 mg/kg/day dissolved in liquid in four divided doses 30 minutes prior to feedings and at bedtime. For infants 6 months to 2 years of age, the maximum dose is 30 mg/kg/day; for those older than 2 years of age, the maximum dose is 40 mg/kg/day. Adolescents may require up to 800 mg/day (as 100-mg capsules dissolved in water in divided doses before meals and at bedtime).

Ketotifen (Zaditen, Sandoz) is a prophylactic medication for allergic disorders that is not yet available in the United States; however, in other countries, it has been shown to be at least partially effective in some patients for control of symptoms related to food allergy. It is a potent antihistamine (H_1 receptor blocker), which has other antiallergic and antianaphylactic properties. Mechanisms of action are not clear at this time. Ketotifen is given in a dose of 1 mg orally twice daily in either tablet, capsule, or syrup form; it frequently requires several weeks or more for maximum effect. Children older than 3 years of age require adult doses, whereas those younger than 3 years of age are given one half the adult dose. It is well absorbed when administered orally.

Hypoallergenic Formulas

Hypoallergenic formulas are valuable tools for the pediatrician in the management of the infant with gastrointestinal symptoms related to diet. Although there are data to suggest that soy formulas are less likely than cow's milk–based formulas to provoke allergic reactions, available data are less convincing that use of soy-based formulas for *initial* feeding is less likely to result in intolerance. Certainly, 30 to 40 per cent of infants sensitive to cow's milk formulas are also intolerant to soy formula.

The availability of protein hydrolysate formulas has made management of infant diet problems easier. Although there are relatively small differences among various hydrolysate formulas, an infant will at times respond to a specific formula better than to the others in that group. *It appears that formulas utilizing caseinate rather than whey protein hydrolysate are better tolerated in sensitive infants.* Formulas based on whey protein may still have a place in prophylaxis of infants suspected of being at risk for development of milk sensitivity, although there is considerable difference of opinion on the indications for the use of such formulas. Sometimes, the rotation of three to five different formulas, one each day, may significantly improve tolerance to feedings by reducing exposure to any one formula. Any formula that is poorly tolerated is eliminated from the group. This principle of a varied diet with reduced reliance on only a few foods may be extended to management of the occasional child who has multiple food sensitivities.

PREVENTION

Prevention of allergic gastrointestinal symptoms has been extensively studied in infants. Mechanisms that appear to predispose some infants to food allergy include persistence of increased mucosal permeability beyond the first few months of life and delay in development of adequate protection by mucosal secretory IgA production. Identification of infants at risk for atopic disease is based on two pieces of information: (1) a positive history of atopic disease in siblings or parents and (2) a concentration of total IgE in cord blood equal to or greater than 1.3 IU/ml.

Knowledge of environmental factors, such as early exposure to antigen and duration of breast-feeding, is also helpful in determining occurrence of allergic reactions to foods. Breast-feeding has been extensively investigated as a primary mode of prevention. Although a number of studies over many years show breast-feeding to have a protective effect, there are still conflicting clinical studies questioning its value in prevention of allergic reactions. Some reports have indicated that limiting foods such as milk, and possibly egg, in the last trimester may reduce the incidence of the infant's sensitivity to these foods

*Tolerex, a synthetic elemental diet (liquid) (Sandoz).

†Nutramigen, a protein hydrolysate formula (Mead-Johnson).

after birth. There is also some evidence that limiting these foods in the mother's diet while the infant is breast-feeding may be helpful in reducing the infant's allergic reactions to the foods. Again, there are data that question these conclusions.

Consultation with a subspecialist should be requested when a child has unusually severe symptoms, is not thriving or is otherwise unable to function adequately in daily life, or is not responsive to usual approaches to management.

ADVERSE DRUG REACTIONS

MATTHEW E. KNIGHT, M.D.

The World Health Organization defines an adverse drug reaction (ADR) as one that is "noxious and unintended and which occurs at doses normally used in humans for prophylaxis, diagnosis, therapy or modification of physiological function." This definition excludes such events as overdoses, medication errors, and problems with administration. This article focuses on the scope of the problem of ADRs in children and provides an overview of mechanisms and examples of ADRs.

SCOPE OF PROBLEM

In the adult population, 5 per cent of admissions to a general internal medicine ward are the result of an ADR.[1] It has been shown that the risk for an ADR in adults is directly related to the number of drugs the individual is taking. A patient taking 1 to 5 drugs has a risk of about 4 per cent for an ADR, whereas someone taking 11 to 15 drugs has a risk of 24 per cent. Of adult patients admitted for any reason, the incidence of ADRs is 6 to 36 per cent, with 3 per cent of those patients experiencing a life-threatening or disabling reaction and 0.7 per cent having a fatal outcome.

It has been more difficult to study ADRs in the pediatric population because children are prescribed fewer drugs. *Recent studies found that, in a general pediatric ward, 2 per cent of admissions were for an ADR.[2] The incidence, as one would expect, is much higher in pediatric cancer patients, that is, up to 22 per cent.* However, only 0.2 per cent of admissions to the neonatal intensive care unit were for an ADR. *In the pediatric outpatient population, the incidence reported for ADRs was 17.1 per cent.[3]* More than half of such reactions were of no clinical consequence, and one half were preventable.

Factors associated with a higher risk for ADRs in children include either the prescriber or the patient/parents increasing the dose; age younger than 12 months; and an increase in the number of drugs taken.[2] The drugs most commonly implicated in pediatric hospital admissions due to ADRs include phenobarbital, aspirin, phenytoin, ampicillin/amoxicillin, theophylline/aminophylline, trimethoprim-sulfamethoxazole, and the diphtheria-pertussis-tetanus vaccine.[2] The symptoms experienced by children with ADRs include gastrointestinal (diarrhea, nausea, vomiting, anorexia, abdominal pain), 75 per cent; cutaneous (urticaria, candidiasis, other rash), 22.5 per cent; central nervous system (hyperactivity/poor attention, hyposomnia), 7.5 per cent; and other, 3.5 per cent (total exceeds 100 per cent because some patients experience more than one ADR).[2]

MECHANISMS

ADRs may be caused by one or more of several mechanisms. Types of mechanisms include pharmacologic or dose-related, drug interaction–related (pharmacokinetic or pharmacodynamic), idiosyncratic, and allergic- or immune-mediated.

Pharmacologic or Dose-Related Reaction

Pharmacologic or dose-related ADRs account for approximately 70 to 80 per cent of all ADRs (Table 1). These reactions involve an excessive response by the individual to the desired pharmacologic effect. An example is symptomatic hypotension due to an antihypertensive medication. A patient may also experience a dose-related toxic effect that is not part of the desired therapeutic effect (e.g., central nervous system irritability with theophylline).

Drug Interaction Reaction

Drug interactions may also account for pharmacologic ADRs. The combined use of erythromycin and theophylline may lead to toxic theophylline serum concentrations as a result of the reduction in theophylline clearance by the presence of erythromycin. This is an example of a *pharmacokinetic interaction.* The combined use of morphine and diazepam puts a patient at higher risk for apnea than does either agent alone. This represents a *pharmacodynamic interaction,* with each agent directly affecting the central respiratory drive mechanisms. This result occurs independent of an effect of either drug on the other's disposition, and is due to a combined effect on central respiratory control.

Characteristics common to pharmacologic and drug interaction ADRs are that they are predictable and dose-related. They may also occur as a result of the presence of *altered organ function,* affecting drug response or drug disposition. For example, renal failure or hepatic failure may allow for accumulation of a drug to toxic concentrations or may alter the disposition of a drug by changing the volume of distribution or protein binding. The presence of respiratory failure or congestive heart failure may mean that the altered physiology in these systems may lead to an enhanced response to the effects of drugs.

In general, these ADRs can be prevented by knowledge of the actions of drugs both under normal conditions and during abnormal organ function. Awareness of clinically important drug interactions will also reduce the risk of ADRs.

Idiosyncratic Reaction

Twenty per cent of ADRs are not dose-related but, rather, idiosyncratic (Table 2). Idiosyncratic reactions are related to an unusual characteristic of the patient that leads to an unpredictable adverse response to the drug. Examples include low serum esterase activity with enhanced response to succinylcholine; hemolytic anemia due to exposure to oxidant

TABLE 1. Mechanisms of Pharmacologic Adverse Drug Reactions

Mechanism	Example
Accentuated dose-related pharmacologic effect	Hypotension during antihypertensive therapy
Dose-related toxic effect	Central nervous system irritability during theophylline therapy
Drug interaction—pharmacokinetic	Reduction of theophylline clearance by erythromycin
Drug interaction—pharmacodynamic	Apnea with combined administration of morphine and diazepam
Toxicity due to altered disposition or elimination due to altered renal or liver function	Digoxin accumulation in renal failure
	Increased unbound phenytoin during renal failure

TABLE 2. Mechanisms of Non-pharmacologic Adverse Drug Reactions

Mechanism	Example
Idiosyncratic—inapparent feature of patient leading to adverse drug reaction	Hemolysis after exposure to antimalarial drugs in patients with glucose-6-phosphate dehydrogenase deficiency Aspirin-induced bronchospasm Prolonged effect of succinylcholine due to low serum esterase activity Phenytoin hypersensitivity due to probable generation of reactive metabolite that may become a hapten
Allergic/immune-mediated	Penicillin anaphylaxis Serum sickness with sulfonamides Stevens-Johnson syndrome with phenobarbital therapy
Anaphylactoid reactions—release of mediators of anaphylaxis without involvement of IgE	Vancomycin-induced cutaneous flushing Radiologic contrast media reactions

drugs, such as antimalarial agents in individuals who are glucose-6-phosphate dehydrogenase (G-6-PD)-deficient; and bronchospasm after aspirin administration in predisposed individuals. The mechanism for aspirin-induced bronchospasm is related to the generation of clinically significant lipoxygenase products after inhibition of cyclo-oxygenase by aspirin. These products include leukotrienes and have been shown to be mediators of anaphylaxis, bronchospasm, and inflammation.

Recent laboratory investigations have shed light on potential mechanisms for idiosyncratic drug reactions. A model has been proposed for the mechanism of phenytoin hypersensitivity.[4] A metabolite of phenytoin found in certain individuals may act to cause cytotoxicity directly and/or become a hapten (see later) and then lead to altered lymphocyte function and dysfunction of the immune system, leading to cell injury and necrosis. There is no information that would allow these individuals to be identified prior to an ADR.

Allergic- or Immune-Mediated Reaction

Allergic and immune mechanisms can also play a role in ADRs. Six to 10 per cent of ADRs are thought to be immune-mediated. Clinical findings that suggest immune-mediated ADRs include urticaria; acute anaphylaxis with bronchospasm, stridor, and hypotension; serum sickness–like symptoms with rash, fever, and joint pain; vasculitis-like rashes, including erythema multiforme, erythroderma, and Stevens-Johnson syndrome; eosinophilia; neutropenia; hemolysis; and thrombocytopenia. Drug-induced immune-mediated ADRs occur if the drug forms a hapten by associating with endogenous proteins. Haptens are compounds that are too small (MW $<$ 5000) to be directly immunogenic but that can serve as an antigenic determinant when attached to larger, immunogenic molecules. Because most drugs have low molecular weights, hapten formation is necessary for an immune-mediated ADR.

All types of immune responses have been shown to cause ADRs. Anaphylaxis (type I) reactions, immediate (0 to 1 hours, immunoglobulin E [IgE]-mediated), accelerated (1 to 72 hours, IgE-, IgG-mediated), or delayed ($>$72 hours, IgE-, IgG-mediated), have been shown to occur with beta-lactam antibiotics. Cytotoxic type II IgG-mediated reactions (e.g., hemolytic anemia with alpha-methyldopa), also have been reported. Penicillins, cephalosporins, sulfonamides, and phenytoin have been shown to cause immune complex type III IgG-mediated reactions leading to clinical serum sickness. Type IV cell-mediated, delayed hypersensitivity has been shown to occur with topical agents containing neomycin, antihistamines, para-aminobenzoic acid, and ethylenediamine.

Penicillin Allergy

The case of penicillin allergy deserves special consideration. An extensive review of penicillin allergy is beyond the scope of this article; however, a few select comments are offered. If a person is thought to be penicillin-allergic, there are lifelong significant implications. Penicillin allergy is potentially life-threatening (1 to 10 per cent risk). Because of this risk and the common use of penicillin, it may be clinically useful to test for allergy to penicillin. Most life-threatening reactions to penicillin are due to the minor antigenic determinant, which is unfortunately unavailable for use in cutaneous (skin prick or intradermal) testing for penicillin hypersensitivity. The major determinant, benzylpenicilloyl (BPO), is available commercially for skin testing and can be used as a screening test in combination with dilutions of penicillin itself.

Anaphylactoid Reactions

Anaphylactoid reactions occur when the mediators of anaphylaxis—histamine, leukotrienes, bradykinin, and others—are released from basophils and mast cells without the participation of IgE. Examples include the acute reactions seen with radiologic contrast media and vancomycin administration. Such reactions may be related to the rate of administration of the agent rather than the use of the agent itself. Vancomycin, if rapidly administered intravenously, may cause symptoms of flushing about the face and neck; yet, if administration occurs over an hour or more, these symptoms are prevented.

PREVENTION

Because the dose-related pharmacologic group of ADRs can be anticipated, prevention of such reactions can be accomplished by careful attention to the pharmacologic, kinetic, and therapeutic properties of these drugs. ADRs must be anticipated in certain high-risk populations (Table 3). For example, critically ill patients in intensive care units are at high risk for ADRs. Factors contributing to the high ADR risk in this group of patients include use of drugs with dramatic, rapid effects on physiology; use of a high number of drugs; and presence of organ system dysfunction, affecting drug disposition and/or response.

In any patient, as the number of drugs used increases, the potential for an ADR increases. The likelihood of drug interactions also contributes to the risk for ADRs. This is especially true for drugs that alter metabolism by induction (anticonvulsants) or inhibition (cimetidine) of metabolism of other drugs.

Oncology patients are also at high risk for ADRs. Factors associated with increased risk of ADRs in this group are critically ill status; use of multiple drugs; organ system failure; and the inherently toxic nature of the drugs used therapeutically. Drugs used in the treatment of cancer have inherently low therapeutic indices (toxicity dose/therapeutic dose) be-

TABLE 3. Patients at Risk for Adverse Drug Reactions

1. Patient taking multiple drugs
2. Critically ill patients
3. Patients with altered renal or liver function
4. Patients taking drugs that alter disposition or metabolism of other drugs
5. Oncology patients

cause of the nature of the disease being treated. These drugs may affect organ system function, which alters, in turn, the response of the patient to the oncology drugs themselves and/or to other drugs.

A careful history regarding the nature of past reactions and associated agents will aid in the determination of future risk for further reactions. Idiosyncratic reactions may also be determined from family history. Conditions such as G-6-PD deficiency and malignant hyperthermia can be suspected on the basis of family history.

The clinical laboratory has limited utility in the evaluation of most ADRs. Confirmation of toxic concentration of drugs may be possible in circumstances in which drug disposition has been altered. Tests may be done for certain idiosyncratic reactions, including reactions due to G-6-PD deficiency or low serum esterase activity. Screening for the presence of antibody-coated red blood cells and circulatory immune complexes can also be done. It is difficult to determine the specific agent involved in these reactions, however. Although such laboratory procedures may aid in the evaluation of ADRs, there is no specific set of laboratory tests that can be used to screen for ADRs. The clinician must be guided by specific clinical information in the evaluation of a patient for an ADR.

REFERENCES

1. Spector R: Evaluation of adverse effects of drugs. *In* Spector R (ed): The Scientific Basis of Clinical Pharmacology. Boston, Little, Brown & Co, pp 27–41, 1986.
2. Mitchell AA, Lacouture PA, Shuhan JE, et al: Adverse drug reactions in children leading to hospital admission. Pediatrics 82:24–29, 1988.
3. Krause MS, Hutchinson TA, Flegel KM, et al: Adverse drug reactions in general pediatrics outpatients. J Pediatr 108:305–310, 1985.
4. Spielberg SP, Gordon GB, Blake DA, et al: Predisposition to phenytoin hepatotoxicity assessed in vitro. N Engl J Med 305:722–727, 1981.

PHYSICAL ALLERGY

JOHN A. ANDERSON, M.D.

Physical factors, such as mechanical pressure, cold, heat, exercise, light, water, and vibration, may result in urticaria/angioedema or systemic signs and symptoms, such as asthma or anaphylaxis, that are usually associated with allergic reactions. As a group, these reactions are referred to as physical allergies. The exact incidence of physical factors resulting in allergic or allergic-like reactions in children is unknown; however, urticaria caused by physical factors accounts for approximately 3 per cent of all patients presenting with urticaria and 10 to 17 per cent of all patients with chronic urticaria (persistent or recurrent symptoms longer than 6 weeks in duration).

Exercise is a frequent trigger of asthma, especially in teenagers and young adults. It is estimated that exercise, particularly running, may trigger wheezing in 90 per cent of all asthmatics in these age groups. Additionally, 40 per cent of all atopics (allergic children) and 3 per cent of "normal" children may have some exercise-induced asthma. Exercise-induced asthma is frequently overlooked in high school and college athletes and has been found to be a problem in 11 per cent of United States olympians.

In all of the common types of physical urticaria/angioedema, chemical mediators, particularly histamine, have been identified as being released from mast cells and basophils. In some cases (dermographism, cold urticaria, solar urticaria), mediator release from effector cells may involve immunoglobulin E (IgE) antibodies, as evidenced by passive transfer experiments.

Nerve pathways may also be involved in producing physical urticaria/angioedema. Substance P release from sensory neurons is involved in the flare response of dermographism and may be involved in heat or cold urticaria.

The stimulus for cholinergic urticaria is thought to involve the release of acetylcholine as well as neuropeptides (such as substance P) from cholinergic afferent fibers in response to stimulants of the autonomic cholinergic pathway for sweating.

The major stimulus for exercise-induced asthma is drying (or increased heat exchange) of the tissues of the upper airway as the patient gulps down large amounts of air through the mouth during exercise. In some of these patients, cold air inhalation (which is usually drier) will also cause asthma. The resulting bronchospasm is caused by reflex to the lower airway.

The therapy used in physical allergy involves either avoidance of the physical agent or pharmacologic therapy designed to block the release of, or combat the effects of, chemical mediators stimulated by the physical agents.

GENERAL PRINCIPLES OF PHARMACOTHERAPY

Table 1 lists the antihistamines used for the treatment of physical allergy and the usual doses for children, beginning with the most commonly effective or commonly used drugs (because of lack of side effects).

Table 2 lists the emergency medicines used in physical allergy, adjutant drugs (to combat resistant cases of urticaria/angioedema), and medications for prevention and management of systemic symptoms caused by exercise-induced asthma or anaphylaxis.

The primary drug used in the emergency treatment of anaphylaxis and urticaria/angioedema is epinephrine (Adrenalin). In most cases of anaphylaxis, and in all cases of simple urticaria/angioedema, subcutaneous epinephrine helps stabilize or reverse symptoms within minutes. In these emergency situations, diphenhyramine (Benadryl) may also be given orally or intramuscularly. Follow-up treatment could include Sus-Phrine, a long-acting form of aqueous epinephrine (4 to 6 hours), and antihistamines to be used at home, such as diphenhydramine (25 mg to 50 mg two to three times daily), terfenadine (Seldane, 60 mg two times daily), or chlorpheniramine (Chlor-Trimeton, 4 mg to 8 mg three times daily). In more severe cases of anaphylaxis and urticaria/angioedema, prolonged observation is advised. If the patient is stable and is released home, a short course of corticosteroids in decreasing doses over the next 5 to 7 days (until follow-up) is advised (e.g., prednisone, 30 mg that day and the next morning (in a single dose), tapering to 25 mg, 20 mg, 15 mg, 10 mg, and 5 mg over the next five mornings).

For prophylactic therapy of urticaria/angioedema or exercise-induced anaphylaxis, the use of a single antihistamine listed in Table 1 might be tried. Hydroxyzine (Atarax) is usually the most effective drug. Because hydroxyzine (as well as diphenhydramine) is likely to produce drowsiness in some patients, other second-generation H_1 antihistamines can be used (e.g., terfenadine, 60 mg two times daily; or astemizole [Hismanal], 10 mg one time daily). Occasionally, symptoms may be better controlled with other first-generation H_1 antihistamines such as clemastine fumarate (Tavist) or either the chlorpheniramines or the brompheniramines. Cyproheptadine (Periactin) has been shown to be particularly effective in the treatment of cold urticaria.

The first-generation H_1 antihistamines (e.g., hydroxyzine, diphenhydramine) may have an increased likelihood of producing central nervous system side effects such as sleepiness, but they have an advantage in that their effectiveness increases with dose used. Therefore, the amount of drug can be titrated to that necessary to control the patient's urticaria/angioedema.

The second-generation H_1 antihistamines (e.g., terfenadine, astemizole) are usually maximally effective at the standard dose. More drug is usually not needed, is costly, and, under rare conditions, can cause other side effects such as cardiac arrhythmias. Astemizole also has a very long half-life and may affect allergy skin test reactivity for 6 weeks or longer. Weight gain has been associated with astemizole use in some patients.

In resistant cases of physical urticaria/angioedema, combinations of antihistamine types may be used, such as hydroxyzine or diphenhydramine during the evening and terfenadine during the day. In the management of chronic urticaria, some success has been achieved with the combination of an H_2 antihistamine receptor drug (e.g., cimetidine [Tagamet] or ranitidine [Zantac]) and one of the H_1 antihistamines such as hydroxyzine. In some resistant cases of chronic urticaria, doxepin (Sinequan), which has been shown to exhibit both H_1 and H_2 antihistamine-like activities, can be used as a single drug. Experience with using doxepin in children is limited, however, and the drug should be used cautiously.

In addition, terbutaline (e.g., Bricanyl) and theophylline compounds (e.g., Slo-bid) have been shown to decrease histamine release in hypersensitivity states. Both drugs decrease chronic urticaria/angioedema in some studies, even though neither drug has been shown to alter the antigen-induced immediate-reacting skin test significantly. We have found that some resistant cases of chronic urticaria/angioedema (physically induced or idiopathic) respond to an addition of either terbutaline (2.5 mg three times daily) or a theophylline compound (enough Slo-bid given three times daily in a divided dose to maintain a blood level of approximately 10 μg/ml) to one of the single or multiple-drug antihistamine regimes.

Short-term corticosteroids may be used for more severe emergency situations in the management of physical allergies. Corticosteroids are not substitutes for antihistamines, however, in the management of physically induced urticaria/angioedema. It is best to manage chronic conditions with antihistamines alone.

The management of exercise-induced asthma differs from that of physically induced urticaria/angioedema and anaphylaxis in that antihistamines are usually not used, and bronchodilators (e.g., albuterol), as well as specific asthma prevention drugs (e.g., cromolyn sodium, corticosteroids, and theophylline), are used.

SPECIFIC THERAPY

Dermographism

Treatment of dermographism consists of avoiding trauma and, when necessary, using an antihistamine. Hydroxyzine is the drug most likely to be helpful in this condition (on an as-needed basis), although other antihistamines and drug combinations may be tried. For persistent problems, especially in patients in whom sedative side effects are an issue, astemizole or terfenadine is usually recommended.

Pressure Urticaria/Angioedema

Treatment of pressure urticaria/angioedema consists of avoiding sustained pressure as much as possible in this rare, usually adult, problem. Delayed pressure urticaria (onset, characteristically 2 to 4 hours after pressure) may coexist with chronic idiopathic urticaria. Antihistamines may be helpful in chronic idiopathic urticaria, but not in delayed pressure urticaria. Corticosteroids, given on alternate days (e.g., prednisone, 5 to 10 mg every other day) may be necessary to control delayed pressure urticaria.

TABLE 1. Antihistamines for Treatment of Physical Allergy

Antihistamine Class (Histamine Receptor)	Drug (Trade Name)	Usual Dose, 27-kg Child (Dose by Weight)
Ethanolamine	Diphenhydramine (Benadryl) (more sedative)	12.5–50 mg 3 × daily (5 mg/kg/24 hr—not to exceed 300 mg/24 hr)
Ataractic (H_1)	Hydroxyzine (Atarax, Vistaril) (more sedative)	10–25 mg 3 × daily for children < 6 yr; 50 mg maximum total daily dose
Piperidine-butanol (H_1) (second generation)	Terfenadine* (Seldane) (no sedative) (less sedative)	60 mg 2 × daily for children ≥ 12 yr; not recommended for children < 12 yr but commonly used
Benzimidazole amine (H_1) (second generation)	Astemizole* (Hismanal) (not sedating)	10 mg q A.M. (1 × daily); not recommended for children < 12 yr
Alkylamine (H_1)	1. Chlorpheniramine (Chlor-Trimeton, Teldrin) 2. Brompheniramine (Dimetane) (less sedative)	2–8 mg 3 × daily
Benzhydryl ether (H_1)	Clemastine fumarate (Tavist) (less sedative)	1.34-mg tablet 2 × daily; not recommended for children < 12 yr of age 0.5 mg/5 ml (syrup) 2–3 × daily—safety confirmed in children 6–12 yr
Piperidine (H_1)	1. Cyproheptadine (Periactin) 2. Azatadine (Optimine)	2–4 mg 3–4 × daily (0.25 mg/kg/24 hr) 1–2 mg 2 × daily; not recommended for children < 12 yr
Phenothiazine (H_1)	Promethazine (Phenergan)	6.15–12.5 mg 3 × daily
Ethylenediamine (H_1)	Tripelennamine (PBZ)	25–50 mg 3 × daily (5 mg/kg/24 hr—not to exceed 300 mg/24 hr)
Thioguanidine (H_2)	Cimetidine (Tagamet)	20–40 mg/kg/24 hr; very limited experience in children < 16 yr
Ethenediamine (H_2)	Ranitidine (Zantac)	Dosage not established in children; see manufacturer's recommendations
Ataractics (H_1, H_2)	Doxepin (Sinequan)	10–25 mg 2 × daily for children ≥ 12 yr as a single drug; not to exceed 75 mg/24 hr; not recommended for children < 12 yr

*Warning: Concomitant use with erythromycin or ketoconazole may raise blood levels and increase risk of cardiac arrhythmias.

Cold-Induced Urticaria/Angioedema

The common form of cold-induced urticaria/angioedema can be confirmed by a positive ice cube test in 50 per cent of cases. That is, after the skin of the forearm is cooled with an ice cube for 10 minutes, a wheal will form upon rewarming.

The mainstay of treatment is to avoid chilling the body.

TABLE 2. Emergency and Adjuvant Drugs for Treatment of Physical Allergy

Drug Type	Drug (Trade Name)	Usual Children's Dosage
Sympathomimetics and β-agonists	Epinephrine hydrochloride 1:1000 (Adrenalin)	0.1–0.3 ml/dose SC (0.005–0.01 ml/kg/dose)
	Epinephrine hydrochloride 1:1000 (Adrenalin) in EpiPen and EpiPen Jr. (Center Laboratories)	0.3 and 0.15 ml (EpiPen and EpiPen Jr., respectively) in automatic doser
	Epinephrine 1:200 in thioglycolate (Sus-Phrine)	0.05–0.15 ml/dose SC (0.005 ml/kg/dose)
	Epinephrine hydrochloride 1:1000 (Adrenalin) in Ana-Kit (Hollister-Stier)	0.3 ml/dose; 2 doses possible
	Albuterol (Proventil, Ventolin)	MDI: 1–2 puffs by inhalation 3 × daily or 2–4 mg 3 × daily; syrup: 1 tsp (2 mg) 3–4 × daily in children 6–14 yr; 0.1 mg/kg 3 × daily in children 2–6 yr
	Metaproterenol (Alupent, Metaprel)	MDI: 1–3 puffs by inhalation—not recommended, but used, in children < 12 yr; syrup: 1 tsp (10 mg/5 ml) 3–4 × daily in children 6–9 yr. Limited published experience in children < 6, but 1.3–2.5 mg/kg/dose 3 × daily well tolerated.
	Terbutaline (Bricanyl, Brethine)	2.5–5.0-mg tablet 3 × daily; not recommended for children < 12 yr
Methylxanthine	Theophylline (Slo-bid 50, 100, 200 mg) (Theo-Dur 100, 200, 300 mg)	Therapeutic blood levels; safe therapeutic blood level approx. 10 μg/ml
Anti-inflammatory	Prednisone (Prednisone 5 mg)	As needed
	Cromolyn sodium (Intal)	MDI: 2–3 puffs by inhalation (800 μg per puff) 10–30 minutes before exercise

Abbreviations: SC, subcutaneous; MDI, metered-dose inhaler.

During the summer, patients should be careful about sudden changes in temperature, especially when swimming (whatever the water temperature). Symptoms and signs usually occur upon rewarming. Hair washing, with resulting evaporative cooling, may be a problem around the head and neck. During the winter, affected individuals should limit outside exposures. Warm gloves and footwear should be worn because the skin of the extremities is already at risk by having a lower ambient temperature than the rest of the body. It is important that an affected individual wear a hat because the head is the major source of heat loss from the body. A facemask can also be helpful.

In one study, cyproheptadine was the superior antihistamine in preventing cold reactions, but hydroxyzine and other antihistamines and antihistamine/alternative drug combinations should be tried in more resistant cases.

Although the "desensitization" method of inducing cold tolerance through serial baths at different temperatures has been tried, it has generally been unsuccessful.

A rare autosomal dominant form of familial cold urticaria exists. In this condition, antihistamines are generally not helpful.

In cases in which cold urticaria/angioedema is a manifestation of an underlying connective tissue disease, possibly associated with the existence of cryoglobulins, cold agglutinins, or cryofibrinogen, treatment of the underlying disease is of particular importance.

Cholinergic Urticaria

The diagnosis of cholinergic urticaria is usually aided by the identification of a morphologically distinct reaction characterized by a marked flare surrounding multiple small (1 to 5 mm) wheals that are extremely pruritic. These lesions usually develop in the "sweat areas" of the body such as the armpits, neck, upper anterior or posterior trunk, and groin areas after a stimulus such as exercise, specific heat exposure or, on some occasions, emotional upset. This condition should be differentiated from exercise-induced anaphylaxis.

"Keep cool" is a good rule for patients with cholinergic urticaria. Antihistamines are usually helpful, beginning with hydroxyzine or diphenhydramine and progressing to other antihistamines or combination therapies in resistant cases. A trial with anticholinergic medication has been advised, but this type of treatment has not been shown to be helpful in most cases.

Another method, that of deliberately producing the rash (by maneuvers such as taking serial warm showers) in order to produce a short refractory period, is also not helpful in most cases.

Localized Heat Urticaria

Localized heat urticaria, a very rare disorder, can be confirmed by carefully placing a heated (45°C) Erlenmeyer flask of water on an area of skin for 5 to 10 minutes. In a positive test, the induced urticaria lesion usually occurs within minutes. Antihistamines such as hydroxyzine have been reported to be successful in the management of some of these cases.

Urticaria/Angioedema Secondary to Light Exposure (Solar Urticaria)

Drug ingestion combined with sunlight exposure may result in either toxic rash (phototoxic reaction) or immunologic contact dermatitis (photoallergic reaction). Drugs implicated in causing a phototoxic reaction include psoralens, topical coal tar, and dimethylchlortetracycline. Agents implicated in causing a photoallergic reaction include phenothiazines, sulfonamides, and griseofulvin. Bacteriostatic agents such as bithionol and halogenated salicylamides, used in soaps and topical medications, may also induce reactions.

Sunlight exposure may also result in sunburn and exacerbate primary dermatologic and systemic disease, including polymorphic light eruption and systemic lupus erythematosus.

Management of solar urticaria is often difficult and consists primarily of avoiding the reaction-producing light wavelengths. In the case of drug sensitivity, the treatment consists of correctly identifying and then avoiding the causative chemical or drug.

Repeated exposure to small, increasing doses of sunlight may induce tolerance in some patients. The patient should wear protective garments wherever possible. Chemical sunscreens can be used to help protect sun-exposed skin in susceptible individuals. These sunscreens, which act by absorbing a specific portion of the ultraviolet light spectrum, are helpful in sunburn prevention and offer skin protection for those patients with primary skin disorders and systemic diseases. These agents are often not helpful in other cases of true solar urticaria, however. Sunscreen with a sun protection factor (SPF) of 15 or above are advised.

Patients with solar urticaria may be classified into groups on the basis of wavelengths of light that experimentally produce the skin reaction. Patients with sensitivity to wavelengths above 320 nm need to avoid light strictly and use physical blockers of light, even though these agents may be less cosmetically acceptable than chemical sunscreens. Some available physical blockers include zinc oxide paste (RVPaque), titanium dioxide (A-Fil cream or Solar cream), and red veterinarian petrolatum (RVP cream or RV Plus).

The 280- to 302-nm ultraviolet light (sunburn range) is filtered by window glass. The higher wavelengths, which can still produce light sensitivity in some patients, are not filtered by ordinary glass.

Oral antihistamines and corticosteroids may reduce the reactions to light in patients with a propensity for solar urticaria. Although the antimalarial drug chloroquine has been used in resistant cases of light sensitivity, the results are disappointing.

Aquagenic Urticaria

Aquagenic urticaria, a rare condition, is the result of water-droplet exposure of the skin, which produces small hive-like wheals on an erythematous base. Water at any temperature may cause this reaction, which must be differentiated from cholinergic urticaria and cold urticaria. It is not induced by exercise or emotional upset.

Antihistamines such as hydroxyzine, as well as other antihistamines or antihistamine and other drug combinations, may help in the management of this condition.

Vibratory Angioedema

Vibratory angioedema, a very rare type of reaction, has been described both as an autosomal dominant condition and as a sporadic condition. The history of reaction to exposure to a vibrating stimulus can be confirmed by skin exposure to the vibration of an electric toothbrush or a laboratory vortex mixer for 5 minutes. Avoidance of the vibratory stimulus is important in the management of this condition. Prophylactic antihistamines and corticosteroids have been shown to prevent the urticaria/angioedema when vibration exposure was unavoidable (e.g., during dental procedures).

Combinations of Physically Induced Urticaria/Angioedema

Cold and cholinergic urticaria may occur in the same patient. The presence of cholinergic urticaria in the patient with exercise-induced anaphylaxis has been described. Any physical urticaria may occur in patients with chronic idiopathic urticaria. The management of patients with combination-type urticaria may be challenging but can usually be handled using antihistamines or alternative drug regimens.

Exercise-Induced Anaphylaxis

Anaphylaxis (urticaria/angioedema or shock) has been shown to be caused by almost any type of exercise in worldwide surveys. Running (e.g., jogging) is the principal cause of this condition in the United States. In some cases, the ingestion of a meal or a specific food in an allergic patient (e.g., celery, wheat, shrimp, fish, peach, or other fruit) within 2 hours of exercise is necessary for the reaction to occur. Care should be taken to differentiate this condition from exercise-induced asthma, cholinergic urticaria, and reactions in atopic patients to environmental allergens (e.g., pollens or mold spores) during outdoor exercise.

Therapy for exercise-induced anaphylaxis involves avoidance of strenuous exercise such as jogging. In some instances, this is not acceptable to the patient. The use of antihistamines, such as hydroxyzine or terfenadine, or other drug combinations prior to exercise may be helpful. For an emergency, patients should be supplied with an adrenalin autodoser (EpiPen or EpiPen Jr., 0.3 or 0.15 ml aqueous adrenalin, respectively). Three units are usually prescribed—one for the home, one for the car, and one for the purse or person—so that a unit is always available when needed. An alternative unit to be supplied for inadvertent anaphylaxis treatment is an Ana-Kit epinephrine syringe (0.3 cc aqueous adrenalin per dose; two doses per syringe). Patients should be instructed to administer adrenalin should anaphylaxis occur during physical exercise, but they should also be instructed to go immediately to an emergency department or a physician's office for further care.

Exercise and Cold-Induced Asthma

Most children with asthma have some degree of symptoms when they exercise. In some asthmatics, exercise is the major reason for wheezing. Children may also wheeze when exposed to cold air, but not all exercise-induced asthmatics wheeze under these conditions. Running is the exercise most likely to produce wheezing, and swimming is the exercise least likely to do so (breathing humidified air caused less drying and thus less of a stimulus to the upper airway).

Therapy in exercise-induced asthma involves avoidance, when possible, of the type of exercise or the degree of exercise that produces significant difficulty. To restrict otherwise normal children from all exercise is not advisable or practical. In some cases, children can "run through" their exercise-induced asthma. Breathing through the nose rather than the mouth while exercising, thus allowing the inhaled air to become properly heated and humidified, has been shown to reduce exercise-induced asthma. The use of an inexpensive, disposable, hard-paper surgical mask that fits over the nose and mouth has been found to reduce exercise-induced asthma by allowing the patient to "rebreathe" a reservoir of warm, humidified air when exercising.

Medication also can be used to reduce or prevent exercise-induced asthma (see Table 2). Cromolyn sodium (Intal) by inhalation (usually through a metered-dose inhaler [MDI] 10 to 30 minutes before exercise) provides significant blocking of the reaction in 60 per cent of affected children and lasts for 2 to 4 hours. β_2-Agonist drugs, usually taken by a MDI (e.g., albuterol), are more effective in blocking exercise-induced asthma when taken immediately before exercise. β_2-Agonists have an additional advantage over cromolyn in that they may be used again if the patient subsequently wheezes or breaks through the prophylactic drug treatment with exercise. Thus, only one drug via MDI needs to be used by the patient. Other asthma-prevention drugs (e.g., theophylline and corticosteroids) usually do not prevent exercise-induced asthma as well as the β_2 agonist or cromolyn sodium.

The management of cold-induced asthma is similar to that of exercise-induced asthma.

ANAPHYLAXIS

PHILLIP A. JACOBSON, M.D.
and P. PEARL O'ROURKE, M.D.

Anaphylaxis is a life-threatening hypersensitivity reaction caused by widespread mast cell degranulation in response to a stimulus. It can be precipitated through various mechanisms, both immune and nonimmune in origin. The most common immune response is immunoglobulin E (IgE)-mediated: the patient becomes sensitized to a stimulus on initial exposure by the binding of antigen-specific IgE molecules to the surface of mast cells, and anaphylaxis then occurs upon repeat stimulus exposure. Penicillin is the prototypic antigen for this pattern. Other examples of immune-mediated stimuli include several foods (e.g., milk products, eggs, nuts, fish, shellfish, and preservatives); both parenteral and oral drugs (e.g., antibiotics, insulin, and vaccines); and hymenopteran stings (e.g., bees, wasps, hornets, and fire ants). IgG-mediated and immune complex–mediated anaphylaxis are other, less common immune mechanisms and are triggered by complement activation.

Nonimmune mechanisms can be direct-acting or mediated by complex biochemical pathways. In the direct-acting type, the stimulus (e.g., contrast media and opiates) acts directly on the mast cell membranes. *Nonsteroidal anti-inflammatory agents can induce anaphylaxis via alteration of arachidonic acid metabolism.*

Idiopathic and exercise-induced anaphylaxis are less common entities. Exercise-induced anaphylaxis occurs in predisposed individuals shortly after the completion of vigorous exercise, which is often preceded by the consumption of a large meal. Its cause is unknown.

In the past, the term anaphylaxis was used to denote an immune-mediated reaction, whereas the term anaphylactoid was used to describe a reaction that was nonimmune in origin. Regardless of the precipitating mechanism, the clinical manifestations are identical. The term anaphylaxis is now used to describe all of these reactions.

Upon degranulation of the mast cells, histamine and other primary and secondary mediators are released. The results are increased capillary permeability and mucous gland secretion, bronchoconstriction, and decreased vascular tone. The integumentary, cardiovascular, respiratory, and gastrointestinal systems are primarily involved. Initially, pruritis and a feeling of impending doom are often reported. This is followed by a generalized flush, which may evolve into an urticarial rash. Shortly thereafter, signs of shock and respiratory distress ensue. Upper airway obstruction secondary to laryngeal edema can occur and present as hoarseness, dysphagia, stridor, and/or dyspnea. Lower airway obstruction, resulting from bronchoconstriction, mucus plugging, and/or pulmonary edema, is common and is manifested by wheezing, rales, and dyspnea. Signs of shock include poor pulses, decreased capillary refill, hypotension, and a diminished level of consciousness. Abdominal pain and/or diarrhea are seen with gastrointestinal involvement. Prompt recognition and treatment are crucial in the management of such patients.

TREATMENT

Removal of the Stimulus

Immediate removal of the stimulus that is suspected of causing a reaction is an important first step in the treatment of anaphylaxis. Intravenous drug infusions and/or blood transfusions should be discontinued. A stinger from a bee or wasp should be removed. If the anaphylactic stimulus enters through an extremity (e.g., parenterally administered drug or bee sting) a tourniquet may be applied proximally to inhibit its circulation. For every 3 minutes of application, the tourniquet should be released for 1 minute.

Respiratory Support

The following respiratory support measures should be taken:

1. Administer 100 per cent oxygen by face mask.
2. Give epinephrine, the "drug of choice," immediately (0.01 mg/kg IV, subcutaneously, or IM). Epinephrine inhibits mast cell degranulation, promotes bronchodilation, and alleviates laryngeal edema. For subcutaneous or intramuscular administration, 0.01 cc/kg of a 1:1000 dilution of aqueous epinephrine is used. For intravenous administration, 0.1 cc/kg of a 1:10,000 dilution of aqueous epinephrine is used. Subsequent doses may be given every 5 to 10 minutes as needed. If several repeat doses are required, an epinephrine drip should be started at 0.1 μg/kg/minute and titrated to effect. A concentration of 2.25 per cent nebulized racemic epinephrine may be used for treatment of laryngeal edema. A volume of 0.25 cc in 2 cc of normal saline can be given every 30 minutes as needed. Some authors recommend the use of subcutaneous epinephrine at the injection site to slow absorption via local vasoconstriction and to attenuate the anaphylactic response.
3. Consider endotracheal intubation for the patient in moderate to severe respiratory distress who does not respond to epinephrine. This is especially important for the patient who shows signs of upper airway obstruction. This airway can be very difficult to manage; therefore, the most experienced person available should perform the procedure. If intubation is unsuccessful and an airway cannot be maintained with a bag and mask, cricothyrotomy should be performed with a 14-gauge intravenous catheter. A patient can be oxygenated this way until endotracheal intubation or tracheostomy is accomplished.
4. Give terbutaline and/or albuterol for the treatment of lower airway manifestations (i.e., wheezing and mucus plugging). These drugs bronchodilate and enhance mucociliary clearance. In inhaled form, the dose of terbutaline is 1 cc in 2 cc of normal saline and that of albuterol is 0.25 cc in 2 cc of normal saline. Each drug may be given continuously for severe bronchospasm or as often as needed.
5. Institute intravenous aminophylline for refractory wheezing. Intravenous aminophylline may even be safely used concomitantly with an epinephrine infusion. Administration is begun with a bolus of 5 to 7 mg/kg given over 20 minutes, followed by 1 mg/kg/hour continuous infusion to achieve serum levels of 10 to 20 μg/L.

Shock

The following measures should be taken to treat shock:

1. Place a large-bore intravenous catheter. A fluid bolus of 20 to 40 cc/kg of lactated Ringer's or other isotonic solution should be given. More fluid may be required based on reassessment of the patient. This step cannot be overlooked

because hypovolemia occurs in every case of anaphylactic shock.

2. Give epinephrine in identical dose to that for respiratory support. It will restore vascular tone and increase myocardial contractility.

3. Use a dopamine drip (10 to 20 μg/kg/minute) if less potent inotropic support is desired.

Adjunctive Therapy

Glucocorticoids are particularly helpful in preventing or attenuating the recurrence of symptoms. They should be administered after more immediate life-sustaining measures have been instituted. Methylprednisolone (2 mg/kg IV) should be given every 4 to 6 hours for 2 days. Equivalent doses of oral prednisone may replace methyprednisolone in a stable patient.

Histamine is a primary mediator of anaphylaxis and contributes to the respiratory and cardiovascular manifestations. *Antihistamines* are a logical choice to treat this entity. They inhibit further action of histamine but do not reverse the physiologic manifestations in progress. Diphenhydramine, an H_1 blocker, is given (1 mg/kg IV every 6 hours). For less severe reactions, oral diphenhydramine (5 mg/kg/day divided every 6 hours, with a maximum of 300 mg/day) or hydroxyzine (2 mg/kg/day divided every 6 hours, with a maximum of 200 mg/day) may be given. The administration of H_2 blockers is controversial. If used, ranitidine is given (1 mg/kg/day IV divided every 6 hours; the oral dose is 2 mg/kg/day divided every 12 hours).

MONITORING

All patients diagnosed with anaphylaxis should be admitted to the intensive care unit (ICU) for at least 24 to 48 hours because the disease process may be protracted or recurrent. In protracted anaphylaxis, clinical manifestations continue for 5 to 32 hours despite ongoing therapy. *In the biphasic (recurrent) form, life-threatening symptoms may recur up to 8 hours after the initial event. Either protracted or recurrent symptoms occur in approximately half of all anaphylactic cases.* They are more common when an oral or potent antigenic stimulus is applied or when the reaction is delayed in onset (>30 minutes).

The level of monitoring in the ICU depends on the severity of the disease. All patients should be monitored by electrocardiograph and have vital signs checked frequently. Those with severe manifestations deserve more invasive monitoring. Placement of an arterial line is helpful for frequent blood gas and continuous blood pressure analyses. A central venous line should be started for infusion of fluid and inotropes and for monitoring central venous pressure. Insertion of a Foley catheter is warranted for evaluation of urine output. A pulse oximeter should also be employed.

PROGNOSIS

The prognosis of anaphylaxis depends on its severity and on the promptness of its recognition and treatment. Death usually occurs within the first hour of the reaction and results from respiratory failure.

PREVENTION

Various measures can be undertaken to prevent the dangerous events of anaphylaxis. The most important measure is to avoid exposure to the offending stimulus. For example, a patient who has had previous adverse reaction to penicillin should receive antibiotics only of other classes. A person who previously developed urticaria from a bee sting should be counseled to avoid areas near bee hives. *One who is prone to exercise-induced anaphylaxis should avoid eating within 2 hours preceding strenuous exercise because eating will increase the risk.*

A careful history is invaluable in identifying potential risks. Medical professionals should thoroughly document any witnessed adverse reactions. The patient should be well informed of drugs or foods to which he or she is allergic. A medic alert bracelet should be worn by one who has had a severe reaction to a drug to warn potential caretakers.

The triggering stimuli of some conditions may be very difficult or impossible to avoid completely. These include exercise, certain food preservatives, and hymenopteran stings. Self-administering epinephrine kits are available for the high-risk patient. The patient should carry the kit at all times and be instructed in its proper use. An individual with exercise-induced anaphylaxis should never engage in strenuous workouts alone.

Occasionally, a patient will have an ambiguous history as to the specific substance that elicited a hypersensitivity reaction. Skin tests and radioallergosorbent tests (RAST) are available to identify only selected agents that cause an IgE-mediated response. These tests are performed under the supervision of an allergist. Positive reactions can alert the patient and physician to which substances need to be avoided. Specific immunotherapy may be administered prophylactically to a patient who is allergic to hymenopteran venom.

Another preventive measure often employed is pretreatment. Glucocorticoids and antihistamines are given prior to the administration of a potential anaphylotoxin to attenuate the anaphylactic response. Methylprednisolone (40 mg IV; 30 mg for children younger than 6 years of age) or equivalent doses of oral prednisone are given 13, 7, and 1 hours before the procedure. Diphenhydramine (1 mg/kg IV or orally) is given 1 hour in advance. This method should not be solely relied upon because it does not fully prevent the reaction nor completely remove the risk. Pretreatment is used for all potential hypersensitivity reactions, although its effectiveness has been proven only in prevention of reaction to intravenous contrast media.

When a known anaphylotoxin must be administered to a patient, a desensitization technique may be employed to prevent a life-threatening response. This involves the administration of very small doses of the offending agent to the patient in gradually increasing amounts. Presumably, a slow degranulation of mast cells and a depletion of mediators result in a weaker physiologic response. This procedure must be performed under the supervision of an allergist or immunologist in an ICU.

Finally, anticipation of the worst is crucial when administering a drug to a high-risk patient. A secure intravenous line should be established. Epinephrine, oxygen, and a bag and mask and other intubation equipment should be immediately available. In addition, the patient should be carefully monitored.

THE IMMUNODEFICIENCIES

BRIAN L. HAMILTON, M.D., Ph.D.
and GWENDOLYN B. SCOTT, M.D.

GENERAL MANAGEMENT CONSIDERATIONS

Antibiotics

The routine use of prophylactic antibiotics for prevention of infection has been found to be beneficial in conditions such as chronic granulomatous disease (CGD) of childhood. However, the benefits of such treatment must be carefully weighed against the risks of predisposing to infections with resistant bacteria or fungi. In general, routine prophylaxis of B cell, T cell, or combined B and T cell immunodeficiencies is not recommended.

Fever in a patient with immunodeficiency should be evaluated promptly. Specimens from appropriate sites should be obtained for culture and inoculated onto media for isolation of aerobic and anaerobic bacteria as well as fungi and mycobacteria. Broad-spectrum antibiotics should be begun promptly pending culture results. Knowledge of the specific immune defect may guide initial therapy; that is, in patients with granulocyte deficiencies, antistaphylococcal coverage should be included; in patients with complement deficiency or antibody deficiencies, initial therapy should include antibiotics effective against *Streptococcus pneumoniae, Haemophilus influenzae* type b, and *Neisseria meningitidis*. When an organism has been identified and its sensitivity pattern to antibiotics determined, a more specific antibiotic therapy should be instituted.

Immune Globulin (Immune Human Serum Globulin, Gamma Globulin)

The immune globulin fraction prepared by cold alcohol precipitation of human serum (Cohn fraction II) is used to treat patients with defective humoral immunity. These preparations contain only the immunoglobulin G (IgG) fraction and are not used to replace IgA or IgM. IgG is prepared from large lots of pooled human serum or plasma. Antibodies to most of the common viral and bacterial pathogens are present, but the titers of antibody vary from lot to lot. It should be recognized that these preparations may not include antibody to pathogens that are not commonly present in the donor population (e.g., dengue) or to pathogens that present a changing serotype each year (e.g., influenza A and B). The standard preparation procedures for immune globulin destroy known pathogens such as hepatitis B virus and human immunodeficiency virus 1 (HIV-1).

The original immune globulin preparations contained sufficient aggregated material to cause severe reactions when given intravenously and thus had to be given intramuscularly. The amount of IgG given by the intramuscular route is limited by the volume required and by the pain associated with the injection. Only modest elevations of the serum IgG levels can be obtained using these preparations. Intravenous immune globulin (IVIG) is prepared by various treatments that stabilize the material and prevent aggregate formation. Most of the preparations currently available contain normal ratios of the four IgG subclasses and retain biologic activity of the IgG (complement fixation, transplacental transfer, etc.). IVIG is preferred by most immunologists because (1) higher serum levels can readily be achieved, (2) it is less painful, and (3) it is more efficacious in preventing chronic pulmonary disease in patients with hypogammaglobulinemia. In addition, high-dose IVIG appears to suppress endogenous immunoglobulin production. This attribute is the basis for using IVIG to treat autoimmune disorders such as idiopathic thrombocytopenia. The disadvantages of using IVIG are the expense (about $100/g infused as compared with about $30 per dose injected for intramuscular immune globulin [IMIG]) and the inconvenience of intravenous access. Intravenous access has typically necessitated monthly clinic visits, but home therapy is now available through several home health care agencies.

Doses for the different immune globulin preparations are as follows:

1. IMIG: A loading dose of 1.5 ml/kg is given, followed by maintenance doses of 0.6 to 0.75 ml/kg usually given every 4 weeks. In general, a maximum of 40 ml per dose is given. The dose is divided between multiple intramuscular sites, usually in 5- to 10-ml volumes. Serum IgG levels are a poor guide to therapy because these preparations do not cause significant elevations. Therapy can be monitored by measuring antibody titers to common antigens such as tetanus toxoid and by clinical response.
2. IVIG: For patients with severe hypogammaglobulinemia/agammaglobulinemia, treatment can be initiated with 400 mg/kg per dose given daily for 4 to 5 days. For mild hypogammaglobulinemia, patients may be started on 200 mg/kg per dose given every 4 weeks. The dose is adjusted to maintain trough levels of IgG above 500 mg/dl. The standard maintenance dose is 400 mg/kg per dose usually given every 4 weeks. Some patients require doses greater than 400 mg/kg to maintain adequate trough levels. Other patients require dosing as frequently as every 2 to 3 weeks to maintain adequate IgG levels and a good clinical response.

Bone Marrow Transplantation

Bone marrow transplantation (BMT) remains the only definitive therapy for congenital disorders of the immune system. All patients with cellular immunodeficiencies (T cell deficiency, severe combined immunodeficiency [SCID]) and severe neutrophil disorders should be considered potential candidates for BMT. The optimal donor is a human leukocyte antigen (HLA)-A, -B, and -DR matched sibling. Recent advances in the field include the use of HLA identical but unrelated donors or haploidentical transplants from HLA mismatched siblings or parents. Allogeneic BMT has proven successful in the treatment of a wide spectrum of disorders, including DiGeorge syndrome, Wiskott-Aldrich syndrome, SCID, CGD, and Kostmann's agranulocytosis.

Enzyme and Growth Factor Replacement

The treatment of congenital immunodeficiencies with appropriate enzymes and growth factors is a promising new approach. This field will grow as additional growth factors and cytokines become available for use in the clinic through biotechnology. Replacement therapy should be considered as an alternative to allogeneic BMT.

Some forms of immunodeficiency may respond to enzyme replacement therapy. Patients with severe combined immunodeficiency resulting from adenosine deaminase (ADA) deficiency have been treated in the past with red blood cell transfusions as a source of normal enzyme with some success. The use of bovine ADA that has been modified with polyethylene glycol (PEG-ADA) has been approved by the U.S. Food and Drug Administration (FDA) for treatment as a weekly intramuscular injection. Many patients have shown marked improvement in their immune function in response to PEG-ADA. Clinical trials of gene therapy for ADA deficiency are also under way.

The use of recombinant granulocyte colony-stimulating factor is currently under investigation in the treatment of congenital agranulocytosis and cyclic neutropenia, with promising results.

Vaccines

Patients with immunodeficiency may safely be given denatured protein, carbohydrate, and killed viral vaccines. However, immunodeficient patients may not always produce an adequate humoral response to standard antigens. Patients should receive routine immunization with diphtheria-pertussis-tetanus (DPT) vaccine, inactivated poliovaccine (IPV), and the newer *H. influenzae* type b (HIB) protein conjugate vaccine. Patients older than 24 months of age should receive pneumococcal polysaccharide (PPS) vaccine. Patients with deficiencies of the terminal complement components (C5, C6, C7, C8,

C9) are more susceptible to infection with *Neisseria* species and may be protected by vaccination with meningococcal vaccine.

Immunodeficient patients should *not* be given live viral or bacterial vaccines (oral polio; measles, mumps, rubella [MMR]; yellow fever; or bacille Calmette-Guérin [BCG] vaccine) because they are at risk of developing clinical disease from the attenuated virus or bacteria. This applies to patients with complement deficiencies and neutrophil disorders as well as those with B and T cell disorders. Patients with X-linked agammaglobulinemia cannot make antibody and should not be vaccinated. Immunologically normal siblings and household contacts of patients with immunodeficiencies should not receive live oral poliovaccine because of the potential for shedding the virus and transmission to immunodeficient siblings. However, siblings and household contacts may receive MMR vaccine because transmission of these vaccine viruses does not occur.

The major exception to these guidelines involves patients with HIV infection. Available data suggest that routine childhood immunizations do not cause serious adverse reactions in either asymptomatic or symptomatic children with HIV infection. However, the efficacy of the various vaccines in this population is unknown, and there are reports of lower rates of seroconversion to some antigens. The current recommendation is to give IPV to all patients. MMR vaccine should be considered for use in all HIV-infected children regardless of symptoms and administered according to the usual schedule. This recommendation is based on the observation that children with HIV infection immunized with MMR have not had adverse effects and on reports of severe and fatal measles occurring in symptomatic HIV-positive children. The authors feel that the use of live viral vaccines in this population should be individualized and that patients with severe immune dysfunction should not receive live vaccines.

Passive Immunization

Immunocompromised children exposed to measles should be given immune globulin. This also applies to children with HIV infection regardless of immunization status. The dose of IMIG is 0.5 ml/kg (maximum dose, 15 ml) given within 6 days of exposure. If a child has been receiving regular therapy with IVIG, additional immune globulin may not be necessary if the exposure occurred within 3 weeks of the last treatment. Immunocompromised susceptible children exposed to varicella should receive varicella-zoster immune globulin (VZIG) within 72 hours of exposure.

HUMORAL IMMUNODEFICIENCIES

Patients with humoral immunodeficiencies tend to develop pyogenic infections, particularly of the lungs and sinuses. These infections are frequently chronic and require aggressive long-term, broad-spectrum antibiotic therapy to suppress infection. Older children and adolescents should have pulmonary function studies done yearly, and their therapy should be adjusted if function is decreasing. Good pulmonary toilet and postural drainage is important for children with sinopulmonary involvement. The goal of therapy is to prevent recurrent bacterial and viral infections.

X-Linked Agammaglobulinemia (Bruton's Disease)

Patients with X-linked agammaglobulinemia or severe hypogammaglobulinemia require life-long replacement therapy. Replacement therapy can be accomplished with IVIG or IMIG. IVIG is recommended because it is less painful and achieves higher serum levels. Use of the intravenous dose is thought to prevent complications such as the chronic lung disease that is common in this entity. Serum IgG trough levels should be maintained at least at or above 500 mg/dl to achieve a good response. The actual dose required varies with each patient and may range from 200 to 800 mg/kg. The frequency of infusion may also vary from every 2 to 6 weeks and should be adjusted depending on the clinical response of the patient. If a serious infection occurs, additional immune globulin may be required. Exposure to varicella or hepatitis B virus necessitates administration of the appropriate hyperimmune globulin. Immunization with live viral vaccines is contraindicated. These patients are at risk for development of vaccine-associated poliomyelitis.

Common Variable Immunodeficiencies

This diagnosis includes a heterogeneous group of disorders. Patients may present with hypogammaglobulinemia at any age—from infancy to adulthood. These patients present with a spectrum of clinical disease because some patients make normal amounts of antibody to specific antigens while others do not. Patients with borderline or low levels of IgG should have quantitation of IgG subclasses and antibody production. Replacement therapy with IVIG must be individualized on the basis of the severity of clinical symptoms. Those with severe, recurrent infections should receive immune globulin replacement therapy. The dose of IVIG is adjusted to control symptoms and to maintain trough levels above 500 mg/dl. The patient with hypogammaglobulinemia should be closely monitored for the development of autoimmune disease.

Transient Hypogammaglobulinemia of Infancy

Transient hypogammaglobulinemia of infancy is a self-limited condition. These patients may present with frequent bacterial or viral infections and are found to have low IgG levels. Patients with this condition usually have normal levels of immunoglobulins by the age of 5 years. Because it is difficult to predict which infants with hypogammaglobulinemia will recover, the diagnosis of transient hypogammaglobulinemia can be made only after the immunoglobulin levels have returned to normal.

Infants with low serum immunoglobulin levels and normal B cell numbers who are asymptomatic do not necessarily require treatment. These children should be followed closely, and serum immunoglobulin levels obtained at 3- to 6-month intervals. One would anticipate that normal levels might be achieved by 3 years of age. However, some children will require a longer period of time to normalize. Infants with severe recurrent infections should receive immune globulin replacement therapy. Therefore, serum immunoglobulin levels should be routinely checked at 3-month intervals in all infants receiving IVIG, and, if normal levels are attained, the infusions may be discontinued and serum IgG levels monitored. In some cases, prolonged therapy might be required. Because immune globulin replacement may suppress the ability to synthesize one's own IgG, young children treated with IVIG for mild hypogammaglobulinemia should be reassessed between 4 and 6 years of age by stopping the IVIG treatments and monitoring monthly serum IgG levels and clinical symptoms.

IgG Subclass Deficiencies

The patient with an IgG subclass deficiency is usually missing one or two of the subclasses but has normal or increased levels of others. Symptomatic patients should be treated with immune globulin injections or infusions, as indicated in the general management discussion.

IgA Deficiencies

At present, no specific treatment is available for IgA deficiency. These patients have a higher incidence of *Giardia lamblia* infection; patients with chronic diarrhea or malabsorption syndrome should be thoroughly investigated for this organism. In a small group of patients, autoimmune disease has been a complication. Some children also have associated IgG subclass deficiencies. In most cases of complete IgA deficiency, immune globulin replacement or blood transfusions are contraindicated. Because the patient has no IgA, there is the possibility that the patient may become sensitized and develop anti-IgA antibodies. However, in some patients with IgA deficiency and associated IgG subclass deficiency, IVIG can be well tolerated and beneficial. In such circumstances, patients should be monitored for the development of antibodies to IgA and should be carefully observed during infusions. Intravenous administration of immune globulin is preferred over intramuscular injection because, if a reaction occurs, the infusion can be terminated immediately. IVIG preparations low in IgA are preferred. A patient with IgA deficiency should be aware that the transfusion of whole blood or blood products may be harmful. If a transfusion is necessary in an IgA-deficient patient, blood obtained from another IgA-deficient donor or washed red blood cells should be given. A Medic Alert bracelet is advised to alert physicians to the fact that a transfusion could be harmful.

IgM Deficiency

IgM deficiency is rare and is associated with an increased susceptibility to meningococcal disease. Because immune globulin preparations do not contain significant amounts of IgM, immune globulin therapy is generally not helpful. Penicillin prophylaxis may be used as an alternative therapy in these patients.

CELLULAR IMMUNODEFICIENCIES

Patients with T cell deficiencies frequently have associated B cell defects. These patients are susceptible to intracellular bacterial infections, viral diseases, and opportunistic infection.

The goal of therapy is to correct the deficiency by enzyme replacement, BMT, or replacement of cytokines if possible. Infectious complications can be minimized by treating with IVIG, trimethoprim-sulfamethoxazole for *Pneumocystis carinii* prophylaxis, chronic antibiotics to suppress bacterial infections, and antiviral agents to suppress viral infections. In addition, all blood products must be irradiated to prevent graft-versus-host reactions.

T Cell Deficiencies

Isolated T cell deficiencies involving thymic hypoplasia can be reconstituted by transplantation of fetal thymic tissue. Fetal thymus fragments implanted in the muscle or injected intraperitoneally have resulted in successful reconstitution of T cell immunity. Thymic tissue is obtained from a 10- to 14-week-old human fetus removed by hysterotomy. The fetus is usually obtained from a therapeutic abortion and is unrelated to the patient and is thus typically an HLA mismatch. The thymus is removed, cut into small fragments, and placed into sterile tissue culture medium. Transplantation should be done within 1 or 2 hours by intraperitoneal injection using a sterile 18-gauge peritoneal catheter, which is removed after the injection.

Cultured thymic epithelial cells also have been transplanted, and partial immune reconstitution has resulted, although more experience with this therapy is needed. Enhanced T cell immunity may also be achieved using immunomodulators such as thymosin, thymopoietin, and other thymic factors. Bone marrow transplantation from a histocompatible sibling has also been successful in reconstitution of T cell function.

Patients with complete DiGeorge syndrome initially require treatment for their hypoparathyroidism. Hypocalcemic seizures need to be controlled and prevented with the use of intravenous calcium gluconate. Calcium supplementation, a low-phosphorus diet, and large doses of vitamin D are important in the treatment of the hypoparathyroidism. Parathyroid hormone injections may also be necessary for control of this complication. Because this is a T cell deficiency, live virus vaccines should not be administered. Blood for transfusion should be irradiated (3000 rad) to prevent graft-versus-host disease and *P. carinii* prophylaxis should be provided (see article on HIV, p. 653). More than 90 per cent of patients with DiGeorge syndrome have associated congenital heart defects such as truncus, interrupted aortic arch, double aortic arch, or aberrent right subclavian artery, for which surgical correction and supportive measures should be provided. Because the incidence of T cell deficiency (complete DiGeorge syndrome) in patients with aortic arch abnormalities is not known, all patients with congenital heart defects should receive only irradiated blood products.

Chronic Mucocutaneous Candidiasis

Chronic mucocutaneous candidiasis is a T cell immunodeficiency characterized by chronic and recurrent infection of the mucous membranes, scalp, skin, and nails with *Candida albicans*. There is a broad spectrum of clinical disease, and a subset of patients will have associated endocrinopathies such as hypothyroidism, hypoparathyroidism, or Addison's disease.

The goal of therapy is to prevent and control fungal infection. The type of therapy needed depends on the extent and location of the infection. For mild infection, topical therapy with mycostatin or clotrimazole may be adequate. Treatment of lesions of the oral mucosa has been facilitated by the development of troches or pastilles containing mycostatin or clotrimazole and has proven to be an effective therapy for the older child. For more extensive oral involvement or esophagitis, oral therapy with ketoconazole, or intravenous therapy with amphotericin B or miconazole, is indicated. Oral fluconazole is an effective newer drug available for use in adults with severe oropharyngeal candidiasis or esophagitis. Iron therapy has proven beneficial in some cases. The child with chronic mucocutaneous candidiasis should be evaluated at least yearly for the presence of an endocrinopathy, and, if documented, appropriate therapy should be given. Various measures have been used as treatment for this disorder. Transfer factor, levamisole, and thymosin have produced variable results.

Wiskott-Aldrich Syndrome

Patients with Wiskott-Aldrich syndrome have thrombocytopenia, eczema, and abnormal T cell function that results in an inability to make antibody responses to carbohydrate antigens such as the capsular polysaccharides of *H. influenzae* type b, pneumococci, etc. These patients, however, may make antibody to carbohydrate antigens that have been conjugated to protein carriers such as the newer HIB conjugate vaccine. Patients with recurrent bacterial infections may respond to monthly infusions of IVIG. IMIG is contraindicated because of the low platelet count and the potential for bleeding in these patients.

Life-threatening episodes of bleeding should be treated with fresh platelet transfusions irradiated at 3000 rad to prevent graft-versus-host reaction. In most cases, episodes of bleeding decrease with advancing age. Splenectomy will usually result in normalization of the platelet count and should be considered for patients who have significant thrombocytopenia and bleeding. Following splenectomy, children should be placed on prophylactic antibiotics to prevent overwhelming infection.

There is an increased incidence of malignancy, particularly lymphoma, in patients with Wiskott-Aldrich syndrome. These patients should be considered for BMT, which has been shown to correct both the platelet and the T cell abnormalities successfully.

Severe Combined Immunodeficiency

Patients with SCID have absent T and B cell immunity, which represents a variety of underlying defects. An evaluation should be done to determine whether an enzyme deficiency such as ADA or purine nucleoside phosphorylase (PNP) is the cause. As mentioned previously, monthly red blood cell infusions have resulted in partial immune reconstitution in some patients with ADA deficiency in the past. Replacement therapy by weekly intramuscular injections of bovine ADA conjugated with PEG-ADA has been approved by the FDA. Such therapy has resulted in clinical improvement in a limited number of patients. Bone marrow transplantation, however, remains the treatment of choice for most forms of SCID. With BMT, some children have shown full reconstitution of both T cell and B cell function, whereas others have had persistence of B cell deficiency. These patients then require full replacement therapy with IVIG.

Other therapies have been attempted in patients with SCID, such as transplantation of fetal liver, fetal thymus, and cultured thymic epithelial cells. A few patients have shown partial reconstitution, but the majority have not. These patients should be placed in strict reverse isolation until appropriate diagnostic testing has been completed and treatment arranged.

Other therapeutic considerations include the use of irradiated (3000 rad) blood to prevent a graft-versus-host reaction. Donor blood seronegative for cytomegalovirus (CMV) should be used if possible. Children with SCID should not receive live viral vaccines. If they are exposed to varicella, they should be given VZIG. *P. carinii* prophylaxis should be given. IVIG therapy should be given until immune reconstitution is accomplished. Fever should be evaluated with aggressive diagnosis, and broad-spectrum antibiotics should be used until culture results are available.

Complement Deficiencies

In general, there are only a few specific therapies available for disorders of the complement system. However, knowledge of the deficiency is important because it can alert the physician to information important in management of the patient. Patients with C3, C5, C6, C7, and C8 deficiencies are susceptible to infection, and, if fever occurs, aggressive diagnosis and treatment should be given. Pneumococcal and meningococcal disease is common with these deficiencies. Immunization with pneumococcal, meningococcal, and HIB conjugate vaccine is recommended for these patients. The use of prophylactic penicillin also should be considered. Patients with C3 deficiency present with severe, recurrent pyogenic infections in a pattern similar to that in patients with severe neutropenia.

Patients with complement deficiencies make poor antibody responses to standard antigens. Thus, patients with recurrent infections should be evaluated for their ability to make antibody. Treatment with IVIG may decrease the incidence of infections in some patients. Patients with absence of an early-acting complement component (C1q, C1r, C2, and C4) may develop autoimmune and collagen-vascular disease and should be closely followed for evidence of these disorders.

Hereditary angioneurotic edema results from an absence of C1 esterase inhibitor. These patients can be treated by avoidance of factors such as trauma that might precipitate an event. Because the patient can present with unexplained episodes of abdominal pain, knowledge of the presence of this deficiency can prevent unnecessary surgery. Semisynthetic androgens (danazol and stanozolol) have been useful in the prevention of acute episodes of swelling. The mechanism of action of these drugs is not known, and they are generally not recommended for use in children. Epsilon-aminocaproic acid (EACA) has also been used prophylactically but has associated side effects. When these patients have undergone elective surgery or have been operated on for presumed appendicitis, which is frequently considered in patients presenting with abdominal pain due to an attack of intestinal angioedema, preoperative administration of EACA has prevented postoperative edema. Patients should be instructed to seek medical help immediately if laryngeal swelling occurs. Tracheosotomy should be performed if needed in patients with laryngeal obstruction. A Medic Alert bracelet is advised to alert physicians to an underlying complement pathyway abnormality.

PHAGOCYTIC DISORDERS

Phagocytic dysfunction is associated with an increased susceptibility to severe, recurrent bacterial infections with a poor response to antibiotic therapy. A spectrum of disorders has been described, including (1) congenital agranulocytosis (Kostmann syndrome); (2) cyclic neutropenia; (3) adherence glycoprotein defects (lymphocyte function–associated antigen [LFA-1]), complement receptor, C3bi and p150); (4) chemotactic defects; and (5) defects of intracellular killing (chronic granulomatous disease, myeloperoxidase deficiency).

Symptomatic treatment of patients with phagocytic disorders includes good skin care with antiseptic soaps and chronic prophylaxis with trimethoprim-sulfamethoxazole (10 mg/kg/day of the trimethoprim component) to decrease the number of infections. Children with fever should be evaluated with appropriate diagnostic tests and treated promptly and aggressively with intravenous antibiotics that includes antistaphylococcal coverage. Granulocyte transfusions are helpful in patients with severe neutropenia (Kostmann syndrome) or with adherence glycoprotein defects. IVIG treatment is usually not necessary because these patients typically have normal humoral immunity.

Chédiak-Higashi syndrome is an autosomal recessive disorder of intracytoplasmic granules that presents with partial albinism, frequent infections due to chemotactic abnormalities of the granulocytes, and depressed natural killer cell activity. Most of these patients undergo a malignant or premalignant transformation referred to as the accelerated phase, usually following infection with Epstein-Barr virus (EBV). These patients should be followed for this complication and considered for BMT after seroconversion to EBV or the onset of marked adenopathy or splenomegaly.

Bone marrow transplantation has the potential to provide definitive therapy for these disorders and should be considered. Marrow transplants from HLA matched siblings has been used successfully to treat Kostmann syndrome and chronic granulomatous disease. Therapy of neutropenia with recombinant granulocyte/monocyte colony-stimulating factor (G/M-CSF) or granulocyte colony-stimulating factor (G-CSF) is currently under investigation for patients with congenital agranulocytosis or cyclic neutropenia and has shown some success in both conditions. Some patients with Chédiak-Higashi syndrome may respond to high doses of ascorbic acid, resulting in normalization of bactericidal activity and decrease in infections during this therapy.

Interferon gamma has been approved by the FDA for the treatment of patients with both the X-linked and the autosomal recessive forms of chronic granulomatous disease (recommended dose, 50 $\mu g/m^2$ for patients with a body surface area $>0.5\ m^2$, and 1.5 $\mu g/kg$ per dose for patients with a body surface area $<0.5\ m^2$). The material is given subcutaneously 3 days a week (e.g., Monday, Wednesday, and Friday). Patients with a history of severe, recurrent infections are good candidates for interferon gamma treatment.

20

Accidents and Emergencies

PREVENTION OF INJURIES*

KATHERINE KAUFER CHRISTOFFEL, M.D., M.P.H.

UNINTENTIONAL INJURIES

Current terminology replaces the traditional term *accidents* with *unintentional injuries* to reflect the fact that they are not unpredictable events. The distinction is not just semantic. Conditions with recognizable patterns of occurrence are more readily subject to intervention than those without such patterns. That injuries have identifiable epidemiologic and clinical patterns means that efforts to control injuries, through a combination of prevention and treatment, can be successful.

Epidemiology

Injuries are the leading cause of death in children and adolescents in the United States after the age of 1 year. Injury death rates in infancy are actually higher than in many later years; injury is not the leading cause of death in the first year only because deaths from several other causes—related to prematurity, perinatal problems, and congenital malformations—are even more common than those from injury.

In 1985, 16,200 individuals younger than 20 years of age died from unintentional injuries. Transportation vehicles are by far the leading cause of fatal injury in childhood and adolescence. On the basis of Centers for Disease Control analysis of 1984 data, we know that victims younger than 15 years old suffered slightly more pedestrian fatalities than motor vehicle occupant fatalities and that both of these amounts exceeded pedalcyclist deaths by almost fourfold. Still, 344 pedalcyclists younger than 15 years old died in 1984. Other types of injuries that caused more than 500 deaths were drownings, burns (most due to house fires), and firearms.

If mortality statistics alone are studied, many prevalent types of injuries that only rarely result in death are hidden. For example, product-related injuries annually cause more than 1 million emergency room visits by toddlers alone; this figure includes more than 50,000 playground injuries. The best estimates are that medically attended nonfatal injuries probably outnumber fatalities by more than 1000 to 1.

Effective prevention approaches must identify and address victim vulnerabilities, exposure patterns, and other factors that contribute to recognized injury patterns. Table 1 summarizes known major risk factors for childhood injuries along with prevention approaches.

Prevention

The design of prevention approaches is based on several principles that have evolved from the conceptual frameworks described earlier and from accumulated experience with both successful and unsuccessful injury-prevention efforts. On the basis of the concept that injury is due to excessive energy transfer, Haddon identified ten points at which the process of damage could be interrupted, the consequence being a potential reduction in injury occurrence, injury severity, or both. Application of Haddon's principles to specific types and circumstances of injury facilitates and organizes the search for prevention options. In Table 2, taken from an actual injury prevention program, Haddon's principles are listed and applied to spill burns that occur in the kitchen and affect young children; the portion of the agent-vehicle-host triad that is affected by each intervention is identified.

Categorical Approaches

Prevention efforts can be characterized as *active* or *passive* in nature. Active approaches are ones that require action on the part of the victim (or the victim's agent, such as the parent or other caretaking adult). Use of seat belts and child passenger restraints are examples of active injury-prevention approaches. Passive prevention approaches are ones that, by contrast, do not rely on victim action. Airbags and other passive passenger restraint systems are examples of these. Because people have habits and preoccupations that interfere with consistent prevention activity, passive approaches are, when available, more successful than active approaches.

Active prevention approaches can be further divided into those that require *single* and those that require *multiple* actions. Use of child passenger restraints requires action on every car trip and thus is a multiple-action approach. Equipping a home with syrup of ipecac is usually required only once and so is a single-action (secondary prevention) method. Single-action

*Adapted from Green M, Haggerty RJ: Ambulatory Pediatrics 4. Philadelphia, WB Saunders Co, 1990, p 144.

TABLE 1. Child and Adolescent Unintentional Injuries: Risk Factors and Prevention Options

Injury Type	Victim Risk Factors	Other Factors Promoting Injury	Promising Prevention Approaches	Proven Prevention Approaches*
Motor vehicle—occupant	· Infancy · Adolescence, esp male and age <18 years —Alcohol —Night exposure	· Car-seat misuse · High school driver education · No curfew · Young drinking age · Vehicle factors · Speed (limit, radar detectors)	· Car-seat loaner programs · Reduce speed limit · Eliminate radar detectors · Tighten vehicle and restraint standards · Increase driving age	· Proper restraint · Eliminate high school driver education · Curfews · Increase drinking age · Passive restraint · Tighter "drinking under the influence" laws
Motor vehicle—pedestrian	· Male —School age—after school, urban —Toddler—driveway play —Adolescent—intoxicated	· Traffic density · Absent play areas	· Supervision · Crossing guards · Reflective clothing · Car back-up buzzers · Play areas away from traffic	(None proven)
Drowning	· Preschool (<5 years) —Whites —Age 2 years—highest in pools —<1 year—highest in tubs · Adolescent —Alcohol —Blacks —Diving —Use of undesignated swimming areas	· Summer · Weekends	· Swimming lessons to school-age children · Risk awareness for parents, adolescents · Raise drinking age · Pool alarms	· Fences with self-latching gates around pool
Burns	Age <5 years · Scald · Housefire —Poverty housing —Winter —Rural —Electrical Age 7–16 years, boys · High voltage	· Cigarettes · Water heater (e.g., coffee pot) design · Makeshift heating · Lack of supervision	· Lower water heater temperature below 130°F · Fire escape plan · Alter propane cigarette lighter · Self-extinguishing cigarettes · Increased supervision · Bury electric cables	· Smoke detectors · Flame-retardant sleepwear · Product modification to reduce spills, insulate wires
Firearms	· Adolescent males · Showing or playing with gun	· Visual similarity of toy and real gun · Family- or friend-owned guns in home, car guns · Media image of gun use · Gun factors: can't tell if loaded, hair trigger, no "safety," repeat firing	· Gun control · Reduce similarity of guns and toys · Increased gun safety features	· (None proven)
Suffocation	<1 year	· Large size of food pieces (e.g., hot dogs) · Size of toy parts · Play with plastic bags or sheeting · Entrapment in crib mattress, bars · Items (e.g., pacifier) around neck	· Alter toddler food portion configuration · Training of parents in Heimlich maneuver · Educate parents re risk factor avoidance · Stricter crib structure regulation	· (None proven)
Poisoning	· <5 years —Exploration · Teens —Risk taking	· Unfamiliar settings · Moves, times of change	· Keep poisons out of reach of young children · Limit medications in home	· Home use of syrup of ipecac · Childproof closures · Limit size of packages
Pedalcycling	· School age · Boys · Evenings	· Riding near traffic · Oversize bikes · Summer	· Separate bikeways · Safe biking education for parents, children	· Helmets
Falls	· Ages 1–4 years · Minorities · Urban	· Tall uncooled buildings · Summer · Infant walker use	· Air-condition tenements · Ban infant walkers	· Window guards

*Proven efficacy in reducing death, injury events, or severity of injury.

approaches are more likely to be carried out and thus to be successful. Single actions that are simplest are the most likely to be carried out and to be successful: parents are more likely to install plug guards (which takes only seconds) than cabinet locks (which takes several minutes).

Prevention approaches can also be categorized as involving modification of the *environment* or the *behavior* (of potential victims or those around them). Efforts to modify behavior can, in turn, be categorized as *persuasive* (educational) or *mandating* (legal) in approach. Road and vehicle improvements that reduce the likelihood of car crashes are examples of relatively pure environmental modifications. Increased stringency in the content and enforcement of driving while intoxicated (DWI)–driving under the influence (DUI) laws are

TABLE 2. Application of Haddon's Principles to Toddler Kitchen Scald Burns

Strategy	Intervention	Means (Focus)
1. Prevent the creation of the hazard	Do not cook food* Eliminate hot water	Educational (vehicle)
2. Reduce the amount of the hazard brought into being	Lower temperature in water heaters Manufacture hot water heaters to heat water only to safe temperatures	Educational (vehicle) Technological/Legislative (vehicle)
3. Prevent the release of the hazard	Create nontip pots, short-cord appliances	Technological (vehicle)
4. Modify the rate of release of the hazard from its source	Install small spouts	Technological (vehicle)
5. Separate the hazard from that which is to be protected by time and space	Cook when children are out of kitchen Do not use hot liquids near children	Educational (host)
6. Separate the hazard from that which is to be protected by a physical barrier	Use gates to kitchen to prevent entry Use counter guards and pot handles that prevent spills	Educational (vehicle) (environment)
7. Modify relevant basic qualities of the hazard	Manufacture appliances that are low conductors of heat	Technological (vehicle)
8. Make what is to be protected resistant	Wear protective clothing	Educational (host)
9. Begin to counter damage done by the hazard	Pour cold water on burns	Educational
10. Stabilize, repair, and rehabilitate the object of the damage	Develop a regional treatment system (prehospital, burn center, and rehabilitation care)	Technological/Legislative

*That is, do not use food that needs to be cooked.
From Micik S, Yuwiler J, Walker C: Preventing Childhood Injuries: A Guide for Public Health Agencies, 2nd ed. San Marcos, Calif. North County Health Services. 1987. p 74. Reproduced by permission.

examples of relatively pure behavior modification. In general, environmental modification has been more effective than behavioral modification, and legal approaches to behavior modification have been more effective than educational ones.

This categorization of prevention approaches is extremely useful for identifying the most promising options when several are available. There is, however, increasing recognition that the categories are oversimplified. For example, the legal changes that are usually needed to bring about environmental modification of the roadway require modification of the behavior of lawmakers. Further, the most successful prevention efforts have been those that use a combination of approaches. For example, deaths due to falls from tenement windows in New York City were dramatically reduced by a program that provided window guards (a passive, one-time environmental modification), education of parents, and enforcement of legislation requiring the installment of such guards by landlords.

Prevention approaches that make sense do not always work as well as expected. For example, "Mr. Yuk" stickers designed to warn toddlers of the dangers in ingesting potential poisons proved, on evaluation, to attract rather than to repel the youngsters. Identification and application of candidate interventions must therefore be followed by evaluation of their efficacy. Sometimes, fine tuning of the implementation is all that is required. At other times, it is necessary to go back to the prevention drawing board.

Specific Interventions for the Leading Injuries

Table 1 lists both proven and promising interventions for the leading causes of mortality from childhood injuries. For some (such as poisoning), the success of prevention efforts (childproof packaging and limitations on the size of packages of baby aspirin) has controlled injuries to the point that they are no longer major causes of mortality. The number of proven specific interventions for preventing serious and fatal childhood injuries is relatively small. Many more are promising but lack proof of efficacy.

For interventions of proven efficacy, advice to use the intervention is not the same as the intervention itself. Although it has been a tenet of most pediatric injury-prevention efforts that pediatrician advice to parents on how to provide for the safety of their young children is a critical component of successful injury prevention, proof of the efficacy of such advice has often been elusive. Some studies have documented clear increases in safe behaviors (e.g., proper child passenger restraint, lowering of water heater temperature, installation of smoke detectors) following educational interventions by pediatricians. However, some of these changes have been modest and of short duration, and several other studies have shown no such benefit. It is likely that the role of anticipatory guidance is more complex than the design of the usual intervention-outcome studies acknowledge. Although counseling by pediatricians about passenger restraints may not lead predictably and directly to increased and sustained use of restraints, it probably does contribute both to a community awareness of the need for restraints and to a receptivity of counseled families to safety-promoting messages from other quarters (e.g., neighbors, media, government officials). With the possible exception of adult counseling of adolescents (who sometimes respond to specific injury-prevention messages with increased risk taking), the pediatric community remains generally confident that its increased attention to injury-prevention education is a good thing, though certainly not all that is needed to prevent childhood injuries.

What Pediatricians Can Do

In the tradition of efforts to control infectious scourges affecting children, contemporary anticipatory guidance increasingly includes efforts to prevent injury. The American Academy of Pediatrics (AAP) has developed the injury prevention program (TIPP), a developmentally oriented counseling schedule designed for use in the context of ongoing health supervision. It includes specific prevention goals, with messages for parents and older children that are reinforced during successive visits. The focus of TIPP is on preventing the leading childhood injuries and on proven interventions, and it utilizes active discussion with families, which many believe is the most effective method for counseling. It has been implemented successfully in a variety of health supervision settings. Pediatricians wishing to introduce or expand their counseling in this area can do so readily with TIPP. It may be most effective to use TIPP in combination with home visiting (to identify specific hazards) and supplying specific devices (e.g., syrup of ipecac, smoke detectors, helmets, child passenger restraints).

Patient counseling, which occurs on a daily basis, is likely to be the most frequent injury-prevention activity in which most pediatricians engage. For maximum effect, counseling must be complemented with other types of activities, such as identification of the most prevalent and serious injuries in the area in which patients live; careful history taking to clarify the risk factors for and mechanisms of injury; efforts to introduce routine use of International Classification of Diseases external cause of injury codes (ICD E-Codes) by local and referral hospitals to facilitate tracking of injury patterns; involvement in local activities that can reduce injuries in small and major ways (e.g., playground design, improved emergency medical services); and participation in lobbying at the state, local, and national levels for legislation and regulation to provide greater protection against childhood injuries (as automobile restraint legislation has). In all of these activities, guidance and support are available from the Injury and Poison Prevention Committee, and the staff of the AAP.*

VIOLENCE

The culture in which children live presents them with problems as well as with sources of strength. One of the problems presented to children in the late twentieth century in the United States is the threat of violence, including homicide, nonfatal assaults, and firearm injuries. To be effective advocates for development and implementation of means to protect children and youth, pediatricians must be aware of current patterns of violent injury.

Homicide

Compared with children in other developed countries, children in the United States have atypically high rates of homicide. As a result of these high rates, homicide is a leading cause of death for U.S. children: among the top five causes for those 1 to 24 years of age and the leading cause for some subgroups of 15 to 24 year olds. The homicide rate has grown during recent decades while rates for other causes of death have fallen; of the leading causes of childhood death in the United States, homicide was the only one that increased during the three decades after World War II.

Homicide particularly affects the youngest children and the oldest adolescents. U.S. Federal Bureau of Investigation data indicate that more than 2000 children and adolescents from birth to 19 years are murdered annually: 60 per cent aged 15 to 19 years and 23 per cent younger than age 5 years. These figures, which are based on police records of murder cases, may underestimate the scope of the problem by as much as one half in the youngest age groups.

Childhood homicide risk is highest for males (after the age of 1 year), particularly for those who live in poor urban black and Hispanic communities. In adults, the increased risk for blacks is largely explained by region (with the highest rates in the north central region and the lowest in the western region) and poverty. It is likely that poverty explains most or all of the risk for blacks in childhood as well. The mechanisms by which poverty and region may affect risk include crowding, alcohol and drug use, feelings of hopelessness, risk-taking behavior, high crime rates, and subcultural patterns (e.g., drug-related violence).

Childhood homicides are of two "types":

1. Infantile: fatal injury by caregivers (child abuse), the overwhelming pattern in very early childhood.
2. Adolescent: fatal injury in the community, the dominant pattern in preadolescence and beyond.

In the infantile pattern, injury is most often due to beatings and, at times, to malnutrition or neglect, falls, burns, and arson. In the adolescent pattern, injury is due to gunshots, hit-and-run automobile accidents, strangulations, and stabbings (the latter often related to home intrusions or time spent in secluded spots, such as in abandoned buildings and near railroad tracks) and includes some deaths related to criminal activity by the victims. Gunshots are the cause of fatal injury in most homicide victims older than 11 years. Children between the ages of 2 and 11 experience the lowest incidence of homicides; those that do occur include both infantile and adolescent types of homicide. In addition to the dominant patterns described, new and hidden patterns of homicide are emerging, including the retributive murder of siblings of adolescents involved in gang and drug activity and the very small proportion of infants who appear to die of sudden infant death syndrome but who may instead be victims of parental asphyxiation or other abuse or neglect.

Nonfatal Assaults

Medically attended nonfatal assaults are estimated to be 100 to 500 times as frequent as fatal homicides. Such assaults are at the severe end of a spectrum of violent interactions that are endemic in our culture. Telephone interview surveys have indicated that 80 per cent of siblings engage in violent interactions each year, with 53 per cent of children attacking a brother or sister to a degree that would be considered assault if it occurred outside the family. Less controversial types of violence also involve children and adolescents to an alarming degree.

Violent Crime

The U.S. Justice Department's National Crime Survey indicates that the highest rates for personal crimes of violence are for victims who are young (12 to 24 years old), black (but not Hispanic), poor, and single. Boys and men are involved in assault about twice as often as girls and women. Victims and offenders tend to be of the same age. For most categories of violent crime, the highest rates are for 16 to 19 year olds, followed by 20 to 24 year olds, and then 12 to 15 year olds. Though their assault rates are highest, adolescents are least likely to report assaults to police and to obtain medical care for their injuries, which may be related to the fact that the youngest victims are least likely to be victimized by strangers.

Sexual Assaults

Detailed information on sexual assaults was obtained in Ageton's 3-year interview study of adolescents, which revealed that 5 to 7 per cent of adolescent females (numbering 700,000 to 1 million) experienced at least one sexual assault annually. Victimization was associated with urban residence and delinquency but not with victim age, race, or social class.

More than 50 per cent of reported assaults involved "verbal force"; less than half involved "minimal physical force"; 15 per cent or less involved beatings or weapons. The more

*The AAP's national office is in Elk Grove Village, Ill. Phone: 1–800–433–9016.

severe force generally was found with older victims, particularly those who were black, lower class, and urban. Women were generally assaulted by dates or boyfriends, who were similar in age to the victims and often deliquent. Interviews indicated that the assault was often encouraged by friends of the assailant, who were frequently intoxicated at the time.

Risk of victimization rose three to four times during the first year after a first assault and is apparently related to deliquent behavior and peers. In follow-up interviews, negative reactions to assaults were lowest at 6 to 12 months, with reactions at 1 year mildest if the victim had successfully deterred the assault. Reactions of depression and fear of being alone were most common 3 years after an assault.

Firearm Injuries

Firearm injuries are due to the energy transferred by a missile fired from a gun, rifle, or other such device. The missile may be a bullet, a BB, a pellet, or another object. The energy may be transferred by exploding gunpowder (powder firearms, including handguns, shotguns, and automatic weapons), pressurized air (nonpowder firearms, including air rifles, BB guns, and pellet guns), or other means (e.g., release of a stretched rubber band in a toy gun with a projectile). The larger the amount of energy transferred, the more serious the injury sustained. Because they are designed as efficient means of human injury, assaults with firearms are more often fatal than are assaults with other weapons.

The Scope of the Problem

It is estimated that there are 150,000,000 or more powder firearms in the United States, including at least 40,000,000 handguns. Approximately half of all U.S. households contain firearms, and most of those contain handguns. In view of the prevalence of firearms in the culture, it is perhaps not surprising that firearms are second after motor vehicles as the most important cause of injury mortality (in the total population) or that U.S. children are affected by the firearm injury epidemic. The scale of gun violence in the United States is unique in the world; its effect on U.S. children and adolescents is growing. Handgun homicide rates increased fivefold during the last three decades; this increase is reflected in rising numbers of surviving siblings and other children. Children are also affected directly; between 1960 and 1990, handgun homicide rates rose fastest for children aged 5 to 9 years. Handguns have become a prevalent problem in high schools. Teenagers have begun using semiautomatic weapons on city streets, and reports of children being killed during street gunfights have become routine in urban newspapers.

Nonfatal powder firearm injuries outnumber fatalities by 40 to 1. Among hospitalized children with firearm injuries, approximately 5 per cent die and an additional 12 to 16 per cent are permanently disabled. Some effects of firearm injuries are unique to children, such as growth arrest secondary to epiphyseal plate disruption by a bullet.

Guns and Boys at Different Ages

Patterns of gun use in the United States are reflected in patterns of gun injuries. Because guns are overwhelmingly the province of boys and men, most injuries are sustained by males. The youngest boys play with toy guns; therefore, gun injuries among the youngest boys are toy gun injuries. The rate of such injuries is fairly low, and most of these injuries are minor. A few, however, are fatal (due to aspiration of projectiles), and some cause blindness. Preteen and teenage boys are the main users of nonpowder weapons and thus predominate among victims of injuries from those devices. Such injuries are more often fatal than are toy gun injuries, but they usually do not result in death. Nonpowder firearm injuries are, however, a leading cause of blindness in school-age and adolescent boys. As they reach adolescence, boys increasingly turn to powder weapons, and the epidemic of firearm death begins. Among all deaths of adolescents and young adults, firearms are the leading cause in some areas, overwhelmingly due to homicide.

Circumstances and Risk Promoters

High firearm injury rates are associated with poverty, minority status, population density, prevalence of guns in the community, and proximity of guns available for purchase.

The prevalence of guns in children's environments undoubtedly promotes injury. Unintentional firearm deaths tend to occur at home, when boys are playing with or examining a gun, often in the company of another child. Thirty per cent of home fatalities among 10 to 14 year olds are due to firearms, as are 9 per cent of such deaths among 5 to 9 year olds. Suicides also tend to occur at home. The danger posed by guns in the home is emphasized by the finding by Kellerman and colleagues that a gun in the home is six times more likely to result in the death of a household member than in the death of an intruder.

Gun play by young boys probably contributes both to firearm injuries during childhood and to the acquisition of the "gun habit" that helps to maintain the gun epidemic in adolescents and adults. The visual similarities between toy guns, nonpowder firearms, and powder handguns and rifles confuse not only children but adults as well. At times, children are fatally shot by police who suspect them of criminal firearm use when they are playing with toy guns. The media image of gun use may, like gun play, promote comfort with and casual use of guns.

Prevention

Prevention approaches can be divided into *primary preventions*, which are designed to reduce incidence of injury and which generally must be aimed at whole populations (or subpopulations), and *secondary preventions*, which are designed to minimize the effects of injuries or reduce recurrence of them (or both) after injury has occurred.

Homicide and Assault

Clearly, only primary prevention approaches can be useful in dealing with homicide; secondary prevention approaches can also be helpful for assault.

Because preadolescent and adolescent homicides tend to occur when youngsters (both boys and girls) find themselves in danger from which they are ill-prepared to escape, training in self-protection skills (e.g., how to assess the risks in a new situation, how to safely avoid and get out of dangerous situations) may be both feasible and life saving for children after the early primary grades. Nonviolent conflict resolution curricula, developed for high school students and now being tested in several cities, may help young people to avoid the arguments that so often lead to assault and homicide in adolescence and early adult life. Self-protection skills should also help to protect girls and young women from sexual assault.

Because substance abuse may contribute to both assault and homicide in adolescence, school curricula that discourage drug and alcohol use may, if effective, assist in both primary and secondary prevention.

Police patrol is a logical, but unproven, primary and secondary prevention approach for assault. A police approach is most likely to be effective for specific kinds of assault, including those in bars and among strangers on the street.

Firearms

Primary prevention of firearm injury can occur at any one of several points: manufacture or importation, sale or transfer, possession, and use. Of these, purchase and possession or storage are the ones most amenable to pediatric anticipatory guidance. Though its effectiveness has not been evaluated, counseling would seem to be imperative if the household contains volatile or depressed individuals, young children, or preadolescent or adolescent boys. Parents can be asked if they have or are thinking of acquiring a gun, and the risks associated with guns in the home can be reviewed with them. If guns are already in the home, and parents resist disposing of them, the need to keep guns and ammunition locked and separate can be stressed.

Several other educational approaches to the primary prevention of firearm injury have been proposed, including training in hunting skills and school-based programs on the dangers of guns. The hunting education approach is not promising because most child and adolescent firearm injuries (including most unintentional firearm injuries) are not related to hunting. Cognitive approaches aimed at young children are likely to be counterproductive: The safety gains are likely to be minimal and any decreased adult vigilance (based on the presumption of such gains) hazardous. Peer-oriented approaches during adolescence make more sense but have not yet been evaluated.

A legal approach to the control of firearms is likely to be an essential component of any effective strategy to reduce firearm injury. Inconsistencies among local jurisdictions have made it difficult to assess the efficacy of existing regulations, which most often address sale and use. There is no evidence that local handgun control ordinances have led to increased firearm injury, as opponents of control have claimed, and there is some evidence that they are associated with lowered rates of injury. Opinion surveys over the last three decades have consistently shown support for increased gun control, even among the majority of gun owners.

The continuing scope of the handgun epidemic makes it clear that current regulations are not sufficient. Several facts suggest that tighter and more consistent gun control would probably lead to lowering the rates of firearm deaths and injuries:

1. Regional handgun ownership rates parallel the proportions of homicides involving firearms.
2. Handguns are more efficient deadly weapons than the usual alternatives (fists and knives).
3. A study comparing Seattle (no gun control) and Vancouver (strict gun control) demonstrated higher rates of assault (sevenfold) and homicide (fivefold) in the city lacking controls, with the increased risk due to crimes involving firearms.

Possibilities for legislation arise at the local, state, and federal levels. Some gun control approaches can assist in primary prevention: permissive or restrictive licensing, registration, and bans. Legal restraints at the point of manufacture and importation could include design requirements that would reduce the ease of intentional or unintentional use of handguns, for example, through built-in safety devices and means to ascertain quickly whether a gun is loaded. Local and federal ordinances have been enacted with the intent of reducing the realism of toy guns. These ordinances have been motivated by the danger such "toys" pose when used in crimes and when they are mistaken for real guns in the hands of playing children. It remains to be seen to what extent legal requirements are effective in this regard and whether reduced verisimilitude of toy guns will impede development of the gun habit.

Background checks as a condition for the purchase of firearms are likely to have limited value as a primary prevention approach. Most firearm homicides and suicides are acts of passion rather than a continuation of a pattern of criminal or deranged behavior. This and several other options for increased gun control (stiffer penalties for firearm violence, prohibition of high-risk groups from owning guns—e.g., very young, alcoholics, mental patients) are most promising for secondary prevention.

School-based secondary prevention educational programs targeted at high-risk students (e.g., those who live in areas in which guns are prevalent or attend schools in which gun carrying occurs) are presently being proposed and are subject to the same reservations as the school-based primary prevention efforts. Applying a passive prevention strategy, some schools now use metal detectors.

The position taken by the AAP on handguns is that guns do not belong in the environments of children. A survey of AAP Fellows indicated strong support for pediatrician advocacy for gun control, even among gun owners. The AAP can assist pediatricians in ascertaining the nature and extent of gun violence and regulation in their areas and in identifying current opportunities for pediatrician involvement in efforts to reduce the effects of gun violence on pediatric patients.

REFERENCES

Ageton SS: Sexual Assault Among Adolescents. Toronto, Lexington Books, 1983.

Alpert JJ, Guyer B (eds): Symposium on injuries and injury prevention. Pediatr Clin North Am 32, 1985.

Christoffel KK: American as apple pie: Guns in the lives of U.S. children and youth. Pediatrician 12:46, 1983–1985.

Christoffel KK: Toward reducing pediatric firearm injuries: Charting a legislative and regulatory course. Pediatrics 88:294–305, 1991.

Christoffel KK: Violent death and injury in U.S. children and adolescents. Am J Dis Child 144:697–706, 1990.

Committee on Accident and Poison Prevention, American Academy of Pediatrics: Injury Control for Children and Youth, 1987 ed. Elk Grove Village, Ill., AAP, 1987.

Kellerman AL, Reay DT: Protection or peril? An analysis of firearm-related deaths in the home. N Engl J Med 314:1557, 1986.

Polen MR, Friedman GD: Automobile injury: Selected risk factors and prevention in the health care setting. JAMA 259:77, 1988.

Public health surveillance of 1990 injury control objectives for the nation: MMWR 37:SS-1, 1988.

Sloan JH, Kellerman AL, Reay DT, et al: Handgun regulations, crime, assaults and homicide: A tale of two cities. N Engl J Med 319:1256, 1988.

Straus MA, Gelles RJ, Steinmetz SK: Behind Closed Doors. Garden City, N.Y.: Anchor Books, 1980.

Swanson JA, Sachs MI, Dahlgren KA: Accidental farm injuries in children. Am J Dis Child 141:1276, 1987.

Wintemute GJ, Teret SP, Kraus JF, et al: When children shoot children: 88 unintended deaths in California. JAMA 257:3107, 1987.

BOTULINAL FOOD POISONING

BARRY H. RUMACK, M.D.

Botulism is most frequently due to improperly home-processed foods, such as vegetables, meats, fruits, pickles, and seafood. Cooking these foods for 10 minutes at 100°C is capable of destroying the formed toxin but does not kill spores. Recent large restaurant outbreaks have involved baked potatoes, sauteed onions, beef stew, and turkey loaf. These foods were not properly refrigerated and not properly reheated. To meet diagnostic criteria, a case of botulism must demonstrate a neurologic illness characterized by descending paralysis, *and* (1) *Clostridium botulinum* must be identified in stool, wound, or an implicated food; *or* (2) a compatible illness in a person who is epidemiologically associated with a laboratory-confirmed case.

TREATMENT

The patient should be hospitalized if there are *any* symptoms (paralysis, ptosis, blurred vision, diplopia, sore throat). Administration of antitoxin must be done under the supervision of the Centers for Disease Control. Patients who receive antitoxin in the first 24 hours after onset of symptoms experience a shorter course and a lower fatality rate. However, the primary treatment is still adequate ventilatory support.

In a series of 308 cases, 68 per cent involved only a single person, 20 per cent two persons, and 12 per cent three or more persons. Restaurant-associated outbreaks accounted for 42 per cent of cases. There was an overall mortality rate of 7.5 per cent. These cases involved *adult botulism*, in which the toxin is preformed rather than produced in vivo, as in *infant botulism*. Recent literature suggests that some cases in patients older than age 4 months may also result from in vivo toxin formation.

ACUTE POISONINGS

HOWARD C. MOFENSON, M.D.
THOMAS R. CARACCIO, Pharm.D.
and MICHAEL SHANNON, M.D., Ph.D.

INCIDENCE

The ingestion of household products by a child is the most common medical emergency encountered in pediatric practice. More than 900,000 such patients are treated in emergency departments annually. There is a biphasic curve to the incidence of pediatric poisonings, with the age groups peaking at 1 to 5 years and at adolescence.

IDENTIFICATION OF THE SUBSTANCE AND TELEPHONE MANAGEMENT

Obtain information regarding the patient's condition. If there are no life-threatening manifestations, obtain a telephone history by asking the reporter's questions: who, what, when, where, how much, action taken, and why.

If symptoms are already present, refer the patient to a medical care facility for further evaluation. *Always remind the caller to bring the container or substance that may have been involved.* Always obtain telephone number and address of the caller. Consult the regional poison control center for updates on the ingredients and management (see Table 54 at the end of the chapter). The "antidote" labels on products are notoriously inaccurate. Proper telephone management, including callbacks, can reduce emergency departments visits.

ASSESSMENT AND MAINTENANCE OF VITAL FUNCTIONS

1. *The first priority is to establish and maintain vital functions.* Immobilize the cervical spine. Establish and secure an airway, and administer 100 per cent oxygen. If the airway protective reflex is impaired, insert an endotracheal tube. Adult pressure cuffed endotracheal tubes are not recommended for those under 8 years of age.

2. *Initiate cardiopulmonary resuscitative measures*, if necessary, and administer 100 per cent oxygen. Establish vascular access, and obtain blood specimens for arterial gases and pH, glucose, electrolytes, blood urea nitrogen (BUN), creatinine, and complete blood count, and take 5 to 10 ml for toxicologic studies. Perform urinalysis, and 50 to 100 ml of urine and gastric contents for toxicologic analysis. Save a portion of blood and urine for additional studies or in case of breakage or loss.

3. Manage hypotension and shock by positioning and by a challenge of isotonic fluids at 20 ml/kg over 1 hour. If these measures fail, give vasopressors. Shock may be caused by heart failure due to myocardial depression, hypovolemia, and decreased peripheral vascular tone due to central nervous system (CNS) depression or adrenergic blockade.

4. *Treat hypertensive crisis* (encephalopathy, heart failure), usually from sympathomimetics, with intravenous therapy, such as nitroprusside, and with continuous arterial pressure monitoring.

5. *Pulmonary edema*, both cardiac and noncardiac, may develop. Noncardiac pulmonary edema may be produced by inhalation or ingestion of substances that may damage the alveolar-capillary membrane. Substances with antidiuretic activity are likely to cause this complication with fluid overload. Other agents increase pulmonary permeability or cause a massive sympathetic discharge resulting in neurogenic pulmonary edema. Minimize fluid administration, diuretics, and oxygen. Respiratory support with mechanical ventilation and positive end expiratory pressure may be required.

6. Obtain an electrocardiogram (EKG) and treat *dysrhythmias* if the patient's condition is unstable. Correction of hypoxia and metabolic derangements spontaneously corrects many dysrhythmias.

7. *Renal failure* due to tubular necrosis may occur as a result of hypotension, hypoxia, or the direct effect of the toxin on the tubular cells. Hemoglobin, myoglobin, and metabolites of ethylene glycol may precipitate in the renal tubules. Dialysis may be required.

8. *Cerebral edema* in intoxications may be produced by many causes, and computed tomography (CT) may aid in the diagnosis. Reduce the increased intracranial pressure by hyperventilation to a P_{CO_2} of 25 mmHg, 20 per cent mannitol (0.5 g/kg) administered intravenously (IV) over 30 minutes and by head elevation.

9. *Metabolic acidosis with increased anion gap* is present in many intoxications. The mnemonic MUDPILES is appropriate: *M*, methanol; *U*, uremia; *D*, diabetic ketoacidosis; *P*, paraldehyde, phenformin; *I*, iron and isoniazid; *L*, lactic acidosis; *E*, ethylene glycol and ethanol, *S*, salicylates, starvation, and solvents (such as toluene). Intravenous sodium bicarbonate may be needed if a pH less than 7.1 persists after correction of hypoxia and establishment of perfusion.

10. *Temperature control* is vital; manage hypothermia or hyperthermia. When hyperpyrexia is due to intoxications, do not give antipyretics.

11. *Chest and abdominal x-rays* may be useful in evaluation for aspiration, foreign bodies, and radiopaque substances. The mnemonic CHIPES is appropriate: *C*, chlorinated compounds; *H*, heavy metals; *I*, iodinated compounds; *P*, Play-Doh, Pepto-Bismol, phenothiazines, packets of contraband; *E*, enteric coated tablets; *S*, sodium and other elements (such as potassium, bismuth, calcium, and solvents that are chlorinated).

12. Classify the state of consciousness and record it with the time of assessment. *The Glasgow Coma Score, originally designed for estimating the prognosis in head trauma, overestimates the depth of coma in intoxications.*

EMERGENCY TREATMENT OF THE COMATOSE OR CONVULSING PATIENT

Poisoning is the largest single cause of stupor and coma of unknown etiology. Obtain specimens for the determinations listed earlier, and immediately perform glucose reagent strip testing and confirmation by laboratory glucose analysis. If the reagent strip shows a glucose value below 100 mg/dl, administer 10 per cent glucose—2 ml/kg in an infant or 25 per cent glucose 1 ml/kg in a child, and 50 per cent glucose 1 ml/kg to an adolescent or adult; record responses. If there is no response, administer naloxone every 2 to 3 minutes (antidote No. 30 in Table 9) and chart the response (change in level of consciousness, pupillary response, and improvement in respirations).

If an adolescent has a history of chronic alcoholism, administer intravenous thiamine (50 to 100 mg) prior to glucose, to avoid thiamine depletion encephalopathy. Anaphylactoid reactions to intravenous thiamine may occur, so be prepared to treat this rare occurrence.

Control convulsions with diazepam intravenously (0.2 to 0.5 mg/kg per dose, slowly at a rate of less than 2 mg/minute, up to a maximum of 10 mg in children or 30 mg in adults). If necessary, give phenytoin (15 to 20 mg/kg, up to a maximum of 1000 mg slowly, at a rate of less than 30 mg/minute) while monitoring for dysrhythmias and hypotension.

PREVENTION OF ABSORPTION AND REDUCTION OF LOCAL DAMAGE

Use appropriate protection for rescuers, attendants, and the environment.

1. Treat *ocular exposure* by immediate irrigation with water for 15 to 20 minutes, with the patient's eyelids fully retracted. Avoid neutralizing agents. All caustic and corrosive injuries should be evaluated by ophthalmologists.
2. Treat *dermal exposure* immediately by rinsing, not forceful flushing—which may result in deeper penetration.
3. For *injected toxins*, such as intramuscular (IM) or subcutaneous (SC) needle injections or envenomation, a proximal constriction band may be required to occlude the lymphatics and veins if there is delay in reaching a medical facility.
4. Remove *inhalation exposures* immediately from the contaminated environment, and administer 100 per cent oxygen. Evaluation may include assessment of arterial blood gases, a chest x-ray, and tests for bronchospasm.
5. *Gastrointestinal exposures* are the most common route of poisoning. Gastrointestinal decontamination is not routine, and the method depends on age, clinical presentation, location of the patient, time of action of the substance, potential toxicity of the substance, and time following ingestion.

Dilutional and Neutralization Treatment

Dilutional treatment with water or milk is indicated for the immediate management of the ingestion of caustics and corrosives (if the patient has no signs of airway obstruction, esophageal perforation, or shock and can swallow). Otherwise, this method is not useful. Use only small quantities of diluting fluid (60 ml in small children and 250 ml in adults) because of the danger of inducing vomiting. Neutralizing solutions are not recommended because of the possibility of an exothermic reaction.

Gastrointestinal Decontamination

In small children, emesis in the home or activated charcoal (AC) orally or via nasogastric tube in a medical care facility is preferred to gastric lavage, especially in cases of ingestion of particulate matter because of the difficulty in inserting a large enough orogastric tube. In an older child or adolescent, gastric lavage is preferred if the child is in a medical facility because it may be accomplished without lag time and will not interfere with retention of AC or oral antidotes. Use both emesis and gastric lavage with caution in patients with dysrhythmias or in those who have ingested cardiotoxic drugs because the vagal response may result in serious dysrhythmias or cardiac arrest. Neither emesis nor lavage is completely effective, removing only 30 to 50 per cent of the ingested substance.

TABLE 1. Contraindications to the Induction of Emesis

1. Ingestions of caustics or corrosives.
2. Loss of protective airway reflexes,* such as in coma or convulsions.
3. Ingestion of substances that are likely to produce early-onset, rapid depression of consciousness, i.e., ethanol, tricyclic antidepressants, short-acting barbiturates.
4. Ingestion of substances that are likely to produce an early onset of seizures, i.e., camphor, isoniazid, strychnine, tricyclic antidepressants.
5. Ingestion of poorly absorbed petroleum distillates. See *Hydrocarbons*.
6. Prior significant vomiting or hematemesis.
7. Age under 6 months because of possible immature protective airway reflex and the lack of data to establish the safe and effective dose.
8. If the patient has ingested a foreign body, emesis is ineffective and there is a risk of aspiration and obstruction of the airway.
9. Neurologically impaired individuals with possible impaired airway protective reflexes.
10. Absence of bowel sounds. When no bowel sounds are present, gastric lavage is preferred.

*The gag reflex may be absent in some normal individuals and does not mean that the airway protective reflexes are lost.

Emesis

Use syrup of ipecac to induce emesis following telephone consultation. Contraindications to the induction of emesis are listed in Table 1, and the dosages of syrup of ipecac are presented in Table 2.

Some studies have safely involved larger doses of ipecac syrup. The dose of syrup of ipecac may be repeated once if the child does not vomit in 15 to 20 minutes. Be sure that the family collects vomitus by having patient vomit into large pot and brings it into the emergency room. The vomitus should be inspected for fragments of pills or the toxin and saved for toxicologic analysis. Note the appearance, color, and odor of the gastric contents.

Gastric Aspiration and Lavage

Plants and large pills are not readily removed by gastric lavage. The best results are obtained with the largest possible orogastric hose that can be reasonably passed. Nasogastric tubes are not large enough for this purpose. In adolescents and adults, use a No. 42 Fr. Lavacuator hose. In children, use a No. 22 to 28 Fr. orogastric tube or a tube approximately the size of the fifth finger.

Lavage is not very effective in children except in the case of liquids. Aspirate first, and save the contents. The amount of fluid used varies with size: in children, use 5 ml/kg of 0.9 per cent saline per lavage until "clear" (no further residue) returns; in adolescents and adults, use 150 to 200 ml per lavage of 0.9 per cent saline until "clear" returns. In some

TABLE 2. Dose of Syrup of Ipecac

Age	Amount
6 to 9 months	5 ml
9 to 12 months	10 ml
1 to 12 years	15 ml
Over 12 years	30 ml

TABLE 3. Contraindications to Gastric Lavage

1. Caustic or corrosive ingestions because of the danger of perforation
2. Uncontrolled convulsions because of the danger of aspiration or injury during the procedure
3. Petroleum products without endotracheal intubation
4. Comatose patients or patients with absent protective airway reflexes, who require insertion of endotracheal tube to protect against aspiration
5. Cardiac dysrhythmias, which must be controlled first, because the insertion of the tube may create a vagal response and cause a life-threatening dysrhythmia

cases, do not continue the lavage "until clear" if it delays the administration of AC or an oral antidote. Contraindications to gastric lavage are listed in Table 3.

Activated Charcoal

In the emergency department, where compliance can be assured. AC may be used alone or after emesis and gastric lavage. Some emergency department personnel use AC as the initial lavage fluid after aspiration. This has the advantage of absorbing any toxin and also serves as marker for completion of lavage "until clear."

The initial oral dose is 1 to 2 g/kg/dose or 15 to 30 g in children and 60 to 100 g in adults. Give AC as a "soupy" slurry suspension in at least 100 ml water with a cathartic. Omit the cathartic from subsequent doses of AC. If the patient vomits the dose, it may be repeated. If AC is used concomitantly with the oral antidote *N*-acetylcysteine (NAC), two loading doses of 140 mg/kg of NAC are recommended or the antidote may be separated from the charcoal by 1 to 2 hours. The substances not absorbed by AC are more easily remembered than the multitude of agents that are absorbed; they are listed in Table 4.

Repetitive doses of 0.5 g/kg of AC are administered orally every 2 to 6 hours, initially with a cathartic. The cathartic may be repeated daily. Repeated doses of AC appear to facilitate the passage of substances from the plasma into the intestine fluid, presumably by creating a concentration gradient. A number of studies have shown that repeated doses of oral AC are effective in reducing the nonrenal half-life of substances and their metabolites even when the substances have been administered intravenously; this has been referred to as "gastrointestinal dialysis." Monitor electrolyte balance and gastrointestinal (GI) motility during therapy.

Table 5 lists some of the products for which repetitive doses of AC have been studied and recommended as effective therapy. Table 6 lists the contraindications to oral AC.

Cathartics

Despite the lack of scientific data on the usefulness of cathartics in poisonings, they continue to be used by most authorities. The saline types are recommended in children; oil-based types are not. Sorbitol, a very potent cathartic, is not recommended for those under 1 year of age and should be used with caution in children under 3 years of age because of possible severe electrolyte disturbances. Dosages are listed in Table 7; contraindications are listed in Table 8.

TABLE 4. Substances Poorly Adsorbed by Activated Charcoal

C—caustics and corrosives (alkali and acids)
H—heavy metals (arsenic, iron, lead, lithium, mercury)*
A—alcohols and glycols (ethylene glycol)
C—chlorine and iodine
O—other substances insoluble in water
A—aliphatic and poorly absorbed hydrocarbons
L—laxatives: sodium, magnesium, sorbitol

*Cyanide: 1 g of activated charcoal binds 35 mg of cyanide. It is recommended that activated charcoal be administered in cases of *ingested* cyanide.

TABLE 5. Substances with Half-Lives Shortened by Repetitive Dosing of Oral Activated Charcoal

Acetaminophen	Nadolol
Carbamazepine	Phenobarbital*
Chlordecone	Phenylbutazone
Dapsone	Phenytoin (controversial)
Digoxin	Salicylates
Digitoxin	Theophylline*
Glutethimide	Tricyclic antidepressants
Methotrexate	Valproate

*The half-life has been shortened even if administered intravenously.

Whole-Bowel Washout

A procedure that involves cleansing the bowel has been used successfully with iron overdose when abdominal radiographs assessed incomplete emptying of ingested iron. Whole-bowel washout has additional implications for gastrointestinal decontamination in other ingestions, such as in sustained-release preparations, contraband "body packers" (persons illegally transporting contraband), and "body stuffers" (persons hiding evidence of an illicit substance). Use a colonic irrigation solution (GoLytely), 0.5 L/hour in children under 5 years of age* and 2 L/hour in adolescents and adults. The end point is when the rectal effluent has the appearance of the infusate. This takes approximately 2 to 4 hours. Do *not* use these measures if there is extensive hematemesis or rectal bleeding, ileus, signs of bowel perforation, or peritonitis.

ANTIDOTES

Systemic antidotes should be highly specific and efficacious with relatively low toxicity. A small number of antidotes have these characteristics. In some cases, the physician may start antidotal therapy on the basis of the history and clinical picture while awaiting laboratory confirmation. Antidotes are not used prophylactically. The antidote formulary (Table 9) is an alphabetical list of commonly used preparations. Contact your regional poison control center (see Table 54) for additional advice and guidance when using an antidote.

ENHANCEMENT OF ELIMINATION

The methods for eliminating the absorbed toxic substances or their toxic metabolites include forced diuresis and osmotic diuresis with or without ion trapping, peritoneal dialysis, hemodialysis, hemoperfusion, exchange transfusion, plasmaphoresis, enzyme induction, and inhibition. The methods for increasing the renal excretion (hemodialysis and hemoperfusion) have been fairly extensively studied, but the others have

*Not approved by the Food and Drug Administration (FDA).

TABLE 6. Contraindications to Oral Activated Charcoal

1. Caustics or corrosives—charcoal ineffective and may obscure or look like a burn
2. Absence of bowel sounds (adynamic ileus)
3. Intestinal obstruction or evidence of peritonitis
4. Inability to confirm location of gastric tube
5. Lack of adequate airway protection, in which case an endotracheal tube should be inserted first

TABLE 7. Cathartics Used in Treatment of Acute Poisonings

Cathartic	Synonym	Pediatric Dose	Adolescent/Adult Dose
Sodium sulfate	Glauber's salt	250 mg/kg/dose	15–30 g/dose
Magnesium sulfate	Epsom salt	250 mg/kg/dose	15–30 g/dose
Magnesium citrate	Citrate of magnesium	5 ml/kg/dose	240 ml (8 ounces)/dose
Sorbitol Conc.		35% (diluted)	70% (standard)
Age		>3 year	
Dose		1.4–2.1 ml/kg	2.8–4.3 ml/kg
Maximum		143 ml	214 ml
Frequency		Once only	Once only

not been well evaluated. In general, the supportive *indications for dialysis* are represented by the mnemonic AEIOU: *A*, acidosis and alkalosis (refractory); *E*, electrolyte imbalance (refractory); *I*, intoxications by a dialyzable poison; *O*, overhydration; *U*, uremia. The use of these modalities is discussed in the management of the specific poisons. See Table 10.

THE TOXICOLOGY LABORATORY

If legal issues are involved, establish a "chain of custody" to ensure the security of the specimen. Always ascertain the units used in the laboratory report. The timing of the blood specimen to determine toxicity should not be in the distribution phase but in the elimination phase of substance (i.e., obtain the specimen for acetaminophen after 4 hours).

MANAGEMENT OF COMMON OVERDOSES AND POISONS*

These agents are presented alphabetically in the following scheme: generic name (common name), toxicity, kinetic data (pharamcokinetic or toxicokinetic), and mechanism of toxicity that has relevance to major manifestations and management, with referral to the antidote in Table 9.

Acetaminophen (APAP, Tylenol, Many Brands)

Toxicity. Child therapeutic dose: 10 to 15 mg/kg every 4 hours for a maximum of five daily doses. Hepatotoxic at 140 mg/kg or more; in adults, at 7.5 g or more. Some studies suggest that hepatoxicity in children may occur at amounts greater than 200 mg/kg. Table 11 presents a calculation of the amounts of commonly used preparations that equal 140 mg/kg.

Kinetics. Absorption time, 0.5 to 1 hour. Vd, 0.9 L/kg. Elimination, 90 per cent in the liver, where acetaminophen is metabolized to inactive glucuronide 65 per cent and inactive sulfate 30 per cent in adults, by two saturatable pathways. Approximately 5 per cent is metabolized by P_{450} mixed oxidase to a reactive toxic agent that is normally inactivated by glucuronidation with glutathione. In children the metabolism is more sulfate than glucuronate, which may be hepatoprotective. If excess reactive metabolite, is produced such as in overdose, the free metabolite, not bound by glutathione, binds to liver protein macromolecules in hepatocytes and causes centrolobular necrosis in liver. Enzyme inhibition by concomitant ethanol ingestion may be hepatoprotective, whereas enzyme induction by chronic alcoholism may increase hepatoxicity.

Abbreviations and terms used in text:

t ½ = Half-life, the time required for the blood concentration to fall by 50 per cent.

Vd = Apparent volume distribution, the theoretical portion of the body mass in which the drug is distributed, or the body burden.

TABLE 8. Contraindications to Cathartics

1. Absence of bowel sounds (adynamic ileus)
2. Evidence of intestinal obstruction
3. Pre-existing electrolyte disturbances
4. Magnesium sulfate in renal impairment
5. Sodium sulfate in conditions requiring salt restriction
6. Evidence of gastrointestinal perforation or peritonitis
7. Evidence of gastrointestinal bleeding

Manifestations

PHASE I. Occurs 7 to 14 hours after ingestion and consists of malaise, nausea, vomiting, and drowsiness for a few hours. Loss of consciousness is *not* a feature; if it is present, suspect another cause.

PHASE II. Occurs 24 to 48 hours after ingestion and consists of a latent period with early signs of subclinical hepatic dysfunction, as reflected in laboratory tests (e.g., an increase in liver enzymes, bilirubin, prothrombin time) and in right upper quadrant pain.

PHASE III. Occurs 72 to 96 hours after ingestion with peak liver function abnormalities, hypoglycemia, and coagulation abnormalities. Consider acetaminophen intoxication in any unexplained case of hepatitis.

PHASE IV. Regeneration and total hepatic recovery may take up to 3 months; if there is extensive liver damage, sepsis and disseminated vascular coagulation may occur and the patient may die in 7 to 10 days. Other organ systems involved include transient renal failure, which develops 1 week after ingestion. In some cases, pancreatitis develops in 3 to 4 days after ingestion.

Management. Because the early symptoms of acetaminophen overdose may be minimal or absent initially, the opportunity to suspect clinically and administer the antidote NAC may be missed.

1. *Avoid* emesis in the emergency department because it may interfere with the retention of AC and NAC. Gastric lavage is preferred. In children, induce emesis in the home if more than 140 mg/kg is ingested. Studies have indicated that AC effectively absorbs acetaminophen. Activated charcoal may be administered concomitantly with the antidote NAC if the loading dose of NAC is administered twice rather than once. Activated charcoal may be continued, separating its administration by 1 to 2 hours from that of NAC. (*Note*: In the past, AC was believed to be contraindicated when NAC use was contemplated.) Saline sulfate cathartics are used because they may enhance the sulfate metabolic pathway and provide hepatic protection.

2. Give oral NAC. NAC is rich in sulfhydryl groups and acts as a surrogate glutathione for hepatotoxic overdose (see antidote No. 1, Table 9). (An intravenous preparation is used in Europe and Canada but is not approved in the United States. NAC has caused fatal anaphylactoid reactions in rare cases intravenously.)

Text continued on page 711

TABLE 9. Antidote Formulary

Medication	Indications and Adverse Reaction (AR)	Comments
1. ***N*-Acetylcysteine** (NAC, *Mucomyst*), Mead Johnson. Glutathione precursor that prevents accumulation and helps detoxify acetaminophen metabolites. **Dose:** *Adult,* 140 mg/kg p.o. of 5% solution as loading dose, then 70 mg/kg p.o. every 4 hr for 17 doses as maintenance dose. *Child,* same as adult. **Packaged:** 10 and 20% solution in 4, 10, and 30 ml vials.	Acetaminophen toxicity. Most effective within first 8 hr (to make more palatable, administer through a straw inserted into closed container of citrus juice). **AR:** Stomatitis, nausea, vomiting. See Acetaminophen p. 703. The full course of therapy is required in any patient whose level falls in the toxic range.	IV preparation experimental. The dose of NAC should be repeated if the patient vomits within 1 hr after administration. Methods to stop vomiting of the NAC are (a) placement of a tube in the duodenum, (b) slow administration over 1 hr, (c) one half hour before NAC dose use metoclopramide (*Reglan*) 1 mg/kg intravenously over 15 min. (max dose 10 mg) every 6 hr. In infants 0.1 mg/kg/dose IM, IV. Droperidol (*Inapsine*) 1.25 mg IV; for extrapyramidal reactions use diphenhydramine (antidote 19).
2. **Ammonium chloride**	Not recommended	
3. **Amyl nitrite**	See 14, Cyanide antidote kit	
4. **Antivenin Black Widow Spider** (*Latrodectus mactans*) **Dose:** 1–2 vials IV infused over 1 hr. **Packaged:** 6000 units/vial with 2.5 ml sterile water and 1 ml horse serum 1:10 dilution.	Black widow spider; all *Latrodectus* species with severe symptoms. Most healthy adults will survive with supportive care. Used in elderly or infants or if underlying medical condition causing hemodynamic instability. **AR:** Same as antivenin polyvalent because derived from horse serum.	Preliminary sensitivity test. Supportive care alone is standard management.
5. **Antivenin Polyvalent** for Crotalidae (pit vipers), Wyeth. IV only. **Dose:** depends on degree of envenomation—minimal: 5–8 vials, moderate: 8–12 vials, severe: 13–30 vials. Dilute in 500–2000 ml of crystalloid solution and start IV at a slow rate, increasing after the first 10 minutes, if no reaction occurs. **Packaged:** 1 vial (10 ml) lyophilized serum, 1 vial (10 ml) bacteriostatic water for injection, 1 vial (1 ml) normal horse serum.	Venoms of crotalids (pit vipers) of North and South America. **AR:** (Shock anaphylaxis) Reaction occurs within 30 min. Serum sickness usually occurs 5–44 days after administration. It may occur less than 5 days, especially in those who have received horse serum products in the past. Symptoms include fever, edema, arthralgia, nausea, and vomiting, as well as pain and muscle weakness.	Consider consulting with regional poison control center and herpetologist. Administer IV. Preliminary sensitivity test. Never inject in fingers, toes, or bite site.
6. **Antivenin,** North American coral snake. Wyeth. IV only. **Dose:** 3–5 vials (30–50 ml) by slow IV injection. First 1–2 ml should be injected over 3–5 min. **Packaged:** 1 vial antivenin, 10 ml. 1 vial bacteriostatic water 10 ml for injection.	*Micrurus fulvius* (Eastern coral snake); *Micurus tenere* (Texas coral snake) **AR:** Anaphylaxis (sensitivity reaction). Usually 30 min after administration. Signs/Symptoms: Flushing, itching, edema of face, cough, dyspnea, cyanosis. Neurologic manifestations—usually involve the shoulders and arms. Pain and muscle weakness are frequently present and permanent atrophy may develop.	Same as for Antivenin polyvalent for Crotalidae. Will not neutralize the venom of *Micrurus euryxanthus* (Arizona or Sonoran coral snake)
7. **Atropine** (various manufacturers). Antagonizes cholinergic stimuli at muscarinic receptors. **Dose:** *Adult,* initial dose 2–4 mg IV. Dose every 10–15 min as necessary until cessation of secretions. Severe poisoning may require doses up to 2000 mg. *Child,* initial dose of 0.02 mg/kg IV to a max of 2 mg every 10–15 min as necessary until cessation of secretions. Use preservative-free atropine if infusion. **Packaged:** 0.3 mg/ml in 30 ml; 0.4 mg/ml in 0.5, 1, 20, and 30 ml vials; 1 mg/ml in 1 and 10 ml vials.	Therapy in carbamate and organophosphate insecticide poisonings. Rarely needed in cholinergic mushroom intoxication (*Amanita, Muscaria, Clitocybe, Inocybe* spp.). Lack of signs of atropinization confirms diagnosis of cholinesterase inhibition. **AR:** Flushing and dryness of skin, blurred vision, rapid and irregular pulse, fever, and loss of neuromuscular coordination. Diagnostic test: child—0.01 mg/kg IV; adult—1 mg total	If cyanosis, establish respiration first because atropine in cyanotic patients may cause ventricular fibrillation. If severe signs of atropinization, may correct with physostigmine in doses equal to one-half dose of atropine. If symptomatic, administer until the end point of drying secretions and clearing of lungs. Hallucinations, flushing of the skin, dilated pupils, tachycardia, and elevation of body temperature are not end points and do not preclude atropine administration. Atropinization should be maintained for 12 to 24 hours, then taper dose and observe for relapse. Atropine has successfully been administered by IV infusion, although this method has not received FDA approval. **Dose:** Place 8 mg of atropine in 100 ml D5W or saline. Conc. = 0.08 mg/ml Dose range = 0.02–0.08 mg/kg/hr or 0.25–1 ml/kg/hr. Severe poisoning may require supplemental doses of intravenous atropine intermittently in doses of 2–4 mg until drying of secretions occurs.

TABLE 9. Antidote Formulary *Continued*

Medication	Indications and Adverse Reaction (AR)	Comments
8. **BAL**	See 17, Dimercaprol	
9. **Bicarbonate**	See 39, Sodium bicarbonate	
10. **Botulism antitoxin,** Connaught Med. Research Labs. **Dose:** *Adult,* 1 vial IV stat then 1 vial IM; repeat in 2–4 hr if symptoms appear in 12–24 hr. *Child,* Check with state health department	Prevention or treatment of botulism.	Contact local or state health department for full management guidelines.
11. **Calcium disodium edetate** (EDTA), *Disodium Versenate,* Riker. **Dose:** *Adult,* max 4 g. *Child,* 1 g max. Moderate toxicity, IM or IV, 50 mg/kg day for 3–5 days. Severe toxicity, IV or IM, 75 mg/kg/day for 4–5 days, divided into 3–6 doses daily. Dilute 1 g in 250–500 ml saline or D5W, infuse over 4 hr twice daily for 5–7 days. For lead levels over 69 μg/dl or if symptoms of lead poisoning or encephalopathy, add BAL alone initially, 4 mg/kg, then combination BAL and EDTA at different sites. EDTA dose: 12.5 mg/kg IM. (See lead text for latest recommendations.) Modify dose in renal failure. **Packaged:** 200 mg/ml. 5 ml amps.	For chelation in cadmium, chromium cobalt, copper, lead, magnesium, nickel, selenium, tellurium, tungsten, uranium, vanadium, and zinc poisoning. **AR:** 1. Thrombophlebitis. 2. Nausea, vomiting. 3. Hypotension. 4. Transient bone marrow suppression. 5. Nephrotoxicity, reversible tubular necrosis (particularly in acid urine). 6. Fever 4–8 hours after infusion. 7. Increased prothrombin time.	Hydrate first and establish renal flow. Avoid plain sodium EDTA since hypocalcemia may result. Procaine 0.25–1 ml of 0.5% for each ml of IM EDTA to reduce pain. Do not use EDTA orally. Limit use to 7 days (otherwise loss of other ions and cardiac dysrhythmias may occur). **MP:** Calcium levels, urinalysis, renal profile, erythrocyte protoporphyrin, blood lead, and liver profile. Contraindicated in iron intoxication, hepatic impairment, and renal failure.
12. (A) **Calcium gluconate** 10% **Dose:** IV 0.2 to 0.5 ml/kg of elemental calcium to max 10 ml (1 g) over 5–10 min with continuous EKG monitoring. Titrate to adequate response. **Packaged:** 10% in 10 ml vial.	Calcium channel blocker poisoning, e.g., nifedipine (Procardia), verapamil (Calan), diltiazem (Cardiazem). It improves the blood pressure but does not affect the dysrhythmias. Hypocalcemia as result of poisonings. Black widow spider envenomation.	Repeat dose as needed. Monitor calcium levels. Contraindicated with digitalis poisoning.
(B) **Calcium chloride 10%** **Dose:** IV 0.2 ml/kg up to max 10 ml (1 g) with continuous IV monitoring. Titrate to adequate response. Rate should not exceed 2 ml/min. (C) **Infiltration of calcium gluconate** **Dose:** Infiltrate each square cm of the affected dermis and subcutaneous tissue with about 0.5 ml of 10% calcium gluconate using a 30 gauge needle. Repeat as needed to control pain.	Hydrofluoric acid (HF) (if irrigation with cool water fails to control the pain). **AR:** IV bradycardia, asystole, necrosis with extravasation.	Infiltration with calcium gluconate should be considered if HF exposure results in immediate tissue damage and erythema and pain persists following adequate irrigation.
Packaged: 10% in 10 ml vial. (D) **Calcium Gel** 3.5 g USP calcium gluconate powder added to 5 oz of K-Y Jelly.	Dermal exposures of hydrofluoric acid less than 20%.	Gel must have direct access to burn area; if pain persists then calcium gluconate injection may be needed. Placing a loose-fitting surgical glove over the gel when the fingers are involved helps to keep preparation in contact with burn area.
13. **Chemet**	See 42, Succimer	
14. **Cyanide antidote kit.** Lilly. Nitrite-induced methemoglobinemia attracts cyanide off cytochrome oxidase and thiosulfate forms nontoxic thiocyanate. **Dose:** *Adult,* amyl nitrite. Inhale for 30 sec of every min. Use a new ampule every 3 min. Reapply until Na nitrite can be given. Then inject IV 300 mg (10 ml) of 3% solution of Na nitrite at a rate of 2.5 to 5 ml/min over 20 minutes. **Alternate:** IV infusion: 300 mg in 50 to 100 ml of 0.9% saline over 20 min. Then inject 12.5 g (50 ml of 25% solution) of Na thiosulfate over 20 minutes. *Child:* Use Chart No. 1 below to determine the dosage of sodium nitrite and sodium thiosulfate. **Packaged:** Two 10-ml ampules Na nitrite injection: Two 50-ml ampules Na thiosulfate injection: 0.3-ml amyl nitrite inhalant.	Cyanide poisoning. **AR:** Hypotension, methemoglobinemia.	*Note:* If a child is given the adult dose of Na nitrite, a fatal methemoglobinemia may result. *Do not use methylene blue* for methemoglobinemia in cyanide therapy. Observe for hypotension and have epinephrine available. Cyanide kits should have amyl nitrite changed annually. Administer oxygen 100% between inhalations of amyl nitrite. Monitor hemoglobin, arterial blood gases, methemoglobin concentration (nitrite given to obtain a methemoglobin of 25%). Some add amyl nitrate to resuscitation bag.

Table continued on following page

TABLE 9. Antidote Formulary *Continued*

Medication	Indications and Adverse Reaction (AR)	Comments
Chart No. 1. This chart should be used to determine the appropriate dose of sodium nitrite and sodium thiosulfate in children based on the hemoglobin concentration in the left column. The average child with a normal hemoglobin concentration will require 0.33–0.39 ml/kg up to 10 ml over 20 minutes.		

Hemoglobin conc.	*Initial Child Dose of Sodium Nitrite 3%* *(do not exceed 10 ml)*	*Initial Child Dose of Sodium Thiosulfate* *(do not exceed 12.5 g)*
8 g	0.22 ml/kg (6.6 mg/kg)	1.10 ml/kg
10 g	0.27 ml/kg (8.7 mg/kg)	1.35 ml/kg
12 g	0.33 ml/kg (10 mg/kg)	1.65 ml/kg
14 g	0.39 ml/kg (11.6 mg/kg)	1.95 ml/kg

If signs of poisoning reappear, repeat above procedure at one-half the above doses. The rate of each agent should be given over 20 minutes.

Medication	Indications and Adverse Reaction (AR)	Comments
15. **Deferoxamine mesylate** (DFOM, *Desferal*). Ciba. Has a remarkable affinity for ferric iron and chelates it. **Therapeutic Dose:** *Adult,* 90 mg/kg IM or IV every 8 hr to max 1 g per injection. May repeat to max 6 g in 24 hr. *Child,* same as adult. IV administration can be given by slow infusion at rate not exceeding 15 mg/kg/hr. **Packaged:** 500 mg/amp (powder).	DFOM is useful in the treatment of symptomatic iron poisoning or serum iron levels greater than 500 μg/dl. If the DFOM challenge test is positive, it is not a definite indication that therapy is necessary in the asymptomatic patient. Oral DFOM is not recommended. Iron intoxication. Therapeutic—see dose in left column. *Diagnostic trial.* Give deferoxamine, 50 mg/kg IM (up to 1 g). If serum iron exceeds TIBC, unbound iron is excreted in urine, producing a "vin rose" color of chelated iron complex in the urine (pink-orange). However, may be negative with high serum iron.† **AR:** Flushing of the skin, generalized erythema, urticaria, hypotension, and shock may occur. Blindness has occurred rarely in patients receiving long-term, high-dose DFOM therapy. Continuous infusions of DFOM over 24 hours has produced severe pulmonary injury manifested as adult respiratory distress syndrome. Contraindicated in patients with renal disease or anuria.	Therapy is usually continued until urine serum iron <100 μg/dl or when positive "vin rose" urine turns clean, or when becomes asymptomatic. DFOM infusion should not be administered for longer than 24 hours. Establish a good renal flow. To be effective, DFOM should be administered in first 12–16 hr. In mild to moderate iron intoxication, IM or IV route. In severe intoxication or shock, IV route only. Monitor serum iron levels, urine output, and urine color.
16. **Diazepam** (*Valium*). Roche. **Dose:** *Adult,* 5–10 mg IV (max 20 mg) at a rate of 5 mg/min until seizure is controlled. May be repeated 2 or 3 times. *Child,* 0.1–0.3 mg/kg up to 10 mg IV slowly over 2 min. **Packaged:** 5 mg/ml, 2 ml, 10 ml vials.	Any intoxication that provokes seizures when specific therapy is *not* available, e.g., amphetamines, PCP, barbiturate and alcohol withdrawal. Chloroquine poisoning. **AR:** Confusion, somnolence, coma, hypotension.	Intramuscular absorption is erratic. Establish airway and administer 100% oxygen and glucose.
17. **Dimercaprol** (BAL). Hynson, Westcott, and Dunning. **Dose:** Recommendations vary; contact regional poison control center. Prevents inhibition of sulfhydryl enzymes. Given deep IM only. For *severe lead poisoning*—see 11, EDTA. For *mild arsenic or gold*—2.5 mg/kg every 6 hr for 2 days, then every 12 hr on the third day, and once daily thereafter for 10 days. For *severe arsenic or gold*—3–5 mg/kg every 6 hr for 3 days, then every 12 hr for 10 days. For *mercury*—5 mg/kg initially, followed by 2.5 mg/kg 1 or 2 times daily for 10 days. **Packaged:** 100 mg/ml 10% in oil in 3 ml amp.	For chelation of antimony, arsenic, bismuth, chromates, copper, gold, lead, and mercury and nickel. **AR:** 30% of patients have reactions: fever (30% of children), hypertension, tachycardia, may cause hemolysis in G-6-PD deficiency patients. Doses greater than recommended may cause various adverse effects: nausea, vomiting, headache, chest pain, tachycardia, and hypertension.	Contraindicated in instances of hepatic insufficiency, with the exception of postarsenic jaundice. Should be discontinued or used only with extreme caution if acute renal insufficiency is present. Monitor blood pressure and heart rate (both may increase), urinalysis, qualitative urine excretion of heavy metal. Contraindicated in iron, silver, uranium, selenium, and cadmium poisoning.
18. **Dimercaptosuccinic acid** (DMSA)	See 42, Succimer	
19. **Diphenhydramine** (*Benadryl*), Parke Davis. Antiparkinsonian action. **Dose:** *Adult,* 10–50 mg IV over 2 min. *Child,* 1–2 mg/kg IV up to 50 mg over 2 min. Maximum in 24 hr, 400 mg. **Packaged:** 10 mg/ml in 10 and 30 ml vials. 50 mg/ml in 1, 5, 10, and 30 ml vials. Caps, tab 25 mg. Elixir, syrup 12.5 mg/5 ml.	Used to treat extrapyramidal symptoms and dystonia induced by phenothiazines, phencyclidine, and related drugs. **AR:** Fatal dose, 20–40 mg/kg. Dry mouth, drowsiness.	Continue with oral diphenhydramine 5 mg/kg/day to 25 mg 3 times a day for 72 hours to avoid recurrence.

TABLE 9. Antidote Formulary *Continued*

<table>
<tr><th>Medication</th><th>Indications and Adverse Reaction (AR)</th><th>Comments</th></tr>
<tr><td>20. EDTA</td><td>See 11, Calcium disodium edetate</td><td></td></tr>
<tr><td>21. Ethanol (ETOH). Competitively inhibits alcohol dehydrogenase.
Dose: Loading—Administer 7.6–10.0 ml/kg of 10% ETOH in D5W over 30 min IV or 0.8–1.0 ml/kg 95% ETOH p.o. in 6 oz of orange juice over 30 min. While administering loading dose, start maintenance.
Maintenance Dose: Volume of 10% ETOH needed IV or 95% oral solution (not on dialysis). [See table of maintenance dose below.] If patient is on dialysis, add 91 ml/hr in addition to regular maintenance dose. See comments to prepare 10% solution if not commercially available.
Packaged: 10% ethanol in D5W 1000 ml; 95% ethanol. May be given as 50% solution orally.
Maintenance Dose:
<table>
<tr><th>Patient Category</th><th>ml/kg/hr using 10% IV</th><th>ml/kg/hr using 50% oral</th></tr>
<tr><td>Nondrinker</td><td>0.83</td><td>0.17</td></tr>
<tr><td>Occasional drinker</td><td>1.40</td><td>0.28</td></tr>
<tr><td>Alcoholic</td><td>1.96</td><td>0.39</td></tr>
</table></td><td>Methanol, ethylene glycol
Ethanol infusion therapy may be started in cases of suspected methanol and ethylene glycol poisoning presenting with increased anion gap and osmolal gap, or if the urine shows the crystalluria of ethylene glycol poisoning or the hyperemia of the optic disc of methanol intoxication.
AR: CNS depression, hypoglycemia.</td><td>Monitor blood ethanol 1 hr after starting infusion and every 4–6 hr. Maintain a blood ethanol concentration of 100–200 mg/dl. Monitor blood glucose, electrolytes, blood gases, urinalysis, and renal profile at least daily. Continue infusion until safe concentration of ethylene glycol or methanol is reached. Ethanol-induced hypoglycemia may occur. Dialysis, preferably hemodialysis, should be considered in severe intoxication not controlled by ethanol alone.
To prepare 10% ethanol for infusion therapy, remove 100 ml from a liter D5W and replace with 100 ml of tax-free bulk absolute alcohol after passing through 0.22 micron filter. 50 ml vials of pyrogen-free absolute ethanol for injection are available from Pharm-Serve 218–20 96th Avenue, Queens Village, NY 11429.
Telephone
718–475–1601.</td></tr>
<tr><td>22. Fab (antibody fragment) (Digibind).
Dose: The average dose used during clinical testing was 10 vials. Dosage details are specified by the manufacturer. It should be administered by the IV route over 30 min. Calculate out on basis of body burden either by known amount ingested or by serum digoxin concentration.
Calculation of dose of Fab:
1. Known amount ingested multiplied by bioavailability (0.8) = body burden. Body burden divided by 0.6 = number of vials.
2. Known serum digoxin (obtained 6 hr postingestion) multiplied by volume distribution (5.6 L/kg) and weight in kg divided by 1000 = body burden. Body burden divided by 0.6 = number of vials.</td><td>Digoxin, digitoxin, oleander tea with the following:
1. imminent cardiac arrest or shock
2. hyperkalemia >5.5 mEq/L
3. serum digoxin >10 ng/ml at 6–12 hr post ingestion in adults
4. life-threatening dysrhythmias
5. ingestion over 10 mg in adults or 4 mg in child
6. bradycardia or second- or third-degree heart block unresponsive to atropine</td><td>Contact regional poison control center.
Preliminary sensitivity test.
Administer through a 0.22 micron filter. Fab causes a rise in measured bound digoxin but a fall in free digoxin. 40 mg binds 0.6 mg digoxin.</td></tr>
<tr><td>23. Flumazenil (Mazicon). Roche Labs. Benzodiazepine (BZP) receptor antagonist.
Dose:
1. Management of BZP overdose: (Caution) 0.2 mg (2 ml) IV over 30 sec may repeat after 30 sec with 0.3 mg (3 ml). Further doses of 0.5 mg over 30 sec. If no response in 5 min and max of 5 mg, cause of sedation is unlikely due to BZP.
2. Reversal of conscious sedation or in general anesthesia: 0.2 mg (2 ml) IV over 15 sec. May repeat in 45 sec. 0.2 ml (2 ml). Doses may be repeated at 60 sec intervals to max dose of 1 mg (10 ml). If resedation, repeated doses may be administered at 20 min intervals to max 1 mg (0.2 mg/min). Max 3 mg should be given in any 1 hour
Packaged: 0.1 mg/ml in 5 and 10 ml multiple use vials.</td><td>1. Reversal of the sedative effects of BZP general anesthesia.
2. Sedation with BZP for procedures
3. Caution in management of overdose
AR: Convulsions, dizziness, injection site pain, increased sweating, headache and abnormal or blurred vision (3–9%)</td><td>No treatment for hypoventilation.
Caution with overdoses.
Flumazenil is not recommended for cylic antidepressant poisoning, if seizures or increased intracranial pressure is present</td></tr>
<tr><td>24. Folic acid</td><td>See 28, Leucovorin</td><td></td></tr>
<tr><td>25. Folinic acid</td><td>See 28, Leucovorin</td><td></td></tr>
</table>

Table continued on following page

TABLE 9. Antidote Formulary *Continued*

Medication	Indications and Adverse Reaction (AR)	Comments
26. **Glucagon.** Works by stimulating production of cyclic adenyl monophosphate. **Dose:** 50–150 μg/kg over 1 min IV followed by a continuous infusion of 1–5 mg/hr in dextrose and then taper over 5–12 hr. 2 mg of phenol per 1 mg glucagon. 50 mg is the maximum amount of phenol recommended; therefore toxicity may result when high doses of glucagon are used. **Packaged:** 1 mg (1 unit) vial with 1 ml diluent with glycerine and phenol; also in 10 ml size.	Beta blockers, quinidine, and calcium channel blocker intoxication. **AR:** Generally well tolerated—most frequent are nausea, vomiting.	*Do not dissolve the lyophilized glucagon in the solvent packaged with it when administering IV infusion because of possible phenol toxicity.* Use 0.9% saline or D5W. Effects of single dose observed in 5–10 min and last for 15–30 min. A constant infusion may be necessary to sustain desired effects.
27. **Labetalol hydrochloride** (*Normodyne*), Schering; (*Trandate*), Glaxo. Nonselective beta and mild alpha blocker. **Dose:** IV 20 mg over 2 min. Additional injections of 40 or 80 mg can be given at 10-min intervals until desired supine blood pressure achieved. Max dose, 300 mg Alternative: Slow IV infusion: 200 mg (40 ml) is added to 160 or 250 ml of D5W and given at 2 mg/min. Titrate infusion according to response. **Packaged:** Solution 5 mg/ml in 20 ml.	Hypertensive crises secondary to cocaine. **AR:** GI disturbances; orthostatic hypotension; bronchospasm; congestive heart failure, AV conduction disturbances, and peripheral vascular reactions.	Concomitant diuretic enhances therapeutic response. Patient should be kept in a supine position during infusion. **MP:** monitor blood pressure during and after administration.
28. **Leucovorin** **Dose:** (for methanol poisoning): 1 mg/kg up to 50 mg IV every 4 hours for 6 doses **Packaged:** 3 mg/ml (1 ml), 5 mg/ml (1 and 5 ml), 50 mg/vial.	1. *Methanol poisoning.* Active form of folic acid used to enhance metabolism of formic acid in animals to carbon dioxide and water. 2. *Methotrexate (MTX) overdose:* supplies tetrahydrofolate co-factor, which is blocked by methotrexate **Dose:** See comments. **AR:** Allergic sensitization	For MTX overdose, initial dose is given IV or IM in MTX equivalent dose up to 75 mg. If MTX blood level is measured 6 hours post ingestion and is above 10 (−8) molar or is unavailable, give 12 mg q 6 hr until the MTX level is below 10–8 molar. Alternatively, if gastrointestinal function is adequate, may give orally 10 mg/m² q 6 hr until MTX levels are lowered to less than 10 (−8) molar. Leucovorin in doses of 5–15 mg/day p.o. have also been recommended to counteract hematologic toxicity from folic acid antagonists, such as trimethoprim and pyrimethamine.
29. **Methylene blue,** Harvey and others. Methylene blue reduces the ferric ion of methemoglobin, to the ferrous ion of hemoglobin. **Dose:** *Adult,* 0.1–0.2 ml/kg of 1% solution (1–2 mg/kg over 5 min IV). Maximum 7 mg/kg. *Child,* same as Adult. Maximum infants 4 mg/kg **Packaged:** 1% 10 ml ampules. May repeat in 1 hr if necessary. Repeat only once.	Methemoglobinemia **AR:** GI (nausea, vomiting), headache, hypertension, dizziness, mental confusion, restlessness, dyspnea, hemolysis, blue skin, urine, burning sensation in vein when IV dose exceeds 7 mg/kg. Treatment is unnecessary unless methemoglobin is over 30% or respiratory distress.	Saliva, urine, and other body fluids may turn blue. *Contraindications:* Renal insufficiency, cyanide poisonings when sodium nitrite is used to induce methemoglobinemia in G-6-PD deficiency patients. Monitor hemolysis, methemoglobin level, and arterial blood gases. Avoid extravasation because of local necrosis.
30. **Naloxone** (*Narcan*). Pure opioid antagonist. **Dose:** *Adult,* 0.4–2.0 mg IV and repeat at 3 minute intervals until respiratory function is stable. Before excluding opioid intoxication on the basis of a lack of naloxone response, a minimum of 2 mg in a child or 10 mg in an adult should be administered. *Child,* initial dose is 0.1 mg/kg IV. **Packaged:** 0.02 mg/ml. 0.4 mg/ml ampule, and 10 ml multidose vial.	1. Comatose patient (not just a lethargic patient) 2. Ineffective ventilation or an adult respiratory rate <12 3. Pinpoint pupils 4. Circumstantial evidence of opioid intoxication i.e., known drug abuser, track marks, opioid paraphenalia. **AR:** Relatively free of adverse reactions. Rare reports of pulmonary edema. Should be administered with caution in pregnancy.	Naloxone infusion therapy should be used if a large initial dose was required, repeated boluses are necessary, or a long-acting opiate is involved. In infusion therapy the initial response dose is administered every hour and may need to be boostered one-half hour after starting. The infusion may be tapered after 12 hours of therapy. Naloxone infusion: Calculate out daily fluid requirements, add initial response dose of naloxone multiplied by 24 to the solution. Divide fluid by 24 hr for naloxone infusion rate per hour. Does not cause CNS depression. Routes: IV or endotracheal are preferred routes. Pentazocine (Talwin), dextramethorphan, propoxyphene (Darvon), and codeine may require larger doses.

TABLE 9. Antidote Formulary *Continued*

Medication	Indications and Adverse Reaction (AR)	Comments
31. **Nicotinamide,** various manufacturers. **Dose:** *Adult,* 500 mg IM or IV slowly, then 200–400 mg q 4 hr. If symptoms develop, the frequency of injections should be increased to every 2 hr (max 3 g day). *Child,* one-half suggested adult dose. **Packaged:** 100 mg/ml: 2, 5, 10, 30 ml vials; 25 and 50 mg tablets.	Vacor poisoning: phenylurea pesticide intoxication. *Note:* Vacor 2% is now available only to professional exterminators. 0.5% Vacor is available to the general public and can be toxic to children if swallowed. **AR:** Large doses—flushing, pruritus, sensation of burning, nausea, vomiting, anaphylactic shock.	Nicotinamide is most effective when given within 1 hr of ingestion. Do not use niacin or nicotinic acid in place of nicotinamide. Monitor liver profile.
32. **Oxygen** 100% **Dose:** *Adult,* 100% oxygen by inhalation or 100% oxygen in hyperbaric chamber at 2–3 atm. *Child,* same as adult.	Carbon monoxide, cyanide, methemoglobinemia. Any inhalation intoxication.	Half-life of carboxyhemoglobin is 240 min in room air 21% oxygen; if a patient is hyperventilated with 100% oxygen, the half-life of carboxyhemoglobin is 90 min, in chamber at 2 atm, half-life is 25–30 min.
33. **Pancuronium bromide** (*Pavulon*). Nondepolarizing (competitive) blocking agent. **Dose:** *Adults and children,* initially, 0.1 mg/kg IV; for intubation, 0.1 mg/kg IV, repeated as required (generally every 40–60 min). **Packaged:** Sol 1 mg/ml in 10 ml 2 mg/ml in 2 and 5 ml containers.	Neuromuscular blocking agent. Used for intubation and seizure control. Acts in 2 min, lasts 40–60 min. **AR:** Main hazard is inadequate postoperative ventilation. Tachycardia and slight increase in arterial pressure may occur due to vagolytic action.	The required dose varies greatly and a peripheral nerve stimulator aids in determining appropriate amount. Should monitor EEG since motor effect may be abolished without decreasing electrical discharge from brain.
34. ***d*-Penicillamine** (*Cuprimine*), Merck; (*Depen*), Wallace. Effective chelator and promotes excretion in urine. **Dose:** 250 mg 4 times daily p.o. for up to 5 days for long-term (20–40 days) therapy: 30–40 mg/kg/day in children. Max 1 g/day. For chronic therapy 25 mg/kg/day in 4 doses. **Packaged:** 125 and 250 mg capsules.	Heavy metals, arsenic, cadium, chromates, cobalt, copper, lead, mercury, nickel, and zinc. **AR:** Leukopenia (2%); thrombocytopenia (4%); GI—nausea, vomiting, anaphylactic shock, diarrhea (17%); fever, rash, lupus syndrome, renal and hepatic injury.	This is not considered standard therapy for lead poisoning after chelation therapy. May produce ampicillin-like rash, allergic reactions, neutropenia, and nephropathy. Contraindication: Hypersensitivity to penicillin. **MP:** Routine urinalysis, white differential blood count, hemoglobin determination, direct platelet count, renal and hepatic profiles. Collect 24-hr urine, quantify for heavy metal.
35. **Physostigmine salicylate** (*Antilirium*), O'Neil. Cholinesterase inhibitor, a diagnostic trial is not recommended. **Dose:** *Adult,* 1–2 mg IV over 2 min; may repeat every 5 min to max dose of 6 mg. *Child,* IV, 0.02 mg/kg over 2 min to a max dose of 0.5 mg. If toxicity persists and no cholinergic effects occur, can readminister at 5 min intervals until a max dose of 2 mg. Once effect accomplished, give lowest effective dose. **Packaged:** 1 mg/ml 2 ml/amp.	Not advised as a diagnostic test or for routine use in treating anticholinergic effects. Reserve for life-threatening complications. **AR:** Death may result from respiratory paralysis, hypertension/hypotension, bradycardia/tachycardia/asystole, hypersalivation, respiratory difficulties/convulsions (cholinergic crisis).	Do not consider for the following: antidepressants, amoxapine, maprotiline, nomifensine, bupropion, trazadone, imipramine. IV administration should be at a slow controlled rate, not more than 1 mg/min. Rapid administration can cause adverse reactions. Can be reversed by atropine. Lasts only 30 min. Contraindicated in asthma, cardiovascular disease, intestinal obstruction.
36. **Pralidoxime chloride** (2-PAM, *Protopam*), Ayerst. Cholinesterase reactivator by removing phosphate. **Dose:** *Adult,* 1–2 g IV infused in 100–250 ml saline over 15–30 min. In severe cases may repeat in 1 hr if needed. Repeat every 8–12 hr when needed; if severe, can give 0.5 g/hr infusion. *Child,* 25–50 mg/kg IV over 30 min, no faster than 10 mg/kg/min; max 12 gm/24 hr. **Packaged:** 1 g/20 ml vials.	Organophosphate insecticide (OPI) poisoning. Not usually needed in carbamate insecticide poisoning. Most effective if started in first 24 hours before bonding of phosphate. **AR:** Rapid IV injection has produced tachycardia, muscle rigidity, transient neuromuscular blockade. IM: conjunctival hyperemia, subconjunctival hemorrhage, especially if concentrations exceed 5%. *Oral:* nausea, vomiting, diarrhea, malaise.	Should be used only after initial treatment with atropine. Draw blood for RBC cholinesterase level prior to giving 2-PAM. The use of 2-PAM may require a reduction in the dose of atropine. **MP:** Monitor renal profile and reduce dose accordingly. ($t\frac{1}{2}$ = 1–2 hours; reversal of OPI effects at 4 μg/ml of 2-PAM. Start early because "aging" of PO_4 on acetylcholinesterase makes it more difficult to reverse.
37. **Protamine sulfate** **Dose:** 1 mg neutralizes 90–115 units of heparin. Maximum dose = 50 mg IV over 5 min at 10 mg/ml. **Packaged:** 5 ml = 50 mg; 25 ml = 250 mg.	Heparin overdose. **AR:** Rapid administration causes anaphylactoid reactions.	**MP:** Monitor thromboplastin times. Doses of up to 200 mg have been tolerated over 2 hours in an adult.
38. **Pyridoxine (Vitamin B_6)** Gamma-aminobutyric acid agonist. **Dose:** *Unknown amount ingested:* 5 g over 5 min IV. *Known amount:* Add 1 g of pyridoxine for each gram of INH ingested IV over 5 min. **Packaged:** 50 and 100 mg/ml; 10, 30 ml.	Isoniazid (INH), Monomethylhydrazine mushrooms. **AR:** Unlikely owing to the fact that vitamin B_6 is water-soluble. However, nausea, vomiting, somnolence, and paresthesia have been reported from chronic high doses. Acutely, up to 52g IV and up to 357 mg/kg have been tolerated.	Pyridoxine is given as 5–10% solution IV mixed with water. It may be repeated every 5–20 min until seizures cease. Some administer pyridoxine over 30–60 min. **MP:** Correct acidosis, monitor liver profile, acid-base parameters. Lethal dose pyridoxine in animals is 1 g/kg.

Table continued on following page

TABLE 9. Antidote Formulary *Continued*

Medication	Indications and Adverse Reaction (AR)	Comments
39. **Sodium bicarbonate** **Dose:** IV 1–3 mEq/kg as needed to keep pH 7.5 (generally 2 mEq/kg every 6 hr). When alkalinization is desired to correct acidosis to a pH of 7.3, use 2 mEq/kg to raise pH 0.1 unit. **Packaged:** 50 mEq per 50-ml ampule.	To promote urinary alkalinization for salicylates, phenobarbital (weak acids with low volume of distribution *excreted* in urine unchanged). To correct severe acidosis. To promote protein-binding and supply sodium ions into Purkinje cells in cyclic antidepressant intoxication. **AR:** Large doses in patients with renal insufficiency may cause metabolic alkalosis. In patients with ketoacidosis, rapid alkalinization with sodium bicarbonate may result in clouding of consciousness, cerebral dysfunction, seizures, hypoxia, and lactic acidosis.	Alkaline diuresis. The assessment of the need for bicarbonate should be based on both the blood and urine pH. Maintain the blood pH at 7.5. Keep the urinary output at 3–6 ml/kg/hr. May use a diuretic to enhance diuresis. Potassium is necessary to produce alkaline diuresis. Monitor electrolytes, calcium, pH of both urine and blood, arterial blood gases.
40. **Sodium nitrite**	See 14, Cyanide antidote kit	
41. **Sodium thiosulfate**	See 14, Cyanide antidote kit	
42. **Succimer** (DMSA) (Chemet McNeil Consumer products). **Dose:** 10 mg/kg or 350 mg/m2 every 8 hr for 5 days, then 10 mg/kg or 350 mg/m^2 every 12 hr for 14 more days (see Chart below). Therapy course lasts 19 days **Packaged:** 100 mg capsule.		

Pediatric Dosing Chart

lb	*kg*	*Dose (mg)*	*No. of Capsules*
18–35	8–15	100	1
36–55	16–23	200	2
56–75	24–34	300	3
76–100	35–44	400	4
>100	≥45	500	5

Medication	Indications and Adverse Reaction (AR)	Comments
	For chelation in children only when blood lead is >45 μg/dl. **AR:** Rashes, nausea, vomiting, an elevation of serum transaminases occur in 6–10% of patients	A minimum of 2 weeks between courses is recommended unless venous lead level indicates a need for more prompt therapy. Patients who have received $CaNa_2$ EDTA or BAL may use succimer after an interval of 4 weeks. In young children, the capsule can be opened and sprinkled on soft food. Monitor venous lead before therapy, on day 7, and weekly for rebound. Monitor the following tests: complete blood count, platelets, ferritin, liver transaminases, renal function tests, calcium, glucose, total protein, albumin, and urinalysis.
43. **Vitamin K** (AquaMEPHYTON), Merck. Promotes hepatic biosynthesis of prothrombin and other coagulation factors. Competitive antagonist of warfarin. It may be administered orally in the absence of vomiting. **Dose:** *Adult,* 2.5–10 mg IV, depending on potential for hemorrhage. Oral dose is 15–25 mg/day. Severe bleeding, 5–25 mg slow IV push. Rate 1 mg/min. Repeat every 4 to 8 hr, depending on prothrombin time. *Child,* 1–5 mg IV, may be given orally when vomiting ceases at a dose of 5–10 mg/day. **Packaged:** 2 mg/ml in 0.5 ml ampules. 2.5 or 5 ml vials. Child oral dose, 5–10 mg.	Warfarin (coumarin), super warfarins, salicylate intoxication.	Fatalities from anaphylactic reaction have been reported following IV route. It takes 24 hr for vitamin K to be effective. The need for further vitamin K is determined by the prothrombin time test. If severe bleeding occurs, fresh blood or plasma transfusion may be needed.

This is for informational purposes and is not intended to substitute for independent judgment. It is always advisable to review the package insert for the most up-to-date information. Contact Regional Poison Control Center for additional details on use.

*This dose may exceed the manufacturer's recommendation.

†The scientific explanation has not been elucidated, although the urine pH and dilution may influence this.

Abbreviations: AR = adverse reactions to antidotes; MP = monitor parameters; FDA = U.S. Food and Drug Administration; EKG = electrocardiogram; CNS = central nervous system; GI = gastrointestinal; EEG = electroencephalogram.

TABLE 10. Dialysis: Indications and Contraindications

Immediate Consideration of Dialysis
Ethylene glycol with levels over 50 mg/dl or refractory acidosis
Methanol with levels over 50 mg/dl or refractory acidosis
Lithium levels consistently elevated over 4 mEq/L
Amanita phalloides

Indications on Basis of Patient's Condition
Alcohol*
Ammonia
Amphetamines
Anilines
Antibiotics
Barbiturates* (long-acting)
Boric acid
Bromides*
Calcium
Chloral hydrate*
Fluorides
Iodides
Isoniazid*
Meprobamate
Paraldehyde
Potassium*
Quinidine
Quinine
Salicylates*
Strychnine
Thiocyanates (certain other drugs also dialyzable)

Indicated for General Supportive Therapy
Uncontrollable metabolic acidosis or alkalosis
Uncontrollable electrolyte disturbance, particularly sodium or potassium
Overhydration
Renal failure
Hyperosmolality not responding to conservative therapy
Marked hypothermia
Nonresponsive Stage 3 or greater coma (Reed Coma Scale)

Contraindicated on Pharmacologic Basis (Except for Supportive Care)
Antidepressants (tricyclic and monoamine oxidase inhibitors)
Antihistamines
Barbiturates (short-acting)
Belladonna alkaloids
Benzodiazepines (Valium, Librium)
Digitalis and derivatives
Hallucinogens
Opioids (heroin, Lomotil)
Phenothiazines (Thorazine, Compazine)
Phenytoin (Dilantin)

*Most useful.

a. Start and give a full course of NAC if a toxic dose has been ingested or if plasma concentrations are above the toxic line (>120 μg/ml *at 4 hours* or >50 μg/ml *at 12 hours*) on the nomogram shown in Figure 1, regardless of subsequent blood values. NAC is most effective when initiated within 8 hours after ingestion. After 24 hours, NAC may not be effective; however, some studies suggest that it may have a role in the treatment of fulminant liver failure. If the initial plasma concentration is in the hepatotoxic range, complete the entire course of therapy regardless of subsequent blood concentrations. Stop NAC if hepatic encephalopathy develops.

b. If the antidote NAC, which has a foul odor and taste, is vomited within 1 hour after administration, give a second dose. If vomiting persists, check that the dilution is appropriate, covering the container. Using tomato juice and a straw may help. It may be necessary to place the nasogastric tube in the duodenum. Administer the antidote by a slow drip into the nasoduodenal tube, over an hour, and/or administer an antiemetic drug, such as metaclopramide (Reglan, 1 mg/kg IV over 1 to 2 minutes) or droperidol (Inapsine, 1.25 mg IV) before the dose of NAC.

Table 12 presents the amount of antidote and the dilution needed to make a less irritating 5 per cent solution for oral administration. Calculation is based on a loading dose of 140 mg/kg. Dividing the loading dose by 200 (for a 20 per cent solution) gives the volume of the solution. Maintenance is half of the loading dose.

3. Treat with dialysis (peritoneal or hemodialysis) and AC. Consider hemoperfusion in severe cases when persistent renal failure occurs.

4. *Avoid* the following agents, which may compete with acetaminophen for the conjugation pathway or, by enzyme induction, may increase the toxic metabolite.

Agents That Decrease Conjugation	Enzyme Inducers
Salicylate	Antihistamines
Phenolphthalein	Barbiturates
Dicumoral	Chronic alcoholism
Testosterone	Phenytoin
Hydroxyzine	Imipramine
Morphine	Chloral hydrate
Chloramphenicol	Ethchlorvynol
Prednisolone	Glutethimide
Tetracycline	Haloperidol
Estrogens	Meprobamate
Salicylamide	Phenylbutazone
Vitamin C	Tolbutamide
Immaturity	Ethacrynic acid

Laboratory Studies. Obtain acetaminophen blood specimens any time after 4 hours following ingestion. Acetaminophen plasma concentrations are recommended in any patient when the overdose substance is unknown so as not to miss the "golden first 8 post-ingestion hours" for antidotal therapy. Use plot levels in the nomogram (Fig. 1) as a guide for treatment. A blood specimen obtained before 4 hours post-ingestion does not influence the therapeutic decision for a full course of NAC therapy. A toxic initial value after 4 hours requires the full course of NAC therapy. Monitor liver and renal profiles, including bilirubin, prothrombin time, and serum amylase, EKG, urine, and serum electrolytes.

Acetone (Dimethyl Ketone 2-Propanone)

Acetone is used in nail polish remover and solvents.

Toxicity. Ingestion of 2 to 3 ml/kg in children; 200 ml in adults has caused central nervous system (CNS) depression.

Manifestations. Drowsiness, coma, and bronchopulmonary irritation if inhalation.

Management

1. Institute GI decontamination procedures, if more than 2 ml/kg has been ingested. Avoid emesis because of rapid onset of coma.

2. Administer 100 per cent oxygen if the patient is comatose, and correct acidosis.

Acids

See Caustics and Corrosives

Alcohols

Ethanol (Grain Alcohol, Cologne, Perfumes)

Toxicity and Kinetics. In general, 1 ml/kg 100 per cent ethanol produces a blood ethanol concentration (BEC) of 100 mg/dl. Alcohol "proof" is double the per cent (e.g., 50 proof

TABLE 11. Toxic Amounts of Acetaminophen Packaging

Age	Weight (kg)	Drops (15 ml 100 mg/ml)	Elixir (60 & 120 ml 160 mg/5 ml)	Chewable Tablets (80 mg)	Tablets (325 mg)	Caplets (500 mg)
<1 mo	3.5	4.9 ml	15.4 ml	6 tabs	1.5 tabs	1 cap
1 mo	4.0	5.6	17.6	7	2	1
6 mo	7.0	9.8	30.8	13	3	2
1 yr	10.0	14.0	44.0	17.5	4	3
2 yr	12.0	16.8	52.8	21	5	3
3 yr	14.0	19.6	61.6	24.5	6	4
5 yr	18.0	25.2	79.2	31.5	8	5
6 yr	20.0	26.2	88.0	35	9	6
9 yr	28.0	39.2	123.2	49	12	8
10 yr	32.0	44.8	140.8	56	14	9
12 yr	34.0	47.6	149.6	59.5	14	10
14 yr	40.0	56.0	176.0	70.0	17	11
15 yr	50.0	70.0	220.0	87.5	21.5	14
Adult	60.0	84.0	264.0	105.0	26	17
Adult	70.0	98.0	308.0	122.0	30	20

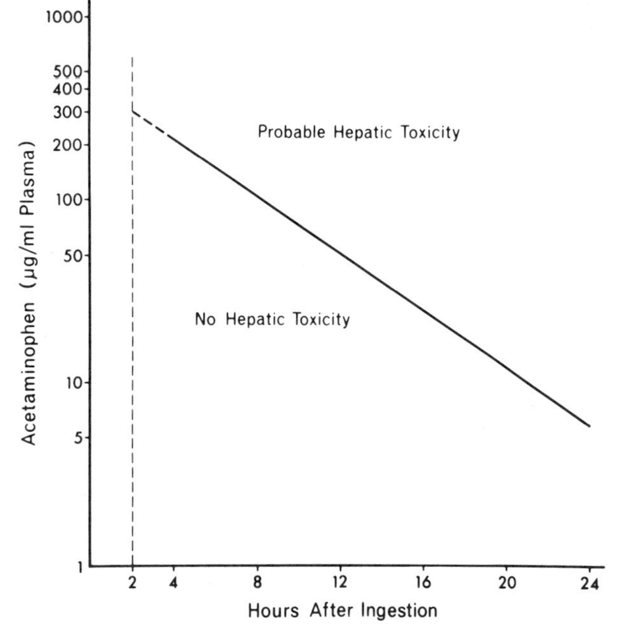

Figure 1. Nomogram for acetaminophen intoxication. Start *N*-acetylcysteine therapy if levels and time coordinates are above the lower line on the nomogram. Continue and complete therapy even if subsequent values fall below the toxic zone. The nomogram is useful only in acute, single ingestions. Serum levels drawn before 4 hours may not represent peak levels. (Modified from Rumack BH, Matthew H: Acetaminophen poisoning and toxicity. Pediatrics 55:871, 1975. Reproduced by permission of Pediatrics, 1975.)

TABLE 12. Dilutions of *N*-Acetylcysteine

Body Weight (kg)	Mycomyst (ml) (20%)	Grams	Diluent (ml)	5% Solution (ml)
140–149	105	21	315	420
130–139	95	19	285	380
120–129	90	18	270	360
110–119	80	16	240	320
100–110	75	15	225	300
90–99	70	14	210	280
80–89	65	13	195	260
70–79	55	11	165	220
60–69	50	10	150	200
50–50	40	8	120	160
40–49	35	7	105	140
30–39	30	6	90	120
20–29	20	4	60	80
10–19	15	3	45	60

= 25 per cent alcohol). Ethanol is metabolized by hepatic alcohol dehydrogenase at a constant rate of 15 to 30 mg/dl/hour by zero-order kinetics. Peak action occurs at 30 to 60 minutes, depending on the last meal. Vd is 0.6 L/kg. Specific gravity (SG) is 0.789. The following equation determines possible BEC from an approximate amount ingested:

$$\text{BEC (mg/dl)} = \frac{\text{amount ingested (ml)} \times \text{\% ethanol in product} \times \text{SG (0.79)}}{\text{Vd (0.6 L/kg)} \times \text{body wt (kg)}}$$

Manifestations. If there is no sign of intoxication by 3 hours, it is unlikely to occur. In small children, a BEC greater than 50 mg/dl may produce the triad of hypoglycemia, hypothermia, and coma. See Table 13.

Management

1. Institute GI decontamination procedures. *Caution*: The rapid onset of CNS depression may preclude the induction of emesis. If a child consumes more than 1 ml/kg of 50 per cent (100 proof), evaluate the child for hypoglycemia, although a recent investigation indicates that the ingestion of up to 105 ml of cologne or perfume (50 to 90 per cent ethanol) did not produce serious symptoms. Activated charcoal and cathartics are *not* indicated unless other drugs ingested.
2. If chronic alcoholism is suspected, give thiamine (100 mg IV) in the comatose adolescent to prevent Wernicke-Korsakoff syndrome.
3. Treat hypoglycemia and hypothermia, and correct ketoacidosis.
4. Consider hemodialysis at potentially fatal BECs (>500 mg/dl) when conventional therapy is ineffective. This is rarely needed.
5. Treat nonhypoglycemic seizures with intravenous diazepam followed by intravenous phenytoin if needed. Repeated seizures, focal neurologic findings, or head trauma warrants CT.

Laboratory Studies. For the BEC, determine the anion and osmolar gap. Each 1 mg/dl of ethanol increases the serum osmolality 0.22 mOsm/kg water.

Isopropanol (Rubbing Alcohol)

Toxicity. Isopropanol is twice as toxic as ethanol. The potentially fatal blood concentration in adults is 120 to 300 mg/dl.

Kinetics. Isopropanol is metabolized by hepatic alcohol dehydrogenase to acetone. Since no organic acids are formed, no metabolic acidosis occurs. Peak action is 30 to 60 minutes. Vd is 0.6 L/kg.

To calculate the blood isopropyl alcohol concentration, use the same equation as the one for ethanol, substituting SG 0.785 of isopropanol.

Manifestations. Ethanol-like intoxication with acetone odor to breath, acetonuria, hyperglycemia, occasionally hypoglycemia, acetonemia often without systemic acidosis, and gastritis, often with hematemesis, occur.

TABLE 13. Alcohol Intoxication

Blood Ethanol Levels (mg/dl)	Manifestations
>30	Euphoria
>50	Incoordination and intoxication
>100	Ataxia (legal toxic level)
>300	Stupor
>500	Flaccid coma, respiratory failure
>500–700	May be fatal

Management. Ethanol is not an antidote.

1. Institute GI decontamination procedures as listed for ethanol.
2. Utilize hemodialysis for a life-threatening overdose (rarely needed).

Laboratory Studies. Osmolal gap: 1 mg/dl of isopropyl alcohol increases the serum 0.176 mOsm/kg water, serum isopropyl alcohol level, and serum acetone level.

Methanol (Wood Alcohol, Nonpermanent Antifreeze, Windshield Wiper Fluid)

Toxicity. One teaspoonful, 100 per cent, is potentially lethal for a 2-year-old and can cause blindness in an adult. The toxic blood level of methanol is above 20 mg/dl; the potentially fatal level is over 50 mg/dL. Methanol is six times more toxic than ethanol.

Kinetics. Methanol is oxidized by alcohol dehydrogenase (ADH) into formaldehyde, which is quickly converted into formic acid—the toxic metabolite—which is further oxidized by a folate-dependent pathway to carbon dioxide and water. Peak methanol blood concentration occurs in 1 to 2 hours. Vd is 0.6 L/kg. Use the same equation as for ethanol for calculating the blood methanol concentration, substituting SG 0.719 of methanol.

Manifestations. Metabolism may delay onset for 12 to 18 hours or longer if concomitant ethanol ingestion has occurred. Methanol produces violent abdominal pain (pancreatitis), blurred vision, and hyperemia of the optic disc; within 3 to 24 hours, the patient experiences a blindness, feeling of "being in a snowstorm," and shock. The odor of formaldehyde on the breath or from the urine may be a clue.

Management. With worsening of acidosis, there is multiple organ failure.

1. Institute GI decontamination procedures up to 1 hour after ingestion. Activated charcoal and cathartics are *not* indicated.
2. Treat acidosis with sodium bicarbonate intravenously.
3. If methanol is suspected because of a metabolic acidosis with an anion gap and/or if the blood methanol concentration is above 20 mg/dl, immediately treat with intravenous or oral ethanol to produce a BEC of 100 to 150 mg/dl (antidote No. 21 in Table 9). Ethanol has 10 to 20 times the affinity for ADH as does methanol. Monitor the BEC every 4 to 6 hours.
4. Folinic acid and folic acid have been used successfully in animal investigations. Use leucovorin (1 mg/kg up to 50 mg IV every 4 hours for 6 doses). See antidote No. 28 in Table 9.
5. Consider hemodialysis if the blood methanol level is greater than 50 mg/dl or if the blood formate level is greater than 20 mEq/L, if there is refractory metabolic acidosis, or if visual or mental symptoms are present. *Note*: The ethanol dose must be increased during dialysis therapy.
6. Continue therapy (ethanol and hemodialysis) until the blood methanol level is below 20 mg/dl and, preferably, undetectable and until there is no acidosis or mental or visual disturbances. Often 2 to 5 days may be needed.
7. Consult with an ophthalmologic specialist.

Laboratory Studies. Each 1 mg/dl of methanol increases the serum osmolality 0.337 mOsm/kg water, causing a delayed metabolic acidosis with an anion gap in 12 to 24 hours. Assess blood methanol and ethanol concentrations every 4 to 6 hours. The blood formate level is a better indication of toxicity if it can be determined.

Amphetamines and Methamphetamine (Diet Pills, Various Trade and Street Names, "Speed," "Ice")

Toxicity. In children, 5 mg/kg, (adult, 20 mg/kg) has been reported to be lethal. These agents act as indirect sympathomimetics stimulating endogenous catecholamine release.

Kinetics. Peak time of action is 2 to 4 hours. Route of elimination is the liver.

Manifestations

1. *Cardiovascular effects.* Tachycardia, dysrhythmias, hypertension.
2. *CNS effects.* Argumentative behavior, hyperpyrexia, convulsions, paranoia, and violence.
3. *Other.* Reactive mydriasis, flushed moist skin, hyperactive bowel sounds.

Symptoms last four to eight times longer than those produced by cocaine (2 hours). The sequelae may include myocardial infarction, cerebral hemorrhage, or hypertensive encephalopathy. Rhabdomyolysis and myoglobinuria may ensue. Chronic use produces dependency and addiction.

Management

1. Institute GI decontamination procedures if the patient is seen less than 1 hour after ingestion.
2. Control extreme agitation or convulsions with diazepam. *Avoid* chlorpromazine, which may be dangerous in impure "street" amphetamine analogues.
3. Treat hypertensive crisis with intravenous nitroprusside.
4. Do not use acidification diuresis with ammonium chloride (antidote No. 2 in Table 9) because of possible myoglobinuria.
5. Treat hyperpyrexia with physical cooling, not antipyretics.
6. If unusual neurologic symptoms are present, perform CT.
7. Observe for suicidal depression, which may follow intoxication.
8. If toxic psychosis is present, treat with haloperidol (Haldol).
9. Significant life-threatening tachydysrhythmia may respond to an alpha-blocker or a beta-blocker, such as labetalol (Normodyne, antidote No. 27 in Table 9) or other appropriate antidysrhythmic agents. In the severely hemodynamic compromised patient with hypotension, shock, or ischemic chest pain, utilize immediate synchronized cardioversion.

Laboratory Studies. Monitor for rhabdomyolysis (creatine phosphokinase), myoglobinuria, hyperkalemia, and disseminated intravascular coagulation. Toxic blood concentration is above 0.1 μg/ml.

Anticholinergic Agents

Examples include antihistamines, antipsychotics (phenothiazines), antidepressants (tricyclics), antiparkinson drugs, over-the-counter sleep and cold medicines, ophthalmic products, plants such as jimson weed (see Plants), and bowel antispasmodic agents.

Toxicity. Potential fatal dose of atropine, 10 to 20 mg in children, 100 mg adults. The toxic dose is 0.05 mg/kg in children and 2 mg in adults.

Kinetics. Atropine: Peak action in 1 to 3 hours, half-life is 2 to 3 hours. Elimination is hepatic; duration of action is only 4 to 6 hours unless very large amounts have been ingested.

Manifestations

1. *Anticholinergic effects.* The following poem is useful: "red as a beet (vasodilation), dry as a bone (anhidrotic), blind as a bat (nonreactive mydriasis), hot as a hare (anhidrotic) and mad as a hatter."
2. *Cardiac effects.* Tachycardia may be preceded by bradycardia, supraventricular tachycardia, hypertension, rarely life-threatening dysrhythmias. The EKG shows a wide QRS and prolonged QT interval.
3. *CNS effects.* Hallucinations, coma, convulsions, and organic brain syndrome.
4. *Other.* Hyperpyrexia, nonreactive mydriasis, flushed skin, dry mucosa, hypoactive or absent bowel sounds, urinary retention, delirium, and leukocytosis.

Management

1. Institute GI decontamination procedures up to 12 hours after ingestion. *Avoid* AC and cathartics if there are no bowel sounds.
2. Control seizures with diazepam.
3. Monitor the EKG. Control dysrhythmias. Treat atrial dysrhythmias only if tissue perfusion is not adequate or if the patient is hypotensive.
4. *Avoid* physostigmine as a diagnostic test or for routine treatment (antidote No. 35 in Table 9). Consider it only for life-threatening anticholinergic effects refractory to conventional treatments. Do not use if EKG abnormalities are present.
5. Relieve urinary retention by catheterization to avoid reabsorption.
6. Control hyperpyrexia by external cooling. Do *not* use antipyretics.
7. Hemodialysis is ineffective.

Anticoagulants

Anticoagulants are used as rodenticides. A very large single dose or repeated small doses of warfarin are necessary to produce toxicity. The more toxic anticoagulant rodenticides, referred to as "superwarfarins," are 40 times or more potent and have a prolonged anticoagulant effect that may last weeks to months.

Toxicity. Amounts greater than 50 g 0.025 per cent warfarin or 25 g or 10 pellets of 0.005 per cent brodifacoum (Talon) as a single dose are considered toxic. The *mechanism of toxicity* involves inhibition of regeneration of vitamin K_1 and damage to the capillary endothelial integrity.

Kinetics. Action continues for 2 to 3 days. Peak hypoprothrombinemia occurs at 36 to 48 hours. The half-life varies: warfarin, 42 hours; brodifacoum, 156 hours or longer in humans.

Manifestations. Hematomas and bleeding result. Hypoprothrombinemia may occur without symptoms.

Management

1. Institute GI decontamination procedures for large amounts, above 50 g of 0.025 per cent warfarin, or over 25 g or 10 pellets brodifacoum, a greenish-blue pellet or 5 to 8 g of indandiones.
2. If a patient requires GI decontamination, obtain a prothrombin time at 24 to 48 hours. Prothrombin times at 24 hours may not detect defects.
3. If bleeding or prothromin time is 10 seconds over control, administer vitamin K_1 only as phytonadione (antidote No. 43 in Table 9) administered orally or intramuscularly. *Intravenous phytonadione may cause anaphylactoid reactions.* It takes 24 hours for vitamin K to be effective.
4. If there is severe bleeding, fresh plasma or blood transfusions may be required.
5. Ascorbic acid (50 mg for a child, 100 mg for an adult) may be administered to limit capillary damage. See Table 14.

TABLE 14. Management of Anticoagulant Rodenticide Ingestion

Product	Contents	Induction of Emesis
Warfarins		Amount = active warfarin
D-Con Ready Mix	Warfarin 0.025%	>50 g = >12.5 mg
D-Con Concentrate	Warfarin 0.33%	>5 g = >16.5 mg
Superwarfarins		Amount = active ingredient
4-Hydroxycoumarins		
Talon, Havoc	Brodifacoum 0.005%	>25 g = >1.25 mg
Super-caid, Maki	Bromodialone 0.005%	>25 g = >1.25 mg
Indanediones		
Caid, Drat, Rozol	Chlorophacinone 0.005%	>25 g = >1.25 mg
	Solution 0.25%	Any amount
	Concentrate 2.5%	Any amount
Pival, Triban, Pivalyn	Pindone 0.025%	>20 g
	Powder 0.025, 0.1, 0.2, 0.5%	Any amount of 0.1–0.5
	Concentrate 0.5%, 1.5%, 2.0%	Any amount
Diphacin, Ramik	Diphacinone 0.005%	>25 g = >1.25 mg
	0.05%, 9.1%, 0.2%	Any amount
	Concentrate 2%	Any amount

Modified from Jaeger and DeCastro: Poisoning Emergencies, St. Louis, Catholic Health Assoc, 1986, p 120; Smolinske SC, et al: Superwarfarin poisoning in children: A prospective study. Pediatrics 84:490–494, 1989; and Katona B, Wason S: Superwarfarin poisoning. J Emerg Med 7:627–631, 1989.

Anticonvulsants

Toxicity. In general, the ingestion of five times the daily therapeutic dose is expected to have the potential for toxicity and ten times the daily therapeutic dose potential for fatality (Table 15).

Manifestations. Nystagmus, ataxia, mental confusion, vertigo, slurred speech, hypotension, hypothermia, alteration of state of consciousness and respiratory depression may be present. Carbamazepine and intravenous phenytoin may cause dysrhythmias. Patients with phenytoin overdose experience nystagmus at blood levels greater than 20 μg/ml, ataxia at 30 to 40 μg/ml, and convulsions at over 40 μg/ml.

Management

1. Institute GI decontamination procedures. Repeated doses of oral AC shorten the half-life of carbamazepine, phenobarbital, primidone, phenytoin, and possibly others.
2. Monitor specific anticonvulsant blood levels.
3. Urine alkalinization enhances excretion of phenobarbital. The effectiveness of hemoperfusion and dialysis has not been established.
4. Naloxone (antidote No. 30 in Table 9) may reverse valproic acid coma.

Antihistamines or H_1 Histamine Receptor Antagonists

H_1 receptor antagonists have anticholinergic properties: Onset of action is 30 minutes; duration of action is 4 to 8 hours, unless the agents are slow-release preparations; and elimination is hepatic.

Toxicity. Potential toxic dose is four times the therapeutic daily dose.

Manifestations. Anticholinergic effects, gastrointestinal upset, tachycardia, drowsiness, ataxia, hyperthermia, and hallucinations may be present. In children, CNS stimulation occurs initially and may produce convulsions followed by depression. Caladryl (diphenhydramine, camphor, ethyl alcohol) has been absorbed through the skin and may produce toxic encephalitis. Terfenadine and astemizole may prolong the Q-T interval and may cause torsade de pointes.

Management

1. Observe the patient at home if there are no symptoms and if less than three times the therapeutic daily dose has been ingested. If between three and four times the daily therapeutic dose has been ingested, treat GI decontamination using emesis at home. If more than four times the therapeutic daily dose has been ingested or if there are symptoms, evaluate the patient in a medical facility. Institute GI decontamination procedures with AC. A cathartic may be useful, but use caution when inducing emesis with large ingestions because of the early onset of seizures.
2. Manage as in anticholinergics poisoning.
3. Dialysis and hemoperfusion are not effective. See Table 16.

Arsenic and Arsine Gas (Some Ant Traps, Rodenticides)

Toxicity. The toxic dose of arsenic trioxide is 5 to 50 mg; the potential fatal dose is 120 mg or 1 to 2 mg/kg. Sodium arsenite is nine times as toxic as trioxide. Organic arsenic (alkyl arsonates in weeding agents) is less soluble and less dangerous. Arsine gas forms when an acid comes in contact with arsenic and releases fumes.

Kinetics. Elimination is renal.

Manifestations

1. *Acute poisoning*: Onset is 1 to 3 hours. Initially, there may be a garlic odor to the breath, severe abdominal pain, radiopaque material in the bowel, hematemesis, diarrhea with "rice water stools" (often bloody), hypotension, shock, seizures, and coma. Later manifestations include exfoliative dermatitis, cardiac abnormalities, or subsequent hepatorenal involvement.
2. *Chronic and subacute poisoning*: Prolonged, low-level exposure produces stomatitis, a pigmented "raindrop" or scaly rash, and sensory "glove and stocking" peripheral neuropathy, alopecia, Mee's white lines in the fingernails, encephalopathy, cirrhosis of liver, and nephritis.
3. Arsine inhalation is characterized by a latent period of 2 to 48 hours and a triad of abdominal pain, hematuria, and jaundice (due to hemolysis).

TABLE 15. Anticonvulsants

Drug	Peak (hr)	VD (L/kg)	$T_{1/2}$ (hr)	Elimination Route	Protein Binding (%)	Therapeutic Dose	Therapeutic Blood Concentration (μg/ml)	Comments
Carbamazepine (Tegretol)	8–24	1.0	18–54 (adult, chronic) 5–25 (adult, single dose) 4–14 (child)	Hepatic	70	10–20 mg/kg/day (max 1600 mg/day)	5–12	
Ethosuximide (Zarontin)	24–48	0.8	36–55	Hepatic	0	20–30 mg/kg/day (max 1500 mg/day)	40–100	
Phenytoin oral (Dilantin)	6–12	1.0	24	Hepatic	90	4–7 mg/kg/day (max 1200 mg/day)	10–20	Has zero-order kinetics above therapeutic concentrations
							20–30	Nystagmus
							30–40	Ataxia
							>40	Convulsions, coma
Primidone	3–4	0.6	3–12	Hepatic	60		8–12	
Phenobarbital metabolite (Mysoline)			30–36		1	<8 yr–125 mg/day >8 yr–250 mg/day	15–40	Massive overdose produces white crystalluria
Valproic acid (Depakene)	1–2	0.4	5–15	Hepatic	20	10–15 mg/kg/day (max 1500 mg/day)	50–100	
Clonazepam (Klonopin)	?		20–60	Hepatic	90	0.05–0.2 mg/kg/day (max 20 mg/day)	0.025–0.075	
Phenobarbital	3–6	0.75	50–100	Hepatic	30		14–40	

Management

1. Institute GI decontamination procedures, followed by abdominal radiographs for radiopaque arsenic. Consider whole-bowel washout if usual methods fail to remove radiopaque arsenic. Activated charcoal is not effective.
2. Use intravenous fluids to correct dehydration and electrolyte deficiencies.
3. Treat shock with oxygen, blood, and fluids. BAL (dimercaprol) alone is ineffective against shock.
4. Administer BAL (antidote No. 17 in Table 9) if an unknown amount or 1 mg/kg of arsenic trioxide has been ingested or if symptoms of arsenic intoxication or toxic concentrations are present. Treat liquid arsenical ingestion until laboratory results prove that it is not necessary. The BAL-arsenic complex is dialyzable.
5. Hemodialysis is effective in acute poisoning and can be used concurrently with chelation therapy in severe cases, especially if renal failure develops. Treat renal and liver impairment.
6. In chronic poisoning, use *d*-penicillamine (antidote No. 34 in Table 9) to chelate arsenic. Continue therapy in 5-day cycles until the urine arsenic level is less than 50 μg in 24 hours.
7. Treat arsine intoxication by exchange transfusion and hemodialysis if renal failure occurs. BAL is ineffective.

Laboratory Studies. A blood arsenic level above 1 μg/ml is toxic, and 9 to 15 mg/L is potentially fatal. Urine arsenic concentrations above 50 μg/L indicate excessive exposure.

Barbiturates

Manifestations. Barbiturates are the prototype of CNS depressants producing ataxia, horizontal nystagmus (plasma phenobarbital > 40 μg/ml), slurred speech, pupil size variations, absent oculovestibular reflexes, depressed respiration, hypotension, pulmonary edema, and flaccid coma. Plasma phenobarbital levels above 120 μg/ml usually produces coma and interferes with cardiorespiratory function. Subcutaneous bullae and dermatographia may be present. Duration of action has no relationship to the duration of coma.

Toxicity. Table 17 lists toxic doses unless the patient is tolerant.

Management

1. Institute GI decontamination procedures. *Avoid* emesis with short-acting barbiturates. Activated charcoal with a ca-

TABLE 16. Common H_1 Antihistamines

Generic Name	Trade Name	Dose—Therapeutic and Toxic
Ethanolamine (diphenhydramine) Caps 25, 50 mg Tabs 50 mg Elixir 12.5 mg/5 ml	Benadryl	Therap 5 mg/kg/day (max 300 mg) Toxic 20–40 mg/kg/dose 2 ounces fatal in 2-year-old Toxic blood conc >5 μg/ml Fatal adult dose 2.8 g
Ethylenediamine (tripelennamine) Tabs 25, 50 mg	Pyribenzamine	Therap 5 mg/kg/day (max 300 mg) Toxic 20–40 mg/kg/dose
Piperidine (cyproheptadine) Caps 25, 50 mg	Periactin	Therap 0.25 mg/kg/day (max 12 mg)
Phenothiazines (promethazine) Tabs 12.5, 25, 50 mg Syrup 6.25 mg/5 ml	Phenergan	Therap 0.5 mg/kg/day (max 40 mg) Not for use under 2 years 200 mg in 2-year-old fatal
Alkylamines (chlorpheniramine) Tabs 4 mg Slow release 8, 12 mg Syrup 2 mg/5 ml	Chlor-Trimeton	Therap 0.35 mg/kg/day (max 12 mg) Toxic 5–10 mg/kg/dose
Piperazine (hydroxyzine) Caps 25, 50, 100 mg Susp 25 mg/5 ml Syrup 10 mg/5 ml Tabs 10, 25, 50, 100 mg	Atarax	Therap <6 yr 50 mg/day >6 yr 50–100 mg/day
Long-acting, nonsedating		
Astemizole	Hismanal	Therap 1 mg/kg/day
Terfenadine	Seldane	Therap 3–5 yr 30 mg/day

thartic initially and in repeated doses has been shown to reduce the serum half-life and increase the nonrenal clearance of phenobarbital by more than 50 per cent. Give repeated doses of AC every 4 hours while signs of toxicity are present.

2. Supportive and symptomatic care is all that is necessary in most cases.

3. Alkalinization with sodium bicarbonate (2 mEq/kg IV) during the first hour, followed by sufficient $NaHCO_3$ (antidote No. 39 in Table 9) to keep the urinary pH above 7.5, enhances excretion of long-acting barbiturates. Use forced diuresis with caution while considering the danger of fluid overload and pulmonary edema.

4. In severe cases with pulmonary edema or high blood barbiturate concentrations not responding to conservative measures, consider hemodialysis (useful in long-acting and intermediate barbiturates) and hemoperfusion.

5. Treat any bullae as local, second-degree skin burns.

Laboratory Studies. Emergency plasma barbiturate concentrations rarely alter management. Order assessments only for confirmation of diagnosis.

Batteries (Disc Type)

A battery usually measures 8 by 23 mm in diameter. Batteries are marked with imprint codes that allow identification of manufacturer and contents. The content varies but usually consists of magnesium, lithium, silver, or mercury as the cathode and zinc as the anode. These elements rarely produce toxicity. An alkali battery is usually 26 to 45 per cent sodium or potassium hydroxide and may cause corrosive injury.

Toxicity. Most batteries negotiate the GI tract without

TABLE 17. Barbiturate Kinetics

	Long-Acting (LA)		Intermediate-Acting (IA)		Short-Acting (SA)
	Barbital	*Phenobarbital*	*Amobarbital*	*Pentobarbital*	*Secobarbital*
Trade name	Veronal	Luminal	Amytal	Nembutal	Seconal
Slang name	—	Purple hearts	Blues	Yellows	Red devils
pK_a	7.74	7.24	7.25	7.96	7.9
Elimination route	Renal Hepatic	Renal 30% Hepatic 70%	Hepatic 98%	Hepatic >90%	Hepatic >90%
Onset IV	22 min	12 min	—	0.1 min	0.1 min
Onset oral	6 hr	20–60 min	15–30 min	15–30 min	10–30 min
Peak oral	12–18 hr	6–18 hr	3–4 hr	2–4 hr	1–2 hr
Protein-bound	6%	20–40%	40–50%	40–60%	40–60%
Fatal dose	10 g 65–75 mg/kg	8 g 65–75 mg/kg	5 g 40 mg/kg	3 g 50 mg/kg	3 g 30 mg/kg
Toxic dose	5–8 mg/kg	15–35 mg/kg 300 mg	3–5 mg/kg 200–300 mg	3–5 mg/kg 200–300 mg	3–5 mg/kg 200 mg
Blood concentrations					
Therap	5–8 μg/ml	15–40 μg/ml	5–6 μg/ml	1–5 μg/ml	1–5 μg/ml
Toxic	>30 μg/ml	>40 μg/ml	10–30 μg/ml	>10 μg/ml	>10 μg/ml
Lethal	>100 μg/ml	>100 μg/ml	>50 μg/ml	>35 μg/ml	>35 μg/ml
Duration	>6 hr	>6 hr	<3 hr	<3 hr	<3 hr
Half-life	56–96 hr	50–120 hr	8–42 hr	15–48 hr	19–34 hr
Vd	—	0.75 L/kg	0.5 L/kg	0.65 L/kg	0.65 L/kg

difficulty, although they may take 14 days to pass. Complications occur with the larger-diameter batteries or if the battery lodges in the esophagus or a Meckel's diverticulum. Complications occur in less than 2 per cent of cases. The mechanism of injury is related to leakage of the alkali and/or direct current electrolysis. An alkaline battery in the auditory canal, nasal cavity, or esophagus may cause corrosive injury.

Manifestations. All reported complicated cases have been associated with overt symptoms of dysphagia, vomiting, and abdominal pain.

Management

1. First, relieve airway obstruction.
2. *Avoid* GI decontamination procedures.
3. Locate the battery on abdominal and chest films. Contact the regional poison control center to identify the ingredients.
   a. If the battery is in the esophagus or respiratory tract, remove immediately with an endoscope.
   b. If the battery appears to be lodged in a Meckel's diverticulum, remove by surgery.
   c. If the battery has passed beyond the esophagus, observe the patient at home for vomiting, tarry or bloody stools, or abdominal pain. Examine all stools to retrieve the battery. Obtain a second radiograph in 7 to 14 days if the battery has not passed. *Lack of movement of the battery is not an indication for immediate surgical intervention.*
   d. Give asymptomatic patients a cathartic.
   e. If battery opens, monitor the blood and urine concentrations for contents of battery (i.e., mercury, lithium). The mercuric oxide in a battery is converted into elemental mercury in the GI tract and is poorly absorbed.
   f. If symptoms of peritoneal irritation develop, perform surgical intervention.
4. Remove batteries from the ears, nose, or other orifices immediately. Magnetic screw drivers may aid removal.

Benzodiazepines

Classification by Duration of Action

LONG-ACTING (>24 hr). Chlordiazepoxide (Librium), chlorazepate (Tranzene), clonazepam (Clonopin), diazepam (Valium), flurazepam (Dalmane), prazepam (Centrex), quazepam (Dormalin).

SHORT-ACTING (3 to 20 hr). Alprazolam (Xanax), lorazepam (Ativan).

ULTRA-SHORT (<10 hr). Temazepam (Restoril), triazolam (Halcion), midazolam (Versed), oxazepam (Serax).

Toxicity. Low toxic potential. Benzodiazepines (BZPs) have an additive CNS depressant effect with other sedatives. Most patients intoxicated with BZP alone recover within 24 hours. The oral therapeutic dose of diazepam is 0.2 mg/kg/dose to a maximum of 10 mg. Five times the therapeutic dose is considered potentially toxic.

Kinetics. Elimination is hepatic. Peak blood concentrations occur 1 to 4 hours after oral administration. Long-acting forms are metabolized into active metabolites.

Manifestations. CNS depression and psychosis can result. Deep coma with respiratory depression and/or cardiac disturbances suggests the presence of other drugs or another cause.

Management

1. Institute GI decontamination procedures.
2. Give supportive and symptomatic care.
3. Flumazenil is a specific benzodiazepine (BZP) antagonist not recommended for treatment of hypoventilation. It is *not* recommended to reverse BZP poisoning if the patient also took a cyclic antidepressant independent of BZP, has seizure history, or has increased intracranial pressure. (See antidote No. 23 in Table 9.)

Laboratory Studies. Document benzodiazepines in the urine.

Beta-Blockers

See Propranolol.

Bleach

Toxicity. Household laundry bleach (e.g., Clorox, Dazzle) is usually 5.25 per cent hypochlorite, which is not caustic. Commercial types of "caustic soda" (10 to 20 per cent) can cause caustic injuries. Other bleach products may be hydrogen peroxide (see *hydrogen peroxide*), perborates (see *Boric acid*). Oxalic acid in some rust removers, metal cleaners and ink irradicators may cause caustic injuries (see *Caustics*).

Manifestations. Household hypochlorite bleach does not produce esophageal burns unless vomiting occurs or very large quantities are ingested. Exposure to gases, produced by mixing hypochlorite bleach with acids or ammonia, is irritating to mucous membranes, eyes, and the upper respiratory tract. Ocular injuries may occur from concentrated or undiluted swimming pool hypochlorite; injuries usually heal in 3 weeks.

Management

1. *Ingestion. Avoid* GI decontamination procedures. Dilute the bleach with water or milk if the patient can swallow.
2. *Esophagoscopy.* Use the endoscope only if the patient is symptomatic or if the product is stronger than household hypochlorite bleach.
3. *Inhalation.* Remove the bleach from the contaminated area. If symptoms persist, observe for pulmonary edema (very unlikely).
4. *Ocular exposure.* Immediately gently irrigate with water for at least 15 minutes followed by fluorescein dye stain to examine for damage.

Boric Acid

One teaspoonful of 100 per cent boric acid powder equals 2.9 to 4.4 g. Borax cleaners contain 21.5 per cent boron by dry weight.

Toxicity. The potential fatal dose is much higher than the quoted values of 20 g in adults and 5 g in children. The majority of exposures are probably nontoxic. There have been no reported deaths since 1928.

Kinetics. Elimination is renal.

Manifestations. Acute gastroenteritis with blue-green vomitus and feces, CNS stimulation, and, in severe cases, seizures and coma may occur. Renal failure may develop. An erythematous rash may appear in 3 to 5 days after ingestion and may desquamate, giving the "boiled lobster" appearance.

Management (Table 18)

A lick or taste of topical powder of less than 5 per cent does not produce toxicity. A teaspoonful of 99 per cent powder in a child should be evaluated in an emergency department. If an approximation of the amount ingested can be made, please see Table 18 for management.

1. Institute initial treatment and GI decontamination procedures.
2. Do not use AC.
3. Treat seizures with diazepam.
4. Treat with hemodialysis if renal failure occurs. Monitor renal function.

TABLE 18. Management of Boric Acid Ingestion

Body Weight	Amount Ingested	Treatment
<30 kg	<200 mg/kg	Observe at home
	200–400 mg/kg	Syrup of ipecac to induce emesis
	>400 mg/kg	Emergency department for gastrointestinal decontamination and evaluation
>30 kg	<6 g ingested	Observe at home
	6–12 g	Syrup of ipecac to induce emesis
	>12 g	Emergency department for gastrointestinal decontamination and evaluation

Botulism

See Section 18, p. 573.

Calcium Channel Blockers (Antihypertensive, Antianginals, Antidysrhythmics)

Toxicity. In adults 3 g and in children 40 mg/kg may produce serious intoxication. Digitalis increases the risk of toxicity.

Kinetics. Elimination is hepatic. The half-life varies from 3 to 7 hours. Vd in 3 to 7 L/kg.

Manifestations. Hypotension, bradycardia within 1 to 5 hours after ingestion, mental status changes, seizures, CNS depression and coma, gastric distress, conduction disturbances, pulmonary edema, and hyperglycemia (calcium necessary for insulin secretion). The first action of verapamil is slowing of conduction through the AV node seen on the EKG as an increase in the PR interval, whereas nifedipine increases atrioventricular (AV) nodal conduction (Table 19). Manifestations are delayed after slow-release preparations. Hypocalcemia does not occur.

Management

1. Institute GI decontamination procedures. Obtain an immediate cardiac consultation. A pacemaker may be needed. Sustained-release preparations should be managed with repetitive doses of AC.
2. Treat hypotension with intravenous calcium gluconate or chloride (antidote No. 12A in Table 9) slowly under EKG monitoring. Calcium elevates the blood pressure but does not affect the tachydysrhythmias. If this fails, use positioning, fluids, and vasopressors (dopamine, norepinephrine).
3. Treat bradydysrhythmias and conduction defects with intravenous calcium gluconate or chloride (antidote No. 12A) slowly under EKG monitorings. If there is no response, try atropine sulfate or isoproterenol (which may aggravate the hypotension) or a pacemaker. If the patient remains unstable, use a pacemaker immediately.
4. Tachydysrhythmias are infrequent, but appropriate antidysrhythmic management is necessary.
5. Insulin therapy is not needed for hyperglycemia.

Camphor

Examples include Vicks VapoRub 4.8 per cent and Campho-Phenique 11 per cent. Five ml of camphorated oil (20 per cent camphor, banned in 1982) or 20 ml of Vicks VapoRub equals 1 g of camphor.

Toxicity. More than 10 mg/kg may cause a seizure. The mean fatal dose is 200 mg/kg. In adults 5 g and in children 1 g have been fatal.

Kinetics. Elimination is hepatic. Pulmonary excretion causes a distinctive odor on the breath.

Manifestations. Onset is 5 to 90 minutes. A specific odor, nausea, vomiting, and burning epigastric pain are present. Seizures may occur suddenly and without warning within 5 minutes of ingestion. Apnea and vision disturbances may occur.

Management

1. *Avoid* the induction of emesis because of possible early seizures. Take the patient immediately to a medical care facility.
2. Remove residual drug by gastric lavage until there is no odor of camphor in the aspirate.
3. Administer AC and a saline cathartic, although there are no scientific data supporting this. *Avoid* oils or alcohol.
4. Treat seizures with intravenous diazepam.
5. Hemoperfusion effectiveness data are controversial.

Carbon Monoxide

Carbon monoxide (CO) is an odorless, nonirritating gas produced from incomplete combustion; it is found as an in vivo metabolic breakdown product of inhaled methylene chloride (paint stripper, solvent). CO binds 210 times more avidly to hemoglobin than to oxygen, interferes with cellular cytochrome oxidase, and shifts the oxygen dissociation curve to the left.

Kinetics. Elimination is pulmonary. The half-life in room

TABLE 19. Properties of Calcium Channel Blockers

	Nifedipine (Procardia)	Verapamil (Calan, Isoptin)	Diltiazem (Cardiazem)
Preparations	10, 20 mg tabs	80, 120 mg tabs	30, 60, 90, 120 mg tabs
Onset oral	<20 min	<30 min	<30 min
Peak oral	1–2 hr	5 hr	30 min
Peak blood conc	30–60 min	90–120 min	120–180 min
Toxic blood conc	>100 ng/ml	>300 ng/ml	>200 ng/ml
Coronary vasodilation	+ + +	+ +	+ + +
Peripheral vasodilation	+ + +	+ +	+
Negative inotropy	–	+	+
Slow AV conduction	–	+ +	+
Slow SA conduction	–	+	+ +
Preload	Decreased	–	Decreased
Heart rate	Increased	Decreased	Decreased
Contractility	—	Decreased +	Decreased

air is 5 to 6 hours; in 100 per cent oxygen, 90 minutes; and in hyperbaric oxygen at 2 atmospheres, 20 minutes.

Manifestations. Time of exposure, oxygen administration, and mental status, are important in analysis of the risk of serious intoxication (Table 20). The skin rarely shows a cherry-red color in the live patient. A frequent clinical complaint is flu-like symptoms. Leukoencephalopathy (poor judgment and concentration) may occur within 3 weeks after exposure and myocardial infarction may occur 1 week after significant exposure. The carboxyhemoglobin (COHb) value in the emergency department may not represent the true insult or peak concentration. *Severe poisoning may involve only mild to moderate COHb levels.*

Management

1. Remove the patient from the contaminated area. Establish vital functions.
2. Administer 100 per cent oxygen to *all* patients until the COHb is 5 per cent or less. Assisted ventilation may be necessary. Keep the exposed pregnant woman in 100 per cent oxygen for several hours after the COHb is zero because CO concentrates in the fetus and oxygen is needed five times longer to ensure elimination of CO from fetal circulation. CO or hypoxia may be teratogenic.
3. Monitor arterial blood gases and COHb.
4. If pH remains below 7.0 after correction of hypoxia and adequate ventilation, give sodium bicarbonate cautiously. Avoid overcorrecting because alkalosis and COHb shift the oxygen hemoglobin dissociation curve to the left, decreasing tissue oxygen.
5. Consider admission and possible therapy with hyperbaric oxygen (controversial) if:
   a. COHb is greater than 25 per cent.
   b. COHb is greater than 15 per cent in a child or a patient with cardiovascular disease.
   c. COHb is greater than 10 per cent in a pregnant female; monitor the fetus by fetal heart rate, uterine contractions, and real-life sonography.
   d. Abnormal or ischemic chest pain or EKG abnormalities occur.
   e. Neuropsychiatric findings are abnormal.
   f. If hypoxia, myoglobinuria, or abnormal renal function is present.
   g. Chest films are abnormal.
   h. There is a history of unconsciousness, syncope, or neuropsychiatric symptoms. A list of hyperbaric chambers may be obtained from Duke University (Phone: 919–684–8111).
6. Treat seizures with intravenous diazepam.
7. Treat cerebral edema with elevation of the patient's head, minimizing intravenous fluid, hyperventilation, and, if needed, mannitol and intracranial pressure monitors.
8. Observe the patient closely, and re-evaluate after recovery for cardiac, pulmonary, and neuropsychiatric sequelae.

Laboratory Studies. Arterial blood gases show metabolic acidosis and normal oxygen tension but reduced oxygen saturation, as measured by co-oximeter, EKG, chest radiograph, and serum creatinine phosphokinase (CPK) levels.

Caustics and Corrosives (Alkalis and Acids)

Acids and alkalis are grouped as caustics, but their pathophysiology differs. *Alkalis* produce liquifaction necrosis and saponification and penetrate deeply. In 80 per cent of the alkali injuries, the esophagus is damaged and the stomach is involved in 20 per cent, usually with liquids.

Acids produce coagulation necrosis and form an eschar, preventing further penetration. They usually do not penetrate deeply (*exception*: hydrofluoric acid). In 80 per cent of the acid injuries, the gastric mucosa is damaged; in 20 per cent, the esophagus is involved.

Manifestations

ALKALIS. Oropharyngeal burns, drooling, pain, dysphagia, stridor, or dyspnea may occur if the respiratory tract is affected. The absence of oral burns does not exclude the possibility of esophageal burns. Esophageal perforation and mediastinitis and shock may develop. The late sequelae are esophageal strictures, usually in 1 to 3 weeks after ingestion. Carcinoma of esophagus has occurred years after original injury.

ACIDS. Symptoms may be similar to those produced by alkalis, but more frequently acids damage the stomach and may produce a "silent" asymptomatic perforation and peritonitis.

Management

1. If the patient can swallow and has no signs of respiratory obstruction, perforation, or shock, dilute the caustic agent with small amounts of milk or water immediately. Administration of more than 5 ml/kg up to 250 ml of dilutent may result in vomiting, which should be avoided. Contraindications to dilution are inability to swallow, signs of respiratory distress, shock, or esophageal perforation. *Avoid* other decontamination measures, induction of emesis, neutralization with acidic or alkalinic agents, gastric lavage, and use of AC.

TABLE 20. Carbon Monoxide (CO) Exposure and Possible Manifestations

% CO in Atmosphere	Duration of Exposure (hr)	Carboxyhemoglobin Saturation (%)	Manifestations
Up to 0.01	Indefinite	1–10	Minimal
0.01–0.02	Indefinite	10–20	Moderate dyspnea on exertion, throbbing headache
0.02–0.03	5–6	20–30	Marked headache, weakness, altered judgment
0.04–0.06	4–5	30–40	Vertigo, weakness, blurred vision
0.07–0.10	3–4	40–50	Confusion, tachycardia, tachypnea, syncope
0.11–0.15	1.5–3	50–60	Above plus Cheyne-Stokes asthma, coma, convulsions
0.16–0.30	1.0–1.5	60–70	Coma, convulsions, respiratory and heart failure, death
>0.40	1–2 minutes	70–80	Death

2. Perform dermal and ocular decontamination immediately by gentle irrigation with copious amounts of water for at least 15 minutes.

3. Give only intravenous fluids following dilution until endoscopic consultation.

4. In acid ingestions, some advocate nasogastric intubation with a small well-lubricated tube, preferably inserted under direct endoscopic vision and aspiration of the stomach contents within the first half hour after ingestion. This time frame is very difficult to accomplish.

5. Consider esophagoscopy at 12 to 24 hours after ingestion to assess severity of the burn. The esophagoscope is introduced to the level of the first lesion.

6. Steroids are controversial. Administer if a second-degree (transmucosal) or circumferential burn is found. However, an 18-year randomized study using steroids has found them to be of no benefit. Steroids are not used in superficial burns because strictures do not develop in patients with this type of lesion. Avoid steroids in transmural burns or if perforation is suspected. The dose is prednisone (2 mg/kg/day) for 3 weeks or more.

7. Antibiotics are not useful prophylactically. Use them if there is evidence of perforation.

8. Esophagrams are not as reliable for diagnosing esophageal damage but may be used after several days. Consider an esophagram and upper GI series at 10 days to 3 weeks after ingestion to assess severity of damage.

9. Consider esophageal dilation at 2- to 4-week intervals if there is evidence of a stricture.

10. For severe strictures, consider surgical replacement if dilation fails to provide an adequate-sized esophagus to consume appropriate nutrients.

11. If a caustic agent has been inhaled, remove the patient from the environment immediately. Perform clinical, x-ray, and arterial blood gas evaluations when appropriate. Oxygen and respiratory support may be required.

Clonidine (Catapres)

Clonidine is an antihypertensive, sometimes used in opiate withdrawal. It is available in tablet form (0.1 and 0.2 mg) and in transdermal patches (2.5 mg).

Toxicity. The toxic amount in children is 0.025 mg/kg; in adults, 4 to 5 mg. It has a central α_2-adrenergic and opioid agonist activity.

Kinetics. Onset is within 30 to 60 minutes, peak in 3 to 5 hours, and duration of 8 hours but in overdose may last up to 96 hours. Elimination is hepatic.

Manifestations. Signs resemble those from an opioid overdose, including CNS depression, hypotonia, hypothermia, and miosis. Apnea and seizures may occur within 8 hours of ingestion in significant poisonings. Cardiovascular effects occur within 1 to 3 hours of ingestion and consist of bradycardia and hypotension. A transient initial hypertension may occur. Atrioventricular block occurs with severe poisonings.

Management

1. Monitor the EKG and blood pressure. Be prepared for intubation and ventilation.

2. Institute GI decontamination procedures with charcoal or a cathartic. *Avoid* induction of emesis because of rapid onset of coma.

Caution: Naloxone may reverse toxicity, but it has been reported to produce hypertension and may be dangerous to hypertensive patients being treated with clonidine.

3. Treat convulsions with diazepam; bradycardia with hemodynamic instability with atropine; hypotension with positioning, fluids, and vasopressors; and hypertensive crisis with intravenous nitroprusside. Phentolamine (5 mg/kg/day orally in four divided doses, or 0.1 mg/kg IV) may be used to treat rebound hypertension after clonidine withdrawal.

Cocaine (Benzoylmethylecgonine)

Toxicity. The potential fatal adult dose is 1200 mg, but death has occurred with 20 mg parenterally. Its mechanism of action involves interference with reuptake of norepinephrine and dopamine.

Kinetics. Cocaine is metabolized in the liver to mostly inactive metabolites that one excreted in urine and serve for detection (Table 21).

Manifestations

1. *Low dose.* Euphoria and CNS stimulation.

2. *High dose.* Anxiety, agitation, paranoid delusions, hypertension, convulsions, hyperthermia, tachycardia, and cardiac dysrhythmias. CNS stimulation is followed by CNS depression.

3. *Sequelae.* Paranoid psychosis, perforation of nasal septa (rare), myocardial infarction, intracranial hemorrhage, intestinal ischemia, suicidal depression, and sudden death.

4. *Perinatal complications.* Spontaneous abortion, abruptio placentae, prematurity, teratogenicity (prune-belly syndrome), and neonatal cerebral infarction. Cocaine is found in breast milk and has caused adverse reactions in nursing infants.

5. *Unusual ingestion types.* Body packers (illicit transport) and body stuffers (hiding of evidence). The packages may leak or rupture and cause sudden death.

Chronic use of cocaine may produce cardiomyopathy, and smoking it may cause bronchospasm, hemoptysis, diffusion abnormalities, pneumothorax, and mediastinum.

Management

1. Institute GI decontamination procedures with AC or cathartic if cocaine is ingested. *Avoid* induction of emesis or gastric lavage because of rapid onset. Do not flush cocaine in the nose; remove with an applicator dipped in a non–water-soluble product (lubricating jelly).

2. Perform cardiac and thermal monitoring. Phenytoin may be effective for ventricular dysrhythmias, whereas *lidocaine may be ineffective and enhance toxicity because lidocaine is often an adulterant.*

3. Consider α- and β-blockers (labetolol, antidote No. 27 in Table 9) and calcium channel blockers (Netredipine in Europe), which are being evaluated to control life-threatening hypertension and tachycardia. Nitroprusside (0.5 μg/kg/minute) may be used in severe hypertension. *Avoid* propranolol.

4. Control seizures with diazepam and, if needed, with phenytoin. Neuromuscular blockers may be needed.

5. Treat hyperthermia with vigorous external cooling. Do *not* use antipyretics.

6. If the patient is pregnant, monitor the fetus (fetal heart rate, uterine contractions, and real-life sonography) and prepare for spontaneous abortion, abruptio placentae, or prematurity. Cocaine use during pregnancy is common, but withdrawal in the newborn is uncommon. Supportive therapy for the complications of prematurity, abruptio placentae, and intrauterine growth failure may be necessary. Rule out hepatitis, gonorrhea, and syphilis in the infant. Conduct careful follow-up of these infants, and involve the family with social services. There may be an increased incidence of sudden infant death, neurobehavioral problems, and child abuse. (See Infants of Drug-Dependent Mothers, Section 21.)

7. Take suicide precautions.

8. Imipramine and dopamine agonists (bromocriptine, amantidine) may aid withdrawal.

TABLE 21. Pharmacokinetics of Cocaine

Type	Route	Half-Life (min)	Onset	Peak	Duration T½ (min)
Hydrochloride	Insufflation	75	1–3 min	30–60 min	60–90 min
	Ingested	49	Delayed	50–90 min	Sustained
	Intravenous	54	<2 min	15–30 min	60–90 min
Free base and crack	Smoked	—	Seconds	10–15 min	<20 min
Coca paste	Smoked	—	Unknown		

9. Establish a drug treatment program.

10. To manage the body packer or body stuffer, administer repeated doses of AC, secure venous access, and have drugs readily available, at the bedside, for treating life-threatening manifestations until contraband cocaine is passed in the stool. Whole-body irrigation without AC has been successful. Surgical removal may be indicated if material does not pass the pylorus. Do *not* use emesis or lavage; endoscopy may be used to remove hard plastic vials containing crack but not the bags. Bags are removed by whole-bowel irrigation, or, if difficulty is experienced in passing, by surgery.

Laboratory Studies. Cocaine is detected in urine up to 12 hours, and its metabolite benzylecognine may be detected 48 to 144 hours, depending on method. Monitor CPK and urine for myoglobinuria.

Cosmetics

Commonly Used Products

Colognes, Perfumes, Aftershave Lotions, Oral Hygiene Products, Suntan Lotions. Toxicity depends on the concentration of alcohol. (See Alcohols earlier.)

Deodorants. Personal preparations of aluminum and zinc are of low toxicity.

Depilatories. These preparations usually contain sulfides or thioglycolates. They are usually irritating to the skin and GI tract. Large doses may produce hypoglycemia and convulsions.

Fingernail Polish Removers. These products usually contain acetone but may contain toluene and aliphatic acetates. (See Acetone.)

Artificial Nail Removers. These products must be differentiated from fingernail polish removers, and they contain acetonitrile, which forms cyanide in the body.

Ointments, Creams, Plain Soaps. These are usually nontoxic.

Hair Products

Dyes and Bleaches. Hydrogen peroxide is a component of bleach. (See Hydrogen Peroxide later.) Metallic hair dyes usually contain small amounts of toxic metals. Large ingestions may necessitate treatment. Vegetable dyes are nontoxic.

Permanent Wave Neutralizers. These preparations may contain perborates (see Boric Acid) or, rarely, the nephrotoxic bromates.

Shampoos. Plain shampoos are nontoxic. Dry shampoos can be dangerous and contain methyl or isopropyl alcohol. (See Alcohols.)

Sprays. Sprays that are chronically inhaled may cause hilar adenopathy and pulmonary infiltrates (thesaurosis).

Hair-Straightening and Hair-Waving Preparations. These may contain 1 to 3 per cent sodium or ammonium hydroxide. (See Caustics.)

Cyanide

Cyanides are found in fumigants (hydrogen cyanide), in some silver and furniture polishes, in the seeds of fruit stones (harmful only if the capsule is broken), and in the antihypertensive agent nitroprusside. Cyanide is released in fires involving the decomposition of silk, wool, polyurethane, and acrylonitrile.

Toxicity. The ingestion of 1 mg/kg or 50 mg of potassium or hydrogen cyanide can produce death within 15 minutes. The volatile hydrocyanic acid permissible exposure limit (PEL) is 10 ppm; 300 ppm is fatal in minutes. Ferriferrocyanide (Prussian blue) is of low toxicity; more than 50 g is toxic in adults.

Kinetics. Elimination is hepatic via the thiosulfate-rhodanese pathway.

Manifestations

1. Early symptoms may mimic the hyperventilation syndrome. The patient may taste bitter almonds, or the odor may be on the breath or be emitted from gastric contents (the threshold of odor is 0.2 to 5 ppm, and only 50 per cent of the population can perceive the odor). If there are no symptoms by 2 hours, exclude *acute* cyanide intoxication.

2. Later respiratory depression and hypoxic symptoms occur without cyanosis. The following may be present: vomiting, seizures, coma, cardiac dysrhythmias, dilated pupils with red retinal veins, bright red venous blood, pulmonary edema, and lactic acidemia. The arterial blood Po_2 is high or normal, and the venous Po_2 is high with decreased arterial-venous oxygen difference.

3. Late cyanosis unresponsive to oxygen.

4. Subacute poisoning may produce neuropathies and thyroid dysfunction.

Management

1. *Do not perform mouth-to-mouth resuscitation* (cyanide is released in the patient's breath). If cyanide is inhaled, remove the patient from the contaminated atmosphere. Immediately administer 100 per cent oxygen and, if needed, assisted ventilation. Continue oxygen and respiratory support during antidote therapy and after it is concluded.

2. Use a cyanide antidote kit (antidote No. 14 in Table 9). *Caution: Children Require Special Doses.* Some investigators have been using only thiosulfate in residential fires when they are suspicious of cyanide intoxication. If symptoms recur, repeat antidotes in 30 minutes as half of the initial dose. Use the antidotes if the diagnosis of cyanide poisoning is suspected, such as in urethane, plastic, or upholstery fires with (a) impairment of consciousness, (b) manifestations not corrected by oxygen and out of proportion to carboxyhemoglobin level, and (c) lactic acidosis and bright red venous blood with high Po_2. Use *caution* with the use of methylene blue to reverse methemoglobinemia in cyanide poisoning because it releases the cyanide ion. Exchange transfusion or hyperbaric oxygen rather than methylene blue may be used if the methemoglobin concentration exceeds 50 per cent.

3. Institute GI decontamination procedures by gastric lavage. *Avoid* emesis. Although AC is not a very effective adsorbant of cyanide, it is recommended.

4. Treat seizures with intravenous diazepam.
5. Hydroxycobalamin, vitamin B_{12a}, which forms vitamin B_{12} cyanocobalamin (investigational), may be a useful antidote if given early after exposure and in very large doses.
6. Hyperbaric oxygen effectiveness is not documented.

Detergents

Soaps (Anionic and Nonionic)

Soaps are salts of fatty acids and are nontoxic. *Anionic* detergents (e.g., Ajax Cleanser, Comet Cleanser, Oxydol, Tide Laundry) and *nonionic* detergents (e.g., Ivory Snow liquid, Joy Dish Detergent) contain sodium phosphates as a water softener and are nontoxic unless they contain more than 50 per cent carbonates, phosphates, or silicates, which may produce alkaline damage to the esophagus and stomach. Polyphosphates ingested in large amounts may produce hypocalcemic tetany. *Granular dishwashing detergents* (e.g., Cascade, Calgonite, Electrosol) may have the potential of caustic properties. (See Caustics.)

Management

1. Immediately dilute with milk or water. Avoid emesis. Irrigate the eyes and skin, and observe for dysphagia, drooling, dyspnea, and stridor with agents that have the potential for caustic injury. For soaps and anionic and nonionic detergent ingestion, only home observation is required.
2. If tetany develops administer calcium gluconate (antidote No. 12A in Table 9).

Cationic Detergents

Cationic detergents are quaternary ammonia compounds such as hexachlorophene (pHisoHex), benzalkonium (Zephiran), and cetylpyridium (Creepryn). In concentrations greater than 2 per cent, they may cause systemic toxicity with convulsions. In concentrations over 7.5 per cent, they may be caustic. Most of these are low concentration (2 per cent or less) and are not toxic unless large quantities are ingested.

Management

1. If the concentration ingested is less than 7.5 per cent, treat by home observation. If it is above 7.5 per cent, dilute with milk or water. *Avoid* emesis. (See Caustics.) There are no data to support that soap will absorb the unabsorbed cationic detergent, and it may produce emesis.
2. Institute supportive and symptomatic therapy.

Digitalis Preparations

Cardiac glycosides are found in medication and plants (Table 22).

Manifestations. Manifestations may be delayed 9 to 18 hours.

1. *Gastrointestinal.* Abdominal pain, nausea, vomiting, diarrhea.
2. *Central Nervous System.* Depression, colored-halo vision, delirium, hallucinations.
3. *Cardiovascular.* Acute poisoning—more likely bradycardia, blocks, atrial dysrhythmia, and hyperkalemia. Chronic intoxication—more likely tachycardia, serious premature ventricular contractions, ventricular dysrhythmias, and hypokalemia.
4. *Electrocardiographic.* No particular dysrhythmia is characteristic of digitalis toxicity.

Management

1. Institute GI decontamination procedures. *Avoid* syrup of ipecac and gastric lavage, which may increase vagal effect.

TABLE 22. Common Digitalis Preparations: Toxicity and Kinetics

	Digoxin	Digitoxin
Trade name	Lanoxin	Crystodigin (0.04 mg/kg)
Onset time oral	1.5–6 hr	5–6 hr
Toxic dose	0.07 mg/kg	NA
GI absorption	50–80%	90–100%
Peak oral	4–6 hr	6–12 hr*
Protein-bound	25%	90%
Vd in neonate	7–8 L/kg	0.6 L/kg
In children	16 L/kg	
Half-life	30–45 hr	>100 hr
Elimination	Renal 75%	Liver 80%
Therap plasma conc	0.5–2.0 ng/ml	17 ng/ml
Toxic plasma conc	>2.4 ng/ml	>30 ng/ml
young infants	>4 ng/ml	
Enterohepatic recirculation	Small	Large
Available tablets	0.125, 0.250, 0.50 mg	0.05, 0.1, 0.15, 0.2 mg
elixir	0.05 mg/ml	

*Maximum therapeutic dose divided by 70.

Activated charcoal is useful and may be administered in repeated doses to interrupt the enterohepatic recirculation.
2. *Avoid* quinidine, bretylium, carotid sinus massage, calcium, and calcium channel blockers.

Caution: Use direct current countershock at the lowest voltage and only as a last resort in threatening dysrhythmias because of tendency to produce ventricular fibrillation in digitalis intoxication.

Treat ventricular premature contractions, including bigeminy, trigeminy, quadrigeminy, ventricular tachycardia, and atrial tachycardia, with phenytoin loading dose (2 to 4 mg/kg IV slowly at a rate of less than 30 mg/minute) with EKG and blood pressure monitoring. Lidocaine also may be administered for ventricular dysrhythmias. Magnesium sulfate (20 ml, 20 per cent solution IV over 20 minutes) has been successful in treating serious ventricular dysrhythmias, including torsade de pointes.
3. Treat hemodynamic unstable bradycardia and second-degree and third-degree AV block with atropine (0.01 mg/kg per dose up to 0.6 mg) or with low-dose phenytoin (1 mg/kg per dose up to 25 mg per dose). Insertion of a pacemaker may be needed.
4. Treat hyperkalemia (above 5.5 mEq/L). *Avoid* calcium to treat hyperkalemia. *If hyperkalemia is present, it is an ominous sign and the availability of fragment-binding antibody for treatment must be sought.*
5. Specific Fab antibody fragments (FAB; Digibind) (antidote No. 22 in Table 9) have been used in immenient cardiac arrest, ingestion of 10 mg in an adult or 4 mg in a child, in hyperkalemia or serum digoxin concentrations above 10 ng/ml, or in life-threatening dysrhythmias.

Laboratory Studies. Monitor EKGs and potassium levels. Obtain digoxin levels 6 to 8 hours after ingestion. An endogenous digoxin-like substance that cross-reacts with most common immunoassay antibodies, as high as 4.1 ng/ml, has been reported in newborns, chronic renal failure patients, and abnormal immunoglobin patients.

Disinfectants

See Detergents (cationic), Pine Oil, Mercury, and Herbicides.

Iodines and Iodophors

See Iodine.

Phenol and Its Derivatives

These have local caustic properties as well as systemic toxicity.

Toxicity. The oral lethal dose is 10 to 30 g.

Kinetics. Elimination is hepatic.

Manifestations

1. *Systemic.* Symptoms develop within 5 to 30 minutes of ingestion and involve the CNS, liver, kidney, and lungs. Early convulsions, coma, acidosis, and shock may occur. Some phenols may produce methemoglobinemia (see Nitrites). Pentachlorophenol has produced transdermal intoxication in infants with perfuse diaphoresis. Phenol disinfectants have caused hyperbilirubinemia in infants.
2. *Local.* Phenol denatures protein and produces dermal and mucosal burns with a coagulum. No esophageal strictures have been reported.

Management

1. Evaluate the patient immediately.
2. Administer AC at once.
3. *Avoid* emesis, alcohol, and oral mineral oil.
4. Institute immediate dermal decontamination measures by copious irrigation with water, followed by polyethylene glycol.
5. Control convulsions with diazepam and phenytoin.

Laboratory Studies. Monitor renal and liver functions.

Ethylene Glycol (Solvent, Permanent Antifreeze, Brake Fluid)

Toxicity. Death has occurred after a 60-ml ingestion; the potential fatal dose is 1.4 ml/kg of 100 per cent solution. Use the same equation as for ethanol (see Alcohols) for calculating blood ethylene glycol concentration, substituting 1.12 as SG and Vd 0.65 L/kg.

Kinetics. Peak blood concentrations occur in 1 to 2 hours. Elimination is hepatic (80 to 90 per cent). Ethylene glycol is metabolized by ADH and other enzymes to the toxic metabolites: oxalate (1 per cent), glycolic acid, and glycoaldehyde by pathways that depend on cofactors thiamine and pyridoxine. Half-life is 3 hours.

Manifestations

PHASE I. CNS depression begins 30 minutes to 12 hours after ingestion with symptoms of drunkness, coma, or convulsions and metabolic abnormalities of lactic acidosis and hypocalcemia.

PHASE II. Cardiopulmonary depression may occur within 12 to 36 hours, resulting in pulmonary edema and congestive heart failure.

PHASE III. Renal failure may develop in 1 to 3 days. (Urine oxalate or monohydrate crystals may be seen in 4 to 8 hours.)

Management

1. Institute GI decontamination procedures up to 30 minutes following ingestion. Activated charcoal and cathartics are not indicated.
2. Treat nonhypocalcemic seizures with intravenous diazepam followed by phenytoin if the patient is unresponsive. Treat hypocalcemia.
3. Correct acidosis with intravenous sodium bicarbonate.
4. Initiate ethanol therapy to block metabolism if ethylene glycol has been ingested, if the blood ethylene glycol concentration is greater than 20 mg/dl, or if the patient is symptomatic but acidotic with increased anion gap or osmolar gap. Administer ethanol as in the management of methanol. Ethanol has 100 times the affinity for ADH as ethylene glycol (antidote No. 21 in Table 9).
5. Early hemodialysis is indicated if the ingestion is greater than 1.4 ml/kg, if the plasma ethylene glycol is greater than 50 mg/dl, if severe acid-base or electrolyte abnormalities occur despite conventional therapy, or if renal failure occurs.
6. Thiamine (100 mg) and pyridoxine (50 mg four times a day for 48 hours) have been recommended but have not been extensively studied.
7. Continue therapy (ethanol and hemodialysis) until the plasma ethylene glycol level is below 10 mg/dl, the acidosis has cleared, creatinine values are normal, and urinary output is adequate.

Laboratory Studies. Urinalysis for oxalate "envelope" crystals and monohydrate "hemp seed" crystals are clues to ingestion of ethylene glycol. Determine plasma ethylene glycol and ethanol levels; each 1 mg/dl of ethylene glycol in the blood raises the serum osmolality 0.17 mOsm/kg water. An ethylene glycol level of 20 mg/dl is toxic. (Levels are difficult to obtain.) The oral mucosa and the urine fluoresce under a Wood's light if ethylene glycol is present.

Fertilizers

Fertilizers contain small quantities of minerals in nontoxic amounts but may contain insecticides and herbicides. In general, noncontaminated fertilizers are of very low toxicity.

Fluoride (Caries Preventative, Insecticide, Rodenticide)

One milligram of elemental fluoride equals 2.2 mg of sodium fluoride or 4.0 mg of stannous fluoride or 7.6 mg of monophosphate fluoride.

Toxicity. Fluoride is toxic above 5 mg/kg; the potential lethal dose is 16 mg/kg of elemental fluoride. Fluoride is a protoplasmic poison that binds intracellular calcium and inhibits enzyme systems.

Kinetics. Peak plasma concentration occurs in 30 to 60 minutes.

Manifestations

1. A low overdose involves intoxication with local gastrointestinal upset, salivation, and metallic taste.
2. A high overdose, in addition to more severe local manifestations, produces systemic symptoms of convulsions, dysrhythmias, acidosis, paresthesias, and coagulation disturbances.
3. Hypocalcemia, hyperkalemia, and dysrhythmias may occur.

Management. For severe ingestions, immediately establish vascular access, monitor EKG, and treat hypocalcemia and dysrhythmias aggressively.

1. To prevent dental caries, if less than 16 mg/kg of elemental fluoride has been ingested, administer milk and observe the patient at home. If symptoms develop, conduct a medical evaluation. If the amount is in excess of 16 mg/kg, administer milk and refer for medical evaluation.
2. For insecticide or rodenticide exposure, administer milk and refer for medical evaluation. Utilize gastric lavage with 0.15 per cent calcium hydroxide 5 ml/L of water or aluminum hydroxide gel (e.g., Maalox). Activated charcoal is not effective.
3. If tetany occurs, use calcium gluconate (antidote No. 12A in Table 9).
4. Hemodialysis is effective but rarely needed.

Laboratory Studies. Monitor EKGs, electrolytes, and calcium and magnesium levels.

Hallucinogens

LSD

Lysergic acid diethylamide is an antiserotonin ergot-like alkaloid.

Toxicity. The Toxic dose is 35 μg.

Kinetics. Peak effect occurs in 1 to 2 hours; duration is 12 to 24 hours; half-life is 3 hours. Elimination is hepatic.

Mescaline/Peyote (Lophophora williamsii)

Toxicity. The toxic dose is 5 mg/kg. Peyote is a species of cactus containing mescaline, an epinephrine-like compound.

Kinetics. Peak effect occurs in 4 to 6 hours; duration is 14 hours.

Psilocybin

Psilocybin, an antiserotonin tryptamine derivative, is found in the "magic mushroom of Mexico," *Psilocybe mexicana*. It is similar in effect to LSD but is short-acting.

Kinetics. Peak effect occurs in 90 minutes; duration is 6 hours.

Marijuana

Marijuana (*Cannabis sativa*, 9-tetrahydrocannabinol [THC]) contains 1 per cent THC but seedless sinsemilla type is 6 per cent THC; when marijuana is smoked, 50 per cent of THC is destroyed.

Kinetics. Oral bioavailability is 5 to 10 times lower than from inhalation. Onset is 2 to 3 minutes smoked, 30 to 60 minutes ingested. Duration is 2 to 3 hours (smoked), more than 5 hours (ingested). Half-life is 28 to 47 hours (shorter for the chronic user). Elimination is hepatic. Enterohepatic recirculation is 15 per cent. Vd is 10 L/kg. Marijuana concentrates in breast milk and is absorbed by the nursing infant.

Manifestations. Visual illusions, sensory perceptual distortions, depersonalization, and derealization occur. The degree of impairment does not correlate with blood concentration. Conjunctival injection occurs at THC blood concentrations of 5 ng/ml, and coma ensues at 180 ng/ml.

Laboratory Studies. A single cigarette allows the metabolite to be detected in the urine for 1 week by screening measures. Chronic use may be detected in urine for a month or longer after cessation of using the substance.

Inhalants

See Nitrites and Hydrocarbons.

Management of Hallucinogens

1. If vital signs are stable, attempt "talk down" rather than prescribing drugs.
2. Arrange drug counseling and psychiatric follow-up. Most episodes are over within 12 hours.

Hydrocarbons

Toxicologically, hydrocarbons fall into six categories.

Petroleum Distillates

Petroleum distillates occur in gasoline (petroleum spirit), 2 to 5 per cent benzene; kerosene (coal oil, charcoal lighter fluid); petroleum naphtha (cigarette lighter fluid, ligroin, racing fuel); petroleum ether (benzine); turpentine (pine oil, oil of turpentine); and mineral spirits (Stoddard solvent, white spirits, varasol, petroleum spirit).

Toxicity and Kinetics. Absorption from the GI tract is poor. A person can tolerate 300 ml in the stomach, but 0.05 ml in the trachea can be lethal. Elimination is hepatic.

Manifestations. Materials aspirated during the process of ingestion produce pneumonitis. Hypoxia, not absorption, is the cause of CNS depression. Myocardial sensitivity resulting in dysrhythmias is produced by inhalation. If a chest film demonstrates pneumonitis, it is usually present within 6 hours of ingestion.

Management. It is unlikely that a child accidentally or an adolescent who is siphoning would ingest a sufficient quantity of petroleum to warrant the induction of emesis. Extremely large amounts above 5 ml/kg, as in suicide attempts, or a product containing dangerous additives warrants emesis within 2 hours of ingestion.

Aromatic Hydrocarbons

Benzene is a solvent used in manufacturing dyes, phenol, and nitrobenzene. The ingested toxic dose for adults is 15 ml. Chronic exposure may cause leukemia.

Toluene is used in plastic cements. The adult ingested toxic dose is 50 ml.

Xylene is used in the manufacture of perfumes. The adult ingested toxic dose is 50 ml.

Manifestations. Hydrocarbons are absorbed from the GI tract and produce CNS depression and asphyxiation, defatting dermatitis, and aspiration pneumonitis. Chronic inhalation of toluene has produced renal tubular acidosis.

Management. A bite into a tube of household plastic cement by a young child does not warrant the induction of emesis. Ingestion of hydrocarbon with a benzene fraction over 5 per cent or 1 ml/kg of aromatic hydrocarbons warrants induction of emesis under medical supervision within 1 hour of ingestion. Endotrachael intubation and gastric lavage are indicated in obtunded patients.

Aliphatic (Straight Chain) Halogenated Hydrocarbons and Solvents

(Table 23)

Manifestations. Myocardial sensitization and irritability, hepatorenal toxicity, and CNS depression may occur. Dichloromethane (methylene chloride) may be converted into carbon monoxide in the body.

Management. Induce emesis with ingestion of any amount under medical supervision.

Dangerous Additives

Ingestion of toxic additives to hydrocarbons, such as heavy metals, nitrobenzene, aniline dyes, insecticides, demothing agents, and methylene chloride, may warrant the induction of emesis.

Heavy Hydrocarbons

Because heavy hydrocarbons have high viscosity, low volatility, and minimal absorption, emesis is unwarranted. Examples are asphalt (tar), machine oil, motor oil (lubricating oil, engine oil), diesel oil (engine fuel, home heating oil), petrolatum liquid (mineral oil, suntan oils), petrolatum jelly (Vaseline), paraffin wax, transmission oil, cutting oil, and greases and glues. No treatment is necessary.

Special Products

Essential oils (e.g., turpentine, pine oil) are treated as petroleum distillates and do not warrant emesis unless large amounts or highly concentrated solutions are ingested.

Mineral seal oil (signal oil), found in some furniture polishes, is a heavy, viscous oil. Ingestion *never* warrants emesis; the oil can produce severe pneumonia if it is aspirated. Absorption from the GI tract is minimal.

TABLE 23. Common Examples of Aliphatic Halogenated Hydrocarbons

	Estimated Fatal Dose (Ingested)	TLV-TWA (ppm)	Synonyms
Trichloroethane 1,1,1	15.7 g/kg	50	Methylchloroform, Triethane, Glamorene Spot Remover, Scotchgard
Trichloroethane 1,1,2	580 mg/kg	10	Vinyl trichloride
Trichloroethylene	3–5 ml/kg ?	50	
Tetrachloroethane	Not known	5	Acetylene tetrachloride
Dichloromethane	25 ml	100	Methylene chloride
Tetrachloroethylene Perchloroethylene	5 ml	50	Tetrachloroethene
Dichloroethane	0.5 ml/kg	200	
Carbon tetrachloride	3–5 ml		

General Management (Table 24)

1. First induce emesis, if necessary, under medical supervision to decontaminate the GI tract. Endotrachael intubation and gastric lavage are indicated in obtunded patients. *Avoid* gastric lavage without endotracheal tubes, AC, oils, and cathartics. If no symptoms have been reported, observe the patient for several hours (at least 6) for development of respiratory distress. Decontaminate the skin.

2. In the symptomatic patient, begin supportive respiratory care for hypoxia. Treat bronchospasm with intravenous aminophylline. *Avoid* epinephrine because of danger of dysrhythmias.

3. If cyanosis is present and the patient does not respond to oxygen, or if the arterial PaO2 is normal, suspect methemoglobinemia, which may necessitate therapy with methylene blue. (See Nitrites.)

4. Steroids have not proved to be beneficial.

5. Antimicrobials are not useful in prophylaxis. Fever or leukocytosis may be produced by the chemical pneumonitis itself.

6. Most pneumonic infiltrations resolve spontaneously in 1 week, except for lipoid pneumonia of mineral seal oil aspiration, which may last for weeks. It is not necessary to treat pneumatoceles, which may develop after the pneumonitis subsides; they clear spontaneously.

Hydrogen Peroxide

Hydrogen peroxide is available as household strength, 3 per cent; as industrial strength, 10 to 20 per cent.

Toxicity. Household strength is nontoxic; industrial strength may be toxic.

Kinetics. Liberation of large amounts of oxygen causes gastric distention.

Manifestations. Industrial strength can result in burns of the exposed tissues and distention.

Management. Do not institute GI decontamination procedures. Administer water to dilute. If gastric distention is present, decompression via nasogastric tube may be necessary.

Insecticides

Pyrethins/Piperonyl (Cypermethrin, Deltamethrin, Fenvalerate)

These compounds are obtained from chrysanthemums and mixed with piperonyl butoxide, which is synergistic. They are an ingredient in common household sprays.

Toxicity. Toxicity is low, greater than 1 gm/kg.

Manifestations. Manifestations usually result from the allergic properties, although CNS excitation may result from very large overdoses.

Management. Institute GI decontamination procedures if very large amounts have been ingested. Treat convulsions and allergic reactions.

Organochlorine

See Organochlorides.

Organophosphates and Carbamates

See Organophosphates.

Rotenone

Rotenone is derived from derris plant roots.

Toxicity. Toxicity is 50 to 3000 mg/kg.

TABLE 24. Initial Management of Hydrocarbon Ingestions

Symptoms	Contents	Amount	Initial Treatment
None	Petroleum distillate only	<5 ml/kg	None
None	Heavy hydrocarbon	Any amount	None*
	Mineral seal oil		None
	Petroleum distillate	>5 ml/kg	? Emesis
None	Petroleum distillate with dangerous additive (heavy metals, pesticide)	Depends on additives' toxicity	Emesis
	Aromatic	>1 ml/kg	Emesis
	Halogenated hydrocarbons		
	A. Trichlor- compound	>1 ml/kg	Emesis
	B. Tetrachlor- compound	Any amount ingested	Emesis
Loss of protective airway reflexes, comatose, seizures	Petroleum distillate with dangerous additive, aromatic, or halogenated hydrocarbon	Gastric lavage	Endotracheal tube prior to gastric lavage

*Emesis may be necessary if machine oil contains triorthocresyl phosphate (TOCP), which causes weakness, sensory impairment, and "partially reversible damage to the spinal cord."

Manifestations. Manifestations of oral ingestion are GI irritation, conjunctivitis, rhinitis, and dermatitis. One death has been reported.

Management

1. Institute GI decontamination with gastric lavage and AC. *Avoid* emesis because of rapid onset of convulsions.
2. Control seizures with diazepam and phenytoin.
3. Treat cerebral edema by hyperventilation and intravenous mannitol.
4. Initiate supportive and symptomatic care.

Insect Repellents

Insect repellents are generally nontoxic with the exception of Diethyltoluamide (DEET) found in Off, Repel, and Deep Woods Off. DEET occurring in high concentrations or sprayed repeatedly on children has resulted in toxic encephalopathy.

Iodine

USP* tincture is 2 per cent iodine and 2.4 per cent sodium iodide in bottles of 15 ml; Lugol's solution is 5 per cent iodine and 10 per cent potassium iodide; organic bound iodide, such as povidone-iodine (Betadine 1 per cent).

Toxicity. The potential fatal dose is 2 to 4 g of free iodine. Food in the GI tract inactivates iodine to harmless iodide salts. Organic bound iodide (Betadine 1 per cent) has one-fifth the toxicity of its iodine base. The mechanism of toxicity is similar to that of an acid corrosive.

Kinetics. Elimination is renal.

Manifestations. A brown stain to the mucosa, GI tract irritation, burns, renal failure, shock, and hypersensitivity reactions may be noted. One case of pyloric stenosis has been reported. Enlargement of the parotid glands has been reported with chronic use.

Management

1. Give milk immediately, followed by 15 g of cornstarch or flour in 500 ml of water; milk may be given every 15 minutes to relieve gastric irritation. *Avoid* GI decontamination procedures. In most instances of household ingestions of tincture or povidone-iodine, only milk and observation are necessary.
2. Perform endoscopy if there are signs of esophageal or gastric damage.
3. If anaphylactoid reaction occurs, treat with epinephrine.
4. Monitor urinary output and renal profile if toxicity develops.

Iron

Accidental iron ingestion is one of the most common poisonings in children. The elemental iron content of some preparations appears in Table 25. Chewable vitamins with iron contain from 12 to 18 mg of elemental iron per tablet and children's liquid from 15 to 18 mg of elemental iron per 0.6 ml or 5 ml. These preparations rarely produce toxicity unless very large quantities are ingested.

Toxicity. The normal serum iron (SI) ranges from 80 to 180 μg/dl (14 to 32 μmol/L) in males and from 60 to 160 μg/dl (11 to 29 μmol/L) in females. Toxic levels usually are above the total iron-binding capacity (TIBC), which is usually 250 to 460 μg/dl (42 to 82 μmol/L). The value of the TIBC in determining toxicity is currently being debated. The free unbound iron causes the toxicity in the body acting as mitochondrial toxin. The presence of signs of intoxication is more important than the estimate of the amount ingested. (See Table 26.)

Kinetics. Peak iron concentration is 3 to 5 hours after ingestion. For excretion there is no normal route except blood loss or GI tract desquamation.

Manifestations. These include the presence of spontaneous vomiting, abdominal cramps and diarrhea, a white blood cell count above 15,000/mm^3, and a glucose level above 120 mg/dl (8.327 mm/L). Radiopaque pills on abdominal films suggest GI toxicity and a more significant ingestion that warrants careful observation. Patients who are asymptomatic for 6 hours rarely experience serious intoxication.

PHASE I. Gastrointestinal mucosal injury may occur, possibly with hematemesis (1 to 6 hours after ingestion). Usually, there is vomiting within 1/2 to 2 hours in 94 per cent of cases if a toxic dose has been ingested. Abdominal pain, diarrhea, and melena may be present. Hyperglycemia may occur. Fever and leukocytosis reflect mucosal damage. In severe cases, hemorrhagic gastritis, intestinal necrosis, perforation, peritonitis, acute blood loss, hypotension, shock, seizures, and coma occur. Iron tablets are radiopaque on x-ray until they dissolve; however, children's vitamins with iron are often not seen because they have small amounts of iron and liquid iron and may not be visible on x-ray at all.

PHASE II. Patients may show a "deceptive" improvement (2 to 24 hours, usually up to 12 hours). In serious poisonings, this phase may be absent and progressive deterioration may occur.

PHASE III. Cardiovascular collapse and severe metabolic acidosis, convulsions, coma, pulmonary edema, cyanosis, coagulopathy, and hepatorenal failure occur at 4 to 36 hours.

PHASE IV. Hepatic injury is due to iron catabolism of lipid peroxidation and is associated with jaundice.

PHASE V. Sequelae of pyloric stenosis, intestinal strictures, and obstruction or anemia (usually appear 2 to 6 weeks after the event but may occur months later). *Yersinia enterocolitica* sepsis may develop.

Management

1. Institute GI decontamination procedures. Induce emesis in ingestions of elemental iron of more than 20 mg/kg in the alert patient unless extensive hematemesis or shock is present. Follow emesis with gastric lavage if large amounts have been ingested (>60 mg/kg).
2. The lavage solutions used for complexation of free iron have not proved to be very effective. Fleet's enema solution is *not* recommended. Use saline 0.9 per cent or 1.0 to 1.5 per cent sodium bicarbonate (prepared by dilution of a sodium bicarbonate ampule with saline). Do *not* use oral AC. The use of oral deferoxamine (DFOM, Desferal) is *not* recommended.
3. Obtain abdominal films for positive postgastric emptying of undissolved tablets and to see whether further GI decontamination is indicated. A negative radiograph does not exclude the presence of iron in the GI tract.
4. Use whole-bowel irrigation if radiopaque pills remain after GI decontamination.
5. Determine serum iron levels at peak absorption within 2 hours of ingestion for liquid and 4 to 6 hours for solid iron preparations before the iron is distributed to the tissues. A serum iron level at 8 to 12 hours is useful to exclude delayed absorption from a bezoar or sustained-release preparations. There is controversy over the value of the TIBC test. It is time-consuming and does not correlate with systemic toxicity. Continue to observe serum iron levels every 4 hours to assess whether iron absorption is continuing.
6. Give deferoxamine (DFOM) (antidote No. 15 in Table

*USP, United States Pharmacopeia.

TABLE 25. Iron Content of Some Preparations

Iron Salt	Elemental Iron Content (%)	Average Tablet Strength (mg)	Elemental Iron Tablet (mg)	Average $FeSO_4$ Strength of Other forms (mg)
Ferrous sulfate (hydrous)	20	300	60	Drp 75/0.6 ml
	20	SR 160	32	Syp 90/5 ml
	20	195	39	Solu 125/ml
	20	325	65	Elixir 220/5 ml
Ferrous sulfate (dried)	30	200	60	
	30	SR 160	48	
Ferrous gluconate	12	320	36	Elixir 320/5 ml
Ferrous fumarate	33	200	67	
	33	SR 324	107	Drp 45/0.6 ml
	33	Chewable 100	33	Susp 100/5 ml

9). About 100 mg of DFOM binds 8.5 to 9.35 mg of free iron in serum (Table 27).

a. *Diagnostic chelation test.* Deferoxamine (50 mg/kg up to 1 g IM) confirms the presence of water-soluble, ferroxamine-chelated iron by producing a red-orange *(vin rosé)* color to the urine within 1 to 3 hours. If results are negative, one cannot reliably exclude high serum iron levels.

b. *Chelation therapy with deferoxamine.* Consider this:

- If the 4-hour serum iron exceeds 500 μg/dl (90 μmol/L) even if the patient is asymptomatic; at levels below 500 μg/dl, start therapy on basis of the patient's symptoms
- If the diagnostic chelation test is positive (*vin rosé* urine) *with* symptoms
- If there are systemic signs of intoxication regardless of serum iron level
- If there are mild to moderate symptoms with radiopaque material on abdominal films, leukocytosis with a serum iron level >15,000 mm^3 within 6 hours after ingestion, and a plasma glucose level above 150 mg/dl (>83 μmol/L)

c. *Dose and administration.* Studies indicate that the intravenous route is preferred and the use of constant intravenous infusion has been recommended on the basis of DFOM pharmacokinetics.

d. *Rate of infusion.* Start continuous infusion at 15 mg/kg/hour (3 ml/kg/hour of 500 mg in 100 ml). Rapid intravenous infusion causes hypotension. DFOM has been administered more rapidly (40 to 50 mg/kg/hour) in severe cases of iron poisoning without adverse reactions. Monitor the vital functions. The intramuscular dose is 50 mg/kg every 6 hours in children or 1 to 2 g every 6 hours in adults until the end point is reached. The maximum dose by either route is 6 g per 24 hours.

e. *End point for DFOM.* Continue chelation therapy until the patient is asymptomatic, the serum iron level is below 100 μg/dl (<18 μmol/L), and the urine shows no orange-red *vin rosé* color if the test result was originally positive.

7. The iron-feroxamine complex is hemodialyzable in cases of renal shutdown and severe poisoning.

8. In significant intoxications, follow up the patient for sequelae of GI strictures and anemia secondary to blood loss.

Laboratory Studies. Serum iron concentrations (normal 80 to 180 μg/dl) correlate to a certain degree with the clinical course.

Isoniazid (INH, Nydrazid)

Isoniazid is an antituberculosis drug.

Toxicity. The toxic dose is 35 to 40 mg/kg, producing convulsions. Severe toxicity is seen at 6 to 10 g in adolescents. One of its mechanisms is to produce pyridoxine deficiency and inhibit the formation of gamma-aminobutyric acid (GABA), the neurotransmitter inhibitor in the brain.

Kinetics. Peak effect occurs in 1 to 2 hours. Elimination is hepatic.

Manifestations. These include visual disturbances, convulsions (90 per cent multiple seizures) that often start within 30 minutes, coma, and resistant severe acidosis.

TABLE 26. Severity of Iron Toxicity Based on Amount Ingested

Severity	Amount Elemental Iron (mg/kg)	Number of $FeSO_4$ 325-mg Tablets	Management
Nontoxic	<20	<3	Observation
Mild	20–60*	4–12	Emesis and medical evaluation
Moderate	>60	>12	Medical evaluation Emesis/lavage Abdominal x-ray Serum iron TIBC not necessary Consider chelation
Severe, symptomatic	180–360 regardless of amount	>30–45 —	Intensive care Medical evaluation

*Some authorities consider 20 mg/kg toxic, 40 mg/kg serious poisoning and 60 mg/kg potentially lethal.
Abbreviations: TIBC, total iron-binding capacity; $FeSO_4$, ferrous sulfate.

TABLE 27. Summary of the Management of Iron Intoxication

Toxicity	Serum Iron 4–6 hr After Ingestion	Shock and Coma Reported	Treatment*
Nontoxic	50–100 μg/dl 8.9–17.9 μmol/L	—	None
Very mild	150–350 μg/dl 26.8–62.6 μmol/L	—	None
Mild	350–500 μg/dl 62.6–89.5 μmol/L	<10%	Administer DFOM+ based on patient's symptoms IV/IM
Moderate	500–700 μg/dl 89.5–125.4 μmol/L	25%	Administer DFOM IV† Supportive care
Serious	>700 μg/dl	50%	DFOM IV, supportive care
Fatal levels	>1000 μg/dl (>179 μmol/L)	75%	Extensive supportive care, DFOM IV†

*If patient is symptomatic, start immediate treatment. Do not wait for serum iron determination.
†Give critical care with hemodynamic capabilities (cardiac output, preload, afterload).
Abbreviations: DFOM, deferoxamine.

Management

1. Control seizures with large doses of pyridoxine (antidote No. 38 in Table 9). Repeat until seizures cease. Administer diazepam with pyridoxine because they act synergistically. *Avoid* phenytoin because it inhibits INH metabolism and INH inhibits phenytoin metabolism.
2. Correct acidosis. Control of the seizures may spontaneously correct the acidosis.
3. *Avoid* emesis because of rapid onset of seizures. After patient is stabilized or if the patient is asymptomatic, other GI decontamination procedures may be carried out. Observe asymptomatic patients for 6 hours.
4. Hemodialysis is rarely needed but may be used as an adjunct for uncontrollable acidosis and seizures. Hemoperfusion has not been adequately evaluated.

Laboratory Studies. Plasma isoniazid levels above 8 μg/ml are toxic. Monitor the blood glucose (often hyperglycemic), electrolytes (often hyperkalemic), and liver function tests. Monitor the temperature closely (often hyperpyrexic).

Lead

See p. 757, Chronic Lead Poisoning in Children.

Lidocaine

Lidocaine is a cardiac antidysrhythmic agent and local anesthetic (2 per cent Xylocaine).

Toxicity. Oral ingestion under 7 mg/kg usually does not produce toxicity.

Kinetics. Peak blood concentration occurs 1 hour after ingestion; oral mucosal absorption is similar to intravenous absorption. Duration is 10 to 20 minutes intravenously. Elimination is by hepatic metabolism into two active metabolites; one (monoethylglycinexylidide [MEGX]) has convulsant properties.

Manifestations

1. *Mild.* Vertigo, drowsiness, dysarthria, perioral numbness, muscle twitching, confusion, and tinnitus (blood concentrations 5 to 9 μg/ml).
2. *Serious.* Psychosis, convulsions, severe bradycardia, sinus arrest, AV block, and respiratory depression (blood concentration > 9 μg/ml).
3. Methemoglobinemia.

Management

1. Treat seizures with diazepam followed, if necessary, by phenobarbital. *Avoid* phenytoin because of its possible synergistic cardiac side effects. Neuromuscular blocking agents, intubation, and ventilation may be necessary. Convulsions may continue with low blood concentrations of lidocaine due to MEGX.
2. Use overdrive pacing and cardioversion for dysrhythmias.
3. Treat methemoglobinemia. See Nitrites.
4. Institute GI decontamination procedures, if lidocaine has been ingested, with AC and a cathartic. *Avoid* emesis because of rapid onset of symptoms.

Laboratory Studies. Obtain lidocaine blood concentrations (therapeutic range is 1.5 to 6 μg/ml). Perform EKG monitoring; if neuromuscular blockers are used, perform electroencephalographic (EEG) monitoring, methemoglobin levels if brown blood or cyanosis occurs.

Lomotil

Each 5 ml or tablet contains 2.5 mg of diphenoxylate. Atropine toxicity may occur within 1 to 2 hours of ingestion, and diphenoxylate toxicity may not occur for 2 to 5 hours. Lomotil may produce, in addition to classic signs of opioid intoxication, convulsions. See Opioids.

Mercury (Table 28)

Toxicity. Elemental mercury is toxic by inhalation. The fatal dose of inorganic mercury salts in adults is 1 g. The ingestion of elemental mercury in thermometers is nontoxic because of poor absorption from the GI tract.

Kinetics. Absorption of alimental mercury is 89 per cent by inhalation, 0.01 per cent of the ingested dose in the GI tract. Route of elimination is renal. Mercury is excreted in the urine and in the bile.

Manifestations. Acute poisoning develops. Mercuric salts, when ingested, act as a corrosive, producing stomatitis, and gastroenteritis with bloody, bluish vomitus within 15 minutes of ingestion, which may lead to dehydration and shock. Within 1 to 3 days, foul breath, a metallic taste, and evidence of hepatic and renal dysfunction develop. Inhalation produces similar symptoms and a pneumonitis.

TABLE 28. Types of Mercury and Mercury Poisonings

Classification	Product Exposure	Absorption and Route	Distribution	Half-life (Days)	Elimination	Manifestations and Comments
Inorganic						
Elemental	Thermometers	Ingestion 0.01%	—	—	—	Nontoxic unless delayed GI passage
	Industry TLV = 0.05 ppm	Inhalation Rapid 80% Chronic	Large	58	Renal	Pulmonary, neurologic, psychologic
	Abuse	Injection Chronic	Large	Long	Renal	Pulmonary, neurologic, psychologic, local abscess
Mercuric salts ($HgCl_2$)	Disinfectant	Ingestion Acute and chronic	Large	40	Renal	Corrosive, nephrotoxic, acrodynia
Mercurous salts (HgCl)	Teething lotion, laxatives	Ingestion/mucosal	Large	—	Renal	Acrodynia
Organic						
Alkyl Short-chained	Methyl: Bioaccumulation Fungicide	Ingestion rapid, complete 100%	Large; passes placenta	52–70	Liver enterohepatic	Neurosensory, developmental (Minamata disease)
(Fish-food chain)	Ethyl. Fungicides	Ingestion rapid	Large	—	Renal	GI, renal, neurologic
Aryl phenyl, methoxyethyl	Diaper rinse	Ingestion very rapid 80–90%	Large	—	Renal	Forms inorganic salts in body
Long-chain thimerosal	Diuretics, antiseptics, agricultural products, contact lens solutions	Ingestion—poorly absorbed	Large	—	Renal	Low toxicity

Management

1. If elemental mercury has been inhaled, remove the patient from exposure.
2. Institute routine GI decontamination procedures for ingestion of mercuric salt.
3. Choose dimercaprol (BAL, antidote No. 17 in Table 9) if there is renal impairment from mercury. BAL enhances mercury excretion, mostly as a complex that is water-soluble at pH 7.5, through the bile as well as the urine. Penicillamine (antidote No. 34) or *N*-acetyl *dl*-penicillamine (investigational use) are oral antidotes that are useful in less severe poisonings or chronic mercury poisonings. BAL in methyl mercury intoxication increases the brain mercury and is contraindicated; penicillamine and its analogue should be used (it decreases mercury in brain). A new investigational chelator, 2,3-dimercaptosuccinic acid (DMSA), holds promise of less toxicity and more specificity.
4. Monitor fluid and electrolytes, renal function, and hemoglobin levels. Determine and monitor blood and urine mercury levels. (Consult the laboratory for proper collection technique and containers.)
5. Early hemodialysis is useful in the symptomatic patient.
6. Perform surgical excision of local injection sites.

Laboratory Studies

1. Blood levels of mercury are normally below 2 to 4 μg/dl and urine levels are below 10 to 20 μg/L in 90 per cent of the adult population. Levels above 4 μg/dl in blood and 20 μg/L in urine probably should be considered abnormal. Blood levels are not always reliable after the first few hours because of tissue binding. Approximately 150 μg/L in urine is equivalent to 3.5 mg/dl in blood.
2. Because methyl mercury is excreted mainly through the feces, mercury urinalysis would not be a reliable measurement.

Monoamine Oxidase Inhibitors

Monoamine oxidase (MAO) inhibitors are prescribed as antidepressants, for example, phenelzine (Nardil), 15-mg tablets; isocarboxazid (Marplan), 10-mg tablets, and tranylcypromine (Parnate), 10-mg tablets. MAO is responsible for the metabolic degradation of the neurotransmitters. MAO inhibitors cause an increase in norepinephrine.

Toxicity. Severe toxicity results from ingestion of 2 to 3 mg/kg, fatalities from 4 to 6 mg/kg.

Kinetics. Elimination is hepatic. Peak activity in overdose occurs in 8 to 12 hours.

Manifestations. Acute overdose results in the following:

PHASE I. The patient is asymptomatic for 6 to 24 hours.

PHASE II. Neuromuscular excitation with tremors and seizures, increased temperature, blood pressure, tachycardia, tachypnea, hyperglycemia, and leukocytosis are seen. In larger doses, masseter spasm, hyperthermia, muscle rigidity, acidosis, and electrolyte abnormalities occur. Nonreactive pupils are a common feature. The EKG may show T wave changes.

PHASE III. CNS depression and cardiovascular collapse occur because the biogenic amines cannot be converted into catecholamines, thus resulting in sympathetic nervous system depression. Symptoms resolve within 5 days but may last 2 weeks.

PHASE IV. Secondary complications from rhabdomyolysis, cardiac dysrhythmias, multiorgan failure, and coagulopathies may occur.

Malignant hyperthermia is characterized by hyperthermia, delirium, convulsions, coma, rigidity; it may occur when tricyclic antidepressants or opioids, especially meperidine and dextramethorphan, are given to patients who are taking or have received MAO inhibitors within the past 2 weeks. *Hypertensive crisis* occurs when patients receiving MAO inhibitors take food or drink that has undergone fermentation and contains large amounts of tyramine, such as cheeses, wines, and beers.

Management

1. Establish and maintain vital functions.
2. Institute GI decontamination procedures, and consider 24-hour hospital admission if the amount ingested is more than 1 mg/kg.
3. Treat malignant hypertension with phentolamine (2 to 5 mg over 20 minutes), then titrated to patient's clinical response. Closely monitor cardiac and intrarterial blood pressure. Nitroprusside may also be used.
4. Control severe hypotension in the course of treatment with norepinephrine infusion. *Avoid* phenothiazines.
5. Manage malignant hyperthermia with external cooling measures, such as dantrolene (20 mg using a 70-ml vial, mixed with 60 ml of distilled water, and administered at 1 mg/kg/minute IV). Average dose is 2.5 mg/kg, with a maximum of 10 mg/kg over 15 minutes. Repeat the loading dose every 15 minutes if necessary. When temperature and heart rate decrease, start infusion of 1 to 2 mg/kg every 2 hours for 3 days, then every 4 hours for 4 days, or until all evidence of malignant hyperthermia has subsided. Watch for thrombophleblitis following dantrolene administration. Give bromocriptine mesylate (2.5 to 10 mg) or amantidine (100 mg twice a day orally or through a nasogastric tube three times a day). Watch for myoglobinemia and renal failure.

Mothballs

See Camphor (no longer used as a demothing agent), Naphthalene, and Paradichlorobenzene. See also Table 29.

Naphthalene

Naphthalene is found in mothballs, repellent cakes, and deodorant cakes.

Toxicity. The ingestion of 250 to 500 mg of pure naphthalene may cause toxicity in patients with glucose-6-phosphate dehydrogenase (G-6-PD) deficiency. Persons without this deficiency require several grams of naphthalene to produce toxicity.

Kinetics. Oil enhances absorption. Skin absorption occurs from clothes stored in naphthalene, particularly if baby oil is applied. Naphthalene's oxidative metabolites (naphthols) are responsible for hemolysis. Elimination is hepatic.

Manifestations. Hemolysis starts on day 1 to 3 after exposure. Other findings may include nausea, vomiting, diarrhea, fever, jaundice, dark urine, renal failure, coma, and convulsions. Rare hepatocellular damage may occur. Recovery begins in 7 to 10 days.

Management

1. Institute GI decontamination procedures, including AC and cathartic. Decontaminate the skin, and discard contaminated clothing. Washing does not completely remove naphthalene from clothes. Monitor hemoglobin or hematocrit level, and obtain a blood smear for Heinz bodies 1 week after exposure.
2. If transfusion is needed in patients with G-6-PD deficiency, use blood from a donor with a normal G-6-PD level. Transfuse to 80 per cent of the normal G-6-PD value. If methemoglobinemia is present, consider methylene blue (antidote No. 29 in Table 9). (See Nitrites.)
3. Establish good hydration, alkalinize, and create a diuresis with furosemide to avoid precipitation of hemoglobin in the renal tubules. Monitor urinary output and renal profile. If renal shutdown occurs, perform dialysis.
4. Consider corticosteroids, reported as helpful in limiting hemolysis, in children showing hemolysis.

Laboratory Studies. Heinz bodies signify impending hemolysis. Eccentrocytes (dense, asymmetric distributions of hemoglobin in red blood cells) are found in active hemolysis. Reticulocyte counts greater than 7 per cent yield normal G-6-PD levels even if deficiency exists. If hemolysis is active, check the parents for G-6-PD.

TABLE 29. Moth-Proofing Agents

Mothballs	Paradichlorobenzene	Naphthalene
Usual form	Crystals, nuggets	Balls, flakes
Appearance	Wet	Dry
Turpentine dissolution test	Dissolves in 60 minutes	Slowly dissolves; 25% remains in 60 minutes
Copper wire test	Produces fleeting but intense green flame in minutes	No green flame
Water test		
Plain water	Sinks	Sinks
Salt water	Sinks	Floats

Nicotine

Nicotine occurs in insecticides (Black leaf 40 per cent solution), tobacco products, and plants (*Nicotiana tabacum* has a nicotine content of 1 to 6 per cent).

Toxicity. Fatal dose is 40 to 60 mg of pure nicotine. A cigarette contains 15 to 25 mg, and cigar has 15 to 40 mg of nicotine. When ingested as tobacco, nicotine is much less toxic than pure nicotine or nicotine insecticide because of poor absorption. Only about 25 per cent of the total nicotine is recovered from cigarette butts.

Kinetics. Route of elimination is hepatic. Onset of action is within 1 hour.

Manifestations

PHASE I. Adrenergic and cholinergic effects results in tobacco odor on the breath, vomiting (2 to 5 mg of nicotine may cause nausea), tachypnea, bradycardia, miosis, hypertension, salivation, abdominal pain, and diarrhea. Early excitation, tremors, and seizures may occur within 30 minutes.

PHASE II. Tachycardia, mydriasis, hypotension (ganglionic blockade), late respiratory muscle paralysis, and coma may ensue. Ileus and urinary retention may occur. If a fatal dose has been ingested, the patient may die within 1 hour.

Management

1. For children who ingest less than one cigarette or three butts, closely observe at home. If a larger amount or liquid nicotine insecticide is ingested, institute GI decontamination procedures with lavage and AC. *Avoid* emesis because of the rapid onset of convulsions. Dermal decontamination may be needed.
2. Control convulsions with diazepam and phenytoin.
3. Use atropine for cholinergic crisis, use β- and α-blockers (e.g., labetolol) for excess sympathetic stimulation.
4. Acid diuresis may decrease reabsorption and may enhance elimination but has not been advocated or investigated.
5. Support respirations, and be prepared for intubation and ventilation.

Nitrites and Nitrates

These salts are readily available in both inorganic and organic forms. Inorganic nitrates and nitrites occur in well water and certain foods (spinach, carrots, cabbage, beets) and may produce methemoglobinemia in infants.

Toxicity. The potential fatal adult doses are as follows: nitrite, 1 g; nitrate, 10 g; nitrobenzene, 2 ml; nitroglycerin, 0.2 g; and aniline dye (pure), 5 to 30 g.

Kinetics. Onset of action of nitroglycerin sublingually is 1 to 3 minutes, with a peak action of 3 to 15 minutes and a duration of 20 to 30 minutes. Other routes are characterized by a slower onset (2 to 5 minutes) and longer duration of action (1.5 to 6 hours). Nitrites are potent oxidizing agents, converting ferrous (Fe^{2+}) of hemoglobin to ferric iron (Fe^{3+}) of methemoglobinemia, which cannot carry oxygen. Elimination is hepatic.

Manifestations

1. *Vasodilation.* Headache, flushing of the skin, sweating, hypotension, tachycardia, and syncope.
2. *Methemoglobinemia.* Slate gray cyanosis with chocolate-colored lips and mucosa, refractory to oxygen therapy, brownish blood that fails to turn red on exposure to oxygen, normal PaO_2, and venous Po_2 with low oxygen saturation. Other causes of methemoglobinemia include congenital factors, oxidizing medications (antimalarials, some local anesthetics, dapsone, nitrites, sulfonamides), and some chemicals (aniline derivates, chlorates, nitrites). Infants are predisposed to the development of methemoglobinemia. See Table 30.

Management

1. Institute dermal decontamination if indicated. Remove aniline dyes with 5 per cent acetic acid (vinegar).
2. Institute GI decontamination procedures if there has been an acute ingestion.
3. Treat hypotension by patient positioning and with fluids. Vasoconstrictors (dopamine or norepinephrine) are rarely needed.
4. If methemoglobinemia occurs, stabilize vital functions; administer 100 per cent oxygen during and after antidotal therapy. Methylene blue (MB) (antidote No. 29 in Table 9) is indicated for methemoglobin levels above 30 per cent, dyspnea, a lactic acidosis, or an altered mental state. Methylene blue reduces the half-life of methemoglobin from 15 to 20 hours to less than 60 minutes. Ascorbic acid is ineffective. *Avoid* methylene blue in G-6-PD deficiency patients because it is ineffective and may precipitate hemolysis. Use a hyperbaric chamber and/or exchange transfusion in symptomatic patients if methylene blue is not effective or is contraindicated, as in G-6-PD deficiency.

Laboratory Studies. Methemoglogin levels and oxygen saturation are measured by co-oximeter, not by pulse oximetry, which does not measure carboxyhemoglobin or methemoglobin and will result in the misreading of saturation in the presence of these compounds.

TABLE 30. Methemoglobinemia

Methemoglobin (%)	Manifestations
10	"Chocolate cyanosis," brown blood
10–20	Headache, dizziness, tachypnea
50	Mental alterations, coma, convulsions
>50	Metabolic acidosis and electroencephalographic changes
70	Pulmonary edema, encephalopathy, shock

Nonsteroidal Anti-inflammatory Agents (NSAIDs)

Kinetics. Peak blood concentration occurs in 1 to 2 hours. Elimination is hepatic. See Table 31.

Manifestations

1. *GI System.* Nausea, vomiting, abdominal pain, bleeding.
2. *Central nervous system.* drowsiness, tinnitus, headache, lethargy. Renal failure occurs with chronic use or massive overdose of NSAIDs. Indomethacin results in neurologic effects; meclofenamate and mefenamic acid produce bloody diarrhea and seizures, phenylbutazone and oxyphenbutazone produce agranulocytosis, aplastic anemia, thrombocytopenia, and exfoliative dermatitis. Sulindac has caused hypersensitivity hepatitis.

Management. See Table 32. If the maximum daily dose is not listed for a child in milligrams per kilogram, calculate this value by dividing the maximum adult daily dose by 70 kg to give the maximum daily dose in a child in mg/kg per 24 hrs. This value is multipled by the child's weight in kilograms to give the estimated maximum daily dose.

1. Observe for GI tract symptoms and CNS symptoms.
2. Monitor vital signs and biochemical, liver, and renal profiles. A metabolic acidosis has been reported in humans with ibuprofen and diflunisal.
3. Initial and repeated doses of AC have been effective in phenylbutazone overdose and merit consideration, although data are limited in regard to other NSAIDs.
4. Test the vomitus and/or gastric aspirate and stools for blood.
5. Treat GI bleeding with iced saline lavage and H_2 blockers and/or antacids.
6. Hypotension is managed with positioning and fluids.
7. Consider alkaline diuresis with sodium bicarbonate (antidote No. 39 in Table 9) Hemodialysis is not useful. Hemoperfusion was successful in one case of phenylbutazone.
8. Treat convulsions with diazepam and phenytoin.

Nontoxic Ingested Items (Table 33)

Criteria for nontoxic ingestion include:

1. Absolute identification of the product.
2. Absolute assurance that a single product has been ingested.
3. Assurance that there is no signal word on the container.
4. A good approximation of the amount ingested.
5. The ability to call back at frequent intervals to determine whether symptoms have developed.
6. A satisfactory explanation of the circumstances, to exclude chemical maltreatment in infants under 1 year and to exclude a "cry for help" in those older than 6 years.

Opioids (Narcotic Opiates)

See Table 34.

Toxicity. *Codeine* may produce minor signs of toxicity at 1 mg/kg. Respiratory arrest has occurred at 5 mg/kg. *Propoxyphene* (Darvon) possesses cardiotoxicity; 10 mg/kg can be toxic, and 35 mg/kg has caused cardiopulmonary arrest. *Dextromethorphan* (10 mg/kg or 90 to 180 mg) has produced symptoms; however, no fatalities have been reported.

Kinetics. The onset of action of most opioids varies between 10 and 60 minutes, the peak is between 30 minutes to 2 hours, and the duration of action is 4 to 6 hours. Elimination is hepatic. Meperidine is metabolized into normeperidine, an active CNS stimulant. The half-life of meperidine is between ½ hour to 5 hours; normeperdine, between 12 and 16 hours;

TABLE 31. Pharmacokinetics of Nonsteroidal Anti-inflammatory Agents (NSAIDs)

Drug	Maximum Adult Dose (mg/24 hr)	Peak (Hours)	Elimination Route	Half-Life (Hours)	Comments
Carprofen (Rimadryl)	600	0.5–4	Hepatic	15	Preparations: Tab 25, 50, 75 mg
Diclofenlac (Voltaren)	200	2	Renal	1.5	Preparations: Tab 100, 150 mg; 30–50% eliminated in bile
Diflunisal (Dolobid)	1500	1–2	>90% Hepatic	8–12	Therap bl conc‡ 120 μg/ml Preparations: Tab 250, 500 mg
Fenbufen	1000	NA	Hepatic	10	Preparations: 300, 450 mg
Fenoprofen (Nalfon)	3200	1–2	95% Hepatic	1.5–3	Therap bl conc 40–70 μg/ml Preparations: 300, 600 mg
Ibuprofen (Children's Advil, Pediprofen, Motrin, Advil, Rufen)	3200 Child 20–50 mg/kg/day or 6 mg/kg/6 hr	0.5–1.5	Hepatic	2–2.5	Therap bl conc 20–30 μg/ml Preparations: Tab 200, 300, 400, 800 mg; Liq 100 mg/5 ml
Indomethacin (Indocin)	200 Child 1–2.5 mg/kg/day in 3–4 doses or 0.2–0.3 mg/kg/dose	1–2	Hepatic	4.5–6.0	Therap bl conc 0.3–4 μg/ml Enterohepatic§ Preparations: Caps 25, 50 mg; SR, 75 mg; Suppos 50 mg; Liq 25 mg/5 ml
Ketoprofen (Oruvail)	300	0.5–2	Hepatic	15	Preparations: 25, 50, 75 mg
Meclofenamate* (Meclomen)	400 Child 4–7.5 mg/kg/day in 3–4 doses	0.5–2	Hepatic	3–4	Active metabolite Therap bl conc 10–20 μg/ml Preparations: 50, 100 mg
Mefenamic acid* (Ponstel)	1000	1–3	Hepatic	2–4	Therap bl conc 0.3–2.4 μg/ml Enterohepatic Preparation: 250 mg
Naproxen (Anaprox, Naprosyn)	750 Child 10 mg/kg/day or 1200–1800 mg/m² in 3–4 doses	1–2	>90% Hepatic	12–15	Therap bl conc 30–90 μg/ml Preparations: Tab 250, 375, 500 mg; Liq 125 mg/5 ml
Oxyphenbutazone* (Oxalid, Tanderil)	400	—	Hepatic	72	Therap bl conc 11–118 μg/ml Preparations: 200, 400 mg
Phenylbutazone* (Azolid, Butazolidin)	400	2	Hepatic	50–100	Active metabolite Therap bl conc 50–100 μg/ml
Piroxicam* (Feldene)	40 Child 0.45 mg/kg/24 hr	2–5	Hepatic	45	Therap bl conc 0.85–13.5 μg/ml Enterohepatic Preparations: 10, 20 mg
Sulindac (Clinoril)	400	1	80% Hepatic	7–8	Therap bl conc 3–6 μg/ml Enterohepatic Preparations: 150, 200 mg
Tolmetin (Tolectin)	2000 Child 15–30 mg/kg/day in 3–4 doses	1–2	80% Hepatic	1	Preparations: Tab 200; Caps 400 mg

*Potentially serious ingestion.
†Withdrawn from U.S. market.
‡Therapeutic blood concentration.
§Enterohepatic recirculation.
Abbreviations: Therap, therapeutic; bl, blood; conc, concentration.

TABLE 32. Management of Overdose with Nonsteroidal Anti-inflammatory Agents (NSAIDs)

Amount Ingested	Treatment
Less than 100 mg/kg ibuprofen (child) Less than maximum daily dose of other NSAID (child or adult)	Observe for symptoms, milk.
Over 100 mg/kg ibuprofen (child)	Induce emesis if delay in reaching hospital; *no emesis* if ingestion of mefenamic acid or >400 mg/kg of ibuprofen.
Over maximum daily dose of other NSAID (child or adult)	Gastric lavage, activated charcoal/cathartic. Observe for 6 hr.
Manifestations already present Over 400 mg/kg ibuprofen (child)	Gastric lavage. Activated charcoal/cathartic. Repeated doses of activated charcoal. Monitor acid base, electrolytes, renal and liver profiles, urinalysis, serial hemoglobin, hematocrit.

methadone, between 15 and 30 hours; and propoxyphene, between 8 and 24 hours.

Manifestations. The classic triad is coma, shallow respirations, and pinpoint pupils.

1. Patients should be observed for CNS depression and hypotension.
2. Seizures may occur with propoxyphene, codeine, meperidine, and diphenoxylate (Lomotil).
3. Pulmonary edema is a potentially lethal complication of mainlining (intravenous use).
4. Most opiate agonists produce miotic pupils. Mydriatic pupils are seen with meperidine, dextramethorphan, and, rarely, Lomotil.
5. Physical dependence and withdrawal are seen.
6. Dextromethorphan, particularly in overdose with long-acting preparations, may cause ataxia, hypertension, tachycardia, restlessness, nystagmus, and lethargy, and naloxone may not be completely successful in reversing these manifestations.
7. Lomotil (atropine and diphenoxylate)—as little as one tablet—may cause serious toxicity. Atropine toxicity rarely occurs; if it does, it starts in 1 to 2 hours. Diphenoxylate toxicity is delayed for 2 to 5 hours or longer. Children exposed to Lomotil should be admitted and monitored in the intensive care unit for 24 hours.

Management

1. Establish vital functions and administer supportive care, particularly with an endotracheal tube and assisted ventilation.
2. Institute GI decontamination procedures with AC and a cathartic initially. *Avoid* induced emesis in an overdose because CNS depression and convulsions occur early.
3. Administer naloxone (Narcan), (antidote No. 30 in Table 9) to improve ventilation and oxygenation. It may be given as a bolus intravenously and followed by repeated intravenous injections or by continuous infusion.

a. Titrate naloxone against the clinical response and precipitation of withdrawal in narcotic addicts. Repeat as often as necessary, because many opioids in an overdose can last 24 hours to 48 hours whereas the action of naloxone lasts only ½ hour to 2 hours. Larger amounts are often needed for codeine, pentazocine, methadone, dextramethophan, or propoxyphene overdose. Signs of naloxone effect include dilation of pupils, increased rate and depth of respirations, reversal of hypotension, and improvement of obtunded or comatose state.

b. The infusion dose is equivalent to the naloxone response dose; administer the response dose as a continuous infusion every hour. Indications for naloxone infusion include:

- The need for a large initial bolus
- The need for repeated bolus
- A very large overdose
- An overdose with a long-acting preparation

4. If the patient is comatose, analyze a glucose reagent strip and administer intravenous glucose if needed. About 3 to 4 per cent of comatose narcotic opioid overdose patients have hypoglycemia. First try naloxone and intravenous glucose to control seizures; if these fail, give diazepam.
5. For pulmonary edema, which does not respond to nal-

TABLE 33. Substances Normally Nontoxic (Unless Ingested in Very Large Quantity)

Abrasives	Laxatives
Adhesives	Lipstick
Antacids	Lubricants
Antibiotics	Lysol brand disinfectant (not the bowl cleaner)
Baby product cosmetics	Magic Marker
Ballpoint pen inks	Makeup (eye, liquid facial)
Bathtub floating toys	Matches (book type)
Bath oil (castor oil and perfume)	Mineral oil
Bleach less than 5%	Newspaper
Body conditioners	Paints (indoor latex acrylic)
Bubble bath soaps (detergents)	Pencil lead (graphite)
Calamine lotion	Perfumes*
Candles	Petroleum jelly (e.g., Vaseline)
Caps (for toy pistols)	Plaster (non-lead containing)
Chalk (calcium carbonate)	Play-Doh
Cigarettes (less than one)	Polaroid picture coating
Clay (modeling)	Porous tip ink marking pens
Colognes*	Prussian blue (ferricyanide)
Contraceptive pills (without iron)	Putty
Corticosteroids	Rouge
Crayons (marked A.P., C.P., C.S.-140)	Rubber cements
Dehumidifying packets (silica or charcoal)	Sachets (essential oils)
Detergents (phosphate type, anionic)	Shampoo (liquid)
Deodorants (spray and refrigerator)	Shaving creams
Elmer's glue	Soaps and soap products
Etch-A-Sketch	Spackles
Eye makeup	Suntan preparations
Fabric softener	Sweetening agents
Fertilizer	Teething rings
Fish bowl additives	Thermometers (mercury)
Fluoride—caries preventative	Toilet water*
Glues and pastes	Toothpaste (even fluoride)
Golf ball core (may cause mechanical injury)	Vitamins (even fluoride)
Grease	Warfarin (single dose)
Hair products (dyes, sprays, tonics)	Water colors
Hand lotions and creams	Zinc oxide
Indelible markers	Zirconium oxide
Ink (blue, black)	
Iodophor disinfectant	

*Depends on alcohol content.

TABLE 34. Opioids (Narcotic Opiates)

Drug	Equivalent Analgesia IM (mg)	Equivalent Analgesia Oral (mg)	Onset (min)	Peak Action (hr)	Elim. Half-Life (hr)	Duration (hr)	Potential Lethal Amount	Therapy
Alphaprodine (Nisentil)	40–60	—	—	—	2	1–2	—	—
Butorphanol (Stadol)	2	—	<10	0.5–1.0	3	2.5–3.5	—	IV, 0.5–2 mg/dose/4 hr; IM, 1–4 mg/dose every 3–4 hr
Camphorated tinture of opium (Paregoric)	—	25 ml	15–30	—	—	4–5	—	Oral, 0.25–0.5 ml/kg/dose (0.4 mg morphine/ml)
Codeine (various)	120	200	15–30	—	3	4–6	800	Oral, 0.5 mg/kg/dose; max 60 mg Toxic dose, >1 mg/kg Fatal dose, 5 mg/kg
Dextromethorphan* (various)	—	15	15–30	—	3–6	3–6	—	Oral, 0.25 mg/kg/dose Toxic dose, 10 mg/kg
Diacetylmorphine (Heroin)	5	60	—	—	0.5	3–4	100	Street heroin is usually less than 10% pure
Diphenoxylate (Lomotil)	—	10	120–240	Delayed by atropine	2.5	14 for active metabolite	300	—
Fentanyl (Sublimaze)	0.1–0.2	—	7–8	0.5	4–6	0.5–2	—	IV/IM, 0.001 mg (1 μg)/kg/dose to 0.1 mg max
Hydrocodone (Hycodan)	—	5–10	—	—	—	3–4	100	
Hydromorphone (Dilaudid)	1.5	6.0	15–30	0.5–1.5	2–3	2–4	100	Oral 1–2 mg/dose/4–6 hr
Loperamide (Imodium)	—	2–4	—	—	5–8	9–14	350	Oral 4 mg/dose 0.1 mg/kg/dose, max 16 mg/24 hr
Meperidine (Demerol)	50–100	75–100	10–45	0.5–1.0	2–5 12–16	3–4	1000	Oral 1–1.5 mg/kg/dose, max 100 mg Active metabolite normeperidine
Methadone (Dolophone)	10.0	20.0	30–60	2–4	22–97	4–12	120	Oral 0.10 mg/kg/dose, max 10 mg
Morphine (various)	10	60	15–60	0.3–1.5	2–3	3–4	200	Oral 0.10–0.20 mg/kg/dose, max 60 mg; IM max 10 mg
Nalbuphine (Nubain)	10.0	—	<15	0.5–1	3–4	3–4	—	IV/IM, 20 mg/dose
Opium tincture	—	7 ml	—	—	—	—	—	—
Oxycodone (Percodan, Tylox)	—	15	<30	—	3–4	3–4	—	Oral 5 mg/dose
Oxymorphone (Numorphan)	1	—	—	1	2–3	4–5	—	Dose, 1 mg IM
Pentazocine (Talwin)	—	30–60	15–60	1	2–6	3–4	—	Dose, >12 yr, max dose 50–100 mg
Propoxyphene* (Darvon)	—	65–100	30–60	2–4	8–24	2–4	500	Dose, >12 yr 65 mg Toxic dose, 10 mg/kg 35 mg/kg 100 mg of HCl salt = 65 mg napsylate salt

*Dose equivalent to 1 mg of IM morphine.

oxone, give respiratory supportive care. Administer fluids cautiously in an opioid overdose because opioids stimulate an antidiuretic hormone effect and pulmonary edema is frequent.

6. If the patient is agitated, consider hypoxia first rather than acute drug withdrawal.

7. Observe for withdrawal (nausea, vomiting, cramps, diarrhea, dilated pupils, rhinorrhea, piloerection). If these occur, stop naloxone.

Laboratory Studies. For drug abusers, consider testing for hepatitis B, syphilis, and (HIV) antibody. (Consent is usually required for HIV testing.)

Neonatal Withdrawal

Neonatal withdrawal mimics colic and usually occurs within the first 24 hours of life.

Management. Supportive care consists of swaddling; small, frequent feedings of a high calorie formula; parental education; and involvement in care.

Only 50 per cent of these newborns require pharmacologic

therapy. Indications for pharmacologic therapy include persistent vomiting, diarrhea resulting in excessive weight loss, failure to gain, dehydration, fever unrelated to infection or dehydration, and convulsions. Tremors and irritability are *not* indications and may persist for months.

The drug of choice is tincture of opium (USP without additives), diluted 25-fold to give equivalent of 0.4 mg/ml of morphine and is stable for only 2 weeks. The dose of the diluted preparation is the same as for paragoric: 0.2 ml orally every 3 to 4 hours and increased by 0.5 ml every 3 hours to a stabilizing dose (i.e., the infant sleeps, eats, and gains weight). Taper the stabilizing dose in 3 to 5 days.

Organochloride Insecticides (DDT Derivatives) (Table 35)

The three groups are:

1. Cyclodienes, used in termite control—chlordane, dieldrin, aldrin.
2. Chlorinated ethane derivatives of chlorophenothane (DDT), which are less acutely toxic than the cyclodienes.
3. Benzene hexachloride (BHC) isomers—lindane, kepone, mirex. These agents do not accumulate in body fat. They are used for centipedes, black widow spiders, and ticks and topically for scabies and lice.

Toxicity. Toxicity varies greatly. Lindane (Kwell) ingestion less than 5 ml in a child or less than 15 ml in an adult has not been associated with toxicity. Prolonged or excessively frequent topical application has been associated with seizures. These insecticides interfere with axon transmission of nerve impulses and produce CNS stimulation.

Kinetics. These agents resist degradation in human tissue and the environment. They accumulate in adipose tissue. Elimination is hepatic.

Manifestations. Manifestations usually develop within 1 to 2 hours, including CNS stimulation, convulsions, late respiratory depression, and increased myocardial irritability. Symptoms may last for 1 week or more. Chronic exposure may cause liver and kidney damage.

Management

1. Provide protective garb for personnel. Institute dermal decontamination procedures, remove contaminated clothing, and discard contaminated leather goods.
2. Institute GI decontamination procedures with AC.

Caution: Be careful with emesis because of rapid onset; do not use oils; many oils are dissolved in petroleum distillates, presenting an aspiration hazard.

3. Do not use adrenergic stimulants (epinephrine) because of myocardial irritability.
4. Cholestyramine (4 g every 8 hours) has been reported to increase the fecal excretion in chronic exposures.
5. Give anticonvulsants if needed.

Organophosphate Insecticides

Organophosphate insecticides (OPIs) are biodegradable cholinesterase inhibitors that may cause (1) irreversible inhibition of cholinesterase, either direct (TEPP) or delayed (parathion or malathion), or (2) reversible inhibition of cholinesterase (carbamates). Examples are presented in Table 36.

Toxicity. The mechanism of toxicity is the phosphorylation of acetylcholinesterase so that it loses its ability to function as an esterase to inactivate acetylcholine. Red blood cell acetylcholinesterase reduced to 25 per cent or less of normal laboratory control may indicate intoxication.

Kinetics. The onset of acute toxicity is usually before 12 hours unless the agents are absorbed by the dermal route or are lipid-soluble (fenthion), which may delay onset for 24 hours. Inhalation produces intoxication within minutes.

TABLE 35. Common Organochlorine Pesticides (DDT Derivatives)

Name	Toxicity Rating	Fatal Dose Adult	TLV (mg/m^3) (Skin)	Elimination Time	Comments
Endrin (Hexadrin)	Highest		0.1	Hours to days	Banned
Lindane (1% in Kwell; as insecticide, Benesan; Isotox; Gamene)	Moderate to high	10 g	0.5	Hours to days	Scabicide; general garden insecticide
Endosulfan (Thiodan)	Moderate		0.1	Hours to days	
Benzene hexachloride (BHC, HCH)	Moderate		0.5	Weeks to months	Banned, produces porphyria (cutanea tarda)
Dieldrin (Dieldrite)	High	3 g	0.2	Weeks to months	Banned 1974
Aldrin (Aldrite)	High	3 g	0.2	Weeks to months	Banned 1974
Chlordane (Chlordan) (10% is Heptachlor)	High	3 g	0.5	Weeks to months	Restricted 1979; termiticide
Toxaphene (Toxakil, Strobane-T)	High	2 g	0.5	Hours to days	
Heptachlor	Moderate		0.5	Weeks to months	Malignancy in rats; banned 1976
Chlorophenothane (DDT)	Moderate		0.1	Months to years	Banned 1972
Mirex	Moderate			Months to years	Banned; red anticide
Chlordecone (Kepone)	Moderate			Months to years	Tidewater, Va., contamination
Hexachlorobenzene	Low				
Methoxychlor (Marlate)	Low			Hours to days	
Ethylan (Perthane)	Low			Hours to days	
Dicofol (Kelthane)	Low	>1 g/kg		Hours to days	
Chlorobenzilate (Acaraben)	Low	600 mg/kg		Hours to days	Banned

High toxicity: LD_{50} <50 mg/kg; moderate toxicity, >50 mg/kg; low toxicity, >500–1000 mg/kg.
Abbreviations: TLV, time-limited volume skin notation.

TABLE 36. Examples of Common Organophosphate Insecticides (OPIs)

Common Name	Half-Life	Synonym	EFD* (g/70 kg)	LD_{50} mg/kg†
Agricultural Products (25–50% formulations, highly toxic; LD_{50} = 1–40 mg/kg)				1–40
Azinphosmethyl		Guthion	0.2	10.0
Chlortriphos		Calathion		
Demeton§		Systox		1.5
Disulfoton§		Di-Syston	0.2	12.0
Ethyl-nitrophenyl thiobenze		PO_4, EPN		
Melvinphos		Phosdrin	0.15	
Methamidophos		Monitor	Delayed neuropathy	
Monocrotophos		Azodrin		21.0
Octamethyldiphosphoramide		OMPA, Schradan		
Parathion		Thiophos	0.10	2.5
Phorate		Thimet		1.1
Terbufos		Counter		
Tetraethyl pyrophosphate		TEPP, Tetron	0.05	1.5
Animal Insecticides (moderately toxic; LD_{50} = 40–200 mg/kg)				
Chlorfenvinophos (tick dip)		Supona, Dermaton		
Coumaphos		Co-ral		
DEF		DeGreen		
Dichlorvos‡		DDVP, Vapona		46
Dimethoate	<24 hr	Cygon, De-fend		>500
Fenthion		Baytex	Long-acting	40
Ronnel		Korlan	10.0	
Leptophos		Phosvel		
Trichlorfon		Dylox		
Household and Garden Pest Control (1–2% formulations, low toxicity; LD_{50} = 200–1400 mg/kg)				
Acephate	1–6 days			>1000
Bromophos				>1000
Chlorpyrifos‖	27 hr	Losban, Dursban, Pyrinex		>500
Diazinon*	12 hr (rats)	Spectracide, Dimpylate	25.0	>400
Dichlorvos‖		DDVP, Vapona (plastic strip)		
Malathion	>92% <24 hr	Cythion	60.0	1375
Merphos			LD_{50}	>1000
Temephos		Abate		>2000

*Estimated fatal dose (g/70 kg); common lawn chemical as 14.3%.
†LD_{50} = dose that is fatal in 50% of animals.
‡Found in flea collars and No-pest strips.
§Most OPIs degrade in the environment in a few days to nontoxic radicals; those OPIs marked by § may be taken up by plants and fruits.
‖Classified as moderately toxic by some.

Manifestations. Garlic breath odor from gastric contents or a container may be a clue.

1. Early muscaric cholinergic crisis: cramps, diarrhea, excess secretion, bronchospasms, bradycardia. Mydriasis may occur early, miosis later.
2. Later, sympathetic and nicotine effects: twitching, fasciculations, weakness, tachycardia, hypertension, convulsions.
3. CNS effects: anxiety, headache, confusion, emotional lability, convulsion, coma.
4. Hypoglycemia or hyperglycemia.
5. Intermediate syndrome of respiratory paralysis. This phenomenon has occurred a few days after successful treatment and does not respond to the antidotes. Ventilatory support may be necessary.
6. Chronic delayed toxicity. This event clinically mimics Guillain-Barré syndrome and has been reported with merphos (Folex), fenthion (Baytex) in humans, and chloropyrifos (Dursban) in animals.
7. Intoxication. In children with intoxication, the scenario is usually house spraying; in a few hours, miosis, salivation, tachycardia, and seizures predominate.

Management

1. Administer basic life support to correct hypoxia (suction, 100 per cent oxygen, intubation, and ventilation). Institute dermal decontamination procedures. Provide protective garb for attending personnel. Continue to suction secretions until atropinization drying is achieved.
2. *If the diagnosis is probable, do not delay therapy while awaiting confirmation.* Atropine (antidote No. 7 in Table 9) is the cornerstone of acute therapy. *Give atropine after cyanosis is corrected because of the danger of atropine producing ventricular fibrillation in the hypoxic patient.* If the patient is symptomatic, adminster atropine every 5 to 10 minutes until drying of secretions and clear lungs. Atropine infusions have been used successfully by adding supplemental atropine to keep secre-

tions dried. Long periods of atropinization may be necessary. Maintain for 12 to 24 hours, then taper observing for relapse. Atropine is both a diagnostic and a therapeutic agent.

3. Give intravenous 2-pralidoxime (2-PAM, Protopam) after atropinization (antidote No. 36 in Table 9) as early as possible before the phosphate bond becomes stable. Its use may require reduction in the dose of atropine as the enzyme regenerates. It is not recommended in mild carbaryl (Sevin) cambamate type poisoning; however, some authorities suggest its use in life-threatening carbamate poisoning. The end point is absence of fasciculations and a return of muscle strength. Its effects are usually seen in ½ to 1 hour.

4. Do *not* use morphine, aminophylline, phenothiazine, reserpine-like drugs, or succinylcholine.

5. Do *not* administer atropine or pralidoxime prophylactically to workers exposed to organophosphate pesticides.

6. Give respiratory support for CNS depression if necessary.

Laboratory Studies. Obtain blood specimen for red blood cell (RBC) acetylcholinesterase values before giving pralidoxime. RBC levels are usually depressed more than 75 per cent for severe symptoms. Monitor acetylcholinesterase weekly.

Carbamates cause partially reversible carbamylation of cholinesterase. See Table 37. The major differences between carbamates and OPIs are as follows:

TABLE 37. Common Examples of Carbamates

Trade Name	Synonym	Half-Life
Pesticides		
Highly Toxic (LD_{50} < 50 mg/kg)		
Ziram		
Temik*	Aldicarb	
Vydate	Oxyamyl	
Isolan	Isolan	
Furadan	Carbofuran	
Zectran	Mexacarbate	
Mesurol	Methiocarb	
Snip fly band	Dimetilan	
Moderately Toxic (LD_{50} > 50 mg/kg)		
Matacil	Aminocarb, Carazol	
Baygon, Unden	Propoxypur	
Ficam	Bendiocarb	
Bux	Befencarb	
Lannate, Nudrin	Methomyl	
Carbamult	Promecarb	
Mesurol, Draza	Methiocarb	
Aphox, Rapid	Primicarb	
Mildly Toxic		
Sevin	Carbaryl	<24 hr (rats)
	Fenethcarb	
	Ambenonium	
	Benzpyrinium	
	Demercarium	
Cholinergic Medications		
Tensilon	Edrophonium	
Prostigmine	Neostigmine	
Antilirium	Physostigmine	
Mestinon	Pyridostigmine	

Modified from Bryson PD: Comprehensive Review in Toxicology. 2nd ed. New York, Raven Press, 1989.

*Some pesticides may be formulated in wood alcohol and have the added toxicity of methyl alcohol.

1. The toxicity of OPIs is less and of shorter duration.

2. OPIs rarely produce overt CNS effects because of poor penetration.

3. Cholinesterase returns to normal rapidly so that blood values are not useful in confirming diagnosis.

Paradichlorobenzene

Paradichlorobenzene is available as deodorant and diaper pail cakes and mothball nuggets, sometimes combined with naphthalene.

Toxicity. The toxic dose is 500 to 5000 mg/kg.

Kinetics. Elimination is hepatic.

Manifestations. Only one report has appeared in the literature of acute toxicity, that of methemoglobinemia and hemolysis developing in a 3-year-old boy. Large amounts may produce GI upset. No fatal cases of human poisoning have been reported.

Management. Institute GI decontamination procedures only if large amounts of OPIs have been ingested, such as an entire mothball or more than one bite of a cake deodorant. *Avoid* milk and oily foods for at least 2 hours after ingestion because they increase absorption.

Paraquat, Diquat

Paraquat is an herbicide rapidly inactivated in the soil by clay particles. Nonindustrial preparations of 0.2 per cent are unlikely to cause serious intoxications.

Toxicity. Commercial preparations, such as Gramoxone (20 per cent 10 ml), have produced death. Ingestion of 20 mg/kg results in vomiting and diarrhea; 20 to 40 mg/kg results in reversible renal failure and pulmonary fibrosis, with death in days to weeks; and more than 40 mg/kg results in multiple organ failure and death in days. Aerosol droplets are too large to produce systemic toxicity. Paraquat on marijuana leaves is pyrolyzed to nontoxic dipyridyl.

Kinetics. Less than 20 per cent of ingested dose is absorbed. The peak is 1 hour after ingestion. The lung concentrates paraquat. Elimination is renal. The mechanism of toxicity is the formation of superoxide radials that destroy the pulmonary cells, resulting in fibrosis.

Manifestations

1. There is a local corrosive effect on the skin and mucous membranes. Acute renal failure occurs in 48 hours (often reversible).

2. Pulmonary effects in 72 hours are progressive, and oxygen aggravates the pulmonary fibrosis.

3. Diquat does not produce effects on the lungs but produces convulsions and GI distention. Long-term exposure may result in cataracts.

Management

1. *Avoid* induction of emesis. Institute GI decontamination procedures by administration of an oral adsorbent, such as AC and a cathartic. Repeated doses of AC are recommended. Whole-bowel irrigation may be used but proof of its effectiveness is not available. Institute dermal and ocular decontamination procedures as needed.

2. Hemoperfusion with AC alone is the present choice; however, the results are still poor. Continue hemoperfusion until blood paraquat levels cannot be detected.

3. *Avoid* oxygen unless absolutely necessary because this aggravates fibrosis. Some use hypoxic air, FiO_2 10 to 20 per cent.

4. Corticosteroids may help to prevent adrenocortical necrosis and suppress superoxide ions. Dexamethasone (8 mg every 8 hours IV for 2 weeks, then orally 0.5 mg every 8

hours for 2 weeks) and cyclophosphamide (5 mg/kg daily IV in three doses to a maximum of 4 g in 2 weeks) reduced mortality in one series. No studies of effectiveness are available.

5. Sepsis often develops within 7 to 10 days after ingestion; treat appropriately.

Laboratory Studies. Blood levels above 2 μg/ml at 4 hours or above 0.1 μg/ml at 24 hours are fatal. Blood analysis and advice may be obtained from the Imperial Chemical Incorporated (ICI) America (Phone: 1–800–327–8633). Crude plasma concentrations and urine detection may be approximated by adding sodium dithionite. A blue-green color develops if paraquat is present. An early negative result should not be considered to be an exclusion of paraquat contamination; continue to test.

Phencyclidine (Angel Dust, PCP, Peace Pill, Hog)

This "drug of deceit" is substituted for many other hallucinogens. Intoxication by inhalation of PCP in a room where adults were smoking has been reported in children.

Toxicity. Phencyclidine is toxic if ingested, snorted, or smoked.

Kinetics. Phencyclidine is rapidly absorbed by all routes. Enterohepatic recirculation is noted. The onset of action, if it is smoked, is 2 to 5 minutes (peak in 15 to 30 minutes), if orally ingested, 30 to 60 minutes. The duration at low doses is 4 to 6 hours, and normality returns in 24 hours. At large overdoses, coma may last 6 to 10 days (waxes and wanes). The adverse manifestions of overdose usually occur within 1 to 2 hours. Elimination is hepatic.

Manifestations. There are sympathomimetic, cholinergic, and cerebellar signs, with early stimulation, later depression. Violent self-destructive behavior or paranoid schizophrenia may develop. Clues to diagnosis are usually miosis with bursts of horizontal, vertical, and rotary nystagmus and coma with the eyes open.

Management. Avoid overtreatment of mild intoxications.

1. Institute GI decontamination procedures. Emesis and gastric lavage may not be effective because phencyclidine is rapidly absorbed. Repeated doses of AC and nasogastric suction may help to remove the drug; recirculation is enterohepatic even if the drug is smoked or snorted.
2. Protect the patient and others from harm. "Talk-down" is usually ineffective. Provide a low sensory environment. Diazepam (Valium) may be used orally or intravenously in the uncooperative patient.
3. For behavioral disorders and toxic psychosis, give diazepam.
4. Control seizures and muscle spasm with diazepam.
5. For dystonia reaction, give diphenhydramine (Benadryl) intravenously (antidote No. 19 in Table 9).
6. For hyperthermia, provide external cooling.
7. For hypertensive crisis, give intravenous nitroprusside 0.3-2 μg/kg/minute. Maximum dose is 10 μg/kg/minute for no longer than 10 minutes.
8. Acid diuresis ion trapping with ammonium chloride (antidote No. 2 in Table 9) is not recommended because of rhabdomyolysis and the danger of myoglobin precipitation in renal tubules.
9. *Avoid* phenothiazines in the acute phase of intoxication because they lower the convulsive threshold. Later they may be needed later to treat psychosis.
10. If myoglobinemia is present, manage with fluid diuresis and alkalinization.

Laboratory Studies

1. Elevation of CPK is a clue to the amount of rhabdomyolysis occurring and myoglobinuria developing.
2. Test urine for myoglobin and pigmented casts.
3. Determine blood phencyclidine concentration and blood glucose levels (20 per cent of patients have hypoglycemia).
4. Test for PCP in gastric juice; values are 40 to 50 times higher than in blood.

Complications and Sequelae. Chronic brain syndrome, intracranial hemorrhage, malignant hyperthermia, schizophrenic paranoia and psychosis, and loss of memory for months may ensue. Delayed toxicity and "flashbacks" occur.

Phenothiazines and Other Major Neuroleptics

Phenothiazine (PTZ) and non-phenothiazine (NPTZ) neuroleptics have similar pharmacologic properties (Table 38).

Toxicity. The toxic dose for chlorpromazine is 20 mg/kg in children and 2 g in adults.

Kinetics. Variable by agent. The phenothiazines are eliminated by the hepatic route into many metabolites, some of which remain in the body longer than 6 months.

Manifestations

ACUTE POISONINGS. Major problems are respiratory depression, cardiac toxicity (quinidine-like), and neurogenic hypotension (antidopaminogenic).

1. Anticholinergic actions are dominant, but miosis, bradycardia and hypotension, hypothermia or hyperthermia and convulsions may also occur.
2. Quinidine-like, membrane-depressant effect on the heart produces depression of the myocardial contractility and impaired conduction. PTZ may produce life-threatening dysrhythmias, including torsades de pointes.
3. Impaired neuronal catecholamine re-uptake produces transient hypertension followed by severe hypotension. Peripheral α-adenergic blockade results in hypotension.
4. CNS stimulation or sedation results. PTZ lowers convulsive threshold and causes neurotransmitter imbalance to produce dystonic reactions or parkinsonian manifestations.

IDIOSYNCRATIC DYSTONIC REACTION. This may occur at therapeutic levels. It begins in 5 to 30 hours after the start of medication and consists of opisthotonos, torticollis, orolingual dyskinesia, akathisia, and oculogyric crisis (painful upward gaze).

MALIGNANT NEUROLEPTIC SYNDROME. This is characterized by hyperthermia, muscle rigidity, and autonomic dysfunction.

Management

1. Institute GI decontamination procedures. If symptoms are already present, some of these agents have antiemetic action, so lavage may be required.
2. Monitor EKG for dysrhythmias, and treat with antidysrhythmic agents.
3. Treat hypotension with positioning and fluid. Vasopressors are used if these fail. *Avoid β-adrenergic agents because of danger of provoking dysrhythmias.* If a pressor agent is needed, use norepinephrine. *Avoid* dopamine (Intropin) because PTZ drugs are antidopaminogenic.
4. Use physostigmine only as a last resort for life-threatening anticholinergic symptoms. *Remember*: Physostigmine produces seizure, and so do phenothiazines.
5. Treat hypothermia or hyperthermia with external physical measures (not antipyretic drugs).
6. Treat idiosyncratic dystonic reaction with diphenhydramine (Benadryl, antidote No. 19 in Table 9), or benztropine

TABLE 38. Pharmacokinetics of Volume Distribution Phenothiazines and Related Compounds

Medication	Metabolism	Dose Equivalent	Absorption	Volume Distribution (L/kg)	Half-Life (hr)	Therapy	Comment
I. ***Alipathic*** (moderate cardiotoxic and hypotensive effects; low sedation; moderate extrapyramidal effects; moderate anticholinergic effects)							
Chlorpromazine (Thorazine)	Hepatic	100 mg	Rapid	10–20	16–30	Oral Child, 2 mg/kg/24 hr max < 12 yr 75 mg/24 hr Adult, 200–2000 mg/24 hr	High sedation Preparations: Tab 10, 25, 50, 100, 200 mg SR caps 30, 75, 150, 300 mg Suppository 25, 100 mg Syrup 10 mg/5 ml, conc 100 mg/ml
Fluphenazine HCl (Prolixin)	Hepatic	2 mg	Rapid	2–12	6.8–9.6 days	Oral; adult 2.5–10 mg/24 hr	Injectible deconate salt Preparations: Tab 1, 2.5, 5, 10 mg Elixir 2.5 mg/ml, conc 5 mg/ml
Promethazine (Phenergan)	Hepatic	25 mg	Rapid	—	12	Oral Child, 0.1–0.5 mg/kg/dose Adult, 12.5–25 mg/dose (25–200 mg/24 hr)	Preparations: Tab 12.5, 25, 50 mg; Suppository 12.5, 25, 50 mg Syrup 6.25, 25 mg/5 ml
II. ***Piperazine*** (least cardiotoxicity and hypotensive effects; very high extrapyramidal effects; moderate anticholinergic effects)							
Prochlorperazine (Compazine)	Hepatic	15 mg	Slow	10–35	8–12	Oral Child, 0.1 mg/kg/dose (not <2 yr) Adult, 10 mg/dose	Preparations: Tab 5, 10, 25 mg Syrup 1 mg/ml
III. ***Piperidine*** (highest cardiotoxic and hypotensive effects; low extrapyramidal effects; high anticholinergic effects)							
Thioridazine (Mellaril)	Hepatic	100 mg	Slow	3.5	26–36	Oral Child, 1 mg/kg/24 hr (not <3 yr) Adult, 150–300 mg/24 hr	Preparations: Tab 10, 15, 25, 50, 100, 200 mg Suspension 25, 100 mg/5 ml, conc 30, 100 mg/ml
IV. ***Butyrophenone*** (low cardiotoxicity and hypotensive effects; low sedation; very high extrapyramidal effects; very low anticholinergic effects)							
Haloperidol (Haldol)	Hepatic	2–15 mg	Rapid	20–30	12–22	Oral Child, 0.1 mg/kg/24 hr Adult, 30–100 mg/24 hr	Preparations: Tab 0.5, 1.2, 5, 10, 20 mg Solution 2 mg/ml
Droperidol (Inapsine)	Hepatic	2.5–10 mg	NA	Large	2.2	IM/IV, 0.1–0.15 mg/kg/dose Adult, 2.5–10 mg/dose Injection, 2.5 mg/ml 2, 5, 10 ml	
V. ***Thioxanthene*** (low cardiotoxic and hypotensive effects, low sedation, high extrapyramidal effects, low anticholinergic effects)							
Thiothixene (Navane)	Hepatic	2 mg	NA	Large	34	Oral Child, 0.25 mg/kg/24 hr Adult, 16–60 mg/24 hr, max 60 mg	Preparations: Caps 1, 2, 5, 10, 20 mg Solution 5 mg/ml
VI. ***Dibenzorazepine*** (low cardiotoxic and hypotensive effects; low sedation; high extrapyramidal effects; low anticholinergic effects)							
Loxapine (Loxitane)	Hepatic	15 mg	NA	Large	3–4	Oral Adult, initially 10 mg twice a day, to max of 50 mg	Preparations: Caps 5, 10, 25, 50 mg Solution 25 mg/ml
VII. ***Dihydroindolones*** (low cardiotoxic and hypotensive effects; low sedation; high extrapyramidal effects; low anticholinergic effects)							
Molindone (Moban)	Hepatic	10 mg	Rapid	Large	1.5	Oral Adult, initially 50–75 mg/24 hr, increased up to 225 mg	Preparations: Tabs 5, 10, 25, 50, 100 mg Solution 20 mg/ml

*Peak levels mainly occur 1 to 4 hours after ingestion and have enterohepatic recirculation. The pharmacokinetics of most phenothiazines resemble those of chlorpromazine. See kinetics for details.

Abbreviations: Therap, therapeutic; Solution, liquid preparation; NA = not available.

(Cogentin), 1 to 2 mg intravenously slowly in adolescents. Continue these drugs orally for 2 to 3 days. This is not the treatment of overdose, only of this reaction.

7. Treat the malignant neuroleptic syndrome with dantrolene sodium or the dopamine agonist bromocriptine mesylate or amantadine. (See malignant hyperthermia under Monoamine Oxidase Inhibitors.)

Laboratory Studies. Two drops of 10 per cent ferric chloride to 1 ml of boiled urine may produce a purple color if there is a sufficient blood level. Non-phenothiazine neuroleptics give a negative test result. Salicylates as cause of purple color are excluded if concentrated sulfuric acid does not cause blanching of the color.

Pine Oil

Pine Sol (19.9 per cent pine oil; old preparation was 35 per cent pine oil) is the most commonly ingested household cleaner that results in hospitalization.

Toxicity. Death from ingestion of 15 ml of 100 per cent solution in a child is reported, although pine oil is alleged to be one fifth as toxic as turpentine.

Manifestations

1. *GI effects.* Odor of violets on the breath, irritation, and occasionally hematemesis.
2. *CNS effects.* Depression, weakness, lethargy, and respiratory depression.
3. *Renal effects.* Anuria.

Management

1. Refer the patient to a medical facility for supervised GI decontamination by AC. Several hours of observation is recommended in children who ingest 30 ml or more of a 20 per cent solution. Patients who ingest more concentrated solutions should be referred to a medical facility.
2. Provide supportive care.

Plants

See Table 39.

Propranolol and Beta-Blockers

These are antihypertensive, antianginal, antiglaucoma, and antimigraine agents. See Table 40.

Toxicity. More than 1 mg/kg of ingested propranolol or a single adult dose may be toxic in a small child and more than the maximum daily dose (propranolol, 480 mg) in an adolescent. These agents act as negative inotropic and chronotropic agents, although some are partial agonists. They also may impair glucose homeostasis, producing hypoglycemia.

Toxicokinetics. Elimination is hepatic for lipophilic agents and renal for hydrophilic agents. Duration is 24 to 48 hours; however, long half-lives prolong toxicity.

Manifestations. Bradycardia, hypotension, bronchospasm, apnea, and convulsions are noted. Hypoglycemia may occur in children. Fat-soluble drugs produce more CNS effects. Partial agonists may initially produce tachycardia and hypertension (pindolol). The EKG shows varying degrees of AV conduction delay or frank asystole.

Management

1. Institute GI decontamination procedures with AC. *Avoid* emesis because of apnea and seizures.
2. Treat hypoglycemia, hyperkalemia, and convulsions.
3. Monitor EKG for cardiovascular manifestations; if signs develop, *glucagon* reverses the negative inotropic effects more effectively than the chronotropic effects (antidote No. 26 in Table 9).
   a. *Bradycardia.* If the patient is hemodynamically unstable or second- or third-degree AV block develops, use glucagon. If there is no response, use atropine. *Caution: Isoproterenol may increase hypotension.* A pacemaker may be required if bradycardia is not easily managed by medication.
   b. *Ventricular tachycardia or serious premature venticular contractions.* Use lidocaine or phenytoin; use cardioversion if the patient is unstable or not easily managed by medication.
   c. *Myocardial depression and hypotension.* Correct dysrhythmias, positioning, and fluids. Hemodynamic monitoring may be required. *Avoid* quinidine, procainamide, and disopyramide (Norpace).
4. If bronchospasm is present, administer aminophylline.
5. Consider hemodialysis or hemoperfusion for unresponsive water-soluble agents, particularly if there is evidence of renal failure. Documentation of effectiveness is limited.

Quinidine and Quinine

These are antidysrhythmic and antimalarial agents.

Toxicity. The toxic dose of quinidine in a child is greater than 60 mg/kg; in an adult, 2 to 8 g. The quinine toxic dose is 15 mg/kg in a child and 1 g in an adult. Qinidine produces more cardiovascular damage, quinine more ocular damage.

Kinetics. The quinidine sulfate peak action is 2 to 4 hours; polygalacturonate, 5 to 6 hours; and gluconate, 3 to 4 hours. Sulfate half-life is 3 to 4 hours; gluconate half-life is 8 to 12 hours. Elimination is hepatic. Quinine kinetics are similar to those for quinidine.

Manifestations

1. Cinchonism (headache, nausea, vomiting, tinnitus, deafness, diplopia, dilated pupils), confusion, dementia, psychosis, and blindness.
2. Myocardial depression and dysrhythmias.
3. Skin rashes and flushing. Hemolysis may occur in patients with G-6-PD deficiency.
4. Respiratory depression, convulsions, coma, acidosis, and hypoglycemia.

Management. Obtain immediate cardiac consultation for electrophysiologic support of the heart with quinidine intoxication.

1. Institute GI decontamination procedures with repeated doses of AC, initially with a cathartic.
2. Monitor EKG. Antidysrhythmic drugs, a pacemaker, and alkalinization may be needed. Glucagon may be useful but has not been evaluated.
3. Acid diuresis is not recommended.

Laboratory Studies. Plasma quinidine above 8 μg/ml—cinchonism; above 14 μg/ml—cardiac toxicity.

Rodenticides

The three major categories of rodenticides in widespread use are anticoagulants (see Anticoagulants), phosphorus, and strychnine. Other rodenticides are available to exterminators, however. Previous purchases may expose children to outdated rodenticides. See Table 41.

Salicylates

Salicylates are NSAIDs with analgesic and antipyretic properties. Salicylic acid and methylsalicylate are used topically as keratolytic agents or rubifacient products. Salicylates act on cyclooxygenase to impair peripheral and central prostaglandin biosynthesis. See Table 42.

TABLE 39. Toxic Plant List*

Common Name/Latin Name	Toxic Class and Parts	Manifestations	Management
Akee (Blighia sapida)	Hypoglycin A: seed, unripe aril, rind	GI upset, hypoglycemia, acidosis biphasic course	S/S†, vigorous hypoglycemic therapy
Apple (Malus sylvestris)	Cyanogenic seeds	See *Cyanide*	
Apricot (Prunus armeniaca)	Cyanogenic seeds	See Cyanide text	
Arum family Caladium (Coladium) Dumbcane (Dieffenbachia) Elephant's Ear (Colocasia) Philodendrum (Philodendrum)	Oxalates insoluble: all parts	Mouth burning, GI upset, no systemic effects, airway obstruction	Rinse out mouth, cold pack to mouth
Atropa (Atropa belladonna)	Anticholinergic: all parts, especially black berries	See *Anticholinergic Agents*	
Autumn crocus (Colchicum autumnale)	Colchicine: all parts	GI upset, coma, convulsions, bone marrow depression	S/S, repeated doses of charcoal
Azalea (Rhododendron sp)	Grayanotoxin I: roots, leaves, honey from flower	GI upset, bradycardia, hypotension, paresthesias, ataxia, convulsions	S/S
Baneberry (Actea pachypoda)	Protoanemonin: all parts	Coumarin-like toxicity	See *Anticoagulants*
Black locust (Robina pseudoacacia)	Phylotoxin (Toxalbumin): seeds, shoots, bark	Delayed GI upset, 1–3 days, hemolysis, convulsions, renal failure	S/S, alkaline diuresis
Bleeding heart (Diecenta cucullaria)	Isoquinolone: all	Ataxia, convulsions	S/S
Bittersweet, European (Solanum duleanum)	Solanine: all	GI upset, bradycardia, diaphoresis, delayed anticholinergic	S/S
Buckeye (horsechestnut) (Aesculis sp)	Coumarin: nuts, twigs	See *Anticoagulants*	
Buckroot (Artium minus)	Anticholinergic	See *Antcholinergic Agents*	
Buttercup (Ranunculus)	See *Baneberry*		
Caladium (Caladium sp)	Oxalates: insoluble, all	See *Arum family* plants	
Castor bean (Ricinus communis)	Phylotoxin (Toxalbumin): bean	See *Black locust* plant	
Cassava bean (Manihot esculenla)	Cyanogenic: bean	See *Cyanide*	
Cherry, wild (Prunus sp)	Cyanogenic	See *Cyanide*	
Chinaberry tree (Melia azedarach)	Neurotoxin: seeds, berries, bark, flowers	GI upset, hallucinations, paresis, seizures, CP arrest	S/S
Christmas rose (Helleborus niger)	Digitalis, saponins, protoanemonim: all parts	GI upset, cardiac toxicity, coumarin-like toxicity	S/S See *Anticoagulants* and *Digitalis*
Climbing lily (Gloriosa superba)	Colchicine: bulb	See *Autumn crocus* plant	
Cocaine (Erythroxylon coca)	Cocaine alkaloid: leaves	See *Cocaine*	
Crowfoot	See *Buttercup*		
Daphne (Daphne mezereum)	Daphnetoxin, mezerein: all parts	GI upset, coumarin-like toxicity	See *Anticoagulants*
Death camas (Zygadenus venenosus)	Zygadenine: all parts	Burning in mouth, bradycardia, shock	S/S
Deadly nightshade (Atropa belladonna)	Anticholinergic: berry, leaves	See *Anticholinergic Agents*	
Dumbcane (Dieffenbachia sp)	Oxalates, insoluble: root, leaves	See *Arum family* plants	
Dutchman's breeches	Another name for bleeding heart		
Elderberry (Sambucus canadensis)	Cyanogenic: unripe berries, roots, leaves, bark	See *Cyanide*	
Elephant's Ear (Colocasia antiquorum)	Oxalates, insoluble: all parts	See *Arum family* plants	
English ivy (Hedera helix)	Hederin, saponin	Burning in throat, GI upset	S/S
Ergot (Clavipus purpura)	Ergot fungus on grains	GI upset, gangrene of limbs, convulsions, abortifacient	S/S, vasodilators, e.g., nitroprusside
False hellebore (Veratrum veride)	Veratrum: all parts	GI upset, hypotension, bradycardia, shock	S/S
Foxglove (Digitalis purpura)	Digitalis: all parts	See *Digitalis*	
Golden chain (Laburnum anagyrodes)	Nicotine: all parts	See *Nicotine*	
Green hellebore (Veratrum veride)	Veratrum	See *False hellebore* plant	
Heliotrope (Heliotropopum arborescens)	Pyrrolizidine: all parts	Hepatotoxic, GI upset, onset delayed up to weeks (carcinogenic)	S/S
Hemlock, poison (Conium maculatum)	Coniune alkoids, nicotine-like: all parts	Resp. paralysis, GI distress, convulsions	S/S, intensive care
Hemlock, water (Cicuta maculata)	Cicutoxin, strychnine-like: all parts	Convulsions	Anticonvulsants; see *Rodenticides*
Henbane (Hyoscyanus niger)	Anticholinergic: all parts	See *Anticholinergic Agents*	
Holly tree, bush (Ilex spp)	Ilicin: berries, leaves	GI upset	S/S
Horse nettle (Solanum carolinense)	Solanine	See *Bittersweet* plant	
Hyacinth (Hyacinth orientalis)	Narcissine: bulb	GI upset	S/S
Hydrangea (Hydrangea sp)	Cyanogenic: all parts	See *Cyanide*	
Indian tobacco (Lobelia inflata)	Lobeline	See *Nicotine*	S/S
Iris (Iris sp)	Irisin: all parts	GI upset	S/S
Ivy, English (Hedera helix)	See *English Ivy* plant		
Ivy, German (Senecio milinoides)	Pyrrolizdine: all parts	GI upset, hepatotoxic	S/S

TABLE 39. Toxic Plant List* *Continued*

Common Name/Latin Name	Toxic Class and Parts	Manifestations	Management
Ivy, ground (Nepeta hederacea)	Essential oils: all parts	Mucous membrane irritants, CNS depression or CNS stimulation	S/S
Jack in the pulpit (Arisaema triphyllum)	Oxalates: fruit, leaves, root	See *Arum family* plant	S/S
Jequirity bean (Abrus precatorius)	Abric acid (Toxalbumins): all parts, especially seeds	See *Black locust* plant	S/S
Jessamine, yellow (Gelseminum sempervirens)	Gelsemine, solanine: all parts	See *Bittersweet* plant. Gelsemine related to strychnine	
Jerusalem cherry (Solanum pseudocapsicum)	Solanine	See *Bittersweet* plant	
Jimson weed (Datura stramonium)	Anticholinergic: all parts	See *Anticholinergic Agents*	
Lantana (Lantana camara)	Lantanine	GI upset, muscle weakness, shock	S/S
Larkspur (Delphinium)	Diterpenoid: leaves, seeds	Onset in minutes, paralysis, bradycardia, seizures	S/S
Laurel, mountain (Kalmia latifolia)	Grayanotoxin I: all parts	See *Azalea* plant	
Lily of the valley (Convallaria majalis)	Digitalis: all parts	See *Digitalis*	
Lima beans (Phaseolus limensis)	Cyanogenic: raw bean	See *Cyanide*	
Marijuana (Cannabis sativa)	Cannabinol: all parts	See *Marijuana* in *Hallucinogens*	
Mayapple (Mandrake) (Podophyllum peltatum)	Podophyllum: leaves, stem, fruit	Severe GI upset, tachycardia, hypotension	S/S
Mistletoe (Phoradendron flavescens)	Unknown: all parts	Bradycardia, GI upset, shock, seizures	S/S
Monkshood (Aconite nappelus)	Aconite: all parts	Paralysis, cardiac dysrhythmias, ataxia, convulsions	S/S
Morning glory (Ipomea tricolor)	Unknown	See *LSD* in *Hallucinogens*	
Mountain laurel	See *Laurel, mountain*		
Nightshade, black (Solanum nigram)	Solanine	See *Bittersweet* plant	
Nightshade, climbing (Solanum dulcamara)	Solanine	See *Bittersweet* plant	
Nightshade, deadly	See *Deadly nightshade* plant		
Oleander (Nerium indicum)	Digitalis	See *Digitalis*	
Peach, pear tree (Prunus persica)	Cyanogenic: pit, leaves, sap	See *Cyanide*	
Pennyroyal oil (Mentha pulegium)	Essential oil, pyrrolizidine	Shock, seizures, hepatotoxic, abortifacient	S/S
Philodendron (Philodendron spp)	Oxalates, insoluble: all parts	See *Arum family* plant	
Poinsettia (Euphorbia pulcherrima)	All parts	Nontoxic unless very large amounts ingested, GI upset	
Pokeweed (Phytolacca americana)	Saponin, phytolacine: roots, berries, leaves	Severe gastroenteritis	S/S
Potato (Solanum tuberosum)	Solanine: sprouts, green tubers, vines	See *Bittersweet* plant	
Privet hedge (Ligustrum sp)	Andromedotoxin: seeds, berries, leaves	GI upset	S/S
Rhododendron (Rhododendron spp)	Grayanotoxin I: leaves, honey from flowers	See *Azalea* plant	
Rhubarb (Rheum rhaponticum)	Oxalates, soluble: leaves, root, stem if eaten raw	Tetany, renal damage, seizures	S/S, calcium
Rosary pea (Abrus precatorius)	Abric acid (Toxalbumins): seeds, stems, leaves	See *Black locust* plant	
Skunk cabbage (Veratrum californicum)	Oxalates, insoluble	See *Arum family* plant	
Star of Bethlehem (Ornithogalum umbellatum)	Cardiac glycoside	See *Digitalis*	
Sweet pea (Lathyrus odoratus)	Curare-like	Weakness, paralysis	S/S
Taxus (Taxus sp)	Taxine alkaloid: all except red aril	GI upset, bradycardia, hypotension, dysrhythmias	S/S
Thornberry (Datura stramonium)	Anticholinergic: all parts	See *Anticholinergic Agents*	
Tobacco (Nicotiana sp)	Nicotinic: all parts	See *Nicotine*	
Tomato (Lycopersicum esculentum)	Solanine: stem, leaves, green fruit	See *Bittersweet* plant	
Wandering Jew (Tradescantia sp)	All parts	Rash, blisters	S/S
Water hemlock	See *Hemlock, water*		
White snakeroot (Eupatorium urticaefolium)	Transmitted through milk	Tremors	S/S
Wisteria (Wisteria sp)	Unknown: seeds, pods, leaves	GI upset (severe)	S/S
Yew (Taxus sp)	See *Taxus*		

*Note: All victims who ingest plants should be observed for airway obstruction. Morbidity and mortality are low from most plant ingestions. The most severe manifestations are generally listed for these plants.

†S/S = Symptomatic and supportive care.

TABLE 40. Beta-Adrenergic Blockers

Agent	Solubility	Half-Life (hr)	Peak (hr)	Elimination	Specificity	Dose	Maximum Daily Dose
Atenolol (Tenormin)	Water	6–9	6–9	Renal	Beta-1	50 mg	200 mg
Labetalol (Normodyne)	Water	3–6		Hepatic	Alpha and beta	400 mg	1–2 g
Metoprolol (Lopressor)	Fat	3–4		Hepatic	Beta-1	50 mg	450 mg
Nadolol (Corgard)	Water	17–23	3–4	Renal	Beta-1	40 mg	320 mg
Oxprenolol (Traiscor)	Fat	1.5–3	1–2	Hepatic	0	80 mg	480 mg
Pindolol (Visken)	Fat	3–4	1¼	Hepatic	Partial agonist	20 mg	60 mg
Propranolol (Inderal)	Fat	2–3	1½	Hepatic	0	40 mg	480 mg
Timolol (Blocadren)	Fat	3	3	Hepatic	0	20 mg	60 mg

Salicylates are available in several forms:

- Aspirin tablets, 65 to 650 mg
- Chewable tablets, 81 mg
- Capsules, 325 mg
- Enteric-coated capsules, 325, 500 mg
- Enteric-coated tablets, 325 to 975 mg
- Slow-release tablets, 650, 800 mg
- Suppository, 60 to 1200 mg
- Liquids
  - Methylsalicylate, 1 ml = 1.4 g of salicylate
  - Pepto-Bismol, 130 mg of bismuth subsalicylate per tablespoonful, which is not completely hydrolyzed and yields 15 per cent less salicylate than aspirin (1 g = 1.19 g ASA), choline magnesium tricyclicate, 600 mg/5 ml.

Toxicity. See Table 43. The usual analgesic and antipyretic dose of acetylsalicylic acid (ASA) for adults is 650 mg per dose, for children 10-15 mg/kg per dose, every 4 to 6 hours or 40 to 60 mg/kg per 24 hours, maximum 80 mg/kg per 24 hours. The maximum single dose in adults is 1 g, and the maximum daily dose 4.0 g.

1. *Acute intoxication.* This occurs in adults from amounts above 10 g or 30 (325 mg) adult aspirins; in children, above 150 mg/kg, or approximately two 81-mg tablets per kilogram or one half of a 325-mg tablet per kilogram. Acute plasma concentrations over 300 μg/ml (30 mg/dl) are associated with toxicity.

2. *Methylsalicylate 98 to 99 per cent (oil of wintergreen).* One milliliter equals 1.4 g of salicylate, and one 5-ml teaspoonful equals 7 g of salicylate or 21.5 adult aspirins or 350 mg/kg for a 20-kg child (5 years of age).

3. *Acetylsalicylic acid.* Unlike other NSAIDs, acetylsalicylic acid produces irreversible interference with platelet function lasting the life of the cell (8 to 11 days). Salicylates without the acetyl group have no antiplatelet effect.

4. *Chronic intoxication.* Because of cumulative kinetics, this occurs when more than 100 mg/kg has been administered for 2 to 3 days.

5. *Bismuth subsalicylate.* Taking 17.5 mg/ml as 1.14 ml/kg every 4 hours, five times a day for 5 days has not produced serum salicylate levels greater than 7 mg/dl.

Kinetics

1. The *GI absorption* of regular ASA is complete and rapid in therapeutic doses. Aspirin is a weak acid with a pK_a of 3.5, (salicylic acid has a pK_a of 3.0). Although it is mostly nonionized in the stomach, it is poorly soluble in the acid gastric juice; therefore, most absorption occurs in the duodenum. In overdose, absorption may be delayed because large amounts interfere with gastric emptying by producing pylorospasm or possibly forming concretions. Absorption of enteric coated tablets is delayed and incomplete, and that of suppositories is slow and erratic. Methylsalicylate, which is highly viscous, is usually very rapidly absorbed but may be delayed for 6 to 8 hours.

2. The *onset of action* after ingestion is 30 minutes with peak in 60 to 120 minutes and a duration of 4 to 6 hours. The plasma concentration is significant in 30 minutes and peaks

TABLE 41. Toxicity of Rodenticides*

Agent†	Mechanism of Action	Manifestations	Onset	Management
Thallium PFD 12 mg/kg Gizmo Rat Killer	Combines with sulfhydryl groups. Interferes with oxidative phosphorylation	GI upset, alopecia, neuropathy, delirium, convulsions	12–24 hr delayed	Oral Prussian blue, hemoperfusion
Strychnine PFD 5 mg/kg El ROY Mouse Bait	Interferes with glycine inhibition of central nervous system	Convulsions	10–20 min	Anticonvulsants, neuromuscular blockers
ZN phosphide PFD 40 mg/kg Field Rat Powder	Releases phosphine gas	Fish breath odor, black vomitus, cardiac pulmonary edema, hepatorenal damage	2–3 hr	Milk, avoid water lavage
Yellow phosphorus PFD 1 mg/kg Yellow, waxy Blue Death Rat Killer	Local burns, hepatorenal damage	Garlic odor, luminescent vomitus and stools, cardiac toxicity, coma, "smoking stool syndrome"	1–2 hr	GI decontamination, anticonvulsants

*See also Anticoagulants.
†These agents are all highly toxic, with LD_{50} < 50 mg/kg. (LD_{50} is the dose that is fatal in 50% of animals.)

TABLE 42. Available Types of Salicylates

Generic Name	Trade Name	% Salicylate
Acetylsalicylic acid	ASA, Aspirin	75
Bismuth subsalicylate	Pepto-Bismol	37
Choline magnesium tricylicate	Arthropan	76
Choline salicylate		56
Homomethylsalicylate	Sunscreens	51
Magnesium salicylate	Mobidin	90
Methyl salicylate (topical)	Oil of wintergreen	89
Salicylic acid (topical)	Mediplast	98–99
Salsalate	Disalcid	96
Sodium salicylate	Many products	84

in 1 to 2 hours but may be delayed 6 hours or more in overdose and with enteric coated or sustained-release preparations or concretions. Peak blood levels occur 1 to 2 hours after ingestion of therapeutic doses.

3. *Vd* is 0.15 to 0.2 L/kg for ASA and 0.13 L/kg for salicylic acid (SA). The spinal fluid (CSF) concentrations may reach 1.5 times the blood level. The lower the blood pH, the higher the CSF concentration. In toxic concentrations, the Vd may be 0.6 L/kg because of increased saturation of protein-binding sites. In acidemia, nonionizable or diffusible salicylate increases and is distributed to the tissues. Salicylate (SA) passes into the breast milk and through the placenta. Mothers who have chronically ingested salicylates have produced intoxications of their neonates and nursing infants.

4. *Protein binding* is extensive, up to 80–90 per cent for salicylic acid mainly to albumin. As serum levels increase, protein binding decreases, sometimes to 50 per cent or less, and free salicylate and Vd increases.

5. *Metabolism.* ASA is rapidly hydrolyzed and deacetylated by plasma esterases to salicylic acid (salicylate), its active metabolite. Salicylate is metabolized in the liver, mainly by two saturable metabolic pathways with glycine and phenolic acid. At high doses, the metabolism follows Michaelis-Menton pharmacokinetics in overdose.

6. The *half-life* at therapeutic doses is 15 minutes for ASA and 2 to 3 hours for SA. The amount ingested increases the half-life; at 1000 mg, the half-life for SA is 5 to 6 hours; at 10,000 mg, the half-life is 20 hours. Chronic administration, as in arthritic conditions and in toxic overdose, lengthens the half-life considerably as a result of saturation of the enzymes for conjugation.

7. The *amount excreted* in the urine is influenced by the urine pH. At acid urine pH (<6.5), 10 per cent free salicylate is excreted; at alkaline urine pH (>7.5), ion trapping inhibits tubular reabsorption and 80 per cent may be excreted. A change of the urinary pH from 6.5 to 7.5 increases the salicylate excretion tenfold. In the kidneys, salicylate undergoes glomerular filtration, active secretion in the proximal tubules, and passive reabsorption in the distal tubules. When hepatic metabolism is saturated, urinary excretion becomes the sole route of salicylate elimination.

Mechanisms of the manifestations in toxicity include:

- Stimulation of CNS respiratory centers
- Inhibition of prostaglandin synthesis
- Uncoupling of oxidative phosphorylation
- Interference with the Krebs cycle
- Irreversible interference with platelet function
- Stimulation of lipolysis
- Bronchospasm

Manifestations

1. *Mild manifestations* are similar to "cinchonism" after an overdose of quinine, resulting in tinnitus (plasma SA 20 to 30 mg/dl or 200 to 300 μg/ml), vertigo, headache, and mental confusion.

2. In more severe intoxication, *vomiting* is usually present within 3 to 8 hours after ingestion of a single overdose.

3. *CNS manifestations* are tinnitus (may be present even at the higher therapeutic concentrations); hyperventilation; and, in severe intoxication, seizures and coma. Patients with convulsions need to be thoroughly investigated because the convulsions may be caused in salicylate intoxication by hypoglycemia, decreased ionized calcium with alkalosis, cerebral edema, intracranial hemorrhage, or hypoxia. Coma is much more common in chronic salicylism. *Altered consciousness is the most important sign of severe intoxication.*

4. *Hyperventilation* is also present early (usually within 3 to 8 hours at plasma concentrations greater than 40 mg/dl or 400 μg/ml) with respiratory alkalosis and later in compensation for metabolic acidosis. The lower the P_{CO_2}, the more serious the intoxication. P_{CO_2} of 10 to 20 torr indicates severe intoxication.

5. The validity of *fever* is difficult to assess if the patient has been ill. Hyperthermia in a previously healthy person with overdose is a sign of serious intoxication.

6. *Hemorrhagic manifestations* are rare (< 1 per cent). They are due to interference with platelet function for the life of the cell. In larger doses, salicylate decreases the production of prothrombin clotting factors II, VII, IX, X and factor VIII and increases capillary fragility. If hemorrhagic manifestations (< 1 per cent), other than GI bleeding, are present, serious intoxication and a plasma SA above 700 μg/ml are indicated.

7. *Metabolic disturbances.*

a. *Acid-base disturbances* in adults and older children usually consist of respiratory alkalosis for 12 to 24 hours with compensatory loss of sodium, potassium, and bicarbonate in the urine. The acutely mild and moderate adult intoxication does not usually progress to metabolic acidosis. The respira-

TABLE 43. Quantities of Aspirin Ingested: Deposition and Manifestations

Toxicity	Amount Ingested (mg/kg)	Toxicity Expected	Gastrointestinal Decontamination Site*	Manifestation Anticipated
Nontoxic	<150	No	No	None
Mild	150–200	Yes	Yes (ECF)	Vomiting, tinnitus, hyperventilation
Moderate	200–300	Yes	Yes (ECF)	Hyperpnea, lethargy, excitability
Severe	300–500	Yes	Yes (ECF)	Coma, convulsions
Very severe	>500	Yes	Yes (ECF)	Potentially fatal

*Intentional ingestions are always sent to an emergency care facility (ECF).
Note: Equation to approximate serum salicylate: mg/dl = dose (mg/0.2) (wt kg/10)

tory alkalosis may be blunted if there is CNS depression or if CNS depressants are ingested concomitantly. In children under 5 years of age, the initial respiratory alkalosis usually changes to metabolic or mixed metabolic acidosis and respiratory alkalosis within a few hours. Metabolic acidosis increases the severity of the salicylate intoxication by allowing for earlier and larger Vd.

b. *Alterations in glucose metabolism* may cause hyperglycemia early in the intoxication as a result of decreased tissue utilization and hypoglycemia late in the course of intoxication. Hypoglycemia occurs early in young children and in chronic salicylism when the glycogen stores are depleted.

c. *Dehydration and electrolyte disturbances* are due to hyperventilation, vomiting, compensation for metabolic disturbances, diaphoresis, and uncoupling of oxidative phosphorylation. Systemic acidemia increases cerebral salicylate levels.

8. Pulmonary edema is more frequent in adults older than 30 years of age. Cerebral edema also may occur in serious intoxications. The mechanisms are not clear, but they may be aggravated by fluid overload in alkaline forced diuresis.

9. *Chronic salicylism* is more serious than acute intoxication, and the salicylate plasma concentration does not correlate with the manifestations. The victims are often young children and elderly adults with therapeutic misadventures. A plasma concentration within the therapeutic range does not exclude chronic salicylism because the salicylates may have already been distributed to the tissues. Chronic salicylism is associated with exaggerated CNS findings, hypoglycemia, mixed acid-base derangements, hemorrhagic manifestations, renal failure, and pulmonary cerebral edema.

10. There is an association between salicylate administration with *Reye syndrome*. Aspirin may increase the risk of Reye syndrome following an acute febrile illness, especially with influenza and varicella. The FDA reports that no association between bismuth subsalicylate (Pepto-Bismol) and Reye syndrome; however, there is a warning on the package insert.

Management. *Do not wait for 6-hour salicylate levels to start treatment of symptomatic patients.*

1. Establish and maintain the vital functions.

2. Institute GI decontamination procedures if ingestion has been greater than 150 mg/kg or 10 g in adults. It may be useful up to 12 hours after ingestion because some factors delay absorption (food, slow-release or enteric-coated tablets, and other drugs); pylorospasm may delay gastric emptying; and concretions may form.

a. Induce emesis in the alert asymptomatic patient in the home if vigorous vomiting or hematemesis has not already occurred. Repeat doses of AC every 4 hours. The data on the effectiveness of repetitive AC are controversial.

b. Concretions and enteric-coated tablets may cause gastric perforation or late-rising plasma salicylate levels; removal may be required by vigorous lavage, whole-bowel irrigation, endoscopy, or gastrostomy. Monitor asymptomatic patients for at least 6 hours, longer if enteric-coated, slow-release preparations have been ingested or if presence of a bezoar is suspected.

3. Give intravenous fluid as an 0.9 per cent saline or Ringer's lactate solution as a bolus for shock in 5 minutes followed by 5 per cent albumin, if necessary. Give saline (0.45 per cent in 5 per cent glucose) in non-shock cases of dehydration as a fluid challenge 20 ml/kg, up 500 ml with 2 mEq/kg sodium bicarbonate (if not alkalotic) over 1 to 2 hours to correct fluid losses, establish urine flow, and achieve daily maintenance fluid. Prompt correction of acidosis is important.

a. Because of the danger of pulmonary and cerebral edema, there is controversy about whether to produce a *forced diuresis* or to just administer sufficient fluids to correct the deficit and achieve daily maintenance. Administer fluids for repair and maintenance and *avoid* diuresis. However, fluid loss may be extensive—up to 200 to 300 ml/kg. Carefully monitor for fluid overload.

b. Give *glucose* because cerebral hypoglycemia may occur in the presence of normoglycemia. Insulin is not necessary to treat the hyperglycemia that may be present.

4. As soon as the patient voids, add *potassium* (1 to 2 mEq/kg/day or 40 mEq/L—more than 40 mEq/L if the potassium is below 3.5 mEq/L). If rapid correction of potassium is necessary, administer potassium chloride (0.25 mEq/kg/hour up to 10 mEq/hour) with EKG monitoring for 2 hours and recheck potassium. An acid urine with alkaline blood profile indicates potassium depletion (more potassium, not alkali is needed). Potassium is essential to produce adequate alkalinization of the urine.

5. *Alkalinization* (antidote No. 39) enhances salicylate excretion and prevents transfer of salicylate to the tissues and the CNS. Give bicarbonate to keep blood pH 7.5 and urine pH ≥8.0. Monitor both urine and blood pH. Do not use the urine pH alone to assess the need for alkalinization. In general, 2 mEq/kg of sodium bicarbonate raises the blood pH 0.1 unit. Perform alkalinization if salicylate concentration is greater than 400 μg/ml (40 mg/dL) in acute poisoning and at lower levels in chronic intoxication. Patients with acidosis may require 2 to 3 mEq/kg of sodium bicarbonate as a loading dose followed by 2 mEq/kg every 3 to 4 hours as needed to keep urine pH above 7.0 and blood pH 7.45 to 7.50 after intravascular volume is established. The sodium bicarbonate is added to 5 per cent dextrose 10.2 per cent saline as 30 to 50 mEg/L. Additional bicarbonate is added as needed to correct pH values. *Caution*: Over-alkalinization may worsen hypokalemia, may precipitate tetany, and cause cardiac dysrhythmias. Too-rapid alkali administration may produce CNS paradoxical acidosis. Elevated urine pH may cause a false-positive dipstick urine protein value. *Avoid* acetazolamide, the carbonic anhydrase inhibitor, because it causes systemic metabolic acidosis as it alkalinizes the urine. Animal studies have shown increased mortality when this agent was used in treatment of salicylism; it enhances distribution of salicylate by causing systemic acidosis.

6. Patients with *pulmonary edema* may require hemodynamic monitoring and assisted ventilation with positive end-expiratory pressure. Treat fluid retention with furosemide (1 mg/kg IM) and fluid restriction.

7. Treat *hyperpyrexia* with external cooling, *not* antipyretics.

8. Treat abnormal bleeding or hypoprothrombinemia with aqueous water-soluble vitamin K_1 (10 to 50 mg IV, [antidote No. 38] at rate of 1 mg/minute). If prothrombin time has not decreased within 8 hours, repeat the dose. If overt bleeding occurs, fresh blood or platelet transfusion may be necessary.

9. *Dialysis*, preferably hemodialysis, or hemoperfusion (which does not correct electrolytes or acid-base disturbances) is indicated because it may reduce the half-life to 2–3 hours. *Consult a nephrologist if intoxication is severe.* The indications are:

a. Persistent, severe acidosis (pH <7.0) and lack of response to fluid and alkali therapy in 6 hours.

b. Persistent, severe electrolyte abnormalities and lack of response.

c. Serum salicylate level greater than 1200 μg/ml (120 mg/dl) at 6 hours after ingestion. Do *not* use the salicylate level as the sole criterion for dialysis; lower serum salicylate levels (such as 60 μg/ml) may be an indication for dialysis in chronic salicylism with altered mental status. Patients with high salicylate levels without complications do not need dialysis.

d. Coma or uncontrollable seizures, congestive heart failure (which limits alkalinization), pulmonary edema, cerebral edema, or acute renal failure.

e. Progressive deterioration despite good management.

10. *Chronic toxicity* is usually a more severe intoxication because of the cumulative pharmacokinetics of salicylates and increased tissue distributions so low plasma salicylate concentration may occur with severe poisoning.

11. Complications and indicators of severe poisoning include noncardiac pulmonary edema, hyperthermia, bleeding diathesis, tetany, and rhabdomyolysis.

Laboratory Studies

BLOOD. Monitor CBC, arterial blood gases, serum electrolytes, blood glucose, coagulation tests (platelets, prothrombin time, partial thromboplastin time), renal function, serial serum salicylate concentrations to determine that the salicylate is decreasing in a logical manner. In methylsalicylate exposure, it is suggested that serum salicylate levels be obtained in 2 hours and monitored every few hours after ingestion to determine the trend.

URINE. Monitor urine pH and urinalysis, urinary output, urine 10 per cent ferric chloride test.

LABORATORY ABNORMALITIES

Metabolic Acidosis. The metabolic acidosis of salicylism features a moderately elevated anion gap and, in significant intoxications, mixed respiratory alkalalosis and metabolic acidosis. Hyperglycemia or hypoglycemia may exist.

Salicylate Level. The severity of the poisoning is not assessed solely by the salicylate blood level. Salicylate blood levels may be very high during the first 6 to 12 hours without significant clinical or metabolic toxicity and slightly elevated or even at "therapeutic" blood levels with chronic intoxications or late in the course of severe acute overdose.

Serum salicylate values used in conjunction with the Done nomogram (Fig. 2) may be useful predictors of expected severity following *acute* single ingestions. In acute overdose, patients with a level lower than 350 μg/ml (35 mg/dl) are usually asymptomatic; at 350 to 700 μg/ml (35 to 70 mg/dl), they have mild to moderate symptoms; at 70 to 100 mg/dl (700 to 1000 μg/ml) they have severe symptoms; and above 1000 μg/ml (>100 mg/dl) results are potentially fatal. There is some question of the nomogram's predictive index for moderate and severe intoxication.

Single serum salicylate determinations are not sufficient to monitor a patient's condition because of delayed absorption from a bezoar or sustained-release or enteric-coated tablets. After large overdoses, the serum salicylate level may continue to rise for 12 hours because of inhibition of gastric emptying by pylorospasm.

The Done nomogram (Fig. 2) is *not* useful (1) in chronic intoxications, (2) in erratic or delayed absorption (such as in methyl salicylate, phenyl salicylate, or homomethyl salicylate ingestions or enteric-coated tablets), or (3) less than 6 hours after ingestion. The salicylate level for use in the Done nomogram should be obtained 6 hours post ingestion after the distribution phase of the medication. Before 6 hours, levels in the toxic range should be treated and levels below the toxic range should be repeated if a potentially toxic dose is ingested. Remember, if the patient is symptomatic, treat.

A delayed peak plasma salicylate concentration for 24 hours or failure of levels to decline may indicate the presence of concretions (tablet bezoar), timed-release tablets, or something delaying passage of the salicylate through the GI tract.

Ferric Chloride Test. Add 1 to 2 drops of ferric chloride 10 per cent solution to acidified urine. In 30 to 60 seconds a purple color develops if any salicylate has been present in the body for more than 30 minutes. The test is nonspecific and findings will be positive with aminoacidurias, acetoacetic acid, phenothiazines, and other products. The addition of concentrated sulfuric acid causes the color to blanch if it is due to phenothiazines; however, the color remains or intensifies if it is caused by salicylate.

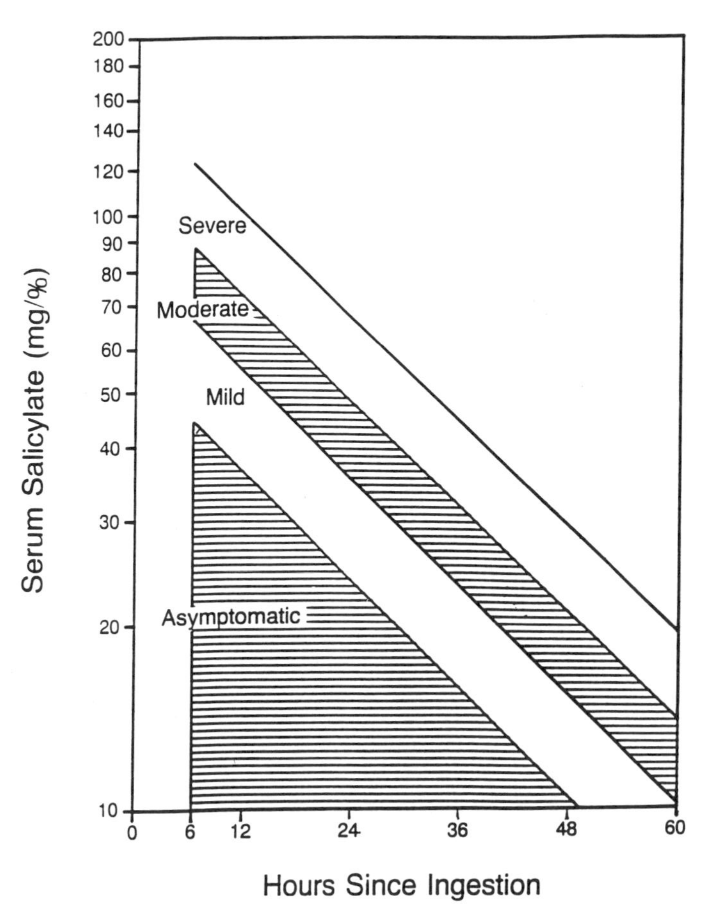

Figure 2. Done nomogram for salicylate poisoning. (Modified from Done AK: Salicylate intoxication: Significance of measurements of salicylate in blood in cases of acute ingestion. Pediatrics 26:800–807, 1960. Reproduced by permission of Pediatrics.)

Prognosis. Persistent vigorous treatment of salicylate ingestion is essential, as recovery has occurred despite decerebrate rigidity. The manifestations of serious intoxication are altered consciousness, metabolic acidosis, hyperthermia, hemorrhage, and low PCO_2. Death is usually due to pulmonary edema, cerebral edema, and cardiac dysfunction. These are more common with chronic intoxications.

Sedative-Hypnotics, Nonbarbiturate and Nonbenzodiazepine

Nonbarbiturate, nonbenzodiazepine sedative-hypnotics are more toxic than benzodiazepines. Overdoses of fivefold the therapeutic dose produce toxicity, and tenfold to 20-fold may be life-threatening. All of these agents have the capacity to cause CNS depression and prolonged coma. A combination of these agents with other CNS depressants makes them extremely toxic in small amounts.

Toxicity and Kinetics. See Table 44.

Management. Therapy is primarily supportive. *Avoid* emesis if rapid onset of convulsions, apnea, and coma has occurred. Concretions may form in the stomach and may require mechanical or surgical removal (meprobamate and glutethimide). Vasopressors may be preferable to large quantities of fluids

TABLE 44. Toxicity and Kinetics of Nonbarbiturate Sedative-Hypnotics

Drug	Absorption Toxic Dose (TD) Fatal Dose (FD)	Peak (hr)	Vd (L/kg)	Elimination Route	Half-Life (hr)	Toxic Blood Concentration (μg/ml)	Comments*
Chloral hydrate (Noctec) Therapeutic dose: 8 mg/kg child, 250 mg adult Onset 30–60 min	Rapid TD 2 g FD 4–10 g	1–2	0.6	Hepatic; active toxic trichloroethanol (TCE) metabolite	8–12	100 (TCE 80)	Pear-like odor, ventricular dysrhythmias, hepatotoxic, GI irritant, radiopaque capsules
Ethchlorvynol (Placidyl) Onset 15–30 min	Rapid TD 2.5 g FD 5.0 g	2–4	3–4	Hepatic 90%; lung elimination gives vinyl odor to breath	10–25 >100 in overdose	20–80	Prolonged coma (up to 200 hr), apnea, hypothermia, pulmonary edema, pink gastric contents, odor of vinyl shower curtain
Glutethimide (Doriden)	Slow TD 5 g FD 10 g or 150 mg/kg	6	10–12	Hepatic; active toxic 4-hydroxyglutanimide metabolite (?)	10	20–80	Prolonged coma cyclic (up to 120 hr), apnea, convulsions, anticholinergic signs, hyperthermia, coma
Meprobamate (Equanil, Miltown)	Rapid TD 10 g FD 12–40 g	4–8	10	Hepatic	6–16	30–100	Coma, convulsions, pulmonary edema, apnea, gastric concretions
Methaqualone (Quaaludes, "love drug")	Rapid TD 0.8 g	1–3	6	Hepatic	10–40	8–10	Hypertonia, hyperreflexia convulsions, apnea, bleeding tendency
Methyprylon (Noludar)	Rapid TD 3 g FD 8–20 g	2–4	1–2	Hepatic	3–6	30	Hyperactive coma (up to 30 hr), miosis, persistent hypotension, pulmonary edema, rare mortality

*Comments include other features besides the typical manifestations of all these agents: respiratory depression, hypotension, hypothermia (except glutethimide hyperthermia), psychological and physiologic withdrawal.

Abbreviations: TD, toxic dose; FD, fatal dose.

when pulmonary edema is anticipated. Consider hemoperfusion or hemodialysis in patients with severe intoxications who fail to respond.

CHLORAL HYDRATE. Institute GI decontamination procedures if more than 25 mg/kg or 1 g in adults has been ingested. *Avoid* emesis because of rapid onset. Activated charcoal with a cathartic is advised. Insert gastric tubes with caution because of corrosive action. *Avoid* use of catecholamines that may produce dysrhythmias. Hemodialysis and charcoal hemoperfusion may effectively remove the chloral hydrate and its metabolite in patients who fail to respond and who have potentially fatal plasma values of 250 μg/ml or greater. Toxic level is 100 μg/ml.

ETHCHLORVYNOL. Institute GI decontamination procedures up to several hours post ingestion. *Avoid* emesis induction because of rapid onset. Ethchlorvynol has a biphasic course as it redistributes from fat stores. Charcoal hemoperfusion is the method of extracorporeal removal when other measures fail in a life-threatening situation with ingestion of more than 10 g or 100 mg/kg and plasma level is over 100 μg/ml in the first 12 hours or 70 μg/ml after 12 hours. Toxic plasma level is 20 μg/ml or greater.

GLUTETHIMIDE. This agent carries the highest mortality of all nonbarbiturate sedative hypnotics. Institute GI decontamination procedures up to several hours post ingestion, but *avoid* emesis because of seizures, apnea, and coma. Repeated doses of AC may be useful for enterohepatic recirculation. The course is biphasic, as the agent redistributes from fat stores. Institute hemoperfusion in life-threatening, protracted coma when the patient has ingested over 5 to 10 g and has a plasma level above 30 μg/ml. Treat hyperthermia with external cooling.

MEPROBAMATE. Institute GI decontamination procedures up to several hours post ingestion. Failure to respond to supportive therapy, prolonged coma with life-threatening complications, or blood concentrations greater than 100 μg/ml require consideration of extracorporeal removal with charcoal hemoperfusion. Toxic blood level is 5 to 30 μg/ml; levels above 200 μg/ml are associated with more fatalities than survivals.

METHAQUALONE. This agent is no longer manufactured in the United States but is imported. Institute GI decontamination procedures. Forced diuresis, dialysis, and hemoperfusion are not indicated. Treat bleeding and convulsions.

METHYPRYLON. Institute GI decontamination procedures. The hypotension usually does not respond to position or fluids alone and may necessitate treatment with norepinephrine. This is a dialyzable drug, but dialysis is usually not necessary. Ingestions of more than 6 g or blood levels greater than 30 to 60 μg/ml have been associated with serious intoxications.

Stimulants

See Sympathomimetics.

Sulfonylurea Agents

The sulfonylureas are oral hypoglycemic agents (e.g., tolbutamide, acetohexamide, tolazamide, chlorpropamide, and second-generation glipizide and glyburide). See Table 45.

Toxicity. Hypoglycemia may occur with therapeutic doses.

Kinetics. Chlorpropamide has the longest half-life and is most commonly reported in accidental and suicidal hypoglycemia. It stimulates the release of insulin, inhibits the release of glucagon, and enhances the utilization of glucose by the peripheral tissues.

Manifestations. Alteration in consciousness, seizures and coma, gastrointestinal upset, inappropriate secretion of antidiuretic hormone (chlorpropamide and tolbutamide) occur. The hypoglycemia may persist for several days, particularly with chlorpropamide, glipizide, and glyburide.

Management

1. Institute GI decontamination procedures with repeated doses of AC; this has reduced the half-life of chlorpropamide.
2. If hypoglycemia is severe or if the patient is unconcious, immediately obtain venous blood for a glucose reagent strip test and laboratory analysis and administer an intravenous bolus of glucose (1.0 ml/kg 25 per cent to a child and 1 ml/kg 50 per cent to an adolescent. Also start an intravenous infusion of 10 per cent glucose and administer at a sufficient rate (10 mg/kg/minute or 0.1 ml/kg/minute of 10 per cent), with adjustments made to maintain a blood glucose level higher than 100 mg/dl. Do not stop the infusion abruptly because of the possibility of rebound hypoglycemia. Administer potas-

TABLE 45. Oral Hypoglycemics

	First-Generation				Second-Generation	
	Tolbutamide (Orinase)	*Acetohexamide (Dymelor)*	*Tolazamide (Tolinase)*	*Chlorpropamide (Diabinese)*	*Glipizide (Glucotrol)*	*Glyburide (Micronase, DiaBeta)*
Availability	250, 500 mg	250, 500 mg	100, 250, 500 mg	100, 250 mg	5, 10 mg	1.25, 2.5, 5 mg
Relative potency	1	2.5	5	5	100	150
Onset (min)	30	30	30	60	60	60
Duration of action (hr)	6–10	12–18	16–24	24–72	16–24	18–24
Half-life (hr)	3–25	3.5–11	7	24–48	2–4	1.36–1.59
Vd (L/kg)	0.1–0.15	0.21	—	0.09–0.27	0.16	0.13–0.57
Protein binding (%)	95–97 Ionic/nonionic	65–88 Ionic/nonionic	94 Ionic/nonionic	88–96 Ionic/nonionic	92–99 Nonionic	99 Nonionic
Metabolism	Hepatic	Hepatic	Hepatic	Hepatic	Hepatic	Hepatic
Metabolites	Inactive	1 Active	3 Inactive	Active and inactive	Inactive	Weakly active
		1 Inactive	3 Weakly active			
	Hydroxy* Carboxy§	Hydroxy† 4-Hydroxy§ Dihydroxy§	Hydroxy‡ Carboxy§ Others§	2-Hydroxy 3-Hydroxy Others§	3-Hydroxy§ 4-Hydroxy§ Others§	3-Hydroxy§ 4-Hydroxy§ Others§
Excreted unchanged	—	10	—	6–20	3–15	None
Diuretic	Yes	Yes	Yes	No	No	Yes
Antidiuretic	Yes?	No	No	Yes	No	No
Antabuse effect	No	No	No	Yes	No	No
Oral bioavailability	Complete	Complete	Complete	Complete	Complete	Complete
Peak plasma levels (hr)	3–6	—	6.8	2–4	1–3	2–8
Dose range (mg)	500–3000	250–1000	100–500	100–500	2.5–30	1.25–20
Frequency of severe hypoglycemia (%)	<1	<1	<1	4–6	2–4	4–6

*Weakly active.
†More active than parent.
‡Moderately active.
§Inactive.

TABLE 46. Sympathomimetics: Kinetics and Actions

	Therapeutic Dose (mg)	Toxic Dose (mg)	Onset (min)	Duration (hr)	Half-Life (hr)	Elimination Route
Phenyl-propanolamine (diet and decongestant over-the-counter drugs) (PPA)	37.5	>150 15 mg/kg	15–60	3	3–6	Renal
Ephedrine	30	>90	15–30	4–8	3–6	Renal
Pseudoephedrine (Sudafed)	60	180	15–30	4–8	7	Renal
Terbutaline (Brethine, Bricanyl)						
Oral	2.5–5.0		30–60	4–8	3	Hepatic
Metered	0.2/puff	NA	5–10	5		
Metaproterenol (Alupent, Metaprel)						
Oral	10–20		15–30	4		Hepatic
Metered	0.65/puff	NA	1–5	3		
Albuterol (Proventil, Ventolin)						
Oral	2–4		30	6–8	6.5	Hepatic
Metered	0.65/puff	NA		4–6		
Caffeine	100/cup	500–1000	15–30	3–4	3–10	Hepatic
Phenylephrine (Neo-Synephrine)	15	60 mg	1–5	3–6		
Imidozolines						
Naphazoline (Privine)			1–5	3–6		
Oxymetazoline (Afrin)			1–5	6–12		
Tetrahydrozoline (Tyzine)			1–5	3–6		
Xylometazoline (Otrivin)			1–5	6–12		

sium if there is likelihood of long-term infusion. Symptoms are usually easily reversed unless postictal depression is present.

3. Glucagon is of limited value.

4. In severe hyperinsulinemia, give diazoxide (Proglycem) (3 to 20 mg/kg/day up to 300 mg in 2 divided doses orally). The intravenous use is investigational.

5. Corticosteroids have no immediate effect.

6. Alkalinization of the urine with sodium bicarbonate reduces the half-life of chlorpropamide when hypoglycemia is produced.

7. Monitor until the blood glucose level has been normal for 24 hours on oral intake. Delayed, prolonged, or relapsing manifestations may occur even after apparent recovery.

Laboratory Studies. Capillary glucose reagent strips are inaccurate at low blood glucose concentrations and in shock.

Sympathomimetics

These drugs include the amphetamines, β-adrenergic agonists (isoethraine, metaproterenol, terbutaline, albuterol), catecholamines, cocaine, ephedrine, and phenylpropanolamine (PPA). Imidozolines are used in eye and nose preparations. See Table 46.

Manifestations. These include nausea, vomiting, hypertension, pallor, tachycardia (initially PPA produces a reflex bradycardia), dysrhythmias, CNS excitation, tremors, convulsions, and coma. Toxic psychosis, anginal pain, myocardial infarction, rhabdomyolysis, and intracranial hemorrhage have been reported sequelae with PPA. Imidazolines produce effects similar to those of clonidine. Hyperglycemia and hypokalemia may occur with β-agonists.

Management

1. Institute GI decontamination procedures for decongestants (ephedrine, pseudoephedrine, PPA). If the patient has ingested three to four times the daily therapeutic dose and is asymptomatic, watch the patient at home for symptoms. Any sign of toxicity precludes the induction of emesis. If amounts over four times the therapeutic daily dose have been ingested, institute GI decontamination procedures only if it can be immediately accomplished; evaluate these patients at a medical facility with blood pressure and cardiac monitoring for 4 to 6 hours.

a. Do *not* induce emesis for the imidazolines. The ingestion of 2.5 ml of 0.05 per cent tetrahydrazoline has resulted in respiratory depression. Give AC.

b. There are no data on agonists. If ingestion is above the therapeutic dose, medical evaluation and AC are recommended.

2. Control agitation and seizures with diazepam.

3. Treat dysrhythmias with appropriate antidysrhythmic agents.

4. For hypertensive crisis, give intravenous nitroprusside (antidote No. 33).

5. Acid diuresis is not recommended.
6. Naloxone (antidote No. 30) may be useful in treating imidozoline overdose.

Theophylline

Theophylline (1,3-dimethylxanthine) is widely used to relieve bronchospasm in asthma and neonatal apnea, and it is frequently involved in iatrogenic overdose.

Toxicity. Approximately 1 mg/kg of theophylline increases serum theophylline levels 2 μg/ml.

Kinetics. Peak levels occur within 1 hour after ingestion of liquid preparations, 1 to 3 hours after regular tablets, and 3 to 10 hours or longer after slow-release preparations. Half-life is 3.5 hours average in a child and 4.5 hours in an adolescent (3 to 9 hours). In neonates and young infants, the drug's half-life is much longer. Overdose increases the half-life. Elimination is hepatic. Factors that influence metabolism table are presented in Table 47.

Manifestations. Acute toxicity generally correlates with blood levels; chronic toxicity does not.

1. *Metabolic disturbances*: dehydration, metabolic acidosis, respiratory alkalosis, hypokalemia (diuretic action), hypophosphatemia, hypocalcemia, hyperglycemia, elevation of amylase and uric acid, rhabdomyolysis, and myoglobinuria.
2. *Slow-release versus Regular Preparations*: Few or no gastrointestinal symptoms are seen with high levels. Peak concentration times may be 10 to 24 hours post ingestion. Onset of seizures may occur 10 to 12 hours after ingestion.

Management. Chronic intoxication is more serious and more difficult to treat than acute intoxication.

1. Institute GI decontamination procedures in acute overdose, up to 4 hours with regular preparations and up to 8 to 12 hours with slow-release preparations. Test aspirate or vomitus for blood. Give AC initially with a cathartic, then repeat every 4 hours until the serum theophylline level is less than 20 μg/ml. *Avoid* inducing emesis (it interferes with charcoal administration). If there is intractable vomiting, use the antiemetic droperidol (2.5 mg IV every 6 to 8 hours for two doses [may cause extrapyramidal symptoms]) or ranitidine (50 mg IV [never cimetidine]).
2. Obtain theophylline levels every 4 hours until they fall below 20 μg/ml.
3. Control seizures with diazepam. If coma, convulsions, and vomiting exist together, intubate immediately.
4. Treat dysrhythmias with appropriate antidysrhythmic agents, but *avoid* nonselective beta-blockers in asthmatic patients because of bronchospasm (i.e., propranolol).
5. Treat hypotension with positioning and fluids; if attempts are unsuccessful in controlling hypotension use vasopressors. Correct fluid and metabolic disturbances.
6. Manage massive hematemesis with iced saline lavage and blood replacement if needed.
7. Consider charcoal hemoperfusion when:
   a. Complications are present.
      1. Seizures lasting more than 20 minutes despite adequate anticonvulsant therapy.
      2. Dysrhythmias are intractable.
   b. Serum theophylline concentration (STC) is known to be extremely dangerous (varies with age and health); the patient is symptomatic and oral AC cannot be retained.
      1. Acute intoxication: STC > 80 to 100 μg/ml.
      2. Chronic intoxication: STC > 40 μg/ml.
      3. Toxic concentrations with liver disease, chronic heart failure, viral disease, and constant fever.
   c. Good supportive medical management fails (Table 48).

TABLE 47. Factors That Increase Serum Theophylline Levels

Age and Disease	Medication, Substances
Under 6 months	Macrolid antimicrobials, e.g., erythromycin
Over 60 years	Oral contraceptives
Liver disease, heart failure	Cimetidine
Viral infections with respiratory syncytial virus	Beta-blockers
Pneumonia	Carbamazepine
Sustained fever >102°F	Caffeine

TABLE 48. Theophylline Toxicity

Plasma Concentration (μg/ml)	Toxicity	Manifestations
10 to 20	Mild	Therapeutic range, nausea, vomiting, insomnia, nervousness, and irritability.
20 to 40	Moderate	Gastrointestinal complaints and central nervous system stimulation, agitation, restlessness, and convulsions. Transient hypertension, hyperthermia, tachypnea.
Over 40	Severe	Convulsions and dysrhythmias may occur at lower levels and without gastrointestinal symptoms. Children tolerate higher serum levels.

Laboratory Studies. Monitor serial STC until a plateau is reached, especially in long-acting preparations.

Thyroid Preparations

Toxicity. See Table 49.

Kinetics. Elimination is hepatic.

Manifestations

1. CNS stimulation—fever, agitation, irritability, insomnia, convulsions.
2. Adrenergic—tachycardia, hypertension, cardiac dysrhthmias.
3. Nonspecific—vomiting, diarrhea, abdominal pain, flushing, fever.
4. Symptoms may last 2 weeks or longer.

Management

1. Repeat doses of AC for large ingestions or if symptoms occur because of enterohepatic recirculation.
2. Treat hyperactivity and insomnia with mild sedative.
3. Use beta-blockers (propranolol) to interfere with T_4 to T_3 conversion (0.5 to 1 mg/kg per 24 hours orally), and increase to control adverse manifestations, up to 2 mg/kg per 24 hours. Adolescent dose is 40 to 160 mg per 24 hours.
4. Control hyperthermia with external cooling.

Laboratory Studies. A thyroxine level at 6 hours post ingestion above 12 μg/ml suggests daily assessment for 10 days. The T_3 may not rise for 2 to 3 days.

Tricyclic and Cyclic Antidepressants

Tricyclic and cyclic antidepressants (TCADs) cause the greatest number of deaths in overdose.

Toxicity. The toxic dose of imipramine is 10 mg/kg in a

TABLE 49. Management of Children Ingesting Thyroid Preparations

Medication (Amount)	Equivalent	Treatment
Levothyroxine (T_4)	100 μg (0.1 mg)	
<2 mg		Home observation
2–4 mg		Emesis, home observation, observe contact for 10 days
>4 mg		Emesis, activated charcoal/cathartic; follow-up visits for 10 days, thyroid tests
> 7.5 mg		Thyroid tests
Triiodothyronine (T_3), any amount	25 μg	Emesis, activated charcoal/cathartic; hospitalize and monitor for 24 hr
Desiccated thyroid <600 mg	65 mg (1 gr)	Emesis, activated charcoal/cathartic; observe contact for 10 days

child; in adults, as little as 500 to 750 mg has been fatal. The following dosages of imipramine may serve as a general guide to the degree of toxicity, although the amount ingested may not correlate with toxicity (Table 50).

Kinetics. Onset varies from less than 1 hour to 6 hours after ingestion. Protein binding is high and decreases with decreasing pH. The half-life varies from 10 hours for imipramine to 100 hours for nortriptyline. In an overdose, the half-life may be much longer. Elimination is hepatic metabolism to active secondary amine metabolites, then by hydroxylation over several days to give rise to inactive metabolites. See Table 51.

Manifestations. Onset rarely occurs after 24 hours, although some suggest 6 hours post ingestion may be sufficient observation for toxicity. However, sudden death has infrequently been reported up to 6 days following ingestion. The phases of intoxication are as follows:

1. Initially, effects are anticholinergic: dry mouth, mydriasis, ataxia, increased deep tendon reflexes, hyperthermia, and tachycardia; CNS effects occur early, and seizures occur in 20 per cent, often just before cardiac arrest.
2. Coma with hypertension, tachycardia above 160 beats per minute, mydriasis, and supraventricular tachycardia.
3. Coma with hypotension, heart rate under 120 beats per minute, respiratory depression, tonic-clonic seizures, and ventricular dysrhythmias. Some studies have shown that EKG with a QRS greater than 0.1 second is associated with a major overdose and seizures and greater than 0.16 second is associated with life-threatening dysrhythmias and seizures.

In general, most antidepressants possess anticholinergic activity. The tricyclics produce dysrhythmic, hypotensive, and convulsant effects; the tetracyclics (amoxapine and maprotiline) are associated with severe convulsive effects that may result in rhabdomyolysis and renal dysfunction. The newer agents (trazadone and fluoxetine) appear to result in mild sedation and little cardiotoxicity, although orthostatic hypotension, vertigo, and priapism have been reported.

Management

1. In significant ingestions, continue intensive care until patients are asymptomatic and there are no EKG abnormalities for at least 24 hours (some studies suggest that 6 hours may be sufficient). If the patient is symptomatic, obtain cardiac consultation.
2. Institute GI decontamination procedures. *Avoid* emesis because of the rapid onset of convulsions and cardiotoxicity. Perform gastric lavage with caution and after correction of any dysrhythmia. Intact pills have been recovered up to 18 hours. Give AC initially with a cathartic, and repeat every 4 hours if bowel sounds are present.
3. At risk are the elderly, children, patients with preexisting heart disease, or patients showing sinus tachycardia or any other sign of overdose. *Any potential pediatric overdose should be examined, observed, and monitored for 24 hours.*
4. Monitor EKG, with the QRS measured periodically on a printout.
5. Control convulsions with intravenous diazepam.
6. Physostigmine is not recommended.
7. Cardiovascular effects (dysrhythmias, blocks, and hypotension) usually begin within 6 hours and are rare after 24 hours.

   a. Treat with alkalinization by sodium bicarbonate (antidote No. 39) over 10 to 15 minutes or by hyperventilation or both to a blood pH of 7.5. Alkalinization is believed to increase the protein binding of the cyclic antidepressants and the sodium ion may inhibit the TCAD effect on the rapid sodium channel. *Avoid* type Ia antidysrhythmics (procainamide, quinidine, disopyramide), β-adrenergic blockers, and physostigmine.

   b. Hypotension that fails to respond to positioning, intravenous fluids, and alkalinization is associated with significant mortality. Treat with norepinephrine. If norepinephrine fails, try inotropic agents (such as dobutamine).

   c. Hypertension may occur early and usually should not be treated.

   d. Manage bradydysrhythmias and serious conduction defects with phenytoin, which improves conduction; however, the usefulness of phenytoin needs further confirmation. A temporary transvenous pacemaker may be used in unresponsive second-degree and third-degree heart block. *Avoid* atropine.

   e. For ventricular tachycardia, use synchronized cardioversion if alkalinization, lidocaine (for one dose only), or phenytoin fails or if the patient is unstable.

   f. For supraventricular tachycardia with hemodynamic instability (shock, ischemic chest pain, hypotension, or pulmonary edema), employ immediate synchronized cardioversion (0.25 to 1.0 watt-seconds/kg) after sedation.

   g. Treat torsades de pointes with magnesium sulfate (2 g in adults or 25 to 50 mg/kg in children as a 20 per cent

TABLE 50. Imipramine Toxicity

Amount Ingested (mg/kg)	Manifestations
10	Light coma, mydriasis, and
20	tachycardia dysrhythmias, respiratory depression, convulsions; patients usually survive
30	Fatalities may result
50	High mortality rate
>70	Patients rarely survive

TABLE 51. Kinetics of Cyclic Antidepressants

Antidepressant	Absorption	Peak (hr)	Vd (L/kg)	Half-Life (hr)	Protein Binding (%)	Elimination	Toxic Level* (ng/ml)	Therapeutic Plasma Level	Comments
I. *Tricyclic Tertiary Amines* (metabolized to active metabolites)									
Amitriptyline (Elavil)	Slow	2–12	8–10	15–19	82–96	Hepatic	>500	50–250	Tab: 10, 25, 50, 75, 100, 150 mg Usual adult dose, 75–300 mg; child, 1.5–2.0 mg/kg/24 hr
Imipramine (Tofranil)	Rapid	1–2	5–20	8–16	76–96	Hepatic	>500	150–250	Tab: 10, 25, 50 mg Cap: 75, 100, 125, 150 mg Usual adult dose, 75–300 mg; child, 3–7 mg/kg/24 hr
Doxepin (Sinequan, Adapin)	Rapid, complete	2–4	20	15–19	95	Hepatic	>150	150–250	Cap: 25, 50, 75, 100, 150 mg Usual adult dose, 75–300 mg
II. *Tricyclic Secondary Amines* (metabolized to nonactive metabolites)									
Desipramine (Norpramin, Pertofrane)	Rapid, incomplete	4–6	28–60	18–28	73–92	Hepatic	>500	125–300	Tab: 10, 25, 50, 100, 150 mg Cap: 10, 50 mg Usual adult dose, 75–300 mg
Protriptyline (Vivactil)	—	—	—	—	—	Hepatic	NA	70–260	Tab: 5, 10 mg Usual adult dose, 20–60 mg
Nortriptyline (Aventyl)	Slow	7–8	21–57	50–150	93–95	Hepatic	>500	50–150	Cap: 10, 25, 75 mg Usual adult dose, 75–200 mg; child, 1.5–2.0 mg/kg/24 hr
Trimipramine (Surmontil)	Rapid	2	NA	NA	Large	Renal	—	100–200	Cap: 25, 50, 100 mg Usual adult dose, 75–300 mg
III. *Tetracyclic Dibenzoxazepines* (metabolized to major metabolites)									
Amoxapine (Asendin)	Rapid	1.5	Large	8–30	90	Renal and hepatic	NA	200–600	Tab: 25, 50, 100, 150 mg Usual adult dose, 150–600 mg
Maprotiline (Ludiomil)	—	8–24	22.6	27–58	88	Hepatic	>300	200–600	Tab: 25, 50, 75 mg Usual adult dose, 75–300 mg

Table continued on following page

TABLE 51. Kinetics of Cyclic Antidepressants *Continued*

Antidepressant	Absorption	Peak (hr)	Vd (L/kg)	Half-Life (hr)	Protein Binding (%)	Elimination	Toxic Level* (ng/ml)	Therapeutic Plasma Level	Comments
IV. *Triazolopyridines*									
Trazodone (Desyrel)	Rapid	0.5–2	NA	4–13	89–95	Hepatic	NA	800–1600	Tab: 50, 100, 150 mg Usual adult dose, 50–600 mg
V. *Unclassified or Bicyclics* (metabolized to active metabolites)									
Fluoxetine (Prozac)	Rapid	4–6	14–102	24–96	94	Hepatic	>400	NA	Cap: 20 mg Syrup: 20 mg/5 ml 4-ounce bottles
				5–7 days					Norfluoxetine active metabolite peak 76 hr Usual adult dose, 20–80 mg
VI. *Dibenzepin*									
Clomipramine (Anafranil)	Rapid	3–5	12	21 54–77	98	Hepatic	500	—	Cap: 25, 50, 75 mg Dimethylclomipramine (DM) primary active metabolite; available to psychiatrists free of charge to treat patients† Usual adult dose, 25 mg, increasing up to 150 mg 3 times daily
VII. *Aminoketone*									
Bupropion (Wellbutrin)	Rapid, 5–20% bioavailability	2	NA	8–24	80	Hepatic	NA	—	Tab: 75, 100 mg Several active metabolites relate to toxicity Usual adult dose, 100 mg twice a day, increasing up to 150 mg 3 times daily

*Toxic level = toxic serum concentration.
†Phone: 1-800-842-2422.
Source: Med Lett 30:102–104, 1988.
Abbreviations: NA, not available; Vd, volume distribution.

TABLE 52. Recommended Daily Allowances of Vitamins

	Unit	Infants 0–12 months	Children <4 years	Children >4 years and Adults	Pregnant and Lactating Females
Vitamin A	IU	1500	2500	5000	8000
Vitamin D	IU	400	400	400	400
Vitamin E	IU	5	10	30	30
Vitamin C	mg	35	40	60	60
Folic acid	mg	0.1	0.2	0.4	0.8
Thiamine	mg	0.5	1.7	1.5	1.7
Niacin	mg	6.0	9.0	15.0	20.0
Riboflavin	mg	0.6	0.8	1.7	2.0
Vitamin B_6	mg	0.4	0.7	2.0	2.5
Vitamin B_{12}	mg	2	3	6	8
Biotin	mg	0.05	0.15	0.30	0.30
Pantothenic acid	mg	3	5	10	10

Most commercial vitamins are in amounts not to exceed 150 per cent of the Recommended Daily Allowance.

TABLE 53. Toxic Doses of Vitamins

Vitamin	Dosage	Manifestations
Fat-Soluble		
A	Acute: >25,000 IU/kg per dose, child; 1.5 million IU units, adult.	Increased intracranial pressure in 8–12 hr; desquamation of skin, hepatosplenomegaly, stomatitis, bone pain in a few days.
	Chronic: >4000 IU/kg/day for 6–12 months, child; >25,000 IU/day for 8 months, adult; above 8000 IU/day in pregnancy is *not* recommended.	Increased intracranial pressure; bone pain; alopecia; hyperostosis; hypercalcemia; edema of lower limbs; scaly, orange discoloration of skin. X-rays of bones show cortical hyperostosis, pseudotumor cerebri may be sole manifestation; hepatitis and hypercalemia noted. Prolonged prothrombin times and epistaxis. Vitamin A is teratogenic.
D	10,000 IU/day for 4 months or 200,000 IU for 2 weeks, child; 60,000 IU for weeks to months, adults.	Hypercalcemia, muscle weakness, apathy, nausea, vomiting, diarrhea, bone pain, ectopic calcification, polyuria, hypertension, renal failure, nephrocalcinosis, cardiac dysrhythmias.
E	300–800 IU/day, adult.	Muscle weakness, headache, nausea, intestinal cramps, large doses antagonize vitamin K, hypertension. Intravenous preparations have resulted in death in premature newborns from benzyl alcohol preservative.
Water-Soluble		
B_6	2–6 g/day for >2 months, adult.	Reversible peripheral neuropathy. Perioral numbness, ataxia and clumsiness. Fetal-neonatal dependency and seizures.
C		Diarrhea and minor gastrointestinal upset. Uricosuria, potential for urinary oxalate stones, hemolysis in G-6-PD deficiency, rebound scurvy in neonates, decreased effectiveness of oral anticoagulants. Increased serum concentrations of estrogen. False-positive result for glucosuria and hematochezia.
Niacin	Acute: 100 mg, adult.	Flushing, burning of the face and upper trunk; 3 g increases uric acid and blood glucose and may produce hepatic damage. Hypotension and tachycardia, asthma, and pruritus—usually not serious.
	Chronic: >1–2 g/day.	Myopathies, myalgia, hepatic enzyme (>3 g/day), hepatotoxicity and cholestasis, ocular changes (>4–5 g/day), duodenal ulcers (>3 g/day). Niacin is diabetogenic.

TABLE 54. Regional Poison Control Centers in the United States*

State	Name	Phone Number
Alabama	Alabama	800–462–0800; 205–345–0600
	Children's Hospital	800–292–6678; 205–939–9201
Arizona	Arizona (Tucson)	602–626–6016
	Samaritan (Phoenix)	602–253–3334
California	Los Angeles County	213–484–5151
	San Diego	800–576–4766; 619–543–6000
	San Francisco	800–523–2222; 415–476–6600
	University of California, Sacramento	800–342–9293; 916–453–3692
Colorado	Rocky Mountain	800–332–3073; 303–629–1123
District of Columbia	National Capital	202–625–3333
Florida	Tampa Bay	800–282–3171; 813–253–4444
Georgia	Georgia	800–282–5846; 404–589–4400
Kentucky	Kosair Children's Hospital	800–722–5725; 502–589–8222
Louisiana	Louisiana	800–535–0525; 318–425–1524
Maryland	Maryland	800–492–2414; 301–528–7701
Massachusetts	Massachusetts	800–682–9211; 617–232–2120
Michigan	Blodgett Children's Hospital	800–632–2727; 616–774–7851
		800–462–6642; 313–745–5711
Minnesota	Hennepin Minnesota	612–347–3141
		800–222–1222; 612–221–2113
Missouri	Cardinal Glennon Children's Hospital	800–392–9111; 314–772–8300
Nebraska	Mid Plains	800–642–9999; 402–390–5400
New Jersey	New Jersey	800–962–1253; 201–923–0764
New Mexico	New Mexico	800–432–6866; 505–843–2551
New York	Long Island	516–542–2323
	New York City	212–340–4494
North Carolina	Duke University	800–672–1697; 919–681–4574
Ohio	Central	800–682–7625; 614–228–1323
	Southwest	800–872–5111; 513–538–5111
Oregon	Oregon	800–452–7165; 503–279–8968
Pennsylvania	Delaware Valley	215–386–2100
	Pittsburgh	412–681–6669
Rhode Island	Rhode Island	401–277–5727
Texas	North Texas	800–441–0040; 214–590–5000
	Texas State Houston	800–392–8548; 713–654–1701
	Austin	800–392–8548; 409–765–1420
Utah	Intermountain	800–662–0062; 801–581–2151
West Virginia	West Virginia	800–642–3625; 304–348–4211

*List of centers obtained from American Association of Poison Control Centers.

solution slowly over 2 minutes) and ventricular overdrive pacing to shorten the Q-T interval.

8. Observe serum potassium levels because the alkalinization may aggravate or precipitate hypokalemia.

9. Dialysis and hemoperfusion are not recommended.

Laboratory Studies. A blood level of 500 ng/ml is usually associated with toxic symptoms, and a value of 1000 ng/ml or greater is generally associated with serious toxicity and a QRS interval usually greater than 100 milliseconds.

Vitamins

Toxicity. The toxicity of vitamins is largely due to their iron content, which in chewable children's vitamins do not usually constitute a risk. Water-soluble vitamins are readily excreted by the kidneys, but fat-soluble vitamins are stored and are more likely to cause toxicity when taken in excess. The excessive doses are usually ten times the daily recommended allowance. In general, vitamins B, E, C, K and the minerals can be considered benign. Recommended intakes are presented in Table 52. Toxicity of vitamins are shown in Table 53.

Management

1. Institute GI decontamination procedures by emesis if more than 50 to 100 chewable children's multivitamins have been consumed. The fillers and the sugars in the vitamins act as a cathartic.

2. With vitamin D overdose, severe hypercalcemia can develop. Prescribe a low-calcium diet, calcitonin, prednisolone, mithramycin, and saline infusions. Monitor fluids, serum calcium levels, and EKG. Treat cardiac arrhythmias. Initiate dialysis if renal failure occurs.

3. Treat hypervitaminosis A, which may produce increased intracranial pressure, with mannitol and dexamethasone.

4. Monitor niacin overdose for hypotension, which may necessitate positioning and rarely fluids. Usually, symptoms resolve spontaneously in a few hours.

5. Discontinue vitamins, since they are stored in the body.

POISON CONTROL CENTERS

A list of poison control centers throughout the United States is presented in Table 54.

CHRONIC LEAD POISONING IN CHILDREN

HOWARD C. MOFENSON, M.D.
THOMAS R. CARACCIO, Pharm.D.
and JOHN W. GRAEF, M.D.

Although lead is a useful metal, it serves no useful purpose in the human body. Lead poisoning (plumbism) is usually chronic, occurring most often in children 6 months to 6 years of age who are exposed to the metal in the environment. Children are the barometer of environmental lead; they are at higher risk because of mouthing behavior (putting objects and hands into their mouths) and absorb more lead than adults because of their developing nervous system.

HISTORY AND THRESHOLD OF CONCERN

Lead poisoning was often lethal to children before the advent of chelation therapy after World War II. Today, lead poisoning most frequently occurs as a subtle condition characterized by elevation of the metal in the blood. This elevation is usually, but not always, accompanied by biochemical evidence of toxicity, such as derangement of heme synthesis.

Prior to 1960, venous blood lead concentrations (VBPb) of >60 μg/dl were considered to be of concern. This value was lowered to 25 μg/dl in 1985. In 1991, the Centers for Disease Control (CDC) in Atlanta and their advisors considered 10 μg/dl (0.483 μmol/L) to be the threshold for concern and promulgated new guidelines for defining childhood lead poisoning.

SCREENING

The screening schedule for lead exposure in 1991 was based on concern about irreversible neurologic developmental damage to infants and young children and the knowledge that children's blood lead levels increase rapidly at 6 to 12 months and peak at 18 to 24 months of age. Guidance regarding childhood prevention of lead poisoning and assessment of the risk of lead poisoning should be part of pediatric care. The CDC recommends that all children 6 months to 72 months be periodically screened for excessive lead exposure by blood lead determinations, with values of 10 μg/dl or greater to be reported to public health departments and followed up. In high-risk situations, this program should begin at 6 months of age. Priorities for lead screening are presented in Table 1; classification and recommended actions are given in Table 2.

In 1984 it was estimated that 17 per cent of all American children, or 3 to 4 million children, had blood lead levels in the neurotoxic range—above 15 μg/dl. About 74 per cent of the privately owned housing built prior to 1960 contained lead-based paint. Blood lead levels higher than 15 μg/dl for white children was 7 per cent in higher socioeconomic groups and 25 per cent in poorer communities; for black children in poverty, the prevalence was 55 per cent.

SOURCES OF LEAD EXPOSURE

Deteriorated lead-based paint, either directly or indirectly, is the major source of exposure to children. It contaminates both the soil and household dust, which are important contributors to childhood lead exposure. Lead contamination of drinking water from improperly soldered pipe joints or lead plumbing has received attention as another important source of lead exposure. Pediatricians should counsel parents on sources of lead.

TABLE 1. Priority Groups for Lead Screening

1. Children aged 6–72 months (was 12–36 months) who live in or are frequent visitors to older, deteriorated housing built before 1960.
2. Children aged 6–72 months who live in housing built prior to 1960 with recent, ongoing, or planned renovation or remodeling.
3. Children aged 6–72 months who are siblings, housemates, or playmates of children with known lead poisoning.
4. Children aged 6–72 months whose parents or other household members participate in a lead-related industry or hobby.
5. Children aged 6–72 months who live near active lead smelters, battery recycling plants, or other industries likely to result in atmospheric lead release.

Centers for Disease Control: Preventing Lead Poisoning Statement, October 1991, Public Health Service, p 95.

The upper safe limit of consumption of lead a day is believed to be 60 μg in adults or 5 μg/kg of body weight.

Housing and Paint

White house paint used freely in dwellings prior to 1955 contained as much as 50 per cent lead. About 70 per cent of the houses built prior to 1960 contained lead paint. In 1977, lead in indoor paint was further reduced to 0.06 per cent. Plaster does not contain lead, but lead seeps into it. A lead paint chip of 2 g (the size of a fifth fingernail) can contain 50 to 200 mg of lead. A chronic dose of 0.5 mg a day increases the body burden, 2.5 mg a day results in toxicity in a few years, and 3.5 mg a day causes toxicity in a few months. *"Yuppie lead poisoning" has occurred from renovation of older dwellings. Sanding and abrading lead in the process of renovation makes the lead that was sealed in paint immediately bioavailable. Safe lead removal is a vital part of any lead abatement program.*

TABLE 2. Recommended Actions in Childhood Lead Poisoning

Class	Venous Blood Lead Concentration (μg/dl)	Action
I	<9	1. Consider as low risk for high exposure 2. Rescreen periodically 3. Consider as high risk for high exposure 4. Rescreen more frequently
IIA	10–14	1. Rescreen every 3–4 months 2. If many children older than 10 years, utilize community intervention
IIB	15–19	1. Rescreen every 3 months 2. Take history to identify high-dose sources 3. Educate parents about cleaning 4. Test iron deficiency 5. Consider environmental investigation and lead hazard abatement if levels persist
III	20–44	1. Conduct medical evaluation 2. Identify and eliminate lead sources
IV	45–69	1. Begin medical treatment and environmental remediation within 48 hours
V	>70	1. Begin medical treatment and environmental assessment; remediation immediately

Centers for Disease Control: Preventing Lead Poisoning Statement, October 1991, Public Health Service, p. 95.

Soil and Dust

Lead is not biodegradable and is thus a long-term source of potential contamination. Traces of lead occur naturally in soil and dust at 50 parts per million (ppm). As the paint deteriorates or is improperly removed, the soil and house dust become contaminated. Soil within 25 meters of roadways, adjacent to houses painted exteriorly with lead paint, alongside smelters or industrial plants used in the manufacture of processed metals, storage batteries, artist paint pigments, and refineries is often highly contaminated (up to 60,000 ppm). The VBPb increases 3 to 7 μg/dl for each 1000 ppm increase in soil or dust lead. House dust may be controlled with wet mopping and cleaning with high-phosphate (5 to 8 per cent) detergents and placing grass or plant barriers alongside contaminated soil.

Drinking Water

Lead pipes were used in the 1920s; copper pipes soldered with lead were common in the 1950s. Acidic "soft" water (low mineral content of cations calcium and magnesium) may leach out lead, particularly when the water is hot. Lead is better absorbed from drinking water than from food. In 1992, the Environmental Protection Agency (EPA) goals for household drinking water from taps were to reduce lead levels from 50 ppm to 15 μg/L (ppb). It is estimated that 20 per cent of lead exposure comes from drinking water. To reduce lead intake, the water for drinking and making infant formula should be used only after cold water has been fully flushed by allowing it to run for at least 2 minutes.

Food

Acidic drinks (e.g., orange juice) that are stored in lead-soldered cans, antique pewter, or ceramic pottery containers may leach lead into the beverage. Lead-soldered cans comprised 1.6 per cent of cans in 1989, although imported cans may contain lead solder. The FDA Compliance Policy Guide 1988 set the limits for the amount of lead leached from ceramic foodware; however, foreign foodware that is not inspected may exceed these levels.

Urban garden plants may feature an elevated lead content if the soil, atmosphere, or water is high in lead content. Wine stored in crystal decanters elutes lead; red- and yellow-labeled plastic bread containers when used as lunch bags cause lead contamination of foods. Natural calcium supplements from animal bone contaminated with lead may be a source of toxicity.

Lead exposure in infants from inappropriate formula preparation has been described, including (1) first-drawn morning water in a lead plumbing circuit; (2) the extensive use of boiled tap water for 5 minutes, which increases the lead concentration; and (3) the use of lead vessels for boiling water.

Occupations and Hobbies

Workers in industries using lead may bring home lead dust on their clothes ("fouling the nest") (Table 3). Hobbies, such as casting ammunition, making lead fishing weights and lead toys, and lead glass art work may be sources of contamination.

"Remedies"

Traditional or ethnic folk remedies that contain lead include Mexican "azarcon por empacho" (lead tetraoxide), and "greta" (lead monoxide), Northern Laos "pay-loo-ah," and some Chinese herbal remedies. The names of other folk remedies containing lead are "alarcon," "alkohl," "Bali," "Goli," "coral," "ghassad," "liga," and "rheda."

TABLE 3. Occupations Associated with Lead Exposure

Lead production or smeltering	Demolition of ships and bridges
Production of illicit whiskey	Battery manufacturing
Brass, copper, and lead foundaries	Machining or grinding lead alloys
Radiator repair	Welding of old painted metals
Scrap handling	Thermal paint stripping of old buildings
Sanding of old paint	
Lead soldering	Ceramic glaze mixing
Cable stripping	
Instruction or maintenance at a firing range	

Modified from Rempel D: The lead exposed worker. JAMA 262:533, 1989. Copyright 1989, American Medical Association.

Retained Lead Foreign Bodies

There have been reports of lead poisoning from retained bullets and after ingestion and retention of a lead foreign body (curtain weights).

Other Sources of Lead

Childhood lead poisoning is a worldwide problem, and children coming to the United States from other countries should be assessed for lead.

NUTRITIONAL STATUS

Poor nutrition increases lead absorption. Nutritional status also plays a role, particularly iron, calcium, magnesium, and zinc deficiencies. Infants and young children absorb more lead than do adults and iron-deficient children may absorb as much as 40 per cent more lead than adults.

ENVIRONMENTAL LEAD EXPOSURE INQUIRY

A clinical history and environmental inquiry, although important, do not offer as much sensitivity for determining lead exposure as does a blood lead test. If the history suggests that exposure to lead has increased, a blood lead test should be performed (Table 4).

KINETICS

Absorption

Approximately 10 to 15 per cent of the ingested lead is absorbed in adults; in children up to 40 per cent may be

TABLE 4. Clinical History and Environmental Inquiry for Lead Poisoning

1. Behavior such as mouthing and pica of plaster, paint chips, dirt or dust, and window sills
2. Age and type of dwelling where child spends most of the day
   a. Live in or regularly visit a house with peeling paint built prior to 1960? This should include day care center or home of baby sitter.
   b. Live in or regularly visit house built prior to 1960 with recent or ongoing or planned renovation or remodeling?
   c. Live with another person being observed or treated for lead poisoning? (Venous blood lead concentration >15 μg/dl)
   d. Live with an adult whose job or hobby involves exposure to lead?
   e. Live near an industry likely to release lead?
3. Nutritional history, formula preparation, food containers.
4. Parents and other members of household, occupation, and hobbies.

absorbed, especially by those with iron deficiency. Absorption occurs by inhalation of organic particles, but inorganic lead particles are too large a percentage to be absorbed. Deficiencies of essential metals in the diet such as iron, calcium, zinc, and copper, and low-protein or high-fat diets enhance lead absorption.

Distribution

Lead is distributed in the blood, soft tissue, nervous tissue, and bone. In the blood, 95 per cent occurs on erythrocyte cell membranes. For a short time after absorption, lead is present in the soft tissues (kidney tubules, liver, testes, bone marrow) and probably the nervous system. Brain and liver lead concentrations are five to ten times those in blood. The final distribution is to teeth, hair, nails, and (95 per cent) bone as lead triphosphate, which is inert. The half-life in the blood is 27 to 30 days; in the bone, it is 10 years. Diet influences lead deposition. Calcium, phosphate, or vitamin D in the diet favors bone deposition, whereas parathyroid hormone, dihydrotachysterol, and acidosis mobilize lead from the bone. Lead enters human breast milk at 20 μg/dl blood lead, and 0.1 μg/g is present. It passes the placental barrier and reaches levels in the fetus almost equal to the maternal blood.

Metabolism

Organic lead is metabolized in the liver to inorganic lead.

Elimination

The total excretion of lead in the absence of poisoning is 9 per cent/day, or about 24 μg/day—8 μg by the fecal route and 16 μg in the urine. When increased absorption occurs, there is increased excretion; however, the increase is not of sufficient magnitude to compensate and lead accumulates.

MANIFESTATIONS IN CHILDREN

Ninety per cent of children are *asymptomatic* in the "classic" sense. Almost all children with a VBPb level below 50 μg/dl are asymptomatic. Symptoms are usually associated with a VBPb level above 70 μg/dl. If the VBPb level is less than 50 μg/dl, other causes for the symptoms should be sought.

Skeletal System

Bone metaphyseal "lead lines" are not really lead but indicate a period of arrested cartilage growth and are nonspecific. In children who have been immobilized for fractures or other reasons and who have a history of lead exposure, VBPb and erythrocyte protoporphyrin (EP) should be measured weekly.

Nervous System

Encephalopathy is seen at VBPb levels above 70 μg/dl blood lead test (BPb) or as a result of organic lead gasoline sniffing. It is more likely to occur in the summer months. The seizures are refractory to anticonvulsants. Signs of encephalopathy are persistent, forceful vomiting; ataxia; intermittent stupor and lucidity; coma; and convulsions. Even when encephalopathy is identified and promptly treated, severe and permanent brain damage results in 70 to 80 per cent of patients. Other nervous system disorders include cognitive deficits, neurobehavioral disorders, loss of a developmental skill, attention deficit syndrome, headaches, lethargy, and neurosensory deafness resulting in delays of language acquisition. Peripheral neuropathy is seen in adults but is rare in children.

TABLE 5. Timetable for Confirming Capillary Blood Lead Results with Venous Blood Lead Test

Blood Lead Level (μg/dl*)	Time of Confirmatory Blood Lead Test
<10	Not applicable
10–14	Not applicable
15–19	Within 1 month
20–44	Within 1 week
45–69	Within 48 hours
>70	Immediately

Centers for Disease Control: Preventing Lead Poisoning Statement, October 1991, Public Health Service, p. 95.

Hematopoietic System

Hypochromic, and normocytic or microcytic anemia, basophilic stippling in only 20 per cent (nonspecific), derangements in excretion of porphorins precursors in the urine. Sickle cell and iron deficiency anemias may coexist with lead intoxication. Eosinophilia from parasitic infection may be a clue to pica and lead poisoning. Lead toxicity may masquerade as sickle cell crisis.

Renal System

Renal damage and adult hypertension may result from childhood lead exposure.

Gastrointestinal System

Nausea, epigastric discomfort, anorexia, weight loss, abdominal cramps, constipation, colicky abdominal pain, and intestinal ileus may occur as a result of lead overexposure. Blue "lead" gum lines are rarely seen in children.

Reproductive System

Infertility and sterility, menstrual disorders, and, in severe cases, testicular atrophy may occur. Infants born to lead-contaminated mothers are of low birth weight, with intrauterine and postnatal growth failure, and may have neurobehavioral disorders. Sperm count and morphologic abnormalities occur at greater than 40 μg/dl (1.930 μmol/L).

In pregnancy, the cord blood lead level is 80 per cent of the maternal blood lead level. The development of children born with cord lead levels above 10 μg/dl has been found to lag behind controls. Mental retardation may occur at higher blood lead levels. The Occupational Safety and Health Administration (OSHA) standard for workers who intend to have children is below 30 μg/dl, but the safe threshold is unknown.

LABORATORY STUDIES

Blood Lead Test

The lead screening test is the blood lead test (BPb). A capillary fingerstick microlead specimen (CBPb), obtained by trained personnel using vigorous skin cleaning, and good blood flow or a venous blood specimen (VBPb) are the screening tests for lead. The risk classification is determined by the blood lead level (see Table 2). A positive CBPb greater than 9 μg/dl should be confirmed by a VBPb because of the possibility of contamination. The VBPb may vary by 4 to 6 μg/dl. The VBPb level reflects recent exposure during the past 3 to 4 months. The schedule for confirmation of results is presented in Table 5.

A VBPb specimen should be obtained using nonlead equipment for the collection. A lead-free blood collection kit or stainless steel needle with polypropylene shank, a syringe, and a purple top blood collection tube are used. The VBPb levels are within 4 to 6 μg/dl of target value. VBPb levels and their possible effects are listed in Table 6 (see also Table 2).

The VBPb influences the management: Surveillance of children should begin at VBPb of 10 μg/dl; management of individual children at 15 μg/dl; and medical work-up, developmental assessment, and management at 25 μg/dl or greater. See Tables 7 and 8.

Erythrocyte Protoporphyrin Test

The erythrocyte protoporphyrin (EP) tests are capillary samples not affected by contamination. These tests had been the most widely used for screening since 1970 but are no longer considered sensitive or specific enough to use as lead screening tests. The sensitivity of the EP test for VBPb above 25 μg/dl was 73 per cent and at 15 μg/dl it was reduced to 37 per cent. However, EP tests are useful in combination with the VBPb in determining the success of interventions and deciding on pharmacologic therapy. The EP reflects disturbance of heme synthesis that is reversible; however, brain damage may not be reversible. All elevated EP test results should be followed by VBPb testing to determine whether lead poisoning is responsible for the elevation.

MEDICAL WORK-UP

The medical work-up begins at a confirmed VBPb level of 20 μg/dl or greater.

History

Inquiry should be made regarding the nature of housing, pica behavior, use of folk remedies, imported ceramics, hobbies and parental occupations, nutritional status, dietary habits, family history of lead exposure, potential sources of exposure (including home renovation or remodeling) and previous lead measurements.

Physical Examination

Neurologic, psychosocial, language, and reading development is assessed. A neurobehavioral assessment is made in children receiving chelation shortly after the diagnosis and as the patient approaches entry into school. If abnormalities are found, the child is referred to appropriate programs.

Environmental Intervention

The local health department should be contacted. Referrals are made for appropriate environmental investigation and abatement of paint, dust, soil, and water at a VBPb level of 15 to 20 μg/dl. Environmental exposure includes places outside the home where a child spends time. The public health department should keep physicians informed about results of the investigation.

TABLE 6. Blood Lead Concentration and Potential Effects in Children

Blood Lead Concentration (μg/dl)	(μmol/L)	Effect in Children
8–15	0.4–0.5	Average urban resident
10–14.5	0.5–0.7	Intelligence score (IQ) changes
>15	0.72	Interferes with hemoglobin synthesis and neurobehavioral effects
>25	1.20	Neurobehavioral changes Subtle and minor symptoms
25–50	1.20–2.41	Renal abnormalities and decreased nerve conduction*
>55	2.64	Overt manifestations
50–70	2.41–3.34	Gastrointestinal symptoms, hematologic effects*
>70†	3.34	*Medical Emergency:* major symptoms; encephalopathy may develop

*In adults.

†There has not been a case of encephalopathy reported below a blood level of 70 μg/ml. Blood lead concentrations are subject to a 10–15 per cent variation in the space of 24 hours, or about ±5 μg/dl, depending on blood lead level.

TABLE 7. Screening Tests Based on Age and Environmental Questionnaire

Age: 6–36 Months

1. *Low risk for lead exposure:* Initial blood lead test at 12 months. If <10 μg/dl, retest at 24 months. If two consecutive values <10 or three <15 μg/dl, retest in a year. If 10–14 μg/dl, retest every 3–4 months. Any lead test above 15 μg/dl needs individual case management and retesting every 3 months.
2. *High risk for lead exposure:* Initial blood lead test at 6 months. If <10 μg/dl, rescreen every 6 months; otherwise procedure is same as for low-risk patient.

Age: 36–72 Months

1. *High risk:* Any child at high risk not previously tested should be tested. All children with blood lead values above 15 μg/dl should be screened once a year until 72 months or later. Rescreen any time history suggests increased exposure.

Iron Status

Iron deficiency can enhance lead absorption and toxicity; it often coexists with lead poisoning. If the VBPb level is above 20 μg/dl, serum ferritin levels are measured to check for iron deficiency. The other tests are not sufficiently sensitive, and the EP is not specific. Iron deficiency can occur in the absence of anemia. A ferritin value of less than 12 μg/dl indicates iron deficiency.

Treatment for iron deficiency should not be started until chelation therapy is completed. Iron should not be given with BAL* (nephrotoxic), $CaNa_2$ EDTA† (decreases effectiveness), or D-penicillamine. The dose of elemental iron to treat a deficiency is 6 mg/kg/day with 200 mg of vitamin C for each 30 mg of iron to enhance absorption.

Principles of Diet

For children with an increased lead body burden, the diet should be high in iron, zinc, calcium, magnesium, and copper and supplemented, if necessary. Fat, which promotes absorption and retention of lead after 2 years of age, should be limited. Storage of acidic foods in cans, pottery, and pewter (even certified) should be avoided.

Follow-up

Follow-up care by a lead center should be established if lead levels exceed 20 μg/dl.

Other Diagnostic Procedures

Many tests for the presence of lead that were done in the past are no longer necessary. Abdominal films are useful only in an acute ingestion; radiographs can indicate ingestion only 24 to 36 hours previously.

"Lead" lines on bone radiographs and basophilic stippling may be associated with chronic, high-level exposure (best seen in proximal fibula); however, they are not specific and can be negative in the presence of serious poisoning. They should not be obtained routinely in lead poisoning.

The testing of the fingernails and hair, which are exposed

*BAL = British antilenisite.

†$CaNa_2$ EDTA = Calcium disodium versenate or ethylene diaminetetraacetic acid.

TABLE 8. Therapy for the Child with Lead Poisoning

Class I

Blood lead level 9 μg/dl (0.434 μmol/L) or below

No action is necessary.

Class IIA

Venous blood lead level 10–14 μg/dl (0.483–0.675 μmol/L)

This level is an indication for surveillance. The recommended threshold of concern is a capillary or venous blood lead level of 10 μg/dl or greater in children. *This is a borderline indicator of recent absorption.* Some of these children may have a blood lead (BPb) level <10 μg/dl because variability of 4–6 μg/dl of the lead laboratory tests. It does not indicate increased body burden or excessive stores of lead in the body.

An environmental history, but not a full home inspection, is advisable. Follow-up determinations of BPb are recommended every 3–4 months. If two consecutive lead tests show <10 μg/dl, retest in a year. No special medical evaluation or developmental assessment is necessary. If large numbers of patients are found in this category, communitywide education, nutritional counseling, and environmental intervention campaigns are prudent. Early detection and control can prevent intellectual and behavioral disturbances.

Class IIB

Venous blood lead level 15–19 μg/dl (0.724 μmol/L)

Individual case management is recommended. A confirmatory venous blood lead level is determined within 1 month. If it is 15–19 μg/dl, take a careful environmental history concerning sources of lead exposure and offer guidance about interventions (control of paint, dust, water, and soil; nutritional counseling; renovation; occupational and hobby contamination) to reduce lead levels. Follow-up venous blood lead levels every 3–4 months are indicated. If a level of 15–19 μg/dl persists at two consecutive examinations at 3-month intervals, conduct environmental investigation and intervention if resources permit.

If three consecutive levels <15 μg/dl occur, retest annually. Ferritin levels should be ascertained to determine whether iron deficiency exists. No special medical evaluation or developmental assessment is necessary. Test other children in the dwelling.

Class III

Venous blood lead level 20–44 μg/dl (0.97–2.12 μmol/L)

This level warrants individual case management. Ascertain a confirmatory venous blood lead level within 1 week. If it is 20–44 μg/dl, the patient needs full medical evaluation and detailed environmental and behavioral history is indicated. Physical examination should include a neurologic examination and evaluation of language development. Tests (usually ferritin) should be done for iron deficiency. Refer the patient to lead center if a lead mobilization test (LMT) or chelation therapy is needed. The patient and family need educational, nutritional counseling and environmental investigation and interventions. Follow-up venous blood lead levels need to be determined within 3–4 months or more often as indicated. Test other children in the dwelling.

Some authorities perform an LMT to determine the need for chelation therapy. Calcium disodium versenate ($CaNa_2$ EDTA) pharmacologic therapy may be used if the LMT has a positive ratio >0.6. If chelation therapy is indicated, follow up every other week for 6–8 weeks, then monthly for 4–6 months. Developmental assessment is necessary.

Class IV

Venous blood lead level 45–69 μg/dl (2.12–3.33 μmol/L)

Individual case management is warranted. A confirmatory venous blood lead determination is needed within 48 hours. If the level is 45–69 μg/dl, the patient needs urgent medical care, including a medical evaluation with detailed history, physical examination, and test for iron deficiency. The patient needs pharmacologic therapy—either ($CaNa_2$ EDTA) parenterally or dimercaptosuccinic acid (DMSA) orally. Refer the patient to a lead center with a staff experienced in dealing with lead intoxication. The patient and family need education, nutritional counseling, and environmental investigation and intervention. Follow-up venous blood level testing is indicated every other week for 6–8 weeks, then monthly for 4–6 months and through at least one summer. Developmental assessment should be performed.

Class V

Venous blood lead level >70 μg/dl (>3.34 μmol/L)

Individual case management is warranted. A confirmatory venous blood lead level determination is required immediately. If the patient is asymptomatic and the level is >70–100 μg/dl, the patient requires emergent hospitalization and chelation initially with dimercaprol (BAL) and 4 hours later with combination of dimercaprol and $CaNa_2$ EDTA. A full medical evaluation, detailed history, and thorough physical examination (including neurologic) are in order. The patient and family need education, nutritional counseling, immediate environmental investigation, and intervention; tests (ferritin) for iron deficiency; and weekly follow-up venous blood lead tests. Developmental assessment should be performed until below 44 μg/dl.

Lead encephalopathy is almost always associated with blood lead concentrations >100 μg/dl, although it has been reported at levels as low as 70 μg/dl. Patients should receive BAL and $CaNa_2$ EDTA and should be managed by a multidisciplined team in intensive care unit.

Symptomatic lead poisoning without encephalopathy is usually associated with concentrations >70 μg/dl, although rarely it may occur with levels as low as 50 μg/dl. Patients should have intensive therapy with BAL and $CaNa_2$ EDTA and should be managed by a multidisciplined team in an intensive care unit.

to external environmental contamination, is not recommended.

A recent testing tool is the Line X-ray Fluorescent Ray (LXFR), which permits noninvasive assessment of metals in bone by measuring the energy emitted similar to that in atomic absorption. The LXFR predicts the outcome of the lead mobilization test (LMT) in most cases. L-line and K-line x-ray fluorescence can be used to measure the lead in the dwelling.

Lead Mobilization Test or Provocative Chelation Test

The LMT provides an index of the "mobile," or potentially toxic, fraction of the total body lead level. Some authorities do not use the LMT. The LMT is performed only in asymptomatic children with VBPb concentrations between 25 and 44 μg/dl to determine whether $CaNa_2$ EDTA chelation therapy is indicated.

Procedure

A baseline VBPb specimen is obtained. After the bladder is first emptied, $CaNa_2$ EDTA (500 mg/m^2 with 0.5 per cent procaine in equal parts [1:1] is administered deep IM or 500 mg/m^2 in 250 ml of D5W is infused over 1 to 2 hours IM. The urine (at least 100 ml) is collected for 8 hours in lead-free equipment, and the volume is carefully measured.

TABLE 9. Venous Lead Levels (VBPb) and Positive Lead Mobilization Test

VBPb (μg/dl)	Positive Test %
<25	4
25–34	35
35–44	76
>45	88

Interpretation

The ratio is determined by the equation

$$\frac{\text{micrograms } (\mu g/ml) \text{ lead excreted} \times \text{volume in milliliters}}{CaNa_2 \text{ EDTA administered in milligrams}}$$

The urine lead level is usually reported in micrograms per milliter by the laboratory and must be divided by 1000 to be used in the equation. A negative or low lead excretion ratio is below 0.6. If the ratio is above 0.6, a 5-day course of $CaNa_2$ EDTA is administered. If LMT results are negative, the VBPb is observed every 1 to 3 months; if elevation of lead persists, a second LMT can be performed. The test should not be done until the child is iron-replete because iron deficiency may affect the outcome of the test. The per cent of LMT-positive tests at various VBPb levels is presented in Table 9.

TREATMENT (Table 8)

Principles of Management

"Get the children out of lead, then get the lead out of the children":

- Remove lead from the environment
- Improve nutritional status

Pharmacotherapy

There are no controlled data showing that chelation has any value in reversing neurotoxic effects of lead; however, this procedure does reverse the symptoms of plumbism, the effect on hematopoietic enzymes, and the biosynthesis of vitamin D. Indications for chelation should include patient age, duration of exposure, and iron status. Chelation is not recommended if the VBPb level is below 25 μg/dl. Chelation does not alter neurotoxicity; abatement does.

Four pharmacologic chelating agents are available (Table 10). The risks of using chelating agents are mainly associated with excretion of essential minerals, particularly calcium and magnesium, and the metal zinc.

Dimercaprol (BAL)

BAL (100 mg/ml in peanut oil) should not be used with iron because it forms a BAL-metal (mercapturide) complex, which is nephrotoxic. BAL must be used with extreme caution in hepatic and renal impairment. It may precipitate glucose-6-phosphate (G-6-PD) deficiency hemolysis; therefore, it is administered only in life-threatening circumstances in these patients. BAL should not be used *in children who are allergic to peanuts or peanut butter.* Because the BAL complex breaks down in acid urine, one must attempt to keep the urine alkaline.

Side effects are experienced in 30 to 70 per cent. Fever occurs in more than 30 per cent of children. Nausea and vomiting may be severe.

Mechanism of Action. BAL is a dithiol, and two of its sulfhydryl molecules combine with one atom of the heavy metal to form a heterocyclic stable ring complex. It interacts extracellularly and intracellularly. Combined with $CaNa_2$ EDTA, BAL reduces the blood lead level by 50 per cent in 15 hours.

Administration. Indications for BAL include encephalopathy, a VBPb level above 100 μg/dl, or symptoms and a VBPb level above 70 μg/dl. BAL (75 mg/m^2 per dose) is given undiluted, deep IM, initially alone and followed in 4 hours by a combination of BAL, deep IM and $CaNa_2$ EDTA IM every 4 hours (not in same syringe) or by $CaNa_2$ EDTA IV infusion over 6 hours daily for 5 days.

Calcium Disodium Edetate

$CaNa_2$ EDTA (calcium disodium versenate), 200 mg/ml, should not be confused with sodium EDTA (disodium edetate), used to treat hypercalcemia, which can produce severe hypocalcemia and tetany. To be effective, $CaNa_2$ EDTA requires adequate renal function. It may aggravate symptoms when the VBPb level is above 70 μg/dl or if overt symptoms of lead poisoning are present. Therefore, one dose of BAL is given 4 hours before BAL-EDTA combination therapy.

Renal toxicity is a major adverse reaction. If acute renal disease not due to lead is present or if the patient is anuric, $CaNa_2$ EDTA is withheld.

Mechanism of Action. $CaNa_2$ EDTA is an extracellular chelator. The calcium is displaced by divalent and trivalent heavy metals, forming a soluble complex that is excreted in the urine. This chelator reduces the blood lead by about 50 per cent and increases the elimination of lead 20- to 50-fold. $CaNa_2$ EDTA is not metabolized, and its half-life is 20 to 30 minutes. A rebound is usually to 65 to 85 per cent of the previous pretreatment lead level and occurs within 2 weeks.

Administration. First, adequate urine flow must be established. The preferred route is intravenously. If the VBPb level is 45 to 69 μg/dl, the daily dose is 1000 mg/m^2, diluted to less than 0.5 per cent concentration, with 0.9 per cent saline or D5W and administered as a continuous infusion or in two divided doses through a heparin lock over 30 to 60 minutes. If $CaNa_2$ EDTA is administered intramuscularly, it is mixed with procaine to reduce the pain, so that the final concentration of procaine is 0.5 per cent. The mixture is administered for 5 days, and a second course is given if the VBPb rebounds to 45 μg/dl within 5 to 7 days after treatment.

TABLE 10. Chelating Agents Used in Treatment of Lead Poisoning in Children

Product Name	Generic Name	Chemical Name	Abbreviation
BAL* in oil	Dimercaprol	2,3-dimercapto-1-propranol	BAL
Calcium disodium versenate	Edetate disodium ethylenediamine calcium	Tetraacetate	$CaNa_2$ EDTA
Cupramine	D-Penicillamine	3-mercapto-D-valine	*d*-Penicillamine
Chemet	Succimer	Meso-2,3-dimercapto-succinic acid	DMSA

Centers for Disease Control: Preventing Lead Poisoning Statement, October 1991, Public Health Service, p 100.
*BAL, British antilewisite.

In general, a minimum of 5- to 7-day intervals is allowed between courses. The intramuscular injection is painful.

If the VBPb level is above 70 μg/dl (with or without symptoms), the daily dose is 1000 to 1500 mg/m²/day. A second course may be required if VBPb *rebounds* to about 45 μg/dl within 5 to 7 days after treatment. Some prefer to administer $CaNa_2$ EDTA IM in divided doses every 4 hours for 5 days to avoid excess fluid in encephalopathy. $CaNa_2$ EDTA is not administered IM in the same syringe as BAL.

Interactions. Corticosteroids increase nephrotoxicity, and $CaNa_2$ EDTA modifies the effect of zinc insulin. Iron should be stopped during therapy because it binds chelating sites and decreases effectiveness. Fluid intake and output, blood urea nitrogen (BUN), creatinine, liver transaminases (transient elevation), electrolyte levels (EDTA may cause hypokalemia and hypercalcemia), urine, serum calcium, and phosphorus are monitored before initial therapy and on the 3rd and 5th days. Proteinuria, hematuria, formed elements in the urine with rising BUN, and creatinine may signal renal failure. The infusion should be discontinued 1 hour prior to obtaining a VBPb specimen.

If the VBPb level is 25 to 44 μg/dl, the clinician may use the $CaNa_2$ EDTA LMT to determine whether chelation is necessary. Others use *d*-penicillamine treatment; still others use chelation only if the VBPb level is above 40 μg/dl.

D-Penicillamine

D-Penicillamine (dimethylcysteine, Cupramine, Depen Titratabs) is available in 125- and 250-mg caps and 250-mg tabs. *Do not administer to a patient with penicillin allergy.* It is considered investigational in lead poisoning by the U.S. Food and Drug Administration (FDA). Adverse reactions, including leukopenia (if the absolute neurophil count is below 1200/μl, discontinue), thrombocytopenia, angioneurotic edema, Steven-Johnson syndrome, and acute hemolysis, occur in 25 to 33 per cent of patients. The environment must be lead-free because penicillamine enhances the absorption of lead. Penicillamine is not recommended in the *acute* treatment of chronic lead poisoning but is used in long-term therapy if VBPb levels are 25 to 45 μg/dl; it is contraindicated in renal disease.

Mechanism of Action. The mechanism is not well defined, but penacillamine forms stable soluble complexes with heavy metals and enhances the urinary excretion of lead.

Administration. The patient should take penicillamine on an empty stomach, at least 1 hour before meals and on retiring for bed. The oral dose is initially 25 to 40 mg/kg per 24 hours, divided into four doses. The dose is increased 25 per cent as tolerated over 3 weeks (i.e., 25 per cent of the desired dose first week, 50 per cent the second week, and the full dose the third week. The maximum dose is 1 g per 24 hours. The entire course is 6 to 8 weeks, with blood lead levels observed every 2 to 4 weeks and monthly monitoring for renal and hematologic effects.

Meso-2,3-Dimercaptosuccinic Acid (DMSA)

Available in 100-mg capsules, DMSA is an *oral congener* of BAL. It has less effect on the essential metals, is less toxic, and is more effective than $CaNa_2$ EDTA. It has an unpleasant, mercaptan odor. It was approved by the FDA in 1991 for the treatment of lead poisoning in children (but not in adults) whose VBPb level was above 45 μg/dl. The environment must be lead-free, and the patient must be asymptomatic.

Mechanism of Action. DMSA forms water-soluble chelates and increases the urinary excretion of lead. It mobilizes lead from the soft tissue without redistribution. $CaNa_2$ EDTA redistributes lead to target organs (i.e., brain). In one study, the VBPb level fell an average of 78 per cent but rebounded to 60 per cent of original value. The VBPb level should be monitored weekly during and after therapy.

Toxicity. Massive animal overdoses (300 to 2400 mg/kg) have produced renal damage, pancreatic islet cell damage, gastrointestinal toxicity, renal failure, ataxia, convulsions, labored respirations, and death. DMSA is dialyzable. A few cases of reversible neutropenia have been reported.

Kinetics. The elimination half-life is 2 days. There is no effect on elimination of iron, calcium, or magnesium; however, zinc excretion doubles, although this is less than that of $CaNa_2$ EDTA.

Administration. All patients undergoing treatment should be adequately hydrated. The oral dose of DMSA is 10 mg/kg or 350 mg/m² every 8 hours for 5 days, followed by every 12 hours (two-thirds the initial dose) for an additional 2 weeks of therapy (total therapy 19 days). A minimum of 2 weeks' rest period between courses is recommended. Patients who have received $CaNa_2$ EDTA, with or without BAL, may use DSMA for subsequent treatment after an interval of 4 weeks' "washout." In young children, the capsule is opened and the medicated beads are sprinkled on a small amount of soft food.

Table 11 presents recommendations for pediatric dosing.

TABLE 11. Pediatric Dosing Chart

Pounds	Kilograms	Dose (mg)	No. of Capsules
18–35	8–15	100	1
36–55	16–23	200	2
56–75	24–34	300	3
76–100	35–44	400	4
>100	≥45	500	5

Severe Lead Poisoning with or without Lead Encephalopathy

Treatment is best given in a lead center with a pediatric intensive care unit. A multidisciplinary team effort, including critical care, toxicology, and careful monitoring of neurologic and fluid status, is required.

1. *Fluids.* Avoid oral intake if airway protective reflexes are compromised. Initiate a good urine flow with an IV fluid challenge of 20 ml/kg D10W over 30 to 60 minutes. Monitor urinary output with an indwelling catheter. Use mannitol (1 to 2 g/kg of a 20 per cent solution) to decrease the intracranial pressure, and attempt to establish renal flow. A urine specific gravity of 0.1010 is desirable. Subsequent fluid is limited to maintenance plus repair because of the danger of cerebral edema.
2. *Cerebral edema.* Use hyperventilation, elevation of the head 30 degrees, and mannitol. To reduce cerebral edema, *avoid* surgical decompression and/or corticosteroids.
3. *Bowel lead.* Therapy for removal of bowel lead.
4. *Chelation.* While waiting for adequate urine flow, administer BAL only. Start with 75 mg/m² deep IM; 4 hours later, start a combination of BAL (75 mg/m² every 4 hours, or 450 mg/m² per 24 hours) with IV infusion of EDTA (1500 mg/m² per 24 hours at 0.5 per cent or less concentration. If it is necessary to restrict fluid because of cerebral edema, give $CaNa_2$ EDTA IM every 4 hours. Treat for 5 days.
5. *Monitors.* Check fluids, renal, hepatic function, electrolytes, calcium, and phosphorus levels. Although reactions are rare, monitor the EKG when administering IV $CaNa_2$ EDTA in these circumstances. A computed tomographic (CT) scan of the head to detect cerebral edema and an x-ray of the abdomen to detect presence of lead are helpful.
6. *Second course of chelation.* A second course of chelation with $CaNa_2$ EDTA alone may be required if the VBPb level

rebounds to 45 μg/ml or greater within 5 to 7 days after treatment. (Some clinicians give a second course after a 3-day rest period if post-treatment VBPb levels are 35 μg/dl or greater.) Give the second course of $CaNa_2$ EDTA combined with BAL if the VBPb level is 70 μg/dl or greater. Wait at least 2 days before giving a second course. For second and subsequent courses, supplement with oral zinc acetate (5 mg) and copper acetate (0.5 mg three times a day).

7. *Third course of chelation.* Give a third course only if the VBPb level rebounds to 45 μg/dl or greater within 48 hours after the second course of treatment. Unless there are compelling reasons, wait at least 5 to 7 days before administering the third course.

8. *Renal failure.* Use chelators with dialysis.

9. *Seizures.* Give diazepam followed by phenytoin.

10. *Serial Blood Lead Measurements.* Obtain levels on days 3 and 5 and then weekly. Stop intravenous infusion at least 1 hour before obtaining blood lead specimens during chelation therapy. Determine the effectiveness of chelation and the need for rechelation therapy by follow-up VBPb concentrations. See Post-chelation Follow-up next.

POST-CHELATION FOLLOW-UP

At the end of each treatment cycle, VBPb levels decline. Within a few days, however, requilibration among the body compartments takes place and usually results in rebound. The blood must be checked weekly after therapy to determine whether re-treatment is necessary. In general, most children who undergo chelation therapy must be closely observed for a year or more. With enormous exposures to lead, it may take years to eliminate the metal. All children undergoing chelation treatment should be seen and VBPb levels checked weekly for a month, then every other week for 8 weeks, and then monthly for 12 months, depending on rebound lead levels. At each clinic visit, housing information must be updated. If history suggests exposure or if blood lead levels are rising, the dwelling must be reinspected. Dietary counseling should be reviewed. The source of exposure must always be identified prior to discharge from hospital. All cases should be reported to the health department.

REFERENCES

Agency for Toxic Substances and Disease Registry: The nature and extent of lead poisoning in children in the United States: A report to Congress. Atlanta, U.S. Department of Health and Human Services, 1988, 1990, 1992.

Centers for Disease Control: Preventing Lead Poisoning in Young Children. Atlanta, U.S. Department of Health and Human Services, 1991.

Graef J: Lead poisoning. Part I. Clin Toxicol Rev Vol 14, No. 8, May 1992.

Graef J: Lead poisoning management. Part II. Clin Toxicol Rev Vol 14, No. 9, June 1992.

Graef J: Lead poisoning. Part III. Therapeutic protocols. Clin Toxicol Rev Vol 14, No. 12, September 1992.

Markowitz ME, Rosen JF: Assessment of the lead stores in children: Validation of the 8-hour $CaNa_2$ EDTA provocation test. J Pediatr 104:337, 1984.

Piomelli S, Rosen JF, Chisolm J Jr, et al: Management of childhood lead poisoning. J Pediatr 105:523–532, 1984.

INSECT STINGS

GILBERT A. FRIDAY, JR., M.D.

Allergic reactions to insect stings range in severity from local inflammation to systemic anaphylaxis. Stings of insects of the order Hymenoptera (honeybee, yellow jacket, hornet, polistes wasp, and fire ant) affect nearly 3 per cent of children systemically. Systemic manifestations may be only pruritus, erythema, or urticaria; however, angioedema or life-threatening symptoms involving the respiratory tract and cardiovascular system, such as laryngeal edema, bronchospasm, and vascular collapse with possible cardiorespiratory arrest, can occur. Fortunately, fewer than 50 deaths from insect stings are recorded in the United States each year, only one or two of which are reported in children.

TREATMENT OF ANAPHYLAXIS[3] (Table 1)

Respirations and blood pressure should be carefully and rapidly assessed. The child is placed in recumbent position, and the lower extremities elevated. Epinephrine is injected subcutaneously. This may be repeated in 20 minutes if necessary. Epinephrine is often sufficient to terminate a reaction; however, one must be prepared to establish an airway if laryngeal edema is present. Supplemental oxygen may be necessary. Diphenhydramine or other antihistamines may be given to lessen urticaria or angioedema. Occasionally, further treatment of bronchospasm may be enhanced by the administration of aminophylline.

Late-phase reactions should be anticipated and prevented by the administration of corticosteroids. Severe reactions may require intravenous fluids and pressors to maintain the blood pressure.

TREATMENT OF LOCAL REACTIONS

For treatment of immediate immunoglobulin E (IgE)–mediated local reactions, ice and antihistamines should be included. To prevent (or, occasionally, to treat) the delayed hypersensitivity reactions (lymphocyte-mediated), a short course of prednisone (0.5 to 1 mg/kg/day) can be given and continued for 72 hours or longer to relieve discomfort, especially in those who have experienced such reactions previously.

PREVENTION

Avoiding Stings

Hives and nests near the home should be eliminated. Children should wear shoes when running in the grass. Stinging insects are attracted to brightly colored or flowered clothing. Children with a history of a previous sting should be dressed in a manner that will not attract stinging insects. Perfumes, sweet drinks, and foods also attract stinging insects and should be considered when children are playing outdoors.

TABLE 1. Treatment of Anaphylaxis

1. Assess rapidly.
2. Place patient in recumbent position and elevate lower extremities.
3. Inject epinephrine 1:1000 (0.01 ml/kg [maximum, 0.3–0.5 ml] subcutaneously q 20 minutes three times).
4. Establish airway; racemic epinephrine via nebulizer or endotracheal tube may be required.
5. Provide supplemental oxygen if needed.
6. Give diphenhydramine (0.5 to 1.0 mg/kg [maximum, 50 mg] p.o., IM, or IV over 3–5 minutes).
7. Establish venous line to maintain blood pressure with IV fluids (saline or volume expanders), pressors (dopamine hydrochloride, 2–5 μg/kg/minute; or norepinephrine bitartrate, 0.05 to 0.1 μg/minute).
8. Give aminophylline (5 mg/kg IV over 20 minutes; then 0.5–0.9 mg/kg/hour) for severe bronchospasm if blood pressure and pulse are stable.
9. Provide hydrocortisone succinate (5 mg/kg [maximum, 100 mg]) or methylprednisolone (1 mg/kg [maximum, 100 mg]) IV q 6 hours.

Identification

Children who have a known hypersensitivity to Hymenoptera should wear a bracelet or necklace indicating anaphylactic hypersensitivity.

Emergency Kits

Emergency epinephrine should be available for administration by the parent or responsible adult, or, in the case of an older child, self-administration. The emergency kits Ana-Kit and Ana-Guard (both distributed by Miles, Inc., Pharmaceutical Division, Allergy Products, Spokane, Wash.) contain a preloaded syringe that can deliver epinephrine doses of 0.3 ml or less. For those who fear needles, the EpiPen syringe (Center Laboratories, Port Washington, N.Y.) offers a recessed needle and a pressure-sensitive spring-loaded injection device. EpiPen delivers 0.3 mg (0.3 ml) of epinephrine 1:1000, and EpiPen Jr. delivers 0.15 mg 1:2000 (0.3 ml) IM.

Planning

When a child is stung, he or she should be carefully observed for signs of a systemic reaction. The first sign is usually itching, redness, and hives distant from the sting site. Epinephrine should be administered immediately, and the child transported to the nearest emergency facility. A single injection of epinephrine may be totally ineffective in reversing severe anaphylaxis, and the other measures noted in Table 1 may be best given in an emergency facility. Parents should be aware of available emergency facilities when traveling or on vacation.

Venom Immunotherapy

The treatment of patients allergic to insect stings with insect venom injections has been shown to be 97 per cent effective in reducing the risk of sting-induced anaphylaxis.[1] Fortunately, venom immunotherapy is unnecessary for most children who are allergic to insect stings (Table 2).[2] Large local reactions do not require immunotherapy but are lessened by immunotherapy. Only approximately 10 per cent of patients younger than 16 years of age with generalized cutaneous reactions have systemic reactions upon repeat stings, and there is no progression to a more severe reaction. However, those children who exhibit life-threatening, immediate respiratory and cardiovascular symptoms should be referred to an allergist for skin testing to identify the culprit (honeybee, yellow jacket, yellow hornet, white-faced hornet, or paper wasp). Fire-ant stings are not a diagnostic problem. Radioallergosorbent test (RAST) may be useful in detecting venom hypersensitivity in instances of questionable Hymenoptera sting reactions, although it is 20 per cent less sensitive than skin tests.

If a sting results in a life-threatening reaction and if venom testing results are positive, immunotherapy with the appropriate venom(s) is started immediately. Increasing amounts of venom are given weekly for several weeks (15+) until a dose of 100 μg (equals two stings) is reached. Maintenance injections are given at 4-week intervals the first year and every 6 weeks thereafter for approximately 5 years. Immunotherapy causes a decrease in the serum level of venom-specific IgE and IgG blocking antibody increases. The development of negative skin test or RAST results after immunotherapy suggests when therapy can be safely discontinued. If a child is stung during this time, epinephrine should be at hand but should not be given unless there are signs of anaphylaxis. Immunotherapy for fire-ant hypersensitivity can be accomplished by whole-bodied extracts rather than the venom, which is not commercially available.

TABLE 2. Selection of Children for Venom Skin Testing and Immunotherapy

Classification of Sting Reaction by History	Venom Skin Test	Venom Immunotherapy
Local	+/−	No
Large local	+/−	No
Systemic (<16 years)		
Life-threatening	+	Yes
Cutaneous alone	+/−	No
Toxic	+/−	No
Delayed (24 hours)	+/−	No

REFERENCES

1. Hunt KJ, Valentine MD, Sobotka A, et al: A controlled trial of immunotherapy in insect hypersensitivity. N Engl J Med 299:157–161, 1978.
2. Valentine MD, Schuberth KC, Kagey-Sobotka A, et al: The value of immunotherapy with venom in children with allergy to insect stings. N Engl J Med 323:1601–1603, 1990.
3. Morris FC. Anaphylaxis. *In* Levin DL, Morns FC (eds): Essentials of Pediatric Intensive Care. St. Louis, Quality Medical Publishing, 1990, p 103.

ARTHROPOD BITES AND STINGS

BERNARD COHEN, M.D.

Arthropod bites and stings are a major cause of morbidity in infants and children and account for 65 per cent of all deaths from venomous animals in the United States. These ubiquitous organisms are elongated invertebrates with segmented bodies, true appendages, and chitinous exoskeletons. Arthropods of importance to physicians include millipedes and centipedes, eight-legged arachnids (scorpions, spiders, ticks, and mites), and six-legged insects (lice, blister beetles, bedbugs, bees, wasps, ants, fleas, moths, butterflies, flies, and mosquitoes).

MILLIPEDES (DIPLOPODA) AND CENTIPEDES (CHILOPODA)

Although superficially similar, millipedes are vegetarian feeders whereas centipedes are carnivorous. When handled, millipedes exude a defensive fluid, which may produce immediate burning, erythema, and edema that progresses to vesicles, bullae, and erosions.

Although all centipedes contain poison glands and some bites result in severe systemic symptoms, in the United States, reactions to envenomation are limited to a transient sharp pain at the site.

Treatment. Irritant reactions and bites can be treated with cool tap water compresses or topical steroids. In severe reactions, prednisone (1 mg/kg/day tapered over 10 to 14 days) can be used.

ARACHNIDS

Arthropods of this class are recognized by their fused cephalothorax and four pairs of legs. Medically important orders include scorpions, spiders, ticks, and mites.

Scorpions

Scorpions are nocturnal tropical arachnids and are readily identified by their stout pinching claws, elongated abdomen, and narrow tail, which ends in a conspicuous bulb-like stinger that it swings over the head to attack prey. Poisonous species in North America are restricted to the deserts of the American Southwest and Mexico. They remain hidden in garages, basements, closets, crevices, and gravel. When accidentally provoked, they will bite, producing a hemolytic reaction consisting of localized burning, swelling, purpura, necrosis, and lymphadenitis. Occasionally, a more severe neurotoxic reaction results in nausea, lacrimation, diaphoresis, abdominal cramps, restlessness, and, rarely, in small children, shock, seizures, and death. Children under 3 years of age account for 75 per cent of all deaths from scorpion stings.

Treatment. In mild reactions, cool compresses, topical steroids, and antihistamines will provide symptomatic relief. In severe reactions, local measures, including the application of ice to the bite and a tourniquet proximal to the sting, may be helpful until a specific antiserum can be administered. In infested areas, creosote or other repellants may be applied to basements, garages, and out buildings; and shoes, boots, and clothing should be inspected carefully before dressing.

Spiders (Araneae)

Spiders are distinguished from other arthropods by their compact cephalothorax and large bag-like abdomen. The majority of encounters in North America occur with the black widow *(Latrodectus mactans)*, a web spinner that prepares its trap across privy seats and cool dark sites in vacant buildings. The female is very aggressive, attacking humans with little provocation, and may be recognized by her red ventral hourglass markings. Local reactions to bites may be painful but are often unnoticed and sometimes followed within 30 minutes by dizziness, nausea, diaphoresis, lacrimation, muscular rigidity, tremors, paresthesias, and headaches. The number of bites is estimated at 500 each year, with a mortality rate of 1 per cent overall and approaching 5 per cent in small children. Symptoms in nonfatal cases increase in severity for several hours, perhaps a day, and slowly dissipate in 2 to 3 days.

Treatment. Prompt treatment with specific antiserum is required for relief of symptoms, especially in children (Antivenin, Merck Sharp & Dohme). After a skin or conjunctival test for horse serum sensitivity, one vial of antivenom reconstituted in 2.5 ml of diluent is administered intramuscularly, or the antivenom may be given intravenously in 10 to 50 ml of saline over 15 minutes.

Other supportive measures include warm baths, intravenous injections of 10 ml of 10 per cent calcium gluconate, morphine, and barbiturates as needed for control of muscle pain and cramps. In healthy adults and older children, antivenom may be deferred pending results of therapy with muscle relaxants and analgesics. Methocarbamol* (Robaxin injectable and tablets) is a useful alternative muscle relaxant, and 10 ml should be administered over 5 minutes followed by 10 ml in 250 ml of 5 per cent dextrose in water at 1 ml/minute. When the patient is improved or if the reaction is mild, methocarbamol (800 mg every 6 hours) may be given orally.

Brown Recluse *(Loxosceles reclusa)*

Slightly smaller than the black widow, the brown recluse spans an overall diameter of 3 to 4 cm with a body 10 to 12 mm long and 4 mm wide. It abounds in the south central United States, where it can be distinguished from other brown spiders by its characteristic dark-brown violin-shaped band extending from the eyes to the end of the cephalothorax. Although occasionally producing a fatal systemic reaction in young children, loxoscelism is characterized by a gangrenous slough at the bite site. Local pain appears 2 to 8 hours after the attack followed by an area of erythema, which develops a necrotic central bulla surrounded by an irregular area of purpura. Over 7 to 14 days, necrosis progresses from a well-demarcated eschar to ulceration up to 20 cm in diameter.

Treatment. No specific antivenom is available in the United States for treatment of brown recluse spider bites. Antihistamines should be used to treat urticarial reactions, and antibiotics may be initiated if secondary infection develops. The use of steroids is controversial, but some experts recommend immediate administration of systemic corticosteroids as soon as the diagnosis is entertained. Intralesional steroids (4 mg of dexamethasone) may be helpful and can be repeated if the lesion continues to increase in size. Large ulcers usually require excision and skin grafting. Semipermeable or occlusive dressings (Duoderm, Vigilon, Opsite) may be applied to facilitate healing.

Ticks (Acari)

Ticks are blood-sucking arachnids with short legs and a leathery integument. They are important vectors for a number of rickettsial and viral disorders and erythema chronicum migrans. Tick bite pyrexia and tick paralysis are produced by a toxin elaborated by the female tick and are promptly relieved by removal of the tick.

Typically, tick bites go unnoticed for several days until a pruritic red papule with a red halo develops at the site. These lesions may resolve in several weeks unless the tick mouth parts are left in place, resulting in a foreign body reaction, which may persist for months. Erythema chronicum migrans is a peculiar eruption produced by a spirochete transmitted by the bite of the *Ixodes dammini* tick. Three to 20 days after a bite from an infected tick, an expanding indurated annular red plaque with central clearing up to 20 cm in diameter appears at the site. Lesions may be multiple and widely disseminated by hematogenous spread from the primary lesion. The rash occurs most commonly in children and may be associated with a rheumatoid factor–negative oligoarticular arthritis (Lyme arthritis; see article on Lyme disease, section 18), meningoencephalitis, and myocarditis.

Treatment. Individuals who have spent time in infested wooded and grassy areas should be carefully inspected daily and all ticks removed immediately. Once the ticks have become embedded in the skin, techniques for removal include application of a hot unlighted match, petrolatum, liquid nitrogen, chloroform, nail polish remover, ethyl chloride spray, and mineral oil. Residual mouth parts are readily removed by skin punch biopsy.

Persistent symptomatic bite reactions will improve with intralesional steroid injections of triamcinolone (0.1 ml of 5 to 10 mg/ml). Erythema chronicum migrans and its associated symptoms may be aborted with oral amoxacillin or tetracycline* (250 mg four times daily for 3 weeks).

Insect repellents, particularly those containing diethyltoluamide (DEET), may provide some protection in endemic areas. However, toxic side effects have been reported with repeated applications to the skin, especially in young children. This risk may be minimized by applying the product only to clothing or by using new low-concentration products with 7 to 10 per cent DEET (Skedaddle).

Mites (Acari)

Infestations with the human *Sarcoptes scabiei* mite have reached epidemic proportions in some communities. The mite spares no age or socioeconomic group and has been identified as a significant medical problem in schools and day care centers and among promiscuous teenagers and adults. The

*Safety and efficacy for use in children under 12 years of age have not been established except in tetanus.

*Use of tetracycline in children younger than 8 years of age may cause discoloration of permanent teeth.

eruption is asymptomatic for weeks to months until the individual becomes sensitized to the mite or its waste products. Papules, vesicles, pustules, and burrows are characteristically found on the wrists, finger webs, axillae, genitals, breasts, and buttocks. The scalp, palms, and soles are also involved in infants and toddlers. A generalized eczematous eruption may occur in sensitized individuals and overshadow the characteristic lesion, making diagnosis difficult. Diagnosis requires demonstration of mites, eggs, or fecal material from skin scrapings.

Treatment. The treatment of choice is 1 per cent permethrin cream (Elimite). Elimite is comparable in efficacy to gamma benzene hexachloride 1 per cent lotion (Kwell, Scabene) and probably provides better ovicidal effect. It has a better safety profile than Kwell and has been used safely in children as young as 2 months. The only drawback to Elimite is the relatively high cost of the product compared with Kwell and generic gamma benzene hydrochloride. As a consequence, when cost is an issue, children can be treated with Elimite, and adolescents and adults with Kwell.

Elimite should be applied to the entire skin surface from the neck down in older children and adults and to the scalp as well in infants. A single overnight application without a preceding bath is usually curative. Treated individuals should bathe thoroughly in the morning. If active lesions are still present in 1 week, a second application may be necessary. All members of the household should be treated, and 1 to 1½ ounces per person per treatment is adequate. Kwell should be used similarly. However, in small children, applications should probably be restricted to 6 to 8 hours.

Neither Elimite nor Kwell is approved for use in pregnancy. The treatment of choice in this setting is 5 per cent precipitated sulfur in petrolatum. Although sulfur appears to be effective, the product is messy (malodorous, stains clothing) and must be applied for 3 to 5 consecutive days.

Crotamiton cream (Eurax) applied for 3 days has also been touted as a safe alternative therapy. However, studies have demonstrated that the failure rate with this product may exceed one third of those treated. Moreover, studies on toxicity and percutaneous penetration of crotamiton are lacking.

Clothing and bedsheets should be laundered in hot water, but extensive treatment of fomites is not necessary, because the mites are dormant at room temperature.

Pruritus, which may last for weeks despite adequate therapy, should be treated with cool baths, emollients, and antihistamines such as hydroxyzine (2 to 5 mg/kg/day divided every 6 hours) or diphenhydramine (5 mg/kg/day every 6 hours).

Other Mites

Children are also commonly infested with animal mites from dogs, cats, mice, and birds. A self-limited itchy papular eruption appears on exposed areas of the arms, legs, and trunk. Harvest mites (red bugs, chiggers) are frequently encountered in parks and grassy areas. Pruritic red papules and nodules with central hemorrhagic puncta appear at sites where the mite larvae are caught in clothing, such as at the waist band, sock bands, and underwear. The larvae are removed inadvertently by scratching, and pruritus wanes over 5 to 7 days.

Treatment. Symptomatic therapy includes topical corticosteroids, shake lotions (calamine), cool compresses, antihistamines, and, in severe cases, systemic corticosteroids (prednisone, 0.5 to 1 mg/kg/day tapered over 10 to 14 days).

Effective prophylaxis can be achieved with insect repellents sprayed onto clothing, including DEET, ethyl hexanediol, dimethyl phthalate, dimethyl carbate, and benzyl benzoate.

INSECTS

Insects are ubiquitous six-legged arthropods with well-defined body segments, including a head, thorax, and abdomen. Organisms of medical significance include bees, wasps, and ants (Hymenoptera), lice (Anoplura), blister beetles (Coleoptera), bedbugs and kissing bugs (Heteroptera), fleas (Siphonaptera), moths and butterflies (Lepidoptera), and flies and mosquitoes (Diptera).

Pediculosis

Human lice are a major public health problem, especially in areas of overcrowding or where facilities are inadequate for keeping people and clothing clean. Pediculosis occurs in three clinical forms: head and body lice infestations produced by two interbreeding varieties of *Pediculus humanus* with characteristic elongated abdomens, and pubic lice caused by *Phthirus pubis*, or the crab louse, which has a short hairy abdomen and two pairs of crab-like claws anteriorly. Lice are acquired through close contact with infested individuals or fomites.

Pediculus Humanus Capitis

Head lice are seen almost exclusively in school-aged boys and girls and in older, long-haired individuals. Lice may be identified on the scalp, and nits are seen about 1 inch from the surface, particularly in the postauricular and occipital areas. Pruritus is intense, and secondary infection is common.

Treatment. Patients should be instructed to lather the scalp and adjacent hairy areas vigorously with 1 per cent gamma benzene hexachloride (Kwell) shampoo for 5 minutes and then rinse thoroughly. Remaining nits may be removed with a fine-tooth comb. The nits may be loosened by application of a solution of equal parts white vinegar and water. Retreatment may be necessary in 1 week because some nits may survive the initial application. Pyrethrins (Rid, R & C shampoo) are effective over-the-counter alternatives, and generally re-treatment is not required.

In 1986, an over-the-counter 1 per cent permethrin creme rinse (Nix) was released for treatment of head lice. Permethrin should be applied to the hair after shampooing and left in place for 10 minutes before being rinsed out. Although it is at least as effective as lindane and has a superior safety profile, the safety of permethrin in pregnant women, nursing mothers, and infants under 2 years has not been established.

Malathion 0.5 per cent lotion (Ovide lotion) is another highly effective agent with marked ovicidal activity. The preparation binds to the hair shaft after application for up to 4 weeks, permitting extended residual activity. As a result, whereas other pediculocides may require a second treatment 7 to 10 days later, only one application is necessary. Patients should be cautioned to avoid hair dryers, open flames, and other heat sources because the product is prepared in a flammable base. As with other pediculocides, its safety in pregnant women, nursing mothers, and young infants has not been established. Step 2 (formic acid) can be used after treatment with malathion. Formic acid loosens the nits and facilitates easy removal with a fine-tooth comb.

Pediculus Humanus Humanus

The body louse hides in the seams of clothing and produces tiny itchy papules and wheals, particularly in the interscapular, shoulder, and wrist regions.

Treatment. Infestation is effectively treated by laundering of clothing and bedding with hot water.

Phthirus Pubis

Crab louse infestation has become epidemic among promiscuous teenagers and adults. The insects are readily identified as grayish spots clinging to the skin in the genital area. Lice and nits may also spread to other hair-bearing areas, including the chest, axillae, and eyelashes. Maculae caeruleae are greenish-blue patches produced by bites on the chest, abdomen, and thighs of infested individuals.

Treatment. One per cent gamma benzene hexachloride lotion should be applied to involved areas, except for the eyelashes, left on for 8 to 12 hours, and then thoroughly rinsed. Pyrethrin lotions should be massaged onto infested areas and then rinsed after 10 minutes. Pediculosis of the eyelashes can be safely treated with petrolatum applied twice daily for 7 to 10 days followed by mechanical removal of nits.

Blister Beetles (Meloidae)

Blister beetles contain cantharidin, a volatile substance that produces an intraepidermal vesicle when the insects alight on the skin or are inadvertently crushed. Blister beetle dermatosis consisting of a linear vesicular eruption is common during the summer months, when the insects are most plentiful.

Treatment. Lesions should be left intact to heal spontaneously in 3 to 4 days. Large lesions (> 1 cm) may be drained and dressed with a compressive bandage soaked with aluminum acetate (Burow's, Blueboro) solution.

Bedbugs *(Cimex lectularius)*

Bedbugs are reddish-brown blood-sucking insects that hide in crevices in floors and walls and feed on unsuspecting victims at night. Although they are a disappearing nuisance, they are still seen occasionally in older, less affluent areas. Although most individuals sleep through the attack, sensitive victims awaken during the bloodmeal, which lasts 5 to 10 minutes. The bite is followed by an urticarial plaque, which may persist for weeks and become reactivated by subsequent bites at other sites. Lesions appear most commonly on the face and other areas not protected by clothing.

Treatment. The bugs are effectively eradicated from the home with insecticides such as chlordane, gamma benzene hexachloride, or hexachlorocyclohexane. Symptomatic relief may be obtained from cool compresses, topical corticosteroids, and oral antihistamines.

Kissing Bugs (Reduviidae)

Although most of these insects prey upon other insects, earning them the name "assassin bug," 75 species attack man. Bites occur frequently on the face, particularly at a mucocutaneous juncture, and result in various reactions, including red papules, giant urticaria, grouped vesicles, and hemorrhagic nodular lesions.

Treatment. Treatment is symptomatic. Insecticides and repellents are not effective.

Fleas (Siphonaptera)

Fleas are a common nuisance for humans and animals. Although there are only two parasites that are consistently associated with man, *Pulex irritans* and *Tunga penetrans*, fleas are only partially host-specific, and cat and dog ectoparasites commonly attack man. The bite may go unnoticed, but sensitized individuals may discover pruritic urticarial wheals with a central hemorrhagic punctum. Multiple lesions in a linear or roseate pattern are typical.

Papular urticaria, a pruritic urticarial eruption at sites of fresh and old reactivated flea bites, occurs almost exclusively in children. Individual papules persist for 1 to 2 weeks and are found on exposed areas of the arms, legs, and trunk, sparing the buttocks and genitals. Lesions tend to recur in spring and summer but may persist year round for 3 to 4 years.

Treatment. Acute reactions are relieved with shake lotions (calamine), topical steroids, cool tap water compresses, and oral antihistamines. Impetiginized lesions should be treated with topical or oral antibiotics if necessary. Fleas may be eliminated by the removal or treatment of infested pets and by vacuuming and spraying carpets, floors, and other infested areas with 5 per cent malathion powder or 1 per cent lindane dust. Despite these measures, fleas may survive in the household for months.

Moths and Butterflies (Lepidoptera)

Contact with the hairs of the brown-tail moth, indigenous to the northeastern United States, and the puss caterpillar, found in the southeastern states from Virginia to the Gulf of Mexico, may produce a burning papular eruption and, occasionally, a severe systemic reaction.

Treatment. Tape stripping to remove embedded hair reduces local reactions. Systemic reactions with symptoms such as muscle cramps, headache, tachycardia, restlessness, and, rarely, shock and seizures require supportive therapy with antihistamines, systemic steroids, and parenteral calcium gluconate.

Flies and Mosquitoes (Diptera)

These ubiquitous insects are important vectors in the transmission of viral and parasitic diseases. Mosquitoes (Culicidae) attack exposed sites on the face and extremities, producing pruritic urticarial plaques that persist for hours. Sandflies, moth flies, or owl flies (Psychodidae) bite silently, seeking out the ankles, wrist, knees, and elbows, and produce white wheals, which resolve over several days. Black flies (Simuliidae), horseflies (Tabanidae), and houseflies (Muscidae) attack silently and inflict a painful bite.

Treatment. Bite reactions are relieved with antihistamines, cool tap water compresses, and topical steroids. Sensitive individuals should wear protective clothing and insect repellents (Cutter, 6-12, Off).

REFERENCES

Frazier CA: Allergic reactions to insect stings: A review of 180 cases. South Med J 57:1028, 1964.

ANIMAL AND HUMAN BITES AND BITE-RELATED INFECTIONS

MORVEN S. EDWARDS, M.D.

Animal and human bite wound injuries are common. It is estimated that 1 to 2 million dog bites, 400,000 cat bites, and 45,000 snakebites occur yearly in the United States. A number of nondomesticated animals, including "pet" ferrets, skunks, squirrels, rats, and monkeys, inflict wounds that constitute approximately 1 per cent of the estimated yearly total "bite wound burden" of $30 million. Although a minority of victims seek medical attention, bite wound assessment accounts for an estimated 1 per cent of all visits to emergency departments during the summer months.

NONHUMAN MAMMALIAN BITES

There are approximately 70 million pet dogs and cats in the United States. Bite wound injuries are most often inflicted by large dogs with weights exceeding 50 pounds. Injuries are usually provoked, and, in the majority of instances, the animal is not the family-owned pet but is known to the victim. A minority of bites (< 10 per cent) are inflicted by stray dogs. The peak incidence of animal bite wounds is in children aged 5 to 14 years; boys are victims more often than girls. Approximately 70 per cent of wounds are to the extremities. Although facial wounds account for a minority of bites (10 per cent), these usually are sustained by young children, and death may occur due to exsanguination.

The bite of a dog is likely to cause crushing and tearing, producing lacerations of varying severity. Bites from pit bull breeds, which tend to be multiple and to pulverize tissue, can exert a force of 1500 pounds per square inch. Over the past decade, pit bull breeds have become the species most likely to cause the 10 to 20 dog bite–related fatalities reported yearly. Cat bites are often puncture wounds, whose benign external appearance may mask injury and inoculation of bacteria into tendon sheaths, joints, or bones.

HUMAN BITES

Human bites occur ten times less commonly than animal bites but are more likely to cause infection. Human bites are sustained by young children at play, adolescents engaged in contact sports, residents of mental institutions, and victims of sexual assault. One series estimates that 42 per cent of human bites involve the upper extremities, 33 per cent the face and neck, and 22 per cent the trunk. Clenched-fist injuries are a distinctive traumatic laceration, usually involving the third and fourth metacarpophalangeal joints of the dominant hand, which results from a clenched fist striking teeth. The apparently benign external laceration may mask injury to the joint capsule or spread of infection along deep tissue planes.

SNAKEBITES

Approximately 20 per cent of snakebites are inflicted by poisonous snakes, and one half of these 8000 injuries annually are sustained by children. The two families of venomous snakes found in the United States are the pit vipers or Crotalidae, which include water moccasins, copperheads, and rattlesnakes, and the Elapidae, represented by the coral snake. Pit vipers may be distinguished from nonvenomous snakes by the features listed in Table 1. Coral snakes may be identified by the pattern of bands, in which red and yellow are adjacent, distinguishing them from king snakes, in which black bands separate the red and yellow bands. Approximately 25 per cent of pit viper bites and one half of coral snake bites are "dry" and result in no envenomation. Diamondback rattlesnakes account for 95 per cent of snakebite-associated fatalities, numbering 10 to 15 yearly, although they account for only 10 per cent of bites.

BITE WOUND MANAGEMENT

Human and Nonhuman Mammalian Bites

The first step in wound care is irrigation and cleansing. The wound may be anesthetized with 1 per cent lidocaine without epinephrine. Cleansing is accomplished by high-pressure syringe irrigation using a 25- or 35-ml syringe and 19-gauge needle and at least 1 L of normal saline or a 1 per cent povidone-iodine solution. Puncture wounds should not be irrigated. All devitalized tissue should be débrided. Radiographs should be performed as indicated, to assess injury to the periosteum or retained foreign material.

The extent to which primary closure influences infection-related morbidity is controversial. When promptly evaluated (< 6 hours) and appropriately cleansed and débrided, most nonpuncture animal bite wounds, except those involving the hand, can be treated by primary closure without significantly enhancing the risk for infection. Puncture wounds should never be sutured. Suturing of nonmutilating human bite wounds, other than those involving the face, should be avoided. In particular, hand wounds should be left open. When potentially serious or disfiguring hand or face wounds are encountered, consultation should be sought with a hand or plastic surgeon.

An immunization history should be obtained. If more than 5 years has elapsed since administration of tetanus toxoid, a booster dose should be provided. In the event that tetanus immunization has not been carried out, 250 units of human immune tetanus globulin should be given and an immunization series with tetanus toxoid initiated.

Venomous Snakebites

On-site first-aid measures for venomous snakebite[1] include the following:

1. Reassurance of the victim.
2. Limb immobilization to minimize spread of venom.
3. Use of a *properly* applied constricting band, placed 15 to 20 cm proximal to the wound to restrict lymphatic but not arterial or venous flow. (This should be accompanied by close observation to ensure that the peripheral vascular status is not impaired by the constricting band should swelling intensify.
4. *Prompt* transportation to a medical facility.

The use of incision is mentioned only to be condemned, except in settings when medical care is unavailable for a number of hours. In this setting *only*, incision of fang marks with a shallow single incision of 3 mm maximum depth and 6 mm maximum length in a plane parallel to the longitudinal body axis *may* reduce envenomation if *initiated* within 5 minutes of injury and suction continued for 30 to 60 minutes.

Definitive medical management of pit viper bites involves determining, on the basis of clinical findings, if envenomation has occurred and its extent. The initial swelling from pit viper bites is always evident within 30 minutes. On the basis of the following assessment, antivenin (Crotalidae) polyvalent (Wyeth), a horse serum product, should be administered—*after* skin testing (as per package insert)—in 5 per cent dextrose in water or in normal saline at a maximum rate of 20 ml/kg/hour:

- *Minimal envenomation*: fang marks and local swelling without systemic reaction (3 to 5 vials antivenin)
- *Moderate envenomation*: swelling extending beyond bite size with laboratory abnormalities or systemic symptoms (6 to 10 vials antivenin)
- *Severe envenomation*: marked local and systemic reaction such as disseminated intravascular coagulopathy (DIC), shock, or respiratory distress syndrome (at least 15 vials antivenin)

It should be noted that antivenin dosage is *not* dependent on age or weight but on extent of envenomation; that its efficacy is inversely proportional to the time elapsed since the

TABLE 1. Features Distinguishing Pit Vipers (Crotalidae) from Nonvenomous Snakes

Feature	Pit Viper (Crotalidae)	Nonvenomous Snake
Shape of head	Triangular	Rounded
Pit midway between eye and nostril bilaterally	Present	Absent
Shape of pupil	Elliptic	Round
Fangs	Present	Absent
Subcaudal scales	Single row	Double row

bite and is maximal when initiated within 4 hours; and that, because reactions to horse serum may occur despite a negative skin test, life-sustaining equipment should be available.

Coral snake bites evoke little local reaction. Tongue fasciculations, disturbed phonation and swallowing, bulbar paralysis, and respiratory distress are signs of envenomation. The treatment of coral snake envenomation is *Micrurus fulvius* antivenin (Wyeth) (5 vials administered intravenously at a rate of 20 ml/kg/hour).

Snake venoms are among the most complex of proteins, eliciting a variety of hematotoxic (primarily pit viper) or neurotoxic (coral snake and Mojave rattlesnake) effects, including increased vascular permeability, tissue destruction, DIC, cardiotoxicity, and respiratory failure. Baseline laboratory testing should include assessment of hematologic and clotting parameters, urinalysis, blood urea nitrogen and creatinine, and type and cross-matching of blood. Patients requiring antivenin should be managed in an intensive care unit. Circulatory and respiratory status and urine output should be monitored, and intravenous access for plasma expanders established. The majority of patients requiring antivenin *will* have a serum sickness reaction, and a subset of these will have symptoms sufficiently severe to warrant use of prednisone (1 ml/kg/day initially) for 1 to 2 weeks of total treatment.

MANAGEMENT OF INFECTION

Patients seeking medical attention for a bite wound within 12 hours of injury generally have noninfected wounds requiring repair or tetanus or rabies prophylaxis, whereas those arriving more than 12 hours after injury often have established infection. The pathogens most frequently encountered in bite wound infection are summarized in Table 2. Signs of bacterial infection may occur within hours, heralded by development of intense pain, swelling, and cellulitis, especially when *Pasteurella multocida* is the infecting organism. *P. multocida* is implicated as a pathogen in up to 50 per cent of infections associated with dog bite wounds and 80 per cent of those associated with cat bite wounds. The onset of staphylococcal or streptococcal wound infection, observed following dog, cat, or human bites, typically develops as swelling, erythema, and cellulitis within days rather than hours. Following rat bite, streptobacillary rat-bite fever occurs after an incubation period of 1 week, whereas spirillary rat-bite fever has a longer (2-week) symptom-free interval (Table 2).

It is estimated that 3 to 5 per cent of dog bites, 20 to 50 per cent of cat bites, and 10 to 30 per cent of human bites for which medical attention is sought become infected. Literally hundreds of aerobic and anaerobic microorganisms composing the oral flora of the biting species may cause infection. Specimens often yield a mixture of aerobic and anaerobic bacteria on culture. The microorganisms listed in Table 2 include the most frequently implicated pathogens.

Although the initiation of antimicrobials as prophylaxis in bite wound infections is a controversial issue, and its efficacy has not been established unequivocally by a controlled prospective study, the following guidelines are proposed for initiation of antibiotics for prophylaxis of noninfected-appearing wounds[2]:

1. All cat bites.
2. Dog bites older than 8 hours.
3. All hand bites.
4. Deep puncture wounds.
5. Wounds in which primary closure is delayed.
6. Wounds occurring in immunocompromised individuals.
7. All human bites involving the hand or face.
8. Snakebites with envenomation severe enough to warrant hospitalization.

TABLE 2. Pathogens Isolated Frequently from Animal and Human Bites

Species	Common Microorganisms
Dog	*Pasteurella multocida*
	Streptococci*
	Staphylococcus aureus
	Coagulase-negative staphylococci (CONS)
	Bacteroides species
	Fusobacterium species
Cat	*P. multocida*
	S. aureus
	Streptococci*
	CONS
	Corynebacterium species
Rat	*Streptobacillus moniliformis*
	Spirillum minor
Human	*Eikenella corrodens*
	S. aureus
	Streptococci*
	Bacteroides species
	Fusobacterium species
Snake	*Pseudomonas aeruginosa*
	Proteus species
	CONS
	Clostridium species
Alligator	*Aeromonas hydrophila*
	Proteus vulgaris
	Pseudomonas species
Shark	*Vibrio* species

*Includes viridans streptococci, group A streptococci, and β-hemolytic streptococci.

A specimen from an apparently clean wound will reflect the normal oral flora of the biting animal on culture and thus does not need to be obtained routinely. In contrast, for overtly infected wounds, a specimen processed to yield aerobic and anaerobic bacteria on culture should be obtained; the laboratory should be alerted as to the specimen's source because *P. multocida* may be confused with other organisms, particularly *Haemophilus*.

Suggested antimicrobial regimens for animal and human bite wounds are shown in Table 3. The availability of penicillins incorporating an inhibitor of beta-lactamase activity permits monotherapy of wound infections encompassing the commonly implicated aerobic and anaerobic pathogens, including *Staphylococcus aureus*. When the pathogen is identified, a penicillin is the preferred antibiotic for streptococci, *P. multocida*, and most anaerobes that cause bite-associated infection. There is no entirely satisfactory regimen for the penicillin-allergic patient. Tetracycline is a good alternative agent for older children. Erythromycin is inactive against 50 per cent of *P. multocida* strains; clindamycin and penicillinase-resistant penicillins are even less active.[3] In serious wound infections due to *P. multocida* in the penicillin-allergic child, desensitization to penicillin should be carried out where feasible. An alternative regimen might include cefuroxime axetil, which shows good activity against *P. multocida*. Rat-bite fever, whether due to *Spirillum minus* or *Streptobacillus moniliformis*, should be treated parenterally with penicillin in the dosage provided in Table 3. In the penicillin-allergic patient, tetracycline is an alternative antibiotic.

Empiric antibiotic therapy, adjusted in accordance with results of cultures, should be continued for 7 to 14 days, depending on clinical response.

TABLE 3. Initial Antibiotic Therapy for Mammal, Reptile, or Human Bites

Indication	Antibiotic Regimen (kg/24 hr)	
	Intravenous Regimen	*Oral Regimen*
Suspected infection Mammal or human bite	Ticarcillin-clavulanate (200–300 mg of ticarcillin component in 4–6 doses)* *or* Aqueous penicillin G (200,000 units in 4–6 doses)* *plus* Nafcillin (150 mg in 4 doses)	Amoxicillin-clavulanate (40 mg of amoxicillin component in 3 doses) *or* Penicillin V (50,000 U in 4 doses) *or* Penicillin V (50,000 U in 4 doses) *plus* Dicloxacillin (50 mg in 4 doses)
Snakebite†	Ticarcillin (300 mg in 4—6 doses)* *plus* Gentamicin (5 mg in 3 doses)‡	Not indicated
Penicillin-allergic patient	Vancomycin (40 mg in 4 doses)§ *plus* Cefotaxime (150–200 mg in 3–4 doses)* *or* Vancomycin (as above) *plus* Chloramphenicol (75 mg in 4 doses)#	Erythromycin (30–50 mg in 4 doses) *or* Tetracycline (25–50 mg in 4 doses)‖
Prophylaxis—see text for indications	As above, for suspected infection—mammal or human bite	As above, for suspected infection—mammal or human bite

Adapted from Edwards MS: Infection following a bite. *In* Nelson JD (ed): Current Therapy in Pediatric Infectious Disease 2. Philadelphia, BC Decker, 1988, p 110.
*Employ the larger dosage and/or more frequent interval for severe infections.
†Infection should be suspected in all cases of moderate or severe envenomation.
‡Monitor serum concentrations to maintain a peak of 5–10 μg/ml and trough less than 2 μg/ml.
§Monitor serum concentrations to maintain a peak of 25–40 μg/ml and trough less than 12 μg/ml.
‖Avoid use in children younger than age 8 years.
#Monitor serum concentrations to maintain a peak of 20–30 μg/ml and trough less than the peak.

COMPLICATIONS OF BITE WOUND INFECTIONS

Complications of bite wounds may be classified as those resulting from direct extension and those serving as inoculation wounds for generalized infections. Among the former, extensions of puncture or extensive wounds to involve the adjacent bone, joint, or, in the case of clenched-fist injuries, synovium or tendon sheath are the most common. Tenosynovitis due to *P. multocida* may develop within hours or may be delayed until symptoms of persistent swelling, tenderness, or tendon sheath mass suggest the diagnosis. In addition to clinical assessment, a radionuclide joint-bone scan is recommended to establish the extent of deep wound infection. Consultation with an orthopedic surgeon to establish appropriate drainage and to obtain specimens for culture is then appropriate. Depending on the isolate(s), parenteral or a sequential parenteral-oral regimen extended for 2 to 4 weeks may be required to eradicate deep infections.

A number of generalized complications, including endocarditis, meningitis, sepsis (especially among patients immunocompromised by splenectomy), and infections of joint prostheses are associated with complicated bite wound infections. Therapy in these patients should be provided parenterally, and management should be assisted by an infectious disease consultant.

Rabies may occur as a consequence of an animal bite, most commonly when the biting species is a wild animal (skunk, raccoon, bat, fox, coyote, or bobcat) or, rarely, a rabid cow, cat, or dog. Consultation with local rabies control health authorities should be sought in the decision to initiate or withhold rabies immunization. As feasible, domestic animals should be observed for 10 days and wild animals sacrificed for fluorescent antibody examination of the brain. When rabies immunization is started, the patient receives 1 ml of human diploid cell (HDC) vaccine intramuscularly as soon as possible after exposure and 3, 7, 14, and 28 days later (some experts recommend a sixth dose at 90 days). Rabies immune globulin (20 IU/kg) should be given intramuscularly at a site different from the first dose of HDC vaccine; up to half the dose is infiltrated in the area around the wound.

REFERENCES

1. Kurecki BA III, Brownlee HJ Jr: Venomous snakebites in the United States. J Fam Pract 25:386–392, 1987.
2. Trott A: Care of mammalian bites. Pediatr Infect Dis J 6:8–10, 1987.
3. Goldstein EJC: Bites. *In* Mandell J, Douglas RG, Bennett W (eds): Principles and Practice of Infectious Diseases. Philadelphia, WB Saunders Co, 1990, pp 834–837.

BURNS IN CHILDHOOD

JOHN T. HERRIN, M.D.

Thermal injuries are very common. The epidemiology is generally well known, and attention to preventable factors could result in the avoidance of as many as 75 per cent of injuries.

PROPHYLAXIS

The pediatrician and pediatric nurse practitioner should undertake the major role in educating parents, children, and community and school groups in preventive measures, coordinating with the various stages of child development. Appropriate clothing, smoke detectors, and planned routes for emergency exit from the home are simple, efficient, and cost-effective prophylactic measures.

CARE STRATEGIES

Treatment of the burned patient aims at

1. Fluid resuscitation.
2. Prevention of infection.
3. Wound coverage.
4. Nutritional support.
5. Rehabilitation, physical and psychologic, through prevention of functional limitation and prevention of behavior-related problems.

Early institution of appropriate monitoring, fluid and electrolyte therapy, and care of the burn injury has increased survival with improved wound healing, more cosmetic scars, and protection of blood supply to the extremity. Adequate early measures facilitate long-term reconstruction and improved rehabilitation.

The general guidelines of life support in the burn patient are well defined. A rapid examination of the patient aims at detection of potential traumatic injuries, determination of the degree and extent of the burn injury, and assessment of adequacy of the airway. During this examination, constricting clothing and jewelry (particularly rings and/or bracelets) are removed. The wound is covered with clean sheeting until it can be cleansed and dressed in an appropriate emergency care center.

In the patient who has been burned in an enclosed space, special care is given to examination of the facial area, nares, and pharynx because facial burns, singed nasal hairs, and carbonaceous sputum or saliva suggest inhalation injury, which necessitates constant care during the triage phase. If inhalation injury is suspected, oxygen (100 per cent) is administered and observation is undertaken for the changes described with (1) smoke inhalation (hypoxia and hypercapnia, local swelling, edema of pharynx or larynx) or (2) carbon monoxide poisoning. Early intubation is necessary if facial swelling is extensive or developing rapidly. Blood carbon monoxide levels should be determined if the burn was sustained within an enclosed space.

Upon admission, a throat specimen is obtained for culture while the pharynx is being inspected for potential burn or inhalation injury. Penicillin is administered prophylactically and continued in patients with a known cardiac anomaly or in those with concomitant streptococcal infection (positive culture).

TRIAGE AND OUTPATIENT CARE (Tables 1 to 3)

Initial therapy should include:

1. *Removing the patient or the affected area from the source of burn.* Degree and area of burn are proportional to the duration of exposure (time of contact) and to the intensity of the heat source. Simple measures such as removing clothing in contact with an injured area, smothering flames, copiously irrigating chemical burns, and preventing panic are extremely important in minimizing further damage.

2. *Ensuring patency of the airway.*

3. *Placing an adequate intravenous access.* Infants with a 10 per cent body surface area (BSA) burn or adolescents with a 15 per cent BSA burn should have a large-bore intravenous catheter placed as soon as practical. Oral fluids are withheld in these patients because ileus and gastric dilatation are so common in the first 48 hours that prophylaxis against vomiting and aspiration is required. Chemical pneumonitis superimposed on a pulmonary burn injury may be lethal. A nasogastric tube should be placed prior to transfer to a treating facility.

4. *Covering the burned area.* The burn area is wrapped in towels or clean sheeting, preferably saturated with ice water. Be sure that the ice does not contact the burn area because cold damage may be superimposed.

5. *Transferring the patient to a burn care facility if appropriate (Table 1).* Patients with major burns or critical burn injury should be transferred as soon as stabilized to a specialized regional burn center. Providing early advice and support by telephone to the regional burn center is recommended.

TABLE 1. Triage of the Burn Patient

Category	Injury Area	Treatment Site
Critical	>30% BSA Inhalation injury Burn injury + aspiration	Specialized burn center
Major	10–30% BSA	Hospital Consider burn center
Minor	<10% BSA	Outpatient

Abbreviation: BSA, body surface area.

ESTIMATION OF THE DEGREE OF BURN AND DEPTH

The varying proportions of head, trunk, and extremities throughout childhood make it necessary to use a surface-area diagram such as the modified Lund-Browderer burn chart used at the Burns Institute, Shriners Hospitals, Boston (Fig. 1). The arbitrary rules such as the rule of nines commonly used in adults are inaccurate in the younger child and can lead to marked discrepancies in estimated fluid needs.

Estimation of depth of injury and area of burn (i.e., approximation of the volume of burn tissue) is important in assessment of the potential for healing and the need for early surgical treatment to provide closure. A clinical guide to the depth of burn may be made by considering the causative agent, appearance of the burn area, pain, and color (Table 4). Even very experienced clinicians have difficulty in differentiating second- and third-degree burns, and a period of dressings and observation may be necessary to allow the area to declare itself as to definitive classification of depth and need for grafting.

Minor Burns

Burns covering less than 10 per cent of BSA or involving less than 2 per cent full-thickness injury may be treated on an outpatient basis after an assessment of the family's ability

TABLE 2. Early Burn Care

First Aid	1. Remove patient and affected area from burn source 2. Ensure patent airway 3. Cover affected area with clean sheet or towel (saturate with ice water)
Assessment	4. Burn surface area and depth
Transport	5. Infant with burns covering >10% BSA Adolescent with burns covering >15% BSA
Specialized Care	6. Pulmonary burn 7. Full-thickness burn >2% BSA 8. Burns of hands, feet, face, neck, or genitalia 9. Inadequate home situation

Abbreviation: BSA, body surface area.

TABLE 3. Preparation for Transport

1. Ensure patent airway Intubate if necessary	Facial edema
2. Place large-bore IV line early Stabilize for transport	10% BSA burn, infant 15% BSA burn, adolescent
3. Administer oxygen	Burn in enclosed space Pulmonary burn Potential carbon monoxide poisoning
4. Provide IV sedation if necessary	
5. Place NPO	
6. Insert nasogastric tube	
7. Commence charting fluid, drugs, and output	
8. Telephone burn center	

Abbreviations: IV, intravenous; BSA, body surface area; NPO, nothing by mouth.

to cope with the burn injury and with needed dressings. Occasionally, a patient will require observation in the hospital to complete this evaluation adequately and to obtain adequate wound dressings.

The first-aid treatment of minor burns includes covering the burn with sheeting and applying water, ice water, or iced towels to the area until full evaluation is carried out. The burn is then gently cleansed with sterile saline. Blebs and blisters are left intact; a closed, bulky, wide gauze dressing is applied after a thin layer of silver sulfadiazine has been applied.

Tetanus prophylaxis is instituted by booster dose if the child has not had recent immunization. For those previously immunized (two prior doses of diphtheria-pertussis-tetanus [DPT] vaccine), 0.5 ml DPT is administered. If no prior immunization has occurred, the wound should be reviewed for potential need of tetanus immune globulin if risk of tetanus is high.* The parents are instructed to return for a dressing change in 2 to 3 days, or earlier if the dressing becomes dislodged, soaked, or malodorous or if the child develops a temperature above 39°C (102°F). Prophylactic antibiotics are not necessary, but antibiotic cover may be needed if fever develops, if dressing is not maintained, or if cellulitis or obvious infection develops.

Fluid Resuscitation

As a general guideline, the Parkland formula (4 ml/kg/per cent burn per 24 hours) is the average amount of lactated Ringer's solution necessary for maintenance of circulation and urine output. Younger children more often require 5 ml/kg/per cent burn per 24 hours, and adolescents (or adults) need 3 ml/kg/per cent burn per 24 hours to maintain circulation as measured by blood pressure, pulse, and urine output. The volume needed varies with the degree of injury and the lapse in time before receiving therapy. This guideline for therapy is modified on the basis of the urine flow rate and review of simple laboratory tests—hematocrit, serum bicarbonate concentration, urinary sodium concentration, serum and urine osmolality—together with frequent review of clinical status.

Day 1. As soon as an intravenous line is placed, resuscitation is commenced with isotonic fluid, usually lactated Ringer's solution using the Parkland formula for initial guidelines. Thus, on day 1, replace combined losses and maintenance fluid as isotonic fluid (4 ml/kg/per cent burn per 24 hours as lactated Ringer's solution). When vital signs, urine flow rate, and acid-base parameters remain within the normal range, adequate circulation is assumed. The estimated regimen is continued, aiming at a urine output of approximately 1 to 1.5 ml/kg/hour with a urine sodium concentration of 40 mEq/L (Table 5). (One half of the calculated fluid volume is given over the first 8 hours post burn injury in order to compensate for early fluid shifts, and the second half is administered evenly over the next 16-hour period.)

Late institution of fluid therapy necessitates higher initial rates of fluid administration and close monitoring. Modifications of fluid rate and type are indicated if target levels are not maintained. In the initial 24 to 36 hours, colloid administration has limited use (a tendency for colloid to leak into the interstitial spaces minimizes effects on circulatory stability). A falling urine output, together with a rise in hematocrit and serum osmolality and a falling concentration of serum protein and serum albumin, indicates deficient colloid replacement. On the other hand, a rise in hematocrit, serum protein, and osmolality with increasing acidosis suggests inadequate crystalloid replacement.

Central monitoring lines are required

1. In the patient with pre-existing cardiac or renal disease.
2. In the patient with refractory shock requiring cardiotonic agents.
3. In the patient in whom circulation remains poor or oliguria persists despite otherwise appropriate fluid intake and rate (Table 6).

Days 2 to 3. On day 2, the patient should receive 10 to 20 ml/kg/day as colloid or lactated Ringer's solution as replacement fluid to maintain circulation and urine output plus 1600 to 2000 ml/m^2/day of 5 per cent dextrose solution as the maintenance fluid allotment.

TABLE 4. Assessment of Burn Depth

Degree	Color	Appearance	Pain	Common Cause
First	Red, blanching	Dry	+ + +	Sunburn Flash burn
Second	Mottled red-white, blanches	Moist/blistered	+ +	Scald Chemical
Third	Charred black, nonblanching	Dry/leathery	±	Immersion Flame Chemical
Fourth	Charred black	Leathery/exposed tendon	−	Electrical Flame

Note: Common causes may lead to overlapping degrees of injury. Degree and area of burn are determined by time of contact and intensity of heat source.

TABLE 5. Guidelines for Adequate Therapy

Indicator	Target
Blood pressure	Normal for age
Pulse	Normal for age
Urine flow	1.5 ml/kg/hr
Urine sodium	40 mEq/L
Urine osmolality	150–300 mOsm/L
Hematocrit	30–35%
Serum protein	4.5–5.5 g/dl
Serum osmolality	280–290 mOsm/L

*A tetanus-prone wound is one that was sustained more than 6 hours before treatment; results in association with crush injury, missile injury, or thermal injury; or shows signs of infection or devitalized or contaminated tissue.

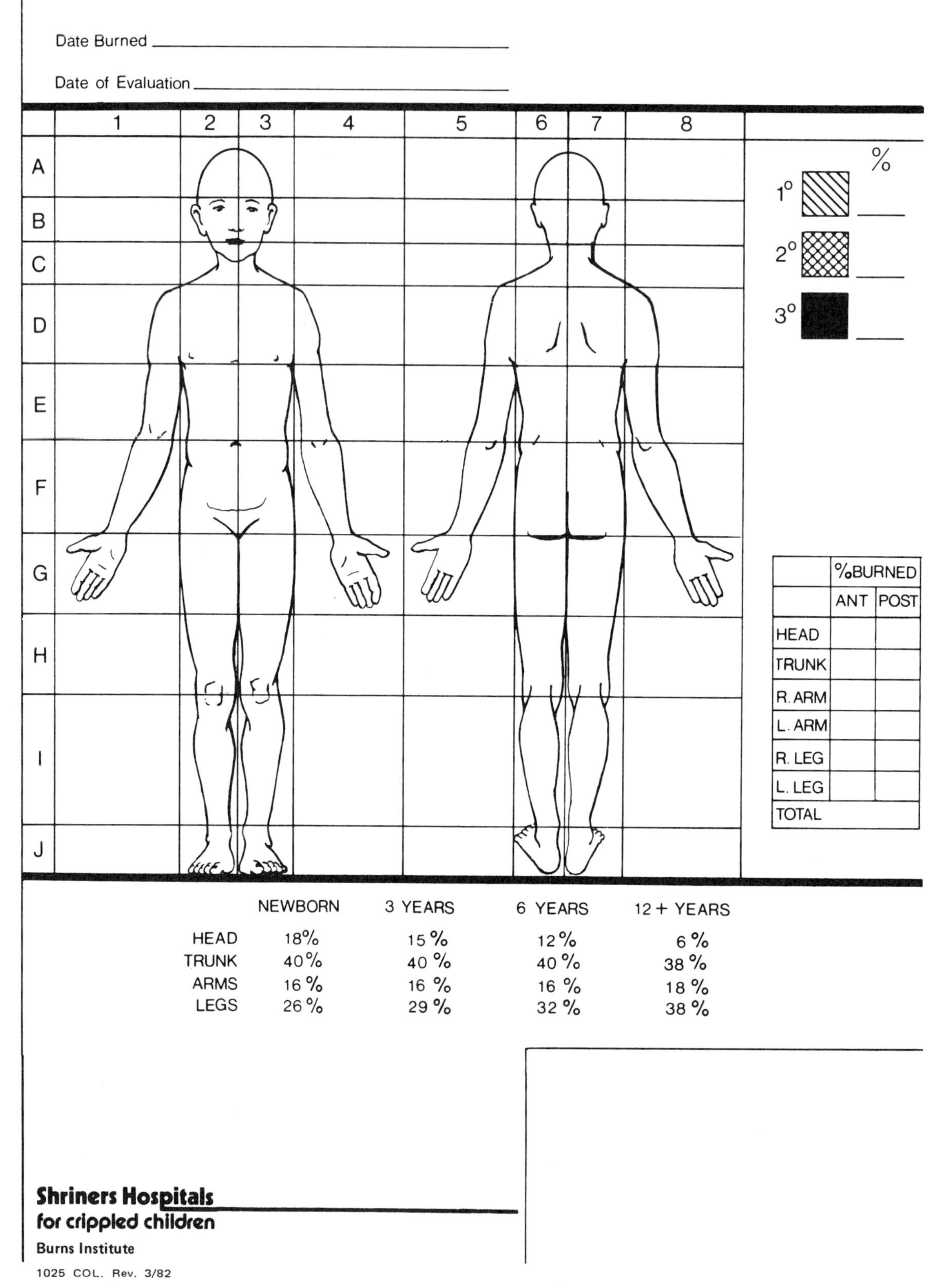

Date Burned ______

Date of Evaluation ______

	1	2	3	4	5	6	7	8
A								
B								
C								
D								
E								
F								
G								
H								
I								
J								

	%
1°	___
2°	___
3°	___

	%BURNED	
	ANT	POST
HEAD		
TRUNK		
R. ARM		
L. ARM		
R. LEG		
L. LEG		
TOTAL		

	NEWBORN	3 YEARS	6 YEARS	12+ YEARS
HEAD	18%	15%	12%	6%
TRUNK	40%	40%	40%	38%
ARMS	16%	16%	16%	18%
LEGS	26%	29%	32%	38%

Shriners Hospitals
for crippled children
Burns Institute

1025 COL. Rev. 3/82

Figure 1. Form for estimating degree and depth of burns. (Courtesy of the Burns Institute, Shriners Hospitals.)

TABLE 6. Indications for Central Monitoring in Burns

1. Pre-existing cardiac or renal disease
2. Shock requiring pressor therapy
3. Refractory shock or oliguria despite appropriate fluid management

On the second day, there is normally a decrease in fluid required for replacement. As the patient regains capillary integrity, there is less fluid loss to muscle and extracellular fluid space. Approximately one half of the day 1 requirement is usually adequate to sustain the circulation (i.e., approximately 1 to 2 ml/kg/per cent burn per 24 hours modified to maintain appropriate urine output).

Colloid infusion may be used when capillary integrity is restored (12 to 24 hours), if serum total protein falls below 2 g/dl, or if the circulation cannot be maintained with infusion of 300 ml/m^2/hour (10 ml/kg/hour).

Maintenance fluid and nutrition are provided orally at 48 hours if circulation is stable. Nutrition is provided enterally after the first 24 hours if ileus is not present or parenterally via a central vein in the patient with major or critical burns, because the metabolic and energy stresses are high. The aim is to provide 2.5 g/kg protein (3 g/kg for infants weighing $<$20 kg) and calories at twice the predicted metabolic requirements.

Fluid mobilization from burn tissue commences on the second to third day, and a diuresis follows. It is not necessary and, in fact, is dangerous to match the urine output at this stage because there is significant extracellular fluid overload and reduction of the edema is necessary for the appropriate wound healing. Close monitoring of weight, circulation, and fluid balance is necessary until the excess sodium and water have been excreted.

Major Burns and Burns Requiring Special Care

Patients with major burns should be hospitalized in a regional burn center, as should patients with burns to hands, face, genital areas, or perineum; with electrical burns; with full-thickness burns greater than 2 per cent of BSA; or with burns suspected of being part of a pattern of child abuse. Guidelines for recognizing child abuse are included in Table 7. The pattern of burn and patient and parental behavior should be noted during evaluation. An experienced social worker, preferably with experience in patients with burns, can be a major help in providing support to the family and in fully assessing the circumstances surrounding a burn. Failure to recognize and report child abuse from thermal injury places the child at severe risk. Patients with questionable home situations or parental care are best admitted to the hospital for a short period. This allows the staff to provide support while teaching dressing techniques, and observation of parent and child will allow assessment and ensure safety of home dressings.

Burn wound care differs in the patient with major burns. Loose skin is débrided, and the area adequately cleaned using sterile techniques before dressings are applied. Analgesia using intravenous doses of morphine sulfate (0.05 to 0.1 mg/kg), meperidine (0.5 mg/kg), or general anesthesia may be necessary for adequate débridement. Morphine is preferred because meperidine metabolites after repeated dosing can produce undesirable side effects such as irritability, hallucinations, or seizures. In patients with limited areas of full-thickness burns, total excision and grafting are performed at a very early stage.

Escharotomies may be needed to protect the blood flow to extremities, fingers, and toes in patients with circumferential burns or to allow full expansion of the chest wall. Clinical assessment of blood flow to the extremities—cyanosis, poor circulatory return, decreasing pulse pressure, deep tissue pain, or paresthesia—should be supplemented by assessment of Doppler flow pulsation and/or direct pressure measurements in compartment areas. If escharotomy is necessary, incisions are made through the entire thickness of the burn on the lateral aspects of the extremity in the area of least blood supply. Local anesthesia is usually not necessary because burns that necessitate escharotomy are generally full-thickness burns without pain. It is necessary to excise through the full thickness of the burn injury and occasionally through the fascia to obtain adequate relief of pressure. Fasciotomy may be necessary in the presence of compartment syndromes.

In patients who require escharotomy or fasciotomy, prophylaxis to maintain urine flow is wise. Sodium bicarbonate (2 to 3 mEq/kg) is given intravenously with mannitol (0.5 to 1 g/kg over 30 to 60 minutes) prophylactically against potential release of the products of rhabdomyolysis.

Occlusive dressings with silver sulfadiazine, sulfamylon, or silver nitrate are used as prophylaxis against wound infection. Choice of local agent for burn wound care depends on the philosophy and facilities of the treating unit. Use of silver nitrate (0.5 per cent), although a very effective agent, is time-intensive; furthermore, silver nitrate has a tendency to leach out sodium and calcium, with the attendant problems of hyponatremia and hypocalcemia, in patients who do not receive adequate replacements.

Early excision of burned tissue and grafting now constitute the most common treatment for major burns. The advantages of such treatment are a reduction in catabolic response, restoration of immunocompetence, and an increased resistance to infection. Antibiotics, although effective in eradicating organisms in small partial-thickness wounds, have more of a supporting role in extensive and deep burns. In extreme or deep burns, control of infection requires excision of the infected tissue.

Critical Burns

In the patient with burns covering more than 30 per cent of BSA or with significant electrical injury or inhalation injury, transfer to a regional burn center for most appropriate care is mandatory. Telephone contact with the burn center is established, and appropriate measures for stabilization of the patient and timing of transfer are arranged. Individualization of the resuscitation plan may be necessary (Table 8) when burn injury involves inhalation or aspiration, circumferential injury, pre-existing medical condition, or delay in the initiation of therapy.

TABLE 7. Recognizing Child Abuse in Thermal Injury

History
- Inadequate supervision
- Delay in seeking treatment ($>$12 hours)
- Burn attributed to child/sibling
- Previous serious injury
- Age 12–24 months
- Poor parent–child interaction
- Lack of preventive care

Examination
- Burn pattern incompatible with story
- Symmetric extremity burns
- Localized burn of perineum, buttocks, genitalia
- Burn incompatible with age-related activities
- Unrelated injuries—lacerations, scars, bruises
- Unsuspected fractures of long bones, ribs, skull

TABLE 8. Situations in Which Individualized Resuscitation Is Required

1. Electrical injury
2. Inhalation injury
3. Large burns not responding to standard therapy
4. Delayed or inadequate initial therapy
5. Circumferential burns to limbs
6. Burn injury plus aspiration injury
7. Pre-existing medical conditions (cardiac, pulmonary, renal)
8. Renal or respiratory condition developing during therapy

PREPARATION FOR TRANSPORT (Table 3)

An airway is established. A large-bore intravenous line allows fluid resuscitation with lactated Ringer's solution to be started using the Parkland formula guidelines. A urinary catheter is placed to monitor urine flow and guide fluid therapy. A nasogastric tube is placed as prophylaxis against vomiting secondary to gastric dilatation or ileus. The burn wound should be covered in sterile dry sheeting. A monitoring chart is prepared, and fluid, drugs, and interventions are accurately recorded during the time of transfer to facilitate continuing care.

Medical Problems Requiring Special Review

Medical problems that require special review include

1. Ileus, inhalation injury (early problems).
2. Sepsis, fever, metabolic stress, nutritional deficiency (ongoing problems).
3. Burns to special sites (face, neck, hands, feet, or genital area).

Ileus and Gastric Dilatation

Ileus and gastric dilatation are common following extensive burns. Nasogastric decompression is necessary until the function of the gastrointestinal tract is established. Vomiting and aspiration may produce a potentially lethal pneumonitis.

Inhalation Injury

Inhalation injury is suggested by facial burns, singed nasal hairs, and carbonaceous sputum. Early bronchoscopy may be necessary to establish a diagnosis and to plan therapy. Oxygen (100 per cent) is then administered, and the clinical phases of pulmonary injury are carefully reviewed.

Phase 1 (1 to 12 Hours After Burn). During this phase, there is a risk of laryngeal edema, bronchospasm, and lung consolidation with progressive hypoxic course. Therapy is endotracheal intubation for laryngospasm; humidity antispasmodics and steroids for bronchospasm; and full respiratory support for lung consolidation.

Phase 2 (6 to 72 Hours After Burn). In this phase, pulmonary edema follows capillary leakage. Careful management of fluid replacement, positive pressure respiratory support, and diuretics (furosemide, 1 to 2 mg/kg IV) are often required.

Phase 3 (3 Days After Burn, and Beyond). Adequate pulmonary toilet and bacteria-specific antibiotics are required in this phase.

Sepsis

Sepsis is the major cause of death in the patient with extensive or deep burn injury. *Pseudomonas aeruginosa* is the major invasive organism. Topical burn care—silver nitrate, sulfamylon, silver sulfadiazine, early débridement, excision, and grafting—are all used in an effort to prevent local invasion. Wound surveillance cultures provide guidelines for systemic antibiotic cover in the event of burn wound sepsis (signs of local tissue invasion, cellulitis, or necrosis) in the presence of fever and toxicity. Polymicrobial sepsis is relatively common, and empiric cover with antibiotics needs to be modified on the basis of a given patient's culture results.

Fever

Fever is a frequent and vexing problem in the burn patient. Although fever may represent a metabolic response to injury (particularly in the patient with eschar present or open wounds), wound sepsis, intercurrent infective syndromes, and pulmonary infection are possible. Removal of eschar and burn wound coverage produces significant decrease in fever. Search for a separate cause of the fever—(1) wound infection, (2) intercurrent throat-ear infection, (3) gastroenteritis, (4) line sepsis, or (5) pulmonary infection—is initially undertaken by inspection of wounds, dressing changes, examination of throat and ears, stool culture (bacterial, rotaviral cultures, rotazyme testing), and chest x-ray films. Blood cultures, ophthalmologic review, and cardiac ultrasonography are indicated in patients with temperatures in excess of 40°C (104°F) or persistent fevers or in the presence of fever with toxicity or shock.

REHABILITATION

For maximal cosmetic and functional independence, physical and occupational therapy should begin upon admission and continue through discharge to the years beyond. Measures used include (1) splinting, (2) exercise (passive, active, and even under anesthesia), and (3) special pressure garments aimed at preventing contracture. Multiple plastic surgical release procedures are necessary for maximal cosmesis and function over the ensuing years.

The pediatrician, social worker, and psychiatrist have a role in the rehabilitation process in helping the treating team to understand the child's regression and manipulation during early therapy and depression at the time of hospital discharge (particularly in adolescents).

Schooling must be continued throughout the long and difficult phase after the initial burn. Increased work and evaluation are necessary before return to a normal classroom. Integration to normal school and social activities is difficult, and the patient, parents, peers, and teachers all require support, discussion, assurance, and understanding. The pediatrician at the burn center can provide advice and back-up as the child returns to the community. Although scarred, the child can partake fully in school activities, social activities, exercise, and sports. Providing constant reassurance that the child is fully recovered and support to the family and school is necessary for acceptance of the child at the local community level.

NEAR-DROWNING

MARK W. UHL, M.D.
and RICHARD A. ORR, M.D.

Drowning is a leading cause of death in children and, in some states, the number one cause of accidental death in children younger than 5 years of age. Near-drowning is defined as survival for at least 24 hours after a submersion accident and is associated with significant morbidity. The age groups at particular risk of drowning are toddlers, aged 1 to 3 years, and teenagers. In both groups, male victims of near-drowning outnumber female victims approximately three to one.[1] Of those victims who arrive at the emergency department comatose and unresponsive, approximately 50 per cent die; of the survivors, 50 per cent remain severely neurologically impaired despite aggressive cardiopulmonary resuscitation (CPR) and attempted cerebral salvage.

Emergency field management should follow established CPR protocols and consists of immediate ventilation and, if necessary, restoration of circulation. The airway should be cleared and mouth-to-mouth ventilation begun immediately, if necessary, even before the child is removed from the water. Use of the Heimlich maneuver to clear water from the lungs is unnecessary and may increase the risk of aspiration of stomach contents. Control of the airway should always include measures to protect the cervical spine because associated spinal cord injury is possible. The circulatory status should be evaluated by auscultation of heart sounds and palpation of central pulses as soon as the victim is removed from the water. In children, cardiac arrest is usually precipitated by a respiratory arrest with resultant hypoxemia and may be reversed by adequate oxygenation and ventilation. If CPR is required, it should be continued until the patient has been transported to the nearest hospital facility and a full evaluation has been performed. The ability to revive an arrested pediatric heart far exceeds the current ability to resuscitate the brain; consequently, hypoxic-ischemic brain injury remains the major determinant of morbidity and mortality after near-drowning.

Emergency management should be focused on the child's pulmonary, circulatory, and central nervous systems. Information, including the child's age, events precipitating the accident, estimated time of submersion, delay in institution of CPR, temperature of water, and pre-existing medical conditions (e.g., seizure disorder), should be obtained. The physical examination should focus on airway patency, respiratory sufficiency, and circulatory status. All patients should receive continuous monitoring of the electrocardiogram (EKG), core temperature, and oxygen saturation by pulse oximetry (S_pO_2). Initial laboratory tests should include chest and cervical spine radiographs, arterial blood gases, hemoglobin and hematocrit, serum electrolytes, blood urea nitrogen, creatinine, glucose, prothrombin and partial thromboplastin times, toxicology screen, and blood alcohol level, if appropriate. The volume of fluid aspirated during human drowning rarely causes life-threatening electrolyte abnormalities or clinically significant hemolysis, despite these theoretic concerns.

Respiratory failure is a frequent occurrence in near-drowning. Aspiration of fluid into the lungs disrupts pulmonary surfactant, causing increased surface tension and alveolar instability. Capillary and alveolar membrane damage allows fluid to leak into the alveoli, with subsequent pulmonary edema and intrapulmonary shunting, leading to hypoxemia. Efforts should be made to maximize arterial oxygen tension (Pao_2) and oxygen delivery to vital organs. Spontaneously breathing patients should be given 100 per cent oxygen by mask; after full assessment, oxygen concentration may be adjusted according to S_pO_2 or arterial blood gas values. If the Pao_2 cannot be maintained above 60 mm Hg in 60 per cent oxygen, or if ventilation is compromised such that arterial carbon dioxide tension ($Paco_2$) is greater than 50 mm Hg, endotracheal intubation and mechanical ventilation should be started. Continuous positive airway pressure (CPAP) or positive end-expiratory pressure (PEEP) is used to maintain adequate oxygenation while allowing further reductions in the inspired oxygen concentration. Placement of a nasogastric tube and use of cricoid pressure (Sellick maneuver) may reduce the risk of further aspiration.

Cardiovascular support should include volume resuscitation with intravenous infusion of isotonic crystalloid solutions (normal saline or lactated Ringer's solution) until the heart rate, blood pressure, and, most important, capillary refill time have returned to normal. Only after hemodynamic stability has been achieved is it appropriate to consider restricting the volume of fluids infused. If the child is hypothermic with a core temperature below 30°C (86°F), active rewarming measures should be undertaken (warmed, humidified gases from the ventilator; peritoneal lavage; or extracorporeal circulatory support). Cardiac resuscitation and adequate neurologic evaluation are impossible at temperatures below 30°C. Above this temperature threshold, *passive* rewarming is most appropriate.

Patients who are apneic, pulseless, and unresponsive have suffered a long period of anoxia and inadequate vital organ perfusion and have profound metabolic acidosis that should be corrected with sodium bicarbonate. Once spontaneous circulation has been restored, efforts should be made to avoid further hypoxemia, hypotension, hyperthermia, or seizures. The use of an inotropic agent such as dopamine, dobutamine, or epinephrine may be required to maintain adequate systemic blood pressure and to improve cerebral perfusion. However, the need for such pharmacologic support portends a very grim prognosis.[2]

Insult to the central nervous system (CNS) is the most devastating consequence of near-drowning. Neurologic outcome after near-drowning falls into one of three categories:

1. Normal function.
2. Death due to anoxic encephalopathy.
3. Neurologic impairment ranging from spastic quadriparesis to a persistent vegetative state.

A major concern has been that the ability to resuscitate hearts and support respiratory function will lead to an increasing percentage of survivors with serious neurologic impairment. Although great effort has been made to identify early indicators of neurologic outcome, no predictive factor is absolutely reliable. Factors that are *not* prognostic include age, sex, duration of submersion (too unreliable), initial arterial pH (reflects ventilatory and circulatory status as well as drugs given during resuscitation), and core temperature on hospital admission. The most positive predictors are recovery of spontaneous respirations and good or improving mental status. All children who reach the emergency department alert and responsive after a submersion accident should recover fully and be discharged neurologically intact. It is still appropriate to admit and observe these patients for 24 to 48 hours because of the remote possibility of pulmonary deterioration. On the other hand, children who are comatose (Glasgow coma score ≤ 5), with fixed and dilated pupils, and who require continuing CPR in the emergency department are unlikely to recover full neurologic function (approximately one in four do).[3]

In the past decade, efforts have focused on cerebral resuscitation after near-drowning. The widely adopted "HYPER" therapy approach has been used to counteract the tendency of near-drowning victims to be hyperHydrated, hyperVentilating, hyperPyrexic, hyperExcitable, and hyperRigid. Management protocols have included fluid restriction and forced diuresis, paralysis and controlled hyperventilation to an arbitrary $Paco_2$ of 25 to 30 mm Hg, intentional hypothermia, corticosteroid therapy, sedation, and intracranial pressure (ICP) monitoring with aggressive control of increased ICP using osmotic agents (mannitol, diuretics) and barbiturate coma. Recent evidence, however, suggests that many of these therapies are ineffective or even counterproductive.[4]

Although ICP is commonly increased for 2 to 4 days after near-drowning, control of ICP has failed to improve neurologic outcome. This suggests that increased ICP and cerebral edema after severe anoxic brain injury result from irreversible neuronal injury (unlike CNS trauma or CNS tumors, in which increased cerebral blood flow and increased brain capillary permeability are prominent factors causing increased ICP). This may explain the lack of demonstrated benefit in near-drowning of ICP monitoring, therapeutic hypothermia, barbiturate coma, controlled hyperventilation, intravenous steroids, and osmotic therapy.[4, 5]

ICP monitoring may be of some prognostic value and may help in deciding to limit resuscitative therapy, because patients with persistent ICP greater than 20 to 30 mm Hg are likely to die or have a very poor neurologic outcome despite therapy. Therapeutic hypothermia has been shown to be of no neurologic benefit for flaccid, comatose victims of near-drowning and appears to increase the risk of infection by inducing immune suppression. Whether mild hypothermia (33 to 34°C) or isolated brain cooling is beneficial remains to be determined. Barbiturate therapy is of value only to suppress postanoxic seizures; barbiturate-induced electrocerebral silence has not improved outcome. Arbitrary hyperventilation to reduce cerebral blood flow may be harmful, especially during postischemic hypoperfusion. Evidence suggests that subsequent hyperemia is due to loss of the normal coupling between brain metabolic rate and cerebral blood flow. In this setting, hyperventilation is unlikely to be of any benefit. Acute hyperventilation to control ICP and prevent herniation is an effective temporary measure. No benefit of intravenous steroids has been shown for the pulmonary or the neurologic complications of near-drowning.

Extraordinary outcomes have been reported for several victims of near-drowning in near-freezing water. The longest reported submersion time with normal neurologic recovery is 66 minutes in a 2½-year-old girl.[6] The publicity such cases generate has obscured the evidence that, in general, hypothermia increases the mortality rate of submersion accidents. The cerebral protection provided by controlled hypothermia *before* an ischemic event is well known and provides the basis for operative repair of complex congenital heart defects under profound hypothermia and circulatory arrest. Whether hypothermia *after* a hypoxic-ischemic injury can be of benefit remains unproven. Most hypothermic near-drowning victims seen in the emergency department are cold because hypothalamic and brain stem injury from anoxia has led to poikilothermic equilibration of body and environmental temperatures. The admonition that no patient is dead until warm and dead still applies, but medical personnel must be prepared to deal with the likelihood of poor neurologic outcome. It is appropriate to maintain cardiovascular function until the difficult decisions regarding discontinuation of life support, and the possibility of organ donation in the case of documented brain death, can be resolved.

With current techniques of CPR, stabilization, transportation, cardiorespiratory support, and neurologic intensive care, one can expect to revive about 15 to 25 per cent of all children who arrive at the hospital in full cardiac arrest with no apparent neurologic function. Similar rates are associated with other types of out-of-hospital cardiac arrest in children. Brain resuscitation measures have had little impact on this survival rate. Nevertheless, a 15 per cent salvage rate justifies continued recommendations to attempt resuscitation of all victims of near-drowning accidents.

REFERENCES

1. Wintemute GJ: Childhood drowning and near-drowning in the United States. Am J Dis Child 144:663–669, 1990.
2. Nichter MA, Everett PB: Childhood near-drowning: Is cardiopulmonary resuscitation always indicated? Crit Care Med 17:993–995, 1989.
3. Orlowski JP: Drowning, near-drowning, and ice-water submersions. Pediatr Clin North Am 34:75–92, 1987.
4. Nussbaum E, Maggi JC: Pentobarbital therapy does not improve neurologic outcome in nearly drowned, flaccid-comatose children. Pediatrics 81:630–634, 1988.
5. Smyrnios NA, Irwin RS: Current concepts in the pathophysiology and management of near-drowning. J Intensive Care Med 6:26–35, 1991.
6. Bolte RG, Black PG, Bowers RS, et al: The use of extracorporeal rewarming in a child submerged for 66 minutes. JAMA 260:377–379, 1988.

SUDDEN INFANT DEATH SYNDROME AND APPARENT LIFE-THREATENING EVENTS

DANIEL C. SHANNON, M.D.

Parents, physicians, and investigators need to know the facts about sudden infant death syndrome (SIDS) and infant apnea, generally called an apparent life-threatening event (ALTE). This review focuses on this need so that all may fulfill their obligations more effectively.

SIDS is the death of a previously well infant between the ages of 29 days and 1 year in whom no cause is found at autopsy or after thorough investigation of the case history or the death scene. Until the past few years, an autopsy was considered sufficient to exclude identifiable causes. Recognition of intentional or accidental smothering or of overheating has led to additional exclusion criteria. This implies that such cases were previously identified as SIDS, that SIDS cases include more than one mechanism of death, and that SIDS is a final common pathway rather than a disease.

An ALTE is characterized by apparent cessation of air exchange associated with pallor or cyanosis and change in muscle tone. The observer believes that the infant would have died were it not for intervention.

COUNSELING PARENTS OF SIDS VICTIMS

Parents need to know that SIDS generally occurs without warning while the infant sleeps, that they are without blame, and that investigators are working hard to find its causes. Despite this reassurance, parents blame themselves for perceived faults of omission or commission and may benefit from association with other families of SIDS victims organized by the National SIDS Foundation. They need to know that even though epidemiologic studies have identified risk factors for SIDS, these factors singly or in combination lack sufficient predictive value to target a high-risk group that might receive special attention during infancy. There is not yet general agreement among investigators regarding the mechanisms responsible for SIDS.

A task force of the American Academy of Pediatrics has recently reviewed several studies from other countries, the results of which suggest an association between placement for sleep in the prone position and the occurrence of SIDS. The task force has recommended that even though these studies have methodologic limitations, the supine position should now be recommended for infants in the United States. I think that this recommendation is premature for a number of reasons. All of the reported studies come from countries in which the incidence of SIDS has been higher than that in the United States and where the reported incidence remained at or above that in the United States following an advertising campaign advising parents to use the supine position. These studies were not adequately controlled for other factors that might have coincidentally affected the incidence of SIDS. Although the position at sleep onset was noted, the position at death was not systematically examined. Finally, this recommendation is certain to arouse considerable anxiety in parents whose infant is old enough to roll over while sleeping as well as guilt from insufficient vigilance in those whose infants die of SIDS regardless of position. One wonders if pediatricians might also be prompted to evaluate more infants for gastroesophageal reflux in an attempt to avoid recommending the supine position for such infants.

The physician should anticipate that parents of SIDS victims may be even more overwhelmed than parents whose children die of another, better understood disease because (1) the SIDS death was sudden and unexpected and (2) SIDS is shrouded by an air of mystery. It is thus of key importance to emphasize and reassure the parents that (1) SIDS is not a definite disease entity and (2) because SIDS can neither be predicted nor prevented, they are in no way responsible for the child's death. It is important to work with surviving siblings about any guilt feelings and to assess family coping. It may be helpful to contact the National SIDS Foundation because contact with other families may be of comfort.*

Physicians should know that parents will need special counseling prior to and during subsequent pregnancies. Parents will anticipate from literature and hearsay that the new infant will be at special risk. The best epidemiologic study examined the birth and death records of nearly 1 million infants born over a 10-year period in the northwestern United States; whereas the incidence of SIDS was the expected 2 in 1000, there were recurrences in only five families. These numbers were too small for the investigators to say with confidence to what extent the risk of SIDS was increased.

The physician who counsels such parents should recall that the population with an average risk of 2 in 1000 is composed of subgroups with widely varying risks. At one end of the spectrum is the unmarried mother younger than 20 years of age who smokes cigarettes and delivers a preterm infant whose risk for SIDS is about four times the average risk. At the other end is the intact family with at least one parent employed, neither parent smokes, who produces a full-term infant whose risk is about one fourth that of the average. I have found that this information is especially reassuring to parents in the latter group. It presents special dilemmas, however, in counseling those at increased risk. Should any special evaluation be done on the next infant? Regardless of the results of such an investigation, should electronic monitoring be recommended given an anticipated risk of 1 in 125? What should be done if the mother is deemed incapable of coping with both a new infant and a monitor? The answers should depend on the particular case and require the best judgment of the physician.

PATHOGENESIS AND CHARACTERISTICS

Investigators want to know what mechanisms can account for the epidemiologic facts and the findings of the pathologist. Without doubt, one of the key problems is that SIDS has multiple causes whereas investigators focus hypotheses based on assumed homogeneity. Thus, statistical associations between SIDS and a particular observation are likely to be confounded from the start. Nevertheless, any hypothesis that explains even a few cases of SIDS must account for silent cessation of vital functions (i.e., gas exchange in the lung, heart, or brain). For example, failure of neural regulation of upper airway muscles such as the abductors of the vocal cords would result in failure of opening of the cords with each inspiration, obstruction to airflow, and failure of pulmonary gas exchange with consequent cardiac and cerebral hypoxia. On the other hand, the primary event could be inadequate regulation of cardiac depolarization or repolarization, failure of perfusion to supply oxygen to the brain, and resulting cessation of ventilation. In either case, our knowledge of the chemical regulation of these events is rudimentary.

The most consistent feature of pathologic investigations is petechiae on the visceral pleural surfaces. These are found in increased numbers in about three quarters of patients that otherwise qualify as SIDS victims. Their presence suggests airway obstruction as a component of the pathophysiology, but they are also consistent with continued perfusion of damaged capillaries.

ALTE

The acronym ALTE was proposed as a general term to characterize episodes in which parents or caretakers thought that infant death was likely had they not intervened to terminate the episode. With careful attention to affected infants over the past 15 years, certain generalizations can now be stated. The majority of episodes reported by caretakers or parents cannot be classified as an ALTE because the events lack one or more significant features. For example, we would not consider an episode of apparent apnea life-threatening if it was observed, lasted for an uncertain duration, and terminated spontaneously.

An identifiable cause for an ALTE is found in about one third of infants after thorough evaluation. These causes include seizure, gastroesophageal reflux, respiratory infections such as respiratory syncytial virus (RSV) and pertussis, and a number of less frequent conditions. The latter include various congenital defects that can obstruct airflow such as vocal cord paresis, tachy- or bradyarrhythmias, congenital central hypoventilation, and factitious or fictitious events.

It is still difficult to decide whether to employ home monitoring for infants who have experienced an ALTE (or, as mentioned above, for subsequent children of parents of a SIDS victim). Generally, monitors are indicated

1. After a particularly severe ALTE requiring prolonged stimulation and mouth-to-mouth resuscitation, or in especially high-risk groups.
2. When the parental anxiety concerning infant death is so marked that the family cannot cope.

Although controlled clinical trials do not currently prove the efficacy of monitoring, its judicious use still plays a role in following certain infants.

The choice of electronic monitoring of vital functions at home should be determined based on the anticipated likelihood of another ALTE. The interpretation of that likelihood by parents will vary with their circumstances and will strongly influence their perception of the need for monitoring; therefore, no strict guidelines can be recommended.

There is general agreement that most of the diseases that cause an ALTE are capable of causing SIDS. What is not known is the extent to which each is responsible for the deaths that occur each year. There is also general agreement that most deaths are probably not the result of this set of diseases and that the mechanism of death in those cases has not yet been identified. A variety of theories continue to be proposed, only to be rejected after further investigation. The physician should continue to be highly skeptical of any retrospective study, of any study lacking an adequate number and type of controls, and of any study that proposes a mechanism that does not clearly threaten to terminate vital functions.

*National SIDS Foundation, 10500 Little Patuxent Parkway, No. 420, Columbia, MD 21044. Phone 1–800–221–SIDS.

PENETRATING KNIFE AND GUNSHOT WOUNDS IN CHILDREN

BARBARA A. BARLOW, M.D.

Pediatricians are now faced with an alarming increase in the number of children presenting with penetrating injuries from bullets or knives. The National Pediatric Trauma Registry's 1988–1990 report on 13,321 pediatric trauma cases, which were admitted to 30 pediatric trauma centers in the United States and Canada, revealed that 13 per cent of cases were caused by penetrating injuries.[1] Gunshot wounds caused 5.5 per cent of the injuries, and stab wounds 5.1 per cent. Although common belief is that gunshot and stab wounds to children usually occur unintentionally, 71.8 per cent of the gunshot wounds and 25.4 per cent of the stab wounds were intentionally inflicted. In the combined pediatric trauma data base, 88 per cent of the injuries were unintentional, 0.5 per cent were suicide attempts, and only 7.1 per cent were intentional.

ADMISSION POLICY

All children with gunshot or stab wounds should be admitted to the hospital for observation, wound care, antibiotics, social evaluation, and psychologic assistance, even when there is no indication for operative intervention. When a child is intentionally injured, the initial history is rarely correct; however, during hospitalization, the child will often volunteer the information as they receive postinjury counseling. Allowing a child to return to the same situation in which injury occurred may mean that the child will be injured again, sometimes more seriously. Hospital admission ensures that there will be time to evaluate the situation surrounding the injury and that proper counseling and support will be arranged for the child and the family.

All children who have been shot or stabbed require support to recover psychologically from the trauma, even if the injury was unintentional. Recurrent nightmares, inability to sleep, regression, school problems, and fear of leaving home are just a few of the symptoms that these children may exhibit. In addition, family members are traumatized when a child is shot or stabbed. Both parents and siblings may develop the symptoms associated with post-traumatic stress. When children have been injured by a family member, intentionally or unintentionally, the entire family needs counseling, with particular help given to the individual who caused the injury. Other children who witnessed the shooting or stabbing often need emotional support to avoid symptom formation. The majority of gunshot and stab wounds are caused by children; these children and their families also require counseling.

Many children in our series of penetrating injuries previously lost a member of their nuclear family to violent death, which is not true for children admitted for other types of injury. It appears that a violent incident in the nuclear family places the children in the family at risk for later violent injury to themselves.[2]

ASSESSMENT AND MANAGEMENT

Immediate surgical evaluation is essential for children presenting with gunshot and stab wounds because the most innocent-looking wound can be associated with life-threatening internal injury. This includes BB gun and pellet gun wounds, which can produce major injuries through penetration of the abdominal wall, the chest wall, and the skull. Because protocols for preoperative evaluation and operative intervention in penetrating wounds vary among centers, the responsible surgeon must be involved in the decision making. Pediatricians who work in areas experiencing an increase in penetrating wounds should work with their surgical colleagues to develop evaluation and treatment protocols for penetrating injuries that are appropriate for their medical center.

The initial assessment of the child presenting with a penetrating injury follows the same steps as the assessment for a blunt injury. The Advanced Trauma Life Support course, developed by the Committee on Trauma of the American College of Surgeons, is excellent preparation for the physician who is called on to manage children with major trauma. This course provides the framework for the initial assessment and management of the child with the penetrating injuries discussed in this article.[3]

Primary Survey

The primary survey involves the ABCs:

A—airway maintenance with intubation, if needed, using cervical spine control for penetrating injury to the head and neck.

B—breathing with chest tube insertion for tension pneumothorax or hemopneumothorax.

C—circulation with hemorrhage control by direct pressure on accessible sites.

D—disability or brief evaluation of neurologic status.

E—exposure by completely undressing the child because there may be multiple penetrating sites that could be missed.

Immediate management is initiated for any life-threatening condition encountered.

Resuscitation

During the next phase, resuscitation, intravenous access is established and volume replacement is initiated when required. In children with major blood loss, two large-bore intravenous lines should be placed, preferably in the upper extremities. Intravenous lines should not be placed in injured extremities. Children with major injury should receive oxygen and continuous monitoring of both vital signs and electrocardiogram. Nasogastric tubes and urinary catheters are used for children with major injury and for children who require laparotomy, unless they are contraindicated. Gastric distention in injured children is common and prevents adequate evaluation of the abdomen. Monitoring urinary output is essential in children requiring volume replacement.

Secondary Survey

At this juncture, the secondary survey can be undertaken, which involves thorough evaluation of the entire child: "a head-to-toe look, listen, and feel examination." All known and suspected injuries are evaluated in order to establish treatment priorities and plan required diagnostic studies. Estimated bullet and knife trajectories are used to suggest possible internal injury. Multiple penetrating sites may indicate multiple bullets or through-and-through injury. In general, the entrance wound is smaller than the exit wound, and close-range wounds have powder burns at the entrance site.

During this phase, laboratory and radiologic studies are obtained. Chest radiograph is a priority study both to evaluate chest tube placement and lung expansion and to diagnose injury missed on physical examination. All hemo- or pneumothoraces caused by penetrating injury necessitate insertion of a chest tube for re-expansion of the lung in order to seal the lung laceration against the chest wall and to provide monitoring of air leak and blood loss. Spinal injury is not uncommon in children with gunshot penetration of the neck and torso. Therefore, spinal radiographs should be obtained as priority studies in these children. Because bullet trajectories may be altered by contact with bone or by deformation of the bullet, which causes tumbling, radiographs should be taken of body areas above and below the entrance wound to avoid missing a retained bullet.

Definitive Care

In the definitive care phase, children requiring immediate operative intervention are triaged to the operating room. Children who are unstable should not be sent for radiographs, and those with major injuries should be accompanied by a physician and monitored carefully during these studies. Children who do not need immediate surgery should receive radiographic evaluation dictated by the wounds sustained. Fractures should be stabilized and splinted and then considered for operative débridement, because fractures caused by penetrating injury are, by definition, "open fractures." In institutions equipped for pediatric angiography, this study can be used to evaluate penetrating wounds of the neck or wounds close to major arteries. Other studies that can be useful in the evaluation of selected penetrating injuries are esophagoscopy, bronchoscopy, proctoscopy, barium swallow, and ultrasonography. Some institutions are now using computed tomography scan in the evaluation of selected penetrating injury. This study can be useful in determining the exact location of a retained bullet or shotgun pellets.

Most trauma centers have sufficient staff and intensive care facilities to manage penetrating wounds selectively. This method allows the patient, who does not have symptoms and signs mandating surgery at the time of admission, to be carefully observed until such signs appear or until it is clear that the patient will not require surgical intervention. In centers that cannot provide the careful monitoring needed for selective management, patients with penetrating wounds should be explored for immediate evaluation and treatment. Penetrating gunshot and stab wounds of the neck, chest, and extremity and stab wounds of the abdomen are often managed selectively. However, few centers selectively manage abdominal gunshot wounds because most require immediate operative intervention. Peritoneal lavage, which is used to evaluate both blunt and penetrating abdominal wounds in some adult trauma centers, is not used as frequently in injured children and is never used for evaluating penetrating injury at our institution. Traditionally, neck injuries penetrating the platysma were surgically explored, but the practice of selective management, with the diagnostic assistance of angiography and endoscopy, is gaining in popularity.[4]

Probing of the wound for depth and direction should be done only by the surgeon managing the child. Wound probing can be dangerous, particularly in the neck, in the chest, or over major vessels. Dye studies of penetrating wound tracts have been abandoned because of the high incidence of tract infection after this procedure and the small but significant incidence of false-negative studies.

Penetrating injuries result in dirty wounds. Infection of the wound tract and abscess formation around a retained bullet are common complications. Therefore, the wound tract is not used for a chest tube site and is not included in the operative incision. Superficial wounds can be irrigated with saline and cleansed. Wound tracts are left open unless wound size or location demands closure. Major wounds should be closed in the operating room, where proper evaluation and débridement can be performed. Tetanus immunization must be up to date, and a booster shot is indicated if the wound is heavily contaminated. A broad-spectrum intravenous antibiotic (such as Keflin, 100 mg/kg per 24 hours in divided doses) is given to all patients to treat the contaminated wound. Operative cases may require a more intensive antibiotic regimen, particularly if bowel was penetrated. Changes in antibiotics are based on wound cultures.

Daily wound care should be done in the hospital. A specimen of wound drainage should be taken for culture. Bullets can push foreign material such as bits of skin, hair, and clothing deep into the tissues, which will lead to late abscess formation. Palpable bullets should be removed on presentation, and the tract cleaned. If swelling initially obscures superficial bullets, these can be removed when the swelling subsides. Bullets located in areas where removal would require a major operation are left in place; removal is undertaken only if the lead level begins to rise and no other source of lead poisoning can be identified. Lead levels should be followed when there is a retained bullet, particularly when the bullet is in contact with bone or joint fluid. The family must be told that lead poisoning can occur from retained bullets and that the risk is lifelong.[5]

Discussion of selective management protocols and operative technique for specific injuries is beyond the scope of this article. Children with gunshot and stab wounds should be treated in a trauma center that has the proper facilities and an appropriately trained staff to evaluate and care for children with this type of injury.

The pediatrician must ensure that the child and family receive the proper support and counseling and that the circumstances surrounding the incident are fully understood prior to discharge. Some children who were intentionally injured may not be able to return to their homes when the circumstances that led to the penetrating injury have not been resolved. Placement with relatives in another community may offer these children protection.

REFERENCES

1. National Pediatric Trauma Registry Biannual Report. Boston, Research and Training Center, Tufts University School of Medicine, 1991.
2. Advanced Trauma Life Support Course. Committee on Trauma, American College of Surgeons, 1992.
3. Barlow B, Niemirska M, Gandhi R: Ten years' experience with pediatric gunshot wounds. J Pediatr Surg 17:927–932, 1982.
4. Cooper A, Barlow B, Niemirska M, Gandhi R: Fifteen years' experience with penetrating trauma to the head and neck in children. J Pediatr Surg 22:24–27, 1987.
5. Dillman RO, Crumb CK, Lidsky MJ: Lead poisoning from a gunshot wound. Report of a case and review of the literature. Am J Med 66:509–514, 1979.

21

Special Problems in the Fetus and Neonate

DISTURBANCES OF INTRAUTERINE GROWTH

M. DOUGLAS CUNNINGHAM, M.D.

Normal fetal growth may be altered at any point in gestation by adverse maternal, placental, or fetal conditions. Newborn infants with birth weights greater or less than two standard deviations from the mean for gestational age are considered to have had abnormal intrauterine growth. Three distinct clinical entities are associated with fetal growth disturbances: intrauterine growth retardation, postmaturity (post-term infant), and large for gestational age (LGA). Although intrauterine growth disturbances have many causes, they present with similar complications and therapeutic requirements.

INTRAUTERINE GROWTH RETARDATION

Fetal growth retardation is most often referred to by obstetricians and perinatologists as intrauterine growth retardation (IUGR). Some confusion of terms exist because of the use by pediatricians and neonatologists of the term small-for-gestational-age (SGA) infant. The latter is simply more clinically descriptive of the undergrown newborn, whereas IUGR is more descriptive of the circumstances of the pregnancy with advancing gestation and limited fetal growth. Infants described as SGA are below the 10th percentile for body weight but may have body length and/or head circumference above or below the 10th percentile.

These variations in body proportions have led to the additional descriptive terms of symmetric versus asymmetric IUGR. An infant with symmetric IUGR is depicted as having body weight, length, and head circumference uniformly below the 10th percentile. The causes of symmetric IUGR are often intrinsic to the fetus and reflect genetic factors, congenital anomalies, effects of toxic substances (drugs, alcohol), or congenital infections.

Asymmetric IUGR is most often the result of factors extrinsic to the fetus and reflect placental abnormalities or maternal illness (Table 1). Typically, the head circumference of the infant with asymmetric IUGR is near the 25th percentile, with body length and weight at or below the 10th percentile. These infants are said to exhibit "brain-sparing" growth in the face of adverse maternal conditions, or uteroplacental insufficiency.

Complications

Immediately upon birth and throughout the postnatal period, SGA infants face a number of complications. Both term and preterm SGA infants require careful assessment and stabilization in the delivery room. A disproportionate body mass-to-surface ratio leads to their rapid loss of body heat and the additional complications of metabolic acidosis, hypoglycemia, and hypertension. Heat conservation in the SGA infant includes use of a radiant warmer or double-walled incubator, a knit cotton cap, and prewarmed blankets.

Hypoglycemia

Hypoglycemia is the most frequent metabolic complication of preterm or term SGA infants. Blood glucose levels decline soon after birth and require close monitoring with bedside screening aids (glucose oxidase test strips) at 20- to 30-minute intervals during the first 2 hours of life. Values of 40 mg/dl or less necessitate administration of intravenous glucose. Laboratory confirmation of hypoglycemia by serum glucose values is recommended if low blood glucose is detected by screening.

Glucose administration at a rate of 6 to 8 mg/kg/minute (100 to 115 ml/kg per 24 hours of 10 per cent dextrose in water) will suffice in most instances until enteral feedings provide adequate caloric intake. If overt symptoms of hypoglycemia appear, miniboluses of 10 per cent dextrose in water (2 ml/kg per dose) may be required until a continuous intravenous infusion of glucose is established.

Occasionally, term SGA infants will be refractory to increased levels of intravenous glucose (12 to 15 mg/kg/minute) and will require short-term adjunct glucocorticoid therapy (hydrocortisone sodium succinate, 5 mg/kg/day IV, or prednisone, 2 mg/kg/day orally). More persistent hypoglycemia (3 to 5 days of life) requires determination of serum insulin levels and an expanded endocrine evaluation.

Hypocalcemia

Hypocalcemia is an occasional finding in SGA infants. Serum total calcium levels of less than 7 mg/dl if symptomatic and 6 mg/dl if asymptomatic require treatment.

Intravenous calcium gluconate is the preferred treatment

TABLE 1. Causes of Intrauterine Growth Retardation

Symmetric	Asymmetric
Genetic	***Uteroplacental Insufficiency***
Trisomy 13, 18, 21	Pregnancy-induced hypertension
Turner syndrome	Chronic renal disease
Multiple sex chromosomes: XXX, XYY	Cyanotic congenital heart disease
Bone and connective tissue achondroplasia, chondrodystrophies, osteogenesis imperfecta	Hemoglobinopathies
	Collagen vascular diseases (lupus erythematosus)
Fetal Infections	Thyrotoxicosis
Cytomegalovirus	***Placenta***
Rubella	Multiple infarcts
Syphilis	Partial, chronic abruptio
Toxoplasmosis	Circumvallate
Herpes simplex	Hemangiomas
Malaria	Chorioangioma
Drugs or Substance Abuse	Single umbilical artery
Heroin (and other opiates)	Multiple gestation
Ethyl alcohol (fetal alcohol syndrome)	Twin-to-twin transfusion
Tobacco (smoking)	
Phencyclidine (PCP)	
Methamphetamines	
Cocaine	
Caffeine (excessive intake)	
Therapeutic Drugs	
Antimetabolites (aminopterin)	
Anticonvulsants (phenytoin or trimethadione)	
Steroids	
Environment/Nutrition	
Excessive exercise	
Chronic malnutrition	
Hyperthermia	
Radiation	

(200 to 500 mg/kg per 24 hours in divided doses for maintenance). If the SGA infant is symptomatic with hypocalcemia, 1 to 2 ml/kg of 10 per cent calcium gluconate solution may be infused slowly over 10 minutes. Calcium gluconate infusions require special precautions, including

1. Slow infusion.
2. A well-functioning and monitored intravenous site.
3. Electrocardiographic monitoring for bradycardia or dysrhythmia.
4. Avoidance of the simultaneous infusion of sodium bicarbonate.
5. Selection of infusion site other than the umbilical artery catheter in order to avoid vasospasm.

Polycythemia

Placental dysfunction may cause chronic fetal hypoxia with resultant polycythemia. Capillary hematocrit determinations of 65 per cent or greater suggest the possibility of hyperviscosity and poor perfusion. Hematocrit (Hct) values must be validated by venipuncture of a peripheral vein. A peripheral venous hematocrit of 65 per cent or greater and signs of central nervous system irritability, demarcating of digits, hypoglycemia, early jaundice, or priapism in males are an indication for partial exchange transfusion.

Symptomatic polycythemia is treated in the newborn period by partial exchange transfusion using saline, 5 per cent albumin, or plasmanate and the following formula:

$$\text{Volume of partial exchange fluid} = \frac{(\text{observed Hct} - \text{desired Hct})}{\text{observed Hct}} \times \text{blood volume (80 ml/kg)} \times \text{weight (kg)}$$

Nutritional Needs

Small-for-gestational-age infants have increased nutritional needs in the neonatal period. Once complications have been cleared and regular oral feedings are established, caloric intake can be increased to 120 cal/kg per 24 hours. By 2 weeks of age, many SGA infants will require 130 to 140 cal/kg per 24 hours to sustain a daily growth pattern of 20 to 30 g of weight gain. Isotonic 24 cal/ounce formula has been particularly useful for feeding these infants once 20 cal/ounce formula has been well tolerated.

These feeding guides are not meant to preclude breast-feeding. If initiation of breast-feeding is successful, the mother can be encouraged to nurse as often as the infant demands, even if seemingly continuous suckling is at times desired. For some mothers, this will be trying and supplemental feedings will be required. Accelerated caloric intake for the breast-feeding SGA infant may be difficult to achieve in the early postnatal weeks. Use of a breast pump and breast milk fortifiers may provide some feeding alternatives.

POSTMATURITY

Extended gestation, usually 42 to 44 weeks, may result in altered fetal growth. The neonate may appear long and thin and be covered by loose, desquamating skin. Meconium staining of amniotic fluid is not uncommon in postdate pregnancies. The fingernails may be strikingly long and yellow-stained, as is the umbilical cord. The head circumference is normal for term to slightly increased, and the length is usually above the 50th percentile. Conversely, the infant's weight is between the 10th and 50th percentile. Because of limited placental nutrition during the extended gestation, subcutaneous wasting takes place. As in the SGA infant, temperature instability and excessive body heat loss can take place.

Complications

Birth Asphyxia

Frequently, postmature infants have fetal distress and birth asphyxia manifested by low Apgar scores. Intrauterine distress, presumably due to chronic hypoxia secondary to advanced placental aging and involution, leads to meconium passage into the amniotic fluid.

At birth, steps must be taken to suction the upper airway before the first breath is taken. Examination of the hypopharynx for meconium by laryngoscopy is recommended. If meconium resides at the level of the vocal cords, endotracheal suctioning is recommended. Anticipation of birth asphyxia and providing supportive measures at the time of birth are key to preventing complications of cold stress, acidosis, and meconium aspiration.

Birth Injury

Birth injuries are common in postmature infants as in LGA infants. In part, this is related to the increased length and advanced bone age in postmatures. The extended intrauterine age leads to increased bone mineralization and hardness.

Hypoglycemia

Hypoglycemia is encountered in postmature infants; it is less frequent and somewhat less pronounced than in SGA infants. Frequent bedside screening, as for SGA infants, is required. Because of the frequency of birth asphyxia and uncertain neurologic status, oral feedings for hypoglycemia should be approached with considerable caution in the first 24 hours. Glucose replacement should follow the guidelines noted for SGA infants.

Hypocalcemia

Hypocalcemia may complicate postmaturity, especially in the face of birth asphyxia and/or meconium aspiration. Calcium replacement and maintenance should follow the guidelines noted for SGA infants.

Polycythemia

Polycythemia and hyperviscosity are of special concern in postmature infants with possible central nervous system compromise and meconium aspiration. Prompt documentation of the central venous hematocrit value is important. In the compromised infant, early partial exchange transfusion to adjust the hematocrit to a level between 50 and 55 is recommended. Serial hematocrit determinations at 4-hour intervals following the first partial exchange transfusion are suggested because some infants show a tendency for rebound polycythemia.

LARGE FOR GESTATIONAL AGE

Infants with birth weights more than two standard deviations above the mean for gestational age are typically associated with diabetic mothers or constitutionally large parents. Infants who are LGA may also be seen with transposition of the great vessels and with syndromes such as cerebral gigantism and Beckwith Coombs syndrome.

Complications

Most LGA infants are susceptible to hypoglycemia, and screening tests for glucose should be done early. Treatment of birth depression, polycythemia, hypocalcemia, and hypoglycemia follows as described previously. Large for gestational age infants of diabetic mothers may prove to have hypoglycemia that is difficult to control. Treatment with glucagon (0.3 mg/kg/dose, up to total dose of 1 mg/kg, subcutaneous, IM, or IV) can be beneficial and can allow for more controlled intravenous glucose administration.

PROGNOSIS

The long-term neurologic outcome of infants with intrauterine growth disturbances is unclear because of the many maternal and neonatal complications. A greater number of neurologic limitations are generally attributed to symmetric SGA infants as a group because of the genetic and congenital infection factors. But specific identifying factors and predicting circumstances are lacking in asymmetric SGA, postmature, and LGA infants. Nevertheless, increasing numbers of reports indicate that all infants with intrauterine growth disturbance are at some risk for adverse long-term neurologic and developmental outcome, for which they all require special consideration in follow-up care.

BIRTH INJURIES

RICHARD A. POLIN, M.D.
and ROY SCHNEIDERMAN, M.D.

Birth injury refers to trauma sustained during the process of labor and delivery. In many instances, birth injury may be unavoidable despite optimal obstetric care. Even though the incidence of birth injuries has decreased in recent years (as a result of increased use of cesarean sections and decreased use of vacuum extractions for difficult vaginal deliveries), the clinician must be aware of the full spectrum of birth injuries, as some are serious and potentially lethal.

SUPERFICIAL BIRTH INJURY

Petechiae

Petechiae that occur following a traumatic delivery are usually the result of an increase in venous pressure. An infant born with a tight nuchal cord may have petechiae limited to the head and neck, whereas infants undergoing a rapid increase in intrathoracic pressure during delivery frequently have petechiae distributed over the entire chest and back.

When the petechiae are distributed in a more generalized fashion, it is essential to rule out thrombocytopenia as the cause. A low platelet count ($<150{,}000/mm^3$) must always be evaluated further. When the petechiae are secondary to a systemic problem and not due to birth injury, the infant is often ill and frequently displays other clinical findings.

Ecchymoses

Ecchymoses are often associated with traumatic and/or breech deliveries and are usually observed over the presenting body part. They are more severe in premature infants, and, in some instances, they may be associated with signs and symptoms of acute blood loss (see discussion of subgaleal hemorrhage later).

Healing occurs without treatment; however, hyperbilirubinemia requiring phototherapy can occur, especially in the premature infant.

Subcutaneous Fat Necrosis

Subcutaneous fat necrosis is primarily due to excessive extrinsic pressure during the birth process. Superficially, the lobules of fat necrosis are raised and violaceous or red. Fat necrosis has also been observed following exposure to cold and in infants of diabetic mothers. The lesion is usually localized to an area of trauma.

No specific treatment other than observation is needed, and resolution usually occurs over days to weeks. The lesions may, on occasion, become calcified and result in the development of hypercalcemia.

Scleral Hemorrhages

Scleral hemorrhages are common, benign, and resolve in 1 to 2 weeks.

HEAD INJURY

Hemorrhage occurring during the birth process can occur in an intracranial or extracranial location.

Extracranial Hemorrhage

Extracranial hemorrhage is divided into three types: caput succedaneum, subgaleal hemorrhage, and cephalhematoma. These lesions are differentiated by their tissue plane of origin and their clinical manifestations.

Caput Succedaneum

Caput succedaneum refers to hemorrhagic edema of the scalp, which is due to compression of the head during vaginal delivery. The edema is soft, superficial, and crosses suture lines. No specific intervention is required, as a caput usually diminishes after the first few postnatal days.

Subgaleal Hemorrhage

Subgaleal hemorrhage, although not as common as a caput succedaneum, carries a greater clinical significance. This form of extracranial hemorrhage is due to bleeding beneath the aponeurosis of the scalp, which connects the frontal and occipital portions of the occipitofrontalis muscle. In some infants, an underlying bleeding disorder can precipitate the hemorrhage.

Subgaleal hemorrhage presents as a firm, ecchymotic, fluctuant mass that can increase to dissect down the posterior neck. Careful attention to hemodynamic support is important, as shock secondary to blood loss can occur. After initial stabilization, the lesion usually resolves over a few weeks.

Cephalhematoma

Cephalhematoma is a subperiosteal hemorrhage occurring in up to 2 per cent of births. The incidence is higher in infants of primipara, male infants, and infants delivered with the aid of forceps. The cephalhematoma is limited by the suture lines of the underlying bone. The parietal bone is most commonly involved. An underlying linear fracture is present in 10 to 25 per cent of infants with cephalhematomas. The elevated periosteal bone at the cephalhematoma's margin often gives a false impression of a depressed skull fracture.

No specific intervention is required unless the cephalhematoma is complicated by a depressed skull fracture or intracranial bleeding. Aspiration is contraindicated because of the risk of introducing a secondary infection. Most cephalhematomas resolve in weeks to months; however, on occasion, some of them become calcified, leading to formation of bony protuberances. These growths gradually disappear over months with skull growth and remodeling.

Intracranial Hemorrhage

The common sites of intracranial hemorrhage following trauma in the perinatal period include epidural, subarachnoid, subdural, and intracerebellar. Intraventricular hemorrhage, although the most common type of intracranial bleeding, is usually a complication of prematurity and not due to birth trauma. The risk factors for traumatic intracranial hemorrhage include prolonged or rapid labors; use of midforceps; breech extractions; foot, face, and brow presentations; and relative cephalopelvic disproportion. The incidence of traumatic hemorrhage is relatively low because of the liberal use of cesarean section for cephalopelvic disproportion and the decreased use of forceps for difficult deliveries.

Epidural Hemorrhage

Epidural hemorrhages are exceedingly rare and are due to lacerations of branches of the middle meningeal artery or bleeding from major venous sinuses. Bleeding occurs in the plane between the bone and the periosteum on the inner aspect of the skull. Most epidural hemorrhages are associated with linear skull fractures, and the majority of infants present with signs of increased intracranial pressure.

Treatment requires surgical intervention and appropriate supportive measures.

Subarachnoid Hemorrhage

Subarachnoid hemorrhage is more common in the preterm infant, in whom it is usually associated with an anoxic event. In full-term infants, subarachnoid hemorrhages are frequently associated with birth trauma.

The neurologic syndromes associated with subarachnoid hemorrhage include (1) minimal or no clinical signs (most common); (2) seizures in an otherwise well-appearing infant; and (3) catastrophic deterioration (rare). The clinical course of subarachnoid hemorrhage is usually benign, and most infants require only observation. An occasional infant will develop posthemorrhagic hydrocephalus.

Subdural Hemorrhage

Subdural hemorrhages are infrequently observed in the neonate. Table 1 lists the major varieties of subdural hemorrhage, presenting signs, and recommended management. Infants with lacerations of the falx and tentorium, as well as those with overt occipital osteodiastasis, exhibit a poor prognosis. The outcome for infants with smaller posterior fossa subdural hematomas is variable. Fifty to 80 per cent of infants with convexity subdural hemorrhages develop normally. Subdural hemorrhages are principally observed in full-term infants who are critically ill.

Treatment of posterior fossa subdural hematomas requires prompt surgical intervention. Infants with minor convexity subdural hematomas may be observed unless signs of increased intracranial pressure or craniocerebral disproportion develop (Table 1).

Intracerebellar Hemorrhage

Intracerebellar hemorrhage usually occurs in the preterm infant and is associated with both asphyxia and trauma. Infants with intracerebellar hemorrhage have usually experienced a difficult labor or delivery. Although the time of presentation is variable (days to weeks), small, sick premature infants tend to present sooner. The clinical syndrome usually includes signs referrable to brain stem compression (apnea, skew deviation of eyes, facial paresis, intermittent tonic extension of limbs, and flaccid quadriparesis). In some infants, there may be obstruction to cerebrospinal fluid flow, resulting in hydrocephalus.

The prognosis for affected preterm infants is poor, whereas term infants tend to do better. However, neurologic deficits are commonly observed in survivors. The indications for surgery are not well delineated unless the neurologic deteri-

TABLE 1. Subdural Hemorrhage

Site	Signs	Management
Tentorial laceration (straight sinus, vein of Galen, lateral sinus, and infratentorial veins)	Major bleed Bradycardia Coma Nuchal rigidity Opisthotonos or retrocollis Skew deviation of eyes Unequal pupils, progressing to: Signs of lower brain stem compression (fixed dilated pupils and respiratory arrest)	Surgical evacuation if possible
	Minor bleed Asymptomatic period (hours to days) Signs of increased intracranial pressure (full fontanelle, lethargy) Respiratory and oculomotor abnormalities, skew deviation of eyes, facial paresis	

oration is rapid. A ventriculoperitoneal shunt is necessary for those infants developing hydrocephalus (approximately 50 per cent).

Skull Fracture

Skull fractures are relatively uncommon and result from compressive forces to the head during labor and/or delivery. Linear fractures are often observed in infants with cephalhematomas and are benign unless they occur at the base of the skull, where they can be associated with excessive bleeding.

No therapy is indicated for a linear skull fracture other than observation. A second skull film should be obtained several months after birth to make sure the fracture has healed. Children with depressed fractures (i.e., "ping-pong" fracture) may be observed initially if the fracture is small and the child is asymptomatic. If spontaneous elevation does not occur, a number of nonsurgical interventions (e.g., breast pump or obstetric vacuum extractor) can be employed. If the infant is symptomatic or the fracture fails to elevate by nonsurgical manipulation, surgical intervention is indicated.

SKELETAL INJURY

The clavicle is the most commonly fractured bone during the birth process. Crepitus over the fracture site is usually present. No treatment is required, although pinning of the arm to the affected side will minimize pain. Occasionally, there is an accompanying brachial plexus nerve injury (see later). Fractures of the humerus and femur occur much less frequently; both carry an excellent prognosis.

Fracture of the spinal cord can occur with stretching of the cord during a difficult breech delivery. The lower cervical and upper thoracic regions are most commonly affected. Edema, hemorrhage, and transection of the cord can occur. Affected infants present in one of three ways: (1) stillborn; (2) with severe respiratory failure during the first few days of life leading to death; and (3) with weakness and hypotonia during the neonatal period with eventual survival. Treatment during the neonatal period is supportive, and long-term sequelae are almost always observed.

VISCERAL INJURY

Birth trauma to intra-abdominal organs, although rare, must be recognized because of the potential for rapid deterioration. Perinatal asphyxia and coagulation disorders are contributing pathogenetic factors. The liver, adrenal gland, and spleen are the most commonly affected organs.

Liver

The liver is vulnerable to injury because of its anatomic position, relatively large size, and soft consistency. Trauma usually results in a subcapsular hematoma. The incidence of hepatic injury has been found to range from 1.2 to 5.6 per cent among stillborns and infants who have died during the neonatal period. Clinical signs vary with the amount of blood loss; however, the infant may appear well for 24 to 48 hours and then go into shock. Abdominal distention is a common finding in affected infants.

Treatment is supportive (volume replacement as needed); however, any underlying bleeding disorder should be promptly corrected. When the capsule of the liver ruptures, surgery is always required.

Adrenal Gland

The adrenal gland is predisposed to birth injury because of its relatively large size and increased vascularity during the neonatal period. The incidence is increased in preterm infants and those born following prolonged labors. Microscopic hemorrhages frequently occur without clinical signs or symptoms. Larger adrenal hemorrhages may present as an intra-abdominal mass; however, more often than not, hemorrhage into the adrenal glands is diagnosed in later years, when calcified adrenals are observed on routine radiographs or at autopsy. Severe bilateral adrenal hemorrhage may lead to clinical symptoms suggestive of blood loss and adrenal insufficiency.

Surgery is indicated if supportive therapy is inadequate.

Spleen

The incidence of splenic rupture, although rare, is increased in infants with enlarged spleens (e.g., those with hemolytic disease). Splenic rupture can occur in healthy full-term infants following a traumatic delivery or after exchange transfusion. Accurate diagnosis is imperative, as shock can ensue rapidly.

Emergency surgery with attempted preservation of the spleen may be life-saving.

NEUROMUSCULAR INJURY

Brachial Plexus Injury

Brachial plexus injury is the most common peripheral nerve injury due to birth trauma, with an incidence of 2.6 in 1000 live full-term births. The frequency of brachial plexus injury is increased in infants with abnormal birth presentations (e.g., breech delivery), in large infants, and in infants delivered following prolonged or difficult labors. The lesion results from stretching or tearing of the spinal roots of the brachial plexus, which are anchored to the cervical cord. There is often an accompanying fracture of the clavicle.

Erb-Duchenne, or upper arm, paralysis occurs in 90 per cent of cases and results from injury to C-5 to C-7 cord segments (Table 2). The infant displays the classic "maitre d'" (waiter's tip) sign. The diaphragm is involved in 1 to 5 per cent of cases of Erb's palsy if the injury extends to nerve roots C-3 to C-4. Isolated Klumpke's, or lower arm, paralysis is rare and indicates involvement of nerve roots C-7 and T-1 (Table 3). More commonly, total plexus palsy occurs, resulting in complete arm paralysis. Horner syndrome occurs in one third of these infants as a result of interruption of sympathetic outflow from T-1.

Electromyographic studies may be useful adjunctive tests to identify diminished motor unit potentials and to detect signs of denervation. Diaphragmatic paralysis can be confirmed by fluoroscopy, and recovery can be assessed serially using ultrasonography. Management of affected infants includes immobilization of the affected extremity during the first 1 to 2 postnatal weeks, followed by gentle physical therapy and splints to prevent contractures. Approximately 90 per cent of infants show complete recovery by 4 months of age. Lower

TABLE 2. Major Pattern of Weakness with Erb's (Proximal) Brachial Plexus Palsy

Weak Movement	Cord Segment	Resulting Position
Shoulder abduction	C-5	Adducted
Shoulder external rotation	C-5	Internally rotated
Elbow flexion	C-5, 6	Extended
Supination	C-5, 6	Pronated
Wrist extension	C-6, 7	Flexed
Finger extension	C-6, 7	Flexed
Diaphragmatic descent	C-4, 5	Elevated

From Volpe JJ: Neurology of the Newborn, 2nd ed. Philadelphia, WB Saunders Co., 1987.

TABLE 3. Major Additional Pattern of Weakness with Total Brachial Plexus Palsy

Weak Movement	Cord Segment	Resulting Position
Wrist flexion	C-7, 8; T-1	Extended
Finger flexion	C-7, 8; T-1	Extended
Finger abduction	C-8; T-1	Neutral position
Finger adduction	C-8; T-1	Neutral position
Dilator of iris	T-1	Miosis
Full eyelid elevation	T-1	Ptosis

From Volpe JJ: Neurology of the Newborn, 2nd ed. Philadelphia, WB Saunders Co, 1987.

arm paralysis, although less common, carries a poorer prognosis.

Diaphragmatic Paralysis

Diaphragmatic paralysis due to phrenic nerve injury may occur as an isolated finding or in association with brachial plexus injury. Most infants with unilateral injury recover spontaneously within 6 to 12 months of birth, although careful respiratory surveillance is necessary during the interim. Bilateral diaphragmatic paralysis carries a poorer prognosis.

Infants with bilateral involvement and infants who require ventilation should be considered candidates for surgical plication of the affected diaphragm (or the more severely affected hemidiaphragm) after age 2 months.

Acquired Facial Nerve Palsy

Acquired facial nerve palsy must be differentiated from the congenital facial nerve palsies (e.g., Möbius syndrome, hemifacial microsomia, hypoplasia of the depressor anguli oris muscle). The acquired type is often observed following forceps delivery and is more common in infants born following term gestations. This injury results from narrowing of the vertical segment of the facial canal by pressure of the head against the sacral promontory or by direct trauma from a forceps blade.

No treatment is necessary, and recovery is the rule. Administering artificial tears and taping the involved eye to protect the cornea are recommended until recovery occurs. If facial nerve palsy persists, surgery may be necessary to prevent synkinesis.

MANAGEMENT OF THE INFANT IN THE DELIVERY ROOM

RONALD S. BLOOM, M.D.
and H. WILLIAM TAEUSCH, M.D.

Most of the time, the transition from fetal to neonatal life goes smoothly and without incident. However, in about 10 per cent of cases, the active intervention of a skilled individual or team is necessary to minimize the risk of asphyxia.

Although many of the principles regarding a resuscitation are agreed on, there is significant variation in the way specific components are implemented. Until further research provides answers to areas of question or controversy, guidelines for resuscitation will legitimately continue to vary. Guidelines such as those of the American Academy of Pediatrics and the American Heart Association, published in *Textbook of Neonatal Resuscitation,* represent a workable compromise among various viewpoints, not a complete consensus.

Because the need for resuscitation cannot always be anticipated, an important goal is to have at least one person skilled in neonatal resuscitation in attendance at every delivery. An additional skilled person should be readily available, as a complete resuscitation requires more than one person. Individuals jointly engaged in a resuscitation should be capable of working together as a team, with each person understanding his or her own responsibility and that of each colleague.

APGAR SCORE

The Apgar score was developed to define objectively the state of the infant after birth. Because an asphyxial process may begin in utero and continue into the neonatal period, waiting 1 minute before initiating a resuscitation may increase the chances for asphyxial damage. Thus, the Apgar score is not used to determine whether or not a resuscitation should be initiated but, rather, to define the state of the infant at various times during and after the resuscitative process (i.e., at 1, 5, 10, and 15 minutes).

EQUIPMENT

Every delivery room should be fully equipped to resuscitate an infant. There should be a radiant warmer, adequate suction equipment, an oxygen source, a bag capable of delivering high concentrations of oxygen, varying sizes of masks and endotracheal tubes, a laryngoscope with extra bulbs and batteries, appropriate medications, and miscellaneous supplies, such as tape, syringes, needles, and catheters.

Of prime importance is that the equipment not only be available but also be in good working order. No one should have to leave a delivery room, with the attendant delay, to obtain equipment normally used in a resuscitation.

COMPONENTS OF A RESUSCITATION

A resuscitation consists of a series of components: initial steps (thermal management, positioning, suctioning, and tactile stimulation), positive pressure ventilation (PPV), chest compression, and medications (Fig. 1). How far one goes in the process is based on an ongoing evaluation of the infant. The initial steps are all that is needed for most infants. Of those that need further intervention, the vast majority will respond to PPV with 100 per cent oxygen. It is the unusual infant who requires chest compression and medications.

Initial Steps

Upon delivery, the infant should be placed in a preheated radiant warmer and dried to reduce evaporative heat loss. The mouth and then the nose should be suctioned to clear the airway. These steps will create enough stimulation for most infants to cry and breathe normally. If an infant does not breathe normally, further stimulation with a foot flick or back rub should be done quickly and the infant's respirations, heart rate, and color evaluated. If the infant is apneic or gasping or the respirations are inadequate to sustain the heart rate above 100, PPV should be initiated. In those circumstances in which the respirations and heart rate are adequate and the infant continues to experience central cyanosis, free-flow oxygen should be provided.

Positive Pressure Ventilation

Positive pressure ventilation can be provided using either a bag and mask or a bag and endotracheal tube; the choice depends on the skills of the resuscitator. If an endotracheal tube is used, it should be inserted quickly. If attempts at intubation are unsuccessful, the effort should be abandoned and bag and mask ventilation provided. Prolonged attempts

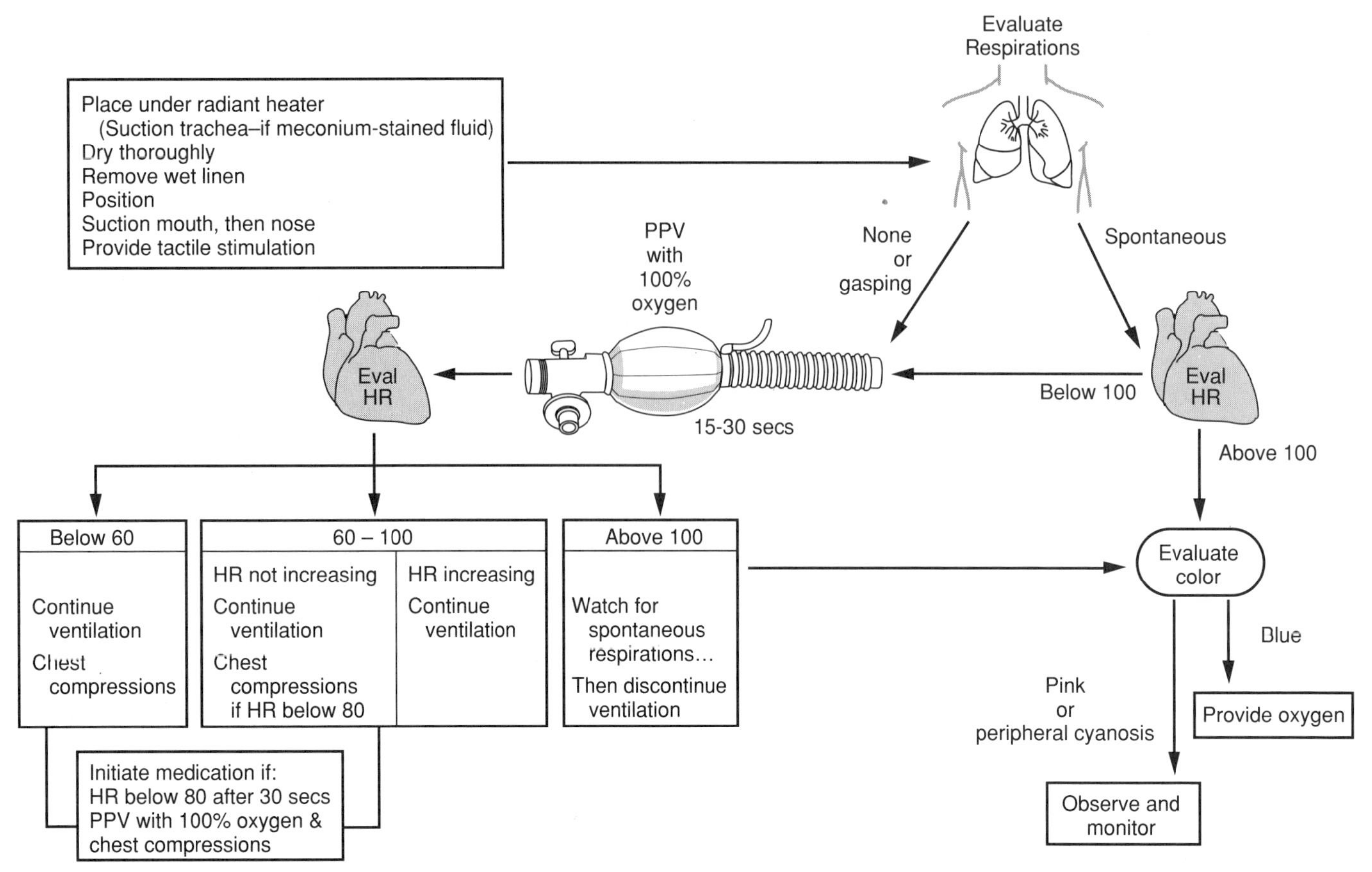

Figure 1. Overview of resuscitation in the delivery room. (Redrawn with permission. From Bloom RS, Cropley C: *In* Chameides L, ed. Textbook of Neonatal Resuscitation, 1987, 1990. Copyright American Heart Association.)

at intubation may extend the asphyxial period and complicate the resuscitation.

Either a self-inflating bag or a flow-inflating (anesthesia) bag can be used to ventilate most infants adequately. Some health care professionals prefer a flow-inflating bag because they feel that it tends to be more responsive and to provide control. However, a flow-inflating bag requires more practice and time to learn to use well. In a delivery room where there are a variety of individuals resuscitating infants, if the entire group does not feel comfortable using an anesthesia bag, self-inflating bags should also be available.

Any bag used for PPV should be capable of providing a high concentration of oxygen (90 to 100 per cent). To attain these concentrations, a self-inflating bag must have an attached oxygen reservoir. Although adequate pressure for ventilation should be determined primarily by chest movement, the bag should have either a pressure relief valve or a pressure gauge. The infant's head should be in moderate extension; hyper- or hypoextension tends to limit passage of air or oxygen into the trachea.

The rate of ventilation should be about 40 to 60 breaths/minute. The initial breath may require 30 to 40 cm H_2O pressure, with subsequent breaths needing only 15 to 20 cm H_2O pressure. If an infant has a disease that limits compliance of the chest, pressures from 20 to 40 cm H_2O may be needed. If ventilation with a bag and mask is to be prolonged, an orogastric feeding tube (8 French) should be inserted to vent gas entering the stomach.

During bag and mask ventilation, insufficient rise and fall of the chest are most commonly the result of an inadequate seal, incorrect positioning of the head, an airway blocked with secretions or meconium, or insufficient positive pressure.

After 15 to 30 seconds of adequate rise and fall of the chest, the heart rate should be evaluated. If the heart rate is below 60, or between 60 and 80 and not rising, chest compression and medications are necessary.

Chest Compression

Before chest compressions are begun, it is essential that the infant be ventilated with 100 per cent oxygen, preferably via an endotracheal tube. The lower third of the sternum should be compressed approximately ½ inch about 100 to 120 times a minute while ventilations are occurring 40 to 60 times a minute. Much discussion has occurred as to whether the ventilations should be interposed between compressions or whether the two should occur simultaneously. Current recommendations are that compressions occur at the rate of one every one-half second with a ventilation replacing every fourth compression. Three compressions of the chest and one ventilation occur in a two second period, with the ventilation interposed between compressions. This results in a rate of 90 chest compressions and 30 ventilations per minute.

Medications (Table 1)

Medications should be used if the infant has not responded to at least 30 seconds of PPV with 100 per cent oxygen and chest compressions. Many physicians feel that if there is no response to PPV, medications should be started simultaneously with chest compressions. Depending on the medication, the umbilical venous, subcutaneous, intramuscular, or endotracheal route may be used.

The first drug that should be given is epinephrine (see Table 1). Epinephrine stimulates β-adrenergic receptors, re-

TABLE 1. Medications for Neonatal Resuscitation

Medication	Concentration to Administer	Preparation	Dosage and Route	Total Dose per Infant			Rate and Precautions
				Weight (kg)	*Total Dose*	*Total ml*	
Epinephrine	1:10,000	1 ml	0.1–0.3 ml/kg IV or ET	1		0.1–0.3	Give rapidly. Make dilute with normal saline to 1–2 ml if giving ET.
				2		0.2–0.6	
				3		0.3–0.9	
				4		0.4–1.2	
Volume expanders	Whole blood 5% Albumin Normal saline Ringer's lactate	40 ml	10 ml/kg IV	1		10	Give over 5–10 minutes
				2		20	
				3		30	
				4		40	
Sodium bicarbonate	0.5 mEq/ml (4.2 % solution)	20 ml *or* two 10-ml prefilled syringes	2 mEq/kg IV	1	2 mEq	4	Give *slowly*, over at least 2 minutes Give only if infant being effectively ventilated
				2	4 mEq	8	
				3	6 mEq	12	
				4	8 mEq	16	
Naloxone	0.4 mg/ml	1 ml	0.1 mg/kg (0.25 ml/kg) IV, ET, IM, SQ	1	0.1 mg	0.25	Give rapidly IV, ET preferred IM, SQ acceptable
				2	0.2 mg	0.50	
				3	0.3 mg	0.75	
				4	0.4 mg	1.00	
	1.0 mg/ml	1 ml	0.1 mg/kg (0.1 ml/kg) IV, ET, IM, SQ	1	0.1 mg	0.1	
				2	0.2 mg	0.2	
				3	0.3 mg	0.3	
				4	0.4 mg	0.4	
					Total μg/minute		
Dopamine	$\frac{6 \times \text{weight (kg)} \times \text{desired dose } (\mu g/kg/minute)}{\text{desired fluid (ml/hr)}} =$	mg of dopamine per 100 ml of solution	Begin at 5 μg/kg minute (may increase to 20 μg/kg/minute if necessary) IV	1	5–20		Give as a continuous infusion using an infusion pump Monitor HR and BP closely Seek consultation
				2	10–40		
				3	15–60		
				4	20–80		

Adapted from Textbook of Neonatal Resuscitation. American Heart Association, 1990.
Abbreviations: IV, intravenous; ET, endotracheal; IM, intramuscular; SQ, subcutaneous; HR, heart rate; BP, blood pressure.

sulting in both an inotropic and a chronotropic effect on the heart. It also stimulates α-receptors in the peripheral vasculature, increasing peripheral resistance and enhancing coronary blood flow and myocardial perfusion. Because epinephrine can be given intratracheally, it can be given very rapidly.

If epinephrine does not produce the desired effect, volume expanders should be considered especially if there is evidence of blood loss or hypovolemia is suspected. Use of sodium bicarbonate should be discouraged during brief CPR but may be beneficial during a prolonged arrest that does not respond to other therapy.

Finally, dopamine can be used, beginning at about 5 μg/kg/minute.

Drug-depressed Infants

If an infant is suffering from respiratory depression as a result of a narcotic being given to the mother, naloxone (0.1 mg/kg) should be given to the infant as soon as ventilation is established. Because the half-life of naloxone is shorter than that of the narcotic, naloxone may have to be readministered.

It is important to understand that if the infant of a mother using cocaine has respiratory depression at birth, it is not due to cocaine, as cocaine is not a narcotic; thus, naloxone will have no effect unless there has been recent narcotic use. Also, naloxone in the infant of a mother who is a chronic narcotic user may trigger acute withdrawal and seizures in the infant.

MANAGEMENT OF MECONIUM

If an infant has passed meconium in utero, the obstetrician should suck out the oropharynx and nasopharynx upon delivery of the head, before the chest is delivered and breathing begins. If the meconium is thin and watery and the infant is vigorous, no further suctioning is needed. If there is thick, particulate meconium or the infant is depressed, the glottis should be visualized as soon as the infant is placed on the radiant warmer and any remaining meconium should be suctioned out. This can best be done with suction applied to the end of an endotracheal tube.

Repeated passes may be necessary to clear the trachea of meconium. In this circumstance, clinical judgment must determine whether PPV should be applied before the trachea is completely cleared of meconium. If an infant has passed thick, particulate meconium and is vigorous and crying, there is some controversy as to whether or not tracheal suctioning should take place.

AFTERCARE

Any infant who has required tracheal suctioning or PPV at birth should be closely observed for at least several hours. Of special concern would be signs of hypoglycemia, acidosis, apnea, hyperventilation, pneumothorax, respiratory distress from other causes, or hypoxic-ischemic encephalopathy.

TREATMENT OF RESPIRATORY DISTRESS SYNDROME

FREDERICK C. MORIN III

Respiratory distress syndrome occurs when the lungs of the newborn are not mature enough to adopt to breathing air.

At birth, the neonate's previously liquid-filled lungs become air-filled. This produces an air-liquid interface along the air spaces. The surface tension thus created tends to collapse the alveoli and small bronchioles. The type II pneumocytes of the lung synthesize and secrete into the airways a surface active material referred to as pulmonary surfactant, which adsorbs onto this air-liquid interface and lowers the surface tension, thereby preventing collapse of the air spaces. The lungs of the prematurely born infant have fewer type II cells, which synthesize less surfactant and secrete less into the air spaces. Thus, the small bronchioles and alveoli of these infants tend to collapse following birth. This collapse causes intrapulmonary shunting and hypoxia. In addition, the lack of surfactant and the atelectasis cause the lung to be noncompliant and therefore difficult to ventilate, leading to hypercarbia. The hypoxia and the hypercarbia together produce a mixed respiratory and metabolic acidosis.

The high surface tension causes leakage of fluid and protein into the alveoli forming the hyaline membranes, for which the disease is also named (hyaline membrane disease). The deep negative deflections in intrapleural pressure produced by the infant attempting to inflate his or her stiff lungs cause overdistention of the alveoli, which remain open, causing air leaks that produce interstitial emphysema and pneumothorax. This barotrauma is accentuated by mechanical ventilation. Toxicity from high fractions of inspired oxygen used in therapy also causes lung damage. Untreated, the disease progresses in severity over the first 2 to 3 days of life. In infants who survive, the type II cells multiply and increase their synthesis and secretion of surfactant, and the lungs recover.

PREVENTION AND TREATMENT

The well-known physician-writer Lewis Thomas has said that there are three stages in the treatment of any disease. In the first stage, no therapy is available. In the second stage, only supportive care can be given. In the third stage, there is direct treatment to prevent or cure the disease.

In the past, treatment of respiratory distress syndrome was aimed at supporting infants until they began to produce their own surfactant and the disease resolved. Initially, this therapy consisted of increasing the inspired oxygen content. Later, intravenous glucose was added and then bicarbonate for treatment of metabolic acidosis. Next, continuous positive airway pressure and, finally, mechanical ventilation were employed. The treatment of respiratory distress syndrome is now making the transition into the third stage, that of the correction of the underlying abnormality by administration of surfactant.

Respiratory Therapy

Supportive care is still necessary in the treatment of respiratory distress syndrome in those infants awaiting surfactant therapy or in those who have an incomplete response to surfactant therapy. This care consists primarily of respiratory therapy. In general, the first element is to increase the inspired oxygen by using a head hood. If this is ineffective in preventing hypoxemia or if there is substantial clinical respiratory distress consisting of grunting, flaring, and retracting, continuous positive airway pressure is the next step. It is given either by nasal cannula or by endotracheal tube. A pressure of 4 to 6 cm of water is generally used. If this is still unsuccessful in maintaining oxygenation and relieving the respiratory distress, or if there is superimposed hypercarbia, the patient is begun on ventilation. Because of the relative weakness of the respiratory musculature, mechanical ventilation is generally begun immediately in infants of less than 28 weeks' gestation with respiratory distress syndrome.

In the vast majority of intensive care nurseries, time–cycled, pressure–limited ventilators are employed. Reasonable initial settings for mechanical ventilation of an infant with moderate respiratory distress syndrome are an inspiratory pressure of 20 cm H_2O, an expiratory pressure of 4 cm H_2O, an inspiratory time of ½ second, and a rate of 20 to 40 breaths per minute. The FiO_2 is generally kept at that which was used prior to mechanical ventilation. If mechanical ventilation is begun immediately following birth, 60 per cent oxygen is a reasonable starting point. The inspiratory pressure is then adjusted to maintain perceptible but not dramatic upward motion of the chest during inspiration.

After initiation of ventilation, hypercarbia is controlled by increasing the rate or increasing the tidal volume. The tidal volume is increased by increasing the difference between inspiratory and expiratory pressures. Hypoxemia is treated by increasing either the FiO_2 or the mean airway pressure. The mean airway pressure is increased by increasing inspiratory pressure, expiratory pressure, or the proportion of time spent in inspiration.

Drugs

One approach to prevention of respiratory distress syndrome has been to attempt to cause the type II cells in the lungs of the fetus about to be born to synthesize and secrete more surfactant. Corticosteroids mature the type II cell, causing it to synthesize more surfactant and also mature the parenchyma of the lung, increasing its elasticity. Giving corticosteroids to pregnant women in the days prior to premature delivery decreases the incidence and severity of respiratory distress syndrome in their newborns. Beta-mimetics increase the secretion of already synthesized surfactant into the air spaces and may also prepare the lungs for air breathing by causing absorption of the fetal lung liquid. Other examples of this approach include current attempts to use thyroxin-related compounds to mature the fetal lung.

Surfactant Therapy

The major advance in prevention and treatment of respiratory distress syndrome has been the direct administration of exogenous surfactant into the lungs of prematurely born infants. Over the past decade, investigators from around the world have found that therapy with exogenous surfactant decreases the incidence of respiratory distress syndrome and improves morbidity and mortality in the prematurely born infant. Questions that remain include: What is the optimum surfactant composition? When should surfactant be given following birth? How often should surfactant be given?

Surfactant Composition

It is known that the major component of lung surfactant is dipalmitoyl phosphatidylcholine (DPPC). However, DPPC alone does not have all of the properties of intact surfactant. It does lower surface tension, but it does not adsorb to the air-liquid interface and does not spread on this interface.

The surfactants currently in use are of two basic types: synthetic and natural. The synthetic surfactants are composed principally of DPPC along with other agents to enhance adsorption to the surface and spreading on the surface. Two such products have been tested. Exosurf, which is DPPC plus tyloxapol and hexadecanol, has been tested in the United States; ALEC, which is a mixture of DPPC and phosphatidylglycerol, has been tested in Europe.

The natural surfactants are obtained from animal lungs by lipid extraction either of lavages of the airways or of minced lung tissue. These surfactants are complex compounds of DPPC, other lipids such as phosphatidylglycerol, and small amounts of lipophilic proteins. In the United States, Infasurf is prepared from lipid extraction of the lavage of calf lungs. In Germany, SF-Rl1 is prepared similarly from cow lungs. In the United States, Survanta is prepared from lipid extracts of minced calf lungs. Curosurf is prepared similarly from pig lungs in Europe.

In animal experimentation comparing the physiologic effects of these agents, the natural products have generally proved to be superior to the synthetic products. Trials to determine whether these physiologic differences hold up in premature infants and whether they translate into differences in morbidity and mortality are now under way. To date, the only agents that have been approved by the U.S. Food and Drug Administration for therapeutic use in neonates are Exosurf and Survanta.

Timing and Rate of Administration

The question of timing and frequency of administration of surfactant is stimulating much study. Surfactant replacement should prevent the development of respiratory distress syndrome but might not ameliorate injury that the lung has sustained because of pre-existing surfactant deficiency. Thus, one approach is to treat all premature newborns at birth in an attempt to prevent respiratory distress syndrome. However, this approach exposes all prematures to whatever unknown risks this therapy has. The risks most commonly raised to date are the risk of intubation, as the surfactants are given via the endotracheal tube, and the potential risk of developing an immune reaction to the surfactant-associated protein of the animal from which the surfactant comes. Antibodies to this protein may have been detected in a small proportion of neonates of greater than but not less than 30 weeks' gestation treated with surfactant. However, no indication of a clinical problem has been found.

Another approach is to wait until a child has developed the syndrome before instituting therapy. However, by this point, the lungs may have already been damaged and complete resolution of the disease may not occur even with appropriate surfactant treatment.

Approach

In order to give the reader a concrete picture of one method of surfactant therapy that has been effective, I describe here the methods that we have used at the Children's Hospital of Buffalo, with the caveat that this is only one of several potential approaches and that not all aspects of this approach have been proven to be optimal by clinical study.

The timing of treatment depends on the risk of the disease versus the risk of therapy. With this in mind and knowing that respiratory distress syndrome becomes progressively more common with decreasing gestational age, we have treated all infants born at Children's Hospital of Buffalo less than or equal to 28 weeks' gestation with surfactant extracted from a lavage of calf lungs (Infasurf). The surfactant suspension is given as a single bolus down the endotracheal tube immediately following birth. In more mature newborns or outborns, we have waited until the diagnosis of respiratory distress syndrome requiring intubation was made. In these infants, we have given the surfactant via a catheter inserted to the end of the endotracheal tube in four divided doses with the infant lying prone, right lateral decubitus, left lateral decubitus, and supine.

We have found this approach to be very effective at preventing respiratory distress syndrome in the infants treated at birth and in ameliorating the syndrome in infants treated after development of respiratory distress syndrome. Unlike treatment at birth, treatment after the development of respiratory distress syndrome does not return lung function to normal. For instance, FiO_2 may be decreased by half, but usually it cannot be reduced to room air. In addition, in those treated after development of the disease, re-treatment is often necessary 8 to 24 hours after the previous dose and several treatments may be required in an individual patient.

NEONATAL PNEUMOTHORAX AND PNEUMOMEDIASTINUM

JON F. WATCHKO, M.D.

Of the extra-alveolar air syndromes known to occur in neonates, pneumothorax and pneumomediastinum are two of the most common. They may occur spontaneously or, more frequently, in the context of positive pressure ventilatory support and underlying parenchymal lung disease (e.g., hyaline membrane disease, meconium aspiration). Pneumothorax and pneumomediastinum result from alveolar overdistention and rupture and are thus often preceded by the appearance of pulmonary interstitial emphysema. Attempts should be made to minimize barotrauma when providing assisted ventilation to reduce the risk of these complications. In this regard, the use of surfactant therapy in the management of hyaline membrane disease has been documented to reduce the incidence of pulmonary interstitial emphysema and pneumothorax by at least one third.

PNEUMOTHORAX

The diagnosis of a pneumothorax can frequently be made on the basis of clinical criteria alone. A spontaneous pneumothorax should always be considered as the cause of respiratory symptoms (tachypnea, grunting, flaring, retractions) in the neonate, particularly when the infant is delivered in a meconium-stained amniotic fluid environment or when positive pressure ventilation is used as part of the delivery room resuscitation. Confirmation of a spontaneous pneumothorax should be made with a chest radiograph. A lateral decubitus view of the infant may be necessary to make this diagnosis when the pneumothorax is small.

Spontaneous pneumothoraces in the term infant can frequently be treated using 100 per cent oxygen for a few hours. This therapy leads to resolution of the pneumothorax as accumulated nitrogen in the extra-alveolar space is "washed out." Moreover, the hyperoxic environment protects against pulmonary vasoconstriction and persistent pulmonary hypertension, which can complicate the clinical course of term infants with spontaneous pneumothorax.

In contrast to the often subtle clinical signs associated with spontaneous pneumothoraces in nonventilated infants, an acute cardiorespiratory deterioration often heralds the development of a pneumothorax in the infant on positive pressure ventilation. Such pneumothoraces are frequently under tension and need to be evacuated quickly with a chest tube to avoid the development of profound hypoxemia and/or hypercapnia, as well as adverse hemodynamic changes. In such instances, the diagnosis can be made clinically (without radiographic confirmation) when asymmetric breath sounds and a shift of heart sounds related to mediastinal displacement are auscultated, and when the hemithorax in question transilluminates with a high-intensity fiberoptic probe.

Chest tube insertion techniques vary. We currently use the recently described percutaneous technique for placement of a pigtail catheter for the treatment of pneumothoraces in neonates. (Blind chest tube insertion with a trochar is dangerous and should be avoided.) We have used the Fuhrman Pleural and Pericardial Drainage Set (pigtail catheter)* for this purpose. The following technique with this drainage set causes minimal trauma to the chest wall, and the pigtail catheter, with its multiple side holes and curved tip, more frequently ensures adequate evacuation with a single placement. The pigtail catheter is inserted as follows:

1. An 18-gauge angiocatheter is placed through the chest wall over the upper rib margin at the desired intercostal space, and its needle is removed (the upper half of the chest wall is preferred in order to avoid damaging subdiaphragmatic solid organs).
2. A guide wire is inserted through the 18-gauge angiocatheter into the thorax, and the angiocatheter is removed.
3. A plastic dilator is inserted over the guide wire, and the insertion site is dilated.
4. The dilator is removed, taking care to keep the guide wire in place.
5. The pigtail catheter is inserted over the guide wire into the thoracic cavity, and the guide wire is removed.
6. The pigtail catheter is connected to a stopcock, and suction is applied to evacuate the pneumothorax.

This technique can be performed in a timely fashion, allowing re-expansion of the underlying lung and avoiding adverse pulmonary and hemodynamic sequelae. Care should be taken when placing any chest tube to avoid puncturing the lung (with possible resultant bronchopleural fistula development) and/or lacerating an intercostal artery (with potential for significant hemorrhage).

PNEUMOMEDIASTINUM

Most neonates with a pneumomediastinum are asymptomatic; the diagnosis is made incidentally on chest radiograph. Given the almost uniform anterior mediastinal location of a pneumomediastinum in the neonate, muffled or distant heart sounds may also lead one to suspect this diagnosis. Radiographically, one sees a marked retrosternal hyperlucency and the typical "spinnaker sail" sign on the lateral chest view; the anteroposterior projection may look spuriously normal.

The spontaneous pneumomediastinum does not appear to be functionally significant in the otherwise normal newborn. It is rarely under tension and usually does not require treatment in the infant on positive pressure support. Iatrogenic tracheal and esophageal perforations, when they occur, are often associated with pneumomediastinum.

BRONCHOPULMONARY DYSPLASIA

BEVERLY S. BROZANSKI, M.D.

Bronchopulmonary dysplasia (BPD) is the chronic lung disease of premature infants who require mechanical ventilation for respiratory failure. It occurs in about 20 per cent of infants weighing 1500 g or less at birth and in 60 to 80 per cent of infants born weighing 1000 g or less. The diagnosis of BPD is based on clinical and radiographic characteristics, but there are no confirmatory pathognomonic signs or laboratory tests. Previous studies have defined BPD as clinical signs of respiratory distress, oxygen dependency at 28 days of life, and specific chronic changes on chest radiographs. A more contemporary definition of BPD includes only those infants who remain oxygen-dependent at 36 weeks' corrected gestational age, because this subgroup of ventilator survivors is most at risk for significant lung disease in infancy. Bronchopulmonary dysplasia is the most frequent cause of respiratory morbidity in premature infants, and its prevention is an important research and clinical goal in neonatology.

The disruption of lung function, characteristic of BPD, is due to airway obstruction, fibrosis, emphysema, and focal atelectasis. The mechanisms responsible for the physiologic and pathologic abnormalities in BPD are, to date, unknown; development of the disease involves a complex interaction of oxygen toxicity, barotrauma, and lung immaturity. Other factors that may contribute to the development of BPD include poor nutrition, acute and chronic infection, and pulmonary edema secondary to excessive fluid administration or secondary to a patent ductus arteriosus (PDA).

PREVENTION

Reducing the incidence of premature birth would be the single most effective way of decreasing the prevalence of BPD. Strategies aimed at preventing BPD through the prevention of respiratory distress syndrome (RDS) have not been successful. Multiple trials with artificial and natural surfactants have demonstrated a marked improvement in both mortality and morbidity of infants with RDS but have not resulted in a decreased incidence of BPD in the smallest infants, who are at the greatest risk. Furthermore, a large multicenter trial designed to prevent barotrauma and perhaps BPD with the use of high-frequency oscillation (HFO) in neonates with RDS showed no benefit of HFO over conventional ventilation.

Enhancing antioxidant protection of the lung with exogenous superoxide dismutase may offer some protection against the development of BPD, but this has not yet been thoroughly evaluated. One recent study suggested that maternal glucocorticoid therapy will decrease the incidence of BPD. The number of infants who developed chronic lung disease was significantly less in the group whose mothers received a complete course of antenatal steroids than in the group whose mothers received no steroids at all.

TREATMENT

Treatment of the ventilated infant is aimed at maximizing oxygenation and ventilation with a minimum of ventilator support. Several uncontrolled studies have indicated that the early use of nasal continuous positive airway pressure may prevent the need for intermittent positive pressure ventilation and, therefore, result in a lower incidence of BPD.

Relative fluid restriction during the first few days of life, as well as prompt treatment of a clinically significant PDA, may decrease the incidence of BPD in surviving infants. Undernutrition has deleterious effects on lung growth, and close attention to the nutritional state of infants with BPD is therefore important. Growth failure is common in these patients and may be related to increased metabolic demands, chronic hypoxemia, and suboptimal caloric intake due to feeding difficulties and fluid restriction.

Drugs (Table 1)

Diuretics

Controlled trials have shown that diuretics can improve respiratory function in patients with BPD. Furosemide is the

*Cook, P.O. Box 489, Bloomington, IN 47402.

TABLE 1. Drugs Commonly Used in the Treatment of Bronchopulmonary Dysplasia

Drug	Dosage
Diuretics	
Furosemide	0.5–2.0 mg/kg/dose IV, IM, p.o. q 12 hours (give only once daily in infants <31 weeks' postnatal corrected gestational age because plasma half-life may be up to 24 hours)
Chlorothiazide	5–20 mg/kg per dose p.o. q 12 hours (May give q.o.d. to prevent electrolyte imbalance)
Spironolactone	0.9–1.5 mg/kg per dose p.o. q 12 hours (May give q.o.d. to prevent electrolyte imbalance)
Bronchodilators	
Aminophylline	Loading dose: 5–7 mg/kg per dose IV Maintenance dose: 1.25–2.5 mg/kg per dose IV q 8–12 hours
Metaproterenol	0.3–0.5 mg/kg per dose p.o. q 8 hours
Albuterol	0.02–0.04 ml/kg per dose (aerosol) 0.5% solution (diluted to 1.5–2.0 ml with normal saline solution)
Steroids	
Dexamethasone*	0.5 mg/kg/day IV, p.o. divided q 12 hours for 3 days; decrease to 0.3 mg/kg/day for 3 days; decrease by 10% every 3 days; at 0.1 mg/kg per dose, give alternate-day therapy for 1 week, then discontinue

*See Cummings et al. N Engl J Med 320:1505–1510, 1989.
Abbreviations: q, every; q.o.d., every other day; p.o., by mouth.

initial drug of choice; in addition to its diuretic effect, it also acts directly on the pulmonary vascular smooth muscle to decrease pulmonary vascular resistance. Side effects include hypochloremia, hypokalemia, metabolic alkalosis, hypercalciuria, and renal calculi.

Hypercalciuria can be minimized by substitution with a thiazide diuretic. The combination of a thiazide and spironolactone in infants with BPD has also demonstrated short-term improvement in pulmonary mechanics.

Bronchodilators

Bronchodilator therapy is the mainstay of pharmacologic treatment of lower airway obstruction and/or bronchospasm. Aminophylline has been shown to improve lung compliance, reduce airway resistance, and facilitate early weaning from the ventilator. The clinical response to theophylline is variable. Some infants will experience a therapeutic benefit with a serum level of 10 mg/ml, whereas others will require levels in the range of 15 to 20 mg/ml. Side effects of methylxanthines include tachycardia, irritability, anorexia, and emesis.

Bronchodilation can also be obtained with systemic or aerosol administration of β-adrenergic agents. Albuterol is the most commonly used β-mimetic because of its specificity to β_2-receptors. Side effects include tachycardia, dysrhythmia, tremor, hypertension, and hyperglycemia. Tolerance can develop with excessive administration. Long-term efficacy of β-agonist therapy has not been established.

Steroids

The use of steroids in the management of BPD remains controversial. Recent reports have documented marked improvement in oxygenation and lung function and a shortened duration of mechanical ventilation during the period of dexamethasone therapy. The theoretic benefits of systemic steroids for lung function include a decrease in pulmonary edema, an increase in surfactant and antioxidant activity, and an inhibition of prostaglandin and leukotriene synthesis. Side effects of dexamethasone include hypertension, hyperglycemia, sepsis, growth failure, and suppression of the hypothalamic-pituitary-adrenal axis. A recent report from our institution linking the development of concentric cardiac hypertrophy to long-term treatment (≥42 days) with dexamethasone for BPD suggests that close monitoring with echocardiography is warranted.

Complications

Pulmonary artery hypertension and subsequent development of cor pulmonale can occur in infants with BPD, reflecting the combined effects of hypoxic vasoconstriction and medial smooth muscle hypertrophy of the pulmonary vasculature. Treatment with oxygen may prevent these changes, and most studies recommend that the clinician maintain an arterial Po_2 of 50 to 55 and oxygen saturation of 90 to 95 per cent in patients with BPD. Recent reports suggest that treatment with nifedipine, an orally administered calcium channel blocker, can decrease pulmonary vascular resistance and improve cardiac output in a subset of these patients. The long-term safety and efficacy of nifedipine therapy for BPD remain to be established.

Follow-up

Infants who have stable arterial oxygen saturations on low levels of supplemental oxygen (via nasal cannula or tracheostomy) can be discharged to home when a well-coordinated home-care program is in place for medical follow-up and family support. Early discharge will decrease both the expense of hospitalization and the emotional and social isolation associated with care in an intensive care unit. Because more than 50 per cent of infants with BPD may also suffer neurologic problems and/or developmental delay, it is important to coordinate treatment with a good neonatal follow-up center.

REFERENCES

Cummings JJ, D'Eugenio DB, Gross SJ: A controlled trial of dexamethasone in preterm infants at high risk for bronchopulmonary dysplasia. N Engl J Med 320:1505–1510, 1989.

NEONATAL ATELECTASIS

JON F. WATCHKO, M.D.

Neonatal atelectasis is a common clinical problem that may manifest itself as a diffuse process (as in hyaline membrane disease) or as a focal phenomenon (as in lobar collapse). Lobar atelectasis in newborns is primarily a complication of endotracheal intubation and may develop as a result of malposition of the endotracheal tube (e.g., right main stem intubation) or, more frequently, during the immediate post-extubation period as a result of poor pulmonary toilet. Post-extubation atelectasis occurs in up to 40 per cent of all intubated infants and serves as the focus of the following discussion.

PATHOPHYSIOLOGY

The pathophysiology of lobar collapse following extubation in neonates is uncertain but likely reflects airway inflammation and ciliary dysfunction in the context of an endotracheal tube in the airway. This inflammation and loss of adequate ciliary function result in airway edema, increased bronchial secretions, and airway obstruction. Focal atelectasis increases the work of breathing and worsens oxygenation by increasing intrapulmonary shunting, thereby leading to recurrent respiratory failure and a need for reinstitution of assisted ventilation. Preventive and, at times, therapeutic measures need to be taken in the intubated neonate to reduce the incidence of focal atelectasis.

PREVENTIVE MEASURES

Preventive measures, such as providing good pulmonary physiotherapy while the infant is on assisted ventilation and using techniques for the adequate fixation of the endotracheal tube itself (thus ensuring a reduced frequency of reintubations), will promote drainage of secretions from the lungs, diminish airway trauma, and reduce the incidence of postextubation complications. Moreover, chest physiotherapy prior to and after extubation, including postural drainage and vibration with an emphasis on the right upper lobe, reduces the chances that post-extubation atelectasis will occur.

Other important preventive measures include

1. Ensuring satisfactory humidification of inspired ventilator gases.
2. Using an endotracheal tube with an appropriate external diameter for a given-sized infant.
3. Keeping the duration of intubation as short as possible (methylxanthines may be effective in this regard in the extremely low birth weight infant).
4. Utilizing an endotracheal suctioning protocol that minimizes suctioning complications. It is important to use an appropriate-sized suction catheter, to utilize negative pressures of no greater than 60 to 80 cm H_2O, and to suction at an individualized frequency based on the amount and character of the airway secretions and the infant's respiratory status.

Some institutions have empirically utilized dexamethasone in infants prior to extubation in an attempt to reduce upper airway (tracheal and laryngeal) edema and thus atelectasis. This practice as a routine, however, has not been demonstrated to be effective and should be used only in selected infants in whom prior failed attempts at extubation were complicated by evidence of upper airway narrowing (e.g., stridor or difficult reintubation secondary to glottic or subglottic narrowing).

If post-extubation atelectasis should occur despite these preventive measures, chest physiotherapy should be continued. Nasal continuous positive airway pressure and/or gentle, intermittent bag and mask ventilation may also be helpful in re-expanding the atelectatic segment but are adjuncts to good pulmonary toilet and should be used with caution. Close monitoring of the infant, clinically and by determination of periodic blood gases, allows the clinician to anticipate recurrent respiratory failure and to intervene in a timely fashion.

Recurrent or persistent focal atelectasis suggests that a congenital anatomic abnormality intrinsic to the airway or compression from a mass or blood vessel extrinsic to the airway is the cause of the lobar collapse; flexible bronchoscopy and surgical and cardiac consultation may be necessary to define the lesion.

LOBAR EMPHYSEMA

DAVID G. OELBERG, M.D.

Lobar emphysema is not a specific disease, but rather it is a symptom complex distinguished by overdistention of pulmonary air spaces. The spectrum of diseases associated with its development can be subdivided into congenital and acquired forms of disease. In congenital forms, males are affected twice as frequently as females and the estimated incidence is approximately 1 in 80,000 children. Congenital lobar emphysema accounts for the third most common cause of neonatal bronchopulmonary malformations, after pulmonary cysts and congenital adenomatoid malformations. The incidence of acquired lobar emphysema is unknown, but its association with other diseases is being recognized with escalating frequency.

ETIOLOGY

Bronchial obstruction, limited deflation of distal airways, and progressive hyperinflation characterize the pathogenesis of lobar emphysema. Obstruction occurs from either intraluminal bronchial lesions or extraluminal bronchial compression. Although the etiology of congenital lobar emphysema remains undetermined in approximately half of all cases, abnormal or deficient cartilaginous bronchial support is the most common identifiable cause. Less frequent causes include bronchial compression by aberrant vessels, bronchogenic cysts, or intralobar pulmonary sequestrations. Other infrequent congenital causes include intraluminal obstruction by redundant bronchial mucosa and bronchial stenosis. Polyalveolar lobes differ from obstructive causes of lobar emphysema because emphysema develops from increased alveolar number rather than increased alveolar size. As with congenital causes of lobar emphysema, the acquired form is primarily intraluminal in origin. Intraluminal sources of obstruction arise from infection, foreign body aspiration, aspirated mucus, and other causes of inflammatory exudate. In infants with bronchopulmonary dysplasia, bronchial scarring, stenosis, and plugging produce lobar hyperinflation in as many as 20 per cent of patients, a small percentage of whom require eventual surgical treatment. As many as 8 per cent of patients with pulmonary interstitial emphysema acquire secondary lobar emphysema. Rare mediastinal tumors (teratoma, neuroblastoma, or mediastinal cyst) provide extraluminal sources of acquired bronchial compression.

DIAGNOSIS

In the most severe cases of lobar emphysema, respiratory distress occurs within the first minutes of life. Although neonatal development of the disease usually presents as a true emergency, mild to moderate respiratory distress is occasionally experienced. In the absence of neonatal symptoms, lobar emphysema usually presents by 6 months of age as recurrent chest infection or intermittent wheezing precipitated by feeding, crying, or excitement. In these cases, respiratory distress is characteristically less severe and diagnosis is often masked by associated infection.

Presenting signs and symptoms include tachypnea, dyspnea,

retractions, expiratory wheezing or grunting, and cyanosis. On physical examination, localized decrease of breath sounds and hyperresonance are noted over the affected hemithorax, particularly in older patients. Chest asymmetry and contralateral shift of the point of maximal impulse may be present.

Chest radiographs are the examination of choice for confirmation of diagnostic impressions. In clinical series, anteroposterior and lateral views of the chest are sufficient for diagnosis of lobar emphysema in 80 to 95 per cent of cases. Typical findings include localized overdistention or hyperlucency of affected segment(s); flattened or inverted ipsilateral hemidiaphragm; compression atelectasis of adjacent ipsilateral lung, apparent as triangular paracardiac densities; mediastinal shift to the contralateral hemithorax; and anterior herniation of emphysematous lung to the contralateral hemithorax on lateral view.

TREATMENT

The therapeutic approach to lobar emphysema depends primarily on the severity of respiratory distress. Surgical excision of emphysematous lung is the treatment of choice for moderate to severe respiratory distress. If associated with congenital heart disease, this should be repaired during the same procedure. Although elective lobectomy for mild, intermittent respiratory distress carries a low operative mortality, alternative trials of supportive medical therapy are justified. Preoperative or elective echocardiograms are indicated in all patients for diagnosis of unsuspected heart disease.

Success of alternative or preoperative medical support relies on optimal oxygenation, ventilation, pulmonary toilet, and nutrition. Frequent arterial blood gas sampling or continuous monitoring by pulse oximetry or transcutaneous oxygen and carbon dioxide transducers is essential for predicting impending respiratory failure. Values of Po_2 should be maintained at 50 to 60 torr with supplemental oxygen as needed.

Intermittent mandatory ventilation should be employed conservatively for maintenance of respiratory status because positive pressure ventilation is associated with rapid hyperinflation of the emphysematous lobe, clinical deterioration, and cardiac arrest. If mechanical ventilation is necessary, ventilate at minimal mean airway pressures. In an attempt to minimize applied mean airway pressure, high-frequency jet ventilation has been employed during surgical resection of emphysematous lung. Although unsuccessful for management of congenital lobar emphysema or acquired lobar emphysema secondary to bronchopulmonary dysplasia, selective intubation of the contralateral main stem bronchus has produced successful resolution of lobar emphysema secondary to pulmonary interstitial emphysema. Intermittent decubitus positioning to promote ventilation of the contralateral lung may improve overall ventilatory status. Bronchodilators are administered for relief of bronchospasm, and corticosteroids are employed specifically for treatment of lobar emphysema secondary to bronchopulmonary dysplasia.

Chest percussion and postural drainage facilitate optimal pulmonary toilet. Although bronchoscopy should be considered whenever the possibility of foreign body aspiration or bronchial plug obstruction is present, particularly in older patients, the procedure should be performed in the operating room with careful anesthetic management and anticipated need for emergency thoracotomy. Bronchoscopy of symptomatic infants is dangerous, and risks should be carefully weighed. Needle aspiration and tube thoracostomy of emphysematous tissue are contraindicated.

PROGNOSIS

In general, postoperative recovery of pulmonary function is excellent. Operative mortality of 7 per cent is highest for patients with congenital heart disease or those requiring emergency procedures. Failure to operate on symptomatic neonates is associated with high mortality rates in some series. In selected patients whose clinical condition permits supportive medical therapy alone, spontaneous resolution occasionally occurs during adolescence or early adulthood.

Postoperative morbidity is variable. Although tissue regeneration does not occur, early pulmonary volume loss resulting from lobectomy is frequently accompanied by compensatory overdistention of remaining lung by later childhood or early adulthood. Recurrent cough, wheezing, or related symptoms occur postoperatively in a minority of patients, but redevelopment of emphysema in remaining parenchyma suggests the presence of residual disease.

MECONIUM ASPIRATION SYNDROME

IAN R. HOLZMAN, M.D.

The passage of meconium into amniotic fluid occurs in anywhere from 10 to 15 per cent of deliveries. Although meconium appears in the fetal ileum between the 10th and 16th week of gestation, it is only infrequently passed from the fetal intestine until the 36th week. The relationship between meconium passage and fetal distress is controversial because the event triggering meconium release may have occurred prior to the onset of labor. Nevertheless, the presence of meconium in amniotic fluid should alert the health care team to the potential for problems.

It is also controversial as to when meconium is actually aspirated into the lower airway. There is evidence that infants suffering severe in utero asphyxia may inhale amniotic fluid and meconium into their lung well prior to delivery. These infants would be less likely to benefit from attempts to remove meconium from the airway at the time of delivery. Because present therapy appears to have decreased the incidence of meconium aspiration syndrome (approximately 5 per cent of infants born with meconium-stained amniotic fluid develop respiratory complications), it would suggest that the majority of infants have not aspirated meconium in utero.

The aspiration of meconium causes a syndrome characterized by marked and prolonged tachypnea, air trapping, and emphysema, which can lead to both a pneumomediastinum and a pneumothorax. Although the inability to ventilate these infants adequately can be life-threatening, the most severe cardiopulmonary complication seen with meconium aspiration is persistent pulmonary hypertension of the newborn. In its severest form, pulmonary hypertension can lead to rapid death from hypoxemia and hypercarbia.

TREATMENT

Peripartum Management

Prevention of in utero asphyxia with resultant meconium passage is obviously the most important management goal, but this is not always possible. A keen awareness of the settings most likely to be associated with meconium passage and aspiration can ensure the presence of a team skilled in peripartum management. Pregnancies that have gone beyond 42 weeks, especially if the volume of amniotic fluid is decreased, result in a disproportionate number of cases of meconium aspiration. Similarly, deliveries near term in which fetal oxygenation may be compromised, such as those involving severely pre-eclamptic women, are at risk for problems with meconium.

Once it is recognized that the amniotic fluid contains meconium, it is important that the pediatric team be made aware of an impending problem delivery. An individual trained in airway management of the newborn must be present during and after delivery. In a vaginal vertex delivery, after the delivery of the head but prior to the exit of the thorax from the birth canal, adequate suctioning of the infant's mouth and nares must be performed. This can be done by the obstetrician or pediatrician using a pressure-regulated source of suction. A bulb syringe is not as efficient a remover of meconium particles as is a suction catheter. With careful attention to removing as much meconium as possible prior to the infant's beginning to breathe, the likelihood of significant perinatal aspiration should be decreased. A similar maneuver can be performed at ceasarean section, but, in this setting, the lack of compressing forces on the infant's thorax makes breathing more likely.

Postdelivery Management

Once the infant is delivered, the team responsible for pediatric care must make a number of decisions. The first of these relates to the quality of meconium present (is it thin or thick?). Watery, nonparticulate meconium-stained amniotic fluid is not frequently associated with neonatal problems. The great majority of such infants are active, crying, and pink within moments after birth. These infants can have their oropharynx cleared of any residual meconium and can then be dried and observed. Once the infant is stable, an orogastric tube can be inserted into the stomach and the contents aspirated. This will eliminate later concern about aspiration and may improve the tolerance for feeding. There is no indication for laryngoscopy and/or intubation in an active, pink neonate born with thin meconium-stained amniotic fluid.

If the meconium is thick and particulate ("pea soup"), the likelihood of neonatal problems is significantly greater and the chances much less that the infant will be crying and vigorous. In this setting, immediate attention to the airway takes precedence over any other manipulation, including drying. A well-lit radiant heater with a resuscitation table should be immediately adjacent to the delivery bed. A reliable source of suction and oxygen dedicated for use by the pediatric team, as well as a working laryngoscope and a selection of endotracheal tubes, is essential. It is also helpful to have ready for use one of the commercially available devices designed for the direct suctioning of meconium from an endotracheal tube.

Laryngoscopy should be performed immediately in a depressed infant with particulate meconium in the oropharynx, and an endotracheal tube (in most cases, a 3.0- or 3.5-mm uncuffed neonatal tube) should be inserted into the trachea. Suction should be applied to the tube, and the resuscitator should observe if meconium is removed. Unless the endotracheal tube is clearly plugged with meconium, it is not necessary to remove the tube and reintubate with a new tube. The initial intubation and suctioning usually require 30 to 60 seconds, during which time the infant may be quite depressed and bradycardic. By 1 minute, it is usually possible to dry the infant rapidly and to begin resuscitative procedures. If the infant has a 1-minute Apgar score of 5 or less, the endotracheal tube should remain in place to ensure adequate oxygenation and ventilation.

If an infant is born with thick meconium but is active and crying, the optimal management is less clear-cut. Many, but not all, neonatologists recommend laryngoscopy and tracheal suctioning if meconium is seen at the level of the vocal cords.

An infant with profound in utero asphyxia and massive meconium aspiration can be quite difficult to manage, often requiring cardiac massage; epinephrine (0.3 ml/kg of 1:10,000 directly into the endotracheal tube); volume expansion with either crystalloid or colloid (10 to 20 ml/kg); and the insertion of an umbilical venous catheter.

Because particulate meconium can cause a ball-valve obstruction, there is a high incidence of pneumothoraces during early management. It is important to be aware of this possibility and to be prepared to insert chest tubes as needed. During delivery room resuscitation, an inequality of breath sounds or a failure to oxygenate is an indication to needle aspirate the chest to rule out a pneumothorax. This is best accomplished with an over-the-needle polytef (Teflon) catheter inserted into the second intercostal space, midclavicular line. The needle can be removed immediately and the flexible catheter left in place. With positive pressure ventilation being applied, the open catheter does not pose any risk. Once the infant is stable, a radiograph can be obtained and a more permanent chest tube can be inserted.

The postdelivery management of infants born with thin meconium in the amniotic fluid and no asphyxia need not differ from that of other infants of similar gestational ages and weights. On occasion, such infants may have a period of tachypnea lasting for 1 to 3 days with minimal, if any, radiographic findings. It is unclear whether this represents mild meconium aspiration or delayed clearance of lung fluid. In either case, observation and an initial intravenous of 10 per cent dextrose and water at 60 to 70 ml/kg/day followed by gavage feeding and minimal intervention suffice for therapy. Unless there is some other reason to suspect infection, antibiotics are not required routinely.

Infants with clear signs and symptoms of meconium aspiration, on the other hand, require management in an intensive care unit. The cardinal finding is a radiograph showing diffuse patchy infiltrates interspersed with areas of emphysema. All varieties of air leaks can be seen, including mediastinal and intrapleural air. The most important goal of therapy is to prevent hypoxemia, which is thought to trigger the syndrome of persistent pulmonary hypertension. The use of a continuous noninvasive measure of oxygenation (pulse oximetry or transcutaneous oxygen pressure) is most helpful. A ready access to arterial blood via an umbilical arterial catheter or a peripheral arterial catheter is also often required.

The therapeutic aim is to keep the arterial Po_2 higher than 80 to 100 mm Hg, with less concern about hyperoxia than one would have with a less mature infant. Alkalosis (pH = 7.50), either by ventilation (Pco_2 = 25 to 30 mm Hg) or by bicarbonate infusion, is also preferred because this has a vasodilatory effect on the pulmonary vasculature.

Although some of these infants can be managed with increased ambient oxygen, many are intubated and ventilator-controlled. Management of the ventilator requires an understanding of the adjustments that can improve ventilation and oxygenation without increasing air trapping and the risk of a pneumothorax. This usually necessitates low end-expiratory pressure and a rapid rate. The use of high-frequency (either jet or oscillatory) ventilation may have a place in the management of these neonates.

In some centers, the addition of paralytic agents (pancuronium, 0.02 mg/kg per dose IV initially and then 0.03 to 0.09 mg/kg every 2 to 4 hours as needed) to improve ventilatory control and the infusion of vasodilators such as tolazoline (1 to 2 mg/kg/hour IV) are part of therapy. Sedation with fentanyl (1 to 3 μg/kg IV over 2 minutes every 2 to 4 hours) is helpful and certainly indicated if an infant is to be paralyzed. The use of these agents often results in significant hypotension, requiring volume expansion with both crystalloid and colloid and the infusion of dopamine (2 to 5 μg/kg/minute IV).

For those infants who develop intractable pulmonary hypertension confirmed by echocardiographic evidence of a right-to-left shunt and a significant oxygen saturation gradient between the pre- and postductal circulation, the use of extracorporeal membrane oxygenation (ECMO) may be considered. Because the number of centers providing this therapy is limited and each has its own criteria, it is essential to consult with a local ECMO center before the neonate becomes too ill to be transferred safely.

COMPLICATIONS

Although respiratory management is obviously crucial, infants with meconium aspiration syndrome are at risk for a multitude of complications. Many of these complications relate to the antecedent asphyxia. Multisystem organ damage can be seen, including cerebral edema and seizures, acute oliguric renal failure, myocardial ischemia, hepatic damage, and gastrointestinal mucosal damage.

Fluid restriction (40 to 60 ml/kg/day) is often indicated for both the cerebral edema and the renal damage, but this may be difficult to achieve because of hypotension from the underlying asphyxia and the use of vasodilators. Careful monitoring of fluid balance and frequent determinations of glucose, electrolytes, blood urea nitrogen, and creatinine are all standard.

The routine use of antibiotics is not required for the aspiration of sterile meconium, although it is important to investigate whether the asphyxia and passage of meconium might be secondary to chorioamnionitis, a condition that would require antibacterial therapy in the neonate.

Some infants may also have postnatal polycythemia; a central hematocrit above 70 is usually an indication for a partial exchange transfusion. Repeated aliquots of 10 ml of blood can be removed via the umbilical vein and replaced with normal saline. Usually, a total exchange of 50 to 75 ml is the calculated quantity to lower the hematocrit to between 50 and 60.

PROGNOSIS

The course of severe meconium aspiration can be prolonged because of both the severity of the lung damage and the pulmonary hypertension. Infants may require intubation and ventilation for 1 to 2 weeks and have a prolonged period of recovery. During the acute and convalescent phases, attempts should be made to provide nutrition, realizing the difficulty of this in the setting of multiorgan damage.

For the majority of infants with meconium aspiration, the long-term outlook is good. Although there can be significant lung damage, the lungs tend to return to near normal during the first year of life. In a minority of infants, there may be an increased risk for future reactive airway disease. Of greater concern is the risk for developmental delay in those infants who may have suffered severe intrauterine asphyxia and postnatal hypoxemia. Careful developmental follow-up is a necessity.

DISORDERS OF THE UMBILICUS

SAMUEL D. SMITH, M.D.

In fetal life, the umbilical ring contains two umbilical arteries, the umbilical vein, the urachus, and the vitelline duct. Failure of these umbilical structures to develop and/or to be obliterated in normal sequence results in vessel, alimentary, urachal, and abdominal anomalies, as summarized in Table 1.

SINGLE UMBILICAL ARTERY

At birth, the umbilical cord has two arteries and one vein arranged in a spiral and supported by Wharton's jelly. Congenital absence of one umbilical artery occurs in 1 per cent of all births and is associated with other congenital anomalies in 50 per cent of affected newborns. The systems most commonly involved are the cardiovascular, gastrointestinal, genitourinary, and central nervous system. Trisomy is also frequently encountered.

Infants found to have a single umbilical artery at birth should be evaluated for other anomalies before discharge from the nursery. The umbilical arteries and ductus venosus remain patent for 3 to 4 days following delivery, allowing potential vascular access.

UMBILICAL GRANULOMA

Umbilical granuloma, the most common umbilical anomaly after umbilical hernia (see later), is not a congenital abnormality but represents a low-grade infection of the cord stump

TABLE 1. Characteristics of Umbilical Anomalies

Diagnosis	Age at Presentation	Presentation	Treatment
Umbilical granuloma	1–6 weeks	Small cherry-red swelling of umbilicus	Several applications of silver nitrate
Patent urachus	0–12 years	Clear umbilical discharge or mucosal swelling	Excision
Urachal cyst	10 months–12 years	Lower abdominal mass midline	Drainage if infected, then elective excision
Persistent omphalomesenteric duct	0–3 months	Feces or flatus from umbilicus; prolapse of the ileum through the umbilicus	Excision
Umbilical polyp	0–2 years	Red swelling; brown weeping drainage	Excision after treatment with silver nitrate
Umbilical hernia	After detachment of cord stump	Reducible skin-covered swelling	If persists, repair after 4 years
Omphalocele	Birth	Transparent membrane covering abdominal contents	Repair primarily or with silo
Gastroschisis	Birth	Protrusion of loops of bowel from small defect to right of umbilicus	Repair primarily or with silo

with resultant formation of granulation tissue, which may weep or produce a discharge.

Treatment consists of several applications of silver nitrate. If no improvement occurs after several applications, probing and or sinography may disclose overlooked communication to the bowel or bladder. Surgical excision is required in these cases.

URACHUS

See article on urachus, Section 12.

VITELLINE DUCT

In the embryo, the midgut is connected to the yolk sac, an early nutrient source, by the vitelline duct or yolk stalk. If the vitelline duct does not degenerate, a vitello-intestinal fistula may occur. Partial degeneration results in the persistence of a sinus, cyst, or fibrous band. Continued growth of the duct at the intestinal wall produces a Meckel's diverticulum. If a patent omphalomesenteric or vitelline duct persists, the presentation depends on the width of the fistula. In the case of a narrow duct, only a clear discharge may be noted.

The diagnosis is obvious if there is passage of meconium or flatus from the umbilicus. With a short, wide duct, the ileum can prolapse through the duct, creating the alarming "horned appearance" of the everted afferent and efferent ileum limbs. It is important to reduce this prolapse by gently squeezing the tips of the "horns" to allow the duct to invert. Venous congestion may cause incarceration and strangulation.

Of cases involving vitelline duct remnants, 82 per cent are Meckel's diverticulae, 10 per cent are a solid cord between the ileum and umbilicus, 6 per cent involve a patent duct between the ileum and umbilicus, and 2 per cent are polyps or sinus tracts involving the umbilicus only. Umbilical polyps are differentiated from umbilical granulomas by failure to resolve with silver nitrate.

UMBILICAL HERNIA

An umbilical hernia represents failure of closure of the fascial ring. Because the peritoneum and skin are intact, this is the mildest form of abdominal wall defect. An umbilical hernia may not be apparent until obliteration of the umbilical vessels and umbilical stump occurs.

The diagnosis is confirmed by noting a fascial defect through which the hernia bulges when the patient is standing, straining, or crying. The incidence of umbilical hernia is higher in premature infants. It is more common in black children. Incarceration or strangulation is rarely encountered. The natural history is gradual reduction in the fascial defect with spontaneous closure by 6 to 9 years of age. If the fascial defect is greater than 2 cm and is not decreasing in size at 2 years of age, surgical closure will probably be necessary. Incarceration in adulthood is increased with pregnancy or obesity.

ABDOMINAL WALL DEFECTS (OMPHALOCELE AND GASTROSCHISIS)

See Section 6, Malformations of the Intestine, pp. 205–207.

NEONATAL ASCITES

ROY PROUJANSKY, M.D.
and JOHN NOSEWORTHY, M.D.

Ascites in the newborn period may occur as the most prominent manifestation of generalized edema or hydrops or as an isolated abnormal collection of fluid in the peritoneal cavity. Rational management is based on determination of the likely site of origin of the fluid and elucidation of the pathologic process leading to its accumulation. After separating out the conditions that are associated with generalized edema or hydrops, the remaining causes can be divided logically based on the character of the ascitic fluid (Table 1). Abnormal fluid accumulation may be urinary, amniotic, bilious, or chylous. In addition, fluid may accumulate as the result of abnormal portal hemodynamics or from peritoneal irritation.

DIAGNOSIS

Initial evaluation of the infant with ascites should be aimed at detecting symptoms and signs associated with pathology in specific organ systems. Generalized edema should lead to an evaluation for immune, cardiac, and other nonimmune causes of hydrops. Abnormalities of the external genitalia, size of the kidneys on abdominal palpation, or alterations in urinary output should lead to a pursuit of the genitourinary causes of ascites. Significant feeding intolerance may suggest associated gastrointestinal tract obstruction. Hepatobiliary pathology may be suggested by jaundice or hepatic or splenic enlargement.

Subsequent laboratory and radiologic evaluation should be guided by the initial diagnostic impression. In the setting of generalized edema, hematologic evaluation should be undertaken to differentiate between the causes of hydrops. Additional testing should evaluate renal function, alterations in electrolyte and serum albumin levels, serum transaminase levels, total and conjugated bilirubin values, and coagulation function.

TABLE 1. Causes of Neonatal Ascites

Causes
Generalized Edema or Hydrops
Immune
Cardiac
Parvovirus infection
Genitourinary Tract Abnormalities
Urethral valves or atresia
Neurogenic bladder
Obstructing tumor (neuroblastoma)
Iatrogenic bladder perforation
Vesicoureteral reflux
Ureteral valves or stenosis
Ureterocele
Hydrometrocolpos
Ruptured ovarian cyst
Renal vein thrombosis
Gastrointestinal Tract Obstruction
Meconium peritonitis
Ileal atresia or volvulus
Intussusception
Malrotation with volvulus
Imperforate anus
Hepatic and Biliary Abnormalities
Bile duct perforation
Galactosemia
Neonatal iron storage disease
Niemann-Pick disease
Congenital infection (cytomegalovirus, toxoplasmosis, syphilis)
Echovirus
Hepatitis B
Herpes simplex
Lymphatic Obstruction
Lymphangioma
Lymphangiectasia
Intestinal malrotation
Mesenteric cyst
Idiopathic

Chest and abdominal radiographs may be helpful for elucidating cardiac and gastrointestinal pathology. Ultrasonography, however, is usually the single most useful study because it allows evaluation of the kidneys, bladder, internal genitalia, and hepatic parenchyma.

Additional imaging modalities are then indicated based on the course of the evaluation. Contrast enema may be used to localize the nature of gastrointestinal obstruction and the possible location of a perforation. Voiding cystourethrography, intravenous pyelography, and renal scintigraphy may also be useful, both to demonstrate anatomic abnormality and, possibly, to delineate the source of a communication of the urinary tract with the ascitic fluid. Suspected bile duct perforation can be evaluated similarly using scintigraphic techniques (PIPIDA, DISIDA scans), which demonstrate the extrahepatic biliary tree.

After this initial approach, there will still exist a number of patients in whom the cause of ascites remains obscure. In this setting, further clarification is often obtained after sampling the ascitic fluid. A urinary character to the fluid may suggest underlying renal or urinary tract disease, although urea nitrogen and creatinine values may be misleading because of rapid equilibration of these constituents with serum. Detection of the normal constituents of amniotic fluid may be due to meconium peritonitis or to the accumulation of amniotic fluid following gastrointestinal perforation. Bilious fluid usually results from bile duct perforation. The presence of chylous fluid (milky fluid with increased triglyceride and lymphocyte content) should suggest obstructed or abnormal lymphatics. Lymphatic leakage may have less of a chylous character in infants who have not been fed.

Although paracentesis is usually performed for diagnostic purposes, there will be a small group of newborns with ascites who as a result of their ascites, have significant diaphragmatic restriction that compromises respiratory function. *Rapid removal of ascitic fluid to lessen this restriction is usually associated with significant fluid shifts from the vasculature and may precipitate hemodynamic collapse.* However, the slow removal of ascitic fluid in small volumes by paracentesis can be accomplished safely with simultaneous replacement of intravascular volume with colloid (5 per cent albumin) through a secure central venous catheter. This, however, is usually a short-term solution, and therapy should primarily be aimed at treating the underlying condition.

MANAGEMENT

Genitourinary Tract Abnormalities

Specific management of ascites resulting from urinary tract pathology is dependent on the location of obstruction and the associated leakage. Intraperitoneal urine may derive from direct rupture of the collecting system into the peritoneal cavity or as a result of primary retroperitoneal rupture with secondary translocation of fluid into the peritoneum. Obstruction resulting from urethral valves or other urethral abnormality can be relieved by catheter drainage of the bladder. Bladder rupture due to a neurogenic bladder, obstructing lesion, or iatrogenic cause can be managed with a suprapubic cystostomy or cutaneous vesicostomy.

Management, however, needs to be individualized, with the overall medical stability of the patient taken into account. Selected patients who are in otherwise good condition may be candidates for a primary surgical repair with associated catheter drainage. Upper tract obstruction may require ureterostomy or nephrostomy, depending on the location of the obstruction. In facilities where endourologic techniques are available, percutaneous drainage is an acceptable alternative.

The outcome of urinary ascites, in terms of subsequent renal function, is based on the nature of the obstruction and how long it was present prior to the development of ascites. Obstruction that was relieved early in embryogenesis, with the associated development of ascites, may result in good renal function and relatively little dysplasia. Initial urea nitrogen and creatinine values may not be reliable predictors of subsequent renal function, as previously noted.

Gastrointestinal Tract Obstruction

Management of gastrointestinal tract obstruction requires demonstration of the level of the obstruction and, subsequently, laparotomy and surgical correction. Spontaneous bile duct perforation requires external biliary drainage to allow the perforation to seal. If perforation is associated with obstruction or stenosis in the distal common bile duct, permanent relief may be achieved with a cholecystojejunostomy or choledochojejunostomy to bypass the obstruction.

Hydrometrocolpos is effectively relieved by surgical attention to the obstructing vaginal atresia or membrane.

Hepatic and Biliary Abnormalities

Hepatic causes of ascites in the newborn period are conditions that are associated with either significant hepatic fibrosis or fulminant hepatic failure. The primary management of these conditions is usually supportive for the consequences of hepatic failure, except in the cases of infectious and metabolic conditions, for which specific medical and dietary therapy is available.

Supportive measures include fluid restriction to 60 to 80 ml/kg/day and diuretic therapy. Spironolactone (200 mg/1.73 m^2/day in four doses) can effect a diuresis, although it may take several days for the clinical effect to be observable. This dosage can be doubled if an initial response is not seen. Furosemide (1 to 2 mg/kg per dose IV) may also be used for a more rapid response, although the potential for creating a disturbance in serum electrolyte values is likely to result from repeated use. Associated coagulopathy in the setting of hepatic failure may preclude the utilization of percutaneous liver biopsy for diagnostic purposes and may make paracentesis of ascitic fluid much riskier.

Lymphatic Obstruction

Chylous ascites usually results from a diffuse abnormality of lymphatic development or, less frequently, from localized obstruction, as may occur with intestinal malrotation and volvulus of the mesentery. Demonstration of the latter should lead to corrective surgery. More commonly, however, the former is present and should initially be approached with dietary therapy aimed at reducing or eliminating long-chain fats and increasing the content of medium-chain triglycerides. This approach may result in a slow but steady decrease in the degree of abdominal fluid accumulation. Over prolonged periods of time, this treatment has occasionally been associated with the development of essential fatty acid deficiency.

Some patients will ultimately experience spontaneous resolution of lymphatic obstruction and may then tolerate a liberalized diet. Persistent accumulation of ascitic fluid can be managed more aggressively with prolonged total parenteral nutrition. Resistant cases have occasionally been managed with shunting procedures aimed at redirecting the chylous fluid back into the vascular system. This approach has had variable success with a high rate of shunt occlusion.

Significant hypoalbuminemia is often seen in association with the hepatic causes of neonatal ascites or when lymphatic obstruction is associated with significant protein-losing enteropathy. The mobilization of ascitic fluid in these settings may improve with correction of hypoproteinemia with 10 ml/kg of fresh frozen plasma or 5 per cent albumin followed by intravenous furosemide. Long-term correction of the hypoproteinemia is dependent on treatment of the underlying disease process.

INFANTS OF DRUG-DEPENDENT MOTHERS

ENRIQUE M. OSTREA, JR., M.D.

In 1985, a survey by the National Institutes on Drug Abuse showed that about 23 million people in the United States use illicit drugs. A sizable number of these drug users are women who are of childbearing age or who are pregnant. In a recent survey of 36 major hospitals, the prevalence of drug abuse among pregnant women ranged from 0.4 to 27 per cent. These figures are probably underestimated.

The drugs that are abused during pregnancy can be subdivided into the narcotics and the non-narcotics. Narcotics commonly include morphine, heroin, codeine, methadone, dextropropoxyphene (Darvon), pentazocine (Talwin), meperidine (Demerol), and hydromorphone (Dilaudid); non-narcotics include alcohol, cannabinoids, amphetamines, and the hypnosedatives (commonly, barbiturates, benzodiazepines, ethchlorvynol, chloral hydrate, bromides, glutethimide, and meprobamate). In the past decade, cocaine has been the most frequently abused drug and is commonly ingested by smoking (crack cocaine). It is not uncommon, however, for the drug-dependent woman to abuse multiple drugs during pregnancy.

Drug abuse during pregnancy is a major health problem because the associated perinatal complications are high. In the antenatal period, complications include a high incidence of stillbirths, meconium-stained fluid, premature rupture of the membranes, maternal hemorrhage (abruptio placentae or placenta previa), and fetal distress. In the newborn infant, the mortality as well as the morbidity rates are high. Besides neonatal withdrawal, there is a high incidence of asphyxia, low Apgar scores, prematurity, low birth weight, intrauterine growth retardation, infections, aspiration pneumonia, congenital malformations, and, at times, cerebral infarction. Aspiration pneumonia is frequently associated with meconium aspiration and complications of persistent fetal pulmonary circulation. Congenital malformations, particularly of the genitourinary system, have been noted. The risk of infection is high, particularly of the sexually transmitted diseases such as syphilis, chlamydia, herpes simplex, gonorrhea, hepatitis B, and, lately, human immunodeficiency virus (HIV).

Long-term problems and sequelae in these infants are not uncommon and include delays in physical growth and mental development, abnormalities in motor tone and reflexes, abuse and neglect, sudden infant death syndrome, hyperactivity, and learning disabilities. Cocaine-exposed infants, in particular, have been shown to score poorly on developmental tests that measure ability to concentrate, interact with others, or cope with an unstructured environment.

Because of these immediate and long-term problems, infants born to women who have abused drugs during pregnancy should be identified soon after birth to ensure that the mother and infant receive appropriate intervention and follow-up.

DIAGNOSIS

Unfortunately, the identification of the drug-exposed mother or her neonate is not easy. Maternal admission of drug use is not frequent and is often inaccurate because of fear of the consequences stemming from such an admission. Even with maternal cooperation, information regarding the type and extent of drug use is often inaccurate. Furthermore, many of the infants who have been exposed to drugs in utero appear normal at birth and do not show any manifestations of drug effects. Thus, the identification of the drug-exposed mother or her infant requires a high index of suspicion. In some populations, a characteristic maternal profile has been shown to be strongly associated with drug use. This profile includes the mother who is a service (nonprivate) patient, single, and multigravida (>3) and who has had little or no prenatal care.

TREATMENT

Initial management of the infant is directed toward the antenatal and neonatal complications that are associated with maternal drug abuse, such as asphyxia, fetal distress, prematurity, meconium aspiration, and congenital malformation. In addition, the following should be included in the routine assessment of the infant: (1) serologic test for syphilis, HIV, and hepatitis B; (2) observation for drug withdrawal; (3) drug screen; and (4) social service referral.

Treatment of Withdrawal

The infant of a drug-dependent mother should be closely observed for withdrawal. The severity of the withdrawal can be assessed by several clinical scoring systems. We employ a system that evaluates the infant specifically on the basis of manifestations that are life-threatening: vomiting, diarrhea, weight loss, irritability, tremors, and tachypnea (Table 1). With this system, drugs are used to treat the withdrawal if there is (1) moderate vomiting, diarrhea, or weight loss or (2) any severe manifestation.

Both narcotic and non-narcotic drugs have been used to treat the withdrawal syndrome. The drugs commonly used are shown in Table 2. Although both types of drugs have been shown to be effective in treating withdrawal manifestations, the narcotics are preferred because their action is more physiologic for an abstinence state. The neurologic manifestations of withdrawal may be successfully controlled by the drugs listed in Table 2, but the narcotics are more effective in relieving the non–central nervous system manifestations (e.g., diarrhea).

Among the narcotic drugs, paregoric, laudanum, and, sometimes, methadone are used. We prefer to use tincture of opium or laudanum (USP) over paregoric because paregoric contains camphor, which is a central nervous system stimulant. (*Caution:* Laudanum, USP, is available in the pharmacy as a 10 per cent solution and contains 1.0 per cent morphine. Laudanum must be diluted 25-fold to a concentration of 0.4 per cent to reduce its morphine content equivalent to that present in paregoric. At this dilution, 0.4 per cent laudanum can be given at the same dose as paregoric [3 to 6 drops every 4 to 6 hours]).

The aim of treatment with drugs is to render the infant comfortable but not obtunded. Thus, the drug should be titrated, starting with the smallest recommended dose and increasing accordingly until the desired effect is achieved. Once the infant is asymptomatic, the drug can be slowly tapered until it is completely discontinued. This usually takes from 4 to 6 days. The infant should still be observed for a day or two after discontinuance of the drug for possible recurrence of symptoms (rebound phenomenon). When the infant is discharged from the nursery, the mother should be instructed to anticipate some mild jitteriness and irritability

TABLE 1. Assessment of the Clinical Severity of Neonatal Withdrawal

	Mild	Moderate	Severe
Vomiting	Spitting up	Extensive vomiting for 3 successive feedings	Vomiting associated with imbalance of serum electrolytes
Diarrhea	Watery stools <4 times/day	Watery stools 5–6 times/day for 3 days; no electrolyte imbalance	Diarrhea associated with imbalance of serum electrolytes
Weight loss	<10% of birth weight	10–15% of birth weight	>15% of birth weight
Irritability	Minimal	Marked but relieved by cuddling or feeding	Unrelieved by cuddling or feeding
Tremors or twitching	Mild tremors when stimulated	Marked tremors or twitching when stimulated	Convulsions
Tachypnea	60–80/minute	80–100/minute	>100 breaths/minute and associated with respiratory alkalosis

that may persist in the infant for 8 to 16 weeks, depending on the initial severity of the withdrawal.

In view of their hyperirritability, infants manifesting withdrawal should be swaddled, placed in a prone position, and cuddled more often. Swaddling, particularly with the infant's extremities flexed and hands placed before its mouth, seems to enhance the infant's own hand-to-mouth facility, which is soothing. A similar soothing action can be achieved with a pacifier.

The frequency of diarrhea and vomiting should be noted, and the infant's weight should be checked at least every 8 hours. Temperature, heart rate, and respiratory rates should be taken every 4 hours. Laboratory examinations to detect serum electrolyte or pH imbalance should be done, as indicated.

Social Service Referral

All infants of drug-dependent mothers should receive a social service referral to assess the adequacy of parenting and care of the infant at home. The discharge of the infant to the mother's care is the primary objective unless serious conditions dictate otherwise. The care of the infant by the mother (with the help of a support person, usually the grandmother or a relative) has, in our experience, been the best situation for a favorable outcome of the infant. The discharge of the infant to a person other than the mother (foster parent) or to an agency should be resorted to only when it is apparent that the infant will be neglected, poorly cared for, or abused. Most mothers hesitate to admit to the use of drugs during pregnancy because of fear that their infants will be taken away from them. They should be assured otherwise; in fact, they should be encouraged to be responsible for the primary care of their infants. The social worker and physician should also advise the mother on the availability of medical and social services in the community for both mother and infant, especially substance abuse counseling and family planning.

Under the child protection laws that are operative in many states, infants born to drug-dependent mothers are considered potentially abused and must be reported to child protective agencies. Many of these agencies require a positive drug screen in the infant before they will take action on the reports. The precautionary measure of referring a drug-exposed infant to a child protective agency is useful if the intent is to ensure the adequacy of care of the infant at home. However, when punitive measures are taken against the mother, the outcome may be counterproductive or even opposite to the law's original intent.

TABLE 2. Treatment of Neonatal Withdrawal Syndrome

Drug	Dosage
Paregoric	3–6 drops every 4 to 6 hours, p.o.
Laudanum (0.4%)	3–6 drops every 4 to 6 hours, p.o.
Chlorpromazine	2–3 mg/kg/day every 6 hours, p.o.
Phenobarbital	3–6 mg/kg/day every 6 hours, p.o.

Follow-up

The infant of the drug-dependent mother is at risk for many long-term problems. These include the risk for child abuse, delays in physical, mental, and motor development, and learning disabilities. The infant is also at risk for ongoing exposure to the drugs in the household as a result of accidental ingestion or passive exposure, particularly to crack cocaine. Follow-up of these infants should be planned not only to assess their medical well-being but also to ascertain the occurrence of these possible complications and the initiation of appropriate interventions.

MATERNAL ALCOHOL INGESTION: EFFECTS ON THE DEVELOPING FETUS

CATHARINE JEAN HARRIS, M.D.

The adverse effects of alcohol on the fetus have been recognized since ancient times. A unique phenotype, fetal alcohol syndrome (FAS), has been related to alcohol teratogenesis. Alcohol and its metabolites freely cross the placenta, reaching concentrations in the fetus at least as high as in the mother's blood.

SCOPE

It is estimated that 10 to 20 per cent of mental retardation (intelligence quotient [IQ] 50 to 80) and up to ⅙ of the cases of "cerebral palsy" are due to maternal alcohol consumption during pregnancy. *Fetal alcohol syndrome is believed to be the third leading cause of mental retardation* (behind trisomy 21 and neural tube defects) and the number one cause of preventable mental retardation. Studies in Seattle suggest an incidence of FAS in live-born infants of 1 in 750 to 1 in 1000.

FEATURES

Alcohol, like other teratogens, has a spectrum of effects. Women who abuse alcohol are at risk for pregnancy complications, including spontaneous abortion, premature labor, perinatal death, and fetal growth retardation. Fetal alcohol syndrome is characterized by a combination of growth retardation, facial abnormalities, mental retardation, and occasional other congenital anomalies. The syndrome varies in the extent and severity of features expressed in each individual.

Infants with FAS are often retarded in their growth and have disproportionally small heads. Many have specific deficits in sucking and require the skill of a speech pathologist for success at oral feeding. Continued postnatal growth failure often leads to a diagnosis of failure to thrive syndrome despite adequate caloric intake in the infant and toddler. Long-term follow-up studies suggest that stature and head circumference remain below the 10th percentile. Although many individuals with FAS remain underweight for height throughout childhood, there is a suggestion that, at puberty, weight gain in females may become excessive.

Infants with FAS may be irritable and jittery, especially if the mother has consumed alcohol around the time of delivery. Such infants may be treated by swaddling and placing them in a dimly lit room. Neonatal seizures are rarely seen in the infant exposed to alcohol alone. Many children with FAS are hyperactive and have poor attention spans. The average IQ is 63, placing them in the mildly mentally retarded range. However, profound mental retardation has occasionally been observed in children with FAS. Few individuals with FAS have normal intelligence. Unfortunately, most available studies have shown no improvement in IQ in children with FAS in foster care. Fine motor and gross motor dysfunction is typically seen in young children with FAS.

Because mental retardation and growth deficiency are uniform features of many genetic syndromes, the diagnosis of FAS rests on the clinician's recognizing the unique facial phenotype. The facies of FAS may include short palpebral fissures, long flat mid face, long flat philtrum, and thin upper lip. Other minor anomalies that may be observed in FAS include hirsutism, ptosis, epicanthal folds, posterior rotation of the ears, micrognathia, short or webbed neck, sacral dimple, radioulnar synostosis, clinodactyly, and hypoplastic nails. At 10-year follow-up, many individuals with FAS show persistence of these facial features.

Major malformations have been described in most organ systems. Congenital heart disease, cleft lip and palate, renal anomalies, ophthalmologic abnormalities (strabismus, myopia, corneal opacities, cataracts, and microphthalmia), vertebral and rib anomalies, scoliosis, and central nervous system anomalies (hydrocephalus, spina bifida, holoprosencephaly, and migration defects) are a few of the more common anomalies that the treating physician must consider in the patient diagnosed with FAS. Dental malalignments, malocclusions, and eustachian tube dysfunction have been reported.

Partial or milder FAS phenotypes exist and are often referred to as fetal alcohol effects (FAEs). These effects are estimated to be twice as common as FAS, occurring in 1 in 300 live-born infants. Because FAE is characterized by isolated growth deficiency, mild mental retardation, or behavior abnormalities, it may be extremely difficult to diagnose without a supporting history of maternal alcohol abuse.

PREVENTION

The diagnosis of FAS or FAE is made easier by a history of alcohol abuse in a pregnant woman, but this history is not always available. There is no accepted safe level for alcohol consumption during pregnancy. Current recommendations include complete abstinence during pregnancy and even immediately prior to conception. However, this rarely occurs, and many women report mild to moderate alcohol use in early gestation prior to recognition of pregnancy. These women should be counseled to refrain from continued alcohol use and should be reassured of a likely normal pregnancy outcome.

There is no clear dose-response relationship between maternal alcohol intake and FAS. The offspring at highest risk appear to be those whose mothers drink greater than 56 to 84 g of absolute alcohol (equivalent to four to six beers, four to six glasses of wine, or four to six mixed drinks) each day. Of this group, it is estimated that 30 per cent of the infants will have FAS and 50 to 70 per cent will have FAS or FAE. Because alcohol is not an obligate teratogen, some women will have unaffected children. In attempting to predict the effects of alcohol abuse in a pregnancy, actual amounts of alcohol use must be considered along with maternal weight, genetic makeup, pattern of consumption (binge versus chronic drinking), and nutritional status, as well as other substances abused. Because the effects of most of these factors are unknown, an accurate prediction of the effects of alcohol abuse is impossible. It is well known that smoking in alcoholic women further decreases the birth weight of the infant. The effects of alcohol appear to be potentiated with increasing maternal age, gravidity, and years of alcohol abuse. The youngest child is usually the most severely affected. The incidence of FAE may be increased in children born to women who drink two to three beers, glasses of wine, or mixed drinks each day.

No method offers reliable diagnosis of FAS or FAE prenatally. Prenatal ultrasonography may be used to screen for serious anomalies and severe growth retardation, but even this study does little to predict the level of mental functioning or behavioral problems. Prevention must depend on educating the public to the effects of alcohol on the unborn child. This has been attempted in some states through television public service announcements, posters in prenatal clinics, warning labels on alcoholic beverages, and signs posted in establishments serving alcoholic beverages warning of the danger of alcohol use during pregnancy. The efficacy of these methods is untested. For the chronically alcoholic woman, the best hope for prevention rests on early identification in prenatal clinics, counseling, and, if necessary, enrollment in an alcohol abuse treatment program.

TREATMENT

Once a diagnosis of FAS or FAE is suggested, the physician must make a careful search for the birth defects, including congenital heart disease and renal, central nervous system, and ophthalmologic anomalies. Weight and growth should be monitored closely. If the weight gain fails to meet expectations, a caloric count and feeding evaluation should be undertaken.

The child should be referred to early intervention programs if there is evidence of developmental delay. Speech, physical, and occupational therapy, behavior modification, and special educational programs should be recommended when indicated. Individuals with FAS should be routinely followed by a dentist and audiologist and should receive preventive health care. It is imperative to offer parents psychologic support and family counseling services when appropriate.

PREPARATION OF THE NEONATE FOR TRANSFER

CHARLES V. BENDER, M.D.

The transport of a critically ill neonate from one hospital to another is an inherently stressful process that can be complicated by the simultaneous and potentially conflicting needs of the infant, the infant's family, the staff of the referring hospital, and the transport team. Ideally, each case would present with adequate opportunity to allow for prenatal transport of mother and fetus, with delivery at a tertiary neonatal intensive care unit (NICU). In those situations in which the ideal is not possible, planning, preparation, cooperation, and communication can do much to ease the strain and to ensure a safe and successful neonatal transport.

PLANNING

Each hospital must perform a realistic self-evaluation of its strengths and weaknesses and the level of care that its staff can provide. The medical staff can then determine in advance which clinical problems and levels of intensity of care will mandate transfer of an ill neonate to another hospital. It may be appropriate to transport most infants to the nearest NICU and to have identified a second, more distant, center for referral of infants who may require extracorporeal membrane oxygenation (ECMO) or other sophisticated care not available at the closer center.

The staff of the primary hospital and of the receiving NICU should discuss in advance the logistics of optimal transport and the capabilities of the receiving institution. These discussions may be formalized by a contract guaranteeing a commitment by the NICU to accept and transport infants whenever needed. *In any case, the step-by-step mechanism for arranging a transport should be codified as a written procedure, including details as elementary as telephone numbers to avoid confusion when the occasion for transport arises.*

In addition to this general needs assessment, there is the opportunity for anticipation in specific cases. A timely telephone call directly from the obstetrician to the pediatrician, instead of a belated cry from the delivery room for help "stat.," enables the pediatrician to initiate communication with the tertiary center and to seek advice in the early management of expected problems. An early call to the receiving NICU staff alerts them to a potential transport and allows the transport team to postpone elective activity and to stand by for mobilization.

INITIATING THE TRANSPORT

The steps of the referral process should be initiated as soon as possible after it is recognized that transport is indicated. The first but often missed step is discussion with the infant's family, giving them a chance to begin to deal with their inevitable anxiety. The physician initiating the call should be prepared to give an accurate history and assessment of the infant, including pertinent laboratory data, to the receiving physician. He or she should then continue stabilization of the infant and, unless the infant is stable and the transport is elective, remain with the patient. *The referring physician's responsibility continues at least until the arrival of the transport team—it does not end with the placement of the call to arrange transport.*

STABILIZATION

The success of a neonatal transport depends greatly on the prevention or adequate treatment of the major ultimate causes of morbidity and mortality: hypothermia, hypoglycemia, hypotension, hypoxia, and acidosis.

Maintaining a normal *body temperature* (36.5°C) is critical to minimizing consumption of oxygen and glucose. Either a radiant warmer or an incubator can provide an adequate thermal environment once the infant is stabilized, but resuscitation and other procedures can usually be done more effectively under a prewarmed radiant warmer. It is essential that the infant's temperature be taken regularly, even when it is being servo-controlled, to prevent hypothermia.

Open lesions such as meningomyelocele or abdominal wall defects can cause both heat and water loss. Covering open lesions with a sterile dressing moistened with warm saline, which, in turn, is covered with a sterile occlusive barrier, will minimize both heat loss and bacterial contamination.

The critically ill infant who requires transport is at risk for *hypoglycemia,* and even the infant who is stable will not be fed during transport. Therefore, intravenous access for administration of glucose is mandatory. Ten per cent dextrose in water (100 ml/kg/24 hours) will provide adequate water and glucose for most infants. Estimation of the blood sugar by a glucose oxidase strip will confirm that glucose intake is adequate. If the blood sugar is less than 40 mg per cent, a bolus of 2 ml/kg of 10 per cent dextrose should be given. Enteral feedings cannot be relied upon to treat a hypoglycemic infant.

Blood pressure is an important measure of cardiac function and vascular tone, but severe volume depletion can cause vasoconstriction adequate to maintain blood pressure with markedly diminished perfusion. Therefore, estimation of perfusion by capillary refill time is an equally important measure of vital signs in the ill newborn. Evidence of decreased perfusion, either by low blood pressure or by capillary refill time greater than 2 to 3 seconds, should be treated by intravenous infusion of 10 ml/kg of crystalloid or colloid solution. If there is a history of significant blood loss resulting in hypoperfusion, packed red blood cells may be given. In emergent situations, O-negative cells may be used until type-specific blood is available.

Because the majority of neonates are transported for management of respiratory disorders, *hypoxia* is a frequent problem prior to and during transport. Any suggestion of respiratory distress mandates evaluation of the need for treatment. During the evaluation and stabilization of the infant with respiratory distress, oxygen should be supplied until it can be demonstrated unnecessary by blood gas or transcutaneous monitoring. A Po_2 between 60 and 80 mm Hg or a saturation between 92 and 94 per cent should prevent hypoxic damage without risking oxygen toxicity.

If significant distress is present or the infant is apneic, assistance with bag and mask breathing must be given until endotracheal intubation can be performed. *Perhaps the single most important message regarding pretransport stabilization is that there should be no hesitation to initiate bag and mask breathing if it appears to be indicated. The only exception to this rule is the infant with a diaphragmatic hernia, who requires immediate insertion of an endotracheal tube to prevent gastric distention and worsening distress.*

The physical examination of the infant with respiratory distress is complemented by a chest radiograph done to rule out diaphragmatic hernia or pneumothorax and to ascertain positioning of an endotracheal tube. Finally, the infant with respiratory distress, whether breathing spontaneously or being assisted, requires a nasogastric or orogastric tube to vent the stomach and prevent gastric distention.

In addition to these general measures for managing respiratory distress, three situations warrant specific mention. First, any significant pneumothorax in a baby with respiratory distress must be drained, either by needle aspiration or by placement of a chest tube, prior to transport. Simply increasing the concentration of oxygen is not adequate treatment of a symptomatic pneumothorax. Second, the role of artificial surfactant in pretransport stabilization of the infant with hyaline membrane disease is controversial. There is probably little to be gained in early administration of surfactant by staff who do not give it frequently and are therefore not skilled in its use. Third, profound cyanosis along with generally decreased opacity on chest radiograph, with or without a heart murmur, may indicate the presence of a ductal-dependent cardiac lesion. The use of a prostaglandin infusion to maintain ductal patency while awaiting transport should be discussed with the receiving neonatologist or cardiologist.

The critically ill infant requires a blood gas not only to determine oxygenation but also to document his or her *acid-base status*. A metabolic acidosis may reflect hypoperfusion, hypoxia, hypothermia, or a metabolic disorder. A severe or persistent metabolic acidosis (pH < 7.28 to 7.3 and base deficit > 5) requires both specific treatment of the underlying cause and treatment of the acidosis with an infusion of sodium bicarbonate (See table, p. 789). A respiratory acidosis (pH $<$ 7.28 to 7.3 and $P_{CO_2} > 50$ to 60) is an indication for intubation and ventilation during transport and is a relative contraindication to the administration of bicarbonate.

Because of the protean manifestations of neonatal *sepsis* and, specifically, the inability to distinguish group B streptococcal sepsis from respiratory distress syndrome, antibiotics are frequently indicated in the neonate to be transported. Treatment should be started with intravenous ampicillin (100 mg/kg) and gentamicin (2.5 mg/kg) after blood and urine specimens are obtained for culture. Lumbar puncture should be deferred if the infant has significant respiratory compromise or is otherwise unstable. The culture specimens may be kept at the original hospital or may accompany the infant to the tertiary center.

Essential routine care measures can be easily overlooked amid the events of pretransport care. The usual protocols for identification, vitamin K administration, and eye prophylaxis must be followed for all infants.

Thorough charting by all caregivers will help the staff at the referral center in reconstructing the infant's course. Copies of all documentation, especially laboratory values, electrocardiograms, consultations, and x-ray films, should be included with a legible copy of the chart. Although written interpretations of the x-ray films may be helpful, the films themselves or at least good copies must be included. The placenta and clotted specimens of the mother's blood and cord blood should also be sent.

PREPARING THE PARENTS

The stresses that the critically ill infant's family feels cannot be overestimated. Even when a problem is detected prenatally and there has been an opportunity for an anticipatory visit to the NICU, the family will experience separation anxiety and feelings of helplessness. Compassion and communication will help in alleviating their discomfort.

The need for transport should be discussed with the parents by a physician as soon as it is anticipated. The parents will benefit from as many specific details as can be included: which hospital the infant will go to, who will accompany the infant in transport, and which physician the infant is being referred to. Oral consent for the transport is obtained at the time of this discussion, with written consent obtained by the transport team during their visit with the family. The team will exchange telephone numbers with the family and tell them to expect an initial call from one of the physicians at the tertiary care center after the NICU staff has had an opportunity to evaluate and stabilize the infant.

The most important event in the transport from the parents' standpoint is a chance to touch the infant once more before the baby leaves the hospital. Only in the most extreme circumstances should this contact be abbreviated, and even less often may it be omitted. This could potentially be the last opportunity for the family to see their child alive. Even when the possibility of death is not likely, it may nonetheless weigh heavily on the parents' minds. *They may wish to have the infant baptized in their presence. A set of footprints and an instant photograph of the infant gives them tangible evidence that they do in fact have a child.*

The final phase of transport is the planning for back transfer when there is no longer a need for intensive care. Introducing this idea to the parents at the time of the initial transport may give them a sense of hope and may help them anticipate the infant's recovery. If the infant dies before the mother has been discharged from the delivery hospital, the option of bringing the infant's body back to the mother's room should be explored. *A chance to hold the child's body privately before the funeral may be helpful to the family's grieving process.*

BREAST-FEEDING

LAURA S. HILLMAN, M.D.

This article provides the primary care practitioner with a background to discuss the advantages and disadvantages of breast-feeding.

ADVANTAGES OF BREAST-FEEDING

Nutritional Factors

The production of human milk represents a compromise between the nutritional needs of the mother producing the milk and the nutritional needs of the nursing infant consuming the milk. Limited quantities of some nutrients are in human milk, but they are exceptionally bioavailable to the infant. Iron, zinc, and calcium are good examples. On the other hand, a number of "nutrients" such as taurine, carnitine, and nucleotides are found in high concentrations in human milk. Accordingly, these substances have been added to infant formula.

All macronutrients in human milk differ from those in other milks with the exception of sugar; all milks contain similar amounts of lactose. Most term infants tolerate lactose whether or not they have lactase; however, if an infant is truly lactose-intolerant, human milk will not be better than a lactose containing formula. The fatty acid composition of human milk is different from that of formula, and human milk contains more monounsaturated fatty acids. The sodium content of human milk is lower than that of most formulas.

The biggest difference between human milk and formula is the protein composition. Human milk is at least 60 per cent whey and 40 per cent casein, whereas cow's milk is 18 per cent whey and 82 per cent casein. The high whey content in human milk results in a softer, more digestible curd that does not stay in the infant's stomach as long as that from formula. Thus, the breast-fed infant requires more frequent feedings and produces more liquid stools, which either are expelled in the middle of each feeding or are stored for 3 to 5 days and then expelled as a single, very large stool. Human milk stools do not have an offensive odor. If milk production is adequate and the infant does not become dehydrated, breast-fed infants usually do not become constipated. All of the major formula companies have duplicated the whey-to-casein ratio in human milk. However, just changing the whey-to-casein ratio does not make cow milk protein the same as human milk protein.

Immunologic Factors

The mother provides the infant a wide variety of immunologic protection through breast milk. Immunoglobulin A (IgA) is specifically secreted into human milk. In addition, human milk contains intact immune cells that may be locally active in the infant's intestine and may even enter the infant's blood stream intact to provide additional immunity. It has been suggested that the high nucleotide content in breast milk provides additional protection. Human milk alters the intestinal pH and establishes a unique bacterial flora that helps resist invasion from other pathogens. Furthermore, human milk comes in a "sterile package." In underdeveloped countries, studies clearly show that human milk protects against diarrheal disease in infants. However, in industrial countries, this benefit is difficult to show. Some data supporting a reduction in upper respiratory infections in infants do exist.

Hormone and Growth Factors

There are a variety of hormones and growth factors present in human milk. Some of these growth factors, usually proteins, get absorbed intact and produce a systemic effect, whereas others probably act locally on the intestine. For example, thyroxine is absorbed in adequate quantities to modify congenital hypothyroidism significantly. Intestinal cells contain receptors for the insulin-like growth factors in human milk.

Emotional and Practical Factors

In developed nations, the most important advantage of breast-feeding may be the emotional effect. Breast-feeding mandates frequent close physical contact with the infant. The let-down reflex assures that the nursing mother does not ignore the cry of her hungry infant. Furthermore, the protein quality of human milk mandates frequent feedings and frequent diaper changes. Clearly, the mother and infant need to be continuously in proximity.

From a practical standpoint, breast-feeding is convenient and economical. The parents do not have to buy, store, fix, warm, or discard formula, nor smell formula stools. The infant can be fed essentially any time or any place. In the middle of the night, the ease of nursing an infant can be greatly appreciated.

DISADVANTAGES OF BREAST-FEEDING

Nutritional Factors

Although rare, nutritional deficiencies or excesses do occur in breast-fed infants. The pediatrician needs to know that these exist in order to evaluate infants who are not thriving at the breast. Deficiencies can result from either maternal nutritional deficiencies or abnormalities in milk secretion.

Extreme protein deficiency in the mother usually does not decrease the protein content of the milk but, rather, decreases total milk production; this may result in a generalized protein-calorie malnutrition in the infant. Although rare in industrial nations, decreased milk production is not uncommon in women in the Third World. Although the fatty acid composition of the human milk reflects the fatty acid composition of the maternal diet, adequate supplies of essential fatty acids are usually preserved. The lactose content also appears quite stable. Thus, most of the deficiencies that may be encountered involve vitamins and minerals.

Of the macrominerals normally present in human milk, phosphorus is the most limited; however, under normal conditions of adequate vitamin D and unlimited volume, human milk is adequate for normal bone mineralization. True vitamin D–deficiency rickets (serum 25-OHD < 6 mg/ml) is rare in the United States; however, when seen, it is almost always in the exclusively breast-fed infant. It is much more common in black infants because serum and milk concentrations of vitamin D *per se* may be lower in black women as a result of decreased skin production due to pigmentation. Other populations at risk are those who, usually for religious reasons, maintain extensive skin coverage. Vitamin D–deficient diets such as those used by strict vegetarians also contribute.

Because vitamin D–deficiency rickets in infancy may be a lifelong crippling condition, it is imperative that pediatricians be alert to these high-risk situations and educate mothers and/or supplement infants. Most infants born in the United States at lower latitudes and where vitamin D supplementation of the food supply is abundant probably do not need additional supplementation. However, in countries such as France, where low maternal 25-OHD levels are the rule, supplementation is probably advisable, as it is in infants born in the northern United States in winter to mothers whose diets may be marginal. There are data to suggest that maintenance of normal versus marginal serum 25-OHD levels by supplementation results in improved bone mineralization.

Zinc-deficient breast milk has been reported in the absence of maternal zinc deficiency and probably represents a secretory abnormality. Similar problems with other trace elements could exist. The selenium content of human milk and cow's milk depends on the selenium content of the maternal diet, which reflects the selenium content of the soil. Although this is not a significant problem in the United States, it is a problem in some areas of the world, especially parts of China and New Zealand. However, the form of selenium found in human milk appears to be very bioavailable. Excesses of selenium in human milk may be possible in areas where selenosis is a problem.

Rarely the sodium content of breast milk may be abnormal. For example, the breast milk of mothers with cystic fibrosis may be very high in sodium chloride, and both the content of the breast milk and the serum electrolytes of the infant need to be monitored if breast-feeding is attempted. We recently encountered an infant with hypertonic dehydration (serum sodium 174 mg/L) secondary to the ingestion of human milk with a markedly elevated sodium content from a woman who did not have cystic fibrosis. The sodium content of the milk decreased over time, and, indeed, the infant was able to resume nursing after a few weeks.

In exclusively breast-fed infants of strict vegetarians not receiving vitamin supplements, deficiencies of vitamin B_{12} and folic acid have been reported, presenting as anemia in the infants.

Toxic Substances

Much has been reported in the media about contamination of human milk by environmental toxins. Although the data may be strong enough to encourage us to clean up our environment, they probably do not indicate a significant health concern for the breast-fed infant. In contrast, illicit drugs that enter the maternal blood stream can pose significant but largely unknown risks for the infant. Women using cocaine should probably be restricted from nursing. Marijuana use is equally disturbing because of its greater prevalence, but its effects are far less clear. Certainly, women should be advised to refrain from smoking marijuana, if only to avoid the detrimental effect on the infant of passive smoking.

The use of prescribed drugs in nursing women provides the greatest number of questions for pediatricians. All drugs enter human milk to some degree but usually in low enough concentrations and with mild enough effects not to pose a problem for infants. However, some drugs are actively secreted or concentrated in human milk and thus exist in large enough concentrations to produce drug effects. Each drug must be individually evaluated, and the referenced textbook on drugs during pregnancy and lactation should be available to all obstetricians and pediatricians.[1]

Emotional Factors

Whereas breast-feeding probably increases maternal-infant interaction, it may decrease paternal-infant interaction. Indeed, some fathers may feel significantly left out. It is important that alternative paternal-infant interactions be encouraged.

If nursing is not a totally comfortable situation for the mother, the job of "producing adequate nutrition" may provide an extra strain. The nursing mother must be supported and helped to relax. If she is unable to relax, milk production may be severely compromised because of decreased let-down reflex. There are situations in which emotional stress makes nursing wrong for both the mother and the infant. The pediatrician must be sensitive to those situations in which support proves inadequate and in which "permission" to stop nursing is indicated.

MEDICAL ISSUES OF BREAST-FEEDING

Breast Milk Jaundice

Breast milk jaundice is a real entity that occurs in about 3 per cent of breast-fed infants. It is very important that a distinction be made between breast milk jaundice and physiologic jaundice. If nursing is temporarily stopped (24 to 48 hours) to treat true breast milk jaundice, an effort should be made to ensure continued adequate milk production. Phototherapy may be necessary if hyperbilirubinemia is sufficient to require temporary cessation of breast feeding.

Breast milk jaundice is usually distinguished from physiologic jaundice by its later onset (4 days to a few weeks after birth). In some infants, the bilirubin will rise very rapidly; in others, bilirubin will remain in the low to mid teens for several weeks. The blood smear will not show signs of hemolysis, the reticulocyte count will not be elevated, and anemia will not be present. The two other common causes of late hyperbilirubinemia—hypothyroidism and infections (usually a urinary tract infection)—need to be ruled out.

Various theories regarding the etiology of breast milk jaundice have been considered and discarded. Most recently, a number of investigators have demonstrated that human milk contains significant amounts of β-glucuronidase. Beta-glucuronidase is an enzyme capable of converting bilirubin monoglucuronides (the predominant bilirubin glucuronide in neonatal bile) to unconjugated bilirubin, which can be easily reabsorbed. Researchers have shown that serum bilirubin levels in breast-fed infants are directly related to the concentration of β-glucuronidase in breast milk on postnatal days 3 and 21 and to levels of fecal β-glucuronidase on postnatal day 21. Similarly, others have reported that β-glucuronidase concentrations in stool samples are higher in icteric infants than in nonicteric infants.

In summary, it is safe to say that the pathophysiology of breast milk jaundice syndrome remains unclear. Although the presence of β-glucuronidase in some breast milk specimens offers a plausible explanation, other theories have seemed equally likely in the past. It is important to remember that this syndrome is a diagnosis of exclusion and that other, more common diseases must be considered first, before the breast is labeled as a villain.

Failure to Thrive

Failure to thrive at the breast requires that the pediatrician carefully evaluate the infant. Nursing from the breast requires strong, coordinated suck and swallow; infants with neurologic problems or respiratory problems may not do well. Careful evaluation for standard failure to thrive problems (congenital heart disease, renal disease) is appropriate. As discussed previously, abnormal breast milk composition is possible but unusual. More commonly, the problem is inadequate production. If the infant has a normal suck, failure to thrive may reflect the mother's inability to relax and experience good let-down reflex. The mother needs to be encouraged to nurse frequently in a quiet environment and to drink large amounts of fluids. A true inability to produce milk adequately is very unusual.

Feeding the Low-Birth-Weight Infant

Premature infants can benefit from the multiple advantages of human milk; indeed, a good case can be made that all premature infants should be fed human milk. However, the nutritional requirements of the premature infant are increased in general and human milk may not be adequate. Both the protein and the sodium content of human milk is increased in the milk of women delivering prematurely; however, these increases may last for only a few weeks. The problem of hypoproteinemia with decreased growth and edema may present in the infant after several months.

Unfortunately, the calcium and phosphorus content of human milk is not increased by premature delivery. The exclusive feeding of unsupplemented human milk to the very premature infant, especially one weighing less than 1000 g, is very likely to result in classic phosphorus-deficiency rickets. Although calcium is well absorbed, it is excreted in the urine because it cannot be accreted by bone without the phosphorus. Supplementation with phosphorus will improve mineralization as well as calcium retention. However, it is recommended that human milk be supplemented with both calcium and phosphorus to levels comparable to those in premature formulas and that protein also be supplemented because mineral supplementation may increase growth rate. Supplementation of trace elements reduces the chances of deficiency due to rapid growth or inhibition of absorption by macromineral supplementation.

Human milk should be supplemented with vitamins, although the effects of supplementation need to be evaluated. It is likely that supplementation allows the infant to have the benefits of human milk without the deficits.

PRACTICAL PROBLEMS

Initiating Breast-Feeding

The secret to prevention of sore and cracked nipples, poor infant nursing, and the inability of the mother to relax lies in prevention of breast engorgement. Unfortunately, in this day of early hospital discharge, the nursing staff has very little time to work with the mother and infant, and the milk will probably "come in with a vengeance" after the mother has gone home.

During the colostrum period, the infant is provided with some major immunologic and nutritional benefits, but it is primarily a time for the infant to "learn to nurse." The new mother will need help achieving a comfortable position and getting the infant on the breast. At first, nursing the infant while lying down is easier than while sitting. In order to suck smoothly on the nipple, the infant must get the entire areola into the mouth, and this requires that the breast be soft. It is often helpful to express milk manually while the infant is nursing, especially early on, before good let-down reflex begins. The infant will often let the mother know that he or she is not getting a good milk flow by rapidly chomping, and it is helpful to express milk manually until a slow, comfortable sucking resumes. Chomping and engorgement lead to sore and cracked nipples, which are painful and make relaxed, pleasant nursing almost impossible. Conversely, an infant who is nursing well is the best guard against engorgement.

Plugged ducts are also a source of discomfort and may be the origin of breast infections. It is a good idea for the mother to check her breasts for lumps and to work them out by manual expression while the infant is nursing before infection occurs. Once true infection occurs, nursing on the infected side is probably contraindicated and manual drainage is imperative. If the breast develops an area that is red or hot, medical attention is needed and antibiotics may be necessary.

Expression of Milk

If engorgement occurs that requires expression of milk before nursing, it can best be done in the shower. Warm water markedly facilitates relaxation and let-down reflex. Manual expression will be helpful later on when the mother is away from the infant for several hours; however, it is probably wise to advise the mother to buy a small hand pump for times when it is necessary to express enough milk for several days or if the milk is to be saved. The pediatrician must identify if an infant is premature or sick and is not going to be able to breast-feed initially. A mechanical pump should be available to the mother so that frequent, adequate stimulation can be provided to start and maintain lactation.

Frequency and Timing of Feedings

Besides a comfortable, relaxed mother, the secret of nursing is a hungry, awake infant. Because no two infants maintain the same nursing schedule, nursing makes rooming-in imperative. The mother needs to be ready when the infant is, and frequent nursing, every 2 to 3 hours, should be the rule, especially initially. It is not crucial to time nursing, but it is important to monitor the quality of the nursing. The feeding should be stopped or the infant switched to the other breast when he or she ceases to obtain milk easily and the breast is comfortably emptied. The mother should always alternate the breast that the feeding is started on to ensure good drainage of both. Once breast-feeding is well established, nursing with only one breast per feeding and alternating from one feeding to the next are possible.

Milk Production At Home

Infants increase their milk requirements in spurts, and there will be a number of times when the mother will be sure that she cannot produce enough milk. During these periods, the mother should nurse frequently, drink large amounts of fluid, and have a quiet environment. The need to drink large amounts of fluid cannot be overemphasized.

Supplements By Bottle

It is best if one can avoid using bottles too early because "nipple confusion" is a real entity. Different muscle coordination is needed to suck and swallow from the breast than from the bottle, and breast-feeding requires more energy. However, hydration is important, and, occasionally, water supplementation is needed early in the infant's life.

After several weeks, when nursing is established, it is helpful to teach the infant to drink from a bottle to give the mother increased flexibility, especially if the mother will be returning to work. Most infants do well drinking from the bottle while the mother is at work and nursing the rest of the time and on weekends. With the excellent formulas available, it is certainly not necessary to provide breast milk for the time when the mother is at work. One does need to be prepared for stool changes if a breast-fed infant is switched to formula for several days.

Returning to Work

Most women do not need to use a pump while at work and yet they have plenty of milk ready as soon as they return home (making breast pads a necessity) and on weekends. Unfortunately, many women plan ahead to give up nursing when they go back to work because they assume that it will be too inconvenient. The pediatrician can do the mother a great service by encouraging her to try nursing and working. Pediatricians need to work on increasing the length of time that a woman nurses her infant.

Solid Foods

After the infant is 4 to 6 months of age, the pediatrician may need to encourage the introduction of other foods by spoon or fingers, because the infant needs to learn to explore his or her world with both fingers and mouth. Some long-term exclusively breast-fed infants can pose later feeding problems. As in all areas of pediatrics, the mother must be taught to use the infant's stage of development as the guide.

Weaning

Milk production decreases when it is not needed. Most infants slowly wean themselves over the course of several weeks or months. Breast-fed infants can easily be weaned directly to the cup at 6 to 9 months. Weaning must be a slow, gradual process for both the infant and the mother and must be viewed in the positive context of infant development. However, most mothers who nurse their infants will have fond memories and some regret for the loss of a very special period of their lives.

REFERENCES

Briggs G, Freeman R, Yoffe L (eds): Drugs in Pregnancy and Lactation. Baltimore, Williams & Wilkins, 1986.

Lawrence RA: Breastfeeding, A Guide for the Medical Profession, 2nd ed. St. Louis, CV Mosby, 1985.

FEEDING THE LOW-BIRTH-WEIGHT INFANT

DAVID BROWN, M.D.

The feeding and nutrition of the low-birth-weight (LBW) infant (birth weight <1500 g) have assumed greater importance as a result of the survival of smaller and smaller premature neonates. With the improving outcome of LBW infants who have respiratory difficulty, the importance of feeding and nutrition problems as sources of morbidity will assume an even more prominent relative position among the clinical problems of the LBW neonate. Any consideration of feeding of the LBW infant implies consideration of nutrition, which, in turn, implies both enteral and parenteral nutrition. The following discussion is divided into enteral and parenteral nutrition, although they are usually not completely separable because most LBW infants will experience both early in life in the clinician's effort to maximize nutrition.

ENTERAL NUTRITION

The ultimate goal in terms of enteral nutrient intake is to have the patient ingest between 100 and 120 cal/kg/day. With the standard formulas, this means that the patient will receive 2.5 to 3.0 g of protein/kg/day and 45 to 50 per cent of the calories as fat. This level of intake will usually result in steady growth.

In the term neonate, this feeding goal is usually accomplished without much difficulty by the end of the first week of life. However, in the LBW infant, achieving this goal is complicated by prematurity. Prematurity implies primary maturational problems such as delayed gastric emptying and lack of mature intestinal enzyme function, as well as the problems that occur secondary to respiratory failure and its treatment. The attempt to overcome these problems has led to alterations in what is fed, how it is fed, and how often it is fed, as well as to the development of the technology required to supply essential nutrients parenterally.

Types of Food

The choice of what to feed is breast milk or formula. Breast milk is usually limited to the infant's own mother's milk. The choice of formula is from among those specially designed for premature neonates. These modified formulas are available from all three major formula manufacturers. The standard formulas with iron supplementation should be used only when the LBW neonate is ready for discharge from the hospital.

Breast Milk

Breast milk has the advantage of containing cellular and humoral infection-fighting elements missing from formula. It also contains lipase, which may aid in fat digestion. The opportunity for a premature neonate's mother to participate in her infant's care by furnishing the child's nourishment may also have psychologic benefits to one or both members of this dyad.

However, there are a number of concerns about the nutritional adequacy of human milk as the sole source of nutrition for the LBW neonate. Human milk is relatively low in minerals (sodium [Na], calcium [Ca], and phosphorus [P]) and protein. There is also concern about the adequacy of the vitamin D content of human milk. Mothers who wish to supply milk for their neonates should be encouraged to do so, especially if the baby is able to feed during the first 7 to 10 days of life, the time when human milk has its greatest cellular content. However, if human milk is to be a LBW neonate's primary food for a prolonged period, it is important either to supplement the milk with protein and minerals or to monitor the neonate for such deficiencies (serum Na, Ca, and P, blood urea nitrogen [BUN], and weight gain) and to respond to deficits as they arise.

Formula

Commercially available formulas specifically tailored to the needs of the LBW neonate have the advantage of being a more nutritionally complete diet, although they lack the immunologic advantages of human milk. These formulas have been modified to supply adequate protein in a form (casein-to-whey ratio) that mimics human milk and to contain adequate minerals. Formula tends to have more polyunsaturated fat than human milk, with the nutritional result being a theoretic increase in vulnerability of cell membranes (e.g., the red blood cell) to oxidative damage. With these formulas, there is no need for vitamin supplementation, although many nurseries still give vitamin supplements routinely. There is probably no danger in this supplementation because the amounts of fat-soluble vitamins in standard vitamin supplements are not excessive, although the use of iron may predispose to increased hemolysis.

Supplementation

No matter which food type is chosen, the option of supplementation is available. As noted, human milk may need to be supplemented with protein and minerals. Acceptable supplements are available from the formula manufacturers. In addition, caloric supplements are available as glucose polymers and medium-chain triglyceride preparations. They are both low-osmolarity additives, which are of unproven value but which are frequently used and apparently safe. As noted, the use of vitamin supplements is not necessary for formula-fed neonates but may be of some value for those fed human milk to avoid the risk of vitamin D deficiency.

Once the food type has been selected, there are a number of other decisions that have to be made. These include how to get the food into the gastrointestinal tract, how much to give per feeding or per unit time, how fast to increase these amounts, what caloric density to feed, and when to begin introducing enteral nutrition.

Feeding Methods

Gavage Feeding

Most LBW neonates will not be able either to nurse directly from their mother's breast or to feed by nipple directly from a bottle. These means can be tried when the patient weighs about 1700 g and may be successful in smaller patients, especially if there was intrauterine growth retardation.

The usual means of first introducing food into the gastrointestinal tract is through a gavage tube. The routine once the tube is in place in the stomach is to draw back with a syringe attached to the tube to determine if there is any volume remaining from the prior feed. If there is a small amount or none, formula can then be introduced by gravity flow through the tube. If residual volumes prior to feeding are more than 2 or 3 ml or represent more than 20 per cent of the volume of the feed, the patient should be examined to ensure that there is no gastrointestinal pathology that would contraindicate continued feeding. The usual feeding frequency is either every 2 or every 3 hours. The shorter interval is used for smaller infants because it allows a smaller volume per feeding for a given daily intake.

Continuous Infusion Feeding

The other means of introducing food into the gastrointestinal tract is by continuous infusion either into the stomach or into the duodenum. These methods have the disadvantage of making feeding intolerance and the presence of "prefeeding" residuals harder to determine. In the case of transpyloric feeds, there are difficulties in placing the feeding tube and there may be disadvantages of bypassing the stomach. These methods offer no particular advantage over intermittent gavage feedings in the typical patient and should be reserved for the patient who seems unable to tolerate bolus feeding.

Concentration and Rate of Volume Advancement

The issues of concentration and rate of volume advancement are dependent on the health of the patient. There are some data to suggest that starting with a dilute formula promotes feeding tolerance. If the patient has no respiratory problems, the feeding concentration can be advanced fairly rapidly from 10 cal/ounce to 20 cal/ounce, and, after an adequate volume is well tolerated, to a 24 cal/ounce formula. This more concentrated formula is commonly used because it allows a smaller volume per feed.

A rapid rate of advancement would be one that would have the patient taking enough nutrition enterally to avoid the need for parenteral fluid by 4 to 7 days after initiating feedings. This rate of advancement should be lower with decreasing patient size and increasing medical problems. A patient weighing 500 to 1000 g at birth should not have feeding volumes increased rapidly. The goal with such tiny premature neonates is to introduce feedings early but to increase feeding volumes very slowly, limiting intake to even as little as 12 to 24 ml/kg/day for the first week. There is evidence that the introduction of even this small amount of enteral nutrition will improve later feeding tolerance.

Any patient with respiratory difficulties should have feedings introduced later in life, preferably not until he or she shows considerable improvement in pulmonary function. Such a patient should have feeding volumes increased more slowly because respiratory function deteriorates following a feeding.

The reasons for delaying feeding are concerns about complications. These are primarily fears of necrotizing enterocolitis (NEC) and of aspiration. Although NEC is not caused by feeding, most neonatologists feel its prevalence can be increased by overly aggressive feeding practices. As noted, respiratory function can be compromised by feeding, and the danger of aspirating gastric contents may be increased under these unfavorable circumstances.

The reasons for not delaying feeding are the obvious growth and development failure that will occur in the absence of adequate nutrition. Although parenteral nutrition can offer a temporary substitute for enteral feeding, it is best used as a supplement to enteral nutrition because its prolonged use is associated with numerous serious complications.

PARENTERAL NUTRITION

Short Term

Almost without exception, all infants born weighing less than 1500 g will require initial parenteral fluid and nutrition. Except for an occasional severely growth retarded neonate, LBW infants are born between 6 and 14 weeks prematurely. Even if they have no respiratory problems, LBW infants are still at increased risk for hypoglycemia and, when fed, are attempting to use an organ system that has not been programmed to begin functioning as a digestive organ for more than a month, even in the most favorable cases. In the patient with significant respiratory disease, there is added stress to overcome if feeding is considered. Thus, the LBW neonate should start life with an intravenous (IV) infusion.

The goals for parental nutrition are: (1) prevention of hypoglycemia, (2) sparing of nitrogen (i.e., giving enough caloric intake to prevent the patient from using his or her body as a fuel source), and (3) growth. The nature of the particular goal dictates the composition of the IV fluid chosen and, to some extent, the route of administration.

The first goal suggests that all LBW infants should receive IV therapy for at least some time early in their neonatal course. For patients with no major medical problems, feeding will be initiated at 24 to 48 hours of age, and, as feedings increase, IV therapy can be decreased at a rate to give the patient the desired total fluid intake. The specific goals in the healthy LBW neonate are to stabilize weight at about 10 per cent below birth weight as the early contraction of the extracellular volume is occurring; to maintain electrolyte balance by adding Na and potassium (K) to the fluid sometime after the first or second day of life; and to prevent hypoglycemia without inducing hyperglycemia, glycosuria, and further weight loss and disturbance of electrolyte balance.

The specific choices to accomplish these goals are an initial IV rate of 60 to 80 ml/kg/day, which is adjusted upward in response to weight loss. This should be higher (80 to 100 ml/kg/day) in extremely low birth weight infants (birth weight <750 g). The maximum rate toward the end of the first week of life may be as high as 250 ml/kg/day in the very smallest neonates but is typically about 150 ml/kg/day. The fluid should initially be 10 per cent dextrose in water (D10W), although D5W may be selected for infants weighing less than 750 g because the more premature the patient, the greater the glucose intolerance.

Serum electrolyte concentrations should be measured daily beginning on the second day. If the serum Na is in the normal or low range, sodium chloride (NaCl, 30 mEq/L) should be added to the IV solution. This will usually give the patient a net intake of 2 to 3 mEq/kg/day, which should meet the Na requirement. However, this amount may need to be increased or decreased, depending on what the serum Na is each day. Potassium chloride (KCl) should also be added (15 to 20 mEq/L) when NaCl is added *if the patient is urinating* and has lost some weight. If all else is normal (including an electrocardiogram rhythm strip), a slightly elevated serum K should not cause the omission of KCl from the IV fluid because serum K values measured in blood obtained from heel puncture are frequently artifactually elevated.

Long Term

For LBW patients with respiratory or other medical problems who are not going to be fed until the end of the first week of life or longer, initial IV therapy is as described previously. However, without enteral nutrition, or with only token, enzyme-inducing enteral nutrition, adding more nutritional support parenterally should be considered. When the infant is 5 to 7 days of age, amino acids can be added to the IV solution. The weight ratio of protein to glucose should never exceed 1:5. Excessive protein intake does not increase growth and can lead to azotemia, dehydration, acidosis, and liver damage.

Of these complications, liver disease is the most difficult to avoid. If enough protein is given for long enough, an obstructive liver disease will develop. This is thought to be caused by abnormal elevations in the serum concentration of a number of amino acids, which occurs with the use of many of the commercially available parenteral amino acid preparations. On the positive side, once the amino acid infusion is discontinued, the obstructive jaundice usually clears without permanent sequelae.

To minimize complications, a 2 per cent solution is usually sufficient for a patient who is going to be fed within the first 2 to 3 weeks of life and has no intrinsic gastrointestinal disease. A 2 per cent solution will result in an intake of 3 g/kg/day at an IV rate of 150 ml/kg/day. This intake is approximately the amount of protein required for growth and, because there will usually be at last a small amount of enteral intake, should be more than adequate.

If parenteral nutrition is to be the sole nutritional source, a major difficulty is achieving an adequate caloric intake. Glucose concentrations above 10 per cent are not initially well tolerated by these patients, although insulin production can be induced in most patients by slowly increasing the glucose and amino acid concentration. At the theoretic IV rate of 150 ml/kg/day, a D10W solution will furnish 60 cal/kg/day as glucose. This can be increased to 75 with D12.5W and to 90 with D15W. At higher glucose concentrations, rapid sclerosis of veins will occur and IV access will quickly become a problem. In addition, the highest concentration some of the more immature patients can tolerate is D7.5W, which will provide only 45 cal/kg/day. The solution to this problem is to add a lipid emulsion to the parenteral regimen.

Intravenous lipid preparations are primarily linoleic acid. At intakes of 5 per cent of total calories, they will prevent essential fatty acid deficiency, and, at higher intakes, they will supply a concentrated source of calories that will not cause hyperglycemia. Eleven calories per gram are available from IV lipid preparations, and up to 4 g/kg/day can safely be infused. The total IV lipid intake should not exceed 40 per cent of total caloric intake, and this total should be approached in increments of 0.5 g/kg/day, with assurances that serum free fatty acids (FFA) and triglycerides (TG) are not grossly abnormal.

As with any therapy, the benefits must be weighed against the risks. With IV lipid preparations, the gain is caloric intake and essential fatty acid intake; the hazards are microscopic pulmonary fat embolization, sepsis, hyperlipemia, and, possibly, kernicterus. Almost all who have studied the problem have found some degree of fat deposition in the pulmonary circulation in patients who are on IV lipid preparations, and others have found respiratory decompensation of some degree with lipid use. The risk of infection caused by *Malassezia furfur,* a fat-requiring species of fungus, is greatly increased by the use of lipid preparations, as is sepsis caused by any bacterial or fungal species. Increases in FFA and TG are to some extent unavoidable but can be minimized by decreasing the infusion rate and by decreasing the total intake in gestationally less mature patients. *The risk of kernicterus is theoretic and related to the displacement of bilirubin from albumin by FFA. This theoretic risk can be avoided by not giving IV lipid preparations until after any jaundice problem has been resolved.*

Once a commitment to long-term parenteral nutrition has been made, it is usual to add a multivitamin preparation to the IV fluid as well as Ca, magnesium (Mg), and P in quantities that can stay in solution. These amounts of minerals will provide lower intakes than can be achieved orally or than would be occurring transplacentally but should be enough to prevent bone disease. Each patient who is receiving a parenteral solution containing protein and/or fat should be monitored for complications. A suggested program of laboratory tests includes FFA, TG, total and direct bilirubin, BUN, Na, K, and Cl weekly and liver enzymes, Ca, Mg, P, and alkaline phosphatase biweekly.

If it is necessary to give higher concentrations of glucose and amino acids for a prolonged period, a central line will probably be required in order to maintain reliable venous access to the patient. Maintenance of IV access is especially important if a hyperinsulinemic state has been induced by high glucose intake, because hypoglycemia is a distinct possibility if a high glucose intake is abruptly stopped. The choices in the LBW patient are umbilical arterial, umbilical venous, surgically inserted central venous, or percutaneously inserted central venous lines.

Because of the high probability of contamination of the umbilical lines (either arterial or venous) secondary to bacterial or fungal growth in Wharton's jelly, the umbilical line is not usually the route of choice. A more usual choice is a central venous line inserted in the brachial or external jugular vein. Such lines can be inserted either percutaneously or surgically. The longevity of these lines is dependent on preventing clotting, accidental removal, and infection. Preventing the first two complications depends on the usual nursing care for any IV line. Preventing infectious complications depends on strict aseptic technique when disconnecting the line to add new IV solutions and on not using the line for any purpose but administration of parenteral alimentation solutions.

The chances of accidental dislodgement of the central line can be decreased by securing it in a number of places or, in the case of the surgically placed line, by tunneling the line subcutaneously from the point where it enters the vein to a distal point where it exits the skin; attaching a cuff to the line will further secure its placement by anchoring it at the point of exit from the subcutaneous tunnel. Protection against infection can be enhanced by placing a millipore filter in the IV line at a point just before the line enters the skin.

Even with the best of technique, placement of a central venous line markedly increases the risk of sepsis, usually from fungus or coagulase-negative staphylococcus. Other complications that occur less commonly now that Silastic catheters are used are vessel perforation by rigid catheters and vena caval obstruction resulting from coagulation at the tip of the catheter.

SUMMARY

Nourishing the LBW neonate involves a combination of enteral and parenteral intake for optimal results. All patients should begin with parenteral support while feedings are being slowly introduced. As feedings are advanced, parenteral intake can be reduced. In cases in which the ideal goal of having a patient on only enteral nutrition by the end of the first week cannot be achieved, there is the option of enriching the parenteral fluid with amino acids, fats, minerals, vitamins, and trace elements to allow the patient an acceptable source of nourishment during the delay in feeding.

NEONATAL INTESTINAL OBSTRUCTION

EUGENE S. WIENER, M.D.

Intestinal obstruction that presents in the newborn period is most often caused by Hirschsprung's disease; a myriad of functional obstructions caused by meconium plugs, prematurity, and diabetes; meconium ileus; intestinal atresia; and malrotation, with or without volvulus.

Bilious vomiting, abdominal distention, and/or lack of spontaneous passage of meconium in the first 24 to 48 hours of life suggest intestinal obstruction until proven otherwise and warrant further patient evaluation and consultation with a pediatric surgeon. Gestational and familial history may provide clues, such as polyhydramnios associated with high obstructions, maternal diabetes seen in infants with small left colon syndrome, and cystic fibrosis or Hirschsprung's disease in family members.

Initial plain radiographs of the infant's entire chest, abdomen, and pelvis (babygram), including decubitus views, should be obtained before nasogastric decompression. After consultation with the pediatric surgeon and radiologist, contrast studies may be obtained. When malrotation is suspected, upper gastrointestinal contrast may be diagnostic. Rectal enema is used, with barium to distinguish the transition zone of Hirschsprung's disease, or with water-soluble agents to differentiate distal atresias and to treat meconium plugs, small left colons, and meconium ileus.

The initial management of the neonate with intestinal obstruction is nasogastric decompression using a 10 French sump-type catheter. The Replogle tube is the ideal catheter for neonates because its holes are closer to the tip and it provides more effective gastric decompression. Reliable intravenous access should be obtained, remembering that, because these infants often need long-term intravenous infusions, each site is precious. Blood should be drawn for routine evaluation and for transfusion, although it is rarely necessary intraoperatively. If the infant has been vomiting for more than a few hours of life or if the abdomen is distended with a significant amount of free fluid, intravenous resuscitation is required and a urethral catheter may be necessary to monitor urine output. Significant abdominal distention that is not relieved by gastric decompression will interfere with ventilation; tracheal intubation before sending such a neonate to a darkened radiology room is often prudent. Antibiotics are administered before operation.

Suspicion of volvulus warrants immediate laparotomy without waiting for complete fluid resuscitation and extensive work-up. Most other neonates can be evaluated and prepared in an orderly fashion before proceeding with an urgent operation.

HIRSCHSPRUNG'S DISEASE (AGANGLIONOSIS)

The lack of spontaneous passage of meconium within 24 and certainly by 48 hours of birth should be considered to be Hirschsprung's disease until proven otherwise. These infants usually have significant abdominal distention from birth, frequently associated with bilious vomiting, and abdominal radiographs show multiple loops of gas-filled bowel with fluid levels, and absent gas in the anorectum. Hirschsprung's disease is rarely seen in premature infants, is more common in males, and has an increased incidence in infants with Down syndrome.

An initial digital rectal examination may distort the transition zone seen on a contrast enema and is therefore best delayed until after abdominal radiographic examination. The enema should be performed by a radiologist experienced in such studies, avoiding the introduction of more contrast agent than necessary to fill the first dilated intestinal segment. Barium is the best contrast agent to reveal the transition zone; this zone may be visualized in some affected infants only after delayed passage of barium in 12 to 24 hours. The diagnosis is confirmed by suction rectal biopsy, performed at the bedside, revealing the absence of ganglion cells in the submucosa and increased acetylcholinesterase staining. Operation may not safely wait for confirmatory biopsy in the occasional infant with marked abdominal distention who does not decompress after contrast or subsequent rectal examination or irrigation.

As soon as the diagnosis is established, a colostomy is performed at the site of transition as proven by intraoperative biopsy, although loop right transverse colostomy is preferred by some surgeons. The subsequent pull-through procedure of choice is usually performed at 3 to 6 months of age. Occasionally, a newborn will decompress so well after irrigation and digital rectal examination, that a primary pull-through without a preliminary colostomy can be performed in the first weeks of life. Children with Hirschsprung's disease do well after pull-through, except for a cohort with recurring enterocolitis or chronic constipation in spite of an appropriate operation.

FUNCTIONAL OBSTRUCTIONS

Meconium plug syndrome, small left colon syndrome, and physiologic obstructions of the premature infant may all mimic Hirschsprung's disease. Meconium plugs are seen on contrast enema without a typical transition zone. If barium was used initially, the contrast material should then be changed to a water-soluble agent, which should fill the colon. Typical white meconium plugs will be followed by explosive, large, normal meconium stools and gas. Suction rectal biopsy should be performed subsequently because Hirschsprung's disease will be present in as many as a third of these infants.

Small left colon syndrome typically occurs in large infants of diabetic mothers. In some cases, the maternal diabetes had not been previously diagnosed or other siblings have been similarly affected. These infants frequently have very severe abdominal distention, and plain radiographs reveal very dilated intestinal loops, especially the cecum. Water-soluble contrast enema reveals a small left colon with a transition at or near the splenic flexure and is usually therapeutic. Occasionally, decompression does not occur promptly and temporary colostomy in the dilated colon is required to avoid cecal perforation. Suction rectal biopsy should be done to exclude Hirschsprung's disease. These infants recover promptly without intestinal sequelae.

Small premature infants may have delayed intestinal function manifested by delayed meconium passage and visibly dilated intestinal loops. Radiographs generally show intestinal loops of equal size without air-fluid levels, and air down to the anus. Gentle, warmed saline irrigations will be followed by meconium stools. These irrigations may need to be repeated on several occasions. Contrast studies and rectal biopsies are needed only if findings persist or the presentation is atypical.

MECONIUM ILEUS

Meconium ileus generally presents as a distal ileal obstruction, although sometimes the obstruction is in the jejunum. The obstruction is due to inspissated meconium, which, in the simple form, is manifested by small pellets in the collapsed distal ileum and by sticky, adherent meconium in the dilated, more proximal intestine. In complicated forms, the dilated intestine may twist, resulting in an atresia, or may perforate, resulting in meconium peritonitis.

When simple meconium ileus is suspected, a contrast enema using a slightly hyperosmolar water-soluble contrast agent is successful in relieving the obstruction in more than half of these infants. Usually, there is rapid decompression with passage of liquefied meconium. Occasionally, a repeated enema or upper gastrointestinal contrast is necessary to achieve complete resolution. If the contrast does not reflux into dilated intestine and/or if meconium fails to pass promptly, meconium ileus complicated by atresia or volvulus is not excluded and immediate operation is required. Throughout the enema examination, additional intravenous fluids are administered to replace the fluid drawn into the intestine by the hyperosmolar contrast agent.

In simple meconium ileus that does not respond appropriately to intestinal contrast studies, and in all complicated cases, urgent operation is required. Depending on the findings, the obstruction may be relieved by enterotomy with irrigations of hyperosmolar or proteinolytic agents, localized resection with reanastomosis, or temporary ostomy. The procedures in infants with complicated forms are more complex and extensive and usually require resection and a temporary ostomy.

Postoperative management includes nutritional and pulmonary support and parent counseling concerning the diagnosis, which may be established from pathologic examination of the removed intestine or appendix but which should always be confirmed by sweat test and, perhaps, chromosome analysis. In a rare infant, meconium ileus may occur without cystic fibrosis. The long-term outlook depends on the nonintestinal disease manifestations, although some children have recurrent inspissated stool obstructions.

INTESTINAL ATRESIA

Atresia may occur in any portion of the intestine, the most common being the duodenum and jejunoileum. The duodenum may be obstructed by a true atresia, a diaphragm or web, a stenosis, or an annular pancreas, causing a picture of a complete or partial obstruction. The ampulla may be distal to the obstruction; the vomitous may be nonbilious, although usually it is bilious. Almost a third of the infants have Down syndrome; associated biliary anomalies may subsequently be noted in infants with annular pancreas. The embryology of these atresias or stenoses is probably related to an error of recanalization, whereas annular pancreas follows abnormal fusion of the pancreatic anlagen.

Complete duodenal obstruction can be diagnosed from a plain abdominal radiograph showing the classic double-bubble sign. This sign may be obscured by excessive fluid in the stomach or duodenum or by prior decompression with a nasogastric tube. Re-establishment of this sign requires only simple insertion of air into the decompressed stomach and does not require other contrast studies. Incomplete obstruction may require contrast studies to establish the diagnosis and rule out malrotation, especially if operation is to be delayed. When the diagnosis is clear, operation can await evaluation of associated anomalies and correction of fluid and electrolyte disturbances. The operation of choice is duodenoduodenostomy for atresias and annular pancreas and duodenoplasty, with or without web excision, for the webs or stenoses. Gastrostomies are rarely needed, and fine Silastic transanastomotic feeding tubes avoid the need for parenteral nutrition. Oral alimentation can be anticipated within 10 days in many infants.

Jejunoileal and colon atresias are most likely due to intrauterine vascular insults or volvulus of the intestine. The clinical and radiographic findings vary with the level of obstruction: the high obstructions have less distention, and plain radiographs show one or two dilated loops beyond the stomach; the distal obstructions have more abdominal distention and multiple loops with air-fluid levels. There may be calcification, suggesting meconium peritonitis. Oral contrast serves no purpose, but rectal contrast is useful to determine whether the colon is patent and to exclude simple meconium ileus, Hirschsprung's disease, and functional distal obstructions.

Operation involves resection of the bulbous, poorly vascularized, dilated segment, where possible, with reanastomosis in a modified, end-to-end fashion. This may be difficult when there is marked discrepancy between the proximal and the distal segments. Tapering or plication of the proximal segment may expedite the anastomosis and promote earlier return of postoperative intestinal function. Colon atresias have the most discrepancy and often require temporary ostomy. Jejunal atresias typically require prolonged parenteral nutrition, whereas ileal atresias resume normal gut function after a few days. This may be related to the inability to resect the entire dilated segment in higher atresias.

Multiple atresias, atresia with volvulus and deficient bowel length, and apple-peel or Christmas-tree atresias involve complex operative and postoperative management problems that frequently require long hospitalizations and long-term parenteral nutrition and gut adaptation.

MALROTATION

Intestinal rotation is a complex process that begins during the extracoelomic phase and is completed during the 10th week of gestation. Alterations of this process can take different forms, resulting in a variety of malrotations, nonrotation, or mixed rotation. Although nonrotation, seen in infants with diaphragmatic hernia, gastroschisis, and omphalocele, rarely causes obstruction, incomplete rotation can obstruct the duodenum by peritoneal (Ladd's) bands or by volvulus of the midgut.

The classic symptoms and signs in infants with malrotation and volvulus are bilious vomiting and bloody stools. The infants may appear ill, be hypovolemic, and have a metabolic acidosis; the abdomen may be tender, and a palpable mass of intestine may be present. These are late signs, and their absence does not exclude volvulus. Plain radiograph may show the sign of a high duodenal obstruction (double-bubble sign), a gasless abdomen, or partial duodenal obstruction. In the sick infant, further delay is not justified; however, in the stable infant, upper gastrointestinal contrast will confirm the diagnosis, which should lead to urgent operation. Neonatal obstruction always requires urgent intervention, but the potential of vascular compromise, reversible in its early stages, is always an emergency.

The operation requires complete evisceration of the intestine, division of Ladd's bands, careful counterclockwise untwisting of the intestine, and unfurling of the mesentery so that it has a wide base. Normal rotation cannot be accomplished; instead, nonrotation is achieved, with the duodenum, unkinked, descending on the right side, the colon and appendix-free cecum in the left upper quadrant, and the mesentery flat and untwisted transversely across the abdomen. Obviously, necrotic intestine should be removed; however, ischemic bowel will frequently recover, although sometimes with strictures that can be handled secondarily. Second-look operations in 12 to 24 hours may be helpful. The guiding principle is always bowel preservation.

When intestinal viability is not affected, early postoperative gut recovery occurs within days of operation. When gangrene occurs, long-term parenteral nutrition and gut adaptation may be required, depending on the length of involved intestine. Recurrent volvulus after an appropriate operation is rare, although adhesive intestinal obstruction may occur.

HEMOLYTIC DISEASES OF THE NEONATE

RICHARD P. WENNBERG, M.D.

Erythroblastosis fetalis due to rhesus factor (Rh) isoimmunization is the prototype of hemolytic disease in the newborn, but the administration of Rh_o(D) immune globulin to nonsensitized pregnant women has reduced the incidence of severe hemolytic disease dramatically over the past two decades. The relative incidence of hemolytic disease due to other causes, such as maternal sensitization to other fetal red blood cell antigens, enzyme deficiencies such as glucose-6-phosphate dehydrogenase deficiency, and hereditary red blood cell morphologic abnormalities, has concurrently increased. In these latter situations, the pediatrician frequently has no warning that a newborn might be affected until the infant presents with jaundice and/or anemia.

Rh ISOIMMUNIZATION

Rh isoimmune disease may be prevented by administration of Rh_o(D) immune globulin (300 mg) to an Rh-negative woman within 72 hours of delivering an Rh-positive infant. Treatment is about 98 per cent effective in preventing sensitization of the mother to Rh antigen. Efficiency may be improved to greater than 99 per cent if an additional dose is administered at 28 weeks' gestation, following amniocentesis in an Rh-negative woman, following abdominal trauma, and following spontaneous or therapeutic abortion. The dose of Rh_o(D) immune globulin (300 mg) may be ineffective if a fetal-maternal hemorrhage exceeds 30 ml of Rh-positive blood. *Pediatricians should be alert to warn obstetricians if a nonsensitized Rh-positive infant is born anemic, as this might represent a larger than usual fetal-maternal transfusion and require a larger dose of immune globulin.* Rh_o(D) immune globulin is ineffective once antibodies appear in the mother's serum.

Destruction of antibody-coated red blood cells in the fetus can produce severe anemia, resulting in chronic hypoxemia, heart failure, massive edema, and intrauterine death. Postnatal death may occur from similar causes, from pulmonary complications of hydrops and prematurity, or from bilirubin toxicity. Hyperbilirubinemia is a major complication in the neonate; high serum bilirubin values are associated with irreversible brain damage, resulting in deafness, choreoathetosis, ocular abnormalities, and mental retardation.

Management of Rh isoimmune hemolytic disease requires close collaboration between the primary care physician, the perinatologist, and the neonatologist for optimal management of the affected fetus and newborn. The timing of delivery is based on assessment of the risks of intrauterine death from anemia or intrauterine transfusion versus the risks of neonatal death from hydrops, kernicterus, or complications of prematurity. If a pregnant woman is Rh-negative, anti-D antibodies should be measured on the first prenatal visit and rechecked at 28 weeks' gestation or sooner if vaginal bleeding or abdominal trauma occur. If the antibody titer is 1:16 or greater, amniocentesis should be performed at 26 to 28 weeks' gestation to evaluate the concentration of bilirubinoid pigments in the amniotic fluid, and at 3- to 4-week intervals thereafter. Earlier amniocentesis, at 22 to 24 weeks' gestation, is indicated if the titer is high or a previous infant was affected.

The amniotic fluid optical density at 450 nm (ΔOD_{450}) provides a reasonably good prediction of anemia or risk for fetal death but is less accurate in predicting the postnatal course of hyperbilirubinemia. We use a modification of the technique developed by Liley. If the amniocentesis indicates that the fetus is moderately to severely affected (Liley high zone II or zone III), cordocentesis is performed, providing direct measurement of fetal hemoglobin and bilirubin. We recommend intrauterine transfusion if the gestational age of the fetus is less than 33 weeks and fetal hematocrit is less than 30 to 35 per cent or ultrasonography reveals evidence of early hydrops. If the fetus is severely affected and the lung profile indicates immaturity, we would administer steroids to the mother for 2 days and deliver the infant. Administration of phenobarbital (125 mg/day) to the mother for 3 to 7 days prior to delivery facilitates fetal liver processing of bilirubin and has been shown to decrease the number of exchange transfusions required after birth.

Delivery Room Management

The immediate goals in caring for erythroblastotic infants at birth are to establish adequate ventilation, minimize oxygen consumption, and assess (and correct if necessary) oxygen-carrying capacity. Resuscitation of a hydropic infant frequently requires assisted ventilation from birth, often at high inspiratory pressures. In severe hydrops, paracentesis is often required to remove excess ascites, which, in combination with hepatosplenomegaly, may mechanically inhibit effective ventilation. Thoracentesis is occasionally needed if large pleural effusions are present. Close attention must be given to drying the infant and maintaining an effective radiant heat source to minimize cold stress with its attendant increase in oxygen consumption.

Cord blood samples should be obtained for determination of hematocrit/hemoglobin, total and direct bilirubin concentrations, and albumin concentration and for Coombs' test and bilirubin binding tests (if available). If the infant has received an intrauterine transfusion, the cord blood may be direct Coombs' test–negative and typed as O-negative. The Kleihauer-Betke acid elution technique may be used to estimate the percentage of donor cells in the circulation. The hematocrit (and occasionally bilirubin) in cord blood may be quite different from values obtained from the infant after stabilization and should be repeated from a venipuncture or indwelling catheter after admission to the nursery. The latter values should be used as a baseline for subsequent management decisions.

Anemia

Kernicterus is not a threat to the infant in the first hour of life. Immediate exchange transfusion, except with packed red blood cells to correct anemia, is not indicated until after stabilization of temperature and respiration has been achieved. If amniocentesis or cordocentesis indicates that the fetus is severely affected, packed type O cells compatible with the mother's blood should be available at the time of delivery. These may be mixed later with AB plasma to reconstitute whole blood if immediate red blood cell exchange is not indicated. Indications for immediate transfusion include inadequate oxygenation or metabolic acidosis in the presence of anemia. Anemia *per se* is not an indication for emergency intervention at birth. However, we would perform a limited exchange transfusion with packed red blood cells in patients with hemoglobin concentrations less than 8 to 10 g/dl. Exchange transfusion with 12 ml/kg packed red blood cells will usually raise the hematocrit by about 0.1.

Delayed anemia is often encountered in hemolytic disease of the newborn, especially when exchange transfusion is not necessary to treat hyperbilirubinemia. Close follow-up of all patients is required for several weeks, and the need for a subsequent transfusion of packed red blood cells at 3 to 4 weeks of age is not uncommon.

Hyperbilirubinemia and Kernicterus

Hyperbilirubinemia is the second major threat to infants with hemolytic disease of the newborn. Phototherapy has little impact on the early rise in bilirubin but may be useful in decreasing the number of exchange transfusions required or in preventing the need for blood replacement in mildly affected infants. In patients with confirmed hemolytic disease, phototherapy is usually initiated if the bilirubin level exceeds 6 to 8 mg/dl. Phenobarbital therapy has been shown to decrease the early rise in bilirubin and the number of transfusions required, but it is most effective if given to the mother prior to delivery. When the bilirubin concentration reaches hazardous levels, exchange transfusion is the only acceptable therapy.

Serum bilirubin concentrations should be determined on cord blood immediately following stabilization and at 4- to 8-hour intervals thereafter until the concentration declines. Total and direct bilirubin fractions should be obtained daily. If the direct-reacting bilirubin is less than 1.2 mg/dl, total bilirubin values may be equated with unconjugated bilirubin concentration. With hepatic overload, the direct fraction may be elevated, reflecting conjugated as well as unconjugated bilirubinemia. If conjugated bilirubin is elevated, the urine will test positive for bilirubin. In such cases, the need for exchange transfusion should be assessed using the indirect bilirubin fraction.

Cord blood hemoglobin and bilirubin values are unreliable predictors of the subsequent course of hyperbilirubinemia. Therefore, we recommend early exchange transfusion only when the cord bilirubin concentration exceeds 6 mg/dl or when the 1-hour bilirubin concentration exceeds 7.5 mg/dl. In most cases, it is better to monitor the rise in serum bilirubin, with immediate attention focused on stabilization and clinical assessment of the infant. If the rise in serum bilirubin exceeds 0.5 mg/dl/hour over a 12- to 18-hour period, exchange transfusion should be performed. Early exchange transfusion has the advantage of removing some antibody as well as antibody-coated red blood cells before hemolysis and bilirubin formation occur.

The concentration of bilirubin that poses the threat of brain damage varies with the condition of the patient and with the concentration and binding characteristics of serum albumin.

The traditional indication for exchange transfusion at an "indirect" bilirubin concentration of 20 mg/dl has been supported by experience (and medical-legal decisions) in stable term infants (>37 weeks' gestation), but appropriate indications for exchange transfusion in sick or prematurely delivered erythroblastotic infants are less well defined; kernicterus may occur at bilirubin concentrations below 10 mg/dl in small sick newborns.

At least three factors must be considered in making a clinical judgment to perform exchange transfusion. First, acidemia may potentiate the development of kernicterus by increasing tissue deposition of bilirubin (irrespective of albumin binding state). Tissue uptake of bilirubin appears to be determined by the concentration of unbound bilirubin acid (BH^- or BH_2). Second, disruption of the blood-brain barrier (e.g., with hydrops, asphyxia, sepsis, or meningitis) may facilitate transfer of bilirubin to susceptible neurons. Third, any insult that compromises brain metabolism may render cells more susceptible to bilirubin toxicity (e.g., by lowering local pH or decreasing tissue energy reserve). Other than by measuring blood gases, there is no method available to assess precisely the contribution of these three factors to the risk for kernicterus. The presence of an abnormal brain stem auditory evoked response (BAER) may provide additional evidence of incipient bilirubin encephalopathy. If available, a BAER should be performed when considering exchange transfusion and before discharge of any infant with severe jaundice.

Because bilirubin is tightly bound to serum albumin and because the uptake of bilirubin by tissue most likely depends on pH and the non–protein-bound bilirubin concentration, assessment of the "free" bilirubin concentration, serum albumin concentration, and binding characteristics of the protein should provide better predictors of risk than serum total or indirect bilirubin. A clear relationship between unbound bilirubin concentration, pH, and cell toxicity has been established in vitro, but clinical application has been insufficient to establish the precision with which measurement of unbound bilirubin or other serum bilirubin binding tests can predict bilirubin encephalopathy in patients. Thus, we recommend multiple criteria for exchange transfusion in infants with hemolytic disease, as listed in Table 1.

Exchange Transfusion

Exchange transfusion should be performed with fresh donor blood compatible with both mother and infant. Packed O-negative cells mixed with AB plasma may be used if blood is prepared prior to delivery. Freshly drawn heparinized blood or blood preserved in citrate-phosphate-dextrose and less than 72 hours old may be used. Blood stored longer than 72 hours may have an unacceptable serum potassium concentration, increased acid load, and decreased 2,3-DPG content.

Exchange transfusion may be performed through an umbilical venous catheter, preferably placed in the inferior vena cava (above the level of the diaphragm), or by simultaneous infusion through a venous catheter and withdrawal from an umbilical arterial catheter. Location of the tip of the catheter should be verified radiographically before exchange transfusion; placement in the liver, heart, or pulmonary arteries should be avoided. Infusion through the umbilical artery should be avoided because retrograde flow may perfuse the brain with hypoxic and acidotic exchange blood.

A two-volume replacement transfusion (infant's weight in kg × 180 ml) will remove about 90 per cent of the circulating fetal red blood cells. The postexchange bilirubin concentration will usually be about one half the preexchange value and will typically rebound to about two thirds of the initial concentration. If the postexchange bilirubin concentration is higher than two thirds of the preexchange level, a large extravascular reservoir of bilirubin probably exists and an additional exchange will almost always be required within hours.

Particular care must attend exchange transfusions in hydropic infants or newborns with marked hypoproteinemia because exchange blood provides a relatively high colloid osmotic gradient that can acutely increase the plasma volume and overload an already stressed myocardium. These infants require monitoring of central venous pressure and careful adjustment of vascular volume, which may necessitate leaving a volume deficit.

TABLE 1. Acceptable Indications for Exchange Transfusion in Hemolytic Disease of the Newborn (HDN)

All Patients
Cord hemoglobin concentration < 8 g/dl
Cord bilirubin concentration > 6 mg/dl
Rise in bilirubin concentration > 0.5 mg/dl/hr over 12–18 hr
Uncomplicated HDN
Indirect bilirubin concentration > 20 mg/dl
Indirect bilirubin concentration (in mg/dl) > 6 times the albumin concentration (in g/dl)
Sephadex staining 1+
Complicated HDN (e.g., hydrops, prematurity with RDS)
Indirect bilirubin concentration (in mg/dl) > 4.5–5.5 times the albumin concentration (in g/dl). Use lower multiple for newborns with hydrops, asphyxia, or vulnerability for developing respiratory acidosis.
Clinical Deterioration
Lethargy, poor nippling, abnormal brain stem auditory evoked response

Abbreviations: RDS, respiratory distress syndrome.

Other Problems

Erythroblastotic infants may manifest evidence of cardiorespiratory failure at birth. In hydropic infants, pulmonary edema may lead to severe pulmonary failure. Hyaline membrane disease complicates the course of many prematurely delivered erythroblastotic infants. Cardiac output may be compromised, and severely affected infants should be monitored for life-threatening cardiac arrhythmias. Infants with intrauterine hemolysis may have a blunted glucagon response as well as beta-cell hypertrophy with resulting hyperinsulinemia. These infants are similar to infants of diabetic mothers and are at risk for developing reactive hypoglycemia, especially following exchange transfusion. Blood glucose must be monitored closely.

Erythroblastotic infants may have low folate levels, and folate supplementation may facilitate both recovery from anemia and subsequent growth. Thrombocytopenia is common in Rh isoimmune disease and is frequently observed following exchange transfusion. Severely affected infants are usually small for gestational age, although this is frequently not appreciated until the edema has resolved.

Obstructive jaundice may result from bilirubin overload to the liver. Conjugated (direct-reacting) bilirubin frequently increases and may herald a peak in the unconjugated bilirubin level, as excretion of the conjugated pigment rather than conjugation becomes the limiting step in liver maturation. More severe and prolonged obstructive jaundice (inspissated bile syndrome) may be caused by bilirubin toxicity to the liver. Phototherapy will not be effective in these patients and may result in the accumulation of a bronze-colored pigment in the serum and skin. The complication is usually self-limited but, rarely, may lead to severe and prolonged hepatic damage.

UNSUSPECTED HEMOLYTIC DISEASE OF THE NEWBORN

On occasion, an infant can be born with unanticipated hemolytic disease due to (1) maternal sensitization to other red blood cell antigens, (2) inherited enzyme deficiencies, or (3) abnormal red blood cell morphology. In most cases, these patients will present with severe jaundice rather than anemia. However, severe erythroblastosis fetalis as well as hydrops fetalis may rarely occur in ABO incompatibility or sensitization to minor antigens, such as Kell or little c from the Rh complex, possibly as a result of a large fetal-maternal transfusion during pregnancy.

Any infant with marked or persistent hyperbilirubinemia (e.g., >14 to 15 mg/dl) should be evaluated for possible hemolytic disease. Evaluation should initially include hematocrit or hemoglobin and screening for isoimmune antibodies. Direct Coombs' test is often only weakly positive in ABO incompatibility, although antibodies may be detected in the infant's serum. If no antibodies are detected, evaluation on red blood cell morphology can be very helpful in identifying the presence of a nonisoimmune hemolytic process. Similar evaluation should be performed in an infant presenting with pallor and anemia. If an anemic newborn has normal erythrocyte morphology and a negative antibody screen, severe perinatal blood loss or, rarely, inherited metabolic disease should be considered. Fetal-maternal transfusion can be diagnosed by examining maternal blood for fetal red blood cells using the Kleihauer-Betke technique.

Management of anemia and jaundice in these infants is similar to that in Rh isoimmune disease. However, it should be remembered that guidelines for "safe" bilirubin levels in hemolytic disease were established from observations in Rh isoimmune disease. Appropriate intervention guidelines for infants without severe intrauterine hemolysis have not been determined by outcome studies. As with Rh incompatibility, the potential for delayed severe anemia requires close follow-up until the infant is 4 to 8 weeks of age.

NEONATAL POLYCYTHEMIA AND HYPERVISCOSITY

VIRGINIA DELANEY-BLACK, M.D.

DIAGNOSIS

Normal term newborns have a mean cord blood hematocrit value of 50 per cent, with a range of 40 to 60 per cent. If the venous hematocrit is 65 per cent or greater, the infant is often referred to as polycythemic; however, some authors have preferred to use a hematocrit level of 70 per cent or greater in diagnosing polycythemia. Identifying the polycythemic newborn is complicated by variations in the venous hematocrit during the immediate newborn period. Studies have suggested that the hematocrit at term will rise from cord levels to a peak at 2 hours of age and then drop slowly over the next several hours. When considering routine screening procedures for newborn hematocrit, it is important to recognize this natural variation. The infant whose hematocrit level makes him or her "polycythemic" at 2 hours of age may, without any intervention, have a normal level at 6 to 8 hours following delivery. Routine hematocrit screening in the well infant is best done after the peak hematocrit at 6 to 8 hours of age. In the child with distress, the timing of initial hematocrit screening should be determined by his or her signs.

One of the most common pitfalls in defining polycythemia is to use a heel- or finger-stick hematocrit without a confirming venous sample. Peripheral sampling overestimates the venous hematocrit in newborns. The difference between the two sites may be minimal if the extremity is warm and peripheral perfusion is good. However, in the immediate newborn period or even later in the infant with problems, there may be very poor correlation. Although the peripheral hematocrit level may be used to screen for polycythemia, one should confirm the diagnosis with a venous sample.

NEONATAL HYPERVISCOSITY SYNDROME

The major contribution to whole blood viscosity in newborns is hematocrit value. Hence, most infants with elevated viscosity will also be polycythemic. A few infants with high normal hematocrits may have abnormal whole blood viscosity because of altered plasma proteins or lipids or abnormal red blood cells. Because viscosity is not measured in the clinical setting, a high index of suspicion may be required.

ETIOLOGY AND COMPLICATIONS

It is commonly believed that cord blood hematocrits are higher than normal adult hematocrits because of the lower arterial oxygen concentration to which the fetus is exposed during intrauterine life. Increasing the fetal hematocrit increases the oxygen-carrying capacity. Factors that may interfere with placental oxygen concentration have all been associated with increased newborn hematocrits to varying degrees. For example, high altitude, maternal diabetes, and intrauterine growth retardation have all been associated with an increased risk of neonatal polycythemia, whereas maternal smoking typically results in only a small but measurable increase in hematocrit.

Even under these adverse intrauterine conditions, not all infants will develop polycythemia. At sea level, as few as 1 to 2 per cent of infants will have elevated hematocrit values; at 5000 feet, as many as 4 to 5 per cent may be affected. Conversely, not all newborns with neonatal polycythemia have been exposed to prolonged oxygen deprivation. Many may have acute or chronic placental transfusions. The earliest descriptions of neonatal polycythemia were in monozygotic twins with arterial-venous anastomoses. The donor twin on the arterial side was anemic, and the recipient twin on the venous side was polycythemic. Because the transfusion is chronic, both twins may have relatively normal blood volumes. Infants with more acute placental transfusions following delayed cord clamping or fetal distress may have an increased blood volume at delivery. In most infants with polycythemia, there is no obvious cause identified.

A variety of newborn problems have been identified in association with neonatal polycythemia (Table 1). Fortunately,

TABLE 1. Neonatal Findings and Diagnoses Associated with Neonatal Polycythemia

Cardiorespiratory	Hematologic
Tachypnea	Hyperbilirubinemia
Cyanosis	Disseminated intravascular coagulation
Apnea	Thrombocytopenia
Cardiomegaly and increased pulmonary vascularity	**Metabolic**
Gastrointestinal	Hypoglycemia
Poor feeding	**Neurologic**
Regurgitation	Lethargy
Abdominal distention	Hypotonia
Diarrhea	Seizures
Necrotizing enterocolitis	Tremulousness
Pneumatosis intestinalis	

even when these problems appear, most polycythemic infants do well. Careful observation and symptomatic treatment for hypoglycemia, feeding difficulties, and cardiorespiratory problems usually suffice. If signs persist or if the signs are serious, treatment with partial plasma exchange transfusion may be warranted to reduce the neonatal problems. It is important to use caution in determining who should undergo this procedure, which has its own inherent risks. Postnatal treatment of polycythemia, particularly if it has been present for some time prior to delivery, will not eliminate sequelae. Furthermore, when sequelae do occur, it is often difficult to determine if they are related to the polycythemia or to the cause of the polycythemia.

TREATMENT

When a partial plasma exchange transfusion is warranted by the child's condition, appropriate preparations will reduce the risk. To calculate the volume of exchange, the following formula can be used:

Estimated blood volume × (current hematocrit [Hct] − desired Hct)/(current Hct)

or, in a term infant:

Weight (kg) × 80 ml/kg × (current Hct − 50%)/(current Hct)

A typical volume of exchange for a 3-kg term infant would range from 48 ml (initial hematocrit of 65 per cent) to 80 ml (initial hematocrit of 75 per cent).

The diluent is often Plasmanate because it will remain in the intravascular space. Fresh frozen plasma, because of its coagulation factors, is not a good choice. The initial procedure is similar to a two-volume exchange and requires a warmer, a monitor, a sterile exchange tray, and an individual to supervise and record. The infant should be restrained. The stomach can be aspirated if the infant has fed or if secretions are present. The umbilical site should be prepared and draped. A slow pull-push procedure through the umbilical vein is the most common technique. Following the exchange, the infant should be given nothing by mouth (NPO) and vital signs should be monitored. Careful observation for hypoglycemia is needed, especially if the infant is to be without feedings for several hours. With appropriate calculation of the volume for exchange, the need for a second procedure is extremely unlikely.

CONGENITAL DIAPHRAGMATIC HERNIA

CRAIG W. LILLEHEI, M.D.

Congenital diaphragmatic hernia remains one of the most common yet lethal newborn surgical emergencies. The reported incidence varies from 1 in 2000 to 1 in 5000 live births. Most (85 to 90 per cent) of the hernias are left-sided. Although the size of the defect varies, it is typically posterolateral, through the so-called foramen of Bochdalek. An anterior rim of diaphragm is usually present, but, posteriorly, the rim may be very narrow or absent. With left-sided hernias, the stomach, spleen, small intestine, colon, or left lobe of the liver may herniate into the chest. On the right, the hernia usually contains liver but may also involve small intestine or colon. A hernia sac is present in only about 20 per cent of cases. The ipsilateral lung is hypoplastic and frequently does not immediately expand to fill the hemithorax. The number of airway generations, arterioles, and alveoli is substantially reduced. There is also increased muscularization around peripheral arterioles. These changes are often seen in the contralateral lung, although they are not as severe.

CLINICAL PRESENTATION AND DIAGNOSIS

Increasingly, diaphragmatic hernia is recognized in utero by prenatal ultrasonography, either done routinely or to evaluate polyhydramnios. Nonetheless, the most common presentation remains respiratory distress within the first few hours of life. Notable on physical examination is a scaphoid abdomen with an increased anteroposterior diameter of the chest. Breath sounds are absent on the side of the hernia, although bowel sounds can occasionally be heard. The cardiac apex is displaced away from the hernia. The chest radiograph is virtually diagnostic, demonstrating gas-filled intestinal loops within the chest and displacement of the cardiac silhouette.

TREATMENT

Preoperative Procedures

The extent of respiratory difficulty depends on the volume of herniated viscera and degree of pulmonary hypoplasia. Early insertion of a nasogastric tube is important to minimize gastrointestinal distention within the chest. It may also aid in radiographically confirming the intrathoracic position of the stomach. If the infant requires ventilatory assistance, prompt endotracheal intubation is essential to avoid further gaseous distention. Monitoring of arterial blood gases may be accomplished by an umbilical artery catheter to measure postductal gases, or by a right radial arterial line to measure preductal gases. Supplemental oxygen is usually required. Rapid, gentle ventilation is used to optimize gas exchange yet avoid excessive barotrauma. *One needs to be constantly aware of the risk of an acute pneumothorax, particularly if high ventilatory pressures are needed.* Many favor prophylactic placement of a chest tube in this setting.

Although, historically, prompt reduction of the hernia and repair of the diaphragmatic defect have been advocated, attention has recently been focused on preoperative stabilization. Extracorporeal membrane oxygenation (ECMO) has been used if necessary. Various predictors of survival have been studied, but precise prognostication remains elusive.

OPERATIVE PROCEDURES

Most pediatric surgeons favor a transabdominal rather than a transthoracic approach.

The entire abdomen as well as both chests are prepared and draped. A subcostal incision is preferred to allow optimal exposure of the diaphragmatic defect. When the peritoneal cavity is entered, the herniated viscera are reduced through the defect by gentle traction. A chest tube is inserted. The hypoplastic lung is inspected, but no attempt is made to hyperinflate this remnant. The posterior rim of the diaphragm is identified and unrolled. Barring excessive tension, primary closure of the diaphragmatic defect is achieved using interrupted, nonabsorbable sutures. Even if the hernia is quite large, it can often be closed medially, adjacent to the esophagus. The remaining defect is closed using a prosthetic patch or muscle flap. Although the intestinal fixation is often abnormal, a formal Ladd's procedure is not routinely performed. A gastrostomy may be inserted to facilitate postoperative gastrointestinal decompression and feeding. If closure of the abdominal fascia requires excessive tension or intra-abdominal pressure, the skin alone is approximated. The resulting ventral hernia can be repaired at a later date, after the infant recovers.

Repair of a diaphragmatic hernia while the infant is on ECMO is feasible but necessitates meticulous hemostasis given the requisite anticoagulation.

Postoperative Procedures

Postoperative management of an infant with congenital diaphragmatic hernia can be exceedingly difficult. Initially, a "honeymoon" period may be seen during which oxygenation is satisfactory. However, the increased pulmonary vascular resistance resulting from a hypoplastic and reactive pulmonary bed typically produces pulmonary arterial hypertension. Right-to-left shunting may occur at the foramen ovale and/or ductus arteriosus, delivering desaturated blood to the systemic circulation. This hypoxemia and acidosis further aggravate pulmonary vasospasm, and a vicious cycle ensues.

The key elements in management are to optimize oxygenation and avoid acidosis. Hyperventilation may be useful, but excessive barotrauma should be avoided. Unfortunately, surgical repair of the diaphragmatic defect may acutely worsen pulmonary compliance, compromising effective ventilation. Intravenous bicarbonate or tromethamine (THAM) is used to correct acidosis. Vasodilators such as tolazoline may be used to reduce pulmonary hypertension, but they invariably cause systemic vasodilatation as well. Moderate fluid restriction is desirable to optimize oxygenation, yet systemic blood pressure must be maintained. High-frequency ventilation has been used with limited success. ECMO is very effective cardiopulmonary support. However, ultimate survival depends on successful weaning from the ECMO circuit with maintenance of satisfactory hemodynamics and gas exchange.

RESULTS

Despite dramatic advances in neonatal intensive care, the mortality rate of infants presenting with symptomatic diaphragmatic hernia within the first 6 hours of life remains nearly 50 per cent. Those who present after 24 hours of age almost invariably survive. *Repair of the diaphragmatic defect has been successfully accomplished in utero, which offers promise for those most severely affected but without other life-threatening anomalies.*

22

Special Problems in the Adolescent

EATING DISORDERS

GEORGE D. COMERCI, M.D.

The likelihood that a primary care practitioner will encounter a patient with an eating disorder is substantial. A decade ago, when such patients were not being treated in large numbers outside of psychiatric facilities, such a statement could not have been made. Today, general pediatricians and family physicians see patients with eating disorders in their offices and clinics and are expected to make the diagnosis of anorexia nervosa and bulimia nervosa. Moreover, they are expected to manage patient care on an ambulatory and often inpatient basis and to assume responsibility for posthospital care and monitoring. Although not responsible for initiating and implementing the *entire* treatment program, the primary care physician, as attending physician or consultant, may be called on to treat medical complications and to design, initiate, and implement behavioral and medical programs directed at weight gain and the resumption of normal physiologic homeostasis.

Effective treatment depends, of course, on an accurate diagnosis with full awareness of those medical and psychiatric disorders that may simulate an eating disorder. Furthermore, the diagnostic assessment must consider the origins and evolution of the condition, the presence of or potential for medical complications, and the role that family relationships, attitudes, and other dynamics have played and are playing in the development and perpetuation of the disorder.

Patients with eating disorder, especially those with anorexia nervosa, are often distrustful of their physicians. They believe the physician's only goals are to make them eat again, force them to gain weight and become obese, and take from them the only means by which they have so effectively controlled their body weight and appearance. They perceive the physician as wanting them to relinquish the sense of special uniqueness that they have achieved at such high cost and with so much hard work, self-sacrifice, and discipline. As long as mistrust of the physician and the treatment team persists, progress will be impeded and truly successful outcomes will be elusive, if not impossible, to achieve.

A prerequisite, therefore, and an essential component of good treatment, is the establishment of a *trusting* working relationship or therapeutic alliance with patients *and* parents. The physician must convey a sense of empathy, a feeling that he or she understands what patients (and parents) are experiencing and wants to help. Just as important is the physician's need to maintain a positive regard for patients with eating disorders, regardless of how they behave or what they say. It is essential that patients come to believe that their physician is and will be in their corner, working to help them recover. From the start, as with any partnership, the physician should warn that there will be difficult times ahead when patient *as well as doctor* and treatment team feel anxious, frustrated, angry, and helpless. By his or her actions and the manner used to enforce program guidelines, the physician gives the message that one can be firm, angry, disappointed, and frustrated but still provide unconditional support—an important lesson for a patient with an eating disorder to learn. Patients must hear the message that, regardless of what transpires, the physician will stand by them throughout the treatment process. *The goal of treatment is not to control patients, not to "show them who's boss," not to "fatten them up," not to punish them for "losing weight and causing so much trouble and expense" but, rather, to relieve them of their pain and suffering and to restore them to normal physical, psychosocial, and emotional health.* This message must be heard by the whole treatment team as well as by patients, their parents, and their families.

TREATMENT

Anorexia Nervosa

The patient should be fed at regular intervals, and surrounded by persons who would have more influence over them [sic], *relatives and friends being generally the worst attendants.*

Sir William Gull, 1874

Although much research and a vast literature has amassed over the past three decades on the treatment of anorexia nervosa (AN), it must be acknowledged that the basic tenets put forth over a century ago, recommending isolation from family and coerced feeding, are still held today.[1] Furthermore, it is not known what constitutes "best" treatment nor the extent to which our current treatment affects long-term outcomes.

Outpatient Treatment

Ambulatory management of the AN patient includes the care provided at the time of and shortly after the initial diagnosis; the care following initial hospital treatment and between hospitalizations; and the long-term care of patients with chronic AN. This article emphasizes outpatient treatment of the patient recently diagnosed as having AN.

The newly diagnosed AN patient should, if her* condition permits, have a trial of outpatient management. Rarely can patients with classic AN avoid intensive inpatient therapy; those that respond to outpatient management are usually atypical or less severely affected. To be considered for outpatient therapy, the patient must be medically stable (Fig. 1); should have lost no more than 30 per cent of body weight; should have had the illness for less than 4 months; and should not be binging and purging.[2] The patient who is clinically depressed and/or suicidal is not a candidate for outpatient management. Clearly, there is a selection bias, which has made a comparison of initial inpatient versus initial outpatient treatment difficult.

Establishing Goal Weights and Nutritional Needs. Adequate time must be spent with the patient to establish rapport and trust. An agreement should be reached with the patient that she will maintain her weight for 1 week and then gain at least ½ pound (227 g) or more every week until the goal weight (to be determined) is achieved. *As with inpatient treatment, a typewritten and signed agreement is helpful.* A weight is established, below which the patient and her parent(s) agree she will be hospitalized. This minimum allowable weight is usually the patient's weight at the time she signs the agreement; less often, a lower "safe" weight is chosen.

A target weight at which body fat equals 22 per cent (weight necessary for ovulation to occur, the physiologic ideal) may be chosen as a goal weight. Some practitioners prefer to use a minimum target weight at which body fat equals approximately 17 per cent. Frisch has suggested that, at 17 per cent body fat, there is adequate estrogen production to allow withdrawal uterine bleeding but not ovulation.[3] These weights can be determined using the graph shown in Figure 2. The weight midway between the minimum (17 per cent fat) and the ideal (22 per cent fat) "safe" target weights is usually used as one of the criteria ("goal weight") for discharge of hospitalized patients (Fig. 2).

The ultimate (final) goal weight should be within a range determined by the physician and the dietitian. This range of ideal weight is best estimated after determining the patient's frame size (large, medium, or small). This is accomplished by applying wrist measurements to standardized charts. The dietitian should provide this information as well as estimates of lean body mass and fat content. Less optimally, standardized growth charts are used. These use height and age to determine weight. They are population-based and do not take into consideration the patient's race, ethnic background, or frame size. If a standard growth chart is employed, one may use 90 to 95 per cent of the patient's average weight (based on the patient's corresponding percentile for height) as a final goal weight for complete weight recovery.

The patient's daily caloric intake at the time of diagnosis will help to determine the recommended initial caloric intake. One can begin with about 250 kcal above baseline, increasing by about 200 to 300 kcal/week until a daily intake of about 2500 kcal is achieved. A slow rate of caloric increase is important if medical complications associated with too rapid refeeding are to be avoided. These complications include gastric dilatation and rupture, pancreatitis, edema, fluid overload with congestive failure, and others. A slow approach also helps avert nonmedical problems, including panic regarding too rapid weight gain, distrust, and the tendency to binge.

Psychologic Care. Ambulatory management does not lessen the need for a multimodal approach, including individual and

*Because females constitute 90 to 95 per cent of patients with eating disorders, feminine pronouns are used to refer to patients in this article.

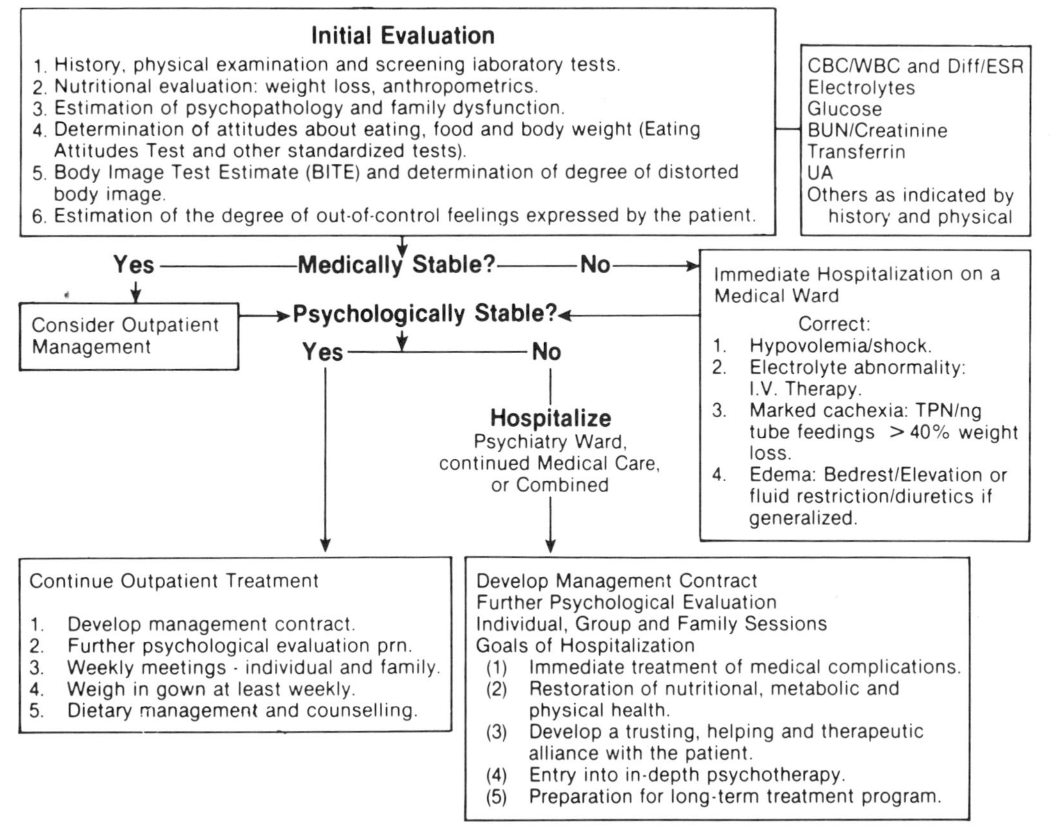

Figure 1. Initial triage and management of the patient with an eating disorder. prn, as needed; CBC, complete blood count; WBC, white blood cell count; ESR, erythrocyte sedimentation rate; BUN, blood urea nitrogen; UA, urinalysis; IV, intravenous; TPN, total parenteral nutrition; ng, nasogastric. (From Comerci GD, et al: Eating disorders in the young: Anorexia nervosa and bulimia. Curr Probl Pediatr 15:17–38, 1985.)

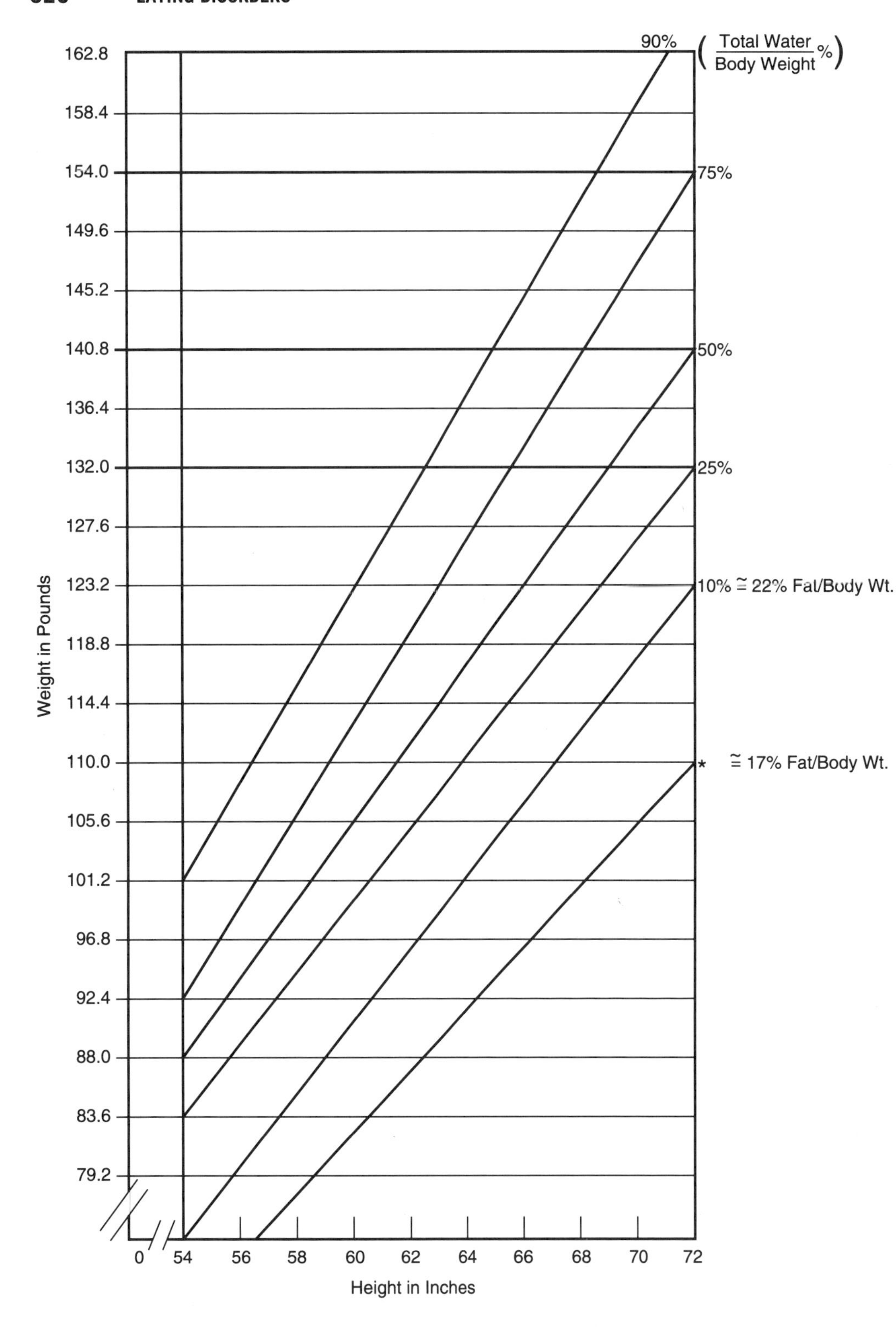

Figure 2. Graph indicating per cent of body weight equal to fat (17% and 22%) used for establishing "safe" and "ideal" goal weights. See also Comerci et al,[2] Frisch et al,[3] Barnes,[11] and Golden and Shenker.[12] (Modified from Frisch RF, McArthur JW: Menstrual cycles: Fatness as a determinant of minimum and weight for height necessary for their maintenance or onset. Science 185:949, 1974.)

family therapy and nutritional counseling. Efforts should be made to address issues of guilt and feelings of responsibility among parents and siblings and to reduce stress within the family.[1] The team should strive to increase the patient's and her parents' understanding of the factors that may have contributed to the development of AN and the harmful effects of self-starvation. There should be reassurance that help is available. The goals of individual therapy are to increase the patient's awareness and recognition of her feelings, to give control back to the patient, and to stop her reliance on food restriction and body thinness to validate herself.

Pharmacotherapy. There is little role for drugs in the outpatient treatment of AN. Rarely, antidepressants may be employed, but there are no data to support their use unless the patient is clinically depressed, in which case the AN patient should be hospitalized.

Post-hospital and Ongoing Care. Post-hospital management of the AN patient is primarily aimed at monitoring weight and continuing counseling and psychotherapy. The patient should be weighed at least once a week until the final goal weight is achieved and weight is stable. The chronic AN patient requires ongoing supportive care, counseling, and guidance with attention to weight maintenance, school, career, and, later, marital and other relationships. Such patients are often depressed, and their risk for suicide is high.

Estrogen therapy may be indicated to prevent osteopenia with periodic induction of withdrawal bleeding, to lower the risk of endometrial cancer.

Inpatient Treatment

Inpatient management demands that there first be early restoration of normal nutritional and physiologic status. Involvement of the family in the treatment regimen and a team approach, or "therapeutic partnership," is essential. Hospitalization allows the development of trust by the patient in the eating disorder team; a time-out (isolation) from a self-perpetuating disturbed home environment; patient education regarding nutrition and eating habits; and the provision of structure, giving the patient an opportunity to establish realistic priorities and to achieve a feeling of being in control. Ideally, the team should include a medical and psychiatric physician, psychologist, social worker, nutritionist, and skilled nurses experienced in working with AN patients, occupational and physical therapists, teachers, and an expressive art therapist. Unfortunately, most programs do not meet the ideal, and various functions must often be assumed by existing staff professionals.

Indications for hospitalization include the criteria listed in Figure 1. Absolute indications for immediate hospitalization include suicidal ideation; abnormally low serum magnesium, phosphorus, and/or potassium concentrations; uncompensated metabolic alkalosis or acidosis; impending cardiovascular collapse or failure; and evidence of severe malnutrition (usually a weight loss of 40 per cent or more). For the severely emaciated patient, confinement to bed may be necessary in order to monitor behavior, keep accurate accounts of intake and output, and avoid further medical compromise. It may be impossible to begin psychotherapy while the patient is malnourished. Too rapid refeeding and weight gain may result in disastrous medical consequences.

Establishing Goal Weights and Nutritional Needs. Unless the patient is severely compromised, the first 2 to 3 hospital days should be devoted to establishing a baseline of behavior, food selection, and daily caloric intake. A review of prehospitalization diet and activity levels provides an estimate of the level of energy intake and output. Anthropometric and laboratory data (transferrin and prealbumin levels) help determine energy needs and other nutrient deficiencies. Finally, the level of caloric and nutrient requirements is influenced by the severity of undernutrition. Because of the marked decrease in basal caloric requirements with starvation, needs based on the patient's present or ideal weight, height, age, and sex will be greatly overestimated. This *must* be taken into account when determining the AN patient's basal energy (calorie) needs.

Most patients requiring hospitalization are able at least to stabilize their weight if asked to consume 75 per cent of their calculated maintenance caloric needs. As the basal metabolic rate normalizes (i.e., increases), the pulse rate, temperature, and blood pressure will also rise toward normal. Maintenance energy needs, influenced by hospital level of activity, will return toward normal as well (usually 1.5 × basal metabolic rate, or about 30 to 40 kcal/kg of body weight).[2] Early in refeeding, most new tissue has a low fat content. As reserves are replaced, the new tissue contains more fat. The energy requirement for early weight gain is about 5 kcal/g of new tissue gained; later, it is 7.5 kcal/g.[2] Thus, in addition to the marked decrease in the emaciated patient's basal metabolic rate, there are less calories needed for early tissue building. The upper limit of relatively lean body tissue that can be gained daily is about 350 g. Therefore, a reasonable daily weight gain early in hospitalization is between 100 g (about ¼ pound; usually "the best the patient can do") and 300 g (about ¾ pound; "the best the body can do"). If the patient is gaining more than 300 g/day, she is either retaining fluid, voluntarily taking extra fluid or salt, or is adding extra weight to her clothing (gown pockets, etc.). If she is gaining less than 100 g/day despite adequate prescribed calories, one must suspect that she is discarding food, purging, or exercising (Fig. 3).

Depending on the AN patient's medical status, her estimated basal metabolic rate, and her level of anxiety and ability (or willingness) to cooperate, the initial diet could be the same as what was estimated she was taking at home, or as high as 1500 kcal (about 1½ basal needs). Patients are usually started at about 250 kcal above the estimated prehospitalization daily intake. Generally, the goal is to provide a daily caloric intake necessary to maintain the patient's admission weight (usually about 50 to 75 per cent of maintenance, depending on the severity of the starvation) plus about 50 per cent of maintenance if the patient is not limited to strict bedrest. Daily intake is then increased by 50 per cent every 5 to 7 days, depending on weight gain and the patient's level of anxiety. Most hospitalized AN patients will, in the early weeks of hospitalization, maintain their weight taking 1000 kcal/day or even less if severely emaciated. As caloric intake is increased, the patients usually gain between 1½ and 2 pounds/week. The staff must observe for attempts at "exercising away" calories. When this kind of obsessional thinking abates, the patient is given more control over her activities.

Nutritional counseling should begin on the day of admission and is important as a means of establishing the patient as an active member of the team who has input and control over some of the decisions being made about her care. These include the option of selecting "safe" foods within a reasonable range and providing *or* giving input regarding goal weights.

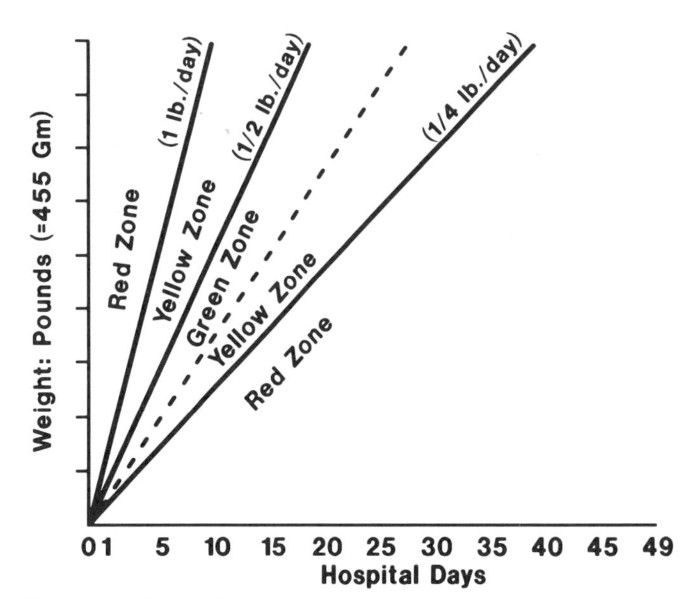

Figure 3. Daily weight graph used to monitor patients' weight gain. (From Comerci GD, et al: Eating disorders in the young: Anorexia nervosa and bulimia. Curr Probl Pediatr 15:17–38, 1985.)

The patient may choose whether to be weighed in a gown after voiding each morning before breakfast or only three times a week. The patient also may choose not to be told her weight, or she may or may not like a chart of her weight gains posted in her room.

For the patient who is extremely phobic and distrustful, it is often advisable to offer, as an alternative to a "regular" menu, a formula containing 1 to 2 kcal/ml. Preparations such as Isocal, Sustagen, Ensure, or Sustacal contain vitamins, minerals, protein, fatty acids, and carbohydrates, making the administration of a balanced diet easy and efficient for both the patient and the physician. The patient should have her choice from a variety of such beverages, keeping in mind that it is often preferable to use a low-fat, low-lactose diet in order to minimize gastrointestinal discomfort and bloating, which are so upsetting to AN patients. The total volume may be divided into 6 to 8 feedings a day. Once the patient is gaining weight, it can be expected that the variety of foods she eats will expand and that her ability to select independently from a menu will improve; these behaviors should be encouraged. A high-calorie beverage can also be used to "make up" calories that were not consumed from the selected menu. This may be prescribed at the end of the day or the following day in divided portions.

Nasogastric (NG) tube feedings and total parenteral nutrition (TPN) may be necessary when weight loss has exceeded 40 per cent and there are signs of severe malnutrition associated with protein, electrolyte, and trace mineral deficiencies. Such feedings may be indicated when the patient has not responded to reasonable corrective measures. TPN, either by central or peripheral line, has the advantage of providing rapid correction of electrolyte imbalance and protein and mineral deficiencies, especially in patients who have impaired absorption from the gastrointestinal tract. Moreover, AN patients often accept TPN with less anxiety and resistance than NG tube feedings, probably because it is not directly related to oral food intake. *TPN is, however, associated with a high morbidity and occasional mortality and should never be considered routine treatment in AN.*

The use of NG tube feedings is associated with problems as well, not the least of which is the perception by the patient that the insertion is an assault or hostile act, this at a time when trust is just beginning to be established. The use of tube feedings may contribute further to the patient feeling out of control and worthless and is a direct intrusion into the gastrointestinal tract of someone who is already preoccupied and misguided about her gut and bodily functions.

Overly rapid oral or NG feeding may result in serious vitamin, mineral, and trace metal deficiencies. If significant hypokalemia exists (more often encountered in the bulimic patient), one must be cautious not to induce further hypokalemia by administering a high carbohydrate load, which can "push" potassium into cells. The NG tube is ineffective if paralytic ileus is present and may be associated with medical complications such as pancreatitis and ulcer formation with perforation.

Psychologic Care. Behavioral modification is the mainstay of inpatient therapy. The program should be sensitive to the special needs of individual patients, firm yet reasonably flexible, nonpunitive, and adaptable to a medical setting. Weight gain, rather than daily caloric intake, and other behaviors should determine privileges. Such an approach minimizes conflict between patient and staff and among staff members themselves. Care must be taken that the behavioral program contributes to the patient's sense of effectiveness and that she not submit to the rules merely to earn her discharge from the hospital. The patient must be convinced of the benefit of temporarily relinquishing control to the eating disorder team but should be reassured that, eventually, control will be given to her.

Family therapy, as espoused by Minuchin and others,[5] is a vital part of inpatient therapy, especially for the young AN patient. However, family dysfunction should not be assumed merely because a family member has an eating disorder. On the contrary, an important goal of therapy is to relieve parental guilt and to reintegrate the patient into an appropriate position within the family. The physician or psychiatrist must make regular *and frequent* contact with the parents in order to forestall the patient's attempts at sabotaging the program, angering the parents, and achieving a premature discharge.[6]

Group therapy is helpful in forcing the patient to deal with confrontation, to identify and express her feelings, to learn more about how others perceive her and her behaviors, and to provide the patient a sense of competence. Through these guided interactions, the patient will learn to trust others, realize that relations are not so fragile, and realize that she can be assertive without losing approval, love, and respect.

Patients with AN may continue to exert control in the hospital, thereby splitting the staff and, through manipulative behaviors, undermining the program. The patients are very effective at turning parents against the program and the staff; their major defense against feelings of incompetence and helplessness is control over their eating and their bodies but involves control over the staff as well. Yates puts it very well: "The turning point in therapy often occurs when the patient cannot exert control and must face how powerless she really is."[7] Successful inpatient hospitalization, even when there is progressive weight gain, usually takes at least 6 to 12 weeks.

Pharmacotherapy. Many of the symptoms of AN are related to chronic malnutrition and resolve when normal weight is achieved. Spontaneous improvement is seen, especially in obsessional thinking, depression, and withdrawal, making drug efficacy studies difficult. Although there have been anecdotal reports of success with different drugs, no one agent has proved to be effective in AN and controlled studies are lacking. There is a potential for serious side effects from many of the drugs used, and therefore the decision to use an agent should not be made lightly. See Table 1.

ANTIDEPRESSANTS. Tricylic antidepressants have not proved effective in the treatment of AN. As stated, the depression associated with AN often subsides spontaneously as weight is gained and malnutrition corrected. Nevertheless, these agents are used frequently because starved patients are depressed. Amitriptyline is used frequently, as are other tricyclics, but *controlled* studies have not shown them to be effective.

ANXIOLYTICS. There is some advantage of the anxiolytics over other agents. They can be used for brief periods and result in few serious medical complications. They can reduce the patient's panic prior to eating and the fear of anticipated obesity. Lorazepam (0.5 to 1.0 mg) may be given 1 hour prior to meals.

CYPROHEPTADINE. Cyproheptadine (Periactin) is an antiserotonin and antihistamine well known among pediatricians to increase appetite. It is a safe drug, free of important side effects and shown to allow a faster weight gain when used in anorexics who have not binged and purged. It is also helpful in decreasing symptoms of depression. It must be used in an adequate dose (4.0 mg two or three times a day).

ANTIPSYCHOTICS. Although indicated in select AN patients, there is little basis for the use of these agents in AN. The side effects, particularly in young undernourished adolescents and preadolescents, are reason to avoid their use. The phenothiazines reduce anxiety and increase appetite, but they also

TABLE 1. Drug Therapy in Anorexia Nervosa and Bulimia Nervosa

I. Drugs used to decrease gastrointestinal signs and symptoms
  A. Parasympathomimetics
    1. Bethanechol: 5 mg three times per day, before meals for bloating (enhanced effectiveness with metoclopramide)
  B. Dopamine antagonists/phenothiazine-like drugs (*Caution:* dystonic reactions, especially preadolescents)
    1. Metoclopramide: 10 mg three times per day, before meals for bloating (enhanced effectiveness with bethanechol)
  C. Antiflatulents/stool softeners
    1. Simethicone: antiflatulent
    2. Mineral oil (heavy): stool softener
    3. Dioctyl sodium sulfosuccinate: stool softener
    4. Hydrophilic colloid with fiber: stool softener
  D. Colonic stimulants
    1. Bisacodyl suppository (preferable to oral dose)
    2. Psyllium seed husks: a natural fiber-bulking agent
    3. Glycerin suppository
  E. Antinausea/antivomiting—limited usefulness
    1. Thiethylperazine: 10–30 mg/day
    2. Metoclopramide (Reglan): 10 mg (as above); may contribute to depression
    3. Domperidone (Motilium): Not available in United States; does not cause extrapyramidal reactions
  F. Antacids
    1. Magaldrate: low-sodium antacid (also available with simethicone)
    2. Sodium-free Tums: also good source of calcium

II. Drugs used to reduce anxiety or to sedate (use in consultation with psychiatrist)
  A. Phenothiazines/butyrophenones—individualize dosage
    1. Clomipramine (Anafranil): for obsessional thinking and compulsive behavior
    2. Haloperidol: for out-of-control feelings
    3. Perphenazine: for out-of-control feelings
  B. Benzodiazepines: for pre-meal anxiety and for sleep; individualize dosage
    1. Diazepam
    2. Lorazepam: 0.5 to 1.0 mg 1 hour before meals
    3. Chlordiazepoxide
    4. Alprazolam
    5. Flurazepam: 15 mg at bedtime for insomnia

III. Drugs used to treat depression (use in consultation with psychiatrist)
  A. Tricyclic antidepressants
    1. Imipramine
    2. Amitriptyline
    3. Desipramine
    4. Trazodone: adolescents
    5. Protryptaline: adolescents
  B. Other antidepressants
    1. Fluoxetine (Prozac): decreases carbohydrate craving
    2. Sertraline (Zoloft): decreases appetite, less toxicity
  C. Monoamine oxidase (MAO) inhibitors: for older, chronic anorectics or for atypical depression when other antidepressants have failed. (*Caution:* no "diet pills" or other dietary precautions)
  D. Lithium carbonate: limited usefulness: for bipolar affective disorders and selected eating disorder patients
  E. Stimulant drugs (use in consultation with psychiatrist)
    1. Sympathomimetic drugs
      a. Methylphenidate: if refractory to tricyclics or as adjunct to tricyclic
      b. Pemoline: as adjunct to tricyclics
      c. Amphetamines should *not* be used
  F. Pyridoxine HCl: especially if patient on oral contraceptives: 50 mg/day with B vitamins

IV. Appetite suppressants (bulimia) and stimulants (anorexia): use in consultation with psychiatrist. Do *not* use amphetamines or phenmetrazine.
  A. Fenfluramine: 120 mg/day, decreases carbohydrate craving
  B. Phentermine resin: appetite control
  C. Mazindol: less stimulating anorectic
  D. Tryptophan: suppression of carbohydrate craving, 1500 mg three times per day with B vitamins
  E. Cyproheptadine (Periactin): "appetite stimulant," helpful in anxious and obsessional anorectics (4.0 mg two or three times a day)
  F. Opioid blockers: as for cyproheptadine (individualize dose)

V. Adjunctive and miscellaneous drug therapies
  A. Diuretics (bulimics/fluid retention)—use with caution. *Do not use* ethacrynic acid
    1. Thiazides: watch for potassium depletion, short use in menses-related fluid retention
    2. Furosemide: may be useful for edema secondary to overrehydration; watch calcium levels and other precautions
    3. Aldosterone antagonists: for secondary hyperaldosteronism
      a. Spironolactone: drug of choice in patients with chronic vomiting and laxative abuse to "wean" off laxatives
      b. Triamterene: as with spironolactone
  B. Potassium supplements (for purgative behaviors)
    1. Intravenous: 20–60 mEq/L, electrocardiogram monitor may be necessary over 40 mEq/L
    2. Oral: up to 80 mEq/day if necessary
    3. High-potassium foods: tomato or orange juice, bananas, dried fruits (raisins)
  C. Hormones—*Do not use* adrenocorticotropic hormone, cortisone, or insulin
    1. Anabolic steroids—very select cases
  D. Anabolic agents
    1. Anabolic steroids—very select cases
  E. Anticonvulsants
    1. Phenytoin: for select bulimics after other drugs have failed
    2. Carbamazepine: for select bulimics after other drugs have failed
  F. Miscellaneous
    1. Acne medications: topical or systemic
    2. Dysmenorrhea: Nonsteroidal anti-inflammatory agents
    3. Dental enamel protectants: acrylic sealant
    4. Multivitamins with minerals (especially prenatal vitamins) zinc, and folic acid
    5. Calcium carbonate (or Tums)
    6. High-calorie supplement beverages (with vitamins)

reduce blood pressure and temperature, both of which are associated with AN.

LITHIUM CARBONATE. There have been uncontrolled clinical reports of weight gain in AN patients treated with lithium carbonate. Without documentation of effectiveness, and considering the neurologic and cardiac toxicity in a vulnerable population, these agents should not be used unless other specific indications coexist.

OPIOID BLOCKERS. Because endogenous opiates are elevated in the cerebrospinal fluid of underweight AN patients, uncontrolled studies of opioid blockers have been done. These agents may increase weight gain and may reduce anxiety, resistance to treatment, obsessive preoccupation with dieting, and euphoria associated with weight loss.

AGENTS USED TO DECREASE GASTROINTESTINAL SIGNS AND SYMPTOMS. AN patients frequently experience abdominal fullness and bloating early in the course of refeeding. These sensations may significantly interfere with their progress. Gastric emptying is slowed after months of minuscule oral intake. Helpful medications include parasympathomimetics, such as bethanechol, metoclopramide (Reglan), domperidone (Motilium), and stool softeners, such as dioctyl sodium sulfosuccinate.

Metoclopramide and domperidone both shorten gastric emptying, but metoclopramide may contribute to depression. Dystonic reactions to metoclopramide are dose-related; special care must be taken when the agent is used in young patients and when the patient's weight is below the adult range. Extrapyramidal reactions are not caused by domperidone. Bloating and abdominal fullness may also be relieved by antiflatulents such as simethicone. (See also pharmacotherapy of bulimia nervosa.)

Laxatives and enemas are generally contraindicated in patients with eating disorders. However, many AN patients complain that their ability to eat is impaired by the feeling of fullness and that the early satiety they experience is aggravated by the constipation. For this reason, the judicious use of rectally administered glycerin or bisacodyl suppositories is acceptable practice in the hospitalized patient. Rectal administration avoids systemic absorption as well as intestinal colic, producing relatively normal stools—an important benefit when one is treating patients who are prone to abuse stimulant cathartics.

MULTIVITAMINS AND MINERALS. Multivitamins with minerals should be used routinely. Zinc should be added if the patient has an aversion to red meat and other zinc-containing foods or if a zinc deficiency is documented.

Bulimia Nervosa

Bulimia nervosa (BN) is often possible to manage on an outpatient basis. The treatment is not as well established as it is in AN. Although BN was described as early as the second century A.D., its recognition as a major health problem and the development of treatment modalities have only occurred over the last few decades. In BN patients, the problem is regulation of food consumption rather than weight loss. The basic tenets of treatment are self-monitoring of binging behavior; establishing obstacles to binge eating once triggering cues are recognized; controlling vomiting following the consumption of "forbidden" foods; and directing other efforts at interrupting the binge-purge cycle.

The knowledge that ingested foods may be vomited (i.e., the "license to binge") drives, in part, the binge-eating behavior. BN patients demonstrate a wide range of psychopathology; no one treatment works for all patients. Most therapists employ a variety of concurrent treatments. *Therapists and primary care physicians must be aware that suicidal behavior, often impulsive, is not an uncommon occurrence in BN patients.*

Outpatient Treatment

The majority of BN patients are treated on an ambulatory basis. Most outpatient programs utilize group therapy or a combination of group and individual therapy. These programs often include keeping a diary of eating behaviors and feelings that lead to bulimic episodes; analysis of such feelings; guidance from the group leader concerning methods of avoidance; stress management; and assertiveness training. The patient is instructed to avoid foods that may lead to a binge. Pleasurable alternatives and distractions to binging are suggested, and the patient is helped to develop a substitute "positive addiction." Because there is often a history of fasting between binging episodes, the patient is urged to eat three moderate-sized meals and two or three small snacks each day. This provides structure to an erratic eating schedule and often chaotic lifestyle, reducing the hunger that develops after fasting (although most bulimics deny hunger prior to binging).

Normal-weight BN patients are at less risk than the patient who both restricts and purges. Patients involved in compulsive vomiting and chronic laxative abuse (frequently 40 to 60 or more laxative doses per day) initiate a vicious cycle of hypovolemia, secondary hyperaldosteronism, and hypokalemia. The physician providing ambulatory care for such patients should anticipate the need to administer intravenous fluids and electrolyte replacement therapy on an ambulatory basis. The details of such therapy are beyond the scope of this article, and the reader is referred to detailed descriptions of the pathophysiology and parenteral treatment of BN.[8]

Pharmacotherapy. Medication has an important role in the treatment of BN, but drugs are often difficult to administer. Erratic retention and absorption as a result of vomiting and laxative abuse may occur, and cardiac and other side effects are more common because of hypokalemia and other fluid and electrolyte abnormalities. Borderline patients are more apt to abuse medications or refuse them because of their untoward effects; depressed patients are more likely to hoard drugs, especially antidepressants, and use them to attempt (and complete) suicide. Nevertheless, a variety of agents have proved effective in treating BN patients.

ANTIDEPRESSANTS. The major medications used for ambulatory BN patients are the antidepressants. The mechanism by which they reduce binging and purging and reduce anxiety and obsessional thinking about food and eating is not entirely clear. All BN patients are not candidates for antidepressant therapy; some therapists restrict its use to patients who meet criteria for a major depression. On the other hand, because some patients show dramatic improvement following the initiation of tricyclics, including clomipramine (Anafranil), and other agents such as fluoxetine (Prozac) and sertraline (Zoloft), it seems unreasonable to withhold such drugs if there is no improvement with behavioral approaches. Fluoxetine and sertraline have the advantage over other antidepressants of decreasing appetite. If the patient continues to deteriorate and there is no response to antidepressants, some recommend the use of carbamazepine or lithium.

AGENTS USED TO DECREASE GASTROINTESTINAL SIGNS AND SYMPTOMS. Both metoclopramide (Reglan) and domperidone (Motilium) are used in BN patients to reduce bloating by stimulating gastric emptying. Bethanechol (see pharmacotherapy of AN) may enhance the effect of metoclopramide by providing cholinergic (acetylcholine) substrate. Domperidone has the advantage of not crossing the blood-brain barrier, and extrapyramidal side effects are therefore rare. Both drugs are dopamine antagonists and have antiemetic effects that may be helpful in reducing spontaneous or reflex vomiting in some bulimic patients. The drugs may aggravate the effects of abused laxatives in BN patients.

APPETITE SUPPRESSANTS. A number of nonamphetamine stimulants have been used in BN patients (see Table 1). Uncommonly, a BN patient will report binging episodes associated with hunger. In such patients, fenfluramine (120 mg/day) has been reported to reduce carbohydrate craving. With the availability of fluoxetine, the use of such drugs should decrease. Amphetamines and phenmetrazine should not be used in BN patients.

DIURETICS. Diuretics may constitute a valuable adjunctive therapy in certain carefully selected BN patients. Fluid retention may occur as a result of secondary hyperaldosteronism due to the hypovolemia associated with vomiting and laxative abuse. Moreover, BN patients tend to more often retain fluid with menstruation, and some have idiopathic edema. In such cases, an aldosterone antagonist, such as spironolactone or triamterene, used with extreme care, may be helpful. Only patients who have dedicated themselves to recovering from BN should be treated with these agents, and then only for very short periods while they reduce their vomiting and laxative abuse. Prescriptions should be given only for small amounts and without refills.

For other drug therapies used for ambulatory BN patients, see the subsequent discussion of inpatient pharmacotherapy and Table 1.

Inpatient Treatment

The physician has no greater responsibility to the BN patient than to understand the metabolic derangements that complicate purgation and to be able to recognize and treat them. Often hypovolemic and in electrolyte imbalance, the BN patient is in a more precarious physical state than the AN patient. The complications can be life-threatening, often requiring immediate action. The hospitalized BN patient is, in many ways, more difficult to maintain in a controlled environment than is the patient with AN. Surreptitious vomiting is common, and covert laxative and diuretic abuse is difficult for the staff to monitor and control. Unlike the food restrictor, whose condition deteriorates only gradually, the purger is in a perilous pathophysiologic condition that may suddenly escalate to include one or more of the following acute life-threatening complications: (1) impending or frank shock, (2) severe hypokalemia, (3) a cardiac dysrhythmia, (4) acute heart or renal failure, (5) hypochloremic alkalosis, (6) convulsions, and (7) acute gastric dilatation and rupture. More complete descriptions of the fluid and electrolyte abnormalities and their analysis and management are available in other publications.[9]

The inpatient treatment of BN is, in some respects, more complex than that of AN. The approach to treatment is less standardized, in part because bulimic patients are less uniform but also because there are fewer outcome studies documenting effective treatment regimens. Although BN patients have much in common, they may or may not be severely depressed or suicidal, have problems with impulse control, or resist treatment. Some patients have severe character disorders and low self-esteem; some abuse drugs; and some are highly successful, competent individuals. Inpatient psychologic management is based on the same principles as ambulatory management (see earlier). The goals of inpatient therapy are the control of binging and purging; the recognition of cues, emotions, and situations that lead to binging or purging; modification of responses to feelings and dysfunctional perceptions; and attempts at teaching ways to maintain such changes following discharge. Regular meals, the introduction of "forbidden" foods without vomiting, and impulse control are essential components of inpatient programs.[10]

Pharmacotherapy

ANTIDEPRESSANTS. As discussed above for outpatients, antidepressants have improved the BN patient's preoccupation with food, body, and weight. Double-blind, controlled studies have shown that imipramine, desipramine, amitriptyline, and other tricyclics reduce binging and purging. Both patients who are clinically depressed and patients who are not may respond to antidepressants with improvement in bulimic symptoms. Although monoamine oxidase inhibitors suppress appetite and probably are effective, the necessary precautions for their use and the unreliability of many BN patients limit their use. The BN inpatient is a more likely candidate for the use of monoamine oxidase inhibitors as well as fluoxetin, sertraline, and clomipramine.

ANTICONVULSANTS. Phenytoin and carbamazepine have been touted as effective agents in BN. The underlying rationale is that the compulsion to binge followed by vomiting and the urge to sleep may constitute a complex partial-seizure phenomenon. Associated electroencephalogram (EEG) abnormalities have not demonstrated this, and there have been no studies documenting anticonvulsant effectiveness in BN. Nevertheless, in patients who are not helped by antidepressants and who do not respond to currently acceptable treatments, carbamazepine, which has a tricyclic structure similar to the antidepressant imipramine, may be a reasonable second-line drug.

LITHIUM CARBONATE. Uncontrolled studies have shown a decrease in bulimic symptoms when other treatments failed. However, because the risk of cardiac dysrhythmia is markedly increased in patients with hypokalemia and other acid-base abnormalities, this drug should be used only when other agents have failed and only in the absence of electrolyte abnormalities.

Because increased levels of plasma β-endorphins have been found in BN patients, opiate blockers have been tried but without great success. See Table 1.

OUTCOME AND FOLLOW-UP

Anorexia Nervosa

The course and outcome of AN are variable, and the prognosis is always guarded. Current methods of treatment do not seem to alter outcome, and at least one study showed no difference between treatment in a general hospital without psychotherapy and that in a psychiatric setting. Moreover, spontaneous recovery is experienced by some AN patients. Even patients who quickly respond to intervention and who are considered successfully treated often relapse within a year.

Indicators of a poor prognosis include binge eating and purgation, premorbid obesity, obsessive-compulsive and neurotic personality traits, and somatic complaints. Good prognostic signs are a younger age and short duration of illness, relatively high self-esteem, acceptance of illness and acknowledgment of it as a problem, motor hyperactivity prior to and during the illness, and a return of hunger during the early phases of treatment.

Despite treatment, patients tend to do poorly socially and in interpersonal and marital relationships. Surprisingly, most AN patients function at a high level in school and career. Fully half of AN patients continue to have difficulties, many requiring repeated hospitalizations in order to prevent death. *The mortality rate, even with appropriate treatment, is between 5 and 10 per cent, with suicide being a major cause of death.*

Bulimia Nervosa

The outcome for patients with BN is not clear. Long-term studies are lacking, and little is known about the outcome for those who receive intensive therapy versus those who receive none. Many studies have shown improvement in eating behaviors and purgation, but it is not known whether the underlying psychopathology improves. There is indication that, in some, the illness improves over time, and, in others, there is a steady worsening of their condition. Some individuals improve without treatment, and some improve when a stressful time of life passes or when there is a separation from parents or spouse. Those with high self-esteem do better.

PREVENTION

Eating disorders are complex, and their cause is multifactorial. Risk factors are difficult to define, and a method to prevent eating disorders is unknown. Sociocultural and biologic factors play an important part in the cause of eating disorders, neither of which can be influenced to any significant degree by the practitioner. Characteristic child-rearing practices, family dynamics, parent-child relationships, and early developmental factors seem to be important, all of which may be affected to some extent by physicians who counsel young parents, children, and adolescents.

Parents should be unconditionally nurturing but, at the same time, encourage autonomy and independence. Children should be expected to perform well, not for the benefit of their parents but for their own gratification, satisfaction, pride, and sense of accomplishment.

A relaxed attitude toward food and eating should be encouraged. Meals should be scheduled but relaxed and enjoyable. Parents and children should be taught what is a normal and acceptable daily caloric intake and body weight. Exercise should be reasonable and should play an appropriate but not dominant place in the lives of children and families.

Parents should be encouraged to set firm but appropriate limits on behavior and should be willing to state their opinions on important and controversial issues. Children should have license to express their feelings, both negative and positive, and family peace and harmony must not be achieved at the expense of total conflict avoidance. The way that the family appears to the outside world should not take priority over a relaxed family atmosphere and home environment.

Prevention cannot be better defined until key questions regarding the biopsychosocial causes of eating disorders are answered.

REFERENCES

1. Anderson AE, Morse CL, Santmyer KS: Inpatient treatment for anorexia nervosa. *In* Garner DM, Garfinkel PE (eds): Handbook of Psychotherapy for Anorexia Nervosa and Bulimia. New York, The Guilford Press, 1985, pp 311–359.
2. Comerci GD, Kilbourne K, Carroll AE: Eating disorders in the young: Anorexia nervosa and bulimia, part II. Curr Probl Pediatr 15:7–38, 1985.
3. Frisch RF, McArthur JW: Menstrual cycles: Fatness as a determinant of minimum weight for height necessary for their maintenance or onset. Science 185:949, 1974.
4. Dwyer J: Nutritional aspects of anorexia nervosa and bulimia. *In* Emmett SW (ed): Theory and Treatment of Anorexia Nervosa and Bulimia. New York, Brunner-Mazel, 1985, p 22
5. Minuchin S, et al: Psychosomatic Families: Anorexia Nervosa in Context. Cambridge, Harvard University Press, 1980.
6. Garner DM, Garfinkel PE: Anorexia Nervosa: A Multidimensional Perspective. New York, Brunner-Mazel, 1982.
7. Yates A: Current Perspectives on the Eating Disorders: II. Treatment Outcome and Research Directions. J Am Acad Child Adolesc Psychiatry 29:1–9, 1990.
8. Comerci GD: Medical complications of anorexia nervosa and bulimia nervosa. Med Clin North Am 74:1293–1310, 1990.
9. Comerci, GD: Fluid and electrolyte and drug therapy considerations in the management of eating disorders. Semin Adolesc Med 2:37–46, 1986.
10. Rosen JC, Leitenberg H: Bulimia nervosa treatment with exposure and response prevention. Behav Ther 13:117–124, 1982.
11. Barnes HV: Physical growth and development during puberty. Med Clin North Am 59:1316, 1975.
12. Golden NH, Shenker IR: Amenorrhea in anorexia nervosa: Etiology and implications. Adolesc Med: State of the Art Rev 3:503–518, 1992.

HOMOSEXUALITY IN ADOLESCENTS

LAWRENCE S. NEINSTEIN, M.D.
and ERIC COHEN, M.D.

DEFINITION

Homosexuality is an emotionally charged issue for the adolescent and his or her family and physician. The need for physician involvement is stated by the American Academy of Pediatrics in a 1983 committee paper: "The American Academy of Pediatrics recognizes the physician's responsibility to provide health care for homosexual adolescents and for those young people struggling with problems of sexual expression."

It is important for the physician to be able to handle both the concerns of adolescents with a homosexual orientation and the worries of heterosexual teenagers who are experimenting with homosexual behaviors. Physician involvement should also include counseling of the teenager's parents as they struggle with the sexual orientation of their child. For those physicians who have personal beliefs that interfere with their management of these individuals, appropriate referrals should be made available.

A *homosexual* can be defined as a person who has a persistent, erotic attraction as an adult to members of the same sex and who usually, but not always, engages in sexual relations with them. In 1974, the American Psychiatric Association dropped its classification of homosexuality as a mental disorder and labeled it as an alternative form of sexual expression.

In discussing homosexuality, many authors refer to it as an alternative "choice" of sexual behavior. The use of this term implies that homosexuals have control over the gender of their object of sexual desire. With very rare exception, this is not true. The homosexual person has as little control over the gender of his or her sexual partner as does the heterosexual. By using the term choice, the physician subtly allows others to blame the individual for having made a wrong decision. This can be harmful in helping both adolescents and their families understand homosexual behavior.

Several points are important in applying the definition of homosexuality to an individual, particularly to teenagers.

1. Sexuality is a continuum. Kinsey developed a seven-point scale (0 to 6) for rating sexual behavior on the basis of psychologic reactions and overt sexual practices. A "0" is a person who is exclusively heterosexual, whereas a "6" is a person who is exclusively homosexual. Kinsey recognized that it is possible for a heterosexual whose expressed sexual behavior is "0" to have some fantasies that are more mixed or homosexually oriented (e.g., "3" on the fantasy scale). Understanding this helps the physician counsel teenagers who may be having disturbing thoughts about homosexual experiences but have not yet consolidated their sexual identity. Having homosexual fantasies, although an early indicator of possible homosexual orientation, does not necessarily mean that the teenager is homosexual.

2. Some homosexual experimental behavior is common for many teenagers. In most adolescents, this genital play appears to be part of a developmental process leading to a heterosexual identity. However, in some adolescents, such behavior can

lead to confusion, anxiety, and even panic. When not expressed outwardly, the teenager may act out these feelings in a number of dyssocial ways. In counseling such teenagers, it is important to remember that reacting with one of the mentioned behaviors to this early genital play does not predict either future heterosexuality or homosexuality.

3. Sexual behavior during early adolescence may or may not parallel one's form of sexual expression as an adult. Young girls, in particular, may display same-sex behaviors such as petting and kissing but have a heterosexual orientation. Conversely, some adolescents cover up their homosexuality by involving themselves primarily in heterosexual behavior.

4. Some adolescents whose true sexual orientation is heterosexual will become involved in homosexual behaviors under certain circumstances. These may include noncoeducational boarding schools, summer camps, the armed services, or prison settings. Most of these individuals engage in heterosexual behavior after leaving such an environment.

The definition of *transvestite* is an individual who derives pleasure by dressing in the clothing of the opposite sex. *Transsexuals* are individuals who believe that the body they were born with does not match the sex they feel they are.

ETIOLOGY

Although there is controversy over the factors involved in homosexual and heterosexual identity, the determining factors remain unknown. The influences of genetics, intrauterine hormone levels, and environment have all been studied. Although compelling evidence that any one of these factors is exclusively responsible for determining orientation is lacking, it seems likely that sexual orientation is influenced by a combination of these factors.

Four stages of acquisition of homosexual identity have been described:

Stage I—*sensitization.* In this stage, the child feels a sense of being different, without understanding the reason for these feelings. The child may become aware of feelings of a homosexual orientation.

Stage II—*identity confusion.* During stage II, the individual uses different defense mechanisms to try to ignore homosexual feelings and activities. There may be same-sex arousal and limited same-sex sexual experiences associated with guilt and withdrawal.

Stage III—*identity assumption,* or the "coming out" phase. In this stage, which may not take place until adulthood (if ever), individuals identify themselves as homosexual.

Stage IV—*commitment.* At this point, the individual experiences satisfaction, self-acceptance, and an unwillingness to alter sexual identity.

The average ages at which individuals experience typical events in the "coming out" process are presented in Table 1. In a study of gay adolescent males, 31 per cent were attracted to men during childhood and the remainder were aware of their attraction to men in mid-adolescence. The mean age of gay self-identification was 14.

TABLE 1. Average Ages At Which "Coming Out" Events Are Experienced

Event	Male (Age)	Female (Age)
Same-sex interest	13	14–16
First same-sex activity	15	20
First same-sex love relationship	21–24	22–23
Disclosure to nonhomosexuals	23–28	28

Adapted from Troiden RR: Homosexual identity development. J Adolesc Health Care 9:105, 1988.

MYTHS

The following myths have long been associated with homosexuality:

1. *Homosexuality is a mental disorder.* Homosexuality is not a mental disorder but, rather, a sexual form of expression. Homosexual adolescents may have problems identifying or adjusting to their sexuality, leading to other fears and anxieties. The exposure of most homosexual adolescents to a society with hostile attitudes, lack of positive role models, and lack of family support can lead to a lowered self-esteem and behavior problems.

2. *Homosexuals are child molesters.* Most child molestation acts are committed by heterosexual males, not homosexual males.

3. *Homosexual males are effeminate and wish to be female.* Most homosexual males cannot be differentiated from heterosexual males and have no desire to be female.

PREVALENCE

Males

The 1970 Kinsey-NORC (National Opinion Research Center) survey indicates that at least 20 per cent of adult males have had an experience with another male ranging from sexual contact to orgasm at some time in their life. This experience occurred before the age of 19 in 90 per cent of these individuals. Kinsey has reported that 37 per cent of males have a history of a homosexual experience that occurred between adolescence and old age. Approximately 10 per cent of males are exclusively homosexual during at least 3 years of their lives, and 4 per cent of males are exclusively homosexual for their entire lives.

Females

The prevalence of homosexuality in females is more difficult to determine because many more homosexual females than males maintain privacy regarding their sexual preferences. Most studies indicate that the prevalence rates are about half that indicated for males.

COUNSELING

It is important to provide teenagers and their parents with factual information. This includes the prevalence of adolescent homosexual experimentation, the continuum of sexual behavior, and the fact that many teenagers worry about their sexual identity. Adolescents and their families must be aware that it is often difficult to assess and predict adult sexual behavior on the basis of adolescent sexual behavior.

Physicians should encourage strong family ties because acceptance from the family is extremely important to the adolescent. They should discourage families from blaming themselves or the teenager for his or her sexual identity and attempt to alleviate guilt in all concerned. The physician, by clarifying the issues, helps support the integration of the teenager into his or her family and social system regardless of sexual preference. The adolescent is a son or daughter who is a homosexual, not a homosexual who is a son or daughter.

Counseling Teenagers

Given a supportive environment, the majority of gay and lesbian youth have no more serious mental health problems than other adolescents. Rather, it is often the effects of homophobia that may lead to psychologic problems in these populations. The physician should not be concerned that discussing homosexuality will cause an adolescent to become homosexual, just as discussing suicide will not create a suicidal adolescent. In fact, discussing sexual orientation issues may allay some of the teenager's anxiety. The physician must also assure confidentiality, even if the parents are aware of their teenager's concerns.

The physician should clearly convey that the adolescent's sexual orientation will not affect the physician's feelings about him or her. By clearly stating one's acceptance, an atmosphere of trust is established. A number of basic concepts should be explored early in the counseling relationship. Discussing the notion that homosexuality is a nonpathologic variation of sexual behavior that is probably established in childhood may help to diminish the teenager's guilt feelings. The physician should communicate the notion that homosexuality is not a problem of making a wrong choice, as choice is rarely a factor. The word *preference* should also be avoided in this context, as it also implies choice. The physician should not trivialize the teenager's concerns about sexual orientation. Also, comments such as "it's just a phase" should not be used, as they may increase the adolescent's confusion.

The teenager should be informed that, in general, attempts to alter one's sexual orientation have been largely unsuccessful. In addition, these attempts may lead to a lowered self-esteem and psychologic problems. However, if the adolescent is requesting help with a change in sexual orientation, a referral to a nonbiased psychologic practitioner is recommended. The teenager should be aware that there is no urgency in deciding on one's sexual orientation. The adolescent may be reassured that the answer to the question "am I or am I not?" will emerge naturally over time.

If the gay adolescent is comfortable with his or her sexual orientation and behaviors, it is still important to present general factual information. However, for males, regardless of whether or not they are concerned about their sexual orientation, the physician must give accurate, clear, and specific information about safer sexual practices and risk-reduction techniques to try to prevent human immunodeficiency virus (HIV) infection. This may be one of the most important reasons in the 1990s to ask about sexual behaviors of male patients.

Counseling Parents

The parent(s) of a homosexual adolescent may have many different feelings, including guilt, shame, fear, and anger. For example, parents may feel that they caused their teenager's homosexuality. Mothers of homosexual male adolescents may feel that they were too overbearing when raising their child, or fathers may feel that they were absent too often to provide an appropriate role model. Parents should be reassured that such fears are not warranted, as the origins of homosexuality are far too complex for such simple explanations.

Homosexual adolescents may have psychologic problems similar to those of heterosexual adolescents that have little or nothing to do with their sexual orientation. Thus, parents should be aware that not every emotional problem their teenager may experience is a consequence of his or her homosexuality. Another important area to explore is the parents' religious beliefs. If appropriate, counseling in this area should be encouraged.

Referral to a parent support group can also be of benefit. One such group is Parents and Friends of Lesbians and Gays (P-FLAG).*

*The mailing address of the national headquarters of P-FLAG is: Federation of Parents and Friends of Lesbians and Gays, P.O. Box 20308, Denver, CO 80220.

The adolescent's major need before and after disclosure of homosexuality is love and acceptance. The parents should be reassured that their adolescent is the same individual who lived with them before such disclosure was made.

MEDICAL CONCERNS

There is an epidemic of sexually transmitted diseases (STDs) among the male homosexual population. This is a consequence of the high prevalence of asymptomatic carriers of STDs; of engaging in sexual activity with multiple partners; and of the anonymity of sexual contacts and thus the difficulty in treatment of contacts. Although there has been an increase in the use of barrier methods (condoms) in the adult homosexual community, this has not occurred to the same degree in the adolescent population.

Sexual History

When evaluating medical problems among gay adolescents, the physician must first be able to obtain the correct information regarding the teenager's sexual practices. Helpful approaches in eliciting this "sensitive" part of the history include establishing confidentiality, outlining why it is important to know this information, and asking questions in a nonjudgmental fashion. The adolescent should know that although these questions are personal, honest answers will help the practitioner give the best care possible.

Physicians need to know if a teenager has begun to have sexual relations and whether those relations are with members of the same sex, opposite sex, or both. They should also inquire about specific sexual practices, determining the adolescent's risk for specific STDs. This information also furnishes an opportunity to provide appropriate education regarding STD prevention. Specifically, physicians should ask about fellatio, anal intercourse (inserter or insertee), anilingus (oral-anal sex or "rim" or "scat"), number of sexual partners, use of condoms, frequency of sexual contact, prior history of STDs, and HIV status (if known).

Documentation of this information must be considered carefully. Access to the adolescent's chart by health professionals, allied health care workers, insurance companies, the courts, and parents carries both legal and ethical ramifications. The physician needs to consider himself or herself as a patient advocate protecting confidentiality. The physician should also be knowledgeable about local state laws governing documentation, particularly in regard to HIV infection.

Examination

In the gay adolescent male who is either not sexually active or sexually active with one partner and consistently using condoms, a simple routine physical examination and syphilis serologic profile would be adequate. If the gay adolescent male is engaging in sexual activity with multiple partners, a more thorough screening is needed.

The physical examination should include close inspection for lymphadenopathy, skin rashes, oral lesions, and anal trauma. The laboratory evaluation should include a gonorrhea culture and chlamydial direct fluorescent antibody test or culture. These should be done on all appropriate sites of sexual contact (oral, anal, and pharyngeal). Additional screening tests include syphilis serologic profile and hepatitis B surface antigen and antibody. Discussion of HIV screening is appropriate. If HIV screening is being considered, appropriate pre- and post-test counseling is mandatory.

Gonorrhea

Anorectal and pharyngeal gonorrhea is often asymptomatic. If symptoms do occur in the anal area, they may include rectal burning, tenesmus, and mucopurulent discharge. Complications include fissures, abscesses, fistulas, and strictures. The preferred therapy for rectal and pharyngeal gonorrhea is ceftriaxone (250 mg diluted in 1 per cent lidocaine [Xylocaine] IM) plus doxycycline (100 mg orally twice a day for 7 days, covering a possible concomitant chlamydial infection). Spectinomycin can be used for rectal gonorrhea in patients allergic to penicillin but is not recommended for pharyngeal gonorrhea. Patients with pharyngeal gonorrhea who cannot be treated with ceftriaxone can be treated with ciprofloxacin (500 mg orally as a single dose). However, ciprofloxacin should be used with caution in growing individuals. Sulfamethoxazole-trimethoprim (9 tablets daily as a single dose for 5 days) can also be used in pharyngeal gonorrhea as an alternative to ceftriaxone.

HIV Infection

Evidence exists that HIV infections may modify infections with syphilis, leading either to accelerated courses of syphilis or to failure to respond to traditional therapy. Cases have also been reported of HIV infection with evidence of syphilis but with negative syphilis serology. HIV-positive adolescents infected with syphilis should be evaluated carefully for late or unusual manifestations of syphilis, including cerebrospinal fluid evaluation. These individuals may also require more intensive treatment with penicillin.

Hepatitis B Infection

Hepatitis B infections are prevalent in homosexual males, with antibody positivity occurring in 37 to 51 per cent of these individuals. A successful vaccine is now available for hepatitis B and should be used in homosexual males with multiple partners who have negative hepatitis B serology.

Cytomegalovirus

Up to 80 per cent of homosexual males who are engaging in sexual activity with multiple partners become infected with cytomegalovirus each year. Although this infection is largely asymptomatic, it may cause a severe mononucleosis-like illness, particularly in the immune-suppressed, HIV-positive teenager.

Anal Problems

Teenagers who engage in unprotected passive anal sex and/or active anilingus risk becoming infected with several enteric pathogens. Such pathogens may include *Giardia lamblia, Shigella, Entamoeba histolytica, Neisseria gonorrhoeae, Treponema pallidum, Chlamydia trachomatis,* human papillomavirus (warts), and herpes simplex virus.

Anal problems can include anorectal trauma secondary to anal intercourse or the use of foreign objects or "fisting" (the practice of using the hand in anal sex); proctitis and inflammation of the perianal area secondary to allergies caused by contactants such as lubricants and infectious agents; pruritus ani secondary to oil-based lubricants and blockage of anal pores leading to inflammation; anal condylomata; hematochezia secondary to anal lacerations caused by anal intercourse; anal ulcers secondary to herpes (painful; usually seen in clusters) or syphilis (painless; a single lesion); and anal discharge secondary to bacterial STDs. The evaluation of the rectum and anus in a symptomatic teenager should include anoscopy, gonorrhea and chlamydial testing, and routine culture of stool for ova and parasites. Treatment is directed at the etiologic agents.

Veneral Warts

Venereal warts, often asymptomatic, are common in the rectal area of individuals engaging in rectal intercourse. External warts are best treated with podophyllin, trichloroacetic acid, or a combination of both. In trained hands, electrodesiccation is also very successful. Internal warts can be treated with electrocautery or lasers. Patients with internal warts are best referred to physicians familiar with their treatment, as overly aggressive therapy can lead to strictures and excessive pain.

AIDS

Acquired immunodeficiency syndrome (AIDS) is the disease causing the most concern among homosexual males. The cause is HIV, a retrovirus. Because of the long incubation period, teenagers infected with HIV may become ill only after adolescence. However, HIV positivity is becoming more common in the adolescent population. Studies suggest seroprevalence rates between 0.3 and 3 per cent, depending on the risk profile of the population being studied.

Although all individuals need to be informed about AIDS, it is especially important in the homosexually active adolescent male.

A discussion should take place between the physician or a qualified HIV counselor and the teenager about HIV testing. One hundred per cent use of condoms for all forms of intercourse should be encouraged among all sexually active teenagers, but particularly in the homosexually active male. The adolescent should understand safer sexual practices, which include limiting sexual partners (abstinence or monogamy); avoiding sexual practices that involve the exchange of body fluids such as blood or semen; avoiding the sharing of needles, if used; using latex condoms and not those made from natural lamb skin; and using water-based lubricants, because oil-soluble ones can damage latex.

SEX EDUCATION

ESTHERANN GRACE, M.D.

Many youngsters enter adolescence with a knowledge base inadequate to understand either the pubertal changes they experience within their bodies or their own subsequent sexual behaviors. Failure to comprehend rudimentary reproductive physiology, coupled with normal adolescent denial mechanisms and risk-taking behaviors, contributes to the high teenage pregnancy rate and rising incidence of sexually transmitted diseases (STDs).

One in ten adolescent females will be pregnant by the age of 17 years. Adolescent pregnancy is a multifactorial problem. Certainly, failure to use contraception consistently significantly contributes to the problem. Life goals, self-esteem, socioeconomic status, and cultural expectations also have an impact on the unplanned pregnancy rate in this age group. In the process of risking possible pregnancy, sexually active teenagers are also potentially exposing themselves to STDs. The adolescent population (ages 13 to 19 years) has experienced the greatest rise in the incidence of STDs, and it is the adolescent female who is at greatest risk of exposure to human immunodeficiency virus (HIV) via heterosexual activity. Because the inherent morbidity and mortality of STDs threaten this population with ever-increasing frequency, adolescents need factual information to avoid these life-threatening consequences of their sexual activity.

How a teenager matures sexually is an individual process influenced by genetics, family expectations, and peer pressure, both positive and negative. The teenager eventually incorporates all of these factors in the final product—namely, the mature sexual identity. The process of achieving this goal is an arduous one and necessitates clear factual input from the adults responsible for sex education. Unfortunately, for 1 in 4 women and 1 in 7 men, sex education appears to have involved some type of sexual abuse during childhood and adolescence. The long-term sequelae of sexual abuse can persist throughout an individual's life. (A more recent medical complication has been the exposure to HIV from sexual abuse.) It appears that the incidence of abuse is rising, but this may reflect an increase in reporting by victims. The safety of the victim must be ensured before he or she will offer prompt disclosure. In many cases, the abuse is revealed years after its cessation for fear of retaliation by the perpetrator. The majority of abusers are known to the victim; they are frequently family members. Sadly, the potential threat to the family structure frequently silences the victim (see also the article on child abuse, Section 2.)

Confusion over gender identity is not infrequent during adolescence. There is a psychic fluidity at this time as teenagers come to terms with their own sexuality as well as the gender preference of their future sexual partners. The majority of adolescents are aware of their sexual preference by their late teens or early twenties. Most fall into the expected grouping of heterosexual or homosexual, although some are bisexual and remain so throughout their lives. (Some individuals are bisexual by availability, e.g., prison confinement.) There is no scientific unifying theory to explain sexual preference, but recent research suggests that the intrauterine bathing of the brain with androgenic hormones may influence the final behavioral outcome. The family and home environment are also thought to have an impact on sexual preference. Reaching the final resolution of sexual identity and partner gender preference requires anticipatory guidance if inadvertent disasters are to be avoided. This guidance, in the form of sex education, is provided by the adults and peers in an adolescent's life.

SCHOOLS

In the United States, only 17 states and the District of Columbia have mandated sex education in schools. Consequently, only 10 per cent of American children are exposed to a structured course in sexuality. This deficit is dramatically contrasted to school policy on driver education courses; 90 per cent of adolescents participate in school-sponsored driver education programs. According to polls of parents on their views concerning sex education in schools, 85 per cent agree that school is an appropriate setting for such a program. Only 3 per cent of parents refuse to allow their children's participation in sex education classes.

A variety of sex education programs have been developed and implemented throughout the United States. The content of the material is geared to age and grade level. Typically, the courses begin in junior high school; however, some start as early as the fourth grade or as late as the eleventh grade. Given the early mean onset of sexual activity of adolescents (16 years for whites, 15 years for hispanics, and 14 years for blacks), delay in sex education could have a significant impact on their future reproductive health. Parental involvement in school sex education contributes to the success of these programs. Most schools require the written permission of the parents and provide them a summary of the material to be covered. This allows a degree of parental control and recognizes religious restrictions in individual families.

Factual information concerning reproductive physiology and sexuality and guidance about responsible decision making within interpersonal relationships make up the content of the courses. To delete any one part reduces the value of the entire program. In most courses, participants are encouraged to keep a journal and discuss their questions in the supportive environment of the classroom. For the shy, reticent youngster, submitting written questions avoids escalating discomfort regarding these sensitive issues. The gender distribution of the classroom setting is a point of controversy. Some educators recommend a single-sex class, whereas others prefer a coeducational classroom. Proponents of the single-sex class generally feel that the freedom of communication among the participants is enhanced, allowing for a more open exchange of information, whereas a mixed class fosters inhibitions. In contrast, those educators advocating shared classes view the integration of the setting as a more realistic view of life. The youngsters in the coeducational class are exposed to both the male and the female points of view, which is often an enlightening experience for all.

The development of school-based clinics provides another source of sex education information because such clinics are frequently staffed by health educators skilled in this area. School-based clinics provide a resource where youngsters can obtain sexual information, often on a one-to-one basis. The beneficial effects of the clinic encounters include a delay in the sexual debut and a modest reduction in teenage pregnancy rate. Most school-based clinics are not authorized to dispense contraception; their success is based on the interpersonal relationship of the staff and student, leading to more responsible decision making.

PARENTS

Sex education has traditionally been considered the responsibility of parents. Unfortunately, many parents are unprepared to teach factual information about the sexual changes their children are experiencing in adolescence. This inability coupled with the typical adolescent reluctance to discuss sexual issues with parents, limits the effectiveness of parental efforts. Nevertheless, parents play a crucial role in their children's sexuality, and they should be encouraged to pursue communication despite the adolescent's discomfort. The parent is in the unique position of presenting the physical, emotional, and moral aspects of sexual behavior. They are also the earliest role models their children observe. How parents interact with each other affects the child's perception of sexual roles.

The diversity of cultural attitudes toward human sexuality precludes a single dictum of appropriate sexual behavior. Consequently, within families, there is a range of tolerated sexual activity from casual dating to sanctioned intimacy. Parent-child conflict results when the family's bounds are exceeded. A clear statement of parental expectations concerning sexual issues provides the guidelines. Unfortunately, for many adolescents, the parent as sex educator is absent. The media, particularly television, assume the role in this absence. Daytime soap operas appeal to large numbers of adolescent females. The sex on these television programs is often impersonal, exploitative, and rarely, if ever, "safe." Furthermore, music videos portray women in demeaning roles, the victims of their own and their partner's lust. Continually titillated by sexual innuendos in popular music, commercials, movies, and television, adolescents experience confusion over the appropriateness of their feelings and behaviors. Parental guidance about responsible sexual decision making facilitates the resolution of such confusion.

PEERS

Regardless of other available sources of sex education, adolescents turn to their peers as a valued information resource. The inaccuracy of the facts their friends expound does not impede their perceived veracity; sexual myths sustained through generations of adolescents account for much of the confusion about human sexuality. Failure to correct these misconceptions in the face of the present epidemic of STDs may prove fatal to the current generation of teens.

Peer counseling programs in schools and communities have been an effective sex education method. Peer counselors are perceived as available, reliable, and trusted sources of information. In community outreach programs, peer counselors have been accessible to school dropouts, who otherwise do not have access to the system. Training of peer counselors requires minimum effort (i.e., a 4- to 6-week course on human reproductive health). The critical aspect of the program is ongoing adult input to monitor the competence of the counselors and the impact of the program on adolescent sexual behavior. Unless behavior is changed (e.g., safer sex practices with the consistent use of condoms), this population remains at risk for increased morbidity and mortality of STDs.

The peer counselor is also a potential proponent of the acceptability of abstinence. Although there is tremendous emphasis on sexually active teenagers, there are also significant numbers of adolescents who abstain from sexual activity. The pervasive presumption that all teenagers are engaging in sexual activity distorts the normalcy of the abstainers. For abstainers to hear that they are normal and not "the last virgin on the planet" is extremely reassuring to their self-esteem. It also diffuses the pressure to be prematurely intimate. Delaying the sexual debut becomes an acceptable alternative. The consequences of the delay are a reduction in the teenage pregnancy rate and a decrease in the incidence of STDs. These beneficial outcomes are also the result of more effective contraceptive use typical of the older teenager. The younger adolescent is a poor contraceptive complier who engages in risky behavior without thought to the long-term consequences of pregnancy and STDs. Reaching adolescents remains a challenging problem; utilizing teenage peer counselors to disseminate the facts ensures teenagers' own role as part of the solution.

THE PHYSICIAN

Physicians have both the knowledge and the opportunity to be sex educators; unfortunately, they rarely fill this role in their patients' lives. The usual reason given is a lack of time within the context of a standard office practice. Yet, when dealing with children and adolescents, to avoid their sexuality is to deny them adequate health care.

A simple explanation commensurate with the child's age of what is appropriate physical contact alerts the child and parent to the physician's willingness to address these issues. Because the mean age of onset of child abuse is 5 years, physicians caring for young children have an obligation to teach them the difference between "good touching and bad touching." Later, monitoring the sexual development and the onset of puberty provides the physician the opportunity for anticipatory guidance to both the child and the parent. Once entering puberty, every young patient requires private time with the physician to address confidential sexual issues. Although all life-threatening medical concerns continue to be discussed with the parents, confidential relationship should be established with the teenager, ensuring access to medical care for developmental and sexual needs.

With the establishment of a confidential physician-patient relationship, young patients will gain information with which they can avoid risk-taking sexual behavior. The physician is the ideal person to dispel myths and correct misinformation. A brief review of sexual activity, contraceptive needs, menstrual function, and sexual concerns, when included within the context of a routine office visit, desensitizes the teenager's reluctance to discuss sexuality. The comfort of the physician with adolescent sexuality is conveyed to the youngster, who eventually views the doctor as a resource person. (This applies to all teenagers regardless of their sexual identity. Homosexual youths frequently find themselves alienated from a doctor who has presumed that they were heterosexual. The physician can play a supportive role facilitating the homosexual youth's adjustment in society.)

Parents frequently consult physicians when concerned about their child's potential sexual activity. A clear, concise definition of confidentiality provided to the parent when their child initiates puberty (Tanner stage 2) should avoid parent-physician conflict. However, despite the doctor's best efforts, some parents demand to know their child's sexual status. Each case is best addressed individually; however, in general, adolescents are considered emancipated minors in sexual issues. Thus, the physician is not obliged to divulge confidential material. Adolescents, when aware of the doctor's constraints on sharing sensitive information, appear more willing to discuss sexual concerns and contraception options before initiating sexual activity.

Physicians play a critical role in educating their patients about the perils of STDs. For those doctors caring for adolescents, preventing STDs via counseling about the value of safer sex (and how to practice it) or about the option of abstinence is essential. With society's awareness of the consequences of STDs, the majority of parents are grateful that the doctor has discussed sexual issues with their child. For those physicians who choose not to address their teenage patients' sexual health needs, providing a referral source in their community is recommended.

SUMMARY

A person's sexuality is an integral part of his or her human nature. Factual information concerning this aspect of humanity provides the basis for responsible decision making on sexual issues. Avoidance of risky sexual behavior is essential in the present epidemic of potentially lethal STDs. Sex education implemented through schools, home, peers, and physicians can meet this very human need.

CONTRACEPTION, PREGNANCY, AND ABORTION

PAMELA J. MURRAY M.D., M.H.P.

CONTRACEPTION

A sexual health history is an essential component of the routine adolescent health maintenance visit and may be indicated at episodic visits, depending on the complaint. This interview should be conducted with the adolescent alone and in private. Guidelines for consent, confidentiality, and financial obligation should be established and shared with the patient.

The sexual history provides a unique opportunity to assess and educate the adolescent about normal reproductive anatomy and physiology and the strong romantic and sexual feelings that emerge in adolescence. Sexual responsibility, including pregnancy and sexually transmitted disease (STD) prevention, should be emphasized. In addition to the practitioner's formal history, responses to written questionnaires and a trained nursing staff may identify important sex education and health care needs. Adolescents or their parents may initiate the request for a "pelvic exam" or for a contraceptive method or education, and such requests should always be addressed or referred. Pamphlets displayed in the waiting area reinforce discussed information and provide further education for the adolescent and his or her parents.

Counseling about contraceptive options should involve a nondirective discussion reviewing potential contraceptive choices as well as their use, risks, side effects, and benefits. Consideration must be given to the age and developmental stage of the adolescent in relationship to the ability to comply with the chosen method and recommended follow-up.

Individual and family religious and moral belief systems, myths and misinformation, and ambiguities about sexual behavior and relationships should be evaluated. Normal developmental risk taking and peer pressure may interfere with compliance with contraceptive use. An explanation of these issues will help the adolescent choose a contraception method that best meets his or her needs.

See also the article on adolescent gynecology at the end of Section 22.

Contraceptive Options

Abstinence

Abstinence from sexual intercourse is practiced by many teenagers. Some adolescents limit their sexual intimacy or select behaviors without risk of pregnancy, such as manual, oral, or anal-genital contact. Identification of these sexual practices is important to ensure detection and to discuss protection from STDs. Supporting adolescents in their choices and providing information to plan knowingly about future sexual activities are essential.

Withdrawal

Withdrawal, or coitus interruptus, is practiced frequently by adolescents at their first and subsequent sexual encounters. Many teenagers who say that they are not using any contraception will then specify that the male partner regularly "pulls out" before ejaculation. Although withdrawal, in contrast to uninterrupted coitus, reduces pregnancy risk, the pre-ejaculate often contains sperm. In addition, it may be difficult for the partner to withdraw completely in sufficient time and withdrawal offers no protection against STDs. Unfamiliarity with one's own and one's partner's sexual response and the often clandestine and rushed nature of adolescent sexual encounters further limit the effectiveness of this method.

Natural Family Planning

Natural family planning and the rhythm method are rarely used correctly by adolescents. Adolescents acquire many misconceptions about the fertile and infertile times of the month, often resulting in significant risk of pregnancy. In general, pregnancy risk is underestimated early in the menstrual cycle and overestimated in the second half of the cycle. It is a very rare teenager who keeps careful records of menses, basal body temperature, and cervical mucus quality and quantity for the suggested 1 to 2 years needed to establish the regularity of one's menstrual cycle and to predict ovulation. For some mature 18- or 19-year-old adolescents in stable relationships, natural family planning may be a reasonable contraceptive choice when adequate initial education, ongoing support, and a committed partner are available.

Barrier Methods

Condoms. Condoms are essential for protection from most STDs and can be a highly effective contraceptive method when used consistently at every intercourse with a vaginal spermicide.

Lubricated condoms made from latex are widely used, inexpensive, and reliable. For individuals allergic to latex, natural-membrane condoms provide contraceptive benefit but less protection from STDs. Condoms are intended for one use only and must be stored where they are not exposed to excessive heat. They are widely available over-the-counter to adolescents and are commonly found in pharmacies, supermarkets, and 24-hour convenience stores. Condoms treated with the spermicide nonoxynol-9 are available, as are extra-large condoms and more durable condoms intended for anal intercourse.

Spermicides. Spermicides, usually containing nonoxynol-9, must be used with condoms to provide highly effective contraception. Nonoxynol-9 may also decrease the risk of transmission of some bacterial and viral STDs. Spermicides are available without prescription and are safe to use. Each preparation of spermicide has instructions that specify the proper insertion technique and the onset and duration of effectiveness. Vehicles include foams, gels, creams, sponges, suppositories, and vaginal contraceptive film. Some individuals are sensitive or allergic to either the spermicide or the base. Changing brands or preparations may avoid further irritation.

Spermicide use near conception has not been shown to cause adverse fetal outcomes. Spermicides must be reapplied with each act of intercourse, except with vaginal sponges, which may be left in place to provide continuous protection for 24 hours.

Diaphragm and Cervical Cap. These barrier methods, in conjunction with spermicide, provide effective contraception. Each must be fitted by a trained practitioner who can verify that the young woman can successfully place and remove the contraceptive device. A 1- or 2-week trial of use at home (in vivo) is recommended before a final choice is made. Older adolescents who are comfortable with touching their own genitals and the devices and who have personal or medical reasons for not choosing hormonal contraception may select these methods.

"Female Condoms." Female condoms may soon be marketed by two companies. One is a latex "bikini" that provides extensive perineal coverage and may decrease STD transmission between partners. A second style is a tubular polyurethane "condom" that has an inner circular rim with a diaphragm-like fit, and an outer ring that is positioned externally against the labia. When sexual activity is associated with any drug use, including alcohol, the effectiveness of coitally related contraceptives is decreased.

Combined Oral Contraceptives

The combined oral contraceptive (COC) pill is the most common contraceptive choice among sexually active adolescents. When taken properly, it provides very effective contraception by suppressing ovulation and by altering the physiology of the female reproductive tract with the influence of both estrogen and a progestogen (see also article on adolescent gynecology at the end of Section 22.) In teenagers using "the pill," the failure rate is higher than in the general population, as it is with all contraceptive choices.

Common indications for use of the pill include contraception, dysmenorrhea, other cyclic menstrual problems, and endometriosis. The COC may be indicated for therapy after appropriate diagnostic measures have been taken in young women with abnormal vaginal bleeding or irregular menses. Concern that COCs should not be started until 6 to 12 months of regular menses have occurred has not been substantiated. The young menarchal girl who is sexually active is at extremely high risk of unintended pregnancy. The consequences of a small theoretical risk of accelerated closure of the epiphysis must be weighed against the social disadvantage and medical risks of an unintended pregnancy.

The absolute contraindications to starting COCs are relatively rare in adolescents and include the following conditions: a history of *clots* (cerebrovascular accident, myocardial infarction, pulmonary or thromboembolism, or phlebitis); *cancer* of estrogen-influenced tissues (breast or reproductive regions); *cholestasis* (of pregnancy, liver tumors, or impaired liver function); or *conception* (pregnancy). Strong relative contraindications likely to be found in adolescents include severe *headaches,* particularly migraines exacerbated by COCs; *hypertension* (>140 systolic, >90 diastolic confirmed on repeated examination); *hepatitis* (proven infection or acute mononucleosis); *hospitalization* (major surgery requiring immobilization in the next 4 weeks or serious injury and immobilization); and *hematologic* concerns of undiagnosed abnormal vaginal bleeding.

Careful consideration of contraceptive choices should be presented and weighed against risks of pregnancy in young women with chronic medical problems. Such problems include diabetes; sickle-cell, gall bladder, collagen vascular, cardiac, and renal disease; and lipid disturbances. Cognitive, behavioral, or psychiatric difficulties in complying with contraception present additional challenges to the practitioner. In the immediate (10 days) postpartum period, throughout lactation, and during a depressive illness, alternatives to COCs may be needed.

Noncontraceptive benefits of COCs should be explained. These include relief of cyclic problems, including dysmenorrhea, *mittelschmerz,* and some premenstrual symptoms. Overall, COC users experience less risk of severe pelvic inflammatory disease, decreased risk of ovarian and endometrial cancer, fewer functional ovarian cysts, fewer nonmalignant breast cysts and fibroadenomas, fewer ectopic pregnancies, and less iron-deficiency anemia. Other benefits include improvement in acne and manipulation of the timing of menses when it would pose unusual personal inconvenience. Menstrual regulation can be used to decrease the frequency of menses to only three or four times a year, in young women with developmental delay and hygiene problems associated with menstrual flow.

Many low-dose COCs are available. Young women should be started on one of these preparations. The most commonly used low-dose COCs contain between 30 and 35 μg ethinyl estradiol, available as a fixed-dose or triphasic preparation. Progestational agents and doses vary among pill formulations. Access to an up-to-date edition of *Contraceptive Technology* is recommended for any practitioner prescribing contraception.

Minor side effects of physical discomfort (nausea, breast fullness and tenderness, mood changes, and breakthrough bleeding) are common in the first few cycles and tend to diminish over the first three cycles. Lower progesterone doses are also associated with increased risk of breakthrough bleeding and very scant (or even absent) menstrual flow. Persistent side effects of nausea, mood changes, and headaches may be dose-related, and changing the pill formulation or time of day that the pill is taken may alleviate these unpleasant symptoms.

With the lower-dose formulations, the risk of accidental pregnancy following one or more missed pills increases. A single missed pill that just precedes or follows the normal 7-day hormone-free week (days 22 to 28) carries a significant increase in the risk of ovulation. Therefore, 28-day pill packages, rather than 21, are strongly recommended in order to maintain the pill-taking habit. Condoms and foam, or another barrier and spermicide method, should be explained and supplied or prescribed, to be used as back-up for the entire first month's cycle of pills when pills are not taken regularly, or if antibiotics are taken.

Ideally, a complete physical evaluation, including pelvic and breast examinations, is performed before COCs are initiated. At the same time, a Papanicolaou (Pap) smear, gonococcal culture, *Chlamydia* determination, rapid plasma reagin (RPR), and wet preparation should be obtained. Attention should be given to the need for human immunodeficiency virus (HIV) testing. In the case of not yet sexually active adolescents or adolescents who refuse to be examined, a plan should be made and documented to perform the examination after 1 to 3 months on the pill. In non–sexually active teenagers, the STD evaluation is not needed. In teenagers who continue to refuse pelvic examinations but who are sexually active, the relative risks of pregnancy should be balanced against the recommended regimen.

A routine for starting pills should be explained and accompanied by written instructions that are reviewed with the patient. Sunday-start or flexible-start regimens are both acceptable as long as the instructions are clear. Pills may be started at other times in the menstrual cycle if one can be certain that the patient is not pregnant.

Return visits may be scheduled after one full cycle of pills to address any problems, encourage compliance, and re-educate about alternative methods if needed. A "pill check" appointment at 3 months is scheduled to review weight and blood pressure changes and to assess side effects and satisfaction with and understanding of pill use. Minor side effects usually abate over three cycles. Three months later, the 6-month follow-up appointment will reinforce the previous issues. In most sexually active adolescents, another examination and STD evaluation at 6-month intervals are routine, as sexual partners often change as frequently.

Common misconceptions that may need to be addressed include the belief that the pill causes cancer, impairs fertility, or is bad for one's health if taken for too long. These issues may need to be reviewed at initial educational and follow-up sessions. At all visits, the necessity of additional barrier protection to decrease exposure to STDs should be emphasized.

Postcoital Contraception or "Morning After Pill." Neither contraception nor human behavior is perfect. Events such as rape, broken condoms, missed pills, and poor judgment may place a woman at risk of an unwanted pregnancy. In case of such emergencies, postcoital contraception can decrease the risk of pregnancy to 1.5 per cent or less. (The "Yuzpe" regimen consists of 100 μg of ethinyl estradiol and 1.0 mg of *dl*-norgestrel or 2 tablets of Ovral taken orally within 72 hours of unprotected intercourse and repeated 12 hours later.) This therapy is most effective if initiated within 24 hours of intercourse.

Although the Yuzpe protocol is much better tolerated than a 5-day course of high-dose estrogen, nausea and occasionally vomiting are reported side effects. Usually, a menstrual period will occur within 21 days, but all patients should be seen for follow-up by the 3rd week. This is a prime opportunity to reinforce ongoing contraceptive plans.

Progesterone-Only Pills or "Minipills." These pills consist of a small dose of progesterone and are taken every day without a hormone-free interval. Even under ideal conditions, progesterone alone is less effective than other hormonal methods and produces irregular bleeding patterns. It is most often used for lactating women, older women of reproductive age, and individuals with unacceptable side effects from higher-dose pills or for whom COCs are contraindicated because of hypertension, migraine, or other conditions.

Depot Medroxyprogesterone

Medroxyprogesterone acetate (Depo-Provera) may be given as a 150-mg intramuscular injection every 3 months, which provides very effective contraception. It is often accompanied by irregular menstrual bleeding, and most young women develop amenorrhea after a series of injections. After injections of "Depo" are stopped, it may take up to 2 years until fertility returns.

Norplant Implants

Norplant implants consist of six Silastic-coated capsules of levonorgestrel that provide 5 years of highly effective contraception. Norplant has been licensed in the United States since 1990. It provides a continuous "ultra-low" dose of progestin. The effect is reversible, but only by removal through a minor surgical procedure.

Both irregular menstrual bleeding and amenorrhea occur in Norplant users. Early trials have suggested that the risk of pregnancy increases in women weighing more than 70 kg. Indications include those mentioned for the minipill and women who have difficulties with compliance with other regimens and who desire long-term contraception. Norplant can be used in some women in whom the COC is contraindicated and offers an attractive option for some adolescents and their families when medical conditions, psychiatric illness, or cognitive disabilities contraindicate pregnancy or parenthood.

Pre-Norplant counseling, insertion, and removal should be provided by a practitioner with specific training.

Intrauterine Devices (IUDs)

The IUDs currently available in the United States include the TCu-380A and the progesterone T device. IUDs are absolutely contraindicated in women with active, recent, or recurrent pelvic infection or suspected pregnancy. It is strongly not recommended for individuals at high risk for future STDs, including women with multiple sexual partners or with partners who have multiple partners. Thus, the IUD is rarely a preferred contraceptive choice for adolescents because they, in general, change partners move frequently and they have a high prevalence of STDs.

As with the implantable progesterone contraceptives, a skilled counselor and trained practitioner are required to obtain informed consent and perform the insertion and removal procedures.

Sterilization

An option sometimes requested by parents of developmentally disabled adolescents and by teenage mothers with several offspring is sterilization. Whereas voluntary surgical contraception, including tubal ligation and vasectomy, provides contraception for many older women and men, it has little place, if any, in the choices for adolescents. Federal and state funds usually cannot be used to support sterilization in individuals younger than 21 years of age; use of these funds usually requires informed consent, documentation of mental competence, and a 30-day waiting period. When there are extenuating medical reasons to consider sterilization in an adolescent, legal counsel and court involvement are advised.

Impending Developments

New developments in contraception include other progestin-containing implants and vaginal rings, new COC formulations, and variations in barrier contraceptives and spermicide delivery options. Adolescents are often eager to try these new products. Practitioners should be prepared to offer them accurate information about reliability and efficacy with respect to the adolescent lifestyle.

PREGNANCY

Approximately 1 in 10 female high school seniors becomes pregnant each year. Pediatricians are often faced with concerns about the possibility of pregnancy. Familiarity with the signs and symptoms, including a late menses, fatigue, nausea, breast enlargement and tenderness, abdominal or pelvic discomfort, weight gain, and urinary frequency, and an awareness of the prevalence of inadequate contraceptive practice among teenagers, should lead one to consider the diagnosis. The date of the last menstrual period may be helpful, but a recent period should not dissuade the physician from suspecting pregnancy. Anxiety, depression, and suicide attempts may also be presenting symptoms.

Urine pregnancy kits for office use provide accurate and low-cost confirmation that can usually be made within 10 days of conception and before the first missed menses. Knowledge of the exact date of the last sexual intercourse is critical to interpret the results and evaluate any risk of undiagnosed pregnancy. Very early or ectopic pregnancies or dilute urine may produce a false-negative result.

If pregnancy is confirmed or remains a possibility, a pelvic examination, including a Pap smear and STD assessment, is necessary. In the pregnant teenager, additional screening procedures should include RPR, HIV titers, hematocrit, rhesus factor (Rh) determination, urinalysis or dipstick, weight, blood pressure, and an estimate of gestational age by history and examination. Discrepancies between the latter may indicate a need for uterine ultrasonography or quantitative serum human chorionic gonadotropin-beta (β-hCG) determination.

Common adolescent behaviors that present specific risks to the mother and fetus should be discussed. The negative consequences of drug use, STDs and other infections, inadequate nutrition, and the lack of prenatal care should be stressed. Genetic risks of relatively common problems, such as sickle cell disease and cystic fibrosis, deserve mention.

Pregnancy counseling should be provided by an individual skilled in nondirective pregnancy options counseling who is also familiar with local resources. Components of pregnancy counseling include confirmation of pregnancy, an understanding of the pregnant adolescent's reaction and circumstances, and identification of individuals who will be available for discussion, decision making, and support, as well as a presentation of options. It is useful to explore the teenager's image of pregnancy and parenthood and to consider the same developmental issues and personal values mentioned earlier under contraception. The adolescent's own family, her partner, and her partner's family may all influence the subsequent events and decision making.

The adolescent's perception of parenting, her family support systems, the experience of her peers, her current achievement level and future plans, and the duration of the pregnancy are likely to influence her immediate decision. These factors will influence her long-term socioeconomic and educational outcome. Pregnancy options to be discussed include continuing the pregnancy with the prospects of single parenting, parenting with a partner (with or without marriage), or adoption, or terminating the pregnancy with a safe and legal abortion. Referral should be made to a facility providing quality prenatal care or abortion services in a timely manner. Continuous surveillance of federal and state legislation regarding access to abortion, maternal and fetal rights in regard to substance abuse, and paternity disclosure may be critical to an individual's perceived choices. Referral for "expert" pregnancy counseling may be needed because of these issues, family conflict, or differences of opinion.

Adolescent anxiety about informing parents of a pregnancy is common. In most cases, the younger the adolescent, the greater the need to involve the parents. Usually, the adolescent's consent is needed to inform and involve the parents, who are often more aware of their adolescent's sexual activity than is perceived by the teenager. After their initial shock, parents are usually supportive and are able to see the longer-term implications of the pregnancy. Their willingness to provide child care and financial support for their children's children deserves serious consideration by the pregnant adolescent.

Access to ongoing secondary education for pregnant teenagers has improved dramatically in the past decades. Unfortunately, tertiary education rarely provides on-site or subsidized child care. Teenage parents are more likely to have further unplanned teenage pregnancies, failed marriages, and less educational, vocational, and economic accomplishment. Their own children are at risk of the same difficulties and at increased risk of neglect and behavioral problems.

Many of the negative medical consequences of teenage pregnancy are accounted for or caused by poverty, the lack of prenatal care, and primiparousness, not by younger chronologic age alone. Nonetheless, the higher incidence of premature labor, premature and low-birth-weight infants, and maternal and infant morality all argue strongly for efforts to prevent teenage pregnancy.

ABORTION

Safe and legal abortions have been available to pregnant adolescents without parental consent for the past two decades in most states in the United States. State laws regarding access, including parental consent, mandatory waiting periods, and indications for legal abortions, are rapidly being challenged and changing at the state and federal level in referendums, legislatures, and the court system. Knowledge of state regulations and local options is critical.

For adolescents considering abortion, another session of pregnancy counseling should include a discussion of the procedure, including risks and complications. For some teenagers, the risks of pregnancy include depression, suicide, and attempts at self-induced trauma, poisoning, and abortion. STDs should be treated before any procedures are performed. However, financial and time constraints often heavily influence the available options and decision-making process; abortions are not covered by public and many private health insurance policies. Planning for postabortion contraception and attention to postabortion grief issues are part of quality abortion services.

Procedurally, most first-trimester abortions are performed in outpatient settings using dilatation and evacuation. Second-trimester abortions are more emotionally difficult and procedurally complex. Local or general anesthesia options and predilatation of the cervical os with laminaria may be offered. Follow-up should be coordinated between the services providing abortion and ongoing primary care.

RU 486, a progesterone antagonist, and prostaglandins are used as a pharmacologic abortifacient for limited indications outside the United States. There is no suggestion that it or any related compounds will be submitted for approval to the U.S. Food and Drug Administration in the near future.

REFERENCES

Hatcher RA, Stewart F, Trussel J, et al: Contraceptive Technology 1990–1992. New York, Irvington Publishers, 1990.

MANAGEMENT OF A DRUG-USING ADOLESCENT

RICHARD H. SCHWARTZ, M.D.

Adolescents of any socioeconomic group anywhere may be adversely affected by drug or alcohol abuse, the symptoms or social consequences of which include adolescent turmoil, unpredictable explosive temper, conduct disorder (chronic lying, thievery, aggression, and/or promiscuity), venereal disease, truancy, serious academic underachievement, depression, involvement in motor vehicle accidents, running away, personality disorders, chronic argumentativeness and disrespect for others, amotivation, low sense of goal direction, and suicide attempts. It appears that drug use is the "Great Imitator" during adolescence and must be considered as a primary cause of, and not merely a secondary effect of, such mood disturbances and behaviors. Because endogenous depression, serious non–drug-related mental illness, and life with a physically or sexually abusive parent may lead to some of the same symptoms as found with drug abuse, pediatricians or their consultants must carefully evaluate each adolescent who exhibits these symptoms in order to reach the correct diagnosis. However, drug use should be a primary consideration.

EVALUATION

The first step in evaluating a teenage patient is to be alert for "red flag" behaviors, such as the combination of two or more D or F grades, cigarette smoking beginning prior to age 16, and serious risk-taking behaviors, such as riding in motor vehicles when the teenage driver has been drinking alcohol. It is less threatening to address some of the initial questions about the adolescent patient's best friend's behaviors. One can ask if the peer group smokes heavily, performs poorly in school, and gets drunk every now and then.

To elicit more information about possible drug abuse, the physician should ask the patient a few nonthreatening questions about school, family relationships, jobs, friends, recreational activities, academic performance subject by subject, vocational aspirations, frequency of conflicts with parents, participation in drinking games at parties, and how many cans of beer the adolescent who drinks alcohol may consume before he or she "catches a buzz."

Drug-using adolescents often become proficient in techniques of denial or minimization of their own role by blaming others, selective muteness, and overt hostility when threatened by references to drug use. Therefore, a more thorough drug and alcohol assessment, if the pediatrician's suspicions are aroused, should be done by a professional with expertise and experience in the field of substance abuse rather than by a well-meaning but naive pediatrician who may easily be manipulated and misled ("conned") by a drug-using adolescent.

The physical examination is unlikely to provide any hard evidence regarding drug use, although some indications of the adolescent's sympathy with the drug culture may be provided by his or her attitude toward the physician and attire. Lack of sustained eye contact, lack of spontaneity, a flattened affect, and an attitude of hostility, secretiveness, or persistent evasiveness should alert the physician to the possibility of drug use, especially when combined with a preference for the hairstyles and clothing favored by drug users. These are "soft signs" and require correlation with the history and laboratory findings as in the diagnosis of any other disease. It is usually more fruitful to concentrate on the adverse social consequences of drug use and avoid threatening direct questions about such use. Intoxicated behavior or concrete evidence of drug use is not often witnessed by parents of a drug-using adolescent until fairly late in the progressive stages of drug use.

LABORATORY DIAGNOSIS

Because it is so difficult to diagnose drug use, any array of factors in the history combined with the attitudes just described should raise the suspicion that an adolescent has this disorder. And because of the potentially life-threatening consequences of continued drug use, the physician should order laboratory tests to assist in further evaluation of such a patient.

Metabolites of marijuana (cannabis) and cocaine persist in the urine for several days after last use of these drugs and may be detected by laboratory analysis. Permission should always be obtained from the parent(s) of minors and from the adolescent patient, unless the physician believes that the adolescent's life is in serious danger because of the drug/alcohol abuse, or the adolescent's parent asserts that such disclosure would precipitate a violent scene or runaway attempt. The half-life of marijuana is 72 hours. Casual or infrequent users of marijuana will have a negative (clean) urine by immunoassay methods after 48 to 72 hours of abstinence. If the adolescent is using cannabis every day, evidence will be detectable in the urine up to several weeks after the beginning of a period of complete abstinence.

A urine specimen collected for analysis of these substances should be obtained, if possible, from a first voiding on a Monday morning (because most adolescents use drugs on Friday and Saturday evenings), preferably under direct surveillance to avoid possible deliberate substitution or adulteration of the urine specimen by the adolescent. Most frequent users of illicit drugs are well aware of procedures for adulterating a specimen for laboratory analysis of such use, including substituting urine of a non–drug-using friend, diluting the specimen with tap water, drinking large quantities of water, swallowing vitamin C tablets or a homeopathic preparation called Golden Seal before voiding, and purposely adding household bleach, salt, or an acidic substance to the specimen. Thus, when direct observation is not possible, the urine specimen should be checked for color, pH, specific gravity, and freshness (warmth of the specimen when obtained in the physician's office or at home).

Testing urine specimens serially (consecutive Monday-morning urine specimens) for the presence of cannabinoids is more informative than a single test for such substances. If cannabinoids are present in two midweek urine specimens obtained several days apart, or if three weekly spot-checked Monday-morning specimens are positive, it is likely that the adolescent is using marijuana frequently enough to warrant a more complete drug evaluation. Such an adolescent may well need immediate intervention and treatment of his or her drug abuse disorder.

ALCOHOL USE

The patient should be questioned carefully about the number of times, if any, that he or she has been drunk and the number of rapidly consumed beers that it takes to get drunk. If initial probing questions elicit positive responses, the adolescent should be asked about citations for driving while intoxicated and about motor vehicle accidents after having had too much to drink. Binge drinking or frequent use of alcohol is more difficult to detect by analysis of body fluids than is marijuana use. A simple colorimetric test strip, which semiquantitatively detects alcohol in the saliva, is available for use in emergency departments and for home monitoring by parents of known adolescent alcohol abusers. If alcohol use has been heavy, damage to the parenchyma of the liver may be present and detected as elevation of the hepatic enzyme gamma glutamyl transpeptidase. This test, however, is relatively nonsensitive and nonspecific for adolescent alcoholism.

Acute alcohol ingestion may also be detected by administration of a Breathalyzer test or immunoassay of a urine specimen obtained within 6 hours of ingestion.

SERIOUS DRUG/ALCOHOL ABUSE

Either persistent, frequent use of mood-altering, pleasure-producing drugs or indulgence in prolonged binges of such drug use characterizes the adolescent who has lost control of his or her use of drugs. Such an individual has a preoccupation with a self-perceived need to obtain a euphoric "high" not reached by other means, usually in the company of peers who have the same mind-set. Because these adolescents may develop a tolerance to their drug(s) of choice, they require ever-increasing quantities of the drug to achieve the same degree of euphoria. Furthermore, because the chemically dependent young person obtains much of his or her pleasure in life from the social use of drugs, he or she cannot or will not stop using these substances. Thus, even though the adolescent may have tried one or more times to remain abstinent, and despite being apprised of the many adverse consequences of drug use (academic underachievement, family conflicts, internalized shame and guilt, legal complications, acute toxic reactions), it must be recognized that the chemically dependent adolescent usually cannot break free of his or her disease without intensive and prolonged professional help.

Outpatient Management

The adolescent who is strongly suspected or known to be abusing drugs or alcohol should be evaluated by an expert in adolescent drug and alcohol abuse. At the initial assessment session, the goal is for every family member of an identified adolescent drug abuser to agree to a drug-free lifestyle and for the parents to state unequivocally that they are prepared to do anything and everything to accomplish this goal. Behavioral changes that will be necessary for the drug user include:

1. Total abstinence from all illicit drugs and alcohol.
2. Dissociation from drug-using friends, as failure to adhere to this is the major reason for continuing drug use.
3. Cooperation in the provision of periodic urine and saliva specimens to monitor compliance with the plan.
4. Participation in family meetings on a regular basis to share concerns and to assess progress.
5. Compliance with a mutually agreed upon contract, including house rules, the breaking of which will have fair but definite and clear consequences.

Activities in which the more advanced drug user should participate include attendance at a peer-support group such as Alcoholics Anonymous (AA) or Narcotics Anonymous two or three times a week for the first month, two times a week for the second month, and once weekly for the next 3 months. A sponsor from the support group should be assigned to act as role model for the drug-using adolescent and to monitor attendance and participation at meetings. The adolescent and family may need psychotherapeutic or pastoral counseling.

It is important for the adolescent and for the professionals who are helping him or her to manage the drug problem to communicate on a regular basis with school guidance counselors, teachers, the pediatrician, the group therapy sponsor, and interested others.

Pediatricians should have a roster of local consultants who specialize in the assessment of drug-using adolescents. It is also helpful to know the names and locations of affordable drug abuse treatment facilities in the community. These range in intensity from afterschool programs to the most intense type of inpatient programs of 1 to 12 months' duration. Pediatricians who care for adolescents recovering from drug or alcohol dependency must also be aware of a long list of medications that contain alcohol or mood-altering drugs, which might trigger a relapse back to drug abuse.

The adolescent's parents would do well to attend a parent support group such as Al-Anon or Toughlove. Parents of drug-using teenagers often feel embarrassed, guilty, insecure, and alienated from parents of "successful" teenagers. Lastly, if the drug that the adolescent has heavily abused is alcohol, a medically supervised trial of disulfiram (Antabuse, 250 mg/day in a single dose for 2 to 3 months) may be considered. Antabuse requires an intensive education as to the reasons for use and its effects if alcohol is ingested, and it should not be prescribed unless it is part of a comprehensive plan of management including regular attendance at AA meetings.

If this necessarily authoritarian plan of therapy is repeatedly unsuccessful, the young person dependent on drugs (including alcohol) should be admitted to an adolescent-oriented drug rehabilitation program with or without his or her consent unless the age of majority has been reached.

Inpatient Management

The basic principles of managing drug abuse are the same, regardless of which of the following drugs is abused: alcohol, marijuana, cocaine, stimulants, depressants, hallucinogens, PCP, or inhalants. Antabuse has been found to be helpful in the treatment of some alcoholics, and phenothiazine or trifluoperazine may be required to treat subacute or chronic drug-related PCP or LSD psychosis as part of the overall treatment plan. Antidepressant medication may be a necessary adjunct in the management of selected severely endogenously depressed and chemically dependent adolescents.

Detoxification is almost always unnecessary for adolescent drug users unless the dependence is on an opiate, barbiturate, or diazepam, or unless the patient had attempted to withdraw from alcohol dependence previously and had shown severe acute symptoms. When necessary, such detoxification can usually be accomplished in 3 to 7 days (unless the drug is diazepam).

Drug rehabilitation programs for adolescent drug users should meet six criteria:

1. No drug use should be permitted in the program, including alcohol, cigarettes, and tranquilizers.
2. Peer-group support should be encouraged.
3. Some staff members should be ex–drug users or alcoholics.
4. Intense family participation should be mandatory.
5. The program must have an aftercare program that includes a large enough group of graduates close enough geographically to the patient that they form an easily accessible peer group of drug-free supporters.

Pediatricians play a crucial role in the identification and treatment of drug-dependent adolescents. By familiarizing themselves with the symptoms of chemical dependency, the techniques of the assessment of a drug-using adolescent, and the resources in their areas to help rehabilitate drug users, they will be much better able to serve their adolescent patients and their families.

REFERENCES

Schonberg SK (ed): Substance Abuse: A Guide for Health Professionals. Elk Grove Village, Ill., American Academy of Pediatrics, 1988.

Schwartz RH: Urine testing in detection of drugs of abuse. Arch Intern Med 148:2407–2412, 1988.

Schwartz RH, Cohen PR, Bair GO: Identifying and coping with a drug-using adolescent: Some guidelines for pediatricians and parents. Pediatrics-in-Review 7:133–139, 1985.

ADOLESCENT GYNECOLOGY

JOAN MANSFIELD, M.D.

SEXUALITY

Adolescence is a period of transition in the patient-doctor relationship. The pediatric office visit usually focuses on the concerns of the parent about the health and needs of the child. As the child enters adolescence, she becomes a patient in her own right with concerns that she may have difficulty sharing completely with her parents. It is important for the physician to encourage communication between the parents and the teenager about sexuality but, at the same time, provide the opportunity for her to bring her sexual concerns to her physician for advice and adult guidance in confidence. If the physician is not able to counsel her confidentially on issues of sexuality and contraception, he or she may prefer to refer the patient to a setting where these services are available.

Because patient and parent often have different perspectives on the medical problem at hand, it is important for the teenager to be seen by herself at some point during the visit, usually during the physical examination. The physician can then address any confidential concerns and, together with the patient, develop a plan that can be shared with the parent. Frequently, the adolescent will present with a minor complaint unrelated to gynecologic issues when she is in fact concerned about pregnancy or contraception. The review of systems therefore becomes a valuable tool for uncovering the real reason for the visit and for teaching the adolescent the variety of health-related concerns that can be addressed during a visit with a physician.

Counseling should begin early in adolescence with basic information on the expected course of pubertal growth and development and reproductive function, the importance of contraception in preventing unplanned pregnancy, and the use of condoms to reduce the risk of sexually transmitted diseases (STDs). Two thirds of teenagers have had at least one experience of sexual intercourse by age 18 years. One in 10 adolescent women becomes pregnant each year. STDs are of epidemic proportions in this age group. Many teenagers are unaware of the risks of sexual activity, including unwanted pregnancy, STDs, and loss of self-esteem. It is appropriate to review these risks in an objective, nonjudgmental fashion. The patient may be reminded that many teenagers choose not to be sexually active for these reasons. If she chooses to be sexually active, she may be encouraged to act responsibly to reduce these risks by using contraception effectively and getting regular gynecologic care. This includes a pelvic examination with a Papanicolaou (Pap) smear to detect cervical dysplasia at least annually and testing for asymptomatic STDs at 6-month intervals.

PREGNANCY

Pregnancy is the most common cause of secondary amenorrhea in adolescents. Any teenager who expresses concern about a period being slightly delayed should have a urine pregnancy test, because many adolescents who are at risk for pregnancy will deny sexual activity. Often, the alleged reason for the office visit is a minor physical complaint such as sore throat or fatigue, and the delayed period is appreciated only on review of systems. The newer urine human chorionic gonadotropin (hCG) office pregnancy tests such as ICON HCG (Hybritech) use monoclonal antibodies to hCG and enzyme-linked radioimmunoassay. The detection level varies with the kit. The ICON HCG is positive above 20 to 50 mIU/ml hCG. The urine specific gravity should be 1.015 or above for greatest sensitivity. Thus, pregnancy can usually be diagnosed 7 to 10 days post conception, even before the period is due. (For additional discussion, see earlier article on contraception, pregnancy, and abortion in Section 2.)

Ectopic pregnancies have become increasingly frequent in young women and now compose 0.5 per cent of all pregnancies in women younger than age 25. Abdominal pain and amenorrhea or abnormal vaginal bleeding suggest the consideration of this diagnosis. A pelvic examination sometimes reveals an adnexal mass. If an ectopic pregnancy is suspected, a quantitative serum hCG should be obtained and repeated in 48 hours if the diagnosis remains in question. The normal doubling time of serum hCG levels is approximately 2.3 days at 5 to 8 weeks' gestation. In ectopic pregnancy, hCG levels are usually lower than normal and the rate of rise is slower.

If the serum hCG is greater than 6000 mIU/ml (IRP) (about 5 to 6 weeks' gestation), an intrauterine gestational sac should be visible on abdominal ultrasonography. Transvaginal ultrasonography may detect a gestational sac at 1500 mIU/ml hCG. Absence of the gestational sac on ultrasonography suggests a possible ectopic pregnancy. A patient with a suspected ectopic pregnancy should be referred immediately to a gynecologist. The pregnancy may be removed surgically, often by laparoscopic salpingostomy preservation of the fallopian tube. Medical treatment with methotrexate followed by citrovorum factor has been used in some centers as an alternative to surgical treatment for ectopic pregnancies less than 3 cm in diameter (hCG $<$ 1500 mIU/ml).

CONTRACEPTION

Contraceptive information is a basic part of health education for the adolescent. Confidentiality has been shown to be an important factor in determining whether the sexually active adolescent obtains and uses contraception. The physician who elects to provide oral contraceptives for adolescents in his or her practice should be able to perform pelvic examinations, including Pap smears, screening for asymptomatic gonococcal and chlamydial infections, and treatment of STDs.

Oral contraceptive pills containing estrogen and a progestin remain the most popular and most effective form of contraception for adolescents. Although the theoretic failure rate of oral contraceptive pills containing estrogen and progestin is 0.3 to 0.5 pregnancies per 100 women years of use, the actual failure rate in adolescents is much higher because many teenagers use the pills incorrectly or sporadically or discontinue use within a few months.

Oral contraceptive pills containing 30 to 35 μg of ethinyl estradiol are appropriate for most adolescents. A fixed-dose pill containing 35 μg of ethinyl estradiol in combination with 1 mg of norethindrone (Norinyl or Ortho-Novum 1/35) is one commonly used oral contraceptive. Ortho-cyclen (norgestimate/ethinyl estradiol) contains a progestin with a longer half-life. Triphasic combinations with ethinyl estradiol and norethindrone (Ortho-Novum 7/7/7) or levonorgestrel (Triphasil, Trilevlen) are similar in efficacy. Levonorgestrel triphasics have less breakthrough bleeding. Ortho Tri-cyclen (norgestimate/ethinyl estradiol) is another alternative.

Within the group of pills containing 30 to 35 μg of ethinyl estradiol, some are relatively more progestin-dominant and some more estrogen-dominant. An estrogen-dominant pill such as Modicon or Demulen 1/35 is a good choice for a patient who has hirsutism, acne, or polycystic ovary syndrome. A pill containing 30 μg of ethinyl estradiol with 0.3 mg of norgestrel (Lo/Ovral) can be useful when breakthrough bleeding is a problem, as can short courses (3 months) of pills containing 50 μg of mestranol (Ortho-Novum, Norinyl 1/50).

Prolonged use of pills containing 50 μg of estrogen is avoided, when possible, in adolescents. A 28-day packet is preferred to a 21-day packet to increase compliance. Pills containing 20 μg of ethinyl estradiol are associated with more breakthrough bleeding and less efficacy if pills are omitted and are therefore reserved for patients who are unable to tolerate doses of 30 to 35 μg of estrogen.

(See also article on contraception, pregnancy, and abortion.)

Progestin-Only Pills ("Minipills")

Oral contraceptives containing small amounts of progestins alone, such as Ovrette (0.075 mg of norgestrel) or Nor-QD or Micronor (0.35 mg of norethindrone), are an alternative for patients who have a medical contraindication to estrogen. Menstrual irregularity, both amenorrhea and irregular bleeding, is a very frequent side effect of these pills. Because pregnancy rates are higher in patients taking minipills, particularly if pills are omitted, periodic pregnancy tests often become necessary in this population.

Implantable Contraceptives

Norplant, a contraceptive device consisting of six small Silastic rods containing levonorgestrel that are implanted in the skin of the arm under local anesthesia and sterile conditions, has recently become available in the United States. The implant provides 5 years of contraception. This appears to be an attractive option for patients who have demonstrated poor compliance with oral contraceptives (especially teenage parents). The expense of the initial implantation and the frequency of menstrual irregularity as a side effect may limit the usefulness of this method. The rods must be removed after 5 years.

Depot medroxyprogesterone acetate (150 mg IM every 3 months) is now approved as a contraceptive method in the United States. It may be an alternative to consider in patients who are unable to comply with oral methods due to mental retardation or mental illness. Amenorrhea is common.

Barrier Methods

Barrier and other contraceptive methods are discussed in the article on contraception, pregnancy, and abortion earlier in Section 22.

GYNECOLOGIC DISORDERS

Vulvovaginitis

Physiologic Leukorrhea

Physiologic leukorrhea, a white, mucoid, homogeneous, nonirritating desquamation of squamous cells, begins before menarche in all pubertal adolescent females. Squamous cells alone are seen on saline wet-mount slide. Patients can be reassured that this is a normal part of adolescent development.

Candidal Vulvovaginitis

Candidal vulvovaginitis may occur in sexually active or virginal females in adolescence, although it is more common in sexually active teenagers. It occurs frequently in patients on broad-spectrum antibiotics, in diabetics, in patients on glucocorticoids, in obese patients, and in pregnant patients. The discharge is pruritic; the vulva and vagina are inflamed, with red papular satellite lesions on the vulva and a lumpy white vaginal discharge revealing candidal hyphae and buds on potassium hydroxide preparation.

Treatment. The imidazole medications are the basis of the many treatment regimens for candidal vaginitis. Vaginal suppositories are less messy than creams but may not treat vulvar involvement as well. Treatment regimens include

- Clotrimazole, 100-mg vaginal suppository for 7 nights
- Clotrimazole 1 per cent cream, 1 applicatorful for 7 nights
- Clotrimazole, 500-mg vaginal suppository for 1 night
- Clotrimazole, two 100-mg vaginal suppositories for 3 nights
- Miconazole, 200-mg vaginal suppository for 3 nights
- Miconazole, 100-mg suppository for 7 nights
- Miconazole, 2 per cent cream, 1 applicatorful for 7 nights
- Terconazole, 0.4 per cent cream, 1 applicatorful for 7 nights
- Terconazole, 80-mg vaginal suppository for 3 nights
- Terconazole, 0.8 per cent cream, 1 applicatorful for 3 nights
- Butoconazole, 2 per cent cream, 1 applicatorful for 3 nights
- Nystatin, 100,000-unit vaginal suppository for 14 nights

Although a longer course of treatment is required, nystatin is an alternative if patients develop an allergic vaginal irritation on imidazole preparations. Imidazoles should be avoided, if possible, in the first trimester of pregnancy.

Bacterial Vaginosis

Bacterial vaginosis is another cause of vaginal discharge. Although it has been associated with the presence of the bacteria *Gardnerella vaginalis,* it probably represents an overgrowth of mixed anaerobic bacteria. Normal lactobacilli are absent. It occurs more commonly in sexually active adolescents. The discharge is gray, white, or yellow and homogeneous, adheres to the vaginal walls, and is usually malodorous. Saline preparations reveal squamous cells coated with bacteria. The vaginal pH is above 4.5.

Treatment. Treatment is with metronidazole (Flagyl, 500 mg orally twice a day for 7 days). Metronidazole gel or Clindamycin cream 2 per cent, intravaginally for 7 days. The side effects of oral metronidazole are nausea, headache, a metallic aftertaste, and rare blood dyscrasias. The patient should be instructed to avoid alcohol during treatment because alcohol in the presence of metronidazole results in emesis. If the infection recurs repeatedly, it may be helpful to treat the partner of the sexually active patient as well.

Trichomoniasis

Trichomoniasis is an STD presenting with a yellow, frothy vaginal discharge, sometimes with dysuria. The cervix may appear inflamed and friable. Saline preparation shows many polymorphonuclear leukocytes and active, wriggling trichomonads.

Treatment. Treatment is with metronidazole (2.0 g orally in one dose). The sexual partner should be treated simultaneously. Alcohol should be avoided during treatment, and intercourse should be postponed until the partner is also treated. The single-dose treatment is effective in 86 to 95 per cent of patients. If the infection recurs more than once, a 7-day course of metronidazole (500 mg twice a day) may be used. Metronidazole should be avoided during pregnancy. Clotrimazole (Gyne-Lotrimin, Mycelex, 1 per cent cream or 100-mg vaginal tablets for 7 nights) may be used in the pregnant patient after the first trimester.

Nonspecific Vulvitis

Nonspecific vulvitis may be caused by heat, nylon underpants, poor hygiene, or sand. Hydrocortisone cream 1 per cent may be applied three times daily to the vulva for 3 to 5 days and the precipitating causes eliminated.

Chlamydia trachomatis Cervicitis and Urethritis

Chlamydia trachomatis is present in 5 to 18 per cent of asymptomatic sexually active teenage women, 40 to 50 per cent of patients with a vaginal discharge, and about a third of patients who have gonorrheal infection. Although the infection is frequently asymptomatic, the classic presentation is a mucopurulent cervical discharge with white cells present on wet preparation. Symptoms often include a vaginal discharge, dysuria, and sometimes the abdominal pain and systemic symptoms of pelvic inflammatory disease (PID) (see later). *C. trachomatis* is also a common cause of perihepatitis, presenting with right upper quadrant pain and tenderness as a complication of PID. Symptomatic or asymptomatic pyuria in the adolescent female may be caused by chlamydia or *Neisseria gonorrhoeae,* and STDs should always be considered in the adolescent female with these findings.

Endocervical chlamydia cultures have a specificity of 100 per cent but a sensitivity of only 80 to 90 per cent. A Dacron swab is used to obtain a specimen for culture. A number of less expensive screening tests for chlamydia based on laboratory examination of direct smear with fluorescein-labeled antibody (MicroTrak), enzyme immunoassays (Chlamydiazime, CellTech), DNA probes, and office-based tests (Testpack CHLAMYDIA) are practical alternatives to culture with somewhat lower sensitivities. Because *Chlamydia* is an intracellular organism, proper techniques must be used in obtaining the specimens to maximize yield. The symptomatic patient with a purulent discharge should be treated immediately at the time of testing, and treatment should be completed even in the absence of a positive test result.

Treatment. Regimens for cervical and urethral infections include:

- Doxycycline, 100 mg orally two times a day for 7 days
- Tetracycline, 500 mg four times a day for 7 days
- Erythromycin base or stearate, 500 mg four times a day for 7 days
- Ofloxacin, 300 mg two times a day for 7 days (in patients 18 years of age or over)
- Erythromycin ethylsuccinate, 800 mg four times a day for 7 days

Tetracyclines and ofloxacin should not be used in the pregnant patient. Amoxicillin (500 mg three times a day) appears effective in pregnant patients. Partners should also be treated. Rescreening in 3 to 6 weeks is useful in the adolescent sexually active patient who is at high risk for re-exposure.

Gonococcal Cervicitis and Urethritis

Neisseria gonorrhoeae is another frequent cause of a purulent vaginal discharge in teens. As in chlamydia, colonization with *N. gonorrhoeae* may be asymptomatic, and sexually active teenage women from high-risk populations should be screened with endocervical culture on Thayer-Martin medium at least twice a year. Patients with gonorrheal infection often have chlamydia as well, and treatment should cover both organisms. Cervical Gram stain may reveal intracellular gram-negative diplococci within polymorphonuclear leukocytes, but this finding is less common and less sensitive than in males with *N. gonorrhoeae* urethritis. Urethral infection with *N. gonorrhoeae* may be asymptomatic or may present with urinary frequency, dysuria, and pyuria. A Bartholin's gland abscess may be caused by *N. gonorrhoeae,* chlamydia, or other organisms and presents with labial pain and swelling. Treatment should include both antibiotic treatment covering *N. gonorrhoeae* and *Chlamydia* and, in most cases, surgical drainage.

Treatment. Treatment of asymptomatic infection, cervicitis, urethritis, or sexual contacts of patients with *N. gonorrhoeae* infection should include coverage for chlamydia because both organisms frequently coexist. Penicillin-resistant *N. gonorrhoeae* has been identified with variable frequency throughout the United States. Chromosomally mediated resistance to penicillin may include resistance to tetracycline. The currently recommended treatment of gonorrhea cervicitis or urethritis is:

1. Ceftriaxone (250 mg IM once; plus doxycycline, 100 mg orally two times a day for 7 days). The ceftriaxone may be mixed with 1 per cent lidocaine without epinephrine to reduce the pain of injection.
2. In the patient with a history of immediate or anaphylactic reaction to penicillin, spectinomycin (2 g IM) followed by doxycycline should be used as an alternative, although cross-reactivity between third-generation cephalosporins and penicillin is uncommon.

Ofloxacin (400 mg orally) has recently been approved for gonococcal treatment. Other regimens with less data available on efficacy include ciprofloxacin (500 mg orally once with 1 g probenecid); norfloxin (800 mg orally once); cefuroxime axetil (1 g orally with 1 g probenecid); cefixime (400 mg orally); cefotaxime (1 g IM); and ceftizoxime (500 mg IM), all followed by doxycycline.

Ciprofloxacin, ofloxacin, and norfloxin should not be used in patients who are pregnant or who are younger than 18 years of age.

A serologic test for syphilis should be sent at the time of treatment. Sexual partners should be treated. A test of cure should be done 7 to 10 days post completion of treatment regimens other than ceftriaxone/tetracycline. Rescreening 1 to 2 months post treatment is of value in all cases because reinfection is common.

Gonococcal Pharyngitis

Gonococcal pharyngitis can be diagnosed by pharyngeal culture on Thayer-Martin medium and treated with ceftriaxone (250 mg IM) or cefixime (400 mg orally). Nonpregnant patients who are at least 17 years of age may be treated with ciprofloxacin (500 mg orally once) or ofloxacin (400 mg orally) if they cannot tolerate ceftriaxone. Another specimen should be obtained for culture after treatment.

Gonococcal Proctitis

Gonococcal proctitis may present with discharge of blood and purulent material or, less acutely, with pain on defecation. Gonococcal proctitis may be diagnosed by culture of rectal swab specimen on Thayer-Martin medium. Treatment is the same as for cervicitis.

Gonococcal Arthritis

Gonocococcal arthritis is often associated with asymptomatic gonococcal infection or with mild cervicitis or pharyngitis. The mild form is associated with migratory polyarthralgias, tenosynovitis, fever, and skin lesions consisting of papules, sometimes progressing to purpuric vesicopustular lesions.

Fluorescent antibody staining of biopsy specimens reveals *N. gonorrhoeae* infection in half of these patients. Blood cultures may be positive if taken within 2 days of the onset of symptoms. The late form consists of a monarticular arthritis, often in the knee. Synovial fluid culture is positive in 20 to 50 per cent of patients, whereas blood cultures are negative and systemic symptoms are not present. Patients who are unreliable or who have purulent joint effusions should be hospitalized.

Treatment. Regimens for gonococcal arthritis include:

- Ceftriaxone, 1 g IM or IV once a day
- Ceftizoxime, 1 g IV every 8 hours
- Cefoxatime, 1 g IV every 8 hours

In patients who are allergic to cephalosporins, spectinomycin (2 g IM every 12 hours) may be used. A specimen should be obtained for chlamydia culture as well. The joint should be immobilized. Aspirations of the joint may need to be repeated. Hip arthritis requires open drainage. Parenteral treatment should be continued until the patient has been asymptomatic for 24 to 48 hours; the patient may then be discharged to complete 7 days of antibiotic treatment with oral cefuroxime axetil (500 mg twice a day), amoxicillin (500 mg with clavulanic acid three times a day), or ciprofloxin (500 mg twice a day) if not pregnant and if older than 16 years.

Pelvic Inflammatory Disease

Pelvic inflammatory disease refers to infection of the upper genital tract, including the fallopian tubes. Of the 1 million women treated each year for acute salpingitis, 16 to 20 per cent are adolescents. Adolescents are at higher risk for PID than adults because of the high prevalence of gonococcal and chlamydial infection among sexually active teenagers. One third to one half of patients with PID have positive endocervical cultures for *N. gonorrhoeae.* The prevalence of positive chlamydial cultures in acute PID is similar. Patients with recurrent episodes are less likely to be culture-positive for these organisms. Other associated organisms are coliforms, *Gardnerella vaginalis, Haemophilus influenzae,* group B streptococci, *Bacteroides* sp., peptostreptococcus, peptococcus, and *Mycoplasma hominis.*

The patient with PID classically presents with lower abdominal pain, vaginal discharge, and fever, often within 7 days of the onset of menses. Irregular vaginal bleeding may also be a symptom of PID. Symptoms of chlamydial PID may be somewhat less acute. The diagnosis of PID is often difficult to make because many patients do not have a classic presentation. The diagnosis is likely if the patient has the following symptoms and signs: a history of lower abdominal pain and cervical motion tenderness or uterine tenderness with adnexal tenderness, along with either purulent cervical discharge, elevated sedimentation rate (> 15 mm/hour), elevated white blood cell count (> 10,500/mm^3), or pelvic abscess detectable by bimanual examination or ultrasonography. The differential diagnosis includes acute appendicitis, ectopic pregnancy, ovarian abscess, corpus luteum rupture, and endometriosis. Laparoscopy may be necessary if symptoms are acute and the diagnosis is in doubt. A pregnancy test should be obtained as well as a complete blood count, sedimentation rate, and serologic test for syphilis, and specimens should be obtained for gonococcal and chlamydial cultures.

Treatment. Incompletely treated, late treated, and recurrent PID are associated with tubal occlusion, ectopic pregnancy, infertility, and chronic pelvic pain. Because compliance with oral antibiotic therapy is often poor in teenagers, many centers admit all adolescents with PID. As a minimum, patients with uncertain diagnosis, suspected pelvic abscess, right upper quadrant pain suggesting perihepatitis complicating PID, peritoneal signs, temperature above 38°C, vomiting, pregnancy, or a history of poor compliance should be admitted to the hospital for treatment.

Many regimens have been used for the treatment of PID. The current Centers for Disease Control guidelines for inpatient treatment of PID are either of the following:

1. Cefoxitin (2 g IV every 6 hours) or cefotetan (2 g IV every 12 hours) plus doxycycline (100 mg orally or IV every 12 hours for at least 48 hours after the patient clinically

improves). The patient is then continued on doxycycline (100 mg orally two times a day for 10 to 14 days). Ceftizoxime, cefotaxime, and ceftriaxone are acceptable alternatives to cefoxitin, *or*

2. Clindamycin (900 mg IV every 8 hours [or 600 mg IV every 6 hours]) plus gentamicin (2 mg/kg IM or IV followed by 1.5 mg/kg every 8 hours [if renal function is normal]). Tobramycin may be substituted. This should be continued until 48 hours after the patient has improved. The patient should then be continued on doxycycline (100 mg two times a day for 10 to 14 days). Clindamycin (450 mg four times a day) is an alternative.

The usual outpatient treatment regimen is ceftriaxone (500 mg IM [or cefoxitin, 2 g IM with probenecid, 1 g orally]) followed by doxycycline (100 mg orally two times a day for 10 to 14 days). Erythromycin (500 mg four times daily) is an alternative for patients who cannot take doxycycline. The patient should return in 48 to 72 hours for a follow-up pelvic examination to determine whether symptoms are improving. The patient's partner should be treated, and the patient should not have intercourse for 3 to 4 weeks.

Sexually Transmitted Viral Infections

Human Papillomavirus

Human papillomavirus (HPV) has become an increasing concern to those providing health care to adolescents. HPV infection is common in sexually active teens. It is a DNA virus with more than 50 subtypes. Some of these subtypes, particularly 6 and 11, are associated with the typical "cauliflower"-like genital warts found on the vulva, vagina, cervix, urethra, and anus. A flat condyloma is usually types 16 or 18. These subtypes are also associated with cervical dysplasia and genital cancers. Genital warts typically appear within 4 to 6 weeks of exposure, but the incubation period is up to 8 months or more. Findings may be subclinical and detectable only by typical HPV changes on Pap smear (koilocytes or cervical intraepithelial neoplasia) or on biopsy using DNA probes.

Treatment. Exophytic warts are treated with application of locally destructive agents in the office. Trichloroacetic acid (TCA) is used in strengths from 25 to 85 per cent. To avoid burns, 85 per cent TCA must be applied just to the lesions. Normal saline may be applied after TCA to reduce the burning sensation. TCA is reapplied weekly. This regimen appears to be less problematic and more effective than 25 per cent podophyllin.

If the lesions fail to respond, the patient may be referred for cryocautery or laser treatment. Carbon dioxide laser treatment requires general anesthesia and is associated with considerable post-treatment discomfort and sometimes with scarring or bleeding. New experimental treatments of genital warts include 5-fluorouracil cream and injections of interferon-α_{2b}. The effectiveness of these regimens is currently being evaluated.

Patients with abnormalities on Pap smear consistent with HPV infection should be referred for colposcopy and biopsy. If biopsy reveals cervical dysplasia, cryotherapy, laser, or cone biopsy is a commonly used therapeutic modality. Follow-up at 3 months is required, with subsequent Pap smears at frequent intervals. A patient whose biopsy findings reveal HPV without dysplasia may be treated with locally destructive therapies or observed closely with repeated Pap smears because the natural history of this infection and the likelihood of subsequent dysplasia or genital cancer in this population are not yet known. Partners of patients with HPV should be examined for genital warts. Wrapping the penis in a cloth soaked with vinegar (acetoacid) or 5 per cent TCA prior to examination improves the chances of detecting warts.

Human Immunodeficiency Virus

Human immunodeficiency virus (HIV) infection is discussed in detail elsewhere in this volume. Adolescents currently account for only 1 per cent of patients with acquired immunodeficiency syndrome (AIDS), with considerable geographic variation in prevalence. However, many of the women who present with AIDS as adults presumably acquired HIV infection in adolescence. This is of special concern because they may pass the infection on to their children before they themselves experience symptoms.

HIV infection may be more easily acquired by patients with genital lesions caused by other STDs. Adolescents with multiple partners are at increased risk. Condom use, reducing the number of sexual partners, and, if possible, abstinence should be encouraged to reduce the likelihood of acquiring HIV infection. Voluntary testing for HIV infection is an option that should be considered carefully and accompanied by supportive counseling in the adolescent because considerable anxiety and depression may result.

Genital Herpes

Genital herpes infection is usually associated with herpes simplex virus type 2 (HSV-2), although up to 15 per cent of primary genital infections are type 1. Of patients with HSV-2, 60 per cent will have recurrence of symptoms over the year following their first episode. Recurrence occurs in 14 per cent of HSV-1 genital infections. In primary infections, vesicles appear on the vulva, labia, and/or cervix, rupturing to produce painful ulcers associated with burning, dysuria, inguinal adenopathy, and often systemic symptoms of fever, headache, and malaise. Urinary retention due to dysuria is a possible complication. Symptoms improve in 10 to 21 days. Recurrences are generally milder and last 3 to 5 days. Itching or burning sensations may precede the appearance of vesicles. Viral culture of the vesicle or ulcer is often used to confirm the diagnosis.

Treatment. Treatment with acyclovir (orally 200 mg five times a day for 10 days) can reduce symptoms and shorten the course of primary herpes. Local treatment measures include sitz baths in tepid water or Burow's solution, dry heat from a hair dryer set on low, and lidocaine (Xylocaine) jelly 2 per cent applied to genital lesions. If dysuria is severe, voiding in a shower or sitz bath may help to avoid urinary retention.

Candidal vaginitis may accompany herpes. Severely ill patients may occasionally require hospitalization and intravenous acyclovir.

Recurrences of genital herpes can usually be treated with local measures. Acyclovir (200 mg five times a day for 5 days) can be begun with the first sign of symptoms but is usually not necessary.

Patients should not have intercourse while genital herpes lesions are present. Although condoms can help to prevent transmission of herpes, they do not provide complete protection. Transmission is most likely when active lesions are present and during the prodromal period; however, viral shedding in asymptomatic patients may also transmit the virus to sexual partners.

Pediculosis pubis (Crabs)

Pubic lice are usually transmitted by sexual contact, although they may be acquired by contact with infected blankets, sheets, towels, and clothing. The primary symptom is pruritus. Adult lice may be visible on the pubic hair. Nits appear as small white bumps firmly attached to pubic hair.

Treatment. Treatment is with 1 per cent lindane (Kwell) shampoo lathered into hair and left on for 5 minutes. A second treatment in 1 week may lessen the likelihood of recurrence. Blankets, sheets, towels, and clothing should be laundered in hot water or set aside for 2 weeks. One per cent permethrin creme rinse (Nix) applied for 10 minutes is a newer and very effective alternative treatment. Other pyrethrin preparations (RID, A-200 Pyrinate) may also be used.

Vulvar Ulcers

The most common causes of vaginal ulcers are HSV (discussed earlier), syphilis, and chancroid. Primary syphilis presents as a painless hard ulcer. The rapid plasma reagin (RPR) is usually positive by the 7th day. Therapy is discussed in Section 12. Chancroid, although still rare in the United States, is increasing in prevalence. Multiple purulent, irregular ulcers are seen with tender inguinal adenopathy.

Treatment. Patients with ulcers associated with tender adenopathy who do not have syphilis or herpes may be treated with erythromycin base (500 mg orally four times a day for 7 days) or ceftriaxone (250 mg IM) for suspected chancroid. Nodes may require drainage if they become fluctuant. Other causes of genital ulcers are inflammatory bowel disease, Behçet's disease, lymphogranuloma venereum, and mononucleosis.

Primary Dysmenorrhea

Primary or physiologic dysmenorrhea is characterized by pelvic pain on the first day or two of menses. The pain is related to increases in prostaglandin secretion. Associated systemic symptoms related to prostaglandins include nausea and vomiting, dizziness, syncope, and diarrhea. Patients who have mild symptoms on the first day of menses should undergo a general physical examination, including examination of hymenal patency. These patients usually respond well to mild over-the-counter analgesic regimens such as ibuprofen (200 to 400 mg). A pelvic examination should also be performed in the patient with severe dysmenorrhea because uterine anomalies leading to partial obstruction and endometriosis may present with similar pain.

Treatment. Nonsteroidal anti-inflammatory drugs (NSAIDs) are usually quite effective in primary dysmenorrhea. Many different NSAID treatment regimens exist, including naproxen sodium (Anaprox, 550 mg to start then 275 mg every 6 hours); naproxen sodium (Anaprox DS, 500 mg twice a day); naproxen (Naprosyn, 250 to 375 mg two to three times a day); ibuprofen (800 mg followed by 400 mg every 4 to 6 hours up to 800 mg three times a day); mefenamic acid (Ponstel, 500 mg to start then 250 mg every 6 hours); and flurbiprofen (ANSAID, 50 mg every 6 hours or 100 mg every 12 hours).

If the patient does not respond to intensive NSAID therapy, oral contraceptives may be prescribed for 3 to 6 months. Pills containing 30 to 35 μg of ethinyl estradiol (e.g., Norinyl 1+35, Ortho-Novum 1/35, Triphasil, Tri-Levlen, Tri-Norinyl, Ortho-Novum 7/7/7, or Ortho-cyclen) are usually prescribed.

Endometriosis

Endometriosis is a common cause of chronic pelvic pain in adolescents. Most severe symptoms are typically just before and during menses, but acyclic pain is also a common presentation. Pain tends to increase with time. In contrast to functional dysmenorrhea, the pain of endometriosis persists and gradually increases despite treatment with antiprostaglandins and oral contraceptives. Patients whose symptoms persist or increase on this regimen should be referred to a gynecologist for possible laparoscopy to diagnosis endometriosis. Most adolescents with endometriosis have normal findings or only mild or moderate tenderness on pelvic examination, without detectable masses or nodularity.

Treatment. Multiple treatment regimens for endometriosis have been used. All are directed toward suppression of ectopic endometrial tissue in hopes of preserving fertility and eliminating pain. Regimens include treatment with progestins (e.g., daily or depot medroxyprogesterone acetate); treatment with androgens (e.g., danazol); continuous oral contraceptive use with a progestin-dominant pill (e.g., Lo/Ovral); and, most recently, use of gonadotropin-releasing hormone analogues to suppress ovarian function completely. All of these regimens are associated with frequent side effects.

Pelvic Masses

A pregnant uterus is a common cause of a lower abdominal mass in an adolescent, even in the absence of a history of sexual activity. Included in the differential diagnosis of the patient with a positive urine test for hCG and a pelvic mass in addition to intrauterine pregnancy are ectopic pregnancy, miscarriage, gestational trophoblastic neoplasia (choriocarcinoma, molar pregnancy), and some ovarian tumors containing germ cell elements that secrete hCG.

Etiology. Causes of adnexal masses include ectopic pregnancy, benign persistent follicular or corpus luteum cysts of the ovary, dermoid cysts, hydrosalpinx, endometriomas, and ovarian tumors. An ovarian tumor, although rare in an adolescent, can occur and is often discovered as an asymptomatic pelvic mass or as a cause of enlarging abdominal girth. Ovarian masses may be associated with chronic pelvic or periumbilical pain. Severe pain similar to that associated with appendicitis may represent torsion of an ovarian mass, infarction, or perforation of a cyst or tumor. Granulosa cell tumors or ovarian cysts that secrete estrogen may present as irregular vaginal bleeding or amenorrhea in the adolescent. Corpus luteum cysts secreting estrogen and progesterone may also present with amenorrhea or with vaginal bleeding as they degenerate and hormone levels fall. A congenital anomaly of the uterus or vagina that obstructs menstrual flow presents with pain and a pelvic mass consisting of the obstructed uterus or uterine horn.

Diagnosis. Pelvic ultrasonography is helpful in the diagnosis of the pelvic mass, although findings may occasionally be misleading. Physiologic developing ovarian follicles reaching a size of 1 to 3 cm are a normal finding, and small amounts of fluid may be seen in the cul-de-sac with ovulation. Fluid can also be a sign of bleeding, infection, or a ruptured cyst. Simple ovarian cysts are generally 3 to 6 cm in diameter and unilocular. Primarily solid masses such as dermoids, which are palpable on bimanual examination, may be missed on ultrasonography; thus, a bimanual or rectoabdominal examination should not be omitted in the adolescent with pelvic pain. Transvaginal ultrasonography provides greater detail in evaluation of the adnexal region than abdominal ultrasonography. Computed tomography and magnetic resonance imaging scans are also used in the evaluation of pelvic masses when the diagnosis has not been established by pelvic examination and ultrasonography.

Treatment. If a simple ovarian cyst of less than 6 cm in size is documented by bimanual examination or ultrasonography in an adolescent, the patient may be followed by monthly pelvic examinations or ultrasonography until the cyst resolves. Monophasic oral contraceptive pills are often prescribed for 3 months to suppress the hypothalamic-pituitary-ovarian axis and prevent the formation of new cysts. If the cyst develops while the patient is taking triphasic pills, many physicians will switch to monophasic pills. If the cyst is greater than 6 cm in size or is causing symptoms, the cyst may be aspirated laparoscopically and the fluid obtained for cytology. Often, the patient is then given oral contraceptives. If the cyst recurs after aspiration or surgery is required, attempts should be made to preserve as much ovarian tissue as possible and minimize periovarian adhesions. Solid or mixed cystic and solid ovarian masses are generally approached surgically.

Abnormal Vaginal Bleeding

Abnormal vaginal bleeding may be due to pregnancy complications, hormonal abnormalities, blood dyscrasia, infection, local lesion, anatomic abnormality, or local trauma. Because adolescents frequently have anovulatory cycles in the first 2 years after menarche, painless cycles at irregular intervals are frequent. Patients who have bleeding at intervals of less than 22 days, whose menses last longer than 7 days, or who have heavy bleeding with clots are considered to have excessive bleeding. Although most adolescents are initially anovulatory after menarche, they usually do have cyclic variations in estrogen levels resulting in cyclic vaginal withdrawal bleeding at variable intervals between 28 and 39 days. Teenagers whose anovulation is characterized by an acyclic pattern, often with intervals of amenorrhea followed by prolonged bleeding, are said to have "dysfunctional" uterine bleeding as a cause of their prolonged heavy menses. This is a common cause of excessive vaginal bleeding but remains a diagnosis of exclusion.

Evaluation. Evaluation usually begins with a careful history of the character and time course of the bleeding, past menstrual history, and history of prior difficulty with bleeding tendencies in the patient or family members. A physical examination should include postural vital signs and careful attention to findings that might suggest a clotting abnormality such as bruising or petechiae, or an endocrine abnormality such as hirsutism or hypothyroidism. Whether or not the patient is actively bleeding, a pelvic examination with visualization of the cervix and vagina should be performed.

Initial laboratory tests should include a urine and serum hCG and a complete blood count. Clotting studies, including a platelet count, prothrombin time (PT), partial thromboplastin time (PTT), and bleeding time, are usually obtained if significant menorrhagia occurs with fall in the hematocrit value or if abnormal bleeding started at menarche. If the patient is bleeding heavily, a type and cross-match should be obtained because transfusion is sometimes necessary. Cervical specimens for gonorrhea and chlamydial cultures are obtained in the adolescent who might possibly be sexually active, and endocrine tests such as luteinizing hormone (LH), follicle-stimulating hormone (FSH), prolactin, and thyroid function tests may be included if the patient has a history of apparent anovulatory bleeding.

Treatment. Treatment varies with the severity of the problem.

MILD BLEEDING. Patients with mild dysfunctional bleeding—normal hemoglobin and monthly menses lasting more than 7 days or cycles of less than 21 days for 2 months or more with only moderately increased flow—may be asked to keep a menstrual calendar and may be given iron supplements to prevent anemia.

MODERATE BLEEDING. Patients with moderately severe dysfunctional bleeding have moderate to heavy flow and menses every 1 to 3 weeks, often with bleeding lasting more than 7 days. Mild anemia is often present. Either medroxyprogesterone or oral contraceptives may be prescribed. Medroxyprogesterone (10 mg once or twice a day for 10 to 14 days) may be started on the 14th day after the period began or on the day of the visit. Repeated cycles of medroxyprogesterone (10 mg for 12 to 14 days each) are begun either beginning on day 14 after the first day of withdrawal bleeding or for the first 12 to 14 days of each calendar month. This latter method is simpler for patients to remember. If the patient begins to have bleeding even before she reaches the 14th day of the cycle, medroxyprogesterone may be started on day 12 or she may be switched to oral contraceptives. If patients do not tolerate medroxyprogesterone, the dose may be decreased temporarily to 5 mg/day. Norethindrone acetate (Norlutate, 10 mg daily for 10 to 14 days) may be used as an alternative to medroxyprogesterone. Cycling should be continued for 3 to 6 months. If the patient does not begin to cycle on her own within 2 months after stopping the treatment, she should again be treated with medroxyprogesterone or oral contraceptives to prevent further dysfunctional uterine bleeding.

SEVERE BLEEDING. If the patient has a history of prolonged or heavy dysfunctional bleeding, or if she has milder irregular bleeding and is in need of contraception, oral contraceptives should be used as the initial treatment. Ovral, Lo/Ovral, or Norinyl (Ortho-Novum) 1/50 or 1/35 may be chosen. Ovral is most effective in stopping heavy bleeding because it consists of a strong progestin norgestrel coupled with 50 μg of ethinyl estradiol. Initially, the patient takes one Ovral twice a day for 3 days until the bleeding stops, and then continues one pill a day to complete a 21-day cycle. Lo/Ovral is often the choice for younger adolescents because the estrogen dose is lower than Ovral. Lo/Ovral may have to be given three or four times a day initially until the bleeding stops, then decreased to once a day.

If the bleeding is initially quite heavy and the patient is mildly anemic (hemoglobin 9 to 11 g/dl), Ovral may be begun four times a day. Bleeding should slow promptly and stop within 24 to 36 hours. Ovral may be continued four times a day for 4 days total, then three times a day for 3 days, then twice a day for 2 weeks. Cyclic oral contraceptives are then continued for 3 to 6 months. Patients who initially require a pill containing 50 μg of ethinyl estradiol can usually be decreased to a pill containing 35 μg of ethinyl estradiol after the first cycle. The physician must be in close contact with the patient during the initial phase of the treatment to be sure that the bleeding is slowing and that the patient understands how to taper the medication. Nausea is a frequent side effect of large doses of estrogen, and an antiemetic is often helpful. After the first month, it is usually convenient to switch the patient from 21-day to 28-day pill packages. The proper use of 28-day packages should be reviewed to avoid confusion. Oral iron and folic acid (1 mg/day) should be given to treat the anemia.

The patient who has a history of prolonged heavy bleeding with a hemoglobin count less than 9 g/dl is considered to have severe dysfunctional bleeding. She may have clinical signs of blood loss. If the initial hemoglobin value is less than 7 g/dl, or if she is orthostatic with heavy bleeding and a count of less than 10 g/dl, she should be hospitalized. Clotting studies and a pregnancy test should be done. A transfusion is occasionally necessary. Ovral is given every 4 hours until the bleeding stops (4 to 8 tablets), then four times a day for 4 days, three times a day for 3 days, and twice a day for 2 weeks. Norinyl (Ortho-Novum) 1/50 may be used in a similar regimen. In patients with acute severe hemorrhage, Premarin (25 mg IV) has been used every 4 hours for two to three doses. Intravenous estrogen increases clotting at the capillary level, which is quite effective at stopping the hemorrhage; however, this method carries a higher risk of blood clots. Ovral is begun at the same time because the effect of the intravenous estrogen is short-lived. Antiemetics are used to reduce nausea in all these high-dose estrogen regimens.

If estrogen is contraindicated, norethindrone acetate (Norlutate, 5 to 10 mg) or medroxyprogesterone (10 mg) can be given every 4 hours and decreased to four times a day for 4 days, three times a day for 3 days, and twice a day for 2 weeks.

If hormone tablets given every 4 hours do not control bleeding within 24 to 36 hours, an examination employing anesthesia and dilatation and curettage may occasionally be necessary.

Withdrawal flow should begin 2 to 4 days after the last hormone tablet is taken; the patient then receives Ovral 28 for 3 to 6 months after an interval of 4 to 7 days from the last pill of the initial cycle. Iron with folate replacement is begun in the first cycle.

Patients with low platelet counts, leukemia, or aplastic anemia may require prolonged therapy to suppress menses. Continuous Lo/Ovral 21 may be used for several months. Medroxyprogesterone (10 mg) may be given daily for months. When platelet counts improve, the patient should be cycled with a low-dose progestin-dominant pill such as Lo/Ovral.

Amenorrhea

Amenorrhea can be primary and secondary. There is considerable overlap in the differential diagnosis; however, it is still helpful to use these terms to distinguish patients who may have an anatomic abnormality preventing menstrual flow, such as absent uterus or obstructed vagina ("primary" amenorrhea), from those who have established that they have a uterus and vaginal outflow tract because they have had menses at some point in the past ("secondary" amenorrhea).

Primary Amenorrhea

By definition, the patient who has primary amenorrhea has not had her first menstrual period within 4 years of the onset of breast development or by age 15 (2 standard deviations beyond the norm). This may be caused by delayed puberty, interrupted puberty, hormonal imbalance causing anovulation, or an anatomic abnormality preventing menstruation. *Delayed puberty,* that is, the absence of secondary sexual development by age 13½ in girls, is discussed in Section 9, p. 300.

A patient who has had breast development but has not gone on to have menarche within 4 years has *delayed menarche.* Evaluation should include a careful history, including symptoms suggestive of chronic disease interrupting the progression of puberty; hormonal imbalance such as hypothyroidism, androgen excess, or hyperprolactinemia; timing of breast and body hair development; athletic activity; and dietary intake. A history of cyclic lower abdominal pain suggests an obstructed uterus. Review of height and weight charts is very helpful because chronic disease, malnutrition, or endocrinopathy often presents with abnormalities of growth.

Physical examination of patients with primary amenorrhea and secondary sexual development includes height and weight measurements. Skin is examined for evidence of endocrinopathy, or excessive body hair. Quantitation of secondary sexual development is done by Tanner staging of breast and pubic hair development and measurements of areolae and glandular breast tissue dimensions. An attempt should be made to express galactorrhea, suggesting the diagnosis of hyperprolactinemia. A neurologic examination, including visual fields by confrontation, is useful because pituitary and hypothalamic mass lesions may interrupt the progression of puberty. The external genitalia are examined for signs of estrogenization (pale pink vaginal mucosa, developed labia minora, fimbriated hymen) and evidence of hymeneal patency. Clitoromegaly suggests androgen excess.

An assessment of internal pelvic structures should be done with the patient in the lithotomy position. If the vaginal opening comfortably admits a single finger, a speculum using a thin Huffman speculum may be inserted to visualize the cervix. A vaginal bimanual examination of the uterus and adnexae should also be performed. If the hymenal opening does not admit a finger, the depth of the vagina can be assessed using a saline-moistened cotton swab and the pelvic structures can be examined by rectoabdominal examination. If the pelvic structures cannot be assessed adequately on this examination, pelvic ultrasonography may be helpful.

Laboratory evaluation may be focused by the differential diagnosis suggested by findings on history and physical examination. A complete blood count, sedimentation rate, LH, FSH, prolactin, thyroid function tests, and radiograph of the left hand and wrist for bone age are useful initial screens. A quantitative assessment of estrogen effect on the vagina using a vaginal smear for maturation index is also helpful.

Secondary Amenorrhea

The adolescent who has established menstrual cycles and then ceases menstruation for 3 months or more is said to have secondary amenorrhea. Because the most common cause of adolescent amenorrhea is pregnancy, any teenager who expresses concern about a period that is even slightly delayed warrants prompt attention. She should be interviewed alone and given a chance to discuss her concerns privately. Many teenagers will not acknowledge that they are sexually active even when carefully questioned. A urine screen for hCG is therefore a fundamental part of the evaluation of any adolescent with a delayed period. The focus of the history and physical examination is the same as in the patient who presents with primary amenorrhea because the diagnostic possibilities overlap. A pelvic examination is appropriate to assess estrogen effect on the vaginal mucosa and to assess the size of the uterus and ovaries.

The adolescent who has persistent *oligomenorrhea*—no established pattern of regular menstrual cycles within 4 years of menarche—often has a hormone imbalance causing chronic anovulation. Some of these patients have chronic ovarian androgen excess (polycystic ovary syndrome) and may show the classic triad of obesity, slowly progressive hirsutism, and oligomenorrhea. Not all patients with this hormonal pattern have obvious signs of androgen excess on examination. Other patients may have partial disruption of the hypothalamic-pituitary-ovarian axis as a result of intense exercise, stress, chronic illness, or limitation of food intake. Sometimes there is no obvious reason for their persistent anovulatory state. Because women with chronic anovulation have an endometrium that is chronically exposed to unopposed estrogen, they are at risk for endometrial hyperplasia, dysfunctional bleeding, and even endometrial cancer with time. It is therefore necessary that patients who do not have what appears to be an ovulatory period at least every 3 months be cycled with medroxyprogesterone acetate or oral contraceptives.

The initial laboratory evaluation includes a urine pregnancy test and LH, FSH, prolactin, and thyroid function tests. If the pregnancy test is negative, a progestin challenge is a useful way to assess the estrogen state of the patient. Medroxyprogesterone (Provera, 10 mg) is given daily for 10 days. If this is followed by withdrawal bleeding, the patient is estrogenized. Sometimes, a medroxyprogesterone challenge is not followed by spontaneous cycling. If the patient does not have cyclic menses on her own, she should be cycled with medroxyprogesterone (10 mg a day for 12 to 14 days every 1 to 3 months) to prevent endometrial hyperplasia. If she is sexually active, it is preferable to use oral contraceptives to avoid exposure to medroxyprogesterone early in an undiagnosed pregnancy. The patient usually returns to the office 2 to 3 weeks after her initial visit to discuss her response to the progestin challenge and the results of her initial laboratory evaluation.

If the patient's LH-to-FSH ratio is 3:1 or more or if there is evidence of androgen excess on examination, she may have polycystic ovary syndrome. The next step is a determination of testosterone level, possibly including adrenal androgens as well. Patients with polycystic ovary syndrome usually have adequate to high estrogen levels and should be cycled to prevent endometrial hyperplasia. Oral contraceptives are the treatment of choice because they can usually lower free androgen levels and prevent progression of hirsutism. A pill containing a nonandrogenic progestin, such as norethindrone, is preferable. Modicon (35 μg of ethinyl estradiol with 0.5 mg of norethindrone) or Ovcon-35 (35 μg of ethinyl estradiol with 0.4 mg of norethindrone) may be used. Ortho-Novum (Norinyl) 1/35 or Demulen 1/35 is an alternative if breakthrough bleeding is a problem. If the patient is opposed to or is not a candidate for oral contraceptives, cycling with medroxyprogesterone (10 mg for 12 to 14 days a month) can result in regular menses and prevent endometrial hyperplasia in these patients; however, hirsutism and acne may progress.

A low-estrogen state may be the result of low levels of LH and FSH due to hypothalamic or pituitary dysfunction or to an inability of the ovary to respond to high levels of gonadotropins. If LH and FSH are elevated into the menopausal range, ovarian failure is a cause of the low estrogen state. If the initial LH and FSH levels are elevated, tests are usually repeated to confirm the diagnosis. A karyotype and antiovarian antibodies can help to determine whether a chromosomal abnormality or autoimmune process underlies the ovarian failure.

The optimum dose of estrogen replacement in adolescents has not been clearly established. The usual menopausal dose of conjugated estrogens (Premarin, 0.625 mg/day) may not be adequate to allow the normal adolescent increase in bone density to take place. If growth is not yet complete, estrogen replacement is begun at low doses to maximize the growth response. One regimen is to begin at 0.3 mg of Premarin and increase to 0.625 to 1.25 mg as growth slows in the second year of treatment. Once the dose of Premarin has reached 0.625 mg/day, the replacement is given cyclically on days 1 to 25 each month, and medroxyprogesterone (10 mg/day) is added initially 5 days/month for 3 months, increasing to 12 to 14 days/month.

A low-dose oral contraceptive containing 30 to 35 μg of ethinyl estradiol is an alternative approach to estrogen replacement once breast development is satisfactory. Other forms of estrogen replacement include ethinyl estradiol (30 to 35 μg), transdermal β-estradiol patches (Estraderm), or micronized estradiol (Estrace, 2 mg). All are used with cyclic progestin for 12 to 14 days/month.

Index

Note: Page numbers in *italics* refer to illustrations; page numbers followed by t refer to tables.